D1758565

Cardiac Catheterization in Congenital Heart Disease: Pediatric and Adult

Cardiac Catheterization in Congenital Heart Disease: Pediatric and Adult

Charles E. Mullins, MD
Professor of Pediatrics
Baylor College of Medicine
Texas Children's Hospital
Houston, Texas
USA

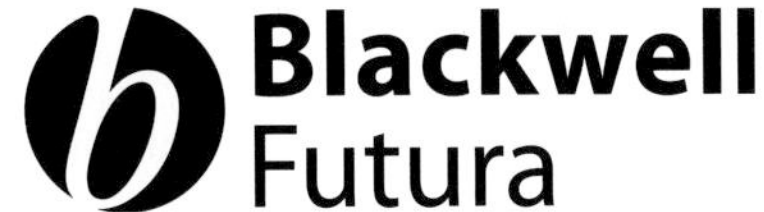

Published by Blackwell Publishing
Blackwell Futura is an imprint of Blackwell Publishing

Blackwell Publishing, Inc., 350 Main Street, Malden, Massachusetts 02148-5020, USA
Blackwell Publishing Ltd, 9600 Garsington Road, Oxford OX4 2DQ, UK
Blackwell Publishing Asia Pty Ltd, 550 Swanston Street, Carlton, Victoria 3053, Australia

First published 2006
4 2007

ISBN 978-1-4051-2200-9

Library of Congress Cataloging-in-Publication Data

Mullins, Charles E.
Cardiac catheterization in congenital heart disease : pediatric and adult / Charles E. Mullins.
p. ; cm.
Includes bibliographical references and index.
ISBN 978-1-4051-2200-9 (hardback : alk. paper)
Cardiac catheterization in children. 2. Congenital heart disease in children—Surgery. 3. Cardiac catheterization. I. Title.
[DNLM: 1. Heart Defects, Congenital—diagnosis. 2. Heart Defects, Congenital—therapy. 3. Heart Catheterization—methods. WG 220 M959c 2005]
RJ423.5.C36M85 2005
618.92'120754—dc22

2005022329

A catalogue record for this title is available from the British Library

Acquisitions: Steve Korn
Development: Simone Dudziak
Set in 9.5/12 Palatino by Graphicraft Limited, Hong Kong
Printed and bound in India by Replika Press Pvt. Ltd

For further information on Blackwell Publishing, visit our website:
www.blackwellcardiology.com

The publisher's policy is to use permanent paper from mills that operate a sustainable forestry policy, and which has been manufactured from pulp processed using acid-free and elementary chlorine-free practices. Furthermore, the publisher ensures that the text paper and cover board used have met acceptable environmental accreditation standards.

Notice: The indications and dosages of all drugs in this book have been recommended in the medical literature and conform to the practices of the general community. The medications described do not necessarily have specific approval by the Food and Drug Administration for use in the diseases and dosages for which they are recommended. The package insert for each drug should be consulted for use and dosage as approved by the FDA. Because standards for usage change, it is advisable to keep abreast of revised recommendations, particularly those concerning new drugs.

Contents

Preface

This text is intended for all individuals who are involved with the cardiac catheterizations of infants, children and older patients with congenital heart disease. The catheterization of a patient with congenital heart disease requires a thorough background knowledge of the normal and abnormal cardiac anatomy, a skill at catheter manipulation and an additional "feel" for that anatomy. The skill necessary for maneuvering a catheter is acquired with experience but the use of these skills also involves some individual intuition. Hopefully, this text will help in attaining the acquired skills, while the experience in using these techniques will provide the "feel"!

The material in this text emphasizes the *minute details and fundamentals* of catheter manipulations and procedures, which are required for the correct and efficient acquisition of the data necessary for meaningful calculations during diagnostic catheterizations. As always has been the case, diagnostic catheterization still only is as good as the accuracy of the data and the interpretation of the data from that catheterization. This text also provides the details of techniques necessary for effectively and safely accomplishing most of the complex therapeutic catheterization procedures that are available currently.

The information contained in this text does have a definite bias as it represents the accumulation of knowledge, techniques and procedures learned, utilized and/or developed by the author during the continued learning, practice and teaching of cardiac catheterization procedures during the past, extremely exciting, four decades in the field. Although much of the past 35 years of this experience has been at Baylor College of Medicine/Texas Children's Hospital, the opinions that are expressed are not necessarily those of the institutions.

The "free hand" drawings in this book were provided by Jeremy Rountree. Jeremy is a senior art student in college and a long-time patient of mine. All of the "computer generated" drawings as well as a few modifications of some of Jeremy's drawings were the responsibility of the author.

Charles E. Mullins, MD

Dedication

This book is dedicated to Arlene, who has stuck by me and been tolerant of me for five decades in spite of my "competing love" of medicine and the cardiac catheterization laboratory. She has been remarkably patient and supportive while awaiting the conclusion of this particular project.

And to Dr Weldon Walker, my mentor in cardiology at Walter Reed General Hospital, who not only taught me cardiology and the techniques and the art of cardiac catheterization, but instilled in me the concepts of perfection and "never taking anything for granted".

And to Dr Dan G. McNamara, my close friend, my associate, my chief and my continuing mentor for the first twenty-five years at Texas Children's Hospital. Dan not only tolerated my activities in the catheterization laboratory, but supported and encouraged me no matter how outlandish my projects may have seemed.

Introduction

There is no "standardized" cardiac catheterization procedure for any pediatric and/or congenital heart patient and/or lesion, any more than any of the complex lesions in these patients are standardized. For the catheterizing physician, each cardiac catheterization procedure is an individualized, totally new experience—some far more so than others—on each new patient and even for repeat catheterizations on the same patient. As a consequence *every* catheterization procedure is a *learning experience* for the catheterizing physician. As procedures are performed repeatedly, the operator becomes more comfortable with the technique and with the limits of the particular procedure. Often this results in "extending" the limits of old procedures and when modified logically and methodically, to the development of new procedures. Almost all of the diagnostic and therapeutic procedures utilized in the catheterization laboratory have developed and/or were perfected through such an evolution.

The procedures and techniques that are described in detail in this text, may not be the "quickest" way to perform a procedure, but rather, the techniques emphasize *reliability* and *safety*, often at the expense of "speed". During the performance of any catheterization procedure, when some specific step and/or part of a safe and established procedure is abbreviated or bypassed in order to "save time", the "short cut" is more likely to result in errors in the data that are acquired, to increased risks for the patient and/or even to result in the total failure of the procedure.

Much of this information will be mundane and of little use to the pediatric cardiologist who is experienced in therapeutic catheterization procedures, however, the goal of this text is to cover the *minute details* of most available cardiac catheterization techniques and procedures. With the avalanche of new devices, procedures and techniques that are being developed, many procedures and devices used in the cardiac catheterization laboratory have come and gone, and will continue to come and go. All of the devices and procedures that remain in use have been modified and/or improved over the years. Undoubtedly, before this text even is published, some of the information will be obsolete. On the other hand, the basic techniques of catheter manipulation and therapeutic procedures are sound, very well tested and should be valid as long as cardiac catheterizations are being performed. Hopefully there will be some information of value for physicians performing cardiac catheterizations at all skill levels.

The demise of diagnostic cardiac catheterization was predicted three decades ago with the introduction of echocardiography, magnetic resonance imaging (MRI) and computed tomography (CT) imaging. With the subsequent evolution of these non-invasive diagnostic modalities over the past three decades all of these modalities individually have been designated to replace diagnostic cardiac catheterization. On the contrary, the need for very detailed and accurate diagnostic cardiac catheterizations in pediatric and congenital heart patients actually has increased. The extremely complex and sophisticated surgery being undertaken for the more and more complex and very bizarre congenital heart defects demands accurate diagnoses that are even more precise.

Although many lesions are diagnosed and referred directly to surgery on the basis of the non-invasive studies, there are innumerable occasions, particularly in the very complex lesions, where more specific details about the anatomy and/or hemodynamics are necessary in order for the surgeons to be able to embark on the more exotic repairs. In 2005, cardiac catheterization still remains the "final court" for the definitive anatomic and hemodynamic diagnoses for most of the very complex lesions where the very precise and very complete information about *all* of the anatomy and physiology still is obtainable only from a thorough, accurate cardiac catheterization. At the same time, the more information from the clinical data and the non-invasive studies that is available prior to the catheterization procedure, the more organized and expedient is the catheterization and the more valid are the data obtained from the catheterization.

In addition to the essential diagnostic information that still only can be acquired from a precise and detailed cardiac catheterization, definitive *therapy in the catheterization laboratory* has become the major indication for cardiac catheterization for many of the lesions in pediatric and congenital heart patients. The numerous therapeutic procedures performed in the cardiac catheterization laboratory have generated an even more essential and often, more challenging, need for extremely precise and purposeful maneuvers with cardiac catheters. The catheters for the delivery of balloons and/or devices must be positioned in very precise locations, not just into the general vicinity of the lesion.

In order to proceed with the appropriate and expedient therapeutic catheter intervention, the accurate diagnosis must be acquired, a decision must be made on the basis of that information during the procedure and then, immediately, the information is acted upon therapeutically. In most cases, the therapeutic procedure is performed during the same catheterization procedure without a decision by "conference". The therapeutic catheterization procedures have resulted in the development of new equipment along with entirely new procedures and techniques, which catheterizing physicians not only must become familiar with, but also must be experts in performing.

The therapeutic catheterization procedures also have stimulated a new collaboration between the interventional cardiologist and the congenital heart surgeon. In progressive institutions, the catheterizing interventional cardiologist plans his diagnostic and therapeutic catheterization interventions based on the stage of surgical repair, which is to be performed subsequently in the operating room. The surgeon also can plan his procedure based on the knowledge that a subsequent therapeutic intervention to "complete the repair" may be performed more expediently in the catheterization laboratory. More and more frequently, therapeutic catheter interventions are performed in conjunction with the surgeon *in the operating room.* Therapeutic catheterizations that are performed in the operating room overcome some access problems for the catheter intervention and at the same time allow better myocardial protection with shorter, or even *no* cardiopulmonary bypass and/or arrest times during the operative procedure.

This text is intended to provide detailed instructions for most of the therapeutic catheterization procedures presently in use for congenital heart defects. Although many of these specific catheter maneuvers are useful during intracardiac electrophysiologic procedures, the specific electrophysiologic diagnostic and therapeutic interventions represent an entirely separate specialty and are not discussed in this text.

1

Organization of a pediatric/congenital cardiac catheterization laboratory

Introduction

The recommended equipment and the arrangement and organization of the space and equipment for the pediatric/congenital cardiac catheterization laboratories which are discussed in this chapter are a culmination of my own experience in cardiac catheterization laboratories over the past 40+ years. During that time I have had the privilege/opportunity of performing catheterizations in some 180 different catheterization laboratories in 120 different institutions throughout the US and much of the rest of the world. During that time I also had the experience of directing several catheterization laboratories for more than 25 years and of having a significant role in, and part of the responsibility for, building 14 different cardiac catheterization laboratories in several different hospitals over those years. The equipment, space and personnel requirements described in this chapter meet *or* exceed all published standards for pediatric/congenital cardiac catheterization laboratories[1,2]. The cardiac catheterization rooms/suite described in this chapter are in operation at Texas Children's Hospital.

The total space requirement for a twenty-first century pediatric and congenital cardiac catheterization room (laboratory) and the accompanying support area or "suite" is significantly greater than for the catheterization laboratory of even one decade ago. The increased requirement for space is a consequence of the physical dimensions of the modern, biplane X-ray equipment, which is capable of compound angulation of both X-ray tubes, the sophisticated ancillary electronic equipment which is required and the increased complexity of the procedures which are now performed in these laboratories. Many of the therapeutic catheterization procedures require additional, large pieces of ancillary equipment (anesthesia machines, transesophageal and intracardiac echo, equipment for partial or total cardiac support, etc.), which not only must be in the catheterization laboratory, but often must be positioned immediately adjacent to the catheterization table. Significant *additional* space also is required to "park" each of these pieces of equipment in the immediate vicinity of the laboratory, if not actually within the catheterization room, when they are not actually in use.

With the longer, more complex procedures and particularly with the frequent use of implants in the catheterization laboratory the cardiac catheterization *room* should be considered a "sterile" environment similar to an operating room. The catheterization room should operate with the doors to adjacent areas (except the control room) closed and it should have a separate, filtered air input which maintains a "positive pressure" circulation within it[3]. At the same time, because of frequent equipment maintenance and other outside support, the entire catheterization *area* or *suite* adjacent to, but outside of the actual catheterization room, is considered a "clean", rather than sterile, area.

The exact location of the catheterization area in relation to other hospital facilities often is dependent upon overall space availability and requires considerable pre-planning. Optimally, pediatric/congenital cardiac catheterization laboratories are located immediately adjacent to, and have easy access to the pediatric/congenital cardiac operating rooms and cardiac intensive care areas. Although the need for surgical intervention during a cardiac catheterization is still very rare, when surgical support is needed, it is needed immediately. "Open chest", operative intervention is preferably performed in the operating room, not in the catheterization room. Having the surgical suite immediately adjacent to the catheterization laboratory and accessed through a sterile corridor allows a patient to be transported very rapidly and expediently from the catheterization laboratory to an operating room even when the patient is on external support or his chest is opened.

The requirements for, and the optimal arrangement of, the modern catheterization laboratory space are detailed in the following section.

The cardiac catheterization room itself

A current cardiac catheterization laboratory ideally should be at least 32 feet long by 24 feet wide. In addition to the large length and width requirements of the catheterization room, the ceiling height must be at least 14 feet in order to accommodate the suspension system of the X-ray tubes and intensifiers from any manufacturer. The *only* "fixed" equipment in the actual catheterization room should be the catheterization table and the suspension systems for the X-ray systems along with the X-ray and physiologic monitors, with no fixed cabinets and none of the X-ray generating equipment included within the actual catheterization room. The arrangement of the catheterization table in the room and the "connections" or "communications" to the room from adjacent areas depend upon the "real estate" which is available immediately adjacent to the catheterization room. The control room for the physiologic and X-ray systems must be adjacent to the catheterization room and have at least a doorway access to the laboratory. The control room can be positioned at the end or at the side of the catheterization room, but in either location the operators in the control room should have a clear view of the patient on the catheterization table. The storage for the majority of the expendable catheterization equipment should be immediately adjacent to the catheterization room with a readily accessible doorway. The catheterization room should have a one-and-a-half or even a double-width doorway for patient access. Even though the patient may arrive on a narrow hospital stretcher, there must be the capability of leaving the room easily with "attached" equipment and personnel adjacent to or alongside of the bed/stretcher during a resuscitation or emergency transfer to an operating room.

The scrub sink(s) for the catheterization laboratories should be located *outside* of the actual catheterization room in an adjacent "clean" corridor or room. It is essential that all personnel in the laboratory scrub before working in the room and that the physicians scrub between each case. At the same time, scrubbing, which is a relatively short task, is performed before the catheterization procedure. It has nothing to do with the procedure itself, it actually can have "dirty" fluids splashing away from the sink and, as a consequence, there is no justification, nor logic for having the scrub sink occupy valuable space within the catheterization room.

During the course of an interventional catheterization procedure the catheterization room can become very crowded with equipment and personnel. The location and arrangement of each piece of *fixed equipment* become critical for the most efficient and safe completion of the procedure.

X-ray equipment

The basic equipment in a catheterization laboratory for pediatric and congenital heart patients includes a biplane X-ray system with compound angulation capabilities, an extra-long catheterization table and dual (quadruple!) CRT or flat panel monitor screens. This basic equipment requires a very large "footprint" of floor space in the room for just the catheterization table and the suspension systems for the X-ray tubes/intensifiers. The catheterization table needs to be "extra long" or have a long extension at the foot end in order to prevent the contamination of the very long catheters, delivery systems and exchange length wires which are introduced and undergo multiple exchanges through the femoral vessels. The footprint of the catheterization table and the suspension system for the X-ray tubes/intensifiers should include enough width to allow unimpeded rotation of the X-ray tubes and support arms without bumping into or having to move other equipment. There must be significant space towards the head of the table to allow clear cephalad–caudal movement of the suspension system, space for physicians working from the head-end of the table, adequate space for relatively large anesthesia/respiratory equipment adjacent to the head *and* room to have a transesophageal echo console adjacent to the patient's head. It is often necessary to have all of this space occupied at the same time! Additional floor space cephalad to, and away from the working areas is required to "park" the lateral X-ray suspension gantry a distance away from the head of the catheterization table in order to allow room for transferring the patient to and from the table.

The catheterization table

The spacial orientation of the catheterization table within the room helps to optimize the usable space. When the catheterization table is placed at an angle, somewhat diagonally across the room, this opens up a large area on one side of the table at the head of the table and an equally large area on the opposite side at the foot of the table. When the larger space at the head of the table is on the side of the access doorway for the patient, this allows a more convenient access to the table for a patient on a stretcher. As an added bonus, the extra space in this area opens up an area for a transesophageal echo machine working from the head of the table. The larger open area at the foot and on the opposite side of the table allows more working space for the physicians on that side of the table. A straight alignment of the table along the long axis in a slightly narrow room compromises the space on both sides of the table and for its entire length.

Work space for the physician/operators

In addition to the large space requirement for the X-ray equipment and the catheterization table, there must be liberal space adjacent to, and all around, the catheterization table/X-ray equipment to allow access to the table for other large pieces of support equipment. This space should allow unrestricted movement of the X-ray tubes and intensifiers as well as the free movement of the personnel within the laboratory around all of this equipment regardless of the positions of the X-ray tubes. The monitor screens are grouped together as a bank of monitors on a large ceiling mounted support, which is on tracks and is movable about the table. The operating physician must have a clear view of all of the monitors while looking *forward* (not over his shoulder or behind him), regardless of the site of catheter introduction into the patient. A very satisfactory arrangement is to have the bank of monitors mounted on a *long* swivel arm which, in turn, is on ceiling tracks aligned *across* the catheterization table at the foot of the table. With this configuration, the monitors can be moved directly over the foot of the table when vascular access is from either side of the neck or even the arm, and completely across the table when vascular access is totally from the left side of the patient. A *long* support arm on a swivel base for the bank of monitors allows sufficient movement of the monitors along either side of the table. With the multiple locations which are possible for the monitors, the operator can always be located across the table and facing the monitors with an unobstructed view of them without any body contortions or having to look round structures or behind him/herself.

The exact configuration of the catheterization table varies from laboratory to laboratory. Most catheterization tables are orientated for a right handed operator—i.e. with any extra space for the scrubbed physician(s) predominately on the right side of the patient's trunk. The person who operates the controls for the movement of the table and X-ray tubes and the person who operates the pressure/flush manifolds and the flush lines, all vary from laboratory to laboratory and affect how the catheterization table is configured. There must be adequate space for two, or possibly three, *scrubbed* operators on either side of the catheterization table particularly during complex therapeutic interventional procedures, when as many as four individuals may be scrubbed with several personnel on both sides of the table when the vascular access is from both sides. It also should be possible for at least two operators to work together from either side of the head and neck area while other operators are working from the femoral areas.

In the catheterization laboratories at Texas Children's Hospital, the table position/movements, the movement of the C-arms suspending the X-ray tubes, the collimation of the X-ray tubes and the control and replay functions of the angiograms all are controlled by the catheterizing physician(s). As a consequence these controls are all maintained sterile with sterile covers/drapes and are positioned on the same (right) side of the patient as the operator, but nearer the foot of the table. In some laboratories these table/cine controls are operated by a separate technician or even a radiologist, in which case the controls are at the foot of the table or even physically away from the table on a separate stand.

In addition to the space for the table controls, an additional length of the table "real estate" along one side or the end of the catheterization table is required for the pressure transducers, pressure/flush manifolds and the flush/pressure lines. The manifold is a series of three or more, three-way stopcocks to which each transducer and the tubing to both the fluid reservoirs and to the patient are connected. In addition, the transducers are attached to electrical cables which run from the transducers to an electrical connection on the table and eventually to the physiologic recorders. When three or four transducers are used simultaneously during a case, the manifolds holding the transducers occupy a meter, or more along one edge of the table. Three-way stopcocks on the manifold allow "opening" the transducer to environmental pressure for balancing, as well as additional connections for the flush tubing to the transducers and separate tubing for flush/pressure lines to the patient from each transducer. In some catheterization laboratories where multichannel pressure recording is not used routinely, the manifold and even the transducers themselves are positioned on the catheterization "field" and operated by the catheterizing physician. Specifically arranged manifolds including the stopcocks, transducers and tubing are available commercially (Merit Medical Systems, Salt Lake City, UT). The exact positioning of the manifold on the surface or along the side of the table will depend upon which personnel operate the manifold during the case.

During the catheterization procedure, the manifold with the transducers ideally is fixed to the catheterization tabletop at a specific height on a stand which allows an initial adjustment in the height of the manifold to compensate for the "height" of the heart within the patient's chest above the tabletop. The exact level (height) for the pressure transducers varies and is determined for each individual patient according to the anterior–posterior (AP) diameter of the chest. The height for the transducer is the measured distance from the tabletop to the mid level of the posterior–anterior chest diameter, or the exact location of the heart is determined on the lateral fluoroscope. The height from the tabletop to the heart should be measured accurately with a ruler and then this exact measurement is transferred to the transducer stand to determine the height of the transducers on the stand. When the transducers are attached to the table at the correct level on a stand, the transducers then move up and down *with the patient* when the table is raised or lowered and, in doing so, the reference height to the heart for *accurate* pressure measurements always remains exactly the same.

In the catheterization laboratories at Texas Children's Hospital, there are usually four transducers with as many as six to eight color-coded flush/pressure lines passing to the patient from pressure/flush manifolds. Each color-coded pressure line corresponds to a similar colored pressure curve which is displayed on the monitors. The entire manifold is operated by a designated nurse/technician who has no other *assigned* duty during the procedure. In this circumstance, the optimal position for the transducers is on the opposite side of the catheterization table as far as possible toward the foot of the table away from the operating physicians, but still within the sight of the catheterizing physician. Since the majority of catheter manipulations by the catheterizing physicians are performed through the femoral vessels and from the right side of the patient, regardless of whether the catheter is introduced from the right or left femoral vessels, the transducers optimally are fixed, semi-permanently, on the left (opposite) side of the table and as far as possible toward the foot of the table.

In some laboratories where one, or at most two transducers are used, the catheterizing physician operates the manifolds including the transducers, the stopcocks, and all of the fluid/pressure lines. In this circumstance, the manifold is fixed on the catheterizing physician's side of the table or actually laid on the patient's legs on the catheterization field. This arrangement is more suited when the catheterization laboratories are used predominately for adult (coronary) catheterizations where less sophisticated hemodynamics usually are necessary.

Regardless of which vascular access site is used, there must be space located immediately behind the catheterizing cardiologist for at least one 30″ × 60″ work table to hold flush solutions, a container of contrast solution, needles, catheters, wires, instruments and other expendable equipment. The work table should have enough room around it to allow the "circulating" personnel and the operators to have access to and around the table without bumping into, or contaminating, it. *Two* large (30″ × 60″) work tables placed end to end behind the operators are optimal for interventional procedures where multiple long balloon catheters or very long delivery systems for device implants are utilized. The additional length of the two tables positioned end to end allows sufficient workspace for the preparation of the long balloon dilation catheters and device delivery catheters. The very long table prevents these long items from hanging over the ends of the table and from being contaminated when they are stretched out lengthwise during their preparation or loading procedures.

Anesthesia space requirements

The anesthesiologist, along with the space for the anesthesia machine, requires access to the patient's head from either the right or left side of the patient. The anesthesia access is *cephalad* to the lateral X-ray support ("C") arm and must allow a convenient connection of the anesthesia machine/tubing to the patient's airway. Connections for oxygen, gas and suction lines usually come through the anesthesia machine from a separate ceiling- or wall-mounted console near the head of the catheterization table. It is essential that the oxygen, gas, suction console also is somewhat mobile and can be moved close to the patient's head for situations where general anesthesia and an anesthesia machine are not being used.

When general anesthesia is being used, the anesthesiologist controls the patient's airway while simultaneously operating the anesthesia machine. This requires a close proximity of the anesthesia machine to the head of the catheterization table. Anesthesiologists usually prefer the right side of the patient's head; however, when vascular access for the catheterization is available only from the right neck, it is preferable that the endotracheal tube connections to the anesthesia machine approach from the patient's left side. In rare circumstances, where vascular access and a complex procedure are to be from the right side of the patient's neck, it is desirable to have the anesthesia machine on the patient's left, as well.

A mobile, floor anesthesia machine provides more flexibility than a ceiling-mounted anesthesia machine when changes in the orientation of the room may be necessary to adjust for different access sites to the patient. At the same time, the floor anesthesia console does occupy considerable floor space.

This same need for sufficient room for access from a particular side of the head holds true for the patient who is on ventilator support without general anesthesia where the ventilator and the connecting tubing need a specific area and room for access. With or without a ventilator, a suction line/apparatus must always be adjacent to the patient's mouth and airway and must be immediately accessible.

Transesophageal echo

Although the transesophageal echo (TEE) console may not be "parked" permanently in the catheterization laboratory, the increasing frequency of use of TEE during congenital cardiac catheterizations has created an additional semi-permanent space requirement very close to the head of the catheterization table. The connecting cable between the TEE probe and the echo console is relatively short, and the person manipulating the TEE probe frequently operates the console while manipulating the probe. As a consequence, the large TEE console is positioned very close to the head of the table. It must be possible to have access to the patient with the TEE probe *and the TEE machine* from either right or left side of the *head* of the table. The location of the TEE depends upon whether vascular access for the catheterization is from either the arm or neck and, in addition, on which side of the head the anesthesia access is located. The current TEE consoles also have a large footprint and necessitate a large amount of space cephalad to the head of the catheterization table, regardless of which vascular access to the patient is used.

The TEE machine is usually operated with the echo console positioned cephalad to the support arm for the lateral X-ray tube and intensifier and to the left of the patient's head. This places the echo console with its monitor and the operator cephalad to (and behind) the lateral image intensifier and out of the view of the catheterizing physicians. An additional mobile "slave" monitor away from the TEE machine will then be necessary in order for the operating cardiologist to see the TEE image. The remote monitor can be positioned away from the TEE console and directly in front of the *catheterizing physicians*, in order to allow the TEE image to be visualized continuously, no matter where the catheterizing physicians are positioned around the table relative to the TEE console. Ideally the slave TEE monitor is mounted with the other ceiling suspended (X-ray and physiologic) monitors. Another alternative is to have the slave monitor of the TEE mounted on a mobile floor cart, which can easily be moved to any open, viewable position around the table. Some X-ray systems allow a "picture in picture" positioning of the TEE image within the image of one of the X-ray monitors. This is not as satisfactory as may be perceived. If it is large enough to be usable the superimposed TEE image occupies approximately one-fourth of the X-ray image and always extends into, and compromises, the critical, *central area* of the X-ray image.

Whenever either X-ray tube is in an LAO-cranial position, the TEE console and the TEE operator physically compete with the location of the image intensifier. This requires good communication and, usually, some displacement of the TEE operator and the console when the X-ray tube/intensifier are rotated into, and remain in that position.

Adjunctive equipment required within the catheterization room

There is a considerable amount of additional, essential, but at the same time, usually mobile equipment in the modern catheterization laboratory. This equipment, although mobile, remains in the catheterization room and takes up a finite, and often a significant amount of additional floor space there. This equipment includes the emergency medication/defibrillator cart, often a separate medication cart, the apparatus for blood oxygen saturation determinations, a patient-warming system, a cardiac output computer, and space for the mobile storage of very frequently used, consumable supplies. In some laboratories the angiographic injector, radiographic protective equipment, suction equipment and adjustable "operating field" lights are on floor-mounted, mobile stands, in which case they require additional floor space.

Emergency cart/defibrillator

Each cardiac catheterization room must have a mobile cardiac defibrillator and an "emergency cart" containing medications and resuscitative equipment. The defibrillator should have a rechargeable battery source of power in addition to a fixed source of (wall) electrical power. Often the emergency cart and defibrillator are combined into one mobile cart. The emergency cart contains items to establish an oral or nasal airway, equipment for endotracheal intubation, equipment to start intravenous or intra-arterial lines, suction catheters and the accessories for the defibrillator. Whenever a patient is in the room, the items on the emergency cart and the defibrillator must be available immediately and conveniently to the personnel in the room and to the patient. This, however, does not require that the emergency cart and defibrillator always be *immediately* adjacent the patient. However, the supplies on the emergency cart are organized in such a way that the location of each item on the cart is known instinctively and each item is available immediately to *all personnel* in the room. The defibrillator is turned on with the appropriate paddles for the patient attached to it and the paste for the paddles readily available. The correct voltage according to the size of the patient is set and the defibrillator is placed in a location from which there is immediate and unobstructed access to the patient during the procedure.

Medication tray/cabinet

In addition to the emergency and defibrillator cart(s), each catheterization room has a separate, readily accessible, medication tray or cart. The medication cart contains all of the emergency drugs, sedatives, and other medications used both in emergencies and more routinely in the cardiac catheterization laboratory as well as a variety of intravenous fluids. The details of the medications which are maintained in the medication cart are discussed in Chapter 2. This medication tray is located in close proximity to the manifold containing the transducers and flush lines. When a nurse is operating the manifold, this nurse has immediate access to the medication cart and usually is responsible for administering medications from the cart.

Operating lights for the catheterization table

Movable or widely adjustable, focused lights over the operating field are essential in the catheterization laboratory. Free-standing floor lights, mounted on a mobile stand and with a long neck that extends over the catheterization table, were the standard for years and are still used in some institutions. These floor lights take up additional floor space immediately adjacent to the catheterization table, they often do not permit the light source to shine from the correct direction on the specific field, creating shadows rather than light over the working areas, and they are a constant potential for contamination of the sterile field. Ceiling-mounted operating room lights on long movable arms are the standard in most catheterization laboratories at the present time. Ceiling-mounted lights conserve floor space and allow the light to be directed more appropriately, but, when there are other ceiling-mounted accessories (angiographic contrast injectors and radiation protection screens), the ceiling-mounted lights add to the congestion in the area immediately above the catheterization table due to the multiple suspension arms. This congestion of the arms creates a problem in the optimal use of the other accessories.

The ideal lights for the catheterization laboratory are a set or group of recessed, high-intensity, focused, ceiling lights, which can be directed toward a specific spot on the catheterization table with a remote apparatus. The lights are adjusted by a small hand-held strobe light or "light wand", which is positioned immediately over the catheter introduction site. The strobe light positioned over the puncture site, in turn, directs each individual ceiling light to that specific spot on the catheterization table. With one, or several, of the lights mounted in the ceiling cephalad to the image intensifier (and the lateral tube X-ray suspension arm) and with the remainder of the lights mounted caudal to the image intensifier, excellent lighting is available to any area of the head, neck or arms as well as to the inguinal areas. These recessed lights do not interfere with other ceiling-mounted equipment and take up "no real estate", but do represent a very expensive initial investment.

Blood oxygen saturation analyzer

The oximeter apparatus for the analysis of blood samples for the immediate determination of oxygen saturations is situated in the catheterization room and in very close proximity to the catheterization table. Most oxygen analyzers are located on a very small, mobile table or cart. The physician should be able to hand the syringe with the blood specimens for analysis directly to the technician/nurse for insertion into the analyzer and, at the same time, the technician should not have to take more than one or two steps between receiving the sample and inserting it into the analyzer. The results from most oxygen analyzers are displayed digitally on a very small screen on the analyzer. A read-out of the saturation results also should be clearly visible to the operator immediately, conveniently and on a large display in the catheterization laboratory. A large, immediately available display of the digital read-out of the oxygen saturation, the time of the sample and the location of the sample can be accomplished with some "hard wiring" from an A-Vox™ Oxygen Analyzer (A-VOX Systems, Inc., San Antonio, TX) to a "slave" computer with a large CRT or flat panel display, which utilizes special computer software which is now available from Scientific Software Solutions (Scientific Software Solutions, Inc., Charlottesville, VA). This provides a large, timed, instantaneous display of each oxygen saturation and its location as it is analyzed. The developed table of saturations, their time and location can be printed and used to verify the data that have been verbally transmitted to the computerized catheterization record.

Ideally, these same data could also be transmitted directly from the oxygen analyzer to the electronic record on the catheterization laboratory computer and be logged into the timed computer record without any verbal (shouted!), hand-written or manually typed transmission of the information. Unfortunately the small pediatric/congenital market has not been enough of an economic stimulus for any of the large manufacturers of physiologic equipment for the catheterization laboratory for them to provide the communication necessary to incorporate this already available, digital information into their physiologic monitoring/recording equipment.

Patient-warming equipment

Equipment for warming the patient is mandatory. Most cardiac catheterization laboratories operate in a very "cool" ambient environment. When the drapes on the patient become wet and room temperature (cold) flush solutions are continually running into the patient, most patients require supplemental support of their body temperature. The most effective means of maintaining the body temperature of the patient is to increase the environmental temperature of the catheterization room. For infants or debilitated patients, this requires an environmental temperature of up to 80° Fahrenheit. Such a high temperature is uncomfortable for most personnel within the room, but at the same time is absolutely necessary for very small or debilitated patients regardless of the use of other supplemental warming systems. High environmental temperatures also interfere with the cooling of any X-ray generating equipment which happens to be positioned within the room and provide another strong argument for a separate equipment bay for this machinery.

There are several separate patient-warming systems commercially available for the catheterization laboratory. Separate, supplemental warming systems for the patient are attached directly to the table or the warming component is actually positioned on the catheterization table. The Bear Hugger™ hot-air warmers currently appear to be the most suitable system for cardiac catheterization procedures and they require a relatively fixed amount of floor space immediately adjacent to the catheterization table. The heating mechanism with its blower is usually positioned at the foot of the catheterization table. A connecting tube from the blower attaches to a very long U-shaped, sterile and disposable "paper tube", the arms of which run, unobtrusively, under the sterile drape and along each side of the length of the patient. The warmed air is blown through these tubes around the patient under the drapes. The tubes do not interfere with access to the patient nor do they show up on fluoroscopy or angiograms.

Several other patient-warming systems are available which take up less fixed space around the table, but in general, are less satisfactory for use in the catheterization laboratory. The K-Pad™ heating system utilizes a plastic pad through which warm water is circulated. The pad, which is positioned under the trunk of the patient, is attached by tubing to a small heater/pump, which is placed on the catheterization table, under the drapes at the foot of the table. The K-Pad™ is not available nor suitable for patients of all sizes and the tubing within the pad is slightly radio opaque and, in turn, shows up on the fluoroscopy and angiographic images, particularly in smaller infants.

Another, even less satisfactory alternative for warming a patient is a floor-mounted "heating lamp". These take up less space on the table and are very mobile, but they must be positioned immediately adjacent to, and over, the trunk of the patient, which always positions the lamp in the working area of either the operator or the fluoroscopy. Like the lights on a floor-mounted stand, the heating lamp extending over the trunk of the patient represents a constant potential for contamination of the sterile field. Of even greater concern is it that, in order to warm a patient through a very focused heat source from above, the heating lamp must generate a relatively high heat and must be positioned fairly close to the patient's skin, the combination of which creates a real potential for actually burning the latter. The use of this type of lamp must be monitored very closely to prevent this occurrence.

Angiographic injector

The angiographic injector should be capable of being attached to the angiographic catheter from either side of the catheterization table, from the top or bottom end of the table and from any catheter introduction site. The injector syringe must always be angled *downward* when it is connected to the hub of a catheter or connecting tubing for an injection. The downward angle forces any air which might be trapped in the injector tubing or injector syringe to rise to the back end of the injector syringe. When the injector syringe is attached directly to the catheter hub, the injector head is *always* positioned above the level of the hub of the catheter in order to assure that the *tip* of the injector syringe is pointing downward.

Fortunately, the "injector head" of the modern MedRad (MedRad, Inc., Indianola, PA) and Liebel-Flarsheim (Mallinckrodt Inc., Hazelwood, MO) angiographic injectors can be separated from the large, bulkier, control apparatus of the injector. This allows the injector head to be mounted separately and away from the control unit. Mounting the injector on a long, movable, ceiling-mounted arm positions the injector head well above the surface of the catheterization table and allows it to be moved to any location about the table. A ceiling-mounted injector does not occupy any floor space and there is less danger of the sterile field or the operator being contaminated when the injector is being attached to, or while it is attached to, the catheter. The separate control unit can be positioned across the catheterization room away from the catheterization table or, preferably, even in a separate, but adjacent control room.

A less satisfactory arrangement is to have the separate injector head mounted on a mobile floor stand. However, the floor stand occupies valuable floor space wherever it is positioned and it must also be moved about the room and positioned immediately adjacent to the catheterization table for injections. This positions the stand very close to the side of the patient and necessitates that the injector extends over, and very close to, the sterile field. With a rigid attachment to the floor stand, the injector head cannot be raised much above the level of the catheter hub in order to keep the tip pointing downward. Some of these disadvantages can be obviated by the use of very long connecting tubes between the injector syringe and the catheter.

Adjustable radiation protection screens

In addition to the regular use of lead aprons and optimal X-ray techniques, supplemental X-ray protection screens should be used during every catheterization procedure. Most of the radiation to the operating physician originates from the scatter, which emanates out of the patient's body *above* the catheterization table. The most effective way of minimizing this radiation to the operator is by the use of a leaded glass screen placed between the patient's body and the operating physician. The preferred screen for the protection of the operating physician is suspended on a long articulated arm from the ceiling above the catheterization table. In this way the screen, covered with a sterile, transparent drape, is moved between the patient and the operator without occupying any "real estate" on the floor of the room and without contaminating the field.

Similar protective leaded glass screens are available on floor mounted stands, which move on casters; however, the floor screens occupy valuable floor space and when used near the catheterization table, interfere with angulation of the X-ray tubes. Large, free standing, transparent, leaded glass X-ray screens, mounted on casters, are useful for the protection of personnel not working directly at the table. The additional personnel who benefit the most from these screens include the anesthesiologist, the circulating nurse/technicians and respiratory therapists.

Cardiac output computer

Determination of the cardiac output is often required during the catheterization of pediatric and congenital heart patients. Although a precise cardiac output is not necessary for calculating *relative* shunts and obvious gradients, when the calculations of absolute flow and resistances are necessary, an accurate cardiac output becomes mandatory. Our cardiac catheterization laboratories now use a thermodilution technique with a small, dedicated, Dualtherm™ Cardiac Output Computer (B. Braun Medical Inc., Bethlehem, PA) designed specifically for calculating thermodilution cardiac outputs. The thermodilution apparatus is relatively small and is mounted on a small mobile cart. When a cardiac output is to be determined, the computer is connected to the specific thermodilution catheter (B. Braun Medical Inc., Bethlehem, PA) on the catheterization table with a sterile, reusable cable, which extends directly from the computer to the catheter. This small cart is moved close to the table for cardiac output determination and is parked well away from the catheterization table when not in use.

"In-room" consumable equipment storage

The great bulk of the consumable equipment, including the back-up supply of the most frequently used items, is stored in a *separate*, dedicated storage room, which is situated immediately adjacent to the actual catheterization room. At the same time, a limited supply of multiple sizes of very frequently and repeatedly used sterile consumable items including percutaneous needles, a variety of guide wires, sheath/dilator sets, syringes, the most frequently used catheters and even gloves are stored directly in the catheterization room, but in mobile carts. While all of the consumable equipment could be stored in the adjacent storage room, the repeated retrieval of very frequently used items from a separate, even though adjacent room, during the case, reduces the functional efficiency of the laboratory very significantly.

Storage of the "high use" expendable materials actually within the room maximizes the efficiency for the frequent retrievals. Specifically configured, mobile storage carts provide the most effective vehicle for this in-lab storage of the frequently used consumables. These can be moved in and out of the room for cleaning, for restocking with new supplies or when the particular items on that cart are not being used at all. These carts can also be moved easily to accommodate a reconfiguration of the arrangement of the room according to the various introductory sites for the catheters or according to the type of procedure being performed.

The mobile storage carts maximize the usable space of the room as opposed to the traditional, fixed cabinets along the walls of the room. Any fixed, built-in cabinets for storage within the catheterization room represent "wasted" floor space, which is lost permanently and cannot be "adjusted". Each row of fixed cabinets or counters reduces the functional width or depth of the catheterization room by at least three feet and reduces the total floor space of the catheterization room by this width times the length of the wall(s) covered with cabinets! Built in cabinets do not allow even minor reconfiguration of the room for different procedures.

"Mobile" equipment stored outside of the catheterization room

There are other pieces of mobile equipment that are shared between several catheterization rooms and stored within the general area of the catheterization laboratory, but preferably just outside of the actual catheterization room. Each piece of this equipment requires space for storage outside of, but adjacent to, the actual catheterization room and, when the equipment is in use, additional space must be provided for it in the catheterization room itself. Among this ancillary equipment are included a separate, but constantly available, 2-D echo machine, a radio frequency generator, an oxygen consumption apparatus with its constant air withdrawal system and several "hoods", an echo console for intravascular ultrasound (IVUS), transesophageal echo (TEE) and/or intravascular echo (ICE), a Laser™ generator and possibly a cardiac "mechanical assist" device. When used, most of these pieces of equipment must be positioned immediately adjacent to the catheterization table. At the same time, the location of this equipment while it is being used should not interfere with the catheterizing physician's access to the patient or the overall mobility within the room. This requires a greater overall planned width or depth to the room in order to prevent severe side-by-side crowding at the tableside.

2-D Echo machine

A 2-D echo machine capable of transthoracic scanning of the pericardial space should be available in the catheterization laboratory immediately for emergency situations. This does not have to be the latest nor the most sophisticated echo machine available but it must be functional. This echo machine is required in addition to, and separate from, the TEE/ICE console, which usually is a special console utilized specifically for TEE and/or ICE and is brought to the catheterization laboratory only when TEE and/or ICE is/are used. Much of the time, the TEE/ICE machine may be needed elsewhere in the hospital and, in turn, may not be available for some time or be physically far from the vicinity of the catheterization laboratory. The separate, always available 2-D echo machine is primarily for screening patients who deteriorate either acutely or unexpectedly. This is particularly important when screening for suspected cardiac tamponade. The added time needed to transport an echo machine to the catheterization laboratory from an area outside of, and remote from, the immediate catheterization area represents a delay in confirming a diagnosis, which could easily represent the difference between a successful and an unsuccessful resuscitation.

Radio frequency generator

Pediatric cardiac catheterization laboratories now require a dedicated radio frequency (RF) generator, which is designed specifically for the perforation of tissues. Although this unit may be used only 6–12 times per year, the infants in whom an RF generator is used are not "scheduled" and often have a critical time window for their treatment. The BMC Radio Frequency Generator (Baylis Medical Co. Inc., Montreal, Canada), specifically for perforation, is quite small and can be stored outside of the actual catheterization room when not being used. When used in any particular procedure it is placed on a small, temporary cart adjacent to the catheterization table and connected to the RF catheter (Baylis Medical Co. Inc., Montreal, Canada) with a sterile reusable cable.

Oxygen consumption apparatus

The MRM-2 Oxygen Consumption Monitor (Waters Instruments Inc., Rochester, MN) for measurement of oxygen consumption is a gas analyzer in conjunction with several different hoods and a vacuum pump/blower used to draw air through the hoods. In most laboratories, the apparatus is used infrequently and, as a consequence, is (should be) stored in an adjacent area, out of the catheterization room. The apparatus is cumbersome; it covers the patient's head, neck and upper thorax and is fairly disruptive to the usual catheterization procedure. When an oxygen consumption determination is to be performed on a patient during a catheterization procedure it is planned ahead of time and the specific arrangements are made for the oxygen consumption measurement when the patient is being placed on the catheterization table. The patient's head and neck are positioned on a flat surface on the catheterization table with no pillow beneath their head. There can be no catheter lines entering the neck and the patient cannot be intubated or receiving oxygen or general anesthesia while oxygen consumption is being measured.

Intravascular ultrasound and intracardiac echo equipment

Currently intravascular ultrasound (IVUS) and intracardiac echo (ICE) imaging are used frequently in many pediatric and congenital catheterization laboratories. The particular consoles from Acuson, Mountain View, CA or Boston Scientific, Natick, MA, which are used for this imaging are quite large. The consoles are usually stored out of the actual catheterization room and brought into the laboratory only when needed for a specific case. The catheter for ICE is a 10–11-gauge French catheter and usually is introduced from a femoral vein, while the catheters for IVUS are smaller and can be introduced into a vein or artery from a femoral or jugular access site and can be introduced from either arm. The catheters are usually attached to their respective console with a long connecting cable within a long sterile sleeve. The physician operating the console is not necessarily the catheterizing physician who is maneuvering the catheter. As a consequence, the machines (consoles) for these procedures usually do not have to be immediately adjacent to the catheter introduction site, but do require a relatively large space, relatively close to the catheterization table in the general area where the imaging catheter is introduced. Like the TEE, a remote or slave monitor is usually necessary in order for the catheterizing physician to visualize the intravascular echo images conveniently.

Laser™ generator

A Laser™ generator (Spectranetics, Colorado Springs, CO) is used for lead extractions and some purposeful perforations. It is another very large piece of equipment, which is used in a pediatric/congenital cardiac catheterization laboratory only occasionally and, when moved into the room, requires significant additional space adjacent to the catheterization table. The Laser™ generator is stored outside of the catheterization room or even away from the laboratory as a shared piece of equipment between several services or even institutions. The use of the Laser™ is scheduled well ahead of time and the generator is moved into the laboratory for the specific procedure. Special precautions for eye protection are required for all personnel who are, or might be, in the room for the procedure. Considerable rearranging of the equipment in the room is required during these isolated and rare circumstances.

Extra cardiac membrane oxygenator (ECMO) or other left ventricular assist device (LVAD)

An even more rarely used piece of very large and cumbersome adjunctive equipment which may become more common and even essential in the future catheterization laboratory is one of the cardiac assist devices including an ECMO apparatus, an intra-aortic balloon pump or even an LVAD. When an assist device is necessary, it likely would be as an emergency. Although the equipment for these procedures would have to be moved from the operating room or intensive care area, it would not be expedient to have to move other equipment which is being used in the catheterization laboratory out of the laboratory, or to have to rearrange the catheterization laboratory very significantly in order to bring these large pieces of emergency equipment to the patient rapidly during such an emergency. A potential physical "corridor" to the table, and place for this equipment, should be considered ahead of time when a catheterization is planned on a patient who might be a potential candidate for such therapy.

Electrophysiology equipment

The pediatric/congenital electrophysiologic (EP) laboratory contains additional very large pieces of equipment which, unlike the catheterization table itself, are not fixed structures in the room, but, at the same time, are not particularly mobile and take up considerable additional fixed space. This equipment varies with each EP laboratory, but at a minimum includes a separate computer and monitor, a separate recorder, a stimulator, a radio frequency generator for ablations, multiple additional CRT monitors and additional mobile storage cabinets for the frequently used, special EP consumables. The Laser™ generator for lead extractions is more likely to be used and stored in the EP laboratory. The extra EP "capital" equipment often has a space requirement equivalent to the space of a separate control room. Usually this equipment is housed in, and used directly within the catheterization room. This extra space should be included in the basic design of the catheterization room which is to be used for electrophysiologic procedures.

Support areas for the catheterization room(s)

The actual cardiac catheterization room is not a "free standing", independent or isolated room, which can be placed randomly at the convenience of any available space. Each catheterization room requires a significant amount of space which must be immediately adjacent to the catheterization room, for the logistical, mechanical and personnel support for the operation of the actual catheterization room. This support space plus the catheterization room(s) make up the catheterization suite. The support space occupies more square footage than the catheterization room(s). The support space ideally includes a separate control room for each catheterization room, a large room for the storage of the majority of the consumable equipment, a separate electrical equipment room or "bay" for the X-ray generators, controls and high-tension switches, a patient holding/preparation area, an administrative support area, a record/angio review/work area, an on-site storage area for "active" patient records and angiograms, a biomedical service/supply area and a separate procedure room for procedures other than X-ray which require monitoring (e.g. phlebotomies, thoracocentesis, transesophageal echocardiograms).

Control room

The control room houses the physiologic monitoring equipment, computer recorder and the controls for the X-ray system for each specific catheterization room. In addition, each control room contains remote monitors of the CRT screens which are in the catheterization room, the controls for the angiographic injector, the computer(s) which is/are connected to the hospital system, the digital X-ray recording system, a digital disk copier, printers for physiologic records, the computer log of the procedure, and hard-copy printers for X-ray images, all with adequate space for at least two nurses/technicians to function comfortably. An area 10 to 11 feet wide and as long as the width of the catheterization room (e.g. 10 × 24 feet) provides a reasonable sized control room with room for some fixed counters and cabinet space in addition to the monitoring equipment. In addition to a good view of the entire catheterization room, including the entire catheterization table, and clear voice communication between the catheterization room and the control room, the personnel in the control room should have direct and easy physical access into the catheterization room.

The control area preferably is *not* situated *within* the actual catheterization room. The control/monitoring/recording equipment takes up a large amount of valuable floor space, which should not be taken from the actual catheterization room. The control room equipment generates noise, accumulates dust and is operated more effectively in a clean, but non-sterile, environment. In addition, when the control room equipment is located within the catheterization room, it exposes the nurses/technicians who operate it to extra and unnecessary radiation. At the same time, the control room must be *immediately* adjacent to the catheterization room. The orientation of the catheterization table diagonally across the catheterization room facilitates a view of the entire length of the patient on the table whether the control room is directly at the end or along the side of the catheterization room. The control room usually is *not* a sterile area and can have additional space in it, which serves as an observation area for consultants/visitors.

A shared central control room between two or more catheterization rooms is seen occasionally, but is not an optimal arrangement. Except for a questionable economy of space, there is no justification for a combined or shared control room. None of the actual electronic control equipment in the control room is shared between separate catheterization rooms. Much of the communication between the separate catheterization rooms and the control room and within the control room is verbal. When the control equipment and personnel from two or more laboratories are grouped together in one room, there are continual distractions, the communication becomes confused and the working environment becomes very congested and noisy.

Consumable equipment storage room

The *majority* of the consumable equipment (catheters, introducers, wires, dilation balloons, special devices, etc.) is stored outside, but immediately adjacent to, the actual catheterization room. For a laboratory performing therapeutic catheterizations on pediatric and adult congenital heart patients, this requires a huge amount and variety of consumable equipment which, in turn, requires a very large storage space, which is equal in size to the optimal sized catheterization room (roughly 32 × 24 feet). Fortunately two, or even three, separate catheterization rooms do not require significantly more consumable equipment and additional storage space for the consumable equipment than a single laboratory. If there is more than one catheterization room, it is most efficient to have a single storage room for the consumables adjacent to, and connected to, all of the separate catheterization laboratories (rooms) with convenient access to each of the laboratories. Because of the large amount of very expensive consumable material required for a pediatric/congenital catheterization laboratory, the storage area must be absolutely secure.

The storage room requires an organizational plan or arrangement for inventory control which (1) keeps track of each item used to facilitate the expedient reordering of used items and, (2) obligates the use of the older items before newer, more recently acquired items in order to avoid the problem of having to discard new and unused items because of material or sterility expiry dates. This organization of the inventory is even more critical when several or more catheterization rooms are drawing supplies from the same storage source.

A catheterization laboratory should have both a blood gas analyzer such as an ABL 700 Radiometer (Radiometer, Copenhagen, Denmark) and an activated clotting time (ACT) machine (Hemo Tec, Inc., Englewood, CA). Both of these machines can be shared between several or more catheterization rooms. These machines are fixed in location and when shared, they are housed conveniently in a central consumable storage area, which is adjacent to all of the actual catheterization rooms. This equipment must be in close proximity to each catheterization room but, preferably, must not be within the catheterization room itself. Under usual circumstances this equipment is used only two or three times during an entire catheterization procedure. Both the blood gas and ACT machines require regular maintenance and calibration by biomedical personnel who normally function more proficiently in a non-sterile environment. When these machines are not in the actual catheterization room, any maintenance/calibration can be performed on them while a catheterization is in progress. Rarely, blood gas machines are used to calculate all of the blood oxygen saturation determinations. In that situation, the blood gas machine should be physically in the catheterization laboratory.

A separate, X-ray equipment room or "bay"

It is now *essential* that modern X-ray generators and X-ray power supplies are housed in a dedicated equipment room, which is completely separate from the catheterization room. There no longer is a place for the cabinets for the X-ray generators, controllers and high-tension "switches" to be located within the actual catheterization room. In addition to the physical space occupied by the high-tension generators and other X-ray electronic equipment, this equipment requires a separate and efficient refrigeration/air conditioning unit to allow continuous, extra and extreme cooling of the X-ray and other electrical components in order to counteract the excessive heat generated by it. The cool environment is essential for the day-to-day stability and operation of the sensitive equipment and in order to maintain the durability of the very expensive electrical equipment. When the electrical equipment is situated in the catheterization room, an environmental temperature which is cool enough to keep the equipment adequately cooled is far too cold to maintain the body temperature of a patient.

Although the "equipment bay" is a separate room, because of the limitations of the maximal lengths of the high-tension cables connecting the X-ray tubes to the generators, it must also be in close proximity to the actual catheterization laboratory. Assuming the "geometry" can be solved for situating more than one catheterization room adjacent to the equipment bay, a single equipment bay can house the generators and power supplies of two or more catheterization rooms while using the same additional cooling system. The equipment bay needs a lot of wall space for the modern digital electronics so that a relatively long but narrow room, for example 10×32 feet, will suffice to hold the heavy electronic equipment for two biplane catheterization rooms (Siemens Medical Systems, Inc., Iselin, NJ) as well as the extra cooling equipment.

In addition to the cooling requirements, even the latest digital and computerized catheterization laboratory X-ray generating equipment still takes up a large amount of space and, if positioned within the actual catheterization room, would reduce its functional width by at least two feet in depth along one entire, long wall. When the generation equipment is within the sterile catheterization room, access to the equipment for maintenance or even minor resetting of circuits is restricted to times when the room is not in operation. Like the electronic equipment in the control room, the X-ray generating equipment has huge areas for attracting and collecting dust, which is not acceptable in a "sterile" working catheterization room.

Preparation, holding and recovery area(s) for patients

Patients do not enter directly into the cardiac catheterization laboratory from "outside", nor do they go directly home after a catheterization. With many pediatric and congenital heart cardiac catheterizations now being performed as outpatient or "day-surgery" procedures, an area is required for the admission of the patients for the catheterization procedure, their preparation for catheterization and the administration of premedications. When the catheterization laboratories operate adjacent to, or in conjunction with, the cardiovascular operating rooms, the same preparation/holding area can be used to admit the patients for both the catheterization laboratories and the operating rooms. The total size of the "holding area" depends upon the number of procedure rooms (catheterization labs or operating rooms), which are being supported.

Each bed space in a "holding/admitting" area should be capable of monitoring and recording several leads of an electrocardiogram, a pulse oximetry display, a display of the patient's body temperature and the capability of displaying at least one pressure monitoring line. The physical space of each "holding bed" must comply with standards for recovery room beds. Each bed requires piped in oxygen, compressed air and suction. The holding area must have a separate "crash cart" including emergency cardiac medications, intubation and temporary ventilation equipment as well as a cardiac defibrillator. All of the facilities and equipment for drawing blood samples as well as starting and maintaining intravenous lines must be available in the holding area. All of the beds can be in one open area, but must be separated from each other by at least curtains or screens. Since some patients may remain in the area for a relatively long period of time awaiting their catheterization or surgery, a television or "play station" is made available for at least half of the beds.

The number of beds and the size of this area, obviously, depend upon the number of catheterization rooms (and operating rooms if the area is shared), any function of the area besides admitting and holding, and the total number of patients expected through the area per day. For patient preparation and premedication, one bed per catheterization procedural room *and* one bed for each operating room are sufficient. This allows for the simultaneous preparation at the beginning of the day of all of the "first" patients for each of the procedural rooms and allows each procedural room to start at approximately the same time when desired. Patients who are scheduled for catheterization (or surgery) as second, third or later cases are scheduled to arrive at the holding area later according to a staggered schedule. This allows a bed for each patient, time to admit each patient comfortably, prepare them for the procedure and to have them totally prepared and sedated by the time the procedure room is ready to start.

A four to six hour recovery/observation period is mandatory immediately post-catheterization for cardiac catheterization patients. The patient should have close monitoring by experienced nurses during that time immediately after a cardiac catheterization. Ideally, this monitoring is accomplished in a cardiac recovery area or cardiac intensive care unit. However, if the cardiac catheterization laboratory is in a location remote from the cardiac recovery/intensive care units, the holding area can be adapted to serve as an observation/recovery area for the patients post-catheterization. With an adequate number of beds and the space and monitoring equipment to be used for patient recovery post-catheterization already established, the same area used for the patients' admission can be expanded to a recovery area. In that circumstance, because of the overlap of the patients arriving for their procedures with the patients who are recovering, the "recovery" beds in the area should be separated from the "admission" beds more solidly than with just curtains. A recovering patient who is uncomfortable, vomiting or having more serious problems, is extremely upsetting and frightening to a patient who is about to undergo "the same" procedure! When the holding area is used for post-catheterization recovery, the nursing staff is larger, the nurses need additional training and experience in the recovery of catheterization patients and the functioning "hours" of the holding area must be extended and very flexible according to the anticipated procedures for the day.

Administrative and general support areas

A liberal amount of additional space is required *within the general catheterization area* for the general administrative support of the catheterization laboratory. This support area includes the working areas for the catheterization laboratory manager and secretarial/administrative assistants. They should be located in close proximity to the actual laboratory in order to support the minute-to-minute activities of the laboratory including the changes in scheduling and assignments during each day. The administrative support area also provides a work area for the nurses, technicians and physicians to review and compile the catheterization records and angiograms, space and the equipment for copying these materials and space for the temporary storage of, at least, the most current and "active" catheterization records and angiograms. For the support of two or more laboratories, this requires working space for two or more personnel. This area can be relatively long and narrow in order to be positioned immediately adjacent to the catheterization laboratories, for example 10 to 11 feet by 32 feet in length.

The catheterization laboratory area must have adequate and convenient toilet facilities, which include sinks and a shower along with secure lockers and changing space for all of the personnel working in the catheterization area. The personnel should not have to leave the general area of the catheterization laboratories to use the toilet or changing facilities. Easy access to a supply of "scrubs" in a convenient changing/locker area within the catheterization suite encourages the personnel to change into scrubs while in the catheterization laboratories, but, at the same time, encourages them *not* to wear the scrubs out of the hospital.

The overall cardiac catheterization area needs a separate break or relaxation area for all of the personnel who work there. The personnel in the catheterization laboratory work in a continually stressful atmosphere and, frequently, at a continual and frantic pace. At least a short intermittent break out of the catheterization room improves the working atmosphere in the room. When this "break room" is still within the area of the catheterization suite, it allows the personnel to have time out of the actual rooms without loosing "transit" time to and from a break area and without the personnel having to change out of their laboratory scrubs.

Cine/angio/data review area

Each catheterization suite requires an area for the physicians to review and analyze the data and the angiograms from the current catheterizations. The review area should have space to accommodate up to four or five physicians at a time as well as a large counter space for the review and measurement of the paper tracings of the recorded pressures, which when stretched out extend for several meters. The review area requires at least one computer, which is in communication with the catheterization laboratory as well as the information systems of the hospital including the hospital X-ray and echo systems. This (or these) computer(s) also should be in communication with the on-line, digital storage system for the digital angiograms from the catheterization laboratory.

The review room requires specific and usually separate equipment for the review of "outside" angiograms as well as those generated in the catheterization laboratory itself. The common transferable, digital media at the present time is the DICOM encoded compact disk (CD). This requires a digital viewer/review station, which can read all medically encoded DICOM digital data. Although all major medical manufacturers supposedly comply with a single DICOM standard, occasionally separate software is required in the CD reader or a completely separate computer/review station is necessary to read CDs from different systems/manufacturers. Since many of the previous, older, angiographic studies on the current patients were recorded on cine film and some existing cardiac catheterization laboratories are still recording on cine film, the reviewing area requires a functioning cine film viewer (Tagarno of America, Inc., Dover, DE).

The review area must have some space designated for the storage of the catheterization reports and angiocardiogram of patients who are currently hospitalized, or who will be hospitalized in the near future. A copying machine for records, catheterization diagrams and digital angiograms improves the efficiency of the area and helps to keep permanent records intact.

Biomedical support area

With the total dependence in a modern catheterization laboratory upon the large variety of both simple and very complex electro-mechanical equipment, all cardiac catheterization laboratories are equally and totally dependent upon biomedical support being readily available in order to operate the cardiac catheterization laboratories daily and continuously. Ideally the biomedical personnel for the cardiac catheterization laboratory are a part of the catheterization laboratory personnel, and their primary responsibility is to the catheterization laboratory. There should be adequate space in the vicinity of, or actually in, the catheterization laboratory suite for the biomedical personnel to work on the mobile equipment. The biomedical area must include space to store the testing and repair equipment as well as pieces of frequently needed and essential "spare" equipment. When there is more than one catheterization laboratory or other "high-intensity electrical areas" (operating rooms, intensive care areas) in close geographical proximity, there is adequate justification for specific biomedical engineers who are knowledgeable in that particular equipment to be assigned to the catheterization laboratories.

Any delay in the investigation and repair of an equipment malfunction, no matter how minor, results in an equivalent "down", or "inactive time" for the room, which includes three or more salaried nurses/technicians and one or more physicians who would be working in that room. A malfunction of a piece of equipment often requires a "repair" which is as simple as resetting a relay or switch and actually takes only seconds for a knowledgeable person to correct. At the same time, the relay may be located in a "high-tension" cabinet containing very complex electronics and, as a consequence, should be manipulated only by experienced biomedical personnel. An otherwise short delay is prolonged unnecessarily when the biomedical support who is capable of the simple "repair" or "resetting" is located any distance (and time) from the catheterization area. An active, fully scheduled, cardiac catheterization laboratory cannot afford any significant "down time". Any equipment failure during operating hours results in the rescheduling of the patients with a frequent "domino" effect on other patients and services throughout the hospital, in addition to the obvious costs in personnel "down time".

A separate "minor procedure" room

Depending upon the size of the cardiology service, there are a variable number of procedures which require monitoring, sedation and, occasionally, even general anesthesia. These procedures include phlebotomies with colloidal volume replacement, "tilt table" and other vaso-motor electrophysiologic testing, transesophageal echocardiography under general anesthesia, pleural taps and drainage with or without chest tube insertion, some pericardial taps and even some difficult intravenous or intra-arterial lines. The "interventional", "intensivist" or "catheterizing" physicians frequently perform these procedures. Although these procedures have been, and can be, performed in catheterization laboratories, they generally do not require *all* of the elaborate equipment and personnel of a catheterization laboratory.

Ideally, a separate "procedure room" is available in the immediate area of the catheterization laboratories/holding area. This room needs to be large enough to accommodate the procedure table, a sterile work table for the physician, any ancillary large equipment (e.g. a TEE machine, an anesthesia machine) and area for personnel to function in the room. The procedure room should have monitoring available with the capability of permanent recording of the ECG, pulse oximetry, a periodic recycling cuff blood pressure apparatus and at least one pressure transducer and recording channel for an indwelling line when desired. Piped in oxygen, compressed air and suction are essential. The procedure table in this room is an operating type of table, capable of tilting or there is a separate "tilt table" which can be moved into the room. The procedure table is lit with a high-intensity, ceiling-mounted, mobile "operating room" light. This room should have a mobile equipment cart to hold the consumables for any procedure being performed. The procedure room must have immediate access to a separate "crash cart" with intubation equipment, resuscitative drugs and fluids and a defibrillator. If the procedure room is *immediately* adjacent to the "holding" area, the emergency cart is shared with the holding area. Patients who are treated in this procedure room need admitting and frequently a recovery time similar to a catheterization patient.

Film processing room

A film processing room (area) is no longer necessary in a cardiac catheterization laboratory with digital X-ray equipment. A film processing room is still necessary in laboratories with older X-ray equipment which are using cine film as the recording medium. Although the image is produced by X-ray energy, cine-angiography film is a photographic film and is processed in a separate processor and with completely different techniques from the processing of X-ray film. Cine film processing is complex, time consuming, space occupying and environmentally polluting, all of which justifies upgrading cine film X-ray equipment to a digital system.

A film processing area includes not only a room for the film processor, but also a dark-room and a separate room to store the processing chemicals. The film processors are fairly compact but very complicated and require plumbing attachments from the chemical tanks and separate attachment to a special drainage system for the highly acidic and toxic developing chemicals. The processor requires constant maintenance in order to obtain the optimal processing of each roll of film. The daily maintenance includes adjusting the composition and temperature of the chemicals, assurance that all of the pumps and drives are functioning properly, and the cleaning of the multiple separate tanks and rollers in the processor. In addition to being consumed by the processor, the processing chemicals deteriorate with time and must be changed regularly regardless of the use of the processor. Possibly by the time this book is published, film processing in the catheterization laboratory will be delegated to the historical annals!

Catheterization laboratory personnel

Physicians

The medical director of the pediatric/congenital cardiac catheterization laboratory should be a pediatric cardiologist who regularly performs procedures in the catheterization laboratory. The ultimate responsibility for the proper equipment and the necessary personnel in the laboratory and, in turn, the smooth operation of the laboratory, is that of the medical director of the laboratory. The physician director must have the full support of the hospital. The number of cardiologists who perform catheterizations and their qualifications depend upon the number and type of procedures being performed in the catheterization laboratory.

A "simple" diagnostic catheterization procedure in a congenital heart patient can be performed by a single pediatric/congenital cardiologist with well trained and experienced support staff. The physicians and staff, for a diagnostic catheterization, do not have to have special training in *therapeutic/interventional* catheterization procedures, but should be experts in the anatomy and hemodynamics of congenital heart disease.

Most complex interventional (therapeutic) catheterization procedures performed on congenital heart patients should be performed by pediatric cardiologists with extra training in interventional catheterizations or with extensive experience in the catheterization laboratory and particularly with these procedures. New devices/procedures being introduced require even experienced interventional cardiologists to have some special individualized mentoring by a physician experienced in the procedure before beginning to use the new device/procedure. Most pediatric cardiologists who are entering the field of interventional/therapeutic catheterizations should and do take at least a year of additional and specific training in interventional catheterization procedures[2].

The more complex the catheterization procedure which is to be performed is, the more highly trained the physician(s) and catheterization laboratory staff must be for performing that procedure. Also the more complex the procedure is, the more experienced physicians and highly trained support nurse/technicians are required to be scrubbed and circulating during each procedure. For example, to perform complex catheter manipulations or even a "simple" balloon dilation procedure, there are multiple exchanges of catheters and wires with long lengths of guide wire extending out of the catheters which must be controlled to prevent their falling off the table. During the single balloon inflation a knowledgeable individual controls the position of the catheter/wire while a second knowledgeable individual inflates and deflates the balloon. The implant of two stents simultaneously represents an extreme of additional staffing needs for skilled staff. Two knowledgeable physicians maintain the stent/balloons precisely in place while two additional, trained individuals simultaneously control the inflation of the two balloons—i.e. four skilled individuals *scrubbed* for one procedure. Working with insufficient numbers of personnel or inadequately trained personnel prolongs a procedure significantly and increases the likelihood of adverse events or serious complications. The same procedure *can* be accomplished with fewer and less well-trained personnel scrubbed, but only with the substitution of a great deal of luck for skill and with an increase in the likelihood of an unsuccessful procedure or a procedure which results in serious complications! The problems encountered are in inverse proportion to the skill of the personnel and the number of skilled personnel involved with the procedure.

Non-physician catheterization laboratory personnel

Most pediatric/congenital cardiac catheterization laboratories require three, if not four, professional nurses or catheterization laboratory technicians to operate a catheterization room *efficiently*. The total number of nurses/technicians for an entire catheterization service must include not only the precise number of skilled individuals to operate each catheterization room, but enough extra personnel to account for illness, vacation, educational and compensatory time of the regular staff. Because of the extensive extra training each individual requires to function effectively as a catheterization nurse/technician in a pediatric/congenital cardiac catheterization laboratory, extra personnel cannot be pulled from other areas or from a general "pool" of personnel in the absence of one of the regular catheterization laboratory nurses/technicians. The laboratory itself must have its own pool of trained nurses/technicians to pull from. This is easier to accomplish when two or more catheterization rooms are operating in the overall pediatric/congenital cardiac catheterization unit.

The nurses/technicians who work in the cardiac catheterization laboratory have a background of registered nurses, practical nurses, radiographic or pulmonary technologists or have graduated from specialized cardiac catheterization or cardiopulmonary technician schools. Regardless of their background, almost all nurses/technicians starting in a pediatric/congenital cardiac catheterization laboratory require *at least six months* of orientation (on the job training) working in the catheterization laboratory under the supervision of the already experienced personnel in the laboratory. To work in a pediatric/

congenital cardiac catheterization laboratory further, extensive training/orientation is necessary, even for a nurse/technician who has extensive catheterization laboratory experience in an adult catheterization laboratory.

All of the nursing/technician personnel in the pediatric catheterization laboratory should be "cross trained" to perform all of the nursing/technician functions within the catheterization laboratory. In that way, any combination from all of the individuals in the laboratory pool can be on call together and in the unexpected absence of any one individual, any other nurse/technician is trained in, and can assume, the missing person's functions. This requires additional in-house training of new personnel in order to make them experts in areas and procedures which were not included at all in their pre-pediatric catheterization laboratory, background training.

Because of all of the extra training, the complex and potentially dangerous procedures performed daily on very sick patients and, in turn, the very high degree of responsibility and stress imposed on each individual, the cardiac catheterization laboratory personnel represent an elite, special group. The efficient completion of every procedure depends upon each nurse's/technician's skills, on their cooperation with each other and the physicians and on their willingness to work together as a team.

The minimum number of nurses/technicians required for each cardiac catheterization room is determined by the physical layout of the laboratory, the organization of the personnel, and the amount of nurse's or technician's work which the physicians themselves perform. Reducing the required or even optimal number of nurses/technicians available during a case represents a false *economy of bodies* at the increased expense of *an inefficiency of function*. When one nurse/technician is missing in a catheterization laboratory, that individual's particular jobs are performed by one of the remaining personnel in the room who, however, already has their own, assigned jobs and functions. The two or three nurses/technicians and the one to three physicians still in the room performing a procedure when one of the support personnel is missing, must wait several or more minutes for a particular procedure to be performed or for an item to be procured while the individual who normally performs that procedure or function is now performing the job of the missing person. Each delay of two minutes as a result of the absence of one individual results in a minimum of 12 minutes of total personnel time lost during the operation of the catheterization laboratory!

For example, in the absence of a circulating nurse, the nurse who operates the manifold must leave the manifold to retrieve an item of consumable equipment in the adjacent storage room. During the time the manifold nurse is out of the room, the operator cannot flush the catheter if he draws a sample, cannot switch to or from the pressure/flush line or balance the transducer to record a pressure and cannot administer medications until the manifold nurse returns. These lost segments of time for all of the personnel performing the case are multiplied many fold during every case when one essential person is missing. The repeated waiting time of the multiple individuals adds up to much more than enough time to account for the salary of the "extra" individual who is missing!

Emergency and off-hour cardiac catheterizations still occur quite frequently in a busy pediatric or congenital cardiac catheterization laboratory. A full complement of nurses/technicians for one catheterization room must be available on call. Although most emergency catheterizations are not as extensive or as prolonged as the usual scheduled procedures, emergency cases are performed on the very sickest and most precarious patients. These patients require the most intensive medical and most *timely* management. As a consequence, the emergency cases should not be undertaken short handed with less than a full complement of nursing/technician personnel in the room during the emergency procedures.

The "on-call" personnel may need to stay late in the laboratory for a prolonged or delayed scheduled case or have to return to the catheterization laboratory in the case of an emergency at any time, twenty-four hours a day and seven days a week. The on-call nurses/technicians are compensated financially for their time on call. In addition, they receive overtime salaries when actually called into the laboratory. In spite of this compensation, the on-call status requires a definite sacrifice for the personnel. They must have a commitment to either no other activities when on call or being able to interrupt *any activity* at *any time* when called. With a fully cross-trained staff of nurses/technicians, this allows the rotation of individuals within the "on-call teams" and allows some distribution of the call to suit the schedules of each of the individuals working in the catheterization laboratory.

The extra on-call duty is not the only sacrifice a pediatric catheterization laboratory nurse/technician makes. In a dedicated, busy, pediatric/congenital cardiac catheterization laboratory, a "normal", *scheduled* day does not exist. Cases frequently extend beyond their scheduled duration as well as beyond the normal working day. The individual cases frequently are longer than scheduled, the pediatric patients often need stabilization by the catheterizing physician between the catheterization procedures, which delays the start of the next case, and there are frequent "add on", urgent cases which appear regularly in the busy pediatric cardiovascular service. All of these factors very regularly extend the hours of the pediatric/congenital catheterization laboratory beyond the "8-hour day".

Rare or occasional extra time added to the regular work day is satisfactorily solved by merely having the involved personnel remain beyond the hours of their work day while receiving overtime compensation in the form of extra overtime salary or compensatory time off. However, in a busy pediatric/congenital catheterization laboratory where the extra hours are a regular occurrence, having each employee working extra hours *regularly* is not a solution. The cost of regular, repeated overtime pay becomes prohibitive to the hospital and there is never time available for the individuals to have compensatory time off. Of even greater importance, the strain on the employees of never having a fixed or dependable finish time to the working day results in employee dissatisfaction and a high employee turn-over. Besides the inconvenience of hiring and retraining new nurses/technicians, the retraining of new personnel is very expensive and time consuming.

As a consequence, in a busy pediatric/congenital catheterization laboratory it is necessary to provide a flexible working schedule for the nurses and technicians. There must be a sufficient total number of nurses/technicians to allow for staggered working hours and to allow additional scheduled time (or days) off to compensate for hours worked overtime. When the catheterization laboratories do finish the scheduled cases early, the personnel are allowed to leave without penalty. In a busy laboratory they still will work their minimal hours! The physicians working in the laboratory must also use some consideration when adding extra or "urgent" cases which could possibly be worked into the regular schedule.

The multiple duties of the nurses/technicians in a pediatric/congenital cardiac catheterization laboratory are divided into three or four different "job descriptions" during the catheterization:

Recording nurse/technician

One or two nurses or technicians operate the monitor/recording and the X-ray equipment in the control room (or area) of the catheterization room. The recording nurse or technician enters the time of the patient's entry into the laboratory, all of the patient's demographics, and the patient's vital signs and overall status upon arrival in the laboratory into the data system of the catheterization laboratory. In the integrated laboratory these data are distributed electronically to the physiologic recorder, the data recorder and the X-ray system, otherwise they must be entered into each of these systems separately. When the data have been entered, the nurse/technician begins a running, timed and detailed record of every event during the catheterization procedure. These detailed records document every event of the procedure with enough detail to become the critical information for a defense in a court of law!

The recording nurse/technician "balances" the pressure transducers electronically and numbers and identifies each recording. At the request of the operating physician the recording nurse/technician sets the scale or "gain" of each of the pressure tracings or changes the gain of all, or individual, channels. When requested, the recording nurse/technician creates a paper recording of the pressure tracings and events occurring on the monitor screen. Most current physiologic recorders also time the events and recordings automatically in the computer record and on any paper recordings. The recording nurse/technician starts the paper recorder at the onset of a major or unusual event occurring to the patient in the catheterization laboratory. A well trained, experienced and attentive recording nurse/technician will begin this recording automatically, without specific instructions and before joining in any emergency efforts.

The data recording person places notations or comments on the *timed record* in the computer record of any changes in the patient's status and for all events occurring during catheterization. The values of the saturations obtained from the oximeter in the laboratory are entered into the running, timed record. In most laboratories these data are transmitted verbally from the nurse/technician in the actual catheterization room to the recording nurse/technician in the control room, who then enters the numbers manually into the computerized, timed record. The timed record also includes all medications and the dose and route of their administration. The introduction, exchanges, and specific manipulations of catheters, wires, sheath/dilators and special devices are all recorded. These recorded data include the type, size, and entry vessel through which the item is introduced.

The recording nurse or technician keeps the operating physician in the catheterization room constantly apprised of the patient's hemodynamic status during the procedure. The recording nurse/technician keeps track of, and records changes in pressures and the electrocardiogram throughout the entire case and watches particularly for any significant changes or *trends* in the patient's vital signs. Although the catheterizing physician can see the physiologic tracings on the monitors in the catheterization room, he or she usually is concentrating on the catheter manipulations directly on the table or on the fluoroscopic screen and cannot watch the physiologic tracings constantly.

When angiograms are obtained, the time, the site of the injection, the type and the amount of contrast, the pressure and rate of injection and the angles of the X-ray tubes are recorded on the continuous flow sheet. In the electronically integrated laboratory the X-ray settings are automatically inserted into the timed record of events, otherwise these values are inserted manually. In addition to recording all of the angiographic related information, a nurse/technician in the control room also adjusts the major settings for exposure rate on the X-ray equipment, the settings for amount of contrast, pressure of injection, flow rate and delay or "rise" time on the injector, "arms" the injector and then initiates the injection during the angiogram. In some laboratories the nurse/technician in the control area also operates the start–stop of the angiographic equipment.

At the conclusion of the procedure, the time the various catheter lines are removed, the time hemostasis is achieved, the type of pressure bandages applied, the vital signs and overall status of the patient, the time the patient leaves the catheterization laboratory and who is accompanying the patient out of the room, are all recorded.

After the patient is removed from the catheterization room, the control room nurse/technician makes printed copies of the catheterization laboratory recorded data for the patient's chart and for a hard copy "catheterization folder" for each patient. When the catheterizing physicians have finished all measurements of the images on a digital system, the images are transferred onto the central storage computer for archiving and a copy onto a back-up storage system is performed by the control-room personnel.

Whenever possible it is desirable, if not absolutely necessary, to have at least two recording/operating nurses/technicians in the control area. During a complicated, difficult case and even with many pre-entered abbreviations and "pre-entered comments" in the recorded data of the catheterization laboratory computer program, the responsibilities in the control room exceed the capabilities of a single person.

Circulating nurse/technician

The third essential person in the catheterization laboratory is the circulating nurse/technician, who performs his/her activities predominantly within the catheterization room. This nurse/technician, along with the "manifold nurse/technician", sets up the catheterization room for the particular patient. This includes opening and arranging the sterile "catheterization pack", which includes the table drape, sterile protective drapes for adjacent equipment, towels, "operating gowns", flush bowls, specific monitoring lines, and, for each particular patient, the needles, wires, and introducers. Any other special or particular catheters or other consumable items specified by the catheterizing physician are added to the tray by the circulating nurse/technician. The circulating nurse/technician sets up any other special or unique equipment necessary for the particular patient including the patient-warming system, intravenous perfusion pumps, cardiac output computers, etc. The circulating nurse/technician may assist the manifold nurse/technician in setting up the manifold and in his/her duties when the manifold person is tied up with other duties.

When the patient arrives in the catheterization room, the circulating nurse/technician helps to position the patient on the catheterization table and secures them in a comfortable position with tape or straps. This same nurse/technician connects the ECG leads, the pulse oximeter, and a cuff blood pressure cuff to the monitor. If the patient requires a Foley™ urinary catheter, this is inserted at this time by the circulating nurse/technician. When there is an intravenous (IV) line, the fluid connection to the line is secured. If there is no IV line and the procedure is being performed under deep sedation without an anesthesiologist, the circulating nurse usually starts a separate IV line once the patient is secure on the table. In such a circumstance, if the patient requires additional sedation, the circulating nurse administers it, either through the IV line or, when no IV is available, intramuscularly.

After the physician has infiltrated each potential vessel entry area with local anesthesia, each area is "scrubbed" thoroughly and widely by the circulating nurse/technician. The circulating nurse assists the physician in draping the patient to isolate all of the sterile fields with the drape and in draping all adjacent equipment which might come in contact with the operator or catheters and wires.

Once the catheterization procedure begins, the circulating nurse/technician takes the syringes with the blood samples for oxygen saturation determination from the physician, verbally notifies the recording nurse/technician in the control room of the location where the blood sample was obtained, injects the blood sample into an oximeter cuvette, places the cuvette in the oximeter device, reads the digital read-out to the physician/operator and to the recording nurse/technician, and makes a record of the result from the oximeter. The results from the oximeter are transmitted verbally to the operating physician and the recording nurse/technician in most laboratories.

There now is the capability of the digital read-out from an A-Vox™ oximeter to be transmitted electronically to a separate computer for a large display and a site-specific, timed, permanent record. This "communication" between the oximeter and the computer requires a special software program from Scientific Software Inc™ (Scientific Software Solutions, Charlottesville, VA). The site where the sample was obtained is selected in the program in either the oximeter or the computer directly by the circulating nurse/technician while the time of the reading and the oxygen saturation of the sample are recorded and displayed automatically on a computer screen. A timed, accurate record of the oxygen saturations and their specific sites from the entire catheterization can be printed at the end of the procedure. Eventually, with a small amount of additional effort on the part of the major manufacturers, these data should go directly to the recording computer in the control room without the current verbal/manual transmission!

In addition to running the oximeter samples, the circulating nurse/technician runs the blood gas analysis or

ACT tests on samples received from the physicians and assures that the operating physician, the anesthesiologist and the recording nurse/technician have the results of these tests. The same circulating nurse/technician is responsible for retrieving additional catheters, wires and devices as needed during procedure from the "in-room" or adjacent room storage. The circulating nurse/technician also has the responsibility for periodically loosening the restraints on the patient's arms and "exercising" the arms by putting them through a full range of motion to prevent brachial plexus injury. If the catheterization laboratory does not have a separate "runner" to retrieve supplies, blood, etc., from sites remote from the catheterization laboratory, the circulating nurse/technician performs that function.

This nurse/technician checks the crash cart for its stock of expendable supplies and drugs before the procedure begins and the defibrillator is pre-set according to the patient's weight and then checked for function. The circulating nurse/technician may be called on to introduce a nasogastric tube or a nasopharyngeal airway into the patient electively during the procedure. During the procedure, in the event of an emergency, the circulating nurse/technician is responsible for bringing the defibrillator to the bedside, "arming" the defibrillator and giving the paddles to the physician. The nurse/technician, however, should be capable of confidently applying the paddles and administering the current him/herself.

At the end of the procedure, the circulating nurse/technician assists the physicians in removing the table drapes and then applies the pressure dressings to the various puncture sites after hemostasis has been achieved. In a laboratory still using cine film, the circulator removes the film cassettes and makes sure the film gets to the person responsible for processing.

"Manifold nurse/technician"

The fourth essential person in the catheterization room is the "manifold nurse/technician". As the name implies, the manifold nurse/technician controls the "manifold"— i.e. the stopcocks, transducers and flushing of the pressure/flush lines connected to the patient. The manifold nurse/technician prepares and sets up the plastic pressure bags of flush solution, sets up and balances the pressure transducers on the manifold, and connects the pressure bags/flush system to the "manifolds". The pressure transducers are mounted on a stand attached to the side of the catheterization table, which is adjustable vertically to allow for the "mid-heart" position according to the patient's size. The manifold nurse/technician physically measures the patient's anterior–posterior chest diameter with a ruler/caliper and then adjusts the height of the transducer stand so that the transducers are *exactly* at the level of the *mid* chest. The exact site of the "mid-heart" height can be determined by a brief look at the lateral fluoroscopy while measuring the chest with a ruler. The accuracy of *all* of the subsequent pressure measurements during the catheterization is dependent on this height measurement and the positioning of the manifolds/transducers!

The pressure bags of flush solution are "spiked" with the bags upside down so that the vent/connecting tubes are positioned upward. Once spiked through the vent/ connecting tubes, the bags are squeezed until ***every last bit*** of air is evacuated from the bag as well as out of the "spiking" tube. Once the bag and tubing are emptied *completely* of air, three units of Heparin/cc of flush solution are injected into the injection port of the bag and mixed with the flush solution. Once the Heparin is added, the pressure/flush bag is turned right side up with the vents and tubing now at the bottom of the bag. The bag is rechecked for *any* residual air in it. When the pressure bag containing the flush fluid unequivocally is empty of air, the bag of fluid is inserted into a pressure cuff, pressure is applied to the cuff and the *tubing* is flushed of any remaining air. Once this bag and tubing system are emptied *completely* of *all* air, there is no possible way for air to enter that part of the system even when the fluid bag is squeezed totally empty or turned upside down again! The pressure bags are maintained with enough pressure to flush any or all parts of the manifold system and against any intravascular pressures (including systemic arterial pressures) with a good, steady flow of fluid.

Once the pressure flush lines are cleared, they are attached to the manifolds and the entire system including the manifolds, the stopcocks on the manifolds and the transducers are flushed while "tapping" each plastic joint/ connection sufficiently to dislodge any micro bubbles, which invariably are trapped on the poorly "wettable" plastics. This assures that the system is completely free of even micro air bubbles and that quality pressure curves are obtained through this part of the system.

Once the patient is prepped and draped, the manifold nurse/technician takes one end of each sterile pressure/flush line from the physician and attaches it to the manifold of the appropriate pressure transducer. Each line is placed on a pressure flush to the table while the physician "taps" that end of the line and the in-line stopcock until it is free of air and any "micro cavitation". Each pressure curve displayed on the physiologic monitor is color-coded to match a specific transducer. Each pressure/flush line on the table is also color-coded and is attached to the transducer with the corresponding colored pressure tracings on the screen. The colors on the monitor screen can be switched or changed completely in the recording computer so that the colors of the flush tubing attached to the transducer and the monitor tracing always correspond. This synchronization of the colors between the flush/pressure tubing and the monitor tracings easily and precisely identifies each pressure/flush line with a specific pressure transducer and tracing on the monitor, and greatly simplifies and increases the accuracy of the communication between the operating physician, the manifold nurse/technician, and the recording technician when requesting flushing, balancing or changing "gains" of any particular pressure curve.

The manifold nurse/technician flushes and "zeros" strain gauges at the beginning and as necessary during the procedure. During the catheterization procedure, the manifold nurse/technician turns the pressures lines on and off *at the manifold* and flushes the system and the catheters from the manifold as directed by the catheterizing physician. The catheterizing physician draws blood samples from a stopcock close to the catheter/line in the patient and, when sure that there is no air in the system, returns the stopcock to the flush/pressure position and requests the manifold nurse/technician to flush the line. The manifold nurse/technician should anticipate and be ready for the physician's next move or request whenever a sample is drawn or a line is disconnected. For example, when a catheter is disconnected from the pressure line in order to withdraw a blood sample, it *always* will need flushing when the line is reconnected to the catheter. At the same time it cannot be flushed until the physician is sure it is clear of air or clot. As the line *is being reattached* to the flush system, the manifold nurse/technician should have his/her hand on the flush stopcock/device awaiting the request for a flush. The physician should never have to request the flush a second time!

The manifold nurse/technician is trained to recognize poor and artifactual pressure curves and should be aware of what causes particular abnormalities in the curves. Any abnormalities noted in the pressure curves should be pointed out to the catheterizing physician if he/she has not noticed the problem. The most common problems with the pressure curves are a result of "micro-cavitation" in the fluid with the creation of micro bubbles as the fluid warms. The almost "non-wettable" nature of the plastics in the manifold, transducers, stopcocks and tubing allows for the progressive accumulation of these micro bubbles until they create an artifactual "over shoot" in the tracing. These artifacts in the pressure curves are eliminated by the meticulous "tapping" and flushing of all of the plastic areas of the tubing and connectors as the system is flushed with the stopcock open and away from the patient.

The other major responsibility of the manifold nurse/technician is the administration of intravenous drugs and solutions during the procedure, particularly when it is performed under sedation without an anesthesiologist. Supplemental sedation is the most frequent medication administered. At the time of very critical maneuvers, often the manifold nurse/technician will have the specific amount of the additional sedation for the particular patient drawn into a syringe in advance and will already have the syringe attached to the manifold in anticipation of the necessary dose. In that situation, the additional sedation can be administered within seconds of when it is needed and requested. The manifold nurse/technician also administers other medications/solutions through the catheters, including supplemental narcotics, heparin, electrolyte and glucose solutions and supplemental fluids as ordered by the operating physician.

The manifold nurse/technician also assists the circulating nurse/technician in setting up the catheterization laboratory and securing the patient on the catheterization table. The manifold nurse/technician may assist the circulating nurse/technician in his/her duties during the procedure; however, the manifold nurse's/technician's primary responsibility is the manifold and he/she should not be away from the manifold for any significant length of time.

Extra "float nurse/technician"

During a very complicated case in the catheterization laboratory, particularly when multiple samples are obtained or where many different wires, catheters and devices are used, a minimum of three nurses/technicians is not sufficient to keep up with the pace of the case, much less operate the room efficiently. This is even truer when a complex therapeutic intervention is performed. When a complicated case is anticipated, the full complement of four nurses/technicians is assigned to the room. The fourth person helps with retrieving the multiple pieces of consumable equipment, may perform the blood saturation, blood gas or ACT determinations, and assists with the data recording in the control room. During a very long case, the "extra" nurse/technician trades duties temporarily with one, or more, of the other personnel in the room to allow them a transient break. The time saved by utilizing this fourth person easily justifies the additional salary.

In cardiac catheterization laboratories which still use cine film, the nurse/technician in the "float position" frequently is the person responsible for processing the cine film. In a cine film laboratory either this person, the technical director or the biomedical engineer turns on the film processor each morning. Turning on the processor includes running a quality control, test filmstrip through the processor at the start of each day.

At the end of each procedure the cine film cassettes are collected from the cine cameras in the catheterization laboratory. In the processing room of the catheterization laboratory, the film is threaded from the cassettes into the photographic film processor and the processor started.

After the film is processed, it is transferred by the nurse/technician from the processing reels to spools for viewing on cine viewing machines.

Technical director

One nurse/technician of the "catheterization team" functions as the technical leader/director of the catheterization laboratories. The technical director is responsible for maintaining the inventory of consumable items, arranging for the preventive and emergency maintenance of all of the equipment, and the scheduling of all of the catheterization laboratory personnel. With one laboratory, the time commitment for the technical director for just these administrative obligations is approximately half of the working time of one of the other catheterization laboratory nurses/technicians. With two or more catheterization laboratories, the technical director's position is a full time job and represents an *additional* full-time employee equivalent (FTEE) for the catheterization laboratories.

In addition to the technical director, one nurse/technician is designated as the leader in each room, at least during each case. The "room" leader for the particular case is responsible for assigning the specific duties to each of the personnel in the room during the case and supervising their activities during the particular case, in addition to his/her assigned duties.

Catheterization laboratory support personnel

Each catheterization laboratory is dependent upon considerable additional support outside of the actual catheterization room. This includes a nurse for admitting and preparing the patient for the catheterization, administrative/secretarial support, environmental services/custodial support, biomedical support and "out of lab" engineering support.

Admitting/holding area nurse/technician

The primary responsibility of the catheterization holding area nurse is to facilitate getting the patient safely into the catheterization laboratory in the most timely manner possible so that there is no delay in the function of the catheterization laboratory. Most cardiac catheterization procedures are performed as an outpatient or "day case", followed by an extended period of close observation. The patients are admitted directly to an admissions/holding area in the cardiac catheterization suite where the patient's demographics and eligibility are verified, the administrative admission to the catheterization laboratory is performed, and the patient is prepared for catheterization. The catheterization admissions area may be exclusively for admissions to the cardiac catheterization laboratory, but it is often shared with admissions for the cardiac operating rooms. When sharing is possible, considerable duplication of equipment and personnel can be avoided.

The admission procedure is relatively extensive. This includes administratively documenting the patient's pre-admission eligibility for the procedure, assigning or verifying the patient's medical record number, placing the patient's identity bracelets on them, and the preparation and organization of the patient's chart. Medically, the pre-admission history and physical examination are verified or obtained, the previous laboratory work is checked for its results and its completeness, and samples for any necessary additional laboratory work are obtained. When the use of blood during the procedure is considered a possibility, a blood sample is obtained for type and cross match or the availability of blood from a previous cross match is verified. Finally, it is assured that the procedure is understood by the patient/their family and that the "operating permit" is understood and signed by the appropriate person(s).

Even patients already admitted to the hospital, but coming from other areas of the hospital, are "admitted" to the catheterization laboratory through the catheterization laboratory admitting/holding area. This assures that the patients are completely ready for the procedure both physically and mentally and that they are physically in close proximity to the catheterization laboratory as soon as the catheterization room is ready for them. Having the patients prepared by the catheterization laboratory personnel and close to the laboratory facilitates a rapid "turn around" time in the catheterization room between patients.

The patient is dressed in a hospital gown and is encouraged to void before being placed on a stretcher/bed. The potential introduction sites for catheters are scrubbed (and shaved if necessary), a peripheral intravenous line is started and the patient is given their pre-medication at the appropriate time. If the patient is to receive general anesthesia, the anesthesiologist is informed of the patient's presence and consults with the patient and family if they have not seen them earlier.

A nurse who is very familiar with the catheterization procedures performs the admission procedures and the preparations of the patient. This nurse is usually one of the catheterization laboratory nurses/technicians or, at least, is assigned to the catheterization laboratory and is *responsible to* the catheterization laboratory. The "holding area" nurse is responsible for the efficient and timely movement of the patients to the catheterization laboratory. The logistics of moving several patients through the holding area when there are two or more catheterization rooms with both rooms starting at the same time requires some assistance, temporarily, from one or more of the "in-room" nurses/technicians.

Ideally the patient is ready to enter the catheterization room as soon as it is ready for the patient. The holding area nurse/technician keeps the physicians in the catheterization room notified of the status of the patients in the holding area, keeps the patient/family informed of their potential starting time and, in doing so, helps to explain any delays from the originally scheduled time. When there are significant delays, the holding area nurse can arrange for a change in the patient's "nothing by mouth" status.

Administrative/secretarial support

In addition to the nursing/technician staff actually operating the catheterization rooms, each catheterization room requires significant administrative and secretarial support.

The extended schedule of the catheterization laboratory, the daily schedule of the patients, the schedules and the assignments for each of the laboratory personnel within each room as well as the schedules for the time off, holidays and "on call" for each of the personnel, all have to be created, maintained and "published". The time sheets for each of the personnel are maintained on a daily basis. Purchase orders for all of the consumable materials are completed and submitted expeditiously. As all consumable items are received, the original orders are compared with the items received and verified. The catheterization laboratory director is informed of any delays/discrepancies in the orders received. The administrative secretary prepares the billing sheet for the procedure, which includes each procedure performed and each piece of consumable equipment that is used in the catheterization laboratory during a procedure. This is submitted to the hospital billing office for the hospital charges.

A new cardiac catheterization record and folder are created for each patient, and for each time they undergo a procedure in the catheterization laboratory. This patient catheterization laboratory folder contains copies of the pressure tracings, a printout and tabulation of all of the hemodynamic data from the procedure, the diagram(s) of the particular heart, a descriptive summary of the important maneuvers and procedures performed during the catheterization procedure, a description of the angiographic technique during each angiogram along with a description of the findings from the angiograms, and a summary of the diagnoses and recommendations as a result of the procedure. Ideally, the catheterization summaries are transcribed by a transcriptionist, who is assigned to the catheterization area and who, in turn, understands the terminology and information in the summaries. When the transcriptionist is a member of the catheterization team, any questions about, or peculiarities of the catheterization summary can be clarified directly and in a timely manner by the physicians or personnel in the catheterization laboratory. The more detailed and specific the catheterization report, the more necessary is this close working association. In laboratories where the complex anatomy is transferred to an individualized diagram, this close cooperation is even more essential. Copies of the finalized catheterization report are included in the patient's hospital record and sent to the referring physicians by the catheterization laboratory secretary.

The catheterization folders are stored in, or in the immediate area of, the catheterization laboratory, separate from the central hospital records, and are maintained by the catheterization laboratory administrative personnel. The catheterization records must be available for rapid retrieval whenever old information on the particular patient becomes necessary for subsequent catheterizations in the future. As many of the most recent catheterization records as possible are stored in the immediate catheterization laboratory area and the remaining (the majority) of the folders must be stored in "off-site" storage. When it is possible to reproduce a hard copy conveniently and *reliably* from an entirely electronic record, the catheterization records are maintained entirely in a computer storage system with a separate electronic backup.

In addition to the hemodynamic data, all angiograms are cataloged with permanent copies stored so they can be retrieved easily and expeditiously. This requires a monumental amount of organization and filing space. With a completely digital laboratory, a digital copy of the angiogram is stored on readily accessible, large "Raid" disks in the cardiac catheterization laboratory/hospital computer system. A separate hard copy of the digital angiogram is maintained as a separate archive. This separate archive copy is stored on either a digital tape, an optical disk or separate compact disks. In any case, these copies are cataloged and physically stored so that they can be retrieved readily or copied back into the electronic system.

Cardiac catheterization laboratories which still use cine angiography have the additional logistical and space problems of a cine-angiogram storage system which is useable yet conserves as much space as possible. Large "rolling files" of the cataloged cine films, which are maintained by the administrative personnel of the catheterization laboratory, are very efficient, but at the same time occupy large amounts of space in the catheterization area.

Biomedical support

The "in-house" biomedical engineer(s) for the catheterization laboratories is/are committed full time to the catheterization laboratories or, at least, they have their time prioritized for the catheterization laboratories. The complexity of the equipment in the modern cardiac catheterization laboratory no longer allows for the laboratory to be dependent only on outside or manufacturers' engineers for the minute-to-minute support of the catheterization laboratory. Each minute of down time in an operating catheterization laboratory adds up to hours of extra, uncompensated expense to the hospital. The in-house biomedical engineers must be intimately familiar with all of the catheterization laboratory equipment, capable of repairing most of the electrical/mechanical equipment, and at least "resetting" major X-ray computer "lock-ups". The in-house biomedical personnel should be able to change common "boards" on the X-ray equipment and of equal, or more, importance, expediently identify major problems with the equipment which do require out of hospital manufacturers' support.

The in-house biomedical engineers must also have a good working relationship with the engineers from the manufacturers/distributors of all of the catheterization laboratory equipment in order to have good "out of hospital" and in-depth support. No in-house biomedical personnel are expected to be experts in each of the infinite types or the continual upgrades of the varieties of capital equipment in a catheterization laboratory. Similarly, no catheterization laboratory, no matter how large or how many catheterization rooms, can maintain a complete inventory of spare parts for all of the electronic, X-ray and mechanical equipment in the laboratory.

The catheterization laboratory equipment usually is extremely dependable; however, when it does fail, rapid *quality* service is indispensable. When service cannot be accomplished expediently by the in-house engineers, manufacturers' support that is immediately available and reliable is essential for the repair of malfunctioning equipment or replacement of defective equipment in the catheterization laboratory. A busy cardiac catheterization laboratory relies upon the manufacturers' local representatives to maintain an inventory of repair/replacement parts within a reasonable access to each laboratory. The availability of this manufacturers' support should play an essential part in the decision as to which type of equipment to purchase.

In 2005, no piece of equipment, no matter how large or where it is manufactured, is more than 24 hours away from a major city! Entire catheterization laboratories routinely are shipped around the world *and assembled* within a day for a *sales display*! The care of patients should receive at least as much priority as a sales exhibit!

A "down" catheterization laboratory is not just an idle piece of "real estate". Inoperable equipment interferes with the timeliness of the remainder of the medical therapy for the particular patient—for example the cancelation of surgery which is already scheduled for that patient following the catheterization. In addition to the huge inconvenience and disappointment, the patient or their family incur extra expenses for their travel, the associated costs for lodging and feeding the remainder of the family, the lost work time for the "provider" or lost school time for the patient plus the additional hospital expenses of an extra stay.

A "down" catheterization laboratory also incurs significant ongoing expense for the hospital while the laboratory is out of function. The personnel on the catheterization laboratory staff still receive a salary, but are idle. There is a necessary rescheduling of any other patients in the catheterization laboratory (and possibly in the operating rooms and other hospital schedules to accommodate the canceled patient(s)). The physicians involved are not optimally productive and require urgent rescheduling of their own, as do many other persons'/patients' activities.

Housekeeping/environmental services

A cardiac catheterization laboratory is considered a sterile environment like an operating room. In order to maintain this environment, the walls of the room and each piece of equipment in the room require frequent scrubbing or wiping down to prevent dust from accumulating. The entire floor requires a thorough antiseptic mop scrub at least once a day as well as localized scrubbing between each case.

In order for a catheterization laboratory to have a rapid turn around for multiple patients during the day, the catheterization room must have a very rapid but thorough cleaning between cases. This includes scrubbing down the catheterization table with a disinfectant and actually scrubbing the floor of the room with a mop. All biologically contaminated materials must be gathered and disposed of properly in "bio-hazard" containers before a new patient can be brought into the room. Usually these custodial services are performed by individuals from an "environmental services" department. When the environmental services personnel are not part of the catheterization laboratory team, but are assigned from other areas of the hospital to help occasionally in the catheterization laboratory, there is frequently a significant delay in getting them back to the catheterization area at the critical times.

The nurses/technicians can (and often do) perform the between-case cleaning. However, these same nurses/technicians have numerous other absolutely necessary duties at the end of one case and just before the next case, but that incurs an obligatory delay while the nurses/technicians perform the extra custodial duties instead of their nursing duties. A catheterization laboratory service with two or more active laboratories justifies a separate employee from environmental services who is assigned to the catheterization laboratories. The environmental services person then becomes very familiar with the operation of the laboratories, is always available in the laboratory area and, as a consequence, is able to anticipate the end of cases and facilitate the cleanup between cases. The employee from environmental services who is assigned to the catheterization area and becomes part of the functioning team also takes more pride in their individual area and tends to perform better.

Catheterization laboratory nurse clinician

Although often not included as part of the catheterization laboratory support personnel provided by the hospital, one, or more, nurse clinician(s) working with the physician(s) is/are an indispensable part of a catheterization laboratory team. The nurse clinician provides continuous contact/communication with the family or patient before, during and after the catheterization. This ongoing communication is invaluable in maintaining a solid rapport with the patient and their family.

The nurse clinician answers questions pertaining to the catheterization and checks on the patients when the physician is occupied in the catheterization laboratory or elsewhere and is not available. The nurse clinician can arrange for and schedule the necessary laboratory work pre- and post-catheterization. The nurse clinician actually performs the patient scheduling for the catheterization laboratory and coordinates support from anesthesia, echocardiography, respiratory therapy and other specialty services. The nurse clinician prepares the patient for discharge and arranges for their follow-up care following the catheterization. When the patients are on "protocol" studies with follow-up visits required at specific times and with specific tests, the nurse clinician arranges these and assures compliance with the protocol. All of these activities *could* be performed by the cardiologist; however, the catheterizing physician is far more productive as a patient care provider and for "income generation" while actually performing catheterizations.

References

1. ACC/AHA. A.C.o.C.A.H.A.A.H.T.F.o.C.C. ACC/AHA guidelines for cardiac catheterization and cardiac catheterization laboratories. *J Am Coll Cardiol* 1991; **18**: 1149–1182.
2. Allen HD *et al.* Pediatric therapeutic cardiac catheterization: a statement for healthcare professionals from the Council on Cardiovascular Disease in the Young. American Heart Association. *Circulation* 1998; **97**(6): 609–625.
3. Dehmer GJ *et al.* Lessons learned from the review of cardiac catheterization laboratories: A report from the laboratory survey committee of the Society for Cardiac Angiography and Interventions. *Cathet Cardiovasc Intervent* 1999; **46**: 24–31.

2 Medications used in or in conjunction with the cardiac catheterization laboratory and patient preparation for cardiac catheterization

Introduction

The most commonly used medications in the catheterization laboratory are sedatives, analgesics and anesthetics. These medications are discussed in the beginning of this chapter along with the overall preparation of the patient for catheterization. In addition to these common medications there is a very large and heterogeneous conglomerate of relevant medications which are used in conjunction with the catheterization or which the patient may be receiving, with which the cardiologist performing the catheterization must be very familiar. The medications important to the catheterizing physician include those medications which the patient may be taking before the procedure which, in turn, affect the hemodynamics or interact with the emergency or supplemental medications which are used during the procedure; those emergency or supplemental medications which are used during the procedure; and, finally, those medications which are needed following the procedure. The medications which are relevant before, during or after pediatric and congenital cardiac catheterization procedures are listed in a large "formulary" section as the final section of this chapter. This compendium of catheterization laboratory medications lists the information about the functions, indications, dose and significant adverse effects of most of the various medications used in or in conjunction with the cardiac catheterization laboratory[1,2].

The medications administered in the catheterization laboratory are required for sedation/analgesia, for the control of the baseline hemodynamic stability and for the treatment of major, and often acute, emergency changes in the patient's hemodynamics or cardiac rhythm. These medications are used frequently enough that they must always be available in the catheterization laboratory for immediate use.

At Texas Children's Hospital, we have found that a printed table of emergency medications, which is *individualized for each separate patient* and made available in the catheterization laboratory, is a very valuable asset particularly during an emergency situation. This medication table is pre-programmed into the cardiac catheterization laboratory computers. The table is produced on a standard Excel™ computer spreadsheet. The *basic* medication table, which is in the catheterization laboratory program, lists the commonly used emergency or supportive medications along with their *per kilogram* doses. As each patient arrives in the catheterization laboratory and is logged into the catheterization laboratory computer, the patient's most recent weight from their precatheterization physical examination is retrieved from the database and placed into the table. The Excel™ program then automatically calculates the ***exact dose*** *of each individual medication*, which is in the spreadsheet, in milligrams and milliliters for that specific patient and places this dose in an adjacent column in the table. The table of medications, which is specific for the individual patient, is printed and is posted by the medication cart/cabinet during the catheterization procedure. At the end of the catheterization procedure, the individualized medication table is taken with the patient to the recovery area and posted with the patient's chart at the bedside. The medication table does not preclude the necessity of calculating each individual dose, but does eliminate the several, or often many, seconds necessary to double check the dose of a medication during an emergency and provides a "safety check" for all of the doses which are calculated for every drug administered during the procedure.

CATHETERIZATION LAB DRUG FORM

NAME	DATE	HOSPITAL NUMBER

WEIGHT (KG)	

MEDICATION	DOSE/KG	mg(mcg)/ml(liquid preparations)	PATIENT'S DOSE

Precatheterization preparation of the patient

The preparation of the patient for a cardiac catheterization is an individualized process for each patient and each cardiac catheterization laboratory. There are no hard and fast rules, but there are volumes written on the subject[3]. Patient preparation begins as soon as the decision is made to perform the procedure. All patients beyond infancy, including young children and regardless of the type of sedation or anesthesia which is used, do need, at the very least, a general explanation about the procedure and the reason why the procedure is being performed. This should include at least a description of the portions of the procedure of which the patients themselves will be aware. There are very few things which can make a child or older patient more anxious, more distrusting or more uncooperative during a cardiac catheterization, than for them to be told ahead of time that "nothing will hurt". For a child undergoing a catheterization, there is nothing worse than for the child to believe that nothing more than a routine "office visit" is going to occur when they arrive at the hospital!

The exact details provided to the patient, of course, depend upon the age, understanding and "interest" of the patient and must be "tailored" according to the response of the patient during the explanation. The information given to the young patient must be truthful, although *not necessarily in enough detail* to induce even more anxiety. The discussion should include information about the necessary pre-procedure laboratory studies including the inevitable "needle stick" for the blood work and premedications/intravenous lines and, for younger children, mention of the transient separation from their parents—emphasizing the *transient*! Older children, adolescents and adult patients are also informed about the length of the procedure, the expected stay in the recovery area, any peculiarities of the recovery (IV lines, bladder catheters, etc.) and the length of the expected total stay in the hospital. The patient is made familiar with the general hospital environment, the catheterization laboratory itself, and the post-catheterization recovery area.

Older patients and the patients' families need a more detailed explanation of the catheterization procedure. This greater detail still is "tailored" to the particular capabilities and understanding of the patient and family. Parents or patients who are in a decision-making position are informed in detail of the risks of the procedure. However, unless the patient is at an unusually high risk (e.g. very high pulmonary vascular resistance), the *emphasis* of the discussion about the catheterization should be about the reason for the catheterization, the technical aspects of the catheterization within the understanding of the patient/family and not just about the risks. Although providing the full details of all of the potential risks of the procedure may make the operator feel "medico-legally" more comfortable, such discussions only increase the patient's/family's anxieties further and do *not* help in a court of law.

No infants, and almost no children, need sedation or medications to "relax them" on the day, or even the night before, the procedure. On the other hand, the adolescent, the adult congenital patient and, occasionally, the *parents* of the patient, can often be inordinately apprehensive. In that circumstance, both the patient and the parent benefit from a mild sedative given to the *parent* the night before the procedure!

In addition to the explanation and psychological preparation for the catheterization, there is other information/instruction provided to the patient when the decision is made to proceed with a cardiac catheterization. Their "administrative" admission preparations with the hospital, with the patient's insurance carrier or payer are arranged as soon as the need for catheterization is determined. Patients who need pre-treatment of any sort are given an admission date sometime before the day of the catheterization. However, since most catheterization procedures are "day admission" procedures, the patients need *detailed* instructions about *where* and at *what time* they are expected to arrive at the hospital before the procedure. Most cardiac catheterization laboratories have a specific admitting/holding area for the admission and preparation of patients for catheterization. Obviously the time varies according to when the patient is scheduled for the catheterization during the day. A patient who is "pre-admitted" administratively arrives at least one-and-a-half to two hours prior to the scheduled procedure. There is no reason to have patients who are scheduled for the catheterization later in the day arriving early in the morning! This will only aggravate the patients and make them more apprehensive.

Older patients are given instructions on preparation of the catheterization site(s) including scrubbing and shaving the area(s) themselves. When the femoral approach is used, the patient should shave each inguinal area from side to side, from iliac crest to iliac crest ("hip bone to hip bone") and from above to below, from the supra pubic area to just above the knees. Particularly "hairy" patients are instructed to shave around their entire thighs and up onto the lower back above the hips when "pressure" bandages are to be applied after the procedure.

For the very "needle shy" child or adolescent and with knowledgeable parents, EMLA™ cream is prescribed and instructions are given for the application of the cream at home to several potential areas for *intravenous* needle punctures before the child arrives for the catheterization[4]. To be effective, the EMLA must be applied one-and-a-half or, preferably, two hours prior to the needle puncture.

Nutritional and fluid requirements precatheterization

The patient is encouraged to have regular meals and an increased amount of oral fluids up to 6 hours prior to the procedure. Often, nothing by mouth (NPO) is ordered for the patient for eight, ten or more hours prior to the onset of the procedure. In actuality, it rarely is necessary and even can be detrimental to have the patient NPO for *more* than six hours before the beginning of the procedure. The child who is ordered "NPO after midnight" and who was put to bed at 8:00 or 9:00 pm the evening before the procedure, may well have had nothing by mouth for 12 or more hours by the time they arrive in the catheterization laboratory the following morning! If a long period of time is anticipated between the patient's last oral intake and the beginning of the procedure (e.g. all night), the patient should be ordered or given oral, clear liquids within six or seven hours of the expected start of the procedure. This should be encouraged, even if it means waking the patient during the night. This fluid intake is even more important in very young, cyanotic or polycythemic patients. In these circumstances, it is preferable to start an intravenous line and the patient is given intravenous fluids to maintain their hydration while waiting for the catheterization, particularly if there is a delay in the start of the catheterization procedure. One-quarter normal saline or Ringer's lactate is administered at a maintenance rate according to the patient's size.

Infants and small children have different fluid/nutritional needs from older patients. The emptying time of their stomach normally is much faster than in an older child, the emptying time of the stomach is not as affected by anxiety about the impending procedure, and they become dehydrated and hypoglycemic faster than an older patient. As a consequence, infants only need to be restricted from oral feeding for four hours prior to the procedure, and a specific effort must be made to insure clear fluids are provided to them just before they are made "nothing by mouth". This becomes even more important in chronically ill, cachectic infants. Parents are encouraged to wake the infant during the night within five hours of the procedure and to feed the patient at least clear liquids at that time.

Immediate precatheterization preparation

If it was not applied at home and it is to be used, EMLA Cream™ is applied locally over the sites for the possible intravenous punctures as soon as the patient arrives in the holding/admitting area. EMLA™ cream appears to be effective at reducing the discomfort from the punctures for starting peripheral intravenous lines and even for the percutaneous catheter introductory sites, however, the EMLA™ cream must be applied at least one, and preferably two, hours prior to the skin and vessel puncture to be at all effective. When the patient has had previous catheterizations and has any "memory" of the catheter puncture sites, EMLA™ cream also is spread over the potential percutaneous sites.

In the "holding area" or on a ward, any infant who has more than a four-hour delay before the start of the catheterization and after being placed nothing by mouth (NPO), should have intravenous fluids running or started. In infants, the intravenous fluid should contain 5% dextrose in quarter normal saline to prevent hypoglycemia as well as maintaining the patient's hydration. At the same time, only an individual who is very skilled at starting intravenous lines should introduce this intravenous line in infants. This is particularly true in small infants or cachectic patients, where it often is very difficult to introduce a line into a vein. In spite of the multiple advantages of the indwelling intravenous line, the presence of such a line ***never*** justifies extensive trauma or the exhaustion of the patient from the crying and fighting created by prolonged or multiple "sticks" during unsuccessful attempts at starting an intravenous line.

In the extremely anxious or combative child, where starting an intravenous line is out of the question, an *intramuscular* dose of 1–2 mg/kg of ketamine provides a very effective and very rapid sedation for the child prior to starting the intravenous line or catheterization. In the worst-case scenario, where an intravenous line cannot be started, the entire premedication is given intramuscularly. In infants and small children, intranasal midazolam in a dose of 0.25 mg/kg is effective and fairly rapid at producing sedation sufficient for starting the intravenous line. If problems are anticipated, or in a very anxious patient, midazolam in a dose of 0.2 to 0.6 mg/kg, administered orally 30 to 45 minutes prior to starting the intravenous puncture, is effective in calming the patient enough to introduce the intravenous line. Midazolam, by either route, is not as predictable or as effective as ketamine. Following the administration of either midazolam or ketamine, the patient should be observed very closely and placed on an ECG monitor.

In addition to the fluids and intravenous lines, there are several additional preparations for the catheterization in the holding area before the patient enters the catheterization laboratory. Any necessary laboratory work (blood CBC, chemistries, urinalysis, X-ray, ECG or type and cross match), which was not completed previously, is carried out at this time. The patient is dressed in a hospital gown and when old enough to cooperate, asked to empty their bladder. If the start of the catheterization is delayed significantly after the patient arrived in the holding area, the patient is asked to empty their bladder again just before they are taken to the catheterization laboratory.

The patient's catheterization sites are cleaned. If the catheterization sites were not shaved adequately by the patient him/her self, the areas are shaved (again) while in the admitting/holding area. The final paper trail leading to the cardiac catheterization, including the "informed consent" forms, are completed and verified.

Polycythemia/anemia

Patients with significant polycythemia or anemia require additional preparation for a cardiac catheterization. Both of these problems negate the validity of any hemodynamic measurements and significantly increase the risk of all cardiac catheterizations.

Polycythemia occurs in cyanotic patients and is particularly common in the older cyanotic patient. A patient is considered polycythemic with a hematocrit over 65%. Problems from the polycythemia increase with the increasing severity of the condition, particularly when the hematocrit is over 75%. Although polycythemia increases the oxygen carrying capacity of the particular aliquot of blood, it *decreases* the overall cardiac output and the localized blood flow along with oxygen delivery to the tissues, and significantly increases the risk of thrombosis and emboli because of the thickened blood. Polycythemia is treated by a phlebotomy, which includes the replacement of the blood withdrawn with a colloidal fluid. The patient undergoing cardiac catheterization has the phlebotomy performed in the catheterization laboratory, after the venous and arterial lines have been introduced, but before the actual catheterization procedure is performed. The details of a phlebotomy procedure are discussed in Chapter 34.

At the other extreme, anemia decreases the oxygen carrying capacity of the blood, falsely increases the cardiac output, and aggravates congestive heart failure. Any measurements of blood flow are falsely elevated by significant anemia. Any pre-existing anemia is *always* made worse during a cardiac catheterization by both the accepted, obligatory blood loss, which occurs during the required blood sampling for blood oxygen saturation, clotting studies and blood gas determinations, along with the additional inadvertent blood loss occurring at vascular puncture sites, around catheters/wires and during sheath/catheter exchanges. When starting with less than 8–10 gm of hemoglobin in a small patient, none of the hemodynamic measurements will be valid. Of equal or greater importance, such an infant can easily reach a point of cardiovascular collapse from the cumulative blood loss.

Any significant anemia should be identified and corrected before the catheterization procedure. Preferably in an elective situation, the anemia is diagnosed weeks before the catheterization and treated with oral iron supplements. If the anemia is not recognized until the time of the catheterization and the catheterization is urgent, the patient's hemoglobin/hematocrit is corrected in the catheterization laboratory with a slow transfusion of 10 ml/kg of packed red blood cells and before any catheter manipulations or hemodynamic measurements are carried out.

Premedication for cardiac catheterization

Some premedication to sedate the patient before the catheterization is utilized by most pediatric/congenital cardiac catheterization laboratories. The goal of the premedication is to have the patient arrive in the catheterization laboratory calm, sleepy, and cooperative but, at the same time, not so obtunded that they need to be lifted onto the catheterization table or need ventilator support. The premedication usually is administered to the patient in the admitting or holding area of the catheterization laboratory or on a hospital ward before the patient enters the catheterization laboratory. Premedication can be administered orally, intramuscularly, or intravenously, although intravenously is preferred. Intravenous medications can be titrated or repeated without disturbing the patient.

Regardless of the route of administration of the initial premedication, it is desirable to have a secure intravenous (IV) line functioning in the patient prior to receiving the premedication and certainly before entering the laboratory for the catheterization procedure. If the intravenous line is not in place prior to the patient's arriving in the holding area for the procedure, it is put in place in the holding area while the patient is being prepared for the procedure. The intravenous line provides a direct route for the administration of the initial premedication, a route for supplemental medications preceding and during the procedure and, if necessary, for emergency and resuscitative medications. When administering the premedication through an intravenous line, the dose of the medication can easily be titrated up or down or supplemented with additional medications without traumatizing the patient further.

When general anesthesia is *not* used, virtually all infants, children, adolescents and even adults undergoing a cardiac catheterization for a congenital heart lesion, require some sedation and systemic in addition to local analgesia. There *are* a very few patients who are stoical enough that they do not need, nor desire either sedation or general anesthesia for a short catheterization procedure. All patients undergoing *long* catheterization procedures should receive systemic analgesia with sedation and/or general anesthesia. Although after the skin puncture the cardiac catheterization procedure *per se* usually does not cause pain, the patient undergoing catheterization is in an unfamiliar, frightening environment, is required to lie very still on an uncomfortable "table" and to remain still for a long period of time. During a long procedure, an indwelling Foley™ catheter is placed in the urinary bladder in order to prevent the extreme discomfort of a very full urinary bladder. Either the Foley™ catheter itself or the full bladder will add to the patient's overall discomfort. The majority of patients usually are "restrained" on the catheterization table, which adds further to their anxiety and discomfort.

Regardless of the age of the patient, under-sedation or no sedation results in a patient who is uncomfortable, anxious, straining, moving, hyperventilating or even crying throughout the procedure. This not only is cruel to the patient and to the staff of the catheterization laboratory, but also produces very significant changes in the physiologic "steady state" of the patient, which introduce marked, artifactual variations in any of the measured hemodynamic parameters. When the patient is not in an absolute steady state, the artifacts make all of the measurements of these parameters *totally useless* and the calculations from these measurements totally *invalid*. Adequate sedation is even more critical in the infant where, proportionately, a huge amount of energy is expended in crying or straining with a resultant, very significant stress placed on the myocardium.

The premedication is given thirty to sixty minutes prior to the anticipated onset of the procedure. Most premedications contain a combination of an analgesic and a sedative. Often, an anxiolytic medication is mixed with the sedative/analgesic for its added "tranquilizing effect" on the patient. Because of the variable response between individual patients, the markedly different ages of the patients in a congenital cardiac catheterization laboratory, and the complexity of the hemodynamics seen in congenital heart patients, no single medication, particular combination of medications, or single dose of medication is satisfactory for all patients.

When any premedication is administered, the operator or another qualified physician must be available within close proximity to the area of the patient when the premedication is given. This precaution is necessary in the event of an unexpected adverse reaction by the patient to the premedication. Additionally, any patient who receives premedication is monitored with, at least, an ECG, pulse oximetry and frequently recycled, cuff blood pressure determinations. This monitoring begins just prior to receiving the premedication and is continued until the patient is attached to the monitoring systems in the catheterization laboratory. The interval of time immediately after the patient has received their premedication and before the procedure actually starts is the most vulnerable time for complications to occur from premedication in these patients. During this time, the patient often has very little external stimulation and, as a consequence, experiences a more profound sedative and respiratory depressive effect from the premedication than during the time when they are actually in the laboratory during the procedure. This same circumstance holds true after the procedure is completed when the sedation is still in effect but, at the same time, all lines are out and all other external stimulation is stopped. The patient often lapses into a deeper level of sedation when all activity about the patient has stopped and after a pressure dressing has been applied to the puncture site(s). The patient should have continual monitoring until they are fully awake and intelligibly conversant following the catheterization.

In infants and very small children, it is particularly important that blood glucose levels and body temperature are monitored during any period of sedation. Hypoglycemia develops very rapidly in the small or sick infant who has had restricted oral intake for any period of time. In addition to being potentially very dangerous to the central nervous system, hypoglycemia initially makes an infant uncomfortable, irritable and impossible to sedate. Unaccounted for irritability in a small infant undergoing catheterization immediately should suggest hypoglycemia.

A drop in body temperature of all patients is anticipated in the cardiac catheterization laboratory. The patient has most (all!) of their clothing removed and the environment of the hospital/cardiac catheterization laboratory is always cool, if not actually cold. In the laboratory, the patient is scrubbed and prepped so that the cold ambient environment is aggravated by the moisture and surrounding wet drapes. The core temperature of infants and debilitated patients in particular, drops precipitously unless specific measures are taken to maintain their body temperature. The hypothermic patient becomes acidotic and very irritable from the hypothermia alone.

General management in the catheterization laboratory

Immediately upon entering the catheterization laboratory and while being secured on the catheterization table, monitoring of the sedated patient is transferred to the monitoring systems of the catheterization laboratory. Monitoring in the catheterization laboratory includes two, or preferably three ECG channels, a pulse oximeter with a display on the central monitor and, until an indwelling arterial pressure line is available, a frequently recycled, cuff blood pressure determination is displayed on the monitor. In addition, *infants* are attached to a respiratory monitor and an esophageal or rectal temperature probe. The esophageal or rectal temperature probe provides a core temperature and is far more secure and reliable than a skin temperature probe, which can easily be dislodged from moist skin. Even when in place skin temperature probes do not provide a true or reliable core temperature because of skin moisture, evaporation and restricted skin blood flow from vasoconstriction.

Even when a patient has "only sedation" or no sedation is anticipated for a catheterization procedure, the catheterization laboratory must always be prepared for all hemodynamic and ventilatory emergencies. All cardioresuscitative, anti-arrhythmic and other supportive equipment and medications must be available immediately in the cardiac catheterization laboratory. The equipment and expertise for orotracheal or nasotracheal intubation for any age or size patient must also be available immediatly in the catheterization laboratory. This includes an entire spectrum of laryngoscope blades, endotracheal tubes, suction equipment and the medications necessary to perform the intubation including supplemental sedation and paralytic agents.

Endotracheal intubation and controlled ventilation implies that the patient is receiving general anesthesia. Although it is convenient to have an anesthesiologist controlling the airway when the patient is intubated and ventilated, it is not always necessary unless an inhalation anesthetic is being used. Endotracheal intubation and controlled ventilation do allow complete control of the patient's respiration. This is a great advantage in patients with underlying airway problems or respiratory distress from congestive heart failure. In a catheterization laboratory, which is staffed with trained nurses and skilled pediatric cardiologists, endotracheal intubation can be performed by the pediatric cardiologist and the control of the ventilator can be managed by a trained respiratory therapist when the patient is on room air or oxygen. This is particularly true with infants and smaller children. The respiratory therapist adjusts the ventilator according to the desires of the primary operator and performs additional tasks such as the administration of oxygen or nitric oxide.

When a long procedure is anticipated (or even possible!), a Foley™ bladder catheter is placed in all patients past infancy. During a long case, the patient frequently receives a large volume of flush solution and, in addition to the fluid, a large volume of contrast material. The combination produces vigorous diuresis and usually a very large volume of urine. The past-infancy patient, may not be able, or may be unwilling to void spontaneously on the table and, in turn, develops a markedly distended and very uncomfortable bladder. No amount of sedation/analgesia, short of very deep general anesthesia, can overcome this discomfort. The Foley™ catheter in the bladder also allows accurate monitoring of the patient's urine output during the procedure, which, in turn, is a rough reflection of their systemic cardiac output from minute to minute.

Local anesthesia

Once the patient is positioned, secured on the procedure table and attached to the monitoring and warming systems, local anesthesia is administered to *all sites* where catheters or indwelling monitoring lines will be introduced.

Emla cream™

Emla cream™ applied to the expected puncture sites several hours before injecting the local anesthetic, appears to be effective in reducing the discomfort from the needle punctures for the local anesthesia and the subsequent percutaneous needle and sheath/dilator introductions. With or without the use of Emla™ cream at the site, the injection of the local anesthetic usually arouses the sedated patient from their "tranquil", premedicated state.

Xylocaine

The preferred local anesthetic is 2% xylocaine *without epinephrine*. All skin sites where it is anticipated that a catheter or indwelling line might be introduced during the catheterization procedure are infiltrated with the local anesthetic at the onset of the procedure. A maximum total dose of 5 mg/kg (0.25 ml/kg) in infants and 7 mg/kg (0.33 ml/kg) in older children is recommended for all sites combined. By infiltrating all anticipated sites at the onset of the procedure, the patient is not "re-awakened" during the procedure by the needle "stick" with local anesthesia for a new site. Often, once the cutaneous injection of the local anesthetic takes effect, the patient returns to sleep, even as the remainder of the local anesthetic is introduced subcutaneously or the needle punctures for the catheter introduction are performed. Occasionally, supplemental sedation is necessary to complete the local anesthetic infiltration, particularly if there has been a delay between the time when the premedication was administered and when the punctures are started for the local anesthesia.

The local anesthesia will last only 2–3 hours. During any catheterization lasting more than 3 hours, the local anesthetic, arbitrarily, is re-administered around each sheath/catheter introduction site. *Any time* a patient arouses during a cardiac catheterization, the adequacy of the local anesthesia should be the *first* thing checked. Most of the time, when a patient awakens during the procedure, it is because of pain from the local cutaneous manipulations outside of the original area of local anesthesia at the introductory site, or because of pain as the local anesthesia wears off. It is much safer and more effective to administer additional *local* anesthesia at a skin site which is painful than to try to overcome that pain with *systemic* analgesia or sedation.

Sedatives, analgesics and anesthesia in the catheterization laboratory

Most cardiac catheterization procedures are performed using a controlled deep sedation/analgesia or total, general anesthesia. The goals of premedication, sedation and anesthesia before and during a cardiac catheterization are very similar. These medications primarily are intended to alleviate the patient's anxiety and to eliminate any discomfort to the patient from the procedure. A secondary goal of these medications is to maintain the patient in a very still "steady state" and totally "cooperative" during the procedure. The necessity of keeping the patient *perfectly* still at certain stages of the catheterization has become increasingly important with the implant of intravascular devices. At the same time, optimal safety and the patient's stable physiologic status must be assured during all phases of the sedation/anesthesia.

General anesthesia is *not required* or necessary for *most* cardiac catheterization procedures. At the same time, there certainly are patients or particular catheterization procedures where general anesthesia is very desirable, if not essential. Additionally, there is often only a very fine line between controlled, deep sedation and general anesthesia. The same medications or combinations of medications, used in different dosages, may be used for both controlled, deep sedation and general anesthesia. With the exception of several of the specific intravenous (IV) anesthetics and the inhaled anesthetics, the major distinction between sedation and general anesthesia is which physician is administering the sedation/anesthesia.

When the cardiologist who is performing the procedure administers the medications for the sedation, the procedure is being performed under what is considered *controlled, deep sedation*. In this circumstance the cardiologist is, unequivocally and totally, responsible for the level of sedation, the patient's respiration, the monitoring of all of the vital signs, and the administration of any medications during the procedure. When the sedation/anesthesia is administered by the anesthesiologists, it is considered general anesthesia. In addition to administering the medications, the anesthesiologist assumes control of the patient's respirations, the administration of intravenous medications, and some of the monitoring of the patient's vital signs and hemodynamic parameters. In spite of this shift in responsibility for the ventilation and sedation of the patient, the operating cardiologist is, ultimately, still responsible for the patient.

There are many different regimes utilized for premedication, sedation and analgesia during the cardiac catheterization of pediatric and congenital heart patients. Many of the sedation regimes utilized during the catheterization procedure are continuations or repeat doses of the original premedication. Most premedication and "sedation combinations" used in the laboratory include both a sedative and an analgesic. Often an anxiolytic medication is added to the sedative and analgesic mixture to maintain the patient "tranquilized". When a patient "doesn't care", often far lower doses of sedatives and analgesics are required. All of the medications have potential problems in any patient, but they are particularly hazardous in patients with complex congenital heart lesions. It is imperative that the physiologic and hemodynamic effects of each separate medication and combination of medications are understood by the primary operator in the catheterization laboratory.

Specific premedication, sedation and analgesia for cardiac catheterization

All of the premedications, sedative and anesthetics mentioned in the text of this chapter are listed in a detailed "Formulary of Specific Medications used in, or in Conjunction with, the Cardiac Catheterization Laboratory" which is included at the end of this chapter. The details of the indications, doses by various routes of administration and for different indications as well as the adverse effects relating to the catheterization laboratory environment are included in the listing (or table) and are not duplicated in the general discussion.

For newborns and small sick infants, often minimal, or occasionally even no, premedication is necessary before beginning the procedure. After administration of the local anesthesia is completed, the catheterization procedure itself is not painful. When the infant has adequate local anesthesia, an environmental temperature which is warm and comfortable for the patient, a normal blood sugar, adequate ventilation and the infant is "comfortably" restrained, the very young infant often remains quiet during the procedure with minimal, or even without any, systemic sedation.

"Sugar nipples"

Many young infants in the past underwent cardiac catheterization with the use of a "sugar nipple" as the only supplemental sedative/analgesia. The "sugar nipple" is a standard rubber or latex nipple off a baby bottle, which is stuffed with cotton and then soaked with a mixture of glucose solution and brandy. The infant's emotional sucking needs, the sugar needs and, presumably, some sedation, are all supplied by the nipple/glucose/brandy combination. The cotton is re-saturated with the solution as needed, although usually the infant sucks on the nipple only very intermittently and re-saturation of the cotton is not necessary very frequently, if at all. The sedation is effective and there are never any over-doses or toxic issues. The brandy, of course, creates "controlled substance" and "moral" issues, but there still are occasional institutions which are progressive enough to utilize this very safe and simple sedation for infants in the cardiac catheterization laboratory.

There are many other more conventional medications or combinations of medications used as premedication in catheterization laboratories. Most of the individual medications and combinations are useful for infants, older children and adults. Some of the more common premedication combinations and sedation/analgesia used in the catheterization laboratory are covered in the following paragraphs.

"DPT Cocktail"

The "DPT cocktail" combination of meperidine (Demerol), promethazine (Phenergan), and chlorpromazine (Thorazine) has been used in a ratio of 2:1:1 mg per kilogram (up to 50 kg) as a premedication for cardiac catheterization for three and a half decades and is still a useful premedication/sedative for cardiac catheterization. The effectiveness of the combination relies upon the cumulative effects of the three drugs with each other, allowing lower doses and, in turn, fewer side effects of each individual drug. The DPT combination is popular because of its effectiveness in providing sedation, analgesia and "tranquility", which puts the patient to sleep from the sedative and anxiolytic effects without significantly depressing their respiration by the opioid.

Thorazine does have a very strong alpha blocking effect with resultant systemic vasodilation, which can result in systemic hypotension. Because of this vasodilation and hypotension effect, the Thorazine is *contraindicated* in the premedication combination in any patient with "tetralogy" physiology, Eisenmenger physiology or any type of significant left ventricular outflow tract stenosis.

D & P (Demerol & Phenergan)

In patients in whom Thorazine cannot be used because of the dependence of the pulmonary or coronary circulation on the maintenance of the systemic resistance, Demerol and Phenergan together, but *without Thorazine*, are used as the premedication/sedation to start the procedure. The Phenergan provides some sedation and allows a lower dose of Demerol for effective analgesia. However, the two together without Thorazine are not as effective as DPT, and must be used in larger doses to provide equally effective premedication/sedation.

Morphine

Morphine is a powerful opiate analgesic with an anxiolytic as well as a *mild* sedative effect. The anxiolytic effect makes up somewhat for the minimal sedative effect. It provides good premedication in infants and children but alone, it does not provide sufficient sedation for a procedure unless it is given in very high, "anesthetic" doses. Morphine is a powerful respiratory depressant in the higher doses and in high doses provides general anesthesia. Usually a benzodiazepine or a short-acting barbiturate is used in conjunction with the morphine to provide sedation without the need for a higher dose of morphine. Narcan provides an effective antagonism to the action of the morphine.

Fentanyl

Fentanyl is a potent opiate analgesic, with a fast onset of action and minimal respiratory depression. It has become very popular as a premedication for catheterization, alone or in conjunction with phenergan or thorazine. In infants fentanyl is frequently supplemented with the benzodiazepine midazolam. Fentanyl has the same side effects as morphine but, in general, to a lesser degree. Fentanyl, like the other opiates, is counteracted with narcan.

Midazolam (Versed)

Midazolam is a benzodiazepine which can be given orally, intramuscularly, intravenously or intranasally. Administered by any of these routes, midazolam provides a very effective sedative prior to a procedure. The oral or nasal routes are more "comfortable" for the patient but the effects are less predictable by these routes. Midazolam also is a good parenteral supplement to other premedications including Fentanyl, the Demerol/Phenergan/Thorazine "cocktail" (DPT) or Demerol/Phenergan (DP) in older patients.

Ketamine

Ketamine is a very effective sedative, with a very rapid onset and short duration of action. It can be used either intravenously or intramuscularly. Ketamine is *not* strictly an anesthetic or analgesic, but it "dissociates" the patient from pain. It has a very rapid action, very little respiratory depression and, if anything, enhancement of blood pressure which makes it an ideal "sedative" prior to a catheterization procedure—including even the insertion of an intravenous line. Ketamine can be used in small infants as well as older patients up to late adolescence.

Morphine and midazolam or fentanyl and midazolam

In order to avoid respiratory or blood pressure depression and provide more sedation, morphine or fentanyl is used in conjunction with midazolam but with a lower dose of the opiate as well as the midazolam. Half of the usual doses of morphine or fentanyl and then half the usual dose of midazolam are infused sequentially intravenously. The combinations provide excellent sedation/analgesia for cardiac catheterization.

Diazepam (valium)

Diazepam is an effective sedative, anxiolytic and amnesic with a moderate duration of activity. It can be given orally, intramuscularly or intravenously. It is a moderate respiratory depressant and also produces pulmonary arteriolar vasoconstriction, particularly when delivered directly into the pulmonary arteries. It should not be used in patients with even the suggestion of pulmonary vascular disease or pulmonary vasoreactivity. Midazolam has replaced diazepam in most cases as a premedication or supplemental sedative in the catheterization laboratory.

There are many other medications and combinations of medications that are utilized throughout the world for premedication/sedation for cardiac catheterization. For the most part, these contain the minimum of a sedative and an analgesic. The particular medicine which is used is not as important as is the necessity that the responsible physician is very familiar with each and every medication which is used in any particular circumstance, in or in conjunction with, the catheterization laboratory.

Supplemental sedatives/analgesics during the catheterization

Most of the supplemental medications utilized *during* the catheterization are the same medications given for premedication, but usually with some variations in the dose. The specific supplemental medications which are used during the catheterization procedure vary depending on the needs of each individual patient. Some patients require very little supplemental sedation while others inexplicably require even double the usual amount or more frequent administration of the supplemental medications. There also are variations in the medications used in different institutions and even between individual operators within the same institution.

When patients still remain restless or apprehensive at the *onset* of the procedure even after they have received the appropriate premedication and the local xylocaine has had time to take effect, other possible causes of the patient's irritability should always be investigated before adding supplemental systemic sedation/analgesia. The operator is responsible for investigating all other possible causes of the patient's discomfort/irritability. There are some particularly suspect areas as the causes of patient discomfort and restlessness.

The most common area of discomfort is the area of the needle puncture or the sheath/dilator introduction. The operator must be sure that the skin area being manipulated is not "outside of the area" of the local anesthesia. Additional local anesthesia in both the cutaneous and subcutaneous tissues is often more effective than even a supplemental full dose of the patient's premedication.

After inadequate local anesthesia has been eliminated as the source of discomfort and restlessness, there still are other causes of discomfort to be ruled out before any additional systemic sedative/analgesia should be added. The tape or restraints securing the patient on the table can be too tight, can bind the patient's extremities tightly or fix the extremities in an uncomfortable position. The environmental temperature in the room should be comfortable *for the patient*—this is particularly important with the small, thin or debilitated patient. The patient's bladder should have been emptied before the patient was premedicated and must have adequate drainage during the procedure. The discomfort of a full bladder cannot be overcome with sedation or analgesia. The blood sugar of all infants should be checked, particularly after any duration of being "nothing by mouth" or when an intravenous line is not in place with supplemental glucose running. Finally, it is essential that the patient's hemodynamic parameters are stable before the administration of additional sedation is considered. It is mandatory to have the arterial monitoring line in place before supplemental sedatives are given. In addition to providing a continual and *accurate* display of blood pressure, the arterial line provides access for obtaining arterial blood oxygen saturations and blood gases at any time throughout the procedure.

Additional supplemental sedatives or analgesics should be administered during the procedure in response to the patient's needs. Just as with restlessness at the onset of the catheterization, when a patient and particularly an infant on the catheterization table becomes restless or begins crying *during* the procedure, the patient again is investigated critically for a source of discomfort as just described. Again, the first supplemental medication to be considered is usually additional *local anesthesia* at the site of the catheter introduction. If there is adequate local anesthesia at the introductory site, the catheter manipulations within the vascular system and heart do not cause pain. Once all treatable sources of the patient's restlessness are excluded, only then is the patient re-sedated.

Supplemental sedation is also added arbitrarily and periodically during *very long* cases to preempt the patient's waking and becoming anxious and uncooperative. Supplemental sedation is given prophylactically just before particularly delicate or critical procedures are performed—for example, extra sedation is given just before the precise positioning of intracardiac devices (atrial septal defect (ASD) occluder devices, stents). Extra analgesia is given just before an interventional procedure that is expected to produce pain (particularly large vessel dilations).

Following the administration of even small doses of sedative, patients, particularly infants, are observed and monitored very carefully for signs of respiratory depression. In the event of transient respiratory depression, any type of physical stimulation—even minimal—of the patient or a few breaths with an Ambu™ face-mask is often enough to reverse it. In the event of prolonged respiratory depression, intubation and controlled ventilation may be necessary.

There are at least as many regimens for supplemental sedation of patients during the procedure as there are premedication regimens. No one supplemental sedation regimen is satisfactory for all patients or even for the same patient under different circumstances. The exact medications which are used vary according to the size and hemodynamics of the particular patient, the established, safe routines in a particular cardiac catheterization laboratory and the individual preferences/experiences of the operating physician. Some of the more common supplemental sedation regimes are as follows.

Demerol, phenergan, thorazine (DPT)

A smaller (usually one half or less), repeat dose of the original premedication combination is very effective as supplemental sedation/analgesia. This is particularly useful if the patient has discomfort or pain or the procedure has lasted for a prolonged time. The respiratory depressant effect of the original Demerol may persist and be cumulative with the supplemental dose. The patient should be watched expectantly for an adverse reaction following the administration of supplemental DPT.

Ketamine

Ketamine, with its very rapid and predictably short action, along with very little respiratory depression, has become one of the primary supplemental sedatives in the catheterization laboratory. It has little analgesic effect but its dissociative effect overcomes this. Ketamine is particularly useful when a patient unexpectedly, suddenly or violently wakes during the procedure. It can be given rapidly through the catheter or, in the absence of venous access, intramuscularly. It is extremely fast acting and doses as small as 0.5 to 1 mg/kg intravenously or through the catheter are effective instantly in most patients. Because of its short activity, it requires repeated doses every 10–20 minutes for continued sedation.

Midazolam (Versed)

Versed, given through the catheter or intravenously, is a very effective and safe supplemental medication for use during the procedure. Its sedative, anxiolytic and amnesic effects have a fairly rapid onset of action, little respiratory depression and little effect on either the systemic or pulmonary vascular resistance.

Morphine sulfate

Morphine is used as a supplement to the sedation primarily when the patient is suspected of having *pain* as a result of catheter or device manipulations. Because of its strong tendency to cause respiratory depression in a "sedative" dose, morphine is not a good drug used alone for supplemental sedation. When the patient is suspected of having pain *and* is in need of sedation, it is better to use morphine in combination with a benzodiazepine.

Morphine and midazolam

In order to avoid respiratory depression and provide more sedation, morphine is used in its anxiolytic dose in conjunction with a half dose of midazolam given intravenously and sequentially to the morphine. The combination provides excellent supplemental sedation/analgesia during cardiac catheterization.

Fentanyl

As a potent, short-acting narcotic *analgesic* without any *significant* effects on respiration, Fentanyl is an ideal analgesic for supplemental use during the procedure as well as for its premedication use in the cardiac catheterization laboratory. As a supplement for pain, it is given in its lowest dose either through the catheter or intravenously. It can be repeated in 30–60 minutes as necessary. Fentanyl is frequently used in conjunction with a low dose of midazolam.

Diazepam (valium)

Valium is another supplemental sedative frequently used during cardiac catheterization procedures. It is a very effective sedative, anxiolytic and amnesic. However, it is avoided in patients when pulmonary vascular disease is known or even suspected because of its pulmonary vaso-spastic effect. Valium is particularly useful given at the end of the procedure as a "chaser" to prevent post-catheterization hallucinations in adolescent and older patients who received ketamine earlier during the procedure.

The precise doses of the separate premedications which are discussed above are outlined in detail in the "formulary list" of catheterization laboratory medications at the end of this chapter.

General anesthesia for pediatric cardiac catheterization

There are institutions where general anesthesia is the routine for all cardiac catheterizations for congenital heart patients. General anesthesia has significant advantages and is safe and effective in those institutions where it is performed by pediatric cardiac anesthesiologists. General anesthesia is used in all institutions occasionally for selective cases. Very well administered general anesthesia produces a very quiet and usually stable patient regardless of the length of the catheterization procedure being performed. For premedication, the anesthesiologist often uses a separate fast acting intravenous sedative/analgesic in anticipation of replacing it with an inhaled anesthetic agent or may begin with the same combination of intravenous medications for the premedication which, in higher doses, provides the general anesthesia.

The anesthesiologist assumes the care of the patient's state of consciousness, ventilation, monitoring of blood pressure and regulation of blood gases. Subconsciously, but not in actuality, the use of general anesthesia shifts the responsibility for the patient's hemodynamic and respiratory stability from the catheterizing cardiologist to the anesthesiologist. The catheterizing cardiologist as well as the anesthesiologist must be aware of all of the effects on the hemodynamics of each particular anesthetic drug alone and in combination.

In spite of its several advantages, general anesthesia does alter the patient's physiologic and hemodynamic parameters significantly. The degree of alteration in the patient's hemodynamics depends upon the patient's underlying condition, the anesthetic agents used, and the amount of oxygen in the inhaled mixture. Calculations of shunts, cardiac outputs and valve areas are, at best, questionable with a patient under general anesthesia, especially if the patient is breathing more than 21% inspired oxygen with an inhaled anesthetic. When the patient is ventilated under general anesthesia, the "passive" phase of the respiratory cycle is during the expiratory phase of respiration and must be used for the measurement of intravascular pressure. General anesthesia with endotracheal intubation potentially introduces separate airway and ventilation problems in addition to the changes in the hemodynamic parameters. Although the pediatric cardiologist performing the catheterization is not administering the anesthesia, the operating cardiologist must constantly be aware of the effects on the patient's hemodynamics of *all* of the medications and of each change in respiratory settings administered by the anesthesiologist. General anesthesia administered by a certified pediatric cardiac anesthesiologist also adds to the overall cost of the catheterization procedure.

The anesthesiologists who administer anesthesia for pediatric and congenital heart patients must be as familiar with the bizarre combinations of abnormal hemodynamics which occur with the multiple varieties of congenital cardiac defects as is the pediatric cardiologist. The effectiveness of both the intravenous and inhaled anesthetics is affected by both right to left and left to right shunts. In the presence of *right to left* shunts, intravenous anesthetics bypass the lungs and go directly to the brain and, in turn, have a more rapid and occasionally more intense or prolonged effect. Inhaled anesthetics, on the other hand, are exposed to less pulmonary blood in the presence of the right to left shunt and, as a consequence, take *longer* to take effect. If the anesthetic is cleared by ventilation at the end of the procedure, it takes longer to be cleared from the circulation in the presence of a right to left shunt.

In the presence of *left to right* shunts, intravenous anesthetics continue to recirculate through the lungs and are diverted away from the systemic circulation. As a consequence, they initially are less effective, require a larger dosage and, once effective, they last considerably longer. Inhaled anesthetics are absorbed into the pulmonary venous blood from the alveoli. In the presence of a left to right shunt, the pulmonary venous blood is recirculated over and over back through the pulmonary circulation. This decreases the effectiveness of the inhaled anesthetic markedly by allowing a smaller percentage of the pulmonary venous blood with the absorbed inhalation anesthetic to reach the systemic arterial circulation. The continued high concentration of anesthetic in the pulmonary venous blood also prevents further transfer of the anesthetic from the alveoli across the capillary membranes into the blood.

In the catheterization laboratory, a patient's hemodynamics change very suddenly and very dramatically. These changes occur as a result of inherent progressive deterioration in myocardial function or even myocardial depression secondary to the anesthetic agent. The patient's pulmonary vascular and/or systemic vascular resistance changes during the procedure as a result of pharmacological manipulations or injection of contrast solutions. Changes in either systemic or pulmonary vascular resistance alter the degree/direction of shunting which, in turn, affects the effectiveness of the anesthetic agent.

The anesthesiologist frequently uses the additive effects of a combination of an inhalant anesthetic with a narcotic or a muscle relaxant (a "balanced" anesthesia) in order to obtain the desired effects of the particular medications, while at the same time minimizing the adverse effects of each of the separate drugs. Supplemental anesthetics administered during general anesthesia are handled by the anesthesiologist and often are simply variations in the dose of the initial anesthetic which was used.

Some of the more common "general" anesthetics used in the catheterization laboratory are mentioned in the paragraphs which follow. The same medications are discussed individually and in more detail, including dosage and potential side effects, under the formulary of specific medications used in, or in conjunction with the cardiac catheterization laboratory which is found later in this chapter.

"General" anesthetics for cardiac catheterization

General anesthetics, when administered in *anesthetic doses* in the catheterization laboratory, are administered only by qualified anesthesiologists who, in turn, maintain total control over the patient's respiration.

Morphine

One of the simplest and safest "general anesthetics" for the catheterization laboratory is morphine administered as a slow intravenous bolus, but in a much larger dose than that used for premedication. In these high doses and used in conjunction with a muscle relaxant, it provides general anesthesia without significant myocardial depression. The strong respiratory depressant effect of these high doses is of no consequence when the patient is intubated and their respiration is totally controlled. It does produce some vasodilation and can result in hypotension, particularly if the patient is volume depleted.

Fentanyl

Fentanyl, like morphine in high doses administered intravenously, produces anesthesia without myocardial depression. Used with muscle paralyzers, it produces even less change in the patient's hemodynamics than morphine. Also like morphine, fentanyl produces respiratory depression, which is of little consequence when used as a general anesthesia when respiration is controlled totally.

Propofol

Propofol is a sedative/hypnotic and general anesthetic. It has a very short duration of action, rapid clearance and minimal respiratory depression at lower doses. It is administered as a rapid intravenous bolus followed by continuous infusion to maintain the anesthesia. Propofol almost always produces some hypotension. This is exaggerated by hypovolemia and is very apparent in all patients who have been restricted from oral intake for any length of time. Propofol is a severe tissue irritant and must be given through a large, free-flowing intravenous line.

Amidate (etomidate)

Amidate, given as an intravenous bolus over a few seconds, is an ultra short acting intravenous anesthetic with rapid onset of anesthesia action with an equally rapid recovery from the effects. Anesthesia is maintained with a continuous intravenous infusion. Amidate reportedly has minimal cardiovascular or respiratory depression, but does increase airway reflexes leading to laryngeal spasm and can cause myoclonus, spontaneous muscular movements, nausea and vomiting. Like propofol, etomidate is locally painful and is administered through a large bore, free-flowing intravenous line.

Ketamine

Ketamine in higher doses is a very effective intravenous general anesthetic. It has a very rapid onset of action and a short duration of action, which makes it good for relatively short catheterization procedures. Ketamine increases heart rate and peripheral vascular resistance, which, in turn, elevates systemic blood pressure. It causes some myocardial depression and at anesthetic doses causes marked respiratory depression. At sea level, even at the higher anesthetic doses, ketamine has no effect on pulmonary vascular resistance, however, it appears to increase pulmonary resistance at higher altitudes. In older patients (teenagers and older), many patients experience bad dreams, hallucinations and even deliriums upon awakening from ketamine anesthesia.

Barbiturates

Barbiturates are potent central nervous system depressants with marked sedative effects. In large enough doses and with controlled ventilation, the barbiturates are occasionally used alone or in combination with a narcotic for very deep sedation/anesthesia for a catheterization procedure. These have been supplanted for the most part by the benzodiazepines as adjuncts for premedication and sedation.

Inhalation anesthetics

All of the inhalation anesthetics are administered by a qualified anesthesiologist/anesthetist with the anticipation of endotracheal intubation of the patient. All inhalation anesthetics used at present are non flammable.

Halothane

Halothane produces deep general anesthesia in a very low concentration of the inspired gases. The low concentration of halothane required for deep anesthesia allows for the administration of very high concentrations of concomitant, inhaled oxygen. Halothane causes a moderate depression of myocardial contractility, decreases heart rate, and is a mild vasodilator.

Enflurane

Similar to halothane, deep anesthesia is achieved with a low concentration of the inspired gases. Enflurane also causes a moderate depression of myocardial contractility, decreases heart rate and is a vasodilator, the combination of which results in a decrease in vascular resistance and overall decrease in cardiac output.

Nitrous oxide

Nitrous oxide (dinitrogen oxide) is an inhalant anesthetic that has little or no effect on cardiac function or vascular resistance, but does require a high concentration of the inspired gas to produce deep anesthesia. The very high concentration of nitrous oxide required for deep anesthesia limits the amount of oxygen that can be administered concomitantly. For this reason, nitrous oxide is usually used in combination with an intravenous agent or a muscle relaxant.

Antithrombotic/anticoagulation

One additional medication which is used regularly in pediatric/congenital catheterization laboratories is heparin.

The frequency of use and the dosage vary immensely from laboratory to laboratory. Many catheterization laboratories administer heparin in all cases, while other, equally reputable laboratories, only administer heparin for special procedures. The purpose of the heparin is the prevention of thrombi during (and after) the catheterization procedure, while hopefully not incurring any excessive bleeding. Some laboratories administer the heparin according to the patient's partial thromboplastin time (PTT) or activated clotting time (ACT), while many laboratories administer an arbitrary, per kilogram dose.

Heparin was initially used in the pediatric catheterization laboratory in an attempt to prevent thrombi at the arterial entrance/puncture sites, however, the reported data are not convincing that heparin has a significant benefit in this use. This author believes that the "tender care and handling" of the artery at the time of the puncture, during the catheterization procedure, and immediately after the withdrawal of the sheath/catheter is more important than the use of heparin. The management of arterial sites is covered in Chapter 4, Catheter introduction.

Whether or not heparin is important in preventing peripheral arterial thrombosis, it is important in preventing central clotting and embolizations from catheters, wires and devices during catheter manipulations anywhere within the circulation. Because the consequences are usually more obvious and devastating in the "systemic" circulation, the major emphasis has been on preventing thrombi and embolization during retrograde or prograde "left heart" catheter manipulations in the systemic circuit. Most operators administer heparin more or less routinely for any "left heart" or "systemic" cardiac catheterization.

Although the consequences usually are less obvious or dramatic, thrombosis or embolization in the "venous" or "right heart" circulation—including the peripheral veins—is equally important. Since "venous" clots in any congenital heart patient with right to left shunting represent potential systemic emboli, most operators instinctively use the same precautions for preventing "systemic" emboli in venous catheter manipulations in cyanotic patients as they do when they are manipulating catheters in the "systemic" circulation. Anticoagulation during "right heart only" catheterizations is not as routine, but at the same time most operators who have extensive experience in a pediatric/congenital catheterization laboratory have witnessed thrombi on catheters, wires, or devices in the strictly "venous" circulation or have withdrawn large clots from indwelling venous sheaths all without any *recognizable* adverse events. Even though "not causing a problem", when a venous thrombus is visualized it is treated aggressively with heparin, thrombolytics or even mechanical thrombectomy. The presence of thrombi in the venous circulation does not represent an "all or nothing" circumstance and probably occurs to some degree on any catheter, wire or device in the venous circulation. The small thrombi strictly in the systemic venous circulation possibly (or probably) result in "silent", very small, pulmonary emboli. Although venous clots rarely result in recognizable adverse events, the use of systemic heparin is recommended for the prevention of any venous clotting during all catheterization procedures in congenital heart patients.

Central venous thrombi/emboli are not the only problems in the venous circulation. When sheaths and catheters are introduced into a peripheral vein, not only is the vein traumatized significantly, but with large catheters/sheaths or any venous spasm, the flow in the vein is obstructed at the entrance site for the duration of the procedure. These circumstances create a prime opportunity for venous thrombus formation and subsequent occlusion of the particular vein or venous system. Complete occlusion of these peripheral veins occurs without obvious immediate clinical sequelae, but becomes painfully obvious to the operator when the vein is found to be totally occluded during an attempt at repeat catheterization through the same site.

There is some good, but anecdotal and "non-controlled", evidence supporting the routine use of heparin for the prevention of these peripheral venous obstructions in all cardiac catheterizations. For many years heparin was not administered routinely in strictly venous catheterization procedures in the catheterization laboratory at Texas Children's Hospital. As with most laboratories, occasional obstructed veins were encountered at subsequent catheterizations. Because of the frequent use of very large sheaths as well as the extra "hardware", and manipulations in the circulation during the implant of intravascular devices, it became routine to heparinize patients fully during the interventional procedure. Most of these implanted devices were in protocol studies and, as a consequence, these patients usually underwent re-catheterization. In spite of the very large sheaths required for the device implants, particularly with the Rashkind™ patent ductus arteriosus (PDA) occluding devices and intravascular stents, very few of these patients had venous obstruction at the previous venous entry site during a subsequent or even multiple, subsequent catheterization(s).

Heparin is now administered routinely to most patients undergoing cardiac catheterization. Many catheterization laboratories arbitrarily administer somewhere between 50 mg/kg and 200 mg/kg of heparin at the beginning of the catheterization. In our laboratory, a baseline activated clotting time (ACT) is drawn as soon as the first vascular access is established. Once *all* vascular access is secured and unless the ACT is very prolonged to begin with, the patient is given 75–100 mg/kg of heparin intravenously. The heparin dose is cut in half when a very short, "right heart" only catheterization such as a cardiac biopsy is anticipated. The ACT determination is repeated after 15–30 minutes. The goal is to adjust the ACT with additional heparin to between 275 and 300 seconds as necessary. The ACT determination is repeated when the catheterization procedure lasts more than two hours and at the end of the procedure. Unless the ACT is above 450 seconds or there is continued bleeding from the puncture sites *and* the ACT is above 300 seconds, the heparin usually is not reversed at the end of the procedure.

Although the potential for bleeding into any body organ including the brain is possible, there are very few reports of significant systemic complications from the use of systemic heparin with any of the described regimens. The most common adverse event from heparin is local bleeding or hematoma formation at the vascular entry site, which may or may not be totally attributable to the heparin. With careful attention to the area of the vascular entry after the sheaths/catheters are removed, even the occurrence of this relatively minor problem is minimized. With continued bleeding at the puncture site and with a persistent significant elevation of the ACT, protamine is administered to reverse the heparin except after the implant of atrial septal/patent foramen ovale occluding devices. The dose for reversal of heparin with protamine is 0.5 to 1 mg of protamine for every 100 mg of heparin previously administered. The protamine dose is reduced by *half* for every *half hour* since the most recent administration of heparin, or is adjusted according to the ACT determination.

Formulary of specific medications used in, or in conjunction with, the cardiac catheterization laboratory

Most of the medications used in, and in conjunction with, the pediatric and congenital catheterization laboratory are tabulated in some detail in the following section of this chapter. The indications, doses and the major adverse effects of each of these medications, particularly as their use pertains to the catheterization laboratory, are described[1,2]. The medications are grouped according to the major categories of use. The order of the groups or categories is, more or less, in the ordinary frequency of their use. Specific antidotes to any particular medications and category of medication are grouped with the particular medication or group of medications for which it is the antidote. The sedatives, analgesics and anesthetics which are mentioned very briefly earlier in this chapter are repeated in more detail in this tabular form as a reference source. In the following formulary section, there is a more detailed discussion of their uses, doses and adverse effects as they apply to the catheterization laboratory.

Index of specific medications used in, or in conjunction with, the cardiac catheterization laboratory

Table 2.1 Specific medications used in, or in conjunction with, the cardiac catheterization laboratory

Local anesthetics
- EMLA cream
- Xylocaine (Lidocaine)
- Bupivacaine (Marcaine, Sensorcaine)

"Sugar nipple"

Opiate analgesics
- Morphine
- Fentanyl (Sublimaze)
- Meperidine (Demerol, Pethidine)
- Hydromorphone (Dilaudid)
- Sufentanil (Sufenta)

Opiate antagonist
- Naloxone (Narcan)

Non-opiate sedatives/tranquilizers
- Phenothiazine tranquilizers
  - Chlorpromazine (Thorazine)
  - Promethazine (Phenergan)
- DPT (Demerol, Phenergan, Thorazine)
- Ketamine (Ketalar)
- Benzodiazepines
  - Midazolam (Versed)
  - Diazepam (Valium)
  - Lorazepam (Ativan)
- Benzodiazepine antagonist
  - Romazicon (Flumazenil)
- Chloral hydrate
- Barbiturates
  - Pentobarbital (Nembutal)
  - Thiopental (Pentothal)
  - Methohexital (Brevital)
  - Phenobarbital (Luminal, Phenobarbitone)

General anesthetics
- Intravenous anesthetics
  - Morphine
  - Fentanyl (Sublimaze)
  - Propofol (Diprivan)
  - Etomidate (Amidate)
  - Ketamine (Ketalar)
  - Barbiturates
- Inhalation anesthetics
  - Halothane
  - Enflurane
  - Nitrous oxide

Neuromuscular paralyzers
- Succinylcholine
- Pancuronium
- Vecuronium

(Continued p. 39)

Table 2.1 *Continued.*

- Atracurium (Tracrium)
- Neuromuscular paralyzer antagonists
  - Neostigmine (Prostigmin)
  - Edrophonium (Tensilon)
- Antiepileptics
  - Diazepam (Valium)
  - Lorazepam (Ativan)
  - Phenobarbital (Luminal, Phenobarbitone)
  - Diphenylhydantoin (Dilantin, Phenytoin)
- Antihistamine
  - Diphenhydramine (Benadryl)
- Adrenocortical steroids
  - Dexamethasone (Decadron)
  - Hydrocortisone (Solu-Cortef, Hytone, Cortef)
  - Methylprednisolone (Solu-Medrol, Depo-Medrol)
  - Prednisone (Deltasone, Meticorten)
- Anti malignant hypertension
  - Dantrolene sodium (Dantrium)
- Antiemetics
  - Ondansetron (Zofran)
  - Promethazine (Phenergan)
- Inotropics
  - Phenylephrine (Neo-Synephrine)
  - Epinephrine (Adrenaline)
  - Norepinephrine (Levophed, Noradrenaline, Levoartenolol)
  - Isoproterenol (Isuprel)
  - Dopamine
  - Dobutamine
  - Milrinone (Primacor)
  - Amrinone
- Alpha adrenergic blockers
  - Phentolamine (Regitine)
  - Tolazoline
- Beta adrenergic blockers
  - Esmolol
  - Propranolol (Inderal)
  - Labetalol (Normodyne, Trandate)
  - Metoprolol (Lopressor)
  - Sotalol
- Vasodilators
  - Nitroglycerin (Nitrostat)
  - Hydralazine (Apresoline)
  - Diazoxide (Hyperstat)
  - Fenoldopam (Corlopam)
  - Nitroprusside
  - Tolazoline (Priscoline)
  - Nitric Oxide (NO)
  - Prostaglandin E 1 (Prostin, Alprostadil, PGE1)
  - Prostacyclin (PGI2)
  - Flolan
- Cardiac glycoside
  - Digoxin (Lanoxin)
- Anti arrhythmic
  - Atropine
  - Lidocaine IV (Xylocaine IV)
  - Adenosine (Adenocard)
  - Bretylium (Bretylol)
  - Procainamide (Procamide, Pronestyl)
  - Verapamil (Calan, Isoptin)
  - Amiodarone (Cordarone)
  - Phenytoin (Diphenylhydantoin, Dilantin)
  - Esmolol (Brevibloc)
  - Propranolol (Inderal)
- Anticoagulants
  - Heparin
  - Heparin reversal—Protamine
  - Low molecular weight heparins (LMWHs)
    - Enoxaparin (Clexane, Lovenox)
    - Dalteparin (Fragmin)
    - Innohep (Tinzaparin)
    - Ardeparin (Normiflo)
  - Warfarin (Coumadin)
  - Warfarin reversal—Phytonadione (Mephyton, Vitamin K)
  - Direct antithrombins-hirudins
    - Lepirudin (Refludan)
    - Bivalirudin (Angiomax)
    - Argatroban (Novastan)
  - Anti platelet aggregating
    - Aspirin (Acetylsalicylic acid, ASA)
    - Clopidogrel (Plavix)
    - Tirofiban (Aggrastat)
    - Eptifibatide (Integrilin)
    - Abciximab (ReoPro, Centocor)
- Thrombolytics
  - Streptokinase (Streptase)
  - Anistreplase (APSAC)
  - Activase (Alteplase, t-PA)
- Thrombolysis reversal—Fresh Frozen Plasma (FFP)
- Diuretics
  - Furosemide (Lasix)
  - Ethacrynic acid (Edecrin)
- Intravenous fluid supplements/electrolytes
  - Normal saline (0.9% NS, NS)
  - Ringer's lactate
  - Sodium bicarbonate (Bicarbonate)
  - Calcium chloride
  - Dextrose solutions
    - D5W
    - 50% Dextrose
- Volume expanders
  - Whole blood
  - Packed red blood cells (PRBC)
  - Fresh frozen plasma (FFP)
  - Human albumin (Albumisol, Albuminar-5, Buminate-5)
  - Plasmanate (Pooled plasma proteins)
  - Hetastarch (Hespan)
  - Mannitol (Osmitrol)
- Bronchodilators
  - Albuterol (Ventolin, Proventil)
  - Terbutaline (Brethaire)
  - Theophylline (Slo-bid)
- Antibiotics
  - Cefazolin (Ancef, Kefzol)
  - Cefuroxime (Zinacef, Ceftin)
  - Amikacin (Amikin)
  - Vancomycin (Vancocin)

Catheterization laboratory formulary local anesthetics

EMLA cream

EMLA™ cream is a eutectic emulsion of 2.5% lidocaine and 2.5% prilocaine. It is used as a topical anesthetic to numb the area to be punctured with a needle. EMLA™ cream appears to be effective at reducing the discomfort from the puncture for starting a peripheral intravenous line and from the punctures for the introduction of needles and sheaths at the catheter introductory sites. EMLA™ cream appears to be most effective in patients who have had previous catheterizations and unpleasant memories from the administration of local anesthesia. It is only used in areas where the skin is totally intact with no associated open wounds, injuries or dermatologic conditions, which might enhance absorption.

Dose
EMLA™ cream is applied in a fairly thick layer to the immediate and surrounding area of the proposed puncture at least one, and preferably two, hours prior to the skin and vessel puncture and the area is covered with an occlusive dressing. The dressing is removed and the cream is wiped away just before the intravenous puncture.

Adverse effects
EMLA™ cream causes contact dermatitis, angioedema, burning or stinging very rarely. If absorbed EMLA™ can cause bradycardia, central nervous system disorientation or seizures.

Lidocaine hydrochloride (Xylocaine)

2% Xylocaine is preferred in the catheterization laboratory. It is infiltrated locally at each site as local tissue anesthesia. It is used *without* adjunctive epinephrine. With 2% xylocaine, half the volume of the local anesthetic, compared to a 1% xylocaine solution, is required to provide the same amount of local anesthesia. The smaller volume of the 2% local solution results in less dilation and stretching of the cutaneous and subcutaneous tissues, which are the major source of pain from the local anesthetic.

Dose
5 mg/kg (0.25 ml/kg of 2%) for infants less than 6 months old or 7 mg/kg (0.35 ml/kg of 2%) injected subcuticularly and subcutaneously. This is the total dose for the combination of *all* sites being infiltrated. (When using 1% xylocaine, 0.5 ml/kg for infants less than 6 months and 0.7 ml/kg for patients over 6 months).

Adverse effects
Given intravascularly or in excessive doses xylocaine causes seizures.

Bupivacaine hydrochloride (Marcaine, Sensorcaine)

0.25% (= 2.5 mg/ml) solution is infiltrated locally for local tissue anesthesia. Also used for peripheral nerve block, sympathetic block and epidural anesthesia.

Dose for local anesthesia
1.6 mg/kg (0.65 ml/kg) for infants less than 6 months and 2.5 mg/kg (1 ml/kg) for patients over 6 months total dose of marcaine for the combination of all sites being infiltrated.

Adverse effects
Bradycardia, hypotension, cardiac arrest and seizures can occur with an overdose or when administered intravenously.

"Sugar nipple"

The "sugar nipple" is a standard rubber or plastic nipple off a baby bottle, which is stuffed with sterile cotton. The cotton is soaked with a solution of glucose and brandy and the infant allowed to suck on the nipple as desired throughout the procedure.

Dose
A 1:1 dilution of 50% glucose solution and commercial brandy in a volume enough to soak the cotton in the nipple. The cotton is resoaked *pro re na'ta* (PRN) if it dries out, but this is usually unnecessary (or necessary no more than once during a cardiac catheterization).

Adverse effects
There are no reported physiologic adverse effects, but the brandy does create a "moral" issue with some individuals and institutions.

Opiate analgesics

Opiates are the primary central analgesics used in the field of medicine in general and in the catheterization laboratory in particular. The beneficial analgesia effects of the opiate are weighed against the side effect of each opiate. All of the opiates are habit forming and their continued use must be closely supervised and limited.

Morphine sulfate

Morphine is a strong central opiate analgesic which increases the patient's tolerance to pain and decreases their perception of pain. Morphine also acts as a mild sedative. Given intravenously, morphine has a half-life of 2.5–3 hours and when given intramuscularly it has a half life of 4–5 hours.

In very small doses, morphine is useful as an anxiolytic for infants and small children prior to starting any procedure including even the starting of a difficult intravenous line. The "relaxing effect" in this dose is useful in treating infants with impending pulmonary edema or hypoxemic cyanotic spells.

When used in combination with sedatives, benzodiazepines, or tranquilizers, the dose of morphine is reduced to half while still maintaining its analgesic effect.

Dose—anxiolytic
0.025–0.05 mg/kg subcutaneously or intramuscularly.

Dose—premedication
0.025–0.1 mg/kg is given slowly intravenously or 0.05–0.1 mg/kg intramuscularly or subcutaneously.

Adverse effects
When given as a rapid infusion, morphine causes vasodilation and hypotension. The sedative effect is additive with barbiturates and phenothiazines. Morphine is a strong depressant of respiration and the cough reflex. It should not be relied upon for total sedation unless extrinsic respiratory support is utilized. It causes biliary and urinary tract spasm and often causes drowsiness, clouded mentation, nausea and vomiting as after effects.

Fentanyl citrate (Sublimaze)

Fentanyl is a potent narcotic analgesic with a fast onset of action with the advantage of producing minimal respiratory depression. The rapid action and minimal respiratory depression have led to its recent popularity as a very effective premedication and for continual analgesia/sedation throughout cardiac catheterization procedures.

Dose—analgesia/sedation
1–3 mcg/kg given intravenously. The dose can be repeated intravenously every 30–60 minutes for maintenance of the analgesia (and some sedation) during the procedure.

Dose—anesthesia
Induction with 5–10 mcg/kg of fentanyl given intravenously and maintained with 1–10 mcg/kg/hr infused intravenously.

Adverse effects
Fentanyl fairly consistently produces hypotension and bradycardia.

Meperidine hydrochloride (Demerol, Pethedine)

Demerol is a moderate strength opioid analgesic and mild sedative (approximately 1/8th the strength of morphine). In addition to its analgesic and sedative effects, demerol also causes disorientation, which may contribute to its overall therapeutic effect. Demerol is used intravenously or intramuscularly. Orally it is not reliably effective. Demerol is much faster acting (less than one minute) and of shorter duration than morphine. Demerol peaks in activity in 10–15 minutes and lasts 2.5 to 3 hours. Because of its continued use in the "lytic cocktail", demerol is still probably the most commonly used analgesic in the catheterization laboratory.

Dose
1–2 mg/kg up to 75 mg (100 mg in *very, very* large patients) given intravenously or intramuscularly. The dose is reduced when used with the phenothiazines in the "lytic cocktail" (see under DPT).

Adverse effects
Demerol depresses respirations and causes circulatory depression which can result in hypotension, particularly in higher doses and in the presence of any volume depletion of the vascular bed. It also results in headaches, nausea, vomiting and euphoria and can have long after effects.

Hydromorphone hydrochloride (Dilaudid)

This is a strong narcotic analgesic (8–10 times the strength of morphine) with a mild sedative effect. It has a fast onset of action and is very long lasting (in hours!). Dilaudid is used more for unusual or excessive pain than as a premedication.

Dose
0.01–0.015 mg/kg given very slowly intravenously (up to a maximum of 2 mg). It can be repeated every 3–4 hours.

Adverse effects
Dilaudid produces vasodilation with resultant hypotension, tachycardia, respiratory depression, and like other opiates it can produce biliary & urinary tract spasm.

Sufentanil citrate (Sufenta)

Sufenta is a very potent narcotic analgesia (5–8 times more potent than fentanyl) with a shorter half-life of action. The effect is longer in neonates.

Dose—sedation
1–2 mcg/kg intravenously and maintained with 0.1–0.3 mcg/kg/hr intravenously.

Dose—anesthetic
When used as the major, deep anesthetic drug, the dose is 10–15 mcg/kg given intravenously over several minutes, while the dose for supplemental maintenance to another anesthetic is 0.1–0.3 mcg/kg/hr.

Adverse effects
Sufenta causes bradycardia, hypotension, nausea and vomiting and causes chest wall rigidity in a small percentage of patients.

Opiate antagonist

The opiate antagonist is a specific and effective antagonist to *opiates*, but is not effective against any other sedatives or depressants.

Naloxone (Narcan)

Narcan is used for the reversal of a *narcotic* effect or overdose. It is very effective at reversing opiates, but has no effect on *other* sedatives/tranquilizers.

Dose
0.1 mg/kg given as an intravenous bolus. The same dose is repeated every 15 minutes (up to three doses) until effective reversal of the opiate is obtained.

Adverse effects
The sudden withdrawal of opiate effect by the effective action of the antagonist can result in hypertension, tachycardia and arrhythmias. The duration of action of narcan is shorter than the duration of the opiate. As a consequence, a rebound opiate narcosis can occur as the effect of the narcan wears off.

Nonopiate sedatives/tranquilizers

Phenothiazine tranquilizers

The phenothiazine group are primarily tranquilizers. They do, however, have some associated sedative effects. Both their anxiolytic and sedative effects are used in the catheterization laboratory as supplements to the analgesics and other sedatives.

Chlorpromazine hydrochloride (Thorazine)

Thorazine is a subcortical psychotropic, sedative and effective antiemetic drug. It is very good at relieving apprehension. In addition to its tranquilizing effect, it intensifies and markedly prolongs the action of narcotics and other sedatives. The dose is reduced when used in conjunction with these. Thorazine also has a strong alpha adrenergic blocking effect which makes it useful in patients where high systemic vascular resistance is a problem.

Dose
0.5–1 mg/kg intravenously or 1 mg/kg intramuscularly. The lower dose is used when thorazine is used in the "DPT cocktail".

Adverse effects
Thorazine causes a central nervous system depression which can result in respiratory depression, cough suppression and severe drowsiness. Occasionally thorazine causes extrapyramidal movements. After intramuscular administration the half-life can be up to 7.5–31 hours in adults and up to 2 days in infants.

The alpha blocking of thorazine results in significant systemic vasodilation and systemic hypotension. Thorazine is *absolutely contraindicated* in patients whose overall circulatory balance is dependent upon a high systemic vascular resistance. For example, patients with "tetralogy of Fallot" and Eisenmenger physiology depend totally upon the systemic resistance and a good systemic blood pressure to perfuse their lungs. A drop in systemic pressure (resistance) in these patients results in a catastrophic drop in pulmonary perfusion with resultant hypoxemia, acidosis, further vasodilation, hypotension and even death. The other patients who should not receive thorazine in their premedication are those with aortic stenosis of any type. These patients already have compromised coronary perfusion. The coronary perfusion is dependent on the systemic diastolic pressure and, in turn, the systemic resistance. A drop in systemic pressure can lead to decreased coronary perfusion and myocardial ischemia in an already compromised myocardium.

Promethazine hydrochloride (Phenergan)

Phenergan is a sedative, antiemetic, antihistaminic (it competes with, but does not block, histamine) and an anticholinergic. It does *not* depress respiration significantly. Phenergan peaks in action in 1.5 hours and lasts 2–3 hours. The half-life of phenergan can be up to 12.5 hours.

Dose
0.5–1 mg/kg given slowly intravenously or *deep* intramuscularly. The lower dose is used when phenergan is used in the "DPT cocktail".

Adverse effects
In addition to over sedation when given in large doses or in particularly sensitive patients, phenergan can cause extrapyramidal reactions. This effect is aggravated by a large dose and in the presence of monamine oxidase

(MAO) inhibitors. Phenergan is a strong local tissue irritant and can cause vasospasm (with pain) and even endothelial necrosis of veins and (especially) arteries when given in superficial vessels.

Demerol–Phenergan–Thorazine (DPT, "lytic cocktail")

Although not an individual medication, the "lytic cocktail" combination of demerol, phenergan and thorazine (DPT) is used so very commonly for both premedication and supplemental sedation during catheterization procedures that the combination is discussed as one medication. The usual "lytic cocktail" is a combination of demerol, phenergan and thorazine in a ratio of 2:1:1 mg/kg, respectively. DPT has a long history of very safe use. The additive effects of the three medications used in the combination allow the use of lower doses of each of the individual drugs which, in turn, decreases the side effects of each medication individually.

Demerol provides analgesia and some sedation. It also disorientates the patient, which actually may contribute to its therapeutic effect in the mixture. Phenergan provides moderate sedation and a strong antihistaminic activity and is a mild, centrally mediated, antiemetic. Although it is a moderate sedative, it does not depress respiration significantly even in combination with demerol. Thorazine has little if any analgesic effect and a very slight sedative effect, but it does provide a strong "tranquilizing" or anxiolytic effect. This effect markedly reduces the need and dose of both the analgesia and/or the sedative by creating an "indifference" to the pain. The DPT combination is popular because of its effectiveness in providing analgesia and "tranquility", which puts the patient to sleep through the sedative and anxiolytic effects without significantly depressing their respiration by the opioid.

The DPT combination is preferably, and usually, used intravenously. Intravenously the effect is almost instantaneous with no cumulative or delayed additional sedative effect. The intramuscular route has the disadvantages of being somewhat painful and being unpredictably longer at taking effect. The intramuscular premedication is given 60 minutes prior to the start of the procedure. The effective sedation from the DPT usually lasts two to three hours.

Although the DPT combination has been used for decades, there is still no commercially available combination of the three drugs, so each catheterization laboratory must mix their own combination of the three drugs, which creates a greater potential for errors in dosage.

Dose—intravenous

Demerol, 1 mg/kg (up to a maximum of 75 mg); Phenergan, 0.5 mg/kg (up to a maximum of 35 mg); Thorazine, 0.5 mg/kg (up to a maximum of 35 mg).

Dose—intramuscular

Demerol, 2 mg/kg (up to a maximum of 75 mg); Phenergan, 1 mg/kg (up to a maximum of 35 mg); Thorazine, 1 mg/kg (up to a maximum of 35 mg).

Dose—supplemental sedation during the procedure

Half of the original intravenous dose is given intravenously or through the catheter.

Adverse effects

The thorazine component of the "cocktail" is absolutely contraindicated in patients whose pulmonary or coronary circulation is dependent upon systemic blood pressure. This effect has been discussed previously in this section on thorazine by itself.

The three drugs are additive in their respiratory depression and sedative effects. Transient "over sedation" resulting in respiratory depression is not uncommon with DPT, particularly when given as a supplement during the catheterization procedure. Usually, gentle, general stimulation of the patient or a few breaths with an Ambu™ bag reverses this respiratory depression.

DPT can have a very long duration of adverse, systemic after effects, with confusion, abnormal behavior, mental debilitation, nausea and vomiting lasting for up to 19 ± 15 hrs, which, therefore, can maintain the effect well into the day following the catheterization. This is more pronounced after intramuscular administration! These effects can last days in infants.

Ketamine (Ketalar)

Ketamine is a phencyclidine that produces a "dissociative" anesthesia. Although it is not an analgesic in the usual sense, it causes a patient to be "dissociated" from pain. It increases sympathomimetic action and, in turn, elevates heart rate and systemic blood pressure. Ketamine in a sedative dose has little effect on pulmonary artery pressure at an altitude at, or close to, sea level. As a consequence, ketamine is useful for the sedation of patients with elevated pulmonary pressures as long as they are not at high altitudes.

Ketamine has a very rapid onset of action and a short duration of action. At doses well below the usual anesthetic doses, it is an extremely effective sedative *without* causing significant respiratory depression. These characteristics make ketamine an ideal preliminary or supplemental sedative in the catheterization laboratory. Ketamine is used either intravenously or intramuscularly and is used in small infants as well as older children up to late adolescence.

Dose—sedation

1 mg/kg intravenously or 2 mg/kg intramuscularly. The dose is repeated in 10–15 minutes as needed.

Adverse effects
Ketamine produces hypertension, tachycardia and, in susceptible patients, myocardial depression. Very rarely, tonic–clonic movements and involuntary muscle spasms, including laryngospasm, occur. Central nervous system reactions, including hallucinations and delirium, occur as long as 18–24 hours after the ketamine is administered.

The hallucinations or delirium on waking are more apparent in patients over 15 years of age. In order to prevent (suppress or outlast) the hallucinations, particularly in older children, ketamine, when used in the catheterization laboratory, is usually "chased" near the very end of the procedure by a longer-acting sedative such as versed or valium.

Benzodiazepines

The benzodiazepines are a group of minor tranquilizers with sedative, hypnotic and anxiolytic effects. These characteristics make them very useful for both premedication and supplemental sedation in the catheterization laboratory.

Midazolam hydrochloride (Versed)

Midazolam is a strong benzodiazepine, which is short acting and water soluble. It has sedative, anxiolytic and amnesic effects. Midazolam is given intravenously, intramuscularly, orally or intranasally, but it is preferentially used intravenously. It has a rapid and dependable onset of action in less than one-and-a-half minutes intravenously while intramuscularly the onset is in 5–15 minutes or even longer. The oral and intranasal routes are more comfortable and do have an advantage in a very apprehensive patient, but the effects are less predictable by these routes.

There is a fairly fast recovery (within 4–6 hours after administration) from the sedative effects, but with persistence of amnesia for the events during the effective period of the drug. Midazolam is an excellent supplement without apparent cumulative effects to most of the other analgesics and sedatives in premedication combinations including morphine, fentanyl, the demerol–phenergan–thorazine cocktail and demerol/phenergan.

Dose—intravenous
In infants & children, 0.05–0.2 mg/kg is titrated intravenously over 2–4 minutes. As an intravenous premedication, it is given 30 minutes before the procedure.

Dose—for continuous sedation
0.06–0.12 mg/kg/hr is given as a continuous infusion administered intravenously or in increments, up to a maximum of 5 mg in adult-sized patients.

Dose—intramuscular
For premedication, 0.07–0.10 mg/kg of versed is given intramuscularly 30–60 minutes prior to the procedure.

Dose—oral
0.2–1 mg/kg (up to a maximum of 20 mg) given 30–45 minutes prior to the procedure.

Dose—intranasal
0.2–0.3 mg/kg.

Adverse effects
Versed can cause hypotension in patients who are stressed and have high circulating levels of catecholamines. Respiratory depression, delayed metabolism and clearance can occur especially in the presence of impaired liver function (for example, severe liver congestion).

Diazepam (Valium)

Valium is a benzodiazepine sedative, anxiolytic, antiepileptic and amnesic similar to versed. The same dose can be administered intravenously, intramuscularly or orally. Given intravenously it has a very rapid onset of action and a moderate duration of activity, with the desired effects lasting for several hours.

Dose—in infants and young children
0.1–0.2 mg/kg is titrated intravenously "for effect" over 2–5 minutes, up to 3 mgs total dose.

Dose—in children over 5 years of age
1 mg is given intravenously every 2–5 minutes up to a total dose of 10 mg. It can be repeated cautiously and with half the dose in 1–3 hours.

Adverse effects
Valium can cause very heavy sedation, respiratory depression, diminished reflexes and hypotension. In larger or cumulative doses, it results in deep sedation to the point of coma.

Valium is a strong *tissue irritant* and must be given directly into a *large* vein. When given through an intravenous line, it is introduced close to the venous puncture site and *not* mixed in the intravenous solution (as it precipitates most intravenous solutions). For the same reason, it is not mixed with other drugs.

Valium is a strong *pulmonary vasoconstrictor*, especially if given directly into pulmonary arteries. *It is not used in patients with known or suspected pulmonary vascular disease.*

Lorazepam (Ativan)

Ativan depresses all levels of the central nervous system. As such, it has a mild sedative, anxiolytic, antiepileptic and strong amnesic effect with minimal respiratory and minimal analgesic effects. Ativan has a slow onset, and a prolonged duration of action. For this reason, it is not a good "in-lab" sedative and is used predominantly for its antiepileptic effect. It can be given orally as well as parenterally.

Dose
0.05–0.1 mg/kg intravenously or intramuscularly and repeated in 15 minutes, times two if necessary. It is effective within 10 to 20 minutes when given intravenously.

Adverse effects
Ativan produces tachycardia, some myocardial depression, hypotension, amnesia, occasional paradoxical excitement, ataxia and chest pain. It has a *long duration* of action in children, with a half-life greater than 14 hours. Unsteadiness is noted for as long as 24 hrs. Ativan has predominantly renal excretion so its action is prolonged in the presence of renal dysfunction.

Benzodiazepine antagonist

Romazicon (Flumazenil)
Flumazenil is a specific antagonist of benzodiazepines. It is used to counter the sedative effects of the benzodiazepine drugs only.

Dose
0.01 mg/kg (up to 0.2 mg total) is given intravenously over 15 seconds. If there is no reversal of the sedation, the same dose is repeated after one minute up to *four more times* or up to 0.05 mg/kg or 1 mg total, whichever dose is lower. The total dose can be repeated after 20 minutes. Romazicon is mixed in 5% glucose or Ringer's lactate.

Adverse effects
The half-life of romazicon is as short as 20 minutes so patients must be observed for *re-sedation* as the romazicon wears off. The major side effect of flumazenil is seizures, which occur primarily in patients who are *chronically dependent* on a benzodiazepine drug.

Chloral hydrate

Chloral hydrate is a sedative and hypnotic but with *no* analgesia effect. It is used occasionally as premedication for cardiac catheterization particularly in extremely anxious, small children. In its sedative dose it has minimal respiratory depression. It is used more often as a sedative for non-invasive procedures.

Dose
75–100 mg/kg orally (PO) or rectally (PR). It is effective in approximately 30 minutes and lasts 1–2 hours.

Adverse effects
Chloral hydrate is unpredictably absorbed, is a gastric irritant, and frequently causes paradoxical agitation, particularly during recovery from the medication. Major cardio-respiratory depression occurs only with significant overdoses or in patients with renal and/or hepatic disease.

Barbiturates

Barbiturates are sedatives with little analgesic effect (they can actually *increase* reaction to pain at subanesthetic doses). The barbiturates have a lower margin of safety for sedation versus respiratory depression than other medications which are now used for primary sedation. The barbiturates are used as adjuncts to general anesthesia and they have an antiepileptic effect, which is discussed later under that category of medication. The barbiturates become addictive with prolonged use.

Pentobarbital sodium (Nembutal)

Nembutal is a sedative with a relatively fast onset of action but it also has a long duration of action (2–4 hours). Nembutal can have a half-life of 25+ hours after intravenous administration. It is effective as an anticonvulsant drug to produce a "nembutal coma" to stop status seizures.

Dose
3–5 mg/kg intramuscularly or intravenously. Intravenously, it is given slowly, working up to the total dose. It is effective in one minute!

Adverse effects
Nembutal causes respiratory depression, coma or hypotension and, at the other extreme, paradoxical excitation and laryngeal spasm.

Thiopental (Pentothal)

Pentothal is a short-acting barbiturate that is used as a sedative or an anesthetic depending upon the dose. It has a rapid onset of action (< 30 seconds) and a short duration of action (< 30 minutes). Pentothal can be administered per rectum in an extremely anxious child.

Dose—sedative
0.5–2 mg/kg is used intravenously for sedation.

Dose—premedication per rectum
For premedication, a dose of 15–30 mg/kg per rectum (PR) is used.

Dose—anesthesia (with respiratory support)
3–5 mg/kg is given as a slow intravenous bolus and followed by repeated 1 mg/kg doses intravenously for maintenance anesthesia.

Adverse effects
Pentothal depresses myocardial function and pooling of venous blood from decreased venous tone, the combination of which can cause hypotension and low cardiac output.

Methohexital sodium (Brevital)

Brevital provides sedation with a very quick onset of action and a short duration of action. It is mostly use for mild, quick sedation as a premedication, especially used rectally when an intravenous route is not available.

Dose
0.25–2 mg/kg intravenously or 15–30 mg/kg per rectum. (Absorption and effectiveness are unpredictable when given rectally.)

Adverse effects
It can cause respiratory depression leading to apnea or seizures, depression of myocardial function and venous pooling.

Phenobarbital (Luminal, Phenobarbitone)

Phenobarbital is a sedative and hypnotic with a slow onset and extremely long duration of action. It is occasionally used to supplement analgesics and other sedatives during catheterization, but its primary use now is as an antiepileptic.

Dose
Hypnotic/sedative: 3–5 mg/kg intravenously or intramuscularly.

Adverse effects
Respiratory depression to point of apnea and bradycardia, which if not treated can lead to cardiac arrest.

General anesthetics

Medications used for deep anesthesia which are *administered by a qualified anesthesiologist* who, in turn, during the anesthesia, also totally manages the patient's respiration.

Intravenous general anesthetics

There are some medications which are classified as intravenous anesthetics only and which are administered only by a qualified anesthesiologist. However, many of the other "intravenous anesthetics" merely consist of larger doses of some of the previously discussed sedatives and analgesics, which are then administered by an anesthesiologist. Since respiration is totally controlled by the anesthesiologist when the patient is receiving general anesthesia, the respiratory depressant effect of the larger doses is of no consequence and, in fact, the intravenous anesthetics are frequently used in conjunction with muscle paralyzers, which totally eliminate any respiratory effort on the part of the patient.

Morphine sulfate

Morphine used in high dose and in conjunction with a muscle paralyzer provides deep general anesthesia without myocardial depression. Patients must be under complete respiratory control with this combination.

Dose—anesthesia
1–3 mg/kg given intravenously as a slow bolus. Maintenance anesthesia with 25–50 mcg/kg/hour of morphine infused intravenously.

Adverse effects
Morphine causes vasodilation, which leads to hypotension. The hypotension is managed readily with volume administration. Morphine produces marked respiratory depression; however, this is of no consequence when it is used as a general anesthetic and where respiration is otherwise totally controlled.

Fentanyl (Sublimaze)

Fentanyl is a very strong synthetic opiate which penetrates the blood–brain barrier very rapidly. In high doses, like morphine, fentanyl produces anesthesia without myocardial depression, but with little, or no, change in hemodynamics.

Dose
10–15 mcg/kg intravenously for induction of anesthesia with a continued infusion of 2–4 mcg/kg/hr.

Adverse effects
There are few or no cardiovascular effects from fentanyl. It causes deep anesthesia and respiratory depression, which is of little consequence when used as a general anesthetic when respiration is controlled totally.

Propofol (Diprivan)

Propofol is a strong sedative with deep hypnotic properties. As such, it provides good intravenous general anesthesia. It has a very short duration of action and a rapid clearance, both of which are desirable characteristics for anesthesia in the catheterization laboratory. It causes minimal respiratory depression, which allows the rapid return of spontaneous respiration as its effects wear off. Propofol produces hypotension in most patients.

Dose—sedation
2–3 mg/kg given as a rapid intravenous bolus and followed by a continuous infusion for maintenance.

Dose—maintenance anesthesia
0.1–0.2 mg/kg/min by intravenous infusion.

Adverse effects
Propofol produces complete apnea in most patients, but this is of no consequence when respiration is controlled by the anesthesiologist. Propofol *decreases systemic vascular resistance* and is a direct myocardial depressant, the combination of which leads to *hypotension*. Volume depletion in the patient exaggerates the hypotension. Supplemental intravenous fluid is almost always administered along with propofol anesthesia. Propofol is a severe tissue irritant causing severe local pain when introduced through a small intravenous site. Seizures or "posturing" of patients occasionally occur with the use of propofol.

Etomidate (Amidate)

Amidate is an ultra-short-acting intravenous general anesthetic, with very rapid onset of action and rapid recovery. It causes *minimal cardiovascular* as well as minimal respiratory depression in spite of producing a very deep level of sedation

Dose—sedation
0.2–0.6 mg/kg as an intravenous bolus given over a few seconds.

Dose—maintenance sedation
5–8 mcg/kg/minute given by intravenous infusion and titrated to the degree of sedation required.

Dose—maintenance anesthesia
10 mcg/kg/minute by intravenous infusion and titrated to the degree of anesthesia required.

Adverse effects
Amidate increases airway reflexes, which can cause laryngeal spasm. It also causes nausea, vomiting, myoclonus and spontaneous muscular movements. It is locally painful unless administered in a large, free-flowing intravenous line.

Ketamine (Ketalar)

Ketamine is a phencyclidine, which produces a "dissociative" anesthesia by direct action on the cerebral cortex. Although it is not an analgesic in the usual sense, it causes a patient to be completely "dissociated" from pain. It increases sympathomimetic action and, in turn, elevates heart rate and systemic blood pressure. At the lower, sedative doses, ketamine has little effect on pulmonary artery pressure at altitudes near to sea level. At higher doses and/or at high altitude, the pulmonary effects are unclear. As a consequence, ketamine is useful for the sedation of patients with elevated pulmonary pressures at sea level but probably should not be used for anesthesia in these patients at high altitudes.

Ketamine has a very rapid onset of action and short duration of action. By itself it produces a deep, extremely effective anesthesia. At "anesthetic" doses, it causes very significant respiratory depression, however, with controlled respiration the respiratory depression is of no consequence. Ketamine is used either intravenously or intramuscularly and is used in small infants as well as in older children up to late adolescence.

Dose—general anesthesia
Only when complete control of ventilation by an anesthesiologist is available: 5–6 mg/kg intravenously or 5–10 mg/kg intramuscularly.

Adverse effects
Ketamine produces hypertension, tachycardia and, in susceptible patients, particularly at the higher anesthesia doses, myocardial depression. Very rarely tonic–clonic movements and involuntary muscle spasms including laryngospasm can occur. The central nervous system reactions including hallucinations can occur as long as 18–24 hours after the ketamine was administered.

Ketamine has a high incidence of postanesthetic hallucinations and deliriums. The hallucinations or deliriums are more *apparent* in children over 15 years of age and all adults. In order to prevent (suppress or outlast) the hallucinations, particularly in older children, when ketamine is used in the catheterization laboratory it is usually "chased" near the very end of the procedure by a longer-acting sedative such as versed or valium.

Barbiturate anesthesia

Barbiturates are potent CNS depressants with marked sedative effects. In large enough doses and with controlled ventilation, barbiturates are occasionally used alone or in combination with a narcotic for very deep sedation/anesthesia for a catheterization procedure. The barbiturates have been supplanted for the most part by the benzodiazepines as adjuncts for premedication and sedation. The more common barbiturates were listed and discussed above under "sedatives", and are not repeated here.

Inhalation anesthetics

All of the inhalation anesthetics are administered by a qualified anesthesiologist/anesthetist who maintains total control of respiration, usually with the anticipation of endotracheal intubation. All inhalation anesthetics used in the catheterization laboratory at the present time are non flammable.

Halothane

A very low inhaled concentration of halothane is required for deep general anesthesia. This allows for very high concentrations of concomitant inhaled oxygen.

Dose
0.5–2.5% of inspired gases administered through an anesthetic machine.

Adverse effects
Halothane causes a moderate depression of myocardial contractility and a decrease in heart rate and is a mild vasodilator. The myocardial depression and vasodilation cause hypotension, which must be anticipated and treated with volume supplement.

Enflurane

Similarly to halothane, a low inhaled concentration of enflurane is required for deep anesthesia. This allows a high concentration of oxygen to be delivered concomitantly.

Dose
0.5–2.5% of inspired gases administered through an anesthetic machine.

Adverse effects
Enflurane causes a moderate depression of myocardial contractility and decreases heart rate and systemic vasodilation. The combination of these effects results in a decreased cardiac output and a decrease in vascular resistance which, in turn, causes hypotension, which, as with halothane, is countered by volume infusion.

Nitrous oxide

Nitrous oxide is an inhalant anesthetic agent which has little or no effect on cardiac function or on vascular resistance. It requires a very high concentration of inhaled gas to achieve *deep* anesthesia, which does not allow concomitant administration of a high percentage of oxygen. Because of that, it is almost always used in combination with an intravenous anesthetic agent or a muscle relaxant.

Dose
50–70% of inspired gases administered through an anesthetic machine!

Adverse effects
Very high concentrations of nitrous oxide are required for deep anesthesia, and these high concentrations limit the amount of oxygen that can be administered concomitantly, which is a serious disadvantage in hypoxemic patients.

Muscle paralyzers (neuromuscular blocking agents, "muscle relaxants")

In the catheterization laboratory, the neuromuscular paralyzers are used primarily for the "total relaxation" of patients during endotracheal intubation and for maintaining them in a "quite", immobile state while they remain intubated.

All neuromuscular paralyzers *must* be used in conjunction with a heavy sedative and/or a tranquilizer. General, and in particular respiratory, paralysis without anesthesia or heavy sedation is a petrifying experience for any patient and represents unacceptably cruel treatment. Deep sedation and the capability of providing complete respiratory support must be available *before beginning* the administration of any of the paralyzing agents. The paralysis rapidly causes hypoxia if respiration is not supported totally. The hypoxia usually results in bradycardia, which can rapidly progress into cardiac arrest. Loss of swallowing reflexes with the paralysis can result in aspiration with any of the muscle paralyzers. Some of the adverse effects of the paralyzers are created from the patient's anxiety when the patient has not been adequately sedated before being given the paralyzer. The hypoxia is treated with vigorous respiratory support and the bradycardia is treated with the administration of atropine.

Succinylcholine

Succinylcholine is the only *depolarizing* muscle paralyzer in clinical use. It has a rapid onset of action and provides a short-acting paralysis. This makes it useful for acute intubation, particularly when it is desirable for the patient to breath on their own shortly after insertion of the endotracheal tube has been completed. The duration is only a few minutes.

Dose—intravenous
1–2 mg/kg infused rapidly. The onset of action is in 30–60 seconds, with a duration of action of 4–6 minutes.

Dose—intramuscular
Twice the intravenous dose is given intramuscularly, i.e. 2–4 mg/kg. The onset of action intramuscularly is in 2–3 minutes, with a duration of action of 10–30 minutes.

Adverse effects
There are ***no*** antagonists or reversal for the effects of the *depolarizing* muscle relaxant. The paralyzing effects must wear off with time while the patient's ventilation is being supported. The paralysis causes hypoxia if respiration is not supported totally. Fortunately, the effect usually lasts only for several minutes. Without adequate respiratory support, succinylcholine results in hypoxia, bradycardia and even death. Bradycardia from succinylcholine is treated by concomitant support of respiration and the administration of atropine. The loss of the swallowing reflexes, which occurs with any of the muscle paralyzers, can result in aspiration.

Succinylcholine can cause an increase in intracranial pressure so it is contraindicated in patients with known or suspected *central nervous system* problems. It may cause hyperkalemia and precipitate cardiac arrest in the presence of neuromuscular diseases, crush or other extensive injuries and is not used in patients with any of these conditions. Succinylcholine is also contraindicated in any patient with any history (patient or family) of malignant *hyperthermia*.

Pancuronium

Pancuronium is a non-depolarizing muscle paralyzer. It has a slower onset and longer duration of action than succinylcholine, and it is used for maintaining muscle paralysis for longer periods of time.

Dose
0.05–0.1 mg/kg intravenously. It is repeated every 30–60 minutes to maintain the paralysis.

Adverse effects
If respiration is not supported, the respiratory paralysis leads to hypoxia, which can eventually cause cardiac arrest. Pancuronium can cause tachycardia and hypertension, but this may be secondary to lack of sufficient concomitant sedation.

Vecuronium

Vecuronium is another non-depolarizing paralyzing agent which is even longer acting. It is useful for the maintenance of paralysis for very long periods of time. Vecuronium, *per se*, does not cause tachycardia.

Dose
0.05–0.1 mg/kg intravenously. The same dose is repeated as needed to maintain paralysis (approximately every hour).

Adverse effects
Hypoxia occurs if respiration is not supported. Vecuronium causes a long persistence of the paralysis, particularly after a long infusion or in patients with renal or hepatic dysfunction.

Atracurium (Tracrium)

Tracrium is a non-depolarizing agent which undergoes spontaneous hydrolytic degradation in the body. As a consequence, it is the paralyzer of choice in patients with renal or hepatic disease.

Dose
0.5 mg/kg intravenously and maintained with an infusion at 2–15 mcg/kg/minute intravenously.

Adverse effects

Hypoxia results if respiration is not supported. Tracrium can cause an *unpredictably long* neuromuscular blockade and paralysis. Occasionally it causes flushing and increased bronchial secretions.

Reversal of non-depolarizing neuromuscular blockade

The following medications are used specifically for the reversal of the paralysis due to a *non-depolarizing* neuromuscular paralyzer.

Neostigmine (Prostigmin)

Neostigmine is a specific reversal/antidote for the non-depolarizing neuromuscular paralyzers.

Dose
0.025–0.1 mg/kg/dose intravenously. It is given in conjunction with 0.015–0.02 mg/kg of atropine, which prevents the side effects of the neostigmine.

Adverse effects
Neostigmine causes nausea, marked salivation, hyperperistalsis, diarrhea, bladder contraction and, rarely, bradycardia.

Edrophonium (Tensilon)

Tensilon is a specific reversal/antidote for the non-depolarizing neuromuscular paralyzers.

Dose
1 mg/kg intravenously given over 10–15 seconds. Atropine 0.015–0.02 mg/kg should be prepared and

ready to administer to counter the adverse effects of the edrophonium.

Adverse effects
Excessive salivation and bronchial secretions, diarrhea, abdominal cramps, ureteral constriction and polyuria.

Antiepileptics

Antiepileptic medications are used in the cardiac catheterization laboratory for the control of seizures. These same medications frequently have other effects and are also listed elsewhere.

Diazepam (Valium)

Valium is an effective antiepileptic as well as a sedative, anxiolytic and amnesic. Because of its rapid onset of action, valium is now the primary drug for the initial treatment of acute seizures in the catheterization laboratory.

Dose—infants and young children
0.05–0.3 mg/kg titrated intravenously for effect over 2–5 minutes, and given up to 5 mg total dose.

Dose—children over 5 years
0.05–0.3 mg/kg intravenously, repeated every 2–5 minutes for effect up to 10 mg total. It can be repeated in 2–4 hours.

Adverse effects
Valium can cause very heavy sedation, diminished reflexes, coma, respiratory depression, myocardial depression and hypotension. It is a strong tissue irritant, so it must be given directly into large veins or through intravenous lines close to the puncture site (at the "needle"). It precipitates with intravenous fluids and many medications, so it should not be mixed with fluids or other drugs in the IV line.

Valium is a strong pulmonary vasoconstrictor, especially if given directly into the pulmonary arteries. It should be avoided in patients with known or suspected pulmonary vascular disease.

Lorazepam (Ativan)

Ativan is a very effective benzodiazepine antiepileptic as well as sedative. It is slower to take effect than valium, but has a long duration of action.

Dose
0.1 mg/kg infused slowly intravenously. It is repeated with a dose of 0.05 mg/kg intravenously in ten minutes if no effects are observed with the initial dose.

Adverse effects
Ativan is a myocardial and central nervous system depressant and can cause hypotension or deep sedation to the point of coma.

Phenobarbital (Luminal, Phenobarbitone)

Phenobarbital is an anticonvulsant as well as sedative. It is fairly rapid in onset in seizure doses and very long acting, so it is also effective as a chronic antiepileptic.

Dose—for seizures
15–20 mg/kg given intravenously as a loading dose. For persistent seizures, an additional 5–10 mg/kg intravenously is repeated in 20 minutes. This dose can be repeated up to a total of 40 mg/kg while monitoring the patient carefully for respiratory depression.

Adverse effects
Bradycardia, hypotension, respiratory depression, paradoxical agitation and hallucinations. Phenobarbital can cause a prolonged "hangover" with somnolescence and irritability.

Diphenylhydantoin (Dilantin, Phenytoin sodium)

Dilantin is a central antiepileptic. It has a fairly slow onset of action and should not be the primary drug for acute seizures in the catheterization laboratory. Dilantin is added when seizures persist after a patient has received valium and/or phenobarbital.

It also has some anti-arrhythmic effect, which is discussed under that category of medication.

Dose
5–10 mg/kg given at rate of 3 mg/kg/min, intravenous loading dose and then continued orally at 2–5 mg/kg/day in 2–4 divided doses per day.

Adverse effects
Dilantin has a very slow build-up (days) until optimal action, so it is not the primary drug to treat acute seizures. It also interacts with innumerable drugs including narcotics, benzodiazepines, barbiturates, steroids and antibiotics. Given chronically, it causes gingival hyperplasia.

Antihistamines

Antihistamines are used in the catheterization laboratory for the prevention and treatment of acute allergic reactions. The most commonly used of the antihistamines also provide some degree of sedation.

Diphenhydramine hydrochloride (Benadryl)

Benadryl is a well established, very effective antihistaminic which also has *sedative* and anticholinergic (drying) effects. It is the first-line medication for acute allergic reactions in the cardiac catheterization laboratory. With its associated sedative effect, benadryl is an excellent supplemental *premedication* for any patient with a history of prior, or even suspected, allergic reactions to contrast materials.

Dose
1–1.5 mg/kg infused intravenously over 1–2 minutes or given *deep* intramuscularly.

Adverse effects
Sleepiness (which can be a *benefit*), CNS depression (or excitability), rare hypotension and thickening of bronchial secretions. It is a destructive, local tissue irritant. Benadryl has an *additive* effect with other CNS depressants.

Adrenocortical steroids

Adrenocortical steroids are used in the cardiac catheterization laboratory for both their anti-inflammatory and anti-allergenic effects. They are used to prevent and treat allergic reactions (including rashes, bronchospastic reactions and anaphylaxis) and to treat local myocardial tissue traumatic injury in the cardiac catheterization laboratory. All steroids mask underlying infections and, in long-term use, can cause sodium retention.

Dexamethasone sodium phosphate (Decadron)

Decadron is a synthetic adrenocortical steroid. It has a rapid onset and long duration (half-life greater than 36 hours) of action. It has a very potent anti-inflammatory and anti-allergic action. With its rapid onset of action, decadron is the most useful steroid for the treatment of acute allergic reactions and acute intracardiac traumatic events (for example acute heart block secondary to catheter manipulation) in the cardiac catheterization laboratory. Decadron is also useful for prophylaxis, even given *on the day* of the procedure, in patients with a newly discovered past history or even suspicion of an allergy to the contrast medium.

Dose—for allergic reactions or myocardial trauma
0.1–0.2 mg/kg intravenously or intramuscularly. The same dose can be repeated in 6 hours for persistence of symptoms.

Dose—for shock
2–6 mg/kg as single intravenous bolus. Continued intravenous infusion of 4 mg/kg/24 hours.

Adverse effects
Adverse effects are rare with acute doses and short-term therapy. The major long-term effects are the masking or aggravation of underlying infections and sodium retention, which can aggravate heart failure.

Hydrocortisone (Solu-Cortef, Hytone, Cortef)

Solu-Cortef is a weak anti-inflammatory, anti-allergenic steroid. It is relatively short acting with a half-life of 8 hours.

Dose
1–5 mg/kg/24 hrs intravenously (divided in two doses).

Adverse effects
Rarely have any adverse effects occurred with acute doses or short-term therapy. Solu-Cortef can cause insomnia and nervousness. Steroids can mask or aggravate infections, and long-term therapy can cause sodium retention, which aggravates heart failure.

Methylprednisolone sodium succinate (Solu-Medrol, Depo-Medrol)

Solu-Medrol is a moderate anti-inflammatory and anti-allergenic steroid. It has an intermediate onset and short duration of action.

Dose—acute
15–30 mg/kg (up to 1 gram) intravenously over 30 minutes.

Dose—maintenance
0.5–1.7 mg/kg/day intravenously divided into 2 or 4 doses per day.

Adverse effects
Insomnia and nervousness can occur with short-term therapy. Long-term use can cause sodium retention.

Prednisone (Deltasone, Meticorten)

Prednisone is an oral corticosteroid for chronic and prophylactic use. It has moderately potent anti-inflammatory and anti-allergic actions with intermediate duration of action (half-life, 24 hrs). Prednisone is used precatheterization for prophylaxis and post-catheterization for follow-up treatment of patients who are *known* to be allergic to or have had a reaction to contrast agents.

It is important in the catheterization laboratory to be aware of patients who have been on long-term, large-dose prednisone therapy in order to supplement the chronic adrenogenic suppression by the steroid with a faster-acting intravenous steroid in the catheterization laboratory.

Dose—oral only
1–2 mg/kg/24 hrs (divided in 4 doses). The prednisone is started *several days* before the scheduled catheterization of a patient with a known or suspected allergy to iodine, or more specifically to contrast agents, when it is anticipated that a contrast agent may have to be used.

Adverse effects
Fluid retention and aggravation of heart failure. Like the other steroids, it can mask underlying infectious processes.

Anti malignant hypertension

Dantrolene sodium (dantrium)

Dantrium is used in the catheterization laboratory exclusively for the treatment or prevention of malignant hyperthermia. Malignant hyperthermia is a dominantly inherited disease and is precipitated when halothane anesthesia or succinylcholine relaxants are used. Malignant hyperthermia is manifest by a rapid increase in and extremely high body temperature associated with tachycardia, tachypnea, cyanosis, acidosis, muscle rigidity and elevation of serum creatine kinase (CK) levels.

Dose—acute
1 mg/kg infused rapidly intravenously, increasing the dose up to 10 mg/kg and continuing the infusion until the reaction subsides. Patients with a past history of malignant hyperthermia are infused with 1 mg/kg of dantrium intravenously prior to the procedure regardless of the intended sedation/anesthesia. The drug is supplied in vials of 20 mg of dantrium in solution with 3000 mg of mannitol, partially buffered with sodium hydroxide to produce a pH of 9.5 when diluted with *60 ml of sterile water*. Other diluents (dextrose, sodium chloride) cause the dantrium to precipitate.

Adverse reactions
Because of its alkalinity, dantrium will necrose tissues if it extravasates from the intravenous line. If exposed to light or mixed with the wrong diluent, it will precipitate out of solution.

Antiemetics

The antiemetics are used primarily to prevent and treat nausea and vomiting following the catheterization procedure. Nausea and vomiting following cardiac catheterization occur primarily as a result of the medications given before or during the catheterization procedure. Antiemetics are often given prophylactically in the catheterization laboratory at the end of the procedure in anticipation of the nausea or vomiting following certain sedatives, anesthetics or analgesics.

Ondansetron hydrochloride (Zofran)

Zofran is a strong antiemetic with a half-life of 3–4 hours. It is administered 30 minutes before the conclusion of the catheterization, particularly in patients who have received DPT, patients who have received general anesthesia and any patient with a history of nausea/vomiting after previous cardiac catheterizations. It is also given prophylactically to patients who have had a device implant which might be dislodged by heavy retching (for example an atrial-septal occluding device in a large defect) before they awaken from sedation/anesthesia.

Dose
0.15 mg/kg (up to 4 mg) intravenously over 1–2 minutes or as an intramuscular injection. It is effective in 5–10 minutes intravenously. Zofran can also be given orally, but is questionably effective by this route in a patient who is likely to vomit before it is absorbed. Increasing the dose, or re-dosing the patient within 3–4 hours has little, or no, beneficial or additional effect.

Adverse effects
Zofran has minimal significant adverse effects, though rare idiosyncratic reactions are reported.

Promethazine hydrochloride (Phenergan)

The phenothiazine phenergan has a moderate antiemetic effect, in addition to its sedative, antihistaminic (competes with histamine, but does not block histamine) and anticholinergic effects. It does *not* depress respiration significantly and has a half-life of up to 12.5 hours.

Dose
0.5–1 mg/kg given as a slow intravenous bolus or *deep* intramuscularly. Presumably, the phenergan in premedication combinations has some persistent antiemetic effect after a procedure.

Adverse effects
In addition to causing over-sedation in large doses and in sensitive patients, phenergan can cause abnormal extrapyramidal movements. These reactions are aggravated by large doses and by the presence of MAO inhibitors. Phenergan is a strong local tissue irritant (vesicant) and can cause vasospasm and endothelial necrosis and thrombosis of veins and (especially) arteries.

Inotropic drugs

The inotropics are used to initiate or stimulate myocardial activity. Depending upon the degree of alpha or beta adrenergic stimulation, the inotropics also affect vascular tone, blood pressure and renal flow. The inotropics are used in conjunction with other medications and mechanisms for improving cardiac function and/or blood pressure.

Phenylephrine hydrochloride (Neo-synephrine)

Neo-synephrine is a potent alpha-adrenergic stimulant with a weak beta adrenergic effect. It causes systemic arterial vasoconstriction, which makes it very useful in the treatment of acute hypotension/shock. The resultant acute increase in *systemic* vascular resistance and *systemic* blood pressure also makes it effective in the treatment of hypoxemic "tetralogy" spells.

Dose—intravenous
5–20 mcg/kg intravenously as a bolus which can be repeated in 10–15 minutes or infused at 10 mcg/kg/minute intravenously until the desired effect.

Dose—subcutaneous (SC) or intramuscular (IM)
When there is no intravenous access, neo-synephrine can be given SC or IM in a dose of 0.1 mg/kg/ up to a total of 5 mg.

Adverse effects
The adverse effects of neo-synephrine are an exaggeration of the desired effects, and the drug can cause undesirable tachyarrhythmias, hypertension with precordial pain, headaches, dizziness or excitability and visceral vasoconstriction with abdominal pain. Locally, it can lead to skin and subcutaneous necrosis and slough of tissue.

Epinephrine (Adrenaline)

Epinephrine is an endogenous catecholamine. It is an alpha, $beta_1$ and $beta_2$ stimulant (adrenergic agonist). Adrenaline is used primarily for the treatment of cardiac arrest and undefined causes of hypotension. Its vasoconstrictor effects are dose dependent. It is also effective in the treatment of bronchospasm and other acute allergic reactions.

Dose—acute intravenous
0.01 mg/kg intravenously (0.1 ml/kg of 1:10,000 solution). For persistent asystole, epinephrine is repeated *with the dose increased* in increments up to 0.1 mg/kg (0.1 ml/kg of 1:1000 solution), i.e. 10 times the original dose!!

Dose—maintenance
0.05–2 mcg/kg/min intravenously.

Dose—acute intratracheal
0.1 mg/kg (or 0.1 ml/kg of a 1:1000 solution).

Adverse effects
Adrenaline causes palpitations, tachycardia, hypertension, irritability, and can precipitate ventricular tachycardia or ventricular fibrillation.

Norepinephrine (Noradrenaline, Levarterenol, Levophed)

Levophed is a very strong alpha adrenergic agonist. It also stimulates $beta_1$ adrenergic receptors. Levophed causes a marked vasoconstriction and an increase in afterload with a resultant increase in blood pressure. The increased peripheral resistance and systemic blood pressure result in a secondary increase in coronary blood flow. It is used to treat very resistant hypotension and shock.

Dose
0.01–1 mcg/kg/min infused intravenously initially. The infusion is continued, increasing the amount up to 2 mcg/kg/min and titrating the dose according to the response.

Adverse effects
The adverse effects are an exaggeration of the desired effects. Initially they include excessive hypertension, bradycardia, headaches and restlessness. More significantly, levophed can result in generalized vascular constriction with significant obstruction of blood flow to vital organs with loss of function (kidneys) or distally resulting in tissue necrosis or even limb loss. This occurs especially in volume depleted patients. Locally, levophed is a vesicant and must be administered through a large, free-flowing intravenous line.

Isoproterenol hydrochloride (Isuprel)

Isuprel is principally a beta adrenergic agonist. It is a particularly good inotropic stimulant *when chronotropic response is limited*. Isuprel is used to accelerate AV node conduction or increase ventricular rate, particularly in the presence of heart block and in transplanted hearts. It acts as a pulmonary vasodilator in some patients, relaxes bronchial smooth muscle and can be used to treat acute bronchospastic conditions in the catheterization laboratory.

Isuprel is used as a test for hypertrophic left heart obstructive lesions. The increase in myocardial contractility combined with the systemic vasodilation results in an exaggeration of the hypertrophic left ventricular outflow tract obstruction.

Dose
0.05–0.2 mcg/kg/min infused intravenously. The isuprel is repeated, increasing the dose for effect up to 1 mcg/kg/min intravenously.

Adverse effects
Isuprel causes sinus tachycardia and can precipitate atrial tachycardias or even ventricular arrhythmias, including ventricular tachycardia and/or fibrillation.

Dopamine

Dopamine stimulates alpha and beta adrenergic receptors. The exact response varies with dose. Dopamine is used for the treatment of decreased cardiac output, hypotension and decreased renal function secondary to hypoperfusion.

Dose—renal
2–4 mcg/kg/min given as a continuous intravenous infusion results in renal arterial dilation. This results in increased renal flow and improved function. There is little chronotropic or arrhythmia effect at this dose.

Dose—inotropic
4–8 mcg/kg/min continuous intravenous infusion results in an inotropic and lusitropic effect.

Dose—vasoconstriction and increased afterload
8–20 mcg/kg/min continuous IV infusion is more of an alpha-1 agonist. At this dose, dopamine results mostly in peripheral vasoconstriction and a resultant increase in afterload. This increases the blood pressure as long as cardiac function is good.

Adverse effects
Dopamine can increases pulmonary vascular resistance, especially in the face of hypoxia. It can also depress respiration. Dopamine is inactivated by alkaline solutions (bicarbonate)!

Dobutamine

Dobutamine produces a good inotropic stimulation and a lusitropic effect. It is effective at treating low cardiac output in association with poor systolic ventricular function by stimulating cardiac $beta_1$ receptors. This increases contractility and heart rate. Dobutamine causes a mild peripheral vasodilation at doses greater than 10 mcg/kg.

Dose
2–20 mcg/kg/min given as a continuous intravenous infusion.

Adverse effects
The primary adverse effect is marked tachycardia.

Milrinone lactate (Primacor)

Milrinone is a bipyridine derivative phosphodiesterase inhibitor that acts as an adrenergic agonist. Milrinone causes significant vasodilation and afterload reduction but it does have some inotropic effect, particularly in a failing heart. It has gained popularity in the intensive care setting but with a very long (several hours) onset of action and long (2–4 hrs) duration of action, it is not useful for the acute management of "pump failure" in the catheterization laboratory. Patients may arrive in the laboratory already on milrinone and it may be added in the lab for continued support after the procedure.

Dose
50 mcg/kg/min given over 10 minutes by continuous infusion pump followed by 0.375–0.75 mcg/kg/min infusion.

Adverse effects
Remarkably few, but hypotension, headaches and arrhythmias can occur.

Amrinone

Amrinone is an earlier bipyridine derivative phosphodiesterase inhibitor. It has a predominately vasodilator effect with only questionable inotropic effect, especially in newborns. The onset of action and duration of action are very long (longer even than for milrinone).

Dose—by continuous infusion pump
Amrinone cannot be mixed with dextrose solutions! Loading dose of 1–3 mg/kg over 30 minutes, followed by an infusion of 5–10 mcg/kg/min.

Adverse effects
Minimal, but can produce hypotension which can be very long lasting. Has been known occasionally to cause thrombocytopenia.

Alpha receptor blockers/antagonists

Alpha receptor blockers are used to counter alpha agonist effects. They are particularly useful for reducing vascular tone and causing peripheral vasodilation.

Phentolamine mesylate (Regitine)

Phentolamine is a powerful systemic vasodilator. It is useful for acutely reducing peripheral resistance or afterload. As an alpha adrenergic blocker, phentolamine is used to block the hypertensive effects of a pheochromocytoma and, in turn, is used for the diagnosis of pheochromocytoma. It is also useful for treating local extravasations of alpha adrenergic stimulants (neosynephrine, levophed, adrenaline) which are developing tissue sloughs.

Dose—for systemic vasodilation
0.05–0.1 mg/kg intravenously, up to 5 mg in a single dose or given as a continuous infusion of 2.5–15 mcg/kg/min.

Dose—for treatment of local extravasations of alpha adrenergic agonists
Phentolamine is used with 5–10 mg diluted in 10 ml of normal saline, and the diluted solution is infiltrated locally into the involved area.

Adverse effects
In excessive doses or in the presence of volume depletion, phentolamine produces hypotension, anginal pain and arrhythmias.

Tolazoline (Priscoline)

Tolazoline is an alpha adrenergic receptor blocker, which reduces catecholamine-induced smooth muscle spasm in vessel walls by transient antagonism of circulating epinephrine and norepinephrine. Tolazoline was principally used as a diagnostic/therapeutic pulmonary arteriolar vasodilator with direct infusion into the pulmonary arteries for pulmonary hypertension in neonates. It has been replaced by nitric oxide in the management of persistent fetal circulation in the newborn.

Dose
1–2 mg/kg intravenously over ten minutes or an infusion of 1–2 mg/kg/hr intravenously.

Adverse effects
Tolazoline can produce hypo or hypertension, bradycardia, arrhythmias and rapid tachyphylaxis. It also stimulates gastric secretions and causes abdominal pain. Because of the unacceptably high incidence of significant adverse effects and the favorable experience with nitric oxide in the diagnosis and treatment of pulmonary hypertension, tolazoline is rarely used any more in the cardiac catheterization laboratory.

Beta adrenergic blockers

Esmolol hydrochloride (Brevibloc)

Esmolol is a very rapid acting, *very short duration*, nonselective beta blocker. It is used in the catheterization laboratory to interrupt hypercyanotic tetralogy spells very rapidly, to acutely relieve dynamic hypertrophic subaortic obstruction and to treat acute hypertension. It is the beta blocker of choice for intravenous use.

Dose
200–500 mcg/kg as an intravenous bolus infused over 1–2 minutes, increasing the dose in increments of 50 mcg/kg/min up to 1 mg/kg/min.

Adverse effects
Esmolol produces bradycardia and hypotension and decreases the cardiac output, all of which are exaggerations of the desired effect. All of the effects of esmolol are very transient and require only time for their resolution.

Propranolol hydrochloride (Inderal)

Inderal is a beta adrenergic blocker which causes a decrease in myocardial contractility, bradycardia and vasodilation. It is used to stop hypercyanotic "tetralogy" spells, to relieve hypertrophic subaortic stenosis and to treat acute and chronic hypertension. Intravenously, inderal *begins* to act in 30 seconds, but can last up to 3–4 hours.

Inderal also functions as a class Ib & class II antiarrhythmic, and will be discussed more under the category of antiarrhythmic drugs. As such, it is useful for the control of both atrial and ventricular arrhythmias.

Dose
0.01–0.02 mg/kg ***very slowly* (*over several minutes!*) *intravenously*** with the patient on continuous ECG and blood pressure monitoring. The dose can be repeated every 10 minutes (each time given *very slowly*) × 4 depending upon effect. Patients to be treated with intravenous inderal are volume loaded with intravenous fluids before receiving the inderal.

Adverse effects
Inderal causes hypotension and bradycardia. The bradycardia can even progress to *asystolic cardiac arrest*, which persists as long as the inderal is circulating. It also causes decreased myocardial contractility and mental confusion, and can aggravate bronchospastic conditions.

Labetalol hydrochloride (Normodyne, Trandate)

Labetalol is an alpha and beta adrenergic blocker with strong vasodilating effects, which make it very effective for the acute treatment of hypertension.

Dose
0.3–1 mg/kg/bolus dose, followed by an infusion of 0.4–1 mg/kg/hr.

Adverse effects
The most prominent adverse effect is exaggeration of the desired effect by excessive lowering of blood pressure. Significant postural hypotension persists for several hours after administration. As with other beta blockers, labetalol aggravates bronchospastic conditions.

Metoprolol (Lopressor)

Lopressor is a beta adrenergic blocker. Although it provides an excellent treatment of acute hypertensive crises in older children, adolescents and adults, lopressor has not been tested sufficiently in small children.

Dose
In *older* children/adolescents, 5 mg of lopressor is administered as an intravenous push. This same dose can be repeated for the desired effect in two minutes and for two subsequent doses.

Adverse effects
Similarly to the other beta blockers, lopressor results in drowsiness and bradycardia. It exacerbates congestive heart failure and causes bronchospasm.

Sotalol (Betapace)

Sotalol is an oral beta adrenergic blocker, which is *not used* in the cardiac catheterization laboratory, but it is a drug which many patients are taking for management of arrhythmias when they arrive in the catheterization laboratory. The effects of the sotalol must be considered during the hemodynamic assessment and when giving the patient other medications.

Dose
Patients are on 80 to 200 mg/kg/day in two or three divided doses (although the maximum dose in adults is 640 mg/day). This dose can slow heart rate or result in hypotension while treating the arrhythmia.

Adverse effects
Sotalol blunts the effects of beta adrenergic drugs. Like the other beta blockers, sotalol can aggravate bronchospastic problems.

Vasodilators

Vasodilators are used as afterload reducers or more specifically as antihypertensive medications. The vasodilators have variable function on different vascular beds. Their primary use is determined by which vascular bed (systemic arteriole, pulmonary arteriole or systemic venous) the particular vasodilator has the most effect on.

Nitroglycerine (Nitrostat)

Nitroglycerine is a pulmonary and systemic vasodilator. It also causes systemic *venous* vasodilation and venous pooling. Nitrostat is a particularly good coronary artery dilator and is particularly useful in pediatric and congenital patients in the case of coronary spasm secondary to catheter manipulations in, or about, a coronary artery. The effect of intravenous nitroglycerine begins within 1–2 minutes and usually disappears within 5–10 minutes.

Dose—intravenous or intra-arterially
1 mcg/kg/min infusion through the cardiac catheter, increasing up to as much as 20 mcg/kg/min for desired effect versus the onset of side effects.

Adverse effects
Nitrostat causes flushing, hypotension, headaches, dizziness and syncope, any of which may last longer than the effective vasodilation effect.

Hydralazine (Apresoline)

Apresoline is a vasodilator with predominant effect on the systemic arterioles. It is a potent systemic vasodilator, but does have some effect on the pulmonary arterioles. It is most useful for afterload reduction in the treatment of hypertension or low cardiac output. It is used for the dilation of pulmonary arterioles to diagnose/treat pulmonary hypertension.

Dose—intravenous
0.1–0.5 mg/kg intravenously up to 20 mg for single intravenous dose. It can be repeated intravenously every four hours.

Dose—oral
0.75–3 mg/kg/24 hours (divided into 3 or 4 doses) for maintenance of its antihypertensive effect after the catheterization procedure.

Adverse effects
Hypotension with dizziness and fatigue. Prolonged high doses cause a lupus erythematosus-like syndrome.

Diazoxide (Hyperstat)

Hyperstat is a benzothiadiazine, which relaxes smooth muscles in systemic arterioles and produces marked peripheral vasodilation very rapidly after intravenous administration. Hyperstat (Diazoxide) is the drug of choice for the emergency management of hypertensive crises.

Dose
1–5 mg/kg intravenously given slowly over 30 minutes up to a maximum of 150 mg/dose. The dose is titrated to the desired level of blood pressure. The same dose may be repeated times two. For a *hypertensive crisis* and in a *supine* patient, it can be given fast as an intravenous push of 5 mg/kg and repeated times 2 or until the desired effect is achieved.

Adverse effects
Diazoxide can produce marked hypotension with shock and decreased cerebral perfusion, particularly in the presence of other antihypertensive medications.

Fenoldopam mesylate (Corlopam)

Corlopam is a dopamine D_1-like agonist and as such is a rapid-acting vasodilator. The vasodilation is dose related when infused intravenously, and with a rapid infusion produces a rapid drop in blood pressure.

Dose
Corlopam is infused *at a constant intravenous infusion* at a rate of between 0.01 and 1.6 **mcg**/kg/min, starting with the lower dose and increasing the infusion rate at intervals of 15 minutes. The solution of corlopam comes as a concentrate of 10 **mg**/ml, which must be diluted in 250 ml of 0.9% sodium chloride for injection per ml of concentrated corlopam. This dilution produces a solution of 40 mcg/ml. Once an acute response has been achieved, the corlopam is usually replaced with an oral antihypertensive agent.

Adverse reactions
Hypotension and tachycardia in proportion to the infused dose is expected and can be controlled by a lower rate of infusion. Hypokalemia has been noted after infusions of as little as 6 hours and should be monitored during long infusions. Glaucoma has been aggravated in patients with known pre-existing increased intraocular pressure, but resolves with the withdrawal of the corlopam.

Nitroprusside sodium (Nitroprusside)

Nitroprusside is a potent smooth-muscle dilator, which acts on the muscles of systemic arteriolar and systemic vein walls as well as pulmonary arteriolar walls. Nitroprusside is used in the treatment of hypertension or low cardiac output. Given directly into the pulmonary artery, it is used to diagnose or treat pulmonary hypertension.

Dose
Continuous intravenous infusion, starting with 0.5 mcg/kg/min and increasing for effect up to 6 mcg/kg/min in neonates (pulmonary hypertension) or 12 mcg/kg/min in children for pulmonary or systemic hypertension. *A solution of nitroprusside must be protected from light, especially while the solution is infusing.*

Adverse effects
Hypotension, palpitations, disorientation, weakness and, in excessive doses, thiocyanate toxicity.

Tolazoline (Priscoline)

Tolazoline is an alpha adrenergic blocking agent, which produces vasodilation by blocking catecholamines and causing vascular smooth muscle relaxation. It is discussed in detail previously under the alpha adrenergic receptor antagonists.

Nitric oxide (NO)

Nitric Oxide is a gaseous, pulmonary vasodilator, which acts directly on the pulmonary endothelium. Inhaled nitric oxide selectively decreases pulmonary vascular resistance and, in turn, pulmonary artery pressure without affecting systemic vascular resistance due to its rapid (one pass) metabolism in the lungs.

Dose
NO is inhaled starting at 40 parts per million (ppm) and increased in 20 ppm increments until effect or 100 ppm are reached. NO is usually given following the inhalation of, or in conjunction with, high concentrations of oxygen.

Adverse effects
NO must be administered to an intubated patient through an inline, closed inhalation–expiration system with specific venting of the exhaust gases. Prolonged use of nitric oxide at higher concentrations can lead to an increase in methemoglobin. The adverse effects of high concentrations usually respond to merely adjusting the NO concentration down slightly.

Prostaglandin E-1 (prostin, alprostadil, PGE_1)

Prostaglandin E1 is a naturally occurring potent dilator of reactive smooth muscle of the ductus arteriosus and is used most often to dilate the ductus arteriosus in neonatal infants. It also has a strong vasodilator effect on pulmonary arterioles and is used in the acute treatment of pulmonary hypertension. It is cleared almost completely from the circulating blood by a single pass through the lungs and, as a consequence, it has a very short half-life in the circulation.

Dose
30–200 ng/kg/min intravenous infusion.

Adverse effects
Prostaglandin can cause apnea, hypotension and fever. A patient who is started on prostaglandin should have the capability for endotrachial intubation and a respirator should be immediately available, or be electively intubated before the infusion.

Epoprostenol (Flolan, Prostacyclin, PGI_2)

Prostacyclin is another naturally occurring and very potent pulmonary and systemic vasodilator, which is used for the treatment of pulmonary hypertension in the presence of pulmonary vascular disease. As opposed to prostaglandin, prostacyclin is metabolized in the liver, so it does have more systemic vasodilation properties. It also has a very short half-life in the circulation.

Dose
Prostacyclin must be administered as a continuous intravenous infusion using a very accurate infusion pump. The starting dose is 1 ng/kg/min, increasing the infusion rate in 2 ng/kg/min increments until adverse effects are reached. Then the infusion dose is reduced by 4 ng/kg/min for the chronic rate.

Adverse effects
Prostacyclin is an equal, or better, systemic vasodilator than prostaglandin. This can result in uncontrollable systemic hypotension, shock, heart failure and multiple lesser symptoms of every body system at doses effective for pulmonary vasodilation.

Because of the increased risk of thromboembolism, combined administration of an anticoagulant is recommended. Prostacyclin is contraindicated in pulmonary veno-occlusive disease and in the presence of severe left ventricular disfunction.

With any abrupt drop in the infused dose of prostacyclin, there can be a severe rebound pulmonary hypertensive crisis with hypoxia and even death.

Cardiac glycosides

Cardiac glycosides increase the force-velocity of myocardial systolic contractions. This effect increases almost proportionate to an increasing dose, up to the therapeutic level, however, with the availability of other inotropes, the glycosides no longer are "pushed" to their maximum dose. The cardiac glycosides also have an arrhythmia effect by slowing sinus node automaticity, slowing atrio ventricular (AV) nodal conduction and prolonging AV node refractoriness.

Digoxin (lanoxin)

Digoxin is the primary cardiac glycoside used in pediatric and congenital heart disease. Digoxin is still occasionally used in the catheterization laboratory for patients with refractory congestive failure or to slow the ventricular response in supraventricular tachycardias. The onset of action of digoxin is slow, even when given intravenously, and the therapeutic dose to toxic dose ratio is very low.

Dose—initial digitalizing
0.01–0.02 mg/kg (10–20 mcg/kg) given slowly intravenously. The Digoxin dose is *not* repeated for 6–8 hours.

Adverse effects
Digoxin can cause high degrees of AV block, supraventricular and ventricular ectopy and even cardiac arrest. Non-cardiac adverse events include nausea, vomiting, confusion and visual changes. The adverse effects are intensified by renal dysfunction, hypokalemia, myocardial inflammation and the drugs quinidine, amiodarone and verapamil in particular.

Anti-arrhythmic medications

There is a huge, and almost daily growing number of "anti-arrhythmic" medications used in pediatric and congenital heart patients. A detailed description of all of these is beyond the scope of even a textbook devoted entirely to arrhythmia management. At the same time there is a select group of anti-arrhythmic medications which are available intravenously and are absolutely essential for the management of acute arrhythmias in the cardiac catheterization laboratory.

Atropine

Atropine is an anticholinergic agent, which blocks acetylcholine at parasympathetic sites. Atropine is used primarily to treat or prevent bradycardia in the catheterization laboratory. It speeds up the heart rate by countering the vagal action of the body or vagal reaction as a result of other medications. Atropine is a drug which must be available immediately in the catheterization laboratory and in the specific dose necessary for the particular patient.

Dose—acute bradycardia
0.02 mg/kg (*minimum* of 0.1 mg and maximum up to 1 mg in children!) as an intravenous bolus. This dose is repeated in 5–10 minutes as needed for persistent bradycardia.

Dose—prophylactic against vagal effect (e.g. intubation, valve dilation)
0.01–0.02 mg/kg intravenously to block the vagal effect caused by the intervention/medication.

Adverse effects
Atropine causes tachycardia, flushing and the sensation of dryness. The effects of atropine wear off rapidly and need no antidote.

Intravenous lidocaine hydrochloride (Intravenous Xylocaine)

Intravenous lidocaine is an IB anti-arrhythmic agent used to prevent and treat acute ventricular ectopy and tachycardias. Lidocaine alters ventricular depolarization and automaticity in Purkinje fibers. It has a rapid onset of action and it is very rapidly metabolized, making repeat infusion necessary for continued effectiveness.

Dose—anti-arrhythmic

1–1.5 mg/kg intravenous bolus (preferably through a catheter directly into the ventricle). The same dose is repeated in 2–5 minutes as needed up to 5 mg/kg. With a very irritable myocardium or recurrent ventricular arrhythmia, a maintenance intravenous infusion of 20–50 mcg/kg/min is started.

Adverse effects

Intravenous lidocaine can cause hypotension and bradycardia as well as vertigo, tremors, confusion and even seizures—especially at high doses.

Adenosine (Adenocard)

Adenosine is a class VI anti-arrhythmic which decreases the sinus node rate and slows or blocks atrioventricular (AV) conduction to the point of a transient (1–5 second) asystole. Adenosine now is the *primary treatment* for supraventricular tachycardia. It has no effect on intra-atrial re-entry, flutter or ventricular tachycardia. The half-life of adenosine is 1–5 *seconds* so it must be given as a very rapid, *central*, intravenous bolus (preferably through a catheter positioned in the heart).

Adenosine is also used electively to *stop* the heart *purposefully* and very temporarily during some interventional procedures (for example during balloon aortic valve dilation and systemic arterial stent implants)!

Dose

0.1–0.2 mg/kg (up to a total of 18 mg) is given as a *rapid* intravenous bolus. It is *given within 1–2 seconds and as centrally as possible*—preferably through a central cardiac catheter in the heart and followed by a push of saline flush.

Adverse effects

Adenosine causes chest discomfort and flushing, and can cause the exacerbation of underlying asthma. Adenosine is completely antagonized by theophylline; a much higher dose is necessary in a patient who is receiving theophylline.

Bretylium tosylate (Bretylol)

Bretylium is a class III anti-arrhythmic drug, which is used for the treatment of ventricular arrhythmias especially ventricular fibrillation. Bretylium is given immediately before, along with, or after electrical defibrillation for ventricular fibrillation. Bretylium is usually used after lidocaine has failed.

Dose

5 mg/kg undiluted is infused intravenously over one minute. If arrhythmia persists, the infusion is repeated with a 10 mg/kg undiluted bolus over one minute. This dose is repeated every 15 minutes up to six times or until the arrhythmia is converted. Its effect is maintained with repeated boluses of 5 mg/kg diluted in normal saline (NS) and given intravenously every six hours.

Adverse effects

Usually, there are minimal overall side effects, but bretylium can cause hypotension, bradycardia, nausea and vomiting. Locally, bretylium is a tissue vesicant and must be given through a catheter or a large, free-flowing intravenous line.

Procainamide hydrochloride (Procamide, Pronestyl)

Procainamide is a class IA anti-arrhythmic, which suppresses normal and abnormal automaticity and is mildly vagolytic. It is used in the catheterization laboratory for treating supraventricular and ventricular tachycardias and in the chemical "conversions" of atrial fibrillation and flutter. Procainamide can aggravate AV block, prolong the Q-T interval and augment the effects of cardiac glycosides.

Dose

10–15 mg/kg intravenous bolus is given at a maximum rate of 0.5 mg/kg/min. The blood pressure is monitored closely for the onset of hypotension—in which case the infusion rate is slowed. For maintenance control of the arrhythmia, a continuous infusion is given intravenously at a rate of 30–80 mcg/kg/min.

Adverse effects

Rapid infusion results in hypotension. High doses depress the myocardial contractility. Procainamide also causes nausea, vomiting, headache, fever, rash, myalgia, insomnia and psychosis. It occasionally causes pancytopenia/agranulocytosis or a lupus erythematosus-like syndrome.

Verapamil hydrochloride (Calan, Isoptin)

Verapamil is a calcium channel blocker. It is a class IV arrhythmic agent. Occasionally it is used in the catheterization laboratory to block or slow AV conduction acutely in the presence of *supraventricular tachycardias*. Verapamil is also a vasodilator, especially of the coronary arteries.

Dose
0.1–0.3 mg/kg bolus pushed intravenously, repeated in 15 minutes up to two times or 5 mg/kg. Maintain with 2.5–5 mcg/kg/min.

Adverse effects
Verapamil causes headaches, dizziness, nausea, vomiting, bradycardia, hypotension and AV block. It has a strong negative inotropic effect in infants. Verapamil shortens the refractory period of aberrant pathways and can accelerate tachycardia through aberrant pathways.

Amiodarone Hydrochloride (Cordarone)

Amiodarone is a class III arrhythmic agent, which prolongs repolarization by inhibiting adrenergic stimulation and prolonging the action potential and refractory period in myocardial tissue. It also prolongs AV conduction and decreases sinus node function.

It has the ability to slow or stop life-threatening tachyarrhythmias such as atrial and junctional ectopic tachycardias, atrial flutter, ventricular tachycardia and fibrillation, which are resistant to other therapies. It is useful especially *in the catheterization laboratory* and the postoperative patient. Amiodarone is contraindicated in patients with significant sinus node disfunction or high degrees of AV block.

Dose
5 mg/kg given intravenously over 15 minutes (up to 150 mg total). This dose can be repeated twice. Amiodarone is maintained at 10–15 mg/kg/day. The initial 5 mg/kg bolus can be repeated for "break-through" tachycardia in addition to ongoing maintenance therapy.

Adverse effects
Amiodarone causes depression of myocardial function and bradycardia, which is atropine resistant, as well as sinus arrest, electromechanical dissociation, hypotension and asystole. Other more chronic adverse effects are ataxia, headache, photophobia, staining of skin and thyroid dysfunction. The pulmonary fibrosis seen in adults has not been reported in children within the recommended doses. The half-life for the elimination of amiodarone is *1–2 months*!

Phenytoin sodium (Dyphenylhydantoin, Dilantin)

In addition to its better known antiepileptic effect, phenytoin is a class IB anti-arrhythmic. Phenytoin prolongs the effective refractory period and suppresses ventricular automaticity in the myocardium. It is used predominately for the control of ventricular arrhythmias, particularly those in postoperative patients and those associated with prolonged Q–T interval, and is seldom used acutely in the catheterization laboratory.

Dose
5–10 mg/kg is given at rate of 3 mg/kg/min as an intravenous loading dose. It is continued orally at 2–5 mg/kg/day in 2–4 divided doses.

Adverse effects
Phenytoin takes days to achieve its optimal action. It also interacts with innumerable drugs including narcotics, benzodiazepines, barbiturates, steroids and antibiotics.

Acutely phenytoin can cause hypotension, bradycardia or cardiovascular collapse, particularly with rapid infusion. With prolonged use it can cause gingival hyperplasia, hypertrichosis and even lupus erythematosus.

Esmolol hydrochloride (Breviblock)

Esmolol is a class II anti-arrhythmic. It is a beta blocker with a very fast onset of action (1–2 minutes) and short duration of action (5–10 minutes). Its arrhythmic effects are slowing of the sinus-cycle length, prolongation of sinus node recovery time and slowing of AV nodal conduction. As an arrhythmic, it is used to slow supraventricular tachycardias and slow the ventricular response to atrial flutter/fibrillation.

Dose
500 mcg/kg intravenous loading dose administered over less than 30 seconds. The loading dose is *repeated and increased* by 50 mcg/kg increments every 3–5 minutes until effect is achieved. The drug loading is followed by a 50–200 mcg/kg/min intravenous infusion for maintenance of effect if necessary.

Adverse effects
Exaggerated bradycardia and/or hypotension. These effects are very short in duration and wear off almost immediately with no additional therapy.

Propranolol hydrochloride (Inderal)

In addition to its hemodynamic effects, propranolol is a class II anti-arrhythmic. It is a potent, but non-selective beta blocker, which has a unique electrophysiologic effect on membrane stabilization similar to that of quinidine. Inderal has a fairly slow onset of action and a medium duration of action, with a half-life of 3.5–6 hours.

Propranolol is used to slow sinus node and AV nodal activity, particularly in the face of very fast atrial tachycardias. It will also suppress ventricular ectopy. Because of its slow onset of action, even slower elimination from the system and potential for severe adverse effects from the slow elimination of propranolol, esmolol has replaced propranolol for most acute indications in the catheterization laboratory.

Dose

0.01–0.05 mg/kg up to a maximum of 10 mg total is given *very slowly* intravenously (over thirty minutes).

Adverse effects

Sinus bradycardia and AV block, which can even lead to irreversible asystole. Myocardial contractility can be depressed leading to an exacerbation of heart failure. Propranolol aggravates bronchospastic conditions. Propranolol is contraindicated in any patient with a significant degree of any of the above conditions.

Sotalol

Sotalol is an oral beta blocker which is used very commonly for refractory atrial and ventricular tachyarrhythmias and although it is *not administered* in the catheterization laboratory, the catheterizing physician must be aware of its use in a patient and familiar with it because of its widespread usage. Sotalol is discussed in more detail in the section on beta blockers.

Anticoagulants/hemostatic controls

Anticoagulants interfere with, or block various steps in the blood clotting cascade and, in turn, interfere with the formation of clots in the blood stream. In the catheterization laboratory, anticoagulants administered intravenously are used to prevent the formation or extension of thrombi/emboli. The anticoagulants have little or no fibrinolytic activity so they do not lyse organized thrombi.

Heparin

Commercial or unfractionated heparin is derived from animal tissues and as such is heterogeneous in molecular size, anticoagulation activity and pharmacokinetic properties. The major anticoagulation effect of heparin is achieved by approximately one-third of the administered heparin, which first must bind with antithrombin III (ATIII). The heparin bound to the ATIII converts it from a slow to a very rapid inhibitor of thrombin, factor X and activated factors IX, XI and XII. Through these actions, heparin is a strong inhibitor of coagulation. However, heparin does *not* bind to thrombin which *is already incorporated into a clot and/or bound to fibrin* so it, *per se*, does *not dissolve* clots. Heparin has an anti factor Xa to anti factor IIa ratio of approximately one to one.

Heparin is used to prevent and to block the extension or progression of thrombi and emboli. In the catheterization laboratory heparin is administered directly to the patient and additional small amounts are added to "flush" and to contrast solutions with the intent of preventing the accumulation of clots on the foreign materials (sheaths, catheters, wires and devices) within the circulation, preventing the development of thrombi in areas of low blood flow or blood stasis and to help prevent the formation of thrombi at the sites of catheter trauma to the tissues including the sites of catheter introduction. Heparin is also used to help prevent the further growth of acute thrombi or thrombotic emboli which have occurred in spite of the heparin prophylaxis.

In the catheterization laboratory, 3 units of heparin are added to *each ml of flush solution* and to *each ml of non-ionic contrast medium*. These extra sources of the drug can add up to a significant amount of additional heparin administered to the patient, particularly when one or more lines/catheters are on a continuous flush or when multiple angiograms are being performed. This extra heparin also needs to be considered when the separately administered heparin is being supplemented during the procedure and when there is a consideration to reverse the heparin at the end of the catheterization.

Dose—added to fluids

3 units of heparin are added to each ml of all flush solutions and to each ml of all non-ionic contrast medium—i.e. 3,000 units of heparin are added to each 1,000 ml container of flush solution and 150 units of heparin are added to each 50 ml bottle of contrast solution.

Dose—prophylaxis

100 units/kg are given intravenously as an acute bolus at the start of a catheterization procedure. An attempt is made to achieve and maintain the blood activated clotting time (ACT) at 275–350 seconds. Depending upon the measurement of the ACT, approximately one half of the initial dose is repeated two hours after the initial dose.

Dose—in the event of a thrombus/embolus

Supplemental heparin is administered in these circumstances to prevent extension and growth of the thrombus/embolus. The same initial heparinizing dose is used for the initial intravenous infusion and then a continuous maintenance dose of 15–25 U/kg/hr is maintained intravenously (or a bolus of 50–100 U/kg intravenously is repeated every four hours). The continuous infusion is monitored with measurement of blood partial thromboplastin time (PTT) and/or ACT.

Adverse effects
Prolonged local bleeding does occur at the vessel entrance sites. This is usually controlled with even longer local pressure and patience. Bleeding internally into any body organ (especially the brain!) can, and rarely does, occur. This more serious complication must always be considered in a patient receiving heparin. Heparin induced thrombocytopenia (HIT) occurs in approximately 6% of patients, particularly with prolonged or repeated therapy.

Acute heparin reversal

Protamine

Protamine, which is a strongly basic compound, binds with the strongly acidic heparin and produces a stable, neutral salt, which has no active anticoagulation effect. Protamine is ***not*** effective *reliably* against the fractionated or low molecular weight heparins (LMWH).

Dose
A 0.25–0.5 mg intravenous *test dose* is given initially to test for allergy/unusual sensitivity. After 3–5 minutes of no reaction (hypotension, bradycardia), 1.0 mg of protamine is give intravenously for every 100 U of heparin previously administered. The protamine dose is cut in half for each intervening half-hour since the most recent dose of heparin was given.

Adverse effects
Rare sensitivity reactions to the protamine include acute, severe bradycardia and hypotension. Protamine by itself without the heparin to react with is itself an anticoagulant.

Low molecular weight heparins (LMWHs)

Low molecular weight heparins (LMWHs) have gained popularity for chronic anticoagulation, but ***not*** yet for acute or routine use *in the catheterization laboratory*. LMWHs are depolymerized (fractionated) heparin compounds with a molecular weight of approximately 1/3 of standard unfractionated heparin. Like unfractionated heparin, the LMWHs act by combining with antithrombin III. The LMWHs act primarily by the inactivation of factor Xa, but they have a longer half-life than unfractionated heparin.

The LMWHs are most useful for maintaining long-term anticoagulation for the *prevention* of thrombotic/embolic complications in high-risk situations. The long half-life of their activity allows them to be given subcutaneously twice a day (and occasionally even once a day) without the need for the careful blood coagulation monitoring required with heparin or coumadin. This appears to be the only advantage over conventional unfractionated heparin. Like unfractionated heparin, the LMWHs have *no* fibrinolytic activity and, as a consequence, do *not* lyse pre-existing thrombi.

The activated partial thromboplastin time (aPTT) and the celite-activated clotting time (ACT) are ***not*** useful for monitoring activity of the LMWHs. The Heptest™ is useful at predicting *gross* over and under dosing with the LMWHs. In general, unless the patient has an underlying debilitating condition (chronic lung, renal, liver or end-stage heart disease), an empirical, per kilogram dose of each of the LMWHs is used. Even with an empiric regimen, when adjusted for body weight, the LMWHs are relatively safe compared the unfractionated heparin.

There are now many varieties of the LMWHs from many different manufacturers. Each manufacturer has a different method of fractionation, and, as a consequence, the LMWHs are even more heterogeneous than unfractionated heparin. Each LMWH has its specific characteristics and dose so that they cannot be considered as a homogeneous group and are *not* interchangeable during use in an individual patient. All of the LMWHs do have a cross antigenicity with unfractionated heparin so they also are capable of causing heparin-induced thrombocytopenia.

Many patients now present for catheterization having been on maintenance LMWH for weeks or months. The LMWH should be discontinued 24–36 hours before the catheterization procedure. Only a few of the many LMWHs are listed here.

Enoxaparin (Clexane, Lovenox)

Enoxaparin is a commercially available LMWH with a molecular weight of approximately 4,400 and an anti factor Xa to anti factor IIa activity ratio of 3:1.

Dose
1 mg/kg intravenous bolus or 1 mg/kg deep subcutaneously followed by 1 mg/kg deep subcutaneously every 12 hours.

Adverse events
Hemorrhage into any organ system (rare at this dose). In a very low percentage of patients, enoxaparin can cause heparin-induced thrombocytopenia.

Dalteparin (Fragmin)

Fragmin is another commercially available LMWH, with a molecular weight of approximately 5,800 and an anti factor Xa to anti factor IIa activity ratio of 2:1. Fragmin has not been used in the catheterization laboratory. It only has been used to maintain the anticoagulation state chronically after a procedure.

Dose
120 IU/kg given subcutaneously *twice a day*.

Adverse events
Hemorrhage into any organ system (rare at this dose). In a very low percentage of patients, fragmin also causes heparin-induced thrombocytopenia.

Innohep (Tinzaparin sodium)

Innohep is a LMWH that has been used extensively in the prevention and treatment of deep venous thrombosis.

Dose
175 U/kg subcutaneously (it is used *only* SC). Concomitant treatment with oral coumadin is usually initiated within several days of starting the innohep.

Adverse events
Hemorrhage into any organ system (rare at this dose). In a very low percentage of patients, innohep also causes heparin-induced thrombocytopenia.

Ardeparin (Normiflo)

Ardeparin is a LMWH with a molecular weight of approximately 6,000 and an anti factor Xa to anti factor IIa activity ratio of approximately 2:1. Like the other LMWHs, ardeparin has been mostly used for the *prevention/treatment of deep venous thrombosis* and is not used acutely in the catheterization laboratory.

Dose
50 anti Xa U/kg subcutaneously twice a day.

Adverse events
Hemorrhage into any organ system (rare at this dose). In a very low percentage of patients, ardeparin can cause heparin-induced thrombocytopenia.

Warfarin sodium (Coumadin) anticoagulation

Coumadin is an anticoagulant that is ***not*** used ***in*** the catheterization laboratory, but because of its frequent use in congenital heart patients who have had and/or are at high risk of thromboembolism, it is a drug with which any physician performing cardiac catheterization procedures must be very familiar. Coumadin is used prophylactically to maintain *chronic* anticoagulation in patients at high risk of spontaneous thrombi and chronically *after* a catheterization when there has been a problem with thrombosis/embolization during the procedure.

Coumadin acts *indirectly* on the clotting mechanism by interfering with the production of vitamin K in the liver. Vitamin K is an essential catalyst in the normal clotting cascade. The first measurable effects of coumadin occur in 8–12 hours, with the peak effect in *5–7 days* after it is administered. The half-life for the blood level is *42 hours*! When patients have received coumadin even days prior to the catheterization, it can still be active and, as a consequence, it potentially can have a disastrous effect on hemostasis during the catheterization if not taken into account. This long duration of action of coumadin must be considered and coumadin therapy stopped 2–4 *days* before an *elective* catheterization. Exactly how long before the catheterization the coumadin should be stopped depends upon each individual patient, their last PT/INR and the urgency of the catheterization. It is not totally unreasonable to begin a catheterization with a PT of 15–16 seconds or an INR of 1.5–2 on the morning of the procedure when the procedure is necessary either medically and/or logistically.

Vitamin K should not be used to reverse the action of coumadin *except* during an extreme, active bleeding, life or organ threatening emergency. The administration of vitamin K results in an acute cessation of the anticoagulation effect of coumadin and, in turn, results in an immediate, *hypercoagulable* state.

Dose
0.2 mg/kg up to 10 mg total loading dose orally (PO). The coumadin dose is adjusted according to the prothrombin time (PT) and INR measurements. Maintenance doses can vary between 1 and 20 mg/day and are adjusted according to PT and INR with the goal of keeping them between 17 and 20 seconds and 2.5 and 3, respectively. Slightly higher levels of PT and INR (20+ and 3–3.5, respectively) are maintained in patients with mitral valve prostheses.

Adverse effects
Prolonged local bleeding at the catheterization site and the possibility of internal bleeding at the site of any internal vessel/organ damage.

Acute coumadin reversal

Phytonadione (Mephyton, Aqua-mephyton, Vitamin K)

In most circumstances the anticoagulant effects of coumadin are allowed to reverse themselves with time. The blocking of the production of vitamin K, and in turn the effects of the coumadin can be overcome by the direct administration of vitamin K. Vitamin K reverses the anticoagulation effect of coumadin totally and within 1–2 hours. Vitamin K is used only in the circumstance of acute, life or organ threatening bleeding due to coumadin overdose or acute, emergent injury/surgery while on coumadin. Once vitamin K has been administered, re-administered coumadin is not effective for *days* (until the vitamin K has been metabolized).

Dose
1 mg, *very slowly* intravenously. For reversal of catastrophic bleeding: 1 mg intravenously, increasing cautiously up to 10 mg total dose intravenously. Vitamin K can be administered subcutaneously as well as intravenously.

Adverse effects
Vitamin K given intravenously can cause anaphylaxis. Acute "rebound" thrombosis can occur as a consequence of the sudden cessation of the warfarin anticoagulation effect!

Direct antithrombins (Hirudins)

Recombinant hirudins are polypeptides obtained from leech salivary glands. Hirudin is a *direct thrombin* blocking agent and, unlike the heparins, has the potential to combine with *thrombin bound to clot* and/or *clot degradation products*. This specific thrombin inhibition has a dramatic inhibitory effect on platelet aggregation and fibrinogen deposition during the *growth* of mural thrombus. Hirudins also have a strong affinity for platelet thrombin receptors and can displace thrombin bound to platelet receptors.

Because of their direct action on thrombin in all locations, hirudins actually seem to be more effective than heparin in preventing the further growth of thrombus on pre-existing thrombi and in preventing re-thrombosis following thrombolytic therapy. Hirudins do not cause significant hemorrhagic side effects when used in their effective antithrombotic doses.

Recombinant hirudins do not induce platelet aggregation and, in turn, do not cause heparin-induced thrombocytopenia (HIT). Hirudins are now recommended in the treatment of HIT and in disseminated intravascular coagulation (DIC).

Lepirudin (Refludan)

Lepirudin is a recombinant hirudin which has no cross reactivity with heparin antibodies. Lepirudin is FDA approved and used for anticoagulation instead of heparin in patients with active, and/or a prior history of, heparin-induced thrombocytopenia. Lepirudin is predominately excreted through the kidneys and dosages are reduced in patients with renal impairment. Lepirudin is itself antigenic. The antibodies to lepirudin actually *enhance* its potency, requiring a *lower* dosage in the face of an antigenic response. The anticoagulant effect can be controlled, approximately, by maintaining the aPTT at 1.5–3 times normal.

Dose—intravenous
0.4 mg/kg bolus followed by 0.15 mg/kg/hr intravenously.

Dose—subcutaneous
0.2 mg/kg intravenously and then 0.5 mg/kg subcutaneously bid.

Adverse effects
Overdose of any hirudin can result in local or systemic organ system bleeding.

Bivalirudin (Angiomax)

Bivalirudin is a commercially available, synthetic peptide derivative of hirudin. Bivalirudin has FDA approval for use in coronary angioplasty. It is as effective as high-dose heparin with repeatedly demonstrated lower risks of bleeding. It has been used mostly in conjunction with thrombolytics to prevent re-thrombosis. Bivalirudin has no cross reactivity with heparin antibodies. Bivalirudin earlier underwent clinical studies under the name of "Hirulog".

Dose—intravenous
1 mg/kg intravenous bolus followed by a 2.5 mg/kg/hr intravenous infusion. When used concomitantly with a platelet glycoprotein inhibitor (see later in this chapter), the dose is lowered to an initial bolus of 0.75 mg/kg and followed with an infusion of 1.75 mg/kg/hr.

Dose—subcutaneous
0.6 mg/kg subcutaneously every 8 hours with monitoring of the aPTT 2 hours after administration of the bivalirudin—the goal is to have the aPTT no more than 1.5 times the control value.

Adverse effects
Adverse effects are rare. An overdose of any hirudin can result in systemic or local bleeding. Bivalirudin is *not* specifically *approved* for the treatment of HIT.

Argatroban (Novostan)

Argatroban is a synthetic direct thrombin inhibitor, which is metabolized primarily in the liver. This makes it a very useful thrombin inhibitor in patients with renal dysfunction. Argatroban has no reported cross reactivity with heparin, so it is useful in patients with HIT. It has a short half-life and is associated with rebound thrombosis if it is discontinued acutely. Argatroban has FDA approval.

Dose
0.125 mg/kg bolus infusion followed by a 0.2–0.3 mg/kg/hr infusion. The argatroban should be tapered very slowly when it is to be discontinued.

Adverse effects
Adverse effects are similar to the bleeding complications of the hirudins, where an overdose can result in systemic or local bleeding. Argatroban appears to have a greater propensity for thrombotic rebound when it is withdrawn.

Anti platelet aggregating drugs

Anti platelet aggregating drugs block the aggregation of platelets during the initiation of the clotting process. The anti platelet aggregating drugs do *not* inhibit the *continued growth* of thrombus on an already formed thrombus, since platelet aggregation no longer is involved with the process at that stage of thrombus formation. The anti platelet aggregating drugs are gaining an increasing use in adult interventional cardiology for the *prevention* of thrombosis on implanted devices. There has been extensive experience with the platelet-blocking drugs in the coronary occlusion and coronary interventional arena. Some of this experience may be applicable in certain congenital heart patients undergoing cardiac catheterization and, in particular, interventional catheterizations where intravascular devices are being implanted.

There are at least three "groups" of anti platelet drugs, which appear to block at different levels of platelet activity in the clotting cascade. There are the drugs which block the arachidonic acid-induced platelet aggregation, those which block the adenosine diphosphate (ADP)-induced platelet aggregation, and those which block the final platelet glycoprotein GP IIb/IIIa pathway of aggregation.

Blockage of platelet aggregation by inhibition of platelet and endothelial cyclo-oxygenase

Aspirin (Acetylsalicylic acid, ASA)

Aspirin is *not* used *in the catheterization laboratory*, but rather as prophylaxis against clotting before and after the procedure in patients at high risk for thrombus formation. Superficial endothelial injury exposes the circulating platelets in the blood to several factors, including collagen, which, in turn, stimulates the platelet aggregation. Circulating aspirin selectively inhibits the platelet cyclo-oxygenase stimulated platelet aggregation. The aspirin effect on blocking platelet aggregation is time dependent, reaching a maximum effect at about six hours, but lasts for the "life" of the affected platelets. Aspirin also has an effect on blocking the deposition of fibrin, which is not time dependent and apparently is separate from the effect on the platelets. The anti platelet aggregating effect of aspirin has been shown to be complementary and additive in effect to other platelet aggregating drugs as well as to other anticoagulants.

Dose
1–4 mg/kg *orally* once a day. In a patient at high risk for thrombus formation and/or a patient who is to undergo a device implant, aspirin electively is started one to two days (or a minimum of 6 hours) before the anticipated procedure. A maintenance dose of 1–4 mg/kg/day is continued for six months following a device implant and indefinitely in the patient who otherwise is at high risk for spontaneous thrombi.

Adverse effects
A very small increase in the tendency to bleeding/bruising. Gastrointestinal irritation due to aspirin ingestion occurs very rarely at this dose. Also, there are very rare allergies to aspirin.

Blockage of adenosine diphosphate (ADP)-induced platelet aggregation

Several thienopyridine derivative drugs are very strong blockers of ADP-induced platelet aggregation. The blocking of ADP-induced aggregation is complementary to, and additive with, aspirin blocking of the collagen-induced aggregation of the platelets. The thienopyridine drugs have been used for their platelet-blocking capacity to prevent acute occlusion or re-occlusion of vessels in several large adult coronary studies.

There is now interest in these drugs for the prevention of thrombosis on implanted devices in congenital heart patients, particularly in older patients and those at high risk for spontaneous thromboembolic phenomena. Of the two medications used in the largest trials, the original thienopyridine, ticlopidine, had a significantly larger number of, *and more serious*, side effects (especially *lethal* neutropenia and thrombotic thrombocytopenia purpura). As a consequence, ticlopidine has been replaced clinically almost completely by the less toxic and, apparently, even more effective thienopyridine clopidogrel.

Clopidogrel (Plavix)

Clopidogrel inhibits the binding of ADP to its platelet receptors and, in turn, blocks platelet aggregation. Clopidogrel can be used concurrently with heparin and in patients who have undergone thrombolysis.

Dose
An *oral* loading dose of 4 mg/kg is given prophylactically before the catheterization procedure or is begun

immediately after implant of a device. Clopidogrel is continued at a dose of 1 mg/kg/day orally for four weeks following the implant. Clopidogrel is more effective than, and is usually used in conjunction with, aspirin (as described above). The *combination* of aspirin and clopidogrel has an onset of significant action within approximately 90 minutes, with a maximum effect after six hours after the oral doses. Clopidogrel *alone* has a significantly longer onset of action.

Adverse effects

The appearance of a significant rash and/or diarrhea has occurred in a very small number of patients. There has been a 0.02% incidence of agranulocytosis reported in patients on clopidogrel, so these patients do require hematological monitoring while on the drug. Otherwise the complications are similar, but usually milder and to a lesser degree, than those of the other anticoagulants. Bleeding usually is milder and superficial.

Platelet glycoprotein IIb/IIIa (GP IIb/IIIa) inhibitors

The platelet glycoprotein GP IIb/IIIa inhibitors are a third, even more potent, group of inhibitors of platelet aggregation. The GP IIb/IIIa inhibitors block the final pathway leading to platelet aggregation. Three different GP IIb/IIIa inhibitors have undergone extensive adult clinical trials and have received FDA approval as adjuncts to inhibit thrombosis during interventions in the cardiac catheterization laboratory. All three of these medications are administered intravenously in the catheterization laboratory. They can be used *in conjunction with* aspirin, heparin, and thrombolytic therapy. When used in combination with heparin during the procedure, the heparin dose is reduced.

The GP IIb/IIIa inhibitors have not been used in the pediatric/congenital population, but have very appealing features for those patients who are at high risk for thrombi and embolization from these thrombi.

Tirofiban (Aggrastat)

Aggrastat is a non-peptide tyrosine derivative, GP IIb/IIIa inhibitor of platelet aggregation.

Dose

4 mcg/kg intravenous bolus of tirofiban over 30 minutes followed by 0.1 mcg/kg/min infusion for up to 24 hours. The tirofiban is administered along with a bolus of 50 U/kg of heparin.

Adverse effects

Local bleeding at the catheter introduction site is the most common complication and may be more related to the concomitant heparin therapy. There has been a very low incidence of significant thrombocytopenia. As a consequence, these patients require hematological monitoring for at least a week after they last receive aggrastat.

Eptifibatide (Integrilin)

Integrilin is a cyclic heptapeptide GP IIb/IIIa inhibitor of platelet aggregation.

Dose

An initial 180 mcg/kg stat bolus of integrilin followed by 2 mcg/kg/min for up to 24 hours. The integrilin is administered along with a bolus of 70 U/kg of heparin.

Adverse effects

As with tirofiban, local bleeding is the only commonly occurring complication. There has been a very low incidence of thrombocytopenia. As a consequence, patients receiving tirofiban require hematological monitoring for at least a week after they last receive integrilin.

Abciximab (Reopro, Centocor)

Reopro is a chimeric monoclonal antibody GP IIb/IIIa inhibitor of platelet aggregation.

Dose

An initial 0.25 mg/kg intravenous bolus followed by 10 mcg/kg/min intravenous infusion for 12 or more hours. The reopro is administered along with a bolus of 70 U/kg of heparin.

Adverse effects

Severe delayed thrombocytopenia, which is more than an exaggeration of the expected effect. Patients who have received reopro should have a scheduled platelet count one week following the initiation of therapy and weekly as long as the drug is continued.

Thrombolytics

Thrombolytics are used to break up and/or dissolve emboli and thrombi that have already formed. They act by converting plasminogen to plasmin which, in turn, degrades the fibrin within a formed clot. Since the thrombolytics cause fibrinolysis at *all* sites of fibrin deposition, all of the thrombolytics have the potential to cause unwanted bleeding, particularly at vascular entry sites and in internal organs where there has been recent tissue trauma. One difference between the currently available thrombolytic drugs is their decreased effect on free circulation plasminogen versus their selectivity for the plasminogen primarily in clots. The later, or "second generation" thrombolytics are more clot specific and cause less generalized or systemic lysis (and bleeding).

All of the thrombolytics appear to be more effective if administered through a catheter directly into, or immediately proximal in the blood flow to, the embolus/thrombus, but they all have some effect when given intravenously from a more peripheral site. The thrombolytics are very effective in recent thrombi/emboli, with their beneficial effects decreasing the older the thrombi are. The thrombolytics have *very little* anticoagulation (preventive) effect and are used in conjunction with parenteral heparin (or hirudin) *and* an anti platelet aggregating drug to prevent re-formation/re-accumulation of the thrombus.

In pediatric and congenital heart patients thrombolytics are used for treating thrombi/emboli in central and peripheral arteries, in central and peripheral systemic venous channels, in cardiac chambers and on prosthetic valves.

First generation thrombolytics

These thrombolytics activate free circulating plasminogen equally as well as plasminogen associated with fibrin in clots.

Streptokinase (Streptase)

Streptokinase is a thrombolytic agent which activates plasminogen to plasmin, and in doing so degrades and liquefies thrombi both from within and from outside of the embolus/thrombus. Streptokinase has been clinically available and has had extensive use for over two decades.

Dose—directly into lesion
50–2,000 U/kg infused over 30 minutes through a catheter directly into the thrombus/vessel followed by a 2,000 U/kg/hr infusion.

Dose—peripheral intravenous
2,500–4,000 U/kg (up to 1.5 million units) administered into a peripheral intravenous line over 30–60 minutes, followed by a continuous intravenous infusion of 1,000–1,500 U/kg/hr until the resolution of the thrombus.

Adverse effects
Streptokinase causes local bleeding at puncture and recent surgical sites, and since it is *not* "clot selective" can cause internal bleeding into any organ system. It can cause hypotension, particularly with rapid infusion.

Because streptokinase is a bacterial protein, it can cause allergic reactions (including anaphylaxis) especially following recent streptococcal infections or with repeated use. If the streptokinase is used for more than 24 hours, monitoring of the fibrinogen and fibrinogen biproduct levels may be useful in preventing unwanted bleeding.

Anistreplase (Apsac, Acylated plasminogen–streptokinase-activator complex)

Anistreplase is a chemically synthesized, thrombolytic combination of streptokinase and lys-plasminogen which was custom designed to overcome the perceived disadvantages of streptokinase. It can be injected *more rapidly* without causing hypotension, it binds semi-selectively to fibrin, where it is activated gradually and continuously, and it has a much longer half-life of activity than the other thrombolytics.

Dose
0.5 U/kg intravenously over 3–5 minutes.

Adverse effects
Unwanted bleeding similar to that induced by the other thrombolytics. No anaphylaxis has occurred. Anistreplase is approximately 10 times more expensive than streptokinase.

Second generation clot-specific thrombolytics

These thrombolytics preferentially activate the plasminogen *bound* in the fibrin and, as a consequence, have less of a generalized or "circulating" thrombolytic effect.

Activase (Alteplase, T-Pa)

Alteplase or tissue plasminogen activator (t-PA) acts by the activation of plasminogen *which is bound to fibrin* into plasmin which, in turn, acts to dissolve the fibrin in the thrombus. Because it is more "clot selective" than the first generation thrombolytics, t-PA is more effective for dissolving established thrombi, and produces less systemic bleeding. The half-life of alteplase is between 3 and 9 minutes, so it must be infused continuously to achieve a continuing effect. At the same time alteplase does not prevent thrombi, so the dose of alteplase is followed by an infusion of an anticoagulant for at least 12–24 hours to prevent re-thrombosis.

Dose
0.2 mg/kg bolus intravenously or (preferably) through a catheter proximal to the site of the thrombus, followed by 0.5 mg/kg/hour intravenous infusion over the next 120 minutes (up to 50 mg total dose). If the thrombus has

not resolved after two hours, the bolus and the infusion are repeated up to two more times. Alteplase is given to a patient receiving heparin or on aspirin or other antiplatelet drugs to prevent re-thrombosis.

Adverse effects
Like the other systemic thrombolytics, t-PA causes local or systemic bleeding. Alteplase is also very expensive—it costs more than *ten times* as much as streptokinase.

Thrombolytic reversal

The thrombolytics are relatively short lived, however, in the event of an acute life-threatening hemorrhage (intracranial), acute reversal of the thrombolytic effect is attempted by using an infusion of plasma and cryoprecipitate.

Fresh frosen plasma (FFP)

FFP is utilized to replace clotting factors in patients who have known clotting deficits or extensive, continuing bleeding following thrombolytic therapy. FFP also serves as intravascular volume replacement.

Dose
10–15 ml/kg given intravenously over 30 minutes.

Adverse effects
Excess volume expansion and aggravation of myocardial failure may occur once the concomitant blood loss has stopped. FFP is a blood product with the potential for the transmission of blood-borne infections.

Diuretics

Acute intravenously-administered diuretics are utilized in the catheterization laboratory to treat acute or threatened circulating volume overload in either the pulmonary or systemic vascular bed. The volume overload may be generalized owing to progression of the patient's underlying failing myocardium, and/or iatrogenic owing to extra fluid received through flush solutions, contrast agents and purposefully administered extra volume. Very localized fluid overload occurs owing to sudden shifts in fluid volume as a consequence of the relief of a severe intravascular obstruction (an obstructed branch pulmonary artery) or, just the opposite, the creation of an intravascular obstruction (acute closure of a large atrial septal defect).

Furosemide (Lasix)

Lasix is a very rapid acting loop diuretic. Because of its rapid onset of action, lasix is extremely useful in the catheterization laboratory for the treatment of acute volume overload and pulmonary edema.

Dose
1–2 mg/kg given slowly intravenously or through an intravascular catheter. The same dose can be repeated within several hours.

Adverse effects
Lasix causes an acute volume depletion and, when the administration is repeated, eventually hyponatremia and hypokalemia.

Ethacrynic acid (Edecrin)

Edecrin has similar effects and indications to furosemide.

Dose
1–2 mg/kg given very slowly intravenously. It is given only as a single dose intravenously.

Adverse effects
Acutely, edecrin can cause hyponatremia and volume depletion. Rapid and/or repeated intravenous boluses cause tinnitus, vertigo and even permanent deafness.

Bumetanide (Bumex)

Bumex is a loop diuretic which inhibits reabsorption of sodium and chloride in the ascending loops in the kidney. It is useful as a diuretic and/or antihypertensive in patients who cannot tolerate furosemide.

Dose
0.015–0.1 mg/kg/dose given intravenously. The dose can be repeated in 6–8 hours.

Adverse effects
Commercial preparation contains bisulfite and may cause allergic reaction in patients allergic to sulfides. It is a strong vesicant so must be delivered in a large, free-flowing intravenous line. As with other diuretics, it can cause hypovolemia, hyponatremia and hypokalemia.

Dyrenium (Triamterene)

Dyrenium is an old, fairly potent, potassium-sparing diuretic, but it is not available parentally so is not used in the catheterization laboratory. It is important, however, for the catheterizing physician to be aware of its possible use in a patient before the patient arrives in the catheterization laboratory, because of the resultant high serum potassium levels which often are created in patients who are receiving dyrenium.

Dose
1 mg/kg administered once or twice a day is the usual dose.

Adverse effects
With prolonged use and as the only diuretic being used, significant hyperkalemia develops.

Spironolactone (Aldactone)

Spironolactone is another potassium-sparing diuretic which is only available in an oral form. Spironolactone is a very weak diuretic, however, it does cause potassium retention very effectively and has a very long duration of action. Spironolactone is often used in conjunction with other more effective "loop" diuretics to counter their potassium losing effects. Spironolactone is not used in the catheterization laboratory, but its potassium-retaining effects persist for days (weeks!) in patients who were receiving it before the catheterization.

Dose
0.5–1 mg/kg/24 hours is the usual dose. The half-life of spironolactone is greater than 48 hours, so administering it any more often than *once a day* is totally unnecessary for it to be effective.

Adverse effects
Alone, spironolactone is not an effective diuretic. An exaggeration of its potassium-sparing effect can result in hyperkalemia.

Intravenous fluids and blood volume expanders

Electrolyte solutions

Normal saline (Ns, Ins)

Normal saline is a solution of 0.9% sodium chloride (NaCl) with no other electrolytes in the solution. Half normal saline (0.45% NaCl) is also available and is exactly that—normal saline diluted to half its concentration. The concentration of the two ions in normal saline is 154 mEq/l. Both the sodium and chloride ion levels are higher than in normal circulating plasma. Normal saline, with or without other additives or diluents, is the predominate solution used for acute volume replacement, "flush solutions" and as a diluent for other intravenously administered medications.

Dose
For acute volume supplement or replacement, 10–20 ml/kg intravenously over five minutes. Repeat once for continued volume loss. For less urgent replacement the rate of infusion is slowed. If further repeat infusions are necessary, Ringer's lactate or an osmotic volume expander should be considered instead of, or in addition to, normal saline solution.

Adverse effects
Normal saline infusions easily produce volume overload and symptoms of congestive heart failure, particularly in a patient with compromised myocardial function or a patient who is already "volume loaded" with a large left to right shunt. The high chloride content of normal saline aggravates pre-existing acidosis.

Ringer's lactate

Ringer's lactate is a more physiologic replacement electrolyte fluid, which is more consistent with the electrolyte content of normal plasma. Each liter contains 130 mEq sodium, 109 mEq chloride, 4 mEq potassium, 3 mEq calcium and 28 mEq bicarbonate. It is also used as a "flush" solution or a diluent with most other infusions.

Dose
For acute volume replacement the dose is 10–20 ml/kg infused intravenously over 5–10 minutes. The "rapid infusion" can be repeated once.

Adverse effects
Acute volume overload can be a problem in a patient with compromised myocardium or in patients with large left to right shunts. Also, potassium and calcium are contained in Ringer's lactate and potentially can aggravate pre-existing hyperkalemia or hypercalcemia.

Sodium bicarbonate

Sodium bicarbonate is an alkalizing agent used for the treatment and/or prevention of metabolic acidosis—as determined by the pH and base deficit from the blood gas analysis and used in the acute treatment of hyperkalemia.

Dose
0.5 mEq/kg × base deficit (mEq/l) infused slowly intravenously (e.g. mEq infused = 0.5 × patient's wt (in kg) × base deficit in mEq/l). The dose is repeated according to the correction of the blood pH. Bicarbonate for infusion is available in 4.2% solution, which equals 0.5 mEq/ml, and 8.4% solution, which equals one mEq/ml.

Adverse effects
Rapid infusion pushes potassium into the cells, which can result in arrhythmias, reduced oxygen dissociation from hemoglobin and even cardiac arrest. Repeated doses can lead to volume overload and agitation of congestive heart failure.

Calcium chloride

Calcium chloride is the form of calcium used in the catheterization laboratory because it provides ionic calcium more readily than calcium gluconate. Calcium chloride is used to treat absolute or relative hypocalcemia caused by the calcium binding by the citrates in transfused blood or by calcium channel blockers. It is also used for the emergency treatment of hyperkalemia and digitalis toxicity. Ionic calcium has an inotropic effect when hypocalcemia exists.

Dose
10–20 mg/kg/dose given slowly intravenously and the same dose is repeated in 10 minutes for a repeat of the problem, e.g. repeat hypocalcemia secondary to repeat transfusion.

Adverse effects
Calcium chloride can cause vasodilation, hypotension, cardiac arrhythmias and cardiac standstill when given rapidly. Calcium chloride is a strong tissue vesicant and can cause vascular spasm to the point of total occlusion and tissue necrosis.

Dextrose solutions

Dextrose is used to prevent or treat hypoglycemia. Hypoglycemia is common in small and/or debilitated infants, especially after they have been "NPO" for any length of time. Hypoglycemia can result in irritability to the point of seizures. Dextrose is available as a 5% solution as D_5S intravenous solutions, as a 10% solution and as a 50% solution of dextrose only. The 5% dextrose solution (D_5S) is used in most maintenance intravenous fluids for infants and children. The 50% solution is very viscous and is usually diluted 1:1 to 1:4 with normal saline or Ringer's lactate for an intravenous bolus when treating hypoglycemia.

Dose—for maintenance intravenous solutions in infants
D_5S in 1/4 normal saline. The maintenance infusion rate is 150 ml/kg/24 hours in infants.

Dose—for significant hypoglycemia
0.5–1 g/kg/min infused intravenously. Usually the 50% dextrose is diluted 1:1 with normal saline to produce a 25% solution (or 0.25 g/ml) before intravenous infusion, and infusions of 2 ml/kg of this solution are given initially.

Adverse effects
Essentially none. Dextrose causes transient hyperglycemia if administered to a patient with normal serum glucose.

Osmotic volume expanders

Whole blood and packed red blood cells (PRBC)

Whole blood or packed red blood cells (PRBC) are the logical volume replacement "fluid" for acute blood loss. These are the only volume expanders that *replenish the oxygen-carrying capacity* of the blood that is lost. The PRBC replace the maximal oxygen-carrying capacity without adding extraneous volume and usually are the preferred volume expander/replacement in cardiac patients following blood loss. ***Fresh*** whole blood does add the plasma clotting factors and platelets as well as the oxygen-carrying capacity of the lost blood but, at the same time, increases the extra cellular volume.

Dose
Usually 10–20 ml/kg of either PRBC or whole blood is administered by intravenous push depending upon the rate and amount of blood loss or hypovolemia.

Adverse effects
Unless planned, whole blood or PRBC is not instantly available. It must be specifically cross-matched for the individual patient, which takes pre-preparation or incurs a significant delay in availability.

Patients with marginal cardiac reserve can be pushed into overt cardiac failure by the volume load. Any blood product infusion carries the potential of blood-borne infection.

Fresh frozen plasma (FFP)

Fresh frozen plasma is frozen whole human plasma which contains most of the clotting factors of the plasma in fresh whole blood. As such, when thawed, it is an excellent volume expander. FFP is used primarily to replace clotting factors when there is a bleeding diathesis associated with blood loss.

Dose
10–15 ml/kg infused over 30 minutes or as a ml for ml volume replacement for active blood loss.

Adverse events
FFP must be thawed and cross-matched before use so it is not instantly available without prior planning. FFP replaces clotting factors, but has no oxygen carrying capacity. As a blood product, it has the potential for transmitting blood-borne illnesses.

Human albumin (Albumisol, Albuminar-5, Plasbumin-5, Buminate-5)

Albumin is a blood product derivative utilized as an

acute volume expander, especially when oxygen-carrying capacity is not a problem. It does not require blood cross-matching so is readily available before whole blood or PRBC are available. In the catheterization laboratory it is used for emergency volume replacement and for volume replacement during plasmapheresis (phlebotomy) performed for polycythemia. Albuminar-5, plasbumin-5 and buminate-5 are iso-oncotic with blood/plasma and are given directly to the patient, while albuminar-25, plasbumin-25 and buminate-25 are concentrated solutions which must be diluted 1:5 with normal saline.

Dose—acute volume replacement
10–20 ml/kg given intravenously over 30–60 minutes in the absence of continuing blood loss. The continued rate of administration depends upon the status of the patient and concomitant blood loss from the vascular space.

Dose—plasmapheresis
The polycythemic blood which is withdrawn is replaced ml for ml with Albuminar-5.

Adverse effects
Acute volume load can precipitate congestive heart failure in susceptible patients. Idiosyncratic reactions include chills, fever and tachycardia as well as pulmonary edema. Albumin is a blood product capable of the transmittal of blood-borne infections to the recipient.

6% Hetastarch (Hespan)

Hetastarch is a synthetic polymer of colloidal starch that is diluted with normal saline and used as a volume expander. It is not a blood product nor does it have oxygen-carrying capacity. The 6% solution is roughly iso-oncotic and is available in 500 ml plastic bag containers ready for administration.

Dose
Approximately 10–20 ml/kg of a 6% solution of hespan in normal saline is administered intravenously over 30 minutes (or more rapidly to compensate for continuing, acute blood loss). It is administered in equivalent volumes to albumin for volume expansion. Hespan is now the preferred replacement fluid for plasmapheresis (phlebotomy) performed for polycythemia. It expands and maintains the circulating volume without the potential adverse effect of transmitting blood-borne disease.

Adverse effects
It can precipitate congestive failure from the acute volume overload in susceptible patients. Itching, chills, bleeding and myalgia can result from a hypersensitivity to hespan.

Plasmanate (Human plasma protein fraction-5%)

5% plasmanate is an iso-oncotic solution of *pooled human* blood plasma proteins utilized as a volume expander similar to human plasma. The plasma is collected from carefully screened donors, tested for infectious agents and heated to inactivate certain viruses.

Dose
Plasmanate is used exactly like plasma as a volume only replacement. Like albumin and hespan it has no oxygen-carrying capacity and contains none of the blood clotting factors. It is used volume for volume for acute blood replacement and during phlebotomies with colloid replacement.

Adverse events
If given too rapidly plasmanate can cause *hypotension*. Plasmanate is a blood derivative and in spite of its careful preparation, still has the potential for transmitting blood-borne infections.

Mannitol (Osmitrol)

Mannitol is a hyperosmotic volume expander utilized in the catheterization laboratory exclusively to re-establish urine output in the presence of acute renal failure.

Dose
250 mg/kg intravenous push administered over 3–5 minutes. The same dose is repeated in five minutes until renal flow has been established. When urine output has been established, the infusion can be continued until a maximum of 1.5 gm/kg/6–8 hrs is reached.

Adverse effects
The acute expansion of the extracellular space aggravates pre-existing congestive cardiac failure. If urine output is not established, mannitol creates a hyperosmotic intravascular fluid.

Bronchodilators

Bronchodilators are used in the catheterization laboratory primarily for the management of acute, reactive, laryngeal and/or bronchospastic problems occurring during catheterization. They are used prophylactically in patients with a history of asthma or other reactive airway problems.

Albuterol sulfate (Ventolin, Proventil)

Albuterol is an inhalant bronchodilator. Albuterol is an adrenergic and beta-2 agonist which relaxes bronchial smooth muscle and, in turn, acts as a bronchodilator. It is utilized in the catheterization laboratory in patients undergoing catheterization who have concomitant active bronchospastic disease.

Dose—metered inhaler
2 puffs every 5 minutes for up to 12 treatments.

Dose—Nebulization
0.1–0.3 mg/kg diluted in 2.5–3.0 ml normal saline for each nebulization treatment; this may be repeated every 20 minutes.

Adverse effects
Tachycardia, palpitations, hypertension, headache and agitation.

Terbutaline sulfate (Brethaire)

Terbutaline is an intravenous adrenergic and beta-2 agonist which results in the relaxation of bronchial smooth muscle and bronchodilation. It is used in the catheterization laboratory to treat acute bronchospastic conditions and bronchial asthma.

Dose
Bolus of 10 mcg/kg infused over 5–10 minutes and followed by an infusion beginning with 0.4 mcg/kg/min and working up to 5–6 mcg/kg/min.

Adverse effects
Tachycardia, hypertension, headaches, nervousness and trembling. Continued use can result in paradoxical bronchoconstriction.

Theophylline (Slo-Bid)

Theophylline is a phosphodiesterase enzyme inhibitor which, among its many effects, relaxes the smooth muscles of the airway, reduces the response of the airway to stimulation and increases contraction of the diaphragmatic muscles. Theophylline is used in the catheterization laboratory for the intravenous treatment of intractable bronchospastic problems.

Dose
Intravenous loading dose with an infusion of 6 mg/kg over 15–20 minutes and maintain with 0.4–0.7 mg/kg/hr.

Adverse effects
Stimulates the release of catecholamines with tachyarrhythmias, hypertension and central nervous system stimulation.

Antibiotics

Although not "catheterization laboratory medications" *per se*, antibiotics are used extensively in the cardiac catheterization laboratory primarily for "antibiotic prophylaxis". Although most catheterizing physicians do not give antibiotic prophylaxis for standard diagnostic catheterizations, antibiotics are given to patients during complicated and/or prolonged catheterization procedures and in those procedures involving the implant of a permanent intravascular device.

Cefazolin sodium (Ancef, Kefzol)

Cefazolin is a first generation intravenous cephalosporin which is effective against the usual skin contaminants from the inguinal area.

Dose
50–100 mg/kg/day divided into four doses at six-hour intervals. The first dose is usually administered during the procedure when the decision is made to implant an intravascular device in the catheterization laboratory.

Adverse effects
Cefazolin has cross sensitivity to other cephalosporins or penicillins. Otherwise, it has minimal or very rare side effects.

Cefuroxime (Zinacef, Ceftin)

Cefuroxime is a second generation intravenous cephalosporin.

Dose
100 mg/kg/day intravenously, divided in four doses. The first dose is usually administered during the procedure when the decision is made to implant an intravascular device in the catheterization laboratory.

Adverse effects
Causes local irritation. May have cross reactivity to patients who are sensitive to other cephalosporins or to penicillin.

Amikacin sulfate (Amikin)

Amikacin is a synthetic aminoglycoside antibiotic which is used in patients who are allergic to cephalosporins and penicillin.

Dose
7.5 mg/kg intravenously through a central intravenous line. The dose is repeated every eight hours times three doses. The first dose is usually administered during

the procedure when the decision is made to implant an intravascular device in the catheterization laboratory.

Adverse effects
Amikacin can cause auditory, vestibular, renal and neuromuscular toxicity.

Vancomycin hydrochloride (Vancocin)

Vancomycin is a very potent antibiotic, particularly against Gram-positive organisms. It does *not* have cross sensitivity to cephalosporins or penicillin, so it is an effective antibiotic for patients with definite allergies to these antibiotics.

Dose
10 mg/kg intravenously every six hours for four doses, all doses administered through a large bore, very free-flowing intravenous line. The first dose is usually administered in the catheterization laboratory during the procedure when the decision is made to implant an intravascular device.

Adverse effects
Vancocin is an endothelial irritant and is very painful given intravenously. In addition, it can cause hypotension, tachycardia, extreme flushing and, rarely, toxicity of virtually any organ system.

References

1. Goldwire M (ed). *Texas Children's Hospital Drug Formulary-6th Edition*. ed. P.D.a.T.C.-T.C. Hospital. Vol. VI. 2001, Lexi-Comp Inc. Hudson, Ohio: Houston, Texas.
2. Sifton D. *Physicians Desk Reference*. Vol 57. 2003, Montvale, NJ: Thomson PDR. 3550.
3. LeRoy S *et al*. Recommendations for preparing children and adolescents for invasive cardiac procedures: a statement from the American Heart Association Pediatric Nursing Subcommittee of the Council on Cardiovascular Nursing in collaboration with the Council on Cardiovascular Diseases of the Young. *Circulation* 2003; **108**(20): 2550–2564.
4. Nilsson A *et al*. The EMLA patch—a new type of local anaesthetic application for dermal analgesia in children. *Anaesthesia* 1994; **49**(1): 70–72.

3 Cardiac catheterization equipment

Introduction

The equipment in the cardiac catheterization laboratory for pediatric/congenital procedures has become more and more sophisticated, complex and expensive. This applies both to the consumable materials as well as to the capital or permanent equipment. It is the obligation of the cardiologist involved with cardiac catheterization to be familiar with the details of each bit of equipment and keep constantly aware of changes or problems with equipment. The physician–director of the catheterization laboratory must be involved with the decisions concerning which equipment is preferred for use and, in turn, which equipment is purchased. This is true for both the capital and the consumable equipment. The cost of equipment certainly must be a consideration but, at the same time, the cost is secondary to the quality, efficacy and safety of the equipment.

Personnel requirements for the operation of cardiac catheterization laboratory equipment

The day-to-day operation of the highly sophisticated, extremely complex, capital equipment, the assistance and participation in the extremely complex catheterization procedure and a familiarity with the large volume of very specialized consumable equipment require very specially trained nurses or technicians for the operation of a pediatric/congenital cardiac catheterization laboratory. Of equal importance, highly qualified engineers capable of fine-tuning and maintenance of the equipment are required almost continuously in the catheterization laboratory. The details of the personnel requirements of the catheterization laboratory are covered in Chapter 1—Organization of the Catheterization Laboratory.

Permanent (capital) catheterization equipment

The fixed permanent capital equipment is the essential operational equipment of the catheterization laboratory and represents a major initial expense for any cardiac catheterization laboratory. The fixed capital equipment is "built into" the catheterization laboratory, and when this equipment is changed, it usually requires some, and often, major physical renovation of the catheterization room. All of this fixed equipment requires additional, on-going maintenance. Although most of the capital equipment usually is very stable and reliable, at the same time it is very complex and is not self-sustaining. With the current advances in technology in these areas, this equipment becomes obsolete quickly and needs to be replaced, often, before it actually wears out. The major components of the fixed capital equipment are the X-ray equipment with its imaging system, the cine or, now, digital angiographic system, the physiologic recorder, the catheterization laboratory computer, the display monitors for the X-ray and the physiologic information and the angiographic injector.

There are numerous other items of capital equipment which are an essential part of the reusable equipment in each catheterization laboratory, but at the same time, are far less "fixed" and do not require renovation in the building structure to exchange or replace. This equipment also is covered in this chapter.

X-ray equipment

The core of a pediatric/congenital catheterization laboratory is the X-ray equipment, its imaging and its recording chain. The absolute necessity of extremely high-quality fluoroscopic imaging and recording of very high-quality permanent images at the lowest possible doses of radiation has made it necessary to upgrade or replace the permanent, high-cost X-ray equipment quite frequently.

X-ray systems now should be amortized over no more than five to six years.

For precise diagnostic angiography in complex congenital defects and in order to perform all of the potential therapeutic catheterization procedures, the pediatric laboratory or any laboratory performing cardiac catheterizations on congenital heart patients must utilize a *biplane* X-ray system with the capability of biplane compound angulation of both of the X-ray planes[1]. The X-ray tubes must have dual focal spots, high-frequency switching and a minimum of 150 kV output. The image intensifiers or flat panel detectors must be capable of high-gain and high-resolution image capture and processing. The television imaging chains should be high resolution with 512 × 512 digital matrixing or the equivalent of 4–5 line pairs per mm on analog film.

The imaging chain is coupled to a very high-resolution recording and playback system preferably at least with digital enhancement capabilities. Digital recording, playback, and archiving have become the standard and certainly are more user friendly than the older cine systems. A digital image at 512 × 512, or even better at 1024 × 1024 matrixing, provides diagnostic images which in several "blinded", controlled studies, provided comparative "diagnostic" information. At the same time these images do not have the detailed resolution of *perfectly exposed, perfectly processed* and *optimally viewed* cine film. The fine details of the anatomy or the individual pictures reproduced from digital angiographic images still are not of equal *esthetic* quality to *perfectly executed* cine film, however, the *diagnostic* information on the digital imaging is the equivalent of, or probably better than that on the cine images, particularly since cine film was seldom *perfect* at all steps of its creation.

Digital imaging

The almost universal acceptance of the Digital Imaging Communication in Medicine (DICOM) standard for digital output is on the way to solving the problems of compatibility between digital systems from different manufacturers. DICOM serves as a standard for transfer of information from one X-ray system to another. As these problems with digital image compatibility are solved completely, digital systems are rapidly replacing film as the recording and archiving medium for cardiac catheterization laboratories. With digital recorders, instantaneous, fixed, clear replay images are consistently and repeatedly displayed as "road maps" for therapeutic interventions. Digital enhancement and manipulations of the fluoroscopic images are available to complement and enhance the viewing of the "on-line" images. All of the digital enhancements still do not improve the actual resolution of the image. However, the improved quality of digital *recording* and *instantaneous digital replay* compared to older tape or disk replay systems do make digital recording essential for therapeutic cardiac catheterization laboratories. As reliable and more reasonably priced means of storing the large amounts of digital data become available, digital systems are replacing cine angiographic recording systems. Certainly, as new catheterization laboratories are installed, totally digital systems replace the earlier analog systems.

Cine (analog) angiography

For the past three decades, the end of the imaging chain for the permanent recording of the angiographic images was cine-angiographic film. Although acquired from an X-ray image, cine-angiographic film is a photographic film and must be handled and developed differently and separately from the X-ray film. For imaging in congenital heart defects, one or more structures frequently must be seen "through" or "behind" another image (e.g. the branch pulmonary artery behind the aorta). This requires different and specific films and techniques for pediatric and congenital heart imaging separate from the usual coronary angiography catheterization laboratories, where higher contrast images with precise edge definition are more important. The cine film for congenital heart lesions requires a longer gray scale (or "longer range") in density than the higher contrast film usually found in primary coronary laboratories. To achieve these qualities from any cine film, a high quality photographic developing system is required. Because of the differences in final desired images, developing the pediatric/congenital film is carried out separately not only from the X-ray film, but also from the cine film in the adult catheterization laboratories.

The final cine images obtained are the net result of the film used in addition to each step and part of the film recording and developing processes. The net process is monitored daily with quality control (QC) strips recorded with the cine system and developed using the chemicals to be used that day. Any variation in the QC strip readings is investigated for the cause and the problem corrected immediately before any cine-angiograms are recorded on patients.

Cine replay

In addition to having the film as the permanent recording medium for the images, the laboratory must have a reliable and high-quality back-up system for all recorded angiographic information. Videotapes were traditionally used as the back-up system for analog cine recording. Even high-definition video recording does not have the image quality of properly recorded and developed cine film and is not relied upon as the only source of recording.

However, on the rare occasion when a problem developed with the filming during the procedure or processing of the cine film after the procedure, the video tape served as a "back-up" for the angiographic information which otherwise would have been lost totally. If the video recording system is of high enough quality and has a quality stop frame system, it can also serve as the medium for the instant replay of images or sequences of images during the catheterization procedure. Video-tape systems, however, are very cumbersome and time consuming to use and are not of sufficient quality or reliability for stop or "freeze" framing of individual images.

Separate optical disks or digital freeze-frame systems have replaced most video replay systems even in the catheterization laboratories still using cine-angiography. These systems provide much higher quality images and are much more convenient to use. Individual frames can be "grabbed" and displayed as a roadmap. Just as these systems became more popular, they were replaced by totally digital imaging, recording and archiving systems. X-ray imaging systems are discussed in more detail in Chapter 11 (Angiography).

Physiologic recorders

In addition to the X-ray equipment, the catheterization laboratory for congenital heart patients requires very accurate physiologic recording equipment. In the modern catheterization laboratory these recorders contain very sophisticated, solid-state electronics and are usually integrated with a computer recording system. The basic physiologic recorder is able to display and record 10 channels or more simultaneously and records at speeds in increments between 5 and 200 feet per second. The recording channels are interchangeable between ECG, pressure and direct DC output channels.

At least two and preferably three leads of the patient's ECG are displayed continuously from at least *four* skin electrodes/leads on the body. This guarantees a continual display of at least one ECG tracing even if one, or even two, skin leads are lost temporarily (e.g. pulled off because of the patient's moving or dropping off from the patient's sweating) during the case. For the adequate recording of pressure in complex diagnostic or therapeutic catheterization procedures, a minimum of four, if not five (or more) pressure channels are used. Each pressure channel should be capable of being displayed and recorded on the same gain and at the same time, with *all* of the pressure tracings being capable of being overlapped with each other and at the same zero baseline. Each pressure channel must be capable of recording at multiple ranges in amplitude (gain) from a full scale of 10 mmHg to a full scale of 400 mmHg and of displaying the pressure curves at multiple different sweep speeds between 10 and 200 mm/second. The physiologic recorder should be capable of printing whatever is displayed on the physiologic monitor and at multiple different recording speeds between 10 and 200 mm/second.

Monitor displays

Color monitoring screens with separate colors for each channel of data are available and have become almost essential when there are multiple channels of data displayed simultaneously and continuously. The three different ECG leads can be displayed in one color while the two to four (or more) separate pressure curves are each displayed in a different color. This allows each channel of data to be identified very rapidly by its color to correspond to its connection to a location in the vascular system. The location of the catheter in the vascular system may not be obvious instantaneously to all individuals in the laboratory, but the color instantly identifies each channel. The scale at which each pressure channel is displayed is labeled along with an analog read-out of the pressure. Both of these numbers are displayed on the monitor screen in the *same color* as the corresponding pressure tracing. In addition, there should be a separate analog read-out of the heart rate and pulse oximetry displayed on the monitor screen. The prominent analog display of these parameters on the monitor allows all of the personnel in the room to be aware of the patient's exact status from instant to instant during the case without having to analyze the individual pressure curves.

Cardiac catheterization laboratory computer

It is now standard to have the physiologic recorder integrated with an on-line cardiac catheterization laboratory computer for the acquisition, analysis and storage of the data. The computer produces a timed record of all procedures performed, medications used and events occurring in the catheterization laboratory. Some of the information which is fed into the computer comes directly from the electronic outputs of the equipment in the catheterization room, while much of the information is still added manually through the keyboard by the recording nurse/technician. The various locations, much of the equipment and many of the procedures can be chosen from a preprogrammed list in the computer program. In a pediatric/congenital cardiac catheterization laboratory, this computer program is specifically designed for the needs of the pediatric or congenital catheterization procedures and must be extremely flexible with the many bizarre locations and great variety of information and procedures performed in these laboratories.

A high quality digital or analog tape recorder with the capability of continually recording and storing the *physiologic* data generated during the case provides a necessary back-up to the physiologic recorder in the catheterization laboratory. This recorder runs continuously in the background from the time the patient enters the room until the case is completed and the patient leaves the room. The continuously running recorder provides a back-up for information missed during the intermittent, "on the go" recording of specific information, and helps to reduce the amount of actual paper recordings performed.

Contrast injectors

An essential part of the angiography is the speed of the injection of the contrast material and, in turn, the injector itself. Modern contrast injectors are capable of injecting very specific quantities of contrast over a specified amount of time or at a specified pressure. The injectors inject as little as two ml and up to 55 ml during a single injection. The amount, rate and pressure variables of the injection are adjustable *independently* from each other. This allows each injection to be adjusted for the pressure and flow limits of the specific catheter, for the specifications of the contrast medium used, and for the particular location of the injection within the heart or vascular system. Variable flow rates within any single injection and ECG triggering of the onset of injections are desirable but not essential components of the power injectors in pediatric/congenital laboratories.

A desirable, if not essential, characteristic of the injector is that the injector unit (head), which contains the pressure/drive motor and injector syringe, is separated from the large, often bulkier, electronic control unit. This allows the smaller injector head to be moved more conveniently as a separate unit to a position immediately adjacent to the catheterization table during each injection. When the head of the injector is separate from the control unit, the control unit for the injector can be positioned even in a separate room. It is also desirable for the injector head to be suspended from the ceiling on an articulating arm over the catheterization table. This keeps any part of the injector from occupying any floor space near the catheterization table. When the injector head is suspended from the ceiling, it is elevated well above the catheterization table, and when connected to the catheter, obligatorily is positioned with the tip of the injector syringe pointing downward. The tip-down position of the syringe provides an additional safety factor by encouraging any air remaining in it to rise to the back of the syringe during the injection which, in turn, reduces the possibility even further of the injection of any air into the circulation.

Most angiographic injectors now have sterile, disposable injection syringes, which fit into a sleeve on the injector head. A new injection syringe is used for each case; however, in the case of multiple repeat injections, the sterile syringe can be refilled during the procedure.

More specifics about contrast agents and the actual injections are discussed in Chapter 11 (Angiography).

Oxygen, compressed air and suction source

Although often considered part of the physical "plant" or hospital construction, each laboratory must have a source of oxygen, compressed air and suction. It is preferable that these gas sources and a vacuum line for suction come from a wall source or a ceiling-mounted source as a part of the physical structure of the catheterization laboratory rather than with separate portable tanks or an electromechanical suction apparatus loose on carts on the floor within the laboratory. To have the gas lines and vacuum source as permanent "wall sources" requires that they are planned into each catheterization room before the physical construction of the room or even the building begins.

An articulated arm suspended from the ceiling provides an extremely convenient location for the permanent gas sources. The arm is mounted on the ceiling toward the head end, and to the side of, the catheterization table. In this way the arm is out of the way of the X-ray apparatus, but with its articulation the sources of gases and vacuum can be moved close to the patient's head for emergencies. The ceiling-mounted arm avoids tubing running across the floor of the catheterization laboratory, which can happen when the gas sources are wall mounted.

Mobile capital equipment

In addition to the fixed or permanent capital equipment, which is built into and actually a part of the catheterization room, a considerable amount of additional expensive, but at the same time mobile, capital equipment is required in each catheterization room. This equipment is equally important for the effective operation of the catheterization room. With regard to repair and replacement, these items of mobile equipment have several advantages over the more fixed equipment. When these pieces of equipment must be repaired or replaced they can be moved in or out of the catheterization room without disturbing the function of the room or without any physical room renovation. These more mobile pieces of capital equipment are not an integral part of any other piece of equipment and, as such, can be repaired/replaced independently. This type of equipment includes defibrillators, crash carts, electrophysiologic equipment, an anesthesia machine, a Site-Finder™ ultrasound machine, a two-dimensional (2-D) echo machine, a transesophageal or intravascular echo machine and a radiofrequency or Laser™ generator.

Cardiac defibrillator

A DC cardiac defibrillator with ECG sensing and synchronization, ECG recording and accurately adjustable output from 1 to 400 watt/second is part of each laboratory. The defibrillator is on a mobile cart, which can be moved readily to a position immediately adjacent to the catheterization table. The defibrillator has paddles of several different sizes in order to accommodate patients of all sizes from tiny infants to large adults. The defibrillator is capable of operating for several hours on an internal, rechargeable battery, however, when not being used portably, the defibrillator remains in the catheterization laboratory attached to the wall power for continual charging. The defibrillator has a set of ECG leads attached to it with skin electrodes for the leads either attached to the leads or immediately and readily available. Paste for the defibrillator paddles is kept on the defibrillator cart. The Medtronic Physio Control Life Pak has been a very reliable and durable defibrillator.

"Crash" (emergency) cart

In conjunction with a portable defibrillator each catheterization laboratory room has a "crash cart" containing all of the items necessary for cardiopulmonary resuscitation. Each laboratory crash cart has the necessary tubing, connections and, if necessary, gauges available to attach to the gas and suction sources. The mobile crash cart holds a complete set of all sizes, and several types, of laryngoscope blades and handles along with a full range of all sizes of endotracheal tubes, oropharyngeal and nasopharyngeal tubes, several sizes of Ambu™ bags, and oxygen masks of multiple sizes. The emergency crash cart also contains needles and the necessary equipment for starting intravenous or intra-arterial lines. The crash cart should also contain several sizes of sterile chest tubes with their trocars. Finally, the emergency cart should have a portable external pacemaker and at least one set of sterile intracardiac temporary pacemaker leads.

The equipment on the emergency cart and the function of all operating equipment are checked and restocked/replaced every day before the first case, and again if any of the equipment is used during a case.

Electrophysiology equipment

Most large pediatric/congenital catheterization services have a dedicated electrophysiologic catheterization room or a single catheterization room which can function as both a diagnostic/therapeutic or an electrophysiologic catheterization room. In *addition* to all of the capital equipment that is necessary for the diagnostic/therapeutic pediatric/congenital catheterization laboratory, there is an extensive amount of additional fixed capital as well as extra consumable equipment required for electrophysiologic procedures.

This text does not intend to cover any of the functions of the electrophysiologic laboratory except to highlight the additional equipment/space requirements for electrophysiologic procedures. For diagnostic electrophysiology studies, twenty or more channels of high frequency, interference free, simultaneous ECG tracings are necessary for intracardiac electrical mapping. Along with this there are special computers and catheters for spatial intracardiac mapping. Computer-controlled electrical stimulators are synchronized with the recorders.

For electrophysiologic ablation procedures the laboratory requires a specific radio-frequency generator with current control and a heat limited cut-off. If the implant, removal and exchange of pacemakers are performed in the electrophysiologic laboratory, the laboratory requires additional sensing/testing equipment along with special surgical instruments and surgical headlamps. The very busy and sophisticated pediatric electrophysiology laboratory has or shares a Laser™ generator for pacemaker lead extractions.

Anesthesia equipment

In a pediatric/congenital catheterization laboratory which uses general anesthesia frequently, or certainly when it is used all of the time, an anesthesia machine and all of its complementary equipment are part of the catheterization laboratory. The "economy" of physically moving an anesthesia machine in and out of the catheterization laboratory and setting it up one, or more, times per day soon becomes illusory. The anesthesia machine is connected to the power, gas and suction lines more or less permanently and is positioned conveniently for the anesthesiologist, yet allows unrestrained movement of the catheterization table and the X-ray suspension arms. The anesthesia machine has its own built-in separate monitoring equipment.

Ventilator

Occasionally a patient requires mechanical ventilation without requiring general anesthesia. Such patients either are intubated once they arrive in the catheterization laboratory, or more often they arrive in the laboratory already intubated, having previously been on a ventilator. The cardiac catheterization laboratory usually does not have a separate permanent ventilator in the room. The ventilator is usually brought into the catheterization laboratory by the respiratory therapy service for the particular case, and is positioned in the area which otherwise would be occupied by the anesthesia machine at the head of the table and cephalad to the lateral X-ray suspension system. The ventilator is connected to the wall oxygen and vacuum, and in turn connected to the patient. A respiratory therapist who remains with the patient throughout the catheterization procedure regulates the ventilator according to the desires of the catheterizing physician. The ventilator is also used when specific concentrations of oxygen and/or nitric oxide (NO) are being administered to patients when they are being tested or treated for pulmonary hypertension.

2-D echo machine

Each cardiac catheterization laboratory or suite of adjacent cardiac catheterization rooms has a 2-D echo machine permanently located in the catheterization laboratory area. This machine is stored in a location convenient to all of the catheterization rooms or the laboratories and in a location which is very familiar to all personnel in the laboratory. The dedicated echocardiogram is necessary primarily for the quick diagnosis of or ruling out of pericardial effusions when cardiac tamponade is suspected as the cause of any rapid, unexplained deterioration of a patient. In that circumstance, time is critical and the time spent in finding, and then transporting, an echo machine which is "remote" from the laboratory can exceed the short window of time during which a patient could be saved by an expedient diagnosis along with an emergent, echo-assisted, pericardial tap.

Site-Rite™ echocardiogram

In a very busy pediatric and congenital catheterization laboratory where compromised vascular access is frequently encountered, a Site-Rite™ (Dymax Corp.) portable 2-D echo machine has become an essential and now standard piece of equipment. The Site-Rite™ is a relatively inexpensive, small and very portable, 2-D ultrasound machine with a small hand-held transducer, which can be used on the sterile field through a sterile sleeve. The probe has the limitation of a maximum depth (or penetration) of 2 or 4 cm into the tissues and has no Doppler capabilities. The Site-Rite™, however, is invaluable for finding vessels in areas where there are no fixed landmarks—for example the internal jugular vein in the neck. The internal jugular vein lies immediately lateral to, but often over the common carotid artery. With the Site-Rite™ the two vessels can clearly be seen in a cross-sectional view and are easily distinguished by their relative sizes, the pulsation of the artery and the compressibility of the vein. With guidance of the Site-Rite™ image the needle can be directed *purposefully* and exactly in line with the internal jugular vein without multiple and essentially "blind" needle sticks into the area of the carotid artery. The Site-Rite™ can also be used to look at the pericardial space in infants and very small children.

Cutaneous Doppler probe

Many pediatric catheterization laboratories utilize a small, portable, "pencil-like" Doppler transducer and console for locating both arteries and veins. The Ultrasonic Doppler Flow Detector, Model 811-B (Parks Medical Electronics, Aloha, Oregon) comes with a reusable (re-sterilizable) Doppler transducer and cable, which attaches to the control unit which is positioned away from the field. The probe distinguishes between artery and vein by detecting and amplifying the different quality of the sound signal between arterial flow and venous flow, while the intensity of the signal increases as the probe is moved *directly* over the specific vessel in order to determine its exact location. It is particularly helpful in locating vessels when the pulses are poor or the landmarks are distorted. The Doppler probe does not help in distinguishing the depth of the vessels within the tissues.

This Doppler probe is useful for finding weak pulses and detecting early return of flow in more peripheral arteries when obstruction to flow is suspected following a catheterization through that artery.

Transesophageal echocardiogram (TEE) machine

Although most cardiac catheterization laboratories do not use a TEE machine enough to justify the presence of the TEE in the laboratory permanently, the active pediatric/congenital cardiac catheterization laboratory performing therapeutic procedures must have frequent and easy access to a TEE machine for use during multiple different therapeutic catheterization procedures. The implant of most (all?) atrial septal occluders requires TEE or intracardiac echo (ICE) guidance. Between the large number of secundum atrial defect occlusions in the catheterization laboratory and the growing number of patent foramen ovale (PFO) closures, the TEE machine is required in the busy catheterization laboratory three to five times per week. TEE machines often are "shared" between multiple catheterization laboratories or cardiovascular operating rooms; however, with the almost routine use of TEE in the operating rooms only one machine between two busy services compromises the scheduling and overall patient care unacceptably.

The TEE probes are cleaned and re-sterilized by soaking in a Cidex™ solution for at least 30 minutes between cases. As a consequence, the TEE cannot be exchanged rapidly between one patient and another unless more than one TEE probe is available. TEE probes have a finite number of uses and if the probe malfunctions, the TEE and the procedures which are dependent on it are out of service for the duration of the malfunction of the probe. Although TEE probes are expensive, it is prudent that a busy catheterization laboratory have at least one spare

TEE probe both for performing multiple procedures on any one day and as a back-up for the whole system.

Intravascular ultrasound (IVUS) and intravascular echocardiography (ICE) are utilized more and more frequently in the pediatric/congenital catheterization laboratory but, in most laboratories, are not considered "routine" procedures and are not used that frequently. Both IVUS and ICE require a large electronic console plus a rather expensive "disposable" catheter. ICE catheters, in general, use the same electronic console as TEE probes. These two items of "semi-consumable" equipment are discussed briefly later on in this chapter.

Capital equipment with disposable consumable components

There are numerous items of capital equipment which come with their own specific consumable equipment. The *specific* consumable items must be available as they are essential for the use of the particular piece of equipment. The capital equipment requires regular maintenance while the consumable components require regular restocking.

Pulse oximetry

Transcutaneous pulse oximetry monitoring is a standard procedure and an essential component in the pediatric/congenital catheterization laboratory. The pulse oximetry system has an adjustable low limit alarm built into it. Pulse oximetry was originally used only for small infants, unstable children, and complex interventional procedures, but the added safety it provided these patients has made it not only routine but essential for all cases. Transcutaneous pulse oximetry allows for a noninvasive *continuous* recording of the patient's oxygenation and provides an early indicator of changes in the patient's status, which is not available by any other technique.

Pulse oximetry probes are disposable while the amplifier is a piece of capital equipment. Most oximeter probes are placed on a digit of an extremity although there are probes which are placed on an ear lobe when the peripheral circulation is compromised. These ear probes have the danger of burning the underlying tissues in small infants when left in place for any duration of time.

Cuff blood pressure apparatus

Although not used for the definitive continuous blood pressure monitoring of the patient during the catheterization procedure, a cuff blood pressure apparatus is available in the catheterization laboratory with the read-out from the manometer displayed on the monitor. The cuff pressure should be available to monitor the patient's blood pressure when the patient arrives in the room and before an indwelling arterial line is in place, and for monitoring the pressure after the arterial line is removed and hemostasis is being obtained at the end of a case. The cuff blood pressure also serves as a back-up should anything happen to the monitored pressure from the indwelling arterial line.

Temperature monitor

Most patients, regardless of size, have difficulty in maintaining their body temperature in the catheterization laboratory. The operating environment of the catheterization laboratory is usually cool (or actually cold), the patients are often wet from the pre-procedure sterile "scrubbing", the drapes over the patient becoming wet from the flush fluids used on the catheterization table, and the patient's core temperature is cooled continuously by the infusion of cool flush solutions. In addition, many patients who are undergoing cardiac catheterization are under-nourished and/or debilitated, which aggravates the core cooling.

As a consequence, all patients have their *core* temperature monitored either with a disposable esophageal or rectal probe, which is connected to a permanent temperature monitor. The core temperature of each patient is displayed continuously on a physiologic monitoring screen within the catheterization room and on the display in the control room. Cutaneous temperature probes are simpler to use, but less reliable at measuring core temperature and much more likely to be dislodged from the moist skin and, in turn, provide no monitoring.

Patient warmer

Along with a temperature monitor, each cardiac catheterization laboratory must have the capability of warming the patient continuously during the procedure. Most catheterization laboratories operate in a "cool" ambient environment. This temperature is comfortable to the personnel in scrub gowns but is *cold* to a non-clothed, wet patient. When the drapes on the patient's body surface become wet and cold flush solutions infusing into the patient are added to this generally "cool" environment, most patients require supplemental support for their body temperature. The smaller, the thinner or more debilitated is the patient, the greater is the need for warming. The apparatus for generating heat may be separated from, or attached directly to, the catheterization table while the actual warming component is on the catheterization table.

The Bear Hugger™ hot-air warmers have proved to be the most suitable mechanism for warming patients of any size in the catheterization laboratory. There is a heating unit and a blower, which are positioned at the foot of the catheterization table. An outlet from the blower attaches to the center of the base of the very long U-shaped, disposable, sterile paper tube. The long arms of the U-tube run along each side of the length of the patient and are immediately adjacent to the patient under the sterile drapes. Warm air is forced through the U-tube, which has multiple tiny holes along the entire length of each of the long side tubes. The multiple holes allow the warm air to escape under the drape which is over the patient and, in turn, to bathe the patient continuously in warm air. The rate of flow and the temperature of the air can be adjusted according to the patient's monitored core temperature. The U-tubing is totally radiolucent and does not interfere with any of the X-ray imaging.

Several other heating systems are available. The K-Pad™ is a series of small tubes imbedded in a plastic pad, in a "switch-back" arrangement, running to and fro and from side to side for the length of the pad. The pad is placed directly under the patient's trunk and warm water is circulated through the tubing by a small detachable electric heater/pump. The heater/pump is small enough that it can be placed on the catheterization table under the drapes at the foot of the table. This system is unsatisfactory for several reasons. The only two sizes of K-Pad™ which are available do not fit all patients and, of more importance, the pad and tubing are somewhat radio-opaque and show up on the fluoroscopy and X-ray images.

The least satisfactory alternative for externally warming a patient is with a floor mounted, movable "heating lamp". This type of heater is very mobile and takes up very little actual floor space. When placed near the patient's head or trunk these lamps do warm patients efficiently. However, when the lamps are close enough to warm the patient there is a great danger of actually burning the skin which is exposed to the warmer! In addition, in order to be positioned close enough to the patient's trunk or head to warm them, the lamp is *always* in the way of the operating field or the posterior–anterior (PA) or lateral fluoroscopy/X-ray tubes or images. The narrow margin of safety for burning the patient and interference with performing the procedure have essentially eliminated the use of mobile lamps for heating in the modern cardiac catheterization laboratory.

Fluid warming apparatus

In order to maintain the patient's body temperature, in addition to externally warming the patient it is often necessary to warm the fluids that are administered intravenously. Most standard flush solutions equilibrate rapidly in temperature with room temperature, which is often 20–25 Fahrenheit degrees below the patient's body temperature. The body can warm a small amount of fluid given over a long period of time enough to compensate for this discrepancy, however, when a large volume of fluid is given over a short period of time or given to a small patient, the body cannot compensate for the temperature discrepancy and the body temperature drops. The smaller or thinner the patient is, the greater is the problem with a cold infusion. This is particularly true when blood, which is usually refrigerated and is very cold until just before use, is administered to a patient.

A partial solution to keeping the patient warm is to warm the particular fluid in its bag in a solution of warm water or a special heater. This technique of warming has the difficulty that the fluid hanging in its container in the catheterization room while awaiting administration cools down again in the cool environment of the room. The optimal solution is a special fluid/blood warmer, the Flo Tem IIe (Data Chem™), which is part of the routine manifold set-up and is interposed in the fluid line between the fluid reservoir and the manifold. These warmers containing a disposable coil of tubing, which is bathed within a circulating bath of warm fluid. In this way the intravenous fluid/blood can be warmed to body temperature shortly before the fluid enters the patient.

Oxygen analyzer for rapid blood saturation determinations

Measurements of blood oxygen saturation are very frequent and critical determinations which are performed during every congenital heart catheterization. A system for rapidly determining blood oxygen (O_2) saturation from small blood samples must be available within the pediatric/congenital catheterization laboratory. Most laboratories use an automated electronic oxygen analyzer, which is based on indirect spectrophotometric techniques and displays the saturation directly. These oximeters are available from Waters, Inc. (Waters Instruments Inc., Rochester, MN) and from A-Vox (A-VOX Systems, Inc., San Antonio, TX). Each catheterization laboratory should have access to an additional blood oxygen analyzing system that uses a *different* technique for analyzing the oxygen content of the blood in order to periodically check the accuracy of the system which is used on a daily basis. The checks and calibrations of the oximeter should be performed at least daily, if not between or even during each case.

In addition to the actual apparatus for determining blood oxygen saturation, there should be a means of displaying the results immediately and prominently to the catheterizing physician. In many catheterization laboratories the results are printed manually onto a diagram of the heart on a chalk board in the room or the result is transmitted verbally (shouted) to the recording nurse who, in turn, types it into the recording system, which displays the result in small print on the monitor screen in the catheterization room. As a much better alternative to these archaic and inaccurate systems, the Avox Oximeter 1000 (Avox Inc., San Antonio, TX) system is now capable of transmitting the result of the oxygen saturation determination as a digital output signal directly from the oximeter through a hard wire connection to a standard PC computer, where a software program from Scientific Software Inc. (Scientific Software Solutions, Charlottesville, VA) displays the data in a timed table on a CRT screen. The A-Vox oximeter times each oxygen sample and the location of each sample is chosen from a table of locations in the oximeter itself or is typed into the computer manually. As the saturation is analyzed and read by the oximeter, the *timed oxygen saturation with its location* is then displayed *directly* and *instantaneously* on a (large) computer screen. This occurs with *no* interposed *"voice transmission"* of the results from one nurse/technician to another and no additional manual input into the system by a second nurse/technician, and provides the physician with a prominent, instantaneous and timed display. The specific spectrophotometric oxygen analyzing systems and the techniques for their use are described in detail in Chapter 10, Data Acquisition and Analysis.

Blood gas apparatus

A blood gas machine that is a part of the laboratory is a requirement for a pediatric/congenital catheterization laboratory. With the frequent determinations of blood gases and the need for immediate access to the results, the blood gas analyzer must be in the catheterization laboratory suite and must be operated by the catheterization laboratory personnel. The ABL 700 Blood Gas Machine (Radiometer, Copenhagen, Denmark) is a very sophisticated but relatively easy to operate blood gas apparatus. It does, however, need fairly frequent and intensive maintenance and calibration.

Many of the patients undergoing catheterization in the pediatric laboratory are very unstable hemodynamically, with their hemodynamics changing markedly from one second to the next. The instability of these patients is compounded by their sedation/anesthesia and is even more common during the prolonged and complex therapeutic catheterization procedures. It is essential that the physiologic status of the patient can be monitored regularly and rapidly with periodic measurements of the blood gases, particularly at the time of any, even suggested, change in the patient's status during the procedure. Because of the frequent and often rapid changes in the physiologic status of these patients and the need for the immediate correction of acid/base abnormalities, the results must be available *within one or two minutes* of obtaining the samples. During an emergency, the result of a blood gas determination is of no value when it is received after the patient already has been treated empirically on the basis of guessing what the blood/gas status might have been!

The blood gas machine also can calculate the oxygen saturation of blood and can serve as a *rough means* of verifying the blood oxygen saturation determinations periodically, albeit not as accurately as with the oximeter.

Activated clotting time (ACT) apparatus

A pediatric/congenital cardiac catheterization laboratory also should have a readily available means of rapidly obtaining an activated clotting time (ACT) on patients in the catheterization laboratory. Three units of heparin are added to each ml of flush solution and to each ml of contrast medium to prevent thrombus formation in these solutions. In addition, most catheterization laboratories administer additional heparin systemically for the prevention of thromboembolic phenomena during some, if not all, catheterization procedures.

The major indication for the use of heparin in the past was for the prevention of systemic arterial thromboembolic events. Now there is also a growing use of additional heparin for the prevention of thrombotic phenomena in the systemic venous and pulmonary arterial systems. Heparin is often administered arbitrarily and in doses varying from 50 mg to 200 mg/kg, with the dose varying primarily according to the patient's weight. The response to heparin is dose related but, at the same time, the response is extremely variable from patient to patient. Occasionally the normal for weight, but arbitrary dose of heparin prolongs the bleeding time dangerously. The patient's response to heparin can be monitored by their activated clotting time (ACT). There are several small ACT machines for measuring the ACT of the blood from Hemo Tec Inc. (Englewood, CO) and Medtronic (Minneapolis, MN). Both ACT machines utilize a very small sample of blood, are very easy to operate, rapid and are fairly inexpensive. An ACT is obtained before administering systemic heparin, periodically during a long case and just before the lines are removed in patients where heparin was administered earlier.

Indicator dilution system and computer

Thermodilution computer/system

A catheterization laboratory should have the equipment to perform quantitative indicator dilution curves for the determination of cardiac output. The thermodilution technique currently is the most—if not the only—available, reliable and reproducible quantitative indicator dilution technique for cardiac output determination, and is the only indicator dilution *curve* still utilized in most (any!) catheterization laboratories. The Dualtherm™ COC (B.

Braun, Bethlehem, PA) cardiac output computer is fairly straightforward to operate and can be calibrated for use with thermodilution catheters from different manufacturers.

A thermodilution curve is a quantitative indicator dilution curve, where the indicator is a precise volume of cold isotonic solution at an exact, known temperature. As the specific amount of cold solution mixes with the circulating blood, it transiently lowers the temperature of the blood in proportion to the amount of cold solution, the temperature of the cold solution, the total amount of the circulating blood and the velocity of flow of that blood (the cardiac output). The cold solution is injected through a proximal port on a catheter and the changing temperature of the blood as the cold solution is diluted in the blood is detected as the mixture passes a thermistor which is located at the distal end of the catheter. The changing temperature is plotted as an indicator curve by the cardiac output computer. The known values of the patient's size and body temperature, the pressures in the area where the solution is injected and the temperature and volume of the injected cold solution are all entered into the thermodilution output computer. From the indicator dilution curve for the injected cold solution, the computer calculates the cardiac output using the Fick™ principal and formula. Assuming that precise, correct information is provided to the computer, the calculations are more accurate than any performed manually.

"Dye" dilution curves

Quantitative cardio-green indicator dilution ("dye") curves were used in the past for the calculation of cardiac output and the quantification of shunts, but they are more complicated to perform and, to be very accurate, require an arterial blood sample to be drawn *through* a sensor at a *very steady rate*. Very few laboratories still have the equipment to perform quantitative cardio-green dye curves. The details of the indicator dilution techniques are discussed in Chapter 10, Data Acquisition.

Although seldom utilized any more, exogenous indicator ("dye") dilution curves still represent the most sensitive techniques for the *detection* of very minute shunts. Densitometers are capable of qualitatively sensing very minute quantities of cardio-green dye in the blood and, in turn, when positioned in the systemic arterial system can be utilized to document very minute right to left shunts. The more recent densitometers are usually built into skin sensors, although earlier systems were available where the blood was actually drawn through a densitometer. When the green dye is injected into the systemic venous blood, normally the bolus of blood/dye mixture must pass completely through the pulmonary circuit before reaching a peripheral arterial sensor. The presence of even a very tiny *right to left* shunt anywhere distal ("downstream") in the circulation to the injection site in a systemic vein, would allow the blood/dye, which was shunted right to left, to reach the peripheral sensor much faster than the remainder of the blood/dye, which follows the normal pathway through the lungs and pulmonary circuit. With the dye dilution technique, even a very tiny amount of right to left shunting which otherwise could not be detected from changes in the blood oxygen saturation, could be detected. With precise recording and calibration of the dilution curves obtained when the blood is drawn through a densitometer, the shunts could actually be quantitated.

Platinized intracardiac electrodes at the tips of catheters are still used for sensing minute shifts in blood pH for the qualitative detection of minute intracardiac *left to right* shunts. A small amount of inhaled hydrogen gas causes a minute, transient shift in the blood pH, which, in turn, can be detected by a platinum electrode positioned distal to the level of shunting in the systemic venous circulation. A very minute shift in the blood pH causes a marked shift in the baseline tracing of an intracardiac electrocardiogram. Hydrogen gas passes through the alveoli walls, is absorbed instantaneously into the pulmonary venous blood, and instantaneously changes the pH in the pulmonary venous blood. When the sensing electrode is distal to an area of left to right shunting in the blood flow within the heart or great arteries, the sensor reacts to the pH change instantaneously, very sharply and markedly. When the sensing electrode is proximal to the level of shunting, the change in the pH does not appear until the blood, which is acidified by the hydrogen, has passed completely through the systemic circulation and then returned to the site of the sensing electrode in the systemic venous system through the normal course of the systemic venous blood. In the absence of a shunt, the sensed pH change and shift in the intracardiac ECG tracing are markedly delayed and attenuated.

Because of the logistics of storing and handling hydrogen gas, the perceived dangers of explosions and the difficulties with the actual precisely timed administration of the gas to the patient, injected ascorbic acid has been substituted for hydrogen gas as the source of hydrogen ions in laboratories which still use pH changes as indicators. Concentrated ascorbic acid is a very acidic solution, which at the same time is very biocompatible. A very small injection of the concentrated ascorbic acid solution acutely shifts the blood pH in a similar way to inhaling hydrogen gas. The same technique for detecting left to right shunts is used except that the hydrogen ions are injected into the pulmonary artery through a catheter rather than absorbed into the pulmonary venous blood.

All of the indicator dilution techniques for cardiac output, shunt detection and shunt quantification are discussed in more detail in Chapter 10, Data Acquisition.

Oxygen consumption apparatus

In order to determine cardiac output *accurately* using the Fick principal, in addition to the very accurate and timely blood samples, an accurately measured oxygen (O_2) consumption determination is necessary. The measured O_2 consumption is not necessary for the calculation of *relative amount of shunting*, since all values for the O_2 consumption cancel each other out in the calculations of shunts, which are based on differences in oxygen saturation in the blood. However, for the accurate determination of the absolute value of the cardiac output, actual pulmonary blood flow, any vascular resistance or valve areas, the actual O_2 consumption must be measured. There are tables of "normal values" which are proportionate to body surface area; however, these do not take into account the variable metabolic states of the patients. In most pediatric laboratories, oxygen consumption is measured by means of a constant flow-through hood in conjunction with a gas analyzer for measuring oxygen content of the air, such as the MRM-2 Oxygen Consumption Monitor (Waters Instruments Inc., Rochester, MN). O_2 consumption is discussed in more detail in Chapter 10.

A source of carbon dioxide

Balloon flow directed catheters are often used in pediatric/congenital cardiac catheterization laboratories, even in those laboratories which utilize torque-controlled catheters predominately. Even when the operator is not concerned about a very small amount of air in the venous system, in the pediatric/congenital population of patients, it is always assumed that any air which enters the blood anywhere can, and will, reach the systemic circulation, where even a small amount of air can be catastrophic. In the pediatric/congenital laboratory, carbon dioxide (CO_2) is always used in the balloons of "floating" balloon catheters. Each catheterization laboratory has a source of CO_2 gas and a means of transferring the CO_2 to the catheterization table and into the balloon catheter.

A disposable tank of CO_2 gas, which has a gas control valve and is secured to a mount on a wall or cabinet, serves very nicely as a reservoir of CO_2. For use in a balloon catheter, the CO_2 from the tank is allowed to flow into a sterile 3 ml syringe through a stopcock, which is closed immediately and tightly once the syringe is filled. CO_2 is extremely diffusable and escapes *instantaneously* into air through *any* opening, including the tiny opening in the tip of a syringe. If the tip of a syringe full of CO_2 remains open, even while transferring the syringe the short distance from the side of the catheterization room to the catheterization table, the CO_2 diffuses out of the syringe and the syringe fills with *room air* before it can be attached to the balloon catheter.

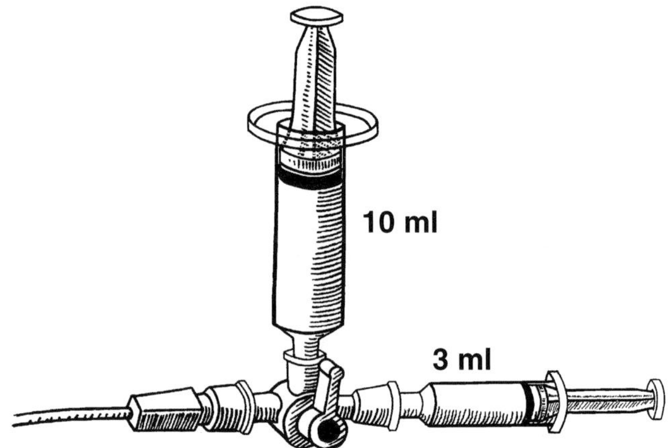

Figure 3.1 Syringes and three-way stopcock arrangement used as a "portable reservoir" for the use of CO_2 on the catheterization table.

The balloon catheter on the catheterization table is attached to the stopcock of the syringe, the stopcock is opened so that the syringe and the balloon lumen are in communication, the balloon is filled from the syringe and the stopcock on the syringe is turned off immediately. CO_2 is very diffusable through the Latex™ of the balloon itself and, as a consequence, empties (diffuses) out of the balloon fairly rapidly. To compensate for this diffusibility, a second 10 ml "reservoir" syringe is attached to the 3 mml syringe through the side port of a three-way stopcock (Figure 3.1). The 10 ml syringe is filled from the CO_2 tank and the stopcock is turned off to the distal opening in the three-way stopcock. This leaves the 10 ml and the 3 ml syringes in communication with each other through the stopcock and, at the same time, closed off to the outside air. Thereafter, once the *distal port* of the stopcock is attached to the lumen of the balloon, the 3 ml syringe can be refilled from the 10 ml syringe while the balloon is refilled from the 3 ml syringe—all through a completely closed system. The smaller, 3 ml syringe provides a means of filling the balloon *more accurately*, but 3 ml only fills the balloon twice at the most. The small syringe is refilled repeatedly from the 10 ml syringe without having to return to the CO_2 canister for each refill of the balloon or 3 ml syringe.

Radio-frequency (RF) generator

With refinements in radio-frequency generators and FDA approval of controlled perforations using radio-frequency energy, a radio-frequency (RF) generator specifically for perforation is now a standard piece of equipment in the pediatric/congenital interventional catheterization laboratory. A small perforating generator (Baylis Medical Company, Montreal, Canada) is designed and approved for perforation of the interatrial septum. An even more important (but "off label") use for the RF energy is the perforation of atretic valves or occluded vessels in congenital defects. With the heat from the RF wire tip, very dense natural tissues can be perforated without the use of significant force.

The perforating RF generator uses a specific fine RF wire and tiny catheter (Baylis Medical Co. Inc., Montreal, Canada), which pass through a preformed, torque controlled, end hole guiding catheter to the desired position to be perforated. When the RF wire/generator is used, a relatively large "grounding pad" is fixed on the surface of the patient's skin to complete the "circuit" during the energy generation.

The RF generator for perforating does not have a maximum temperature limit for the catheter tip like the RF generator used for the ablation of intracardiac electrical pathways. Without some significant internal engineering adjustments within the generator for each case, the perforating RF generator cannot be used interchangeably with the ablation RF generator and, as a consequence, requires a separate RF generator from the ablation RF generator. The perforating generators and equipment are discussed in detail in Chapter 31.

Capital equipment which is desirable but not routinely or necessarily available in pediatric/congenital catheterization laboratories and which also require associated consumable items

A variety of different equipment which requires fairly expensive consumable accessories initially was used primarily in investigational studies in pediatric/congenital catheterization laboratories. At the present time, this type of equipment is being used more regularly in a few pediatric/congenital interventional catheterization laboratories. This equipment includes intravascular ultrasound (IVUS), intracardiac echocardiography (ICE) and the Doppler needles.

Intravascular ultrasound (IVUS)

Intravascular ultrasound (IVUS) has had considerable, but sporadic, use in the pediatric/congenital therapeutic catheterization laboratory. Most of the IVUS is used in studying the walls of vessel before, immediately after and in the long-term follow-up after various balloon dilations or intravascular stent implants. At the same time that pathologic lesions are being studied, the operators are still determining the normal appearance for these vessels by IVUS imaging. The findings have been striking, very interesting, and at times even frightening, however, the IVUS findings seldom significantly influence decisions about the particular pediatric/congenital lesion or patients. The same situation occurs with the study of the coronary arteries in the pediatric cardiac transplant patients—interesting findings but not correlated with management decisions.

Although many feel that the information from IVUS in these lesions is invaluable, the high cost of the dedicated IVUS machine itself, the additional significant cost of each of the disposable IVUS catheters and, finally, the lack of definitive decisions which can be made from the IVUS findings at present has led to the very slow acceptance of the technique. Almost certainly, as experience with IVUS increases, there will be greater correlation of the findings from IVUS with the clinical outcomes and, in turn, the use of IVUS will increase until it becomes an integral part of every pediatric/congenital cardiac catheterization laboratory.

Intracardiac echo (ICE) apparatus

The use of intravascular echo (ICE) for the placement of occlusion devices for atrial septal defects (ASD) has generated significant interest in the use of ICE in the pediatric/congenital catheterization laboratory in the past few years. Intracardiac echo provides dramatic, clear and easily understandable views of intracardiac structures. Intracardiac echo does require a reorientation of thinking about intracardiac images and requires the use of an additional 11-French venous access site. Like the IVUS machine, the basic ICE console is very expensive, but often the console used for the transesophageal echo (TEE) is the same console as for the ICE catheters, which makes the console more available. On the other hand the cost of the ICE catheters is even worse than that of the IVUS catheters, with each disposable ICE catheter being very expensive. At present, ICE images are equivalent to TEE images in most cases although there are situations where the images are very discrepant. The cost of using single-use ICE catheters is calculated to be less than the combined cost of the TEE and associated cost of general anesthesia for ASD implants. There is now the capability of having ICE catheters resterilized commercially and each catheter can be reused three times, reducing the per use cost significantly. Most pediatric institutions at the present time, however, find it hard to justify switching to the use of ICE instead of TEE while still utilizing general anesthesia for the interventional catheterization procedure. If and when ICE probes come down in both size and price, ICE could replace TEE for the placement of ASD occlusion devices.

Doppler needles

To help locate vessels for percutaneous puncture, there is a tiny, disposable Doppler probe, which functions through a special needle and comes as a set—the Smart Needle™. The needle/probe is attached to a disposable sterile cable, which attaches to a small, portable, reusable, Doppler machine. The special needle is filled with saline or flush solution and introduced just barely into the superficial cutaneous tissues and the fluid level in the needle checked and refilled. The needle must remain full of fluid in order to transmit a Doppler signal. The Doppler probe is introduced into the intact fluid column within the special needle while the needle full of fluid is positioned in the very superficial subcutaneous tissues. The angle and depth of the needle/probe are directed toward the desired vessel according to the intensity of the Doppler signal generated from the probe within the needle. The quality of the signal from these Doppler needles distinguishes between arterial and venous flow and can determine the side-to-side location of the particular vessel by the changing intensity of the particular signal. The intensity of the signal does not help to determine depth *per se*, however, as the tip of the needle/probe touches *and compresses* the wall of the vessel, the signal does change significantly.

The Doppler apparatus itself is a capital item, but is used with the special disposable needles and probes, which represent a significant, ongoing expense. There are only two sizes of the needle/Doppler probe combination available, the smaller of which is a 20-gauge, which is not particularly useful for small infants where this technology theoretically could be very useful. The Doppler needles are much more effective for larger vessels where it usually is not as necessary to have a Doppler signal to find the vessel.

Entirely disposable consumable equipment

Each separate piece of expendable equipment in the catheterization laboratory is chosen carefully and specifically for the utility and safety of its use while, at the same time, considering the cost of the item. Because of the complexity of the procedures performed in the modern pediatric/congenital cardiac catheterization laboratory, each procedure has its own requirements for specialized catheters and other pieces of consumable equipment. The requirement for a specialized piece of equipment is frequently unpredictable or changes during any one procedure. As a consequence, a modern pediatric/congenital cardiac catheterization laboratory is obligated to carry a very large inventory of a huge variety of consumable items. The size of this inventory is magnified in the pediatric/congenital laboratory by the large variation in the size of the patients (from a few kilograms to a few hundred kilograms) and the infinite varieties of defects and procedures encountered.

In spite of the huge variety of equipment which is available and used for congenital heart patients, very little of this equipment is designed (or intended) for use in pediatric or congenital cardiac catheterization procedures. The consumable equipment which is developed specifically for the pediatric/congenital heart procedures is often manufactured in very small volumes and then requires even more precision (often hand) manufacturing. This in turn, often results in very high costs for the individual items. In spite of their high costs, almost all of the consumable equipment for use in the catheterization laboratory is for one-off use only and is disposable. These combined factors necessitate a very expensive as well as large inventory for each laboratory performing catheterizations on pediatric/congenital heart patients.

The alternative, which is a common practice outside of the United States, is to have each piece of consumable equipment supplied and delivered individually for each separate case by the equipment vendors. This, of course is dependent upon a *demonstrated, reliable and rapid* source of direct vendor supply to the individual catheterization laboratory and very precise pre-planning of each case. Even with the best of planning, this policy does not take into account unexpected findings which occur every day in catheterization laboratories which are studying and treating congenital heart lesions. Also, with the vendor system, each individual piece of equipment is far more costly to the hospital or the patient. The vendors are reimbursed for maintaining the large inventory of equipment (instead of the hospital) and, in addition, are reimbursed for their time and availability. All of these expenses of the vendors are included in the cost of the equipment to the consumer.

The total inventory of consumable equipment in each laboratory varies with the individual physicians working in the laboratory and with the types of procedures performed in the particular laboratory. There are often many similar items which can be used to accomplish the same result, so the particular piece of equipment which is used varies with the preference and experience of the operators, the economics and the "customs" of the particular laboratory. This technical manual obviously emphasizes those preferred by the author. Because of continual improvements in the consumable equipment and the availability of certain items, the specialty items and even the equipment routinely used in any laboratory change frequently. Most of the specialized equipment (needles, wires, sheaths, dilators, catheter, etc.) mentioned in this section is discussed in detail in later sections dealing with specific techniques or procedures using it.

General consumable items

There is some consumable equipment that is required in every cardiac catheterization procedure and is provided for every case, regardless of what additional, more specific items are necessary for a particular procedure. These include flush solutions, connecting and flush/pressure tubing, "manifolds" (which include stopcocks and pressure transducers), and the catheterization "trays" or "packs" for the catheterization table.

Flush solutions

Each procedure requires a quantity of sterile, physiologic fluid for flushing transducers, connecting tubing and catheters. It is also necessary to have some additional fluid solution on the table, usually in a bowl, for rinsing/flushing pieces of equipment which are not connected to the flush/pressure system.

The safest and most satisfactory sources of fluids for the catheterization laboratories are the 500 or 1,000 ml, *collapsable plastic* ***bags*** of physiologic fluids. The bags are far superior and safer than the older bottles of these fluids. The collapsible bags are emptied *completely* of any air initially and then safely pressurized by an *external* pressure bag. Once the bags have been prepared *properly* and *meticulously*, there is absolutely *no* danger of ever pumping air into the system and/or the patient, regardless of the amount of fluid remaining in the bag or the position of the bag.

The safety of the collapsible bags of fluid is in stark contrast to the constant potential danger of the older *bottles* of flush solution. The bottles were frequently pressurized by pumping air under pressure ***into*** *the bottle of fluid*! If a bottle emptied or got tilted while in use so that the outlet to the tubing was placed toward the top of the bottle, the air under pressure above the fluid level preferentially and very forcefully entered the flush system (and the patient if the tubing was connected to the catheter!).

With fluid bags, a special intravenous tubing set containing a sharp hollow spike is introduced or "spiked" through a tubular port in the bottom of the bag. After the bag has being spiked, it is turned upside down so that the port is situated at the *top* of the bag. Once the tubing is connected into the bag, the bag is squeezed until ***all the air*** rises out of it and is forced out of the connecting tubing to be followed by an intact column of the fluid in the tubing. When the bag is completely empty of air, 3 units of heparin are added to each ml of flush solution through the second, adjacent port on the bag. Once the bag and the connecting tubing are emptied completely of air and the heparin has been added, the bag is turned over to the upright position so the ports (or openings) are oriented at the bottom of the bag. Once the bag and tubing are cleared completely of air with the tubing now coming out of the bottom of the bag, there is no way for air to enter the system passively, even if the bag while still under pressure is placed on its side or even with the ports positioned at the top as the bag empties completely! In order to generate pressure in the bags for flushing, pressure is applied to the *outside of the bags* of fluid with a pressure cuff.

The fluid bags with their tubing are supplied from the manufacturers in sterile packaging and can be maintained sterile if they are to be used directly on the sterile catheterization field.

Connecting and flush/pressure tubing

Each catheterization procedure requires a variety of tubing for fluid delivery to the patient and for the transmission of pressure from the catheter to the pressure transducers. The tubing extending from the fluid bags to the manifold is discussed above. If desired, this tubing is maintained sterile when it is opened and when it is connected to the fluid bags or transducers. The tubing carries the fluid under pressure from bags of flush solution to a system of stopcocks, or "manifold", where the fluid is distributed to the pressure transducers and to the separate pressure tubing, which attaches to indwelling lines and catheters which, in turn, are in the patient.

All tubing that is to transmit pressure for recording must be *non-compliant* tubing in order to transmit the pressure accurately and reproducibly. This requires tubing which is thick walled and non-elastic, but at the same time transparent and flexible. These fluid/pressure lines connecting to the patient's catheters/lines should have small lumens in order to minimize the amount of fluid delivered to the patient when the tubing/catheters are flushed. This becomes particularly important when the entire length of tubing must be flushed thoroughly after a medication is administered through the length of the tubing. Ideally, each separate length of tubing between separate catheters/lines in the patient and each separate transducer is color-coded to correspond to the color of the specific pressure tracing from the transducer as it is displayed on the monitor. This is extremely convenient, or even essential, when more than two pressure lines are being used. The color-coding of each separate tubing facilitates communication between the catheterizing physician, the manifold nurse/technician and the recording nurse/technician and, in turn, increases the accuracy and efficiency of recording, flushing and changing gains on specific lines/transducers. The length of tubing on the field which extends from the catheter in the patient to the manifold, is maintained sterile except for the end which is connected to the manifold of stopcocks, which usually is off the field.

Manifold system

The "manifold" is a system of three-way stopcocks in series. The series of stopcocks allows the connection of the line(s) from the fluid bags to all of the transducers and, in turn, the transducers to the separate pressure lines and allows the lines from the fluid source to be diverted directly to the pressure/flush lines. The manifold can be built individually for each case with a series of three-way stopcocks clamped together in line, however, there are now a variety of commercially available manifolds that are manufactured (Merit Medical Systems, Salt Lake City, UT, and Argon Medical, Athens, TX) to suit almost any desired set-up or number of transducers. The manufactured manifolds not only are more convenient, but are cheaper and more secure than creating one's own with separate stopcocks and separate transducers.

Preferably, the manifold is mounted "remotely" and out of the sterile catheterization field on a stand, which, however, is attached to the side or end of the catheterization table. The manifold stand is adjustable in height. The height of the manifold (and transducers) positioned on the catheterization table is adjusted at the beginning of each case according to the anterior–posterior diameter (thickness) of the chest of different patients. This allows the series of transducers to be positioned at the mid position (mid-cardiac level) in the posterior–anterior diameter of any particular patient's chest. Once fixed on the edge of the table, the manifold, and in turn the transducer remain at a fixed height relative to the patient's heart/chest, regardless of the up or down movements of the table and patient.

Pressure transducers

Pressure transducers are very accurate electromechanical devices for measuring pressure. External transducers are connected to catheters and indwelling lines in the patient through the pressure/flush lines and the manifold. Each transducer, in turn, is connected electrically to the physiologic recorder, where it is calibrated and balanced electronically. Most modern catheterization laboratories utilize relatively inexpensive, but very accurate, disposable transducers designed for one-off use (Merit Medical Systems, Salt Lake City, UT and Argon Medical, Athens, TX). In spite of their disposable labeling, these transducers remain very stable even through multiple uses and frequently are used for several cases before being discarded.

When transducers are connected through a manifold, they are isolated from the sterile field (and any blood/fluid from the patient) by the length of the indwelling catheters or monitoring lines plus the length of the flush/pressure tubing and, in turn, are not contaminated by blood during any one case, unless fluid backs up through the entire length (100–150 cm) of catheter/flush/pressure tubing. As a consequence each transducer, when attached through a remote manifold system, is used several times before being discarded. When reused, the transducers are reattached to new sterile tubing, flushed with sterile flush solution and recalibrated and balanced. The transducers are re-balanced to "air zero", occasionally during each case as well as between cases. When there is any question about the accuracy of a disposable transducer, it is discarded and replaced quickly and easily. Each transducer has its own calibration factor, which usually must be entered into the electronic recording equipment. When a pressure from a single location is transmitted through *two separate lines to two different transducers*, a single pressure tracing (line) should be produced on the monitor (*see* Figure 10.1). This provides a rapid, very easy check of the accuracy of a new transducer which is introduced into the system.

Catheterization "packs"

Every catheterization procedure requires one or more sterile drapes over the patient on the catheterization table, operating gowns for all of the scrubbed personnel, towels, sterile wipes ("4 × 4s"), bowls for flush solution and waste fluids, multiple syringes, several needles, a knife blade, tubing/towel clamps, containers for medications or contrast solution, sterile drapes for the adjacent side-tables, sterile covers for the equipment that is immediately adjacent to the sterile field (X-ray tubes, image intensifiers, radiation screens, etc.) and occasional other items which are unique to a particular catheterization laboratory.

In modern cardiac catheterization laboratories, all of these items are disposable and are set up as a tray on a table adjacent to the catheterization table to suit the preferences and needs of each individual case and operator. Most of these items can be available, packaged together commercially, as a single, sterile "pack" or "set", which is prepared to suit the needs of a particular catheterization laboratory. When the specifically manufactured commercial packs are used, once the pack is opened and arranged on the adjacent (sterile) worktable, for the most part, the case is ready to begin. Usually a few individual, extra disposable items like special introductory needles and wires for the particular case, the color-coded connecting/flush tubing which is used between the catheters and the transducers, gloves and extra gowns for each scrubbed physician/nurse, and any special drapes are added to the materials in the standard pack. Most catheterization laboratories utilize a few reusable/sterilizable metal items like scissors, needle holders and instrument clamps, which are added to the tray during the set-up.

In addition to their convenience, the table set-ups using all disposable items have several other major advantages. The most significant advantage of the disposable "tray and set-up" is the safety factor at the end of the case. Once the very few reusable items and sharps are removed from the catheterization table, the entire table drape containing all of the contaminated consumable equipment and materials is rolled up as one, contained mass of contaminated (bloodied) materials without any of these individual items having to be touched by any individual. The single contained mass is disposed of in a "bio-hazard" trash container with only the one, single handling and that from the *outside* of the mass of contaminated material! As a consequence, the individual contaminated items from the catheterization are not handled by any of the personnel in the laboratory. In addition, none of the materials are handled subsequently by *any hospital personnel* for the purpose of separating and cleaning, as is necessary with reusable items.

An additional advantage in most industrialized societies who utilize accurate cost accounting is that the disposable packs are cheaper than the combined initial cost of all of the comparable reusable items plus the additional costs of the labor for the cleaning, repackaging, sterilizing, stocking and redistributing of all of these items.

Unique consumable items for each particular case

In addition to the "general" consumable items used during every case, each separate catheterization procedure requires some special individualized items depending upon the patient's size, the procedure being performed and the preferences of the individual catheterizing physician(s). These items are requested specifically before or during each particular case.

Needles for percutaneous puncture

The ideal needles are chosen for the single wall puncture technique, which is preferred for the percutaneous entry into all vessels and is discussed in detail subsequently in Chapter 4[2]. The entry technique into the vessels is very similar to the introduction of a needle into a peripheral vein, except that in the catheterization laboratory the vessel usually is not visible, and often not even palpable. The needles which are used for the percutaneous technique using a single wall puncture are small in diameter, thin-walled, short beveled and, at the same time, very sharp needles. When a needle with a *long bevel* at the tip is introduced at any angle to the vessel, the tip and bevel of the needle incise through both the front and back walls of a small vessel while the lumen of the needle is still not within or does not align with the lumen of the vessel. A *short-beveled* needle, on the other hand, allows the lumen of the needle to fit within and align better within the lumen of the vessel once the vessel is punctured. The longer, sharp, cutting edge on the tip of the long-beveled needle lacerates multiple structures, including the vessel, as it enters the tissues. The shorter bevel, on the other hand, tends to dissect through the tissues as opposed to lacerating them. At the other extreme, a needle which has a bevel that is too short or is dull, loses *all* of its cutting ability in penetrating the tissues and/or the vessel and tends to dissect past and push the vessels aside as it is introduced into the subcutaneous tissues.

There *must* be an absolutely smooth taper from the inside of the hub of the needle into the lumen of the needle. There can be no inner ridges, flanges or edges which would interfere with the absolutely smooth passage of a wire from the hub of the needle into the attached shaft/lumen of the needle. It is preferable that the hub of the needle is clear in order to have an immediate, clear view of the fluid/blood returning into the needle. The AMC needles (Argon Medical, Athens, TX) have these ideal characteristics and are available in various sizes (diameters) and lengths. The smallest diameter needle is used, which will accommodate the spring guide wire which is being used for the percutaneous introduction. The shaft of the needle only needs to be long enough to reach the vessel through the subcutaneous tissues. The needle should be significantly *smaller in diameter than the vessel* which is being punctured and entered. With a smaller diameter needle, the entire tip, not just an edge or part of the tip of the needle, enters the vessel cleanly. For infants and small children, a 21-gauge needle approximately 3 cm in length is used. For larger children and young adults of normal body stature, a 19-gauge needle approximately 5 cm in length is used, and for very large or obese patients, an 18-gauge 7–8 cm long needle is used. The correct technique for the use of these needles is described in more detail in Chapter 4 (Needle, Wire, Catheter Introduction).

The true "Seldinger™ technique" is not used for percutaneous puncture into vessels. With the Seldinger™ technique, the needle purposefully passes through *both* the front and back walls of the vessel. A true Seldinger™ puncture technique requires a special, two-component, Seldinger™ needle, which has a solid, sharp trocar within the lumen of a hollow blunt cannula[3]. The special Seldinger™ needle is a thin-walled, absolutely *blunt tipped*, hollow metal cannula with a squared-off tip and a Luer-lock proximal hub. A sharp, solid, metal stylet or trocar fits snugly within the hollow cannula and extends just beyond the tip of the cannula. The blunt tip of this outer metal cannula tapers smoothly onto the surface of the inner stylet/trocar. The combined inner stylet and outer cannula make up the Seldinger™ needle. The solid inner stylet/trocar has a sharp, beveled tip which extends beyond the blunt tip of the hollow cannula. The sharpened bevel *of the stylet* provides the tip for puncturing the tissues and vessel.

The stylet is fixed within the outer squared-off or blunt cannula during the Seldinger puncture. The combined blunt cannula with the contained, beveled stylet is introduced into the tissues and toward the suspected location of the vessel. The tip of the combination trocar/cannula is introduced into the tissues and advanced deep into the subcutaneous tissues, purposefully and completely *through* the *front and back walls* of the vessel. Once the combination stylet/cannula has been introduced well into the tissues and the vessel *presumably* has been transected, the inner, solid, sharp stylet/trocar is withdrawn from the cannula. Obviously, with the Seldinger™ technique, the needle set is purposefully passed completely through both the front and back walls of the vessel. With the stylet completely out of the blunt cannula, the hub and proximal end of the blunt cannula are pressed against and more parallel to the skin surface while the cannula is withdrawn very slowly from within the tissues and (hopefully) back into the lumen of vessel. The Seldinger™ technique and its modifications are described in detail in Chapter 4.

The Chiba™ needle is another very special needle used when the transhepatic technique is used for percutaneous vessel entry. The Chiba™ needle is similar to a Seldinger™ needle but with a very long blunt outer plastic cannula and a long sharp inner metal stylet. The Chiba™ needle is described in more detail in the discussion of vessel introduction by the transhepatic puncture technique in Chapter 4.

Guide wires for cardiac catheterization

There is an infinite variety of guide wires available from multiple manufacturers for use in the cardiac catheterization laboratory. Most guide wires used in the cardiac catheterization laboratory are of spring steel wire construction and consist of a very smooth, hollow winding of a *very fine* stainless steel wire. The central lumen within this outer winding of very fine wire contains a central, relatively stiff straight "core" wire and a soft and very flexible fine, ribbon-like, safety wire. Variations in these three components and how they are used together create the specific characteristics of each individual guide wire. The safety wire extends the entire length of the outer winding and is fixed ("welded") at both ends of the outer wire winding. The core wire is between 1 and 15 cm shorter than the safety wire and the outer winding wire at the distal end. The absence of core wire at the distal end creates the softer more flexible tip of the spring guide wire. Some guide wires have a core wire which tapers to a very fine distal tip and is attached at both ends of the outer wire windings and replaces the separate safety wire.

All spring guide wires should be treated very gently during use. They should never be forced into any location nor should dilators and catheters be *forced* over them. The operator must constantly be aware of the entire length of wire in order to prevent perforation through vascular structures by the tip of the wire, and the formation of kinks or knots in a portion of the wire that happens to be out of the field of view. Sharp kinks or acute bends in wires are to be avoided in all circumstances, as they prevent the wire from moving freely within the catheter or the catheter from passing over the wire, and eliminate any torque characteristics of the wire. When a kink or sharp bend is created in a wire, it is abandoned.

Wires specifically for vessel entry

The most essential criterion for a guide wire which is used for percutaneous vessel entry is that it has a very soft, flexible (or even floppy), but straight, tip. Even a relatively soft-tipped wire, in actuality, is very stiff and straight as the *first 1 to 2 mm* of the tip of the wire protrudes beyond the tip of the needle. A very floppy tip on the wire is imperative when the needle is not exactly aligned or parallel within the long axis of the lumen of the vessel as the wire is advanced out of the needle. The *extra* soft tip of the wire allows the very distal tip of the wire to bend or be deflected into the lumen of the vessel when the needle is aligned or angled more perpendicularly off the long axis of the vessel. Special "extra" or "very" floppy tipped wires are available for percutaneous entry into very small vessels (Argon Medical, Athens, TX). The wires from Argon are specially designed for this purpose, while there are other wires available with very soft tips which were designed for other uses, such as very small (0.014″) floppy-tipped, coronary guide wires. The "extra" floppy tips are created at the expense of thickness and strength of the core and safety wire components. As a consequence, the "extra" floppy-tipped wires are even more fragile and require even gentler handling.

The size (diameter) of the spring guide wire used for any percutaneous introduction should be of a size significantly *smaller* in diameter than the internal diameter of the needle being used, and never the same size and/or an "exact fit" within the needle. For example, a 0.018″ wire is used within a 21-gauge needle or a 0.021″ wire is used in a 19-gauge needle. The smaller diameter of the wire within the larger lumen of the needle allows for slight, additional, side-to-side play of the wire within the needle lumen, which in turn, allows for freer angulation of the tip of the wire as it is advanced past the tip of the needle and enters into the vessel (*see* Chapter 4 for details of this).

"J"-tipped wires are popular for percutaneous vessel entry, particularly for introduction into the larger vessels. They have the advantage that once the J tips of the wires are well within the vessel, they advance more easily through the vessel without catching on or deflecting into, side branches or tributaries off the central vessel. On the other hand, they have the disadvantage that the tip of the wire forms a sharp angle away from, and essentially perpendicular to, the long axis of the needle as soon as the tip of the wire extends initially beyond the tip of the needle. When the J tip of the wire is extruded, the vessel must be large enough for the distal end of the wire and its tip to enter the vessel "sideways" or the angle of the bevel of the needle must be at an exact angle to be in line with the lumen, which requires that the needle is almost perpendicular to the long axis of the vessel. J-tipped wires are *not* recommended for initial vessel entry through the needle in infants and small children with small vessels or in debilitated patients where the venous pressure is very low. J-tipped wires are recommended only for percutaneous entry into very large vessels which are well distended (e.g. in patients with known higher venous pressure and large veins or in larger arteries). Once the initial wire and a plastic cannula or dilator are well within the vessel, then a J-tipped wire is very useful for advancing the wire tip through the central channel of the vessel.

General usage guide wires

Spring guide wires have many other uses in the catheterization laboratory besides percutaneous entry into vessels. When used in the body within or extending out of catheters, all guide wires should be introduced through a wire backbleed/flush port and maintained on a slow continuous flush. The continuous flush facilitates the movement of a wire that is within a catheter and reduces (eliminates) the possibility of thrombus formation around the wire.

Wires made of different materials, in many sizes (diameters), many lengths and configurations and for many different uses are available. The use of soft straight tipped wires and J-tipped wires for vessel entry has been mentioned. An infinite variation in the degree of softness and the length of the distal soft tip is available in all sizes and configurations of the wires. Wires with long, soft tips are used when they are advanced beyond the tips of catheters, for example to enter into more distal vessels or even to pass carefully through valves in either the prograde or retrograde directions. Some of the floppy tips are manufactured from or coated with special materials like platinum to make them more easily visible. Wires of larger diameter or heavier construction are available to support both small and large catheters during various catheter manipulations, particularly when catheters are advanced over wires which have previously been positioned in specific locations. In order for a guide wire that is positioned within the body to allow a relatively long catheter to be introduced over the wire outside of the body, the wire must be very long. Special "exchange length" (260–300 cm) wires allow even very long catheters to be removed entirely out of the body over the wire with the distal end of the wire still fixed in a particular distal location within the heart or vasculature. Whenever an exchange of a catheter over the wire *may* be a possibility during a catheterization, an exchange length wire is used for the initial positioning.

Many of the spring guide wires are available with special coatings (heparin or teflon), supposedly to make them less thrombogenic and to allow them to slide more easily through catheters. The use of these coated wires is helpful or is imperative to keep the wire and catheter from binding together when using a spring guide wire within any of the extruded plastic catheters. The coatings on the wire, however, do seem to make the coated wires slightly stiffer than the comparable size and type of non-coated wire. As a consequence, coated wires are not recommended for the initial percutaneous introduction into vessels. The coatings presumably make the wires less thrombogenic, however this is not proven and certainly does not remove the necessity of keeping the wire on a continuous flush when it is positioned within a catheter in order to prevent clotting. The exchange length wires and the coated wires are special, and usually more expensive, variations of the more standard spring guide wires; however, they are in such common usage that they usually are not considered special or unique. There are, however, some wires of very special design for unique uses. Extra stiff, or Super Stiff™ wires (Medi-Tech, Boston Scientific, Natick, MA) are available in the standard and exchange lengths. The shafts of the stiffest of these extra-stiff wires are actually very rigid. All of these stiff wires do have a segment of various lengths of a soft or "floppy" distal end. When used properly and in spite of their rigidity, these wires actually make the delivery of stiffer catheters and sheaths much safer, and they provide a much better support for balloon catheters during dilation procedures. They are indispensable for some of the more specialized therapeutic catheterization procedures and their use in these procedures is discussed in more detail in the chapters dealing with those techniques. Special, stiffer wires such as the 0.014″ Iron Man,™ the 0.018″ V-18 Control,™ and the 0.021″ Platinum Plus™ wires are available in these smaller sizes and are very useful for supporting small balloon dilation catheters. These wires were developed primarily for use in coronary arteries, but are invaluable in the cardiac catheterizations of infants and small children.

When the core wire is attached to the outer "winding" wire *throughout* the length of a spring guide wire, it allows the entire length of wire to be rotated (torqued) in a specific direction. If the combined wire and core wire are stiff and rigid enough, the wire can be torqued with a 1:1 ratio of the degree of rotation from end to end. With a curved, soft distal end on these wires, a torque wire can then be directed into very specific locations, into particular vessels, branches or orifices by applying purposeful torque on the proximal wire. The rotation or torquing of the wire is facilitated by a small handle or "torque vise" attached on the proximal shaft of the torque wire. Again, this capability is absolutely essential in the performance of some of the more specialized therapeutic techniques, and is described in detail in Chapter 6.

Another wire which is probably the most unique of the special designs and is very effective for entering difficult locations is the Glide™ or Terumo™ wire (Terumo Medical Corp., Somerset, NJ). This is not a stainless spring guide wire but a long, fine, shaft of uniform diameter, Nitinol™ metal with a hydrophilic coating. The Nitinol™ material of the Terumo™ wire makes it very flexible and at the same time, virtually kink resistant. The hydrophilic coating, *when very wet*, makes the wire extremely slippery, however it becomes sticky and resistant to movement as the coating begins to dry. The combination of the springy shaft material, the slippery characteristics and a soft tip allows the wire to follow even small tortuous channels and to make acute turns when extended out of the tip of the catheter. Although these characteristics make a *freely moving, non-constrained*, tip *less* likely to perforate structures, these same characteristics, however, also allow the wire to penetrate through myocardium and vascular walls more easily than standard spring guide wires. When the tip of the Terumo™ wire is exiting a catheter or the shaft of the wire is otherwise constrained because the shaft cannot bow or bend freely away and, at the same time, the tip is forced against intravascular or intracardiac structures, it readily perforates tissues.

Standard, straight spring guide wires can be curved or formed to particular shapes for special uses. A J or even "pig-tail" curve can be formed on the soft tip of a standard straight spring guide wire. The soft or floppy distal end of the wire is pulled gently between a finger and a sharp straight edge of an opened scissors or clamp similar to curling the end of a piece of ribbon. Enough pressure between the finger and the straight edge is applied to curl the wire, yet not so much pressure is applied that the wire is stripped, pulled apart or the safety wire within the outer winding wire is broken. This curving of a soft wire tip is a learned procedure. Once a slight angled curve is formed on the soft tip of a torque controlled wire, the wire can be directed purposefully from side to side.

Curves formed on the stiff ends of wires are very useful for deflecting the tips of catheters, particularly in deflecting the tip in two or more directions (three-dimensionally) simultaneously. The *stiff end* of a wire is always, and only, used completely *within* a catheter and never extended beyond the tip of the catheter. Curves are formed on the *stiff ends* of standard spring guide wires by manually bending a smooth curve with the fingers or wrapping the stiff end of the wire smoothly around a finger or a small syringe. The stiff end ***cannot*** be curved by pulling it between the finger and a sharp edge like the curving of the soft end. In forming any curve on a wire, special care is taken *not* to create any sharp bends or kinks in the wire. A sharp bend or kink creates resistance or even prohibits the passage of the wire through a needle, dilator, or catheter. A bend or kink along the shaft of a wire also prevents any rotation or torquing of the wire within a catheter. The details for forming these curves and the special uses of these wires are discussed in Chapter 6.

In addition to the use of spring guide wires for adding extra support to catheters and for forming compound curves within catheters, there are special, smooth, fine stainless steel wires which are manufactured especially for the purpose of providing extra support for very floppy catheters and for forming specific curves on catheters. The Mullins' Deflector Wires™ (Argon Medical, Athens, TX) are fine, polished stainless steel wires with a very tiny welded bead or micro ball at each tip. The tiny "bead" at each end keeps these wires from digging into the inner walls of the catheters. These wires are available in 0.015″, 0.017″ and 0.20″ diameters. The details of their use are described in Chapter 6.

There are also special active "deflecting" wires with control handles used for actively deflecting or bending the tip of the wire and, in turn, the tip of catheters (Cook, Inc., Bloomington, IN). These are discussed in more detail in Chapter 6, dealing specifically with deflector wires. The standard guide wires and special wires are available from a variety of manufacturers including Boston Scientific, Cook, Argon, Medtronic and Guidant.

Sheath /dilator sets for catheter introduction

Percutaneous introduction and then the use of an indwelling vascular sheath in vessels is the standard technique used for vascular access in the catheterization of pediatric and congenital heart patients. The advantages and the exact technique of this approach as well as the reasons for particular preferences for certain types of sheath and dilators are covered in detail in Chapter 4, "Catheter Introduction". The specifications of the sheaths and dilators and their specific uses are discussed here. As with the needles and wires, the sheaths and dilators are available in many sizes and varieties and from many different manufacturers, including Argon, Cook, Cordis, Medtronic, Daig, Terumo and Boston Scientific.

The French size of the ***dilator***, like the French size of a catheter, designates the ***outer*** diameter of the dilator. At the same time, the French size of the ***sheath*** designates the ***inner*** diameter of the sheath and/or the diameter of the dilator/catheter that the sheath will accommodate. Usually the outer diameter of the sheath is approximately one French size larger than its advertised (inner) diameter, but depending upon the thickness and the materials from which the sheath is manufactured and the tightness of the fit of the sheath over the dilator, the outer diameter of the sheath can be as much as 2–3 French sizes larger than the stated sheath diameter/size. The Association for the Advancement of Medical Instrumentation (AAMI) established the standards for catheters, sheaths and dilators over three decades ago. The manufacturers agreed that sheaths must have precise manufacturing tolerances for the *minimum diameter of their inner* lumens while dilators and catheters must have equally strict tolerances for their maximum *outer* diameters. A catheter of a stated French size *must* pass smoothly through a sheath of the same advertised French size. A *catheter* should never be advertised as being a particular French size if it is even 0.01 mm larger in diameter than the advertised French size, and sheaths should never be advertised as a particular French size if the lumen is 0.01 mm narrower than the advertised French size. At the same time, when the catheter is passing through a sheath of the same French size, there should be no significant slack or extra space around the catheter within the lumen of the sheath and, in turn, no bleeding around the catheter even when there is no back-bleed valve in place on the sheath!

There are some specific requirements for the ideal sheath/dilator sets used in cardiac catheterizations, particularly in pediatric and congenital patients. The distal end of the dilator should have a long, fine and smoothly tapered tip. The inner lumen of the dilator tip should fit tightly over the guide wire designated for use with the dilator, and the tip of the dilator should have a smooth, fine transitional taper onto the surface of the wire. For example, the tip opening of a 4-, 5-, or 6-French dilator fits snugly over a 0.021″ wire, while a 7-French, or larger, dilator fits snugly over a 0.025″ wire. In order to facilitate manipulation *as a single unit* during their introduction into a vessel, the dilator should lock securely into the sheath when the two are attached together. When the sheath and dilator are locked together, the taper of the dilator should begin at least one cm beyond the tip of the sheath; e.g. if the dilator has a 2 cm long taper, the tip of the dilator should extend 3 cm beyond the tip of the sheath when the hubs are together.

Sheaths should be very thin walled, but their walls should be stiff and firm enough that they do not crumple, kink, or "accordion" on themselves when reasonable forward pressure or torque is applied to the sheaths. Most sheaths are now manufactured from thin teflon tubing. The *tip* of the sheath should fit very tightly over the dilator, so that there is no gap or "interface space" between the outside of the dilator and the inner diameter of the tip of the sheath. The very tip of the sheath actually often tapers slightly to accomplish this tight fit over the dilator. The sheath should have a female Lure™ lock connecting hub at the proximal end and should have an available, but *detachable* back-bleed valve/flush port that is not permanently attached to it.

When introduced from the inguinal area, the sheath should be long enough to extend into the common femoral vein and, when in position there, to have the tip aligned parallel with the iliac vein. In small infants, it is preferable for a sheath that is introduced into the femoral vein to *extend proximal* to the bifurcation of the inferior vena cava. When the *tip* of a short sheath only reaches and is positioned in an iliac vein in an infant, the tip tends to orient *perpendicularly* to the opposite iliac vein. This position traumatizes the vein wall unnecessarily, particularly as various catheter tips are advanced beyond the tip of the sheath. Twelve cm seems to be an optimal compromise in the length of the intravascular portion of the sheath (not including the length of the connection to the hub, the hub and the back-bleed valve) for both infants and larger sized patients.

Sheath/dilator sets for special uses

In addition to sheaths of the usual lengths for peripheral percutaneous introduction, there is now a variety of extra long sheath/dilator sets available from several manufacturers including Cook, Daig, Arrow and Medtronic. These are used to circumvent unusual or difficult vessel introduction sites as well as for special diagnostic and many therapeutic catheterization procedures. Most (all?) of the currently available long sheaths come with attached back-bleed valves/flush ports.

When a vein or an artery somewhere beyond the introductory site has sharp bends or is very tortuous, an extra long sheath which extends through or past the bends and through all of the areas of tortuosity is positioned in the vessel at the onset of the procedure to bypass the bend or tortuosity. With the longer sheath in place, the manipulation around a sharp bend or through the tortuosity is performed only the one time during the introduction of the long sheath/dilator. Thereafter, the indwelling, longer sheath directs wires, catheters and devices through and past the sharp angles or tortuosity with no additional manipulations being necessary. Extra long sheaths are used to guide catheters directly and repeatedly to an area within the heart itself (biopsies, blade catheters), for transseptal procedures, to deliver special devices to particular areas within the heart or great vessels (stents, occlusion devices), and for the withdrawal of foreign bodies from the vascular system. There are large, long, special sheaths from Cook and Arrow which have a metal "braid" or winding in their walls to reinforce the sheaths against kinking. All of these special sheaths are discussed in subsequent chapters dealing with the specialized techniques for which they are used.

All of the sheath/dilator sets which are necessary to accommodate the introduction of all sizes and varieties of catheters and devices which are utilized for all sizes of patients should be available in any laboratory performing extensive pediatric/congenital procedures. The diameters range from the very small 3-French to large 20+-French sheaths. Some sheaths are available with special "pre-curved" tip configurations, and most sheath/dilator sets can be specifically formed by using some form of heat to soften the sheath material first. Many of the various French sizes are available in extra long lengths as well as in the standard vessel introductory lengths, and many additional lengths can be obtained by special order.

Hemostasis (back-bleed)/flush valves on sheaths

Back-bleed, or hemostasis, valves prevent blood loss from a sheath when a wire or catheter is/are in the sheath, or from a catheter when a wire is in the catheter. A hemostasis valve allows the use of catheters several sizes smaller than the sheath and the manipulation of wires through catheters or sheaths even when the catheter tip is in a high-pressure area. These valves are of two basic types. The most common type contains either a leaflet or diaphragm-like valve, which in the resting state is totally closed but opens or expands passively to accommodate the catheter or wire as it passes through the valve. The second major type of hemostasis device is the so-called Tuohy™ type valve. This type of back-bleed valve has a compressible, elastic grommet or washer within a screw-tightened hub on the valve. As the hub is tightened on the valve mechanism, the grommet is compressed and flattened, narrowing or even obliterating, the lumen through the grommet.

Most of the valves are available with side ports for flushing and recording pressure. Back-bleed valves *without* flushing side ports should *not* be used for any length of time for either catheters through sheaths or wires through catheters or sheaths! Even with excellent tolerances between the catheter and sheath or the wire within a catheter, blood still seeps back into the sheath around the catheter or into a catheter around a wire. In the presence of a back-bleed valve without the capability of repeated or even continuous flushing through a side port, the blood in the sheath or catheter thromboses. The clotted blood binds the catheter within a sheath or the thrombus is pushed into the vascular system with any subsequent catheter or wire manipulations, exchanges or flushes! A side flushing port on the back-bleed valve allows continual or, at least, frequent intermittent flushing with alternating pressure recording through the sheath. The flushing prevents clotting, lubricates the catheter within the sheath, and allows the use of the sheath as a route for medications. The side port can be used to monitor intravascular pressure through the sheath when the catheter which is in the sheath has a smaller French size than the sheath, or through the catheter while there is a wire in place. The side port may have a connecting plastic tube off the valve apparatus or be as simple as a "Y" port off the side of the valve. To be usable for pressure recording, any tubing off the back-bleed valve must be of *non-compliant* material.

Many back-bleed valves/flush ports are a fixed, permanent part of the sheath. Although the valve mechanisms in many of the attached back-bleed units are quite good, the fixed or permanently attached hemostasis valves have several significant disadvantages. The side flush/pressure arm of the unit prevents the sheath/dilator set from being adequately and/or rapidly rotated while the sheath/dilator is being introduced into the skin, subcutaneous tissues and the vessel. With a fixed back-bleed valve system on the sheath, the catheter must always be maneuvered/manipulated through the back-bleed valve. Even with the very best of these valves, the valve *always* offers significant resistance to the movement/manipulation of any catheter which passes through it and, in turn, compromises the ability to torque the catheter. Of equal, or greater, significance, the back-bleed valve gripping the catheter compromises the tactile sensation transmitted from the catheter (within the vasculature) to the operator's hands during catheter maneuvers. There is no way for the operator to discriminate between the force required to overcome the resistance of the valve or the force required to move or torque the catheter within the heart, or even from the force of a catheter *perforating* a vascular structure! Some of the hemostasis valves are worse than others, with some valves almost totally prohibiting the movement of the catheter through the valve.

Separate, detachable back-bleed valves with side ports are available as separate units from Argon Medical (Athens, TX), Burron OEM Division of B. Braun Medical Inc. (Bethlehem, PA) and Maxxim Medical (Clearwater, FL). A detachable back-bleed valve gives the operator the option of using it attached to the hub of the sheath, a combination of using the valve intermittently attached or not using the valve at all. The detachable valve can be loosened or even removed during the introduction of the sheath/dilator. Loosening or removing the back-bleed valve allows free, rapid rotation or spinning of the sheath or dilator as they are advanced through the skin and subcutaneous tissues. Then, when desired, the hemostasis valve can be reattached to the sheath once it is in the vessel. When a catheter is manipulated within a sheath of the same specified French size as the catheter (and the sheath and catheter are manufactured with proper tolerances), bleeding does not occur around the catheter and out of the sheath even without the back-bleed valve. If the manufacturing tolerances are very precise, the hemostasis valve on the sheath will not be necessary to prevent bleeding around the catheter even in an artery. Ideally, once the catheter is introduced through a detachable valve into the sheath, the back-bleed valve can be detached from the sheath and withdrawn back over the shaft of the catheter and all of the way to the hub of the catheter. In this position, the back-bleed valve is completely out of the way and does not interfere with catheter manipulation. Any time when the catheter is not being manipulated, if unusual bleeding does occur around the catheter or when a catheter is being exchanged through the sheath, the back-bleed valve apparatus is reattached to the sheath. With or without the back-bleed valve attached to the sheath, a moist sponge is kept on (around) the catheter just at the hub of the sheath in order to keep the surface of the catheter lubricated and prevent fine clots from forming on the catheter surface and within the sheath.

Most of the valve-type, catheter back-bleed devices do *not* seal tightly around guide or deflector wires which pass through them, and many of these hemostasis valves on the sheaths are totally unsatisfactory for preventing bleeding around a wire. In those situations, the procedure is planned so that whenever a wire passes through these valves, the wire is always within a catheter or, at least, through a short dilator which fits tightly over the wire.

The Tuohy™ type back-bleed valves are frequently used for wires within catheters, in sheaths and on some very special types of delivery catheters (Cook Inc., Bloomington, IN, B. Braun, Bethlehem, PA, and Meditech/Boston Scientific, Natick, MA). With the Tuohy™ type valves, it is more cumbersome to adjust the optimal tightness around wires or catheters, and frequently there is no satisfactory, intermediate adjustment between leaking significantly or no movement of the wire through the valve at all. When most Tuohy™ valves are tightened enough to totally prohibit leaking, they are closed so tightly that they also prohibit *any movement* of the wire that is passing through the valve. The rigid "Y" side port along with a very tight valve does allow very accurate pressure recording through the side port of the valve even with a wire passing through it. Tuohy™ valves are sturdy enough to withstand high-pressure contrast injections through them without allowing any leakage around the wire. Larger Tuohy™ valves can be used as a detachable back-bleed/flush valve for smaller catheters.

In addition to the previous two types of "official" back-bleed valve/flush ports for sheaths and catheters, there are small, inexpensive, "wire back-bleed" or Hemostasis Valves (Cordis Corp., Miami, FL) with side-flushing tubing, which function extremely well as wire back-bleed valves/flush ports when attached to the hub of a catheter. These back-bleed valves were originally designed to be used on the hubs of indwelling intravenous lines as a port for repeated injections. The valve was punctured with a needle each time medications or fluids needed to be introduced into the indwelling line.

The ports are less than one cm in length and have a distal male slip lock attachment, which fits into the hub of a standard female Luer-lock hub/connector of a catheter. They now have a very thin latex diaphragm across the proximal, unattached end and a flushing port/tubing off one side of the small valve port. A wire introducer or needle is passed through a center hole in the latex diaphragm and the wire is introduced through it. The introducer is removed from the diaphragm over the wire, leaving the wire in place through the diaphragm. The latex diaphragm produces a tight seal around the wire, which prevents any back bleeding and allows a continuous or intermittent flush or pressure recording around any wire passing through the valve and catheter. These valves are not sturdy enough to allow for pressure angiography through them. They are now used routinely whenever any type of wire is used within a catheter.

Catheters

There are innumerable types and an extremely large variety of the many types of cardiac catheter available for diagnostic and therapeutic procedures in the pediatric/congenital catheterization laboratory. Like the other materials used in pediatric/congenital catheterizations, very few of these catheters were designed or intended for use in pediatric/congenital patients. Multiple different cardiac catheters are available from many different manufacturers; often, a large variety of catheters are available from each of the manufacturers, and new varieties appear every month. Some of the major manufacturers of catheters that are used in pediatric/congenital cardiac catheterizations include those from Medtronic (the old USCI™ catheters), Cook, Cordis, Maxim (Argon), Mallinckrodt, NuMED, Arrow and B. Braun. Every catheter has minor or major variations from the catheters of other types or from catheters of similar types from different manufacturers. Each variation is designed to enhance the usability of the catheter for a specific purpose. Catheters vary in the materials from which they are manufactured, whether they are intended to be flow guided or torque controlled, whether they are end hole or closed ended angiographic catheters and whether they are pre-shaped or are shapable. The exact choice of catheter used in any particular situation should be primarily the choice of an experienced individual catheterizing physician, although the medical director of the laboratory is responsible for the total inventory of a catheterization laboratory. The choice of catheter which is used depends upon its specific characteristics, availability and, often, price.

Cardiac catheters are manufactured from a variety of materials. The catheters that were used initially in cardiology were originally manufactured for urologic use. These catheters were constructed of woven dacron with a polyurethane coating (USCI, Billerica, NY). Some of these same catheters with very slight modifications are still in use and available through Medtronic Inc. (Minneapolis, MN). Fine dacron fibers are woven around a hollow nylon core and then coated with polyurethane. This produces a catheter that is relatively stiff, has excellent (1:1) torque qualities and has the unique characteristic of the shaft's smoothly following the tip when advanced through curves. Modifications which have been made in woven dacron catheters include special tips and specific curves at the tips for special uses. These catheters are still in use and still represent the "gold standard" for all subsequent torque-controlled catheters.

Because of the complexity, expense, limited permanent shaping possible with the woven dacron and, at the same time, the exploding market for cardiac catheters, alternative manufacturing techniques were developed and have persisted. The large majority of present-day catheters are constructed from tubing extruded from different plastic materials including polyethylene and teflon. Each material or technique of extrusion imparts a different characteristic to the final catheter. Some of the tubing is extruded over a mesh or weave of wire or fibers in order to enhance the strength or torque capabilities of the final catheter. No combination of materials or added fillings in the extruded material has yet matched the ideal characteristics of woven dacron as a malleable torque-controlled cardiac catheter.

The extruded materials do have the advantage that very specific and fairly permanent curves can be shaped into the distal ends of the catheters, which makes them ideal for certain selective applications where overall maneuverability is not as important. The extruded tubing also can be manufactured containing multiple lumens or can be made softer and more pliable for use in flow-directed or "floating" catheters. The extruded materials have the capability of being coated with other materials to make them less thrombogenic and/or more slippery. Therapeutic catheters are all manufactured from extruded materials where the versatility of the tubing is necessary for some of their unique features.

Diagnostic cardiac catheters are divided into two large, completely different groups—guidable or *torque-controlled* catheters and flow-directed ("floating") balloon catheters. Each of these two types of catheter are subdivided into "end-hole", diagnostic catheters and closed-ended, angiographic catheters. The specific uses of these varieties of catheter are described in detail in Chapters 5 and 7. The characteristics of the various catheters are described here.

The major difference between cardiac catheters is whether the catheters are totally torque-controlled or flow-directed. Torque-controlled catheters generally have a stiffer shaft and have a favorable ratio of torque or rotation of the tip in relation to torque or rotation applied to the proximal end of the catheter, which gives them the capability of being specifically and selectively directed. Flow-directed catheters have a small balloon mounted at the tip, which is intended to pull the catheter along with the flow of blood with minimal directional control. The shaft of flow-directed catheters is usually softer and has little, or no, torque properties. Both flow-directed and torque-controlled catheters have some special advantages or special uses, which are described in Chapter 5—Catheter Manipulation and Chapter 7—Flow Directed Catheters, respectively.

Both torque-controlled and floating catheters are available as end-hole catheter and closed-ended catheters. End-hole catheters have an extension of the central lumen through the *distal* tip of the catheter and usually have several or more side holes close to the tip. They are utilized in diagnostic catheterization procedures when wedge pressures or wedge angiograms are desired. An end-hole catheter is used when there is a need to advance a guide wire out of and beyond the tip of the catheter either for special manipulations into specific areas or when one catheter needs to be exchanged over a pre-positioned guide wire for another catheter.

Angiographic or closed-ended catheters have a closed distal end with several side holes close to the distal tip. The closed end of the catheter helps to prevent recoil of the catheter during rapid, high volume or high-pressure injections of contrast through the catheter. The angiographic catheter with a closed end can be used equally well for blood sampling and pressure recordings except in the "wedge" positions. Some angiographic catheters, in addition to the side holes, do have an end hole. In these catheters the end hole either is narrowed relative to the remainder of the catheter lumen or the end of the catheter is formed into a tightly curved, roughly 360°, loop or "pig tail". The rest of the physical characteristics of end-hole and closed-ended angiographic catheters are very similar. The major differences between them depend upon the materials from which they are manufactured.

There now is a combination or "hybrid" catheter, which combines some of the advantages of the end-hole catheter with some advantages of a closed-ended, angiographic catheter. This hybrid catheter is the Multi-track™ catheter. The main lumen of the Multi-track™ catheter can have either an open or a closed distal tip; however, in addition to this catheter lumen, there is a small, short tube or loop of the catheter material which accommodates a guide wire and is attached to but offset to the side of the distal tip of the shaft of the catheter. The loop or short tube at the tip is passed over a pre-positioned guide wire, which allows the catheter to be advanced along the wire over the short tube at the tip, which, in turn, guides the tip of the catheter over the wire. As a consequence, the wire runs outside of the true lumen of the catheter and adjacent to its shaft, and the true lumen of the catheter is not used or compromised at all by the wire. This allows for larger volume angiography or the passage of an additional wire through the true lumen of the catheter while the original guide wire still is in place and supporting the tip of the catheter through the short tube.

When a Multi-track™ catheter is introduced through a percutaneous sheath, the Multi-track™ does have the disadvantage of the guide wire running *outside* of the catheter and adjacent to the shaft of the catheter within the sheath. This, in turn, requires a significantly larger diameter introductory sheath along with a *very competent* hemostasis valve on the sheath in order to prevent bleeding around the wire, which remains passing through the valve *adjacent* to the catheter. Another significant problem with the Multi-track™ catheters, when compared to a catheter which has the wire passing through its true lumen, is their poorer ability to track or follow a wire within the heart. This is a particular problem when the course of the wire has one or more loops in it. This problem can be partially overcome by placing a second wire within the true lumen of the Multi-track™ in order to stiffen the shaft of the Multi-track™ as it is being advanced.

The preferred general purpose and "universal" diagnostic catheters are the torque-controlled catheters. With a proper curve on the tip of the catheter, the use of guide wires or deflector wires as aids in their manipulation, and with skillful manipulation, these catheters can be maneuvered into all desired locations. The precise maneuverability of these catheters depends on the materials from which they are manufactured as well as how they are used by the individual physician who is performing the catheterization. Most torque-controlled catheters are manufactured with some preformed curve at the tip, which may or may not be suitable for the size of the particular patient or the intended use of the catheter. The curve of the tip usually can be modified or reshaped temporarily if not permanently by softening the tip of the catheter with heat and then manually forming the desired curve which fits the size of the specific patient better or the desired target more precisely. The precise positioning/placement of torque-controlled catheters does not depend upon the patient's cardiac output nor the direction or force of blood flow, but does depend, for the most part, on the experience and skill of the catheterizing physician to manipulate them to the proper location. The details of the techniques for the manipulation of torque-controlled catheters are covered in Chapter 5.

Flow directed or "balloon floating" catheters are the other major type of diagnostic cardiac catheter. In order to achieve their floating capability, flow-directed catheters have a small inflatable balloon at the distal tip of the catheter which, when inflated, serves as a small "sail" to pull the catheter along with the blood flow. Flow-directed catheters have completely different physical characteristics from torque-controlled catheters. The shafts of flow-directed catheters are softer and more malleable in order to achieve their floating characteristics. Like torque-controlled catheters, flow-directed catheters are available as both end-hole catheters and closed-ended, angiographic catheters. Angiographic flow-directed catheters are different from wedge or end-hole flow catheters only in that the lumen of the catheter stops at several side holes that are positioned *proximal* to the balloon rather than extending through a single distal end hole beyond the balloon.

Flow-directed (balloon) catheters have the advantage of floating with the *forward* blood flow without the use of much manipulation or skill on the part of the operator. This is particularly true when the blood flow is *normal* or *vigorous*—i.e. in normal circulation. The tips of flow catheters can be pre-curved with *very slight* heat to enhance their floating around curves or into loops with the course of the blood flow. Flow-directed catheters are particularly useful when the route or channel of the blood flow undergoes one or more 180° turns in its course to a particular location. In this situation, with a curve at the tip of the catheter and good forward flow, the floating catheter is often pulled through the circuitous course of the blood flow without much additional manipulation of the catheter. When the balloon is inflated, the flow-directed catheter also has the advantage of being safer for the operator to manipulate. The inflated balloon covering the tip provides a very large, blunt and soft tip, which, when inflated could not possibly perforate anything.

These same characteristics make flow-directed catheters very difficult to manipulate *purposefully* into many selected locations. They are not satisfactory for use *against* the direction of flow of the blood or in the presence of a regurgitant flow against the course of flow. Some of the unfavorable maneuvering qualities of floating catheters are overcome by the use of guide or other special wires positioned within the lumen in order to support the softer shaft of the catheter and give it some "pushability". Curves formed on the stiff ends of wires or specific deflector wires can be used to turn or deflect the tip of flow-directed catheters while the wire supports the shaft of the catheter. The detailed use of balloon floating catheters is covered in Chapter 7.

In addition to the almost infinite variety of diagnostic catheters, there are many catheters designed for very special techniques or procedures. These include intracardiac and intravascular echo, electrode, pacing, thermodilution, fiberoptic, retrieval, biopsy, balloon dilation catheters, and special catheters for the delivery of devices. Each of these special catheters is discussed in a subsequent chapter dealing individually and very specifically with these many special techniques.

Miscellaneous small consumable items

In addition to the needles, wires, sheaths/dilators, catheters and the basic catheterization packs there is a large number of other small, miscellaneous consumable items used regularly in the catheterization laboratory. Although many of these items are used commonly in other areas of a hospital and are available readily from the central materials supplies of the hospital, a certain number of these items must be considered in the space and inventory requirements of the catheterization laboratory itself in order to ensure that they are always stocked and available to the laboratory. All consumable items now used during a catheterization procedure are disposable. Because of the hazard of breakage, potential lacerations or punctures with the resultant risk of serious contamination/infection of operating personnel, items manufactured of glass are no longer used in the catheterization laboratory.

The largest number and variety of extra consumable items used during any pediatric/congenital cardiac catheterization are disposable plastic syringes. For procedures where the syringe is attached and detached frequently, a slip-lock connector on the syringe is preferred to a Lure-lock™ connector, particularly if the tip of the syringe is connecting to a metal hub on the catheter. Two or three, 5–10 ml capacity syringes are used on the procedure table for drawing samples, flushing needles, catheters and tubing, injection of supplemental local anesthesia, and hand infusions of medications or fluids through the catheters. Small, 1.5 or 2 ml syringes are used to transfer each separate blood sample from the table to the oximeter, blood gas machine or ACT machine. As many as 20, 30 or even more of these syringes can be used during a single, complex, catheterization procedure. Larger, 20 ml or occasionally up to 60 ml syringes are used to inflate sizing or dilation balloons. Special 5 or 10 ml syringes with an *extra hard* barrel and plunger are used when a syringe is used for rapid, "hand" injections of contrast through a catheter where significant pressure on the syringe must be used.

In addition to the extra syringes, extra or special connecting tubing, extra bowls for flushing, extra sterile gloves, extra towels and sponges are frequently required during a case. All of these items are frequently used and should be readily available in the catheterization room. Each therapeutic catheterization has its own separate requirement for special consumable equipment. Each of these items is included in the chapters on those procedures.

Complications of equipment

Although any manufactured product, large or small, can be defective or fail, most complications of equipment are complications in the use of the equipment. When the major or capital equipment fails, it usually results in the interruption or cancellation of the case with no adverse or permanent consequence for the patient. The exception would be the failure of the X-ray/imaging equipment at the precise instant or a critical point in an interventional procedure. A major failure at the precise instant of the intervention could result in a displaced device or the dilation of the wrong area/structure. Fortunately this combination of circumstances is extremely rare and essentially is not a consideration. Both angiographic and physiologic recorders fail, but again very infrequently, and aside from the possible lost data from the procedure, there usually are no sequelae for the patient.

Most of the complications related to the expendable equipment are a result of the improper use of the equipment and are included in the complications of each individual procedure/technique. In spite of the strictest and most rigid manufacturing controls that are imposed on medical devices, with the millions of pieces of consumable equipment utilized in catheterization laboratories throughout the world, occasional manufacturing flaws are inevitable. The more complex the particular equipment, the greater is the likelihood of a defective piece of equipment. As a consequence, more problems are encountered with therapeutic devices/catheters than with routine diagnostic equipment.

Flaws in disposable/expendable equipment which result in breaks or fractures and the loss of catheter tips or pieces of spring guide wire do result in the embolization of a solid particle. Fortunately, most materials designed for intravascular use are radio-opaque so that "errant pieces" can usually be located. The consequence of the embolization of a piece of expendable equipment depends upon the "destination" of the embolized particle and its retrievability. Fortunately such instances are extremely rare and most embolized small pieces of equipment can be retrieved as a foreign body in the catheterization laboratory, as described in Chapter 12.

Catheter hubs coming loose during high-pressure injection result in a failed angiogram, but cause no adverse effect to the patient. Leaks in stopcocks or connecting tubing result in poor pressure transmission and inaccurate pressures being recorded, but when recognized, result in no adverse effect to the patient. An *unrecognized leak* in a stopcock adjacent to the catheter can allow air to be drawn into the system when any negative pressure is applied to it, and if the presence of air in the system is not recognized or the air is not removed from the system, it could result in air being injected into the patient. This, like most of the complications which are a consequence of defective equipment, are avoidable by meticulous observation of all stages of the procedure along with preventive measures when problems exist with the equipment.

References

1. Allen HD *et al*. Pediatric therapeutic cardiac catheterization: a statement for healthcare professionals from the Council on Cardiovascular Disease in the Young, American Heart Association. *Circulation* 1998; **97**(6): 609–625.
2. Neches WH *et al*. Percutaneous sheath cardiac catheterization. *Am J Cardiol* 1972; **30**(4): 378–384.
3. Seldinger SI. Catheter replacement of the needle in percutaneous arteriography. *Acta Radiol* 1953; **39**: 368.

4 Vascular access: needle, wire, sheath/dilator and catheter introduction

Vessel entry

Most catheterization laboratories in the twenty-first century utilize a percutaneous puncture with a needle and guide wire to enter the vessels and then an indwelling sheath within the vessel during catheter manipulations. This certainly is the accepted standard approach in the majority of centers in the United States. However, the time-tested technique of performing a "cut-down" with an incision in the skin extending through the subcutaneous tissues down to the vessel and then with direct introduction of the catheter into the incised vessel is still utilized in some centers, particularly in developing countries of the world where "disposable" supplies are less available. Even when a "cut-down" approach through the tissues and down to the vessel is used, catheters now are usually introduced *into* the vessel and manipulated within the vessel through an indwelling sheath. The wire is introduced into both the artery and the vein through a direct needle puncture and the sheath/dilator is introduced over a wire into the vessel without a separate incision in the vessel.

Percutaneous technique

The percutaneous technique is applicable for the introduction of catheters into both veins and arteries. The percutaneous, indwelling sheath technique performed correctly and carefully results in a very low incidence of venous and/or arterial complications—significantly lower than by utilizing a cut-down approach to the vessel. A "single wall" needle puncture and the subsequent, smooth (delicate!) introduction of a finely tapered dilator through a well anesthetized skin and subcutaneous field is far less traumatic to the vessel than any dissection and eventual incision into the vessel wall which is necessary during a cut-down. The percutaneous entry into the vessel eliminates the dissection of the subcutaneous tissues adjacent to the vessel required during a cut-down and, in turn, eliminates the *extrinsic* irritation to the vessel wall incurred by the dissection of the cut-down. This results in a reduction or elimination of the associated vessel spasm from the dissection during the cut-down with the result that vessels entered percutaneously initially have a much larger effective diameter and lumen. The intrinsic large diameters and the capacity of the deep veins in the groin to dilate to accommodate several large sheaths are much greater when none of the vessel spasm associated with a subcutaneous dissection is present.

An *indwelling* sheath in any vessel prevents the continual irritation to the vessel wall by the movement of the catheter against the vessel wall at the puncture site and, in turn, essentially eliminates vessel spasm around the catheter. Most physicians who have used only a percutaneous indwelling sheath technique, in fact, have never experienced "vessel spasm" around the catheter! When percutaneous catheters and sheaths are removed from vessels, hemostasis is achieved readily by local pressure over the vessel and this usually only requires a short period of time. Following a percutaneous procedure, the area only needs to be kept dry and clean, with no wound to care for, no sutures to remove later, no dressing and essentially a zero incidence of infection at the local entrance sites.

Assuming that a vessel is present in a particular area, and that when present the vessel is patent, with an understanding of the anatomy in the area of the vessel, meticulous preparation of the puncture site, patience, and, finally, skill and practice with the technique, all patent vessels *can* be entered percutaneously. For many reasons, the percutaneous introduction of catheters into the vascular system is the most desirable and the most expedient approach for cardiac catheterizations in infants, children and older patients with congenital heart disease[1].

Although the percutaneous introduction of the needle and wire into a femoral or saphenous vessel occasionally takes longer than a skillfully performed cut-down on the same vessel—especially for operators inexperienced in the percutaneous technique—apart from this very occasional advantage in the time of access, the cut-down technique has *no* other advantages and many disadvantages! The percutaneous approach does not destroy or distort the anatomy of the area around the introductory site and/or subsequently obliterate the individual vessels with large dense scar formation in contrast to a cut-down on the area. Not only is this a consideration for the cosmetics of the area, but it becomes very important during subsequent cardiac catheterizations which are usually required (often frequently) in congenital cardiac patients.

Percutaneous vessel entry

The exact procedure for needle/wire introduction into a vessel varies with the location of the vessel and whether a vein or artery is being entered. At the same time there are many similarities in the techniques for puncturing and entering both veins and arteries which are very important for every percutaneous vessel entry. Knowledge of the vessel anatomy in the area and the identification of the superficial landmarks with their relationship to the anatomy of the underlying vessels are critical to the success of any percutaneous procedure.

Femoral percutaneous approach

The "external" or "surface" anatomy is important particularly for the percutaneous approach in the femoral area where the vessels themselves are not visible and the veins are not even palpable. The landmarks are identified carefully by inspection and palpation *before* the patient is scrubbed and draped. The patient is secured on the table with his/her legs extending straight in line with the trunk and with the feet extending as straight as possible. It is preferable neither to adduct nor to abduct the legs unless the percutaneous procedure is always performed by the particular operator(s) with the legs in the particular position, and the puncture technique and location are always adjusted for the particular rotation of the legs. Any unusual or different positions of the legs and/or rotation of the feet/legs, changes the relationship of the artery and vein to each other as well as to the fixed landmarks in the inguinal area.

Once the patient is secured on the catheterization table with the legs positioned properly, both the *inguinal ligament* and the *inguinal skin crease* are identified and their relationship to each other noted mentally. These two landmarks, although often considered synonymous, have no fixed relationship in their distance from each other[2]. The ligament and the inguinal crease may be very close to each other in a patient with little subcutaneous tissue or, at the other extreme, widely separated. The *ligament* extending from the anterior superior iliac spine to the pubic tubercle is the *fixed* landmark which is used as the *reference structure*. The femoral artery and vein are fairly superficial in the immediate location where they pass *under the inguinal ligament*. At the ligament, both vessels are aligned parallel to the long axis of the extremity as well as relatively parallel to the skin surface in their anterior–posterior relationship (Figure 4.1). As little as one centimeter above (*cephalad*) to the inguinal *ligament*, the iliofemoral vessels both dip into the pelvis and are separated from the skin surface by a caudal fold (or reflection) of *peritoneum* actually within the *abdomen* and, in turn, the vessels cannot be palpated and/or manually *compressed* from over that area (Figure 4.2). As little as one to two centimeters below (*caudal to*) the ligament, both vessels penetrate below the sartorius muscle and deep posteriorly into the tissues of the leg, losing their superficial position and relatively parallel alignment to the surface of the skin.

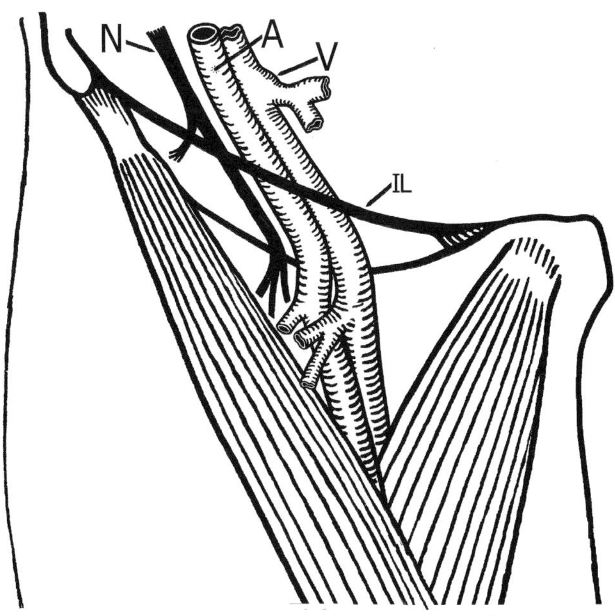

Figure 4.1 Anterior–posterior view of the anatomy of the vessels in the inguinal area. A, artery; V, vein; N, nerve; IL, inguinal ligament.

The femoral arterial pulse is palpated just caudal (distal) to the inguinal *ligament*. The relationships to the rest of the inguinal area including the side-to-side distances from the femoral pulse to the anterior iliac spine and to the tubercle of the pubic bone are noted. The pulse (vessel) usually lies approximately mid distance between the anterior iliac spine and the tubercle of the symphysis pubis. At the inguinal ligament the femoral vein lies adjacent (between 1 cm medial and immediately under) and deep to the artery.

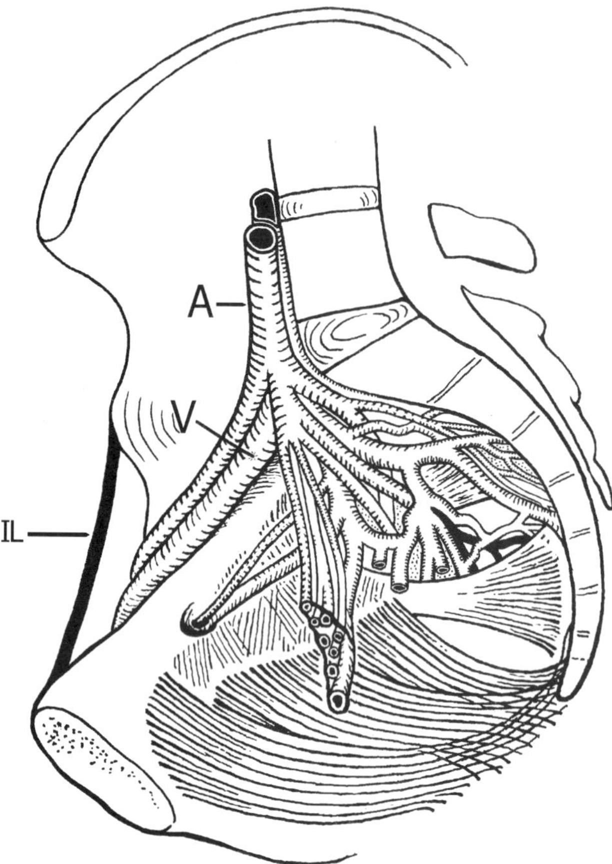

Figure 4.2 Lateral view of the anatomy of the vessels in inguinal/pelvic area. A, artery; V, vein; IL, inguinal ligament.

Local anesthesia

The infiltration of local anesthesia is usually the most uncomfortable part of the entire catheterization for the patient. The local anesthesia procedure often converts a previously calm sedated (even asleep) patient into a combatant, irrational squirming and fighting individual! EMLA™ cream applied locally *60 to 90 minutes before* any needle stick is somewhat effective in reducing the pain from the cutaneous needle stick.

It is preferable to administer the local anesthesia to the inguinal area *before* the patient is "surgically" scrubbed or draped. This allows clear visualization and identification of all of the landmarks even if the patient moves significantly during or after the infiltration with the local or during the sterile draping. Also, even if the patient's movements become extensive during local anesthetic infiltration, but occur before the sterile preparation of the field, the sterile field for the catheterization is not disturbed or contaminated. 2% xylocaine is the preferred local anesthesia in patients of all sizes. Although 2% xylocaine is, potentially, more toxic than 1% xylocaine, half of the *volume* of anesthetic fluid is used for each site of infiltration, which, in turn, causes less stretch or distention of the subcutaneous tissues and less pain locally before the anesthetic takes effect.

Both inguinal areas are infiltrated with local anesthesia at the beginning of the procedure and *before* the patient is draped. This allows the option of using femoral access on either or both sides without reawakening the patient with further needle sticks to introduce a new local infiltration. Having both sides anesthetized is helpful, particularly if a vessel on one side is inadvertently punctured but cannot be cannulated immediately with the wire. Hemostasis in that vessel is achieved with pressure, which has to be applied for several minutes before a repeat puncture can be performed in that area. In that circumstance, during the time while pressure is held over the first puncture site, a separate puncture can be made into the vessel in the opposite, already anesthetized, inguinal area without disturbing the patient.

Prior to xylocaine infiltration, the skin over and around the puncture site is cleaned locally and very thoroughly with an antiseptic (alcohol) sponge. The operator can be gloved with sterile gloves and proceeds with the local infiltration keeping the needle, syringes and general area sterile in the event that it is advantageous to introduce the wire during this stage of the procedure. The initial superficial, epidermal puncture for the xylocaine is made with a 25-gauge needle. This injection is performed directly over the palpated pulse and the expected puncture site for the artery, which should be approximately 1 cm caudal to the inguinal ligament. The 1 cm distance caudal to the inguinal ligament frequently does *not* correspond at all to the location of the inguinal skin crease, which, again, is not the fixed landmark. Only a very superficial skin wheal is created initially with the 25-gauge needle.

If a vessel is entered inadvertently and blood withdrawn into the syringe during the infiltration of xylocaine with the small 25-gauge needle, this needle is withdrawn from the skin and pressure is applied for at least several minutes before either continuing the xylocaine infiltration or starting the purposeful vessel puncture. A punctured vessel, especially an artery, bleeds subcutaneously for a considerable time even if visible bleeding does not make it to the surface of the skin. The more subcutaneous bleeding that occurs, the more the vessels in the subcutaneous area are distorted or compressed by the extravasated blood and, in turn, the more difficult will be the subsequent puncture into the lumen of the vessel. After superficial infiltration with local anesthesia is completed, the tiny puncture site on the skin surface from the puncture with the xylocaine needle serves as a persistent, superficial "landmark" for the subsequent vessel puncture, particularly after the patient is draped and all of the other landmarks are covered or distorted.

After the skin wheal is created, the deeper subcutaneous tissues are infiltrated through the same puncture site but usually with a slightly larger (21- or 20-gauge) needle. During the infiltration with the local anesthetic, an attempt is made to introduce the needle on each side of the femoral vascular sheath without puncturing any of the vessels in the area. Negative pressure is maintained on the xylocaine syringe anytime the needle is actually being introduced into, or withdrawn from, the tissues. The local is introduced only while the tip of the needle is in a fixed position in the subcutaneous tissues and there is no blood return with negative pressure on the syringe from that location. The larger diameter needle not only allows the use of less force and more control on the syringe for the injection of the local anesthetic into the tissues, but, when a vessel is entered inadvertently during the process of the introduction of the needle, the larger needle allows a definite, quick flashback of blood or, if desired, allows the introduction of a guide wire through that same needle.

Catheter field preparation and draping

After the infiltration with xylocaine, both inguinal areas are scrubbed with antiseptic solution over a wide area around the expected puncture site and then dried very thoroughly with a sterile towel. The scrubbed areas should include all of the skin area extending from just below the umbilicus cranially to almost the knees caudally, across the midline medially and laterally to the lateral aspect of the thighs on both sides. In the older patient, this same distribution (with additional extension of the area to the back of both thighs and lower back laterally) is shaved of all hair. It is more expedient if this extensive shaving can be performed prior to the patient entering the catheterization laboratory! Older adolescent and adult patients often prefer to perform the shaving for themselves—particularly if they have had the experience of having tape removed after a previous catheterization!

Both femoral areas are scrubbed and thoroughly dried. The femoral areas are then draped to produce a very large sterile field over the entire patient. The preferable drapes for all catheter procedures are manufactured, composite, paper/plastic single sheet, disposable drapes. The disposable paper drapes are available from many manufacturers, available in both infant and large (adult) sizes and can be used for patients of all ages and sizes. When ordered in quantity, some manufacturers (e.g. Argon Medical Inc., Athens, TX) will custom manufacture the drapes to suit the specifics and desires of the individual catheterization laboratory and the particular configuration of the catheterization table. For the inguinal/femoral approach the preferable drape is a large femoral or "lap" drape with two pre-cut holes which accommodate the two femoral areas. The size of the holes and the distance required between the holes varies according to the size of the patient. Usually, by careful positioning and individually adjusting the two openings before they are stuck to the skin, only two different sizes of drapes are necessary to accommodate the large majority of patients, including all sizes from newborns to adults. The patient's side (underside) of the holes of each femoral area opening is surrounded by adhesive while the working surface (top) has a large extra absorbant area extending widely to both sides, above, below and between both of the femoral openings. These disposable paper drapes have numerous advantages over the old "sheet and towel" systems of draping.

The most important advantage of manufactured disposable drapes is that they provide a far better and a more secure sterile field. In contrast to cloth towels and cloth sheets, the special absorbant surface material along with the plastic backing of the paper drape provides a barrier that is impenetrable to fluid and does not allow fluid seepage through the drape to the patient's skin or to the tabletop. Of even more importance than keeping the patient dry, the plastic backing is much safer for the patient by also providing a complete barrier against contaminants. Disposable, waterproof drapes prevent bacteria from passing through the saturated material of a cloth drape to the sterile field. In addition, the properly applied, one-piece drape provides a very flat working surface over the entire catheterization table and especially in the inguinal areas. This flat surface greatly facilitates the percutaneous introduction of needles and wires into the vessels and subsequent wire/catheter manipulations at the site. This "flat field" is far superior to the traditional, cloth, sheet and towel drapes where the towels, which are bunched-up and folded around the puncture site, create a deep "valley" around the entry site into the vessel.

The large paper drape provides a smooth, flat, contiguous surface, which extends cephalad over the patient's chest to caudal over the patient's feet. The paper drape also eliminates unwanted shadows in the field of the fluoroscopic and cine images which occur from the bunched-up folds in the reusable cloth drapes, which frequently become impregnated with and incompletely rinsed of contrast medium. With the flat field extending over the feet of the patient and past the end of the catheterization table, the field can accommodate long catheters and wires, which tend to overhang the caudal end of the table. No towel clips are in the work area or fluoroscopy field. The adhesive around each area, when correctly applied to a thoroughly dried skin surface, provides a seal around the puncture area and prevents any shifting or sliding of the drapes away from the sterile area should the patient move or be moved.

Of equal importance, properly handled disposable drapes markedly reduce the exposure of the personnel in the catheterization laboratory to contamination from blood and otherwise potentially infected materials and, as a consequence, the disposable drapes are far safer. At the end of the procedure, none of the expendable materials on the catheterization field are handled at all by the personnel in the room. The drape is folded together from the outside edges and around all of the contaminated disposable items on the table. The contaminants which are contained within the drape are then removed from the patient as a single bundle. In this way the transfer of the bloodied drape, catheters and other disposables is performed as one large bundle all rolled together containing all of the soiled disposables from the patient, rather than multiple separate loose pieces being handled separately. The bundle is deposited into a bio-hazard trash container which, in turn, is sealed before being removed from the room. As a consequence, none of this material is handled directly thereafter by catheterization laboratory or any other hospital personnel.

Finally, unless manual labor is extremely cheap in the community where the catheterization laboratory is established, taking into account the initial expense of the cloth materials, their manufacture, maintenance, cleaning, repackaging and re-sterilizing, the disposable drapes are more economical. When true cost accounting is utilized and certainly in the United Stated, disposable drapes are far cheaper to use than reusable cloth towels and drape sheets.

After the patient has been surgically scrubbed from the umbilicus to the knees and dried very thoroughly, the drapes are opened, the cover is removed from the adhesive around the holes and the drape spread over the patient, preferably by the catheterizing physician or at least by a very experienced associate. As the drape is unfolded over the patient, the openings in the drape are centered approximately over the proposed puncture sites of both inguinal areas but the drape is not pressed against the skin nor sealed over the areas at this stage of the draping. Once the drape is completely unfolded over the entire patient, the inguinal areas are visible through the holes in the drape although the drape is still away from the skin and still not adherent to the skin.

At this point in the draping, each opening in the drape is centered individually and precisely over the exact puncture site over each separate inguinal area by the catheterizing physician him (or her) self! Each hole is centered, pressed and stuck to the patient over the respective puncture site individually so that the field is exactly centered in each femoral area. The operator who introduced the local anesthesia has the most accurate knowledge of the catheterization site and the location of the vessels and, as a result, is the most appropriate person to center the drapes accurately over the actual puncture sites. The proper positioning of the drapes is very important for the subsequent vessel punctures. If the drapes are positioned "casually" over the sites without very special attention to the location, the actual puncture sites are often located at the edge of, or even out of the circular, open area of the drape.

Usually the center portion of the precut drape which is between the two femoral openings must be folded up into a smooth, longitudinal ridge between the two openings in order to accommodate the different sizes of patients and yet have the two opening align properly from side to side and exactly over both puncture sites. This longitudinal fold of the drape does not interfere at all with the subsequent puncture and catheter manipulations.

When the holes in the drape are in the exact position with the proposed puncture sites on the skin at the center of the openings, the adhesive tape around each hole is pressed firmly against the dry skin of the legs surrounding the inguinal areas. When the skin has been dried properly and thoroughly, a "watertight" seal is created around each inguinal site. This provides a sterile field extending from the patient's chin, over the working area, past the patient's feet and beyond the caudal end of the table.

One alternative to the pre-cut full table sized paper drape is the use of a plastic Steri-drape™ applied separately over each inguinal area in conjunction with traditional, non pre-cut, cloth towels and drapes. The opening in the Steri-drape™ is placed precisely over the center of each sterile, inguinal puncture site on the skin as described above for the pre-cut drapes. The Steri-drape™ over each opening is surrounded with towels clipped together around each opening and the remainder of the field is covered with one or more, large, cloth, lap drapes.

There are many and very significant disadvantages to the reusable cloth drape. The deep "valley" of towels and drapes created around each femoral area by the overlapping and folded towels has been mentioned. This valley does not allow a flat enough angle to be created between the skin surface and the angle of the needle for a satisfactory needle puncture and a subsequent easy introduction of the wire into the needle/vessel. With cloth drapes, any patient movement results in the entire field sliding, often completely away from the puncture (and sterile) site. The sliding field or the soaking of the cloth towels and drapes with blood and flush solutions results in the total loss of sterility of the operative field. The reusable cloth towels or drapes also become impregnated with small amounts of spilled contrast material over time. This contrast medium does *not* rinse out of the cloth materials completely with subsequent laundering. This imbedded contrast shows up on the fluoroscopy and angiograms whenever a towel or cloth drape is present in the X-ray field during subsequent cases. At the end of, and after the procedure, the bio contaminated, reusable cloth drape or towels must be handled separately and repeatedly in the catheterization laboratory by the catheterization laboratory personnel and again by personnel in the hospital cleaning facility.

All of the problems of reusable drapes are magnified when used during catheterizations in the newborn infant, especially when both the umbilical and femoral approaches are used together. The "mountains" of towels and drapes heaped up on the combined areas of access in the small infant, with the resultant valleys between the towels, compound all of the previously mentioned problems which occur with cloth drapes.

A modification of the usual infant disposable paper drape provides a better solution for newborn patients. The newborn is scrubbed from mid-chest to knees. One side (edge) of a Steri-drape™ (3-M Corp., Rochester, MN), which would otherwise extend caudally over the inguinal area of the newborn, is trimmed along one side of the circular opening. The umbilical area is draped with the modified Steri-drape™ with the new "short" (absent) side directed caudally. With the Steri-drape™ in place over the umbilicus, the still sterile and exposed inguinal areas along with the rest of the infant's body are draped with the infant disposable paper lap drape as described previously for the inguinal areas. Once the paper drape has been positioned precisely with the two holes sealed tightly over the inguinal areas, a third hole is cut in the paper drape cephalad and centrally, directly over the opening in the previously prepared Steri-drape™ over the umbilical area. This allows access to both groins as well as the umbilical vessels but, at the same time, with a flat, non-permeable, non-sliding field.

In many catheterization laboratories, the patient's catheterization site is scrubbed and draped by the catheterization laboratory nurse or technician before the infiltration with local anesthesia. This is satisfactory only if the individual doing the draping is extremely familiar with the precise area for the vessel entry in each of the catheterization sites and pays very careful attention to the location of these sites during the placement of the drapes. Otherwise, the draped, sterile field is often not centered over the desired area, or even over the vessel puncture site at all, making all of the remainder of the percutaneous procedure more difficult and less sterile.

Needle, wire and dilator/sheath introduction

Needle introduction—initial vessel entry

In infants and small children, the needles and wires that are used are designed specifically for the purpose of percutaneous introductions (Argon Medical Inc., Athens, TX; Cook Inc., Bloomington, IN). The needle is thin walled and as small in diameter as possible in order to enter the very small vessels and yet still be able to accommodate the introductory spring guide wire. The tip of the needle for a percutaneous introduction should have a short bevel rather than the more standard, long, sharper, cutting

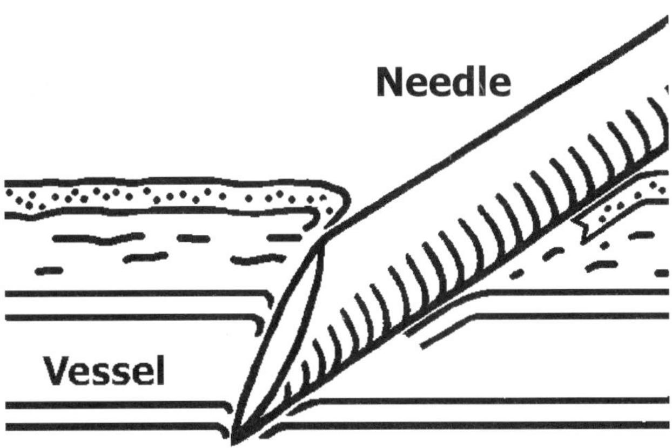

Figure 4.3 Large bore needle "straddling" a small vessel.

bevel found on needles for injections. The hub of the needle must have a smooth taper/transition into the shaft of the needle and preferably be clear. For infants and smaller children, a 21-gauge, thin-walled, short bevel needle is used along with a 0.018'' special, extra soft tipped spring guide wire. For larger children and even most adults, a 19-gauge needle with a 0.021" soft tipped spring guide wire is used. Occasionally, for a *very* large patient, a longer 18-gauge needle with either a 0.021" or 0.032" soft tipped guide wire is used. The larger the needle, the greater the chance of lacerating a side wall of a vessel by the needle's cutting through the side of the vessel or totally straddling the opposite walls of a small vessel with the opposite sides of the needle without actually entering the lumen of the vessel in either situation (Figure 4.3). As a consequence, even though blood return occurs through the needle and appears in the hub of the needle, a wire will not enter the vessel. The smaller the patient and the vessels are in proportion to the needle, the greater is the problem when using larger needles.

As emphasized earlier, it is important that the inguinal ligament connecting the anterior–superior iliac spine with the pubic tubercle is used as the landmark for determining the site of puncture and not the skin crease, which has no fixed relationship. The femoral vessels are in a fixed relationship to the ligament while the skin crease or fold varies according to the patient's superficial subcutaneous tissues. This variation in distance of the skin fold can be as much as 2 cm cephalad or caudal in its relationship to the desired puncture site. The preferred puncture site on the skin in a small infant is 0.5 to 1.0 cm caudal to the inguinal ligament, with the needle angled as close as possible to parallel to the skin, and aligned with the long axis of the extremity. With the proper alignment, the needle enters the vessel under or immediately caudal to the inguinal ligament and parallel to the vessel (Figure 4.4a).

When the skin is punctured too cephalad—i.e. too close to or just at or cephalad to the inguinal ligament—the

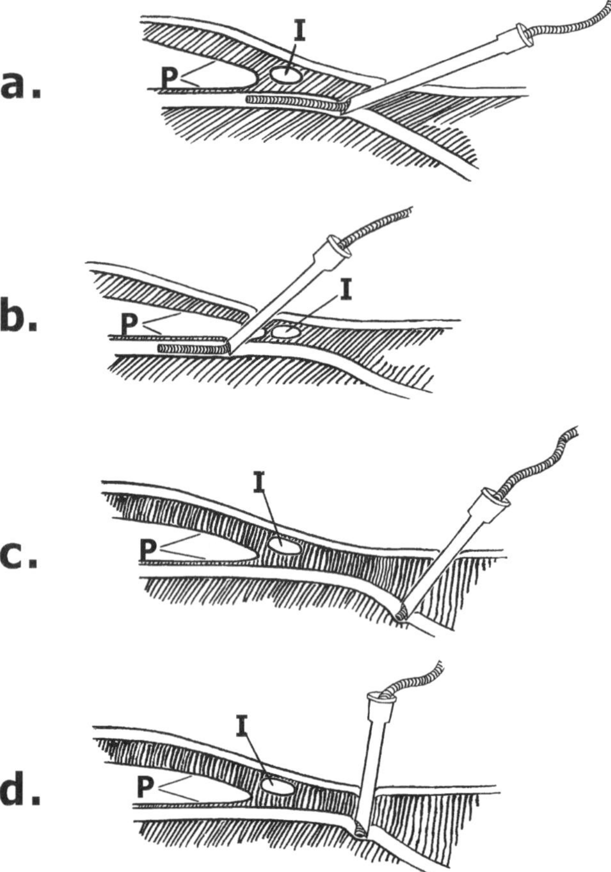

Figure 4.4 Lateral view of different angles of needle introduction into the femoral area. (a) Proper position and angle of needle below inguinal ligament; (b) needle puncture too high and passing into and through peritoneal cavity before puncturing vessel; (c) needle puncture too caudal to inguinal ligament; (d) needle puncture too perpendicular to skin (and vessel). I, the inguinal ligament on "edge"; P, peritoneal reflections above the inguinal ligament.

result is a puncture of the vessel, which actually occurs within the abdominal cavity (Figure 4.4b). Above the inguinal ligament, the subcutaneous supporting tissues, which normally surround the vessel, are separated from the skin surface by the reflection of the peritoneal cavity! When the puncture site of the skin is just at the ligament, the puncture of the vessel becomes even more cephalad and pressure over the skin puncture site cannot prevent bleeding into the retroperitoneal space or abdominal cavity from the puncture site in the vessel. During the catheterization procedure, the vessel is usually sealed by the catheter/sheath in the puncture opening but, after the catheter and sheath are withdrawn, the hole in the vessel, which is within the retroperitoneal space or abdominal cavity, is opened and will be separated from the skin area by the peritoneal cavity. The puncture in the vessel(s) cannot be compressed by pressure over the skin surface even when external pressure is applied more cephalad over the abdomen.

At the other extreme, when the puncture site is too far caudal to the inguinal ligament, it is more difficult or even impossible to introduce a wire into the vessel even after the vessel is punctured and blood return into the needle appears adequate. Immediately distal (caudal) to the inguinal ligament, the femoral vessels leave their very superficial position under the skin and dive deeply and posteriorly beneath the sartorius muscle toward the center of the leg and the femur. When the vessel is in this deep location, the tip of the needle will not even reach the vessel when the needle has been introduced parallel to the skin. In addition, as the vessels penetrate into the deeper tissues, they angle away from their parallel orientation to the skin. As a consequence, when the puncture site is too far caudal from the inguinal ligament (even as little as a few cm caudal to the ligament), the needle must be introduced more vertically to the surface of the skin in order to reach the deep vessels. As the angle of the needle become more perpendicular to the skin, the needle becomes perpendicular to the vessel, which, in turn, prohibits the introduction of a wire into the vessel (Figure 4.4c). Some operators utilize a very long needle, puncture the skin 5–6 cm caudal to the inguinal ligament and create a very long, superficial and "horizontal" subcutaneous "tunnel" beneath the skin in order to traverse the distance within the subcutaneous tissues toward the inguinal ligament before the vessel is to be entered near the ligament. Unless this unusual technique is used, the skin on the leg should *not* be punctured far caudal to the inguinal ligament.

Too steep an angle of the needle to the skin (and vessel), regardless of the distance below the ligament, is equally problematic. When the angle of the needle is too steep (perpendicular) relative to the surface of the skin, the tip of the needle will also be oriented perpendicular (or worse) to the vessel. A perpendicular angle of entry into the vessel will prohibit the introduction of the wire into the vessel because of the totally unsatisfactory needle to vessel angle (Figure 4.4d).

Standard needle introduction—single wall puncture technique for the approach to vessels

Femoral approach

The puncture site on the skin is determined from the prior needle mark from the xylocaine infiltration, from the palpable pulse and/or from the location of the inguinal ligament. These are all used as standard surface landmarks for puncture of the femoral vessels. In the area of the inguinal ligament, the vein lies immediately adjacent to (usually just medial to) and deep to the palpable artery. In the area under the inguinal ligament, both major vessels are surprisingly close to the skin surface (as little as 3 mm in an infant and less than 1–1.5 cm even in most larger children and adults). In the precise area under the inguinal ligament, both vessels run parallel to the skin surface and parallel to the long axis of the leg.

The single-wall puncture technique for the introduction of the needle into the vessel is identical to the technique used for the venepuncture of tiny, superficial, peripheral veins. Before the needle introduction is started, *good* lighting of the proposed *puncture site* is essential. The light should be directed *perpendicularly, from straight above* the hub of the needle during the entire procedure. A light coming from the foot of the catheterization table or from behind the operator creates a shadow from the operator's arm and/or body and is more of a hindrance than a help. A light directed toward the operator *from* the patient's head, and/or *from* the opposite side of the patient, creates glare on the field which interferes with the visualization of the fluid within the hub of the needle.

The needle, especially the hub, is filled with flush solution. The spring guide wire which is to be used for the introduction into the vessel is placed on the table with the soft tip of the wire readily accessible and immediately adjacent to the puncture site. The needle is positioned with the bevel at the tip of the needle facing up while the hub of the needle is held between the thumb and forefinger. The skin at the proper site over the vessel is punctured very superficially with the needle with nothing attached to it. If the fluid in the hub of the needle empties from the hub before, or as, the tip of the needle enters the skin, the hub of the needle is refilled with fluid. The needle is introduced and advanced very slowly into the skin, keeping it as flat and parallel to the skin surface as possible (i.e. the needle should be almost flat against the skin surface of the leg) and as parallel to the direction of the long axis of the leg (not trunk) as possible in order to follow the expected course of the vessel. With the bevel of the needle facing up (toward the skin), the needle is *advanced* into the tissues *very slowly* and *smoothly*, (***not*** in jabs nor as a large, single thrust) while watching the hub of the needle very closely as the needle is advanced into the tissues looking for the first, slight movement or "quiver" of the fluid in the hub. The puncture site over the vessel ***never*** is speared, jabbed or "harpooned" with the needle during its introduction. The needle also is ***not*** rotated or "spun" *at all* during its introduction. "Spinning" the needle as it is introduced results in the bevel of the needle creating a very effective "cutting" or "boring" tool through the tissues *and through the vessel wall*. The purpose of the single-wall puncture technique is to enter only the *anterior wall* of the vein (or artery) during the introduction of the needle (similar to a superficial venepuncture for an IV) and ***not*** to transect the vessel ***nor*** to puncture through the posterior wall at all. The single-wall puncture results in the very least trauma to the vessel and as little blood extravasation into the adjacent tissues as possible.

As the very first sign of movement of the "bubble" of fluid occurs in the hub of the needle as the needle is being advanced, the advancing of the needle is stopped immediately and the fingers holding the needle are released while the operator waits at least several seconds for blood return into the hub of the needle. This allows the needle to assume a "neutral" position in the vessel. In the presence of very low venous pressure, there may be no back-flow of blood from the vein following the initial slight movement of the fluid bubble in the hub. When the fluid column in the hub moves at all, even if blood does not flow back into the hub of the needle, the soft tip of the wire is introduced very gently and slowly into the needle and an attempt is made at threading the vessel very carefully with the wire.

When no movement of the fluid or no blood return is seen in the needle hub, the needle is advanced slowly into the tissues until either movement of the fluid does occur or the hub of the needle reaches the skin. If the needle is introduced fully to the hub, even when there is no detectable puncture into the vessel during the needle's introduction, the needle is withdrawn very slowly and smoothly, a millimeter or less at a time, with *no* rotation or spinning of the needle and, similar to during its introduction, continually observing the fluid in the hub for *any* movement during the withdrawal. It is possible that the needle has punctured the vessel during the introduction, but as it punctures the anterior wall, the needle tip compresses the lumen of the vessel and passes completely through the vessel without any blood return into the needle. During the withdrawal of the needle, with any movement of the fluid or any actual blood return into the hub, an attempt is made at introducing the wire exactly as when the vessel is entered during the introduction of the needle. If the vessel is not entered and no blood is encountered either during the introduction or withdrawal of the needle, the needle is withdrawn completely from the skin and flushed thoroughly and the puncture/introduction begun again using a slightly different direction, depth, angle or location.

If blood actually spurts back from the needle during its introduction or withdrawal, although it is almost instinctive to do so, the hub of the needle is ***not*** covered or blocked with a finger nor is any other attempt made to plug the hub of the needle to stop the squirt of blood! Rather, the soft tip of the wire, which should be available *immediately* adjacent to the needle hub, is introduced rapidly into the spurt of blood from the needle before disturbing the needle with any other movement or manipulation with the fingers. Even a very slight pressure applied to the open end of the hub of the needle when trying to "cap" a squirt of blood with a finger tip can advance the tip of the needle further into the tissues and, in turn, *completely through the lumen* of a tiny vessel and through the opposite (posterior) wall of the vessel. Although the sudden squirt of blood is startling and rather dramatic, when the wire is introduced expeditiously, there is minimal loss of blood even from an artery.

Generally, an attempt is made to introduce the venous catheter first. If, however, the artery is punctured inadvertently and entered cleanly while aiming for the vein during the percutaneous needle introduction, arterial access is established. A guide wire is introduced through the needle and into the artery identically to the technique used for introduction of the wire into the vein as described subsequently in this chapter. Once the wire has passed into the artery some distance, the needle is removed and replaced with the small plastic cannula of a Quik-Cath™ or Leader-Cath™ or even a 4-French dilator. This arterial cannula is attached to the flush-pressure line and is used for continuous arterial monitoring, arterial blood sampling and the possible, later introduction of a retrograde sheath/catheter. The indwelling arterial cannula also prevents bleeding from the inadvertent arterial puncture site without having to hold pressure for 5–10 minutes. The tubing attached to the arterial cannula is clamped to the drape (to prevent inadvertent withdrawal from the artery) and the venous puncture is carried out, with the arterial cannula now also serving as visible lateral "landmark". The arterial cannula usually is *not* sewn to the skin before the venous line is secured. Because of the close proximity of the two vessels, it is often necessary to move the hub of the arterial cannula a few millimeters from side to side away from the vein puncture site during the subsequent attempts at puncturing the adjacent vein. This is particularly important in infants and small children, where the vessels tend to overlap each other. Once the vein has been successfully cannulated, the arterial cannula is sewn to the skin by means of the eyelets on the hub of the cannula.

Often, children who have been fasted after midnight, in actuality have had nothing by mouth (NPO) for 12 or more hours even when a scheduled early morning start of their case has not been delayed. Although the NPO was intended for only four to six hours, when the patient goes to bed at a reasonable evening hour (particularly when they have not been given fluids before going to bed), the patient easily can be NPO for more than twelve hours before their catheterization begins the next morning. If there is an unanticipated delay in starting the case, this interval of NPO approaches 18 hours! This duration of NPO will dehydrate *any* individual and, in turn, significantly empty their vascular space and lower their venous pressure. Any dehydration is aggravated in very small or debilitated patients or in very warm geographical environments or low humidities. Any, or a combination, of these circumstances results in a very low venous pressure and very collapsed veins and makes the percutaneous puncture of the veins even more difficult.

Under these circumstances which create dehydration of the patient, there are several alternatives to circumvent the problem. In the hospitalized patient, supplemental oral fluids should be ordered and administered at specific times throughout the night. In smaller or debilitated patients, maintenance fluids are administered intravenously. If the patient is still dry on arrival at the catheterization laboratory and venous puncture for the catheterization initially is impossible, a 10 ml per kilogram bolus of fluid is given through the pre-existing intravenous line or through a peripheral IV started in the laboratory. A final alternative, particularly if all venous access is a problem, is to enter the artery with the initial percutaneous puncture. Once the cannula for the arterial monitoring is in place, a bolus of 10 ml/kg of isotonic fluid is administered slowly through the arterial line.

Except in some very large patients, it is generally better *not* to have a syringe attached to, nor to apply negative pressure to the puncturing needle while the needle is being introduced into the tissues. A syringe attached to the needle eliminates the ability to see any infinitesimally small movement of fluid in the hub of the needle, interferes with the "feel" of the needle during the puncture and in the presence of a low venous pressure or small vessels, significant negative pressure applied to the syringe/needle can actually collapse the vessel as it is entered. Also when a syringe is attached to the needle, the manipulation required to detach the syringe in order to introduce the wire once blood does appear in the needle/syringe, often displaces the tip of the needle from the small lumen of the vessel. This is an even greater problem in very small patients.

The exception to having nothing attached to the needle is when the patient shows signs of pain and requires more local anesthesia during the attempts at vessel entry. In this circumstance, a syringe containing the local anesthesia is attached to the percutaneous needle which is being used for the attempted percutaneous vessel entry. Negative pressure is applied to the attached syringe full of xylocaine as the percutaneous needle (now being used for the local anesthesia injection), is advanced very slowly into the tissues. Assuming no blood returns during the needle introduction, the area is re-infiltrated through the percutaneous needle exactly as at the onset of the procedure. However, by using the larger percutaneous needle, if, while the area is being re-infiltrated, the vessel is entered inadvertently and blood is withdrawn into the syringe by the continuous negative pressure on the syringe, the syringe is removed without disturbing the position of the needle in the vessel and the wire is introduced through the same needle. After the wire is introduced in this fashion, additional xylocaine is introduced around the puncture site and vessel to alleviate the pain of further manipulations, but now through a separate smaller needle.

"Seldinger" technique of needle introduction

The first technique described for percutaneous vessel entry for cardiac catheterization was the Seldinger™ technique[3]. Although all percutaneous techniques frequently are considered synonymous and interchangeable, the Seldinger™ technique used a very special needle and is very different from the currently used single-wall technique. The true Seldinger™ needle is seldom used anymore, but many operators in cardiac catheterization laboratories still use a crude modification of the Seldinger™ technique. The Seldinger needle™ used in the true or original Seldinger™ puncture consisted of a hollow, blunt-tipped metal cannula which was relatively smooth, with no angled bevel at the tip. The cannula had a tight fitting, solid, sharp-tipped stylet which extended several millimeters beyond the tip of the hollow cannula. The edges of the tip of the blunt cannula tapered to a smooth transition against the outer wall of the contained stylet.

The Seldinger™ needle, and the technique are designed for a through and through puncture of both walls of the vessel during the needle introduction with the intent that the lumen of the vessel is entered during the withdrawal of the hollow canula only. The puncture site is prepared and the intended vessel localized as described for the single-wall puncture technique. The Seldinger™ needle with its enclosed solid stylet is introduced into the skin at a steep angle (45–70°) over the vessel. The needle is advanced smoothly, directly and empirically into the tissues at this angle until the needle stops or the hub of the needle reaches the skin. When the needle has been introduced fully into the tissues (and hopefully has passed completely through the center of the vessel), the sharp, solid stylet is withdrawn completely from the hollow cannula and the angle of the hollow cannula is decreased (flattened) to as close to parallel to the skin surface as possible. With the hollow cannula maintained at this flattened angle, it is withdrawn slowly, while continually watching for blood return in the cannula. Some operators attach a syringe to the cannula after the stylet has been removed and apply negative pressure to the cannula during its slow withdrawal.

The entrance of the tip of the lumen of the blunt canula into the lumen of the vessel is accomplished as the tip of the blunt canula is withdrawn through the back wall of the vessel and before it is pulled out through the anterior wall of the vessel during the slow, meticulous withdrawal of the canula. As the blunt-tipped metal cannula is withdrawn very slowly, the tip is withdrawn through first and, hopefully, only the posterior wall of the vessel, and as a consequence becomes positioned within the lumen of the vessel. When properly within the vessel lumen, blood returns into the cannula (with or without suction with a syringe). When blood return is obtained and while maintaining the cannula in the precise position and as flattened against the skin surface as possible, the blunt cannula is gently advanced further into (hopefully) the vessel lumen. The concept is that when blood return is obtained, the blunt, smooth tip of the cannula (without the stylet) is entirely within the lumen of the vessel. The blunt tip of the cannula, without a sharp tip to puncture or catch on the vessel wall, theoretically advances smoothly within the lumen of the vessel. This technique is effective when the vessel is large and the initial puncture passes centrally through and not off to one side of the vessel. Similar to other percutaneous techniques, a wire can be advanced into the vessel through the Seldinger™ cannula rather than advancing the cannula itself. Unfortunately, neither the Seldinger™ needle nor the technique assures a central puncture of the vessel and even a side nick of the vessel with only a small part of the blunt tip within the lumen of the vessel can allow blood return into the cannula but, at the same time, will not allow the cannula to be advanced nor a wire to be introduced into the vein through the cannula.

The Seldinger™ puncture technique is no longer advocated for vessel entry for cardiac catheterization procedures. The classic Seldinger™ technique has no better chance of accurately puncturing the vessel than the single-wall technique, and when the vessel is punctured both the anterior and posterior walls of the vessel are punctured obligatorily and purposefully. Even when the vessel is successfully cannulated with a wire and then a sheath/dilator, the large posterior puncture of the vessel remains patent and allows continued bleeding into the tissues throughout and after the procedure.

Although the classic Seldinger™ needle is seldom used anymore, a bastardized version of the Seldinger™ technique is, unfortunately, commonly used. With the current Seldinger™ technique the tissues are speared repeatedly and rapidly with a standard, sharp and open-tipped needle. The needle is introduced rapidly and deeply, knowingly and purposefully trying to transect the vessel during its introduction, with the eventual intent of entering the vessel lumen during a slower withdrawal of the needle through the vessel from the deeper tissues. Unfortunately, when the true Seldinger™ needle is not used, each puncture is made with a sharp cutting bevel of the needle, which results in significant trauma to the tissues and vessel walls. Also different from the true Seldinger™ technique, when blood return is observed into the hub of the needle during its withdrawal, rather than attempting to advance the sharp needle itself, a wire is introduced through the needle into the vessel. This technique has no greater accuracy or likelihood for puncturing the vessel, but also produces a through and through puncture of both the anterior and posterior walls of the vessel (Figure 4.5). Often this technique is used by more "impatient" operators

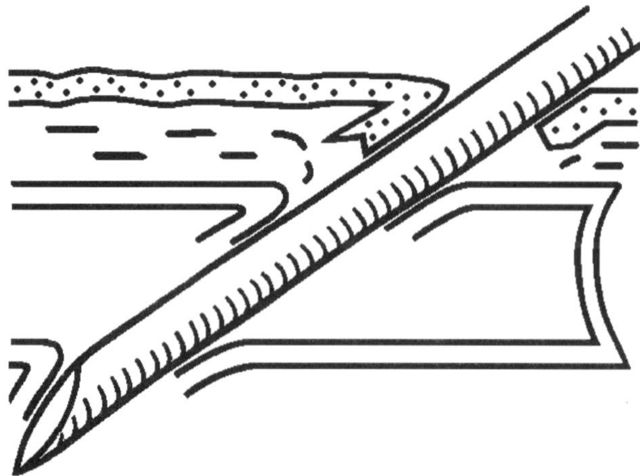

Figure 4.5 Through and through puncture of vessel producing unnecessary and undesirable hole in posterior wall of vessel.

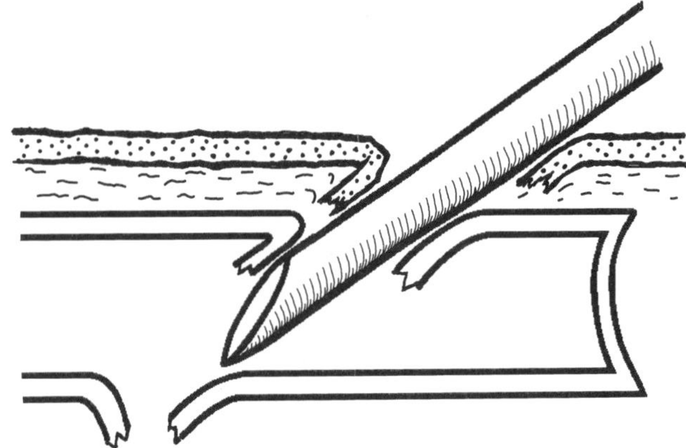

Figure 4.6 Tip of needle withdrawn into vessel lumen after through and through puncture of vessel, but leaving an unnecessary and undesirable open hole in posterior wall of vessel.

who perform multiple, repeated stabs at the vessel in fairly rapid sequence until blood eventually appears in the needle. Unfortunately, this relies on one of a large number of "random" stabs (and vessel punctures!) to eventually enter a vessel, rather than any attempt at entering the vessel precisely with a single-wall puncture. This is a particularly poor technique for infants and small children, where the diameter of the cutting bevel of the needle is close to the diameter of the vessel—particularly when the vessel is in spasm from the trauma of prior unsuccessful stabs.

The through and through Seldinger puncture is occasionally performed inadvertently while attempting a single-wall puncture. During the needle introduction in the attempt at a single-wall puncture, but when no blood is obtained even when the needle is introduced all of the way to the hub, the needle is then withdrawn very slowly while observing for the return of blood into the needle. In this circumstance, occasionally the needle has collapsed and passed completely through the vessel during the needle's introduction with no blood return being observed. At the same time, the needle may have passed exactly through the anterior vessel wall, through the center of the vessel lumen and on through the posterior wall. In this circumstance, as the needle is withdrawn very slowly through the back wall of the vessel, the lumen of the needle enters the lumen of the vessel (Figure 4.6). Although this was not the intended technique for entry into the vessel, when blood returns into the needle during its withdrawal, the wire is introduced similarly to a single-wall puncture technique.

Other modifications of the Seldinger™ technique use the Medi-Cut™ or Quick-Cath™ needles as the percutaneous puncture needles. These needles with a blunt plastic cannula over the sharp tapered metal needle are used to enter vessels in one of two separate techniques. When used to enter very superficial, visible or palpable vessels for intravenous therapy or peripheral arterial monitoring, the needle set is introduced very slowly and meticulously toward the visible or palpable vessel with the needle set as parallel to the vessel and as flat against the skin as possible. As the metal tip of the needle punctures the anterior wall of the vessel, blood returns into the hub of the metal needle. With the central metal needle fixed in this position, the plastic cannula is advanced off the metal needle and, it is hoped, into the lumen of the vessel. Blood should continue returning through the hub of the metal needle while the tip of the plastic cannula is being advanced within the lumen of the vessel. With continued good blood return after the cannula has advanced at least 5 mm off the metal needle, the central metal needle is withdrawn. Blood should continue to return through the plastic cannula at this point. With good blood return, the peripheral intravenous/flush line is attached to the cannula, and with good flow into the cannula from the intravenous or monitoring tubing, the cannula is advanced further into the vessel.

When Medi-Cut™ or Quick-Cath™ needles are used for the introduction of sheath/dilators and then catheters into these more peripheral vessels (radial, brachial), once the plastic cannula has been successfully advanced into the lumen of the vessel, instead of attaching an intravenous/monitoring line, a soft tipped, spring guide wire is introduced into the plastic cannula and advanced well into the vessel. Thereafter, the introduction of a sheath/dilator over the wire and then a catheter through the sheath is the same as the technique described later in this chapter.

The second use of the Medi-Cut™ or Quick-Cath™ needle is to use the plastic cannula of these needles in a similar way to the metal cannula of the Seldinger™ needle during a deep vessel puncture. The Medi-Cut™ or

Quick-Cath™ needle with its covering plastic cannula is introduced into the deeper tissues and punctures completely through the vessel as the set is advanced into the tissues. Once completely into the tissues, the metal inner needle is withdrawn completely from the plastic cannula. After the removal of the metal inner needle, the plastic cannula is slowly and meticulously withdrawn until the tip of the cannula pulls through the posterior wall of the vessel and back into the lumen of the vessel, similar to the technique using the metal cannula of the true Seldinger™ needle. Since the angle of puncture into a deeper vessel is relatively steep, and any flattening of the plastic cannula against the skin merely bends or kinks the cannula at the skin's surface, when blood returns in the plastic cannula it is *not* advanced into the vessel but a soft-tipped spring guide wire is introduced into the plastic cannula *without* advancing the cannula. This technique using the Medi-Cut™ or Quick-Cath™ set still has the sharp cutting edge of the needle transecting both walls of the vessel during the introduction and still does not assure any better chance of entering the vessel centrally, or at all.

Introduction of the wire into the percutaneous needle

The preferred wire for the percutaneous technique is a special, very soft, straight-tipped, spring guide wire (Argon Medical Inc., Athens, TX), which is significantly smaller in its outside diameter than the inner lumen of the needle through which the wire is being introduced. Wires for percutaneous entry into vessels are preferably non-coated in order not to compromise the flexibility of the tip of the wires. There are many satisfactory wires available either as separate wires or as part of percutaneous kits (Cook Inc., Bloomington, IN). Some of the small, special, "torque-controlled" wires have particularly soft, floppy tips and are useful for the percutaneous entry into difficult vessels. These torque wires are very expensive, which makes them inappropriate for routine use.

The introduction of the wire into a needle during percutaneous vessel entry must be a very precise, smooth and gentle procedure. The wire is never introduced nor withdrawn rapidly nor forcefully. The wire should be advanced only when the tip of the needle is in a perfect position and alignment within the lumen of the vessel. When the tip of the needle enters the vessel correctly during either the needle puncture or the needle withdrawal back into the vessel, and when the wire is advanced correctly as it is introduced, the wire passes beyond the tip of the needle and into the vessel without even the slightest change in the tactile sensation to the fingers holding the wire and absolutely no resistance to the wire advancing. There should be no difference in the feel of the wire once it is moving past and then outside of the needle compared to the sensation of the wire advancing within the needle. In addition to no change in sensation as the tip of the wire advances correctly into the vessel beyond the tip of the needle, there is absolutely no resistance to the forward movement of the wire, no bowing or bending of the proximal wire and no extra pressure applied to the wire! If any resistance is felt and/or if the wire actually stops advancing at any distance beyond the tip of the needle, the wire is ***not*** advanced ***any*** *further*. Absolutely no force should be applied to the wire.

In order to prevent any excessive force from being delivered to the tip of the wire during its introduction, the wire is gripped 6–10 cm back and away from the distal tip by the fingers that are holding the wire, as the wire is being introduced into the needle. As the wire is advanced into the needle, the fingers grasping the wire are moved progressively back along the wire proportionate to the distance the wire is introduced. The fingers grasping the wire should *never* be any closer than 6 cm from the hub of the needle during the wire introduction. This very proximal gripping of the fingers on the wire allows the wire to bow or deflect laterally away from the hub of the needle when any resistance is encountered at the tip of the wire or any forward force is applied to the wire against resistance (Figure 4.7). This, in turn, prevents undue force from being delivered to the tip of the wire during its introduction.

When the wire is gripped immediately adjacent to the hub of the needle, enough force can be applied to the wire to dig the tip of the wire into the tissues beyond the tip of the needle and adjacent to the vessel without any tactile recognition of the erroneous location of the tip of the wire outside of the vessel lumen. With continued forward force, a wire which is held close to the hub of the needle will kink at the hub of the needle (Figure 4.8). The undesirable force applied to the wire also becomes obvious when the wire is withdrawn and the wire tip is distorted (mangled). This is only caused by unrecognized or inadvertent extra force applied to the wire.

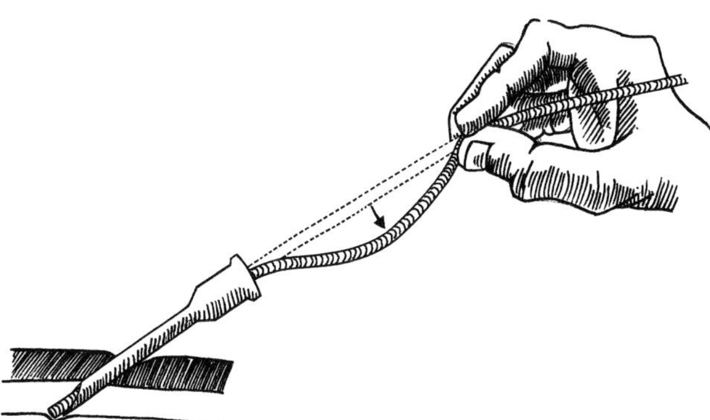

Figure 4.7 Correct position of the fingers on the guide wire away from the hub of the needle during the introduction into the needle/vessel. The wire can bend or "bow" to the side when minimal extra force is applied.

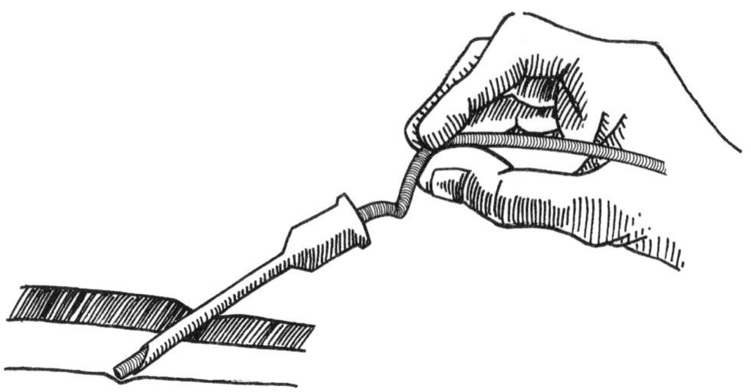

Figure 4.8 Incorrect position of the fingers on the guide wire close to the hub of the needle during the introduction of the wire into the needle. Any force on the wire will kink the wire at the hub.

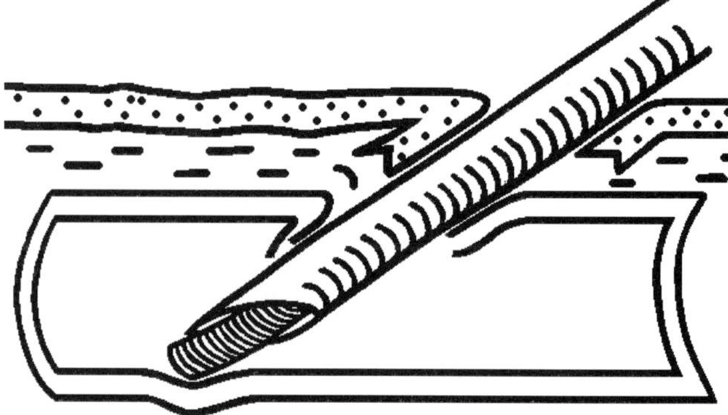

Figure 4.9 Tip of wire advancing from needle with bevel of needle facing down (posteriorly) in vessel, with wire prevented from leaving needle.

When even minor resistance is encountered during the introduction of the wire, it is slowly and carefully withdrawn completely into the shaft of the needle. Again there must *not* be any resistance to the withdrawal of the wire into the needle. If the wire is withdrawn forcefully, a bent or distorted soft tip of the wire can easily be sheered off the distal end of the wire by the sharp tip of the needle. The wire should be withdrawn gently, entirely out of the needle and the tip of the wire examined. If the wire does not withdraw smoothly into the needle and without any resistance at all, the needle and the wire together are withdrawn out of the skin entirely and the percutaneous puncture restarted after complete hemostasis has been achieved.

The *angle* of *entry* of the needle into the vessel is changed by *slight* side to side and/or up and down movement of the hub off the surface of the skin or by an interment ***very slight*** (5–10°) ***slow and partial rotation*** of the needle. These changes in the direction of the needle are made in an attempt to redirect the angle of the bevel at the tip of the needle very slightly within the lumen of the vessel in order to redirect and align it more in line with the lumen of the vessel. When the bevel is facing posteriorly or even laterally, the angle of the bevel actually interferes with the tip of a wire as it advances beyond the tip of the needle, and prevents it from passing into the lumen of the vessel at all (Figure 4.9). A change in the direction of the bevel at the tip of the needle or a slight change in the angle of the needle will align the bevel or the lumen of the needle better within the lumen of the vessel as the shaft of the needle aligns better with the skin and vessel (Figures 4.4a and 4.10). With each very slight redirection of the angle of the needle, a repeat gentle attempt is made at the reintroduction of the wire.

If the fine wire still meets resistance or buckles and even when there is good blood flow through the needle around the wire, it indicates that the tip of the needle is still *not* aligned *correctly* and/or is not completely *within* the *lumen* of the vessel. The wire is withdrawn, but initially the needle should *not* be advanced into, nor withdrawn out of, the vessel any further. First, multiple attempts should be made at changing the ***angle*** of the entrance of the needle into the vessel or the angle of the bevel to the vessel. The vessel in an infant is only one or two millimeters in diameter and even *minimal, in or out movement* of the needle will advance the tip of the needle through the posterior wall or withdraw the tip of the needle completely out of the lumen of the vessel.

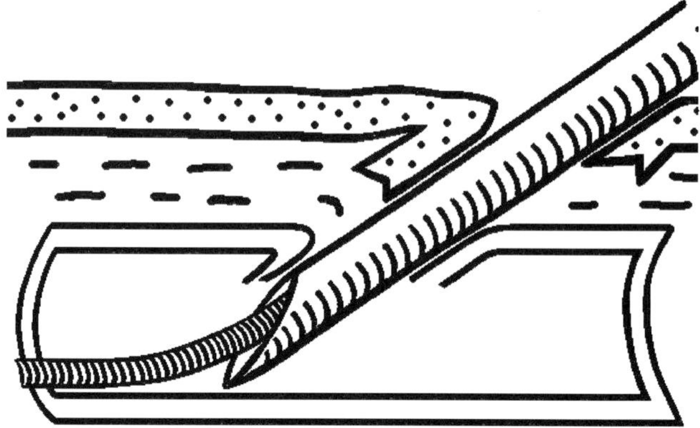

Figure 4.10 Small, soft wire advancing easily out of the tip of the needle with the bevel of the needle facing up (anteriorly).

If, after multiple attempts at introducing the wire, the tip of the wire still does not advance freely past the tip of the needle and into the punctured vessel, or if any extravasation of blood/hematoma begins to form around the puncture site, the wire and the needle are withdrawn completely from the vessel and skin. Firm pressure is immediately applied over the puncture site to prevent visible or subcutaneous oozing from the vessel. If there had been good venous blood return through the needle with the first puncture, the pressure over the site is maintained for three to five ***minutes*** before restarting the puncture. Even when blood does not leak through the puncture site at the surface of the skin, when the needle is removed from the vessel after a vessel has been punctured, bleeding from the vessel will continue beneath the skin into the subcutaneous tissues unless pressure is maintained for sufficient time to achieve hemostasis of the vessel.

Although the bleeding is not apparent at the skin surface, continued subcutaneous bleeding creates a significant subcutaneous hematoma. If a hematoma begins to form visibly around the needle during wire manipulation or during readjustments of the needle, the needle is withdrawn completely and pressure held for 5 minutes (or more, especially if the punctured vessel was an artery!). A hematoma not only eventually creates pain and a cosmetic problem for the patient, but makes all subsequent punctures in the area more difficult. The blood which has extravasated into the subcutaneous tissues and is extrinsic to the vessel, changes the course and location of the vessel and can actually compress adjacent veins making the target for the puncture even narrower. A subsequent puncture into the hematoma creates false blood return into the needle from blood in the hematoma returning into the needle during additional punctures. Before restarting the puncture, the needle is flushed thoroughly and cleared of any small clots.

The wire size relative to the internal diameter of the lumen of the needle makes a difference to the ease of passing the wire from the needle into the vessel. Even the tip of a very soft-tipped guide wire remains straight and relatively stiff for several millimeters as it extends just beyond the tip of the needle. The stiffer and the thicker the wire, the further the wire will continue out of the tip of the needle in a straight direction that is parallel to the long axis of the needle, rather than deflecting even slightly to conform to an even slight angle into the vessel lumen. When there is a discrepancy between the direction of the long axis of the needle and the long axis of the vessel, the tip of a stiffer or thicker wire digs into (and through!) the opposite wall of the vessel rather than deflecting into and passing within the lumen of the vessel (Figure 4.11). The tighter the fit of the wire within the needle (e.g. a 0.021″ wire within a 21-gauge needle) the greater distance the tip of the soft wire remains straight, beyond the tip of the needle, before the wire begins to deflect and follow the course of the vessel lumen.

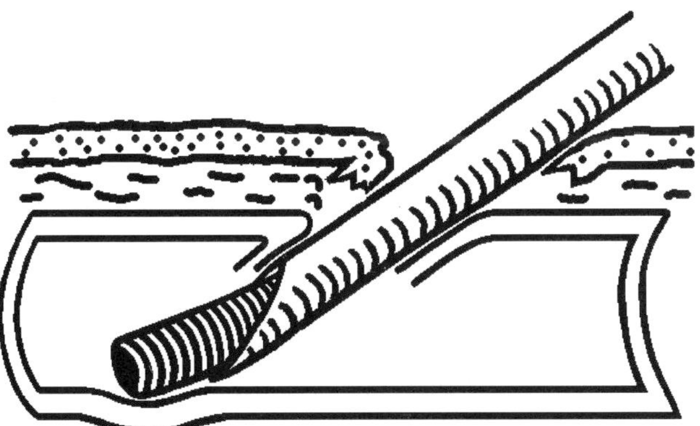

Figure 4.11 Larger diameter wire at anything less than an ideal angle stops in the wall of the vessel just beyond the tip of needle and has no capability of deflecting into lumen of vessel.

When there is any difficulty in introducing the guide wire into the vessel, the wire being used should be downsized. For example, a 0.018″ wire is used in a 21-gauge needle. A wire which has an outside diameter (OD) that is significantly smaller than the inside diameter (ID) of the needle has more flexibility and allows slack at its tip as it exits the needle into the vessel and allows the wire to deflect into the vessel lumen much sooner (Figure 4.10).

When the wire passes freely into the vessel with no resistance and, preferably, no change at all in the tactile sensation as the tip passes beyond the tip of the needle, the wire is advanced into the needle and vessel quickly, smoothly and as far as possible. As soon as the guide wire is well into the vessel and secured, the needle is withdrawn over the wire and out of the vessel and skin. The wire is grasped very securely while firm pressure is applied over the puncture site. While holding pressure over the wire/puncture site, a brief scan is made by fluoroscopy over the thorax and cardiac silhouette in order to visualize the course and movements/deflections of the wire within the thorax, which should help to verify whether the wire is in a vein or an artery. A venous location of the wire is verified by the wire buckling in a wide loop within the cardiac silhouette (e.g. in the right atrium) and passing into the ventricle from the atrium with or without the generation of any premature ventricular contractions. A wire merely passing on the right side of the vertebral column in the area of the cardiac silhouette, by itself, does *not* verify that the wire is in a venous channel passing to the heart. Passage of the wire up a right descending aorta or an azygos vein can appear identical to passage through the inferior vena caval channel to the right atrium! The wire must buckle or be advanced into the right ventricle to verify the venous location. Verification of entrance into a femoral artery is of less importance, since only a small cannula will be introduced into the vessel before the pressure is verified.

Occasionally the wire can be introduced through the needle easily, but advances only a short distance beyond the tip of the needle (several cm) and then stops abruptly. This occurs more commonly with wires introduced into the left inguinal area. In this circumstance, the wire may have entered the initial vein properly but then advanced into a side branch of a vein and/or occasionally has actually exited the lumen of the vessel! Once the wire stops advancing freely, it should ***not be*** advanced any further until the tip of the wire is visualized directly on the fluoroscopy and an attempt is made at redirecting the tip of the wire under direct visualization. If the redirected wire again moves freely within the vessel into the thorax and then to the right heart chambers, the introduction of the sheath/dilator is continued.

When, even under direct visualization, the wire stops moving at all or cannot be advanced freely within the vessel beyond the initial 2–4 cm, the wire is fixed very securely in place in the vessel, the needle is removed over the wire and replaced with the plastic cannula of a Medi-Cut™ or Quick-Cath™. For this maneuver, the tip of the Medi-Cut™ cannula is introduced just to the beginning of the taper of the Medi-Cut™ cannula and the Quick-Cath™ is advanced only half of the length of its cannula. In either case, the plastic cannula should be securely in the vessel, blood returns into the cannula around the wire and the wire is withdrawn from the plastic cannula. If the wire was initially definitely within the vessel lumen, blood returns freely through the plastic cannula following the complete withdrawal of the wire. When blood returns from the vessel, a small "J" curve is formed on the soft tip of the wire or a commercially available "J-wire" is used. The J-tipped wire is reintroduced through the Medi-Cut™ cannula, which is secured well into the vessel. The tightly curved tip of the J-wire usually passes unhindered through the cannula, into the vein and on into the thorax. If not, the wire is removed from the plastic cannula very slowly. If there is still free return of venous blood through the cannula, a small (1 ml), slow and gentle, test injection of contrast is performed through the Medi-Cut™ cannula while recording over the area on biplane angiography or biplane stored fluoroscopy. This angiogram verifies that the tip of the cannula is within the vein and that the vein actually is patent. If the vein is patent and the Medi-Cut™ is well within the vein, the soft J curved wire is reintroduced through the Medi-Cut™ and advanced carefully while the course of the wire is observed under fluoroscopy. In rare circumstances, when the vein is widely patent but there is an unusual branch or turn in the course of the vein, a torque-controlled wire with a curved, flexible tip is used to purposefully follow the angiographically defined course of the proper venous channel.

If there is no blood return when the wire is removed from the Medi-Cut™ cannula, then the Medi-Cut™ cannula is withdrawn very slowly and smoothly (in half-millimeter increments) while watching carefully for a new blood return into the Medi-Cut™ cannula. This withdrawal is similar to the slow withdrawal of the original puncture needle after the initial needle puncture had inadvertently passed completely through the vessel. When the tip of the needle was passing through the lumen of the vessel, blood could return into the needle very transiently. However, once the tip of the needle had passed completely through the vessel, the wire (and subsequent Medi-Cut™ cannula) will be directed into the soft subcutaneous or adventitial tissues behind or adjacent to the vessel. During the slow withdrawal of the Medi-Cut™ cannula, with its squared off non-beveled tip, from "behind" the vessel, the tip of the cannula often pops back squarely into the lumen of the vessel (similarly to the original Seldinger™ vessel cannulation technique), allowing free blood return and easy, proper introduction of the wire. If the wire does not pass easily through the tip of the plastic cannula, the side-to-side or up–down angle of the cannula is changed slightly (similarly to the procedure with the original needle) while gently and repeatedly reintroducing the wire until it passes into the lumen of the vessel.

If the wire does not pass easily and smoothly into the vessel with any of these maneuvers with the cannula, the cannula is withdrawn, pressure held for several minutes and after good hemostasis is achieved, the needle puncture is restarted.

Alternative wires for percutaneous vessel entry

The use of specially shaped or even non-metallic wires has been advocated to assist in percutaneous vessel entry. A J-tipped wire has been used and is often part of a percutaneous kit. J-tipped wires are occasionally used to introduce wires into larger diameter vessels but this requires a fairly large lumen of the vessel. The use of a J-tipped wire also requires that the tip of the needle is positioned precisely in the lumen and that the tip is even more perfectly aligned within the lumen following the puncture.

When the very tip of a J-curved wire exits the tip of the needle, the preformed curve at the tip of the J-wire causes the very tip of the wire to exit essentially perpendicular to the long axis of the needle (and vessel) initially and for the first few millimeters. As a consequence, the needle tip must be positioned very securely and centrally in the vessel with the bevel aligned with the lumen, and the vessel must be large enough in diameter to accommodate the curve of the J-wire backing out of the needle (Figure 4.12).

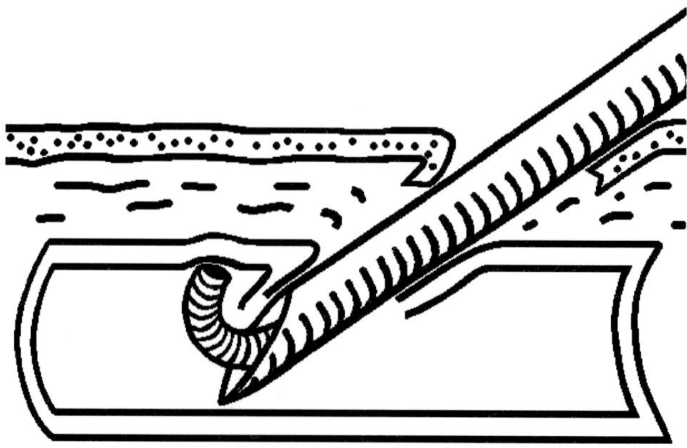

Figure 4.12 J-tipped wire exiting the tip of a needle with the bevel up.

Once the J-tipped wire enters the lumen of the vessel cleanly, the J-curve traverses the course of the vessel without becoming hung up on side branches. In very small vessels, the lumen of the vessel is often not of adequate diameter to accommodate the perpendicular exit of the tip of the wire from the needle unless the bevel of the needle fortuitously is aligned exactly in the direction of the lumen of the vessel. A J-tipped wire does not help with the precise puncture of the vessels and is actually counter productive for the introduction of wires into very small vessels. J-tipped wires are *not* recommended for routine percutaneous vessel entry in infants and children. They are, however, extremely useful for maneuvering through tortuous vessels once the cannula and wire are securely in the vessel.

In the absence of small, very soft tipped wires, fine, filamentous, nylon fishing-line has been used as a substitute for the percutaneous wire. These nylon lines were effective at entering the vessel, but also were prone to being cut in two by the tip of the needle during any attempt at withdrawing the line back through the needle. This was particularly hazardous since the excised segment of line in the vessel produced an intravascular foreign body, which was non-radio opaque. Occasionally nylon lines, even when introduced successfully into the vessel, were not stiff or supportive enough to introduce a sheath/dilator over them. This problem of support for the sheath/dilator is overcome by first replacing the original needle which is over the nylon line with a Medi-Cut™ cannula. Once the Medi-Cut™ is secured, the nylon line, which is well into the vessel through the plastic cannula, is replaced with a standard spring guide wire. Nylon line is not recommended for percutaneous introductions because of the potential for depositing a non-radio opaque foreign body into the vascular system.

"Target"-assisted percutaneous access to vessels

When access to a vessel is not possible by a standard, direct, percutaneous puncture, a catheter or wire that is introduced from an alternative site can be directed into the vessel to be punctured and, in turn, used as a "target" for the puncture. The tip of a catheter or wire introduced into a different vessel is advanced centrally and then redirected peripherally into the target vessel which has been difficult (impossible) to enter by direct percutaneous puncture. The tip of the catheter coming from another introductory site creates a very well defined target within the vessel, which otherwise is difficult to puncture. Target-assisted access to a vessel is used when an additional or better vascular access is necessary and the additional vessel being punctured cannot be entered because of distortion, narrowing or spasm in the vessel. The target technique is usually performed from a contralateral femoral vessel although a "catheter target" for a percutaneous puncture can be created approaching from any other vessel in continuity with the target vessel, e.g. from a jugular vein to a femoral or hepatic vein or vice versa. This procedure is possible from virtually any combination of two vascular introductory sites unless either of the vessels is obstructed or obliterated centrally between the two peripheral sites.

The target technique is useful for any vessel that is difficult to enter for any reason, as long as the target vessel is not totally obstructed and the vessel can be accessed from another vascular introductory site. The target technique is useful in very small patients or when the target vessel has been distorted by a prior indwelling line or prior catheterization procedures. It is also useful when the introduction of several very large sheaths is necessary and the vessel which is already cannulated is considered too small for a "piggy-back" introduction of the second catheter into the same vessel. This technique is used most commonly to introduce additional venous sheaths, but also can be used for difficult arterial access.

Biplane fluoroscopy is essential in order to use this technique effectively. An end-hole catheter is introduced into another peripheral vessel, manipulated from that vessel, first centrally in the circulation and then into the more peripheral target vessel into which the introduction of the additional needle/wire is being attempted. The catheter tip is advanced as far as possible peripherally to the proposed (or attempted) puncture site in the target vessel. Often this requires the adjunct maneuvering of a torque-controlled wire ahead of the catheter and into the more peripheral vessel. The catheter tip is advanced in the target vessel until the tip of the catheter is positioned immediately beneath the skin puncture area of the proposed needle puncture site. This position is verified with biplane fluoroscopy over the needle puncture site. A needle or metal instrument is placed directly over the proposed puncture site on the skin surface to serve as a reference on the fluoroscopy between the proposed puncture site and the tip of the target catheter, which is within the vessel.

The lumen at the tip of an end-hole catheter coming from the other vessel provides the ideal target for the needle puncture. The catheter tip is maneuvered within the target vessel until the lumen at its tip is facing the puncture site on the skin over the vessel. The tip of the end-hole target catheter must be visualized using biplane fluoroscopy in order to have both side by side and depth relationships. When the lumen of the target catheter is larger than the diameter of the percutaneous needle for the puncture (e.g. a 6-French or larger diameter catheter and a 21-gauge needle), the percutaneous needle can be introduced into the lumen at the tip of the catheter. The needle is introduced through the skin, through the subcutaneous tissues and with a small amount of precise manipulation under direct biplane fluoroscopic guidance, the tip of the needle is advanced into the end of the lumen of the end-hole catheter within the vessel. The guide wire is passed through the needle directly into the catheter. As the wire passes from the needle and, in turn, is introduced retrograde into the catheter, it is unequivocally within the target vessel lumen!

Once the wire has been advanced far into the catheter, the needle is withdrawn off the wire and out of the skin. The catheter from the contralateral vessel is withdrawn far enough over the distal end of the wire within the target vessel to allow a sheath/dilator to be introduced into the vessel over the wire from the skin puncture site. The sheath/dilator is introduced over the wire into the skin and advanced into the vessel as the target catheter is withdrawn off the wire.

When a difficult vessel entry is anticipated because of local tissue scaring or vessel spasm, the wire can be advanced retrograde all of the way within the target catheter until the tip of the wire appears at the hub of the target catheter outside of the skin at the introductory site of the target catheter. This creates a through and through wire which can be held very securely while the sheath/dilator is introduced into the target vessel.

Occasionally the percutaneous wire does not enter the catheter tip but enters the vessel cleanly next to the target catheter and passes centrally with some further manipulation. In that circumstance, the central location is documented on fluoroscopy. The target catheter is withdrawn and the sheath/dilator is introduced into the vessel exactly as with any other percutaneous puncture which is performed without a target catheter.

A somewhat more complicated but useful alternative to the use of the tip of the end-hole catheter as the target is to use a small snare and a snare catheter introduced from the alternative introduction site as the target[4]. With this technique, the needle puncture into the target does not have to be quite as precise nor even totally within the vessel lumen. A Microvena™ snare catheter (ev3, Plymouth, MN) with a small (2–4 mm) snare loop is introduced into the original vessel and manipulated distally into the vessel which is being punctured. The snare loop will serve as the target. The snare loop can be introduced through almost any end-hole catheter previously introduced into the original vessel. The snare is opened in the target vessel just beneath the skin puncture site for the target vessel (Figure 4.13a). The open snare creates a slightly larger, "circular target" within the vessel just beneath the expected puncture site. The needle puncture of the area is carried out using biplane fluoroscopic visualization and aiming for the center of the loop of the snare as the target. After the needle passes through the center of the loop of the snare in both fluoroscopic planes, blood is usually seen in the needle and a standard wire introduction is carried out. Even if blood return is not seen in the needle but the needle is definitely through the open loop of the snare, the wire is introduced to the end of the needle and, if possible, beyond the needle tip (Figure 4.13b). The snare is cinched loosely around the needle within the lumen of the vessel (Figure 4.13c). The needle is withdrawn while keeping the wire fixed in place through the snare within the lumen of the vessel. The snare is tightened and, in

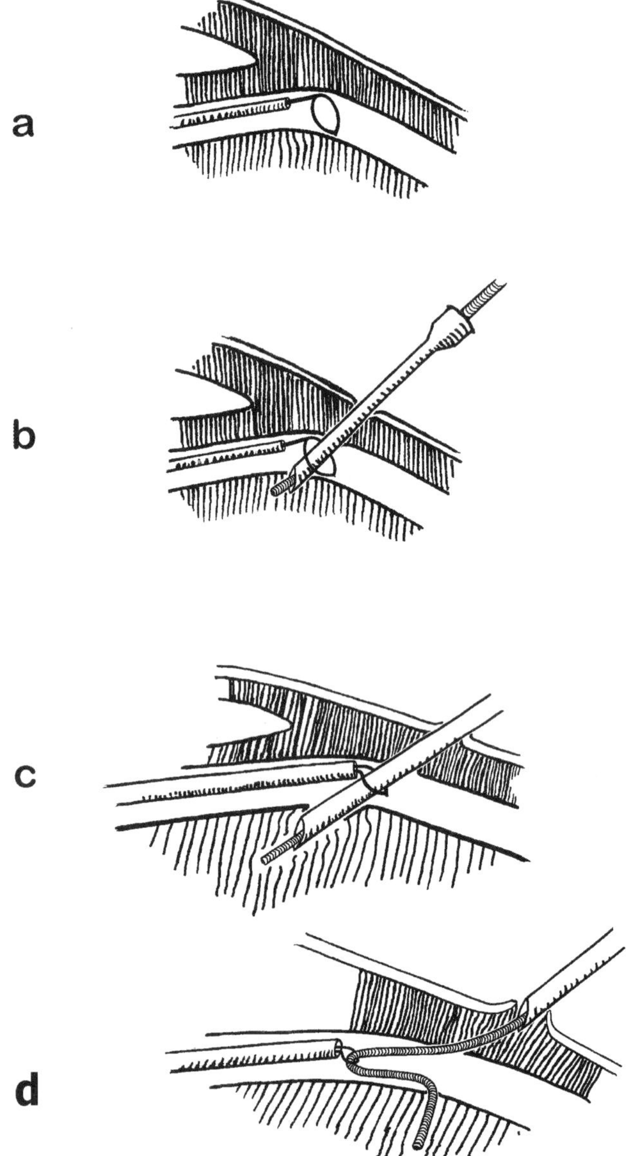

Figure 4.13 Snare assisted puncture: (a) snare opened in "target" vessel after introduction from remote site; (b) needle and wire passing through loop of opened snare within target vessel; (c) needle (and contained wire) passing completely through vessel with snare within lumen of vessel cinched loosely around portion of needle which is passing through lumen; (d) needle is withdrawn off wire and the wire, which is captured by the snare within the lumen, is withdrawn into target vessel after the needle has been withdrawn.

turn, closes around the wire. Once the wire has been grasped securely by the snare, the needle is withdrawn completely. The snare catheter, which is holding the percutaneous wire, is withdrawn along with the "snared wire" toward the central vasculature and away from the original puncture site. This pulls the part of the percutaneous wire which is grasped by the snare into the vessel (Figure 4.13d).

If the wire tip had passed through the posterior wall of the vessel and the tip was not actually in the lumen of the vessel, the snare still grasps the part of the wire where it passes through the snare within the vessel. In this situation the wire is drawn into the lumen when the snare is withdrawn back into the more central vessel. When the tip of the wire is outside of the vessel, the wire folds into the vessel as the tip is pulled out of the surrounding tissues. This is slightly more traumatic to the vessel, producing an unnecessary posterior opening in the vessel. Once the percutaneous wire has been withdrawn and is securely within the vessel, the sheath/dilator is introduced over the wire. Putting tension on the wire with the snare, which is holding the wire from within the vessel, assists in the introduction of the sheath/dilator through dense or scarred tissues.

These target techniques are used to access any difficult-to-enter peripheral vessel or during the training of new catheterizing physicians for a new vascular approach. The target techniques are particularly useful in vessels which are distorted or stenosed by a previous catheterization or indwelling line(s). A catheter introduced from an accessible femoral vein passes readily to an internal jugular, subclavian, axillary or even a hepatic vein to serve as the target for a percutaneous introduction through those entry sites. The opposite is true with catheters introduced from the arm or neck vessels passed into the femoral or hepatics serving as targets for percutaneous puncture into those locations. The same target technique is used successfully for arterial puncture in patients where the particular peripheral arterial pulse is very poor—for example to enter the contralateral femoral artery in a patient with coarctation of the aorta. Catheters can even be advanced to a peripheral arterial site from the central left heart with a catheter that is introduced prograde into the left heart.

Adjunct devices for the identification and localization of the vessels for percutaneous needle/wire introduction

Several systems based on the use of Doppler signals to detect blood flow and echo to image the vessel are available to help locate vessels deep within the subcutaneous tissues. Doppler systems are good for detecting flow and for distinguishing between arterial and venous flow and are fairly accurate for determining the side to side location of both arteries and veins in the deep subcutaneous tissues beneath the skin. The type of vessel beneath the probe is distinguished by the difference in the timing and frequency of the audible flow signals, arteries and veins having distinctly different timing and frequencies. These Doppler-based systems detect only blood flow and do not provide visualization of the lumens, the size of vessels/lumens or extra vascular "spaces" like the signals from an echogram. No precise information about the physical size of the vessel is provided by the Doppler signal. Extravasated blood or fluids in the adjacent subcutaneous tissues do not interfere with the Doppler signal as they do with echo images.

One of these Doppler systems, the Model 811-B, Ultrasonic Doppler Flow Detector (Parks Medical Electronics, Aloha, OR) uses a very thin Doppler probe/transducer, about the size of a pencil, to identify flow in vessels. The probe attaches by a reusable/resterilizable cable to a fairly inexpensive amplifier. The probe and cable can be sterilized repeatedly and are used in the sterile operative field while attached to the amplifier, which is enclosed in a sterile wrap away from the puncture site. The probe scans the subcutaneous tissues beneath it and which are directly in line with it. The side by side location of vessels in the area and type of flow in the vessels are determined from the quality and timing of the Doppler signal. By mentally plotting a straight line into the tissues directly in line with the extremity when the signal from the probe from the desired vessel is of maximum intensity, the probe is pointing at the vessel (within 2–4 mm from side to side). This identifies side to side locations/relationships of vessels but does not provide information about the depth of the vessel. The Doppler signal does not aid in judging precisely how close a puncturing needle is to the vessel until the needle actually compresses the vessel and, in doing so, changes the velocity of flow in the vessel which, in turn, distorts the audible signal being transmitted by the Doppler probe. This system is used to identify the general location of vessels at puncture sites which otherwise are distorted and when no blood return is obtained from the vessels after multiple attempts with the usual puncture procedures. It is also very useful for detecting very faint arterial flow in an artery that is distal to a puncture site when the palpable pulse is absent following a procedure.

Other Doppler devices, such as the P.D. Access Doppler needles™ (Escalon Vascular Access, New Berlin, WI), have a very fine, wire-like, Doppler probe which actually passes through a special percutaneous needle. These needle probes also connect to relatively inexpensive (but reusable) amplifiers by means of a thin disposable sterile cable. The Doppler needle/probes are available as sterile, disposable sets consisting of the special percutaneous needle, the fine Doppler probe and the attaching cable.

The P.D. Access Doppler needles™ are available in three sizes: 18, 20 and 22 gauge (the gauge referring to the size of the percutaneous needle).

The special needle is filled with fluid and introduced superficially into the skin over the anticipated site of the vessel. Once the tip of the needle is under the skin, the needle is refilled with flush solution, making sure that there are no bubbles of air in the column of fluid. The Doppler probe is then introduced into the needle and positioned just within the tip of the needle while the intensity of the Doppler signal is adjusted. The needle with the enclosed probe is angled from side to side and cephalad to caudal within the subcutaneous tissues until either the venous or the arterial Doppler signal is detected. When the appropriate signal is detected for the vessel which it is desired to puncture, the combined needle/probe is advanced into the subcutaneous tissues, angling it to "follow" the intensity of the signal. Theoretically, and most of the time when the needle follows the direction of the maximum Doppler signal, the needle advances to, and punctures the vessel. As the vessel is entered, the Doppler signal increases and changes abruptly, albeit faintly. The Doppler probe is withdrawn from the needle and, hopefully, a column of blood follows the probe out of the needle. Once blood return is obtained, a spring guide wire is introduced similar to the introduction through any other percutaneous needle.

Doppler needle/probe systems superficially appear ideal for introducing needles into the appropriate vessel, however, the vessel is not actually visualized and the change in amplitude and quality of the signal during the transition from the signal in the tissues to the different signal in the vessel is very indistinct. As a consequence, determination of the exact moment of entry into the vessel is difficult. The greater the experience with the system, the easier the subtle changes in the signal are to distinguish as the needle enters the vessel. In addition to the relative inaccuracy, the smallest Doppler needles do not provide as good a signal, and the larger needles with a better signal are too large for the very tiny vessels in infants where help during a percutaneous puncture would provide most advantages. The accuracy of the Doppler guidance certainly improves as the system is used more routinely for percutaneous needle introduction, but routine use also significantly and, probably, unnecessarily increases the expense of the catheterization procedure.

Two dimensional (2-D) echo images are used to visualize the peripheral vessels. The actual lumen of the various vessels within the tissues can be visualized on the 2-D echo image for percutaneous punctures. Whether the vessels are visualized longitudinally or in cross section with the echo depends entirely upon the orientation of the echo transducer on the skin. The echo image distinguishes artery from vein by the distinct pulsation of the artery or by the ease with which the veins are compressed by gentle pressure on the skin with the echo transducer. The actual walls of the peripheral vessels are very indistinct within the subcutaneous tissues as seen on the echo images and, as a consequence, it is difficult to distinguish veins from free collections ("lakes") of fluid within the tissues. For example a pool of extravasated blood from a previous "missed puncture" or a collection of previously injected local anesthesia is hard to distinguish from an intact venous structure. In addition, many standard echo transducers are quite large and bulky. As a consequence, when the vessel is properly imaged, the transducer head occupies most of the area exactly over, and around, the precise puncture site. Most standard 2-D cardiac echo machines are very expensive, making it impractical (impossible!) to use a standard echo machine as a dedicated routine adjunct for all percutaneous punctures in the catheterization laboratory.

The use of a 2-D image to localize vessels has become more routine with the availability of the Site-Rite™ 2-D echo system (Dymax Corporation, Pittsburgh, PA), which is a small, portable, battery operated, and relatively inexpensive echo machine. The Site-Rite™ has a relatively small transducer and is very useful (essential!) for the identification and localization of the vessels during percutaneous punctures, particularly in the neck area. This apparatus is described in detail later in this Chapter in the discussion of the "Jugular vein approach".

Sheath/dilator introduction

As soon as the wire has entered the vein successfully and advanced well into the vasculature (either before or after arterial cannulation), and while continually holding pressure over the entrance site, the needle is immediately removed over the wire from the skin/vessel. A small skin incision is made over the wire utilizing a #11 blade. The skin incision is perpendicular to the long axis of the limb (parallel to the direction of the skin lines) and long enough to accommodate the circumference of the sheath which is to be introduced. When using a dilator with a finely tapered ("feather-tipped") tip and entering a vessel in a patient where the area has not been violated by previous catheterizations, cut-downs or indwelling lines, the sheath/dilator set is introduced over the wire without any further pre-dilation. A "drilling" motion of both the sheath and dilator should be used during the introduction of all sheath/dilator sets as their tips penetrate the tissues of the skin and advance through the subcutaneous tissues and into the vessels. In "virgin" tissues, the sheath dilator set is often introduced with the side arm hemostasis valve still attached to the sheath. In this circumstance, the sheath/dilator is "drilled" into the skin and vessel, using more of a side to side, back and forth rotation of the sheath/dilator rather than a complete, 360° rapid drilling.

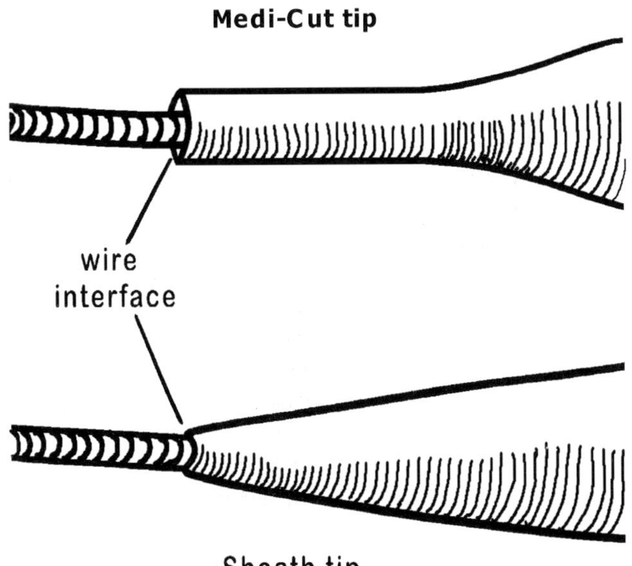

Figure 4.14 Comparison of the tips of feather-tipped dilator and Medi-Cut™ cannula.

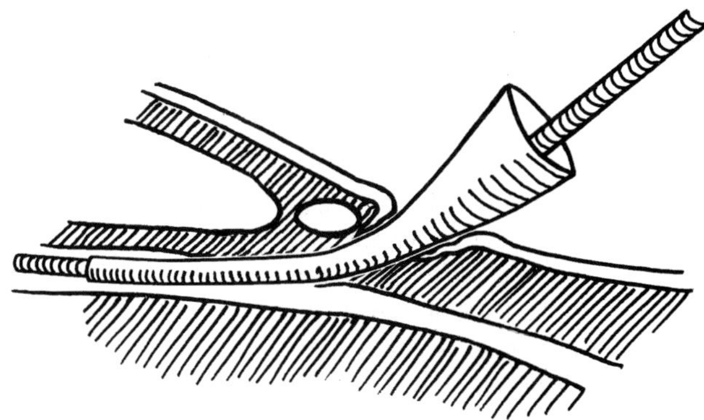

Figure 4.15 Dilation of subcutaneous tract with tapered plastic cannula of a Medi-Cut™.

With the newer, finely tapered pediatric introducing dilators, the earlier technique of pre-dilating with a Medi-Cut™ cannula or creating a subcutaneous "tunnel" with fine-tipped forceps is not only unnecessary but actually counter productive. The tip of the Medi-Cut™ cannula is larger in external and internal diameter than the tips of the new pediatric or feather-tipped dilators and, as a consequence, there is a much greater discrepancy between the lumen of the Medi-Cut™ and the guide wire than between the tip of the dilator and the wire (Figure 4.14). With meticulous, gentle technique, even a 9- or 10-French, fine tipped sheath/dilator can be introduced over a 0.018″ wire!

If, on the other hand, only the older, blunt tipped ("adult") sheath/dilator sets are available, then pre-dilation of the subcutaneous tissues and the wall of the vessel is necessary, using the plastic cannula of a Medi-Cut™. The Medi-Cut™ is introduced over the wire and advanced deeply enough into the skin to enter into the vein. By advancing the Medi-Cut™ as deeply into the tissues as possible (to the hub of the Medi-Cut™), the funnel shaped proximal taper on the Medi-Cut™ cannula enters the skin and subcutaneous tissues and, in turn, dilates the tissues to a diameter which easily accommodates the sheath/dilator set (Figure 4.15).

After the Medi-Cut™ cannula, which is over the wire, has been buried to the hub into the tissues, the Medi-Cut™ is removed over the wire while holding pressure over the wire and the enlarged puncture site. The sheath/dilator set is then introduced over the wire. When there is considerable scarring or very dense tissues are encountered and the initial wire for puncture into the vessel was a 0.018″ wire, the small wire should be exchanged through the Medi-Cut™ cannula for a larger, stiffer wire before removing the Medi-Cut™. The larger diameter, stiffer wire fits better within the lumen at the tips of blunt-tipped dilators, provides a more rigid support for the larger sheath/dilator passing through the subcutaneous tissues and, in turn, facilitates the introduction of the sheath/dilator into the vessel.

While introducing the sheath/dilator through the subcutaneous tissues, pressure is held over the puncture site and along the course of the wire beneath the skin between the skin puncture and the puncture into the vein. This supports the wire beneath the skin and prevents the wire from bending or kinking in addition to preventing subcutaneous bleeding as the sheath/dilator set is advanced over the wire through the skin and subcutaneous tissue into the vessel. A high-speed "drilling" motion of the combined sheath/dilator set is used over the wire while introducing the sheath/dilator into the subcutaneous tissues (Figure 4.16).

This drilling with the sheath/dilator is particularly important in the presence of dense or scarred subcutaneous tissue. The rotation of the tips of the dilator/sheath facilitates their entry into the tissues and vessel by preventing any "flare" or "lip" from forming on the tips of the dilator or sheath (Figure 4.17a). If a lip does form on the tip of the dilator or sheath, the drilling motion rotates the lip into the vessel as the set is rotated and advanced (Figure 4.17b). If the sheath and dilator are not rotated and merely forced forward straight into the tissues, the initial lip which was created at the tip grows into a "shelf" perpendicular to the shafts of the sheath/dilator! Such a large shelf on either the sheath or dilator makes vessel entry very traumatic or, in all likelihood, prevents entry into the vessel at all (Figure 4.17c). Further force on the sheath/dilator will very likely cause kinks in the guide wire. Either occurrence prohibits the successful introduction of a sheath/dilator over the wire into the vessel or unnecessarily traumatizes the vessel. As a consequence,

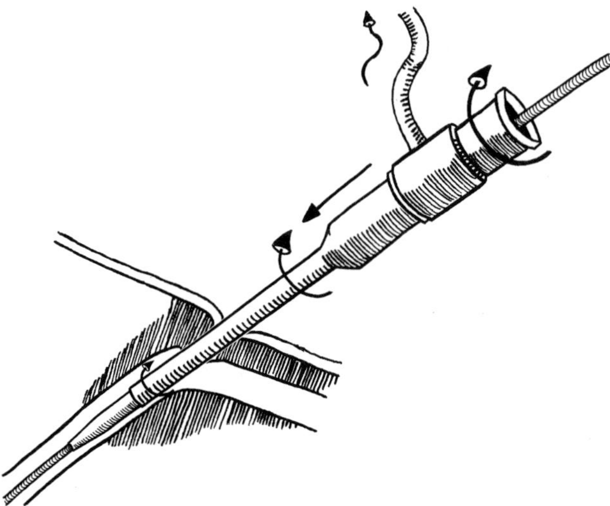

Figure 4.16 Drilling motion of sheath/dilator together as they are introduced through the subcutaneous tissues into the vessel.

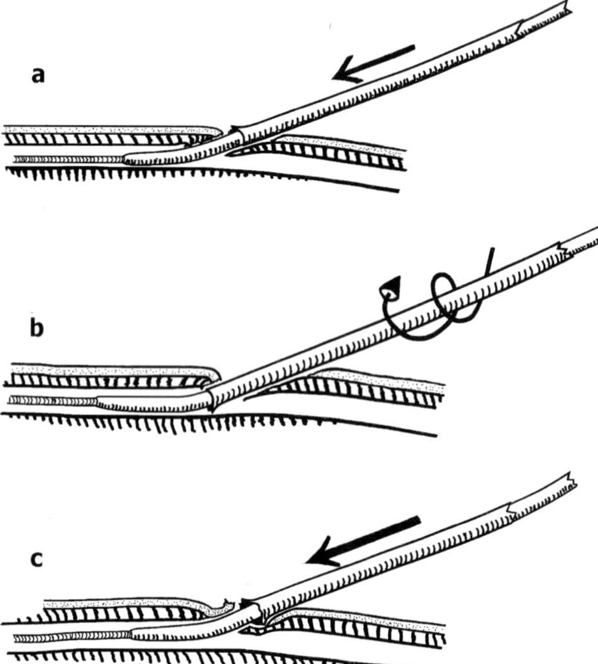

Figure 4.17 (a) "Lip" created at the tip of the sheath during introduction straight into the skin and tissues; (b) lip on sheath introduced into vessel by rotation of sheath during introduction; (c) lip enlarged and vessel/tissues distorted by forcing sheath with lip at tip straight into tissues.

rotation of the sheath/dilator combination is always used to introduce the sheath/dilator set into the tissues and vessel.

The best introducer sheaths have a removable back-bleed/flush device (Argon Medical Inc., Athens, TX). When dense subcutaneous tissues are encountered, the side arm/valve/back-bleed device is loosened from the hub of the sheath before beginning the sheath/dilator introduction. This facilitates an easier and "high-speed" 360° rotation of the sheath alone during its course through the tissues (Figure 4.18). With the back-bleed loosened from the sheath, the side arm of the back-bleed is not rotating and flapping around, catching on adjacent lines or tubing, during the rapid rotations of the sheath. In extreme circumstances the back-bleed valve/flush port housing can be taken completely off the sheath/dilator set before introducing the set into the skin in order to facilitate better "drilling" of the sheath/dilator combination.

If the sheath/dilator cannot be introduced into the vein without excessive force, it is removed over the wire and a 20-gauge Medi-Cut™ cannula is introduced over the wire. The tract is re-dilated by advancing the Medi-Cut™ cannula *all* of the way to the proximal (funneled) hub end of the cannula (Figure 4.15). The 20-gauge Medi-Cut™ is removed over the smaller wire and replaced with an 18-gauge Medi-Cut™ cannula. The larger cannula should be introduced into the vein by a smooth, "high-speed" drilling motion. Once the larger cannula hs been secured deep in the vein, the original (0.018" or 0.021") introducing guide wire is removed and replaced with a 0.035", long, flexible-tip, stiffer (even a Super Stiff™ [Medi-Tech, Boston Scientific, Natick, MA]), straight spring guide wire. Over this heavier wire the tissues are re-dilated by inserting the 18-gauge Medi-Cut™ cannula deep into the tissues and completely up to its hub. The cannula is removed and the sheath/dilator reintroduced over the heavier wire. In order to introduce the sheath/dilator set over the larger wire, the dilator of the set must usually be switched to a blunt-tipped dilator which has a larger lumen at its tip.

In the rare circumstance where the dilator and sheath still cannot be passed into the vessel over the wire—usually in patients who have had surgical acces to the vessels or multiple previous cut-downs with dense scar tissue formation—the sheath/dilator is removed over the wire. The wire is checked for sharp kinks beneath the skin either by withdrawing it carefully for several centimeters, or by brief direct fluoroscopic visualization over the inguinal area. Even if the wire is not kinked and is still well within the vein, if the original wire was a standard spring guide wire it is replaced with an extra-stiff or Super Stiff™ wire before the larger Medi-Cut™ cannula is removed. This provides additional support for the introduction of the sheath/dilator through the skin and dense subcutaneous tissues. This is useful particularly for the introduction of the very large diameter, long sheath/dilator sets used during therapeutic catheter procedures.

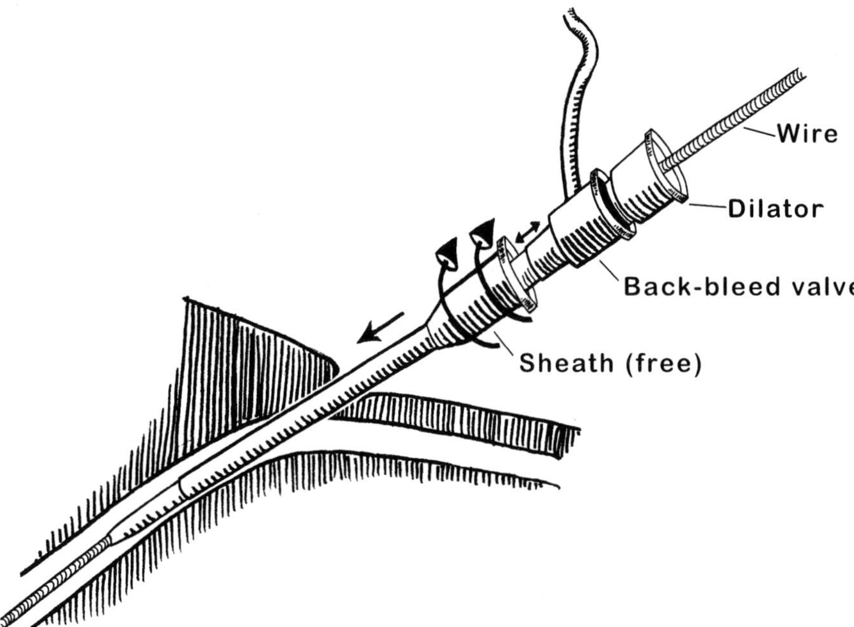

Figure 4.18 Back-bleed valve of sheath loosened and withdrawn with the dilator; allows sheath alone to be rotated rapidly during introduction.

When even the Super Stiff™ wire does not allow the introduction of the sheath/dilator, then only a dilator which is *at least* one French size smaller than the previous sheath/dilator set is introduced over the wire and a progressive, sequential dilation with larger and larger diameter dilators is accomplished. Even with the dilators alone, rapid "drilling" of the dilator through the very dense subcutaneous tissues will be necessary. Once a dilator has been introduced which is larger in outer diameter than the outer diameter of the sheath/dilator combination to be used, the sheath/dilator enters the vessel easily.

A final additional technique for dilating very dense subcutaneous tissues is possible only in catheterization laboratories which still have the old thick-walled USCI™ teflon Desilets-Hoffman venous sheath/dilator sets (United States Catheter, Inc. [USCI] BARD, Glens Falls, NY) in stock. The sheaths of these "venous sheath" sets had a very thick teflon wall. The outside diameter of these sheaths gradually increases four French sizes in diameter from the tip to the hub of the sheath. As a consequence, a Desilets-Hoffman venous sheath/dilator set that is two or three French sizes smaller than the actual sheath that is intended for the procedure, can be used for this pre-dilation. This introducer set is much stiffer, and coupled with its smaller size distally usually passes easily into the veins. As with the introduction of the other introducer sets, a drilling motion through the tissues and into the vessel facilitates the introduction of both the dilator and the sheath. Once the tip of the sheath has entered the vessel, the sheath itself acts as a progressively larger dilator as it is introduced well into the vessel almost to the hub of the sheath. This thicker-walled, smaller lumen sheath/dilator is then removed and a thin-walled, larger lumen, sheath/dilator set is introduced into the now dilated tract and vessel. With one, or a combination, of these techniques, the sheath/dilator can *always* be introduced into the vessel once the guide wire has been introduced successfully and correctly.

Once the sheath/dilator is introduced into the vessel successfully, the wire and the dilator are removed from the sheath very cautiously. The wire is withdrawn first and slowly from the dilator, taking care that there is no resistance to its withdrawal. The wire should never be pulled rapidly or with a jerking motion. With the twisting and "drilling" during the introduction of sheaths/dilators, wires easily become kinked, looped, bent or knotted around/within the vascular system or within the heart itself. A rapid withdrawal of a wire which has a knot or has looped around an intravascular structure can avulse or tear the intracardiac or intravascular structures or break the safety core of the wire, which results in an uncoiling of the spring guide wire. Rapid withdrawal of the wire also creates a vacuum in the dilator, which results in a small amount of air being sucked into the dilator as the wire is withdrawn.

Once the wire has been removed from the dilator, the dilator is withdrawn very *slowly* from the sheath. Rapid withdrawal of the dilator from either a "valved" or open sheath results in a significant amount of air being sucked into the sheath (and vessel) through the lumen of the dilator, between the dilator and the sheath or through the back-bleed valve of the sheath. After the dilator has been removed completely and while observing the tubing on the side port of the back-bleed valve of the sheath very carefully, the side port of the back-bleed valve is cautiously opened and allowed to bleed-back passively to clear the sheath/valve of all trapped air and/or clots. With any sign of the fluid column in the tubing which is attached to the side port flowing toward the sheath, the stopcock on the side port is immediately turned to the off position to the sheath. When a patient has a very low venous pressure or any airway obstruction, the opened side port or an open end of a sheath allows air to be sucked into the sheath rather than blood to flow out of it. After assuring that there is no airway obstruction or, if there is, correcting it, diffuse heavy hand pressure is applied over the patient's abdomen while the side port is again cautiously opened. The external abdominal pressure increases intra-abdominal, intrathoracic and intravascular venous pressure enough to force blood flow out of the sheath and prevent air from being sucked into the sheath. If the patient is intubated, positive pressure is delivered to the airway while the stopcock is opened.

Unless the back-bleed *valve* on the sheath can be capped *very tightly* with a finger, suction is ***never*** applied to the side port of a back-bleed valve. With any obstruction to the flow of blood into the distal end of the sheath, even slight negative pressure on the side port results in air being sucked *through the back-bleed valve* and into the sheath. Once the side arm, back-bleed valve chamber and the length of the sheath are all cleared of any air, the side arm of the sheath is flushed with flush solution and, preferably, attached to a pressure/flush system and placed on a slow continuous flush.

When a sheath/dilator set is introduced which does not have a back-bleed valve attached to the sheath, a separate back-bleed device must be attached to the sheath as soon as the wire and dilator are removed. After the sheath/dilator set has been introduced completely into the vessel, first, the wire alone is removed carefully and slowly from the dilator and blood is allowed to drip from the proximal end of the dilator. Once the wire has been removed, the dilator is withdrawn slowly from the sheath. With non-valved sheaths, this creates direct continuity between the vein and the environmental air at the tabletop! As soon as the tip of the dilator is free of the hub of the sheath, the hub is capped *immediately* with the catheterizing physician's gloved finger or a syringe. The sequence of removing the wire first allows the wire to be completely out of the sheath/dilator before the dilator is withdrawn in order to eliminate the potential large gap between the large lumen of the internal diameter (ID) of the sheath and the tiny outside diameter (OD) of the wire-only passing through the sheath. A wire alone within a sheath without a back-bleed valve allows both excessive blood loss or very direct and easy access for the entry of air into the sheath around the wire. The slow withdrawal of the dilator usually allows blood from the vein to "follow" the tip of the dilator back into the sheath, allowing the sheath to fill with blood as the dilator is withdrawn. After free blood return from the sheath is assured or after attaching a syringe directly to the hub of the sheath and gently withdrawing blood through the sheath, a flush/back-bleed valve system is attached to the sheath. After the back-bleed valve/port is attached, the sheath/back-bleed valve is again passively cleared of air and clots exactly as when a sheath is introduced with a back-bleed valve attached.

Occasionally a catheter is introduced directly into the sheath without a back-bleed valve. In that situation, blood should be flowing *out* of the hub of the sheath, and the catheter should be on a continuous flush as it is introduced into the column of blood flowing out of the hub of the sheath.

Special care is taken to *never* leave the end of the sheath uncapped or a non-valved sheath open without a catheter or dilator within it. All patients are capable of generating huge negative intrathoracic and intravascular pressures during obstructed inspiration and, as a consequence, are capable of sucking *lethal volumes* of air into the venous system through the large lumen of an open, short sheath. A patient with significant airway obstruction can generate as much as *60 mmHg negative intravascular pressure* with a vigorous inspiratory effort.

Pre-curving percutaneous sheaths for special circumstances

When using the femoral veins in small infants, the jugular veins in infants and small children, the left femoral vein, either subclavian vein or the hepatic approach in any sized patient, it is helpful, and occasionally essential, to pre-form a curve on the distal end of the short vascular sheath which is to be used before the sheath/dilator set is introduced.

The curve on the sheath can be formed by repeatedly pulling the distal end of the sheath/dilator combination between the clenched forefinger and thumb while simultaneously forming a curve on the distal end of the combination. A curve also can be formed by heating the sheath/dilator combination (while fitted together) in either boiling sterile water or in the hot air jet of a "heat gun" to soften the sheath/dilator. The desired curve is formed manually on the set with the fingers and then the sheath/dilator is cooled in cool flush solution while manually fixing (holding) the curve on the combination until it has cooled. The preformed curves are useful (essential) in many circumstances.

From the left femoral vein and either subclavian vein access, the more central vein makes an acute curve or angle just distal (central) to the location of the tip of an indwelling short sheath. When a catheter is introduced through the sheath in these locations, the catheter tip is directed straight by a straight sheath. This straight direction results in the catheter digging into the opposite wall of the vein or entering small side branches, which arise at the curve in the vein just as the catheter exits the tip of the sheath. As a consequence, the catheter cannot be advanced further. This requires withdrawal and readjustment of the catheter and sheath and the use of unnecessary fluoroscopy over the area (and the operator's hands!) with each catheter introduction or exchange in order to advance the catheter more centrally. A gentle, 30–90° curve preformed on the distal end of the sheath will conform to the curves in the natural course of the vein and direct the tip of the sheath and the exiting catheter into the lumen of the more central vein, making catheter introduction or replacement essentially automatic.

A standard length sheath introduced from the jugular veins in infants and small children extends from the skin puncture site well into (or even through) the right atrium. A catheter introduced into such a straight, short sheath which is introduced to its hub in the jugular vein, obligatorily is directed toward the inferior vena cava and, in turn, directing a catheter toward the tricuspid (atrioventricular) valve through such a straight sheath is very difficult. It is difficult, if not impossible, to maintain these sheaths only partially inserted into the jugular vein during extensive catheter manipulation. Even if the catheter is manipulated across the atrioventricular valve and into the respective ventricle from the straight sheath, any forward push on the proximal catheter advances the more proximal catheter shaft in the direction of the sheath—toward the inferior vena cava—and, in doing so, can even withdraw the catheter tip from the ventricle. A 45–90° curve, pre-formed at the distal end of the short sheath, conforms to the usual course or direction from the superior vena cava/right atrium to the atrioventricular valve/ventricle. This curve makes the introduction or exchange of catheters into the ventricle simpler and almost automatic. The curve on the sheath also directs any forward push on the proximal shaft of the catheter in the direction of the ventricle.

Catheters introduced from the transhepatic approach make almost a 90° turn in passing from the hepatic veins into the inferior vena cava or right atrium. When the short introductory sheath is straight, making this curve or "forming" curves on the catheter by bending against the tissues of the liver is difficult and potentially dangerous. A 90° curve placed on the distal end of the sheath before it is introduced automatically conforms to the curve from the hepatic vein bending cephalad toward the right atrium, and directs the tip of any catheter cephalad and into the right atrium without any unnecessary or traumatic manipulations.

Pre-curving the sheath and dilator prior to their introduction is very simple and saves many minutes of fluoroscopy time and much unnecessary catheter manipulation. The anatomy and potential need for a curve on the sheath should be considered before the introduction of every sheath.

Multiple needle/catheter introductions

Often with electrophysiologic or therapeutic catheter procedures two, three or more venous catheters are necessary. It is preferable to utilize separate veins for each sheath/catheter; however, for various reasons, a second vessel may not be available or, when available, not provide optimal access to the heart. There are several special techniques for introducing a second needle/wire/sheath/dilator into the same vein when several venous lines are necessary.

Multiple sheaths "piggy-backed" into a single vessel

When obstruction of the venous access of one extremity is documented, and particularly in larger patients, a "piggy-back" technique can be used for the introduction of a second needle/sheath/dilator into the vein which is already cannulated. In patients who are older than one year, a single large peripheral vein can accommodate two (or more) separate sheaths and catheters by piggy-backing the second sheath adjacent to the original. This technique is usually used in the femoral veins, but is applicable to the brachial veins as well. The femoral veins are remarkably large and compliant and will readily accommodate two sheaths which are relatively large in proportion to the size of the patient. The second, or additional needle/sheath is usually introduced into a location in the vein peripheral or "up-stream" to the site of introduction of the initial sheath in the vein (distally in the extremity). The first sheath in the vein serves as an ideal landmark for the subsequent puncture.

The hub and proximal shaft of the sheath which is already in the vein are elevated off the skin and the needle puncture for the introduction of the second sheath is performed 1–2 mm peripheral to (and under) the entrance site of the first sheath. The second needle is introduced parallel to the long axis of the extremity and in a direct line with the first sheath. The first sheath may partially occlude the lumen of the vein and, in turn, dilates the vein "up-stream" in the area of the second puncture. As a consequence, the vein is entered easily with the second needle with very good blood return into the needle. Once blood return in the needle occurs, the wire is introduced as with any other percutaneous introduction.

Occasionally the wire stops advancing after several centimeters of free passage beyond the tip of the needle as it begins to pass the first sheath within the same vein, which presumably is in some spasm or has a restricted lumen. In this circumstance, the course of the wire is visualized directly with fluoroscopy. Usually persistence and small, repeated advances of a soft-tipped wire prevail in passing the wire adjacent to the original sheath. When in doubt as to the exact location of the wire or the reason why the wire does not advance, a Medi-Cut™ cannula is introduced over the wire; the wire is removed and a small (1 ml), minimal pressure, biplane angiogram is performed through the Medi-Cut™ in order to visualize the vessel anatomy in the area. This angiogram demonstrates the exact course of flow around the first sheath. Once the route of blood flow is determined, this course is followed with a torque-controlled wire, which is introduced through the same Medi-Cut™ cannula. Once the wire advances past the first sheath and is well into the thorax, the second sheath/dilator is introduced into the same vein beneath the original sheath exactly as with any other sheath introduction. The second sheath/dilator "dilates" its way past the first sheath as it is introduced.

In the upper extremities, usually the vein with the original sheath and any tributaries into that vein are visible, sticking up from the surface of the skin. Instead of puncturing under the original sheath, the puncture can often be performed in a tributary branch of the larger, more central vein. The same techniques with a Medi-Cut™ cannula, angiogram and torque-controlled wire are used to advance the wire past the original sheath as are used in the lower extremity.

Sheath/dilator introduction during the skin prep of the patient

Occasionally an alternative sequence of introducing the anesthesia and the needle/wire is used to assist in the needle/wire/dilator/sheath introduction during infiltration of the local anesthesia. This technique requires a change in the sequence of draping of the area, puncture of the vein and a very special handling of the sheath/dilator to prevent contamination of the field. The area to be punctured for the vessel introduction is scrubbed thoroughly and widely as for any other preparation of a sterile field for a catheterization. However, only the superficial skin wheal is created with the 25-gauge subcuticular needle and then this needle is withdrawn from the skin. The small initial subcuticular needle on the xylocaine syringe is replaced with a larger 21- or 20-gauge percutaneous needle. The larger needle is used for the remainder of the xylocaine infiltration and for the vessel puncture and wire introduction.

A syringe with a "slip-lock" hub (*not* a Luer-lock™ hub) is used in order to facilitate an easier and smoother removal of the syringe from the needle. The xylocaine infiltration is continued using the larger needle. Whenever the needle is being advanced or the needle tip is moved at all within the subcutaneous tissues, negative pressure is maintained on the syringe. The use of the larger needle is essential for the modified technique. With the continual negative pressure on the xylocaine syringe and with the larger needle, when a vessel is entered as the needle is being introduced blood returns readily into the syringe of xylocaine. The return of blood into the syringe is very brisk and the percutaneous wire can be introduced through the same needle. Obviously, *no* xylocaine is injected if any blood return is encountered! While maintaining the needle position very securely and precisely in the vessel, the syringe is removed very carefully from the needle. Once the syringe has been removed and there is still free blood return through the needle, the guide wire is introduced into the punctured vessel through this needle as described previously for any other percutaneous wire introduction. As with all wire introductions, after the wire has passed well beyond the tip of the needle, the needle is removed over the wire, pressure is applied over the puncture site and the position of the wire in the thorax is checked under fluoroscopy before proceeding any further.

The needle is withdrawn out of the skin over the wire and pressure maintained over the vessel puncture site/wire with one finger. As the needle is removed completely from the wire, the free end of the wire is looped tightly in one hand and held as a loop away from the skin and puncture area. The sterile area immediately around the puncture site (and the hand holding the wire) is draped temporarily with several separate, sterile towels. These sterile towels are not clamped together.

The sheath/dilator set is introduced into the skin over the wire until the hub of the valved sheath is against the skin surface. The wire and then the dilator are removed separately while maintaining the side arm of the sheath sterile by keeping it elevated off the skin and contained within a gloved hand. After the sheath is cleared of air, but before the side arm is attached to the flush system, the whole field is draped with a standard pre-cut catheterization table drape. The draping is accomplished over and around the protruding proximal hub of the sheath. The side arm and the hub of the sheath as it enters the vessel are raised off the skin surface and, as the pre-cut drape is lowered over the patient's skin, the proximal hub and side arm of the sheath are passed through the hole in the drape from underneath to the top, while all the time keeping the sheath and side arm sterile. After the hub of the sheath has passed through the hole in the drape, the hub of the sheath and its side arm are placed on the sterile field (top surface) of the drape, the previous towels are removed from beneath the drape and the hole in the drape is sealed over the sterile skin surface area.

When a vessel is entered inadvertently with a larger needle and the wire is introduced early during the xylocaine infiltration process and *before* the entire area was scrubbed, draped and totally anesthetized, special steps are required to drape the patient and maintain the sterile field before the sheath and dilator are introduced. After the needle is removed and the wire which enters the vessel is looped tightly in one hand, the entire area, including the puncture site and the finger holding pressure, is scrubbed and prepped thoroughly. The area is draped partially and temporarily with towels to provide a localized sterile field around and under the grasped wire. Using a second small needle and syringe, additional xylocaine is infiltrated around the wire/vessel puncture site to prevent discomfort when the sheath/dilator set is introduced over the wire. Once the area is draped temporarily and anesthetized, a valved sheath/dilator set is introduced over the wire. Thereafter, the "permanent" draping of the patient is identical to the procedure for introducing the wire through the local anesthesia needle when it was planned from the beginning.

There are two advantages to entering the vessel purposefully during the xylocaine infiltration. When a vessel is punctured inadvertently during the usual xylocaine infiltration and the needle is removed, pressure must be held for 3–5 minutes. By introducing the wire with this first puncture, the time necessary for holding pressure on the vessel to control bleeding is saved and, once vigorous blood return is obtained during the puncture, access into that vessel is virtually assured. When this technique and sequence are used for routine vessel entry, all of the prepping and draping of the field are performed by the operator, before the infiltration of the local anesthesia and introduction of the wire are started.

Indwelling sheath catheterization technique

An indwelling sheath technique is used routinely and continually for both arterial and venous catheterizations and for all catheter manipulations throughout the duration of the entire catheterization procedure. An indwelling sheath is equally advantageous for catheters introduced into vessels by a percutaneous or a cut-down technique. Although the sheath around the catheter adds 1–2 French sizes to the outside diameter of the combination within the vessel, this one disadvantage is far outweighed by the multiple advantages of indwelling sheaths[1].

Of most importance, the indwelling sheath creates a smooth, atraumatic and fixed channel through the access opening in the vessel wall which has just been traumatized. This lining of the vessel and separation from the wall of the vessel created by the sheath, eliminates the continual friction, irritation and trauma created by the outer surface of the moving and rubbing catheter as the catheter is maneuvered in and out of the vessel against the recently "injured" introductory site and adjacent intima of the vessel. By isolating the catheter from the vessel wall, the indwelling sheath eliminates any vessel spasm on the catheter itself and, in turn, eliminates any resistance to catheter manipulation from the vessel wall. This facilitates catheter movement and reduces the trauma to the vessel even further, which, in turn, stops the vicious cycle of further irritation causing subsequent spasm, resulting in more resistance to movement and more irritation, etc. The overall reduced trauma to the vessel wall reduces the stimuli for spasm and thromboses and, probably, even reduces the incidence of vessel thrombi. During catheter manipulation the outer surface of the catheter at the entry site into the sheath is moistened repeatedly with a sponge to keep drying blood from adhering between the catheter and the sheath. This helps to prevent the catheter from binding within the indwelling sheath, which can cause secondary motion of the sheath within the vessel.

The indwelling sheath also allows the introduction of all types of catheters/devices into the vessel and the rapid, multiple and easy exchange of catheters—all without further trauma to the vessel. Catheters and devices are exchanged as many times as desired or necessary, without difficulty and without further damage to a vessel. With the first exchange of a catheter, especially when using a balloon catheter or a catheter for the delivery of a device, any of the occasional time or speed advantages of direct catheter introduction into vessels are immediately nullified! With the back-bleed valve on a sheath, blood loss during catheter exchange is eliminated.

The rougher the walls or outer surfaces of the catheters, balloons, delivery systems or devices are, the greater is the advantage of the sheath for the protection of the vessel. Indwelling sheaths protect the entry/exit sites of the vessels from the rough, irregular and very traumatic walls of deflated angioplasty balloons or balloons with stents mounted on them. Balloon and balloon dilation catheters passing through sheaths usually require a significantly larger sheath than the shaft size of the balloon catheter. The indwelling larger diameter, but *fixed* sheath in the vessel throughout the duration of the procedure is far less traumatic to the vessel than the rough and larger profile of the deflated dilation balloon being advanced into or removed from the vessel even once.

Ironically, the percutaneously introduced indwelling sheath allows the introduction of larger catheters in spite of the slightly larger external diameter of the sheath. When a catheter or sheath is introduced initially, the vessel will be at its largest diameter in a state of "maximum dilation" (relaxation) before any additional manipulation or trauma to the vessel. A large sheath is easily introduced at this initial stage of the procedure. Thereafter, as the vessel spasms around the sheath, the larger sheath is already in place for larger catheters. There appears to be a lower incidence of iliofemoral vein thrombosis and associated inferior vena caval thrombosis with the use of the percutaneous indwelling sheath approach, and local wound infection is essentially zero following percutaneous indwelling sheath procedures.

When multi-catheter studies are required (e.g. detailed electrophysiologic studies, combined hemodynamic and pharmacologic testing or multi-catheter therapeutic procedures) several sheaths (and catheters) are easily introduced percutaneously into the same vein adjacent to, or in line with, each other as described earlier in this chapter.

Once *all* anticipated vascular access is secured using a percutaneous technique, systemic heparin is administered to the patient as described in Chapter 2. This helps to prevent thrombi formation when there is stasis proximal in the blood flow to, around or adjacent to the indwelling sheaths.

Removable back-bleed valve/flush ports

Introductory sheaths with removable or detachable hemostatic valves/side port flush systems are preferable and are used whenever available for both the sheath/dilator introduction and during subsequent catheter manipulations through the sheath. When the back-bleed/side arm device is permanently attached to the sheath during the introduction of the sheath, an adequate "high-speed" drilling motion of the sheath/dilator or the sheath alone cannot be accomplished during the introduction. As the sheath with the attached side port is rapidly rotated, the tubing of the side port catches on adjacent structures or lines. With a detachable back-bleed valve, the sheath/dilator is introduced into the patient with the back-bleed loosened and stationary away from the hub of the sheath (Figure 4.18) or even totally removed from the sheath. The preferred method is to loosen the back-bleed valve mechanism from the hub of the sheath, but leaving it attached to the dilator during the introduction of the sheath/dilator. In this way the sheath can be rotated rapidly and independently as the sheath and the dilator are advanced during their introduction into the tissues/vessel. The back-bleed valve loosened from the sheath prevents the side arm of the back-bleed valve from flopping around and catching on adjacent structures as the sheath alone is rotated rapidly over the dilator. Once the sheath has been drilled completely into the vessel and before the wire or dilator are withdrawn, the back-bleed/side port is reattached to the hub of the sheath.

An alternate method to allow free rotation ("drilling") of a sheath during its introduction is to remove the back-bleed valve completely from the sheath/dilator set before the introduction is started. The back-bleed valve/flush port is reattached to the sheath after the sheath has been introduced into the vessel and the wire and dilator have been removed from the sheath. This does incur some additional bleeding and a greater potential for the introduction of air during the time the dilator is removed from the sheath and the time the valve is reattached to the sheath. Bleeding from the sheath is minimized by withdrawal of the wire entirely out of the dilator before the dilator is withdrawn from the sheath. There is minimal if any bleeding through the small lumen of the dilator after the wire has been removed, even from an artery. If there is significant bleeding from the dilator after the wire has been removed, the bleeding is easily stopped with the tip of a finger over the hub of the dilator. As soon as the tip of the dilator has been withdrawn from the sheath, the end of the sheath is capped with a finger or the back-bleed device is reattached on the sheath immediately.

Although invaluable for the prevention of blood loss, particularly during the exchange of catheters, the back-bleed valves themselves, when attached to the sheaths, do create some significant problems with the manipulation of catheters. The problems during catheter manipulations and the advantage of detachable back-bleed valves are discussed in detail under Catheter Manipulations in Chapter 5, while the other potential problems of the back-bleed valves are covered here.

Although some blood escapes around a catheter passing through the attached valve, blood loss is minimal during catheter manipulations with the back-bleed valve in place and clinically insignificant even during a prolonged procedure. However, when a *wire by itself* passes through a standard back-bleed valve on a sheath, blood loss is often very significant. In that circumstance, a large quantity of blood can be lost during a prolonged catheter/sheath exchange or replacement process where the wire remains through the valve. If a wire must remain through a back-bleed valve for any length of time, it is useful to reintroduce a dilator, the tip of which fits tightly over the wire, and to reinsert the dilator over the wire and into the valve until the time that either the wire is removed or a new catheter is introduced over the wire.

The attached back-bleed valve/flush devices (hemostasis valves) create a potential hazard through the possible introduction of air whenever they are in place during use. It is *falsely* assumed that when a back-bleed valve is attached to the sheath nothing escapes or enters through the valve. What is not readily apparent, but at the same time is *potentially very hazardous* to the patient, is that whenever negative pressure is generated on a valved sheath, it creates a partial vacuum in the sheath which results in air *being sucked into the sheath through the valve* and trapped within the sheath.

Negative pressure and a partial vacuum in a sheath can be generated by several different mechanisms. Air entry occurs through the valve on the sheath when any suction or negative pressure is applied to the side port of a hemostasis valve in an attempt to clear the sheath of air or clot. Usually this is apparent by the appearance of air being visibly drawn into the clear tubing of the side port! Air is also likely to enter the sheath when either a dilator or a catheter is withdrawn *rapidly* from the sheath. When the tip of a sheath which has only a single end hole is positioned against the wall of a vessel or chamber, or if the tip of the sheath is constrained within a small lumen in a vessel, return of blood into the tip of the sheath is very slow, or often non-existent, as the tip of the dilator/catheter is withdrawn into the sheath. As a consequence, as a dilator or catheter is withdrawn, a partial vacuum is created within the sheath and air is sucked into the sheath through the dilator and/or *through the back-bleed valve* around the dilator or catheter! The more rapidly the dilator/catheter is withdrawn, the greater the partial vacuum which is created and the greater the likelihood of air being sucked into the sheath. In most cases this is ***not*** apparent unless the partial vacuum that is created is extreme and an audible "sucking" sound is produced as the tip of the dilator/catheter exits the valve! Air sucked through the dilator is trapped throughout the length of the sheath but especially near the very tip of the sheath where it is immediately adjacent to the intravascular circulation. Air entry becomes an even greater problem when the catheter which is being withdrawn from the sheath has a smaller size than the sheath and/or has a very loose fit within the sheath. If the tip of the sheath is even partially occluded, air is sucked through the valve more freely around the smaller catheter as it is withdrawn. When the sheath is very long, all of the problems are compounded by its increased capacity.

The other common source of a partial vacuum within a sheath is the introduction of any type of balloon catheter into a sheath! The deflated balloon has a larger diameter than the shaft of the balloon catheter. When a dilation balloon catheter is introduced into a sheath, the balloon material fills the lumen of the sheath around the balloon and acts as a plunger, creating a very effective partial vacuum behind it and around the smaller shaft of the catheter as the balloon is advanced within the sheath. With the smaller shaft of the catheter behind the balloon, this space within the sheath easily and rapidly fills with air, which is sucked in through the valve as the balloon is advanced in the sheath.

In addition to the air within the shaft of the sheath, all hemostasis valves have a small "chamber" or "dead space" within the hub of the valve/side port apparatus (Figure 4.19). When a wire, dilator or catheter tip is first introduced into a back-bleed valve, the valve is vented to room air and the chamber quickly drains of any fluid and *fills with air*. The air is trapped in this chamber and is *not* cleared by simply opening the side flush port to drain the fluid/air without some specific extra effort to remove the air.

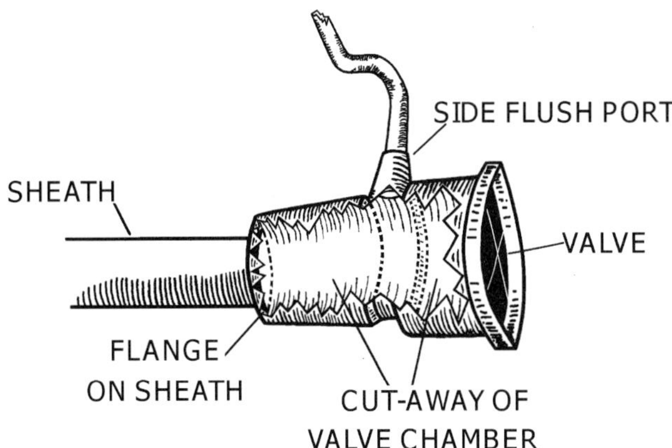

Figure 4.19 Cut-away drawing of back-bleed valve/flush port apparatus, showing the large "dead space" within hub of the back-bleed housing.

The chamber, however, does empty everything in it in the opposite direction and *into the patient's circulation* when the sheath is flushed vigorously without first specifically emptying the chamber! When the sheath containing trapped air in the chamber is flushed or a new catheter is introduced into the sheath, the trapped air is pushed into the circulation. The problems with air trapped within sheaths are magnified when dealing with very long sheaths which can hold very large volumes of air. The seriousness of the adverse events which result from air introduced through the sheath depends upon which location in the circulation the air travels to and the total amount of air that is introduced. The consequence of air in the circulation varies from as "minor" as a bubble that is noted incidentally bouncing around in the right atrium or right ventricle to the other extreme of a catastrophic stroke or cardiac arrest from the air reaching the systemic circulation.

Awareness of the potential problems and the regular, consistent use of a few special techniques and extreme caution in the handling of sheaths, effectively prevent all events related to air entry into the circulation. Whenever dilators and catheters are withdrawn from sheaths using any combination of sheath, dilator or catheter, the withdrawal must be *very slow*. The slow withdrawal of the dilator or catheter is usually sufficient to allow a column of blood to "follow" the tip of the dilator or catheter into the sheath as the catheter or dilator is withdrawn from the sheath and, in turn, prevents the creation of a partial vacuum which would suck air into the sheath. When there is a wire and/or catheter passing through the valve, suction or negative pressure should ***never*** be applied to the side arm of the back-bleed/flush device.

Rather than applying negative pressure (suction) to the side port, the side port is opened very carefully under very close observation, and the blood (and air) is (are) allowed to flow out of the sheath and side port *passively* before the side port is attached to a pressure/flush line or before flushing the sheath. As the stop-cock on the side port is opened, the tubing of the side port must be *observed very carefully* to verify that blood (and air) is (are) flowing ***out*** of the sheath and *not* being sucked back into it from negative intrathoracic pressure! As the side port drains, the valve chamber of the sheath is elevated slightly off the surface of the catheterization table and rotated from side to side in order to position the side port facing up. At the same time, the valve chamber is tapped vigorously to free any trapped air from within it.

In patients with inspiratory airway obstruction, passive drainage of the side port cannot be used. Negative intrathoracic pressure preferentially sucks air *into* the side port rather than allowing the sheath and valve chamber to drain. In the presence of airway obstruction, special precautions and procedures are used to clear the sheath of all air before flushing or the introduction of a new catheter. These techniques are described earlier in this chapter. Although a small "bouncing bubble" in the right heart circulation usually causes no problem, it represents very sloppy technique and certainly the potential for a catastrophic event under slightly different circumstances or anatomy.

Whenever a catheter of a smaller size is used within a larger sheath, a back-bleed valve on the sheath is essential to prevent excessive blood loss around the catheter. The back-bleed valve prevents blood loss around a catheter very effectively, however, the discrepancy between the larger internal diameter of the sheath and the smaller outer diameter of a smaller catheter creates a large dead space within the sheath. The size of this dead space, obviously, depends upon the discrepancy in size between the ID of the sheath and the OD of the catheter and the length of the sheath. The dead space is a potential not only for the entry and accumulation of air as described above, but also for blood stasis and the formation of thrombi. Any thrombus within a sheath represents a potential, solid particle embolus when pushed or flushed out of the sheath. To prevent air entering and thrombosis from occurring, whenever there is a discrepancy between the sheath and catheter sizes and after the sheath has been initially cleared of all air, the side port of the sheath is attached to, and maintained on, a continuous flush.

All of the potential problems of air/clot emboli are magnified with the use of long or large diameter sheaths and especially when there is a discrepancy between the catheter shaft diameter and the sheath diameter. The long sheaths in the larger sizes can hold as much as 12 ml of air or clot! When positioned in the left heart or in the presence of even a potential right to left shunt, this represents a very real life-threatening potential.

Whenever a long sheath/dilator set is to be introduced, the sheath is flushed through the side port while the sheath is prepared *outside* of the body. Once it has been cleared completely of air, the side port of the sheath is turned off. A wire back-bleed device is attached to the proximal end of the long dilator and the dilator is placed on constant flush before and as it is introduced into the long sheath. As the tip of the dilator is introduced into the valve on the long sheath outside the body, the side port of the *sheath* is hand flushed vigorously to prevent air from entering the vented valve of the sheath. Thereafter, as the sheath/dilator is advanced over the wire, the *dilator* remains on a constant flush through the wire back-bleed valve, beginning before the dilator enters the skin and continuing for as long as the dilator remains within the sheath.

When the dilator and/or wire are removed from a long sheath, they are removed separately and the withdrawal of both the dilator and the wire are performed very, very slowly. When the wire is to remain in the sheath after the dilator is removed over the wire from the sheath, the wire back-bleed port on the dilator is maintained on a constant pressure flush during the withdrawal of the dilator *until the tip of the dilator within the sheath reaches the puncture site at the surface of the skin*. In this way any potential vacuum "space" that might be created distal to the tip of the dilator within the sheath by the withdrawal of the dilator will be filled with the flush solution, which, in turn, leaves no space for air to be drawn into the more distal sheath.

As the dilator is being withdrawn from the sheath and before the tip of the dilator approaches the back-bleed valve of the sheath, the flush on the dilator is *stopped* when the tip of the dilator still is *within the sheath* and is palpable at the *skin surface* and/or when the tip of the dilator is approximately 10 cm from the back-bleed valve on the sheath. The position of the dilator tip is easily palpated through the walls of the indwelling sheath as the dilator is being withdrawn. In spite of the above procedures and all precautions, air still often becomes trapped in the chamber of the back-bleed valve/flush port of the sheath. In large sheaths, this amounts to several ml of air! When a wire is still within the sheath, this remaining air must be cleared passively after the dilator has been removed. The dilator is withdrawn slowly out of the sheath. After the tip of the dilator has been withdrawn through the valve, the side port of the sheath is opened and allowed to passively drain while the valve chamber on the sheath is elevated off the table, rotated to position the side port facing up and tapped gently while observing closely to be sure that no air is being sucked into the side port. This technique allows any air trapped in the back-bleed valve chamber and within the sheath to escape and be cleared completely after the dilator has been removed.

Air and/or clots within the sheath are the greatest potential hazards during any use of long sheaths within the circulation. This is an extremely serious problem during the delivery of devices into the systemic circulation through these sheaths. Fortunately, with meticulous attention to the details and the use of the described techniques, this should be a totally avoidable problem.

Exchanging vascular sheaths

Often a larger sized catheter (and, in turn, sheath) is desired for angiography or is necessary for specialized catheters/devices. The exchange of sheaths is accomplished easily and similarly to the original sheath introduction. If the sheath exchange is performed more than one hour after the initial sheath introduction, the area around the vessel is re-infiltrated very liberally with local anesthesia regardless of the type of general sedation/ anesthesia being used. The original catheter is withdrawn slowly from the sheath. If there is no back-bleed valve on the sheath, the catheter is replaced immediately with either a detachable hemostasis/flush valve or with the original dilator containing a spring guide wire. The dilator and the wire or the back-bleed valve on the sheath occlude the lumen of the sheath and prevent excessive bleeding or any air from being sucked into the sheath. The wire is advanced into the thorax, the original sheath—with or without the dilator—is withdrawn out of the vessel over the wire and the new, larger sheath/dilator set advanced over the wire into the vessel exactly as with the first sheath/dilator introduction.

When it is anticipated that a significantly larger sheath will be necessary in a vein later during a procedure, it is preferable to start the procedure with the larger sheath, which will accommodate all anticipated procedures. The trauma of exchanging to a larger sheath during a catheterization procedure is greater than the trauma caused by the presence of a larger indwelling sheath placed at the beginning of the procedure.

Removal of indwelling sheaths and catheters

The care and handling of the vascular puncture sites at the conclusion of the procedure are as important for the preservation of vessel integrity as the techniques with the vessels at any other time during the procedure. As a consequence, in pediatric patients this very non-glorified job is *not* delegated to either inexperienced or uninterested personnel, and certainly not to a mechanical clamp. A lost vessel from improper care during the last few minutes at the end of or after a procedure is no less lost than one lost at other stages of the procedure! The lost vein or artery clinically may not be apparent immediately after the catheterization in the pediatric patient, however, many of these occlusions have long-term clinical consequences and certainly create major problems for future vascular access which is required, more often than not, in congenital heart patients.

At the conclusion of the procedure, before removal of the vascular sheaths, the skin and subcutaneous tissues in the local area around the introductory sites are re-anesthetized very liberally with local anesthesia while the patient is still sedated/anesthetized adequately. The adequacy of the sedation or local anesthesia is tested very easily by pressing firmly on the puncture sites with the tip of a finger. *Any* response from the patient indicates the need for more local anesthesia or sedation before the withdrawal of the catheters and sheaths is begun. A vigorously crying, straining or moving patient generates a very high venous pressure as well as a "moving target", both of which make it impossible to maintain an adequate or steady pressure precisely over the vessels. This is guaranteed to create a hematoma, if not a compromised vessel.

When the patient is calm, the catheter is removed from the sheath, the sheath is allowed to bleed-back slightly through the side port, and then the sheath is removed. The removal of the catheter through the sheath before removing the sheath allows any clot or debris which has formed at the catheter–sheath interface within the vessel to follow the tip of the catheter into, and to flow out through, the sheath and not be stripped off within the vessel at the puncture site. With cyanotic patients and on the withdrawal of any catheter from an arterial sheath at the end of the procedure, slight suction is applied to the catheter as it is withdrawn through the sheath. After the catheter is out of the sheath, the sheath is allowed to bleed one or two spurts of blood and then the sheath is withdrawn. The sheath is withdrawn smoothly from the vessel and pressure is applied immediately over the vessel puncture site.

As soon as the sheaths are removed from all of the vessels, the drapes are removed from all access areas. This allows visualization of the exact puncture site and the entire area surrounding it. Once the drapes have been removed, any extravasation of blood into the subcutaneous tissues of the surrounding area immediately becomes apparent. When the area remains covered except for the hole in the drape and if pressure is applied slightly off the punctured vessels, large hematomas can form in the subcutaneous (or deeper) tissues under the areas covered by the drape.

The pressure is applied directly over the estimated puncture site in the vessel—which is not necessarily the skin puncture site! If pressure is applied too cephalad on a vein, the pressure actually tourniquets the vein "down-stream" from the puncture site and any bleeding through the puncture site "up-stream" in the vein is enhanced rather than controlled. Similarly, pressure applied too caudally over the artery tourniquets the artery beyond or "down-stream", from the puncture site and enhances the arterial bleeding. In the thin, or average sized patient, it is preferable to apply this pressure directly with the gloved finger—not through a pad or wad of dressing. In this way, the arterial pulsation can be palpated continually and the area around the puncture site is observed directly to prevent hematoma formation.

In order to achieve hemostasis with pressure over only a venous puncture, generally only very light (venous!) pressure is necessary. If very firm pressure is applied, arterial flow to the puncture site and entire vascular system distal to the puncture site, and, in turn, venous flow back to the site, is stopped. This does prevent bleeding while still holding pressure, however, it prevents any flow of blood in the vessel with its contained thrombogenic agents to the area and actually increases the amount of time necessary for good hemostasis.

Somewhat more local and heavier pressure must be used to control bleeding from an artery. While holding pressure on an artery, a more distal pulse in the same extremity (dorsalis pedis or posterior tibial) is palpated continually and simultaneously with one hand while holding the pressure over the artery with the other hand. The ideal pressure over the artery is just enough to prevent bleeding or hematoma formation at the puncture site, while at the same time it is light enough to palpate the distal pulse continuously. Too great a pressure applied over the artery stops the bleeding at the puncture/pressure site but, at the same time, obliterates any blood flow through the vessel and precipitates spasm and thrombus formation in the artery.

When both the vein and artery are punctured in the same extremity, it is difficult to apply pressure separately over both vessel puncture sites. In this case, pressure is applied with a tight wad of 4 × 4 sponges. Often, when both the artery and the vein are punctured and being held at the same site, a compromise must be made between the different pressures necessary for control of the bleeding from the vein and the artery. In these circumstances, close observation of the puncture sites while holding the pressure is even more critical. The amount of pressure applied is sufficient to control the arterial bleeding, however, it is adjusted continually according to the type of any residual bleeding which occurs under the direct pressure being applied and, at the same time, to assure there is persistence of the more peripheral pulse.

In very heavy patients or any patient with a great deal of subcutaneous tissue in the inguinal area, pressure over the puncture sites is applied with a large, firmly wrapped wad of dressing. In this type of patient, it is impossible to apply pressure precisely over the puncture sites of the specific vessel(s). A broader, more diffuse area of pressure is achieved with the wad of dressing while still observing for bleeding under the wad and maintaining a more peripheral arterial pulse.

Essentially all percutaneous puncture sites, regardless of the sheath/catheter size used, can be controlled with manual pressure and a great deal of patience. This is one part of the catheterization procedure that cannot be hurried up.

Percutaneous brachial vein catheterization

With multi-catheter techniques or when the venous access from the femoral approach is compromised, a venous approach from an arm is often desirable or necessary. The approach from the arm is usually performed in combination with an approach from the femoral area where, at least, a femoral arterial monitoring/access line is introduced. A percutaneously introduced, indwelling sheath technique is applicable for both venous and arterial catheterizations in the arm. In congenital heart patients the brachial vessels are the preferred area in the arm, but the techniques for the percutaneous arm approach are applicable to other upper extremity sites, including the axillary vessels.

There are several modifications to the previously described femoral percutaneous technique when a percutaneous technique is used in the arm[5]. In the arms the veins that are used for percutaneous entry are generally smaller, more superficial and are palpable or even visible. As a consequence, the ability to access these veins is dependent more on actual feeling and seeing the vein. The veins in the arms do *not* have the fixed relationships to the artery and other landmarks in the brachial area as they do in the inguinal area. As a consequence, if an arm vein is not visible or palpable, entering the vein can be much more difficult, or even impossible. As the arm vessels are usually considerably smaller than the femoral vessels, it is necessary to use smaller sized sheaths and, in turn, smaller catheters than is really desired.

Before attempting a puncture, the vein to be cannulated should be easily visible or palpable in the antecubital space (or other locations on the arm). A tourniquet is placed centrally around the proximal arm (between the puncture site and the trunk) in order to engorge the vein and optimize access to it. Medial veins or at least veins directed medially on the arm are preferable. The medial veins course along the medial aspect of the arm and join the axillary vein. The axillary vein, in turn, joins the subclavian vein and empties directly to the superior vena cava, providing relatively direct access to the heart. The lateral veins of the arm, on the other hand, tend to course posteriorly and up over the shoulder, which creates a very circuitous course to the central venous system, which often cannot be traversed with a catheter. Even if a catheter is maneuvered to the heart through the lateral veins, subsequent catheter manipulations within the heart are more difficult, if not impossible.

When the veins in the brachial area cannot be visualized or palpated because of excessive subcutaneous tissue, a peripheral intravenous (IV) line is started in a hand or wrist vein. An angiogram of the arm veins is performed by injecting contrast into this more peripheral IV line. A percutaneous needle placed on the skin surface over the brachial area before the injection provides a "reference" structure on the angiogram of the arm for localizing the site of the major veins deeper in the arm.

To prevent distortion of the landmarks and loss of the visualization and/or palpation of the vein, the puncture into the vessel is performed ***before any*** infiltration with local anesthesia. Since the initial needle puncture is performed before any local anesthesia is given, the patient is administered a heavy dose of extra systemic sedation/anesthesia before the site is prepared and the puncture with the needle is begun. The area is scrubbed widely around the visible/palpable vein and the site is draped using a disposable, single hole, Steri-drape™ or a larger "brachial" drape, to provide a large flat sterile field.

The technique for venous puncture is similar to the procedure for introducing a peripheral intravenous line except the puncture of the vessel for the introduction of a wire is performed with no syringe attached to the needle. The tourniquet is applied to the proximal extremity, the distended vein is visualized or palpated directly and its course identified. The puncture is performed with the smallest percutaneous needle which will accommodate the percutaneous guide wire to be used. Again, it is emphasized, this phase of the needle introduction is performed *before* the area is infiltrated with local anesthesia. The previously flushed needle, with nothing attached to the hub, is introduced slowly and meticulously into the vein. The needle is directed along the long axis of the vein and as flat against the skin surface as possible while still allowing the needle to enter the subcutaneous tissues. The purpose is to introduce the needle by a single-wall vessel puncture similar to the introduction of a needle for a peripheral intravenous line. Good blood return is obtained as soon as the needle enters the vein properly and with the tourniquet in place. The wire is introduced gently into the needle and from the needle into the vein exactly as with a femoral puncture technique. The wire should pass beyond the tip of the needle with no palpable change in sensation or visible resistance and no buckling of the proximal wire. In the peripheral arm veins, often the wire advances beyond the tip of the needle very easily but for only 1–2 cm and then abruptly stops. This usually happens because the wire encounters a venous valve, which often cannot be passed with the wire alone.

Once the wire is secure within the vessel, even if it is stopped at a valve, the needle is withdrawn over the wire and firm pressure is applied over the wire and puncture site. With the wire fixed in the vessel and pressure held securely over the vein, *then* the area around the wire and vein at the puncture site is infiltrated thoroughly and widely with local anesthesia. After infiltration with local anesthesia, several minutes are allowed for the anesthesia to take effect, all of the time holding firm pressure over the puncture site where the wire enters the skin and vein. Pain created in this area causes venous spasm, which can prevent the introduction of the sheath and dilator or prohibit a catheter from being advanced through the vein beyond the sheath.

While holding the wire, which is still outside of the needle away from the field, the sterile field of a single-hole drape is placed on the arm and is extended onto the patient's head and trunk with towels in order to produce a contiguous sterile field in conjunction with the sterile drape(s) from the inguinal area. This produces one large sterile field over which flush/pressure lines and various instruments and catheters can be passed from the femoral area without becoming contaminated.

Once the field is completely draped and the local anesthesia has had time to react, the wire is advanced as far further into the vein as possible. Once the wire has been introduced further and is secure well into the vein, a small incision is made in the skin across the entrance site of the wire. The sheath/dilator set is introduced identically to the technique used for the femoral approach. If the wire cannot be advanced more than several centimeters beyond the puncture site, even after infiltration with local anesthesia, a Medi-Cut™ cannula is introduced over the wire and into the vein. Blood should return through the Medi-Cut™ cannula around the wire. When adequate blood return occurs, the wire is removed and a small, slow hand injection of diluted contrast solution is performed through the Medi-Cut™ cannula while recording the flow of the contrast along the course of the arm with biplane stored fluoroscopy or angiography. Once the exact course of the vein has been visualized, the vein in the arm can usually be traversed with a torque-controlled, floppy-tipped, wire and maneuvered to the thorax and cardiac silhouette through the patent course of the vein. Once the wire has reached the cardiac silhouette as visualized by fluoroscopy, the sheath and dilator are introduced the rset of the way into the vein over the wire.

An alternative technique when the wire cannot be advanced all of the way to the thorax from the arm, is to introduce the sheath/dilator only as far as the initial secure distance of the wire within the vein. The wire is removed from the dilator very slowly. The dilator is flushed very gently and then continuously with warm (body temperature) flush solution as the dilator is withdrawn very slowly from the sheath. The dilator is replaced in the sheath with a smooth, blunt-tipped (angiographic) catheter. The smoother tipped catheter is manipulated along the known course of the vein that was visualized previously by angiography. As the catheter is introduced into the sheath and as it is advanced through the vein toward the central circulation, the catheter is kept on the slow continuous flush of body temperature flush solution. This infusion of warmed fluid helps to dilate the vein and open the valves of the vein in front of the advancing tip of the catheter. Once the catheter has been advanced well beyond the sheath, the sheath is advanced completely into the vein over the advancing catheter. The course of the catheter along the patient's arm, into the thorax and, finally, into the heart is observed with fluoroscopy to prevent unnecessary (and painful) probing of small, side branch veins. Occasionally intermittent, small, gentle, venous angiograms through the catheter are necessary to verify the true course of the vein. Venous spasm can prohibit further movement of the catheter in spite of all of the previous efforts. In that circumstance a very small amount of intravenous 1% lidocaine is infused through the catheter or sheath into the vein. The patient is observed for five minutes after the infusion before attempting to move the catheter again.

In larger patients, when the large branches of the brachial vein are identified visually or by palpation, side by side or piggy-back sheaths can be utilized in the same vein as for the brachial approach. Instead of trying to introduce the second sheath into the exact venous channel, the second sheath is introduced into a visible or palpable tributary branch of the more central brachial venous channel. The same technique used for the first brachial sheath is used for the additional brachial sheath. When the size of the veins is questionable, it is best to introduce both wires into the separate veins before infiltration of the local anesthesia and before introducing either of the sheaths.

Axillary vein entry

Occasionally the axillary vein is used in order to accommodate a larger sheath and catheter or because of loss of the usable brachial vein from prior catheterization procedures (especially a prior cut-down or indwelling IV lines) or from more peripheral venous spasm. The axillary veins are made more visible or palpable by extending and abducting the entire arm and then bending the forearm up and over the head.

The vein in the axilla lies in a fairly fixed relationship to the palpable artery as the vessels pass over the head of the humerus. The axillary vein lies parallel to, and just inferior (caudal) to the artery with the arm extended over the head. The brachial nerve plexus is in this same area so care is taken not to over-extend the arm and to avoid excessive or deep puncturing in the area. The same techniques are used for axillary vein puncture as for brachial puncture except that the application of a tourniquet to the vein is accomplished by digital pressure across the head of the humerus (and the vein) at the patient's trunk (body) side. The course of the artery is palpated to confirm the course of the vein when the vein does not appear visible or palpable.

The entire axillary area, including down onto the arm and the wall of the chest (and back), is scrubbed widely and draped with a Steri-drape™ or a single-hole brachial drape placed over the head of the humerus. In adolescent and older patients the entire area is shaved before the patient is scrubbed or draped. The percutaneous needle is introduced into the vein after the area has been scrubbed and draped but, again, *before* any local anesthesia is introduced. A very superficial puncture, parallel to the vein and the skin, is usually sufficient to enter the vein with the needle and, in turn, introduce the wire into the vein. Once the wire passes securely into the vein, it usually advances easily and far into the vein. The needle is removed over the wire and the wire position within the thorax or right heart chambers is verified by fluoroscopy. After the wire has been confirmed to be in the proper and secure position, the area around the puncture site and vein are infiltrated thoroughly with local anesthesia. The sheath and dilator are introduced utilizing extreme precautions for the prevention of the entry of any air. With the venous entry site close to the thorax, air can be sucked into the system even more readily than from a peripheral vein.

Jugular vein approach

The jugular venous approach is used very frequently for cardiac catheterizations in congenital heart patients. The jugular vein is used as the preferential approach for some procedures and out of necessity as a consequence of the loss of other venous access from previous indwelling intravenous lines or catheterizations. The jugular vein is usually used in preference to any of the arm veins because the large size of the jugular vein allows the introduction of larger sheaths/catheters, the route to the heart does not have the tortuosity found when approaching from the peripheral veins of the upper extremity, and the jugular vein does not have the frequent problem of venospasm which occurs in the arm veins. The right jugular vein provides a "straight course" to the heart and is used for almost all access from the jugular approach. The straight course to the superior vena cava, right atrium and right ventricle makes the jugular vein an ideal approach for endomyocardial biopsies and the preferred (only) approach to the right ventricle for the closure of apical/mid-muscular ventricular septal defects.

When the jugular vein approach is used and even when there is known or suspected absence of central venous access from below, the inguinal areas are prepped and draped in addition to the prepping of the jugular area. The inguinal area is used for an arterial monitoring line, and often a femoral vein can be accessed peripheral to a more central, deep venous obstruction and is used for fluid and medication administration.

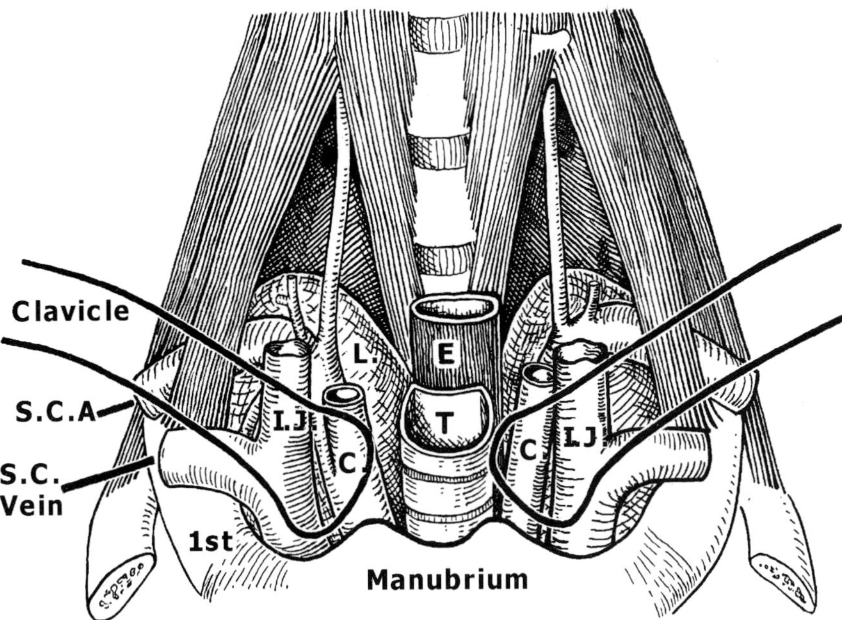

Figure 4.20 Anatomy and structures in the supraclavicular area. Clavicle, outline of clavicle over (in front of) supraclavicular structures; I.J., internal jugular vein; C, carotid artery; S.C.A, subclavian artery; S.C. Vein, subclavian vein; T, trachea; E, esophagus; L., apex of lung.

2-D echographic guidance is now used routinely for all jugular venous punctures. A meticulous, very directed and controlled approach for venous punctures is more important for entry into the internal jugular vein than for any other venous access. There are multiple very critical structures (carotid artery, trachea and apex of the lung) adjacent to, or in the immediate vicinity of, the internal jugular vein, and the adjacent subcutaneous tissues are looser and less constraining than in other areas used for venous access (Figure 4.20).

The earlier technique of attempting to puncture the vein purposefully with a very small needle attached to a syringe of local anesthesia in order to "identify the vein's location" by obtaining blood, while introducing the local anesthesia and then having to repeat the puncture of the jugular vein with subsequent, more or less random and multiple stabs with a larger needle in order to introduce the wire is no longer acceptable. The use of echo guidance for direct visualization of the vessels combined with a very meticulous technique for the direct puncture of the visualized vein makes the introduction of needle, wire, sheath, and dilator into the vein more definitive, less traumatic to the vessels and surrounding tissues and safer for the patient.

General anesthesia is preferably used for the jugular venous approach. Alternatively, the patient must be sedated very heavily and repeatedly. When a patient awakens during a jugular venous puncture or during manipulation from a jugular approach, it is very frightening to the patient and usually results in violent head, neck and shoulder movements, which make it impossible to maintain a sterile field. If patient movement occurs during the percutaneous needle introduction, vital structures that are adjacent to the jugular vein can very easily be punctured or lacerated. If movement occurs during a critical step in the catheter manipulations, control of the catheter is lost in addition to the compromise of the sterility of the operative field. If a patient moves during a therapeutic procedure from the jugular vein, any movement of the patient's neck is transmitted more directly to the catheter/device with the result that the device can be malpositioned easily or even lost within the heart.

Ideally, in order to distend the veins for a jugular venous puncture, the patient should be in a head-down (Trendelenburg) position. Unfortunately, modern cardiac catheterization tables do not have the capability of tilting lengthwise into the Trendelenburg position so it is not possible to accomplish venous engorgement by positioning the table. However, there are ways of producing jugular venous distention, at least transiently. The patient is administered 10 ml per kilogram of body weight of intravenous lactate or 0.25% normal saline through a separate intravenous line. This fluid increases the circulating volume and dilates the venous system transiently. With the patient under general anesthesia, the anesthesiologist can maintain a positive pressure inspiration at the precise time of the puncture and wire introduction. The forced inspiration produces a transient Valsalva maneuver and increases the intrathoracic and venous pressure transiently. It also hyperinflates the lungs, including in the supraclavicular area. Another alternative or adjunct method of achieving distention of the jugular vein is to have a scrubbed associate hold pressure over the vein just above the clavicle and caudal to the puncture site during the needle puncture and the introduction of the wire. The area that is available for this digital compression, however, is often in the exact area where the puncture should be performed. Another alternative technique is to have an associate provide deep, steady compression over the abdomen and particularly the hepatic area during the needle puncture and especially during the exchange of catheters or wires through a jugular venous cannula. Wedges placed under the hips and trunk of smaller patients raise the jugular venous pressure; however, if the femoral approach is used concurrently, this elevation of the hips compromises the sterility and access of the inguinal areas.

Before being prepped and draped, the patient's head is turned away from the expected side of the puncture and is secured in that position. Since the patient's head will be completely beneath the drapes with the jugular approach, it is preferable to have the patient intubated and ventilated. If the patient is not intubated and ventilated, the patient *must* have a secure airway and receive continuous flow, blow-by air or oxygen under the drapes. Before prepping the jugular area, the patient's hair is covered completely with a secure surgical bonnet, tucking all loose strands up under the bonnet and securing the bonnet with tape if necessary. The area is surgically scrubbed from the hairline or bonnet (cephalad), to the infraclavicular area on the chest (caudally), as far posteriorly as the field allows on the involved side of the neck and past the midline anteriorly. A Steri-drape™ is positioned over the expected puncture area with the inferior (caudal) margin of the opening on the cephalad edge of the clavicle. A single-opening, disposable paper brachial drape is preferred for the remainder of the draping. These brachial drapes usually have a single opening placed excentrically in the drape. The longer side of the drape is positioned cephalad over the patient's head (and over the head end of the table) to ensure a sterile field cephalad to the puncture site. With this orientation of the brachial drape, the adhesive around the opening of the drape is attached over the opening in the Steri-Drape™. This results in the long end of the drape extending cephalad and laterally to cover the head and shoulders, while the shorter end extends caudally to overlap part of the sterile lap drape from below. This combination creates a single large sterile field extending from well above the patient's head to below his/her feet!

In addition to the operative field, the AP image intensifier, the collimator of the lateral X-ray tube, the lateral image intensifier and the yoke of the C-arm of the posterior–anterior X-ray tube are covered with sterile drapes. The catheters, flush/pressure tubes, wires, other equipment and the operators themselves repeatedly (continuously!) pass in close proximity to these components of the X-ray equipment.

The right internal jugular vein is preferred, however, the left internal or even a superficial jugular vein is occasionally used when the right internal jugular is inaccessible or occluded. Even though echo guidance is used for jugular vein punctures, the operators must be familiar with the critical structures adjacent to the vein (Figure 4.20) and the palpable landmarks in the area (Figure 4.21)[6].

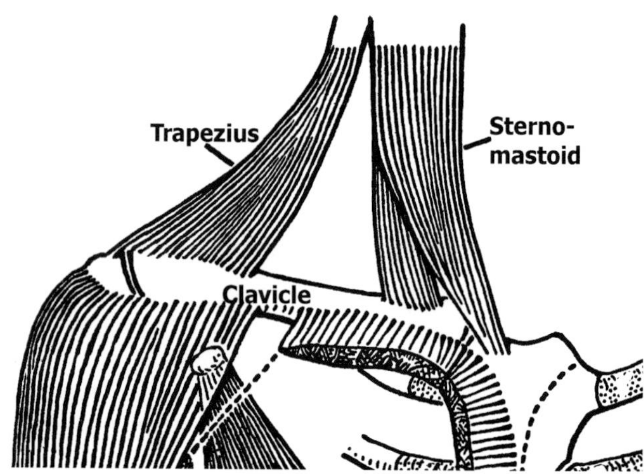

Figure 4.21 Structures defining the supraclavicular triangle in the neck.

The landmarks for the puncture of the internal jugular vein are within a triangle formed by the sternocleidomastoid and trapezius muscles and the clavicle. The top or cephalic apex of the triangle is formed by the fusion of the heads of the sternocleidomastoid muscle anteriorly and the trapezius muscle posteriorly. The base of the triangle is formed by the separate tendonous attachments of the caudal heads of the trapezius muscle laterally and the sternocleidomastoid muscle anteriorly onto the cephalic (upper) edge at both ends of the clavicle. The caudal trapezius head attaches at the middle-lateral end of the clavicle and the caudal clavicular head of the sternocleidomastoid muscle attaches at the clavicular-manubrial junction. The carotid artery pulse is palpable within this triangle. The internal jugular vein lies just lateral to the palpable carotid artery. The preferred puncture site for the vein is at the apex (cephalic end) of the triangle, which is usually several centimeters above the clavicle. Caudally the jugular vein joins the subclavian vein, which turns caudally into the superior vena cava. Caudally the jugular/subclavian veins are very close to the apex of the lung.

Once the landmarks are identified and the patient is prepped and draped for the jugular venous puncture and ***before any*** local anesthesia or other needle punctures, the vessels are visualized with the 2-D echo. It is extremely important to visualize the area with the echo *before **any** punctures* are made in the area. Infiltration with local anesthesia creates "lakes" of fluid in the tissues, which appear on the echo image and are indistinguishable from the veins on the echo image. Likewise, an unsuccessful puncture into the vein which may even nick the wall of a vessel results in extravasation of blood into the very loose tissues of the neck. The extravasated blood also appears on the echo image as fluid lakes that are indistinguishable from the true venous channels. Of equal importance, extravasated fluid/blood can compress the true venous channels and make any subsequent puncture into the jugular vein more difficult.

A small, dedicated Site-Rite™ (Dymax Corporation, Pittsburgh, PA) "vessel finder" 2-D echo machine is now used routinely for the visualization of the jugular vein and to direct the puncture into the vein[7]. The Site-Rite™ machine is relatively inexpensive (for an echo machine!), battery operated, small, portable and has a relatively small transducer. The Site-Rite™ machine is kept in the catheterization laboratory so that it is always available. The Site-Rite™ echo provides a clear visualization of the vessels and tissues in the neck, which can be in a longitudinal view or, preferably, in a cross-sectional view, depending upon the orientation of the transducer. A disposable, sterile sleeve which covers the transducer and transducer cable along with sterile echo gel are available for use with the vessel finder. These provide a means of using the transducer in the sterile field and allow visualization of the vessels not only before but during the actual puncture of the vessel. There is a sterile needle guide which snaps onto the transducer over the sterile sleeve and holds a 19-gauge needle in line with the transducer. This guide reportedly helps to align the direction of the needle with the echo beam although, this has not been very useful in our experience.

The echo visualization of the jugular vein can be performed with a standard two dimensional (2-D) echo machine and transducer, however, standard echo machines are quite large and cumbersome with equally large and cumbersome transducers. Of equal importance, the standard echo machine is a very expensive piece of capital equipment, which cannot be dedicated to remain in the catheterization laboratory for this very selective and once- or twice-a-day usage.

After the scrubbing and draping of the field, the Site-Rite™ transducer is prepared for sterile use. Standard, non-sterile echo jelly is placed inside the transducer end of the long, rolled-up, sterile sleeve. A non-scrubbed associate places the tip of the non-sterile transducer in the puddle of echo jelly within the sleeve. The sleeve is unrolled over the transducer and its attached cable from the outside of the sleeve by the (sterile) operator. The non-sterile cable is threaded inside the sleeve while the sterile field is maintained on the outside of the sleeve. Sterile echo jelly is applied over the end of the transducer on the outside of the sterile sleeve precisely over the site of the enclosed tip of the transducer within the sleeve. The puddle of jelly within the sleeve along with the jelly applied to the outside of the sleeve creates an "echo contact" between the transducer, through the sleeve and to the skin. The transducer within the sleeve is placed directly over the expected puncture site on the skin with the ridge for the needle attachment on the transducer facing cephalad and aligned with the suspected site and direction of the vein. The lateralization for right or left orientation is corrected with the Site-Rite™ controls according to which side of the neck is used. In addition to their relative locations (artery medial to the vein), the carotid artery is identified on the echo image by its pulsations, while the internal jugular vein is identified by its usually larger diameter and its easy compressibility when even very gentle pressure is applied with the transducer to the skin over the area.

Once the patient is positioned, the field draped and the vessel has been located by echo, the patient is given a substantial dose of additional general anesthesia or sedation. The extra anesthesia/sedation helps with the initial, very superficial, skin wheal of local anesthesia and allows for the deeper needle puncture, which is performed before any additional deeper local anesthesia is administered. A generous, but very superficial, skin (only) wheal is made with 2% xylocaine injected through a short 25-gauge subcuticular needle directly over the expected puncture site of the jugular vein. Care is taken ***not*** to extend this local anesthesia into the deeper subcutaneous tissues at all at this time.

A straight, extra-soft-tipped, 0.018″ wire for percutaneous vascular introductions is positioned on the field with the tip placed immediately adjacent to the site of the skin wheal. In patients who, unequivocally, do ***not*** have any respiratory obstruction or other causes of increased inspiratory effort and/or who *are on* positive pressure ventilation with general anesthesia, a standard percutaneous needle, which is *not* attached to a syringe, is used for the jugular puncture. The percutaneous needle including the hub is filled with fluid exactly as with other percutaneous punctures. The needle, with nothing attached to it, is introduced into the skin directly beneath the tip of the needle guide on the Site-Rite™ transducer. The needle is advanced in a direction parallel to the course of the jugular vein but aiming into the tissues at a 45° angle to the skin.

The needle is advanced slowly into the tissues while watching for movement of the fluid bubble in the hub of the needle and also watching the image on the Site-Rite™ echo for directional guidance. During the introduction of the needle, the tip of the needle on the echo image can be seen to indent or compress the tissues that are directly in front of it as the tip of the needle penetrates the tissues in front of it. There is occasionally a black line in the echo image, which represents the echo "shadow" behind the needle. This linear shadow serves as an additional guide for the direction of the needle during puncture. If the needle is introduced deeply without entering the vein and/or is seen to compress tissues that are adjacent to the vein rather than over the vein, the needle is withdrawn slowly while observing for blood return in the needle hub. When no blood return is obtained during the needle withdrawal and while observing the needle continuously on the echo image, the needle is redirected appropriately and re-advanced very slowly. If the patient has any discomfort from the needle, more systemic sedation or more general anesthesia is given to the patient rather than infiltrating with local anesthesia at this stage of the procedure.

This needle introduction is repeated slowly and meticulously until the vessel is punctured. The anterior wall of the vein on the echo image will be seen to be compressed by the tip of the needle as it advances and approaches directly over the vein, and just before the needle punctures the vein. Usually, the "pop", or give, into the vein is visualized clearly on the echo as the tip of the needle enters the vein. With an accurate entrance into the lumen of the vein, blood appears in the hub of the needle. Assuming the return of blood from the needle hub is *not* a *spurt* of arterial blood, the tip of the straight, soft-tipped, spring guide wire is quickly, but gently, introduced into the needle and from there into the jugular vein. As with all other wire introduction, there should be no sensation of resistance at all and certainly no force should be necessary as the wire passes beyond the tip of the needle and into the vein. As soon as the wire is well into the vein, the needle is withdrawn, pressure is applied over the jugular puncture site and the course of the wire is visualized by fluoroscopy. Once the wire is well within the thorax, additional local anesthesia is administered through a separate needle around the site of puncture at this juncture of the procedure.

When the patient has any signs of respiratory obstruction, puncture of the jugular vein is always carried out with the percutaneous needle attached to a syringe partially filled with flush solution. A standard 21-gauge percutaneous needle is attached to a slip-lock syringe that is partially filled with flush solution (but no air!). Mild negative pressure is applied to the syringe while the needle is being introduced cephalad to, and immediately beneath, the Site-Rite™ transducer. Whenever the needle is being manipulated within the tissues, slight suction is maintained on the syringe. When blood return is obtained in the syringe, airway positive pressure is administered by the anesthesiologist or abdominal compression provided by an associate, the syringe is removed quickly but very carefully, and the wire is introduced into the needle immediately but, at the same time, very gently and carefully.

The wire introduction is performed exactly as it is for any other percutaneous venous introduction through a needle. There should be no resistance felt and no bending or bowing of the more proximal wire as the wire tip advances past the tip of the needle into the vessel. If the wire does not pass easily, the angle of the needle is changed or the needle is rotated very slightly and the attempted introduction of the wire is repeated. This combination of maneuvers with the wire and needle is repeated until the wire passes easily beyond the tip of the needle. As soon as the tip of the wire passes easily well beyond the tip of the needle, the position of the tip of the wire in the thorax is verified on fluoroscopy, and when the wire moves freely and unequivocally in the cardiac silhouette, the needle is removed over the wire from the vein and completely out of the skin. Pressure is maintained over the puncture site while the area around the puncture site is infiltrated with local anesthesia. Once the area is well anesthetized with local anesthesia, a skin nick is made over the wire at the puncture site and the sheath/dilator set is introduced over the wire into the vein.

When there is blood return into the hub of the needle, but the wire cannot be introduced into the vein even with gentle repositioning and a slow, stepwise rotation of the needle, the needle is withdrawn and pressure held over the puncture site for at least five minutes. Because of the looseness of the subcutaneous tissues in the neck, even a very small puncture of a vein in the neck causes significant bleeding into the subcutaneous tissues in the area of the puncture. The greater the extravasation of blood adjacent to the vein, the more difficult is the subsequent entry into the vein. If the artery is inadvertently entered during the attempted venous puncture, the area is compressed manually for at least ten minutes after the needle is withdrawn. Even though blood does not exit through the puncture opening in the skin, bleeding from the vessel continues under the skin for several minutes with resultant accumulation of a large "lake" of blood in the adjacent subcutaneous tissues.

When the Site-Rite™ vessel finder or other echo guidance is not available the introduction of the needle into the jugular vein is guided by the visual and palpable landmarks in the neck along with the continual palpation of the carotid artery medial to the vein. When echo guidance is not used for the jugular puncture, a very superficial skin wheal is created just lateral to the palpable arterial pulse over the expected puncture site for the vein. The skin wheal is created with a 25-gauge needle on a syringe filled with 2% xylocaine. As soon as the skin wheal has been completed, the 25-gauge needle on the syringe of xylocaine is replaced with the 21-gauge needle which is to be used for the percutaneous puncture. The percutaneous needle on the syringe of xylocaine is introduced into the neck lateral and immediately adjacent to, the palpable pulse of the carotid artery, angling approximately 45° into the tissues from the skin surface and aiming in the direction of the right, mid clavicular line (toward the right nipple). Negative pressure is applied continuously to the syringe as the needle is advanced deeper into the tissues. With each deeper introduction of the tip of the needle and when no blood return is observed into the needle/

syringe, the area is infiltrated with a small amount of local anesthesia through the percutaneous needle and the process repeated until either the vein is entered or the needle has reached its hub in the tissues. When the needle cannot be introduced further into the tissues, it is withdrawn slowly while maintaining *slight* negative pressure on the syringe until either there is blood return in the needle or the needle comes out of the skin. After the needle has been withdrawn completely out of the deeper tissues, the angle of the needle is changed slightly and the introduction toward the vein is repeated slowly and carefully until the vein is entered.

As soon as blood return from the vein is observed in the syringe, the syringe is removed, the guide wire introduced and advanced into the cardiac silhouette and the needle withdrawn over the wire, all as expeditiously as possible since the open needle can allow air to be sucked into the vein. If the vein was entered during the initial attempt at the puncture and before good local anesthesia was completed, pressure is held over the wire and puncture site while the infiltration of local anesthesia into the surrounding tissues is completed after replacing the percutaneous needle which was on the syringe of local anesthesia with the 25-gauge needle. When the infiltration of the local anesthesia into the surrounding area was completed during the attempts at puncture and the wire has definitely passed into the cardiac silhouette, a small skin incision is made over the wire with the tip of a #11 blade. A fine tipped sheath/dilator set is introduced over the wire and advanced into the superior vena cava or right atrium.

When the local anesthesia is completed and the original wire passes easily into the jugular vein but does not advance into the cardiac silhouette, a Medi-Cut™ cannula is advanced into the vein over the wire. There should be some blood return through the Medi-Cut™ over the wire. The original wire is removed through the Medi-Cut™ cannula and replaced with a J-tipped or torque-controlled wire. This is manipulated well into the cardiac silhouette under direct fluoroscopic visualization, and once it is within the cardiac silhouette the Medi-Cut™ is removed and replaced with the appropriate sheath/dilator set.

Introducing the sheath/dilator from the jugular venous approach is one of the circumstances where the back-bleed device should remain attached to the sheath. The absolute prevention of air being sucked into the venous system unequivocally outweighs the advantage of being able to freely rotate the sheath without the valve attached during sheath introduction. If a non-ventilated patient has any respiratory difficulties, the inspiratory effort generates large negative pressures and the potential for introducing air is multiplied by the immediate proximity of the sheath to the thorax. When a patient does generate deep inspiratory efforts that cannot be overcome or suppressed, it becomes necessary to apply *gentle* suction on the sheath to clear it of air. Whenever suction is applied to a side arm of a valved back-bleed device, the valve of the back-bleed device *must* be capped and closed tightly with a gloved fingertip by pressing the finger tightly over the valve. Once the sheath has been completely cleared of air and clots, the side arm of the sheath is attached to the pressure/flush system and maintained on a slow, continuous flush during subsequent catheter introduction or manipulations.

Any open lumen which is in communication with the venous system in the neck is in direct communication with the potentially very strong, negative intrathoracic pressures. When a wire is removed from a needle, Medi-Cut™ or dilator, the proximal end of any open lumen in the vein is capped immediately with a syringe or finger or another wire is introduced immediately into the open lumen to prevent air from being sucked in through even the tiny lumen of the dilator or plastic cannula. In order to produce an increase in venous pressure at any time when there potentially will be an open lumen into the jugular vein, sustained positive intrathoracic pressure is created either by the anesthesiologist during ventilation or by an associated applying external abdominal pressure.

When using a sheath which does *not* have the back-bleed valve attached during the introduction (which is ***never*** recommended in the jugular area), the wire is always withdrawn completely from the dilator before the dilator is removed from the sheath. Otherwise, as with all wires passing alone through the lumen of a sheath, a large, open space is present between the open lumen of the sheath and the fine wire within the open lumen. At the same time, the wire alone passing through the hub of the open sheath prohibits the effective closing off, or capping of the open end of the sheath. On the other hand, the much smaller, longer lumen of the dilator or Medi-Cut™ does not permit air entry through it after the wire has been removed and during the short period of time while the dilator is being withdrawn. As soon as the dilator has been removed from the sheath, the sheath is capped with a syringe or a back-bleed valve/flush device and cleared of any entrapped air and/or clot by *gentle* negative suction. Passive blood flow from the sheath is possible only when patients are *not* generating negative intrathoracic pressure during their active inspiration.

When a very large and/or long sheath will be necessary in the jugular vein for a specific procedure, but that particular procedure will not be performed until much later during the catheterization, a smaller, short sheath is initially placed in the jugular vein and used until the time when the larger sheath is needed. The smaller diameter sheath allows freer blood flow in the jugular vein around the indwelling sheath until the time when the larger sheath is necessary. In addition the majority of larger sheaths used for the introduction of devices are very long, and once such a sheath is introduced into the jugular vein, the proximal end of the long sheath extends off the sterile field and well cephalad to the patient's head. After the introduction of a long sheath into the jugular venous system, the sheath at the head of the table requires the *full-time attention and care* of a *second operator* and/or very knowledgeable assistant. When a larger sheath is needed later during the case, the area is re-anesthetized locally and the smaller sheath which was present in the jugular vein initially is easily exchanged for the new one.

In addition to the potential problem of all indwelling sheaths of creating venous obstructions, perforations or the introduction of air, internal jugular vein access has the potential for several other, unique complications. The carotid artery lies immediately adjacent to the internal jugular vein (Figure 4.20) and can easily be punctured inadvertently with the needle during attempts to puncture the vein. This should be recognized immediately by the appearance of the arterialized blood or the pulsatile flow from the needle so that the sheath/dilator is *not* introduced into that vessel. If not recognized by the nature of the blood return in the needle, the wrong vessel should be recognized unequivocally by the anomalous course which the wire takes in the artery/aorta when a wire is introduced into the artery, as opposed to the usual course in the vein to the right atrium. This emphasizes the necessity of visualizing the course of the wire fluoroscopically and in both planes whenever a percutaneous wire is introduced into the neck as well as into any other vessel. When a small needle is used for the puncture, and the arterial puncture is recognized, the needle is withdrawn and pressure held for five or more minutes until total hemostasis is achieved, usually without adverse consequences.

The apex of the lung is very close to the junction of the jugular and subclavian veins (Figure 4.20). With a more caudal location in the neck for the puncture of the internal jugular vein or a deeper (more posterior) puncture aiming for the subclavian vein, the pleura and underlying lung are easily entered. If the lung is entered, the patient will very likely develop a pneumothorax and will require treatment with a chest tube. If not recognized quickly the patient can develop severe respiratory distress and can even die from this complication. The best way to avoid this complication is a patient, slow single-wall puncture into these veins and a more cephalad internal jugular or a more superficial subclavian puncture. The more precise puncture is facilitated by the use of a Site-Rite™ portable echo with continuous visualization of the vessel as it is punctured. More definitive management of an acute pneumothorax is covered in Chapter 35 under "Respiratory Complications".

When a catheter is removed from the internal jugular vein, adequate pressure often cannot be applied over the vein without compromising the airway. It is helpful to place these patients in a 45° sitting position while achieving hemostasis over the veins in the neck.

Subclavian vein catheterization

In patients who have had multiple or very complex surgical or prior interventional catheterization procedures, or patients who require a chronic indwelling venous line, the subclavian vein provides an alternative venous access. The axillary vein, as it passes onto the anterior thorax from the arm and past the axilla, becomes the subclavian vein. The subclavian vein passes medially under the pectoral muscles and cephalad toward the mid portion of the clavicle. As the subclavian vein exits from under the medial aspect of the pectoralis muscles, it passes obliquely, in a slightly cephalad and medial direction, passing just caudal to, and under, the mid portion of the clavicle. Along this course from the axilla, the axillary/subclavian vein runs parallel and slightly anterior/caudal to the artery (Figure 4.22).

Under the clavicle, the subclavian vein also leaves its subcutaneous location and enters the thoracic cavity, where it joins the jugular vein and becomes the innominate vein which, in turn, joins the superior vena cava. The area and the surrounding structures in this intrathoracic course of the subclavian vein account for the major complications associated with subclavian vein punctures. Punctures extending into the tissues deep, or cephalad to the vein result in a pneumothorax, while punctures through the subclavian vein or into the adjacent subclavian artery can result in a hemothorax.

During the needle, wire and sheath/dilator introduction for a subclavian vein puncture, it is desirable to have the veins in the upper thorax or neck distended. This is accomplished either with the patient in a Trendelenburg position (when not on a catheterization table), by distention

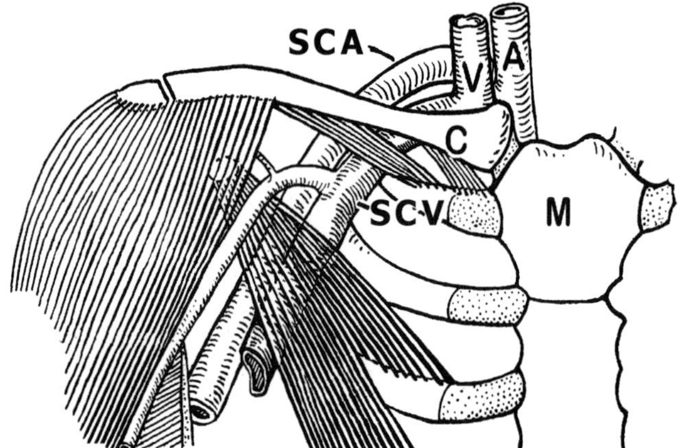

Figure 4.22 Subclavian outlet anatomy. SCA, subclavian artery; SCV, subclavian vein; C, Clavicle; M, manubrium; A, Innominate artery; V, Jugular vein.

of the entire venous system with a large supplemental bolus of intravenous fluid prior to the puncture, by the anesthesiologist producing an increase in intrathoracic pressure with a positive pressure inspiration or by the manual application of external pressure over the abdomen. The entire upper chest wall and neck are scrubbed and the area around the mid portion of the clavicle is draped to produce a sterile field. A disposable single-hole, brachial or extremity drape is most satisfactory for this area. The larger percutaneous needle, which will accommodate the guide wire, is used for the introduction of the deeper local anesthesia during a subclavian puncture. As described previously for the puncture of the jugular vein, this allows a purposeful aim at the vein while the needle for the xylocaine is being introduced and the introduction of the wire through the same needle if the vein is entered.

A skin wheal (only) is created with a 25-gauge local needle. This needle on the xylocaine syringe is replaced with the slightly larger, 21-gauge, percutaneous needle. With the appropriate, extra-soft-tipped wire readily available on the sterile field immediately adjacent to the puncture site, the percutaneous needle, which is attached to a syringe filled with the local anesthesia, is introduced into the skin just lateral to the mid clavicle and just at the lower (caudal) edge of the clavicle. The needle is aimed at the suprasternal notch. A finger pressed deep into the suprasternal notch provides a more defined target direction for the puncture with the needle. Negative pressure is applied to the syringe while the needle is advanced just under the caudal edge of the clavicle and while keeping the direction of the needle roughly parallel to the clavicle with a slightly cephalad angulation toward the finger in the suprasternal notch. Slight negative pressure is maintained on the syringe as the needle is introduced into the tissues.

If there is no blood return into the syringe when the needle has been introduced several millimeters, a small additional amount of local anesthesia is injected through this needle into the tissues. Negative pressure again is applied to the syringe and the needle is introduced further in the same direction. These steps are repeated until blood is withdrawn into the syringe or the needle has been introduced to the hub (of the small needle). In larger patients where larger, and particularly longer, needles are used, the longer needle is not introduced to more than 2/3 of its total length or past the medial 1/3 length of the clavicle.

If the tip of the needle is estimated to be past the proximal one third of the clavicle and as far as the hub without entering a vein, the needle is withdrawn slowly while still maintaining slight negative pressure on the syringe. If blood returns into the syringe during the withdrawal of the needle/syringe, the needle is fixed carefully and securely in this position, the syringe is removed, and the wire is introduced quickly into the needle exactly as when guide wires are introduced into needles in any other vessel. When no blood is obtained as the needle is withdrawn, the needle/syringe is withdrawn out of the tissues and flushed. The puncture procedure is restarted, but now with the syringe which previously was filled with local anesthesia, replaced with a syringe filled with flush solution. During repeat punctures, a slight change in the angle of introduction of the needle is used each time until the vessel is entered.

When blood appears in the syringe during the needle introduction, the needle is fixed in position and the syringe is carefully removed. A soft-tipped spring guide wire is immediately introduced through the small percutaneous needle without first capping or placing anything over the hub of the needle. The wire usually passes easily four or five centimeters beyond the needle tip, but often stops at that point because of the tight curves or tortuous course within the venous system. Once the wire passes easily and a good distance into the venous system, the needle is removed over the wire and pressure applied over the puncture site in the skin as well as up and under the clavicle. The wire is visualized continuously under fluoroscopy while it gently is manipulated into the superior vena cava and from there into the cardiac silhouette. The wire should never be pushed forcefully against any palpable resistance. If the original straight, soft-tipped wire cannot be manipulated around the curves in the venous system even using direct visualization, a Medi-Cut™ cannula is introduced over the wire and the straight wire replaced with a J- or curved-tipped, torque-controlled wire. Either of these wires is manipulated readily around the curves in the veins and into the heart.

Once the wire is well within the cardiac silhouette, the sheath/dilator set (or an indwelling subclavian line) is introduced over a wire similarly to other puncture sites. Before the sheath/dilator is introduced into the subclavian vein, a 45–90° curve is formed on the distal end of the sheath (and dilator) by pulling the two between the fingers or by heating the set in boiling water or in the jet of a heat gun and then forming the curve on the sheath by hand molding. This curve allows the sheath to conform to the acutely curved course from the subclavian vein into the superior vena cava. The wire and dilator are removed from the sheath and the back-bleed system is opened to clear the sheath of air and clots. Clearing the sheath is accomplished very carefully and rapidly as described previously for the jugular vein. As in the case of the jugular vein, any inspiratory negative pressure within the thorax is delivered directly and with a greater vacuum to the sheath than from the more peripheral venous puncture locations.

Transhepatic venous access

As more complex and multiple diagnostic and therapeutic catheterizations are performed and more indwelling venous lines installed, patent venous access sites present an ever-increasing problem. There are now many occasions when the infrarenal inferior vena cava or both iliofemoral venous systems are obstructed, cannot be reconstituted and, in turn, prevent access to the heart from the usual femoral or caudal approach, which is critical for some specific interventional procedures. There are even a few patients in whom all of the major venous access channels, including those in the jugular veins and superior vena cava as well as the infrarenal inferior vena cava, are obliterated by previous indwelling lines or procedures. The transhepatic approach provides a venous access which is possible, repeatable and, at least in the short term, relatively safe[8,9].

Direct percutaneous hepatic punctures were first used for liver biopsies, then for the placement of indwelling intravenous lines, and are now used for diagnostic as well as therapeutic cardiac catheterization procedures. The general preparation of the patient is similar to that for any other cardiac catheterization although, because of the even greater need for a quiet, immobile patient during the transhepatic puncture, general anesthesia is preferred (required!) for these procedures. The patient undergoing a transhepatic catheterization should have a separate, secure and large-gauge peripheral intravenous line. As is the case with other non-femoral venous approaches, in addition to the site for the transhepatic puncture the inguinal area is prepped and draped. This allows the placement of an indwelling femoral arterial line for continual blood pressure monitoring, which should be standard when using the transhepatic approach. The patient undergoing a transhepatic catheterization has a unit of blood typed, cross-matched and available in the catheterization laboratory.

The lateral chest wall together with the abdominal wall on the one side of the body are scrubbed and draped from the mid-line, cephalad at the sternoclavicular junction and caudally at the umbilicus, around posteriorly to the right posterior axillary line (assuming situs solitus) on the chest and to the posterior iliac crest on the back.

The goal with the hepatic puncture is to enter the liver caudal to the most caudal reflection of the diaphragm but, at the same time, above the caudal edge of the liver and posterior (dorsal) to the gall bladder and biliary system. The skin over the tenth intercostal space (approximately half the distance from the dome of the diaphragm to the liver edge as visualized on fluoroscopy) and between the mid and the anterior axillary line is infiltrated with local anesthesia using a long 25-gauge needle. While maintaining the syringe of local anesthesia on negative pressure, the needle is introduced in small increments, perpendicular to the skin, between the ribs, through the subcutaneous tissues and all of the way to the capsule of the liver. The local anesthesia is injected every few millimeters as long as no blood return is obtained in the syringe. Contact with the liver capsule is indicated by a moving sensation of the needle, which corresponds to respiratory movements. The capsule is infiltrated thoroughly with local anesthesia following which the needle and syringe are removed from the tissues.

A long (20 cm), 22-gauge Chiba™ needle (Medi-tech, Boston Scientific Corporation or Cook Inc.), which has a metal stylet, a thin-walled needle and an outer, thin-walled, plastic cannula, is introduced into the anesthetized site. The needle is directed slightly cephalad toward the xiphoid process maintaining it in a roughly horizontal to slightly posterior (dorsal) plane as it is advanced into the liver using biplane fluoroscopic guidance. The needle, with the stylet still in place within it, is advanced within the hepatic shadow observed on fluoroscopy. With PA fluoroscopic guidance the tip of the needle is advanced medially and slightly cephalad to the edge of the vertebral column (2–3 cm before reaching the midline) while with lateral (LAT) fluoroscopic guidance the tip is directed horizontally and toward the anterior edge of the vertebral column. The stylet is withdrawn from the needle with its plastic cannula and a syringe filled with diluted contrast solution (50:50 with flush solution) is attached to the hub of the needle. *Slight* negative pressure is maintained on the syringe as the needle/cannula is slowly withdrawn. When blood returns into the syringe, a ***very small*** and *very gentle* injection of the dilute contrast is performed through the needle while *recording* on biplane stored fluoroscopy or biplane angiography. When the tip of the needle has been withdrawn successfully into a hepatic vein, the contrast flows directly cephalad from within the liver's shadow through the hepatic vein and into the cardiac silhouette. When the tip of the needle is not properly in the lumen of the vein, a very small "stain" or "tag" of contrast is created in the tissues of the liver or the contrast flows in a circuitous course in some other channel (the portal or the biliary system) in which case, the injection is stopped immediately. The needle/cannula is withdrawn very slightly and the gentle injection of contrast is repeated until the contrast flows freely in the hepatic veins. Once good flow from the needle/cannula into the hepatic veins and the heart has been established, the needle/cannula is held securely in this precise position, the syringe is carefully removed and a 0.018″ floppy-tipped, torque-controlled guide wire is introduced immediately into the hub of the needle/cannula (and into the continuing back flow of blood from the needle) without attempting to cap the hub of the needle to stop this flow. While visualizing the tip of the needle/cannula and the hepatic/cardiac shadow on fluoroscopy, the wire is advanced through the needle/cannula and into the vein. As is the case with the percutaneous introduction of all wires, the wire must pass freely and easily beyond the tip of the needle/cannula with no sensation of even slight resistance. During the entire wire introduction, the needle and wire are observed under fluoroscopy to ensure the correct passage of the wire into the cardiac silhouette.

If, after blood returns into the needle/cannula but before the tip is actually in a hepatic vein, the small injections of contrast create small tissue "tags" along the tract in the liver instead of the contrast flowing to the heart. This indicates that the tip of the needle/cannula is not cleanly in the vein, in which case the wire will not pass easily or at all from this location toward or into the cardiac silhouette. In that circumstance, the needle is withdrawn stepwise from the liver all the way to and out of the skin. Once the needle has been completely withdrawn it is flushed, the stylet is reintroduced into the long needle and a new direction for the puncture is determined utilizing the location of the small tags of contrast in the liver parenchyma to redirect the needle introduction. The needle introduction into the hepatic parenchyma is repeated with the needle angled differently (slightly more posteriorly [dorsally], more cranially or even more anteriorly, depending upon the original tract) and again advanced almost to the spinal column. The same process of performing small injections of contrast through the needle/cannula after the stylet has been withdrawn completely and as the needle/cannula is being withdrawn in small increments is repeated until the proper hepatic vein is entered and the fine wire threads easily into the vein and heart.

Once the wire has passed into the right atrium, the plastic cannula is advanced further over the wire, past the hepatic veins and into the right atrial silhouette. The needle is removed from the cannula and the fine wire is replaced with a sturdier, 0.035" wire. A fine tipped sheath/dilator set which is large enough to accommodate the proposed diagnostic or therapeutic catheter is prepared for introduction over this wire.

Before the sheath/dilator is introduced, a curve of approximately 90° is preformed at the distal end of the sheath/dilator to conform to the angle from the hepatic veins to the heart as they course from the puncture angle in the hepatic parenchyma toward the heart. This is accomplished before the introduction of the sheath, as described earlier in this chapter. Once pre-shaped, the sheath/dilator is advanced until the sheath tip is positioned high (cephalad) in the hepatic vein or inferior vena cava (IVC) or even in the low right atrium. The curve on the sheath and the more cephalad positioning of the tip of the sheath prevent catheters from repeatedly becoming lodged in the liver during subsequent catheter introductions or exchanges.

Occasionally, the hepatic vein which is entered creates a very awkward angle of approach to the desired area of the heart. If the preformed curve on the introductory sheath does not make the angle of approach usable, a second transhepatic introduction is performed while the original sheath is still in place to serve as a guide for the subsequent puncture.

When a significantly larger or specialized sheath is required for a transcatheter therapeutic procedure, an end-hole catheter is passed through the original sheath and manipulated to, or past, the location where the larger sheath/device is to be delivered. A 0.035" Super Stiff™ exchange length wire is introduced through this catheter, advanced completely through the liver and cardiac silhouette and to the site of the therapeutic procedure. The long sheath for the therapeutic procedure is preformed to correspond to the course through the liver to the particular area of the heart. The short sheath and end-hole catheter are removed over this wire and replaced with the desired larger, longer sheath/dilator set. The stiff wire helps the larger, stiffer sheath/dilator set to traverse the course through the liver parenchyma and to the desired site.

From a properly placed transhepatic approach, transseptal punctures through an intact atrial septum or even through intra-atrial baffles can be performed safely and quite easily. The angle of the transhepatic approach is more perpendicular to the septum or to the walls of the baffles. This perpendicular angle and the almost straight direction to the septum require that the curve at the tip of the transseptal needle be straightened before the puncture, but the straighter direction allows a stronger forward force to be placed on the needle for the puncture (See Chapter 8—Transseptal Technique—for details). When the transhepatic approach is performed from slightly more laterally in the liver, it provides a relatively straight course to the right ventricle and, in turn, to the pulmonary artery for pulmonary artery angioplasties or stent implants. The transhepatic approach allows the implant of atrial septal defect occlusion devices in the presence of bilateral iliofemoral vein or low IVC interruption or obstruction. The angle of approach from the properly placed transhepatic puncture is almost perpendicular to the atrial septum and this is preferable even to the femoral approach in this respect.

Once the catheterization and/or intervention through the transhepatic route has/have been completed, a specific procedure is employed to remove the sheath from the tract and to achieve hemostasis in the liver from the hepatic puncture. An end-hole-only catheter, which can accommodate a 0.038" coil and which is at least one size smaller than the internal diameter of the sheath that is already positioned in the liver, is introduced into the sheath through a back-bleed valve with a side flush port. The tip of the catheter is advanced to the tip of the sheath, cleared of any air, flushed and then capped with a syringe. A syringe containing diluted contrast solution is attached to the sheath through the side arm of the back-bleed valve and the sheath around the catheter is filled with contrast solution. The sheath/catheter combination is withdrawn in very small increments, and very slightly negative pressure is applied intermittently to the syringe on the sheath. While the tip of the sheath is still within the lumen of the hepatic vein, blood returns into the syringe from the side arm of the sheath. During the withdrawal of the sheath/catheter, as the tip of the sheath reaches intermittent locations which are no longer in the vascular channel, *no blood will be withdrawn* from the sheath into the syringe by this slight negative pressure. At these locations, a minute amount (0.2 ml) of the diluted contrast solution is injected very slowly through the sheath. When the tip of the sheath has been withdrawn out of the lumen of the hepatic vein and into the liver parenchyma, a tag of contrast is formed in the tissues verifying that the tip is no longer in the flowing vein! A repeat, small injection of contrast is performed through the coil delivery catheter to verify that the tip of this catheter has also been withdrawn to a position outside the lumen of the vein at that location. When the catheter tip is confirmed to be in the parenchyma, the tips of the catheter/sheaths are maintained in this position and a 0.035″ or 0.038″ 3×3 or 4×4 Gianturco™ coil is delivered through the coil delivery catheter to this location. As the coil is extruded, the catheter and sheath are withdrawn enough to allow the coil to unravel within the liver parenchyma. A controlled release coil could help to prevent embolization into the central circulation, but in the US the lack of commercially available controlled release coils which are robust enough prevents their use. Once the coil is in place, another small contrast injection is performed through the sheath which was withdrawn slightly before the coil implant. This injection verifies that the coil is in its proper position and that there are no additional vascular communications, either toward the heart or out toward the skin. The sheath is withdrawn back to the edge of the liver and the small injection repeated to make sure that there are no more peripheral hepatic vascular communications and that there is no bleeding out of the liver into the peritoneum.

Once out of the skin, there is no logical need for pressure over the skin because the puncture into the vascular channel is beneath the ribs and presumably within the liver on the visceral side of the hepatic capsule. Skin pressure is useful only if there is associated superficial skin/subcutaneous bleeding. Following a transhepatic procedure patients are maintained sedated for several hours in order to keep them absolutely still. These patients are observed with frequent recording of their vital signs and repeated physical examinations of the abdomen for at least 12 hours before their discharge. Discomfort to palpation or absence of peristalsis to auscultation on an examination of the abdomen may indicate bleeding into the abdomen/peritoneum and is investigated further. The transhepatic approach can be used repeatedly when necessary.

Umbilical vessel approach

The newborn infant offers unique routes for the introduction of both arterial and venous catheters[10]. These routes require a cut-down introduction into the vessels. The umbilical vessels potentially remain patent for a week or more after delivery although the tissues of the umbilical stump appear dried and shriveled by that time. The introduction of an umbilical line after the immediate newborn period should be performed in a cardiac catheterization laboratory with biplane fluoroscopic capabilities. When the introduction of catheters into the umbilical cord vessels are to be attempted, the remnant (or stump) of the umbilical cord is scrubbed vigorously and then amputated by shaving the stump off perpendicularly to it and as close and parallel to the abdominal wall as possible. Within the remaining stump of the amputated cord, the cut ends of the two umbilical arteries and the single umbilical vein are usually easily identified. Unless the infant is immediately post-delivery, these vessels usually do not bleed. The arteries are identified as two similar vessels of smaller diameter but with thicker and smoother vessel walls. The umbilical vein appears larger in diameter with a thinner and slightly undulating vessel wall.

In order to cannulate these vessels, the wall of the particular vessel is grasped with a fine toothed forceps while the occluded lumen of the vessel is probed gently for a short distance with a small, smooth-tipped, metal probe. As soon as the patency of the lumen is established for a short distance and even without blood return in the vessel, the wall of the vessel is still gripped with the small forceps while the probe is replaced with a plastic umbilical catheter or a small, plastic "feeding tube". Plastic umbilical catheters and feeding tubes are relatively soft and have smooth and blunt tips. It is helpful to grasp the umbilical catheter with a separate small forceps very close to where the catheter enters into the stump of the vessel and to push the catheter into the vessel in very small increments with this forceps. The catheter is pushed several millimeters at a time while pulling the stump of the vessel wall in the opposite direction with the separate forceps. When the vessel is still potentially patent, although not actually open, the catheter advances without too much resistance. Eventually, blood return appears in the catheter as it is advanced into the patent lumen of the vessel.

Once an umbilical vessel is entered with the catheter, an activated clotting time (ACT) is obtained and, unless the ACT already is prolonged beyond 200 seconds, the infant is given heparin, 75 units/kg through the catheter. In earlier studies of umbilical artery lines in newborn infants, there was a high incidence of central arterial thrombus related to the umbilical catheters, with a significant number of resultant serious complications[11]. Although there have been improvements in the material of the catheters used and a greater amount of heparin is used in the flush solutions during cardiac catheterization procedures, everything possible should be done to prevent potentially serious complications of the umbilical lines.

The umbilical vein itself frequently remains patent longer than the umbilical arteries. When cannulating the vein, the soft umbilical catheter is directed into the abdomen and toward the heart in a posterior and cephalad direction from the umbilical stump. The major impediment to passage directly into the heart is usually the ductus venosus, which closes very soon after birth. If the umbilical vein catheter does not pass readily into the heart with several repeated probes, a small, slow, hand injection of contrast is performed through the umbilical vein catheter and recorded on biplane angiography in order to define the proper channel in order to cannulate the channel purposefully. When this channel has a very tortuous course, the soft umbilical catheter is exchanged for a smooth-tipped, end-hole, but relatively soft cardiac catheter with a slight curve formed at its tip. This allows purposeful manipulation of a torque-controlled, soft-tipped, guide wire through the positively identified venous channel. Once the wire enters the heart, the catheter is advanced over the wire. With patience and when the umbilical vein is patent, the heart can usually be entered with this approach. Once the end-hole catheter has been advanced into the heart, the fine torque-controlled wire is replaced with a sturdier spring guide wire and the soft probing catheter is removed over the wire.

A small curve is preformed at the distal end of a standard, short sheath/dilator before the sheath/dilator is introduced into the umbilical vein. The curve formed on the sheath is similar to that formed on the sheath for the transhepatic approach, which is described earlier in this chapter. The pre-curved, short sheath/dilator set is introduced over the wire, through the umbilical vein and into the heart. The sheath will remain in place throughout the remainder of the procedure in order to maintain the patency of the umbilical route and obviate re-manipulation through the tortuous, spasmed, ductus venosus channel during subsequent catheter exchanges. All areas of the heart and great arteries are approachable from the umbilical vein in the newborn.

The umbilical arteries are often more difficult to cannulate and provide a much more challenging approach for maneuvers to, and within, the heart. Often, however, the umbilical artery has already been cannulated before the newborn is even considered to have heart disease or for cardiac catheterization. This allows definite access to an artery at least for pressure monitoring and arterial blood sampling. Before an attempt at exchanging an indwelling umbilical arterial catheter is made, all possible information is recorded through that catheter, including even an angiogram when the tip of the umbilical arterial catheter is near, or in, the aortic arch. When the prior arterial catheter is an end-hole umbilical catheter, this facilitates an over-wire exchange of this catheter in the artery for a more usable cardiac catheter. Arteries, including the umbilical arteries, have a much greater tendency to spasm, which interferes with any catheter movement and manipulation. Because of this, infants undergoing umbilical artery catheterization are sedated deeply or receive a systemic analgesic to eliminate any sensation of pain before beginning any manipulation of the umbilical arterial catheter.

From the umbilical stump the umbilical arteries initially pass posteriorly (dorsally) and caudally toward the pelvis, where they join the iliac arteries at the iliofemoral junctions. At the junction with the iliac arteries, there is a 160–180° angle between the umbilical and iliac arteries. A catheter introduced into the umbilical artery must traverse this acute turn before being advanced cephalad toward the heart. After making this turn, the catheter must still be advanced cephalad up the descending aorta and around the aortic arch before entering the heart! This circuitous course and the greater tendency for the arteries to spasm often make purposeful catheter manipulations very difficult. The direction away from the heart between the umbilicus and the iliofemoral junction and the acute turn in the course of the vessels in the pelvic area, both tend to work against attempts at advancing catheters to the heart. The "push" to advance the arterial catheter is directed caudally, away from the heart, hoping that the angle at the junction between the umbilical artery and the iliac artery will redirect or "bounce" this force in a cephalad direction! If a stiffer catheter is used to overcome this problem there is a significant risk of kinking the artery at the acute turn or even tearing the junction of the arteries at the iliofemoral junction.

The preferred technique for catheterization from the umbilical artery is to utilize a soft, end-hole catheter (umbilical artery catheter) or a soft, small "feeding tube". The soft-tipped end-hole catheter is advanced to the aortic root with the aid of a teflon coated spring guide wire with a very floppy tip or a torque-controlled, fine spring guide wire. The wire remains within the catheter to support the body of the catheter or it can be advanced ahead of the catheter to provide guidance and support for the tip of the catheter as the latter is advanced. Once the tip of the catheter reaches the aortic root, the initial guide wire is replaced with a soft-tipped but stiffer, exchange length, torque-controlled, guide wire, which is passed through the length of the catheter and manipulated into whichever ventricle gives rise to the aorta. Once the wire is in place other catheters, including balloon dilation catheters, can be passed over this wire directly into the ventricle.

If the patient already has an umbilical line in place, this line is used as an arterial monitoring line even if it is not used for the introduction of other catheters. With the availability of the new, smaller and more usable diagnostic and therapeutic catheters along with smaller sheaths to accommodate them, the femoral artery is still the preferred route for retrograde arterial catheterization where therapeutic catheter procedures are anticipated, even in the smallest infants who have an indwelling umbilical arterial line. The maneuverability and control over the catheters is significantly better from the femoral approach than from the umbilical approach.

Percutaneous arterial cannulation

An indwelling, arterial monitoring line is used in essentially all pediatric/congenital heart patients undergoing cardiac catheterizations, particularly therapeutic catheterizations. At the same time, an arterial sheath/catheter is often not necessary to obtain complete left heart information and, as a consequence, is not placed in an artery. A small, teflon Quick-Cath™, a plastic Leader-cath™, or a small diameter vessel dilator (in larger patients) is used for the arterial monitoring lines. Small arterial monitoring lines can be placed in any accessible artery, although as the usual catheter access in pediatric/congenital patients is through the femoral approach, the femoral arteries are the most frequently used for indwelling monitoring lines. The arterial monitoring line remains in place throughout the procedure or until it is replaced with an arterial sheath for the performance of a retrograde catheterization or a retrograde therapeutic procedure. When a retrograde left heart procedure is necessary, the arterial sheath/catheter is not introduced until much later in, and closer to the end of, the catheterization procedure. This reduces the duration of time in the artery of a large and potentially occlusive sheath/catheter.

The femoral arteries are the usual access sites for arterial (retrograde) left heart catheterizations in pediatric/congenital patients. Only rarely are there problems with femoral artery access in this population of patients. The femoral arterial approach is described in detail subsequently in this chapter, but almost any other peripheral artery can be (or has been) used for the introduction of retrograde catheters. In the earliest days of cardiac catheterizations, retrograde arteriograms were performed through a needle that was secured in a brachial artery after being placed percutaneously. At that time, the preferential sites for retrograde catheterizations, which all were performed by a cut-down technique, was a brachial artery. The brachial artery still represents a good alternative or secondary site for a percutaneous arterial catheterization. Even the radial arteries have more recently gained some popularity for the catheterization of adult coronary arteries. The techniques for introducing needles, wires and sheath/dilators into the brachial, radial and even the axillary arteries and the handling of the arteries during and after the procedure are identical to the techniques and procedures used with the femoral arterial approach. The carotid arterial approach represents a very special, unique and potentially more hazardous arterial approach, which is used particularly for aortic valve catheterizations/balloon dilations in small infants, and is discussed separately in a subsequent section in this chapter and in Chapter 19.

For a percutaneous arterial introduction into the femoral (or any other peripheral) artery, the same needles and wires are used and they are introduced into the arteries in an identical fashion to the percutaneous venous introductions. The single-wall percutaneous arterial puncture, similar to the percutaneous venous puncture, is even more important in entering the artery than in puncturing the venous system because of the higher pressures and greater likelihood of bleeding from an unnecessary posterior wall opening in the vessel.

Needle/wire introduction

The floppy-tipped, introductory guide wire is placed on the catheterization field with the soft, distal tip of the wire close to the puncture site. The needle is introduced into the skin directly over the palpable pulse with *nothing* attached to it. The needle is directed into the subcutaneous tissues toward the palpable arterial pulse, in line with the extremity, introduced slowly and steadily (not in "jabs") and at an angle of no more than 45° to the skin surface until blood *spurts* out of the needle. When blood return is obtained, the hub of the needle is released from the grip of the fingers and the wire introduced immediately *without touching the needle further* with the fingers, and definitely without placing a finger tip over the hub of the needle to stop the bleeding when the first blood spurt appears. Although the initial spurt of blood is dramatic, if a finger is placed over the hub of the needle to stop it, the needle tip is easily (and usually) advanced through the back wall of the artery and out of the true lumen which, of course, prevents the subsequent introduction of the wire! When, on the other hand, the wire is immediately introduced into the undisturbed needle, the wire in the lumen of the needle reduces or stops the blood flow through the needle and minimizes blood loss occurring from the puncture. When, in spite of a good spurt of blood from the hub of the needle, the wire does not advance easily through and out of the tip of the needle and into the artery, the angle of the needle relative to the skin surface (and vessel direction) is changed very slightly or the needle is rotated incrementally, very slowly and *very slightly* (1/8 to 1/4 turn) while repeated attempts at advancing the wire are performed very gently. The needle is not "spun" and should ***not be*** *advanced or withdrawn* at all as these initial repeated attempts at advancing the wire are performed. When there is good blood return from the needle, slight changes in the angle or very slight rotation of the bevel of the needle is usually sufficient to align the tip of the needle within the lumen of the vessel properly and allow the wire to advance freely into the vessel. (Described and illustrated earlier in this chapter under "venous punctures").

When the wire does not advance, even after repeated attempts at changing the angle and/or with slight rotation of the needle, the needle is withdrawn very slightly and the changes in the angle and/or the slight rotations are repeated with repeat attempts at advancing the wire. If the wire still does not advance or a hematoma begins to form during these attempted gentle wire introductions, the needle/wire is withdrawn and pressure is applied for 3–5 minutes before reattempting the arterial puncture.

During the puncture of the artery and when the needle is introduced to its hub without any blood return, the needle is withdrawn slowly and smoothly with the bevel facing upward while watching for blood return into the needle. Occasionally, as is the case with venous punctures, the needle, on its way into the tissues, compresses the opposing walls of the artery against each other and, in doing so, passes completely through the artery without any blood return into the needle. In this circumstance, vigorous blood return usually does occur as the tip of the needle is withdrawn back into the arterial lumen. When blood does return into the needle as the needle is being withdrawn, the wire is introduced with the identical technique to the procedure when the artery was punctured during the introduction of the needle. If no blood return is obtained as the needle is withdrawn slowly, the needle is withdrawn completely, flushed and the puncture is restarted, aiming the needle tip in a slightly different direction or location.

As soon as the wire passes freely into the artery, the needle is withdrawn and pressure is applied with the fingers over the course of the wire in the subcutaneous tissues from where the wire enters the skin to its entry into the artery. Once the wire has been successfully introduced into the artery and after the needle has been removed, a small skin incision is made over the wire. No additional dilation of the skin or vessel is performed over the wire for the introduction of a monitoring Quick-cath™, Leader-cath™, or small dilator. The cannula/dilator which is to be used for monitoring the line is introduced into the artery directly over the wire by "drilling" the plastic cannula of the Quick-cath™, Leader-cath™, or the small dilator through the skin, subcutaneous tissues and into the vessel as it is being introduced. Repeat, local anesthesia is administered arbitrarily around the arterial puncture site every hour during the catheterization procedure or if the patient exhibits *any* evidence of discomfort during the puncture, cannula introduction or subsequent sheath/dilator introduction into the artery. A Quick-Cath™ or small dilator can be introduced directly over the wire; however, before introducing a sheath/dilator, the course of the wire in the artery within the thorax is checked on fluoroscopy.

Arterial sheath introduction

When the sheath/dilator is introduced initially and immediately after the arterial puncture, the needle is removed over the wire as soon as the wire has passed beyond the tip of the needle and is positioned far into and securely in the artery. Manual pressure is maintained over the wire at the arterial puncture site while a small, horizontal incision is made into the skin with the tip of a #11 knife blade. This incision is made parallel to the skin lines just at the site of the wire entering the skin and should be long enough to accommodate the circumference of the sheath which will be introduced into the artery. With the finely tapered sheath/dilator sets which are now available and even if there is pre-existing dense scar tissue, further dilation of the tract with a Medi-Cut™ cannula is usually unnecessary, and when performed is usually counter productive. If a dilation of the artery with a Medi-Cut™ cannula is performed before introducing an arterial sheath/dilator, the Medi-Cut™ cannula definitely should not be buried to the hub of the cannula during this dilation. When the broad hub of the tapered Medi-Cut™ cannula is introduced too deeply into an arterial puncture, the opening in the arterial wall is dilated to a diameter larger than that of the sheath which is to be introduced. The excessively large opening in the arterial wall will result in a continual ooze of blood around the sheath. If, however, a Medi-Cut™ cannula *is* used to dilate the artery, and while it is still in the artery over the original wire, the original, usually small (0.018″) percutaneous guide wire can be replaced with the largest diameter guide wire which the tip of the dilator will accommodate. The larger wire provides a tighter fit between the tip of the dilator and the wire and provides a stiffer support for the dilator as it passes through the subcutaneous tissues and enters the artery. As in the venous system, an extra-stiff or Super Stiff™ wire of the same size will facilitate a difficult introduction through dense scar tissue. Similar to the introduction of a sheath/dilator combination into a vein, the sheath and dilator are "drilled" into the artery with a "high speed" rotation of the sheath/dilator combination as it is advanced over the wire through the subcutaneous tissues and arterial wall.

When an arterial sheath is replacing an indwelling Quick-Cath™ or other small monitoring cannula, the area around the artery is re-infiltrated liberally and deeply with local anesthesia regardless of the time since the previous application of local anesthesia. This assures total local anesthesia of the entire area with the goal of preventing any pain and the resultant arterial spasm during the sheath/dilator introduction. It is either impossible or very traumatic to the artery to introduce a sheath/dilator into an artery which is in spasm. The sheath/dilator introduction otherwise is the same as when the sheath/dilator is introduced directly after the needle puncture.

As is the case with a cardiac catheterization through a venous access and for the same reasons as in venous access sites, the indwelling sheath remains in the artery throughout all catheter manipulations and device delivery/implants in the arterial system. Although a small arterial *monitoring line* is introduced at the very beginning of cardiac catheterization procedures, in order to reduce the time in the artery with a larger sheath/catheter and, in turn, the overall trauma to the artery, introduction of the arterial sheath or "arterial or retrograde" catheterization is usually not performed until the very end of, or at least very late in, the procedure. There is no advantage in having a larger cannula present in the artery for long periods of time when it is not being used! However, when a larger sheath will definitely be necessary in an artery within a short time after the initial introduction of any sheath into the artery, the larger sheath is introduced initially to avoid the added trauma of exchanging the sheath/dilator in the artery.

Before the arterial sheath is removed at the end of the procedure, the area around the introductory site and artery is again re-infiltrated very liberally with local anesthesia. The catheter is withdrawn from the sheath and the sheath is allowed to bleed back a few drops of blood from the hub or the side port. This allows any fibrin or clot which has formed around the catheter–sheath interface to flow into and out of the sheath, as opposed to being stripped off within the vessel from outside of the sheath as the sheath is withdrawn. As the sheath is being withdrawn, firm pressure is applied with the fingers of one hand over the arterial puncture site. Once the sheath has been withdrawn from the artery, finger pressure is maintained over the arterial puncture site with one hand while palpating the arterial pulse more distally in the same extremity with the other hand. Ideally, the pressure applied is sufficient to prevent bleeding while, at the same time, allowing the pulse in the more distal artery to be palpated continuously.

Immediately after the withdrawal of the sheath from the vessel, all drapes are removed from around the puncture site in order to allow a clear visualization of the tissues surrounding the site. This allows direct observation of the soft tissues surrounding the puncture site, where extravasated blood can easily extend into the tissues adjacent to the actual "pressure point". Manual pressure is maintained for at least ten minutes and preferably for 15–20 minutes. *Pressure over the puncture site is applied by a conscientious, concerned and patient individual*—preferably the catheterizing physician. The person who is holding pressure should be aware of exactly what has been introduced into the artery, any problems with the artery or the introductions into the artery and should be knowledgeable about the mechanisms of arterial flow and the potential for injury. Since the exact site of the arterial puncture does not correspond to the site of the skin puncture, finger pressure is applied over the inguinal area in a fairly broad distribution in the cephalad/caudal direction from the skin to the arterial puncture site. The pulse in the extremity distal to the puncture site is palpated continually with the fingers of one hand while applying pressure over the puncture site in the vessel with the other hand. The amount of pressure applied over the site is continually titrated so that local bleeding at the puncture is prevented, while at the same time the more peripheral pulse is still palpable.

In patients who have been anticoagulated or in whom large arterial sheaths were used, an hour, or more, of carefully applied manual pressure may be required to control bleeding! Meticulously applied pressure is one of the most important aspects in avoiding arterial complications. Once bleeding has stopped completely, the puncture site is covered with a small but firm, light pressure dressing. The area still requires careful and repeated (continual!) observation for an additional 6–8 hours before the patient is allowed to ambulate. Using these techniques and precautions, the incidence of arterial injury requiring any subsequent therapy is reduced to < 1% of all catheterization procedures. The management of an arterial complication that cannot be prevented depends upon the type and severity of the complication, and is discussed at the end of this chapter.

"Unique vascular" access

Direct puncture of the left ventricular cavity

Direct transmural left ventricle (LV) puncture through the apex of the heart at one time was the preferred approach for obtaining left ventricular pressures and even left ventricular angiograms. Although now considered "barbaric" and almost never performed, direct left ventricular puncture remains the only way of obtaining valid hemodynamics from the left ventricle in the presence of mechanical prosthetic valves in *both* the aortic and the mitral positions[12]. Although most mechanical valves ***can be*** crossed, there is the real danger of the catheter's becoming trapped in the mechanical valve and, of equal importance, any pressures obtained with a catheter across a mechanical valve will usually be totally inaccurate and invalid. When a catheter crosses the "central" orifice of a mechanical valve, the valve is always propped open during the valve closure, and/or the valve may be restricted from opening fully by the catheter crossing adjacent to the central orifice of the valve—either of which circumstances invalidates the pressures from within the chamber/vessel on either side of the valve.

Fortunately, enough indirect information is usually available from the echo Doppler to negate the need for the precise measurement of left ventricular pressures in these cases. If the pressure is considered absolutely necessary, for example for a definitive surgical decision for replacing one or both prosthetic valves, the very patients who require a direct transmural left ventricular (LV) puncture are the "safest" candidates for such a procedure. Any patient who has prosthetic valves in both the mitral and aortic positions has a very thick walled ventricle and has had several (or more) prior thoracic surgical procedures. As a consequence, these patients have extensive intrathoracic (pleural and pericardial) scarring and the thick wall of the ventricle will clamp down on, and close off the needle tract after a direct puncture through the wall of the ventricle; all of which reduces (or eliminates) bleeding from the LV puncture. The scarring around the heart and within the thorax reduces (or eliminates) the possibility of either an extensive pneumothorax or of a tamponade from a pericardial effusion.

The area of the apex of the heart is identified by physical examination and verified with biplane fluoroscopy. The wall of the entire left chest is scrubbed and the area over the apex is isolated with a sterile, single-hole adhesive drape. A retrograde catheter is positioned in the aortic root and a venous catheter is positioned in the left atrium (transseptally if necessary) before proceeding with the direct LV puncture. If visualization of the left ventricular cavity is desired, an angiogram is recorded in the LAO/cranial and RAO/caudal (or PA and lateral) projections with injection through the left atrial catheter. The pre-positioned aortic catheter is placed on pressure recording at a 200 mmHg gain while the left atrial catheter is placed on a 40 mmHg gain.

The skin and superficial subcutaneous tissues in the area on the chest wall and in the rib space directly over the apex of the heart are infiltrated through a fine 25-gauge subcuticular needle on a slip-lock syringe filled with 2% xylocaine. A flush/pressure line, which is connected to a third transducer, is attached to a three-way stopcock and then the line/stopcock is positioned on the field adjacent to the puncture site over the apex. If the prosthetic aortic valve is considered the most dysfunctional, the third transducer is placed on a 200 mmHg gain, while if the prosthetic mitral valve is considered to be the worse, the third transducer is placed on a 40 mmHg gain. The fine subcuticular needle on the slip-lock syringe of xylocaine is replaced with a long, 20-gauge, short bevel needle, which is introduced into the subcutaneous tissues over the apex and directed toward the cardiac silhouette. The cardiac silhouette and the needle are viewed on fluoroscopy in the PA and lateral views. The syringe is placed on negative pressure with the fingers as soon as the needle has been introduced under the skin of the chest wall directly over the apex. With the needle/syringe maintained on negative pressure, it is introduced between the ribs while keeping the needle on the cephalad surface of the more caudal rib in the particular interspace where the apex is located. Negative pressure is maintained as the needle is advanced into the thorax directly toward the left ventricular apex. When *no* blood return is obtained after the syringe/needle has been advanced 2–3 mm, the tissues are again infiltrated with xylocaine. Negative pressure is reapplied to the syringe and the needle advanced another 2–3 mm. As the needle reaches the surface of the heart, the tip of the needle rubs against the moving surface with a "scratching" sensation or actually moves in synchrony with the beat of the heart. When this occurs, the syringe is removed from the needle and the needle is attached to the stopcock on the pressure tubing. The needle is advanced further until a left ventricular pressure is visualized. Occasionally the needle enters the left ventricle while it is still attached to the syringe and blood flows (pumps) back into the syringe. In that circumstance, the syringe is immediately replaced with the pressure tubing/stopcock. After the needle enters the left ventricle by either means and before the pressure is recorded the stopcock is vented to air for a brief instant. This allows a brief squirt of blood from the LV pressure to clear any xylocaine or air from the needle/stopcock, and then the needle is flushed briefly.

The left ventricular pressure is recorded simultaneously with the aortic and left atrial pressures, changing pressure gains to correspond to the gains of the aortic and left atrial catheters. Once valid systolic and end-diastolic pressures are recorded along with the pressures in the adjacent vessels/chambers, and the pressure lines are balanced, the needle is withdrawn. No other information is necessary from this approach. The longer the needle remains in the ventricle the greater the chance of a complication. Direct left ventricular angiograms are no longer performed through the left ventricular needle. The necessary and equally valid angiographic data can be obtained from the left atrial or aortic root angiogram. Following a direct left ventricular puncture, the patient is monitored for at least several hours, observing primarily for bleeding into the chest cavity.

The most significant complication from a direct left ventricular puncture in this type of patient, however, is not bleeding into the thorax or pneumothorax but the direct puncture of a coronary artery branch on the apical surface of the heart. Fortunately, there are no major branches over the actual apex, so if the procedure is performed properly with good fluoroscopic guidance, even this complication should be avoided.

Other direct intracavitary cardiac punctures

Direct puncture through the chest wall into a cardiac chamber other than the left ventricle can be performed to obtain specific pressures and anatomic information or to perform therapeutic catheter procedures when all "normal" access to the chambers is absent. The necessity of this approach always occurs in very complex congenital heart patients who previously have had multiple cardiac surgery or procedures. This approach is most essential in patients who have "failing Fontan" type of single ventricle repairs. In this type of patient, non-invasive studies do *not* provide adequate or valid hemodynamic estimates because of the low velocity flows which, in turn, generate minimal or no, gradients or flow velocities. The direct cavity puncture may also be desired or necessary to provide the necessary access to a particular area for a therapeutic catheterization procedure when the usual venous access routes are obstructed.

As with patients who require a direct left ventricular puncture, these patients will have had multiple prior surgeries. Because of their compromised hemodynamics, they also have greatly enlarged cardiac chambers, the atria in particular. With this combination of circumstances, there are large areas of the walls of the atria or ventricle that are "plastered" against, and very adherent to, the inner wall of the thoracic cavity. These chambers are identified from X-rays of the chest, previous catheterization/angiograms and current echo studies. Unless these patients have had a recent (since their last surgery) catheterization with aortic angiography, they should undergo a retrograde arterial catheterization with aortic root plus/minus selective brachiocephalic arterial angiography to identify the arterial supply to the chest wall or any coronary supply that might be in the area of the potential direct puncture. This study can be made just prior to the direct chamber puncture, but because of known access problems the retrograde study is usually performed at the very beginning of the catheterization when a direct puncture of a chamber is to be performed.

The area where the atrium is in closest approximation to the chest wall and which provides the most direct route to the areas of the anatomy in question is chosen for the direct puncture. The area is prepped and draped as described for any other catheterization site. The interspace between the ribs in the area is identified and the skin over the desired interspace for the puncture is infiltrated with 2% xylocaine using a small (25-gauge) subcuticular needle. After the skin wheal has been made, the subcuticular needle is replaced on the slip-lock syringe of xylocaine with a standard, 20-gauge, short-bevel, percutaneous needle.

This needle that is attached to the xylocaine syringe is introduced into the interspace over the site to be punctured, staying along the cephalad edge of the more caudal of the two ribs forming the particular interspace. The needle is advanced with the syringe maintained on negative pressure, alternating with the infiltration of more xylocaine exactly as described for the direct puncture of the left ventricle. When blood returns in the syringe, it is removed and, while observing closely on fluoroscopy, a soft-tipped spring guide wire is passed through the needle and into the cardiac chamber. As soon as the wire is well within the cardiac silhouette and away from the opposite wall of the heart or intracardiac valves (in both PA and LAT X-ray views), the needle is withdrawn. The wire is secured within the heart and a fine-tipped sheath/dilator set is introduced into the chamber while observing the course within the chamber on biplane fluoroscopy. Except for the direct observation, the sheath/dilator set is introduced exactly as it is introduced into a vein or artery. In most cases of direct thoracic puncture, the tract through the interspace and into the chamber will need some sequential dilation in order to introduce a sheath of adequate size to perform a therapeutic catheterization procedure. The necessary pressures, oxygen saturations and angiocardiograms are obtained through the appropriate catheter, which is introduced and manipulated through this sheath. This sheath, which has been introduced in close proximity to (directly into!) the heart and has its tip in a cardiac chamber must be handled meticulously with all precautions against the introduction of air or clots via any sheath within the systemic circulation. This is particularly crucial when larger sheaths or multiple exchanges of sheaths/catheters are required for catheter interventional procedures.

Special procedures, including transseptal punctures through the atrial septum and intracardiac baffles, the implant of stents or occlusion devices and the dilation of structures, can all be performed through direct punctures through the wall of the thorax into cardiac chambers or vascular spaces.

After the necessary information is obtained or the intravascular therapy completed, the sheath is withdrawn from the direct puncture site and hemostasis achieved by direct pressure (prolonged!) over the puncture site or a small purse string suture is applied in the subcutaneous tissues around the site.

Cut-downs on veins and arteries for vascular access

With the exception of catheter introduction into umbilical vessels, in our institution the indications for and the use of cut-downs on vessels are few and far between. Although initially trained only in the cut-down technique, this author personally has not performed a cut-down in the past 30 years of cardiac catheterizations. Obviously, patience and persistence with the percutaneous approach were necessary in some cases. The only possible disadvantage of this experience is that a current generation of pediatric cardiology trainees has absolutely no experience with a cut-down procedure in the catheterization laboratory. Even when a more central vein is occluded, a percutaneous entry into the more peripheral venous system is often possible where a cut-down would aggravate the peripheral venous spasm further and not allow access even into the peripheral veins.

There may be a few absolute indications for a cut-down on either an artery or vein. A cut-down may be indicated in extreme emergency situations where patients present in extremis, peripherally collapsed and where an access line is needed instantaneously. In this circumstance, a cut-down is indicated, but only if a physician who is very experienced in the technique is available to perform it. Another definite indication for a cut-down is for the introduction of a catheter into the carotid artery for balloon dilation of the aortic valve in small infants. At the same time, a vascular or cardiac surgeon who is experienced in microvascular techniques should perform any cut-down on a carotid artery. Still another indication for a cut-down on either an artery or a vein, is the introduction of the massive (20+-French) cannulae which are still necessary for some of the "assist devices" and larger therapeutic devices. However, with the continued refinement of materials and techniques, this latter indication is becoming less frequent and hopefully will disappear.

Cut-downs on the vessels are occasionally necessary on either veins or arteries to extract foreign bodies or errant devices from the vessel after they have been grasped with a foreign body retrieval system and withdrawn to the peripheral vessel, but then cannot be withdrawn out of the vessel. The "grasped foreign bodies" are usually crumpled by the retrieval system rather than folded or compressed into their original configuration and, as a consequence, can be withdrawn only partially into the retrieval sheath. The sheath with the crumpled and partially exposed foreign body is withdrawn to the peripheral entrance site in the vessel, but lodges in the vessel at the entry site and cannot be withdrawn out of the vessel or through the skin without disrupting the vessel. This occurs more commonly when the original sheath which was used for the delivery of the errant device is used for the attempted retrieval of the foreign body rather than using a new, much larger diameter retrieval sheath with the percutaneous retrieval system. The problem of a foreign body lodged within the peripheral vessel can often be avoided by performing the entire retrieval procedure through a long sheath with a significantly larger diameter, or by initially introducing the standard delivery sheath through a larger-diameter, outer, short "recovery" sheath which is placed over the delivery sheath at the onset of the procedure.

Cut-down technique

Femoral vessel cut-down

To perform a cut-down in the femoral area, the preparation of the area, including deep infiltration with local anesthesia, scrubbing and draping, is identical to the preparation for a percutaneous introduction. The incision for the cut-down begins at approximately the same site as a percutaneous puncture, i.e. just at the infiltration site over the artery and 1–3 cm caudal to the inguinal ligament, depending upon the size of the patient. The incision is made completely through the skin, extended medially from the site over the artery and running parallel to the inguinal ligament (and skin lines) for one to three centimeters (depending upon the size of the patient *and* the thickness of the subcutaneous tissues of the particular patient). Once completely through the skin, blunt dissection is carried out straight down (posteriorly) and deep into the subcutaneous tissues below the skin incision. The blunt dissection for the exposure of the femoral sheath and vessels is directed perpendicularly to the skin incision and parallel to the long axis of the extremity and the major vessels. A curved "mosquito" clamp or a small "Kelly" clamp is ideal for this dissection. Unless there is previous scarring from a previous incision, the tissues separate very easily, and unless the patient is very obese the vessels within the vascular sheath become apparent within one-half to two centimeters below the skin surface. With careful, continued blunt dissection, the artery and vein are separated from each other and the branches of the femoral vein and artery are isolated. When there is previous scar tissue in the area, some sharp dissection with tissue scissors becomes necessary.

When the skin incision for the cut-down is in the proper location, the femoral vein is exposed just at, or slightly caudal to, the point where the deep femoral and saphenous veins along with several smaller veins join together to form the femoral bulb and then continue cephalad as the common femoral vein, which passes beneath the inguinal ligament and into the pelvis. The femoral artery in this same area bifurcates into the superficial and deep femoral arteries as it exits the pelvis caudal to the inguinal ligament.

When the femoral vessels are visualized initially before extensive dissection or before any isolation of the vessels is performed, the vessels appear quite large even in small infants. Once the branches of the major vessels are identified, they are isolated with 2-0 silk ties, but not ligated. Ligation of the branch vessels or extensive dissection causes both the veins and the artery to spasm and shrink markedly in size.

The exact site and type of entry into the vessel, even in the era when many cut-downs were performed, was, and presumably still is, an individual operator's choice and varies quite extensively from operator to operator. The site of vessel entry also depends upon the size of the patient and what is being introduced into and/or withdrawn from the vessel. One common characteristic of the many techniques for the direct introduction of catheters into vessels was that all feeding or branch vessels to the vessel in question had to be *controlled* either individually or as part of a ligature around the large vessel.

With the universal availability of very thin walled vascular sheaths, now, even after a dissection through the subcutaneous tissues down *to the vessel*, the exposed vessel is entered with a needle and a wire, and then a sheath/dilator is introduced into the vessel over the wire in a similar fashion to a percutaneous entry, but under direct vision into the vessel. The sheath remains indwelling in the *vessel* during the remainder of the procedure. The use of an indwelling sheath with the cut-down procedure capitalizes on the fact that the vessels are significantly larger before they are disturbed by adjacent dissection or by the introduction of a catheter into them, and that most bleeding can be controlled with a loose tie around the sheath. The sheath used for the introduction and which then remains in the vessel also incorporates all of the advantages of the indwelling sheath for reducing trauma to the vessel and allowing easy exchange of catheters at any time during the procedure.

Once the vessel is isolated and the proximal and distal trunk vessels (as well as any branch or feeding vessels) are controlled with non-tightened ligatures, a needle puncture is performed under direct visualization into the lumen of the vessel. A soft-tipped, spring guide wire is introduced into the vessel through the needle and the needle is removed. With gentle traction applied to the trunk vessel caudal to the puncture, a fine ("feathered") tipped sheath/dilator set is advanced over the wire and introduced into the vessel under direct vision. If the inside diameter of the dilator tip does ***not*** have a very tight fit over the wire, it is necessary to make a *tiny* incision in the vessel wall precisely over the wire puncture site in the vessel wall to allow the dilator/sheath to pass readily into the vessel without tearing it.

For the introduction of a catheter into a vein, this is usually all that is necessary to enter the vein and to maintain adequate hemostasis around the sheath. Once the sheath is completely in the vein, and assuming that any incision into the vein was smaller than the diameter of the sheath, the controlling ties around the branch or feeding veins to the main vein can usually be loosened. This allows flow from the tributaries and more normal flow in the main venous channel. If there is significant bleeding around the sheath, a single purse string suture tie is placed around the sheath just at the entry site into the vein. Additional ties about the sheath or other branches are occasionally necessary, but are performed only if significant bleeding continues. Once the sheath is in place in the vein, this cut-down introduced sheath has the same advantages as the sheath introduced percutaneously in terms of catheter movement and catheter exchanges. With an indwelling sheath in the vein, less attention to the cut-down introductory site is necessary, although the area must still be checked periodically for bleeding.

When a sheath/dilator is introduced directly into an exposed artery, less attention is necessary for the control of the branches of the artery. However, a purse string tie using 5-0 or 6-0 arterial suture material is placed in the arterial wall around the proposed puncture site for the needle before the needle puncture into the exposed artery is performed. The circle of the purse string is made at least as large in diameter as the circumference of the sheath which will be used in the artery. Once the sheath is in place, the purse string is tightened around the sheath to control bleeding. Rarely, when bleeding at the puncture site persists, the purse string must be redone or some branch vessels must be ligated temporarily during the procedure.

With the original cut-down technique using direct catheter introduction into the vessel without a "protecting" sheath, each feeding or branch vessel had to have a suture around it to control bleeding. An incision was made into the vessel wall and, with the use of special forceps or "introducing guides", the catheter was introduced directly into the vessel lumen. With this type of direct vessel entry, vessel spasm around the constantly moving catheter was the rule and created a major problem at the entry site in both veins and arteries. The trauma to and around the vessel resulted in a marked decrease in both the visualized and functional diameter of the vessel. The spasm of the vessels compromised catheter movement significantly and, in the event of a catheter exchange, the spasm with the resultant "thread-like" vessel frequently made the introduction of the replacement catheter(s) impossible or resulted in the total disruption of the major vascular channel.

Once the catheterization procedure is completed after a cut-down on a vessel, the vessel and the cut-down incision are repaired. The repair of the vessel depends on the entry site and which vessel is entered. After a cut-down on a vein, the entire vein where the catheter was introduced was usually ligated at the end of the procedure, particularly if the catheter had been introduced into the saphenous vein or even the saphenous bulb. When the common femoral vein was utilized, an attempt was made to repair the vein after removal of the catheter/sheath. Because of the thin walls of the veins, the spasm of the veins and their resultant friability, salvage of venous flow by repair of the vein was seldom successful. Fortunately, because of the plethora of potential venous channels in the inguinal and pelvic areas and the potential ability to form new collaterals around obstructed veins in the area, there *appears* to be little, if any, long-term clinical consequence from the ligation of these localized veins.

Many articles have been written about the cut-down technique on arteries and the proper incisions in them, the introduction of catheters into the arteries and on the proper technique for the repair of the incision after the catheter has been removed. The general consensus was that a longitudinal incision be performed before the introduction and, when closed, this incision is pulled together from end to end with fine 6-0 to 7-0 arterial suture to create a "transverse suture line" across the artery when repaired. This maximized the lumen diameter and supposedly minimized the scarring of the vessel wall after repair. With essentially universal acceptance of percutaneous techniques for even the smallest arteries, little has been published in the cardiology literature over the past two decades on cut-down techniques or vessel repairs following cut-downs on arteries.

Following a cut-down on either a vein or an artery, the repair of the subcutaneous tissues and the skin incision also varies from operator to operator. Generally the subcutaneous tissues are drawn together from side to side of the incision (cephalad to caudal) over the repaired or ligated vessel using one or two fairly heavy (2-0 or 3-0) resorbable sutures. When the subcutaneous sutures are placed correctly, the opposing skin edges frequently approximate each other almost naturally. The skin is closed with either interrupted "mattress sutures" using 5-0 or 6-0 silk or with a running, subcuticular, resorbable 5-0 or 6-0 suture. A light dressing is applied for 12 to 18 hours and thereafter the area remains exposed. The inguinal area is hard to keep clean and dry and is more prone to infection. An occlusive dressing that remains in place for more than 24 hours retains moisture and contamination rather than protecting the incision. Non-resorbable interrupted sutures require removal in six to seven days. Regardless of the type of skin closure, a medical person should examine the area of the cut-down by that time at the latest.

Brachial cut-down technique

Cut-downs on both the brachial veins and arteries were common before the acceptance of the percutaneous technique, but at present are almost never used. The brachial cut-down was easier and faster because the vessels are more superficial, they are visible even before the incision and there are fewer (no) branching vessels in the area of the cutdown to control. Brachial cut-downs had the disadvantage that the vessels are generally smaller and, as a consequence, they create more problems with vascular spasm during catheter manipulation. The cut-down technique is similar for both the brachial artery and veins.

For a brachial vessel cut-down, the proposed vessel is identified by direct visualization or palpation. The entire antecubital area of the arm around the vessel which is intended for the cut-down is scrubbed and draped. The skin and subcutaneous tissues are infiltrated with xylocaine using a fine (25-gauge) subcuticular needle. The deeper infiltration is performed on both sides of the visible/palpable vessel. If the vessel is punctured inadvertently during infiltration of the local anesthesia the needle is withdrawn and pressure held over the area for at least several minutes before infusing more local or beginning the cut-down.

Once the area is anesthetized, an incision is performed very carefully through the skin, directly over and across the course of the intended vessel (perpendicular to the long axis of the arm and vessels and along the direction of the skin lines). The superficial vessels in the arm may be directly under and very close to the skin and can be incised with the skin incision if care is not taken. Once the incision is through the skin, blunt dissection is carried out in the direction of the vessel and directly over and on each side of the vessel until it is completely exposed. Loose 2-0 ligatures or umbilical tapes are placed above and below the expected site of entry into the particular vessel, but not tightened round it. Once the vessel is exposed and controlled, a needle, wire and then a sheath/dilator are introduced directly into the brachial artery as described for the femoral cut-down technique. When the sheath/dilator is removed from the vessel after a brachial cut-down, the brachial vein is ligated but the brachial artery is repaired.

Carotid artery approach

There is growing evidence that the retrograde approach from the carotid artery is the most expedient and safest approach for balloon dilation of the aortic valve in newborns and very small infants[13,14]. At the same time, the carotid artery approach does have the potential for very serious adverse events. Any embolized particles from the carotid artery entry site obligatorily go directly to the brain and any damage to the vessel at the introductory site compromises blood flow to the brain!

The carotid artery is approached and entered by a cut-down technique. A cut-down on the carotid artery is utilized in order to control the vessel completely, and hopefully to eliminate the chance of embolization of *anything* from the site of catheter introduction. Even when a cut-down on the carotid artery is anticipated, a small line is placed in a femoral artery for the continual monitoring of the patient's systemic pressure, and is used for an instantaneous measurement of the effects of valve dilation without having to abandon access to the ventricle which was achieved from the carotid approach. Usually a prograde venous catheter is advanced into the left ventricle via a patent foramen ovale in order to obtain the initial hemodynamics and to continually monitor the patient's left ventricular pressure before, during and after the dilation through the carotid.

Only operators who are extremely skilled and experienced in microvascular surgery on very small vessels should perform the cut-down on, and the repair of, the carotid artery—i.e. a microvascular or cardiovascular surgeon. As a consequence, the catheterization procedure from the carotid approach must be performed with very close collaboration between the pediatric cardiologist and the microvascular surgeon performing the cut-down. The surgeon performs the cut-down on the artery, exposes the artery and performs the incision in the arterial wall for the wire/sheath/dilator introduction, and controls the carotid artery during the subsequent catheter manipulations. Once the artery is isolated and controlled, a floppy-tipped wire is introduced into it, either through a small incision made by the surgeon or through a needle puncture performed by the pediatric cardiologist. The wire that is introduced must be small enough in diameter and long enough to accommodate the exchange of a diagnostic catheter or the balloon dilation catheter that will be used.

The wire is introduced by the pediatric cardiologist under direct fluoroscopic visualization or transthoracic echo (TTE) guidance, and is advanced into the ascending aorta or the left ventricle. A 4-French sheath/dilator with a back-bleed valve/flush port attached on the sheath is introduced into the artery over the wire through a small incision in the arterial wall over the entry site of the wire into the artery. The sheath/dilator that is used must be large enough to accommodate the proposed balloon dilation catheter that will be used for the aortic valve dilation. The sheath/dilator is advanced under continual fluoroscopic visualization until the tip of the dilator is positioned one to two centimeters above the aortic valve. The sheath is advanced to the tip of the dilator under direct fluoroscopic visualization. When the tip of the sheath is positioned in the ascending aorta, the wire and then the dilator are carefully removed from the sheath and the sheath allowed to "bleed back" passively through the side arm in order to clear it of any air or clot. An end-hole catheter is introduced into the sheath and advanced to the aortic valve. With this almost straight approach to the aortic valve the catheter alone has a good chance of passing through the stenotic valve and directly into the ventricle. If not, the catheter is withdrawn in the aortic root to a distance of 1–2 cm above the valve and a very-floppy-tipped wire is manipulated through the catheter and into the ventricle as described under the retrograde approach in Chapter 9.

Occasionally, as the wire is introduced into the carotid artery, it initially advances directly into the left ventricle before even being visualized on fluoroscopy. This can occur even in the face of very tight aortic valve stenosis. If so, the wire is fixed in place while the sheath/dilator is introduced into the *ventricle*. Assuming that the patient's hemodynamics will tolerate the sheath across the stenotic valve, the dilator *alone* is removed over the wire from the sheath and the sheath is cleared of air by allowing the side port of the back-bleed valve to bleed passively from the sheath. When the initial wire is of a size that the balloon for dilation will accommodate, the balloon catheter is introduced directly over this wire and through the sheath at this time. If this wire is not sturdy or large enough to support the dilation balloon, an end-hole, pigtail catheter is advanced over the wire, through the sheath and into the left ventricle. The original wire is exchanged through the pigtail catheter for a preformed wire that is appropriate in size for the balloon dilation catheter. The pigtail catheter is removed over the new wire *and through the sheath*. The sheath is again meticulously cleared of air, and the balloon dilation catheter is introduced over the wire and rapidly centered across the stenotic valve as observed on fluoroscopy or TTE[14]. If the sheath tip is still across the valve, the sheath is withdrawn well off the balloon and back into the aorta/carotid artery. The balloon is inflated and deflated rapidly while recording on biplane angiography and TTE. The angiogram of the dilation is reviewed and the dilation repeated as necessary in order to position the balloon precisely and abolish the "waist" on the balloon during the inflations. The balloon is withdrawn over the wire and through the sheath. The hemodynamic measurements are repeated using the prograde catheter in the left ventricle along with the sheath in the ascending aorta or the femoral arterial line for the comparative pressures. An angiogram is performed in the left ventricle or the aortic root. If the dilation is unsatisfactory, a new, slightly larger diameter balloon can be introduced over the wire and through the sheath with essentially no new manipulation.

Once a satisfactory dilation is documented or when significant aortic regurgitation is produced, the wire and then the sheath are removed from the carotid artery. Upon removal of the sheath/catheter from the carotid artery, the microvascular surgeon meticulously repairs the cut-down on the carotid artery. Although in children and even in adults, one external carotid artery is often considered "expendable", there are no valid data about the long-term effects on the brain of a child or an adult from the sacrifice of any major artery to the head during infancy. As a consequence, ultimate care is taken to preserve not only the internal carotid but also the external carotid branch off the common carotid during the repair. In skilled hands, this has been done very successfully without acute complications. Good persistent flow has been preserved in all vessels when examined by Doppler interrogation during follow-up months to years after the procedure.

Vascular occlusion devices—vascular seals

In the adult catheterization environment with large numbers of patients, all of whom are essentially large, and where the primary priority is on rapid turnover and rapid ambulation, several types of vascular occlusion devices have become available for the faster closure of vessels after percutaneous access. There are "plugs" of collagen materials, which are implanted in the subcutaneous tissues *over* the vascular puncture sites, combinations of a collagen "plug" and a biological procoagulant, and there are "percutaneous suture" techniques/devices. All of these devices and techniques are better suited for *large* arteries with relatively *small* (6–8-French) puncture sites. Percutaneous suture devices are available for 10-French introducers and, in certain circumstances, are used to close both smaller (brachial) arteries and significantly larger percutaneous arterial punctures (22-French).

The VasoSeal™ is a collagen plug which is pushed through the subcutaneous tract and onto the surface of the arterial puncture site over a wire that is positioned in the vessel. The Angio-Seal™ is a collagen sponge plug, but it is attached to a resorbable polymer intravascular "anchor or foot" with a resorbable suture. The Duette™ system utilizes a collagen plug that is held in place temporarily by a tiny intravascular balloon while thrombin is infused into the collagen plug in the subcutaneous tissues to accelerate the coagulation of the collagen. The tiny balloon is withdrawn after the thrombin infusion. All of these plugs are bioresorbable so that they spontaneously disappear over time and, reportedly, after 6–8 weeks do not interfere with subsequent access to the artery. Angio-Seal™ devices have been used to seal venous puncture sites without demonstrated acute complications, however, there is no information on the long-term patency of the veins which were sealed.

The percutaneous suture closure devices are technically more difficult to use, but in the hands of experienced operators appear to have fewer complications than the plugs. One of these devices/techniques is the Perclose™ Device and technique. These devices actually place tiny vascular sutures percutaneously into the arterial wall around the puncture site. The sutures are placed in the arterial wall at the beginning of the percutaneous procedure before the introduction of the sheath. The sutures are exteriorized and tied down over the puncture in the vessel within the subcutaneous tissues at the end of the procedure. This device has been modified and is in its third generation so that now several sutures are introduced together in order to close large openings. These sutures can fail to catch on the arterial wall or pull through the arterial wall, which actually enlarges the opening and requires direct surgical repair. The suture devices are better suited for larger arteries with smaller punctures, however, two of the Perclose™ Closure systems have been used together to close very large percutaneous sites.

All of these vascular seal/suture devices have complications related to the devices themselves. All of the vascular occlusion devices/procedures have a steep learning curve and all require a continued regular experience with their use for the operator to remain proficient in their use. Most pediatric/congenital catheterization laboratories do not have a sufficient number of suitable patients to justify the learning process and, in turn, the use of the current vascular occlusion/repair devices. The complications from the vascular occlusion devices are significantly higher than the complications of vascular access in our institution when careful, meticulous manual compression following sheath removal is used to control the bleeding. As these devices develop for use in smaller arteries, very large vessel punctures and venous punctures, they may become more appropriate for use in the pediatric/congenital laboratory.

Complications of vascular access

The most common adverse events and complications occurring from cardiac catheterization procedures in pediatric and congenital patients are complications of the vascular access sites. Complications of vascular access sites occur with the arterial, the venous or both vessels. Although these complications can be very serious, many adverse events of vascular access sites are self-limiting and create no permanent sequelae. The complications from arterial access sites are usually more serious and more likely to lead to recognizable, permanent sequelae.

Bleeding at the site of the catheter introduction into the vessel is a very common event, and can occur from the puncture and cannulation of the arterial, the venous or both vessels. This bleeding can occur during the procedure, as well as after the procedure has been completed and the cannulae/catheters have been removed. Bleeding from puncture sites in the vessels can be very extensive if the patient is not observed very carefully for such an event. Bleeding from a vessel can result in external blood loss at the skin puncture site or can result in the creation of a significant hematoma from the extravasation of blood into the subcutaneous tissues due to an unrecognized leaking vessel. Bleeding at the vascular access site may not be totally preventable even with the most conscientious maintenance of pressure over the site, however, when bleeding does occur and is recognized, it almost always can be controlled by continued external pressure over the site.

External, visible blood loss usually produces a more "dramatic" event, however, unless totally unrecognized or non-contained when it does occur, it usually does not require even blood replacement. Deep hematomas are common and are a result of unrecognized or uncontrolled, continuing blood loss beneath the skin into the subcutaneous tissues from a punctured vessel. The thicker and deeper the subcutaneous tissues are, the greater is the chance of a large amount of unrecognized bleeding occurring there. Hematomas are uncomfortable and cosmetically unsightly for the patient, but usually do not lead to any permanent sequelae and only very rarely require drainage.

Peripheral arterial (femoral, brachial, axillary) injury

Arterial obstruction is one of the more serious complications of vascular access. Arterial obstruction is a result of injury to the vessel wall, arterial spasm, thrombosis of the artery or a combination of any of these factors. Total obstruction results in the loss of the pulse and inadequate blood flow distal to the obstruction. When not treated appropriately, arterial obstruction can result in the loss of parts of, or even the entire extremity or even the death of the patient. When arterial obstruction is only partially treated, the residual obstruction can result in the diminished growth or decreased function of the extremity. Occasionally, however, total obstruction of a superficial femoral artery is discovered incidentally during an attempt at a subsequent catheterization study with no other recognizable signs or symptoms.

The primary treatment of arterial obstruction is prevention by the use of proper equipment and very meticulous management of the arterial puncture before, during and after the procedure as described earlier and repeatedly in this chapter. Obstruction of an artery may not be totally preventable but certainly there are numerous steps that can reduce the incidence markedly and minimize the effects. In some therapeutic catheterization procedures, sheaths and catheters that are very large in proportion to the size of the artery must be introduced, in which case arterial injury is more likely to occur. The techniques and care of these particular arterial sites are even more important for the prevention of injury in these arteries and are discussed in detail previously in this chapter and subsequently in Chapter 9.

Manipulation of an artery in any manner results in pain. The pain, in turn, results in vascular spasm, reduced flow and, potentially, thrombus formation. Techniques to reduce the trauma to the artery and to eliminate any pain in the area are extremely important in preventing arterial complications. Adequate local anesthesia around the vessel is imperative. The artery at the puncture site is palpated and local anesthesia infiltrated on both sides of the artery as well as into the tract through the skin and subcutaneous tissues down to the vessel. Two percent xylocaine is preferred. This more concentrated local anesthesia requires less volume and, in turn, less "stretching" of the subcutaneous tissues in the vicinity of the artery. During a long procedure and/or at the time of *any* exchange of sheaths in the artery, the area around the artery is re-infiltrated generously with local anesthesia.

The ***technique*** used for the arterial puncture is extremely important in preventing arterial injury. As the artery is palpated, an appropriately sized needle is introduced slowly and carefully toward the vessel in an attempt to utilize a "single wall" puncture technique. The hub of the needle is observed for the very first return of blood during its introduction to assure that the artery is *not transected purposefully* with the needle. The puncture of the posterior wall of the artery serves no purpose but, potentially, remains open and allows unnecessary bleeding from the vessel throughout the procedure. When a vessel is not entered during the introduction of the needle, however, the needle is still withdrawn very slowly while observing for blood return. Occasionally the needle passes completely through both the anterior and posterior walls of the vessel without the appearance of any blood during its introduction. On a *slow* withdrawal of this needle, its tip is withdrawn through the posterior wall and cleanly into the lumen of the artery producing a spurt of blood and allowing smooth introduction of the wire. Although this is not the desired technique, a small hole has already been created in the posterior wall. When the needle tip has not entered the arterial lumen during either its introduction or withdrawal, it is withdrawn completely from the tissues, flushed and the slow introduction repeated until the vessel is entered and cannulated successfully. Multiple, rapid and "random spearing" or "harpooning" in the direction of the pulse appears faster but, in actuality, has absolutely no advantage and multiple distinct disadvantages over a slow careful needle introduction. The random needle puncturing produces more trauma to the tissues in the area and certainly results in through and through, double wall punctures of the artery.

The ***duration of time*** in the artery *with a sheath and catheter* also is an important factor in causing arterial damage. The longer the time the sheath and catheter are in the artery, the greater the chance of arterial damage. The most effective way of eliminating arterial complications is not to introduce a sheath/catheter into the artery at all! Although continuous intra-arterial monitoring is a requirement for modern cardiac catheterizations in pediatric/congenital patients, this monitoring does *not* have to be with a catheter in the vessel throughout the entire procedure. Very small—21 or 20 gauge—teflon cannulae provide continuous arterial pressures and access to arterial blood samples, and can remain in the artery for hours (days!) without interrupting flow or causing significant trauma to the vessel. Most, if not all, of the information from the left heart can be obtained from the venous approach after passing prograde through pre-existing intracardiac communications or through a purposeful transseptal atrial puncture. When the artery must be catheterized for very specific information or for a specific therapeutic procedure, small arterial cannulae can be exchanged easily and smoothly for a larger sheath/ catheter. This larger sheath/catheter then only has to remain in the artery for a very short period of time. When this arterial catheter is to be used only for a diagnostic procedure, it usually can be very small.

Once the needle and wire have been introduced smoothly into the artery there are several measures that can be used to reduce trauma to the vessel when a catheter is to be introduced. The *proper* ***choice of equipment*** for the arterial cannulation reduces the vessel trauma markedly. A finely tapered dilator with a very fine tip, which fits tightly over the wire, along with a smooth taper between the sheath and dilator allows the sheath/dilator to dilate and slide smoothly through the needle puncture site, through the wall of the vessel and into the lumen. When resistance to the introduction of the dilator/sheath is encountered, the dilator/sheath combination is *rotated* rapidly ("spun" or "drilled") over the wire as the combination is pushed into the vessel rather than bluntly and forcefully pushing the sheath/dilator straight into the vessel (Figure 4.17).

An ***indwelling sheath*** is utilized for *all catheter* introductions and manipulations in the artery. Although the sheath may be one or even several French sizes larger than the catheter being used, once in place it provides a "lining" between the catheter and the arterial wall so that after the introduction of the sheath there is no motion or rubbing against the arterial wall by the catheter. Arterial spasm around the catheter and "binding" of the catheter in the artery do not occur with the use of an indwelling arterial sheath. On the other hand, spasm around catheters that are introduced directly into arteries *without* the use of indwelling sheaths is a common occurrence. Continued attempts at manipulation of a catheter in the presence of spasm can tear or disrupt the arterial wall. Of equal importance, with the use of indwelling sheaths even very rough irregular catheters (balloons) can be withdrawn or exchanged multiple times without the direct trauma (including disruption of the artery) caused by these catheters being pulled directly through an introductory site in the arterial wall. In addition to the reduced trauma to the artery, there is no blood loss when catheters are exchanged through sheaths with back-bleed valves.

Once the sheath is introduced into the artery if the patient has not received heparin previously, systemic heparin is administered at that time. Heparin is particularly important when the sheath is large compared to the size of the artery and when extensive manipulation or a therapeutic procedure within the systemic circulation is anticipated. A sheath within an artery, along with any vessel spasm, occludes blood flow locally around the sheath and leads to thrombosis in the artery adjacent and distal to the sheath. Heparin is also essential when the catheter used is smaller in external diameter than the internal diameter of the sheath. This discrepancy between the outer diameter of the catheter shaft and the inner diameter of the lumen of the sheath creates a dead space in which thrombi form. Any thrombus that forms in the sheath can be dislodged into the artery by the movement of the catheter or exchange of catheters. When the sheath is larger than the catheter or when there is no catheter in the sheath, the arterial sheath is *maintained on a slow continuous flush* to help prevent thrombus formation in the space between the sheath and catheter or within the empty sheath.

Occasionally, unnecessary trauma to an artery occurs when a large *sheath/dilator* is introduced *inadvertently* into an artery while attempting to cannulate the adjacent vein. The larger the diameter of the sheath/dilator that is introduced, the greater is the potential problem with the artery. Inadvertent entry into an artery occurs most frequently in patients who are cyanotic and have a right aortic arch. The needle is introduced smoothly into the vessel and blood returns into the needle; however, the blood return into the hub of the needle appears *non-pulsatile* and/or it may not appear "red" to presumably reflect the appearance of "arterial" blood. The wire is introduced smoothly through the needle into the vessel and when the wire course in the thorax is checked on fluoroscopy, it passes to the right of the patient's spine similar to a normal venous course. If the wire is not advanced all of the way into the thorax and then buckled or looped in the right atrium, there is no way to distinguished the position in the artery with a right aortic arch from a correct position in the vein by fluoroscopy alone. With the cursory appearance of the wire being in the vein, the large venous sheath/dilator is erroneously introduced into the artery. This becomes readily apparent when the dilator is removed from the sheath and/or the sheath is attached to the pressure monitoring system!

A general knowledge of the patient's anatomy before the procedure and precise attention to the details of catheter introduction should prevent the accidental introduction of a large sheath into an artery. When a very large sheath is introduced inadvertently into the artery, particularly at the onset of a catheterization, the sheath is withdrawn from the artery and hemostasis achieved for that artery before proceeding with the remainder of the catheterization. The small arterial monitoring line is introduced percutaneously into the femoral artery in the opposite extremity.

The ***care of the artery at the conclusion*** of the procedure is equally important at preventing arterial complications. At the end of the procedure and before the sheath is removed from an artery, the skin and subcutaneous tissues around the artery are re-infiltrated with local anesthesia. The systemic heparin is *not* reversed unless the ACT is > 275–300 sec. The catheter is withdrawn *completely out* of the sheath *slowly* and *before* the sheath is withdrawn. This allows any thrombi that have accumulated and are "dangling" around the catheter or at the catheter–sheath interface, to "follow the catheter" and flow *into* the sheath rather than being stripped off the sheath/catheter into the vessel. Once the catheter has been removed, the sheath is allowed to bleed back very briefly through the side port and as it is bleeding back, it is withdrawn from the artery. Pressure is applied *manually* with "finger pressure" over the puncture site as, and after, the sheath is withdrawn.

The drapes over the puncture site are removed while still maintaining pressure over the site. The removal of the drapes allows a large area around the puncture site to be visualized. This helps to assure that, even though the site itself is not bleeding, there is no bleeding occurring into the areas adjacent to the puncture site! *Pressure over the puncture site(s) is applied only by a conscientious, concerned and patient individual.* The person who is holding pressure should know exactly what was done to the artery and should be knowledgeable about the mechanisms of arterial flow and the potential for injury. Since the exact site of the *arterial puncture* does not correspond to the site of the *skin puncture*, finger pressure is applied over the inguinal area in a fairly broad distribution in the cephalad/caudal direction between the skin and the arterial puncture site.

It is desirable to apply pressure with the fingers of one hand while palpating a pulse distal to the puncture site in the same extremity with the other hand. The amount of pressure applied over the site is titrated so that local bleeding at the puncture is stopped, while at the same time the more peripheral pulse is still palpable. Occasionally, especially after a very large sheath has been used, a very long compression time over the vessel is required to achieve hemostasis. After all bleeding at the site (through the skin *and subcutaneously*) has been stopped, a pressure dressing is applied, but this should be loose enough so that the more distal pulse remains palpable. Using these techniques and precautions, the incidence of arterial injury requiring any subsequent therapy is reduced to < 1% of all catheterization procedures.

The management of an arterial complication that cannot be prevented depends upon the type and the severity of the complication. Arterial obstruction is one of the most serious complications of vascular access. This occurs acutely with the loss of the pulse and resultant inadequate blood flow distal to the obstruction. Arterial obstruction results from vessel wall injury, arterial spasm, intra-arterial thrombosis or a combination of any or all of these factors. When not treated appropriately, arterial obstruction can result in the loss of parts of, or even the entire extremity and/or even death of the patient. When the obstruction is only partially treated, arterial obstruction can result in the diminished growth and/or function of the extremity although, often, total obstruction of a superficial femoral artery is discovered incidentally during an attempt at a subsequent catheterization study, with otherwise no recognizable signs or symptoms.

The primary treatment of arterial obstruction is prevention by the use of proper equipment and the very meticulous management of the arterial puncture before, during and after the procedure, as described earlier in this chapter. Acute arterial obstruction usually becomes apparent *in* the catheterization laboratory at the end of the procedure. A diminished pulse with a cool or cold extremity following a catheterization procedure is treated immediately and aggressively upon recognition. The *appearance* of the extremity and the ability to palpate a distal pulse is more important than a pulse "detected" by Doppler. Doppler does verify some flow, but it is so sensitive that it can detect even minimal collateral flow around a totally occluded artery.

Initial treatment is with a bolus and then infusion of intravenous heparin. If the patient is already on heparin, an infusion of 15–25 mg/kg/hr of intravenous heparin is continued to maintain the ACT between 300 and 350 seconds. If the patient is not on heparin, or if the heparin has already been reversed, the patient is given a bolus of 100 mg/kg of heparin intravenously and is maintained on 15–25 mg/kg/hr intravenously with the rate of infusion maintained to keep the ACT in the 300–350 second range. The patient is maintained under close observation for the return of a palpable pulse, or for any evidence of excessive bleeding or any clinical deterioration in the flow to the extremity. As long as the extremity definitely *is improving*, heparin is continued for 24 to even 48 hours.

When, on the other hand, the extremity remains extremely cold, there is *any* deterioration in the appearance of the extremity and/or the pulse and color of the extremity have not returned within four hours, a decision is made whether to proceed with a mechanical dilation of the obstruction in the catheterization laboratory, to begin the patient on thrombolytic therapy or to refer the patient to surgery for a thrombectomy. These options are discussed in Chapter 9.

The availability of "micro" vascular balloons and equipment from the armamentarium of the coronary angioplasty arena have made direct re-cannulation and angioplasty of even small arteries more feasible and appealing[15,16]. It is appropriate to begin a mechanical thrombectomy of the obstruction while the patient is still in the catheterization laboratory, although the patient can always be returned to the laboratory for this therapy even many hours later. For catheter treatment of the obstructed artery, the artery is approached with a catheter introduced into an artery in the contralateral limb. In the newborn/

small infant, the obstructed artery can be approached prograde, first with a floating balloon catheter or a catheter/wire combination passed through the atrial septum, through the left heart, out into the aorta and down the descending aorta to a position just above the involved artery. In larger patients the femoral artery can also be approached from a catheter introduced into the brachial artery or prograde through a transseptal atrial puncture.

The damage to the artery is defined accurately with a small, selective, biplane angiogram, injecting contrast just proximal to the puncture site in the artery. Once clearly identified, the area of recent thrombus/occlusion is probed with a torque-controlled, soft-tipped, guide wire or the soft tip of a Terumo Glide™ wire, which is advanced through the catheter in the aorta and manipulated very carefully past the lesion. Once the thrombus or obstruction in the area is crossed with this wire, the arterial catheter is advanced through the area over the wire and the original wire is replaced with a wire that will accommodate and support a small angioplasty balloon. An angioplasty balloon with the same diameter as the comparable, but non-involved, area in the contralateral artery is chosen. The area is dilated with this balloon, repeating the dilation several times with slight forward or backward positioning of the balloon between each inflation/deflation of it. Blood flow should return through the area immediately. This is verified with a repeat, small biplane angiogram, injecting proximal to the lesion. Once the vessel has been opened, systemic heparin is continued for 24 hours. Acute catheter intervention has proven effective and may represent a more definitive solution to acute, post-catheterization arterial injuries.

The experience with thrombolytic therapy for arterial obstruction post-catheterization in pediatric and congenital heart patients is limited (fortunately) and not too well documented. However, the minimal experience reported in the treatment of peripheral arterial obstructions in congenital heart patients has been successful with minimal side effects or complications in the reported usage. As a consequence, the tendency is to begin intravenous thrombolytic therapy sooner rather than later. Thrombolytic therapy is begun when there is an unsatisfactory response to heparin or as an alternative to mechanical dilation of the lesion in the catheterization laboratory. The details of thrombolytic treatment are discussed in Chapter 9 on Retrograde Catheterizations and in Chapter 2 in the discussions of the various anticoagulant and thrombolytic medications.

There are several different thrombolytic agents available that activate plasminogen, converting the plasminogen to plasmin which, in turn, results in the dissolution of clots. There are multiple treatment regimes with each of these agents. It is important that any institution performing cardiac catheterizations should have at least one thrombolytic agent available and be familiar with its use. The thrombolytics have the potential for creating significant bleeding in any or all systems of the body as well as locally at any vessel puncture/introductory site. The use of thrombolytics is contraindicated in patients who have had recent surgery or newborns with intracranial bleeds. Any patient undergoing thrombolytic therapy requires close, intensive care observation.

Streptokinase is available as Streptase, and there is a fairly good history of its use in congenital heart patients[17]. The regime recommended for streptokinase is an initial bolus of 3,500–4,000 units/kg (up to a maximum of 250,000 units) given over 30 minutes, followed by a continuous IV infusion of 1,000–1,500 units/kg/hr and continued until there is resolution of the clot. When the streptokinase can be delivered through a catheter directly into the thrombus, the dose can be reduced. Once the pulse and color return, the infusion of streptokinase is stopped, however the patient is continued on parenteral heparin for an additional 24 hours.

Recombinant tissue plasminogen activator (rt-PA) has a greater specificity and a strong affinity for fibrin in a thrombus. As a consequence rt-PA probably has an advantage when administered systemically. The rt-PA is infused at 0.05 to 0.1 mg/kg/hr and continued until the thrombus dissolves or for up to 12 hours. As with streptokinase, once thrombolysis with rt-PA has been completed, the patient is continued on heparin for at least an additional 24 hours to prevent re-formation of thrombus.

If a total arterial occlusion is not responsive to mechanical dilation or thrombolytic therapy, an obstructed artery should undergo surgical thrombectomy and surgical repair of the artery by a (micro-)vascular surgeon. Ideally mechanical opening of the artery in the catheterization laboratory and/or the less invasive thrombolytic therapy is tried and only if unsuccessful is the patient referred for surgery. Unfortunately, the prolonged duration of the effects of the thrombolytic agent almost prohibits subsequent surgical intervention for at least 36 hours following the use of thrombolytics. As a consequence, surgical repair should be considered as an *alternative*, not a supplement, to thrombolytic therapy. In the current era, surgical repair is generally successful but it still is not 100% successful.

Bleeding at the arterial puncture site can and does occur. This bleeding can occur during the procedure, as well as immediately and/or fairly long after the procedure is over. Bleeding from a high-pressure artery is potentially more serious than bleeding from a venous puncture site. The patient who has had an arterial catheterization is observed in a recovery room/intensive care environment for a minimum of four hours post-catheterization. The puncture site should be examined particularly carefully any time the patient moves the involved extremity, coughs or retches. The pressure bandage is removed 4–6 hours after the procedure and the patient observed in the hospital for at least another four hours. Any pain, *even* without obvious *external* bleeding and/or hematoma formation, should be investigated thoroughly. Bleeding from a femoral arterial puncture site has the potential for "third spacing" in the thigh and/or retroperitoneal in the abdomen without producing any immediate evidence of superficial extravascular bleeding. Continued or repeated external bleeding from the puncture site should be manageable with continued pressure over the site, reversal of excessive anticoagulation and, of most importance, patience. Surgical intervention for continued bleeding has been "necessary" only three times during the past three decades in our institution.

There are now several materials/techniques available for percutaneously closing large holes in vessels in the catheterization laboratory. These devices were discussed previously in this chapter under "vascular seals". They are available for both a pre-planned part of the catheterization procedure and/or are used at the end of the procedure. These techniques are used routinely in the adult interventional setting, however, because of the relative infrequency of *large* arterial punctures in congenital patients, they have not had significant use in this population. They may be more applicable and more frequently utilized as larger devices are used through a percutaneous arterial introduction.

Local bleeding from an artery can produce a "false aneurysm" at the site of puncture. An aneurysm is the potential end result of the formation of a localized, circumscribed hematoma at the arterial puncture site. The hematoma, which remains in communication with the arterial puncture site, becomes liquefied rather than resorbing into the tissues and the cavity which is created, and communicates with the arterial lumen to become the false aneurysm. The aneurysm becomes apparent as a localized, painful, and often pulsatile swelling. Echo/Doppler interrogation of the area confirms the diagnosis. A small, false aneurysm, that is noted early in the follow-up after the catheterization is treated initially with local pressure applied over the aneurysm for 6–24 hours. Pressure can be applied with one of the external "compression clamps" or with "sand bags". Compression therapy should be tried regardless of the time after the catheterization that the aneurysm became apparent; however, the chances of eliminating the aneurysm with pressure alone decrease with increasing time after the catheterization.

When the aneurysm is not controlled by compression and/or is recognized late, in a larger, adult sized patient, it can be treated with catheter-delivered embolization therapy as described subsequently in Chapter 26, by direct subcutaneous injection into the aneurysm with a solution of thrombin while temporarily isolating the neck of the aneurysm with an angioplasty balloon in the feeding vessel or by isolation of the opening of the aneurysm from the feeding vessel with a covered stent. If an aneurysm does not disappear with one of these procedures or if it is progressive, it is treated surgically by direct closure of the opening in the artery and evacuation of the blood-filled space.

A rare and potentially more serious "extension" of an aneurysm is the development of an arteriovenous fistula. These can develop when the vein and artery are punctured side-by-side to each other in the same extremity, and/or when both the artery and vein are punctured with an unrecognized through and through *transection* of the artery and the vein by the needle while en route to the puncture of the desired vessel (Figure 4.23a). This is more common following a Seldinger or "spearing" approach to the vessel where the target vessel is transected and then entered during the withdrawal of the needle from the deeper tissues. The fistula is created when the sheath/dilator passes through the transected vessel. The indwelling sheath seals the punctures in the non-intended vessel for *as long as it is in place* (Figure 4.23b). When the sheath is removed at the conclusion of the procedure, the opening in the inadvertently transected vessel lies in apposition with the puncture site in the purposefully cannulated vessel. A tract (fistula) easily forms between the two large openings in the adjacent vessels during the manual compression of them (Figure 4.23c).

An arteriovenous fistula can also be created when separate punctures of the artery and vein are made in vessels which are adjacent to each other in the same introductory site in one extremity. When pressure is applied over the skin at the puncture sites the external skin bleeding is controlled but subcutaneous bleeding can continue, with the formation of a hematoma around the two vessels and the creation of a channel of communication between the artery and the vein.

As with all other complications, fistulae are treated most effectively by prevention, using meticulous techniques during vessel punctures and meticulous attention to the control of the vessels at the end of the procedure. *Single wall vessel punctures* always are attempted, and through and through punctures of either the artery or the vein are avoided in order to prevent punctures of an adjacent vein or artery during the same needle stick. When only one arterial and one venous line are necessary, the lines are preferentially placed in different extremities in order to avoid having to puncture the two vessels adjacent to each other in the same extremity. When both the arterial and venous lines are placed in the same extremity, care is taken specifically to keep the puncture of the second vessel away from the vessel punctured initially. In spite of the best techniques, arteriovenous fistulae may not be *totally* preventable.

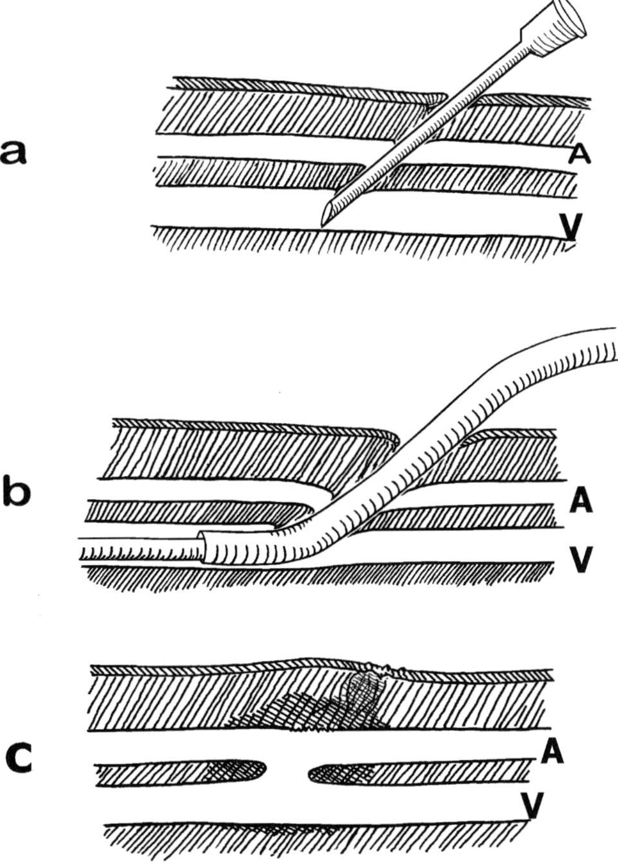

Figure 4.23 Creation of an arteriovenous fistula. (a) Needle puncture through both artery and vein; (b) sheath in vein after passing through artery—the sheath effectively seals both the artery and the vein while it is in place; (c) sheath removed leaving tract (fistula) between the artery and the vein. A, artery; V, vein.

Even a small opening between an artery and a vein creates a large left to right shunt. When an arteriovenous fistula is created, it usually becomes obvious as a painful swelling in the area of the puncture site. Occasionally the first sign of a fistula clinically is seen long after the catheterization procedure, and is found incidentally on examination by the presence of a continuous bruit over a slight swelling or tenderness noted by the patient in the area of an earlier catheterization. There is a bruit and an easily audible, continuous murmur over the area. The fistula is confirmed by an echo/Doppler study over the area. The exact anatomy is defined with an arteriogram in the involved artery with injection of contrast into the afferent artery of the fistula.

When a fistula is recognized, particularly just at the end of the procedure, a tight compression bandage is applied over it in an attempt to stop the flow through the venous channel of the fistula and to allow clotting of the venous "effluent end" of the fistula. This pressure bandage is applied with echo/Doppler control in order to obtain the optimal compression over the precise site to stop the flow through the fistula but, at the same time, not to occlude the arterial flow. This same management should be tried even when a fistula is discovered hours, days or longer after the procedure. In a larger patient such a fistula can occasionally be closed with a small transcatheter-delivered septal occlusion device or a covered stent in the artery, but in smaller patients and even in most larger patients, the fistula usually requires surgical ligation, division and repair by a vascular surgeon.

Peripheral venous (ilio-femoral, brachio-axillary-subclavian, jugular) injury

Complications from significant injuries to veins are probably far more common than arterial complications, however, these injuries often result in no outward signs, symptoms or morbidity and, as a consequence, usually go unrecognized until repeat access through that particular vein is attempted. A vein can be severely obstructed or even totally occluded with no outward signs. In the past, when the cut-down approach was used for the introduction of catheters into veins, the veins were commonly found to be occluded during subsequent attempts at catheterization whether an attempt had been made at repair of the vein or not. Occlusion of the veins at the introductory site is not a common occurrence following the controlled, careful percutaneous entry into veins. Many patients have undergone up to six (or even more) percutaneous catheterizations through the same venous site, have had very large sheaths in place for hours during the catheterization or have had several sheaths within the same vein, all without having any apparent permanent damage to the vein, much less loss of it.

The most severe acute complication with a venous puncture site is a tear or total disruption of a large vein. This occurs most commonly in small patients following attempts at introducing large sheaths or catheters (usually for a therapeutic procedure) into very small veins. Total occlusion of a vein can occur in any sized patient secondary to a traumatic catheter introduction or following a prolonged infusion of fluids or medications through an indwelling venous line. If a tear or disruption occurs below the inguinal ligament or more peripherally in an extremity, local venous congestion or a hematoma develops, but there are usually no more significant *acute* consequences than that. Bleeding from a disruption below the inguinal ligament is controlled by local pressure over the area with no attempt to repair the vein. The main consequence of this type of disruption is the loss of that vein for future access.

Very rarely, acute obstruction of the vein progresses with swelling and congestion of the extremity to the point of compromised flow into and out of the extremity because of the build up of pressure in the vascular spaces. The extremity in these cases becomes markedly swollen, tense and deep blue/purple in color with no capillary refill. This degree of obstruction represents an acute emergency and requires surgical fasciotomies to relieve the pressure and re-establish arterial flow. Decompression of acute "third space syndrome" due to venous obstruction has been treated successfully with the application of medicinal leeches to the extremity. The combination of the withdrawal of the pooled blood and the simultaneous infusion of hirudin by the leeches appears optimal and may avoid the necessity of a fasciotomy.

Tears also occur in the venous system above the inguinal ligament. These occur when the sheath/catheter introduction is too high (cephalad) to the inguinal ligament or too forceful, or during poorly controlled, traumatic catheter manipulations in the iliopelvic areas. When a tear or disruption occurs above the inguinal ligament, retroperitoneal bleeding occurs. Because of the depth within the pelvis, separated from the surface of the skin by the peritoneum, bleeding occurs in an area where there is no possible means of applying pressure over the torn vessel externally. Fortunately, bleeding from even this type of tear is usually self-limiting. When a patient has a retroperitoneal bleed, they develop significant abdominal discomfort. Once a significant amount of extravasated blood accumulates retroperitoneally, the tear usually "tamponades" itself. Occasionally surgical drainage of retroperitoneal blood from a venous tear is required because of pain or obstruction to the remaining intact venous flow. With large tears in veins with significant extravasation of blood, the continuity of the particular torn vein is lost, but collateral flow is sufficient to prevent symptoms or signs of venous obstruction. Very rarely the bleeding from a venous tear extend into the peritoneal cavity, in which case, surgical intervention becomes necessary and urgent to ligate or oversew the disrupted vein/cava in order to stop free bleeding into the peritoneal cavity.

Prevention of retroperitoneal bleeding is the primary treatment. Meticulous attention to the site of puncture in relation to the inguinal ligament should prevent punctures that are too high to control with inguinal pressure. Continued attention to proven techniques for the introduction of needles, wires, sheaths and dilators into vessels and understanding and correcting the causes of "difficult" sheath/dilator introductions will prevent most unnecessary local trauma. Strict attention to the (unnecessary) forces applied to catheters and an understanding of when catheters that are constrained from side to side, as in the iliopelvic vessels, can or cannot be bowed and/or deflected should prevent traumatic perforation of venous structures.

Chronic total obstruction of peripheral (and central) veins is quite common. The most common cause of significant peripheral vein occlusion does not appear to be from the presence of cardiac catheters/sheaths in the veins during a catheterization, but, rather, thrombosis occurring as a consequence of "indwelling lines" that remain in the vein for any length of time. Even the use of large sheaths in small veins, *per se*, has *not* been a *usual* cause of venous damage. The peripheral veins are *relatively* large, very compliant and, usually, easily accommodate a very large sheath, particularly compared to the adjacent artery. On the other hand, the *rough introduction* of *and/or handling* of needles, wires, dilators, sheaths and catheters of any size in the veins, inadequate local anesthesia leading to pain and vessel spasm and the failure to use indwelling sheaths in the veins during the catheterization, can all cause unnecessary trauma, tears or disruption of the veins, resulting in subsequent venous occlusions.

Indwelling lines are often left in place in the central veins through the sites of catheter introduction after the catheterization is completed and/or new lines are placed in these same veins specifically for chronic infusions. Any foreign material within the vascular system is potentially thrombogenic, and the longer it remains in the vessel the greater is this potential. Thromboses and/or occlusions created by indwelling lines are aggravated by "caustic", non-ionic, solutions and medications delivered through those lines. These solutions serve as endothelial irritants or even sclerosing agents. The presence of an indwelling infusion line in a central vein in a small infant or child is almost a guarantee of a subsequent venous occlusion. The sicker and more debilitated the patient is and the longer the indwelling line remains in place, the greater the chance of thrombosis of the vein from the line.

Prevention is the most effective treatment of venous obstruction. ***All*** of the suggestions and techniques for the care and handling of the arteries to prevent arterial injuries are applicable for the prevention of peripheral venous injury. Systemic heparinization, the liberal use of local anesthesia, the use of indwelling sheaths during the manipulation of all catheters and devices in the veins, not leaving indwelling intravenous lines in the access veins and the overall gentle handling of venous access sites, all help to prevent venous obstruction. Although no controlled study of this has been performed, heparinization of the patient is probably even more important for the prevention of peripheral venous thrombosis. Because of the low venous pressure and the inherently sluggish venous flow, a large sheath present in a peripheral vein causes significant stasis or can even produce total obstruction of that vein much more easily than a sheath produces arterial obstruction. The adjacent tissue pressures from the infiltrated anesthetic solution, local subcutaneous bleeding or multiple sheaths in the same area can easily compress and obstruct an otherwise adequate venous channel. This obstruction of the venous channel, combined with the slow flow, leads to the development of thrombi around, as well as both proximal and distal to, the introductory site of the sheath. This is true particularly in patients who are polycythemic and/or dehydrated, and/or when a sheath is in place in the vein for a prolonged period of time.

There is good evidence to suggest that the use of a sheath that is even several sizes larger than the catheter is less traumatic to the vein than a smaller catheter shaft passing directly into the vein without the protection of the sheath, particularly when using balloon catheters. As is the case with sheaths in arteries, the venous sheath provides a protective "channel" and a "lining" extending well into the vein, which prevents its endothelium from touching the moving catheter. Once the sheath is in place, there is no friction against the wall of the vein by the catheter and/or other irritation from the catheter movement. Venous spasm and the "binding" of catheters in veins are non-existent when using indwelling sheaths.

Experience at Texas Children's Hospital with the delivery of intravascular stents has demonstrated a marked reduction in the loss of veins following the *use of indwelling sheaths*. The stents initially were mounted on very large balloons, but all were introduced through *very large sheaths* compared to angioplasties and valvuloplasties which were performed using the same large balloons, but without sheaths. There was a much higher incidence of vein loss following the angioplasties than following stent implants.

When venous obstruction above the inguinal ligament is present, these obstructed veins can frequently be re-cannulated, dilated and maintained open with intravascular stents as described in Chapter 24. Probably, the more recently the obstruction developed from a prior procedure, the greater the chance of re-cannulating and opening the vein permanently with the use of intravascular stents.

A percutaneous puncture presumably into a vein only can result in an arteriovenous fistula when the artery in the same introductory site is punctured during the same procedure. This potentially serious complication has been discussed earlier under the complications of arterial puncture. An arteriovenous fistula is the consequence of both the artery and the vein having an opening created in them, but the fistula probably develops during the manual compression of the vessels (*see* Figure 4.23). When multiple sheaths are introduced into a single introductory site and/or vessel as occurs in many of the interventional procedures, this likelihood is increased. The best treatment of a fistula is prevention. Separate, single wall punctures of each vessel, if possible in separate extremities and, if the punctures cannot be in separate extremities, as far away from the adjacent vessel as possible, all help to prevent the development of arteriovenous fistulae at the puncture sites.

Infections of the tissues around vascular access sites were common problems with the use of cut-down procedures for the introduction of catheters, but they have been essentially eliminated by percutaneous introductions and the use of more rigid sterile techniques for all catheterization procedures. Meticulous cleansing of the percutaneous entrance site, very careful sterile technique in the entire laboratory and cleansing and exposure of the site after the procedure appear to be sufficient to prevent local infection after percutaneous catheter introduction. The percutaneous technique essentially has no open wound during the procedure nor any incision to heal afterward. In the adult catheterization environment, there has been a slight resurgence of infection at the introductory sites with the use of the various percutaneous suture and sealing devices/techniques. This, however, is in a very small percentage of patients and, as yet, is not a problem in pediatric/congenital laboratories.

As with all other complications of cardiac catheterization, awareness of the potential for the complication with prevention by the use of proven and meticulous techniques are the most effective means of treating the complications of vascular access.

References

1. Neches WH *et al.* Percutaneous sheath cardiac catheterization. *Am J Cardiol* 1972; **30**(4): 378–384.
2. Lechner G *et al.* The relationship between the common femoral artery, the inguinal crease, and the inguinal ligament: a guide to accurate angiographic puncture. *Cardiovasc Intervent Radiol* 1988; **11**(3): 165–169.
3. Seldinger SI. Catheter replacement of the needle in percutaneous arteriography. *Acta Radiol* 1953; **39**: 368.
4. Cowley CG *et al.* Snare-assisted vascular access: a new technique. *Catheter Cardiovasc Interv* 1999; **47**(3): 315–318.
5. Hesslein PS *et al.* Percutaneous sheath brachial vein cardiac catheterization in children. *Cathet Cardiovasc Diagn* 1980; **6**(2): 197–205.
6. Daily PO, Griepp RB and Shumway NE. Percutaneous internal jugular vein cannulation. *Arch Surg* 1970; **101**(4): 534–536.
7. Denys BG, Uretsky BF and Reddy PS. Ultrasound-assisted cannulation of the internal jugular vein. A prospective comparison to the external landmark-guided technique. *Circulation* 1993; **87**(5): 1557–1562.
8. Johnson JL, Fellows KE and Murphy JD. Transhepatic central venous access for cardiac catheterization and radiologic intervention. *Cathet Cardiovasc Diagn* 1995; **35**(2): 168–171.
9. Sommer RJ, Golinko RJ and Mitty HA. Initial experience with percutaneous transhepatic cardiac catheterization in infants and children. *Am J Cardiol* 1995; **75**(17): 1289–1291.

10. Linde LM *et al.* Umbilical vessel cardiac catheterization and angiocardiography. *Circulation* 1966; **34**(6): 984–988.
11. Neal WA *et al.* Umbilical artery catheterization: demonstration of arterial thrombosis by aortography. *Pediatrics* 1972; **50**(1): 6–13.
12. Walters DL *et al.* Transthoracic left ventricular puncture for the assessment of patients with aortic and mitral valve prostheses: the Massachusetts General Hospital experience, 1989–2000. *Catheter Cardiovasc Interv* 2003; **58**(4): 539–544.
13. Fischer DR *et al.* Carotid artery approach for balloon dilation of aortic valve stenosis in the neonate: a preliminary report. *J Am Coll Cardiol* 1990; **15**(7): 1633–1636.
14. Weber HS *et al.* Transcarotid balloon valvuloplasty with continuous transesophageal echocardiographic guidance for neonatal critical aortic valve stenosis: an alternative to surgical palliation. *Pediatr Cardiol* 1998; **19**(3): 212–217.
15. Samal AK and White CJ. Percutaneous management of access site complications. *Catheter Cardiovasc Interv* 2002; **57**(1): 12–23.
16. Peuster M *et al.* Percutaneous transluminal angioplasty for the treatment of complete arterial occlusion after retrograde cardiac catheterization in infancy. *Am J Cardiol* 1999; **84**(9): 1124–1126, A11.
17. Kirk CR and Qureshi SA. Streptokinase in the management of arterial thrombosis in infancy. *Int J Cardiol* 1989; **25**(1): 15–20.

5 Catheter manipulations

Introduction

Specific techniques and purposeful manipulation are required for all cardiac catheters, however they are an absolute essential with torque-controlled catheters, which respond only to the maneuvers applied by the catheterizing physician. True torque-controlled catheters are designed to have a one-to-one relationship between motions performed on the proximal catheter and the response at the distal end, and can be directed selectively into specific sites[1]. Skillful manipulation of cardiac catheters combines a certain amount of inherent talent with the learned skills of the techniques. The purpose of this chapter is to provide some guidance about the techniques for maneuvering torque-controlled catheters.

Cardiac catheterization is not a procedure performed strictly according to rules nor by the repetition of previous maneuvers, however, there are some rules of common sense and safety. These rules and techniques apply to the manipulation of all catheters, but are particularly applicable to using torque-controlled catheters. The special catheter manipulations that are applicable primarily to floating balloon catheters are covered in Chapter 7.

Rules for good catheterization technique

General

1 *Plan the pocedure.* It is important to have a plan for the entire catheterization procedure. It is important to determine what is the most critical or essential (and often most difficult to obtain) information and to obtain this information as early as possible during the procedure. It makes no sense to spend several hours during a catheterization obtaining extraneous information and then to end the procedure without the absolutely essential information.

The "memory" of the "preformed" curves of many torque-controlled cardiac catheters is at its very best immediately after the catheter is introduced into the patient. The longer these catheters remain in the circulation, the worse the memory and controllability of the catheter become. This is particularly true for woven dacron catheters. For example, a catheter with a proper, short 90° curve at the tip is maneuvered readily into the right ventricle and from there, into the main and then the right pulmonary artery. However, within a few minutes, these catheters lose the pre-formed curve at the tip and become softer and straighter. As a result, far more extensive manipulation with the catheter or the use of adjuncts such as deflector wires becomes necessary to accomplish what initially was a straightforward manipulation with the properly curved catheter alone. A catheter that becomes straight preferentially passes from the right atrium to the superior vena cava or from the main to the left pulmonary artery with the turns from the right atrium to the right ventricle or from the main pulmonary artery to the right pulmonary artery being almost impossible without the use of an adjunct deflector system in the catheter. When saturation data is the most important information needed from the study, each delay between samples due to unnecessarily prolonged manipulations during attempts at entering critical areas, causes large time intervals between samples and lessens the validity of each of the oxygen saturations obtained.

2 *Innovation.* The catheterizing physician must be capable of instantaneous and innovative changes during each step of the procedure. These changes must be instinctive. While having a plan for the catheterization procedure, the operator must always be aware of unexpected and/or unusual locations and/or fortuitous positions of the catheter, which are reached inadvertently en route to the "planned" or "desired" location and data. The data from the unexpected location are often essential and the same, unexpected location may *be difficult or even impossible* to enter deliberately later in the case. The information from such an area should be recorded permanently or an angiogram should be obtained, even if this was not the next step in the original plan. The operator must often stop and totally replan the procedure when the data from a particular location do not fit into the expected anatomy or hemodynamics. Once the unexpected area is explained and the data recorded, and/or an angiogram obtained from that location, then the original plan can be resumed or a new plan formulated to fit the new or unexpected data.

3 *Never take anything for granted.* Catheter locations, pressures and saturations in even slightly unusual positions and/or with findings that are at all out of the ordinary should always be verified *at that time*. Unexpected areas are rechecked and identified with at least a blood sample for a determination of the oxygen saturation or a hand test injection of contrast with *biplane* stored fluoroscopy or *biplane* angiographic recording. Always determine the significance of an unusual or unexpected finding *when it occurs* and while the catheter *is in that location/position*. When there is *any* question of the location, never assume that a catheter tip is in a particular place, or pressure is recorded from a location without confirming it. For example, a catheter introduced from the inferior vena cava to the right atrium can advance *straight cephalad* to an anomalous right upper pulmonary vein by way of the superior vena cava or *straight cephalad* through a patent foramen ovale/atrial septal defect, into the left atrium and into a normal right upper pulmonary vein. The course of the catheter is identical in both the posterior–anterior (PA) and lateral (LAT) views! The route of the catheter to the possibly anomalous site must be confirmed. No amount of guessing or theorizing once the catheterization procedure has been completed, particularly on the following day, replaces the factual information gained at the time!

4 *Anticipation.* During any stage of the catheterization procedure, the *next* (and next, next!) step should always be anticipated and prepared for. The greatest conservation of time, aside from the technical skill of the operator, is achieved by thinking and moving ahead to the next step in the procedure or to the next bit of information to be obtained. The operator anticipates and begins the next move while directing the laboratory staff accordingly. For example, when a wedge position is achieved and *while the pressure is being recorded*, the next step is planned and begun. If it is to be a "pull back" recording, the recording technician is instructed accordingly and informed of the pressure gain and recording speed to be used. On the other hand, if the next step is a wedge angiogram, the patient is positioned and the field of the X-ray image is set for the angiogram *during* the recording of the pressure. Think, plan and prepare ahead. It is very inefficient to stop, pause and "contemplate" and/or "admire the catheter position" *between* each step of the catheterization procedure!

5 *Speed.* The speed or "short time" of the catheterization procedure is not accomplished by the speed of each individual catheter maneuver, but by the careful *preplanning* and *preparation* for the study and by the deliberate, skillful, thorough and planned progression through the procedure. Rapid, repeated catheter movements make it seem as though the procedure is proceeding more rapidly, but actually are usually purposeless and counterproductive.

Fluoroscopy rules

1 Always adjust the image intensifier (II) to patient distance as close as is physically possible with ***both*** the posterior–anterior (PA) *and the lateral* (LAT) X-ray image intensifiers. This reduces radiation dosage, reduces the scatter and, at the same time, improves the quality of the X-ray image. The PA intensifier is usually and almost automatically positioned close to the patient's chest, while the LAT intensifier often remains many centimeters away from the side of the patient. The distance between the image intensifier and the patient should be the same, or as close to the same as possible in both planes. This requires that, at the onset of the procedure, the patient is positioned on the catheterization table as far to the patient's *left* as possible and that any extra support for the patient's left arm (pillow, "board", etc.) does not extend beyond the left edge of the table in order that the lateral image intensifier can be positioned *against* the side of the *patient's thorax*.

2 Use fluoroscopy only while actually maneuvering a catheter, when "setting the field" for an angiogram and/or when actually performing an interventional procedure. In all circumstances fluoroscopy is used for as short a time as possible. Catheters that are sitting still or are already in the desired position should not be "admired" on fluoroscopy! The radiation dose to the patient *and the operators* is directly proportional to the duration of the X-ray exposure. At the same time, it is preferable to utilize *continuous* fluoroscopy *while the catheter is being maneuvered* rather than to intermittently step on and off the fluoroscopic peddle. Once the catheter has reached its desired position, fluoroscopy is stopped while the next step in the procedure is determined.

3 Collimation, collimation, collimation! A circular image *never* should be seen on the fluoroscopy screen and/or in an angiographic image!! A circular image represents no collimation and usually X-radiation to a large and unnecessary area outside of the useful field (or even beyond the area of the image intensifier input screen). Radiation dose is proportional to the *square* of the area visualized. Reducing the area visualized in half cuts the

radiation to the patient *and to the operator* four-fold. In addition, the better the field is collimated over the exact area of interest, the better is the resultant image.

4 During catheter manipulations, utilize as small a field of view as possible—i.e. keep the heart or area being explored with the catheter in the center of the field and close the "sides, top and bottom" of the field of view to include only the heart or the specific area being explored. The abdomen, neck and/or lungs should ***not*** be visualized while the catheter is being manipulated from the right ventricle and into the pulmonary artery! Radiation to the patient (and the operator!) is proportionate to the *square* of the *area* of coverage. Bear in mind that the radiation dose to the patient occurs only during the single procedure, while to the catheterizing physician it is cumulative from patient to patient, from day to day and from year to year!

A better image with better catheter definition is obtained on the monitor from the smaller field of view on the X-ray. The smaller the field size, the more homogeneous is the density of the image that is viewed and in turn, the better the quality of the image. With a field of uniform density, the automatic brightness control of the system does not compete with itself. For example, if half of the field of view is over the heart while the other half is over a lung field, the automatic brightness controls try to increase the X-ray dose over the heart, but at the same time, decrease the X-ray dose over the lungs, and neither area is visualized optimally.

5 Liberally utilize *lateral plane* or even *biplane* fluoroscopy for obtaining quick images in the lateral (perpendicular) plane in order to check the anterior–posterior position *and the exact direction* in which the tip of the catheter is pointing. For selective, purposeful cannulation of a specific vessel or orifice, frequent intermittent checks in the lateral view are essential. Multiple, quick, one or two second glimpses at the lateral plane utilize far *less radiation* than several minutes of non-productive, "blind probing" with the catheter in only the single, posterior–anterior view.

6 Use the magnify or zoom modes appropriately but sparingly. Each step in the magnification of the fluoroscopic (and cine) image increases the radiation to the patient and the operator approximately two-fold in each plane, except when using the "acquire zoom" setting. If there is a small area of interest where details of the image are critical, then magnification of the area is indicated. Often the increase in radiation from the magnification can be compensated for by tight collimation over the precise area of interest. In the very small infant, when an increase in size of the viewed image is desirable or necessary to obtain a reasonable sized working image of the heart on the monitor, with the "acquire zoom" setting of digital X-ray systems the viewed image can be magnified *without* increasing the radiation exposure to the patient and/or operator. In the acquire zoom mode, the image is zoomed or magnified digitally only. As a consequence, the image is enlarged, but there is some degradation of it. Although the acquire zoom image is not as pleasing aesthetically, the gross outline of the heart without an image with fine details is sufficient for most manipulations of a catheter. True magnification of the image with the finer details preserved is necessary for angiography and precise positioning of devices, etc.

7 Very small, hand, biplane, test injection angiograms to identify the precise location of the tip of a catheter during catheter manipulations, and biplane angiograms of balloon inflations during dilations and/or stent implants and/or during the release of devices during implants are desirable or essential. The biplane images from these test injections and procedures should be recorded *permanently*, either on biplane stored fluoroscopy or on *slow speed* biplane cineangiography. The capability of recording stored fluoroscopy is available in the biplane mode of most modern digital X-ray equipment. Stored fluoroscopy results in a multi-fold reduction in the radiation exposure for those images that need to be recorded with less critical detail. An alternative recording technique is the use of 15 frames per second (fps) or better still 7.5 fps (or even 3.25 fps, which is available on some systems) for the angiographic recording of these events. These particular events in the catheterization procedure are analogous in speed to "grass growing" and although they need recording, they do not need high-speed recording.

Catheter manipulation—general rules

1 *Continual electrocardiogram (ECG) monitoring*. A minimum of two, and preferably, three separate and different ECG leads are displayed simultaneously and continuously while recording from at least four separate skin electrodes. The multiple leads allow for the immediate detection of very subtle, localized changes on the ECG. When a four + lead system is used on the patient, there will always be at least one readable ECG tracing visible on the monitor when a single ECG wire becomes disconnected owing to the patient's movement or sweating.

2 *Pressure monitoring*. The catheter is attached to a pressure monitoring system with a continuous visible display of the pressure curve whenever a catheter is being manipulated. Both the catheterizing physician(s) and the recording technicians or nurses should be carefully and continuously monitoring the pressure curves displayed from catheters and/or any other indwelling lines during all catheter manipulations. A change in pressure may indicate that a new chamber or vessel has been entered, but can also indicate that a catheter has

come loose (with potential blood loss) and/or that a vessel or chamber wall has been perforated.

3 All catheter manipulations and all forward catheter movements are performed using direct fluoroscopic visualization. At the same time, when the catheter is *not* being maneuvered or when the radiographic tubes are *not* being repositioned, the fluoroscopy should be switched off.

4 A catheter (or wire) is never jerked backward rapidly or pulled out of the heart rapidly *unless one intends to tear or evulse* a structure (e.g. a balloon septostomy). Rapid motions during catheter withdrawal are more dangerous than when the catheter is being advanced. A wire that is withdrawn rapidly straightens forcefully as it is withdrawn and, in turn, incises into any convex curved surface of the structures in its path. The potential for evulsing an intracardiac structure around which the catheter has become looped or otherwise entangled is always present during a rapid catheter withdrawal. In addition, a rapid withdrawal will tighten any loop or bend that is present in the course of the catheter and/or wire and convert loops or bends into fixed kinks and/or knots, which can be extremely difficult to untie or remove.

5 *Heparinization.* The use of systemic heparin is covered in detail in Chapter 2 on medications. All congenital heart patients undergoing cardiac catheterization should be heparinized during the procedure. The initial dose and repeated doses of heparin are determined according to the patient's measured activated clotting time (ACT) before and during the procedure. Heparin does not eliminate the necessity for using all other means of preventing clots by the elimination of any stasis in catheters/vessels and keeping catheters thoroughly flushed.

Curves at the tip of cardiac catheters

Cardiac catheters come with many preformed curves and configurations at the distal end and tip. Some of these standard tip configurations are useful, but many more are not only of no use, but are often a hindrance for accomplishing a particular maneuver in the heart of a small patient or one with a complex congenital heart problem. Any single, specific, preformed curve built into a catheter cannot be effective or necessarily even useful for every congenital heart patient or, even, for every maneuver within any one patient's heart. A specific curve is chosen or formed on the tip of the catheter for each different patient, the particular anatomy in that patient, and the specific maneuver that it is necessary to perform.

It is far more efficient and cost effective to hand form individualized, specific curves on the tip of a catheter for each particular heart or location within the heart than it is to try to maintain an inventory of the infinite variety of catheters with multiple different tip curves and sizes which would be needed to accommodate all of the hearts encountered and particular locations/maneuvers necessary in a pediatric/congenital heart catheterization laboratory. At the same time, "hand-formed" curves on catheters seldom are as "permanent" and/or have as good a "memory" as the curves built into catheters by their manufacturers, particularly in the extruded plastic materials of most current catheters. As a consequence, a certain inventory of catheters with "factory" curves will be necessary in all pediatric/congenital catheterization laboratories.

Fairly permanent curves can be formed on almost any catheter while it is outside the body. The distal end of the catheter is softened by heating it in boiling water, in a jet of steam, or in a column of very hot air from a "heat gun". After the material has been softened, the distal tip of the catheter is bent or formed to produce the desired curve. When the curve has been formed or molded on the heated catheter by hand, it is fixed by flushing it with a cool flush solution or by dipping it in a bowl of cool, sterile solution. The amount and duration of heat that are necessary (and possible to use) depend upon the material from which the particular catheter is manufactured. Extruded polyurethane and polyethylene catheters in general take very little heat to soften them and can actually melt if exposed for too long a time to hot air. Woven dacron catheters require more heat, and teflon catheters require even higher temperatures to soften the tips sufficiently for forming. At the same time, both of these latter materials are very resistant to damage by heat. Catheters with reinforcing wire braids within their walls usually cannot be molded or reshaped sufficiently.

Very transient curves can be formed and fixed fleetingly on catheters while they are being manipulated *within* the heart or vessels. When a cardiac catheter is in the warm blood of the circulation, most catheter materials soften to some degree. During the manipulation of a catheter within the heart or vasculature, its tip often catches against, or actually into an intracardiac/intravascular structure. When the catheter is advanced gently with the tip fixed in that location the catheter just proximal to the fixed tip bends or bows into a curve. If the catheter is flushed with the room temperature (cold!) flush solution, this very fleetingly fixes the curve that is created by the bend on the softened catheter material within the heart or vessel. The fixation of the newly formed curve lasts only seconds, but if used quickly and effectively, often this transient curve is sufficient to allow or enhance a specific maneuver of the catheter.

A common example of the use of a "temporary curve" in the catheter is in maneuvering the tip of the catheter from the right atrium to the right ventricle, particularly after the catheter has softened and straightened in the warmth of the circulation. When the straightened catheter is maneuvered to and fro or rotated within the right atrium, its tip eventually catches in the atrial appendage or along the wall of the atrium. A slight forward force or push on the catheter bows the distal end of the catheter, which is just proximal to the tip, into the open area of the atrium. Flushing with cold flush solution for several seconds through the catheter very temporarily fixes the curve that is formed on the catheter within the atrium. The "new curve" on the catheter is maintained for only a few seconds which, however, is long enough to allow expeditious and purposeful maneuvering of the catheter from the right atrium into the ventricle *immediately after* the flush is stopped and the catheter tip is withdrawn out of the fixed position. The technique of temporarily fixing a curve on the catheter is particularly effective when using woven dacron catheters.

Catheter manipulation—fine technical considerations

In spite of the apparent large size of the cardiac silhouette on the fluoroscopic screen, the operator must constantly bear in mind how small is the heart in which the catheter is being manipulated. Manipulations of the catheter are performed with *finger* movements—in millimeter increments —not with gross hand or arm and elbow movements!

The fine to-and-fro and rotational maneuvers performed by the operator's hands on the proximal end of the catheter can, for the most part, be transmitted to the distal end and the tip of the catheter, and the same motions performed proximally are duplicated, approximately, at the distal end and tip within the heart. The distal end of the catheter responds to the operator's *to-and-fro* motions on the shaft of the catheter in roughly a *straight line.* Any rotation of the tip of an *absolutely straight catheter* will not change the direction of its tip! When pushed cephalad, the *straight tip* of a catheter moves only *straight* cephalad regardless of any rotation of the shaft. The catheter *must* have at least a slight curve at the tip for the rotation of the shaft to have any effect at all on changing the direction of the tip of the catheter (Figure 5.1).

Many catheters soften with time when exposed to warm body temperature and, in doing so, straighten and lose any preformed curves and any capacity for them to be directed purposefully. This is particularly true for woven dacron torque-controlled catheters. Unless the catheter maneuvers are performed shortly after their introduction into the body or *immediately* after a new curve is formed, no purposeful changes in direction can be made on the tip of the catheter merely by pushing on, and/or torquing, the proximal shaft of the straightened catheter.

Continuous to-and-fro movements on the catheter while applying torque to it

When attempting to torque and/or rotate the tip of the catheter by applying torque on the proximal shaft of the catheter, the entire catheter must be kept in a *constant, simultaneous*, very slight, ***to-and-fro motion*** while the torque is applied to the more proximal shaft of the catheter (Figure 5.2).

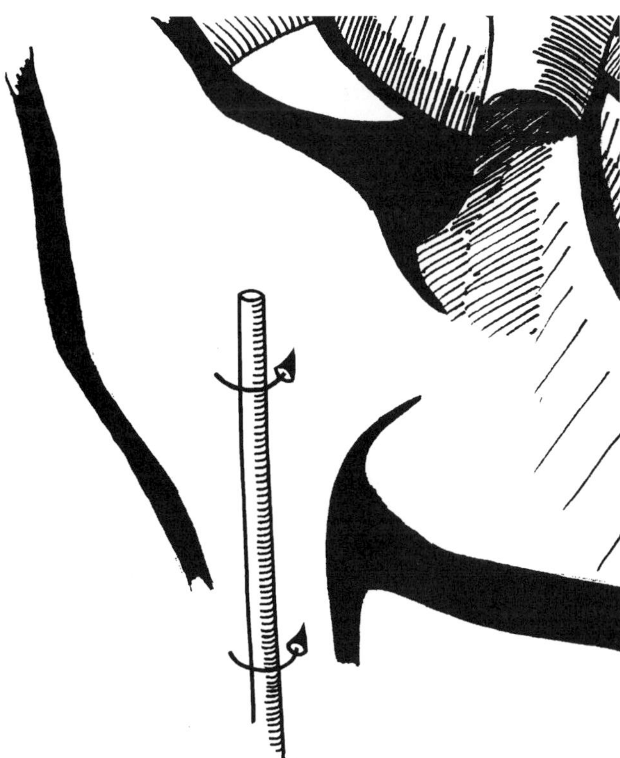

Figure 5.1 Rotation of straight catheter with no curve at the tip produces absolutely no change in the direction of the catheter.

Even when utilizing a properly fitting sheath and *without* a back-bleed valve attached to the sheath, significant resistance to any rotation of the tip of the catheter is always encountered along the entire shaft of the catheter. The resistance to rotation of the catheter is caused by the introductory sheaths themselves as well as the curves and bends within the walls of the vessels and the cardiac chambers. A back-bleed valve fixed on the hub of the introductory sheath adds significantly more resistance to any rotation or movement of the catheter. As a consequence of these multiple areas of resistance to rotation, without *simultaneous* short, *to-and-fro and continuous* movement of the entire length of the shaft of the catheter, the rotation of the proximal shaft of the catheter will *not* be transmitted to the tip of the catheter by an isolated rotation or twisting of the proximal shaft of the catheter. During the simultaneous, to-and-fro motions along with the rotations, the operator also must be sure that the *tip* of the catheter is *free* and moving in direct response to the purposeful to-and-fro movements on the proximal shaft.

When the tip of a catheter is fixed and/or burrowed into a corner, crevasse and/or into the myocardial tissue and does not move out of this fixed location with the to-and-fro motions of the catheter, the shaft of the catheter merely

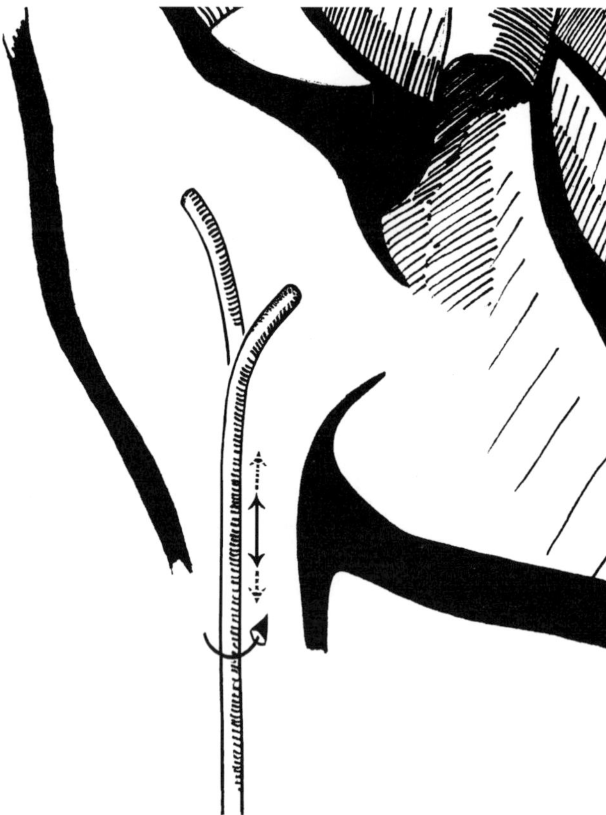

Figure 5.2 To-and-fro motion on shaft of catheter while simultaneously rotating catheter keeps the tip of the catheter free and facilitates transmission of torque or rotation to the tip.

bows or bends with the to-and-fro catheter motions while the tip rotates in *its fixed position* without any actual change in position and/or direction of the tip! (Figure 5.3). A catheter which is twisted or rotated at the proximal end without keeping the shaft in this constant, fine, to-and-fro motion usually does not transmit this rotation to the tip and, in fact, can twist the shaft of the catheter on itself. In that circumstance, when any rotation finally *is* transmitted, the torque is transmitted to the tip in less than a 1:1 ratio and with a "delayed" response. More often, without the simultaneous to-and-fro motion, the *proximal* end of the catheter merely twists on itself, often 360–720° (or even more), without transmitting any rotation to the tip. When the tip of the catheter does catch up to the proximal torque on the shaft, it responds with a "propeller-like" spin as the torque overcomes the resistance against the shaft of the catheter within the sheath and vessels. When the tip that still has *not* been moved out of its fixed, buried location, does rotate, it merely spins while buried in the same place—for example embedded within a trabecula of the right ventricle. Twisting a very soft catheter without the to-and-fro motion can twist or kink its wall structure, resulting in permanent damage or even breaking it.

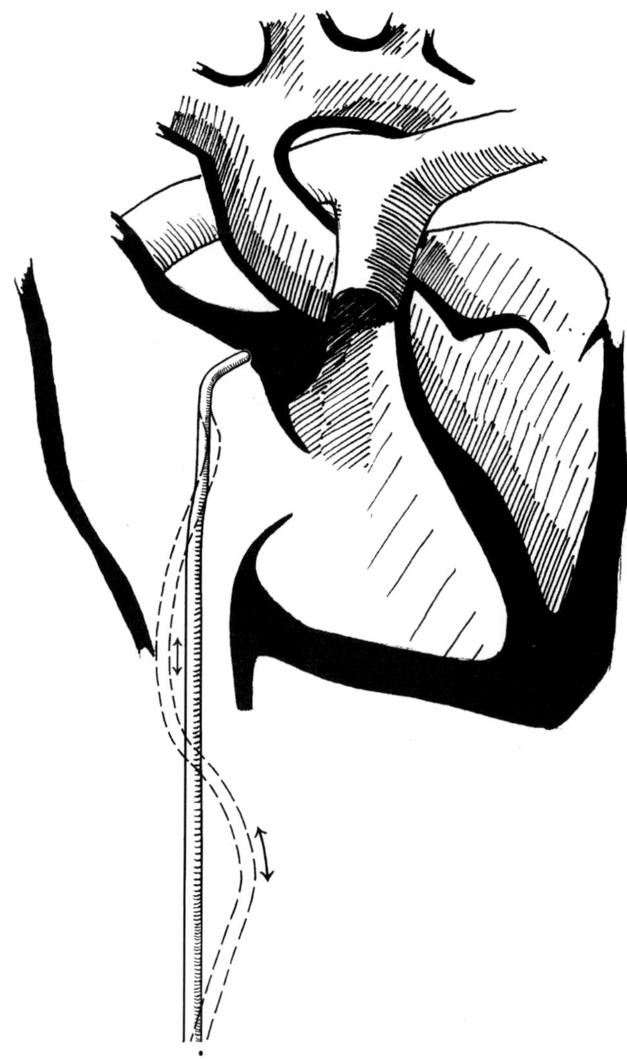

Figure 5.3 The tip of the catheter is caught and cannot move to-and-fro along with the rest of the catheter; to-and-fro movements of the shaft result in side-to-side "bowing" of the shaft of the catheter without movement of the tip of the catheter.

Quick, repeated precise movements

Each catheter maneuver should be fairly rapid, short and well controlled as opposed to slow, meticulous and "tedious". Five or six *quick, but at the same time, gentle,* precise and controlled movements of the catheter toward the proper location are far more effective (and conservative of radiation!) than one, slow, meticulous torque maneuver performed over the same period of time. Repeated, quick rotations with simultaneous to-and-fro movement of the catheter are far more likely to turn or advance the tip of the catheter than slow, methodical, torque applied to its shaft. Quick, repeated movements are also much more productive per unit of fluoroscopy time than slow torquing and methodical pushing of the catheter. The one exception to the quick, repeated movements is when deflector wires or devices are used within a catheter to direct the tip of the catheter very specifically. Techniques with deflector wires are covered in detail subsequently in this chapter and in Chapter 6.

When a specific catheter manipulation is unsuccessful after it has been repeated 4 or 5 times, the same maneuver is not likely to be successful when repeated 5, 10 or more times!! A different maneuver, either with the same catheter, with an adjunct device, a completely different catheter and/or a *different catheter pusher* should be used.

"Lubricating" the catheter

In addition to the to-and-fro and rotational motions of the shaft of the catheter, the catheter should be kept "lubricated" where it enters the sheath. This is important whether with, or without, the use of an attached hemostasis valve. Saline or any other flush solution is applied continuously to the surface of the catheter outside of the sheath with a cotton sponge that is liberally and frequently moistened with flush solution. It is beneficial to actually keep a moistened sponge adjacent to, or even around the hub of the sheath and to moisten this sponge repeatedly during the procedure. Otherwise dried blood collects within the sheath, between the outer wall of the catheter and the inside of the sheath, and begins to "glue" the catheter to the sheath.

Maneuvering through a sheath with or without a back-bleed valve

The various back-bleed valves that were discussed in Chapter 3 (Consumable Equipment) are valuable or essential for reducing blood loss around a catheter, particularly during the exchange of catheters into and out of the vascular system through the sheath. However, *all* back-bleed valves "grip" the walls of the catheter to some degree and, in doing so, create resistance to its free motion. Of equal importance, when a catheter is manipulated through an attached back-bleed valve, the tactile "feel" of the catheter that is transmitted from events occurring within the vasculature to the fingers of the catheterizing physician, is lost completely, and the maneuverability of the catheter is reduced significantly by any attached back-bleed valves. When these valves remain in place and fixed on the sheath during catheter manipulations, the operator has no way of discriminating between the force used to overcome the resistance of the back-bleed valve itself and the force actually being delivered to the tip of the catheter. Some valves are so tight that the catheter cannot be moved without a great deal of additional and significant force being applied to the catheter. When the catheter is moved within these tight valves, the sheath will move in and out of the vessel in synchrony with the motion of the catheter. The continuous motion of the sheath within the vessel obviates the protective effect of the sheath for the vessel.

Because of the interference with catheter manipulation and loss of the tactile sensation of the catheter caused by back-bleed valves, it is always preferable to use sheaths with detachable hemostasis/flush port valves. Catheter sizes are labeled according to their outside diameter (OD), while sheath sizes refer to their internal diameter (ID). When a catheter is used which is the same French size as the sheath (internal diameter of the sheath and external diameter of the catheter) and there are precise tolerances on the part of the manufacturers, the catheter will move freely within the sheath, yet there will be no bleeding around the catheter even without a back-bleed valve on the sheath and even when present in an artery! When a detachable back-bleed valve is present on the sheath, the valve is loosened from the hub of the sheath and withdrawn back onto the proximal shaft of the catheter during all catheter manipulations (Figure 5.4). When both sheaths and catheters are manufactured with precise tolerances, the back-bleed valve can be removed from the hub of the sheath during the procedure, even when the sheath is in an artery. When the catheter is not being manipulated or when a catheter exchange is necessary, the removable back-bleed valve/flush port is placed on a flush and the entire valve is re-advanced over the catheter and reattached to the hub of the sheath.

It is particularly important to avoid the use of back-bleed valves during very fine or delicate catheter manipulations. The tighter the back-bleed valve fits around the catheter, the more the valve interferes with fine motions of the catheter. Those sheaths with back-bleed valves that are permanently attached to the sheath and which fit very tightly around the catheter, should be avoided when any fine catheter manipulations are anticipated.

The manufacturers are very good at assuring that the fit of a catheter within a sheath of the "same" French size never is too *tight*. However, at the other extreme, manufacturing tolerances are more lax and the sheaths often are very loose relative to a catheter of the "same" French size. Occasionally, manufacturers market catheters and/or sheaths of in-between sizes from standard French sizes, in order to overcome the necessity of producing accurate

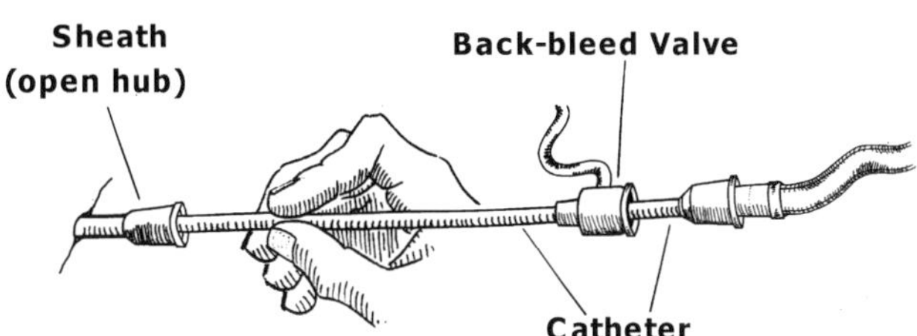

Figure 5.4 Back-bleed valve loosened from hub of sheath and withdrawn back on shaft of catheter during catheter maneuvers.

tolerances. In these circumstances, where manufacturing tolerances are poor and the fit of the sheath over the catheter is very loose, excessive bleeding will occur around the catheter without a back-bleed valve, and the valve must remain attached to the hub of the sheath throughout the entire procedure. This is true particularly in the newborn and small infant, where a steady leaking of even a few drops of blood from the sheath around the catheter is significant and necessitates that the back-bleed valve is attached to the sheath almost continually. However, even with a very loose sheath or in a small infant, when a fine delicate maneuver with the catheter is necessary, the back-bleed valve is temporarily detached from the sheath and withdrawn back on the shaft of the catheter until the maneuver has been completed. The back-bleed valve is then reattached.

Tip deflection and direction

If a catheter cannot be advanced into or through an expected orifice after multiple careful attempts, and after checking the proper direction in both planes of the fluoroscopes, there is little reason to persue the same maneuver even one more time. Repetitive, non-purposeful or forceful movements of the catheter, particularly banging the tip of the catheter around within a chamber, represent poor technique, are nonproductive and potentially dangerous and expose all involved in the catheterization laboratory to unnecessary irradiation. Such maneuvers are far more likely to produce heart block or perforation of the heart than a purposeful, controlled entrance into the desired specific location.

When the catheter tip does not enter the desired location using the presumed appropriate maneuver, the reason for the failure should be determined before pursuing further random manipulations. The pressure and saturation in the area are verified. A small (1–2 ml) hand test injection of contrast is performed while recording on biplane, stored fluoroscopy or on biplane angiography to identify the location of the catheter positively and the exact location of the orifice being sought. If the test injection is not saved initially, in all likelihood it will have to be repeated. Once the anatomy is identified precisely and if the opening or orifice being sought is confirmed to be in the expected location, a change in materials or technique is necessary. A different catheter is used with a newly formed curve on the catheter or the catheter is used in conjunction with a guide wire or a deflector wire.

Often, extruded plastic catheters with preformed curves have relatively stiff shafts, which tend not to "follow" the tip around curves in the vasculature even after the tip has been maneuvered successfully into the desired location. In that circumstance, a relatively stiff, spring guide wire with a very soft tip is advanced through the catheter, passed out of the distal tip of the catheter, and advanced through and distally beyond the desired orifice. The wire is advanced further until both the transition and the stiff portions of the wire are well past the orifice being entered. Even a relatively stiff catheter will usually follow a guide wire when the stiff portion of the wire is positioned well distal to the desired orifice. An alternative, and often preferable, technique is to deflect the tip of the catheter toward, or even into, the orifice with an active deflector wire or a stiff, static deflector wire and then the catheter is advanced into the orifice off the wire.

Once it has been demonstrated that the tip of the catheter is directed precisely toward or into the desired orifice (valve orifice, septal defect, outflow tract, etc.) with a deflector wire, the catheter is advanced off the deflector wire and into and through the orifice while the wire and its curve are fixed in position. Force is never required for these manipulations of the catheter/wires. If the catheter tip does not advance into the orifice, it is because the tip of the catheter is not pointing in the exact direction in one of the planes of view. When viewed in the second (perpendicular) fluoroscopic plane, the erroneous direction or absence of the expected orifice become apparent instantaneously. Whichever type of deflector wire is used, once the proper curve is formed on the catheter by the wire, it is important that the wire tip is held exactly in its position by holding the proximal wire against the table-top outside of the patient while the catheter is advanced off the wire. If the wire is not fixed in position, the curve on the wire/catheter advances as a unit within the lumen of the central vessel and slides the tip of the catheter past, rather than pushing the tip into, the desired orifice. The use of guide and deflector wires in maneuvering catheters is covered in detail in Chapter 6.

Catheter tip rotation relative to the catheter approach

The anterior–posterior and the side-to-side directional effects of the curved tip of the catheter in response to rotation of its proximal end depend upon several factors. Introduction of the catheter from a site cephalad to the heart via the superior vena cava reverses not only the direction of the approach to the heart, but reverses the direction of rotation of the tip of the catheter *in response to the clockwise or counterclockwise rotation of the proximal shaft* of the catheter when compared to the rotation when the catheter is introduced from the femoral approach. The initial direction in which the tip is pointing, either from side to side or anteriorly or posteriorly, also changes the direction of the response of the tip to a particular torque applied to the proximal end of the catheter. Finally, if the overall curve is more than 90° along the course of the catheter, the actual cephalad or caudal direction of the tip of the catheter *in relation to the proximal end of the catheter* changes the direction which the tip of the catheter turns in relation to the direction of torque on the proximal shaft of the catheter.

The *initial* anterior or posterior direction of the tip of the catheter determines whether a catheter turns to the right or to the left with a clockwise or counter clockwise torque on the proximal catheter and, vice versa, the *initial* rightward or leftward direction of the tip determines whether the catheter turns anteriorly or posteriorly with a specific torque on the proximal shaft of the catheter. This absolute dependence on the direction of the tip in the perpendicular plane emphasizes the importance (necessity) of instantaneous biplane fluoroscopy for purposeful, complex maneuvers through the contorted, always different, courses within congenital heart defects. The operator must know unequivocally, in three dimensions and at all times, which direction the tip of the catheter is pointing in in order to perform purposeful and meaningful maneuvers.

Catheters introduced from the femoral approach

From the femoral approach, the catheter enters the heart in a straight line from the inferior vena cava. The rightward or leftward direction in which the tip of the catheter is pointing initially, determines whether a clockwise or a counterclockwise torque on the proximal shaft of the catheter directs the tip *anteriorly* or *posteriorly* (dorsally). When the tip of the catheter initially points *laterally* to the *patient's* right (operator's left), a *clockwise* rotation directs the tip *anteriorly* (Figure 5.5a) and a *counterclockwise* rotation directs the catheter tip *posteriorly* (Figure 5.5b). Conversely, when the tip is initially pointing to the patient's left (operator's right), a clockwise rotation rotates the tip posteriorly and a counterclockwise rotation directs the tip anteriorly.

Similarly, with a catheter introduced via the inferior vena cava whether the tip of the catheter turns toward the right or left with a clockwise torque of the proximal shaft depends upon whether the tip *initially* is pointing *anteriorly* or *posteriorly*. When the tip of the catheter coming from the femoral approach is initially directed anteriorly, a clockwise torque of the proximal shaft directs the tip medially, to the *patient's left* (operator's right) and toward the tricuspid valve (Figure 5.6a), while a counterclockwise rotation would direct the tip in the opposite direction, laterally and toward the patient's right. If the tip of the catheter initially is pointing *posteriorly*, a *counterclockwise* torque (rotation) of the proximal shaft of the catheter is necessary to direct the tip of the catheter to the *patient's left* (operator's right) and the tricuspid valve (Figure 5.6b).

A 360° loop in the shaft of the catheter proximal to the tip does not change the relative response of the *tip* of the

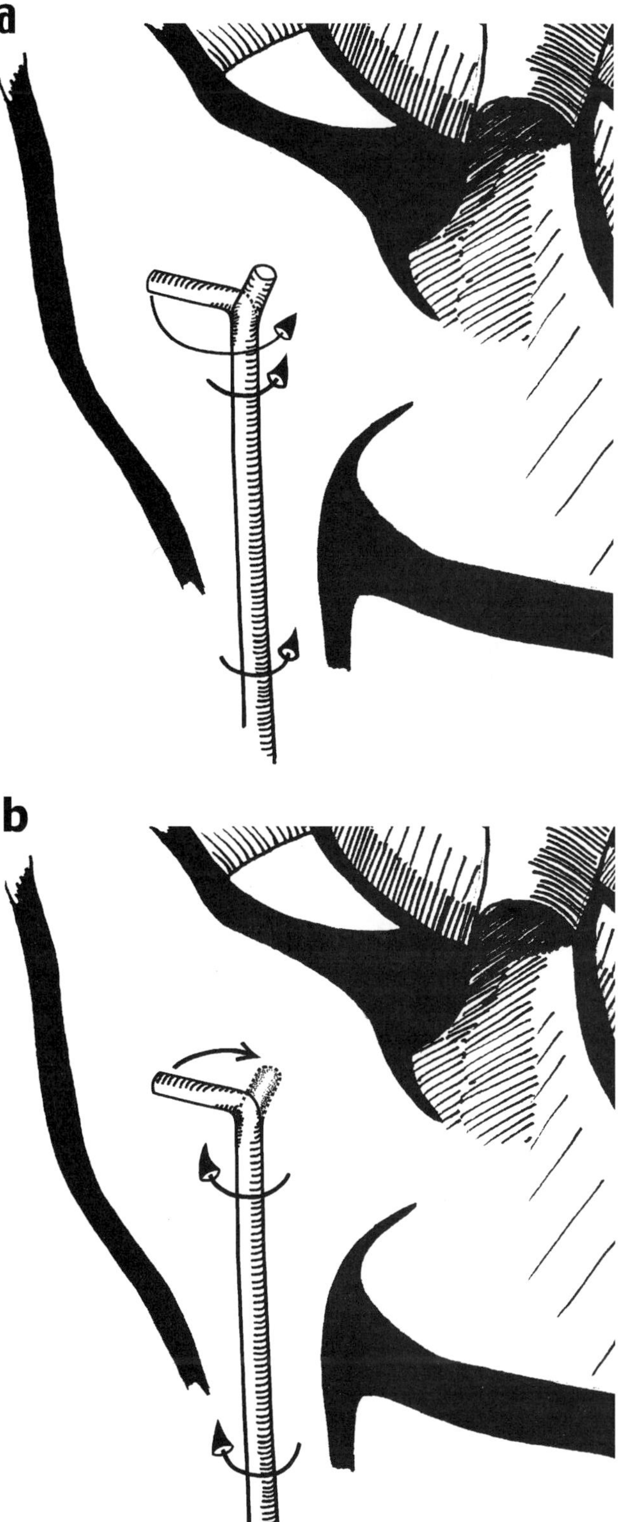

Figure 5.5 (a) When the tip of a catheter is initially directed *laterally* (toward patient's right), a *clockwise* rotation of the shaft of the catheter turns the tip of the catheter *anteriorly*. (b) When the tip of a catheter is initially directed *laterally* (toward patient's right), a *counterclockwise* rotation of the shaft of the catheter turns the tip of the catheter *posteriorly*.

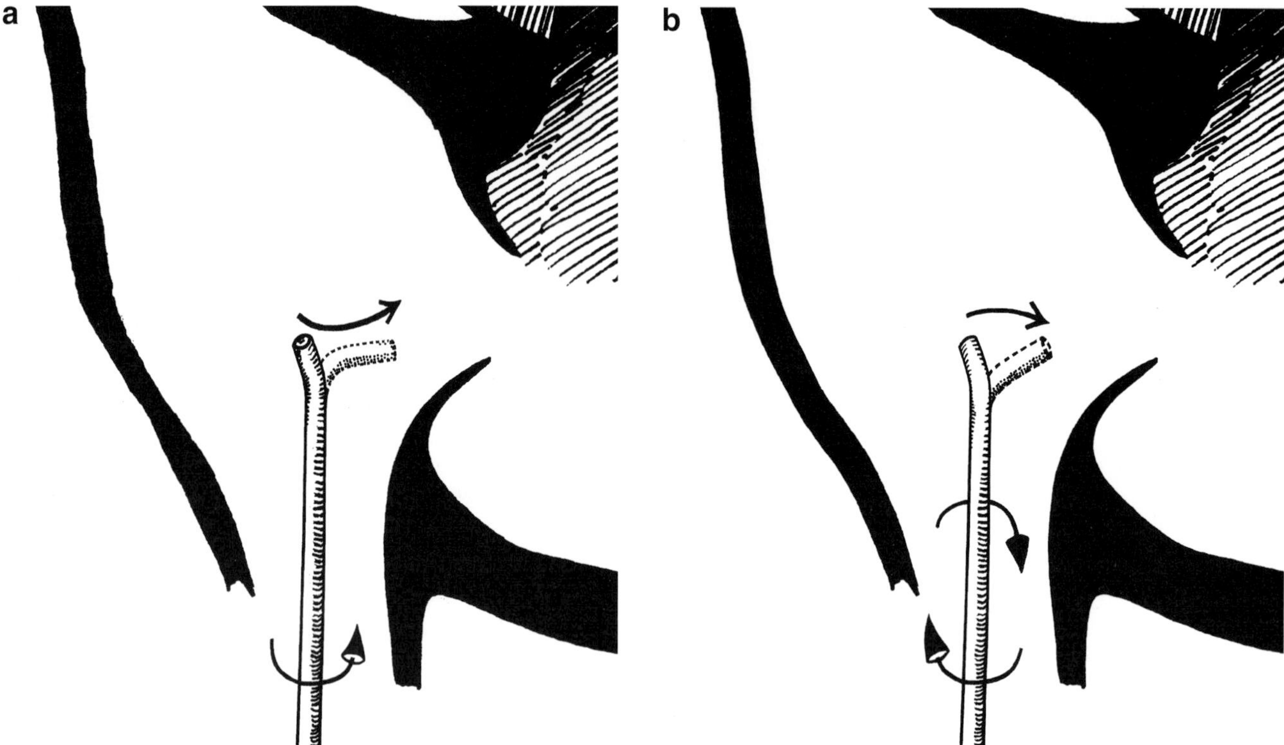

Figure 5.6 (a) When the tip of a catheter is initially directed *anteriorly*, a *clockwise* rotation of the shaft of the catheter turns the tip of the catheter *medially* toward the patient's left and the tricuspid valve. (b) When the tip of a catheter is initially directed *posteriorly*, a *counterclockwise* rotation of the shaft of the catheter is necessary to turn the tip of catheter *medially* toward the patient's left and the tricuspid valve.

catheter to torque on the proximal shaft. The entire, large loop of the catheter tends to turn as though it is a "tip curve", but the tip itself also turns independently from the loop of the catheter. When the long axis of the shaft of the catheter, which is immediately adjacent to the tip of the catheter, is aligned in the same direction as the proximal end of the catheter and regardless of an intervening 360° loop, the *tip* tries to turn in the direction of a proximal torque as though the catheter was straight. This response is regardless of the bends in the rest of the catheter shaft. When the tip points toward the patient's right (operator's left side), a clockwise proximal rotation still rotates the *tip* anteriorly even when there is a 360° loop in the catheter course (Figure 5.7). A counterclockwise rotation of the catheter produces the opposite anterior–posterior effect on the tip of the catheter as well as on the entire 360° loop.

On the other hand, a 90–180° change in the cephalad–caudal direction of the *shaft* of the catheter anywhere proximal to the tip of the catheter, ***reverses*** the expected direction that the tip of the catheter turns as a result of a torque that is applied to the proximal shaft of the catheter. The large, 180° loop or curve in the shaft of the catheter responds like a "large tip curve", while the curve at the *tip* is actually turning in the opposite direction to that which is "expected" from the same direction of torque on a straight catheter. This reversal of the transmitted torque direction occurs with both rightward and leftward as well as anterior and posterior directions and turns of the tip of the catheter. If the catheter has a loop resulting in a *net* 180° change in the direction of its distal end just proximal to the tip—i.e. back toward the introductory direction—the anterior–posterior and the right–left effects on the *tip* are *just the opposite* from the response when the catheter shaft is straight, i.e., when the shaft of the catheter is directed straight and away from the operator. With a catheter that is looped 180+° with the *tip* initially pointing to the patient's *left* (operator's right) but with the distal end of the catheter headed back toward the feet following the 180° loop, a *clockwise* rotation of a catheter results in an *anterior* turn of the catheter tip (Figure 5.8a). With the same 180° loop on the catheter and the *tip* of the catheter initially pointing anteriorly, a *counter-clockwise* rotation will direct the tip *medially* and toward the tricuspid valve, but at the same time will tend to rotate the loop posteriorly (Figure 5.8b). In the presence of a 180° loop in the catheter, the direction in which the *tip* of the catheter turns in response to torque applied to the proximal shaft will be opposite to the expected direction to that in which the tip would turn in response to the same torque in the presence of a straight catheter.

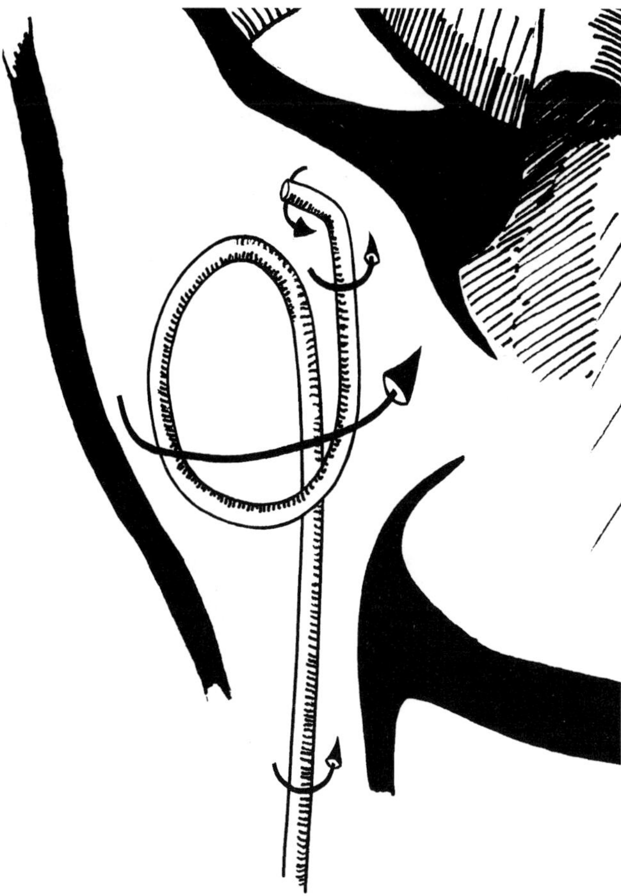

Figure 5.7 In the presence of a 360° loop in the more proximal shaft of the catheter, the tip of the catheter turns in response to rotation of the shaft of the catheter as though the catheter were straight. Clockwise rotation of the proximal shaft of the catheter rotates the loop clockwise and the laterally directed tip anteriorly.

Catheter rotation when the catheter is introduced from the arm or neck (right or left) via the superior vena cava

When the catheter is introduced from a cephalad, superior vena cava (SVC) approach, regardless of whether it is introduced from the right, left arm or neck veins, and whenever the shaft of the catheter just proximal to the tip is directed caudally (toward the IVC or feet) and the tip is pointing anteriorly in the heart, a *counterclockwise* rotation (torque) on the proximal shaft of the catheter will direct the *tip* of the catheter *medially*, toward the patient's left and the tricuspid valve (Figure 5.9). A *clockwise* torque on the catheter from the same entry direction with the tip initially pointing anteriorly directs the tip laterally. On the other hand if the tip is pointing *posteriorly* (to the *patient's back*) with the overall direction of the catheter still directed caudally from the SVC, then a *counterclockwise* torque would direct the tip laterally while a *clockwise* motion directs the tip medially toward the patient's left and the tricuspid valve (Figure 5.10). This re-emphasizes the necessity of biplane imaging in order to know instantaneously the anterior–posterior as well as side-to-side directions of catheters.

When the catheter tip is initially pointing *laterally* with the catheter coming from the SVC, a *counterclockwise* rotation initially rotates the tip anteriorly and eventually, with continued counterclockwise torque and to-and-fro motion on the catheter, the tip turns medially toward the tricuspid valve (Figure 5.11). A clockwise rotation of this same catheter initially would rotate the tip posteriorly, and eventually the continued clockwise torque would rotate the tip 180° and toward the tricuspid valve. If the tip of the catheter is initially orientated *posteriorly* with the catheter entering the right atrium from the SVC, the direction which the tip of the catheter turns in response to the direction of the torque on the shaft of the catheter will be just the opposite from when the tip is pointing anteriorly, i.e. a clockwise rotation on the catheter shaft rotates the posteriorly directed tip toward the patient's left and a counter-clockwise rotation directs the tip toward the patient's right.

When 180° loops are formed on catheters within large chambers or vessels, the response of a curve at the tip of the catheter becomes much more complex and slightly less predictable whether the catheter is introduced from the inferior or the superior vena cava. When a loop is formed on a catheter with a curve (angle) at the tip, usually the acute curve present at the tip of the catheter will face the concave (inner) direction of the loop. When the catheter is approaching from the arm or neck via the superior vena cava and a 180° loop is formed on the catheter so that the distal portion of the catheter *just proximal to the tip* is directed cephalad back toward the patient's head (and/or the pulmonary artery) in the atrium (or ventricle) then the ***exact opposite effect*** on the ***tip*** occurs as a result of torque applied to the proximal shaft of the catheter compared to torque or rotation applied to a catheter entering the atrium straight from the SVC. This applies whether the catheter has looped entirely in the atrium and/or the tip of the loop has flipped into the ventricle.

Thus, when the catheter is introduced via the superior vena cava and looped 180° in the atrium or into the ventricle, the distal part of the catheter will be heading cephalad back toward the head and right ventricular outflow tract while the *tip* of the catheter initially points toward the patient's right (the concavity of the loop). A *counterclockwise* rotation on the proximal shaft will tend to direct the *tip* of the catheter *posteriorly* and toward the pulmonary artery (Figure 5.12). A clockwise rotation on the proximal shaft of the catheter would direct the tip of the catheter anteriorly. Unfortunately, the torque on the shaft of the catheter also tends to rotate the entire 180° loop in the catheter, even to the point of rotating the entire loop out of the ventricle.

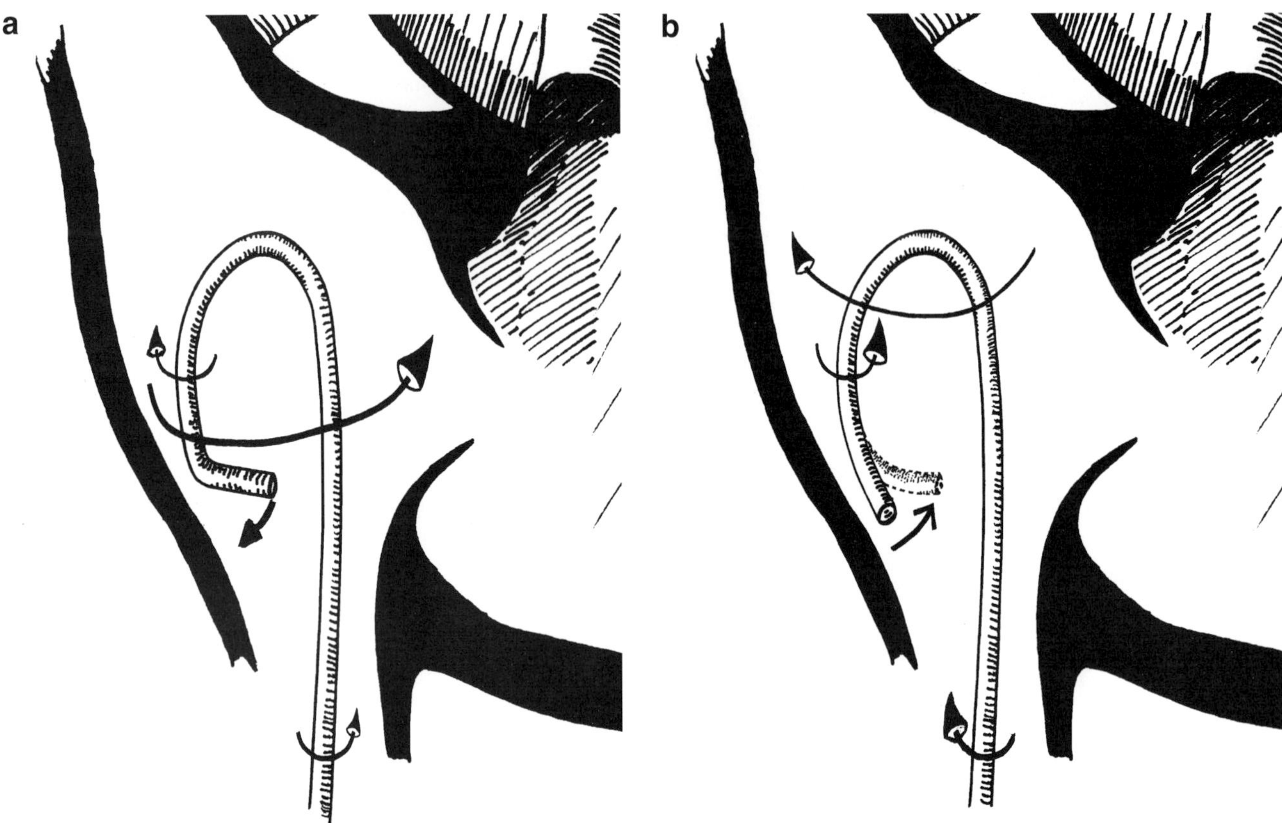

Figure 5.8 (a) In the presence of a 180° loop, a clockwise torque on the shaft of the catheter rotates the loop clockwise but turns a medially directed tip anteriorly. (b) In the presence of a 180° loop and with the tip initially directed anteriorly, a counterclockwise torque on the shaft of the catheter rotates the tip of the catheter medially toward the tricuspid valve, but tends to turn the loop counterclockwise, posteriorly and potentially away from the valve.

If a 180° loop forms in a catheter that is introduced from the SVC into the right atrium, the distal end of that loop will be directed cephalad while the separate "curved tip" of the catheter will be directed "centrally" toward the concavity of the loop. When the 180° loop is directed *posteriorly*, the separately curved tip will face anteriorly. A counterclockwise rotation of the proximal shaft of the catheter rotates the shaft of the catheter and the entire 180° loop toward the patient's right which, in turn, points the curved tip toward the patient's left (toward the tricuspid valve). When the distal end of the 180° loop is pointing *anteriorly*, the separate curved tip initially will point posteriorly (toward the concavity) and the effects on the distal end of the catheter of torque on the proximal shaft of the catheter are just the opposite to when the loop was pointing posteriorly. A clockwise torque on the proximal shaft of the catheter rotates the *anteriorly directed loop* to the patient's right, while the separate curved tip then points medially and toward the patient's tricuspid valve. A counterclockwise torque on the shaft does just the opposite, directing the loop toward the patient's left (and tricuspid valve) but turning the curved tip laterally. When a 360° loop forms in either the atrium or the ventricle, and regardless of whether the catheter approaches from the neck or via the inferior vena cava (from the groin), the *tip* responds to proximal torque on the catheter shaft as though the catheter is straight.

When a 180° loop from the SVC is initially pointing toward either the patient's left or right, then any rotation of the proximal shaft produces either an anterior or posterior rotation of the loop, while the separate acutely curved tip will be directed in the opposite direction—i.e. a clockwise torque on a 180° loop, which is initially directed laterally, will rotate the loop posteriorly with the centrally facing, separate curved tip pointing anteriorly. A counterclockwise rotation of the proximal shaft of a 180° loop which is initially facing laterally (to the patient's right) rotates the 180° loop anteriorly while the tip ends up pointing posteriorly (Figure 5.13).

These "rules" for catheter rotation in relation to the general orientation of the catheter tip become instinctive with experience and are described here only as an introduction to the effects of purposeful torque applied to a torque-controlled catheter.

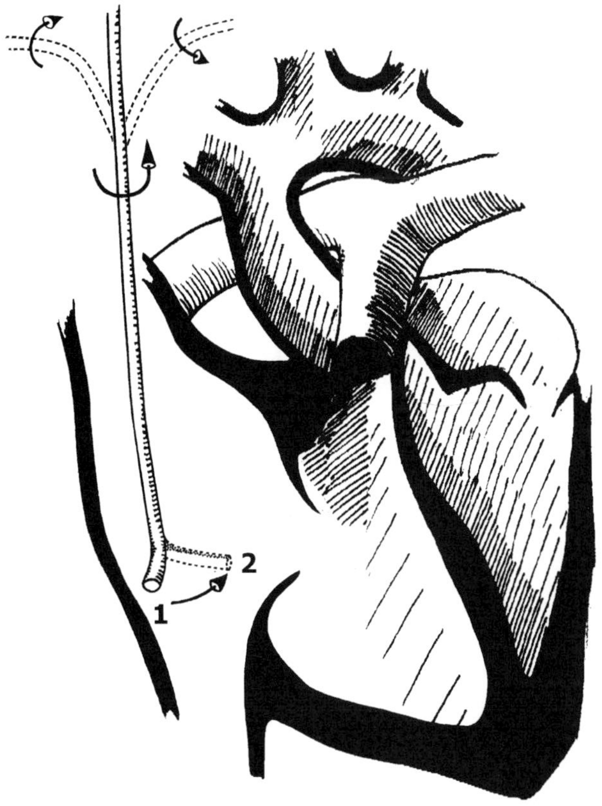

Figure 5.9 Catheter introduced from the neck (superior vena cava) with the tip of the catheter initially directed anteriorly. Counterclockwise rotation directs the tip medially (to patient's left).

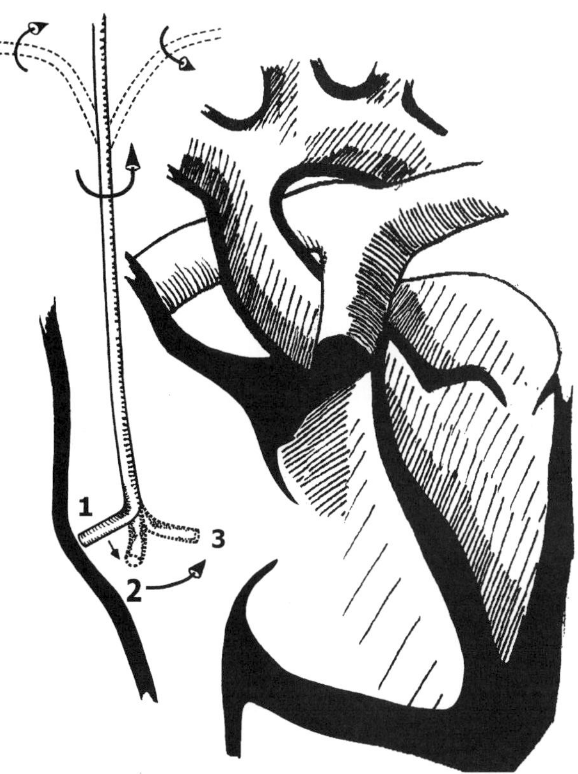

Figure 5.11 Catheter introduced from the neck with tip of catheter initially pointing laterally. Counterclockwise rotation of the shaft of the catheter rotates the tip from lateral to anterior to medial.

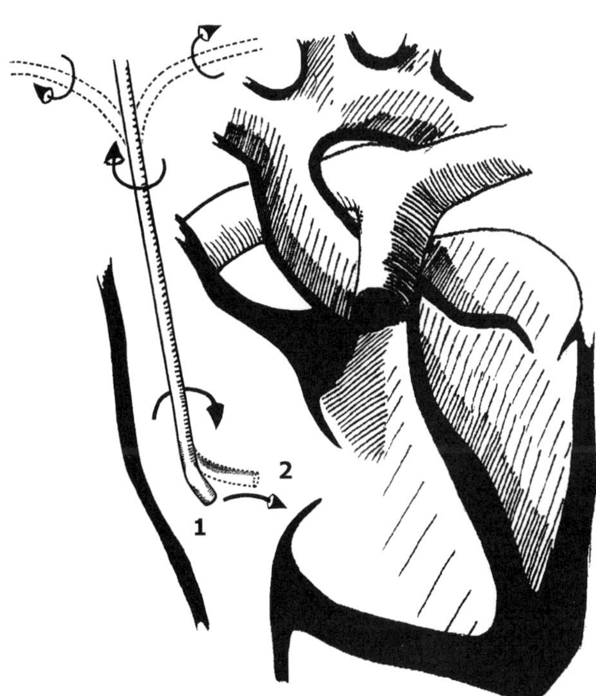

Figure 5.10 Catheter introduced from the neck (superior vena cava) with the tip of the catheter initially directed posteriorly. *Clockwise* rotation directs the tip *medially* (to patient's left and toward tricuspid valve).

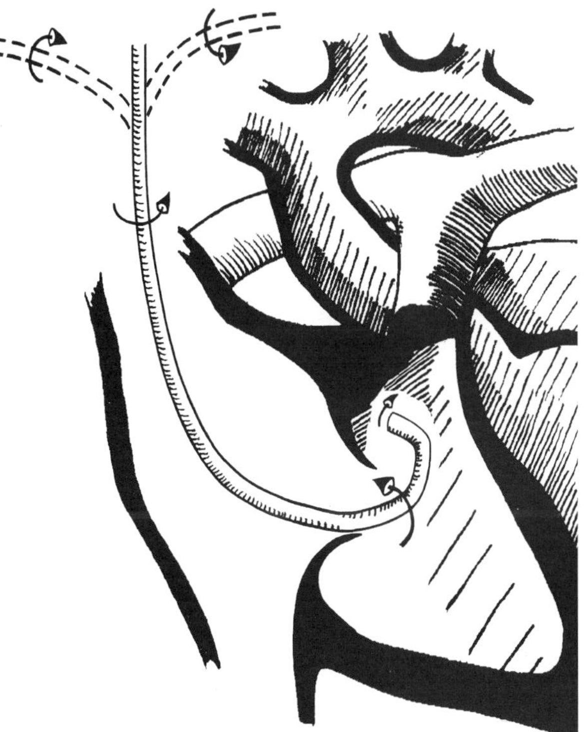

Figure 5.12 Catheter entering the right atrium from the superior vena cava and looping 180° toward the patient's left and into the right ventricle with the tip of the catheter pointing toward the patient's right. A counterclockwise torque on the proximal catheter rotates the tip posteriorly.

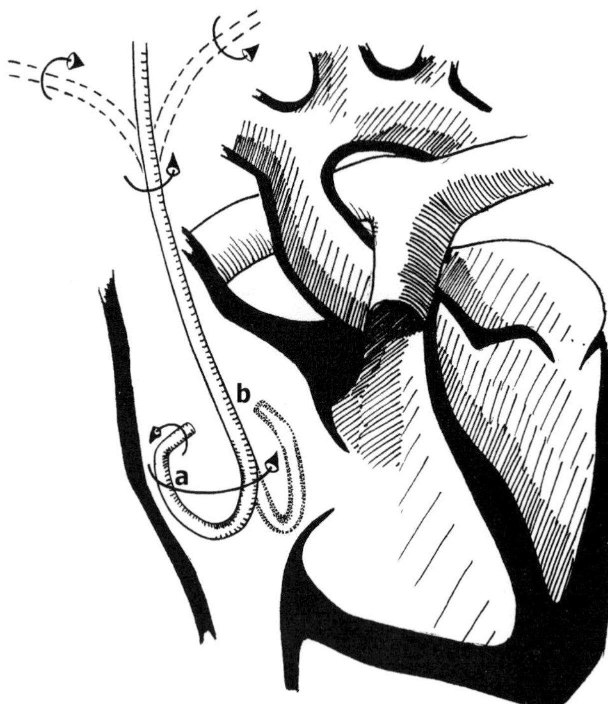

Figure 5.13 A catheter introduced via the superior vena cava with a 180° loop which is initially directed laterally (position a), when torqued counterclockwise rotates the loop medially and anteriorly while the separate curved tip faces posteriorly (position b).

Very common specific catheter manipulations

Right atrium to superior vena cava

A common and simple, but at the same time often one of the more frustrating catheter maneuvers for the novice, is advancing a catheter which is introduced from the femoral approach through the right atrium and into the superior vena cava (SVC). This is simplified by a thorough knowledge of the anatomy of the right atrium, the inferior vena cava (IVC) and the SVC and, in particular, knowledge of where the cavae enter the atrium. The IVC and a catheter entering the right atrium from the IVC is directed slightly anteriorly from a relatively posterior entrance into the right atrium. The SVC enters the cephalad area of the right atrium and posterior to the right atrial appendage. Straight probing with a catheter from the femoral approach directs the catheter anteriorly and into the right atrial appendage. In order to enter the SVC, the catheter with a slight curve at the tip is directed toward the lateral wall of the right atrium (the patient's right). While moving the catheter to and fro gently but rapidly, the catheter is gradually rotated counterclockwise in slight increments as it is advanced forward. This rotates the curved tip of the catheter posteriorly off the anterolateral, and then the lateral wall of the right atrium and into the SVC. The posterior/lateral direction and any unusual or unexpected location of the tip of the catheter are verified intermittently (and repeatedly when in doubt) with very brief "taps" on the lateral fluoroscope. Once a catheter with a slightly curved tip has entered the SVC, the curved catheter is easily directed to the patient's left into the innominate vein, straight cephalad into the right jugular system or to the patient's right into the subclavian and axillary veins. As with other attempted catheter maneuvers, torquing does not turn or direct a *straight* tip of the catheter to either side. After one or two unsuccessful attempts with a straightened catheter, the redirection of the tip is accomplished using a curved, stiff end of a wire, an active deflector wire within the catheter or a new catheter in order to have some curve on its tip.

Crossing from right atrium to left atrium through an atrial septal defect or patent foramen ovale

Although considered a straightforward, almost automatic maneuver for individuals routinely using torque-controlled catheters and particularly with biplane fluoroscopy, crossing the atrial septum, even through a pre-existing defect, can be a challenge for operators who are familiar only with floating balloon catheters or who do not have access to biplane fluoroscopy—i.e. in the adult catheterization laboratory where it becomes necessary to cross the patent foramen ovale. Familiarity with the anatomy of the right atrium and of the atrial septum is essential. The foramen ovale/secundum atrial septal defect is located in the mid to lower half of the atrial septum and on the posterior–anterior (PA) image of the heart, at the junction of approximately the lower and middle thirds of the length (height) of the right atrial shadow. Biplane fluoroscopy makes maneuvers across the septum very simple, safer and much quicker (almost automatic).

As a catheter with a slight curve at the tip enters the right atrium from the inferior vena cava, it is often "automatically" directed posteriorly and toward the patient's left—i.e. directly at the atrial septum, and in the presence of an atrial septal communication, directly into the left atrium, in which case the catheter will advance cephalad and toward the left heart border with absolutely no resistance. The position is checked in both the posterior–anterior and lateral fluoroscopy planes and confirmed with a blood sample for blood oxygen determination. If the catheter does not pass "automatically" from the right atrium into the left atrium, then some specific maneuvers may be required.

Occasionally a catheter that is introduced from the inferior vena cava is initially directed anteriorly, which, in turn, directs the tip toward the right atrial appendage and directly away from the posterior interatrial septum. The catheter is advanced in the right atrium until it stops, which usually happens in the appendage. Even without biplane, the location becomes obvious as the tip of the catheter will move considerably from side to side. Starting from this location, the catheter is simultaneously withdrawn and rotated counterclockwise very slightly with constant to-and-fro movements on the catheter until the tip of the catheter is positioned in the low right atrium. The tip should be facing medially toward the patient's left. If the withdrawn tip ends up directed laterally toward the patient's right, continuous, fairly rapid, to-and-fro movements, along with gentle counterclockwise torque, are continued on the shaft of the catheter until the tip rotates and *just* begins to face medially (toward the patient's left). With the tip maintained facing posteriorly and toward the patient's left, the catheter is advanced cephalad until it either enters the left atrium or until it stops on some structure within the right atrium and begins to bow or buckle. When the advancing catheter stops in the right atrium, the position of the tip is checked on biplane fluoroscopy. When there is no lateral (LAT) fluoroscopy to check the anterior–posterior position of the tip, the catheter is withdrawn and the entire maneuver is repeated until the tip of the catheter does enter the left atrium.

Occasionally, in the presence of a patent foramen ovale with a long septum primum which creates a long tunnel, the tip of the catheter will catch on the limbus of the foramen and begin to buckle or bend rather than "sliding" through the foramen (Figure 5.14a). Continued pushing on the catheter causes its shaft to bow further into the right atrium, which creates a perpendicular angle of the tip of the catheter to the actual tract of the foramen (Figure 5.14b). In the PA view (and LAT view, when available), the tip of the catheter appears to be in the proper location for the foramen. A small, hand injection, angiogram (biplane!) should be performed to confirm the location. When the catheter is caught on the limbus, it is withdrawn very slightly and rotated in order to straighten its shaft slightly and align its tip more cephalad and in line with the "tunnel", rather than horizontally (Figure 5.14c). Then, while the tip is still caught on the limbus, the catheter is torqued clockwise as it is advanced gently. These maneuvers should rotate the tip of the catheter under the limbus and through any "tunnel" in the foramen. Repeat small biplane angiograms are invaluable to verify the position of the tip of the catheter during all of these maneuvers.

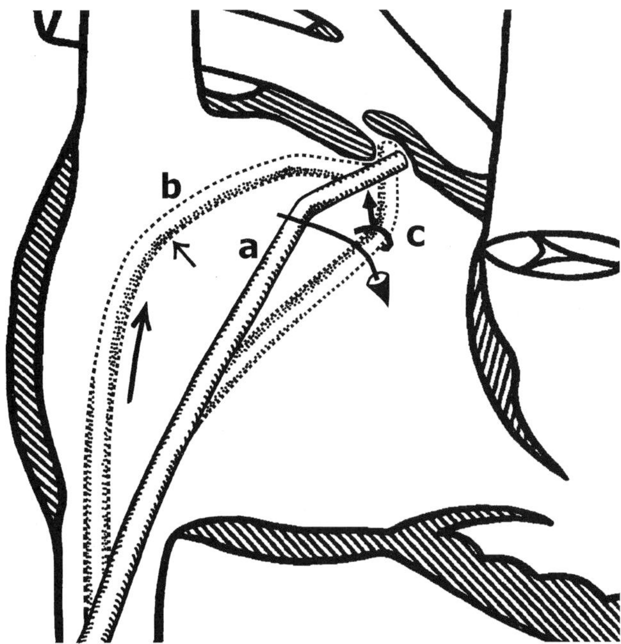

Figure 5.14 Maneuvers to cross a patent foramen ovale. Tip of catheter beneath the limbus but against the septum primum of the foramen (position a); continued straight "push" on the shaft of the catheter bows the shaft into the right atrium and directs the tip of the catheter perpendicular to the "opening" of the tunnel (position b); catheter tip rotated to align tip with tunnel (position c).

Right atrium to right ventricle

Probably the most common catheter maneuver within the heart, but another challenge for the newcomer using a torque-controlled catheter, is the manipulation of the catheter from the right atrium to the right ventricle and from there into the pulmonary artery. In a normal sized heart and with an appropriate, short "right-angle" curve at the tip of the catheter, when the catheter is introduced from the femoral vein and directed anteriorly and toward the *patient's* left, it almost "falls" into the right ventricle. However, if the catheter is straight or becomes straightened in the warm circulation, or when the right atrium is enlarged, this otherwise straightforward maneuver can become a challenge. Remembering that torquing a straight shaft does not redirect the tip at all, the first step is to form some curve on the distal end / tip of the catheter as described earlier in this chapter.

A very fleeting or temporary curve can be formed on the catheter while it is still within the heart. The straightened tip of the soft catheter is caught on, or "embedded" *gently* into, any structure within the right atrium (e.g. the lateral wall, the cephalad roof or even the right atrial appendage) and advanced slightly (and gently) until a slight curve is formed within the right atrium on the distal end of the catheter just proximal to the tip of the catheter. A bolus of room temperature (cool) flush solution, when flushed through the catheter, very temporarily fixes the curve which was formed at the distal end of the catheter. With this new curve formed and fixed by the flush, the flush is stopped, the catheter is withdrawn *rapidly* from its embedded position and redirected toward the tricuspid or other desired orifice. This "fixation" of the curve on the catheter is very fleeting and lasts only 5–10 seconds. As a consequence the new maneuver toward the right ventricle must be performed within the 5–10 seconds before the

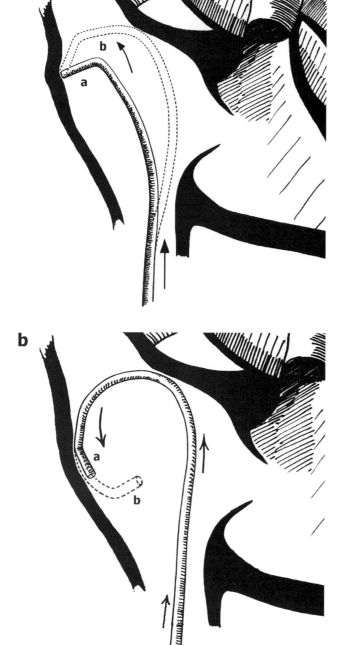

Figure 5.15 (a) Forming a 180° loop in RA from inferior vena cava approach. Tip of catheter purposefully caught on septal wall (position a); catheter advanced with tip caught begins to bow shaft of catheter into broad curve (position b). (b) Final formation of 180° loop in RA. Continued pushing against the initial curve (position a) enlarges initial curve into 180° loop (position b).

catheter loses its new temporary curve and becomes straight again. Multiple quick attempts are more effective than a single methodical, slow maneuver during these 5–10 seconds.

If this technique is not effective and the right ventricle still cannot be entered directly with the straight catheter, another choice is to form a large 180° loop on the catheter within the right atrium. The large 180° loop is formed by catching the tip of the catheter on any structure within the atrium (Figure 5.15a) or even in the liver, and then pushing the soft, straight catheter gently against this resistance within the atrium until the catheter bows and a long 180° curve is formed on the shaft of the catheter within the right atrium (Figure 5.15b). If a 180° loop is not formed with the first attempt, the catheter is flushed, the tip of the catheter is caught again against the lateral wall and bowed again, increasing the size of the loop on the catheter within the atrium. This is repeated until a 180° loop has been formed.

The entire loop, which is directed laterally and caudally (Figure 5.16a), is rotated by *clockwise* torque combined with short to-and-fro motions on the proximal catheter until the distal end of the loop in the catheter, which is still in the right atrium, is pointing medially, to the patient's left and toward the tricuspid valve (Figure 5.16b). The separate, short, curved tip of the catheter is usually pointing caudally, to the patient's right and away from the tricuspid valve. By withdrawing the shaft of the catheter slightly, the loop in the right atrium begins to open and the distal end and the tip of the catheter usually move further medially and drop well into the right ventricle (Figure 5.17).

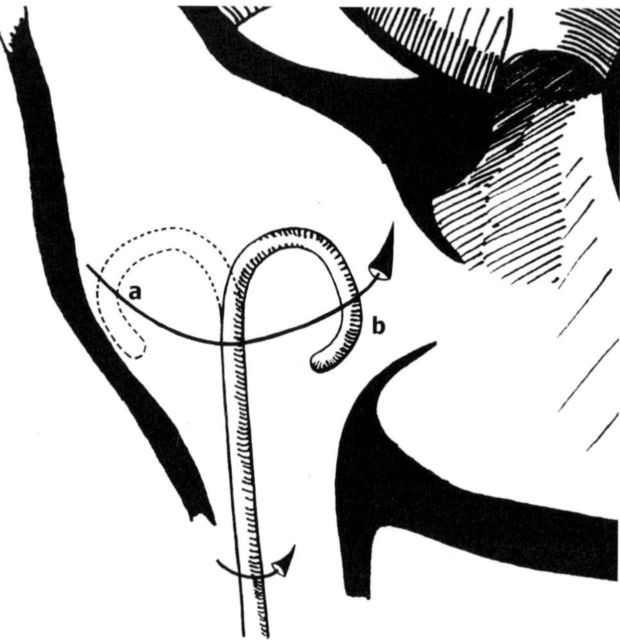

Figure 5.16 Rotation of 180° loop in atrium. Initial lateral direction of 180° loop after forming (position a); position of loop after 180° lateral rotation of entire loop (position b).

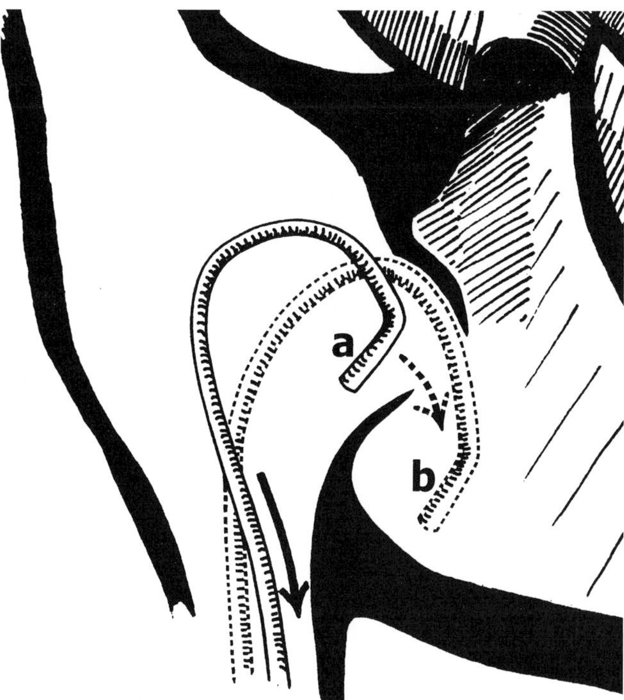

Figure 5.17 Maneuver of loop from right atrium to right ventricle. Loop directed medially with tip of catheter against tricuspid apparatus (position a); careful slight withdrawal of proximal catheter allows loop to open slightly and drop into the right ventricle (position b).

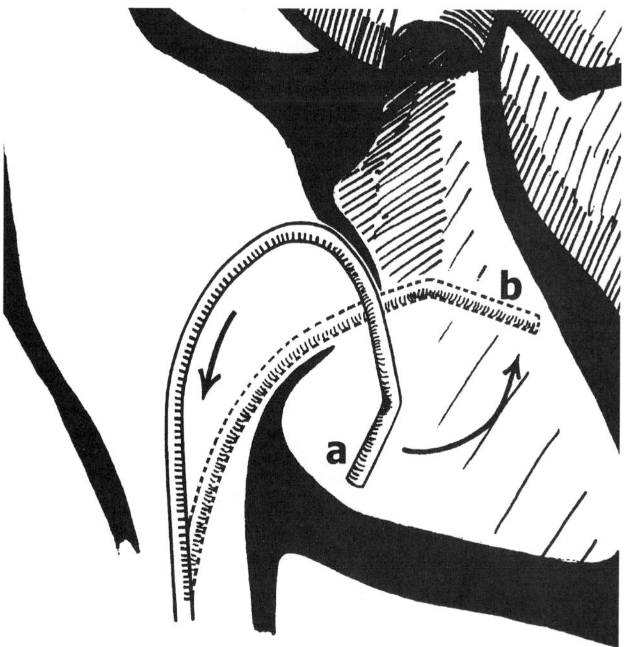

Figure 5.18 "Straightening" the 180° loop in RV. Position of tip of catheter in RV after rotating 180° loop into ventricle (position a); straightening of catheter across RV by withdrawing shaft of catheter (position b).

If none of these maneuvers facilitates entrance into the right ventricle and after no more than two or three attempts, the most reliable means of advancing a catheter from the right atrium to the right ventricle is with the use of a deflector wire as described in the next chapter (Chapter 6). When there is a large dilated right atrium or ventricle or when the catheter is relatively straight to begin with, experienced operators often resort to one of the deflector-wire techniques as the very first alternative in order to accomplish an expedient entrance into the right ventricle before attempting any "flailing" around in a large right atrium.

Right ventricle to pulmonary artery

After maneuvering the 180° loop into the right ventricle, the next step of turning the tip of the catheter cephalad and maneuvering a catheter from the right ventricle into the pulmonary artery is often a very significant challenge, particularly when the tip of the catheter has become straight or soft. Significant dilation of the right atrium and/or the right ventricle also makes this maneuver more difficult. Maneuvering into the pulmonary artery is considerably more straightforward when the catheter has retained some of the stiffness of its shaft and some of the right-angle curve at its distal end.

When the catheter does enter the right ventricle, particularly from the femoral approach and after rotating a 180° loop from the right atrium into the ventricle, the tip of the catheter is usually directed caudally and toward the apex of the right ventricle (Figure 5.18a). This caudal curve can usually be straightened somewhat and directed laterally (patient's left) and toward the septal wall of the ventricle by withdrawing the catheter in small increments while continuing small to-and-fro movements and small rotations of the proximal shaft of the catheter (Figure 5.18b). Clockwise torque is applied to the catheter while all of the time using tiny, to-and-fro motions on the proximal shaft of the catheter. The to-and-fro motions allow the shaft of the catheter within the body to rotate freely and keep the tip moving in and out of the many trabeculations in the right ventricle, while the torquing rotates the curved tip *posteriorly* along the septal wall of the right ventricle (Figure 5.19, a and b). With the tendency of the catheter to straighten and point cephalad, the continued torque along with the to-and-fro motion "walks" a curved tip of a catheter up the posterior, septal wall of the right ventricle, over the crista and into the posteriorly directed pulmonary artery (Figure 5.19c).

Occasionally, with a large and hypertrophied right ventricle or in the presence of an inlet (atrioventricular canal) type ventricular septal defect, the initial rotation of the catheter needs to be *counterclockwise* instead of the usual clockwise. In the presence of a very large crista, the tip of

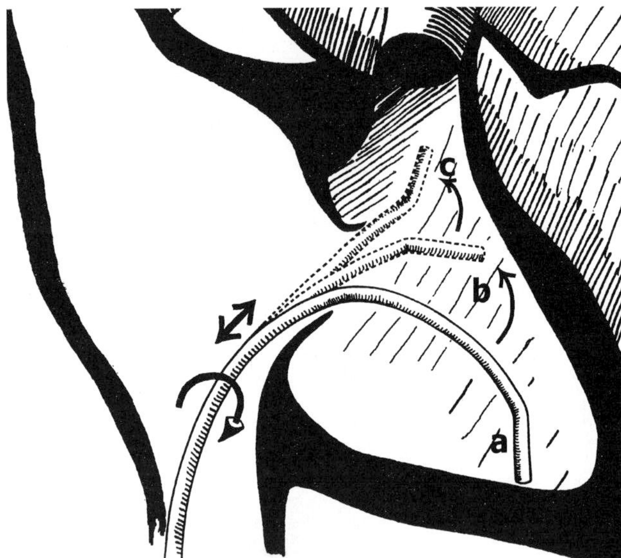

Figure 5.19 "Walking" catheter from IVC up wall of RV. Catheter tip in apex of RV (position a); catheter tip advanced cephalad along septal wall of RV (position b); catheter tip rotated and advanced further cephalad into right ventricular outflow tract (position c).

the catheter must first be rotated anteriorly and out from under the crista with the counterclockwise rotations of the shaft of the catheter. Once the tip of the catheter has "popped" anteriorly and out from under the crista, the catheter is advanced while the rotation of the catheter shaft is simultaneously reversed to a *clockwise* direction. This redirects the curved tip from facing anteriorly to posteriorly and cephalad (and over the crista) toward the pulmonary valve.

In the presence of a significant inlet ventricular septal defect, there is no posterior wall of the right ventricular septum. The usual clockwise rotation of the shaft of the catheter turns the curved tip posteriorly in the right ventricle and, as a consequence, directs the tip back through the atrioventricular valve and usually directly into the left atrium. In the presence of an inlet ventricular septal defect, once the tip of the catheter has been advanced from the right atrium into the right ventricle, the *initial* torque on the shaft of the catheter along with the usual short to-and-fro forward motions should be *counterclockwise*. This maneuver will "walk" the curved tip anteriorly, over the free wall trabeculations of the right ventricle, cephalad and toward the patient's left. Once the tip has advanced as far as possible cephalad and laterally in the ventricle, the torque on the catheter is reversed to clockwise along with the continued to-and-fro motions, in order to redirect the tip posteriorly, over the crista and toward the main pulmonary artery.

When the right ventricle is very large or there is not a good curve on the end of the catheter, then various wires or deflector techniques (Chapter 6) are used to manipulate the catheter from the right ventricle into the pulmonary artery.

Utilizing purposeful loops on the catheter for manipulations

With advanced skill and familiarity with specific catheters, their feel and their characteristics, large loops formed on the catheter can be used to the operator's advantage for entering difficult locations. When loops are formed, the operator must be sure that the shaft of the catheter is *free in the particular chamber* and *has room to bend or loop* within the particular cavity or large vessel when forward force is applied to the proximal end of the catheter. Otherwise, if the shaft of the catheter is constrained, the forward force applied to make the bend or loop will be directed *only in line* with, and *to the tip of*, the catheter (and possibly through the heart or vessel wall!). Several examples of the use of these back loops are detailed:

1 The use of a large 180° loop formed in the right atrium to enter the right ventricle was described previously in this chapter. Starting with the tip of the catheter against the lateral wall of the atrium as described previously, and with care taken that the catheter tip is against a free wall and not burrowed into the right atrial appendage, a loop is formed by advancing a soft catheter against the resist-ance of the wall (Figure 5.15 a, b). Once the loop is formed and using continual, fine, to-and-fro motions of the catheter, the *shaft* of the catheter is torqued either clockwise or counterclockwise until the *whole loop* of the catheter rotates (Figure 5.16). The tip and the whole loop of the catheter are observed intermittently in *both* the PA and LAT fluoroscopic planes during the entire rotation. As long as the tip remains free, the catheter is rotated in small increments until the *loop* rotates 180°, resulting in the distal curve of the catheter's facing anteriorly and to the *patient's* left, and usually, as a consequence, the actual *tip* will be pointing away from the tricuspid valve. Once the distal loop is directed toward the valve, the loop tends to open and direct the distal end and the tip toward the tricuspid valve, in which case the catheter's shaft is alternately advanced and withdrawn slightly, which, in turn, pushes the tip caudally and through the tricuspid valve and into the right ventricle (Figure 5.17). Usually the tip of the catheter continues caudally and anteriorly toward the apex of the right ventricle. Once the tip has been secured in the apex, the shaft of the catheter is withdrawn slowly until the 180° curve in the shaft of the more proximal catheter within the right atrium straightens gradually, while at the same time still keeping the tip of the catheter within the right ventricle (Figure 5.18). As the catheter straightens and courses directly from the IVC to the right

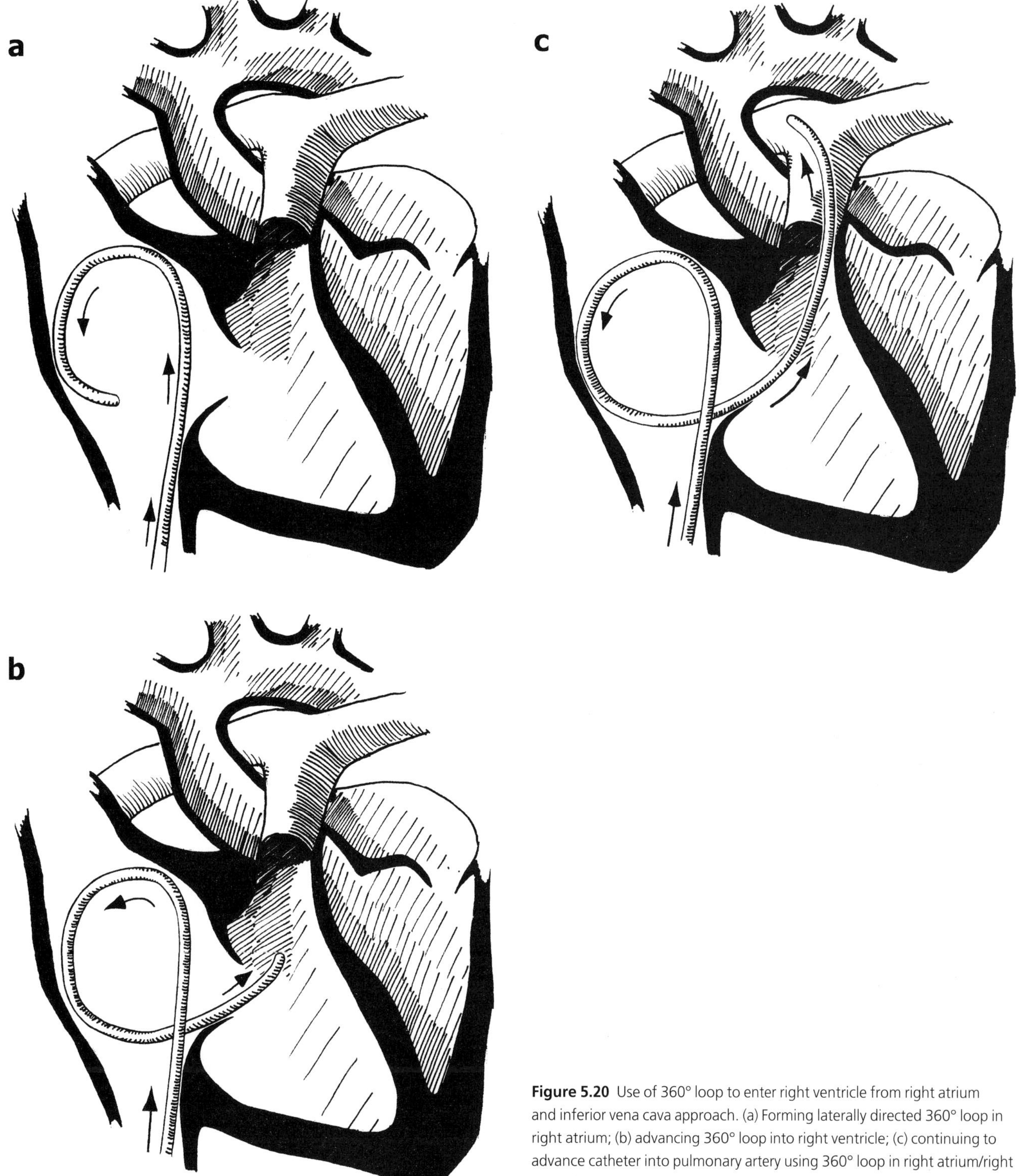

Figure 5.20 Use of 360° loop to enter right ventricle from right atrium and inferior vena cava approach. (a) Forming laterally directed 360° loop in right atrium; (b) advancing 360° loop into right ventricle; (c) continuing to advance catheter into pulmonary artery using 360° loop in right atrium/right ventricle.

ventricle, the tip becomes directed cephalad and more toward the outflow tract (Figure 5.19).

2 A large 360° loop formed on the catheter in a very large right atrium can be used to enter the right ventricle/ pulmonary artery. The tip of the catheter is maintained pointing laterally in the right atrium (toward the patient's right) when forming the atrial loop. By continuing to advance the catheter in the right atrium with this "laterally

directed" loop, the catheter eventually approaches a complete 360° loop within the atrium. This loop, which began heading toward the lateral wall of the right atrium, now directs the distal end of the loop and the tip medially, toward the patient's *left* and roughly toward the tricuspid valve (Figure 5.20a). With the proximal *loop* still directed to the patient's *right* in the atrium, the catheter shaft is moved to and fro further and, if necessary, torqued slightly, in which case the tip of the catheter becomes directed *toward the patient's left, slightly anteriorly* and toward the tricuspid valve. Further simultaneous torque and fine to-and-fro motion on the catheter direct the tip across the tricuspid valve and into the right ventricle, now with the curved tip directed cephalad (Figure 5.20b). By advancing the catheter further, the tip advances directly into the great artery which arises cephalad off the right ventricle (Figure 5.20c).

3 Similarly, the coronary sinus is entered more easily from the femoral approach with a loop formed on the catheter in the right atrium similar to the 360° loop which has just been described. With the tip directed laterally (to the patient's right) and slightly anteriorly when forming the right atrial loop, as the catheter is advanced further in the right atrium, the catheter again completes a 360° loop. However, by reversing the previous torque on the catheter as it is advanced, the torque results in the distal portion of the loop and the tip of the catheter pointing posteriorly. When advanced further with very slight torque and to-and-fro motions, the tip enters the coronary sinus and is directed in the course of the coronary sinus. Lateral fluoroscopy is extremely helpful (essential) in accomplishing this maneuver. The 360° loop is useful as a way of entering the coronary sinus, particularly for performing electrophysiologic procedures. This entry into the coronary sinus may occur inadvertently during attempts at entering the right ventricle with the 360° loop and should be considered when the distal portion and the tip of the catheter are constrained in their lateral movement.

4 When attempting to advance a catheter from the femoral approach, even with the catheter passing straight from the right atrium into the right ventricle and into the pulmonary artery, entrance into the right pulmonary artery is often difficult to negotiate, particularly when the catheter has straightened and/or when there is a large dilated right ventricle. The right pulmonary artery has a more proximal take-off and is even more acutely angled off a dilated or displaced main pulmonary artery. With the tip of the catheter fixed against the wall in the main pulmonary artery, the soft catheter can be carefully and continually advanced against the resistance of the tip until a curve, and eventually a 360° back loop, is formed on the more proximal shaft of the catheter, which is still in the right atrium. This 360° loop on the more proximal shaft of the catheter redirects the tip of the catheter, which, hopefully, is still in the pulmonary artery, toward the patient's right and caudally. Further advancing the catheter with this 360° loop directs the tip from the main pulmonary artery into the right pulmonary artery. A 360° loop formed in the right atrium initially as described above in (2) (Figure 5.20c) often produces the same effect on the tip of the catheter after it enters the main pulmonary artery, directing the tip slightly more rightward and caudally and, in turn, directly into the right pulmonary artery.

5 Although it is safer and more direct to use a preformed, stiff end of a wire to deflect the tip of a catheter from the atrium into the ventricle, occasionally it is desirable to back a loop that is more proximal on the shaft of the catheter, through the atrioventricular (AV) valve. In this way, the tip of the catheter, which is following the more proximal loop into the ventricle, will be facing the opposite direction from the loop entering the ventricle. By "backing" a narrow 180° loop at the distal end of the catheter into the ventricle, the tip of the catheter "follows" the loop into the ventricle and will be directed toward the outflow tract and the semilunar valve. A loop can be backed into either ventricle through either atrioventricular valve from the connected atrium using a relatively soft, easily bendable catheter (any woven dacron catheter after it has been in the body more than 15 minutes).

To create the initial loop in the left atrium, the tip of the soft catheter is directed against the cephalad and either right or left wall of the left atrium. The catheter is slowly and carefully advanced against this fixed tip of the catheter. This creates a slight loop or bow in the catheter shaft just proximal to the tip and within the left atrium. The loop usually forms caudally and toward the AV valve. Further advance of the proximal end of the catheter bows the catheter and pushes the loop through the atrio-ventricular valve into the ventricle. It is usually necessary to stiffen or support the apex of the loop in the catheter with the stiff end of a spring guide wire with a very slight and long curve formed on the stiff end of the wire (see Chapter 6). As the loop that is near the distal end of the catheter advances into the ventricle, the tip follows the loop into the ventricle (with or without the help of a stiff wire) but now with the tip pointing "backward" or cephalad. Once in the ventricle, the loop of the catheter is pushed toward the apex by slight rotation of the catheter or loop while the tip is still directed toward the outflow tract. As the catheter is advanced further into the ventricle or is advanced off the supporting wire, the tip advances away from the apex of the loop and through the more cephalad semilunar valve arising from the ventricle.

6 When the catheter is introduced from a superior vena cava approach, a loop is often formed in the right atrium

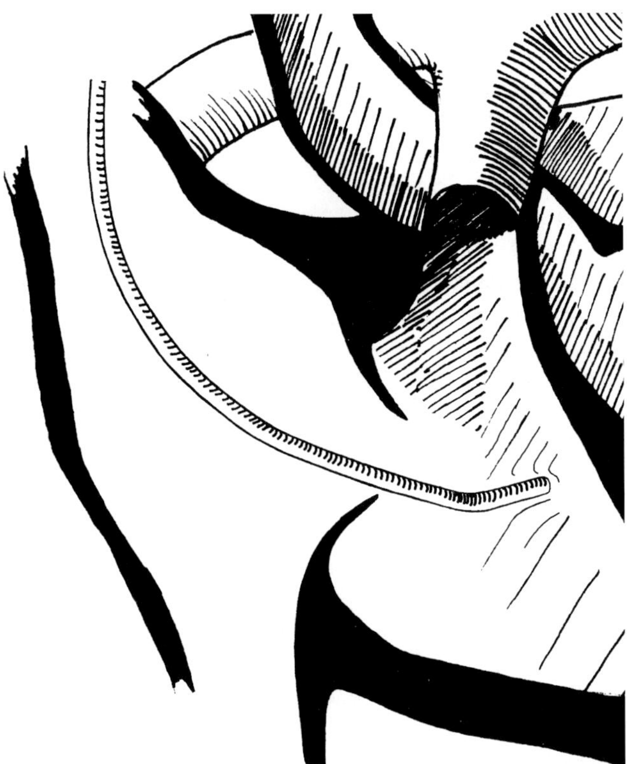

Figure 5.21 Catheter introduced via the superior vena cava passed directly from the right atrium into the right ventricle and apex of the ventricle.

in order to advance a catheter from the right atrium into the right ventricle and, from there, into the pulmonary artery. With a catheter introduced from the jugular, subclavian or brachial vein, it usually passes directly from the superior vena cava, through the tricuspid valve and into the apex of the right ventricle (Figure 5.21). From this position and when directed caudally toward the apex, the tip of the catheter can seldom be manipulated toward the right ventricular outflow tract and into the pulmonary artery without significant or traumatic manipulations or the use of deflector wires. This is particularly difficult when the catheter has straightened or has become very soft.

As an alternative, the tip of the catheter is initially directed from the superior vena cava toward and against the lateral wall of the right atrium. By further advancing the catheter, a large 180+° loop is formed within the right atrium until the tip of the catheter is pointing cephalad (Figure 5.22a). By rotating the whole 180+° loop in the catheter (Figure 5.22b), the tip of the catheter is rotated in the right atrium from laterally to medially and toward the tricuspid valve (Figure 5.22c). With this rotation, the distal end of the loop and the tip of the catheter tend to flop through the tricuspid valve, with the tip of the catheter pointing directly at the right ventricular outflow tract/pulmonary artery (Figure 5.22d). Advancing the catheter with minimal torque or manipulation pushes the tip of the catheter into the main and usually the right pulmonary arteries, usually without the use of deflectors or other wires (Figure 5.22e).

7 Loops are occasionally made in the great arteries in order to redirect the tip of the catheter 180° (or more) for selective entrance into side branches, which arise at very acute angles off the central vessel. Such loops are used for entering the brachiocephalic branches off the aortic arch, for entering collaterals off the descending aorta, and for entering branch pulmonary arteries. Usually, for these purposes, a 180+° loop is formed with an active deflector wire within a very soft catheter as described in Chapter 6. The loop is formed distal to the origin of the branch/side vessel to be entered. Once the loop has been formed, the catheter with the loop maintained in its distal end is withdrawn within the central vessel until the "backward facing" tip is drawn into the side vessel. Once the tip catches in the orifice of the branch vessel, as the catheter is withdrawn further, the tip of the catheter will advance at least for a short distance into the side vessel.

8 Loops in the distal end of a catheter introduced from a retrograde approach can be used to cross the semilunar valve from the aorta. Occasionally, the tip of the retrograde catheter continually drops into the sinus of the semilunar valve and, even without stenosis of the semilunar valve, will not pass readily through the valve. When the catheter has become very soft, often a loop will form at the distal end of the catheter when the tip is pushed into the sinus of the semilunar valve. Such a loop will direct the tip of the catheter cephalad and away from the semilunar valve. In that circumstance, the valve orifice can be probed with the loop in the catheter, which extends several centimeters in front of the tip of the catheter. The apex of this loop now extends across the lumen of the aorta, which centers the apex of the loop across the center of the valve annulus, which, in turn, allows the loop to pass through the central orifice of the valve.

9 A loop that has passed retrograde through the semilunar valve is very useful for purposefully crossing a perimembranous and/or high muscular interventricular septal defect and for entering and crossing the semilunar valve arising from the ventricle on the opposite side of the ventricular septal defect[2]. As a loop at the distal tip of the catheter is backed through the semilunar valve into the ventricle, the tip of the catheter tends to align transversely across the outflow tract. By torquing the catheter and, in turn, rotating the loop very slightly in the outflow tract, the tip of the catheter will flop through the ventricular septal defect while still *tending* to point somewhat cephalad. When the catheter is advanced with the curve at the distal end passing through, and resting on, the lower margin of the ventricular septal defect, the tip is

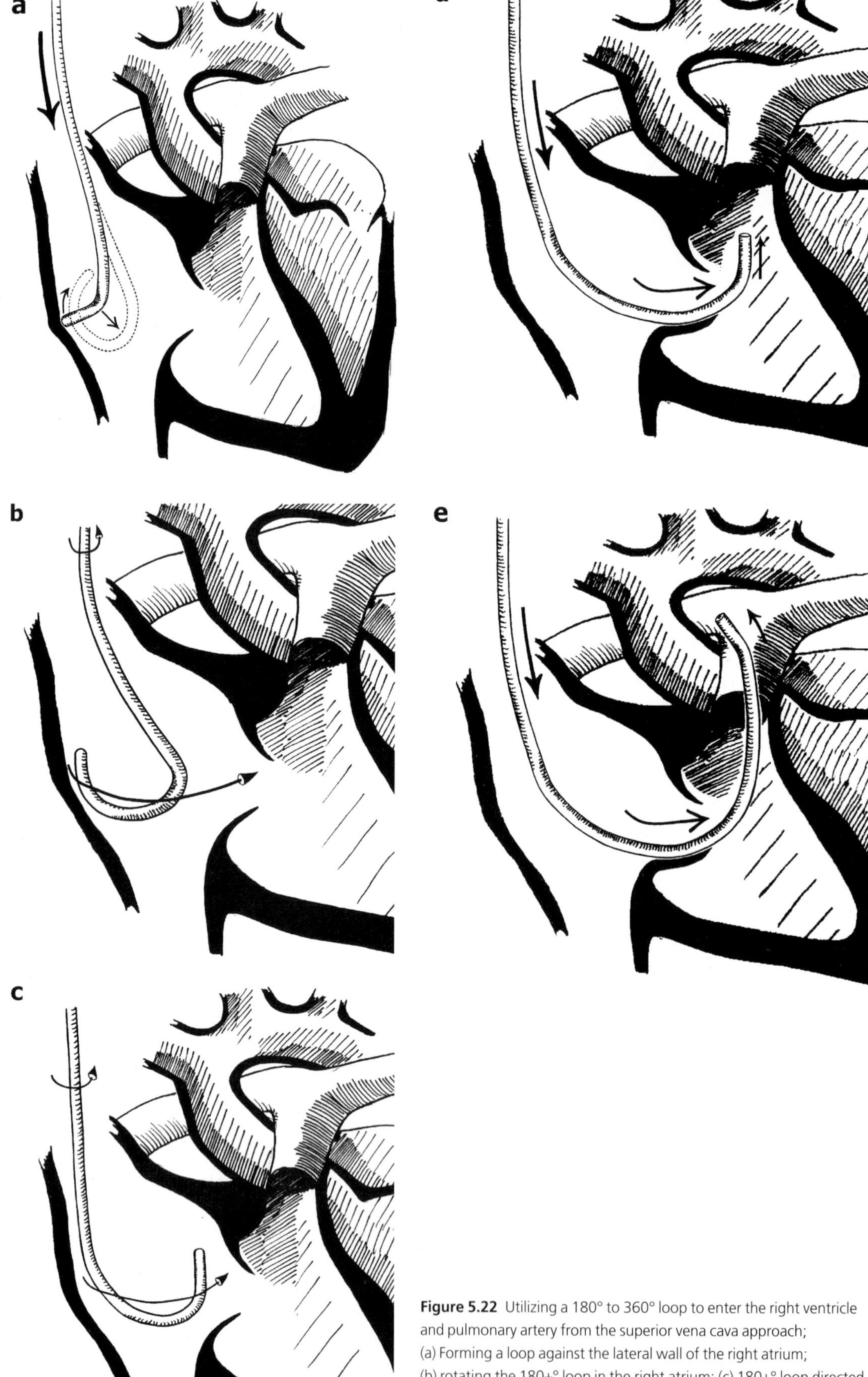

Figure 5.22 Utilizing a 180° to 360° loop to enter the right ventricle and pulmonary artery from the superior vena cava approach; (a) Forming a loop against the lateral wall of the right atrium; (b) rotating the 180+° loop in the right atrium; (c) 180+° loop directed toward tricuspid valve after rotation; (d) loop advanced into right ventricle and directed toward RVOT; (e) loop advanced into main pulmonary artery.

directed further cephalad and into the semilunar valve at the other side of the ventricular septal defect.

If the loop was not backed through the semilunar valve, and in order to manipulate the tip of the catheter through a ventricular septal defect and/or into the semilunar valve on the opposite side of the defect, a loop or curve can be formed at the tip of the catheter with an active deflector wire while the tip of the catheter is in the outflow tract of the ventricle just below the semilunar valve. This is described in Chapter 6, "Guide and Deflector Wires".

Non pressure monitored catheter manipulations

In exceptional occasions and in experienced hands, the catheter can be disconnected from the proximal flush/ pressure line and capped with a syringe, while very specific and complex maneuvers of the catheter are being performed. This removes the additional resistance to torque caused by the connecting tubing at the proximal end of the catheter but, at the same time, removes the protection and reassurance of knowing exactly where the catheter tip is located, which are provided by the monitored and visualized pressure from the tip of the catheter. This technique is most commonly utilized when manipulating the tip of the catheter within large veins or great arteries in order to cannulate side vessels very selectively. It is the preferred technique for the selective cannulation of the coronary arteries. This technique is used only when the catheter is moving very freely within the sheath and vascular system so that all movements and all sensations of resistance are transmitted from the tip and the shaft of the catheter to the fingers which are maneuvering the catheter. The capping syringe on the proximal hub of the catheter is filled with contrast material, which is used to perform small injections of contrast periodically in order to confirm the position of the tip of the catheter. Only very experienced and skilled operators should attempt this technique when it is utilized for manipulation within cardiac chambers.

Since even more precise and difficult maneuvers of the catheter can be accomplished using deflector wires within the catheter, catheters are often detached from the pressure/monitoring system when wires are used in the catheter to deflect the tip. With most catheter/wire combinations, pressures can still be obtained simultaneously while there is a wire in the catheter by introducing the wire through a wire back-bleed valve with a flush port and attaching the flush port to the pressure system. When a tight, Tuohy™ type of valved/side port is used with a Mullins™ deflector wire, very accurate pressures can be recorded while the wire is in place in the catheter. The techniques, advantages and dangers of the deflector wire techniques are detailed in Chapter 6 on "Guide Wires and Deflection Techniques".

Preformed catheters

There are thousands of different catheters available, most of which have very special, fixed, preformed curves at their distal ends for the purpose of selectively cannulating very specific vessels or orifices. Many of these catheters are in the standard armamentarium of the adult catheterization and the vascular radiology laboratories. These catheters are extremely effective for the cannulation of specific vessels and particularly in a usual sized patient where the basic structures and anatomy are located normally and predictably. Unfortunately, none of these prerequisites apply very often in pediatric/congenital heart patients. Preformed catheters are often useful in a pediatric/congenital patient, but are usually used in an entirely different location or for an entirely different purpose than that for which the specific curve was designed and manufactured.

Even preformed coronary catheters, which make cannulation of the coronary arteries in the adult patient an almost automatic and unconscious procedure, are usually not very useful for cannulation of the coronary arteries in children and congenital patients. The different diameters of the aortic root, the markedly different lengths from the aortic sinuses to the aortic arch in younger patients, and the frequent aortic arch and coronary artery anomalies in congenital heart patients compared to the usual adult coronary patient preclude the automatic use for even the coronary arteries in pediatric/congenital patients.

These same selective "coronary curves", however, are often useful for the selective cannulation of branch vessels off the descending aorta and off the main or the right or left pulmonary arteries. A small "right coronary artery curve" is very useful for directing a wire from the right ventricle to the exact center or opening of an atretic/ stenotic pulmonary valve. Once an abnormal and difficult course to an unusual location or a branch vessel is defined, there is often a preformed catheter that can facilitate the selective cannulation of that vessel/location with either the catheter itself or with a wire passed through the catheter. Unfortunately, it is impossible to maintain a complete or even a very large inventory of very many of these very specific catheters.

Complications of catheter manipulations

There are a very few complications that are a consequence of the *manipulation* alone of standard catheters. Certainly, direct perforation of a *vascular* and/or *cardiac structure* is a common fear, but in actuality it is extremely unusual and unlikely[3]. Most cardiac catheters that are manipulated within the heart or vascular system are somewhat "soft" and very flexible. As a consequence, when a catheter tip is forced into or against a structure and/or wall, the catheter shaft bends or bows to one side and dissipates any forward push or force sideways and away from the tip. The exception, when a catheter *can* be pushed through an intracardiac or vascular structure, is when the *shaft* of the catheter is *confined* or *restrained* within a vessel or chamber or has already bowed sideways to the limits of the walls within the chamber or vessel. In that circumstance, all additional forward force on the catheter will be transmitted longitudinally along the shaft of the catheter and directly to the tip of the catheter, which, in turn, can force the tip through a wall.

Perforation of a vessel by a catheter occurs most commonly in the peripheral venous system. In that area, the shaft of the catheter is constrained very tightly by the lateral walls of the small peripheral veins at the introductory site and, at the same time, the veins themselves are very thin walled, almost "friable", they have many small tributaries which arise tangentially, and the tributaries narrow rapidly when they are any distance from the main channel. This combination of factors makes it easy to trap the tip of a catheter in a branch/tributary and to deliver significant forward force to the tip because of the side-to-side restraint of the catheter within the small more central vein.

Other, more serious examples of vascular perforation occur when the tip of a catheter is wedged into an atrial appendage *in conjunction with* a 180–360° loop that has been formed on the shaft of the catheter and already extends around the widest circumference of the atrial chamber, or when the tip of the catheter is buried in a sinus of the aortic valve while the shaft of the catheter is pushed tightly against the outer circumference of the aortic arch. When additional force is applied to advance the catheter forward in either of these circumstances, the shaft of the catheter has no further lateral or side-to-side space to bow away from the force. As a consequence, all of the forward force is transmitted to the tip. These are rare circumstances which can be avoided by awareness of the potential problem, careful observation of the entire course of the catheter during all manipulations, and avoidance of all significant force applied to the catheter during manipulations. The management of cardiac wall perforations is covered in detail in the chapters dealing with specific procedures where perforations are more likely (Chapter 8, "Transseptal Technique" and Chapter 31, "Purposeful Perforations").

Probably the most common adverse event/complication of catheter manipulations is the creation of ectopic beats or sustained arrhythmias. Isolated, or even short, self-limited, runs of ectopic beats are a part of catheter manipulations within the heart! Fortunately most pediatric/congenital heart catheterizations, although in complex defects, are carried out in younger patients who have normal coronaries and *healthy myocardium*. In these patients, when ectopy does occur, it is not sustained nor does even a sustained arrhythmia usually result in a deterioration of the hemodynamics. When older or adult congenital heart patients are catheterized, they do not necessarily have this protection of underlying healthy myocardium and/or a margin of safety in their hemodynamic balance and, as a consequence, far mare attention must be paid to even isolated ectopic beats in such patients. Occasionally, an ectopic beat in a pediatric or congenital patient triggers a sustained run of tachycardia and very, very rarely, even fibrillation and/or heart block, any of which can cause hemodynamic instability. This can occur in any patient but is far more common in patients with myocardial disease, older patients, and patients with defects associated with ventricular inversion.

When a catheter manipulation does result in multiple ectopic beats, the manipulation is stopped and/or changed to allow the heart rhythm to stabilize. The appropriate medications and a defibrillator are always available. A printed medication sheet, which has the exact dose of each emergency medication pre-calculated in both milligrams and milliliters for each individual patient—as described in Chapter 2—certainly facilitates the rapid administration of medications. The defibrillator is preset for each individual patient at the onset of the procedure and is immediately available close to the catheterization table for the conversion of an arrhythmia.

Thrombi and/or air flushed from the catheter during the manipulation of any catheter creates the potential for catastrophic problems, but problems which should be avoidable. In many congenital heart patients, "right heart" catheterizations have the same potential for catastrophic *systemic* embolic phenomena as "left heart" manipulations because of the frequency of intracardiac communications and/or discordances. As a consequence, *all* catheterization procedures in pediatric/congenital heart patients are considered "systemic". Catheters are always allowed to bleed back and/or blood is withdrawn with an absolutely free flow before *anything* is introduced into and/or flushed through a catheter and/or sheath. Wires are always introduced into catheters through back-bleed valves with flush ports, and catheters with wires in them are maintained on a flush to keep thrombi from forming on the wire within the catheter. Pediatric/congenital heart patients undergoing cardiac catheterizations should all be systemically heparinized in order to reduce the likelihood of thrombi formation in catheters and/or on wires. When catheters are manipulated with guide or deflector wires within them, the procedures do become potentially more hazardous. The complications associated with wires are covered in Chapter 6.

Catheters easily can become kinked and even knotted unknowingly whenever loops or bends are formed in them, particularly when they are not observed closely. This occurs most commonly in the inferior vena cava when a very soft catheter is being manipulated against a curve and/or resistance within the heart and the inferior vena cava is out of the field of visualization. Knots and/or kinks occur most commonly with flow-directed balloon tipped catheters and woven dacron torque-controlled catheters, which become very soft in the warmth of the circulation. The treatment of kinks and knots is prevention. The catheterizing physician must always be aware of the presence of and the position of the *entire* catheter. A to-and-fro or rotational movement performed on the proximal catheter outside of the body should always be transmitted to a similar (identical!) movement at the tip of the catheter and in a "one to one" relationship. If the proximal end of the catheter is advanced 6 cm, the distal end and tip of the catheter within the cardiac/vascular silhouette should move forward a comparable 6 cm. When the proximal shaft of the catheter is rotated properly, the tip of the catheter within the heart/vasculature should rotate proportionately. Whenever these "one to one" movements of the proximal and distal ends of the catheter do not occur, the entire length of the catheter/wire should be visualized immediately.

A catheter with a "simple" kink or twist in its shaft usually can be straightened and/or withdrawn directly into and through the introductory sheath. If the kink or twist is the consequence of a prior 360° loop, the shaft of the catheter on one side of the twist becomes offset from the shaft at the other side of the twist, and cannot be withdrawn through a sheath of the same size without first "unwinding" the twist. "Unwinding" the kink or twist is accomplished by re-advancing the catheter and rotating the loop that has formed in the *opposite direction to the initial twist*—all very carefully and under direct vision. The stiff end of a spring guide wire with a slight 30–45° curve preformed at the stiff end is introduced into the twisted catheter and advanced to the area of the twist/kink. This curve on the wire is transferred to the shaft of the catheter and usually helps to begin opening the loop and unwinding the twist.

Usually, if a knot has not been tightened by totally *uncontrolled* maneuvering, it can be untied by advancing a spring guide wire into the catheter while simultaneously advancing the catheter in the area of the kink/knot. Either the soft end or a slightly curved stiff end of the wire, when advanced adjacent to the knot, is often sufficient to change the angle of the shaft of the catheter entering the knot enough to allow the straight portion of the catheter immediately adjacent to the knot to be pushed into, and loosen, the knot enough to begin untying it. If the knot cannot be loosened completely with the wire within the catheter itself, a second sheath is introduced into a separate vein and an end-hole catheter advanced to a position adjacent to the knot. A 0.025" tip deflector wire with a 1 cm curve at the tip is advanced through the second catheter. With the aid of *biplane* fluoroscopy, the tip of the wire is manipulated into and through the loop in the knot. Once the tip of the wire has advanced into the knot, the tip of the deflector wire is deflected tightly. This grasps one edge of the loop of the knot in the catheter, allowing the knot to be teased apart by the combination of pushing on the wire that is within the lumen of the knotted catheter while gently pulling on the loop of the knot with the separate deflector wire[4].

A third alternative for "untying" knots that have become very tight is to use a bioptome as the second catheter instead of the deflector wire. When a wire cannot be passed through a loop in the knot, one edge of the catheter within the knot is grasped with the jaws of the bioptome while pushing the knot apart with a stiff wire within the lumen of the knotted catheter. If a knot cannot be "untied", a significantly larger sheath is introduced into the second vein, the tip of the knotted catheter is grasped with a snare introduced through the larger sheath, and the knotted catheter is withdrawn into the larger sheath. Once the whole knot is within the larger sheath, the proximal end of the knotted catheter must be amputated to allow it to be withdrawn into the venous system and out through the larger sheath.

As with all complications, prevention is the best treatment. With catheter manipulations in particular, the proper handling and maneuvering of catheters can prevent most, if not all, complications.

References

1. Gensini GG. Positive torque control cardiac catheters. *Circulation* 1965; **32**(6): 932–935.
2. Mullins CE *et al.* Retrograde technique for catheterization of the pulmonary artery in transposition of the great arteries with ventricular septal defect. *Am J Cardiol* 1972; **30**(4): 385–387.
3. Lurie PR and Grajo MZ. Accidental cardiac puncture during right heart catheterization. *Pediatrics* 1962; **29**: 283–294.
4. Dumesnil JG and Proulx G. A new nonsurgical technique for untying tight knots in flow-directed balloon catheters. *Am J Cardiol* 1984; **53**(2): 395–396.

6 Special guide and deflector wires and techniques for their use

Introduction

There are numerous times when neither precise catheter manipulation utilizing a torque-controlled catheter or blood flow using a balloon flow-directed catheter will direct the catheter to a specific location. Even when the catheter starts with a preformed curve at the tip, the warm body temperature within the circulation tends to soften and, in turn, straighten the curves at the tip of many catheters. The repeated "pushing" of a *straight* catheter ("straight wire, catheter, anything"!!), even with a balloon at the tip, only results in the linear object advancing in a *straight line*. No matter how many pushes and rotations are attempted the straight tip does not change its direction. There is frequently the need for the tip of the catheter to "reverse" direction as much as, or even more than, 180° in order to cross a valve or enter a branch or side vessel. The importance of selectively entering stenotic, distal or branching vessels is intensified by the added necessity of securing extra stiff guide wires far distally in these vessels, which has become imperative with the advent of balloon dilation and intravascular stent implant in these lesions.

Fortunately, there is now a large variety of special wires to assist in directing the catheter precisely to the specific area, no matter how small and tortuous the course may be. With these special adjunct wires and the specific techniques for their use, there is little excuse for the statement "can't be entered" in the sophisticated biplane pediatric/congenital catheterization laboratory of the twenty-first century.

Back-bleed/flush devices for wires

All wires when used within a catheter should be used in conjunction with a valved wire back-bleed valve/flush device attached to the proximal end of the catheter in order to prevent blood loss and to allow flushing to prevent thrombosis around the wire. This is vitally important when the wires are to remain within the catheters for any length of time. These back-bleed/flush devices not only eliminate blood loss through the catheter and around the wire, but allow continual or intermittent flushing through the catheter. The flushing prevents thrombus formation around the wire within the catheter[1]. This is equally as important when the wire/catheter combination is used in a low-pressure venous system as it is in a high-pressure area (e.g. in a ventricle or great artery), where the blood bleeding back into the catheter around the wire is more forceful and more obvious. The continual flush also lubricates wires within catheters, making any manipulations of them smoother. This is important particularly when using catheters manufactured of extruded plastic materials, when using wires that have a tight tolerance within any type of catheter, and when using any of the hydrophilic coated, "glide" type wires within any catheter.

By interruption of the continual flushing, intermittent pressure monitoring can often be accomplished through the side port, even with a wire within the catheter. Pressure monitoring helps to identify the location of the tip of the catheter when it is in an area that it is essential or particularly difficult to enter. The back-bleed valve/flush system also allows the capability of injecting small amounts of contrast through the catheter around the wire. This is extremely helpful for verification of the location of the tip of the catheter during maneuvers where a wire is being used in the catheter to assist the positioning of the catheter. With the more sophisticated, rigid, "Y"-connectors with Tuohy type of compression wire back-bleed valves, pressure injections of contrast for angiograms can be performed with the wire in place within the catheter. A wire maintained within the catheter is very often essential to stiffen the catheter and to keep it in its exact position during some high-flow pressure contrast injections.

There are several types of specific wire back-bleed/flush devices, which are effective for controlling bleeding while wires are passing through them. Unfortunately, none of the catheter back-bleed valves that commonly are available on the hubs of sheaths are effective at all at preventing bleeding around wires passing through them. The simplest wire back-bleed device is a rubber or latex "injection" port with a "Y" or "T" side arm (Coris Corp., Miami Lakes, FL). These rubber ports are commonly available in neonatal and intensive care units for intravenous injections into existing lines. They were designed to be used attached to the hub of intravenous lines and used primarily for the repeated insertion of needles through the rubber port for the purpose of injections of medications into the lines. At the same time, these injection ports make very simple, inexpensive, yet very effective wire back-bleed valve/flush ports to prevent bleeding around wires and allow the flushing of catheters that have wires within them. The simplest of these wire back-bleed valve/flush ports has a straight slip-lock connector with a proximal rubber valve and a side port of a short length of connecting plastic tubing attached to the side of the valve apparatus.

The wire back-bleed valve apparatus is attached to the catheter hub, the wire is introduced through the rubber port (initially usually through a needle, a wire introducer or "Medicut" canula which has punctured through the rubber valve) and the side arm is attached to the flush/pressure system. This simple device effectively prevents bleeding and allows intermittent pressure recording alternating with the flushing of the catheter. These simple rubber valves do *not* allow pressure injections of contrast around the wire, and occasionally the pressure curves that are transmitted through them are dampened.

A more effective, yet still simple type of back-bleed device is a small "Y" Luer-Lok connector with a Tuohy™-type compression grommet/valve on the straight arm of the Y (Merit Medical Systems, Salt Lake City, UT; B. Braun Medical Inc., Bethlehem, PA; and C.R. Bard, Inc., Covington, GA). This grommet is tightened around the wire to produce a tight seal. This tight seal and the rigid side arm permit very accurate pressure recordings, flushing of the catheter, and, when maximally tightened, allow a pressure injection through the side port with the wire still in place in the catheter. A direct connection of the pressure recording tubing to the female Luer-Lok connection off the side of the Y allows more accurate pressure recordings as well as pressure injections through the side port.

Sophisticated (and expensive) variations of this Y type of Tuohy™ valve with rotating Luer connectors have been developed for coronary angiography and can be used with any of the wire uses that will be described. All of the Y–Tuohy™ systems can be used for pressure injections during angiography while *none* of the ***non***-Tuohy™ hemostasis devices are useful for pressure contrast injections. With all of these valve/side port devices, care is taken that the *side port* and the *valve "chamber"* are flushed free of any entrapped air before the valve/side port is attached to the catheter and that the chamber within the back-bleed valve/flush port is cleared of air and clot before flushing through the valve to the patient. Negative pressure ***never*** should be applied to, nor an attempt made to withdraw blood through the side port of, a hemostasis valve of any type when it is attached to the catheter *and* there is a wire passing through the valve of the back-bleed device. When any suction is attempted through the side port of a back-bleed valve through which a wire is passing, air is preferentially drawn ***in*** *through the valve* around the wire along with any blood that is being withdrawn through the catheter.

In the absence of a commercially available Y or T wire back-bleed device, and in order to prevent massive blood loss during the use of a wire within a large catheter or sheath that is positioned in a high-pressure system, a very simple, makeshift back-bleed device can be improvised. The latex plug taken off an injection port of an intravenous (IV) fluid bag can be used to produce an effective back-bleed plug. The valve from the IV bag is removed from the bag while it is still sterile, when the covering package of the IV fluid bag is first opened. When the fluid bag is not opened on the sterile field, a latex plug from another bag can be used. If the bag is not maintained sterile when opened, the latex plug must be removed from the bag and sterilized separately in a gas sterilization system and saved in a sterile package in anticipation of such a use. The latex plug fits into the female Luer™ hub and folds securely over the rim of the hub of the catheter. The rim or edge of the plug is rolled over the lip of the catheter hub to create a tight seal. The plug allows the introduction of the wire through it and effectively prevents bleeding around the wire.

This make-shift hemostasis plug, however, does *not* allow flushing nor continuous pressure monitoring and, consequently, is *not* recommended for routine use. Since it does not allow flushing of the catheter, the plug should be used only for short periods of time, the wire should be removed every few minutes, and the catheter cleared and flushed repeatedly[2]. The large dead space within the catheter and around the wire when the catheter is not on a flush can, and usually does, result in a large thrombus developing in this space within a short period of time. On removal of the wire when using this or any other plug or back-bleed valve, the system is cleared carefully of air and clots by a thorough withdrawal of blood directly from the hub of the catheter before the catheter is flushed.

Heparin

Because of their "rough" invaginated surfaces, all spring guide wires have the potential to be quite thrombogenic within the circulation. Some spring guide wires have some type of "heparin coating" or binding, which reportedly reduces (but does not eliminate) their thrombogenicity. Teflon coatings, which reduce the "stickiness" of wires within catheters, possibly enhance thrombogenicity[1]. The original recommendations for the use of guide wires in the circulation were that they should never be left in a catheter and/or within the circulation for more than several *minutes* without withdrawing the wire and cleaning it and also clearing and flushing the catheter every several minutes! In the era of complex and very long interventional procedures, which are often performed over hours and require "supporting" spring guide wires during the entire procedure, this recommendation is certainly not reasonable and the notion on which it is based has been disproved clinically, if not scientifically. At the same time thrombi do occur on intravascular guide wires and all possible measures should be used to eliminate the formation of thrombi and embolic phenomena from wires.

Always introducing and using wires through backbleed valves with flush ports and maintaining the lumen of any catheter that contains a wire on a "continual" flush with a heparinized flush solution appears to be sufficient to prevent thrombi from forming around wires within the catheter. Not leaving the wire "bare" in the circulation any longer than necessary by keeping a wire completely within the catheter and on the continual flush whenever possible (e.g. when not actually maneuvering the wire ahead of the catheter or after positioning a wire for a balloon dilation with a guide catheter, but while preparing the balloon and before introducing the balloon) will reduce the "free wire" time in the circulation. Finally, all patients in whom guide, support or deflector wires are used (all patients?) should receive 100 units/kg of intravenous heparin prior to any maneuvers in the circulation with wires.

Standard spring guide wires

Spring guide wires, as their name implies, are tubular spring wires made of an extremely uniform winding of a very fine, usually stainless steel wire. The winding of wire is hollow and the lumen within this tubular winding of wire contains at least one length of very fine flexible ribbon wire, which is welded at both ends of the tubular winding and serves as a safety wire to prevent the windings of the wire from pulling apart. Many spring guide wires have an additional, stiffening or core wire, which also runs most of the length within the outer winding of the wire. At the distal end of the tubular wire the stiffer, central core wire is usually 1–10 cm shorter than the wound wire, or the central wire tapers to a very fine, flexible wire for that distance at the distal end. In either case, the core wire adds stiffness to the length of the wound spring guide wire except at the distal tip, where it either is absent or tapers, which results in its remaining very flexible or even floppy.

Spring guide wires are available in an almost infinite combination of diameters, lengths, stiffness, tip configurations and coatings. The wires that are packaged with percutaneous introduction sets are usually 45–80 cm in length while most wires for use within catheters or the exchange of catheters are between 150 and 400 cm in length. There are wires as small as 0.014″ and as large as 0.045″ and each diameter comes in various degrees of stiffness. Most of the spring guide wires will support the passage of catheters through tortuous courses within the vascular system, at least to some degree. The flexible distal ends of the wires vary in length from 1 to 10 cm and, in addition, vary from slightly flexible to very soft and flexible. Some spring guide wires are coated with teflon or with heparin with the intent of increasing lubricity within polyurethane catheters and decreasing thrombogenicity, respectively[1].

Spring guide wires, including those with special modifications, are probably the most commonly used expendable items in the catheterization laboratory. Spring guide wires are used for the percutaneous introduction of all sheaths/dilators and catheters. They are used extensively for the selective cannulation of side or branch vessels as well as for crossing valves during both prograde and retrograde approaches. Spring guide wires are now used to support diagnostic catheters during complex manipulations, to support the delivery of therapeutic sheaths/dilators, and to support all varieties of balloon dilation catheters during dilation procedures.

Standard spring guide wires have been used in the catheterization of pediatric and congenital heart patients for over three decades. The wires are used for routine catheterization procedures as well as for entering locations where the usual or standard catheter manipulations are unsuccessful[2]. Guide wires are advanced out of the tip of the catheter and into a desired location, after which the wire is advanced over the catheter into the chamber/vessel. Wires of various sizes with straight soft tips, curved tips or J tips are advanced out of the tips of either straight or curved, end-hole catheters and then the wires are directed selectively into specific areas or orifices. Once the wire is secured distally in the area or orifice, the catheter is advanced over the wire into the area[2].

This use of spring guide wires is particularly useful when, after some time within the body, the catheter becomes soft, and even though the catheter is pointing directly at the desired location it forms back loops rather than advancing when forward motion is applied to the proximal catheter. In this circumstance, a standard spring guide wire with a soft or J tip is introduced through a wire back-bleed valve/flush port into the catheter and advanced through the catheter and, from the distal end of the catheter, the tip of the wire is advanced beyond the catheter tip and quite easily into the desired opening. Occasionally some curve at the distal end of the wire is helpful in directing the wire, but usually when using standard spring guide wires, the direction of the wire toward an orifice is accomplished by changing the location/direction of the tip of a slightly curved catheter.

Whenever a wire is advanced *out of the distal tip of a catheter*, only *very soft, flexible tipped and/or J tipped wires* should be used. The shaft of the catheter always *must be free* and able to move away (back) from the direction of the tip as a wire is extruded from the tip of a catheter. If the tip of the catheter is confined within the walls of a vessel or in a small chamber *and* the shaft of the catheter is *constrained* in the vessel/chamber so that the catheter cannot move freely and the tip of the catheter cannot move readily away from a wall or surface, the wire will be forced *through* the wall of the vessel/chamber as it is extruded! (Figure 6.1a). If, on the other hand, the catheter is not constrained and is free to move from side to side in the vessel, the tip of the wire that is pushing against the vessel/chamber wall will push the tip of the catheter away and allow the wire to deflect (Figure 6.1b).

Often the additional stiffness provided to the shaft of a very soft catheter by a wire within its lumen is sufficient to allow the otherwise soft, non-maneuverable catheter to be maneuvered forward purposefully. A short segment of an exposed soft tip of the wire, which is beyond the tip of the catheter, can also add some directional control to the tip, while the presence of the stiffer portion of the wire within the shaft of the catheter allows more of the torque applied to the proximal end of the catheter to be transmitted to the distal end and tip of the catheter. This alone often facilitates the manipulation of the catheter tip into the desired location or to be advanced off the wire into the desired location.

Torque wires

Materials

A torque wire is a special guide wire that has a very rigid core wire, which provides a "one to one" (or very close to "one to one"), rotation or "torque ratio" between the proximal end and the distal tip of the wire. Torque wires all have very floppy distal tips of various lengths beyond their stiff shaft. Torque wires either are spring guide wires with the special core wire or are manufactured of a fine, uniform Nitinol™ metal shaft with a softened tip. Both

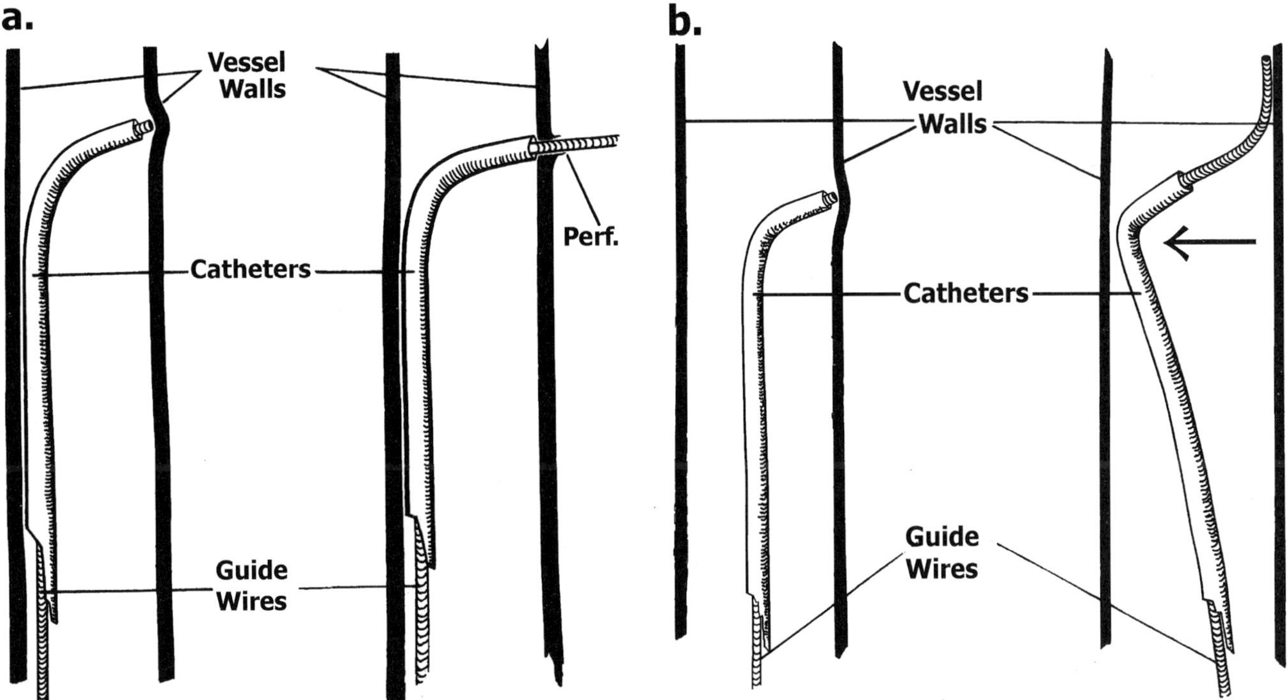

Figure 6.1 (a) Catheter constrained within walls of vessel—wire pushing into and *through vessel wall* when advanced out of catheter; Perf., site of perforation. (b) When catheter is not constrained within walls of vessel, it can push away from the wall as wire is advanced.

types of torque wire are available in various diameters and lengths with a relatively stiff shaft and a long, floppy distal end and tip. The entire floppy portion of these wires is often made of a different material that is extra dense when visualized on fluoroscopy. These extra dense tips allow better visualization of the specific maneuvers of the tip as a result of torquing. The floppy distal segments of spring guide torque wires are initially straight and usually 5–10 centimeters in length, but can vary in length from a few centimeters to 15 cm. A slight curve *must* be formed on the distal tip of a wire before its use as a torque wire, in order that any torque or rotation applied to the proximal straight shaft of the wire has "an angle to turn" at the tip of the wire.

The connection or "transition" portion between the stiff shaft of the spring wire and the floppy distal portion is usually quite abrupt. This abrupt change in stiffness along the wire creates a significant problem with most of these torque wires. While the curved, floppy portion of the wire can almost always be maneuvered into virtually any desired opening or orifice (Figure 6.2a), the stiff portion of the wire proximal to the transition area often will not follow the floppy segment through angles or bends that are at all acute. As the stiffer shaft of a torque or other guide wire that has had the soft tip successfully positioned in a side branch, is advanced further toward the orifice of a side branch, and as the transition area of the wire reaches the orifice, unless this "following" stiff portion of the wire is aligned exactly with (parallel to) the distal softer portion of the wire, the transition and stiff portions of the wire usually will not follow the floppy portion of the wire into the orifice (Figure 6.2b). Usually the stiff portion of the wire continues in a straight direction, which withdraws the previously positioned floppy portion out of the area or vessel (Figure 6.2c).

The wires are supplied with small, finger comfortable, vice-like devices which clamp on the proximal portion of the wire to facilitate the torquing of the wire. The 1:1 torque characteristics of these wires allow a curved tip of the wires to be directed in very specific directions by fine precise rotation (torquing) along with simultaneous, short to-and-fro motions of the proximal wire. As during the maneuvering of all catheters or wires through long channels (vessels, sheaths or catheters), in addition to the torque applied to the proximal end of the wire, the wire must be kept in this constant, slight, to-and-fro motion.

There are many torque wires available. Those most frequently used in pediatric and congenital patients are the Wholey™ wires (Advanced Cardiovascular Systems [ACS], Santa Clara, CA), the Platinum Plus™ and Magic™ wires (Boston Scientific, Natick, MA), the Ultra-Select™ and HyTek™ wires (ev3, Plymouth, MN)) and the Nitinol Glide™ wires (Terumo Medical Corp., Somerset, NJ and Boston Scientific, Natick, MA).

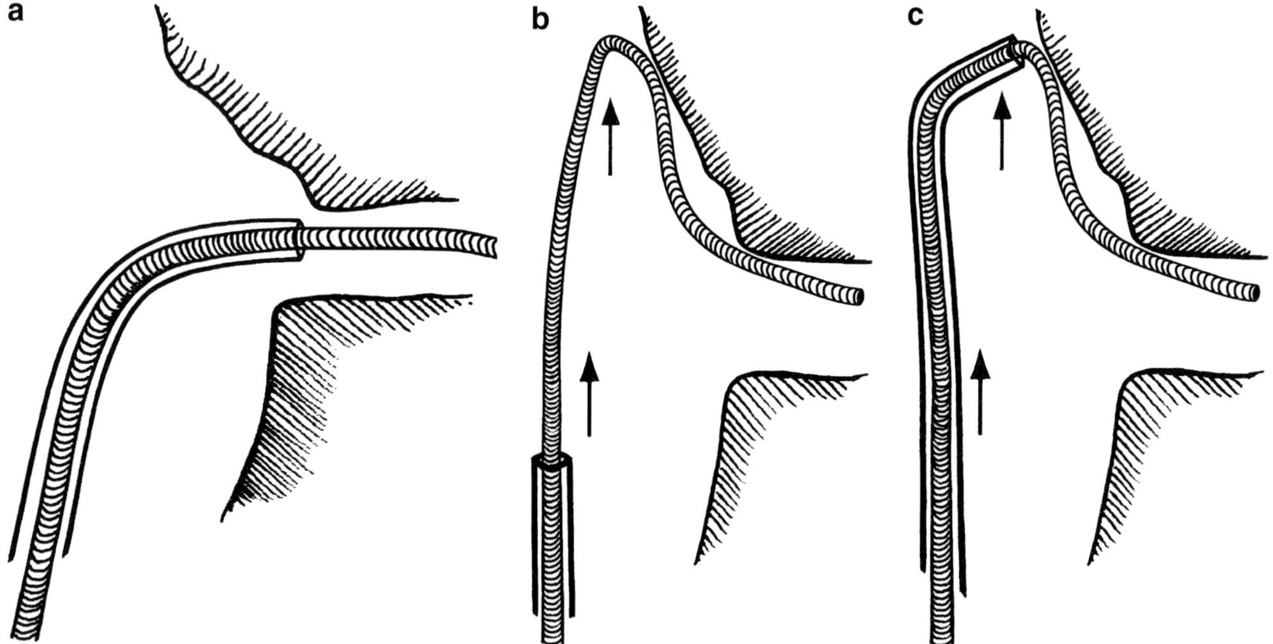

Figure 6.2 (a) Soft wire advanced out of tip of catheter into perpendicular side branch/orifice; (b) "transition" or stiff portion of wire does not follow soft tip of wire into orifice of a side branch when the wire is not advanced directly in the direction of the side branch; (c) curved catheter continues to advance along the wall of the vessel and pulls the soft wire out of the side branch when an attempt is made to advance a stiff curve in the catheter over the soft portion of the wire entering a side branch/orifice.

Technique using torque wires

All torque wires must have at least a slight curve on the distal, soft tip in order to have something to "turn" when the proximal wire is rotated. Rotating a perfectly straight object (or wire) does not alter the direction of a straight tip at all. Torque wires are maneuvered with the soft end of the wire advanced out of and well *beyond* the tip of an end-hole catheter. The wire is then manipulated with its floppy tip totally exposed in a cardiac chamber or vessel. As with other wires used through catheters, it is essential to introduce the torque wire through a wire back-bleed valved/flush device. With the tip of the wire still within the tip of the catheter, the tip of the *catheter* is maneuvered to a position as close as possible to, and pointing in the direction of, the desired orifice or side branch vessel before the wire is advanced out of the catheter. The tip of the catheter should never be forced against or into the wall of the vessel or chamber as the wire is being advanced out of it, as even the soft tip of a torque wire can perforate a wall when the catheter is constrained in the vessel/chamber (Figure 6.1a).

The tip of the wire is advanced out of (beyond) the tip of the catheter and selectively manipulated into the desired side branch or orifice by turning ("torquing") the proximal end of the wire while simultaneously adjusting the position of the tip of the catheter toward the orifice and rotating and moving the wire slightly to and fro. Maneuvering a torque wire is like maneuvering a torque catheter, using fine, short, to and fro, but fairly rapid motions of the wire as it is turned simultaneously within the catheter. Torquing the wire *without* the to-and-fro motion is likely to have no effect on the tip of the wire initially and then suddenly, several rotations of the previously applied torque will be transmitted to the tip of the wire all at once resulting in a propeller-like rapid rotation of the tip of the wire rather than a precise, controlled turning of the tip.

Torque wires are very effective for entering side branches of vessels that arise at an oblique, and not too acute, angle off the main vessel. The *floppy portion* of these wires can almost always be manipulated into the side vessel regardless of the angle of its take-off (Figure 6.2a), however, the stiffer, supporting portion of the wire often will not follow if the angle off the main vessel is at all acute. As much of the distal, soft segment of the wire as is possible (all of it!) is advanced into the side or branching vessel before an attempt is made to advance the catheter over the wire. In order to have all of the soft end of the wire in the branch vessel, the distal end of the soft portion of the wire must often be doubled back on itself or actually wadded up in the side or branch vessel in order to have the stiff portion approach even near the side orifice. Often, as the transition or stiff portion of the wire approaches the take-off of the branch vessel, the straight, stiff portion does not make the bend to angle into the side vessel. Instead, the following, more proximal, stiff portion of the wire continues in a straight direction on past the orifice. As a consequence, instead of the stiff portion of the wire entering the side vessel, the floppy portion of the wire is pulled backward or actually flips out of the side branch. A small, preformed curve on the *transition* portion of the wire between the floppy and straight stiff wire assists in the passage of the stiffer portion around the angle; unfortunately, even a small curve on the stiffer, transition, portion of the wire will compromise the free rotation of the wire severely when torquing it within a catheter is attempted.

A standard end-hole catheter will usually *not* follow over the soft distal portion of the wire even when it will readily follow over the stiffer portion of the same wire. When an attempt is made to advance the catheter over only the soft portion of the wire, the catheter continues in a forward direction along the vessel and will pull the wire out of the side branch/orifice (Figure 6.2c). For this reason, when these wires are used to advance a catheter over the wire into a specific location, a significant length of the stiff portion of the guide wire that is proximal to the floppy tip must be advanced well within the branch vessel before an attempt is made at passing the catheter over the wire. With this one, often very frustrating, exception, these wires are very effective at selectively catheterizing very small orifices which arise at moderate angles away from the main direction of the catheter. Torque wires are also excellent for traversing very circuitous courses through chambers and vessels.

Once the tip of the torque wire is through the orifice of a side or branch vessel, the wire is advanced cautiously until the stiff portion follows the tip and is deep into the side branch. This often requires several different approaches to the vessel and may require that a long floppy portion of a wire be bunched or balled up in the distal vessel. Once the stiff portion of the wire has been advanced at least some distance into the side/branch vessel, the catheter is advanced as far as possible over the wire into the side/branch vessel. Once the catheter has been advanced over the wire to the desired distal vessel location, the original torque wire is removed, leaving the catheter in place in the vessel. With this initial catheter securely in place, then a larger and stiffer wire can be introduced through the catheter in order to guide larger delivery catheters or sheaths into the area for complex interventional procedures.

With all of the torque wires, care must be taken to avoid permanent bends, kinks or even permanent smooth curves on any part of the stiff shaft of the wire. Even a small acute bend or kink on the shaft of the wire causes

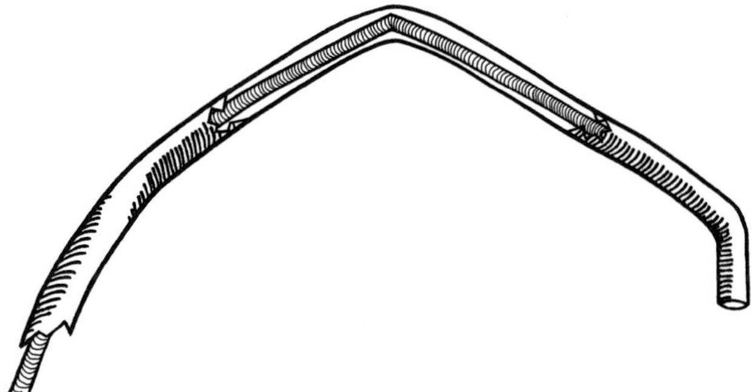

Figure 6.3 An acute kink in a wire within a catheter will compromise/prevent any movement within the catheter and totally prevent any rotation (torque) of wire within the catheter.

that portion of the wire to conform to the curves of the catheter within chambers or vessels through which the catheter is passing, and prevent any purposeful rotation of the tip of the wire (Figure 6.3). If the wire inadvertently develops a bend or kink and further torquing or manipulation is required, the wire should be exchanged for a new one without wasting time and fluoroscopy exposure trying to torque the bent wire.

Terumo™ "Glide wires"

Terumo™ "Glide wires" (Terumo Medical Corp., Somerset, NJ) are not spring guide wires but hydrophilic coated, solid Nitinol™ wires which functions as guide wires. The Glide™ wires are available in four sizes (0.025″, 0.032″, 0.035″ & 0.038″), in multiple lengths including exchange lengths, and in standard and extra stiff versions. The Glide™ wires all have a short soft(er) tip at one end and are available with a straight or very slight curve on this soft tip. The Nitinol™ material is *almost* impervious to additional bending, forming or *kinking* and retains or returns to its straight configuration even after extensive bending or buckling within the heart or vessels. The solid wire construction of the Terumo™ wires gives them an ideal, 1:1 torque ratio. The Nitinol™ is coated with a hydrophilic material that makes the wires extremely slippery *as long as the surface of the Glide™ wires is kept wet*. These two characteristics give these wires the unique property of passing ("gliding") through very small orifices and often through very tortuous courses through the heart and great vessels. These wires follow particularly well when they are advanced in the direction of blood flow and along the course of an existing channel. The Glide™ wires *must* be kept very wet at all times. When the wires begin to dry at all, they become very sticky and bind within catheters, particularly in catheters made of extruded plastic. This binding within a catheter is particularly severe when the internal diameter of the catheter is close to the outside diameter of the wire.

Although generally considered safe and freely maneuverable within vessels and chambers, these wires definitely have the ability to perforate myocardium and even vessel walls easily when the tip of the wire is advanced out of the tip of a catheter that is confined (restricted in its lateral movement) within a vessel or chamber and the tip of the catheter is wedged against, or into, the wall of the chamber or vessel. Because of their "gliding" and smooth characteristics, there may be little or no unusual sensation of force as these wires pass *through* vessel walls, tissues and/or myocardial walls!

Techniques for the manipulation of Terumo™ Glide™ wires

It is imperative that the Terumo™ wire is prepared by thoroughly flushing the entire length of the housing of the wire with saline or dextrose/saline flush solution in order to wet the entire wire while it is still within the tubular housing. The Glide™ Wire is introduced directly from its housing into the catheter as it is withdrawn out of the housing. The wire is introduced through a wire back-bleed valve/flush port on the catheter, which is maintained on continual flush. Terumo Glide™ wires are all manipulated *beyond* the tip of the catheter. The tip of the end-hole guiding catheter is maneuvered to a location in the vicinity and direction of the desired opening or orifice that is to be entered, but at the same time, the tip of the catheter is *not forced tightly against* any structure or surface. The Terumo™ wire is advanced gently beyond the tip of the end-hole catheter and the *wire*, which is free in the circulation, is maneuvered to the desired location.

The Terumo™ wire is maneuvered beyond of the tip of the catheter with gentle, repeated probing with the wire as the catheter and wire are torqued and maneuvered to and fro so that, eventually, the changing directions of the combination will direct the tip of the wire toward the desired orifice. The manipulation of the Glide™ wire is similar to the manipulation of any other torque wire, i.e. frequent gentle, to-and-fro probes while rotating the wire or catheter. With each to-and-fro advance of the wire, the proximal end of a curved tip, Terumo™ wire is rotated with a torque control device attached proximally on the wire outside of the catheter. In addition to changing the direction of the tip of the catheter, entrance into difficult areas is facilitated by torquing the wire with multiple repeated passes, each time changing the angle of both the tip of the catheter and the tip of the curved wire very slightly. Since the orifice to be entered cannot actually be visualized on fluoroscopy, there is still con-siderable random chance to this manipulation. When the target cannot actually be visualized, multiple, rapid, but gentle to-and-fro motions along with the torquing maneuvers are more effective than any attempt with slow precise torquing of either the catheter or the wire.

Once the Terumo™ wire enters the desired orifice, it is advanced as far as possible into the area before attempting to advance a catheter over it. Extra care and attention must be provided to "maintain" the Glide™ wire in any side or branch vessel. Once in a specific location, the wire must be purposefully, continuously and firmly held in place with a conscious effort at maintaining it in its secure location. The characteristics of the Nitinol™ material of the Glide™ wire predispose it to straightening and spontaneously working its way back out of side vessels when they arise at any angle or curve from the straight course of the wire, unless the wire is purposefully held in place.

Like the other types of torque wire, it is often difficult to get a catheter to follow into a desired distal location over a Glide™ wire. With Glide™ wires it is particularly difficult to keep the wire in the distal location if the course to that area is at all tortuous. Sometimes it is worthwhile to "over advance" the wire after it has reached its most distal location and to form a large, 360°, more proximal, back loop in the right atrium or other more proximal chamber. This large proximal loop provides a longer but smoother curve along the course of the wire to the tip and allows support of the free outer circumference of the broad curves of the loops of the wire against the chamber walls.

Another approach to advancing a catheter into a desired distal location over the Glide™ wire is to begin initially with a smaller more flexible catheter over the Glide™ wire. This first requires the removal of the original guiding catheter and replacing it with a smaller more malleable catheter, all of the time maintaining extra special attention and effort to keep the Glide™ wire in place. A 5-French Terumo™ Glide™ Catheter™ (Terumo Medical Corp., Somerset, NJ) is very effective as the smaller replacement/exchange catheter when there are angled or other difficult locations to enter. These catheters are quite soft and flexible and have a hydrophilic internal and external coating similar to the surface coating of the Glide™ wires. Like Terumo™ wires, Terumo Glide™ catheters must be kept wet continuously, both inside and outside. After the smaller, softer Glide™ catheter has reached the most distal location, the Glide™ wire is removed and replaced with a larger diameter, standard or Super Stiff™ teflon-coated spring guide wire. Extreme care must be taken during this exchange of wires. Larger, stiffer wires tend to advance in a straight line at their transition zones and in doing so can easily displace smaller catheters from even a far distal location in a side branch. For a very circuitous location this often requires the repeated exchange of several sequentially larger wires or catheters. Once a sufficiently large or stiff wire is in place, the smaller catheter is removed over the wire and the larger, desired sheath, dilator or therapeutic catheter is passed over the stiffer guide wire.

Deflector wires

Deflector wires, as their name implies, are wires used to bend or "deflect" the *tips of catheters* purposefully and in a particular direction. There are two major types of deflector wire used in the cardiac catheterization laboratory; "active" or "controllable" deflector wires and "passive" or "rigid" deflector wires. When using *any deflector wire*, the catheter is advanced until its tip is in a position adjacent to or just past the desired orifice and then the deflector wire is introduced into the catheter (Figure 6.4a). As the rigid deflector is advanced to the tip of the catheter or a controllable deflector wire is activated at the tip of the catheter, the tip of the catheter is deflected (bent) toward the desired orifice with the deflector wire (Figure 6.4b). The curved deflector wire *then is fixed in position* while the *catheter is advanced off the wire* (Figure 6.4c). If the deflector wire is advanced with the catheter or allowed to move as the catheter is being advanced, this will move the whole catheter and the contained wire. More specifically, the whole fixed curve at the tip of the catheter is pushed forward in the direction of motion of the catheter, and the tip of the catheter is moved *away* from the desired orifice (Figure 6.4d).

All pediatric/congenital heart interventionalists performing cardiac catheterizations, particularly interventional procedures on very complex pediatric or congenital heart defects, should be proficient in the use of both types of deflector wire in order to assure that all catheters and devices can be maneuvered to *all* locations in these complex hearts. When either type of deflector wire is used, it is used *while it remains completely within* the lumen of the catheter. Once the deflector wire has deflected the tip of the catheter toward the proper location, the catheter is *advanced off the wire* into the orifice or opening (Figure 6.4c). In contrast to the use of *torque-controlled guide wires, where the wire is pre-positioned* into an orifice or vessel and then an end-hole (only) catheter is advanced *over* the wire—as described earlier in this chapter—when using deflector wires, any type of *catheter* (including closed-end angiographic catheters) can be directed and maneuvered into difficult areas.

Deflector wires are routinely introduced and manipulated through wire back-bleed valves, which remain attached to the hub of the catheter and which contain a side port for flushing. The wire hemostasis valve prevents excessive back bleeding into and through the catheter, while a continual flush through the side port during the use of the wire prevents thrombosis around the wire *and* "lubricates" the lumen of the catheter to facilitate the movement of the wire within the catheter. When a deflector wire is used within a catheter positioned in the systemic arterial system and/or in a high-pressure chamber and/or vessel, the use of a wire back-bleed valve is

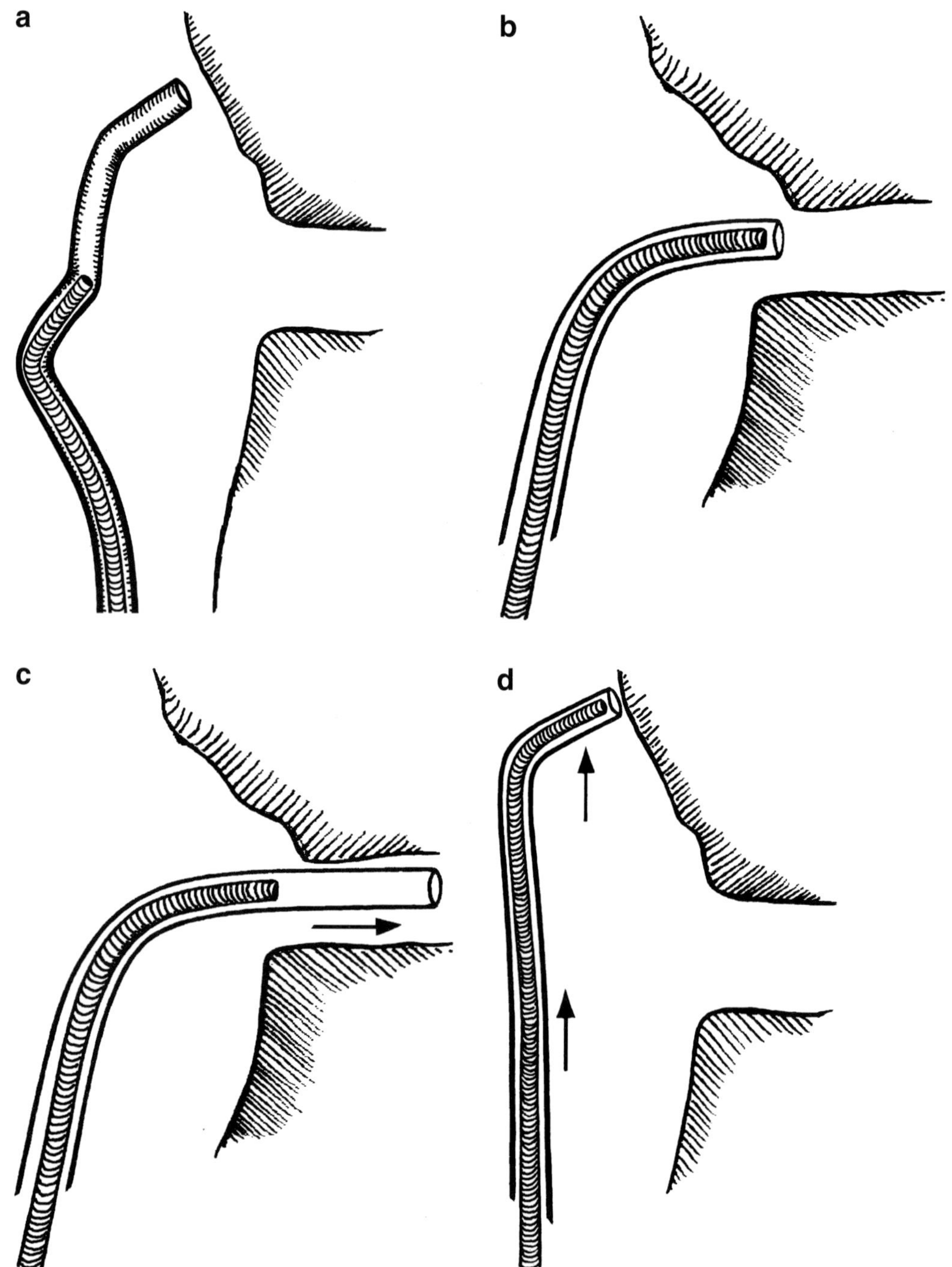

Figure 6.4 (a) The angled tip of a rigid deflector wire distorts and displaces the catheter as the stiff curve is being advanced within the pre-positioned catheter; (b) a curved deflector wire that is positioned properly within a catheter and deflecting the tip toward the desired orifice; (c) the catheter is advanced correctly off the wire and into the orifice while the wire is fixed in position; (d) the catheter and deflector wire are advanced together incorrectly, which merely pushes both the wire and the catheter away from the desired orifice.

even more essential to prevent excessive blood loss around the wire.

Although it is always preferable to use wire back-bleed valves with wires within catheters, there are a few occasions when a "simple deflection" is accomplished without the use of a back-bleed valve/flush system. The catheter should be in the low-pressure, systemic *venous* side of the circulation and only used in patients with no intracardiac shunts, and it should be anticipated that the deflection can be performed rapidly (in less than 1–2 minutes). The ideal situation for the use of a deflector wire without the use of a back-bleed/flush valve is when it is anticipated that the procedure can be performed very rapidly and the wire can be removed and the catheter cleared by withdrawing blood (and air and clots) within a few minutes. However, when deflection of the catheter begins in a low-pressure system, but the catheter is being directed into a high-pressure chamber or vessel (e.g. from left atrium to left ventricle), the deflector wire should always be used through a back-bleed valve. In this circumstance, once the catheter enters the high-pressure area with a wire in it, there otherwise will be excessive blood loss, or the manipulations to position the catheter in the high-pressure system would be compromised because of the urgency imposed by the excessive bleeding.

When any wire is withdrawn completely out of a catheter, whether it is a torque wire used beyond the tip of the catheter or any type of deflector wire, and whether the wire was used with, or without, a back-bleed valve/flush port, blood is *always* and *immediately* withdrawn into a syringe from the hub of the catheter in order to be absolutely sure that the catheter is free of clots and air. Only after the catheter unequivocally has been cleared completely of any air and clots, is it attached to the flush-pressure system and flushed thoroughly.

Amplatz™ ("controllable" or "active") deflector wires

The most commonly used type of deflector wire is the "active", "controllable" or "variable" tip, Amplatz™ deflector wire (Cook Inc., Bloomington, IN). These deflector wires are absolutely indispensable items in the inventory of the pediatric/congenital catheterization laboratory. They are most useful in softer catheters and when it is necessary to negotiate only a single curve to enter a specific location. Active deflector wires will bend or deflect the tip of the wire/catheter purposefully *only* in a single direction. A properly functioning active deflector wire bends or deflects the tip of the catheter only in the direction of any pre-existing more proximal ***concave*** curve on the catheter/wire. The direction of the deflection only will increase the direction of the concave curve toward the concavity and usually only in the one direction of the catheter immediately proximal to the area being deflected and already formed on the catheter from its course through the vasculature. Active deflector wires complement rigid or fixed deflector wires in the catheterization laboratory; the latter, which can produce complex curves on a catheter, are discussed subsequently in this chapter.

Materials

The Amplatz TDW™ (Cook Inc., Bloomington, IN) is an active deflector wire that has a special, flexible spring guide wire with a second, partially movable, stiff, core wire within the outer spring wire. The movable core wire is attached within the tip of the wire distally and to the activator handle proximally. An active curve is formed on the wire in order to deflect the catheter by applying traction to the core wire through the special handle. The angle of deflection can be changed by applying variable degrees of force on the deflecting handle. Tension on the handle reduces the length of the second, inner, core wire, the shortening of which causes the tip of the spring wire to bend or deflect. When the tip of the deflector wire is positioned at the tip of a catheter that is not too stiff, tension on the handle at the proximal end of the deflector wire deflects the tip of the catheter along with the tip of the wire into a predetermined concave curve. Amplatz TDW™ deflector wires are available in multiple lengths, in wire diameters of 0.025", 0.028", 0.035", 0.038" and 0.045", and with three different tip curves—of 5, 10 and 15 mm diameter—which can be formed at the tip of the wires with deflection of the proximal handle. The current Amplatz™ deflector wires are available only as a disposable unit consisting of the wire and a permanently attached disposable handle. The deflector wires of the disposable units supposedly are identical to the original Amplatz TDW™ deflector wires, however, the disposable, plastic and permanently attached deflector handle has replaced the original, detachable, reusable, all stainless steel handles. The disposable units function in the same way, however the disposable handles/wires appear to be slightly less "robust" than the original reusable handles, which were available separately from the individual wires and could be re-sterilized. There may be a few of these reusable handles still available throughout the world, but the separate wires are no longer manufactured for use with them.

The Amplatz TDW™ deflector wire in its non-deflected state has the advantage of being a straight wire with a relatively soft, flexible tip as it is introduced into the catheter. This flexible, soft wire can be advanced easily to the tip of the catheter without displacing the tip of the catheter out of often relatively precarious positions, even when the catheter passes through a very tortuous course. This is particularly important when there is significant tortuosity with multiple curves along the course of the catheter proximal to the area where the curve is to be formed for the deflection of the catheter. Often, a rigid deflector wire (discussed later in this chapter) cannot be advanced to the tip of the catheter through the curves in the catheter without pulling the tip of the catheter out of its critical position. The flexible tip of the Amplatz™ deflector wire can usually be advanced easily through these same curves.

The degree of deflection and the angle of the tip in a single plane are changed by changing the force on the handle. This is accomplished without having to remove, re-form or reintroduce the particular deflector wire. A relatively strong deflection force can be produced at the tip of the catheter with the larger diameter, active, deflector wires. This force and, in turn, the degree of deflection are in direct proportion to how hard the handle is squeezed up to the limits of each wire. In softer catheters (e.g. a floating balloon catheter or a "warmed" woven dacron catheter), a 180° deflection can easily be achieved at the tip of the catheter with the thicker diameter Amplatz™ deflector wires.

Technique

The catheter that is to be deflected is first maneuvered into a position adjacent to the orifice or branch vessel that is to be entered. Assuming that the desired direction of deflection is similar in direction to the most distal and adjacent concave curve that is already present on the catheter just proximal to its tip, the deflector wire with the appropriate diameter curve and of the largest diameter wire which the catheter will accommodate, is introduced into the catheter through a valved wire back-bleed/flush device and advanced to the tip of the catheter. The tip is deflected by a controlled but strong squeeze on the deflector handle. In general and within the limits of each deflector wire, the greater the force on the handle, the more acute is the curve that is formed at the tip. The handle is squeezed until the deflected tip of the catheter is directed exactly at the desired orifice. This curve on the deflector wire is maintained while the proximal wire extending out of the hub of the catheter along with the squeezed handle *is fixed on the tabletop or against the patient's leg*. With the proximal wire fixed securely in this position so that the wire does not move forward or backward, the catheter is advanced *off the wire* into the desired orifice. The degree of angulation of the tip can be controlled and varied somewhat by the strength of the deflection, while the exact location of the tip of the catheter, which is pointing at the vessel or orifice, can be varied slightly by advancing, withdrawing and/or rotating the catheter *and the wire* together very slightly.

Several common applications for deflecting the tip of a catheter with active deflector wires are as simple as deflecting the tip of the catheter from the right atrium toward the right ventricle (in the presence of a very large right atrium or significant tricuspid regurgitation) or even more commonly, deflecting a catheter from the left atrium into the left ventricle. Another very common use of the active deflector wire is when advancing a prograde catheter from the body of the left ventricle toward, and out through, the semilunar valve, which arises off the ventricle. The tip of a catheter entering the left ventricle from the left atrium usually points toward the left ventricular apex, which is 180° *away* from the direction of the outflow tract. Once the catheter is well within the left ventricle, the tip of the catheter is deflected by 180° and pointed toward the semilunar valve arising from the left ventricle—whether it is the aortic valve or the pulmonary valve in a transposition of the great arteries. The active deflector is also invaluable in deflecting catheters into specific side branches or into collaterals that arise at an acute angle off the aorta. A single Amplatz™ deflector wire can often be used for multiple different deflections in different locations during a single case.

There are, unfortunately, several disadvantages to the controllable Amplatz TDW™ deflector wires. The active deflection produces a curve only *in a single direction*—i.e. in the direction of the adjacent, *immediately proximal, concave curve* or course of the catheter. Thus, the adjacent more proximal curve that is created on the catheter (and the contained deflector wire) by their passage through the adjacent more proximal chamber or vessel, determines the only direction in which the tip of the wire/catheter can be directed with the active deflector wire. Also the curve on the catheter/wire formed with the active deflector wire is difficult to torque from side-to-side away from the initial direction of the curve. Both the catheter and the deflector wire (and handle!) within the catheter must be torqued and moved to and fro together. The active deflector wires are not teflon coated, and tend to bind within catheters when the internal diameter of the catheter is even close to the external diameter of the wire. This is particularly true when the active deflectors are used within catheters manufactured from extruded polyurethane materials. Severe binding of the wire within the catheter lumen can prevent the catheter from being advanced off the wire once the tip has been directed accurately toward a particular area.

The most serious potential problem of these wires is a result of one of their advantages—the strong force of the deflection. When applying a strong force on the handle in order to produce the curve at the tip, there is no way of discriminating between the resistance to the deflection, which is due to the stiffness of the catheter, from the resistance that is created by an *intact wall* of a vessel and/or chamber—i.e. whether the active deflection is toward an orifice or actually *through* some intact and critical wall or structure!! This must be considered with every deflection with the Amplatz™ deflectors, but particularly when deflecting within cardiac chambers—for example near an atrial appendage and/or within the trabeculae of a ventricle!

One additional disadvantage of active deflector wires is the higher cost of the controllable Amplatz™ deflector wires compared to the simpler, rigid deflection wires. Some of the current disposable active deflector wires do tend to lose their capability for deflection or actually break after several deflections within the same patient. Even a slight kink along the course of the shaft of the deflector wire can prevent the deflection function, or occasionally the internal wire that creates the tension to produce the curve, will snap after several deflections.

The effective use of active deflector wires requires some experience, but once this is achieved, they represent an *absolutely indispensable* item in a pediatric/congenital catheterization laboratory. Although they represent an extra piece of relatively expensive consumable equipment, the time saved by the judicious use of active deflector wires easily compensates for their extra cost.

Rigid (static) deflector wires

The second type of deflector wire is the rigid or "static" deflector wire. The rigid deflector wire is a much simpler apparatus and is available in every catheterization laboratory as it can be formed from the stiff end of a standard spring guide wire. They are, however, capable of far more complex uses. A rigid deflector wire basically is a stiff wire that is pre-formed outside of the body into specific and often compound curves, which correspond to the desired course and direction of the catheter within the body. The stiff, preformed wire is introduced into the catheter with the purpose of deforming (deflecting) the tip of the catheter into a curve or curves that correspond(s) to the curves on the wire. The preformed wire is advanced within the catheter until the curve in the wire is just within the tip of the catheter where the deflection of the tip is desired. As with active deflector wires, the entire preformed curve of the rigid deflector wire remains *within the catheter* while the catheter is advanced off the wire. These rigid deflector wires are a complement to active deflector wires and are indispensable items in the inventory of the pediatric/congenital catheterization laboratory.

Either the stiff end of a standard spring guide wire or a specialized, straight, stainless steel, Mullins™ wire (Argon Medical Inc., Athens, TX) can be used to form the rigid deflecting curves for this type of deflection. Each curve is preformed on the stiff wire to conform precisely to the size of the patient's heart and the specific direction(s) in which the tip of the catheter is to be deflected. The curves in the stiff wires are formed by manually bending them *smoothly* around a finger or a small syringe. Extra care must be taken not to create any kinks or sharp angles in the wires during the formation of the curves. Even a very slight acute kink in the wire is likely to prevent it from being advanced through the catheter. The curves are formed slightly tighter than the curves that it is desired to form in the catheters within the structures where they will be used. The "tighter" curves on the wire allow for some straightening of the wire and widening of the curve in the catheter due to the stiffness of the catheter itself. Once the pre-curved wire is introduced into the proximal end of the catheter and while the portion of the catheter with the combination catheter/wire is still outside of the body, the curves in the wire can be tightened further or retightened by re-bending the curves in the wire along with the portion of the catheter that is still outside of the introductory site.

Like all other wires, rigid deflector wires are used through a wire back-bleed valve/flush port on the hub of the catheter. When the pre-curved wire is introduced into the catheter and when the curve in the stiff wire is positioned at the tip of the catheter, the stiff, curved wire deflects the distal end and tip of the catheter to conform to the curve of the wire. The stiffer the wire that is used to form the static deflector curves, the more precisely the tip of the catheter will be deflected. However, a tight, stiff curve on a stiff wire is often difficult to advance through a catheter without the wire causing the tip of the catheter to be withdrawn. Often a compromise must be made between the use of a very stiff wire, which would produce the acute, precise deflections, and a slightly softer wire, which would allow the stiff deflector curve to advance to the tip of the catheter but might not deflect the tip as precisely.

Rigid deflector wires do have multiple advantages. Curves away from the concave course of the catheter and purposeful, side-to-side, "three-dimensional" curves can be formed on the wire, and in turn on the distal end of the catheter away from the original direction of the catheter. Thus, curves can be formed which will direct the catheter not only cephalad or caudally, but anteriorly or posteriorly at the same time. This allows very precise deflection of the tip of the catheter to point in any "three-dimensional" desired direction. The stiff ends of the spring guide wires and the straight Mullins™ deflector wires are both shaped and used with similar techniques.

Standard spring guide wires as rigid deflectors

The stiff ends of many spring guide wires make very effective "static tip deflector wires" for catheters. The stiff end of a spring guide wire can be formed into any desired smooth curve, including very acute, compound or three-dimensional curves. Standard 0.035" or 0.038" wires are the most useful for this purpose, although wires of almost any diameter can be used depending upon the size of the catheter that is to be deflected. For large or stiff catheters, even extra-stiff wires are occasionally used, while at the other extreme, smaller (0.025") diameter wires are used for 4- and some 5-French catheters. Spring guide wires that have an antithrombus coating (heparin or teflon) have the advantage of sliding more easily through catheters and, theoretically, of reducing thrombus formation around the wires while they are within the catheter.

Mullins deflector wires™

Mullins™ deflector wires (Argon Medical Inc., Athens, TX) are straight, smoothly polished, relatively stiff, stainless steel wires, which are available in several diameters and all of which have a tiny, polished, welded "bead" at each end of the wire. The tiny bead is only slightly larger than the actual diameter of the wire and serves only to decrease the sharpness or "digging" characteristics of the fine stiff wire itself. Mullins™ wires are available in three sizes: 0.015", 0.017", and 0.020", with 150 cm lengths in all three diameters of the wires.

The use of Mullins™ wires to deflect catheters is identical to the use of a pre-curved, stiff end of a spring guide wire. Mullins™ wires have the advantage of being very smooth, single, stainless steel strands of polished wire, which potentially are less thrombogenic and definitely have a smaller diameter than a spring guide wire of comparable stiffness and deflection capability. With the smaller diameter of the wires compared to a spring guide wire, better pressure tracings can be obtained through the catheter and angiograms can be performed with Mullins™ wires in place. The diameter of the Mullins™ wire that is used, is chosen appropriately for the size, type and stiffness of the catheter that is to be deflected or supported, i.e. a 0.015" wire is used for a 5- or 6-French catheter, a 0.017" wire for a 7-F or thin-walled 8-F catheter, and a 0.020" wire for a standard 8-French or larger catheter.

When used as a deflector, the tip of the wire is selectively shaped or formed exactly as with the formation of the curves on the stiff end of a spring guide wire. Mullins™ wires are also used to stiffen the shafts of very soft catheters (e.g. warmed woven dacron or balloon flow-directed catheters) in order to facilitate catheter maneuvering or to support the position of a soft catheter in order to prevent the recoil of the catheter during a power injection of contrast.

Forming curves on rigid deflector wires

A catheter is manipulated to a site until its tip is adjacent to the orifice or branch vessel that is to be entered or to the valve that is to be crossed. Once it is determined that a rigid deflector wire will be desirable or necessary to enter a particular area, a mental note is made of the "three-dimensional" angles and directions from the tip of the catheter to the desired location. These angles and directions of the eventual curves in the wire are determined from one or more biplane angiograms in the area. The directions and dimensions of the curves that need to be formed in the wire are determined from this angiographic information according to the precise anatomy as well as the body and heart size of the patient.

A smooth, three-dimensional curve, which is *slightly* tighter (smaller), but corresponds to the desired angles and directions, is formed on the stiff end of the spring guide or either end of the Mullins™ wire. This is accomplished by bending the wire manually and very smoothly with the fingers or by winding the wire around a small syringe with a slightly smaller diameter than the diameter of the desired curve(s). The curve(s) in the wire is/are formed in small increments, always being sure to keep them very smooth. The technique of "pulling" one surface of the wire across a sharp surface, which is used to form curves in the floppy tips of spring guide wires and which is similar to "curling" a decorative "holiday ribbon", is ***not used*** for forming curves on the *stiff ends* of either spring guide wires or Mullins™ wires.

The curve formed on the wire is created significantly tighter than the bend or curve desired for the tip of the catheter since the wire within the catheter will be straightened significantly by the stiffness of the catheter. This straightening of the wire by the catheter is over-compensated for by forming the curve(s) on the end of the wire approximately 50% smaller (or tighter) and extending 50% further round the circumference than the anticipated final curve or deflection that is desired for the tip of the catheter. That is, if the desired diameter of the curve within the heart is judged to be 3 cm, the curve on the wire is formed 2 cm or less in diameter. If it is desirable to deflect the catheter 90° off its straight axis, the curve at the tip of the wire is formed so that it curves or bends 130° off the straight or long axis, i.e., somewhat back on itself. When a three-dimensional curve is necessary on the tip of the catheter, the same degree of over-curvature or over-tightening is applied to the secondary anterior–posterior curve as well as to the right or left curve.

It is extremely important that ***no*** *sharp bends, kinks* or *angles* are created anywhere along rigid deflector wires, and particularly not in the newly formed curve(s). Even very small but sharp bends or kinks in the wire will bind the wire within the catheter at the location of the kink as the wire is introduced or is being advanced. *Occasionally* an unwanted kink can be straightened when the wire is outside of the catheter by using two pairs of forceps like pliers on the wire; however, once an acute bend or kink has been formed inadvertently, it is usually simpler and more expeditious to use a new wire. When a sharp kink or bend occurs owing to overaggressive introduction of the wire, the kinked wire is withdrawn, the desired curve is formed in a *new wire* and the introduction is started all over rather than fighting against a kink in the wire within the catheter.

Technique for the use of rigid deflector wires

The catheter being deflected can be either an end-hole or a closed-end catheter since the deflector wires will not be advanced out of, or beyond the tip of, the catheter. The tip of the catheter is positioned adjacent to or slightly past the orifice or side branch to be entered. With the catheter tip in position and the desired curve formed on the wire, the curved, stiff end of the wire is introduced through a back-bleed valve/flush port on the catheter. Because of the tight curve at the tip of the wire and after being introduced into the back-bleed valve, often the tip of the wire will not pass into or through the hub of the catheter even with the use of a "wire introducer". In that circumstance, the wire back-bleed valve is removed from the catheter and the curved, stiff tip of the wire passed all of the way through the back-bleed valve. The back-bleed valve is withdrawn several centimeters back on the wire. The curved tip of the rigid wire itself is then manipulated through the hub of the catheter and well into the catheter. The back-bleed valve chamber is then placed on a continuous flush and re-advanced onto the hub of the catheter.

With or without removing the back-bleed valve from the hub of the catheter, the manipulations that are required to introduce the curved, stiff end of the wire into the catheter often straighten or distort the carefully pre-formed curves on the wire. When this occurs, the remaining curve of the wire is advanced beyond the reinforced hub of the catheter and into the catheter shaft, which is still outside of the body. With the wire now within the lumen of the catheter, the wire and catheter are "re-bent" to re-form the original curve while the "curve" on the catheter and wire is still outside of the introductory site into the vessel. With the wire in the lumen of the catheter, it is often easier to form even tighter, smoother curves than it is to form the same curve on the wire alone.

The properly curved wire is advanced into the catheter in very small increments (1–2 cm at a time) with the fingers pushing the wire while gripping the wire very close to the hub of the catheter. Gripping the wire close to the hub and pushing in small, very careful, increments are necessary to prevent inadvertent "Z-bends" from being created on the wire just proximal to the hub as an attempt is made to push the wire into the catheter with excessive force. Even a single acute kink or sharp bend in the wire makes advancing it through the catheter any further very difficult, if not impossible. If there is significant resistance while advancing the wire with the fingers alone, the tip and entire length of the wire are visualized under fluoroscopy to be sure that the wire has not dug into the wall of the catheter and that the catheter is not kinked somewhere along its course, blocking further advancement of the wire. With tight deflector curves formed on larger diameter rigid wires, and when used within stiffer catheters, a needle holder or Kelly™ clamp is substituted for the fingers and used as a pliers to grip and push the wire in order to introduce and advance it. The wire is advanced through the catheter very carefully and in *very small* (0.5–1 cm) increments.

During the stepwise introduction of the wire, the hub of the catheter is held securely against the surface of the catheterization table or the patient's leg to ensure that the tip of the catheter does not advance or withdraw inadvertently. The shaft of the catheter, which extends from the hub to the introduction site into the skin, should be maintained parallel to the long axis of the body and in as straight a line as possible. Any angle or bend away from the long axis of the body increases the resistance and decreases the forward motion on the wire as it is advanced within the catheter. Keeping the portion of the catheter that is still outside of the body as straight as possible, while allowing the catheter to flex or bend as the curves of the wire pass through any one segment of the catheter, facilitates the introduction of the wire. Slightly greater resistance is encountered as the wire passes through the straight sheath at the skin–vein junction, and as the wire passes through other rigid or fixed and straighter areas of the pelvic or abdominal venous system.

As the bends in the tip of the wire advance through the more proximal shaft of the catheter, the distal end of the catheter within the thorax is checked intermittently to ensure that it is not being withdrawn or advanced by the manipulations on the more proximal shaft of the catheter. As long as the tip of the catheter remains in position, the hub of the catheter remains fixed in place on the tabletop and the wire moves smoothly, it is not necessary, nor desirable, to watch the tip of the wire and shaft of the catheter continuously on fluoroscopy as the curved wire is being advanced through the pelvis and inferior vena cava. This merely increases radiation exposure unnecessarily to the abdominal/pelvic area of the patient. It ***is*** necessary to watch the *proximal* end of the wire visually where it is still outside of the body and proximal to the hub of the catheter, paying very careful attention not to kink, or bend, the wire as it is pushed into the catheter.

Whenever the tip of the wire approaches curves closer to the distal end of the catheter in the course of the catheter, the tips of both the catheter and wire do need to be observed frequently in both the PA and LAT planes. There is a tendency, particularly with soft catheters, for the tight curvature of the wire to pull the tip of the catheter back away from its original position or direction or even out of its original chamber/vessel unless special care is taken during this phase of the introduction (*see* Figure 6.4a). When the catheter had been advanced through tight curves in its course to the desired location, this maneuver with the rigid deflector wire often takes some complicated, combined to-and-fro maneuvering of the wire and the catheter together, particularly with very soft catheters. When an end-hole catheter is being used, care must be taken not to allow the stiff end of the wire to pass *beyond* the tip of the catheter.

Once the rigid deflector wire has reached the tip of the catheter, the catheter tip should point directly at the desired side branch or orifice (*see* Figure 6.4b). When the deflector wire has bent or curved the tip of the catheter toward the orifice or valve to be entered, the *proximal end of the deflector wire*, which still is outside of the hub of the catheter, ***is fixed*** *firmly* against the surface of the catheterization table. While keeping this proximal portion of the wire fixed and straight against the table, the *catheter* ***is advanced off the wire*** into the desired location and as far as possible into the vessel or chamber (*see* Figure 6.4c). When using any type of deflector wire within a catheter, the catheter ***always*** *is advanced off the wire* into the desired orifice! During this maneuver, if the catheter and wire are advanced together without fixing the wire, the entire curve of the catheter (with the enclosed curved deflector wire) will be advanced linearly within the original chamber/vessel in a direction aligned with the vessel. The curved tip of the catheter would then move *past* rather than into the desired orifice (*see* Figure 6.4d).

When the catheter is advanced off the wire that is directed toward the orifice or valve, it goes directly into the vessel/chamber. Once the catheter has entered the target vessel or chamber, it is advanced off the deflector wire into the desired position *within* the vessel or chamber while the wire is still in place supporting the more proximal catheter. The curved deflector wire is then withdrawn very slowly and carefully. The distal end of the catheter should be observed carefully on fluoroscopy until the deflector wire is well out of the field and away from the tip of the catheter to be sure that the acute, rigid curvature of the wire does not displace the catheter tip during the withdrawal of the wire.

Any type of soft tipped wire advanced beyond the end of the catheter and utilizing specifically formed curves or torque control can be used to advance the catheter even further out into the branch vessel or into an even more secure very distal location in a cardiac chamber. Occasionally a deflector wire with a different curve at the tip will be useful or necessary to reposition the tip of the catheter into a more desirable very distal location, particularly when the catheter is *not* an end-hole one. The routine use of a back-bleed/flush device on the hub of the catheter eliminates all rushing and urgency in maneuvering the catheter and wire into the desired location, even a high-pressure location.

With this combination of maneuvers and patience on the part of the operator, *all* branch vessels and chambers should be accessible. The advantage of using a wire with a preformed curve is that it deflects *the tip of the* ***catheter*** directly at and into vessel orifices or at and through valves that are at awkward angles to the long axis of the catheter. The angle to be deflected can be as much as 180° away from the original direction of the tip of the catheter!

The ability of rigid deflector wires to deflect the distal tip of the catheter effectively in three dimensions depends upon the even *more proximal curve(s)* in the *course of the catheter/wire* to hold or force the distal curve into its desired three-dimensional direction. The more proximal curves on rigid deflector wires are formed purposefully to conform to the more proximal curves in the course of the catheter within the heart. For example, creating a long sweeping proximal curve on the wire, which corresponds to the course from the inferior vena cava, through the right atrium and to the left atrium, forces a more distal curve that is angled acutely caudal and anteriorly (toward the mitral valve) to deflect the tip of the catheter caudally and specifically in the anterior direction. A similar (or any) bend on the proximal shaft of a torque wire would prevent the tip of that wire from rotating at all within a catheter.

Rigid deflector wires have several advantages over the "controllable" catheter tip deflector system. As just discussed, they have the ability to actually deflect the tip of a catheter purposefully in three dimensions, i.e. with a rigid deflector wire, the tip of the catheter can be bent or curved not only from right to left or anteriorly and posteriorly, but simultaneously from right to left and *selectively* either anteriorly or posteriorly. Unlike the active deflector wire, which will only accentuate the more proximal concave curve on the wire/catheter, with rigid deflector wires the tip of the catheter can be deflected away from the concave curve of the more proximal course of the catheter.

The rigid deflector system is maneuvered entirely within the catheter. The curve created on the catheter is "passive", allowing the catheter to follow the wire rather than forcing the tip of the catheter, which is very safe. If the tip of the catheter is against a wall or in a fixed "crevice" rather than properly toward an orifice, as the stiff curve on the rigid deflector wire approaches the tip of the catheter to deflect the catheter, the tip of the catheter is merely pushed away from the wall/crevice rather than through it. Likewise, when the catheter is advanced off the wire, the tip of the catheter is relatively soft and blunt and maintains little of the forward force so that the wire and catheter are pushed back and away from any rigid obstruction before the catheter can penetrate any solid structure. For example, a rigid deflector wire with a 180° tight curve formed at its tip and advanced to the tip of a straight catheter that is wedged in the trabeculae of the left ventricular apex, will push the shaft of the catheter away from the apical position and not dig into the trabeculae.

The Mullins™ rigid deflector wire has several additional advantages. It is much stiffer than a spring guide wire with a comparable diameter. The smaller diameter of the Mullins™ wire allows better pressure recordings while the wire is still within the lumen of the catheter and allows for larger volume, faster contrast injections with the wire still in place in the catheter. With its small diameter and polished smooth surface, it presents less resistance while passing through catheters, including catheters with walls of extruded polyurethane materials. The Mullins™ wire, with no spring coiled wire within the catheter has less potential for creating thrombi.

Disadvantages of "rigid" deflector wires
Preformed, "rigid" deflector wires do have some disadvantages. It takes knowledge of the anatomy, experience and practice to form smooth and exactly appropriate curves for each individual location and every size of patient. Even in experienced hands, when complex deflections are required, the wire often has to be withdrawn from the catheter to re-form the curve several times to achieve the ideal curve(s) on the catheter. The precise wire curve is formed outside of the body and must be advanced to the tip of the catheter through the length and various bends in the course of the catheter within the heart and vascular system. The wire easily loses some of its precise preformed curvature and tends to straighten out while being introduced into the proximal end of the catheter or while being advanced through the catheter. When there are tight preformed curves on the wire, it is frequently difficult to advance the curved wire through a tortuous course of the catheter en route to the tip of the catheter. When the tight preformed stiff curve of the rigid deflector wire approaches the tip of the catheter, it can very easily dislodge the tip away from a location, chamber or direction that the catheter was pointing directly at before the introduction of the wire. When the catheter is relatively stiff, the wire may not be strong enough to deflect the catheter sufficiently.

Examples of common uses of rigid deflector wires or unique preformed curves for entering specific locations

Curve #1—stiffening a soft catheter
One of the simplest but very effective uses of rigid deflector wires is to support or straighten, rather than deflect, otherwise very soft or malleable catheters. Because of its small diameter and smooth surface, the Mullins™ wire is particularly useful for this purpose. When used for supporting a catheter, the size of the rigid wire and the appropriate stiffness of the wire are determined according to the size of the catheter. The wire is introduced through a back-bleed valve/flush device attached to the flush/pressure system. When used with the Tuohy™ type back-bleed/flush device, accurate pressures can be recorded through the catheter, and angiograms can be performed through the catheter with the wire remaining in place to support the catheter.

The rigid wire is used to stiffen catheters that have become soft and pliable after being at body temperature for some time. For this use the wire can either be straight, or have a very slight (10–20°), long, gentle curve formed at the tip. Stiffening the catheter with a wire is useful or essential for wedging catheters into the pulmonary arterial or pulmonary vein capillary wedge positions, particularly in the presence of pulmonary hypertension.

The tip of the catheter must be observed very carefully as the stiff wire is being introduced when using these wires in end-hole, wedge type catheters. The end opening of the end-hole catheter can allow a very stiff deflector wire to extend beyond the catheter tip. The correct procedure is to advance the wire so that its tip stops 1–2 mm proximal to the tip of the catheter. The Mullins™ wire adds sufficient support to the remaining shaft of the catheter to achieve and maintain the wedge position, while a Tuohy™ type back-bleed valve with the Mullins™ wire allows very accurate pressures to be recorded and wedge angiocardiograms to be obtained with the wire remaining in the catheter.

Angiographic catheters that have passed through significant curves within the heart or great arteries, have a great tendency to recoil during high-pressure power injections. A Mullins™ wire used with a Touhy™ back-bleed device "stiffens" and straightens these catheters sufficiently to keep them securely in position during pressure injection while not significantly interfering with the flow rate of the contrast.

Curve #2—deflection from descending to ascending aorta
Often the tip of a catheter is too straight or becomes straightened after introduction into the femoral artery and does not advance readily around the aortic arch and all of the way into the aortic root. Even with a great deal of catheter manipulation, extensive and traumatic buckling of the catheter tip against the arterial wall or branch vessel, and excessive fluoroscopy time, a relatively straight catheter often cannot be maneuvered around the arch into the aortic root.

To accomplish the passage of any retrograde catheter easily and very quickly around the aortic arch from the femoral approach, a rigid deflector wire with an acute curve at the tip is used within the catheter to form an acute bend on the tip of the catheter. A relatively short (1–2 cm), smooth, 90–180° curve is formed on the tip of the stiff end of a spring guide wire or on one end of a Mullins™ wire. The curve formed on the wire should be smaller (tighter) in diameter than the diameter of the curve of the aortic arch. With the tip of the straight catheter in the dorsal or descending limb of the transverse aorta, the wire is introduced through a back-bleed valve to the *tip* of the catheter. This "automatically" deflects the tip of the catheter 90+°. In this circumstance, the *wire and catheter* are advanced *together* while rotating the combination slightly. Within seconds, the tip of the catheter/wire falls into the transverse arch and heads toward the ascending aorta or aortic root. From there, the *wire is held in place* and the *catheter only* is advanced off the wire and further into the aortic root. The wire is withdrawn from the catheter, the catheter is cleared of air and clots by a purposeful withdrawal directly from the hub of the catheter and the catheter is re-attached directly to the flush/pressure system. Further manipulations to cross the aortic valve are accomplished after the deflector wire has been removed. Because of the arterial pressures and potential for a large amount of blood loss around the wire in the catheter, a back-bleed device should be used in this situation even when the operator is very dexterous with the technique.

Curve #3—entering a vessel that is perpendicular off a major central vessel

When a side branch arises perpendicularly, or even more acutely, to the long axis of a central vessel, it is often difficult, if not impossible, to manipulate a catheter directly from the central vessel into the side branch. Even when the side branch can be entered with a guide wire, a large or stiff catheter or delivery system for a device often will not follow the wire through the acute angle into the side branch. Access into a side or branch vessel is accomplished easily by a two (or three) dimensional perpendicular deflection of the tip of the catheter with either an active or a rigid deflector wire. With the use of a smooth, relatively tight, right angle (or greater) curve on a rigid deflector wire, the tip of the catheter is deflected according to the curve on the wire. This acute deflection points the tip of the catheter at the orifice of the side branch and allows the stiffer catheter to be advanced off the wire and well into side branches off major central vessels. These right angle deflection curves are useful in deflecting from the main pulmonary artery into the right pulmonary artery, from the right or left pulmonary artery into specific branch pulmonary arteries, or from the descending aorta into renal, collateral, or other branch vessels or shunts off the aorta.

The catheter tip is positioned adjacent to, or slightly past, the orifice to be entered. An appropriate curve is formed on the rigid deflector wire and the preformed, stiff, curved end of the wire is introduced through a back-bleed valve into the catheter and advanced to just within the tip of the catheter. As the curved tip of the wire approaches the distal end of the catheter, the catheter tip bends (deflects) corresponding to the curve on the wire. The catheter/wire combination is rotated until the tip points directly at the desired orifice or side branch. Once the tip of the catheter has engaged in the side branch, the proximal end of the wire is fixed against the top of the catheterization table and the catheter is advanced off the wire into the vessel. Once in the vessel, the technique is the same for carefully removing the wire and then clearing the catheter of any possible air or clots.

Curve #4—deflection from left (or right) atrium into left (or right) ventricle

A specific "three-dimensional" curve on a stiff deflector wire facilitates the passage of any catheter from the right atrium to the right ventricle or from the left atrium into the left ventricle. The capacity to form a "third dimension" to the curve on the wire is where rigid deflector wires have a marked advantage over "controllable" tip deflector wires. Controllable deflector wires form only a two-dimensional curve, which can only be deflected in the direction of the *convex course* of the catheter immediately proximal to the tip.

When the catheter approach is from the femoral vein and crosses the septum into the left atrium, the catheter can usually be backed or "flipped" off the left atrial wall, out of a pulmonary vein or the atrial appendage and into the left ventricle, but only with persistence, traumatic probing, buckling off the atrial wall and considerable time. This maneuvering into the left ventricle often requires a great deal of manipulation, always causes trauma to the endothelium of the left atrium, and almost always requires extensive fluoroscopic time. With the use of a three-dimensional deflector wire the trauma is avoided entirely and the deflection from the left atrium to the left ventricle is performed quickly, reliably and without excessive irradiation of the patient and operators.

The tip of the catheter is positioned, either through an ASD, PFO, or transseptally, into a location well within the left atrium. Before the rigid deflector wire is introduced into the catheter, a smooth 180° curve is formed just proximal to the stiff end of the wire. The diameter of this curve is approximately *one half* of the *transverse diameter* of the cardiac silhouette. This 180° curve will bend the tip of the wire (and catheter) back caudally toward the apex of the heart shadow. This strictly two-dimensional curve/deflection could be accomplished with a controllable deflector wire, but *only* the two-dimensional curve could be formed. With a rigid deflector wire a second, "three-dimensional" curve is readily added to the distal half of the first 180° curve on the wire in order to add purposeful anterior direction to the previous caudal deflection. With the wire manually fixed on the tabletop and with the original 180° curve pointing toward the operator's right (patient's left) as the operator faces the patient, a second, anterior curve is formed on the *distal half* of the original 180° curve. The new distal curve should bend upward, off the table, toward the operator.

As this wire with the "three-dimensional" curve is advanced into the catheter that is positioned in the left atrium, the wire deflects or bends the tip of the catheter from its original cephalad, left and posterior position to a caudal, leftward and anterior direction. The tip of the catheter is now pointing in the direction of the mitral valve (or any left sided A-V valve) arising from the left atrium.

Occasionally, the catheter tip will pass posteriorly into a pulmonary vein and will be relatively fixed in this posterior position. Initially, if the tip of the catheter is relatively deep in the vein, it does not allow any caudal or anterior deflection of the tip of the catheter, even with the curved rigid deflector wire advanced all the way to the tip of the catheter. At the same time, the caudal force applied to the catheter by the wire will not tear or damage the vein or left atrium. From the pulmonary vein, the catheter and wire are withdrawn together, slowly applying counterclockwise torque on the catheter. As the tip of the catheter with the curved rigid deflector wire in it is withdrawn out of the vein, the catheter tip springs free of the pulmonary vein and "automatically" points anteriorly and usually directly toward (into) the mitral orifice! Occasionally the catheter, either with the initial introduction of the wire or after withdrawal from the pulmonary vein, ends up too far anteriorly and in the left atrial appendage—i.e. very far anteriorly and more cephalad in the left atrium. This location is apparent by the very cephalad and anterior position of the tip of the catheter/wire. The tip of a catheter/wire in the appendage has considerable "bounce" in spite of being very cephalad within the left atrial shadow. When in doubt about the location of the tip of the catheter, the location is verified by a gentle, small, hand injection of contrast through the side port of the wire back-bleed valve, around the wire and through the catheter. When the tip of the catheter is in the left atrial appendage, the catheter/wire combination is withdrawn *without* any counterclockwise torque until the tip of the catheter springs free from the appendage and is free in the cavity of the left atrium.

Once the tip of the catheter is free and directed anteriorly and caudally, the proximal end of the wire outside of the catheter (and body) is fixed in position on the tabletop or patient's leg while the catheter is advanced off the wire and into the ventricle. A continued counterclockwise torsion on the catheter/wire while the catheter is being advanced is useful to help direct the tip of the catheter well into the *apex* of the left ventricle and not "just into the ventricle". The *final* catheter positioning necessary for subsequent measurements of pressure or angiocardiograms is accomplished while the wire is still within the catheter rather than after the wire has been removed. With the wire passing through a back-bleed valve, there is no urgency to remove the wire, which is usually very helpful for positioning the catheter precisely for angiograms or manipulation to the outflow tract. Once the catheter is in the desired position, the wire is removed, the system carefully cleared of possible air and clot by purposefully withdrawing blood or fluid from the *hub of the catheter* and then flushed through the side port of the back-bleed system or attached directly to the pressure line.

A similar curve and technique are useful for advancing a catheter from the right atrium into the right ventricle. The use of a pre-curved rigid deflector wire is particularly helpful in patients with a large dilated right atrium or right ventricle or in the presence of marked tricuspid regurgitation.

Curve #5—pushing a back loop through an atrioventricular valve

A straight stiff wire or a stiff wire with a long, slight curve is useful for pushing the apex of an 180° curve or loop that has already been formed on a catheter within a chamber (atrium usually) through an atrioventricular valve. The apex of the loop or curve in the catheter is pushed through the valve in order to "back" the loop through the valve structures *ahead* of the tip of the catheter and, as a consequence, leave the tip of the catheter pointing toward the proximal end of the catheter. This is useful, for example, to back the apex of a 180° loop that is in the shaft of a catheter proximal to the tip of the catheter, through the mitral valve. Once the apex of the more proximal curve in the catheter enters the left ventricle, the tip follows or is pulled behind the curve with the result that, as the curve approaches the ventricular apex, the tip now points backward and toward the semilunar valve.

In order to perform this maneuver through the mitral valve, the tip of a relatively soft catheter is advanced from the right atrium across the atrial septum to near, or actually into, the orifice of a pulmonary vein or the left atrial appendage. Advancing the catheter even further with its tip fixed in this location buckles or bows the shaft of the catheter and produces a larger curve within the left atrium (Figure 6.5a). The apex of the curve in the shaft of the catheter is usually directed caudally and toward the left side of the heart. Without other support and by merely advancing the catheter further, this curve usually loops around within the atrium, making it more convoluted and difficult or impossible to back the loop selectively toward the left atrioventricular valve (or any area) without displacing the tip out of the pulmonary veins.

The stiff end of a spring guide wire or a Mullins™ wire is used to push the apex of the curve in the shaft of the catheter into the ventricle. A long, smooth, slight (10–15°) curve is formed on the Mullins™ wire or the stiff end of a spring guide wire. The curve is given a slight, anterior, "three-dimensional" bend, molding the stiff wire very slightly caudally and anteriorly relative to the position of the catheter in the heart. The stiff, slightly curved wire is introduced into the catheter and advanced within it to the mid portion of the curve within the left atrium so that the tip of the wire is just proximal to the area of maximum curvature in the catheter where the catheter is beginning to buckle or fold caudally (Figure 6.5b). The catheter and wire are advanced together, and the stiff tip of the wire pushes the apex of the loop in the shaft of the catheter as the "leading edge" through the AV valve and to the apex of the ventricle (Figure 6.5c).

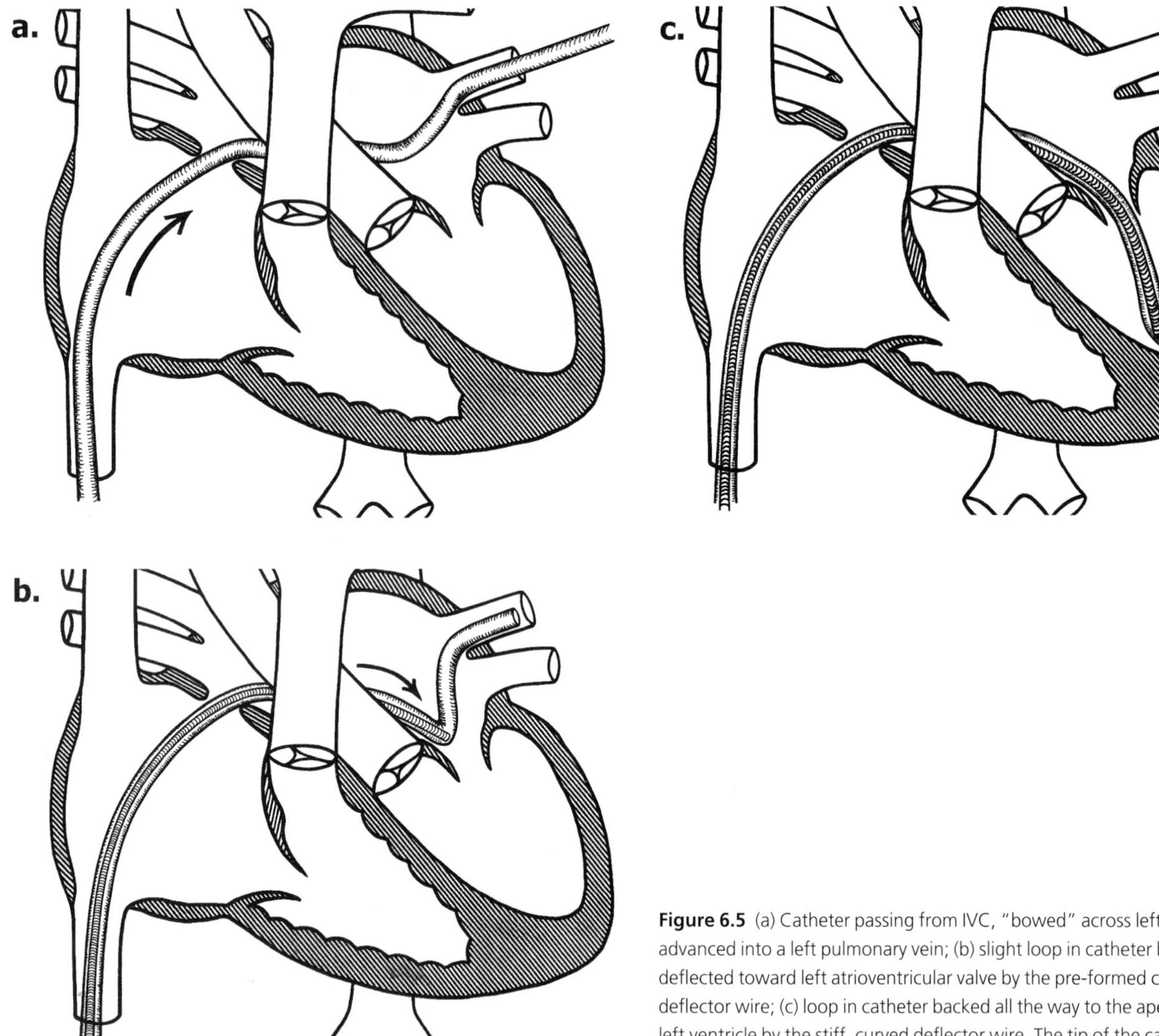

Figure 6.5 (a) Catheter passing from IVC, "bowed" across left atrium and advanced into a left pulmonary vein; (b) slight loop in catheter being deflected toward left atrioventricular valve by the pre-formed curved deflector wire; (c) loop in catheter backed all the way to the apex of the left ventricle by the stiff, curved deflector wire. The tip of the catheter has "followed" the more proximal catheter into the left ventricle.

If the tip of the "curved" catheter does not follow into the ventricle and remains in the atrium, the wire is held in place (or advanced slightly) while the catheter is slowly and carefully withdrawn over the wire. This maneuver withdraws the entire catheter while the fixed wire, which is in the loop of the catheter pushing toward the left ventricular apex, "pulls" the tip of the catheter through the atrioventricular valve and into the ventricle. With the catheter thus backed into the ventricle, the tip of the catheter becomes directed cephalad and often headed for the semilunar valve (Figure 6.5c). Once the tip backs into the ventricle and the ventricular pressure has been recorded, the wire is held in that position while the catheter is advanced off the wire. This maneuver often allows the tip of the catheter to advance through the semilunar valve which arises from that ventricle.

Curve #6—deflection from right ventricle to main pulmonary artery

Fixed curves on rigid deflector wires have the unique capability of being formed into *compound reverse* curves for manipulation of catheters into very specific or difficult locations, particularly with the use of "three-dimensional" or more convoluted curves added to the wire. With a compound reverse curve, the tip of the catheter can be directed away from the direction of the "concavity" of the course of the rest of the catheter. One common use of a combined compound reverse and three-dimensional curve is the use of an "S-shaped" wire to advance a catheter from a large dilated right ventricle into the pulmonary artery. This is particularly useful in patients who are postoperative and have large right ventricular outflow patches, aneurysms of the outflow tract, or significant pulmonary valve regurgitation. Flow-directed catheters obviously are totally useless in these circumstances. In this group of patients a torque-controlled catheter can be manipulated into the right ventricle and even made to point cephalad toward the pulmonary artery. However, because of the large diameter of the right atrium and right ventricle, when the catheter is advanced forward with the usual torquing maneuvers, the tip of the catheter merely moves laterally or the proximal part of the catheter bows into large loops within the right atrium.

To use a rigid deflector wire with a compound reverse curve in this situation, the catheter is positioned with its tip as deep within the body of the right ventricle as possible, and at least against the septal/lateral wall of the right ventricle. An "S-shaped" curve is formed outside of the body on the rigid end of the guide or Mullins™ wire. The bottom (proximal) part of the S is formed to correspond to both the curvature and the distance from the mid-right atrium to the free right ventricular wall. The S curve is formed so that its "height" is somewhat less than the length of the "bottom" curve of the S. Once the S has been formed, the wire is placed on the table so that the S is inverted and the top of the S at the distal tip of the wire is pointing cephalad, and the proximal (bottom) curve of the S is pointing to the patient's right (toward the operator). With the S lying across the patient and reversed in that position, its bottom points caudally while its top is directed to the patient's left and cephalad on the patient. A second *posterior (or dorsal)* curve is formed on the distal (top) "limb" of the reverse S nearest the tip of the wire. The consequence of this particular compound curve is that the *proximal* curve of the reverse S will conform obligatorily to the concave course of the catheter—passing from the patient's right to the patient's left—that is formed as it passes from the *IVC/right atrium into the right ventricle*. This, in turn, *obligates* the distal curve of the reverse S to point cephalad, and the secondary "three-dimensional" curve to point posteriorly!

The reverse S curved wire is introduced into the proximal end of the catheter, which must be maintained as deep in the right ventricle as possible. Once the compound curve is *completely* past the hub and back-bleed valve on the catheter, and several centimeters into the shaft of the catheter, it is useful to re-form the curve on the wire within the proximal portion of the catheter that is still outside the body. As discussed earlier in this chapter, this re-formation assures that the desired, previously formed curve on the wire is still present and is as "tight" as originally formed. As the cardiac silhouette or right ventricle is approached as the wire is being advanced within the catheter, significant extra care becomes necessary in advancing the wire. A relatively rigid, compound, reverse curve on the stiff end of a wire has a tendency to pull the tip of a soft catheter backward and out of the ventricle as the wire is advanced around the curve from the right atrium into the ventricle. When the catheter has become unusually soft, this maneuver is particularly difficult and, occasionally, impossible.

Sometimes, it is helpful to form a 360° curve on the more proximal shaft of a catheter that is still within the right atrium by advancing the catheter that has its tip wedged against the lateral wall of the right ventricle. This very broad loop around the outer circumference of the right atrium does not give the catheter any room to "back" into the atrium as the stiff compound curves are advanced through the loop!

Once a compound reverse S curve in a wire has been advanced to the tip of a catheter, the combined catheter and wire are withdrawn slightly, gently and very cautiously. With this maneuver the bottom, or proximal, portion of the reverse S curve will conform to the curvature of the usual catheter course from the inferior vena cava, through the right atrium, across the tricuspid valve and into the right ventricle. With the proximal curve of the catheter forced into this position by the proximal curve on the wire, the distal and posteriorly directed curve on the wire automatically "flips" cephalad and points the tip of the catheter cephalad and posteriorly toward the right ventricular outflow tract and pulmonary artery (Figure 6.6). With the proximal end of the wire, which is outside the

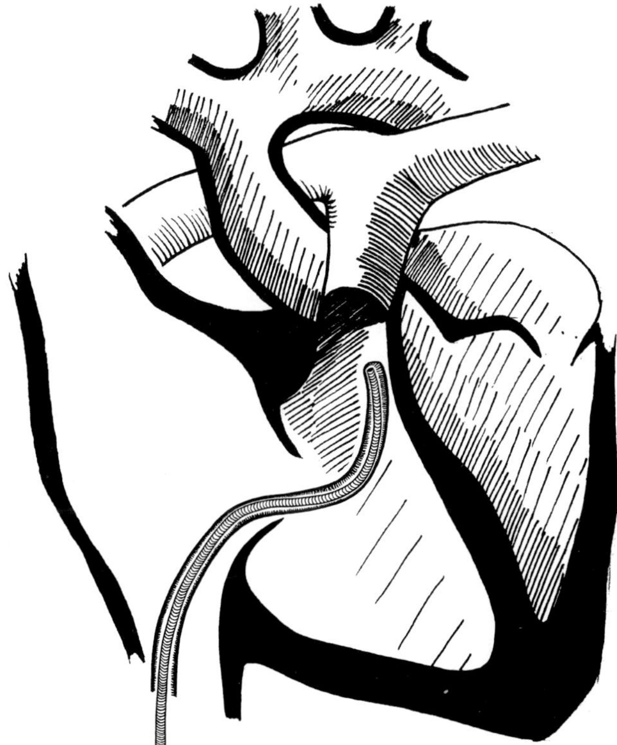

Figure 6.6 Compound reverse "S" curve on a rigid deflector wire obligatorily deflecting tip of catheter toward the pulmonary from the right ventricle.

body, fixed against the tabletop or patient's leg, it is usually very simple to advance the catheter off the tip of the wire and directly into the pulmonary artery. Once the catheter has entered the pulmonary artery, it is advanced off the deflector wire as far as possible into a distal pulmonary artery branch, and if possible the catheter is wedged into a distal branch artery. The position of the catheter must be observed very carefully during the withdrawal of the stiff S wire to ensure that the tip of the catheter is not withdrawn inadvertently from the pulmonary artery.

Curve #7—deflection into an acutely angled take-off of a left pulmonary artery

A tighter, compound true reverse S curve is invaluable for entering left pulmonary arteries which are stenosed or arise at unusual or very acute angles off the main artery or junction of the main and right pulmonary arteries. This anatomy is particularly common in patients who have had previous surgical repair of tetralogy of Fallot, pulmonary atresia/VSD or truncus arteriosus, and is a very common area of proximal branch pulmonary artery stenosis. A floppy-tipped, torque-controlled wire can usually be introduced into such vessels, but very often the stiff portion of the wire or catheter will *not* follow around the sharp curves that are encountered entering the left branch pulmonary artery. The compound curves on the stiff deflector wire are formed according to the size of the heart and the angle of take-off of the left pulmonary artery in each individual patient. The sizing of these curves to match the anatomy is critical for the success of this technique, and the specific curves must often be re-formed after some trial and error in each individual patient. For this deflection, the long proximal curve of the S is created with a secondary slight posterior (dorsal) curve. This proximal and central part of the S is intended to correspond to the course from the right atrium, through the right ventricle and into the right pulmonary artery. The curve on the distal part of the S is formed much shorter and also with a secondary short, posterior curve. In this particular use, the long curve on the *proximal* portion of the S wire obligatorily conforms to the course of the catheter traversing from the right atrium, through the right ventricle inflow, into the outflow tract and toward the main pulmonary artery (RA–RV–RVOT–PA). Once the proximal curve on the S conforms to this intracardiac curve, the tight curve on the distal part of the S obligates the tip to deflect toward the patient's left and posteriorly (into the left pulmonary artery [LPA]).

To utilize this compound deflection, the catheter is first advanced as far as possible into the distal right pulmonary artery (RPA). With a tight, compound, three-dimensional reverse curve on the stiff wire, there is an even greater tendency for the catheter to be withdrawn from its distal location as the stiff, curved wire is advanced into, and through, the right ventricle. The pre-formed wire is advanced carefully all the way to the tip of the catheter while maintaining the latter securely in the distal RPA. Extra patience and multiple catheter maneuvers are often necessary to accomplish this part of the procedure. Often, as the stiff curve in the wire begins to enter the ventricle, the proximal catheter is backed out of the ventricle and the tip becomes withdrawn from the distal right pulmonary artery. As the catheter backs out of the ventricle, a very large loop usually begins to form in the right atrium. It is often useful to allow a complete 360° loop to form in the right atrium by advancing the catheter along with, or slightly ahead of, the wire before the catheter begins to back out of the ventricle. Once the 360° loop is formed and "fills" the circumference of the right atrium, the lateral wall of the right atrium is used to support the outer circumference of the catheter/wire as the wire is advanced through the catheter, around the 360° loop in the atrium, and into and through the continuing loop in the right ventricle.

After the tip of the wire with its compound curve reaches the tip of the catheter, the proximal curve on the S of the wire will correspond to the course through the right ventricle to the distal right pulmonary artery. This curve will force the distal reverse curve at the tip to be directed cephalad and posteriorly. The combination of the catheter and wire together is slowly and carefully withdrawn back toward the main (and left) pulmonary artery. As the combination catheter/wire is withdrawn, the proximal, longer curve on the S conforms more rigidly to the natural curvature of the course of the RV–RVOT–RPA on the proximal catheter, while the secondary (distal), three-dimensional curve in the wire obligatorily deflects the tip of the catheter/wire first cephalad and posteriorly and second—as the proximal curve is pulled more into the right ventricle—posteriorly and to the left and usually directly at or into the orifice of the LPA (Figure 6.7).

Once the tip of the catheter is in or pointing exactly at the orifice of the LPA, the proximal end of the wire outside the catheter (and body) is fixed in place on the tabletop while the catheter is advanced off the wire and as far as possible into the distal LPA. As with the previous compound curves, once the catheter has been advanced into the proper location, the wire is removed very cautiously to prevent the simultaneous withdrawal of the catheter. This particular combination of curves in the stiff deflector wire and the accompanying catheter maneuvers have always resulted in a successful entrance into abnormally positioned left pulmonary arteries, particularly for subsequent interventional procedures such as dilations with or without intravascular stent implants.

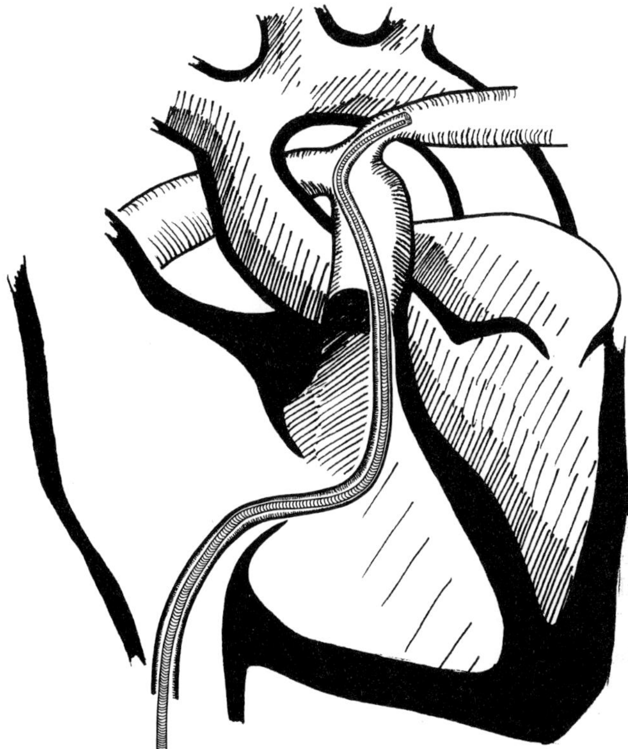

Figure 6.7 Compound reverse "S" curve with tertiary very distal posterior bend in the wire, which will deflect the tip of the catheter almost obligatorily into the left pulmonary artery.

Curve #8—deflection into the pulmonary veins from the retrograde/right ventricular approach following a baffle (Senning/Mustard) venous switch repair of transposition of the great arteries

A similar type of compound S curve is useful for entering the pulmonary veins in patients who have had a venous switch repair of transposition of the great arteries ("Mustard" or "Senning" procedure). When these patients require cardiac catheterization, it is usually imperative that the pulmonary veins are entered as part of the procedure. From a retrograde approach and once the catheter has been manipulated into the right ventricle and from there maneuvered retrograde across the tricuspid valve into the distal chamber of the pulmonary venous atrium (distal part of the original right atrium), the tip of the catheter will be directed *anteriorly and usually caudally*. It is always a significant challenge to redirect the tip of the catheter cephalad and posteriorly toward (and into) the common pulmonary vein channel and from there into the separate pulmonary veins. When the retrograde approach is used and by the time the tip of the catheter reaches the *distal* pulmonary venous atrial chamber (adjacent to the tricuspid valve), there are already *two* 180° curves more proximally in the course of the catheter. As a consequence, most of the torque and/or any other control over the tip of the catheter is lost. In this situation, a different, but still "compound S" curve is utilized to redirect the tip of the catheter. The proximal (or bottom) portion of the S is formed into a long 180° curve. This curve is formed to correspond to the curvature of the catheter as it passes *around the aortic arch* from the descending to the ascending aorta. A slightly longer central "straight" portion of the "S" then is formed on the wire. This straighter central portion of the "S" is formed to correspond to the distance between the *most cephalad portion of the aortic arch* to *the middle of the right ventricular cavity (level of the tricuspid valve)*. The distal part (top) of the "upright S" is formed to correspond to the second 180° curve in the catheter and to direct the tip of the catheter cephalad again as the catheter passes retrograde from the right ventricle, through the tricuspid valve, to the distal part of the pulmonary venous atrium (adjacent to the tricuspid valve). With the "S" thus formed on the wire outside of the body and with the "S" wire positioned on the table with the *distal end (top) of the "S"* now *caudal* with the tip of the "S" (and wire) facing toward the *patient's* right, an additional posterior or dorsal curve is formed on the top or distal end of the "S". This "three-dimensional" posterior curve on the distal "S" is designed to deflect the tip of the catheter from the "distal" pulmonary venous atrium, cephalad, posteriorly and back toward the confluence of the pulmonary veins, which pass laterally and posteriorly around the baffle.

The retrograde catheter is manipulated around the arch, from the aorta into the right ventricle and retrograde through the tricuspid valve into the distal portion of the pulmonary venous atrium. This maneuver often requires multiple attempts and considerable "probing" or the use of floppy-tipped guide wires to cross the tricuspid valve and reach the "old" right atrium. The S curve on the stiff wire, which will be used eventually to enter the pulmonary veins, is occasionally useful in directing the tip of the catheter from the right ventricle into the right atrium. Once the tip of the catheter has crossed the tricuspid valve and is positioned well into the distal pulmonary venous atrium, the pre-formed, curved, stiff deflector wire is advanced carefully to the tip of the catheter. Again, special care is taken as the stiff end of the curved wire is passed through the right heart chambers to prevent the catheter tip from being withdrawn back into the right ventricle by the wire. When the wire reaches the tip of the catheter in the "old" right atrium, the tip of the catheter will be pointing cephalad and posteriorly. The wire is fixed in position and the catheter is advanced off the wire, over the inferior limb of the baffle and into the proximal part of the pulmonary venous atrium. Once the tip of the catheter has been secured in the proximal portion of the pulmonary venous atrium, the compound, curved wire is again advanced to the tip of the catheter. The compound curve of the wire within the tip of the catheter now should direct the tip of the catheter toward the common pulmonary venous channel, which passes laterally around the baffle. The wire is again held in a fixed position against the tabletop while the catheter is advanced off the wire into the common pulmonary venous channel (and back into a pulmonary vein). Obviously, the curves that are formed on the wire to accomplish this deflection must be individually preformed very precisely according to the sizes of the patient and their heart and chamber. As with other compound curves on rigid deflector wires, the wire may have to be re-formed outside the body on several occasions.

Curve #9—tight 180° deflections

Occasionally it is desired to reverse the direction of the tip of the catheter 180° and *simultaneously* to change the direction of the tip anteriorly or posteriorly during the deflection. A fairly tight, but smooth, 1.5–2 cm diameter, 180° to 230° curve is formed on the stiff end of a spring guide or a Mullins™ wire. The distal end of the curve is then bent smoothly either anteriorly or posteriorly—depending upon the proposed use of the curve—to form the "third dimension" of the curve. As with all rigid deflector wires, the wire is pre-shaped outside of the body before it is introduced into the catheter. An active (or controllable) deflector wire (described earlier in this chapter) can be used to reverse the direction of the tip of the catheter by 180°, but provides no anterior/posterior control over the deflected tip.

The 180° curve with a slight, anterior "3-D" component is invaluable for crossing from one iliofemoral vessel to the contralateral iliofemoral vessel. A similar 3-D, but slightly wider, curve is used to enter the pulmonary artery from the right ventricle when the catheter has been introduced into the right atrium/ventricle from the superior vena cava. A 180° curve with a slight 3-D bend at the distal end is extremely useful when the catheter is maneuvered into the ventricle but the tip of the catheter is facing away from the area or vessel to be entered, for example when a catheter that has been introduced into the left ventricle prograde through the mitral valve is to be advanced into the left ventricular outflow tract; or when crossing a ventricular septal defect with a retrograde catheter or manipulating the catheter through a ventricular septal defect and into the great vessel arising from the opposite ventricle.

When a rigid deflector wire is used to deflect the tip of the catheter from the apex of the left ventricle to the left ventricular outflow tract, a relatively tight 180° curve is formed at the stiff end of the wire. The 180° curved wire is positioned on the tabletop passing across the patient from the patient's right to the left and an additional, slight, anterior bend is added to the most distal part of the 180° curve. A long smooth curve, which corresponds to the course from the inferior vena cava, across the atrial septum to the left atrium and left ventricle, is formed on the stiff wire just proximal to the tight distal 180° curve.

Similarly to advancing other rigid deflector wires into pre-positioned catheters, as this tight curve is advanced within the catheter that is pre-positioned in the ventricle, the tip of the catheter is usually pulled back by the advancing curve in the wire. As a consequence, the position of the catheter must be adjusted accordingly to maintain its tip deep within the apex of the ventricle. Once the curve has reached the tip of the catheter (in any of the locations where this curve is used), the tip of the combined catheter/wire is withdrawn slightly in order to free the tip of the catheter from the trabeculae of the ventricle or wall of a vessel. Once the tip of the catheter with the wire has been withdrawn "out of the apical tissues", the tip of the wire/catheter will move freely and will conform to the complete 180° deflection (curve) of the wire. Once the tip of the catheter is moving freely and is pointing toward the outflow tract of the ventricle or other desired area, the wire is fixed in position outside the body against the tabletop or patient's leg while the catheter is advanced off the wire into the desired location. Even with a three-dimensional curve on the stiff end of the wire, usually some rotation and slight to-and-fro motion of the combined wire/catheter are required as the catheter is advanced into the desired location.

Occasionally the tip of the combined wire/catheter remains somewhat constrained and does not deflect the desired 180° even when the tip has moved proximally toward the inflow of the ventricle. In that case, the combination is advanced together very carefully. The combination of the tip of the catheter with the stiff wire within it usually will catch on the wall of the ventricle and begin to curl back on itself into a tighter curve than the 180° curve on the wire, which, in turn, directs the tip of the catheter toward the center of the cavity of the ventricle. The catheter is then advanced off the wire.

Summary—rigid deflector wires

An infinite variety of curves can be formed on rigid deflector wires, and along with the specific maneuvers of the wire/catheter combination, it is usually possible to enter any area that would otherwise be difficult or impossible to access with the usual catheter manipulations. As mentioned earlier, rigid deflector wires have some significant advantages over the active or controllable type of deflector wire. The greatest advantages are that rigid deflector wires have the ability to actually deflect the tip of a catheter in "compound" or reverse directions away from the concave course of the catheter and purposefully in "three dimensions"; i.e. the tip of the catheter can be directed *away* from the convex curve of the more proximal portion of the catheter and simultaneously it can be deflected purposefully not only from right to left or anteriorly and posteriorly, but simultaneously from right to left *and* specifically either anteriorly or posteriorly. While rigid deflector wires purposefully deflect the tips of catheters to very acute angles, they do so without exerting any *forward* force on the tip of the *catheter* and without any possibility of "excavating" tissues within the curve of the wire as the tip is deflected. This makes rigid wires relatively safe against perforation. Another advantage is that a rigid wire deflection system is far cheaper than an active deflector wire. Furthermore the polished straight Mullins™ deflector wires with their lack of a coiled spring wire within the catheter have a lower potential for thrombi.

The major disadvantage of rigid deflector wires is the "learning curve" inherent in forming and then using the curves. Even in the hands of an experienced operator who is familiar with the wires and all the possible curves, rigid wires can cause the catheter to "back out" of its location as the stiff and rigid deflector wire is introduced. This problem usually, but not always, can be overcome with experience and by changing the *stiffness* of the wire used to form the curves relative to the stiffness of the catheter.

Complications of guide/deflector wires

Guide and deflector wires are not immune from potential complications although most, if not all, complications from the wires are preventable by the use of proper techniques. The introduction into and the removal of wires from catheters always generate the potential for introducing air and/or particulate matter into the catheter and, in turn, into the circulation. Meticulous precautions are strictly adhered to in order to clear catheters of air and/or clots before anything is introduced into them. The presence of a wire in the lumen of a catheter compromises the lumen and potentially causes stasis of blood in the lumen whenever the catheter is in the circulation. Blood stasis results in thrombi which, if pushed out of the catheter, become emboli! Wire back-bleed devices with side flush ports, which are maintained on an almost continuous flush, are used whenever a wire is used or through a catheter. The flush is discontinued only when a pressure is being recorded and/or an angiogram is being performed through the catheter and around the wire. Suction or negative pressure ***never*** should be applied to a back-bleed valve/side port that has a wire passing through it in order to draw samples and/or in "clearing the line". Air *preferentially* will always be sucked *through the valve* rather than any blood and/or debris being withdrawn from the long, narrow lumen of the catheter.

Perforation of cardiac structures and/or vessels occurs more commonly during the manipulation of wires separately and/or within catheters than with the manipulation of catheters alone. Perforations are more common when wires are manipulated outside catheters as opposed to their use to stiffen and/or deflect catheters. Perforations of almost any structure can, and do, occur with almost all types of wire. The stiffer the wire and the more constrained the area or structure where the wire is being manipulated, the greater the chance of a perforation occurring with a wire.

The end capillaries of the pulmonary arteries are frequently perforated during the fixation of the tips of Super Stiff™ (Boston Scientific, Natick, MA), spring guide wires far distally out in the pulmonary arteries during various interventional procedures when the wires are purposefully "buried" deep into the capillaries of the peripheral pulmonary arterial bed. Even with precise control of the wire, some capillary disruption appears unavoidable. Usually these very peripheral perforations are of no consequence and often go unnoticed during the procedure, with the patient incidentally mentioning pleuritic pain on the day following the procedure in the area where the distal end of a wire had been during the procedure. If a wire is forced into or through or is repeatedly probed into the distal pulmonary vessels, especially if the particular area of the pulmonary artery has a higher than normal pressure, then significant bleeding can occur following a wire perforation of the very distal pulmonary vessels. In patients who have had previous thoracic surgery, the extravasation of blood is usually contained in the scarred area and appears as a localized density in the lung field on X-ray and/or fluoroscopy. Such an extravasation can present as hemoptysis and/or as an accumulation of blood in the pleural space with or without an associated deterioration in the patient's hemodynamics. When bleeding from a peripheral lung vessel persists, the treatment is to occlude the vessel just proximal to the perforation with a catheter delivered device (coil), and a pleural tap and/or chest tube to drain the pleural space when there is significant bleeding.

Perforation through the wall of a chamber and/or vessel is possible during the manipulation of a wire outside a catheter. This occurs almost only when the tip of a wire is advanced out of the tip of a catheter *when the latter is wedged into or forced against the wall of a structure.* If the remaining, more proximal course of the catheter is fixed or constrained within a chamber or vessel, and the tip of the catheter cannot "back away" as the wire is extruded forcefully out of it, the wire will perforate! An example of this is when a catheter is looped 360° securely around the "outer circumference" of an atrium while the tip of the catheter is wedged into the atrial appendage. If a wire is forced out of the tip of the catheter, the catheter cannot bow or back away into any wider circumference in the atrium, so the wire is forced through the wall of the appendage. Similarly, when a catheter is advanced from the right atrium to the right ventricle and toward the right ventricle outflow tract using a large 360° atrial loop, and the loop in the shaft of the catheter is reinforced by the wire within it, the wire/catheter loop is "confined" within the outer circumference of the right atrium and right ventricular free wall. If, at the same time, the tip of the catheter is buried in the musculature of the right ventricular outflow tract rather than pointing *exactly* at the pulmonary orifice, *any* wire extruded from the tip of the catheter will perforate any structure in front of it. The stiffer the catheter, the stiffer the overall wire and the stiffer the tip of the wire, the more likely this type of perforation is to occur.

Perforations with the tips of wires that are manipulated free within the vasculature are prevented by using wires with very long and very floppy tips, and even with those wires, never attempting to extrude a wire from a catheter where the tip of the catheter is fixed or buried into a wall or tissues. Wires with special, very short floppy tips are used for fixation in the distal lung vessels, but these wires and the stiff ends of any wires should never be advanced out of the catheter when the tip of the catheter is in a chamber or central vessel.

Terumo™ Glide™ wires have a unique potential of their own for perforation. Because of their smooth and fairly rigid characteristics, Terumo™ wires perforate intracardiac structures even more easily than standard spring guide wires when they are being extruded from a catheter. When a straight Terumo™ wire is advanced out of the tip of a catheter, the tip of the Terumo™ wire does not deflect or bend away from its straight direction out of the tip of the catheter for a distance of at least 4–5 mm. If the tip of the catheter is constrained and cannot "back away" from the wall of the structure, the Terumo™ wire easily perforates into or through the structure. This is true particularly when a Terumo™ wire is extruded into the trabeculae of a ventricular cavity. The stiffer shaft of the Terumo™ wire does not tend to bow or bend away from the resistance, and its tip easily burrows into the relatively soft myocardium.

Perforation is also a greater potential problem when a Terumo™ wire is used to cross the aortic valve from the retrograde approach. When the tip of an end-hole retrograde catheter is advanced against an aortic leaflet in the aortic root *and* the more proximal shaft of the catheter is pushed against the outer circumference of the curve of the aortic arch, the catheter or wire cannot back away from the valve as the wire is extruded, and the wire perforates rather than being deflected back into the aortic arch. This is avoided either by not using Terumo™ wires in this circumstance or, if a Terumo™ is used, by always using a curved tipped wire and *always* assuring that the catheter tip is well above the aortic leaflets when the wire is extruded out of the tip of the catheter.

There is an additional, unique and real potential hazard with the use of *active deflector wires*. The deflection of the tip of the wire is accomplished by a very strong force applied manually to the deflector handle, but there is no means of measuring this force and no way of determining what is causing the total resistance against it. One part of the resistance is inherent in the wires themselves, and varies from one wire to another even with deflector wires that are the same size. There is also resistance created by the relatively stiff walls of the catheter as it is deflected from its straight configuration to the desired curve. Finally, if the catheter tip is forced against any intracardiac or intravascular structure during a deflection, resistance to the deflection is created by these structures. As the wire/catheter overcomes this resistance, it can "dig" through the adjacent structure, which, in turn, represents a real potential danger of active deflector wires. When, in addition, the more proximal shaft of the catheter is constrained in a tight area, it does not allow the tip of the *catheter* with the deflecting wire to move away from a fixed structure, and forces the tip ***into*** and/or ***through*** the structure! When the constraint is very tight or the structure very delicate, the wall of the structure can easily be disrupted. This likelihood should always be considered when deflecting in or near an atrial appendage or within the trabeculae of a ventricular chamber. Whenever any unusual force is required, entrapment of the tip of the catheter must be considered as the source of the resistance.

The majority (all?) of the complications of intravascular wires and wire manipulations are avoidable by proper and careful techniques.

References

1. Ovitt TW *et al*. Guide wire thrombogenicity and its reduction. *Radiology* 1974; **111**(1): 43–46.
2. Takahashi M *et al*. Percutaneous heart catheterization in infants and children. I. Catheter placement and manipulation with guide wires. *Circulation* 1970; **42**(6): 1037–1048.

7 Flow directed catheters ("floating" balloon catheters)

Flow directed balloon catheters

The concept of a floating balloon catheter is just that! Balloon-tipped catheters are designed to "float" along with, and follow the course of, blood flow[1]. A small, inflated, latex balloon at the distal end of the catheter acts as a "sail" to pull the catheter along in the blood stream. The shafts of these catheters are manufactured of a thinner wall, softer and more flexible, material in order to provide better "floating" characteristics. As a consequence, balloon floating catheters are dependent almost totally on their floating capability and on being pulled along with the vigorous flow of the blood. Most torque and guidable qualities of the catheters are lost in order to achieve the softer, better floating characteristics. Floating balloon catheters generally require a fairly vigorous flow of blood and, even then, do not float to every desired location. As a consequence, floating catheters cannot be relied upon as the only catheters for a procedure. All physicians who perform diagnostic or therapeutic catheterizations on pediatric or congenital heart patients must be adept at the use of separate, torque-controlled catheters as well as floating balloon catheters.

For optimal floating, the balloon of the catheter is filled with a gas, and in the pediatric and congenital cardiac catheterization laboratory, the gas should always be filtered carbon dioxide (CO_2). Carbon dioxide diffuses instantaneously into blood and, as a consequence, theoretically does not form a discrete bolus or bubble of gas which could obstruct blood flow in small vessels. CO_2 is available commercially and relatively inexpensively. It comes in very high-pressure gas cylinders and is made accessible to the catheter through a gas reduction valve on the cylinder. Most commercial CO_2 contains some particulate impurities and should be filtered before it is used in an intravascular balloon in a patient. CO_2 is very diffusable in air and moderately diffusable *through* latex. Consequently, between the storage cylinder and the catheter the CO_2 must be maintained in an absolutely sealed system. Even a transient opening for a *few seconds* "to air", of a stopcock on a syringe containing CO_2, allows the majority of the CO_2 in even a 10 ml syringe to diffuse out while air flows into the syringe! A 10 ml syringe of CO_2 carried across a room with the tip of the syringe open would be 99+% air by the time it arrives at the catheterization table across the room. CO_2 also diffuses through latex balloon material at a noticeable rate, which results in the balloon filled with CO_2 decreasing in size fairly rapidly when inflated in the circulation. As a consequence, the balloon on a floating balloon catheter requires refilling every few minutes to maintain an effective floating size.

A convenient, sterile, "bedside reservoir" for CO_2 is fabricated for each individual patient from a sterile 10 ml Luer™ lock syringe, a sterile, 3 ml Luer™ lock syringe, and a sterile, air tight, three way stopcock (Figure 7.1). The two syringes are attached very tightly to the female connections of the stopcock and a sterile, disposable, micro gas filter is attached to the male connector of the three-way stopcock. The outlet from the reduction valve on the

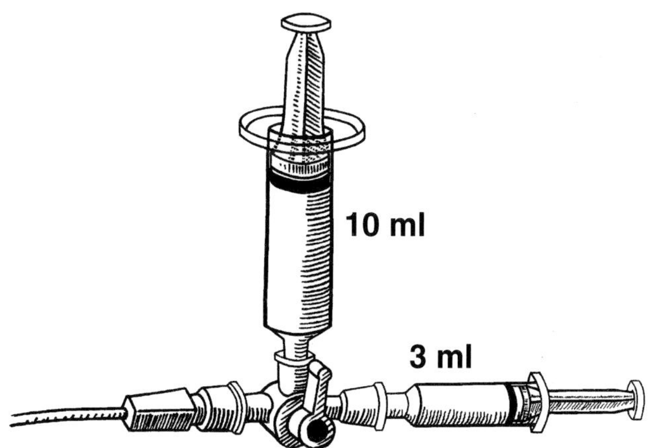

Figure 7.1 Set-up of two syringe and three-way stopcock to create an "on the table reservoir" for CO_2.

CO_2 cylinder is connected through tubing to the filter on the stopcock by a technician. The 10 ml syringe is then filled and emptied several times with CO_2 from the cylinder by the operator while the technician controls the flow of the gas. It takes a little practice to adjust the flow rate of the CO_2 into the 10 ml syringe, without blowing the plunger out of the barrel of the syringe. With the third filling of the syringe, the stopcock is turned to block off the male connection of the stopcock and the attached tubing. With the stopcock in this position, the 10 ml and the 3 ml syringes are in communication with each other, sealed from the "outside" air and, in turn, creating the sealed reservoir filled with CO_2. The filter is removed and discarded.

On the catheterization table the male fitting of the three-way stopcock is attached to the balloon lumen of the catheter, now creating a sealed connection between the reservoir and the balloon on the catheter. The 3 ml syringe is filled with CO_2 from the 10 ml syringe while the balloon on the catheter is filled from the 3 ml syringe with the appropriate volume of CO_2 for the balloon. The small volumes required for the balloon are easier to control accurately from the 3 ml syringe, while the 10 ml syringe provides a larger reserve volume of CO_2 for repeated refilling of the small syringe and balloon without having to go back frequently to the gas storage cylinder.

Ideally, and frequently, balloon catheters actually do float with the blood flow and are extremely useful when they do. There are many cardiac catheterization laboratories where a floating balloon catheter is the standard or only catheter used for "right heart" cardiac catheterizations. Floating balloon catheters are particularly useful in complex anomalies where several 180° curves must be traversed to approach particular areas in the heart. For example, in order to enter the pulmonary artery in a patient with transposition of the great arteries and intact ventricular septum, or to enter any part of the heart in patients with absent hepatic portion of the IVC and "azygous continuation" to the SVC, a 180° curve must be traversed before the pulmonary artery and/or the heart itself is entered.

The *most essential* use of floating balloon catheters is to *ensure that* they, and all wires, catheters and/or sheaths exchanged for them subsequently, pass *through the central, true orifice* of the atrioventricular valves. The relatively large, inflated balloon of a floating balloon catheter will float through the orifice of a valve only if the orifice is as large in diameter as the balloon, while non-floating, totally torque-controlled catheters easily pass or are maneuvered through any small area or part of the atrioventricular valve apparatus, *including small chordal spaces*, while they are being maneuvered through the valve.

When a very small area of the valve is crossed inadvertently and an attempt is made to pass a large delivery sheath and/or an angioplasty balloon through other than the large, true orifice of the atrioventricular valve, the passage of the balloon catheter or the sheath/dilator through the narrow, abnormal opening through the chordae is restricted or blocked completely. In an even worse case scenario, the deflated and smooth, factory folded, balloon angioplasty catheter *does advance through* the abnormal, narrow orifice, but when an attempt is made to withdraw the rough, irregularly deflated balloon through the very narrow abnormal space in the valve, it catches on the valve mechanism and tears or disrupts the valve. The outcome for the valve is even worse if the particular atrioventricular valve itself is being dilated and the angioplasty balloon has passed through other than the true orifice of the valve.

All floating balloon catheters have at least two separate lumens within the shaft of the catheter, for the balloon lumen and the true catheter lumen, each with separate hubs at the proximal end of the catheter. One lumen communicates with the balloon at the distal end of the catheter and is for inflation and deflation of the balloon. The second, catheter lumen, depends upon the type of balloon catheter. There are two basic types of floating balloon catheters—end-hole or wedge catheters and closed-ended or angiographic catheters. In the Swan™ end-hole or "balloon wedge" catheter, the lumen extends completely through the catheter, including the area where the balloon is attached, and exits at the distal tip of the catheter. In the Berman™ or floating balloon angiographic catheter, the second lumen ends at a group of side holes that exit the side of the catheter either just proximal to, or, rarely, just distal to the area where the balloon is attached.

In the end-hole or wedge variety of floating balloon catheter, the lumen, which passes completely through the catheter including the area of the balloon and the distal tip of the catheter, allows pressure recordings and small injections through only the tip of the catheter. This type of balloon catheter is particularly useful for obtaining pulmonary artery wedge pressure recordings and to perform wedge angiograms, and it allows wires to be passed beyond the tip of the catheter to help in entering difficult areas or for exchange with other catheters over the wire. End-hole balloon catheters are *not* useful for large-volume or high-pressure angiography. The single end-hole and the relatively small catheter lumen cause the tip of the catheter to recoil violently when a pressure injection with any volume of contrast is attempted through these catheters.

Thermodilution catheters are a modification of the end-hole balloons, however they have a third lumen within the shaft of the catheter which exits from the side of the catheter approximately 10 cm proximal to the distal tip of the catheter. This third lumen, which is used for the injection of the cold "indicator" solution during a thermodilution cardiac output recording, has a separate hub at the proximal end of the catheter.

The other major type of floating balloon catheter is the angiographic or Berman™ floating balloon catheter. The catheter lumen of the balloon angiographic catheter has no distal end hole but instead, exits at multiple side holes, which are usually positioned just proximal to the balloon at the tip of the catheter. These balloon catheters have a larger catheter lumen and slightly stronger walls, both of which are designed for pressure injections of contrast through the catheter. The Reverse Berman™ catheter is a modification of the standard Berman™ angiographic catheter. It also has a closed distal end, but the side holes of the catheter lumen exit from the lumen from a 1-cm segment of catheter that is just *distal* to the position of the balloon. The Reverse Berman™ catheter is used for occlusion angiographic studies where it is desired to perform the injection of the contrast distal to the occluding balloon—e.g. in pulmonary artery and vein wedge angiograms.

Floating balloon catheters should never be *relied upon* to enter any specific location, even when vigorous blood flow is going to that area. There are circumstances where the blood velocity is not sufficient to "pull" the catheter behind the balloon, where the major volume of blood does not flow preferentially to the vessel or area that it is desired to enter, and/or where the blood does not flow toward the desired area at all. For example, in the presence of valvular regurgitation the balloon does not float forward. When it is desired to enter an obstructed vessel where there is a large shunt lesion or a large non-obstructed vessel that arises proximal to the obstruction, the floating balloon catheter preferentially floats *away* from the obstructed location into the branch vessel or through the shunt.

Floating balloon catheters also usually only "float" with the blood flow when the direction of the tip of the catheter *along with the long axis* of the catheter are pointing at, and are exactly in line with and *parallel to* the exact direction of the blood flow. The force of the blood flow is seldom vigorous enough to pull and/or deflect the balloon with the tip of the catheter perpendicular to the long axis of the catheter. Special techniques and maneuvers are required to align the tip of the catheter in the direction of the flow of blood during manipulations of balloon catheters.

Although floating balloon catheters are designed to "float with the blood flow", they always require some manipulation. Preforming a curve in the distal end of a floating balloon catheter is essential to accomplish any directional control over it. Otherwise the shaft of such a catheter is absolutely straight, which allows nothing to turn as torque is applied to it. The curve at the tip can be formed by dipping the distal end of the catheter *very briefly* in boiling, sterile water or by exposing the distal end of the catheter *very briefly* to the jet of heat from a "heat gun". The brief exposure to heat will soften the catheter material transiently but long enough to allow the manual formation of at least some curve on the tip of the catheter.

Both of the "warming/softening techniques" for floating balloon catheters must be performed *very quickly and very carefully* in order not to *melt* the extruded material of the catheter shaft or destroy the balloon or the bond of the balloon with the catheter. One method of ensuring that the balloon catheter is not "over-cooked" is for the operator to grasp the balloon between the gloved thumb and first finger, form the desired curve on the catheter around the gloved finger, and, with the balloon pinched between the finger and thumb so that the deflated balloon is completely covered and protected by the fingers, dip the distal end of the catheter—with the fingers—rapidly into the boiling water or expose it to the heat of the heat gun. The presence of the fingers in the heat source ensures that the catheter does not remain there too long! Once the tip has been softened, it is shaped into the desired curve and the newly formed curve is "fixed" on the catheter by dipping the tip with the formed curve in cold flush solution.

In addition to forming a curve at the distal end of the balloon catheter, it is helpful to "stretch" the last few centimeters of the shaft (just proximal to the balloon) at the distal end. This maneuver will help to make this end of the extruded shaft more flexible. To stretch the catheter, it is grasped with one hand over the balloon at the tip. The distal end of the catheter just proximal to the balloon is then "pulled" away from the balloon between the thumb and first finger of the other hand while the fingers grip the shaft of the catheter very tightly. This stretching is started from the position where the fingers of the first hand are grasping the catheter shaft over the balloon. The catheter shaft is pulled between the finger and thumb as they are pulled over the catheter shaft for a distance of 4–5 cm away from the balloon. The pulling between the fingers is repeated 3 or 4 times in rapid sequence. This softens the material of the catheter shaft slightly and facilitates the "floating" characteristics of the tip of the catheter.

In maneuvering floating catheters, the major manipulation is to direct the tip of the catheter into the desired or suspected direction of blood flow and then "feed" an adequate length of catheter behind the balloon to provide "slack in the line" for further forward motion of the balloon tip. Small, precise, isolated and/or *slow* torque movements on the proximal shaft of floating balloon catheters are ***not*** transmitted to the distal end of the catheter *at all* and, as a consequence, are a *total waste of time, effort and fluoroscopy*. Large, frequent to-and-fro movements of the shaft of these catheters, with *simultaneous torquing* of the shaft, are necessary to deliver any torque to the tip. Large, simultaneous to-and-fro and torque motions together allow multiple slight redirections of the shaft of the catheter to be transmitted to the tip, and provide plenty of "slack" in the shaft for forward flow once the tip enters the proper blood flow.

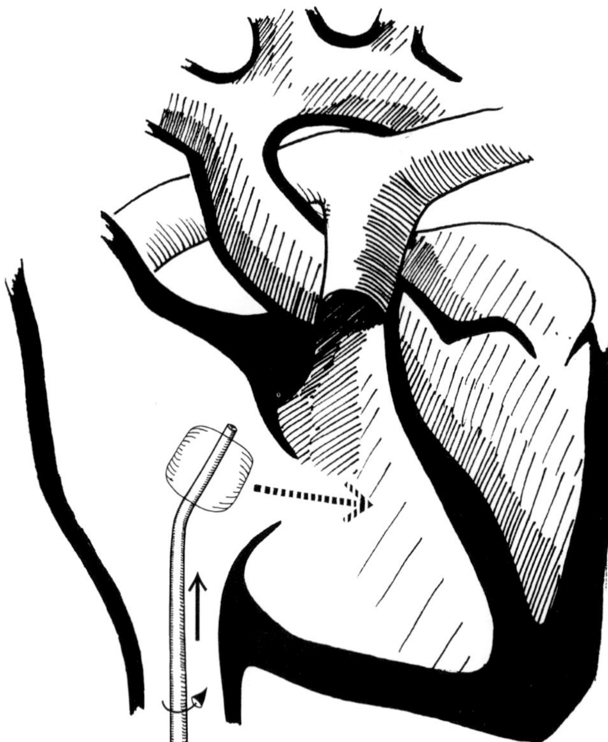

Figure 7.2 Straight balloon catheter when advanced from the inferior vena cava into the right atrium. The direction of the shaft of the catheter is parallel to the tricuspid valve annulus and across (perpendicular to) the direction of the flow of blood. Dotted arrow, direction of blood flow; solid arrows, direction of movement of catheter.

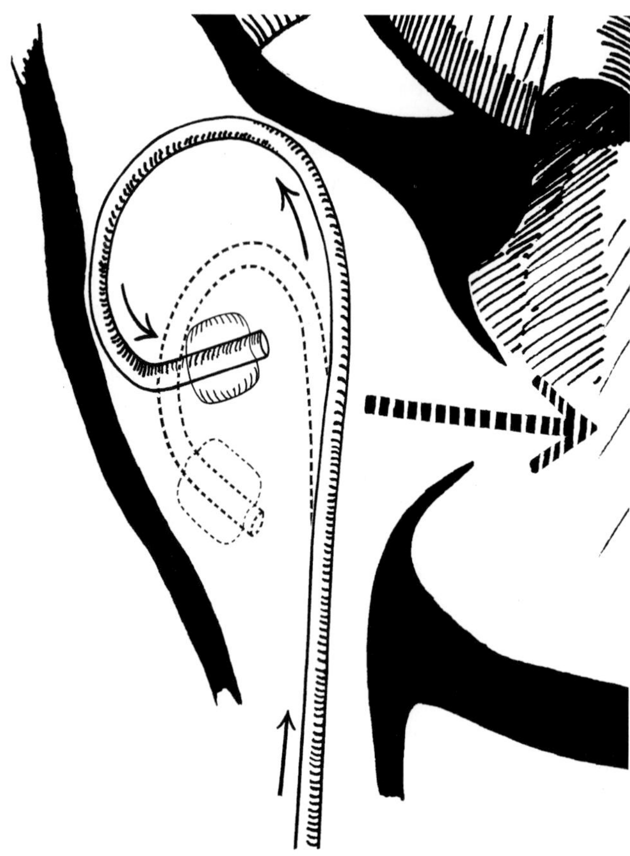

Figure 7.3 A curved balloon catheter looped in the right atrium directs the tip of the catheter toward the tricuspid orifice and orients the balloon and tip of the catheter in the direction of blood flow into the valve and ventricle. Dotted arrow, direction of blood flow; solid arrows, direction of catheter.

Often, as balloon catheters are advanced, loops can be formed on their more proximal shafts. These loops can cause knotting or entrapment in structures[2,3], but if used carefully and with skill, can be used to the operator's advantage to align the tip and distal shaft of the catheter parallel with the direction of blood flow. This is best illustrated by examples.

When the catheter enters the right atrium from the inferior vena cava, the shaft of the catheter is aligned almost parallel with the orifice of the tricuspid valve and perpendicular to the direction of blood flow from the right atrium into the right ventricle (Figure 7.2). It is very unlikely that the force of the blood flow will be sufficient to draw the balloon and the tip of a balloon catheter into this 90° turn. If, on the other hand, a large counterclockwise loop is formed in the right atrium, the tip and distal shaft of the catheter eventually point directly at the valve and in line with the direction of blood flow (Figure 7.3). This loop in the right atrium is formed with the tip of the balloon catheter starting cephalad and toward the patient's right (toward the free wall of the atrium).

As the catheter is advanced cephalad within the right atrium with the balloon inflated, the balloon is deflected off the cephalad roof of the right atrium and away from the blood from the superior vena cava, and begins to loop in the atrium. The loop is torqued so that as the tip of the catheter with the balloon passes inferiorly along the lateral wall of the atrium, the tip naturally loops around medially across the atrium, directing the balloon toward the orifice of the tricuspid valve. The formation and use of this type of loop with a catheter was described and illustrated in detail in Chapter 5.

The use of this loop to enter the right ventricle has the added advantage that once the tip of the catheter with the balloon has entered the right ventricle, continued "feeding" of the catheter and advancing the loop advance the tip of the catheter, which is automatically directed cephalad, toward the right ventricular outflow tract and eventually into the right pulmonary artery. Controlling the loop and the direction of the course of the catheter is often difficult because of the soft nature of the catheter material.

As previously mentioned, the major advantage of the floating balloon catheter is that when it floats through a valve, it floats through the largest and central orifice of that valve. Passage through the center of the valve is imperative in the dilation of atrioventricular valves and in any therapeutic procedures, including balloon dilations, where dilation or other therapeutic catheters must pass through an atrioventricular valve to approach a more distal area for therapy. The floating balloon passes through the largest orifice and *not* through small chordae or small secondary clefts in the atrioventricular valve. Thus, when the floating balloon catheter is replaced with the wire to introduce a dilation balloon or a large sheath/dilator, the wire definitely passes through the central, major orifice of the valve. This is obviously very important during dilation of the mitral valve or the tricuspid valve itself.

When the initial catheter and then the dilation balloon do *not* cross through the true, central orifice initially, the valve can be destroyed very easily by tearing a leaflet or tearing loose the small subvalve chordae. It is equally important during the dilation of a pulmonary valve, branch pulmonary arteries or a prograde dilation of the aortic valve, where stiff wires and large balloons must pass through, and often impinge upon, the atrioventricular valve apparatus, and the rough and irregularly deflated dilation balloon must be withdrawn back through the atrioventricular valve after the inflation/dilation. The atrioventricular valves can be torn during the dilation procedure itself by the straightening of the wires or the milking backward of the inflated balloon into the tricuspid or mitral valve. When the dilation wire/balloon passes through a small orifice or through small chordal attachments of the valve, the valve will often be damaged.

Some of the shortcomings of the materials of floating balloon catheters can be overcome by the use of guide wires or deflector wires in conjunction with them, as described in Chapter 6. In order to reduce the possibility of clotting around the wires and to facilitate the movement of the wires within the catheter, a teflon-coated wire *and* a wire back-bleed valve with a flush port are used whenever a wire is used in a floating balloon catheter. A wire that is not teflon-coated tends to bind with the extruded materials (polyethylene) of floating balloon catheters. With end-hole balloon catheters, J wires or extra soft and long tipped wires can be advanced beyond the tip of the catheter and passed carefully into structures or orifices into which the balloon does not float on its own. Once the wire has been secured distally in the side or branch vessel, the balloon catheter can usually be advanced over the wire with the balloon inflated to assure passage through the proper orifice of the valve.

Stiff wires and active deflector wires are useful to enhance the purposeful manipulation of floating balloon catheters or to direct the tip of the catheter specifically at an orifice. A slight curve is formed at the tip of the stiff end of a standard spring guide wire or a Mullins™ wire. The wire is used within the catheter lumen of the floating balloon catheter to stiffen the entire shaft of the catheter. With the curve at the end of the wire advanced to just within the tip of the catheter, the wire gives the balloon catheter a bit of "guidability" and makes it more responsive to torque and forward push. Unfortunately, a spring guide wire within the catheter lumen usually prohibits simultaneous pressure recordings and injections through the catheter. However, pressures can be recorded and injections can be performed with a Mullins™ wire passing within the catheter lumen to stiffen the catheter when the wire is introduced into the catheter through a Tuohy™ Y adaptor.

Either rigid or controllable deflector wires can be used to redirect or point the tip of the balloon catheter in the direction of blood flow or toward or into any desired location. The deflector wire is introduced into, and advanced to the tip of, the catheter. Either the preformed curve on the rigid deflector wire or the developed curve on the controllable deflector is used to deflect the tip of the floating balloon catheter toward a particular orifice or direction of blood flow. The deflector wire is fixed in position, while the floating balloon catheter (with or without the balloon inflated depending upon the lesion) is advanced off the wire. Deflector wires used in this manner are extremely useful for redirection of the tip of the catheter as much as 90–180° in order to align the direction of the tip with the direction of the flow of blood. For example, a floating balloon catheter that is advanced from the inferior vena cava into the right atrium is deflected 90° in order to redirect the tip to enter the tricuspid valve/right ventricle. A floating balloon catheter that has entered the left ventricle from the left atrium will usually be directed toward the apex of the ventricle. The tip of a balloon catheter that is in the ventricle can be deflected 180° in order to redirect it toward the left ventricular outflow tract.

There are several precautions in the use of floating balloon catheters. The balloon is always inflated with filtered carbon dioxide (CO_2) rather than air. If the balloon is used on the systemic side of the circulation or when there is even the slightest chance of right-to-left shunting, the hazard of an occlusive, air embolus traveling to vital structures is reduced if a balloon ruptures when the balloon is filled with CO_2. The catheter tip and the balloon itself are observed closely on fluoroscopy during the inflation of all floating balloons to ensure that the balloon is not entrapped between trabeculae or in a vessel that is too small to accommodate the balloon. During manipulation, the *inflated* balloon preferentially is *not* withdrawn back across any intact valve and certainly never with any force. Whenever the (deflated) balloon of a floating balloon catheter is withdrawn across a valve, it is observed continually on fluoroscopy and is withdrawn very carefully and gently. Even the rough surface of the deflated balloon can catch transiently on leaflets or between chordae, and with even minimal force can evulse the valve. As mentioned earlier, when feeding "slack" to the balloon catheter as it is introduced into a patient, large loops frequently form along the more proximal shaft of the catheter. Along with the tip of the catheter, its shaft should be observed repeatedly during all maneuvers of the catheter. When loops are formed in the shaft of a balloon catheter, the catheter is never withdrawn (tightened) unless it is being observed constantly, and extra care is taken not to form or tighten a large, loose loop into a kink or even a knot.

When the balloon is not inflated, the catheter tip is relatively "sharp" and when a balloon catheter is first introduced into the vascular system, the shaft can be relatively stiff. When the catheter is first introduced into the vascular system and is being advanced with the balloon deflated, care must be taken that the tip does not wedge tightly into a small branch vessel or even perforate a small, fragile, peripheral branch vessel. To prevent this, the balloon is inflated *as soon as* it passes beyond the distal tip of the sheath and into the vein. The balloon is maintained inflated while the catheter is advanced toward, and into, the heart. The inflated balloon follows (is pulled by) the flow of the venous blood in the larger channel, which keeps the tip from angling into side branches off the vena cava. The inflated balloon is capable of catching in large branches and then bending, looping or kinking on itself if it does become stuck in those vessels.

There are several advantages and special uses for floating balloon catheters besides their flow-directed uses. The inflated balloon at the tip of the catheter is "softer" and blunter and, as a consequence, causes less endocardial stimulation, presumably less trauma and fewer ectopic beats when it bounces against the walls of the cardiac chambers. With the balloon inflated, the catheter tip is very blunt and is on a "soft" catheter shaft. The combination of the balloon and the soft catheter makes floating balloon catheters relatively safe for intracardiac manipulation, and virtually eliminates the possibility of cardiac perforation by the tip of the catheter as long as the balloon is inflated. These characteristics provide a distinct advantage during manipulations in small, critically ill infants with their more delicate and thinner myocardium. However, inflated balloons are relatively large compared to the tiny structures of a small infant's heart, and even these catheter shafts are *relatively* stiff, which, in turn, compromises the floating capability of balloon catheters in these patients.

Another situation where the floating balloons are utilized for "routine" intracardiac manipulations is in all patients with ventricular inversion. In these patients, the atrioventricular conduction bundle runs anteriorly, superficially and on the *left ventricular* (right) side of the septum. As a consequence of this more vulnerable location of the bundle, these patients are prone to complete atrioventricular block during any catheter manipulation in the left ventricle, particularly during attempts at entering the pulmonary artery from the left ventricle. A floating balloon catheter can be manipulated more gently into the pulmonary artery off the inverted ventricle, and appears to be less traumatic to this vulnerable area than the stiffer tips of the usual torque-controlled catheters.

With the balloon of the balloon angiographic catheter inflated during the positioning and during contrast injections for angiocardiograms, it is virtually impossible to produce intramyocardial injections. Even if the balloon itself is erroneously embedded into the myocardium, the holes of the standard Berman™ balloon angiographic catheters are sufficiently proximal to the balloon so that there will not be an intramyocardial stain from the embedded catheter tip.

In addition to the use of floating balloon catheters to assist in entering difficult locations, balloon wedge (end-hole) catheters are commonly used for the measurement of pulmonary arterial capillary wedge pressures. The balloon catheter is advanced to the most distal possible position in the branch pulmonary artery with the balloon inflated. Usually, as the balloon progresses into the vessel, it stops as the vessel narrows sufficiently proximal to the wedge position. Wherever the balloon does stop, it usually occludes the pulmonary artery branch at that location. Frequently the pressure that is recorded and obtained through the lumen passing through the tip of the catheter is from distal to the inflated balloon. With the proximal flow/pressure excluded by the balloon, the pressure reflects the capillary wedge (left atrial) pressure. The characteristic waveform of an atrial pressure curve must be displayed in order to conclude that the recorded pressure does represent a valid capillary wedge pressure. Respiratory variations often cause the recorded pressure to change from a wedge pressure to a pulmonary artery pressure and back with each respiration. Because of the lag in the propagation of these low pressures, this respiratory variation must be eliminated by manipulations of the patient's airway before accurate wedge pressures can be taken. Often, from the position in the distal pulmonary artery with the balloon inflated and the wedge pressure displayed, the balloon can be deflated slowly while simultaneously advancing the catheter further, and the catheter tip will advance into a true, or better, wedge position once the balloon is deflated completely. Occasionally, even with the balloon inflated, it is necessary to introduce a wire into the balloon catheter in order to stiffen the shaft enough to obtain a wedge position. This frequently produces unsatisfactory pressure readings because of air and/or particulate debris remaining in the catheter lumen and/or the catheter withdrawing from the wedge position once the wire is removed.

For all the reasons discussed previously, balloon catheters obviously have some advantages and are safer for intracardiac manipulations, particularly for inexperienced, less skilled or less meticulous operators. However, the floating characteristics of these catheters cannot be relied upon as the only means of catheter manipulation. All physicians performing cardiac catheterizations in pediatric and congenital heart lesions should be skilled in the use of torque-controlled as well as floating balloon catheters.

Balloon catheters have multiple uses other than strictly for the manipulation of the catheter. They are used for test occlusions of various intracardiac and intravascular defects. Often the balloon is filled with very dilute contrast solution instead of CO_2. This results in a less "mobile" balloon, and the contrast solution does not escape from the balloon as does CO_2. The inflated balloon effectively occludes small to moderate sized lumens and orifices and allows measurement of the "occlusion" hemodynamics. Pressures can be measured either proximal or distal to the balloon depending upon the type of balloon catheter used for the occlusion.

For example, with an angiographic type of balloon catheter, a balloon inflated in the aortic end of a patent ductus arteriosus occludes the flow through the ductus while the pulmonary artery pressure is measured through the proximal holes in the catheter. The distal systemic arterial pressure can be measured simultaneously through the indwelling arterial line, thus simulating the effect of ductal occlusion on the two pressures simultaneously. This occlusion pressure in the pulmonary artery is important particularly in the presence of high pulmonary artery pressures without accompanying, high, measured (calculated) pulmonary artery flow.

The balloon angiographic catheter is also very useful for test occlusions of the "fenestrations" between venous channels or chambers following a cavo-pulmonary repair of a patient with single ventricle physiology. The catheter, with balloon deflated, is advanced from the systemic venous channel, through the fenestration and into the left (or pulmonary venous) side of the defect. The balloon is inflated and withdrawn against the left, or pulmonary venous side of the defect. This occludes the defect with the holes of the catheter positioned on the right, or systemic venous, side of the defect. Thus changes in the systemic venous pressure are monitored simultaneously with changes in systemic arterial pressure while determining if the patient's hemodynamics tolerates the temporary occlusion of the defect.

Balloon catheters are useful for the measurement (calibration) of intracardiac defects by the direct passage of the inflated or partially inflated balloon (or resistance to the passage of the balloon) through the defect. The maximum cross-sectional diameter of most inflated floating balloons is less than 1.5 cm, even when inflated with several ml of CO_2 or dilute contrast solution. This small diameter limits the measurements or calibrations with this type of catheter to structures in infants, where all structures are smaller, and to smaller vascular structures in larger patients. There are larger balloon catheters specifically designed to test occlude larger structures such as atrial septal defects and ventricular septal defects. However, these "sizing balloons" have a significantly larger and stiffer shaft and require a much larger introductory sheath. Sizing balloons are discussed elsewhere.

Balloons are used for the temporary occlusion of defects or vessels during angiocardiograms to maximize the flow of blood or contrast to a certain area. Occlusion of the aorta distal to the origin of aortic to pulmonary shunts, branch vessels or collateral vessels maximizes the flow through the vessel(s) proximal to the occlusion. Occlusion of defects through which large shunts are occurring improves the prograde flow that was diverted by the shunt, and allows more contrast and better visualization of structures distal to areas of the previous shunt. For example, in infants with a combination of a large ventricular septal defect and coarctation of the aorta, it is difficult or even impossible to visualize the aortic arch and the area of the coarctation adequately from an injection in the left ventricle. The predominant flow of blood and contrast goes through the ventricular septal defect, into the right ventricle, and away from the aorta. When, in the presence of a large ventricular septal defect with a large left to right shunt, a balloon angiographic catheter is advanced (floated) from the left atrium into the left ventricle, the inflated balloon preferentially floats from the left ventricle, into and through the ventricular septal defect, and into the right ventricle (or pulmonary artery) with little chance of passing into the aorta. By withdrawing the catheter very carefully *with the balloon inflated* or intermittently deflated–inflated, the balloon impinges on the right ventricular side of the ventricular septal defect. With the balloon held firmly against, or within, the ventricular septal defect, the defect is occluded with the injection holes of the catheter located on the left ventricular side of the septum. With the defect occluded, the contrast injection during a left ventricular angiocardiogram fills the ascending aorta and aortic arch selectively from the left ventricular injection. This occlusion technique using a balloon angiographic catheter avoids the necessity of a retrograde catheterization for purely diagnostic purposes in a small infant.

Balloon occlusion angiocardiograms are also useful in demonstrating the anatomy of more proximal central vessels or details of branching vessels off more central vessels. To enhance the visualization of aortic branches, a balloon angiographic catheter is advanced prograde into the aorta and to a location just distal to where the structure to be visualized arises. The balloon is inflated and occludes the aorta just *distal* to the origin of the lesion or branch to be visualized. The angiocardiogram is performed with the balloon inflated during the injection, concentrating the contrast in the aorta proximal to the balloon. Occlusion aortograms are performed with the ascending aorta occluded in order to visualize the coronary arteries in neonatal transposition of the great arteries. Occlusion aortography is often helpful in visualizing systemic to pulmonary collaterals off the descending aorta. The lower thoracic aorta or high abdominal aorta is occluded below the take-off of the collaterals. The aortogram is performed with the balloon inflated, which fills the more proximal structures while eliminating run-off to the distal aorta. Occlusion angiography is used to selectively visualize a right or left pulmonary artery by occluding the contralateral, proximal, branch pulmonary artery opposite to the pulmonary artery that is to be visualized during the injection.

Occlusion angiography does have a disadvantage. The occlusion of the central vessel eliminates the diastolic run-off, which may result in less desirable imaging of the more distal branching vessels. A high-pressure, rapidly injected, non-occlusion angiogram often gives as good, if not better, images in the run-off vessels.

The Reverse Berman™ catheter can be used for standard angiography, however it was designed to perform balloon occlusion angiography with the injection performed distal to the occluding balloon—for example, for pulmonary artery or vein wedge angiography where it is desired to fill a larger segment of the capillary bed. The Reverse Berman™ balloon is very useful for looking at the pulmonary veins from a pulmonary artery wedge angiogram or for looking at the true pulmonary arteries from a pulmonary vein wedge angiogram.

There are definite disadvantages to floating balloon catheters. They certainly do not float *against* the flow of blood, which makes them totally ineffective for advancing against significant valvular regurgitation or for advancing a catheter retrograde. The major disadvantages of balloon catheters, however, result from their "softer" characteristics. In order to achieve their floating abilities, they are softer and more pliable than most other catheters. As a consequence, floating balloon catheters have very poor torque control and maneuvering characteristics. When they do not float to the desired location, they are very difficult to maneuver selectively or purposefully.

Some floating balloon catheters are manufactured from polyvinyl chloride, which provides some stiffness and torque characteristics, but these catheters do not "float" as effectively, if at all. Because of the two (or more) lumens in these catheters each separate lumen is smaller than the catheter lumen in a comparable sized torque-controlled catheter. To make the catheters float better, softer wall materials are used. Because of the smaller lumen and softer material of the walls of the shaft of such catheters, smaller floating balloon catheters transmit pressures less accurately, and it is more difficult to draw samples through them. Because of the extruded plastic catheter materials and the smaller lumen size, when wires are used within the catheters, smaller gauge wires must be used and even then the wires tend to bind within the catheters. When a wire is very tight within a catheter, clotting occurs more readily. Because of the wall material of the catheters, the lumen size, and the catheter length there is a limit to the amount or rate of contrast that can be delivered through a balloon angiographic catheter during angiograms. Finally, with some of these catheters, the outside diameter of the deflated balloon is slightly larger than the catheter shaft, thus a larger sized introductory sheath than the "advertised" size of the catheter must be used to introduce them.

Although balloon catheters are extremely useful, if not essential for some specific maneuvers, they are certainly not universally useful or effective and should never be depended upon for routine procedures or as the only catheter available.

Complications of floating balloon catheters

In addition to the several disadvantage in their use, there are major complications of floating balloon catheters *per se*. The most significant complications are related to balloon rupture. When a balloon from a floating balloon catheter ruptures, there is the potential for the embolization of air or particles of the balloon material. If the balloon is not filled with CO_2 when it ruptures, a bolus of air is released into the circulation. Air remains as a bolus and rises to the "highest point" in the particular circulation. When trapped in the right heart the air floats to the anterior of the right atrium, the right ventricle, or the proximal trunk of the pulmonary artery, and usually bounces around in the area causing no particular problem. In the systemic circulation, on the other hand, the "highest position" is often the right coronary sinus and right coronary artery, with the resultant occlusion of the coronary artery flow by the bolus of air! The patient immediately develops ST-T wave changes and usually becomes hemodynamically unstable. Occasionally the bolus of air divides or bypasses the coronary sinus/artery and some goes to the most anteriorly positioned carotid artery. With a large enough bolus, the patient develops hemodynamic instability, but the true or long-term effects may not be appreciated until the patient does not wake up following the procedure or exhibits localized neurologic signs.

The treatment of air embolization from a balloon is prevention by *always* using CO_2 in it. In the event that air inadvertently gets in, and embolizes from, the balloon, time alone is usually sufficient to allow the air to be cleared or absorbed, however additional management is necessary when there is significant hemodynamic compromise. Air obstructing a coronary artery with cardiovascular collapse is treated by external cardiac compression, which is continued until the signs of cardiac ischemia resolve. This may require as long as 15 to 30 minutes of external compression. Other resuscitative medications or maneuvers are used along with the compressions as necessary. When there are ST-T wave changes only, a selective coronary cannulation with a contrast injection should identify the air, which may be approached with a fine wire in the coronary.

If a latex balloon ruptures, fragments or even the entire balloon may come loose and embolize in the circulation. Latex is not radio-opaque, so the location of the fragment of the balloon can only be determined from the signs and symptoms of an ischemic organ resulting from the obstruction of the artery to that organ by the fragment. Fortunately, there are usually no signs or symptoms and the location of the piece goes undetected. Treatment again is prevention. Balloon catheters should be stored in a controlled environment, which includes no exposure to light. They should not be used past their expiration date and, when used, they should not be over-inflated.

The balloon on a floating balloon catheter very rarely does not deflate. This occurs almost only when the balloon is inflated with dilute contrast for special use. When the balloon cannot be deflated, it is carefully withdrawn out of any areas in the circulation that are immediately proximal to vital structures. The inflated balloon is then punctured using a stylet or a long needle passed through an adjacent catheter and removed from the body.

Floating balloon catheters can become entrapped on intracardiac structures, and if withdrawn forcefully can actually evulse these structures. An inflated balloon catheter passes through the largest orifice of a valve with the prograde flow of blood, but after deflation can be pulled into the edge of a valve leaflet during withdrawal. The deflated balloon catheter can easily be advanced through narrow chordae or clefts in valve leaflets, but because of the rougher surface of the balloon it can become caught very firmly on the same valve structure when it is withdrawn. Awareness of these possibilities and their prevention is the treatment. No catheter should be withdrawn very rapidly across a valve or without observing it very carefully, but this is particularly true for a floating balloon catheter, whether inflated or deflated.

Because the shafts of floating balloon catheters are so much softer than those of most of the torque-controlled catheters, the manipulations of balloon catheters often involves forming large loops in the more proximal catheter shaft either purposefully or inadvertently. If these loops are not observed continuously, kinking or even knotting of the catheter shaft can occur very easily. Again, prevention is the best treatment. The *entire length* of the catheter all the way back to the introductory site must be observed, at least intermittently, during all manipulations of floating balloon catheters. Any push, pull or torque applied to the shaft of the catheter outside the body should be transmitted in both distance and degree of rotation to the distal end of the catheter within the heart or vessel and in a 1:1 ratio. Whenever the tip of the catheter does not advance in proportion to the forward movement applied to the shaft of the catheter, a loop should be suspected, looked for and corrected.

No catheter should *ever* be withdrawn rapidly or forcefully unless the intent is to tear something! This is particularly true of floating balloon catheters, which can easily develop knots in them when an undetected kink or loop is withdrawn rapidly. The catheter must be unlooped while the entire loop is under very close visualization and the catheter must be withdrawn much less rapidly.

When kinks or knots do occur, they can be undone and the catheter straightened with skillful manipulations and patience. Once a knot has formed, the catheter should not be withdrawn any further, as this only will tighten the knot further. A 45–90° curve is formed at the distal end of a Mullins™ wire or the stiff end of a spring guide wire and this stiff curved wire is advanced within the catheter lumen to a position adjacent to the knot. This curved wire changes the angle of the shaft of the catheter as it enters the knot. This allows the catheter to be advanced off the wire and pushed into the knot to loosen it. If the rigid deflector wire does not accomplish this, the same maneuver is attempted using an active deflector wire with a 1 cm deflection curve. The variable curve can often be maneuvered into the knot within the lumen of the floating catheter.

If the knot cannot be loosened with a curved wire advanced within the knotted catheter, an additional end-hole catheter is introduced into the same vascular system and the tip is positioned immediately adjacent to the knot. A 0.025″ active deflector wire with a 1 cm curve is introduced through the end-hole catheter to a position immediately adjacent to the knot. The tip of the deflector wire is maneuvered into and through a loop of the knotted catheter. The deflector wire may pass into the knot when the wire is straight, nearly straight or during the formation of a curve. Once the deflector wire is through a loop in the knot, the wire is deflected tightly. This creates a hook through the loop of the knot and allows it to be teased open as the shaft of the knotted catheter is advanced simultaneously. If the wire cannot be introduced *into and through* the loop in the knot, the end-hole catheter is replaced with a long sheath/dilator set that is large enough to accommodate a 7-French bioptome catheter. The distal curve on the long sheath should be straightened or preformed to be only 20–30°. A similar slight curve is formed on the distal end of a 7-French bioptome and this is introduced into the long sheath. One edge of the loop of the knot is grasped with the jaws of the bioptome and the knot teased loose with the combined pull on the bioptome and push on the knotted catheter.

Occasionally, the knotted catheter is too flimsy to offer enough resistance against the deflector wire or the bioptome in order to untie the knot. In that case the deflector wire or the bioptome must be introduced from the opposite direction in the vessel from the introduction of the knotted catheter. For example, if the knotted catheter had been introduced from the femoral vein, the deflector wire or the bioptome is introduced from a subclavian or jugular vein. In this way more forceful traction can be applied to one strand of the loop of the knot.

When standard precautions are taken in their use, floating balloon catheters are the safest catheters for intracardiac manipulations and the easiest to manipulate in some circumstances. Unfortunately, these advantages do not compensate universally for their major drawbacks. The biggest disadvantages of floating balloon catheters are their lack of consistent forward floating with the forward blood flow in all situations, the inability to use them *against* the blood flow, and their designed lack of torque, which can compromise their entrance into some difficult locations. In spite of the disadvantages, floating balloon catheters should be available in every pediatric/congenital catheterization laboratory.

References

1. Swan H *et al*. Catheterization of the heart in man with use of a flow directed balloon-tipped catheter. *N Engl J Med* 1970; **283**: 447–451.
2. Lipp H, O'Donoghue K and Resnekov L. Intracardiac knotting of a flow-directed balloon catheter. *N Engl J Med* 1971; **284**(4): 220.
3. Foote GA, Schabel SI and Hodges M. Pulmonary complications of the flow-directed balloon-tipped catheter. *N Engl J Med* 1974; **290**(17): 927–931.

8 Transseptal left heart catheterization

Introduction

When pre-existing communications between the right and left heart are not present or, when present, cannot be crossed easily from the right heart, the atrial transseptal puncture technique from the right atrium into the left atrium is the most direct, dependable and safest approach to the left heart[1]. By using a transseptal approach through the atrial septum to the left heart, the potential for compromise of an artery is reduced or even eliminated. When a retrograde study is necessary for specific aortic root or arterial information, it can be performed with a smaller diameter catheter and requires a much shorter time with the catheter in the artery when most of the "left heart" information is obtained by way of the transseptal procedure.

The modified Mullins™ long sheath, atrial, transseptal approach with modern equipment makes entrance into the left atrium and left ventricle safe, precise, dependable and versatile. Biplane fluoroscopic imaging allows a mental "three-dimensional" reconstruction of the intracardiac structures, which provides depth, as well as a simultaneous, side-to-side relationship within the heart during the procedure. Modern X-ray imaging allows precise, clear visualization of the needle as well as the sheath/dilator set and clearly shows the relationships of the sheath, dilator and needle to each other and to surrounding structures during the entire procedure.

Mullins™ long transseptal sheath/dilator sets used with the original Brockenbrough™ transseptal needle add to the safety, versatility and dependability of the transseptal procedure[2]. The tips of the original Mullins™ dilators have a very tight fit and a better, smoother, taper over the fine distal tips of Brockenbrough™ needles. The long, thin-walled sheath should fit very tightly over the dilator. These very tight junctions allow the sheath/dilator combination to pass over the needle and through the septum with minimal force during the puncture of the septum. There are no side holes at the distal end of the Mullins™ dilator so there is no chance of the needle catching on, or actually passing through, a side hole in the dilator during the introduction of the needle or with changes in the needle position during the puncture, as was commonly seen with the original Brockenbrough™ catheter. Additionally, the long sheath positioned in the left heart adds significant versatility to the procedure.

Advantages of the long sheath, Mullins™ transseptal technique

There are numerous advantages to the long sheath transseptal technique[3]. The transseptal approach itself gives dependable, precise and safe entrance into the left atrium and left ventricle, and when desirable, prograde entry into the ascending aorta. All varieties of catheter can be used in any of these areas. The transseptal entrance into the left atrium allows a direct and dependable access not only to the left atrium proper, but also to the pulmonary veins and the area in the left atrium immediately proximal to the mitral valve. True, reliable, *direct* left atrial pressures are obtained. With current catheters and techniques, entry into the pulmonary veins or the left ventricle from the left atrium is easily possible without trauma to the left atrium from any extensive, random manipulation in the left atrium. All of this is accomplished without any compromise of an artery.

Once the long Mullins™ transseptal sheath is secured in the left heart all types and sizes of catheters and catheter-delivered devices can be introduced, maneuvered and easily exchanged within the left heart. A large variety of diagnostic catheters with any desired pre-curves can be used in the left heart. Softer and more malleable catheters, including floating balloon catheters, can be introduced through the sheath and can be manipulated more extensively, yet safely, within the left heart. End-hole catheters are used in pulmonary veins for definitive diagnostic pulmonary venous pressure measurements, selective pulmonary venous sampling, and for pulmonary vein wedge angiograms.

The long sheath allows the introduction of closed ended (either balloon or torque-controlled) and large diameter, as well as relatively short, angiographic catheters, from the venous approach into the left atrium, left ventricle or even the ascending aorta. This allows for high volume, and at the same time, low-pressure injection of contrast for very high-quality left heart angiography, all without any compromise of an artery.

Prograde entry into a great artery arising from the left ventricle is accomplished readily through the Mullins™ long sheaths using a prograde, flow-directed, balloon catheter or a semi-soft, torque-controlled catheter in conjunction with the use of deflector wires. If a retrograde study is considered necessary for selective coronary artery studies, to visualize other specific arterial structures or to evaluate the aortic valve for regurgitation, the arterial entry and manipulation are performed with a smaller, shorter catheter and can be performed using a very short duration of time within the artery after all the other left heart information has been obtained through the prograde transseptal approach.

By using a catheter at least one French size smaller than the long transseptal sheath, simultaneous pressures can be recorded from any two locations within the left heart or great artery arising from the left heart. All this information is obtained through the single venous introductory site and without entering an artery at all. Pressures can be recorded from *three* left heart locations simultaneously using only one retrograde arterial catheter in combination with the transseptal sheath and a prograde catheter. When the catheter tip(s) and the sheath tip are positioned in the same location, the accuracy of the transducers is verified or balanced until the two (or three) simultaneous, overlapping pressure curves are displayed as a *single line* on the pressure tracing. Variation in the baseline pressures, which occur as a result of significant respiratory effort or catheter "fling" during "withdrawal" pressure recordings, are eliminated when two or more separate, simulataneous pressure curves are obtained. Pressures recorded simultaneously through the sheath and the catheter from the two separate locations eliminate the artifacts and discrepancies that occur during "pull-back" pressure recordings. A direct left atrial pressure eliminates the propagation or lag time and the overall question of the accuracy of pulmonary artery wedge pressures as a representation of true left atrial pressures.

Catheters with no lumen at all such as electrode catheters, biopsy forceps, and special, catheter tipped, transducer catheters can be introduced into any area of the left heart through the long Mullins™ transseptal sheath. Single or multiple transducers at the catheter tip of manometry catheters or multiple electrodes on electrode catheters, none of which have any catheter lumen, are easily positioned anywhere within the left heart through pre-positioned long transseptal sheaths. These high-fidelity catheters allow refined physiologic measurements, intracardiac electrical recording or even radio-frequency ablation procedures within the left heart. Left ventricular biopsies are relatively straightforward through a precurved, pre-positioned long transseptal sheath.

There are situations in which the atrial transseptal approach is the only reasonable approach to a particular area of the heart. In patients with compromised or absent arterial access, the transseptal approach provides a very reasonable and safe route to the entire left heart. In the presence of mechanical prosthetic valves in the left heart, the only absolutely reliable means of recording trans-prosthetic valvular gradients or of obtaining quality angiocardiograms through standard catheters in the chambers proximal to the valves is by the transseptal approach. Following complex congenital heart repairs such as a "Mustard" or "Senning" venous switch for transposition of the great arteries, or the lateral tunnel "Fontan" for single ventricle, the most reasonable access to critical locations in the pulmonary venous circulation is by a transseptal puncture through the baffles.

For left heart therapeutic catheterization procedures, the long sheath transseptal approach is even more essential. This technique allows the introduction of all types and sizes of therapeutic catheters and devices into the chambers and vessels within the left heart. The blade septostomy catheter for an atrial septostomy is delivered to the left atrium through a long transseptal sheath. When the atrial septum is totally intact in a patient undergoing a blade septostomy, the sheath is positioned across the septum by a transseptal puncture. Even when there is a pre-existing small atrial septal defect (ASD) or patent foramen ovale (PFO), the blade catheter is introduced into the left atrium through a long sheath, which can be positioned across the septum through a *separate* puncture site away from the original opening.

For the dilation of the mitral valve, direct entry into the left atrium is essential for documentation of the severity of the lesion, for the delivery of the dilation balloons to the mitral valve, and for the immediate documentation of the results of the therapy. With the dilation of the aortic valve or a coarctation of the aorta, the transseptal approach makes the procedures more precise and controllable. Although the dilation balloons for the dilation of both the aortic valve and coarctation of the aorta are usually delivered retrograde from the femoral arteries, the hemodynamic data and the precise anatomy are obtained using a prograde catheter through a transseptal approach prior to the introduction of the arterial catheters. This approach very significantly reduces the necessary duration of time in the arteries with large sheaths/catheters. With the prograde catheter and long sheath that are introduced through a transseptal technique remaining in the left ventricle or in the aorta, the results of dilation of the aortic valve or of a coarctation, are evident immediately without the necessity of first removing the balloon dilation catheters or exchanging the balloons and arterial wires for diagnostic catheters. This, in itself, markedly reduces the trauma to the arteries. The prograde approach has been advocated for the introduction of balloon dilation catheters for the dilation of both aortic stenosis and coarctation of the aorta. In the absence of a pre-existing atrial or ventricular communication, this requires a transseptal puncture procedure.

In the presence of an intact atrial septum, the dilation of pulmonary veins and the implant of intravascular stents into these veins are accomplished through an atrial transseptal approach. Unfortunately in spite of the reliable access to the pulmonary veins, the therapy has not been successful for producing lasting results in these particular lesions.

Equipment for transseptal puncture

Most modern catheterization laboratories use the Brockenbrough™ transseptal needle in conjunction with a Mullins™ transseptal sheath/dilator set as the standard equipment for a transseptal puncture[2,4]. The Brockenbrough™ needle sets include the transseptal needle with a contained fine stylet along with a straight and totally blunt "dummy" needle. The transseptal needles are available in two standard lengths. The pediatric needle has a 62 cm *usable* length (from the distal end of the hub/arrow to the distal tip of the needle) while the adult needle has a 72 cm *usable* length. Brockenbrough™ needles have a one-centimeter section at the tip that is narrower than the remainder of the needle, with the pediatric needle decreasing from a 19-gauge shaft to a 21-gauge tip and the adult needle decreasing from an 18-gauge shaft to a 20-gauge tip. The larger gauge of the adult needles results in their being considerably sturdier.

Both Brockenbrough™ needles have an approximately 30° curve in the last 8 cm of the distal end of the needle. The proximal end of the original transseptal needles had a two-way stopcock incorporated into a female Luer™ lock hub. For some inexplicable and illogical reason, one of the several manufacturers of current Brockenbrough™-type transseptal needles has removed the permanent stopcock from the needle so that the proximal hub always remains open! All the transseptal needles have a flat "arrow" attached between the hub and the shaft of the needle, which is perpendicular to the long axis (the shaft) of the needle. When the needles are new, this arrow points exactly in the direction of the curve at the distal end of the needle. Even during initial use, the direction of the curve of the needle can become distorted and becomes malaligned compared to the direction of the arrow when any torsion is applied to the proximal needle. The arrow still remains useful in indicating the *general direction* of the tip of the needle, but the absolute direction of the tip of the needle must be verified visually on *biplane* fluoroscopy during the positioning of the needle.

The transseptal needles are stainless steel and can be cleaned and reused, however with the expense, difficulty and potential dangers of blood contamination in the handling, cleaning, repackaging and sterilizing of the needles, most centers in the United States now discard them after a single use. Brockenbrough™ needles are now used preferentially with the Mullins™ transseptal introducer sets (MTS™) (Cook Inc., Bloomington, IN). The MTS™ are available in both pediatric and adult lengths. The usable length of the dilator is the distance from the *proximal* end *of the hub* of the dilator to the distal tip of the dilator. This dilator length should be 2 cm less than the length of the corresponding needle in both the pediatric and adult sets, while the sheaths should be 2 cm shorter than their corresponding dilators.

There are a variety of manufacturers of Mullins™ sheath/dilator sets (USCI, Cook, Daig, Arrow, Cordis). The sheaths of most of these sets are now available only with an attached, back-bleed valve/flushing port on the hub of the sheath. At least one version (Cook™) has a built in, radio-opaque band at the distal ends of the long sheaths. This band is very useful for locating the end of the sheath, especially when the dilator or a catheter is positioned within the distal end of the sheath when the "set" is in the heart shadow on fluoroscopy.

Ideally, the tip of the dilator tapers smoothly and tightly over the thin narrow portion of the needle. Unfortunately, the tip of an ideal, finely tapering dilator, which was present on the original USCI™ Mullins™ transseptal sets, only accommodated a 0.021″ or, at most, a 0.025″ wire. These finer wires did not support the introduction of the larger, long sheath/dilator sets very well. As a consequence, most of the dilators that are available in current transseptal sheath/dilator sets have a larger opening in the tip of the dilator, which accommodates a 0.035″ or even a 0.038″ wire. The larger opening makes the tips of the current transseptal dilators much "fatter" and blunter so that they do not fit tightly over the narrower portion of the transseptal needles. During the puncture of the septum with these blunter dilators, the needle must be advanced further into the dilator so that the thicker part of the needle is within the tip of the dilator and even then, more force is necessary to push the tip of the dilator through the septum.

Similarly, the original USCI™ Mullins™ transseptal sheaths were very thin walled teflont sheaths with a very close, tight tolerance to the comparable dilator of the same French size. The thinness and the tight fit over the dilator contributed to an excellent, smooth transition from the dilator to the sheath as well as an easier introduction and transseptal puncture of the septum. Unfortunately the thin material of the sheath kinked very easily and did not support the delivery of larger stiffer devices. Most of the current long sheaths, including transseptal sheaths, are manufactured of a thicker teflon material and, in addition, have poorer tolerances, with the sheaths having some slack in their fit over the dilators. To compensate for this, the sheath is usually tapered at the tip to fit somewhat more tightly over the dilator at the tip of the sheath. The thicker materials are far more kink resistant, which makes them more satisfactory for most uses. The discrepancy between the larger diameters of the sheaths compared with the external diameters of the dilators occasionally causes problems with the passage of the tip of the sheaths through the septum, tough baffles, or through tight and circuitous orifices such as fenestrations in baffles and small ventricular septal defects. This problem with the loose tolerance over the dilators with the Cook™ RB-MTS™ sheath/dilator sets is overcome by using a long dilator that is one French size larger in diameter than the long sheath being used, taken from a separate sheath/dilator set—e.g. a 12-French dilator in an 11-French sheath. By using this larger dilator, a very nice, tight fit is provided for the sheath over the dilator, particularly at the tip of the sheath on the dilator!

It is important to note that the long Mullins™ sheath/dilator sets are also used for many other procedures besides transseptal punctures and, as a consequence, are manufactured in much longer lengths than the standard transseptal sets. These longer sheath/dilator sets are *much longer than the available transseptal needles* and, as a consequence, these longer sets *cannot* be used for the transseptal punctures with the Brockenbrough™ needles. Because of the multiple lengths of the sheath/dilator sets that are available, each sheath/dilator set that is to be used for a transseptal puncture with standard Brockenbrough™ needles, must be ordered specifically in the exact transseptal lengths.

Even when ordered for a transseptal procedure, each Mullins™ transseptal sheath/dilator set should be measured carefully and compared to the needle length before the sheath/dilator set is introduced into the patient. Unfortunately, all the manufacturers of the sheath/dilator sets are not always aware of the purpose of the transseptal sets, and even those labeled as transseptal sheath/dilator sets for use with the needles are occasionally too long for the needle.

The pediatric and adult transseptal sheath/dilator sets and the longer sets are available in many different French sizes. In the pediatric transseptal length, Mullins™ transseptal sets are available in 5- to 8-French diameters, and in the adult transseptal length, from 6- to 9-French. Previously, the adult transseptal length sets were available up to 12-French. Additional diameters of long sheath dilator sets, up to 16-French, are available by special order.

In any individual patient, the shorter of the two available lengths of transseptal needles and sheath/dilator sets which will reach through the interatrial septum *and into the left ventricle* is used whenever possible. The length of the sheath/dilator used corresponds to the length of the needle—e.g. "adult" vs. "pediatric" lengths. The one exception to using the same length needle with the sheath/dilator set is when it is anticipated that the septum and/or structure that is to be punctured is very thick or tough (e.g. through a patch or baffle). In that circumstance, the "adult" needle, which is heavier and sturdier, is used regardless of the length of the Mullins™ sheath/dilator set.

Although the Brockenbrough™ needle is, and has been, the standard for transseptal punctures for the past four decades, there are alternative needles available for atrial transseptal puncture. The original transseptal needle was the Ross™ needle[5]. This was a long 18-gauge needle with no taper at the distal tip, but with both a curved distal end and a female hub with an arrow at the proximal end similar to its successor, the Brockenbrough™ needle. The Ross™ needle was designed to puncture the septum but, following the needle puncture, a fine, polyethylene tubing was advanced *through* the Ross™ needle. Pressures were measured and samples collected through this tubing from within the left heart. This needle and technique had several significant disadvantages. The initial puncture through the septum—or inadvertently through any other structures—was made with the large bore needle. Once into the left atrium, the fine polyethylene tubing was not at all controllable and transmitted pressures very poorly. The Ross™ needle and technique were replaced fairly soon after their introduction by the Brockenbrough™ needle and technique and now are of only historical significance.

To overcome the perceived problems with the transseptal needle impinging on the septum, the Endrys™ needle was developed. This "needle" is actually a set consisting of a long, blunt, outer, metal tubing (cannula or needle), similar to the Ross™ needle with a curve at the distal end and with a proximal hub/arrow. The hollow, distal tip of the outer cannula of the Endrys™ needle set, however, is squared off and blunt. The second component of the Endrys™ needle set is a very long, fine, needle with a sharp tip, which fits very snugly within, and extends completely through and beyond the tip of the larger curved, outer tubing (cannula). When the inner needle is inserted completely into the outer tubing, the sharp end and tip of the fine inner needle extend approximately one centimeter beyond the tip of the outer cannula. When the movable, inner needle is positioned all the way into the outer cannula, the combination has the appearance at the distal end of a Brockenbrough™ needle. The advantage of this needle set with the movable inner needle is that when the outer cannula is placed firmly against the septum, the inner needle can be advanced separately into the septum out of the outer cannula. Some operators believe that more specific curves are easier to form on the outer cannula and that it is easier to impinge on the proper area of the septum with this set. On the other hand, the combination of needles is more delicate and more complex to handle than the Brockenbrough™ needle.

In addition to the alternative needles for a transseptal puncture, there are alternative catheters for introduction into the left atrium. The Ross™ catheters have just been described but are no longer used. The original Brockenbrough™ catheters are still available. These, essentially, are very long, stiff, dilators with side holes near their distal tips in addition to the end-hole. The Brockenbrough™ catheter fits over the needle and is used similarly to the dilator of the MTS™. However, once the Brockenbrough™ catheter is in the left heart, the dilator-like catheter is used to record pressures, draw samples and perform angiograms and is maneuvered to different locations there. The Brockenbrough™ catheter is *rigid and sharp* in order to puncture through the septum and function as a sharp dilator. However, these same puncturing features make it difficult and dangerous to maneuver separately within the left heart. For angiography through the Brockenbrough™ catheter, there is a stylet with a fat, blunt occluder at its tip. When the stylet/occluder is advanced to the tip of the Brockenbrough™ catheter, the blunt occluder fills the single distal hole at the tip and, in doing so, produces a "side hole only", angiographic catheter. The stylet in the Brockenbrough™ catheter is also used to deflect or position the tip of the catheter. Unless the Brockenbrough™ catheter is exchanged over a wire for an MTS™ set with its long sheath, no other types of catheter are usable in the left heart through the transseptal approach.

Although biplane fluoroscopy is recommended very strongly for the performance of atrial transseptal punctures, the procedure can be performed using a single plane fluoroscopic system with a rotating "C-arm" suspension for the X-ray system. This is recommended only under extenuating circumstances and only for operators who are experienced and skilled in the transseptal technique and who have a thorough knowledge of the atrial septum and its variations. In the presence of any of the features that add to the hazards of a transseptal technique, a transseptal puncture should probably not be performed using only a single-plane system.

When a single-plane X-ray system is used, various supplemental techniques are described to assist the transseptal procedure[6]. The most important supplemental procedure is to perform a right heart or a pulmonary artery angiogram, separately, in *both* the PA and lateral projections in order to visualize all of the left heart structures on the recirculation phases of the angiograms. Freeze frames of the left heart phase of the angiograms are stored as "road maps" to be used during the puncture. On both planes of the recirculation angiograms, special attention is paid to the *location* of the left atrium, the *size* of the left atrium (in atrial systole and diastole), the location and size of the *aortic root*, and the relation of all these structures to the fixed, bony landmarks within the thorax. When the actual puncture is performed, the X-ray tubes are positioned in exactly the same positions as when the "road map" images were acquired.

In the presence of a large aortic root, it is advocated that a "pig-tail" catheter be looped in the aortic root in order to help identify its limits. The validity of this in actually demonstrating the limits of the aortic root, of course, depends upon the looped catheter lying against the walls of the aortic root that are closest to the atrial septum and closest to the aortic walls in both planes! Some operators advocate positioning the X-ray tube in a specific but different, oblique angle to aid in the transseptal puncture during the actual puncture. Unfortunately, *no single* view is satisfactory, and any angulation displaces the bony landmarks that are far more familiar to most operators in the PA view. With a single-plane system, the ability to change easily and rapidly from the PA projection completely around to the straight lateral projection by the use of the "C-arm" is far more important.

Echocardiography is used to assist the transseptal puncture. Transthoracic, transesophageal (TEE) and more recently intravascular echo (ICE) have all been recommended to guide the transseptal puncture[7]. With all of these echo modalities, although the needle is seen when it passes through a particular plane of the echo, neither the entire length of the needle nor the entire atrial septum and its surrounding structures are seen together *at any one time* and the total "three-dimensional" relationships are never visible by echo. As a consequence, echo is not particularly useful while the needle is being introduced and being positioned for the puncture. Once the needle impinges on the septum, then the echo modality becomes helpful in determining the exact location on the septum, where the needle is penetrating the septum, and the relationship of other structures near the tip of the needle, and it does demonstrate when the needle actually punctures through the septum. In the absence of a biplane X-ray system, ICE or TEE support during the puncture is more useful. With the use of TEE, the patient should be under general anesthesia, as any movement (e.g. retching) caused by the echo probe at a critical time during the puncture can be catastrophic.

Technique of transseptal needle puncture of the atrial septum using the Mullins™ transseptal sheath/dilator set

For the transseptal procedure, patients are sedated or anesthestized exactly as for any other catheterization procedure. However, just before the moment of the puncture of the septum the sedated patient is given a supplementary dose of sedation in order to ensure no movement of the patient during the actual puncture. When a transseptal procedure is anticipated during a catheterization, systemic heparin usually is *not* administered to the patient until *after* the completion of the puncture and *after* the successful positioning of the sheath in the left atrium. Once the puncture has been accomplished, however, these patients are heparinized fully because of the extensive catheter and wire manipulations that will be performed in the systemic circulation.

After completion of the right heart catheterization and after documentation that there is no foramen ovale or atrial septal defect by exploration of the atrial septum with a torque-controlled right heart catheter, preparation is made for the transseptal puncture. The relationship of the left atrium and interatrial septum to the fixed and visible extracardiac structures within the thorax are amazingly consistent even in the presence of very complex intracardiac anatomic abnormalities. However, until the operator is very comfortable with the transseptal technique and the feel of the atrial septum, transseptal puncture is preceded with a biplane right ventricular (RV) or pulmonary artery (PA) angiogram. The angiographic recording is continued through the recirculation of the contrast through the lungs and the left heart. The recirculation of the contrast through the left heart allows visualization of all of the pulmonary veins, the left atrium, the mitral valve, the left ventricle, the aorta and the relationships of each of these structures to each other and to the fixed intrathoracic (reference) structures. Even in experienced hands, if there is any peculiarity or question about the anatomy in the area, the prograde RV or PA biplane angiocardiogram is recorded before the transseptal puncture is performed. Specific abnormalities looked for on the angiogram include a very small or a very large left atrium, an unusually shaped left atrium—particularly when the bottom of the left atrium in the "double density" on routine fluoroscopy cannot clearly be visualized or in the presence of a left superior vena cava emptying into a (large) coronary sinus—a malpositioned heart or left atrium, or an enlarged or displaced aortic root.

When viewing the recirculation angiocardiogram, special attention is paid to the location of the aortic root, particularly the rightward (patient's right) and posterior (dorsal) most limits of the aortic root as seen on the PA and lateral projections, respectively. The left atrium is visualized paying special attention to the left atrial size and limits, both in atrial systole and diastole. The relationships of the cephalad wall of the left atrium to the left main stem bronchus in the PA view and of the posterior wall of the left atrium to the vertebral column in the lateral view are critically important in delineating the limits of the left atrium when the needle is being advanced after the septum has been punctured. Fortunately, these landmarks and their relationships to each other are very constant in spite of other cardiac anomalies or positional abnormalities. With these landmarks committed to memory or preferably on a "road-map" imaging system, the equipment is readied for use to proceed with the transseptal puncture.

Transseptal needle punctures are commonly approached from a right femoral vein although the left femoral vein, a hepatic vein or, rarely, even the right jugular vein can be used. With the usual approach from the femoral veins, the puncture and passage of the wire/catheter must be through the true iliofemoral system and not through pelvic collateral veins. Pelvic collateral veins, which "detour" deep into the pelvis, usually develop as a consequence of obstruction of the iliofemoral veins and frequently from previous indwelling lines in the femoral veins or previous cardiac catheterizations. The deep pelvic veins may course in the same general direction in the PA X-ray view as the true femoral veins, however, in the lateral view, the collaterals pass acutely posteriorly and deep into the dorsal pelvis. Unless looked for specifically or unless significant resistance was encountered while advancing the wire/catheter through this course, the operator may be unaware of the abnormal pelvic venous connections even after a thorough right heart catheterization and even after the long sheath/dilator set has been positioned in the superior vena cava for the transseptal procedure. The deep pelvic veins usually do re-communicate with the iliac vein or the IVC more centrally. As a consequence, a wire, a diagnostic catheter or even the long transseptal sheath/dilator set may pass through the sharp curves of these abnormal deep, pelvic veins and, in the PA view, appear in a normal course to the IVC and right atrium.

Unfortunately the stiff transseptal needle usually will *not* make the deep bend through the pelvis, but will catch on the wall of the dilator at the depth of the posterior pelvic curve. If the needle is forced as it is being advanced in this circumstance, the tip of the needle can easily puncture through the side of the sheath/dilator. When even slight resistance is encountered during any phase as the needle is being introduced, the area of the tip of the needle is visualized with biplane fluoroscopy and the cause of the resistance/obstruction determined. Even if the needle can be advanced through a deep, acute curve in the pelvis, the subsequent maneuverability of the needle in the heart will be compromised severely by this acutely angled course. This, in turn, can prevent adequate positioning of the tip of the needle on the septum. Even if the transseptal procedure is accomplished and the long sheath is positioned in the left atrium, large or stiff devices (rigid stents, "pods" for large occlusion devices, etc.) will not advance through the acute, deep curves in the posterior pelvis.

The size of the transseptal sheath/dilator set is chosen so that the long sheath will accommodate any catheter that might be used subsequently in the left heart in the particular patient. The needle, the sheath and the dilator are all flushed thoroughly before introduction into the patient. After the needle has been flushed, the stopcock on the needle is positioned in the closed position and is *not* attached to the flush/pressure system at this time. When the needle does not have a built-in stopcock, a separate disposable stopcock is attached to the hub of the needle and this is closed after flushing the needle.

When using transseptal sheaths that do not have a distal, radio-opaque marker band and before being introduced into the patient, the transseptal dilator is introduced into the sheath outside of the body. The dilator is advanced within the sheath until the tip of the dilator exactly reaches the tip of the sheath—still within the tip of the sheath. A mental notation or an actual physical measurement is made of the distance between the hub of the sheath and the hub of the dilator when the tip of the dilator exactly reaches the tip of the sheath. On some of the sets, there are small, calibrated measurements in 2 mm increments on the proximal shaft of the dilator. These marks facilitate this measurement, which can become essential when using sheaths with no distal radio-opaque band since the sheath positioned over the dilator is invisible on fluoroscopy. In order to determine when the tip of the sheath is actually in the left atrium as it is advanced along with or over the dilator and into the left atrium after the atrial septal puncture, the operator must be aware of the distance between the hub of the sheath and the hub of the dilator when the tip of the sheath is at the tip of the dilator.

Once all of the equipment for the transseptal procedure has been inspected and prepared, a long, exchange length of 0.025″ or 0.035″ spring guide wire is introduced into the femoral venous access site. The wire is advanced through the true iliofemoral venous system, through the right atrium, well into the superior vena cava and preferably into the left innominate vein. The wire used is the largest diameter wire over which the transeptal dilator that is being used will pass. It is introduced directly through the back-bleed valve of the short sheath in the groin or through the end-hole catheter that was used for the right heart catheterization. It is preferable to position an end-hole catheter purposefully in the superior vena cava and the left innominate vein and then to introduce the wire through the catheter before the short sheath is removed. The relatively straightforward manipulation of a torque-controlled catheter into the SVC/innominate vein allows fast and precise wire positioning without extensive and often fruitless manipulation of the wire by itself in the right atrium when the wire is introduced separately. The floppy portion of the wire is positioned well into the superior vena cava or, preferably, out in the left innominate vein. The stiff, shaft portion of the wire should be completely through the right atrium and at least partially into the SVC. The tip of the catheter/wire positioned in the innominate vein creates a distinct advantage for the subsequent positioning of the sheath/dilator and needle. When the curved distal end of the transseptal sheath/dilator set is advanced over a wire positioned in the innominate vein, the distal end of the sheath/dilator angles from SVC to innominate vein toward the patient's left side. When the needle is introduced, the curve of the distal end of the needle will follow in the same direction.

Once the exchange wire is in place, the original short sheath or catheter is removed over the wire. Frequently considerable time elapses between the local anesthesia given at the beginning of the case and the beginning of the transseptal procedure. As a consequence, and since the transseptal set is often larger in diameter than the original sheath, the skin area is re-anesthetized with local anesthesia and the patient given additional sedation before the transseptal sheath/dilator set is introduced. The skin incision is enlarged enough to accommodate the transseptal sheath. The transseptal sheath/dilator set is introduced over the wire, through the subcutaneous tissues and into the venous system. As with the introduction of all sheath/dilator sets, if any resistance to the introduction is encountered, the tip of the long transseptal sheath/dilator set is drilled over the wire and through the skin and subcutaneous tissues into the vein.

Once the tip of the long sheath is completely into the venous system, no further "drilling" is necessary. The sheath/dilator is advanced smoothly over the wire through the inferior vena cava and to the level of the inferior vena cava/right atrial junction. From the area of the junction of the inferior vena cava with the right atrium, the tip of the transseptal set is observed intermittently but quite closely on fluoroscopy and in both the PA and lateral views during subsequent maneuvers of the sheath/dilator. The stiffer portion of the wire should, but does not always, support the curved, transseptal sheath/dilator set as it is advanced through the right atrium into the superior vena cava.

If the guide wire is not stiff enough to resist the bend of the curved distal end of the transseptal sheath/dilator set as it is advanced through the relatively straight course through the right atrium, the curved distal end of the sheath/dilator bows, or deflects the wire into the right ventricle or atrial appendage. In doing so the distal end of the wire can be pulled out of the SVC or kinked, and the previously achieved smooth access to the SVC is lost. It often takes some very purposeful torquing and manipulation of the transseptal set with close observation in both X-ray planes, to advance a large transseptal set successfully through the right atrium and well into the superior vena cava, particularly over 0.025″ or smaller wires.

Once the tip of the transseptal sheath/dilator set is well within the superior vena cava or, preferably, into the left innominate vein, and while keeping the sheath/dilator set securely in this position, the wire is removed slowly. The dilator is cleared of any air or blood by *gentle* suction with a syringe on the hub of the dilator. Occasionally, blood cannot be withdrawn easily through the dilator. A strong negative force ***never*** is applied to the syringe, but rather the sheath/dilator set is rotated very gently and very slightly as *gentle* suction is applied to the dilator. If this does not allow the free flow of blood, the set is withdrawn *very slightly* (0.5–1.0 mm) until blood flow is obtained, still with only *gentle* suction. Once the dilator is cleared of air and clot and once blood easily flows out of the dilator, the dilator is attached to the pressure/flush system and flushed.

To introduce the needle, the flush system is detached from the dilator. With the stopcock on the transseptal needle turned *off* and nothing attached to the needle, the needle tip is introduced into the hub of the dilator. The needle hub remains ***not*** attached to the pressure/flush tubing *while the needle is being introduced and advanced* through the sheath/dilator set. When the two separate hubs on the sheath and dilator of the smaller transseptal set are locked together, the two hubs together form a relatively long, straight and ridged length of lumen within the combined hubs. This straight segment can straighten or kink the curved portion of the needle as an attempt is made to advance the curved needle through the straight segment of the joined hubs. To prevent this, the hubs of the smaller sheath and dilator are separated slightly by advancing the sheath 0.5–1.0 cm forward over the dilator, keeping the dilator fixed in its position. This separation of the hubs allows the hub of the dilator to bend and the curved tip of the needle to pass through the two hubs and into the shaft of the sheath/dilator set without distorting the needle. Once the straight portion of the needle is into and through the two hubs, the hubs are reattached to each other by withdrawing the sheath (only) over the dilator. The dilator should never be moved at all.

Once the tip of the needle is past the hubs, it is advanced within the sheath/dilator set, through the pelvis and IVC, through the cardiac silhouette, into the superior vena cava and to the tip of the *dilator*. The hub of the needle still is ***not*** attached to the flush/pressure tubing as the curved distal end of the needle advances within the sheath/dilator set. This allows the needle/hub to rotate freely and bend along with the rest of the needle as the curved tip advances through curves in the course of the veins through the pelvis and to the heart. Often the hub of the needle rotates >360° as the curved tip of the needle advances through the pelvis/IVC area. If the shaft of the needle is not allowed to rotate and bend freely, the tip of the needle can easily be forced into and puncture through the wall of the dilator (and sheath) and even outside of the vessel. For this reason, *nothing* is attached to the hub and the needle and it is allowed to rotate freely while the tip of the needle advances through the *entire length* of the dilator lumen.

The needle is advanced until its tip and the tip of the dilator are approximated, preferably with the tip of the needle no more than one millimeter from the tip of the dilator. When the tips of the needle and dilator have been approximated, the arrow/stopcock/hub at the proximal end of the needle will still be one, or more, centimeters away from (proximal to) the hub of the dilator. If the tip of the needle is positioned more proximally within the tip of the dilator, the latter can bend acutely away from the direction of the tip of the needle and kink the dilator as the needle/sheath/dilator are withdrawn as a unit.

With the needle/sheath/dilator all positioned in the superior vena cava or innominate vein and in position to begin the transseptal procedure, the stopcock on the transseptal needle is opened and the proximal end of the needle is attached to the flush/pressure system. The flush/pressure system should be flowing continuously as it is attached to the hub of the needle. The needle is flushed thoroughly. Because of the small bore of the needle and since the tip of the needle is still within the tip of the dilator, ***no attempt*** is made to withdraw anything through the needle by suction at the hub of the needle. The flush system, which is now attached to the lumen of the needle, is switched to pressure monitoring.

With a properly flushed system, when the tip of the dilator is free in the SVC or innominate vein and in spite of the small lumen of the needle, a very good pressure wave should be transmitted through the needle. The monitored atrial pressure is placed on a full scale (gain) of 20 mmHg. If a good right atrial pressure curve is not visualized, there are several areas to be checked:

- The tip of the dilator must be free in the lumen of the vein. It may need to be withdrawn 1–2 mm or rotated very slightly.
- The entire system from the tip of the needle all the way back to the transducer must be flushed free of air and clots.
- The connecting pressure tubing must have an adequate wall stiffness and lack of compliance to transmit low-amplitude pressures.
- The recording system must be set on the correct amplitude (gain) and frequency to visualize the low-pressure wave forms.

All of these areas, locations and systems are checked and corrected until a good pressure reading is obtained through the needle.

As the positioning of the set for the puncture begins, the tip of the needle/sheath/dilator along with the proximal arrow may be pointing in any direction. The exact direction of the tip of the sheath/dilator/needle is determined by viewing the distal ends of the sheath/dilator/needle directly in both the PA and lateral projections with biplane fluoroscopy. The direction of the arrow on the proximal end of the needle generally corresponds to the direction of the tip of the needle, but should *never* be relied upon totally to represent the precise direction of the tip. Regardless of the direction that the tip of the sheath/dilator/needle is pointing initially, the combination is *not* rotated at this juncture of the procedure. The tip of the dilator is sharp and with the needle in it, very stiff. The combination is designed for *puncturing*! If the dilator is advanced or rotated, even with the transseptal needle still within the tip of the dilator and without the needle protruding, the tip of the *dilator* alone is capable of puncturing or tearing the vessel wall if rotated while in a fixed location.

The proximal end of the needle, along with the approximated, proximal ends of the sheath and dilator, are all grasped together by the right hand of the operator in order to maintain the three components as a single unit in this fixed relationship. The combination is grasped in such a manner that the distance between the hubs of the sheath/dilator and the hub of the needle is fixed in the exact forward–backward position relative to each other. Occasionally it will be necessary to use both hands on the needle in order to keep the needle/sheath/dilator hubs in an exact relative position to each other and to control the direction of the needle/sheath/dilator. This fixed distance between the hub of the needle and the hub of the sheath/dilator set must be maintained continuously in order to keep the tip of the needle *just within* the tip of the dilator as the entire needle/sheath/dilator system is withdrawn to the position for the atrial puncture.

The original grip and the position of the hand(s) on the proximal end of the needle/sheath/dilator often are very awkward and/or in an uncomfortable position. This awkward grip on the needle frequently requires that both hands are grasping the needle/sheath/dilator hubs during the initial steps of the procedure. This is particularly true when the initial direction of the tip of the needle/sheath/dilator in the superior vena cava is pointing anteriorly and/or toward the patient's right as illustrated by position "a" in Figure 8.1. The hubs/arrow of the needle/sheath/dilator should be grasped initially in such a way that *after the needle/sheath/dilator have been rotated to the final direction for puncture of the septum*, the hand(s) holding, and controlling, the direction of the needle then *will be* in a *comfortable* position when the tips of the needle/sheath/dilator are pointing posterior (dorsally) and towards the patient's left scapula as visualized on fluoroscopy.

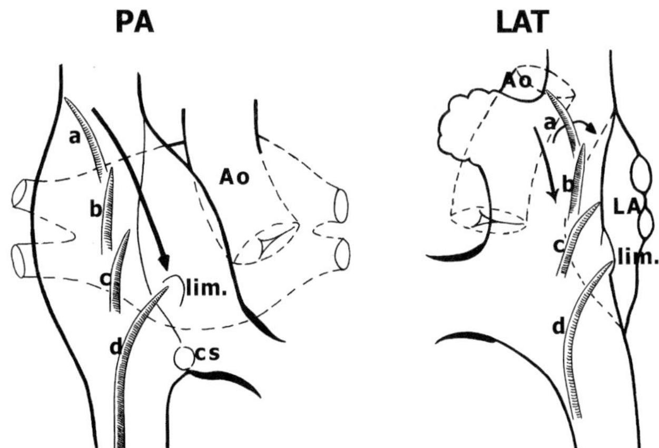

Figure 8.1 Positions of the tip of the transseptal set in the PA and lateral views during the withdrawal and positioning of the set for the puncture. (a) In superior vena cava (pointing anteriorly and laterally); (b) withdrawn into right atrium while being rotated medially (toward patient's left); (c) withdrawn further into right atrium and rotated medially and posteriorly; (d) withdrawn under the limbus, into fossa ovalis and positioned (correctly) posteriorly and toward the patient's left. PA, posterior-anterior; Ao, aorta; lim., limbus; cs, coronary sinus; LAT; laterial projection; LA; left atrium.

Once the proper grip is secured on the proximal end of the needle/sheath/dilator, the combination of hubs along with the arrow *simultaneously* is rotated toward the proper puncture position *as it is being withdrawn* out of the superior vena cava into the right atrium and along the interatrial septum as illustrated diagrammatically in steps "a–c" in Figure 8.1. It is imperative that during the withdrawal of the needle/sheath/dilator along the septum and during the puncture of the septum, the grip by the controlling hand(s) on the proximal end of the needle/sheath/dilator *is not released* nor even *relaxed* from the sheath/dilator/needle hubs during any of these critical maneuvers. This very tight grip on the hubs/arrow is necessary both to keep the hubs of the needle/dilator/sheath in their absolute fixed relationship to each other and to maintain the tip of the needle pointing in the proper direction. In the presence of a high left atrial pressure and/or an otherwise enlarged left atrium, the septum bulges toward the right atrium creating a tense, *convex*, rounded septal surface. As a consequence, considerable and continuous torque must be maintained on the hubs/arrow of the needle/sheath/dilator in order to maintain the tip of the needle at the proper angle to the septum and to prevent side-to-side slippage of the position of the tip of the needle on the septum. Any relaxation of the grip on the hub/arrow of the needle results in loss of the torsion control on the angle of the tip of the needle/sheath/dilator.

For the best visualization of the tips of the needle/sheath/dilator during these manipulations, both the

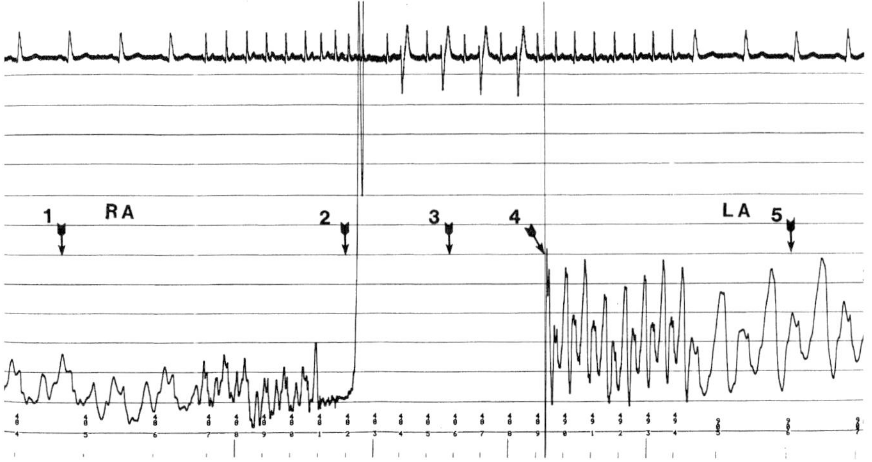

Figure 8.2 Pressures during transseptal puncture. 1, pressure recorded through needle in the right atrium before starting puncture; 2, loss of pressure with the needle tip against the septum; 3, continued lost or "damped" pressure while needle is advanced within septal tissue; 4, appearance of phasic pressure as needle "pops" through septal tissues; 5, good left atrial pressure when tip of needle is free within left atrium. RA, right atrium; LA, left atrium.

posterior–anterior (PA) and lateral (LAT) fluoroscopic images are enlarged in magnify mode in the X-ray system. Magnification of the image allows the tip of the needle to be visualized very clearly even while it is still within the tip of the dilator. Before beginning the maneuvering of the needle/sheath/dilator, the PA X-ray field is positioned to provide a clear image of the entire right and left atrial areas. In the lateral view, the field of view should extend sufficiently posteriorly so that at least the anterior border of the spinal column is seen. With the fluoroscopic fields so arranged, the hand(s) positioned correctly on the proximal ends of the needle/sheath/dilator, and with a continual pressure through the needle visualized on a sensitivity range which will accommodate the anticipated left atrial pressure as seen in Figure 8.2, withdrawal/rotation of the needle/sheath/dilator from the high superior vena cava/ left innominate vein to the atrial septum is started.

The combined needle/sheath/dilator is withdrawn slowly *as a single unit* from the superior vena cava toward the right atrium while ***simultaneously*** rotating the tip toward the desired direction for the septal puncture (toward the left scapula). The rotation of the needle/ sheath/dilator may be either clockwise or counterclockwise from the initial, starting direction of its tip. The direction of rotation depends upon which is safer and more comfortable to achieve the desired direction for the correct puncture of the atrial septum. The needle/dilator/sheath is rotated only while the combination is being withdrawn, and the *entire* rotation that will be necessary to direct the needle/sheath/dilator posteriorly and to the patient's left, should be accomplished *completely* during the withdrawal from the high superior vena cava to the low superior vena cava and *before* the tip of the needle/sheath/ dilator has been withdrawn out of the superior vena cava into the right atrium. As the tip of the needle/sheath/dilator slides into the right atrium from the superior vena cava (Figure 8.1c), the needle should be directed posteriorly and to the left without having to rotate the set significantly any further.

Once the tip of the needle/sheath/dilator is directed properly and while maintaining a firm grip on the hub of the needle with the right hand to control the direction of the needle/sheath/dilator, the left (non-controlling) hand of the operator is shifted to a position on the shaft of the needle/sheath/dilator at the point where the sheath/dilator enter the skin. This hand supports the long shaft of the needle/sheath/dilator and keeps the portion of the transseptal set outside of the body from bending significantly when the needle is advanced into the septum.

The tip of the needle/sheath/dilator should *not be* moved from side to side *at all* when it is *not* being withdrawn simultaneously. The sharp tip of the dilator with the tip of the needle just within it is stiff and designed for perforation! If the sheath/dilator/needle is rotated within a vein or chamber while the tip is not being withdrawn, it can easily tear or perforate the wall of a vein or chamber. Although the pressure through the needle is often lost intermittently and very transiently as the needle rotates or is withdrawn, there should be an almost continual visualization of the right atrial pressure throughout the entire rotation/withdrawal maneuver (Figure 8.2, pressure curve—arrow 1). The withdrawal of the combined needle/sheath/dilator set is continued so that the tip of the combination is actually sliding down the center of the convex interatrial septum. The position of the needle tip is rechecked repeatedly on both PA and lateral fluoroscopy, but most of the withdrawal and positioning of the needle is observed in the PA view. With a large, distended left atrium, the distal end and the tip of the needle/sheath/ dilator are bowed or displaced toward the patient's right. It usually takes significant extra manual effort to maintain the tip directed properly from side to side on the center of a very tense and convex atrial septum.

As the tip of the needle/dilator is withdrawn caudally down the interatrial septum and approaches a position roughly 2/3 of the way down the septum (which corresponds to 2/3 of the way down the body of the right atrium), the needle tip usually slides, or deflects slightly, toward the patient's left and posteriorly as it drops into the fossa ovali (Figure 8.1d). The needle and sheath/dilator set together are withdrawn caudally several millimeters further in order to allow the tip of the needle/dilator to move at least several millimeters below the limbus of the fossa. In this position, the pressure visualized through the needle as seen at the position of arrow 2 in Figure 8.2, usually disappears as the tip of the needle/dilator becomes perpendicular against the wall of the atrial septum. The proper position and direction of the tip of the needle/sheath/dilator are verified on both the PA and lateral fluoroscopy. Although the angle of the arrow at the proximal end of the needle and the tip is directed posteriorly on the lateral view, the tip itself must not be allowed to deflect either far anteriorly to the patient's left (into the groove between the anterior aorta and atrial septum) or far posteriorly to the patient's right (into the groove between the posterior atrial septum and posterior wall of the atrium). The tip of the needle/sheath/dilator should be pointed posteriorly and between 45° and 60° off the horizontal and toward the patient's left (toward the left scapula). In the PA view, the tip should be centered on the septum between the right and left limits of the right atrium. In the lateral view, the tip should be directed posteriorly but still *in front* of the vertebral column. The various steps in the withdrawal of the needle/dilator/sheath are summarized diagrammatically in Figure 8.1, a–d.

With the proper position verified and the direction of the needle fixed in the proper direction so that it cannot rotate, the needle is advanced out of the tip of the dilator until the dilator begins to advance with the needle. There is usually some resistance to advancing the needle, and the monitored pressure definitely disappears as the needle is advanced out of the dilator and into the septum (Figure 8.2, arrow 2). The pressure tracing may go above or below the monitor screen. This direction has no significance and the pressure can be ignored temporarily. Supporting the needle so that the needle/sheath/dilator does not rotate, the needle/sheath/dilator is advanced into the interatrial septum *as one unit*. As the needle/sheath/dilator advances into the septum, the septum is displaced cephalad yet the tip of the needle still may not pop through the septum and into the left atrium. Moderate resistance to the forward motion of the needle/sheath/dilator is often felt, and even some bowing of the shafts of the combination needle/sheath/dilator is encountered with this maneuver. The bowing or curving of the shafts of the needle/dilator/sheath is never allowed to approach a 90° angle to the long axis of the shafts of the set.

If very significant resistance and/or extreme bowing of the needle/sheath/dilator is encountered, the needle tip is withdrawn into the tip of the sheath/dilator set and the entire set with the enclosed needle is withdrawn caudally very slightly into a new starting position for the puncture in the fossa. In the new position, the needle is advanced out of the dilator tip and the entire set is again advanced together. While advancing the needle, even without the sensation of much resistance or bowing of the needle/sheath/dilator, the tip of the needle along with the sheath/dilator often advances as much as one or two interspaces in a cephalad direction without any sensation of "pop" or "give" of the needle passing through the septum. This represents a very common and normal cephalad displacement of the entire interatrial septum!

As the tip of the needle advances *through* the septum, the operator usually feels *and sees* a "give" as the tip of the needle "pops" into the left atrium. Often the tip of the dilator advances through the septum along with the needle. When such a give is seen or felt, a left atrial pressure curve should appear immediately on the monitoring screen (Figure 8.2, arrow 4). If left atrial pressure is *not* visualized, neither the needle nor the sheath/dilator is advanced *any* further. While carefully holding the needle in exactly the same position, the pressure/monitoring line is disconnected and a small syringe containing 1 ml of contrast is attached to the hub of the needle. The hub of the needle should be filled with contrast before and as the syringe is being attached. ***0.1–0.2 ml*** of contrast then is injected *forcefully* through the needle. If the needle successfully and accurately entered the left atrium, a faint, free "swirl" of contrast will be seen there. Because of the very small amount of contrast and the rapid flow of blood in the left atrium, this contrast may be only barely visible. If, however, the needle has not perforated the septum, or has advanced into an abnormal location (e.g. the posterior wall of the left atrium and/or the pericardium!), a small "tag" of contrast extravasates into the tissues of the abnormal location and is visualized very vividly. It usually requires a great deal of force, even with a small, hard syringe, to exude the contrast out of the tip of the needle *into* any tissues. This resistance to the injection is, itself, an indicator that the tip of the needle is not free! The tag of extravasated contrast, once created at the tip of the needle, remains in the tissues for a considerable length of time but causes no problem for the patient. Since any contrast extravasated into the tissues remains in place for a considerable time and a large amount of extravasated contrast would obliterate adequate visualization in the entire area, it is imperative that *very, very minute quantities* of contrast are used for these test injections. If the needle tip is still within the interatrial septum and still in a good position on the septum, but merely has not punctured all of the way through the septum, the pressure/monitoring system is reattached to the needle and the needle is flushed free of contrast by a hand flush from the manifold. Occasionally this flush completes the puncture and the contrast that is flushed out of the needle swirls around in the left atrium! If not, the needle is advanced further until the sensation of "popping through" occurs simultaneously with the appearance of the left atrial pressure. If the sensation of the needle popping through some structure is encountered, but still no pressure is visualized, the injection of a *minute amount* of contrast through the needle is repeated in this location. Again, unless the needle tip is *confirmed* to be free in the left atrium by either a good left atrial pressure curve (Figure 8.2, arrow 5) and/or by free flow of contrast into the left atrium with the repeat, small hand injection, the sheath/dilator set ***never*** should be advanced any further with, and/or over, the needle.

When a needle punctures through the septum, but then passes completely through the left atrium and into the posterior atrial wall or pericardium, no atrial pressure will be visualized through the needle! A tag of contrast injected through the needle, however, identifies the abnormal location exactly. Unless the left atrial pressure is *extremely* high, the tip of the needle alone entering the posterior wall of the left atrium, or even into the pericardial space, does not cause a clinical problem. However, if the tip of the needle that is in such an abnormal location is rotated significantly in that position, or the much larger diameter sheath/dilator combination is advanced along with the needle into one of these abnormal locations, a significantly larger hole is created and the results can be catastrophic.

When the tip of the *needle alone* is in or through the posterior atrial wall, it is withdrawn very carefully and for only a very short distance while observing for the appearance of the left atrial pressure curve. If no pressure curve is visualized after several millimeters of withdrawal, a small injection of contrast through the needle is repeated in order to identify the exact location of the tip of the needle. The next step depends on the needle/sheath/dilator location and position once the needle has been withdrawn.

If the tip of the needle has not punctured *through* the septum, the small tag of contrast through the needle and into the tissues clearly shows the location of the needle on the septum. The tag of contrast usually remains in the atrial septal tissues for many minutes and serves as a good reference marker for subsequent attempts at the transseptal puncture. The tag shows the location on the septum and clearly demonstrates the cephalad displacement of the septum as the needle/sheath/dilator is advanced and before the needle pops through the septum during a subsequent puncture attempt. The tag of contrast on the septum also demonstrates when the needle is too far, either anteriorly, posteriorly (dorsally), or cephalad on the septum. When the needle is in an undesirable location that is too cephalad for a puncture, it is withdrawn into the dilator and the entire set is then withdrawn along the septum, slightly more caudally, while rotating the combination needle/dilator/sheath more onto the center of the lower atrial septum. When positioned correctly, the transseptal puncture is restarted.

When the tag of contrast demonstrates that the tip of the needle is too low (caudal) on the septum, the flush pressure line is detached from the needle, the needle is withdrawn from the sheath/dilator set, the dilator cleared of air and clot and the sheath/dilator re-flushed. The original introducing spring guide wire is re-advanced through the dilator and back into the superior vena cava. The sheath/dilator set is re-advanced back into the superior vena cava over the wire. With the sheath/dilator positioned in the superior vena cava or left innominate vein, the needle is reintroduced and the transseptal procedure is started all over. The previously produced tag on the septum serves as an additional reference point or marker in order to reposition the set with the enclosed needle more ideally on the septum.

Electively injecting a small tag of contrast through the transseptal needle into the tissues of the atrial septum from the very start of the puncture represents an alternative addition to the standard transseptal procedure that occasionally may be helpful. The tag is useful particularly when the operator is unsure about the exact anatomic landmarks. After positioning on the septum and as soon as the needle tip is advanced out of the sheath/dilator set and impinges in the atrial septal tissues, a "micro-injection" (0.1–0.2 ml) of contrast is performed through the needle to produce the tag of extravasated contrast in the tissues on the septum. This tag of contrast produces a distinct, visual landmark in the interatrial septum, which remains there for 10–20 minutes. As the needle and set are advanced, the tag demonstrates any displacement of the septum very dramatically and allows visualization of the needle actually puncturing the septum (through the tag) into the left atrium. It also provides a graphic visualization of when the needle slips out of the septal tissues and merely slides along the septum rather than actually displacing the septum as the puncture is being attempted.

When the needle punctures the septum successfully and advances into the left atrium, and even if no pressure curve is seen, a tiny injection of contrast through the needle demonstrates a tiny "whiff" of free-flowing contrast swirling in the left atrium. When a good pressure curve is seen or there is free flow of contrast from the needle into the left atrium, the needle/system is reattached to the pressure/flush system and *flushed forcefully by hand* from the manifold in order to clear any contrast from within the needle. After flushing, the system is switched to the pressure line to resume the continuous pressure visualization. A good left atrial pressure (Figure 8.2, arrow 5) must be visualized before the needle/sheath/dilator are advanced any further and during all further advances of the needle/sheath/dilator. Once the tip of the needle has advanced through the septum properly, and a left atrial pressure curve is obtained through the needle, the needle/sheath/dilator are rotated to direct the tip of the needle laterally (i.e. in a straight horizontal direction toward the patient's left). This horizontal direction of the tip allows more space for the needle to advance within the cavity of the left atrium before it approaches/touches the posterior or cephalad wall of the left atrium.

With the needle and set directed straight laterally, the *entire system* (*needle/dilator/sheath*) is advanced further into the left atrium. A good left atrial pressure curve *must be* present and must be observed very carefully and continuously during all the time that the needle/set is being advanced. The continually visualized left atrial pressure curve verifies that the left atrium has not been traversed completely and that the posterior or cephalad wall of the atrium has not even been touched by the tip of the needle. If at any time the pressure disappears while the needle/sheath/dilator are being advanced, the advancing of the combined needle/sheath/dilator is *stopped immediately* with *nothing* being advanced further—*not even slightly*! If the monitored pressure is lost, the sheath/dilator are held precisely in the same position while the *needle* alone is withdrawn several millimeters. When the advancing of the needle/sheath/dilator is stopped immediately, an infinitesimal withdrawal of the needle should result in the reappearance of the left atrial pressure. As long as the left atrial pressure tracing is visualized, the entire needle/sheath/dilator combination can be advanced further very slightly. This maneuver is repeated until the operator is reasonably sure that, in addition to the tip of the needle, at least the tip of the dilator has advanced into the left atrium. The tip of the needle is withdrawn to just within the tip of the dilator, but not completely out of the dilator. The needle within the sheath/dilator adds extra support to the system and, of equal importance, still allows the sheath/dilator/needle to be directed purposefully from side to side by rotation of the needle as the dilator or sheath is advanced into the left atrium off the needle.

Once the dilator is positioned securely in the left atrium, the needle and dilator are held together and fixed in position and the *sheath alone* is advanced over the dilator until the tips of the sheath and dilator are approximated within the left atrium. If significant resistance is encountered while the sheath is being advanced over the dilator, the dilator and needle together are withdrawn 0.5–1.0 cm and the sheath/dilator/needle are advanced *together* as a single unit further into the left atrium. The combination can be advanced together as long as the *left atrial pressure* remains visible and undamped.

An alternative technique for advancing the sheath through a tough septum into the left atrium is to hold the dilator and needle in position and to rotate (spin) the shaft of the sheath alone over the dilator while advancing the sheath with, or without, the dilator. The pressure curve through the needle/dilator must be maintained during the rotation and while advancing the sheath. The separate rotation of the sheath will rotate any small flair or flange that may have developed at the tip of the sheath and allow the sheath to pass through the septum more easily, like the introduction of a sheath into a peripheral vessel. In this case there is usually a slight sensation of give as the tip of the sheath passes through the septum into the left atrium.

The separate positions and the relationships of the tips of the needle, dilator and sheath are clearly seen with most modern fluoroscopy equipment. However, when a long sheath that does not have a distal radio-opaque marker band is used, often there is a problem in visualizing the tip of the sheath once it is within the left atrium, particularly when the sheath is positioned over a dilator or catheter. This problem should be anticipated by the type of sheath being used before the sheath/dilator combination was introduced into the patient and the "reference measurements" of the sheath/dilator lengths relative to each other at the hubs should have been made outside the body before the sheath/dilator were introduced. If the various components cannot be seen clearly on fluoroscopy, the relative relationships of the tips of the sheath and dilator can be determined using the prior measurements between the hubs on the separated sheath and dilator before they were introduced into the patient.

Once the dilator is well within the left atrium, the sheath is advanced into the left atrium over the dilator with the dilator fixed in position. The sheath is advanced until the tips of the sheath and dilator are approximated visually or until the hubs of the dilator and sheath are separated the same (3–4 cm) distance that was measured on the proximal shaft of the dilator when the tips of the sheath and dilator were approximated as the transseptal set was being prepared. When this separation has been achieved and a good left atrial pressure is visualized through the dilator, it can be assumed that the tip of the *sheath* is in the left atrium even if it cannot be seen clearly on fluoroscopy. After the tip of a sheath that cannot easily be seen is well into the left atrium, the distance from the skin puncture site to the proximal end of the hub of the sheath is measured. This external distance measurement provides a future reference in order to ensure that the tip of the sheath is still positioned within the left atrium later during the case.

The potentially most *dangerous* part of the transseptal procedure begins *after the needle puncture is completed and the sheath is positioned in the left atrium*! The needle, the dilator and the sheath all provide direct access to the left atrium for air or clot! Very meticulous techniques must *always* be used for clearing the dilator and then the long sheath of all air and/or clot. Extreme and continual caution must be used during the removal and/or reintroduction of the various components of the transseptal system and of any catheters or devices that are used through the sheath.

After completing the transseptal puncture with the sheath successfully advanced over the dilator/needle into the left atrium, the stopcock on the needle is turned to the off position and the needle hub is disconnected from the flush/pressure tubing. Detaching the needle allows it to rotate freely and be withdrawn straight through the transseptal sheath/dilator. The needle should be withdrawn very slowly. Blood should follow the needle dripping from the hub of the dilator adjacent to the needle as the needle is withdrawn from the dilator. If there is no blood return as or after the needle is withdrawn completely from the dilator, a syringe is attached to the dilator and *very gentle* suction applied to the dilator lumen as the dilator is withdrawn several millimeters. If there is still no *easy* return of blood, the gentle suction is released and the *combined* sheath and dilator are withdrawn several millimeters together and gentle suction reapplied. This is repeated until there is a good and easy flow of blood through the dilator.

Following the withdrawal of the needle, and once free flow of blood through the dilator is established, the dilator is withdrawn separately and *very slowly* out of the sheath. The dilator is withdrawn still with nothing attached to the hub of the dilator. As a result, with a slow withdrawal of the dilator, there should be a slow, continuous drip of blood out of the hub of the dilator as the dilator is withdrawn from the sheath. The slow withdrawal of the dilator allows blood to follow the tip of the dilator into the shaft of the sheath and, at the same time, does *not* create a partial vacuum within the emptying space within the sheath. If the dilator is withdrawn more rapidly than the blood can follow the tip of the dilator into the sheath, a partial vacuum is created and the space in the sheath fills with air sucked through the lumen of the dilator or around the dilator! If the distal tip of the sheath (which has only the single distal end hole) happens to be positioned against the posterior wall or roof of the left atrium, or is positioned distally within a pulmonary vein, the tip of the sheath will be occluded completely. When the tip of the sheath is occluded, no blood can follow the tip of the dilator into the sheath and a partial vacuum is created within the sheath as the dilator is withdrawn out of the sheath. No matter how slowly the dilator is withdrawn, if the distal end of the sheath is obstructed, a partial vacuum will be created and the only way this vacuum in the sheath can be vented is by sucking air into the sheath through the dilator, between the sheath and dilator or even through a back-bleed valve on the sheath! This entry of air must be prevented or, if introduced, removed completely when the dilator has been removed from the sheath. If blood does not flow out of the dilator as the dilator is withdrawn or blood cannot be withdrawn from the dilator with a syringe even with multiple changes in the distal position of the sheath/dilator, it is better to withdraw the sheath/dilator back to the right atrium, clear the dilator and restart the transseptal puncture.

Most of the current long sheaths come with a permanently attached back-bleed valve/flush port. This attached back-bleed valve/flush port actually presents a "double-edged sword". The back-bleed valve/flush port very effectively prevents back bleeding from the sheath and allows flushing of the sheath. At the same time back-bleed valve/flush ports all have a chamber within the hub at the proximal end of the sheath, which has a significantly larger internal diameter than the rest of the sheath and a capacity as much as several ml, which exaggerates the problem of trapped air in the long sheath (Figure 8.3).

Even though the sheath, including the back-bleed/flush port, is flushed thoroughly and filled with fluid during preparation for use, as soon as the tip of the dilator is introduced into/through the back-bleed valve as the dilator is introduced into the sheath and before the introduction of the sheath/dilator into the body, the valve chamber is vented to air. Air enters through the lumen of the dilator as well as through the back-bleed valve leaflets around the tip of the dilator. This air fills the *chamber of the back-bleed valve/flush port* apparatus on the sheath. Any air introduced at any time remains in the valve chamber throughout the transseptal procedure or any other manipulations of the long sheath as long as the dilator is still in place. If special maneuvers are not carried out to remove the air from this chamber after the dilator is removed, the

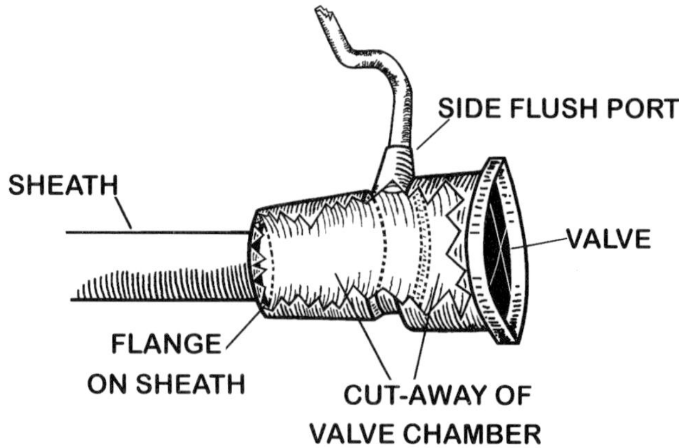

Figure 8.3 Diagrammatic "cut-away" of back-bleed valve/flush port of a sheath showing the "dead space" within the valve chamber.

air from the chamber will definitely be flushed into the body (left heart!!) with the first flush of the long sheath through its side port!

As soon as the dilator is withdrawn completely out of the sheath, the chamber of the back-bleed valve/ flush port of the sheath is very meticulously and very specifically cleared of air to eliminate the possibility of the air in the chamber being delivered to the body. The proximal end of the sheath, including the back-bleed valve chamber, is pressed down against the patient's leg or preferably into the depression in the drapes between or on either side of the legs. This places the back-bleed valve chamber lower than the corresponding horizontal level of the heart. The stopcock on the side port of the hub is opened very cautiously and only partially and with excellent lighting of the area in order to be able to open the tubing to room air while observing the sidearm tubing very closely. Extreme care is taken to be sure that the column of fluid/air in the side arm of the flush port *runs out of* and is ***not*** sucked ***into*** the sheath from the side port when the stopcock is opened slightly and cautiously. When absolutely sure that fluid and/or air is/are flowing freely ***out*** of the side port and stopcock, the stopcock is kept open while the proximal end of the sheath with the *side flush port* on the back-bleed valve is raised slowly and slightly off the tabletop. While ensuring that blood continues to flow freely ***out*** of the sideport, the whole valve system is moved up and down and rotated slightly while the hub is tapped crisply and repeatedly with an instrument. During all of this manipulation of the sheath, the side port must be observed very closely to be sure that the flow *always* is ***out*** *of the side port* even when the proximal end of the sheath is raised slightly. These maneuvers allow air bubbles in the sheath to "rise to the surface" and flow out of the system and passively clear the hub of the sheath of any trapped air after the removal of the dilator.

Preferably, no attempt is made to suck fluid and/or air actively out of the side port of the valve of the long sheath. The back-bleed valve *"leaflets" themselves* represent the path of least resistance, and with even the slightest resistance to flow at the tip of the sheath, when suction is applied to the side port, air will preferentially be sucked in through the back-bleed valve and into the sheath. This is a particular problem when there is anything (a wire, dilator or catheter) passing through the valve and venting it. Occasionally, however, in patients with very low venous pressures or with any respiratory obstruction, active suction must be used on a long sheath to clear it of air or clot. This can and should be performed only when there is *nothing passing through the valve* of the sheath. Before suction is applied to the side port of the back-bleed valve, a gloved finger is pressed firmly over the entire back-bleed valve in order to seal the valve tightly while any suction is applied to the sheath.

Once the air/clot is cleared completely and there is passive flow of only blood out of the side port, the sheath is attached to the flush/pressure system and flushed through the side port, and then the system is switched to the pressure monitor system. A good left atrial pressure should be visualized through the sheath. When the transseptal procedure has been completed and whenever pressures are not being recorded through the sheath, the system is maintained as a sealed system on a constant, slow flush to prevent any back-flow of blood or areas of stasis with possible clotting between the lumen of the sheath and the outer wall of the catheters within the sheath. Each time a catheter is withdrawn from the sheath, the same precautions to remove air and prevent the entry of air are observed.

The problem of clearing the sheath of air is different if the sheath does *not* have an attached back-bleed valve. Once the dilator tip is withdrawn completely out of a long sheath that does *not* have an attached back-bleed valve, the sheath is capped quickly with the flush/pressure system tubing, which is *closed*, or with a detachable, back-bleed valve/flush port, which is closed. In either case, the flush system remains *off* and initially *no* flow is allowed into the sheath. Once the system has been closed with a back-bleed valve/side flush port, the newly attached side port is opened very slightly and very briefly, exactly like an attached valve on the sheath, while observing very closely. There should be back flow out of the sheath or from the side port of any air or blood that has entered the sheath from its distal end. If there is no free or continuous flow of fluid or blood out through the side port, then an attempt is made to withdraw the fluid/air very gently. A syringe is attached to the three-way stopcock on the flush/ pressure tubing on the back-bleed valve, and simultaneously the back-bleed valve is covered (capped) tightly with a gloved finger. With the valve tightly occluded, *very gentle* suction is applied to the syringe until all blood and air are withdrawn from within the sheath and valve chamber. Until there is a free back flow of blood only from the side port or the proximal end of the sheath, the system is *never* flushed and no catheters or devices are introduced into the sheath.

Back-bleed devices should always be used on long sheaths and they should always be attached to a separate flush/pressure system, in order that either continual or frequent, intermittent flushing can be accomplished around catheters and wires within the sheath. If a long sheath is used without a back-bleed valve, there will be continual back bleeding into the sheath around the catheter no matter how tight the fit of the catheter within the sheath. Clot forms in the dead space between the outer wall of the catheter and the inner wall of the sheath. If a back-bleed valve *without* a side arm flush port is used, the free back bleeding from the body is stopped, but clots can still form in the dead space between the sheath and catheter or, as a catheter is withdrawn from a sheath without simultaneous flushing into the sheath, air can be drawn into the sheath around the back-bleed valve.

If free back bleeding is not obtained from the long sheath in the left atrium (with or without a back-bleed valve) by the previous maneuvers, the sheath is withdrawn several millimeters and rotated slightly. Repeated attempts are made to withdraw blood *very gently* from the side port at the proximal end of the sheath while tightly sealing the back-bleed valve with a gloved finger. Strong suction should *never* be applied to the sheath or the side port while the tip of the sheath is in the left atrium. Strong suction is more likely to suck the wall of the left atrium into the tip of the sheath, and in doing so create an even tighter occlusion of the tip of the sheath and an even stronger vacuum within the sheath.

If free flow of blood has still not been achieved, the sheath is again withdrawn several more millimeters, rotated slightly, and the procedure repeated. When the sheath has been withdrawn several times, it may appear that the tip of the sheath has been withdrawn completely out of the left atrium. However, even after the sheath has been withdrawn a centimeter or more, the puncture site in the septal wall tissues is still usually positioned more proximally on the shaft of the sheath and still proximal to the tip of the sheath in the left atrium. During the transseptal puncture of the atrial septum, the sheath/dilator tip displaces the interatrial septum several centimeters into/toward the left atrium and bows the septum in that direction with considerable tension. As soon as the tip of the sheath passes through the bowed atrial septum and into the left atrium, the atrial septum springs, or recoils, back along the shaft of the transseptal sheath until it is positioned in the neutral position of the septum, which is usually several centimeters proximal to the tip of the sheath. The sheath can be withdrawn that far before its tip falls back into the right atrium.

Only after a good free back flow of blood has been established and the sheath is *entirely* free of all air and debris, is the sheath opened to the flush/pressure system and flushed thoroughly. It is better to withdraw the sheath completely into the right atrium, in order to be sure that it is cleared completely, and then to repeat the entire transseptal puncture than to flush even the smallest amount of air or debris into the systemic circulation! These precautions for clearing sheaths of air and thrombotic debris are equally important for all long sheaths positioned within the heart, but especially for sheaths positioned within the left heart.

Transseptal puncture from the left inguinal area

Although technically slightly more difficult, it certainly is possible to perform the atrial transseptal puncture from the left inguinal area. The course of the needle/sheath/dilator set through the left iliac vein is slightly more tortuous, making it more difficult to advance the needle through the sheath/dilator to the level of the right atrium. However, this delivery is possible if the needle is allowed to rotate freely as the tip is advanced carefully through the iliopelvic area. Occasionally it is necessary to allow the sheath/dilator set to be advanced very slightly along with the needle as the needle passes through very tight curves in the pelvis. This is performed very cautiously and while observing the tip of the dilator within the superior vena cava continually as the combination is advanced. The needle tip within the dilator advances readily along with the dilator, but the sharp, unprotected tip of the dilator within the superior cava can easily perforate vascular structures if pushed into them too vigorously.

The angle of approach (or, better, lack of angle of approach) of the tip of the needle against the interatrial septum is the second problem with transseptal needle punctures performed from the left groin. With the approach from the left inguinal area, even the curved tip of the transseptal needle when it reaches the right atrium tends to align parallel with the septum. When the needle/sheath/dilator set is advanced within the right atrium for the puncture into the septum, the tip of the needle slides along the septum instead of engaging into the tissues and puncturing the septum. This problem can be overcome by simply *bending* (not twisting!) the patient's shoulders (and thorax) as far as possible toward the patient's right prior to withdrawing the needle/sheath/dilator from the superior vena cava and down along the interatrial septum (Figure 8.4). This bending of the thorax aligns the interatrial septum on an angle more perpendicular to the angle of the tip of the needle coming from the left leg, and allows the tip of the needle to engage in the interatrial septal tissues (Figure 8.5).

The patient is maintained in the "bent" position until the transseptal puncture has been completed *and* the catheter which was advanced through the sheath has been secured within the left atrium. Straightening the patient's thorax causes the interatrial septum to move toward the patient's left and away from the tip of the needle set or tip of the sheath. Straightening the patient before the sheath/catheter is secure in the left atrium can cause the tip of the needle or the sheath to be withdrawn out of the left atrium or the atrial septum.

Conditions requiring special precautions during transseptal needle punctures

Even with the relative safety and all the advantages of the transseptal procedure, there are some conditions that do add to the risk of the procedure. These conditions do not preclude the use of the transseptal technique but definitely

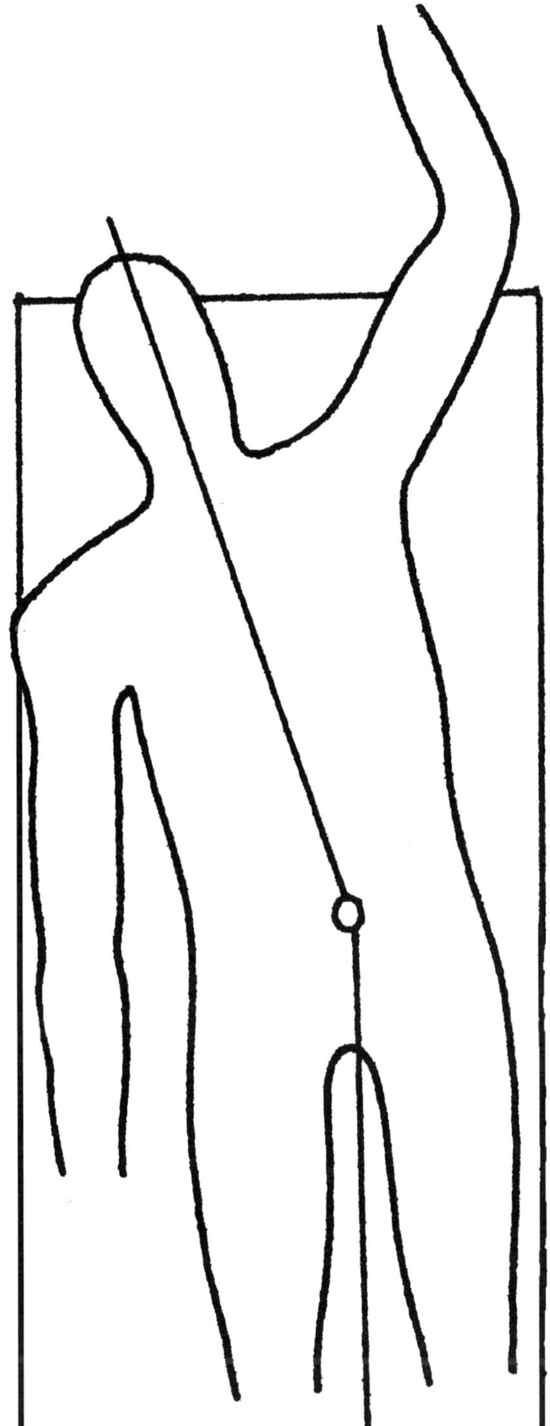

Figure 8.4 Bending the thorax to the right during a transseptal puncture, particularly when approaching from the left inguinal area.

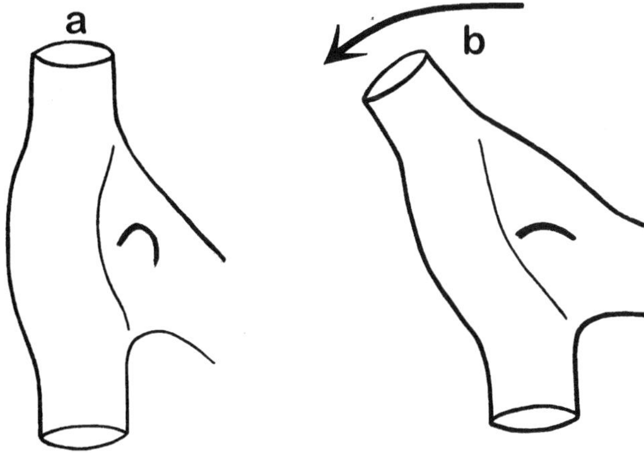

Figure 8.5 Diagrammatic representation of change in angle of interatrial septum in relation to needle by bending thorax.

require special attention when performing a transseptal atrial puncture.

Obviously, a very small left atrium creates a smaller target for the needle puncture through the septum and allows much less room for the sheath/dilator to follow the needle into the left atrium. A low left atrial pressure in association with a small left atrium creates an even greater potential problem. In addition to the more obvious, small side-to-side dimensions of a small left atrium, the anterior–posterior (front to back) diameter of the left atrium in the presence of a low atrial pressure is *very flat* (Figure 8.6a). In this case, as the needle pushes against the atrial septum for the puncture, the atrial septum in the presence of a low pressure in the left atrium is pushed posteriorly (dorsally) and actually can be pushed *flush against* the posterior wall of the left atrium (Figure 8.6b). As the needle pops through the septum, it simultaneously passes into or through the posterior wall of the left atrium (Figure 8.6c)!

When this happens no left atrial pressure is recorded through the needle as the needle pops through the septum and, obviously, the sheath/dilator or the needle *must not* be advanced any further. Instead, when no pressure is visualized in spite of the sensation of popping through something, 0.1–0.2 ml of contrast is injected through the needle. When not free in the left atrium, a small tag of contrast is created in the tissues. This tag demonstrates very clearly the errant location of the needle tip in the tissues or in the pericardium. If the abnormal location of the needle alone is not recognized and the dilator/sheath is advanced, a large hole will be created in the posterior wall of the left atrium with potentially catastrophic results.

When the tip of the needle is recognized to be out of the heart and into or through the pericardium, the position of the dilator or sheath must be determined before any further maneuvers are undertaken. If, during the transseptal puncture and along with the needle, the dilator or sheath did penetrate through the posterior wall of the atrium, it is imperative that this is identified immediately. The patient

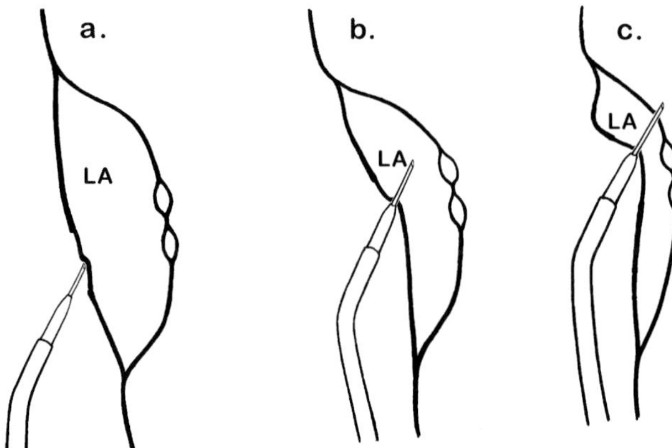

Figure 8.6 Diagram of lateral view of the left atrium. (a) Flat lateral configuration of small, low-pressure left atrium; (b) needle tip compressing atrial septum against posterior wall of left atrium; (c) needle passing into posterior pericardium without ever entering left atrium. LA, left atrium.

will usually remain stable as long as the dilator or sheath remains in position through the perforation.

When the needle alone is withdrawn all the way back into the dilator from the extracardiac position and *no* left atrial pressure reading is obtained, a repeat small test injection of contrast through the needle will extravasate into the pericardium or the mediastinal tissues outside of the pericardium rather than swirling in the left atrium. The sheath and dilator are maintained in position in the extracardiac position with slight forward pressure maintained on them. The needle, still within the dilator, will help to support and maintain the position of the sheath and dilator. The patient is typed and cross-matched urgently for 4–8 units of blood, preparations are made for a pericardiocentesis and the operating rooms/cardiovascular surgeons are alerted and prepared for an immediate, emergency thoracotomy. A transthoracic echocardiogram is performed and the pericardial space is monitored by echo while the other preparations are being carried out. If a pericardial effusion (hemopericardium) develops even with the sheath/dilator still in the perforation, a pericardiocentesis is carried out with the initiation of an auto-transfusion of blood, which is withdrawn before transferring the patient to the operating room. A large left atrial perforation from a sheath dilator has very little chance of sealing spontaneously and unless closed surgically, will probably lead to permanent sequelae (including, potentially, the demise of the patient).

When it is recognized by the tag of contrast that *only the needle* has passed through the posterior wall of the left atrium or into, or even through, the pericardium, the needle is withdrawn very slowly and carefully. If only the needle perforates into the pericardium, on slow withdrawal the tip of the needle usually drops out of the posterior wall/pericardial location and "falls" into the left atrium, and a left atrial pressure will be recorded through the needle. When the tip of the transseptal needle is withdrawn from a location outside the heart and back *into* the tip of the dilator, but no left atrial pressure appears, a repeat tiny injection of contrast through the needle is performed. This contrast injection identifies definitively where the tip of the dilator is located. When a left atrial pressure is recorded through the needle or the injected contrast material swirls in the left atrium, the patient is observed for five to ten minutes to ensure their stability. After the stability of the patient has been demonstrated with no changes in the intracardiac and arterial pressures during the period of observation, the transseptal procedure can be completed.

Often in the presence of a small or low-pressure left atrium, which the needle may or may not have transected, and in order to complete the introduction of the sheath/dilator into the left atrium, the needle must be replaced with a soft-tipped guide wire. The tip of the sheath/dilator is advanced firmly against the septum but not hard enough to kink the sheath/dilator or to push the tip of the needle through the posterior wall of the atrium again, while the needle is withdrawn from the sheath/dilator. In order to replace the needle with a wire, at least the very tip of the dilator must have penetrated the septum and this tip must be maintained in the left atrium. Once the needle has been removed, the dilator is cleared of air and a fine, exchange length, guide wire with a long floppy tip but as stiff a shaft as possible, is advanced into the left atrium through the tip of the dilator. The floppy portion of the wire must be looped around in the small left atrium in order to have the stiff portion of the wire across the atrial septum and well into the left atrium. The introduction of the sheath into the left atrium using this technique is described later in this chapter.

Surprisingly, a very large left atrium is equally problematic for an atrial transseptal puncture. With marked dilation and distention of the left atrium, the interatrial septum becomes tense and creates a large, *convex* bulge into the right atrium. This tense, marked convexity of the septum creates a sloping surface that drops off anteriorly, very steeply into a very deep groove, which occurs at the junction of the atrial septum with the ascending aorta and posteriorly (dorsally) into a sharp, equally deep groove at the junction of the atrial septum with the posterior wall of the atria. As a needle/dilator/sheath set is withdrawn from the superior vena cava into the right atrium, the tense, convex bulge of the septum tends to deflect the tip of the needle/dilator from side to side and off the center of the septum. The tense septum also obliterates the landmarks of the fossa ovalis, making it difficult to judge tactilely and/or visually when the needle is in the proper location in the fossa for the puncture. When the needle slides all the way to the anterior septal-aortic or the posterior wall-septal groove as it is being withdrawn on the septum, it is very difficult to reposition the tip of the needle easily and/or safely back onto the center of the septum from either of these locations.

If the shaft of the needle/dilator/sheath is rotated while the tip of the needle is in one of these grooves, the *angle of the tip* of the needle may *turn*, but at the same time, the tip of the needle *remains in the groove* at one edge or the other of the septum. Along with the turning of the needle, the "arrow" on the proximal end of the needle turns in the direction of the tip of the needle (as visualized on fluoroscopy) and "points" in the approximate direction of the curve at the tip; however, the needle tip can still be fixed in one of the grooves, either far anteriorly or far posteriorly at either extreme *edge* of the septum. These abnormal locations are apparent only when there is a high index of suspicion and the *location* of the needle tip is scrutinized simultaneously and very carefully *on both the PA **and lateral** fluoroscopy*. When there is any question about the position of the tip of the needle, a tiny test injection is performed through the needle. If these abnormal locations are not recognized and the puncture continued at one of these extreme edges of the atrial septum, the puncture results in a catastrophe. If the puncture is carried out with the tip of the needle in one of the lateral grooves, either the aorta, anteriorly or the pericardium, posteriorly will be entered!

Once the tip of the needle slides off a tense bulging septum in the presence of a very large left atrium, it is usually necessary to withdraw the needle from the sheath/dilator, re-pass a guide wire into the superior vena cava, reposition the sheath/dilator back in the superior vena cava and restart the transseptal procedure all over.

Any distortion of the left atrium by other structures can create a potentially dangerous situation for a transseptal puncture. A large coronary sinus, which drains a left superior vena cava, foreshortens the length of the atrial septum in the cephalad–caudal dimension within the right atrium, which shortens the distance the needle/set can be withdrawn down the septum for the puncture. The foreshortened septum decreases the height and depth of the left atrium that the needle has available to traverse in a cephalad direction within the left atrium before the posterior-cephalad wall of the left atrium is reached and even after the successful puncture of the septum.

In addition, as the needle/dilator/sheath is withdrawn down the septum from the SVC, the large orifice of a dilated coronary sinus is displaced cephalad and can easily be mistaken for the indentation of the fossa ovalis. As the sheath/dilator/needle is withdrawn down the septum in the presence of a dilated coronary sinus, the tip of the needle/dilator is deflected medially and posteriorly as it drops off the septum into the coronary sinus. This movement of the tip of the needle/dilator is very similar to the movement of the tip when it slides off the septum correctly into the fossa ovalis.

A transseptal puncture starting from within the coronary sinus and aimed in the proper direction usually does enter the left atrium and even demonstrates a good left atrial pressure. However, the needle (and the subsequent sheath/dilator) has actually passed through the roof of the coronary sinus, *into the pericardial space* (which is in the pericardial reflection posterior to the interatrial groove) and back through the inferior (outer) wall of the left atrium. When this occurs, it results in a tract with *two* openings into the pericardial space from within cardiac chambers. This course may not be apparent as long as the long sheath remains through the abnormal course and, in turn, seals the punctures in the wall(s). However, once the sheath has been withdrawn from the two openings, they will very likely result in pericardial bleeding and tamponade. A large coronary sinus does not preclude a successful transseptal puncture, but the abnormal structure must be recognized and extra precautions taken to make a more cephalad puncture on the septum in order to avoid a puncture through the roof of the coronary sinus.

A very large aortic root or an enlarged, high-pressure transposed pulmonary artery can distort and compress the roof of the left atrium and make the transseptal puncture more hazardous. A very large aortic root encroaches on the cephalad portion of the interatrial septum and the anterior-cephalad portion of the left atrium. If this encroachment is not recognized, a transseptal puncture directed even slightly more horizontally or anteriorly than usual, will enter the aorta. With a high-pressure, transposed pulmonary artery, a slightly high puncture on the atrial septum can enter the main or the right pulmonary artery. A puncture into either very high-pressure arterial system, even with just the tip of the needle, can result in uncontrollable bleeding. When structures encroaching on the septum or the left atrium are recognized, the transseptal puncture can still be carried out safely by slight redirection of the angle or position of the puncture after the encroaching structure has been identified and localized by a prior angiocardiogram. This is a circumstance where transesophageal or intracardiac echo would be beneficial in identifying the location of the tip of the needle just before the puncture.

Displacement of the left atrium and interatrial septum by even severe scoliosis does not significantly alter the position of the left atrium relative to the other intracardiac structures nor does it preclude a safe transseptal procedure. Scoliosis can change the angle of the interatrial septum and make impinging on the atrial septum with the tip of the needle more difficult. These positional abnormalities may require some readjustment of the patient's position on the table or a change in the curvature of the needle as described previously for a transseptal from the left inguinal area.

Dextrocardia with *situs solitus* really does not change the relative positions of the atria and the atrial septum significantly and does not complicate a transseptal procedure. Situs inversus with dextrocardia or levocardia symmetrically reverses the entire anatomy 180° from side to side, thus the transseptal procedure is performed in a 180° direction (from right to left). Otherwise with pure situs inversus the relationship of atrial structures and the procedure are the same except positioned in a mirror image of normal. Complex abnormalities of situs (ambiguous) do displace the right and left atria, however most patients with complex situs abnormalities have pre-existing atrial communications. In the presence of any of these malpositions of the atrial septum and left atrium, the recirculation phase from a preceding right heart/pulmonary artery angiocardiogram identifies the abnormal location and is essential before considering a transseptal puncture. With the abnormal positions identified, modification of the transseptal technique to adjust for the peculiarities allows a safe and successful puncture.

There are probably no absolute contraindications to a transseptal atrial puncture if all of the previously mentioned precautions are observed. Bilateral obstruction of the iliofemoral venous systems or an absent hepatic segment of the inferior vena cava certainly would preclude a standard femoral approach for a transseptal atrial puncture. This can be overcome by using a transjugular or transhepatic approach to the right atrium and proceeding with the puncture from the superior vena cava or transhepatic entry into the right atrium.

A wire through the dilator to replace the needle during a transseptal puncture into a very small left atrium

Needle puncture of the septum can usually be accomplished even in the presence of a very small or peculiarly shaped left atrium. However, in the presence of a small left atrium and after the needle puncture of the septum, but before the sheath/dilator are advanced, often there will be no left atrial pressure visualized through the needle. In this circumstance the needle tip usually has punctured into and/or through the *posterior wall of the left atrium* along with the atrial septum. In that situation, once the needle has punctured the atrial septum, no left atrial pressure is visible and the sheath/dilator definitely are still in the right atrium, the needle is withdrawn several millimeters until the left atrial pressure appears. This phenomenon is particularly likely to occur in a small left atrium, in the presence of a thick or tough interatrial septum or with very low left atrial pressure. The needle tip ends up against or through the posterior-superior wall of the left atrium directly after it punctures the septum (*see* Figure 8.6). Even when the tip of the needle is still in the left atrium, there is insufficient room (depth) there to advance the dilator *and* the sheath completely into the left atrium along with, or over, the needle without the danger of puncturing the posterior wall of the atrium with the needle/sheath/dilator.

The needle is fixed in a position in the left atrium and, while continually visualizing a left atrial pressure through the needle, the sheath and dilator are advanced *over* the needle until the tip of the dilator (only) is engaged in, or preferably just through, the septum. The sheath/dilator is held firmly against (or in) the septum while the needle is withdrawn carefully from the sheath/dilator set. The sheath/dilator is maintained with a firm push against the septum, but with not enough force to kink it or buckle it away from the septum. Blood and air are cleared from the dilator using very gentle suction directly on the hub of the dilator.

Once there is free flow of blood from the hub of the dilator and this blood is confirmed to be left atrial blood, a wire back-bleed valve with a side flush port is attached to the dilator hub and the system is flushed through the pressure/flush system. The side port is switched transiently to the pressure monitor to verify that the dilator tip is still in continuity with the left atrium. A pig-tail curve is formed on the floppy tip of a stiff, 0.025″ or 0.035″ exchange length, spring guide wire (the largest possible wire diameter which will pass through the opening of the tip of the transseptal dilator). This wire is advanced through the dilator into the left atrium. The curved floppy tip of the wire is looped around within the left atrium until the stiff portion of the wire has advanced completely through the area of the interatrial septum. A long, very soft, curved tip of a spring guide wire can be very safely manipulated further into a pulmonary vein, the left ventricle, or into a redundant loop within the left atrium. Usually the stiff portion of the wire beginning to loop around in the left atrium or extending into the pulmonary veins provides enough support and the extra distance within the left atrium to allow the safe introduction of the long dilator and sheath over the wire and into the left atrium.

Once the stiff portion of the wire is across the septum and secured in the left atrium, the combined sheath/dilator is advanced over the wire into the left atrium. A drilling motion of the sheath/dilator set is used to cross the septum if necessary. The tip of the sheath pops through the septum exactly as when it passes over the needle/dilator combination, while at the same time the wire looped in the left atrium prevents the sheath/dilator from popping into and perforating the posterior wall of the left atrium. The wire is watched closely on fluoroscopy during these maneuvers to ensure that the wire or sheath/dilator does not kink at the septum or just within the left atrium.

Once the tip of the sheath is well within the left atrium, the dilator is withdrawn over the wire very slowly, then the wire is withdrawn slowly from the sheath. The wire remaining in place through the sheath within the left atrium while the dilator is being withdrawn helps to keep the tip of the sheath with its end-only opening from becoming occluded against the side of the atrium or distally in a pulmonary vein. The same precautions and techniques for clearing air and clot from the sheath as are used after the standard transseptal puncture where the sheath/dilator is advanced over the needle, are used to clear the sheath after the modified delivery of the sheath/dilator.

Access through prosthetic patches and baffles using the transseptal needle technique

Transseptal puncture through intracardiac patches and baffles is not only possible, but represents a reasonable approach for entering difficult areas in complex postoperative patients[8]. These transseptal punctures through patches and baffles have been accomplished through pericardial, dacron, teflon, and Gore-Tex™ materials. A transseptal puncture through patches or baffles does require a thorough knowledge of the unique anatomy of the particular patient as well as familiarity and skill with the basic transseptal procedure. In general, regardless of the material from which the patch or baffle is made, it becomes very tough and rigid and is very resistant to puncture. To avoid puncturing through the very tough material itself, occasionally the puncture is performed just to one side of the patch or baffle. Often, however, the puncture must be directly through the prosthetic material.

Although a standard transseptal puncture *can* be performed reasonably safely using a single plane X-ray system, because of the complexity of the anatomy, the different nature of the tissues being punctured and the relative infrequency of the procedure, a puncture through prosthetic material should never be attempted without a biplane fluoroscopy/X-ray system. The capability of *simultaneous* biplane fluoroscopy is useful, but not absolutely essential as long as the operator can switch *instantaneously* between the two separate planes of the biplane system.

Because of the toughness of the patches/baffles and regardless of the size of the patient, larger gauge, stiffer adult transseptal needles are used for these punctures. In order to exert more straight and forward pressure at the tip of the needle, the curve at the distal end of the needle is straightened as much as the particular anatomy will allow. However, there must be enough residual curvature on the distal end of the needle to permit the tip of the needle to engage on the septum (patch/baffle) as the puncture is started *and* to allow some directional control of the tip of the needle and the sheath/dilator set. Usually a 10–15° curve remains on the "straightened" needle. When the trans-baffle puncture is performed in a postoperative venous switch patient, the 180° transseptal curve at the tip of the long sheath/dilator set is straightened to a very slight, 20–30° curve off the long axis of the sheath/dilator. The tip of the dilator must have a very fine taper and fit very tightly over the narrower tip portion of the needle for a puncture through a patch or baffle. The original USCI-Bard™ transseptal dilators (Medtronic Inc., Minneapolis, MN) have the optimal tight fit and smooth taper over the needle. Patience, persistence and very great care in choosing the exact positioning and course of the needle are essentials for crossing patches and baffles.

Information that can only be obtained by the catheterization of the pulmonary venous atrium or even the pulmonary veins themselves, is often essential for treatment decisions in patients who have undergone atrial switch ("Mustard" or "Senning") type of repairs to transposition of the great arteries. In the past, lesions in these patients were studied by complex retrograde left heart cardiac catheterization, however, the retrograde arterial approach to the pulmonary venous atria has significant inherent problems. Once the pulmonary venous chambers have been entered from a retrograde approach, there are two 180° curves and a very long distance between the peripheral site of the catheter introduction and the target area. The retrograde approach requires considerable time and very extensive manipulations in the artery and, even then, entering all, or even any, of the desired pulmonary venous locations is often unsuccessful. Even when the desired areas have been entered, transcatheter therapeutic procedures are difficult, if not impossible, to perform from a retrograde approach to the pulmonary venous chambers and pulmonary veins.

A transseptal puncture through the baffle in a postoperative venous switch patient is a safe and far more direct and reliable approach to the pulmonary venous atria and the pulmonary veins than any retrograde approach. All of the precautions of any transseptal procedure are necessary when perforating an intracardiac baffle. When a "Mustard" or "Senning" baffle is approached from the femoral veins, an end-hole catheter is advanced through the inferior limb of the baffle into the "new right atrium" (above the mitral valve in the area of the left atrial appendage). The catheter is replaced with an exchange length guide wire with a long floppy tip. The floppy portion of the wire is looped or coiled in the new right atrium. The specifically prepared transseptal sheath/dilator set is advanced over the wire as far as possible as long as the set maintains a relatively straight course through the IVC and baffle and into the new right atrium. With the long sheath/dilator in this position, the wire is removed, the dilator cleared of air and clot, and the transseptal needle is introduced into the set and advanced to just within the tip of the dilator. The "resting" position of the needle/sheath/dilator set after the needle has been introduced is usually toward the patient's left scapula.

For punctures through the inferior limb of the venous switch baffle, the tip of the needle is directed *anteriorly* and to the patient's right, i.e. in the opposite direction from the standard transseptal puncture. The operator's hands should be positioned on the proximal end of the combination needle/sheath/dilator almost exactly the opposite from the position for a standard transseptal procedure through the normal atrial septum. The grip on the needle must be comfortable when the needle is pointed in the proper direction *for the puncture* without having to reposition the hands or relax the grip on the needle/sheath/dilator during the procedure. This puncture direction is exactly the opposite from the standard atrial transseptal puncture. With the tip of the needle/sheath/dilator starting in the "new right atrium" some distance above the mitral valve and with the hands properly positioned on the needle/sheath/dilator, the tip of the needle/sheath/dilator is observed on fluoroscopy in both PA and lateral views while the combination is withdrawn toward the IVC. If simultaneous biplane fluoroscopy is not available, the PA and lateral views are examined intermittently very frequently. As the combination needle/dilator/sheath is being withdrawn toward the inferior limb of the baffle, it is rotated until the proximal arrow on the needle and the tip of the needle point *anteriorly* and slightly to the patient's *right*. With the needle/sheath/dilator pointing in the direction for the puncture, the combination is withdrawn within the inferior limb of the baffle to approximately the lower third of the channel in the inferior limb. When the set is in the proper position for the puncture, the tip of the needle is pointed at a large area that is anterior and rightward to the lateral (rightward) wall of the inferior atrial baffle. This area represents the distal pulmonary venous chamber in the "neo left" atrium.

With the needle attached to the pressure channel and while continuously observing the tip of the needle on both planes of fluoroscopy, the needle is advanced out of the tip of the dilator and into the baffle. The baffle is usually convex on its systemic venous side, and when it has been in place for many years its surface is often rigid and actually feels hard against the needle. This combination can make it difficult to engage the needle tip into the hard tissues. It often takes several "re-bends" of the distal curve of the needle as well as readjustments in the position and direction of the needle tip before it engages securely. If, during the readjustments, the combination needle/sheath/dilator becomes displaced too far caudally off the desired puncture site, the needle is withdrawn, the sheath/dilator is repositioned over the wire back into the new right atrium and the withdrawal of the needle/dilator/sheath along the baffle started all over again. Occasionally, the tip of the needle will only engage at one edge of the convex surface of the baffle, in which case once the tip of the needle is engaged the entire needle must be rotated to direct the tip toward the open area of the "neo left atrium".

Once the needle is engaged in the baffle, more force or push than is usually used with a standard transseptal puncture is necessary to accomplish this puncture as the needle/sheath/dilator is advanced through the baffle. In spite of the increased forward force, there is little displacement of the rigid baffle as the needle is advanced. When the needle appears to advance forward, but no left atrial pressure is seen, the needle is disconnected from the pressure line and 0.1–0.2 ml of contrast is injected forcefully through the needle. Similarly to the standard transseptal procedure, when the needle tip has not popped free into the pulmonary venous atrium, the contrast creates an opaque tag in the tissues and clearly demonstrates the location of the tip of the needle in the tissues. The tissues are often so dense that the tagging requires considerable force applied with a hard syringe, and in fact, a tag may not be possible. The direction of the needle is readjusted or the needle is withdrawn and the puncture started all over according to the position of the tissue tag.

When the tag demonstrates that the needle is pointing correctly toward the large free area of the distal pulmonary venous chamber, the needle is re-advanced, but applying even more force than during the previous attempt(s). Because of this extra force, when the needle set does penetrate through the baffle, it advances with a fairly vigorous "lurch" and for a significant distance. Fortunately, this "new left atrial area" is quite spacious anteriorly and laterally and usually accommodates a considerable length of needle/dilator/sheath. After the needle set pops through the baffle, the location of the tip of the needle in the new left atrial chamber is verified from the pressure through the needle or with a small angiogram, injecting through the needle. The needle, along with the sheath/dilator, is rotated to point in the direction of the maximum space in the chamber. The combination needle/sheath/dilator is advanced until the tip of the sheath has definitely crossed the baffle. While fixing the needle in this position, the dilator is advanced to the tip of the needle. The needle, still positioned within the sheath/dilator, is used to rotate the combination purposefully to a specific desired direction within the chamber and then the sheath is advanced over the dilator and into the distal pulmonary venous atrium. Once the sheath is at the tip of the dilator, the tip of the combination is rotated posteriorly toward the common pulmonary venous channel, again using the needle to direct the tip of the combination.

As soon as the sheath is well into the "new LA" (the distal pulmonary venous chamber) and directed toward (or into) the common pulmonary venous channel, the needle and then the dilator are removed very slowly from the sheath as described earlier for the standard transseptal procedure. Once the needle and dilator have been removed, the sheath alone passing through the inferior baffle limb usually rotates back to the direction of the puncture or anteriorly and to the patient's right. A catheter passing through the sheath must be redirected almost 180° posteriorly and laterally within the distal pulmonary venous chamber in order to enter the common pulmonary venous channel. This is accomplished using static (fixed) deflector wires within the catheter as described in Chapter 6. The static deflector wires are pre-formed into the appropriate three-dimensional curves before being introduced into the catheter.

Occasionally, it is necessary to puncture the superior limb of the baffle in a patient with a venous switch. The superior limb of the baffle usually makes a fairly sharp turn from the vertical, superior vena cava, medially toward the patient's left and into the "new right" atrium. This curve or angle in the channel creates an almost perpendicular surface for the puncture, which makes it quite easy to engage a transseptal needle in the wall of the superior baffle for a puncture through it. The "manufacturer's" distal curve on the transseptal needle is straightened even more than it is straightened for the puncture through the inferior limb of the baffle. The actual puncture is even more straightforward than crossing the baffle from the inferior vena cava. However, after the puncture of the superior limb of the baffle and once the tip of the long sheath is any distance into the new *distal* pulmonary venous chamber, it is far more difficult to maneuver a catheter back into the common pulmonary venous channel or the pulmonary veins from the cephalad, jugular vein/superior vena cava approach. The only indications for a puncture through the superior limb of the baffle as the approach to the pulmonary venous channel are either an interruption of the inferior vena caval access to the inferior limb of the baffle or the absolute inability to puncture the inferior limb of the baffle.

The superior limb of the baffle is approached from a right jugular vein/superior vena cava approach. An end-hole catheter is advanced from the right jugular vein through the superior limb of the baffle and into the area of the mitral valve in the new right atrium. A catheter from this approach often passes directly into the left ventricle. The catheter is replaced with an exchange length, Super Stiff™ 0.035″ guide wire with a *very long* floppy tip. This tip is pre-formed into multiple loops as, in all likelihood, the wire will advance into the left ventricle where, hopefully, it will loop smoothly around in the ventricle and, in doing so, will not create too much ectopy. Once the wire is in a stable position, the catheter is withdrawn over the wire and replaced with a straightened long transseptal sheath/dilator set. Again, the tip of the dilator may pass through the very straight course and enter the left ventricle, and care must be taken not to allow the tip of the dilator to approach the apex of the ventricle. Once the sheath/dilator combination is stable over the wire, the wire is removed and the straightened transseptal needle is introduced into the sheath/dilator set, advanced to the tip of the dilator and attached to the pressure/flush system. During the introduction of the needle continual care must be taken to ensure that the tip of the dilator is not against or through the ventricular wall.

The direction of the puncture through the baffle from the superior caval approach is anteriorly and to the patient's right. Again, the proximal end of the needle is grasped so the hand(s) will be comfortable when the needle tip is pointing in the direction for the puncture. Under close biplane fluoroscopic observation, the combined needle/dilator/sheath is withdrawn into the superior limb of the baffle while rotating the tip of the needle anteriorly and laterally (toward the patient's right). With this maneuver, the tip of the needle/dilator/sheath usually moves laterally, aligning with the superior vena cava and more or less perpendicular to the more caudal wall of the superior limb of the baffle. With the needle tip pointing anteriorly and slightly toward the patient's right, the needle is advanced into the baffle. Once impinged on the baffle, the needle and the sheath/dilator set are advanced together. Puncturing through the baffle, even with a very perpendicular angle to it, still requires significant force, and when the transseptal dilator and sheath do pop through the tissues, they advance suddenly and for a significant distance into the "new distal left" atrial chamber. Whenever the location of the needle tip is unclear or a good pressure tracing through the needle is not visualized, the location of the tip is identified with a small (0.1–0.2 ml) injection of contrast through the needle. These injections can be performed intermittently during the puncture as well as after the needle and set have popped through the baffle. If the tip of the needle is buried into tissues with no pressure reading obtainable through the needle, the tags of contrast injected into the tissues again identify the exact location of the tip of the needle. The position of the needle/dilator/sheath is readjusted toward the largest open area of the new distal left atrial chamber and the puncture resumed until a good new left atrial pressure is recorded through the needle or the contrast from the test injection through the needle floats freely in the distal new left atrial chamber. Once the tip of the needle has been positioned in a completely free location, the dilator and then the sheath are advanced over/along with the needle into the chamber.

Once the sheath has advanced completely into the new distal left atrial chamber, the needle and then the dilator are removed, again observing all the precautions for clearing any air and clots from the transseptal set. A malleable catheter is advanced through the sheath and maneuvered to the desired location with the use of various active or pre-curved static deflector wires.

Occasionally a puncture through a totally obstructed or otherwise interrupted area of a venous channel is required. These situations occur most frequently in the superior limb of the "Mustard" baffle or in various areas of the venous channels following caval pulmonary or "Fontan" surgical repairs. The perforation of these obstructions with needles, wires and radio-frequency energy are covered in detail in Chapter 31.

Utilizing the transseptal needle for specific directional manipulations

The very precise control over both the side to side and anterior–posterior direction of the curved transseptal needle and the sheath/dilator set when the needle is still within the set has been alluded to in discussions of the maneuvers within the left atrium following a standard transseptal puncture. This same directional control is very useful, not only in the control of the direction of the actual puncture from the very start, but for the more purposeful and controlled redirection of sheaths/catheters once they have entered the left atrial or other chamber.

Because the curved tip of a transseptal needle has a very rigid, 1:1 torque ratio, the needle within the sheath/dilator (or rarely, any other catheter) can be used to direct the tip of the sheath/dilator purposefully in very precise directions. This capability is utilized routinely for directing the tip of the needle/sheath/dilator in a lateral direction after the needle has popped almost straight posteriorly through the atrial septum during a standard transseptal puncture. This same capability of using the needle for directing the tip of the sheath/dilator is used in the initial positioning for, and during the actual puncture through, unusually oriented tissues, as described in the previous section on punctures through atrial baffles.

Once the needle has impinged securely on the septum or baffle, the entire needle/sheath/dilator can be rotated to direct the puncture toward the largest left atrial target area or to a selected area within the left atrium. An example of this is to direct the puncture toward a right upper pulmonary vein as opposed to toward the left pulmonary veins during a standard transseptal puncture. To accomplish this, as soon as the tip of the needle has impinged *securely* in the septum or has even popped through the septum, the needle set is rotated clockwise and toward the right before advancing it to complete the puncture. This, of course, requires extremely close observation of the position of the tip of the needle on biplane fluoroscopy, the pressure curve through the needle and multiple tags of contrast to verify the position at each step during the puncture. Once the needle and sheath/dilator have traversed the septal tissues, purposeful rotation of the needle is used to direct the sheath/dilator to selected areas within the left atrial chamber as the combination is advanced off the needle.

The transseptal needle is also useful for specific directional control of the tip of a catheter in complex intracardiac anatomy with or without a transseptal puncture. For this use a much more acute curve on the distal end/tip of the needle is usually required. When a septal or baffle puncture with the needle is not required or after the puncture has been completed, and once the sheath/dilator or catheter is in the desired chamber where a selective manipulation is required, the more acute curve is formed on the needle outside of the body. When the needle is used only for the redirection of a catheter, sheath or dilator and not for an actual puncture, the tip of the needle remains within the catheter, sheath, or dilator during all the maneuvers.

An example of the use of a needle totally within a catheter to redirect the catheter very selectively is in patients who have undergone cavopulmonary repairs, after a catheter has advanced through the wall of the baffle by means of a puncture or through a pre-existing opening of the baffle into the pulmonary venous chamber(s). When a catheter tip that has crossed into the pulmonary venous chamber must be manipulated away from the atrioventricular valves, the curve of the transseptal needle with its 1:1 rotational control is used within the catheter to direct its tip purposefully away from any particular area or structure, e.g. to direct the catheter tip posteriorly, cephalad and away from the atrioventricular valve structures.

Transseptal puncture from other than the femoral approach

The standard approach for an atrial transseptal puncture is from the inferior vena cava and more specifically from a right femoral vein. The approach from the left femoral vein is not too different and has already been discussed. Occasionally, the approach from either femoral venous system is not possible at all, or entrance into the left atrium from another direction is desirable. The most common indication for an alternative approach is the interruption or occlusion of the iliofemoral veins—usually from prior catheterizations or surgical interventions. Another indication for a non-femoral approach to an atrial transseptal puncture is a congenital interruption of the hepatic portion of the inferior vena cava with azygos or hemiazygos vein continuation to the superior vena cava. Finally, an entry into the left atrium from a cephalad approach is occasionally preferable in order to enter the lower pulmonary veins selectively or to have a more direct approach to the mitral valve. When the femoral approach is not available or not desired, either the right internal jugular vein or a transhepatic venous puncture is used for the catheter and needle introduction for an atrial transseptal puncture.

Transseptal puncture from the jugular vein approach

Transseptal atrial puncture from the jugular vein approach is used when there is no access from the femoral/inferior vena caval approach or for delivering balloons or stents to the lower pulmonary veins[9]. The jugular vein approach to the left atrium also provides a very straight access to the mitral valve for mitral valve dilation. The *right* jugular vein provides the only reasonably straight course to the septum. Access from the left jugular/innominate vein directs the needle toward the lateral wall of the right atrium, which directs the tip of the needle completely away from the septal surface.

A transseptal needle puncture is not always possible even from the right jugular vein. It is desirable that the left atrium bulges into the right atrium at least slightly to allow the needle tip coming from the jugular vein approach to impinge on the cephalic end of the septum. The orientation of the *normal* atrial septum is often parallel to, or even away from, the course from the SVC to the right atrium. As a consequence, the tip of even a very curved needle cannot engage into the tissues of the atrial septum and merely slides along the septum and through the right atrium. A bulge of the septum into the right atrium produces a slight ridge at the cephalad end of the septum. When a ridge at the upper edge of the septum is present, even a fairly straight transseptal needle will engage the septum rather than merely slide along its surface.

When there is *no* bulging of the septum into the right atrium and the jugular vein approach is used, the curve on the distal end of the needle is exaggerated significantly before it is introduced into the sheath/dilator. The curve that is formed on the distal end of the needle is adjusted according to the anatomy of the septum within the right atrium of each patient. Care must be taken not to create such an acute angle on the shaft of the needle that the forward force on the proximal needle causes the needle to bend acutely (or kink) at the curve rather than to push forward to puncture the septum. When a puncture from the superior vena cava is unsuccessful with the initial attempt, the needle is withdrawn, curved slightly more and the puncture reattempted until successful.

To perform an atrial transseptal puncture from the superior vena caval approach, a catheter is introduced into the right jugular vein and advanced through the right atrium into the inferior vena cava. The catheter is replaced with an exchange length spring guide wire and the catheter and short sheath are removed through the sheath, leaving the wire in place.

The 180° transseptal curve on the Mullins™ transseptal sheath/dilator set (MTS™) is modified for the jugular vein/superior vena caval approach and according to the purpose of the transseptal procedure. To enter the left ventricle, the acute sheath/dilator curve is straightened to form a gentle 15–20° curve at the distal tip of the sheath. Once the sheath has entered the left atrium and the needle and dilator have been removed, this curve directs the tip of the sheath almost directly toward the mitral valve. To enter the pulmonary veins, a more acute curve of 90 to 180° is formed on the sheath/dilator, depending upon the particular anatomy.

The preformed MTS™ sheath/dilator set is introduced into the *right* jugular vein over the pre-positioned wire and advanced into the inferior vena cava (IVC). The needle with its preformed curve is introduced into the sheath/dilator set while the latter is still in the inferior vena cava. The needle is attached to the pressure/flush line, flushed and then placed on pressure recording. While watching the tip of the needle carefully on biplane fluoroscopy and the pressure on the monitor screen, the needle/sheath/dilator tip is withdrawn from the IVC into the caudal portion of the right atrium while *simultaneously*, the tip of the needle is rotated toward the patient's left and posteriorly. While maintaining the needle tip pointing *posteriorly* and toward the patient's *left*, the needle/dilator/sheath combination is withdrawn through the right atrium toward the superior vena cava. The needle/sheath/dilator must never be allowed to turn or deviate anteriorly. The aortic root forms the leftward/anterior/superior wall or roof of the right atrium and can easily be punctured by a needle pointing anteriorly.

As the tip of the needle/sheath/dilator approaches the top one-third or one-fourth of the septum, the sheath/dilator set is *withdrawn off* the needle leaving the needle tip bare and hopefully against the septum. The combination sheath/dilator/needle, with the bared needle, is advanced several millimeters, attempting to engage a cephalad "shoulder" of the interatrial septum by the slight advance of the combination, all the time observing the pressure through the needle. If no resistance is encountered or the combination merely slides down the septum, the needle is withdrawn into the sheath/dilator, the needle/sheath/dilator is withdrawn together back to the top of the right atrium, the direction of the needle/sheath/dilator changed slightly, and the puncture reattempted by advancing the needle out of the sheath/dilator. If the puncture fails after several repeated attempts, the needle is withdrawn completely out of the sheath/dilator and the curve on the needle changed to better suit the angle to the septum. After repeated attempts at a slow puncture with the needle bared, an attempt can be made at using a short, quick jab toward the septum with the needle/sheath/dilator with the needle bared.

When resistance to advancing the needle/sheath/dilator is encountered but no pressure is visualized through the needle, an injection of 0.1–0.2 ml of contrast is performed through the needle to verify the position of its tip. This is similar to the tags in the septum during a standard transseptal puncture. When the tag is in the septum and the needle appears to be engaged in the septum, the combination needle/sheath/dilator is advanced further while monitoring the pressure as well as observing the needle/sheath/dilator in relation to the tag on fluoroscopy. If the needle is seen and/or felt to pop through something, a left atrial pressure curve should be visualized on the monitor. If not, or if there is any question about the location of the needle tip, a repeat, small injection of contrast is performed through the needle. This either demonstrates contrast swirling within the left atrium or creates a new contrast tag on the atrial septum (or in an undesired location). In either case, the needle/dilator/sheath is repositioned and the combination re-advanced in a similar step-wise fashion until the tip of the needle is in a free and secure position within the left atrium *and* a good left atrial pressure is visualized.

With the rigid, acutely curved needle still in place within the sheath/dilator, the pressure through the needle still visualized, and with the needle tip pointing away from the atrial walls or any other intracardiac structures, the needle is used to turn and redirect the dilator and then the sheath as they are advanced into the left atrium. Once the tip of the sheath has been secured within the left atrium, the needle and then the dilator are removed slowly, one at a time. The sheath is cleared meticulously of any air and clot and attached to the flush/pressure system similar to all other atrial transseptal procedures. Which catheter is introduced depends upon what procedure is to be performed from the left atrium.

The atrial transseptal puncture from the jugular venous approach is considerably easier in the presence of a large left atrium, as occurs with left atrioventricular valve disease, systemic ventricular disfunction and large left to right shunts distal to the atria. In these circumstances with increased left atrial volume or pressure, the left atrium is dilated, which results in a bulging of the atrial septum into the right atrium. This creates the "shelf" or shoulder of the atrial septum protruding into the cephalad portion of the right atrium just at the entrance of the superior vena cava into the right atrium. This shoulder creates a more "perpendicular" target for an atrial transseptal puncture from the superior vena cava. In the presence of an enlarged left atrium and a "shoulder", the curve on the transseptal needle can usually be straightened from the original "factory curve" to facilitate the puncture from the jugular vein. This usually makes punctures from the superior vena cava even more straightforward.

Occasionally an atrial transseptal needle puncture cannot be accomplished from the jugular vein approach because the tip of the needle cannot be engaged on the septum at all. The use of radio-frequency (RF) energy to "burn" rather than forcefully push through the septum now allows access across the atrial septum from the jugular route in essentially all cases. The RF wire can be positioned against the septum around very sharp curves and does not require significant force against the septum in order to perforate it. The RF transseptal technique is described in more detail in a subsequent section in this chapter.

Transseptal puncture from the hepatic vein approach

Transcutaneous hepatic puncture into a hepatic vein is utilized for venous access primarily when neither femoral venous nor superior vena caval access is available. The transhepatic approach is occasionally used preferentially to provide a more perpendicular approach to the atrial septum, a more direct access to the left atrium after a transseptal puncture, or a more direct access to the right ventricular outflow tract/pulmonary arteries. To use the transhepatic approach for an atrial transseptal procedure, the puncture into the hepatic venous system and wire introduction into the right atrium are exactly as for any other transhepatic puncture as described in Chapter 4.

Because the approach from the hepatic puncture site is almost perpendicular to the surface of the interatrial septum with the resultant perpendicular alignment with the septum, the curves on the needle and the sheath/dilator set are straightened almost completely before being used for transseptal puncture from the transhepatic approach. A slight (10–15°) curve is left on the needle to provide some directional control to the procedure.

The transhepatic wire is passed through the right atrium and preferably well into the superior vena cava. Occasionally the wire makes too acute a turn to pass smoothly from the hepatic veins to the superior vena cava, in which case the floppy tip of a stiff wire is looped in the high right atrium. The transseptal sheath/dilator set is introduced over the wire through the transhepatic puncture site and advanced over the wire to the high right atrium or into the superior vena cava immediately adjacent to the right atrium. The transhepatic approach with the "perpendicular" puncture into the septum allows a wider choice for the exact site of the puncture of the septum. The site on the septal surface can be chosen without concern about the needle sliding along the septum and into other structures before it actually punctures the septum. The needle is introduced and advanced to the tip of the dilator. With continuous biplane fluoroscopic guidance, the tip of the combination needle/dilator/sheath is withdrawn caudally from the high right atrium/superior vena cava junction, down along the surface of the interatrial septum until the tip of the needle/dilator approaches the center of the atrial septum or actually slides, or drops, into the foramen ovale on the atrial septum.

The needle/dilator/sheath set is rotated to the appropriate direction for puncture *as it is being withdrawn* along the septum. In the presence of a very tense left atrium, there may be no visual or tactile sensation when the foramen is reached. In that circumstance, the tip of the needle/sheath/dilator is guided with biplane fluoroscopy very carefully over the convex surface of the atrial septum until it is positioned adjacent to the center of the right atrium and the center of the atrial septum. As the tip of the needle/dilator slides into the foramen or approaches the middle of the septum, the needle is advanced out of the dilator and into the septum. With the transhepatic approach and with the straightened needle aligned perpendicular to the septum, the needle engages the septum and perforates into the left atrium with minimal forward force. As with all transseptal punctures, a good left atrial pressure should be visualized as soon as the needle advances into the left atrium. Once the needle definitely is in the left atrium, the dilator and sheath are advanced along with the needle into the left atrium, guiding the needle/sheath/dilator straight laterally with the needle. Thereafter, the transseptal procedure is the same as when approached from the femoral vein.

Upon completion of the left heart study or intervention, the catheter and sheath are removed from the hepatic puncture exactly as with any other transhepatic puncture. When larger sheaths are used through the transhepatic approach for interventional or therapeutic procedures, the tract definitely should be "plugged" (coiled) as the sheath/catheter is removed.

Radio-frequency perforation of the atrial septum

The use of radio-frequency (RF) energy to perforate the atrial septum is a recent addition to the atrial transseptal procedures[10]. RF perforation of the atrial septum is particularly useful when there is no direct approach or capability for a needle to impinge upon and forcefully be pushed through the atrial septum. This adjunct for perforation of the septum is especially useful when the approach to the procedure is from the jugular vein and there is no enlargement of the left atrium or no bulge of the atrial septum into the right atrium. The use of RF energy for the perforation allows the perforating wire to be positioned against the septum using a preformed guiding catheter, which can be curved acutely as much as 90° to conform to a circuitous approach to the septum. With the use of RF energy and an RF wire, the tip of the guiding catheter does not have to be positioned as forcibly against the septum as a needle for the perforation to occur.

The RF energy is delivered to a very tiny spot of tissue through a very fine insulated wire. The RF wire is advanced to the spot to be perforated through a small, preformed guiding catheter. When the RF energy is delivered through the wire, the wire burns through the tissue at the site of contact with the tissue. Using RF energy to perforate the septum also eliminates the strong and potentially dangerous forward force necessary to push a transseptal needle through tough or thick septal tissues or baffles, although RF energy does not burn through synthetic materials.

Because of the use of a fine RF wire (Baylis Medical Co. Inc., Montreal, Canada) and a relatively small, flexible guiding catheter—as opposed to the straight, stiff, transseptal needle/dilator/sheath combination—perforations can be performed through structures that are in somewhat more circuitous locations and not in a "straight line" from the venous introductory site. Using a specially preformed guiding catheter with the RF wire, a transseptal atrial puncture through a normally orientated atrial septum can be performed readily from the superior vena caval approach.

The RF energy for *perforation* is different from the RF energy that is used for *ablations* to abolish arrhythmia tracts. The ***ablation*** procedure depends upon the generation of heat by a relatively high-power (35–50 watts), low intensity (30–50 volts) electrical current, administered over a relatively long period of time (60 seconds) and through a relatively broad electrical tip (a 6- or 7-French electrode). When the temperature generated is higher than 45°C, it coagulates the tissue. The heat is conducted primarily laterally and circumferentially away from the electrode and is intended *not to* penetrate the tissues deeply.

The energy necessary for ***perforation*** is a low-power (5 watt), high-intensity (150–180 volts) electrical current, which is administered for a very short (0.4 second) duration through a very tiny diameter (1.3-French) electrode. This energy causes breakdown of the tissues that are in contact immediately in front of the electrode, does not spread laterally in the tissues around the electrode tip and, at the same time, does not generate much heat away from the tip.

Radio-frequency generators designed for ablation can be modified to deliver the type of energy for perforation. The energy produced in these modified generators is not ideal for perforation, and the modification requires a fairly complex internal rebuilding of the generator, which cannot be done (and undone) easily or at short notice. RF generators specifically designed for perforation are now available, which have relatively simple controls (Baylis Medical Co. Inc., Montreal, Canada). These generators are available with RF perforation wires and catheters designed to function with the generator. The Baylis™ RF wire is 0.016″ in diameter and is coated with teflon insulation, which gives the wire a functional diameter of 0.024″.

Technique of radio-frequency transseptal atrial septal puncture

The use of the Baylis™ Radio Frequency Perforation System™—which is now available in the United States and is representative of such systems—is described. Before the catheterization begins, a grounding plate, which is attached by an insulated wire to the RF generator, is placed on the patient's back. A pre-shaped guiding catheter is chosen according to the course through the venous system from the introduction site to the site of puncture, and to the area on the atrial septum that is to be perforated. The guiding catheter should accommodate a 0.038″ wire. The guiding catheter can be a commercially available coronary guiding catheter, an individually pre-shaped catheter or, in the presence of a reasonably straight transseptal course to the septum, even a long transseptal sheath/dilator set. The tip of the dilator of the transseptal set, however, must be able to accommodate a 0.038″ wire. There are now specific transseptal sets to be used with RF transseptal perforations (Baylis Medical Co. Inc., Montreal, Canada).

The guiding catheter is advanced to the area of the septum to be perforated and is maneuvered until its tip is positioned at the precise location for the perforation, where it is held and fixed securely against the septum, and the Nykanen™ Radio Frequency (RF) Perforation Catheter™ (Baylis Medical Co. Inc., Montreal, Canada) is advanced through the guiding catheter. The connecting cable is attached between the generator and the electrode at the proximal end of the RF catheter. The RF catheter is advanced out of the tip of the pre-positioned guide catheter as 0.5 seconds of RF perforating energy is delivered through the wire. In most cases, the wire tip passes through the septum as though it was not even there. If not, the energy is re-delivered to the catheter while gently advancing the wire further into or through the septum. The RF energy to the tip is stopped as soon as the tip passes through the septum. Once the wire passes through the septum the tip becomes free, and much more side to side motion of the tip of the wire is seen on fluoroscopy. If there is a question as to whether the wire has perforated, the connecting cable is removed from the proximal end of the RF catheter and a Tuohy™ adapter is advanced over the proximal end of the RF wire and attached to the hub of the guiding catheter. A small angiogram is performed, injecting through the Tuohy™ side port on the guiding catheter and around the wire. This demonstrates the tract through the septum.

Once the RF perforating catheter has entered the left atrium, the RF energy is stopped immediately and the wire is advanced into the left atrium at least several more centimeters while maintaining the guiding catheter in position against the septum over the RF catheter. The connecting cable is removed from the proximal end of the RF catheter and a 0.035″ or a 0.038″ BMC Coaxial Injectable Catheter™ (Baylis Medical Co. Inc., Montreal, Canada) is advanced over the RF catheter, through the guide catheter and through the septum. Once the coaxial catheter is through the septum and is a secure distance into the left atrium, the RF catheter is withdrawn from the coaxial catheter. During all this exchanging over of the RF wire, the guide catheter is maintained firmly against the septum over the RF or the coaxial catheter. A stiff 0.021″ or 0.025″ exchange length guide wire is passed through the guide catheter and coaxial catheter and into the left atrium.

Occasionally, when there is a relatively straight route to the septum, the transseptal sheath/dilator set can be advanced into the left atrium directly over the combination of the stiff exchange guide wire and the coaxial catheter. More often, when RF septal perforation is used, there is either a very tough septum along with a small left atrium or a peculiar angle of approach to the septum. In these circumstances, the coaxial catheter is withdrawn over the wire and a low profile, 3–4 mm diameter coronary balloon dilation catheter is advanced over the wire and into the septum. The septum is dilated with this small angioplasty balloon following which the balloon is withdrawn over the wire. Following dilation of the septum, a long transseptal sheath dilator set is advanced over the wire and into the left atrium (usually with little or no force). Once the sheath is in the left atrium, transseptal left heart catheterization and any necessary left heart therapeutics are performed as described previously in this chapter.

RF energy is sufficient for the perforation of thickened and scarred pericardium and/or other ***tissues*** found in intracardiac baffles and patches. However, there is still very little experience with the attempted use of RF energy for synthetic materials, and RF energy does not penetrate materials that do not have tissue ingrowth into them. The ability to perforate very tough structures without the use of excessive forward force and the ability to achieve better angles of approach to these lesions represent a major advantage of RF perforation over needle perforation for baffles and patches. More experience will determine the efficacy of this technique for these lesions.

Catheter introduction and manipulations in the left heart through long sheaths introduced transseptally

Once a long MTS™ sheath has been introduced into the left atrium, thoroughly cleared of all air or clots and flushed, all varieties of catheter and catheter-delivered devices can be introduced into the left heart via this route. This is the major advantage of this technique. The desired catheter for the left heart studies or procedures is chosen, flushed, attached to a separate pressure/flush system, introduced into the sheath through the back-bleed valve, which is on a continuous flush, and advanced into the left heart. When any catheters are advanced through or positioned in long sheaths, both *the sheath and the catheter* are kept on a continuous slow flush with the pressurized flush solution. As a catheter is advanced within the sheath it acts as a "plunger" and potentially creates a partial vacuum behind it. Unless there is a continual flush through the flush port on the sheath, which is behind the advancing catheter, this vacuum sucks air around the back-bleed valve and into the sheath!

When a balloon catheter is introduced through a long sheath, the plunger effect of the balloon on the catheter is even more pronounced. The sidearm of the sheath is maintained on a vigorous, continual flush as the balloon is introduced very slowly through the valve and advanced through the entire length of the sheath. The rapid flushing into the sheath behind the slowly advancing balloon fills the potential space of the vacuum with fluid faster than a vacuum can form, and in this way prevents the vacuum from sucking air in through the back-bleed device. This vigorous flush is continued until the balloon actually passes beyond the distal end of the sheath into the left atrium or left ventricle.

With either a catheter or a wire remaining in the sheath, the sheath should be maintained on a continuous slow separate flush. Without a continuous flush on the sheath there is always a back-flow of blood at the tip of the sheath around the catheter or wire and into the sheath. Without a continuous flush on the sheath, the blood within the sheath is stagnant, which results in thrombi forming in the dead-space between the outside of the catheter and the inside of the sheath. When the catheter and sheath are the same French size, the thin thrombus between the catheter and the sheath "binds" the catheter within the sheath and prevents easy maneuvering of the catheter. When the catheter has a smaller outside diameter than the internal diameter of the sheath, there is an even greater potential for the formation of thrombi around the catheter and for subsequent embolization of particulate material.

In addition to the sheath and catheter both being kept on continuous flush, suction ***never*** is applied to the side arm of a back-bleed/flush device at any time when either a catheter or wire is passing through the back-bleed valve. The catheter or wire through the valve props it open, and anything positioned through the valve (wire, catheter, needle, device delivery system, etc.) also prevents a finger seal over the valve with a gloved finger while suction is applied to the sheath. Without the capability of manually covering and tightly sealing the valve, any suction on the side port allows air to be drawn preferentially around the catheter or wire and through the back-bleed valve into the contiguous blood/fluid system.

By introducing a long sheath purposefully into the left ventricle, it is possible to position any poorly maneuverable catheter of any variety into any desired, specific site within the left ventricle. This is particularly useful for catheters with no lumen such as catheter-tipped, high-fidelity, transducer catheters, multi-electrode catheters, and bioptome catheters. Positioning the sheath into a specific location in the left ventricle is facilitated by forming a predetermined, three-dimensional curve on the distal end of the transseptal sheath prior to the introduction of the transseptal set for the transseptal procedure. The transseptal procedure is accomplished using the sheath/dilator set with the pre-curved sheath. The sheath is advanced only as far as the left atrium. When the needle and dilator have been removed, a maneuverable, torque-controlled, end and side hole catheter is advanced through the sheath into the left atrium. Using a static deflecting wire with a preformed, three-dimensional curve or a controllable deflector wire, the catheter is manipulated to the desired position within the left ventricle. Both the catheter with the contained deflector wire(s) and the sheath are maintained on a continuous flush. The pre-curved sheath is then advanced over the pre-positioned catheter to the desired location in the ventricle. The sheath is advanced all the way to the tip of the catheter and actually slightly embedded into the ventricular wall at the desired location. The combination of the pre-curving and embedding maintains the tip exactly in the desired location. The catheter is withdrawn out of the sheath *very slowly* while both the sheath and the catheter are flushed continuously and vigorously. If the tip of the sheath is embedded in the myocardium, there will be absolutely no free back-bleed of blood from the sheath as the catheter is withdrawn and it will not be possible to aspirate anything from the sheath. Because of this, in order to ensure that no vacuum is created and no air is drawn into the sheath, a continuous high-flow flush must be maintained through both the end-hole catheter and the sheath as the catheter is withdrawn.

Once the sheath is pre-positioned in the proper location within the left ventricle, any non-maneuverable catheter can be advanced to the precise location in the left ventricle through the sheath. The sheath is withdrawn whatever distance necessary to expose the functional end of the catheter being used. If the non-maneuverable catheter needs to be repositioned within the ventricle, it is preferable to remove it from the sheath, replace it with the end-hole catheter and repeat the positioning of the sheath using the latter catheter along with the deflector wires. The precautions necessary to prevent the introduction of air or debris during every exchange of catheters and wires cannot be emphasized enough!

In order to pass a floating balloon catheter from the left ventricle into the aorta, the transseptal sheath is advanced well into the left ventricle as described above. After clearing the sheath of air and clot, it is placed on a vigorous flush. A balloon catheter with a tight 180° curve preformed at its distal end is introduced through the sheath. The sheath and the balloon catheter are maintained on a vigorous flush while the catheter is introduced. The sheath directs the balloon catheter directly into the left ventricle without unnecessary, redundant manipulations of the catheter within the left atrium. Once the tip of the balloon passes beyond the tip of the sheath, the balloon is inflated. The inflation is observed on fluoroscopy to ensure that the balloon is not embedded in the myocardium of the left ventricle or trapped under a chorda of the mitral apparatus, as indicated by a distorted shape of the inflated balloon or no movement of the balloon-tipped catheter within the ventricular cavity. As the inflated balloon is advanced, the preformed curve on the balloon deflects the tip 180° away from the apex and "floats" the balloon toward the left ventricular inflow or outflow tract. The sheath helps to support the shaft of the balloon catheter, and prevents it from backing up or unwinding into the left atrium as the shaft of the catheter is advanced out of the sheath. Occasionally, the balloon catheter curls around in the ventricle and does not float to the outflow tract, or even floats back into the left atrium. In that circumstance, a controllable deflector wire is used within the balloon catheter to deflect its tip and stiffen its shaft. Once the catheter tip has been deflected toward the outflow tract, the wire and sheath are held in place and the balloon catheter is advanced through the sheath, off the wire and into the outflow tract. It is sometimes helpful to withdraw the sheath slightly within the left ventricle during these maneuvers. The more proximal the tip of the sheath is positioned along the septum, the better the balloon catheter will be directed toward the left ventricular outflow tract as it exits the tip of the sheath.

The transseptal system is very useful for recording simultaneous left atrial and left ventricular pressures or simultaneous left ventricular and ascending aorta pressures, all through the transseptal catheter. This technique is particularly useful in the presence of multiple levels of left heart obstruction. A catheter at least one French size smaller than the sheath is introduced into a long transseptal sheath through a back-bleed valve with a side pressure/flush port. Very accurate pressures can be recorded simultaneously through the lumen of the catheter and from the tip of the sheath, which is connected to the pressure system through the side-port of the sheath. With the tip of the sheath in the left atrium and the tip of the catheter advanced into the left ventricle, accurate and simultaneous left atrial and left ventricular end-diastolic pressures are recorded on identical "gain". With the tip of the sheath in the left ventricle and the catheter manipulated or floated to the outflow tract or into the great artery that rises off the left ventricle, accurate and simultaneous left ventricle (through the sheath) and outflow tract or great artery (through the catheter) pressures are obtained. During all of these left heart manipulations the sheath is maintained on a continual flush except during the brief times when the pressures are actually being recorded through the sheath.

On rare occasions, even with the preformed transseptal curve on the long sheath, the tip of the sheath in the left atrium tends to point posteriorly (dorsally) or toward the patient's head (cephalad). The sheath pointing in these directions interferes with maneuvering catheters that are introduced into the left atrium through the sheath, further into the left ventricle. To facilitate maneuvering the catheter, the sheath with the catheter within it is withdrawn until the tip of the sheath is as close to the interatrial septum as possible. When a catheter is used that is the same French size as the sheath, the sheath can actually be withdrawn back into the right atrium in order to improve the maneuverability of the catheter within the left atrium. With the sheath tip back in the right atrium, this also removes the catheter/sheath "tip–interface" from the systemic circulation and decreases the likelihood of embolization of thrombi from that area.

On the other hand, when the catheter that is introduced through the long sheath is even one French size smaller than the sheath, the sheath should *not* be withdrawn back into the right atrium. The discrepancy between the wider lumen of the sheath and the narrower shaft of the catheter usually prevents later reintroduction of the sheath back across the septum into the left atrium over the smaller catheter.

Complications of transseptal atrial puncture

The greatest potential danger to the patient from the transseptal procedure is not the risk of the puncture as such but rather the risk of air or clot embolization into the systemic circulation after the successful transseptal procedure. The potential for some type of embolization is present many times during each transseptal procedure, but the occurrence may not be apparent until hours after the procedure. There is no real or definitive treatment after an embolic event, even when such an event is recognized. The outcome from an embolization is not predictable, but often leaves permanent sequelae. However, most, if not all, embolic complications are *avoidable*.

Meticulous attention to the details of the technique for removing air and clot from the various components of the system during each step of the procedure, liberal continuous flushing of the system and the liberal use of systemic heparinization should prevent these complications. These techniques and procedures have been described in detail earlier throughout this chapter.

The most feared serious complication of the transseptal procedure is the perforation of the external wall of the heart or the aorta during the puncture. A puncture of the external wall of the left atrium with the transseptal needle alone, when recognized and unless followed by the dilator and/or sheath, *usually* does ***not*** result in significant bleeding and/or any subsequent problems. When a puncture of the left atrial *wall* occurs and is documented to be only by the needle, the needle is withdrawn and the patient's pericardial space examined by echocardiogram for the development of pericardial effusion or tamponade. If an effusion does occur, it is removed with an emergent pericardial tap in the catheterization laboratory using fluoroscopic and echo guidance. If the puncture is due to the needle alone, it is usually self-limiting, seals itself and requires no treatment.

The left atrial wall, appendage or a pulmonary vein can be punctured by guide wires that are used in association with an atrial transseptal procedure. These punctures actually occur after the procedure itself has been completed successfully and uneventfully. Even the "soft tip" of a guide wire is, in actuality, very stiff for the first few millimeters as it is extruded out of the tip of a constrained catheter or dilator. If the tip of the catheter or dilator that has advanced through, and is supported (constrained) by, the long sheath in the left atrium becomes wedged into or forced against a wall or in the appendage, the wire can easily perforate the wall as it is pushed out of the tip of the catheter. To prevent this type of perforation, the tips of the catheter and wire are observed continually for free movement of them both during any manipulations, and when there is doubt about the position of the tip of the catheter/dilator, a small injection of contrast is performed through it.

If *a dilator and/or sheath* is/are advanced into the pericardium over a transseptal needle that has punctured the wall of a cardiac chamber, major bleeding and acute tamponade *usually* follow upon withdrawal of the sheath. Although the hemodynamic consequences of a puncture with the transseptal *dilator* or *sheath* are usually more significant than a puncture with a needle alone, the treatment is well established and, if timely, the event usually results in no permanent sequelae. The management of this type of perforation was discussed previously in the section on transseptal punctures of small left atria. The sheath or dilator remaining in the perforation and "plugging" the hole in the wall of the heart usually prevents rapid or massive acute bleeding while preparations are made to manage the inevitable, larger pericardial bleed. When there is any fluid in the pericardial space, and even with the patient still hemodynamically stable, an elective pericardial tap with the insertion of a large pericardial drainage catheter is performed. Even when the effusion is aspirated and blood replaced, the patient usually needs surgical repair of the hole created by a sheath or dilator, and preparations for this should be made as soon as such a puncture of the vascular structure is recognized.

Once all the preparations for surgical intervention have been completed, a large drainage catheter secured in the pericardium, the surgical team and operating room alerted and prepared for the patient, then the sheath or dilator is withdrawn from the pericardial space back into the heart while continually observing the patient's hemodynamics, the drainage from the inserted pericardial catheter and the pericardial space by echocardiogram. Even if there was no fluid accumulation before the sheath or dilator was withdrawn from the pericardium, and if no pericardial catheter is in place, the patient will probably need a rapid pericardiocentesis and drainage for evacuation of the accumulating effusion even if the chest is to be opened. The pressure from the rapidly accumulating effusion will require rapid relief before the chest can be opened. Because of this, it is always prudent to place a drainage catheter in the pericardium before withdrawal of the sheath/dilator.

Again, attention to the details of the procedure and the utilization of small injections of contrast through the needle when there is a question as to the location of the tip of the needle and *before* the dilator or sheath is advanced should make this an avoidable complication. A possible exception is the patient with a very small, low-pressure left atrium where the atrium is compressed from front to back during the needle puncture, and as a consequence there is a greater risk for the transseptal puncture to perforate the posterior atrial wall (*see* Figure 8.6). Transseptal punctures using radio-frequency energy may obviate this complication in this group of patients.

It is possible to puncture the wall of the left atrium, the left atrial appendage or a pulmonary vein with a wire or sharp dilator manipulated in the left atrium *after* a transseptal puncture has been successfully completed. This is more likely to occur when very stiff wires (which are used to support sizing balloons or for the delivery of devices or angioplasty balloons), are advanced through the transseptal dilator or a catheter is passed through a transseptal sheath. Once the transseptal sheath and/or dilator has/have passed through the tight puncture opening in the atrial septum, the mobility and/or lateral motion of anything passing through the septum is/are lost. As a consequence, when a dilator or stiff wire that is passing through a sheath is advanced within the left atrium, it cannot deflect or "bow" from side to side, and minimal forward push can easily advance a relatively sharp and stiff structure through the wall of the atrium. This potential must always be considered when exchanging dilators, wires and catheters within the left atrium following a transseptal puncture.

Puncture, even with the needle alone, into an adjacent, high-pressure structure such as the aorta or a puncture through the wall of a very high-pressure left atrium results in acute bleeding and can be catastrophic. A puncture into such adjacent high-pressure structures is avoided by understanding the underlying defect, by identifying the location of the abnormal structure definitively on biplane imaging before the transseptal procedure is performed, and by always using biplane imaging when performing a transseptal procedure with complicated anatomy. Whenever there is any question about the location of such structures and unless there is a contraindication to the use of contrast medium, a biplane right heart/pulmonary artery angiogram with a good recirculation phase through the left heart is performed before beginning the transseptal puncture. The recirculation phase of the biplane angiocardiogram demonstrates the anatomy and relationships of "at risk" structures adjacent to the septum or left atrium and allows the use of a "road map" of the structures and adjustments to be made in the transseptal technique in order to avoid them.

If the wall of a high-pressure left atrium or an adjacent high-pressure vessel or chamber is punctured with the *needle only* and when this is recognized, as is the case when a dilator or sheath is advanced through a hole, the needle is left in place while preparations are made to care for an acute pericardial or extracardiac bleed. When punctures do occur into high-pressure vessels or chambers, they usually occur in patients who have the worst underlying heart problems and most complex anatomy and, as a consequence, are more precarious hemodynamically. These patients are not likely to stabilize by leaving the needle or dilator/sheath in the hole. Immediate, aggressive management is necessary. Even with the patient remaining stable, the surgical team and the operating room are informed, preparations are made for an immediate pericardial tap, large intravenous lines are secured and replacement blood or Ringer's lactate (until blood is available) is administered empirically. The patient is stabilized with replacement fluid and blood. A pericardial tap is performed using both fluoroscopic and echo guidance and a large drainage catheter is secured in the pericardial space. Available, typed and cross-matched, banked blood is retrieved from the blood bank while more blood is cross-matched. If blood had not been cross-matched previously, the patient is cross-matched for blood urgently. When there is a rapid accumulation of blood in the pericardial space and before replacement blood is available, the blood can be withdrawn from the pericardium into large syringes and auto-transfused (through a blood filter) back into the patient.

A perforation of the aorta from the right or left atrium creates an acute intracardiac shunt. The magnitude of the shunt depends somewhat on the size of the puncture but, because of the high pressure in the aorta, the shunt is often significant. With a perforation into the aorta, it is usually easier to stabilize the patient in the catheterization laboratory than it is to stabilize patients who have had an extravascular perforation. Unless the puncture site is identified accurately while the needle is still through it and the hole can be closed with a catheter-delivered device, these patients will almost certainly require open-heart surgery to close the puncture site.

The best treatment of the complications of the transseptal procedure is to *prevent them*. Meticulous attention to the details of the proven techniques of the procedure, avoiding known hazards and avoiding the temptation of "short cuts", all contribute to preventing the major complications of the transseptal procedure.

References

1. Duff DF and Mullins CE. Transseptal left catheterization in infants and children. *Cath Cardiovasc Diagn* 1978; **4**: 213.
2. Mullins CE. Transseptal left heart catheterization: experience with a new technique in 520 pediatric and adult patients. *Pediatr Cardiol* 1983; **4**: 239–246.
3. Brooksby IAB *et al.* Long sheath technique for introduction of catheter tip manometer or endomyocardial bioptome into left or right heart. *Br Heart J* 1974; **36**: 908–912.
4. Brockenbrough EC, Braunwald E and Ross J Jr. Transseptal left heart catheterization. A review of 450 studies and description of an improved technique. *Circulation* 1962; **25**: 15–21.
5. Ross J Jr, Braunwald E and Morrow AG. Transseptal left heart catheterization: a new diagnostic method. *Prog Cardiovasc Dis* 1960; **2**: 315–318.
6. Doorey AJ and Goldenberg EM. Transseptal catheterization in adults: enhanced efficacy and safety by low-volume operators using a "non-standard" technique. *Cathet Cardiovasc Diagn* 1991; **22**(4): 239–243.
7. Cafri C *et al.* Transseptal puncture guided by intracardiac echocardiography during percutaneous transvenous mitral commissurotomy in patients with distorted anatomy of the fossa ovalis. *Catheter Cardiovasc Interv* 2000; **50**(4): 463–467.
8. El-Said HG *et al.* 18-year experience with transseptal procedures through baffles, conduits, and other intra-atrial patches. *Catheter Cardiovasc Interv* 2000; **50**(4): 434–439; discussion 440.
9. Joseph G *et al.* Transjugular approach to balloon mitral valvuloplasty helps overcome impediments caused by anatomical alterations. *Catheter Cardiovasc Interv* 2002; **57**(3): 353–362.
10. Justino H, Benson LN and Nykanen DG. Transcatheter creation of an atrial septal defect using radiofrequency perforation. *Catheter Cardiovasc Interv* 2001; **54**(1): 83–87.

9 Retrograde arterial cardiac catheterization

Introduction

A retrograde cardiac catheterization is the catheterization of the heart and/or great vessels with a catheter introduced into a peripheral artery and passed "retrograde" through the systemic arterial system and aorta to the heart—usually the left heart. Although the femoral artery is the entry site that is used most commonly, essentially any "peripheral" artery, including the femoral, umbilical, brachial, radial and even the carotid arteries, are used for the introduction of retrograde arterial catheters. The retrograde approach is the most common, and often, the only approach used in the cardiac catheterization of adult patients where abnormalities of the coronary arteries and of left ventricular function are the main interest.

Indications for retrograde arterial catheterization

When there is necessary information and/or procedures in the left heart and/or systemic great artery that cannot be obtained or carried out from a prograde approach, then a retrograde arterial catheterization procedure is performed. In the pediatric and congenital heart patient, as much of the left heart information as possible is obtained with the venous ("right heart") catheter advanced into the left heart through pre-existing intravascular communications or through an atrial transseptal puncture. The information that can be obtained from the prograde approach to the left heart includes all of the hemodynamics and angiograms from the left heart chambers, pulmonary veins and aorta. The *prograde* approach often provides a more direct access to the left-sided chambers and areas, and, in particular, to the left atrium and pulmonary veins. With direct, safe access to the left heart with a "venous" catheter, much larger diameter angiographic catheters can be introduced safely into the left heart in order to perform high-quality angiography without any concerns about the compromise of an artery.

By utilizing the prograde approach to obtain most of the left heart information—including angiograms—minimal, if any, time is spent in the artery with larger catheters and sheaths. When a retrograde arterial catheter is introduced near the very end of the total catheterization procedure, the retrograde catheterization can be completed with a smaller French sized sheath/catheter than when all of the left heart hemodynamics and angiograms are obtained with a retrograde catheter. When retrograde manipulations are required, the previously placed, indwelling arterial monitoring line is easily, quickly and safely exchanged over a wire for the necessary arterial sheath. When the prograde approach is used for the majority of the left heart study and subsequently, when the retrograde catheter is introduced, the arterial catheter requires much less potentially traumatic manipulation and, very likely, no exchanges of the arterial sheaths in order to complete the retrograde left heart procedures. Since most of the left heart information is obtained from the previous prograde left heart procedure, once the retrograde catheter is placed in the artery, it remains there for only a relatively short period of time.

The retrograde approach provides direct access to the systemic arterial system and usually to the systemic ventricle, which gives rise to the aorta. However, in order to obtain information from the left atrium or pulmonary veins with only the retrograde catheter, significant, extra, complex, long and potentially dangerous manipulations are required within the systemic ventricle. The retrograde approach is *essential* in the evaluation of some congenital heart lesions and occasionally is the *only* approach available to study the intracardiac anatomy and physiology from either side of the heart. Most chambers and central vessels on both sides of the heart in very complex congenital heart lesions can be entered from a retrograde arterial approach, although using only the retrograde approach, it is often difficult to obtain access to the right atrium, the "non-systemic" ventricle or a pulmonary artery which arises from the systemic venous ventricle.

In the catheterization laboratories at Texas Children's Hospital, the primary indication for a retrograde left heart catheterization is the inability to obtain the necessary "left sided" or arterial information from the prograde approach. The routine prograde procedure includes primary access to the left heart through a transseptal atrial puncture when the atrial septum is intact[1]. In the majority of cardiac catheterization studies in pediatric and congenital heart patients, it is rare that all of the left heart information cannot be obtained with the prograde right heart catheter after passing prograde through existing intracardiac defects or entering the left heart transseptally. In patients where the atrial septum has been closed surgically with a patch or an intra-atrial baffle, transseptal puncture is still possible, but slightly more difficult, and occasionally necessitates a retrograde study to obtain the left heart data. Similarly, the presence of bilateral iliofemoral vein obstruction, inferior vena cava obstruction or interruption or congenital interruption of the hepatic portion of the inferior vena cava in association with azygos continuation of the inferior vena cava makes transseptal access to the left heart from a femoral vein approach impossible, and an atrial transseptal procedure is more complicated when performed with the catheter introduced from the jugular vein.

Most patients with azygos continuation of the inferior vena cava to the superior vena cava usually have one or more associated intracardiac communications that allow access to the left heart from the inferior cava/azygos approach. However, in these same patients, because of the very complex or circuitous venous anatomy, it often makes the retrograde approach more expedient and preferable for access to the right heart as well as the left heart.

The retrograde approach is not only desirable but essential in many circumstances. The retrograde approach to the left and the right heart is necessary when there is no reasonable systemic venous route that enters any part of the heart from a peripheral venous access. Total absence of systemic venous access prohibiting any entry into the cardiac chambers from the systemic venous route is usually acquired, and occurs mainly in patients who have lost both the femoral and the jugular venous access from multiple, previous, indwelling and chronic venous lines. The alternative approaches for catheter introduction then are a transhepatic puncture, a direct transthoracic puncture or a retrograde arterial approach through existing intracardiac communications or defects.

There are some areas of the left heart circulation which, although they can be approached (or a particular procedure can be performed) with a prograde catheter from the venous approach, are preferentially approached using retrograde catheterization. The retrograde approach usually gives more direct access to the aorta itself, branches off the aorta and to the systemic ventricle, and is often more expedient and less time consuming than obtaining the same information from the prograde right heart catheter. These procedures include selective catheterization of the coronary arteries with selective coronary angiography, aortic root angiography (particularly when aortic valve regurgitation is being assessed) and the selective cannulation of systemic great arteries, systemic to pulmonary shunts, and collaterals or branch vessels off the descending aorta.

There are many pediatric and congenital cardiologists who preferentially use the retrograde arterial approach to the left heart, even when prograde access with the venous catheter is very readily available.

Retrograde approach to the "right heart"

"Right heart" catheterization is occasionally accomplished entirely from the retrograde arterial approach along with the "left heart" study. This is only possible in the presence of intracardiac or great artery communications. The retrograde approach may be necessary or preferred for entering the pulmonary artery via an interventricular septal defect in patients with all types of transposition of the great arteries with an associated ventricular septal defect[2]. In complex lesions, including atresia of the pulmonary artery or pulmonary valve, and in the presence of discontinuous pulmonary arteries, the only access to one or both of the pulmonary arteries is often by a retrograde approach through a ductus arteriosus, through a surgically created shunt or through another naturally occurring systemic to pulmonary communication. Even in the presence of normally connected great arteries when either no venous access is possible or the prograde approach to enter the pulmonary artery is unusually complicated or even impossible because of the associated intracardiac anatomy, the retrograde approach is used to enter the pulmonary artery. Access in those cases is through a patent ductus, a ventricular septal defect or a systemic to pulmonary artery shunt.

Left heart therapeutic procedures

When therapeutic catheterization procedures are to be performed on the aorta, aortic branches or the aortic valve, the retrograde approach is preferred or required. For balloon dilation of the aortic valve and coarctation of the aorta, the standard approach with the dilation balloon catheter is retrograde from the femoral artery. In attempts to avoid peripheral arterial damage, both the aortic valve and coarctation of the aorta have been dilated using a prograde approach to introduce the balloon dilation catheter, but with far greater complexity to the procedure and frequently resulting in more serious complications. With the current balloon dilation equipment and refinements in retrograde techniques, the prograde approach for balloon dilation of the aortic valve or coarctation of the aorta is used only under very extenuating circumstances, which are discussed in detail in Chapters 18 and 19.

One exception where the prograde approach to the aorta does simplify a left heart therapeutic catheterization procedure is in patients with coarctation of the aorta *and* an associated ventricular septal defect or transposition of the great arteries. With this combination of intracardiac and vascular lesions, the prograde approach with the dilation balloon introduced through the ventricular defect or directly from the right ventricle to the aorta to the coarctation, is the safest and most direct approach for treating this lesion.

Even when a retrograde approach is planned for a therapeutic procedure in the left heart or aorta, the preference at Texas Children's Hospital is to utilize the prograde approach using a venous catheter for the left heart catheterization to obtain all of *the diagnostic information (hemodynamics and angiograms)*. During a therapeutic procedure in the left heart, the prograde venous catheter is left in place and used for monitoring the changes in the hemodynamics instantaneously and for performing follow-up angiography. By utilizing a primary prograde approach to the left heart, most of the left heart information can be acquired, and more direct and often better, left heart angiograms can be obtained. Pressures can be monitored continuously, angiograms can be obtained repeatedly during subsequent interventions *without* the exchange of catheters or wires and, as a consequence, arterial trauma and complications are minimized. When the left heart is not entered directly through naturally occurring intracardiac communications, it is approached safely, reliably and expediently using an atrial transseptal puncture as described in Chapter 8. Using the long sheath transseptal technique, all varieties and sizes of catheters can be introduced reliably, consistently and safely into all areas of the left heart, including the aorta, with no compromise of the arterial system.

Guidelines for retrograde arterial catheterization

A direct, safe and expedient approach for entering the aorta, left ventricle, left atrium and pulmonary veins is obviously essential. Ideally, this approach does not produce any adverse effects for the patient. The retrograde arterial approach provides this direct and *relatively* safe approach to the aorta and, usually, to the left ventricle. However, a retrograde catheterization can be associated with significant potential problems because of the necessity for the introduction of a catheter into an artery and the often extensive manipulations of catheters and wires in the systemic arterial system. Often, the more essential it is to enter the left ventricle or the left atrium to obtain particular information or to perform a therapeutic procedure (stenotic aortic or mitral valves), the more difficult and prolonged is the retrograde catheterization of that area.

There are multiple factors that can contribute to arterial damage. Improper or traumatic vessel entry, the duration which catheters, with or without sheaths, remain in the artery, the use of indwelling sheaths versus direct manipulation of the catheter at the arterial introductory site, the size (diameter) of the catheter/sheath and the type of catheter and sheath (materials) used in the artery, all have effects on and are related to potential damage to the artery.

Local arterial trauma and damage at the introductory site are related and proportionate to many factors, all of which can be modified (minimized) by minimizing the time in the artery and by very gentle care and handling of the artery at the puncture site. The special care and handling of the artery begin with the infiltration of local anesthesia, continue during the introduction of the needle and wire, as well as, before and during the introduction of the sheath/catheter into the artery, during catheter manipulations through the arterial sheath, during sheath and/or catheter exchanges and during and after the removal of the sheath from the artery. The special care and handling of the artery during *every aspect* of the retrograde catheterization procedure are equally important in preventing arterial damage.

The use of systemic heparin during retrograde arterial catheterization probably does not affect the adverse results to the arterial introductory site itself, but does decrease the potential for other systemic thromboembolic events originating from the retrograde catheters and wires. The relative importance of each of these separate variables in relation to their detrimental effects on the artery has not been determined, but probably the adverse effects are cumulative. Fortunately, *all* of these variables are controllable to some degree *by the operator*. By careful attention to *all* of the variables, arterial complications can be minimized and may actually be preventable!

Arterial monitoring

Although a retrograde ***catheter*** often may not be introduced *at all* during a *complete right and left heart catheterization* of a pediatric/congenital heart patient, *all* patients undergoing cardiac catheterization have continual arterial monitoring with an indwelling arterial cannula, which is maintained in place for the duration of the entire prograde catheterization. The indwelling arterial monitoring line does not have to be (and seldom is) a catheter, but instead of a large-diameter catheter, a small, 21-, 20- or 18-gauge, teflon cannula is introduced percutaneously and secured in the artery at the beginning of the procedure.

In much larger patients, a 4- or 5-French dilator only (without the sheath) is substituted for the small teflon cannula as the arterial monitoring line. The arterial line provides *continual* intra-arterial pressure monitoring as well as access for repeated arterial blood sampling. Normally the arterial monitoring cannula is placed in a femoral artery, however, any systemic artery, including the radial or brachial, is adequate for the monitoring line since the cannulae are very small.

The arterial monitoring cannula is introduced into the artery over a small spring guide wire after the needle has been introduced into the artery using a standard, percutaneous, "single wall" vessel puncture technique as described in Chapter 4. The single wall needle puncture and the introduction over a wire prevent unnecessary disruption of the vessel wall in the area of the introduction of the cannula, as often occurs if the cannula is advanced off a needle directly. Once a clean, crisp return of blood is obtained through the needle during its introduction, a very soft tipped, spring guide wire is introduced precisely and gently through the needle and threaded into the artery. The needle is removed and the arterial monitoring cannula is introduced directly over the guide wire. For the introduction of a small, 21- or 20-gauge, indwelling, arterial monitoring canula, it is ***not*** necessary to dilate a "tract" over the wire by any extra, specific dilation through the subcutaneous tissues. The smaller monitoring cannulae are only minimally larger than the external diameters of the needle used for the puncture, and the tips of the cannulae have a very fine and tight taper over the wire. Any extra dilation of the puncture site can easily open it excessively into the artery, which, at the very least, results in prolonged bleeding or hematoma formation in the tissues around the indwelling cannula.

Small, arterial monitoring cannulae and small dilators produce essentially zero trauma to the artery, even when in place for hours (days!). "Sewing eyes" are incorporated on the hubs of many arterial cannulae. When sutures are placed into the skin very close to the puncture site, these sewing eyes provide a secure fixation of the shaft of the cannula in the artery. Once the cannula is sewn in place, further motion of the cannula in the vessel and trauma to the vessel are minimized or eliminated. With the monitoring line sewn in place, the cannula is attached to the flush/pressure line with a Luer-lock connector. Thereafter, less attention to the security of the line is necessary during the procedure. The small indwelling arterial line is easily exchanged for an arterial sheath/catheter at any time later during the procedure when it becomes necessary to introduce a retrograde catheter.

Small arterial cannulae or indwelling dilators provide *continuous*, instantaneous and *accurate* arterial pressure monitoring or recordings, and allow instantaneous access for repeated arterial blood saturations and blood gases. Minute changes in the continuously-monitored arterial pressure provide a very early and definitive indicator of any instability of the patient during the procedure. This early warning *cannot* be achieved from the occasional pressures obtained from an intermittently inflated blood pressure cuff. Of equal importance, the simultaneously recorded arterial pressure provides the necessary, accurate reference, or control, systemic pressure recording for all the other hemodynamic measurements that are recorded during the procedure. Changes in the arterial pressure reflect even the smallest changes in the patient's state as a result of sedation/anesthesia, reaction to discomfort or contrast media or other volume changes. This "reference" systemic arterial recording is particularly important during long procedures or when the patient's hemodynamic status is changed purposefully during the catheterization, for example, during oxygen or drug "challenges". The indwelling arterial line also provides instantaneous and definitive access to the artery for a subsequent retrograde arterial catheterization.

Technique of retrograde arterial catheterization

When retrograde catheterization is to be performed, in order to minimize the time and manipulation in the artery the retrograde study is planned thoroughly before the introduction of the arterial sheath and the retrograde catheter. The information to be obtained is determined, and the procedures and catheter(s) necessary to obtain that information or perform those procedures are decided upon *before* the artery is entered with the sheath. *All* of the equipment necessary to obtain the information is readied—paper loaded in the physiologic recorder, the digital angiographic system is readied or film is loaded in the cine cameras, the injector is loaded with contrast and the particular catheters that are to be used are "pulled" from the supply area and made available in the catheterization room for immediate use. All of these preparations may seem elementary, but, if not arranged purposefully ahead of time, will cause (and have caused!) significant delays during critical periods of a procedure or an overall prolongation of the time in the artery with the sheath/catheter.

When a therapeutic procedure through the retrograde arterial approach is anticipated, the specific wires, catheters, balloons or devices that are necessary are also "pulled" from the inventory and made available in the catheterization room for immediate use. The type of arterial catheter is chosen for the specific information to be gathered or procedure to be performed from the arterial approach. The smallest diameter catheter with which *all* of the particular retrograde procedures can be accomplished, is used, as long as it does not compromise the information gained or the subsequent therapeutic procedure to be performed. If it is anticipated that a larger retrograde catheter will be necessary before the end of the procedure and particularly within a short time after introducing the initial retrograde sheath, then a larger sheath that will accommodate the larger catheters/devices is introduced initially. This will avoid the subsequent trauma to the vessel of changing to a larger sheath.

Indwelling arterial sheaths

Indwelling sheaths are used with ***all*** arterial catheterizations. Although the sheaths are always one (or up to 2.5 in the case of balloons), French sizes larger in outer diameter than the shaft of the catheter itself, the significant protection the sheath provides to the artery far outweighs the disadvantage of the increased diameter of the sheath in the artery. When a catheter is introduced directly into an artery without a sheath, there is continual abrasion of the intima of the artery as a result of the constant rubbing and twisting of the surface of the catheter against the inner wall of the artery near the puncture site. This continual trauma to the arterial wall results in irritation, pain and, as a consequence, arterial spasm around the catheter, which, in turn, results in more pain and more spasm. Once an indwelling sheath is positioned in the artery, all catheter movements that otherwise would have rubbed directly and continuously against the puncture site and wall of the artery, are within the sheath and, essentially, do not touch the wall of the peripheral artery no matter how much the catheter is moved.

Before the routine use of arterial sheaths, arterial spasm was a frequent and often disrupting occurrence during retrograde catheterizations. Arteries as large as the femoral artery can spasm so severely around a catheter that is introduced directly into the artery that the catheter cannot be moved at all within the artery without tearing or disrupting the arterial intima/wall. In addition to reducing the trauma during catheter manipulations, the indwelling sheath eliminates trauma to the artery and all of the blood loss during the exchange of catheters.

Before the indwelling arterial monitoring cannula is replaced with a sheath/dilator for a catheter introduction, the area all around the arterial puncture site is very liberally re-infiltrated with local anesthesia a few minutes prior to the introduction of the arterial sheath/dilator. The repeated and additional local anesthesia is administered regardless of the time since the initial introduction of local anesthesia to the area or the time since the introduction of the small arterial cannula. Without sufficient local anesthesia, the enlarging of the skin tract and the introduction of the sheath/dilator into the skin and artery produce significant pain. The pain of the puncture and "dissection" through the subcutaneous tissues and the discomfort from pressure over the artery result in arterial spasm. The spasm reduces the diameter of the artery, making the introduction of the larger dilator/sheath into the artery more difficult and producing more pain. The additional pain propagates a vicious cycle of pain and spasm, which works against the smooth introduction of the sheath/dilator into the artery. Of more importance, the introduction of a dilator/sheath into an artery in the presence of pain and arterial spasm is more likely to result in tears or disruption of the arterial wall with the potential for permanent arterial damage.

For the introduction of the sheath, it is very important to lengthen the *incision in the skin* around the wire enough to accommodate the circumference of the sheath that is being introduced. An inadequate opening in the skin produces extra resistance to the introduction of the tip of the sheath and is very likely to damage the tip of the sheath during attempted passage through it. For the introduction of the sheath/dilator into the artery, it is particularly important to use a dilator with a long, smooth and finely tapered tip, with the tip's internal diameter as close to the outer diameter of the guide wire as possible. The "transition" from the external tip of the dilator over the wire should be tight, with no gap or space between the wire and the internal lumen of the tip of the dilator. Most of the newer, finely tapered or "feather tipped" dilators taper smoothly and tightly over a relatively small wire and do *not* require additional subcutaneous dilation for their introduction into an artery.

When the subcutaneous tissues are severely scarred or very dense, it is occasionally necessary to pre-dilate the tissues to produce a subcutaneous "tract" before introducing an arterial sheath/dilator that is significantly larger than the previously introduced indwelling arterial cannula. This depends on the density of the scarring in the subcutaneous tissues and the type and size of dilator/sheath that is to be used in the artery. When dilation of the subcutaneous tissues is necessary, the plastic cannula of a 20- or an 18-gauge Med-I-Cut™ provides an excellent dilator for the tissues and the vessel wall. The cannula of the Med-I-Cut™ has a very smooth taper, increasing in diameter from the narrow distal tip, which fits tightly over the wire, to a wide proximal hub. Dilation of the subcutaneous tissues is accomplished by introducing the cannula of the Med-I-Cut™ directly over the wire and into the tissues and pushing the Med-I-Cut™ cannula into the tissues all of the way to the hub of the plastic cannula. This dilation of the subcutaneous tract can also be accomplished using sequentially, larger and larger fine-tipped dilators or even with a small "mosquito" surgical clamp to dissect through the subcutaneous tissues down to the artery.

The sheath that is used in the artery should be thin walled, fairly rigid and fit tightly or taper tightly around the dilator at the tip of the sheath. The tract (course) of the guide wire as it passes from the skin, through the subcutaneous tissues and into the artery is "supported" in the subcutaneous tissues beneath the skin during the sheath/dilator introduction. The fingers of the opposite hand are pressed firmly over the skin along the course of the wire between the puncture site into the skin and the anticipated course to the suspected puncture site in the vessel, which is located deeper and slightly cephalad in the tissues. Pressure is applied continuously as the sheath/dilator is introduced into the tissues. The firm external support prevents the wire in the subcutaneous tissues from bending or kinking between the skin and the arterial puncture site and prevents bleeding around the wire before the sheath/dilator is introduced into the artery.

In densely scarred or otherwise very resistant subcutaneous tissues, an extra stiff guide wire should be used for the introduction of the sheath/dilator set. This requires the exchange of the original, small, floppy, percutaneous introductory wire for a larger and stiffer support wire. The exchange of wires is accomplished through the previous indwelling arterial line, or if a significantly larger caliber, stiff wire is necessary, through the Med-I-Cut™ cannula used to dilate the subcutaneous tract.

A very gentle and very precise technique is always used for entering the artery. *Never* use extreme, direct and/or "jabbing" forces to introduce either the dilator or the sheath. Use the "high-speed drilling" motion to advance both the sheath and dilator over the wire, through the skin, through the subcutaneous tissues and through the arterial wall as described previously in Chapter 4. For the percutaneous introduction of the sheath/dilator into the artery, it is extremely helpful to have a *detachable* side arm/back-bleed valve/flush port on the sheath. With a detachable back-bleed valve, the valve can be loosened from the hub of the sheath, which allows the dilator or the sheath alone to be rotated freely and rapidly. When the back-bleed valve has been loosened from the sheath, the valve apparatus and the dilator are withdrawn a few millimeters back off the hub of the sheath in order to allow the sheath to rotate freely. Alternatively, the detachable valve mechanism is removed completely from the sheath/dilator set before beginning the introduction of the sheath/dilator into the skin. With the back-bleed valve loosened or removed, the dilator or sheath can be rotated ("drilled") rapidly and independently through the tissues without the side arm of the valve flopping around and becoming entangled on adjacent lines, or even itself. Once the sheath is securely in the artery, the back-bleed valve is reattached to the sheath before the wire and dilator are removed. If the valve was removed completely from the sheath/dilator, first the wire, then the dilator are withdrawn from the sheath. There is minimal bleeding from the hub of the dilator but, as soon as the tip of the dilator exits the hub of the sheath, the open end of the sheath, which now creates a large lumen in direct continuity with the lumen of the artery, is capped immediately with a fingertip. The back-bleed valve is quickly reattached to the sheath as the fingertip is "simultaneously" removed from the hub of the sheath. If the back-bleed valve is reattached expeditiously, there is minimal blood loss during this exchange.

The smallest diameter sheath/dilator set which will accommodate the largest catheter that is to be used through the retrograde approach is introduced into the artery initially. If it is anticipated that an even larger catheter will be necessary in the artery within a relatively short period of time, a sheath that will accommodate the larger catheter is introduced at the *beginning* of the retrograde arterial procedure, so that replacing a smaller sheath with a larger sheath will not be necessary. The introduction and exchange of sheath/dilator sets into arteries in themselves produce some trauma to the artery. When all of the left heart diagnostic information has been obtained previously with a prograde catheter, only the one introduction of the larger sheath into the artery is necessary for the therapeutic procedure, thus eliminating all exchanges of arterial sheaths.

During the course of a long, retrograde arterial catheterization or therapeutic procedure, the very liberal administration of local anesthesia is repeated periodically and arbitrarily around the puncture site. Local anesthesia is also repeated should it become necessary to exchange arterial sheaths. Any general reaction or body movement by the patient during catheter manipulations is a strong indicator of the need for more local anesthesia in the area of the puncture—particularly around the artery. The absence of any response by the patient to manipulations in the area of the vessel punctures usually indicates that the local anesthesia is adequate. The patient does not feel movement of a cardiac catheter within the heart; the patient only feels movement of the catheter/sheath at the entry site! Even when a patient is under general anesthesia or is paralyzed, additional local anesthesia should be infiltrated in the area of vessel entry to prevent reflex, local vessel spasm from the local pain.

Once the artery is cannulated successfully with the sheath and dilator, the indwelling sheath remains in the artery for the remainder of the retrograde catheterization. The sheath remaining within the artery for the duration of the procedure reduces (eliminates!) the local, continuous and repetitive trauma from the catheter rubbing at the site of entry into the artery and along the adjacent arterial wall during catheter manipulations. With the sheath in place in the artery, the arterial wall in the area of the puncture has no direct contact with the sliding in and out or rotational motion of the shaft of the catheter, no matter how extensive the catheter manipulations may be. Any theoretical disadvantage of the slightly larger diameter of the sheath (approximately one French size or 1/3 mm larger than the catheter shaft) in the artery is far outweighed by this reduction in trauma. Any arterial spasm that does occur at the puncture site, occurs around the stationary sheath in the vessel and has no effect on catheter manipulation. The reduction in direct contact and trauma to the vessel becomes even more important during catheter exchanges in the artery. When catheters are exchanged through the indwelling sheath, again, any direct catheter contact with the entry site and, in turn, any additional trauma to the entry site into the artery and to the adjacent arterial wall is eliminated by the indwelling sheath.

An indwelling sheath technique is even more important during retrograde balloon dilation or stent implant procedures, even though the indwelling sheath must be several French sizes larger than the shaft of the therapeutic (balloon) catheter. Balloons, particularly after they have been inflated and deflated, all have irregular, rough surface profiles and significantly larger diameters than their shafts. When introduced into an artery without an indwelling sheath, the deflated balloon, which is several French sizes larger than the shaft of the catheter, is forced through the arterial wall, leaving a large traumatized opening in the wall over the following, smaller catheter shaft. This large opening in the wall of the artery results in continual bleeding around the shaft of the catheter at the introductory site into the artery. During all manipulations of the balloon catheter in the artery without an indwelling sheath, the shaft of the balloon catheter passes directly against, and continually irritates, the already traumatized artery wall, particularly at the entry site. After a retrograde dilation procedure without an indwelling sheath, the deflated dilation balloon, which is now even larger and rougher and has very stiff, even sharp, "shoulders" and "wings" (which would be ideal for "vein stripping") must be pulled forcefully through and directly out of the already injured artery.

Occasionally, even when a balloon dilation catheter is introduced through a sheath, the balloon cannot be withdrawn entirely out of the artery through the sheath after it has been inflated/deflated in the body. Even in these circumstances, the sheath still protects the artery during and after the introduction and during the manipulations in the artery before the removal of the balloon. During withdrawal of the balloon, the very rough, proximal "shoulder", along with much of the refolded balloon, can be withdrawn into the sheath, which, in turn, protects the vessel wall from the balloon, even when the sheath must be withdrawn over the wire along with the distal end of the balloon.

Even in the very rare instances when a "cut-down" approach to an artery is used, an indwelling sheath/dilator is introduced into the arterial lumen through the "arteriotomy". Once the indwelling sheath is in place and secured in the artery, there will be no further irritation of the artery by the movements of the catheter at, or near, the introductory site. In turn, there is no spasm of the artery on the moving catheter resulting in further damage. When a catheter exchange is necessary through a sheath that is positioned in the cut-down in the artery, the exchange is very simple and atraumatic to the artery, and requires no additional manipulations of the sutures or clamps on the artery at the entry site.

Heparinization of the patient, particularly for the arterial study, is advocated by most centers. However, conclusive evidence that the use of heparin prevents, or even decreases, local arterial damage has not been demonstrated. Spending minimal time in the artery with the sheath/catheter, the use of indwelling sheaths, the use of small diameter sheath/catheters and the use of careful techniques, all are far more important for the prevention of peripheral arterial injury. When an arterial procedure with extensive manipulation of wires or catheters in the systemic circulation is anticipated, or if a therapeutic procedure is planned with the retrograde catheter, then heparinization is utilized to prevent systemic emboli off the wires and catheters that are indwelling in the systemic arterial circulation.

The use of systemic heparin is probably even more important at preventing venous thromboses, and is mandated if the patient has exhibited any prior tendency for hypercoagulability. The usual dose of heparin is 100 mg/kg. If not administered earlier in the procedure, heparin is given immediately after the sheath/dilator is introduced into the artery and definitely prior to any left heart manipulations with catheters or wires. An activated clotting time (ACT) is obtained in the laboratory and the heparin dose is adjusted according to that value. A desirable therapeutic range for the ACT in the pediatric/congenital patient is 275–350 sec. Repeat ACT determinations are carried out during long procedures and before the administration of more heparin. At the end of the procedure, particularly if it has been a long one or if it has been a long time since the last heparin dose was given, it is usually unnecessary to reverse the heparin before removing the lines. A repeat ACT determination helps with that decision.

The use of detachable back-bleed valves on sheaths is equally as useful for the manipulation of catheters through arterial sheaths as for catheters in venous sheaths. A back-bleed valve attached to the sheath is necessary during the introduction or exchange of catheters into the arterial sheath, however, as with venous sheaths, the back-bleed valve itself "binds" and restricts the movement of a catheter when the latter must be manipulated through the back-bleed valve. The binding of the catheter in the valve attached to the sheath also generates repeated, small movements of the sheath against the arterial wall during the catheter manipulations, which, in turn, defeats some of the advantages of the use of a sheath. When the manufacturing tolerances are precise, and when the sheath that is used in the artery is the same French size as the catheter passing through the sheath, even with the back-bleed valve detached, no significant bleeding will occur around the catheter through the sheath in the artery. The back-bleed valve is loosened from the hub of the sheath and withdrawn back on the shaft of the catheter during catheter manipulations in the artery exactly as with indwelling sheaths in the veins. As in the veins, when the back-bleed valve is loosened from the sheath in the artery, the feel and movement of the catheter through the sheath are facilitated very significantly. The shaft of the catheter where it is adjacent to and as it enters the hub of the sheath, is continuously kept moistened with a wet sponge as the catheter is manipulated in the sheath. This is exactly as with manipulations of catheters through venous sheaths. When a catheter is exchanged or a catheter is being used which has a smaller outside diameter of the shaft than the internal lumen of the sheath (even though the "same" French size), the back-bleed valve is reattached to the sheath.

The retrograde catheter is chosen which is best suited to the particular procedure being performed. For example, a thin-walled, high flow pigtail catheter is ideal for aortograms, aortic root "flushes", or even retrograde ventriculograms, and also allows for "downsizing" of the sheath/catheter diameter. The catheter used should not be significantly longer than necessary to reach the furthermost location planned for the retrograde approach. The resistance to the flow of contrast medium through a catheter is proportional to the length and inversely proportional to the diameter of the catheter. Inventory limitations, however, may prevent using the ideal shortest length in each patient. The exact catheter used for the retrograde approach varies from patient to patient and even within a single patient according to its intended use in the arterial system.

Catheters with specific preformed curves are available, and a specialized curve can be formed manually on the tip of the catheter for a particular procedure. For example, an acute angle at the tip of the catheter facilitates entrance into side or branching vessels. Manufactured, preformed coronary catheters are used for selective right and left coronary artery studies. Deflector wires within arterial catheters are useful to deflect the catheter tip purposefully into side vessels or even around the arch when approached from the descending aorta. The use of a deflector wire is preferable to, and more successful than, random, repeated pushing, pulling and twisting of a retrograde catheter, especially if it has become soft or has little or no preformed curve at its distal end.

When any type of a wire is used within an arterial catheter, a wire back-bleed/flush device is used on the hub of the catheter and is placed on a continual flush. The back-bleed valve prevents external bleeding from the proximal end of the catheter and, along with a continual or frequent intermittent flush, prevents bleeding back into the distal end of the catheter, which, in turn, reduces the chance of clot formation in the catheter and around the wire. The flush through the side port also provides a continual lubrication around the wire, which facilitates wire movement in the catheter. When a wire that is smaller in diameter than the internal diameter of the catheter lumen and that is relatively loose within the catheter is used, pressures can be recorded through the catheter. For the most accurate pressure recordings, the wire is introduced through a Tuohy™ type, pressure, back-bleed device with a side port. The arterial catheter is connected to the pressure monitoring system through the side port of the Tuohy™ valve apparatus. By using a Tuohy™ pressure adaptor, high-pressure angiograms can be performed around the wire within a catheter. Even using a standard, non-pressure, wire back-bleed device, very small, low-pressure, hand injection angiograms can be performed through the catheter around a wire that is loose within the catheter lumen. When a wire is removed from a systemic arterial line, the catheter is cleared very carefully of air and clots by the withdrawal of blood before the catheter is flushed, even if it was previously on a continual flush through a back-bleed valve/flush system.

Retrograde catheterization of the left (systemic) ventricle

Crossing a stenotic aortic valve from the retrograde approach is one of the more challenging, *least predictable* and *least controllable* maneuvers performed in the cardiac catheterization laboratory. It is also a procedure that is required very frequently in a pediatric or congenital cardiac catheterization laboratory, particularly during various therapeutic catheterization procedures. Even crossing an aortic valve that is not stenotic can be challenging, particularly when there is a large, dilated and/or distorted aortic root. The procedure for crossing the aortic valve is different in every patient and will depend upon the patient's size, the length of the ascending aorta, the diameter of the ascending aorta and the aortic root, any distortion of the aortic root, and the amount of stenosis or distortion of the semilunar valve itself. There is no single, ideal catheter, wire, technique or combination of these for crossing the aortic valve in all patients! All varieties of catheters and combinations of catheters and wires are used according to the patient's anatomy, the introductory site and the individual catheterizing physician's preference.

Before an attempt is made to cross a stenotic or distorted aortic valve, the valve is visualized angiographically in at least two views with a biplane aortic root or left ventricular angiogram. The angiogram demonstrates the size and "angle" of the ascending aorta and the location and orientation of the column or jet of blood flow from the valve orifice in relation to the sinuses of the aortic valve. A freeze-frame of both views of a biplane angiogram is isolated and displayed side by side with the fluoroscopic image to use as a "road map" during the attempts at crossing the valve.

A catheter is chosen with a preformed curve at its distal end that will direct the *tip* of the catheter toward the orifice of the valve after the tip of the catheter has been advanced retrograde around the aortic arch and into the ascending aorta. Advancing and withdrawing an angled, preformed curve at the distal end of a catheter changes the side-to-side direction of the tip as visualized on posterior–anterior (PA) fluoroscopy. Torquing the catheter clockwise or counterclockwise changes the anterior–posterior direction of the tip of the same catheter as visualized on lateral fluoroscopy. With the combined use of these two motions, the catheter tip can be directed purposefully in any direction toward the suspected location of the valve orifice. The catheter maneuvers toward the aortic valve are performed while the tip of the catheter is still in the ascending aorta and before the tip has been advanced all of the way into the aortic sinuses.

Unfortunately, the "target orifice" of the aortic valve is actually "invisible"; its location is moving continuously and the valve leaflets are opening and closing with each heartbeat! As a consequence, even visualizing the valve angiographically in biplane views and mentally "knowing where the orifice is" do not localize the valve orifice in reality nor guarantee passage across it. Occasionally, with the fortuitous choice of the ideal curve at the tip of the catheter, the preformed catheter itself when advanced into the aortic root is directed exactly at, and passes across, the orifice in the valve and into the ventricle. Although this is rarely the case, several gentle probes at the valve orifice with the catheter itself are worthwhile. Usually the valve is crossed using a combination of catheters, multiple wires and many maneuvers.

In attempting to cross the semilunar valve retrograde, multiple, rapid and repeated, but at the same time, delicate probes with the very soft tip of a wire are preferable to slow, deliberate attempts at passing through a valve (or any other structure) *that cannot actually be seen*—i.e., in order to advance a catheter or wire retrograde through an aortic valve involves some talent but, in addition, a great deal of chance at "hitting" the "invisible", moving, opening and closing, stenotic valve orifice, particularly while the valve is in the open position during systole. The heartbeat is too fast to time the probes toward the valve accurately and purposefully only during systole. Because of this, ten quick "chance probes" provide a higher likelihood of crossing an aortic valve when it is in the open position, compared to one slow, deliberate, but still chance advancing of the catheter toward the valve. Each of the repeated probes or advances of the catheter or wire should also involve some side-to-side or anterior–posterior redirection of the angle of the tip of the catheter/wire. The change in direction is accomplished by torque or slight to-and-fro motion applied to the proximal end of the curve-tipped catheter while the wire is moved in and out of the precurved tip of the catheter. The same techniques are used for crossing any semilunar valve or the atrioventricular valves from a retrograde approach.

A wire with a very floppy tip, but a relatively short floppy segment, is used for crossing the aortic valve. A wire is chosen that can be directed purposefully yet has a soft enough tip that it will not damage, or possibly even perforate, a valve leaflet or the adjacent tissues when repeatedly "banged" against them. At the same time, the wire tip cannot be so soft that a high-velocity jet of blood through a tight, stenotic orifice will blow the tip of the wire repeatedly away from the orifice. The wire should slide to and fro easily within the retrograde catheter. Depending on the type of wire, and when using a catheter with a fixed curve on its tip, the floppy tip of the wire can be straight or have a very slight curve. The direction of the straight wire is changed by the combined torquing and to-and-fro movement of the curve on the tip of the retrograde catheter. When the wire is torque-controlled, such as a Magic™ or a Platinum Plus™ wire, a slight curve on its tip allows additional changes in the direction of the wire alone by torque on the wire. The direction of the tip of the catheter is changed continuously by the to-and-fro and torque on the shaft of the catheter, while the wire is moved in and out of the tip of the catheter, repeatedly "bouncing" the tip of the wire off the valve and valve sinuses until the wire pops (randomly!) through the valve orifice and into the ventricle.

Regardless of the type of wire used, while it is being advanced in and out of the tip of the catheter, the latter should always be maintained well above (away from) the aortic valve in order that the tip of the wire has room to bounce or loop easily off the valve (Figure 9.1a). The tip of the catheter ***never*** should be positioned *deep* in the aortic root and/or *close* to the valve leaflets and/or the aortic sinuses. When the tip of a retrograde end-hole catheter is positioned and maintained close to the surface of the semilunar valve, even a soft-tipped spring guide or Terumo™ wire initially exits the catheter for the first *several millimeters* as a straight and *stiff* tip. The tip of the wire continues in a straight course as it advances out of the orifice at the tip of the catheter, before it can begin to (or can!) deflect off structures (Figure 9.1b). As a consequence, the wire preferentially ***perforates*** before beginning to deflect. A very *slight* curve on the floppy tip of the wire usually aids in the maneuvers to cross the valve as well as adding some safety to the wire extrusion.

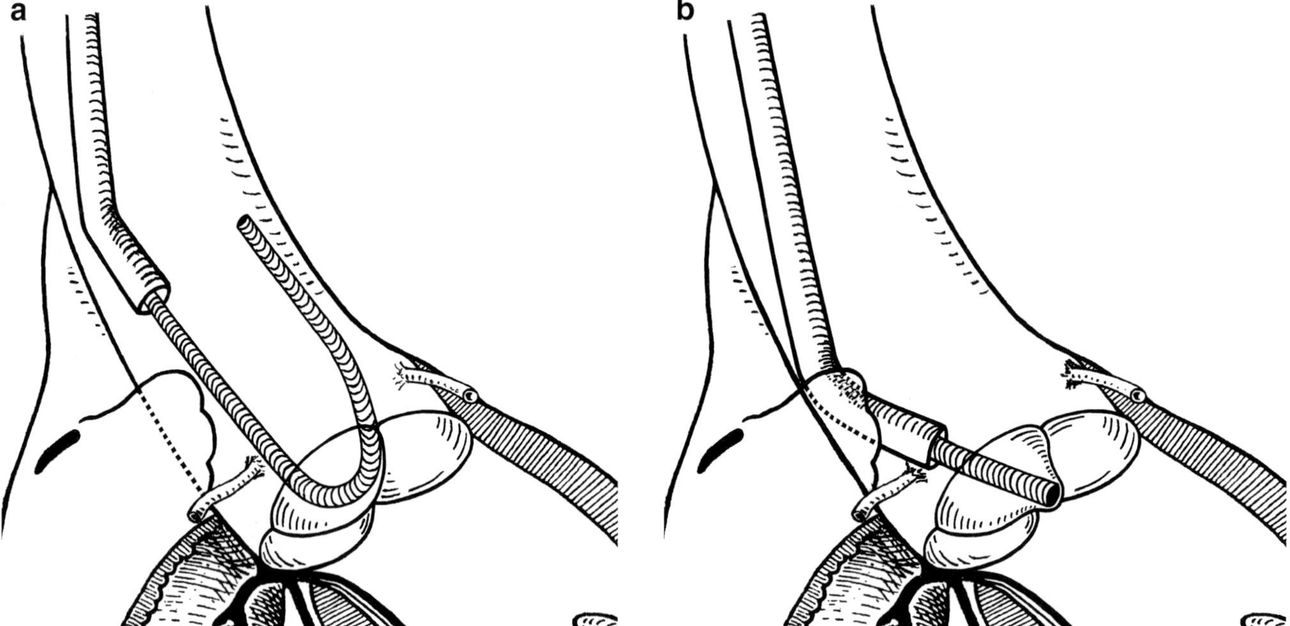

Figure 9.1 (a) Tip of retrograde catheter positioned relatively high in the ascending aorta, allowing the guide wire that is advanced out of its tip to "bounce" or loop off the valve as the wire is advanced into the valve leaflets aortic sinuses; (b) tip of retrograde catheter positioned deep in aortic valve sinus, which does not allow the tip of even a soft wire to "bounce" or deflect away from the leaflet while it is being advanced out of the tip of the catheter.

When a larger gauge or stiffer wire is used, it should *always* have a slight curve or angle at its tip to prevent its "drilling through" tissues instead of bouncing off them. This is particularly true of the Terumo™ Glide™ wires, which are designed to pass through tissues. The wire used to cross the valve must have characteristics that will not allow it to damage structures, but at the same time, be sturdy enough to cross the valve. Once the soft tip of the wire has passed the valve, the shaft of the wire must be stiff enough to support a catheter advancing over the wire into the ventricle.

A preferable alternative to the use of the rapid, repeated and "blind" probing with the wire when crossing the semilunar valve from the retrograde approach is to position a catheter and/or wire passing prograde through the valve prior to the retrograde approach. The course of the prograde catheter or wire through the valve orifice then serves as a guide to be followed with the retrograde wire or catheter. A prograde venous catheter and/or wire is positioned in the systemic ventricle through a pre-existing communication or an atrial transseptal puncture. From the systemic ventricle, a catheter or wire is manipulated prograde into the aorta. A floating balloon catheter facilitates advancing the catheter from the left atrium, to the systemic ventricle and then out into the aorta, as described in Chapter 7. The prograde catheter or wire is left positioned in the aorta, passing through the orifice of the semilunar valve, while the retrograde wire/catheter is introduced. The prograde catheter or wire passing through the semilunar valve provides a visual guide to the exact course through the orifice of the valve and demonstrates by its course exactly where the orifice is located in both planes of the fluoroscopy/X-ray image. The retrograde catheter or wire is then manipulated slowly and purposefully, following the course of the prograde guide catheter/wire to, and through, the orifice of the valve. In this situation continual biplane or rapidly alternating posterior–anterior and lateral fluoroscopy are required. Very precise, deliberate and controlled torquing and to-and-fro motions of the retrograde catheter are used to redirect the tip of the wire in order to follow precisely along the now visible course of the prograde catheter/wire. This technique for crossing the aortic valve represents another huge advantage to performing the left heart study initially with a prograde catheter, even when a retrograde procedure is planned.

Once the tip of the retrograde wire has passed through the valve and into the ventricle, the wire is advanced further into the ventricle and secured in a stable position, and the retrograde catheter is advanced over it. This catheter is usually the one that was used to guide the wire across the valve initially; however, it is usually not the final catheter needed in the ventricle. Once the catheter has entered the ventricle, the wire used to cross the valve can be exchanged for a wire more appropriate for the therapeutic procedure to be performed, or the initial catheter can be exchanged for a catheter more suitable for positioning or redirecting a sturdier wire within the ventricle.

In order to direct the tip of the wire back toward the left ventricular outflow tract or the mitral valve, a pigtail catheter is advanced over the initial retrograde wire, across the valve, and into the ventricle. The initial wire is replaced with a stiffer wire that has a 180° curve manually formed at the transition region between the stiff and floppy parts of the wire and a tight pigtail formed in its soft distal tip. The stiffer wire is advanced through the retrograde pigtail catheter until the 180° curve in the wire is positioned in the pigtail curve of the catheter in the body of the ventricle. This usually directs the distal, softer portion of the wire, which is distal to the 180° transition curve, out of the tip of the pigtail and back toward the left ventricular outflow tract. Once the stiffer wire is in this position, the pigtail catheter is withdrawn over the wire and replaced with any desired diagnostic or therapeutic catheter.

Manipulation within the ventricle with the retrograde catheter

For balloon dilation of the aortic valve from the retrograde approach, it is desirable to have a Super Stiff™ wire (Medi-Tech, Boston Scientific, Natick, MA) with a long floppy tip secured in the ventricle. The retrograde catheter in the ventricle is manipulated until a 180° loop is formed on the catheter within the ventricle, or a pigtail catheter is advanced over the initial wire until its tip is directed back toward the aortic valve. A pigtail loop is formed on the floppy portion and a smooth, but, relatively tight, 180° curve is formed at the transition zone between the floppy and stiff portions of the Super Stiff™ wire before it is introduced through the catheter into the ventricle. The Super Stiff™ wire is advanced through the previously positioned catheter into the ventricle until the 180° loop on this wire is situated in the ventricular apex and the tip is directed back on itself toward the aortic valve. If the patient is to undergo a double balloon dilation of the aortic valve, a second wire, catheter and eventually Super Stiff™ wire are introduced into the ventricle using the same technique.

Occasionally it is necessary to enter into the pulmonary artery through a ventricular septal defect, to pass through a muscular ventricular septal defect, or to cross into one of the atria from the systemic ventricle by the retrograde approach. In order to accomplish this, the retrograde catheter that is positioned in the systemic ventricle needs a distal tip that is fairly stiff and angled 90–180°. This angled catheter is introduced into the left ventricle over a wire as just described or, occasionally, the catheter with the curved tip itself is advanced into the ventricle directly, since lesions where manipulations from the ventricle are required are usually not associated with stenosis of the aortic valve.

Alternatively, a 180° loop is formed at the distal end of a catheter while the catheter is within the aortic root, and the loop is backed across the valve and into the ventricle from the aortic root. The loop in the catheter in the aortic root is formed by pushing the catheter forward with its tip fixed against a structure such as the wall of the aorta or the orifice of a branch vessel. The forward push on the catheter with the tip fixed usually causes the distal segment of the catheter just proximal to the tip to bend on itself. Alternatively, an active deflector wire is used to initiate the curve against the wall or the entire 180° loop is formed with the active deflector wire. A relatively soft tipped catheter is used for all of these "bending" maneuvers and for "backing" across the valve. The bending and backing maneuvers across the valve are performed blindly with multiple probes with the catheter, similar to passing a guide wire across the valve. When this technique is used, the aortic valve is usually normal (not stenotic), which makes it possible to back a loop of the catheter across the valve.

When the retrograde catheter does not loop or the straight catheter passes straight through the semilunar valve, which positions the tip of the catheter pointing straight into the apex of the ventricle, the catheter is withdrawn into the aortic root and a repeat attempt is made at forming a loop in the aorta and backing the *loop* across the aortic valve. When a loop cannot be formed on the catheter in the aortic root, the catheter is removed from the artery and either the same catheter is heated to recurve the tip manually, or a totally new catheter with a different preformed curve is used to repeat the attempt at backing across the aortic valve.

Once the catheter loop has been backed across the aortic valve and into the ventricle, the catheter tip is usually directed 180° back on itself within the ventricle. The goal of backing the loop into the ventricle is to have the distal end of the catheter in the ventricle directed 90–180° on itself, back toward a ventricular septal defect, the other semilunar valve or an atrioventricular valve.

When attempting to maneuver a retrograde catheter that is in the ventricle back through an atrioventricular valve, the most successful approach is by repeatedly turning the loop while moving the catheter slightly in and out within the ventricular chamber in order to redirect the tip with each motion. When the retrograde catheter itself cannot be manipulated through the atrioventricular valve, a floppy-tipped wire or, preferably, a "J-tipped" wire is advanced through the tip of the curved catheter while the distal end of the catheter is being redirected within the ventricular cavity. As the catheter is manipulated in the ventricle, the soft tip of the wire is moved in and out of the catheter very carefully in an attempt to "buckle" the wire back through the atrioventricular valve. Biplane imaging is essential to direct the catheter tip/wire toward the general direction of the valve orifice, but even with this, crossing the valve is somewhat dependant upon chance in conjunction with multiple repeated probes toward the valve.

When the loop at the tip of the catheter cannot be advanced into the ventricle, the alternative is to pass the straight catheter into the ventricle and then to use an active deflector wire to form a 90–180° loop temporarily at the distal end of the catheter once the straight catheter is in the ventricle. A 90+° deflection redirects the distal end of the retrograde catheter across the long axis of the ventricle and toward the desired orifice. With the curve on the deflector wire fixed, the catheter is advanced off the deflector wire toward, and hopefully through, the desired valve or opening arising from the ventricle. The deflector wire technique is more successful for crossing muscular ventricular septal defects than manipulating the catheter "backwards" through the atrioventricular valves.

Occasionally, the catheter cannot be manipulated back through the atrioventricular or the other semilunar valve, even when a loop has been backed into the ventricle and with the use of a floppy-tipped wire along with the catheter. In this situation, a *three-dimensional* curve, which corresponds to the course from the left ventricle to the desired orifice, is preformed manually at the distal end of a *rigid* deflector wire (*see* Chapter 6). With the loop in the distal end of the retrograde catheter still positioned in the body of the ventricle, the preformed rigid deflector wire is introduced into the catheter and advanced to just within its tip. This three-dimensional curve redirects the tip in the "third dimension", which is usually enough to allow the catheter to be advanced off the wire and through the desired orifice. Both maneuvers must be performed very carefully while observing on continual biplane or frequent, intermittent posterior–anterior and lateral fluoroscopy to avoid perforation of a wall or other structure or the entrapment in intraventricular structures.

Since the frequency of arterial complications increases in direct proportion to the time spent in the artery, economy of time should be a primary consideration, particularly for all maneuvers on the arterial side of the circulation. With this in mind, once a particular catheter and/or maneuver is attempted several times and repeatedly has been unsuccessful, the catheter and/or the technique is changed before repeating the same unsuccessful maneuver with any further and futile attempts.

Arterial sheath/catheter removal

When the arterial study/procedure has been completed, special procedures are used for removing the catheter and sheath and caring for the puncture site. Unless the total arterial procedure has taken less than 10–15 minutes, the area around the arterial entrance is again liberally re-infiltrated with local anesthesia. The catheter is withdrawn to a position in the descending aorta adjacent to the tip of the sheath. Suction is applied to the proximal end of the catheter while it is being withdrawn through the sheath and out of the vessel. The suction to the catheter allows any fibrin or clots that have accumulated on the surface of the catheter—particularly at the catheter/sheath interface—to be withdrawn into, and through, the sheath and, in turn, out of the vessel rather than being stripped off into the artery as an embolus. The side port on the back-bleed valve is opened slightly and after a single "spurt" of blood from the sheath, the sheath is withdrawn from the artery while pressure is applied over the puncture site. The blood flow into the sheath, again, allows any clot in the artery at the end of the sheath to flow out of the artery and into the sheath before the sheath is withdrawn.

When applying pressure over a percutaneous arterial puncture site, it is preferable to apply the pressure directly over the puncture site in the arterial wall with the gloved fingers. In this way, the pulse can be palpated continuously while the immediate area around the puncture site can be observed simultaneously for oozing or hematoma formation. Pressure is applied as the sheath is being withdrawn and is continued over the puncture site after everything is out of the artery. As soon as the sheath has been withdrawn from the artery, the drapes are removed from the patient, specifically off the extremities where the sheaths/catheters were introduced. The puncture site and the entire percutaneous area are observed continuously while a pulse in the extremity distal to the puncture site is palpated simultaneously and the distal extremity is observed for color and capillary flow. Too little pressure applied over the puncture site allows continual bleeding through the vessel wall, bleeding through the skin or into the tissues with the development of a large hematoma. At the other extreme, too much pressure applied over the puncture site completely stops blood flow in the artery, resulting in stasis and thrombus formation within the artery. When there is no blood flow to the local area of the vessel, clotting factors do not reach the puncture site and the clotting mechanism externally around the artery is inhibited. The pressure applied over the arterial puncture site should be "balanced" or "titrated" to allow the distal pulse in the extremity to be palpated continually while, at the same time, local bleeding at the puncture site is stopped. This part of the procedure cannot be rushed or delegated to a mechanical device or "uninterested party" in pediatric or adult congenital heart patients! After the bleeding has stopped totally and a good distal pulse has been verified, a *very light* pressure bandage is applied over the puncture site, again being careful that it is not so tight as to reduce or actually eliminate the pulse distal to the bandage or to tourniquet the venous flow.

Often in very large patients with very large thighs, the *precise* site of the arterial puncture is deep within the tissues and cannot be palpated, exactly identified or compressed precisely with the fingertips. In patients with very large thighs or deep adipose tissue in the inguinal area, it is preferable to use a tight, 2–3 cm diameter, roll of "four by fours" for the compression over (and into) the tissues over the area of the puncture site. The entire area around the puncture site should be observed equally vigilantly with the drapes removed, and a peripheral pulse should be palpated continually while holding the pressure over the artery. Since many milliliters of blood can collect within deep, thick, subcutaneous tissues while still not reaching the puncture site at the skin surface, it is a good idea to maintain pressure over the area in this type of patient for an even longer period of time after the "skin bleeding" has stopped.

Usually, the heparin is not "reversed" prior to withdrawing the arterial line. A repeat ACT is done before removing the arterial sheath, particularly if there was any question about the value of the ACT during the case or extra heparin had been administered shortly before the conclusion of the procedure. When bleeding at the puncture site persists in spite of local pressure over it for more than 30 minutes, there is still a good peripheral pulse *and* the ACT remains greater than 300 seconds, then reversal of the heparin with protamine is considered.

Additional arterial access sites

In pediatric and congenital cardiac catheterizations, the femoral artery is the usual arterial access site. The femoral artery is larger than any other peripheral artery and there are reasonably good collateral vessels in the area around the common femoral artery. Occasionally, however, other arterial sites are used for arterial access.

In the newborn infant, the umbilical artery is frequently available and has often been cannulated prior to the infant's arrival in the catheterization laboratory. When already cannulated or when still accessible, the umbilical artery provides, at the very least, a good line for indwelling arterial monitoring. The umbilical arteries themselves are "expendable" and are supposed to clot off and, as a consequence, they can be used for arterial pressure monitoring and blood sampling with very few negative consequences when managed properly. When the umbilical artery is available during a cardiac catheterization in a neonate, a separate, peripheral artery often does not have to be entered at all[3].

However, the umbilical artery is less desirable as an approach for retrograde catheterization procedures. The technique for the introduction and manipulation of umbilical artery catheters is covered in more detail in Chapter 4. There are two major problems with the retrograde approach from the umbilical artery. First, there are two fairly sharp, 180° bends in the course of a catheter traversing from the stump of the umbilicus to the heart and second, there often is significant arterial spasm around catheters introduced through the umbilical artery. Because of acute turns in the arterial course, any forward push on the proximal umbilical arterial catheter must be directed *caudally*, toward the iliofemoral junction, which is exactly away from the direction to the heart. This long and circuitous course and arterial spasm around the catheters compromise all manipulations and maneuvers of the umbilical artery catheter. In spite of these problems, catheters can usually be advanced to the aortic root and even the systemic ventricle from umbilical artery access. This usually requires the combination of soft catheters, exchange guide wires and a great deal of patience with catheter manipulations and exchanges.

Occasionally, the original umbilical arterial line that was already in place, or a replacement, polyethylene umbilical catheter, can be advanced fairly readily at least into the descending thoracic aorta and often as far as the aortic arch or even the aortic root. This catheter is satisfactory for angiography or recording pressures in those areas. Angiograms through an umbilical catheter are satisfactory enough to visualize a coarctation of the aorta, a patent ductus, the aortic root and the aortic valve in the newborn. The pressures and angiograms from the aorta and transverse arch that are obtained through the umbilical artery catheter, combined with the "left heart" hemodynamics and angiograms that are acquired through a prograde venous catheter are usually sufficient to record all necessary *diagnostic* information.

Umbilical artery access has been used for performing retrograde therapeutic procedures, particularly dilation of coarctation of the aorta and/or the aortic valve. The use of the umbilical arterial route for therapeutic procedures is discussed in some detail in Chapters 18 and 19 under 'Dilations of Coarctation of the Aorta and the Aortic Valve'.

A radial or brachial artery is often cannulated as a *monitoring line* in the pediatric/congenital cardiac intensive care unit and occasionally in the catheterization laboratory. The technique for the introduction of wires and small cannulae into these peripheral upper extremity arteries in the catheterization laboratory setting is exactly the same as for their introduction into the femoral artery discussed previously in this chapter. The brachial and radial arteries are more superficial and easier to palpate or even visualize. Although these arteries and even the ulnar artery are frequently used in catheterizations of the coronary arteries in adults, the radial, ulnar and brachial arteries are not used for routine retrograde catheterization procedures in pediatric/congenital patients, except in extremely special circumstances and then, only in larger patients. The vessels are much smaller than the femoral arteries, and once the catheter has been advanced to the heart, complex maneuvering in the congenital heart patient is more difficult from these peripheral, upper extremity approaches.

The carotid artery is now used frequently as an approach for some neonatal aortic valve dilations[4]. This technique, along with its advantages and disadvantages, are discussed in detail in Chapter 19. The carotid artery is approached by a *surgical cut-down* directly onto the artery. A vascular surgeon who is skilled in microvascular techniques performs the cut-down, the introduction of a sheath into the carotid artery, and the eventual repair of the artery. The pediatric cardiologist performs the retrograde catheterization and the balloon dilation of the aortic valve through the indwelling sheath in the carotid artery. At the end of the procedure after the dilation has been completed and the hemodynamics are verified or any angiography repeated, the surgeon removes the sheath, repairs the carotid artery and closes the incision.

Complications of retrograde catheterizations

The most common complication resulting from a retrograde approach for a cardiac catheterization is the compromise of the artery where the catheter was introduced. Arterial complications are reported to occur in somewhere between 0.5 and 10% of cases. With the very selective and, as a result, minimal use of the retrograde approach and with special handling of the arterial puncture sites, the incidence of arterial complications of any sort as a result of cardiac catheterizations at Texas Children's Hospital is less than 0.5–1%.

Arterial complications can vary from a small localized hematoma, to a decrease in the peripheral pulse/pale extremity, to the total loss of arterial flow in the involved extremity distal to the arterial puncture site and even to the reported loss of a limb. The best treatment is prevention; the next best treatment is early aggressive management. Problems with the arterial puncture site usually become apparent while the patient is still in the catheterization laboratory or while hemostasis is being achieved. That is the time that treatment should be started! A persistent weak pulse may be the only physical sign initially, but the weak pulse indicates decreased perfusion to the extremity, and chronic decreased limb perfusion can cause decreased limb growth with, eventually, a shorter extremity of the involved limb. Arterial damage with a lost peripheral pulse can progress to severe limb ischemia and even limb loss on very rare occasions.

When the peripheral pulse distal to the introduction site into the artery is noted to be absent, or the extremity is underperfused even slightly (cooler and/or paler extremity) the patient is re-heparinized at that time regardless of where and when the diminished (lost) pulse is detected. A repeat ACT is obtained before repeating heparin administration. If the patient's ACT has returned to normal, the patient is given a bolus of 100 mg/kg of heparin and then continued on a heparin drip at a rate of 1 mg/kg/hr over the next four hours. If the patient is still heparinized and the ACT is still above 300 seconds, then continuous infusion of heparin is begun without a repeat initial bolus. If the pulse remains absent or very faint or if the color and capillary reperfusion have not returned at the end of three to four hours of heparin infusion, then a decision is made between switching to a "mechanical intervention" to relieve the obstruction or instituting more aggressive medical therapy. If there is any *progression* of the signs of ischemia at any time during the heparin therapy, more aggressive therapy is instituted earlier.

Mechanical intervention utilizes catheter recanalization of the artery with an angioplasty balloon[5], while more aggressive medical management is with the use of intravenous and/or locally infused thrombolytics[6,7]. Both balloon recanalization and thrombolytic opening of traumatic lesions have been very successful, and surgical repair of the arterial introductory site is now seldom required.

For the catheter (mechanical) management of the involved artery, the patient is maintained on heparin therapy. The occluded artery is approached from the contralateral femoral artery, or as an alternative, particularly in infants, with a venous catheter advanced prograde through the left heart, ascending aorta and descending aorta to the involved femoral artery. An end-hole catheter is manipulated to a position just proximal to the lesion in the involved vessel and a biplane angiogram is recorded with a small selective injection performed through the end-hole catheter, which is positioned just proximal (in the direction of blood flow) to the lesion. The angiogram demonstrates the extent of the vascular damage, any extravasation from the lumen, and the presence of associated thrombi in the vessel.

Once the local anatomy has been clearly defined, a fine, soft-tipped, spring guide or a Terumo™ guide wire is maneuvered through, and well past, the lesion while being very careful not to advance the wire out through any defect in the arterial wall. Once the wire has been secured distally in the involved vessel and well beyond the lesion, the catheter is removed and replaced with a low-profile angioplasty balloon. Occasionally, the end-hole catheter is advanced through the lesion in order to exchange the original wire for a smaller or otherwise more satisfactory wire that the angioplasty balloon can accommodate. The diameter of the angioplasty balloon is chosen to be the same as that of the non-involved, proximal or distal adjacent vessel or, if that vessel is in spasm, the diameter of the contralateral vessel at the equivalent location. The lesion is dilated several times, moving the balloon forward or backward slightly in order to ensure that it covers the entire lesion during one or more inflations. The arterial pulse and perfusion distal to the obstruction are monitored during and immediately after the dilation for evidence of improved flow.

In the absence of a second catheter in the area of the lesion, the balloon is withdrawn over the wire and replaced with an end and side hole catheter with an internal diameter slightly larger than that of the wire. The tip of the catheter over the wire is advanced to a position in the artery that is just proximal to the lesion. A Tuohy™ valved adaptor with a side port is advanced over the wire and attached to the hub of the catheter. A contrast injection is performed into the involved artery through the side port and over the wire while recording on biplane imaging. This small selective injection usually provides a sufficient volume of contrast to obtain a usable, selective biplane angiogram that will be adequate enough to determine the success of the dilation of the area. The angiogram demonstrates any residual or adjacent obstruction or any extravasation of contrast through the puncture opening/tear in the artery. If there is renewed leak out of the artery at the initial puncture site, it is controlled with very precise, manual pressure over the puncture site. If there is significant residual obstruction of the artery, the balloon angioplasty is repeated. Once the obstruction has been relieved, heparin infusion is continued for at least another 12 hours while maintaining the involved extremity under very close observation.

The alternative, more aggressive medical management of the lesion is to use a thrombolytic agent administered intravenously instead of the mechanical angioplasty treatment[8]. Thrombolytic therapy avoids the necessity of repeat catheter intervention and, in limited experience, has been very effective at relieving post-catheterization arterial obstruction. Early experience with thrombolytic agents utilized both streptokinase and urokinase. These agents were very successful at revascularizing totally occluded vessels; however, recently there has been a problem with obtaining both of these agents, although streptokinase is now available as Streptase.

Currently a patient with an occluded artery occurring post-catheterization, which has not responded to intravenous heparin, is started on tissue plasminogen activator (tPA) with a bolus of 0.1 mg/kg followed by an intravenous infusion of 0.5 mg/kg/hr along with the heparin infusion for the next two hours. When the pulse returns, the tPA is discontinued while the heparin infusion is continued for 6–8 hours. If the pulse has not returned by the end of the first tPA infusion, the bolus of tPA is repeated with a repeat infusion for four more hours. This sequence can be repeated up to three times, although this has not been necessary in our limited experience with arterial obstructions following cardiac catheterization procedures.

Any patient undergoing tPA therapy must be observed extremely closely in an intensive care/recovery area environment for local or systemic bleeding. The arterial puncture sites (and any other vessel puncture sites) are left exposed with *no dressing* over them. The local puncture area(s) must be well lit during the entire period of therapy and observation. It is common to light the local area with a spotlight with the remainder of the room lights dimmed in order to calm the patient.

If the artery shows absolutely *no response at all* to the heparin and the first tPA course, and particularly if there is progression of the signs of obstruction, the vascular surgeon should become involved before proceeding with continued thrombolytic therapy.

Other complications of retrograde catheterizations

Pseudo aneurysms

Besides occlusion of arteries, occasionally a pseudo aneurysm develops at the arterial puncture site, or a local arteriovenous fistula is created between the arterial and adjacent venous punctures. Pseudo aneurysms develop as a result of a "liquefaction" of a hematoma, which is a consequence of a persistent leak from the punctured artery which, however, is contained in the subcutaneous tissues. Careful, single wall, arterial puncture techniques along with meticulous care of the puncture sites once the sheath(s) is(are) removed, are usually effective at preventing this complication. When an aneurysm does develop, it may be apparent as a painful swelling while the patient is still in a recovery area, but may not be recognized for several days following the procedure. Aneurysms usually present as a painful, discrete swelling at the catheter introductory site. The swelling is not associated with any bruit and is diagnosed by an echo over the vessel or, more definitively, by an arteriogram of the involved femoral artery. Successful treatment usually involves applying enough localized pressure over the area to "flatten" or compress the aneurysm while not totally obstructing the pulse in the involved extremity peripheral to the lesion. Pressure is applied for up to 24 hours. Occasionally these aneurysms have been ligated or evacuated surgically.

Arteriovenous fistulae

Arteriovenous fistulae present as localized painful swellings, which, in addition, are associated with a continuous bruit over the involved area. These result from through and through or very close simultaneous punctures of the artery and the vein in the same introductory site, as described in Chapter 4. Meticulous, gentle, single wall, vessel puncture techniques, keeping the puncture sites between the artery and the vein separated and meticulous care following the withdrawal of the sheaths are usually effective in preventing this complication. When the arteriovenous fistula is recognized early after the procedure, the area is compressed with a pressure dressing which is tight enough to allow only a very faintly palpable pulse distal to the fistula in the involved extremity. The pressure dressing is maintained in place with this degree of compression for at least 24 hours; however, the area is checked at least every 2 hours for persistence of the fistula and persistence of a good pulse in the artery distal to the compression dressing over the fistula. In smaller patients, if the fistula persists surgical division and repair of the fistula is recommended. In a larger patient, with larger vessels, closure with one of the double disk occluder devices is considered.

Perforation or dissection of vascular structures

The other complications related specifically to the retrograde technique involve the perforation or dissection of vascular structures by the retrograde wire or catheter. Perforations of arteries in the inguinal area, which occur cephalad to the inguinal ligament, usually result in a retroperitoneal hemorrhage, which is manifest initially by fairly localized abdominal pain. With an arterial perforation, the pain is usually progressive and is associated with a drop in the patient's hemoglobin/hematocrit. A small perforation may seal itself, however, unless the pain subsides and the hemoglobin/hematocrit stabilizes, the retroperitoneal perforation will require surgical intervention. These perforations usually occur in the iliac artery from percutaneous punctures, which are too cephalad in the inguinal area, or from force applied to catheters/wires being maneuvered in the pelvic arteries.

Perforation of more central vascular structures is likely to occur when a wire is forced out of the tip of a catheter while the catheter is constrained or the tip is wedged into a structure or tightly against the vascular wall, as illustrated in Chapter 6. Similar perforations can occur in the aortic sinuses and in the left ventricular cavity when a wire is pushed either blindly or forcefully out of the tip of a constrained catheter, or when a stiff catheter, which is itself constrained in the aortic arch, is pushed into these areas. Perforations can occur when a catheter is deflected with an active (controllable) deflector wire when the catheter is constrained and the catheter/wire does not have room to form the desired curve that is being created by the active deflector wire. When the distal end of the catheter does not have room to "back away" in order to form a curve/loop and, in turn, the distal tip of the catheter cannot "push away" from the tissues, the wire or catheter is forced to dig into and through the tissues of the chamber/vessel wall.

The treatment of perforations primarily is prevention by avoiding maneuvers that have a higher risk of perforation. Once a perforation does occur, its management depends upon its size and location and its immediate consequences. There is always extravasation of blood and even significant blood loss following an arterial perforation but, occasionally, this is self-limiting because of the small size of the perforation, or the extravasation is constrained by the surrounding tissues. The maneuvers with the catheter that occurred immediately preceding the perforation should provide a strong indication as to the site of the perforation. Regardless of the size of the perforation and the proposed management, the exact site should be identified precisely with an angiogram in, or just proximal to, the suspected area, and the surgeons should be alerted to the problem. When a large amount of blood does escape from a perforation, the extravasated blood must be withdrawn from the space where it has accumulated by either a pericardiocentesis or a thoracocentesis. With large amounts of blood loss, the blood is replaced with previously cross-matched whole blood and/or by auto transfusion with the blood that is recovered from the bleeding site. If the bleeding persists, a decision is made as to whether the perforation/tear can be closed with a catheter-delivered device (occlusion device or covered stent) or whether surgical repair will be necessary. When the perforation is in an artery, often a balloon can be inflated in the artery adjacent to the perforation in order to stop the acute blood loss and, in doing so, to assess whether a catheter intervention may be possible. When surgery is necessary, the patient is taken to the operating room for surgical repair of the hole or tear as soon as the operating room is ready.

Central nervous system

Central nervous system (CNS) injuries, which are presumed to be due to embolizations associated with retrograde left heart catheterization procedures, are very serious complications and are always a possibility during catheterization in the systemic arterial circulation. CNS events are usually a result of the embolization of air or particulate matter to the brain. The consequences of such embolization can be as minor as a slight degree of transient confusion or a short isolated seizure to the other extremes of complete hemiplegia or even death. Again the best treatment is prevention by the use of meticulous techniques to avoid the introduction of either air or clot into the vascular system from the catheters. Patients undergoing catheter/wire manipulations in the systemic (or potentially systemic!) circulation should definitely receive heparin and have their ACT maintained at ~300 sec. The catheters or wires within catheters in the systemic circulation should be maintained on a nearly constant flush. Wires within the circulation should be kept within a catheter and on a vigorous flush for as much of the time as possible.

In the event of a massive cerebrovascular accident, the patient should have an immediate head MRI or head CT scan and a neurology consultation. If, as is usually the case, the etiology is a thrombus, the patient is considered for treatment with tPA under the supervision of a neurologist.

References

1. Mullins CE. Transseptal left heart catheterization: experience with a new technique in 520 pediatric and adult patients. *Pediatr Cardiol* 1983; **4**: 239–246.
2. Mullins CE *et al.* Retrograde technique for catheterization of the pulmonary artery in transposition of the great arteries with ventricular septal defect. *Am J Cardiol* 1972; **30**(4): 385–387.
3. Linde LM *et al.* Umbilical vessel cardiac catheterization and angiocardiography. *Circulation* 1966; **34**(6): 984–988.
4. Fischer DR *et al.* Carotid artery approach for balloon dilation of aortic valve stenosis in the neonate: a preliminary report. *J Am Coll Cardiol* 1990; **15**(7): 1633–1636.
5. Peuster M *et al.* Percutaneous transluminal angioplasty for the treatment of complete arterial occlusion after retrograde cardiac catheterization in infancy. *Am J Cardiol* 1999; **84**(9): 1124–1126, A11.
6. Wessel DL *et al.* Fibrinolytic therapy for femoral arterial thrombosis after cardiac catheterization in infants and children. *Am J Cardiol* 1986; **58**(3): 347–351.
7. Brus F *et al.* Streptokinase treatment for femoral artery thrombosis after arterial cardiac catheterisation in infants and children. *Br Heart J* 1990; **63**(5): 291–294.
8. Balaguru D *et al.* Early and late results of thrombolytic therapy using tissue-type plasminogen activator to restore arterial pulse after cardiac catheterization in infants and small children. *Am J Cardiol* 2003; **91**(7): 908–910.

10 Hemodynamics, data acquisition, and interpretation and presentation of data

Introduction

The purpose of diagnostic cardiac catheterizations in congenital heart patients is to define the *exact* anatomy of the lesions, to define the *exact* hemodynamic abnormalities and to determine, *accurately*, the severity of these abnormalities. The anatomy is defined with selective and appropriate angiocardiograms. The techniques and procedures for obtaining quality angiocardiograms are discussed in the next chapter (Chapter 11, "Angiography"). The hemodynamic information is generated from the intravascular pressures, determination of the oxygen saturations of the blood from all locations, and other indicator dilution studies obtained during the cardiac catheterization procedure.

The scientist in all physicians has a great urge to transform numerical information into formulas that provide mathematical solutions to any particular problem. Most calculations based on the hemodynamic data acquired in the catheterization laboratory are a reflection of this attempt. Most of the formulas used in calculating the hemodynamics in the heart and circulation are derived from mechanical or hydraulic formulas, which were generated in systems made up of rigid tubing (Bernoulli, Poiseuille, Venturi, Gorlin, Hamilton–Stewart). However, because of the complexity and elasticity of the human circulation and no matter how accurate the basic data, none of the calculated hemodynamic data are gospel or irrefutable. The errors in the many calculations, however, can be minimized by the accurate collection of basic data from which the calculations are derived.

The cardiologist performing the catheterization (the "operator") is responsible for the acquisition of accurate and truly representative pressure recordings, meaningful sampling for oxygen saturation determinations, and the performance of accurate cardiac output measurements. The operator determines when, and which pressures are recorded, from which sites oxygen saturations are obtained, the order in which they are obtained and the number of samples which are necessary to validate the calculations. The operator also must distinguish between hemodynamic data that are truly abnormal and those which are erroneous or artifactual owing to the sampling techniques. The operator determines which of the data are valid, important, and to be permanently recorded.

Modern cardiac catheterization laboratories have very sophisticated, accurate and stable physiologic recording systems. The requirements of these recorders are discussed in Chapter 3, "Equipment". Electronic physiologic recording systems in the modern cardiac catheterization laboratory have solid-state electronics and are computer controlled. Physiologic recording systems, all of which have similar basic features, are available from many manufacturers. The combination of the stability of modern, solid-state electronics, the competition between manufacturers for "market share", and the imposed regulatory requirements from the government, has resulted in the availability of extremely accurate and stable recording systems. The differences between the available recording systems are mostly in the extra features ("bells and whistles") and the particular conveniences in the use of each machine. All of the physiologic recorders currently used in modern catheterization laboratories record any data that are transmitted to them very accurately, but neither the recording system nor the computer system can determine which data are to be transmitted or recorded, nor can the equipment distinguish valid from artifactual data. The operator in the catheterization laboratory is responsible for the accuracy of the data that are transmitted to the recorder.

When the operating cardiologist wishes to record the pressure from a particular location, the nurse or technician makes a note on the computer record of the location and physically turns on the recorder to record the pressure curves. An experienced cardiac catheterization laboratory nurse or technician should recognize a poor or unusable pressure tracing and should inform the operating cardiologist if he (she) has not noted and corrected it on his (her) own. The nurse or technician, however, *should not* make the final determination of exactly which pressures are satisfactory, valid or even usable. Nor should the nurse or technician make the decision exactly when to begin the pressure recording; at what gain to record the pressure; nor for how long a particular pressure tracing should be recorded. The validity and accuracy of all of the pressures obtained and recorded, like all of the other data, are the responsibility of the operating cardiologist.

Similarly, during the acquisition of oxygen saturation data in the cardiac catheterization laboratory, a nurse or technician performs the analysis of the blood samples obtained from the patient, reads the oxygen saturation that is displayed on the oxygen analyzer and then transmits or records these data to/on the permanent record. Although the experienced nurse/technician often has valuable input about the catheterization procedure or the status of the patient, they do not maneuver or position the catheter for a sample; they are not responsible for recognizing the exact location where the "sample" is obtained; nor are they responsible for determining whether the value obtained from the sample has any significance or not. The nurse or technician also does not determine how many blood samples are needed for oxygen saturation determinations in order to validate the presence or absence of a shunt. These determinations are all the responsibility of the cardiologist who is performing the catheterization.

The operating cardiologist must be aware of ***every bit*** of data ***as it is acquired***. For *all* of the data acquired from the catheterization procedure, the time to recognize and rule out artifacts or erroneous data is *during the procedure*, while the data are still being collected, and *not* when reviewing the data after the case has been completed! There are several useful rules to consider when obtaining and recording data. Assume that *every bit of data* that is recorded: (1) is critical in determining the outcome of that particular patient; (2) may be published; and (3) may be used in a court of law against the operator!

Pressure recording

As a reflection of the "mechanical" pumping action of the heart, its sophisticated inflow and outflow valve systems and the elasticity of the entire cardiovascular system, multiple, different, and continually varying normal pressures are generated within the heart and vascular system. Deviations from these known "normals" in the pressures provide diagnostic information about the cardiac function and the status of the various components of the cardiovascular system. In order to recognize abnormal pressures, the operating cardiologist must be thoroughly familiar with the "normal" pressure curves and pressure values from every location within the heart and vascular system.

Pressures in the chambers or vessels can be recorded very accurately from directly within the chamber or vessel with a pressure sensor or micromanometer (transducer) positioned at the tip of a catheter or wire. More commonly, intravascular pressures are measured indirectly through hollow tubing and a contiguous fluid column, which is connected to a remote pressure sensor (transducer) outside of the body. With either recording system the *exact* location (height) of the catheter tip micromanometer or the end hole(s) at the tip of the fluid-filled catheter must be identified radiographically at the precise time of the recording.

Remote transducers connected through a fluid column

In the large majority of clinical cardiac catheterization laboratories, "remote" transducers are used for pressure recording. Intracavitary and vascular pressures are transmitted through a long "fluid column" as a pressure pulse wave to remote transducers. The fluid column extends from the distal opening(s) of a catheter that is positioned in the site within the vascular system, through the catheter to a fluid-filled connecting tube outside of the vascular system, and to the transducer, which is positioned on, or adjacent to, the catheterization table. The pressure wave itself is transmitted through the entire fluid column and sensed, measured and recorded at this remote transducer.

The fluid column actually acts as an extension of the fluid in the chamber or vessel where the tip of the catheter is located. Fluid-filled catheters frequently have multiple side holes, which extend for at least a centimeter along the sides at the distal tip of the catheter. As a consequence, the multiple holes have the possibility of "bridging" across several adjacent locations within the vascular system and creating artifactual readings that are "fusions" of two pressures from adjacent areas, with the resultant pressure not being representative of the pressure from either area. For pressure recording from precise areas using a fluid-filled catheter, the catheter must have a single end hole or, at most, two additional openings within 1–2 mm of its tip.

The fluid column between the vascular site and the transducer includes the fluid within the length of the catheter itself, fluid in all connectors and stopcocks and within all connecting tubing between the proximal end of the catheter and the remote transducer, the small amount of fluid in the transducer itself, and the fluid within the connectors of the transducer to the tubing. The pulse wave generated in the chamber or vessel must be transmitted along this long, complex fluid column to the transducer as an identical pulse wave. The absolute integrity of the ***entire** fluid column* and *the tubing containing the fluid* is critical in the transmission of an accurate pressure waveform to the transducer.

The pressure curves display very minute deflections that reflect even the most minor pressure changes. With the proper connecting tubing, proper fluid in the column, meticulous flushing of all segments of the fluid column including that in the transducer, along with properly operating and accurately calibrated transducers, pressures recorded from fluid column systems are crisp, smooth and very accurate, and are comparable with the pressure curves obtained from catheter or wire tipped transducers, which are discussed later in this chapter. At the same time, this pressure measurement/recording system—with the long complex, interposed fluid column—does present the opportunity for many different types of artifacts or erroneous pressure waveforms.

In order to transmit the pressure accurately, the entire length of tubing between the pressure source and the transducer (the catheter and connecting tubing) *must* be non-elastic (non-compliant) and have an adequate and fairly uniform diameter of its lumen. Most cardiac catheters themselves have fairly rigid walls, are very non-compliant and, in general, transmit pressures reliably. Usually the firmer the shaft of the catheter, the better the pressure transmission. There are, however, a few polyethylene catheters and catheters with very small lumens (< 4-French catheters) that transmit pressure poorly, and generally these should be avoided when very accurate pressures are required.

There are many varieties of commercially available, flexible connecting tubing, which are very satisfactory for the connection between the proximal end of the catheter and the transducer. However, any tubing with soft or compliant walls, such as that which is often attached to the side ports of sheaths and back-bleed valves, attenuates the pressure transmission and is not satisfactory for use within the pressure system. Compliant or soft tubing dampens (smoothes or flattens) the pressure curves. However, very "elastic" tubing produces exactly the opposite effect. Because of the elastic recoil of the tubing, a marked "overshoot" (exaggeration) of the pressure curves is created.

The entire fluid column within this tubing must be one continuous, intact column of a non-compressible liquid. It must be completely free of air, blood, clots or contrast material anywhere along the column. Many of the current plastic materials used in the connecting tubing/system are virtually "non wettable" and, as a consequence, tend to trap minute bubbles along their inner surfaces. As the fluids warm, the trapped gases within the fluid effervesce from the fluid into larger bubbles.

There are usually multiple connectors or stopcocks between the catheter and the transducer including the manifold to which the transducer is attached. Each junction in the system or stopcock represents a potential disruption of the fluid column. A loose connection or, more commonly, a trapped micro-bubble of air at one of the junctions totally interrupts the transmission of the pressure wave through the fluid column. It is extremely important that all junctions and stopcocks along the course of the tubing are cleared of even minute bubbles to obtain accurate recordings. Each junction should be tapped *vigorously* with a hard instrument as the fluid system is flushed vigorously into a flush bowl on the table at the onset of the case and again anytime during the procedure when the pressure curves change or deteriorate.

Originally, pressure transducers were small and extremely accurate Wheatstone bridges or "strain gauges". The strain gauge transmitted infinitesimally small movements of a fluid column into small movements of a diaphragm in the transducer. The diaphragm movements changed the distances and, in turn, the electrical resistances between pairs of resistors. These changes were converted into variations in an electrical signal that was passing through the resistors, which was displayed on the screen of a cathode ray tube (CRT) or other monitor as a pressure curve. These pressure curves were electronically attenuated from electrical interference so they were not "flingy" or ragged appearing.

Modern transducers have much smaller and more rigid diaphragms, which move solid state crystals to produce the electrical signal of the pressure curve. These solid state transducers are equally as accurate, and more stable than, Wheatstone bridge transducers. At the same time, solid-state technology has allowed for a much less expensive manufacturing process for these transducers, making them essentially disposable. This allows for the easy replacement of the transducer if there is any question of its accuracy. The electrical signals from the transducers are transmitted and recorded as pressure curves in the physiologic recording apparatus, a tape or disk recording system and/or onto a paper record.

A remote transducer is usually positioned on the rail of the catheterization table at one side of the patient, or occasionally, actually lying on the surface of the catheterization table itself near or on the patient's feet or legs. In order to compensate for different patient sizes, the transducer itself or a reference, "zero point" of an open fluid column, connected directly to the transducer, is positioned at the "mid-chest" level, halfway between the front and back of the thorax[1]. The transducer is calibrated to zero electronically with this zero fluid level opened to the room atmosphere at the mid-chest level. The transducer or "zero level" tubing is attached to the table at this level so that it moves up or down with the patient when the patient and table are moved up or down.

This measured and fixed zero level does not take into account the differences in vertical height between various locations *within* the cardiac chambers and vascular system. Each difference of 2.5 cm in vertical height creates a

1.9 mmHg difference in pressure; however, in the usual anatomy, and particularly in smaller patients, these internal vertical distances and the resultant pressure differences are negligible. In large patients, particularly where pressures are being recorded from the lower-pressure areas (for example the distance in a supine patient between the posterior of the left atrium and the anterior of the right atrium) the pressure difference due to the difference in height between the two locations can lead to erroneous "gradients". When there is concern about this, the actual distances between the catheter tips are visualized and measured accurately using the lateral X-ray system in the straight lateral view. In the biplane pediatric catheterization laboratory, any significant discrepancy in these vertical distances becomes apparent very readily during the normal, intermittent use of the lateral fluoroscopy plane.

In most catheterization procedures involving complex congenital heart lesions, *at least* two, if not more, catheters are used simultaneously. Two catheters with their tips positioned in the same location within the cardiovascular system offer the best opportunity to verify the accuracy of the entire pressure recording system. With properly functioning transducers and properly prepared and flushed fluid lines and connections, the two separate pressure tracings from the two separate catheters positioned in the same location and displayed or recorded at the same pressure gain produce a ***single line*** (Figure 10.1). This almost *single line* tracing from the superimposed tracings from *two separate catheters* and *two separate pressure systems/transducers* verifies the accuracy of the entire system! The lower the gain on the recording apparatus, the more accurate this comparison of the pressure curves will be. For example two venous pressures that are displayed at a maximum pressure gain of 10 mmHg, demonstrate very vividly even tiny differences between the two, supposedly identical pressure curves, while if the same pressure curves are displayed at a pressure gain of 100 mmHg, differences of 1–2 mmHg are easily missed.

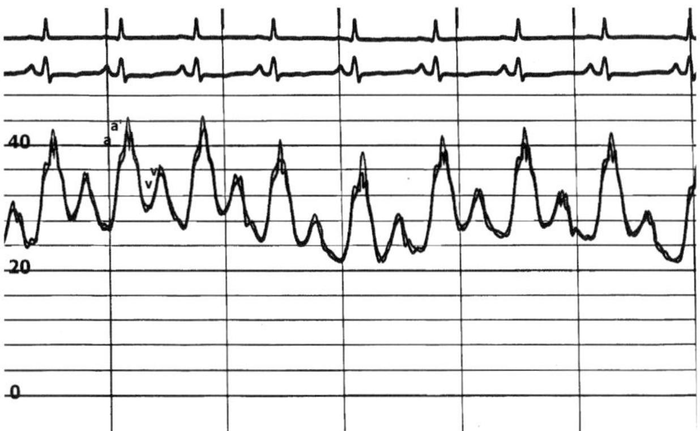

Figure 10.1 "Single" pressure curve from two separate catheters in the left atrium recorded through two separate pressure systems.

When *more* than two catheters are used during a catheterization, it is imperative to check the pressure curve from *each additional* catheter (and pressure system) against one of the other, already verified or corrected, pressure curves from one of the other catheters. Two, three, four or more simultaneous pressures generated from the same location, and displayed at the same gain, should display a *single line pressure curve of all the superimposed curves*! This verifies the integrity of the entire pressure system and of each separate catheter/pressure system. When a pressure curve from any separate catheter or pressure system does not superimpose, the source of error is investigated and corrected before proceeding with any pressure measurements during the catheterization procedure.

During the catheterization, when a pressure measurement or recording is made from any location, a separate "reference pressure" is recorded simultaneously. The usual reference pressure is a peripheral arterial pressure tracing from the indwelling arterial line or catheter. The arterial pressure is displayed continuously and recorded simultaneously along with any other pressure being recorded. If this reference pressure is *not* always present, a difference in pressure between two locations that is recorded at different times and under different physiologic conditions, can be interpreted erroneously as a "pressure gradient" between the two sites, even when no difference actually exists. The simultaneously recorded reference pressure clearly demonstrates changes in *all of the pressures* along with any changes in the patient's "steady state".

As an example of the value of the reference pressure: At the beginning of the catheterization a patient with a suspected large ventricular septal defect has a *right* ventricular pressure of 70/0–3 while a simultaneous femoral arterial pressure of 80/45 mmHg is recorded. As the case progresses, the patient receives a bolus infusion of extra fluid, still more fluid from catheter flushes, and undergoes several right-sided angiograms. Somewhat later in the case, a pressure of 95/0–8 is recorded from the *left* ventricle. This, alone, suggests a 25 mm gradient between the two ventricles and, in turn, a restrictive VSD! In actuality, the femoral systemic pressure now is 105/60 with all of the intravascular/intracardiac pressures increased by the "volume expansion". When rechecked against this systemic pressure, the right ventricular pressure also is 95/0–8! Without the reference arterial pressure, the overall pressure rise in all of the chambers or vessels can go unrecognized and lead to erroneous conclusions.

As with all pressure systems, the pressure tracing from the reference catheter/transducer must also be checked against another catheter/transducer system being used in the patient at the beginning of the case, as described previously. If the arterial line itself is being used for pressure recording (e.g. across an aortic valve or aortic obstruction) a pressure from another catheter, even in a right-sided site, is recorded as the reference for the arterial tracing. The new reference pressure from the catheter has already had its own "steady state" reference against the original arterial pressure recording and any changes in the patient's steady state are reflected equally by changes in any second pressure. With a reference tracing always on the recording, pressures from all locations can be compared to the "original reference" and, in turn, to each other regardless of the differences in the patient's "steady state" at the different times of the actual recordings.

When measuring the pressure difference (gradient) between two locations, *two simultaneous pressures from two separate catheters* are preferable to a "pull-back" pressure tracing using a single catheter. This of course assumes that the two pressure systems are balanced accurately and are identical. Two simultaneous pressure tracings measure and record the actual pressure differences, precisely, on a beat-to-beat basis, with no interposed artifact from catheter movement, hand motion on the catheter and/or respiratory variations to affect the actual *gradient*.

A "pull-back" tracing, on the other hand, measures the pressures *sequentially, not* necessarily under the same hemodynamic conditions and always with superimposed catheter/operator's hand motion artifact(s) on the tracing of the pressure waveforms. When pressures are measured sequentially, there are frequently significant fluctuations in the base-line pressures during the pull back due to the operator's hand movements (tremors), the patient's respirations, the patient's movement due to straining from pain or from extra beats or true arrhythmias (Figure 10.2). When using a a pull-back tracing, the sequential pressures that are recorded must be adjusted to account for these artifacts before the gradient can be *estimated* rather than actually *measured*. When pull-back recordings are used, very long recordings before and after the catheter withdrawal must be recorded in order to visualize, and to be able to adjust for, all of the variations in the base-line pressures. This is particularly important when measuring pressures in low-pressure systems.

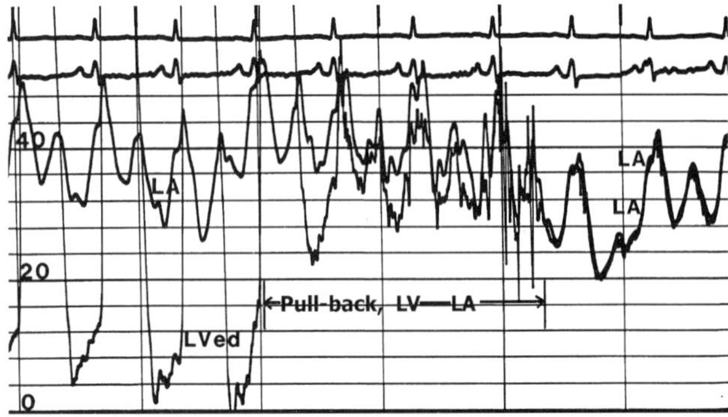

Figure 10.2 "Pull-back" pressure curve from left ventricle (LV) to left atrium (LA) with a simultaneous separate left atrial pressure tracing; LVed, left ventricular end diastolic.

Errors in pressure sensing/recording due to the fluid column when using remote transducers

Errors in the mid-chest, zero level of the transducer or the open zero fluid column create a very common, but, at the same time, easy to recognize and easy to correct abnormality in the pressure tracings. When a cardiac catheter is first introduced into the venous system, a systemic venous (or right atrial) pressure can be obtained through the catheter. With knowledge of the patient's clinical diagnosis, the operator is immediately able to recognize whether the displayed venous pressure correlates with that particular patient's clinical status or is at least close to a "reasonable" value. An atrial mean or a ventricular end-diastolic pressure tracing which registers at or below the zero base-line on the monitor or the recorder, indicates that either the transducer or the zero reference is too high for the particular patient or the patient is extremely volume depleted. The same pressures registering well below the zero line definitely are the result of a transducer zero reference level that is too high. A disproportionately high venous or ventricular end-diastolic pressure, on the other hand, suggests either severe right heart failure, or, more likely, that the zero reference level is too low. The measurement for the height of the transducer should be double checked against a radio-opaque marker positioned at mid chest or even compared to the level of the tip of the catheter in the right atrium on the lateral fluoroscope image.

Other very common abnormalities in pressure tracings occur because of interruptions in the continuity or integrity of the fluid column between the tip of the catheter and the transducer. The interruption can be from inclusions of bubbles or clots within the fluid column or from a mixture of several fluids with different densities (e.g. saline with blood or contrast) within the fluid column. A very tiny gas (usually air) bubble anywhere in the long, complex column of fluid causes a major overshoot or "spike" in the pressure tracing. These spikes result in an exaggeration of both the peak systolic and the ventricular end-systolic pressures (Figure 10.3). An immediate clue to the presence of this artifact is the sharp "spiky" appearance of the peak systolic pressure curve and the presence of end-systole ventricular pressure curves that pass well below the zero base-line. Physiologic pressure curves do not have sharp spikes! Any such pressure curves must be investigated and corrected before any recording is performed. The tiny bubbles accumulate from the effervescence of gas from the flush fluid itself as it warms within the tubing/transducers. These microbubbles can occur

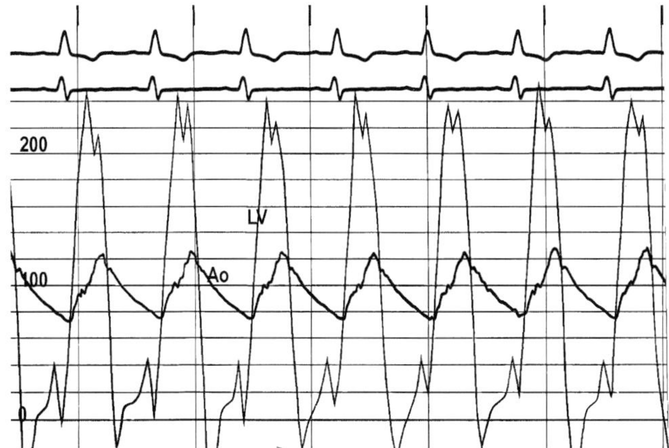

Figure 10.3 The exaggeration of end-systolic and peak systolic left ventricular pressure tracing due to "microbubbles" within the fluid column giving a very "spiky" left ventricular pressure curve.

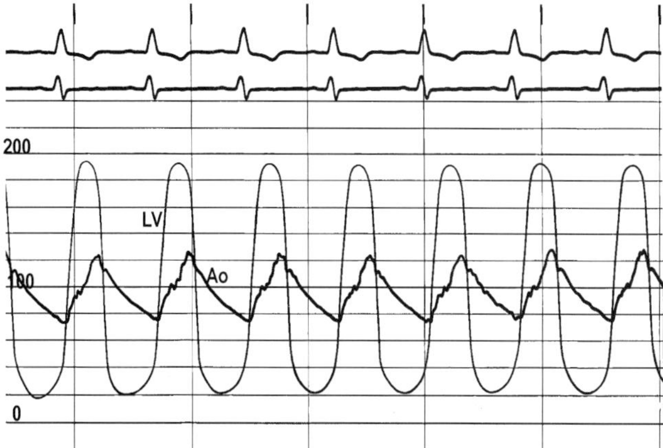

Figure 10.4 Dampened left ventricular pressure curve with blunting and lowering of the peak systolic pressure and blunting and elevation of the end systolic/diastolic pressures.

even if the system was flushed and completely cleared of bubbles previously. They are very elusive, "hiding" and clinging within the catheter, the plastic connecting tubing, in the junctions and stopcocks between the segments of tubing or even in the transducers themselves.

The *only valid* solution to this "fling or spiking" artifact is to remove the offending bubble(s) from the fluid column. The tubing system is first disconnected or diverted away from the catheter which is in the patient. In order to dislodge these "micro bubbles", each of the segments and connections in the tubing/transducer fluid "column" throughout its entire length is tapped *crisply and vigorously* with a metal instrument while the system is flushed thoroughly. Fluid is withdrawn from the separated catheter while the hub is tapped and then the catheter is hand flushed and reattached to the cleared fluid column. These "micro bubbles" can be very elusive and resistant to dislodging, particularly in the virtually non-wettable plastic materials of the tubing, connectors and transducers themselves. If the artifact is not eliminated even after the fluid column (including the fluid in the transducer) is entirely free of bubbles, the transducer should be exchanged.

The *appearance* of the "overshoot" can be erroneously eliminated by the introduction of contrast or blood into the fluid column. This much denser fluid dampens the "overshoot" and smoothes out the curve. However, this, in turn, superimposes a *second* artifact that *obscures*, but does not *eliminate* the original artifact, and produces a doubly erroneous pressure curve. Seldom do two wrongs make a right! This "remedy" may create smoother or "prettier" recordings, but certainly does *not* produce *accurate* pressure recordings.

In contrast to the "micro bubbles", a denser fluid, a *large* bubble of air, or a clot within the fluid column are all inclusions that flatten or "dampen" the pressure waveform. Large gas bubbles create "air locks" which flatten (dampen) the pressure wave significantly. Fluids such as blood or contrast medium, which are significantly denser than physiologic flush solutions, "resonate" at a much lower frequency than the flush solution and dampen the waveform. Very small clots easily compromise or totally occlude the small lumen of a cardiac catheter and dampen or obliterate the pressure wave. Thrombi commonly form at the tips of catheters following wire exchanges through the catheter. Blood that refluxes back into a catheter and is not flushed out, thromboses and compromises or can occlude the lumen of the catheter.

A smoothing, or "rounding-off" of both the top and bottom of the pressure curve indicates an artifact from one of these inclusions in the fluid column (Figure 10.4). In addition there will be no end systolic/diastolic deflections in the ventricular curve and no anacrotic or dicrotic notches on the arterial pressure curves. In addition to the rounding-off of the curve, there is a lowering of the peak systolic pressure and an elevation of the end-systolic and diastolic pressures. In extreme cases of this artifact, the pressure wave appears like a sine wave or even becomes a mechanical mean of the systolic and diastolic pressures. To correct these artifacts, all non-flush solution, bubbles or clots must be withdrawn from the catheter and flushed from the catheter tubing before the catheter and tubing are refilled with an *uninterrupted* column of clean flush solution.

A segment of very compliant or soft connecting/flush tubing interposed as an extension tubing in the pressure/flush system will produce this same artifact of a dampened pressure curve. Similarly, a fluid column that is too narrow to transmit fluid waves also flattens or dampens the waveform of the pressure curve. This usually is the result of using a catheter that is too small in diameter (e.g. 3-French or even some 4-French in some materials). The only solution to this problem is to replace the catheter or tubing. A kink in the catheter or pressure line will also dampen or obliterate the pressure. Usually, however, a kink interrupts the pressure abruptly or intermittently as the catheter is maneuvered. A kink in the catheter is easy to identify by visualizing the course of the catheter under fluoroscopy.

Some catheter materials (e.g. woven dacron) actually swell when exposed to "moisture" at body temperature, as a result of which the internal diameter of the lumen of a very small catheter can be reduced so much as to make it unusable. This problem is recognized by an initially good, crisp pressure curve when the small catheter is first introduced but in which, as the case progresses, the pressure gradually dampens. The "normal" appearance of the pressure may return transiently after the catheter is flushed, only to be re-dampened within minutes (seconds) after each flush. The only solution in order to obtain meaningful data in this circumstance is to exchange the catheter.

A tiny thrombus at the end of the catheter results in a similar intermittent dampening of the pressure. Flushing the catheter often improves the pressure curve for a few cardiac beats, only to have the dampening recur within a few seconds. This is a common occurrence after the withdrawal of a spring guide wire from the catheter where fibrin or actual thrombi are stripped off the wire and withdrawn into the tip of the catheter lumen as the wire is withdrawn into the catheter. In this circumstance, either the clot must be withdrawn completely from the catheter by strong, forceful suction on it or the catheter is exchanged.

There are several logical and fairly quick steps to verify that there actually is an artifact in the pressure curve and then for determining the source of the error when the pressure curve is artifactual. The types of artifactual pressure recordings—as described in the previous paragraphs—provide clues to the source of the abnormal curve. The first step is to open the transducer and fluid line to air zero, flush the lines outside of the body thoroughly, and then "rebalance" the transducer(s). Once these fundamentals have been performed, the pressure recording from the suspect catheter is checked against a pressure recording from the same location through a second catheter with a completely separate fluid tubing system and transducer.

If the two curves are different in amplitude but identical in configuration, even though set to record at the same gain, usually the electronic calibration of one of the transducers is off. Each transducer comes with its own specific electronic calibration factor, which is electronically adjusted, in the recording apparatus. Occasionally this factor is off or drifts in value. The easiest check is to change the transducer for a new one. Modern electronics and manufacturing have allowed the production of very accurate, stable, yet relatively cheap and disposable transducers. This allows for the frequent and easy replacement of transducers.

A more time-consuming alternative to replacing the transducer is to re-calibrate it against a mercury manometer and then reset the calibration factor on the recording apparatus during the procedure. Although this re-calibration of transducers is performed routinely and on a regular basis, the procedure is time consuming and is usually performed by, or at least requires the assistance of, the biomedical engineer, and is performed more conveniently when the catheterization laboratory is not in use.

When there is not only a different amplitude of the pressure curves obtained from the same location, but also a different configuration to the curves, the solution to the problem is a little more complicated. The first step is to electrically balance and calibrate both transducers against zero, while the suspect fluid system is flushed thoroughly. If there are still different pressures, the pressure tubing between the catheters and the transducers are switched at the *catheter hubs*. If the abnormal pressure curve "moves" to the other transducer, the catheter is at fault and needs further clearing, flushing or replacing. If the abnormal pressure curve remains with the original transducer, the original tubing and/or the transducer is/are at fault. The pressure tubing between the catheters and transducers is now switched at the connection to the transducers. If the abnormal pressure is now generated from the other transducer, the connecting tubing is at fault and is replaced. If, on the other hand, the artifactual pressure remains with the same transducer, the original transducer is at fault.

If a transducer is determined to be at fault, that transducer is re-flushed, re-zeroed and its electrical connections are checked. If the pressure tracing still is not correct, the electrical connections from the two transducers to the recording apparatus are switched. If the abnormal pressure "moves channels" with the transducer, the transducer itself is at fault. When all other sources of artifacts in the pressure curves have been eliminated as the source of error, the transducer is replaced. A brand new transducer should be checked against the pressure curve from another transducer, comparing a pressure curve from the new transducer with a curve that was obtained in the same location from another catheter/transducer system.

Catheter and wire-tip micromanometers (transducers)

The most accurate pressure recordings available in the catheterization laboratory are obtained with catheter or wire-tip micromanometers (transducers) (Millar Instruments Inc., Houston, TX). These micromanometers are actually tiny piezoelectric crystals which respond directly to changes in pressure, converting the changes into a proportionate electrical signal. The tiny pressure sensors (transducers) are embedded in, or near, the tip of a catheter or guide wire. The pressure is actually measured within the chamber or vessel by the micromanometer crystal, which is positioned in the chamber. The pressure is converted into an electrical signal and the electrical signal from the catheter or wire-tip micromanometer is transmitted from the catheter tip to an amplifier, monitor and recorder. As a consequence, all of the common artifacts due to the interposed fluid column, which are a part of the system using remote transducers, are eliminated by the use of catheter-tipped pressure transducers.

A high-quality, properly functioning catheter or wire-tip transducer provides pressure curves that are extremely sensitive and accurate. With these catheter/wire-tip transducers, there are no artificial pressures created by a difference in the height of the *transducer* relative to the *chamber*, however, catheter or wire-tip transducers are so sensitive that gradients can be recorded between two catheter or wire-tip transducers which are positioned at significantly different *vertical* heights from each other but are still within the same chamber! The transducers are small enough that two or more transducers can be mounted at different locations on a single catheter or they can be mounted with other additional sensors (flow meters). With more than one micromanometer or a flow meter on a catheter, simultaneous pressures with or without simultaneous flow measurements from different areas within the heart or vascular tree can be recorded using only one catheter. Catheter or wire-tip transducers are invaluable when extremely precise pressure measurements are required. They are useful, particularly, for recording high-fidelity pressure curves in low-pressure areas. When derivatives of the pressure curves (dP/dT) and actual analysis of the wave forms of the pressure are desired, catheter/wire-tip micromanometers are the only type of transducer that should be used.

Pressure recordings from catheter/wire-tip micromanometers are not without some problems. Artifacts in the high-fidelity pressure curves can, and do occur. Artifacts occur when the tip of the catheter/wire (with the transducer) is entrapped in either a trabecula or a small side branch vessel or when the catheter/wire-tip transducer along with the catheter/wire is "bounced" against structures within the heart/vessel as the heart beats. As mentioned above, erroneous pressure gradients can also be recorded when there is a significant *vertical* distance between the transducers within the heart. For example, in the supine patient, if one transducer is positioned anteriorly in the right atrium with the other transducer positioned posteriorly in the left atrium, an electrical adjustment for the difference in vertical distance often must be made to record accurate and comparable pressures. Each 2.5 cm in vertical distance within the heart results in a 1.9 mmHg difference in pressure. This height difference produces large "artifactual gradients" within the low-pressure (venous) system, particularly in very large hearts!

The catheter tip transducer catheters themselves have some inherent disadvantages. Catheters containing catheter-tip transducers are difficult to maneuver compared to the usual diagnostic, cardiac catheters. In addition, most of the catheters with transducers at the tip do *not* have a catheter lumen which would allow passage over a wire, deflection with a wire, or withdrawal of samples or injections for angiograms through the catheter. These problems with the catheters themselves make them impractical for routine diagnostic catheterizations.

Wire-tipped transducers overcome many of the technical problems encountered with maneuvering catheters with tip transducers. The wires are small enough in diameter (0.014″) that they pass through the lumen of very small catheters. In this way, a small, standard, diagnostic, end-hole catheter can be maneuvered into, and through, difficult areas and then the wire with the transducer at the tip can be advanced beyond the catheter. The catheter along with the wire can be torqued in order to direct the wire selectively into very small or tortuous locations distal to the tip of the catheter.

The crystals of the micromanometers on both the catheter and the wire-tip transducers are quite fragile. Before, and repeatedly during, measurements, they require precise and somewhat tedious calibration. Catheter and wire-tip transducers also are very expensive. The expense makes them hard to consider as disposable but, in the current catheterization laboratory environment, it is difficult, or, realistically, impossible, to re-sterilize and reuse them in patients. Because of these negative factors, catheter and wire-tip transducers are seldom used in the clinical cardiac catheterization laboratory.

With their accuracy and in spite of their problems, the pressure tracings from catheter/wire-tip transducers serve as the "gold standard" for absolutely accurate pressure recordings of both amplitude and configuration of pressure curves.

Physiologic artifacts in pressure tracings/recordings

In addition to the previously described artifacts which originate from the catheters, fluid columns and transducers, the intravascular pressures from the human vascular system generate a considerable variety of physiological variation. Significant changes in intravascular pressure tracings commonly occur during even normal respiration due to the physiologic changes in the intrathoracic pressure. These respiratory variations are greatly exaggerated when the patient experiences any respiratory difficulty during the catheterization. During normal respirations, there is a 3–8 mmHg negative pressure deflection with each *inspiratory* (active) respiratory effort. Because of this, pressure measurements from the recordings in a patient who is breathing normally, should be taken at the end expiratory (passive) phase of the respiratory cycle. This is particularly important when measuring the generally lower pressures in the pulmonary arterial, right ventricular, all atrial and any capillary wedge positions.

The most common and significant artifacts in the pressure curves are a result of ventilation problems related to upper airway obstruction, in which case the negative intrathoracic pressure during inspiration can be magnified greatly. Negative intrathoracic pressures greater than minus 50 mmHg can be generated with severe inspiratory obstruction! Obviously, with such extreme sweeps in the base-line pressure, none of the intracardiac recordings, either during inspiration or expiration, are valid. In such circumstances every effort is made at correcting or circumventing the airway obstruction. This type of obstruction is often due to large tonsils or adenoids or a congenitally small posterior pharynx (particularly in patients with Down's syndrome). With such upper airway obstruction, pulling the jaw forward and extending or bending the neck backward or to the side occasionally is sufficient to correct the problem. If not, then an oral-pharyngeal or nasopharyngeal airway is inserted gently in order to "bypass" the obstruction. A relatively large diameter, soft, rubber, nasal "trumpet" is very effective as a "splint" for the nasal airway and is tolerated very well *once it is in place*, though the patient may require some supplemental sedation in order to tolerate the introduction of any airway. Only in rare circumstances is endotracheal intubation necessary to overcome the effects of airway obstruction. However, if the intracardiac pressures are critical for the diagnosis and decisions are to be made from the pressures, then endotracheal intubation is necessary in order to record valid pressures.

Another common, but often subtle, cause of artifacts in the pressure tracings is the result of the patient beginning to waken and becoming uncomfortable. The operator must be cognizant of a patient's experiencing discomfort or pain, which can waken the patient from a deep sleep when apparently under good sedation or even under general anesthesia. Often, the first sign of a patient waking is an increasing heart rate as a result of the patient's rising epinephrine level associated with a moving baseline of the pressure tracings as a result of their unconscious (or conscious) straining or movement.

The patient with pulmonary edema or bronchospastic disease creates another and opposite respiratory artifact in the intravascular pressures. These patients actually generate a high or positive end expiratory pressure (PEEP) from their forceful expiratory effort. This abnormal respiratory effort is recognized on the displayed pressure curves by very high or positive swings in the base-line pressure curve with each expiratory phase of the patient's respirations. If the forced expiration is persistent and cannot be corrected by treating the underlying cause, then the inspiratory phase of pressures is used as the passive or base-line pressures. In severe cases, endotracheal intubation with total control of the respirations is usually necessary in order to manage the patient's respiratory problem and to obtain valid pressure recordings.

When a patient is on a respirator, the various effects of the respirator must be taken into consideration in interpreting the pressure curves. The usual pressure or volume respirators apply positive pressure during the inflation of the lungs (inspiration) and have a passive expiratory phase. The intravascular pressures of a patient on a ventilator are measured during the *passive expiratory* phase of the respiratory cycle. For very accurate recording of intracardiac pressures in patients on a respirator, the patient is detached from the respirator temporarily for a few seconds at a time while the pressure recording is being made.

All of the normal and abnormal pressure waves in the heart are a direct consequence of the electrical stimulation of the cardiac chambers through the electrical conduction system of the heart. The contractility of the various chambers of the heart, and, as a result, each pressure wave have a temporal relationship to the ECG impulse. The atria are normally synchronized by this electrical activation to contract precisely as the adjoining ventricle is "relaxing", and vice versa—to "relax" as the ventricle contracts. This allows the atrio-ventricular or "outlet valve" of the atria to open freely into a zero, or even negative pressure in the ventricle as the atria contracts and to complete their emptying before the ventricle begins to contract. The degree of filling of the ventricle and the volume of the ventricular output are dependent upon this synchronization of contractions. As a consequence, the cardiac rhythm and the integrity of the conduction system have a marked influence on the amplitude and configuration of the pressure waves, particularly of the atrial waves. Normal sinus rhythm is necessary for the generation of normal pressure waves in the heart and vascular system.

Normal intravascular pressures

Each chamber and vessel in the cardiovascular system has characteristic, "normal" pressure waves in both amplitude and configuration. The pressure waves are all related temporally to the electrocardiographic (ECG) events. The operator must be familiar with the normal and the variations in normal pressures and the variations in normal wave forms from each location in the cardiovascular system.

The atria (and central veins) normally have characteristic, positive "a", "c" and "v" waves. The "a" pressure wave corresponds to atrial contraction. It begins at the *end* of the electrical, "p" wave of the ECG complex. At the end of atrial contraction, the "a" wave begins to descend. Its descent is interrupted very early and transiently by the small "c" wave of atrioventricular valve closure. Often the "c" wave is so small and so close to the peak of the "a" wave that it is inseparable and included in the "a" wave amplitude. The "a" or "a-c" wave is followed by a drop in pressure, the "x" descent, which corresponds to atrial relaxation. This "x" descent is interrupted by first a slow and then a rapid rise in pressure, the "v" wave, which corresponds to the filling of the atrium from the venous system against the closed atrioventricular valve. The "v" wave begins at the end of the QRS curve of the ECG and corresponds in time to ventricular systole. The "v" wave is followed by another drop in the pressure curve, the "y" descent, which corresponds to the atrial emptying into the ventricle (and ventricular filling!).

Usually the "a" and "v" waves are of similar amplitude, although the right atrial "a" wave is normally slightly higher than the "v" wave and the left atrial "v" wave may be slightly higher than the "a" wave. The "normal" atrial pressures in childhood are slightly lower than those observed in the older or adult patient. These higher pressures in older patients may well represent a slight deterioration in cardiac function rather than an increase in the true normal pressures. In childhood, the normal right atrial "a" wave is 2–8 mmHg, the "v" wave is 2–7.5 mmHg, with a mean pressure in the right atrium of 1–5 mmHg. In the left atrium, the "a" wave is 3–12 mmHg, the "v" wave is 5–13 mmHg, with a mean in the left atrium of 2–10 mmHg (Figure 10.5).

If there is no naturally occurring access to the left atrium and left atrial pressures are necessary, but the operator is unskilled in or uncomfortable with the atrial transseptal procedure, a pulmonary artery capillary "wedge pressure" can provide an adequate reflection of a left atrial pressure. The pulmonary veins have no venous valves, so a pressure from an end-hole catheter that is "wedged" in the pulmonary arterial capillary bed should reflect the venous pressure from "downstream" (i.e. from the pulmonary veins/left atrium).

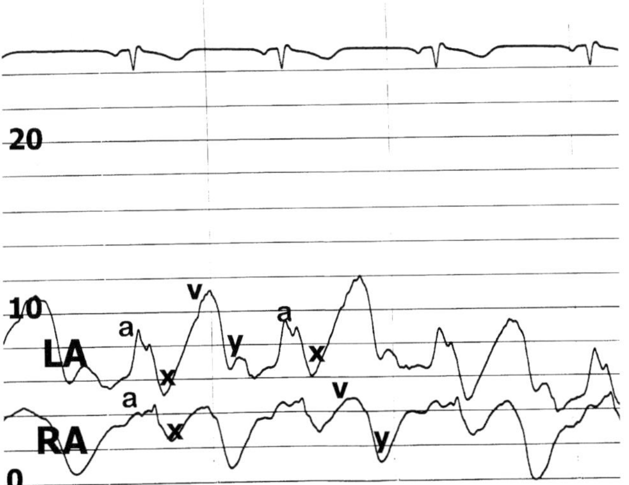

Figure 10.5 Normal right (RA) and left atrial (LA) pressure curves: a, "a" wave; v, "v" wave; x, "x" descent; y, "y" descent.

In order to obtain a pulmonary capillary wedge pressure, an end-hole catheter is advanced as far as possible into a peripheral distal pulmonary artery. This can be either one of numerous types of end-hole, torque-controlled catheters or a flow-directed, floating, "Swan™ Balloon" wedge catheter (Edwards Lifesciences, Irvine, CA). The torque-controlled catheter is pushed forward into the peripheral lung parenchyma as vigorously and as far as possible with the purpose of burying the tip of the catheter into the pulmonary capillary bed. In order to achieve a wedge position, it may be necessary to deliver the end-hole, torque-controlled catheter over a wire and even to record the pressure around the contained wire in order to maintain the tip of the catheter in the wedge position. A standard spring guide wire often fills the lumen of the catheter and does not allow recording of the pressure through the lumen and around the wire, and withdrawing the wire when the tip of the catheter is wedged often dislodges the catheter from the wedge position or leaves debris in the catheter lumen, which dampens the pressure. To overcome this problem of spring guide wires, a 0.017″ Mullins™ wire (Argon Medical Inc., Athens, TX) is used within the catheter through a wire back-bleed valve to help obtain a good wedge position. The fine stainless steel wire will add stiffness to and support the catheter without compromising its lumen.

The end-hole, floating balloon catheter is floated as far as possible distally in the pulmonary artery, deflated slightly while still advancing the catheter, and finally partially reinflated. Either the shaft of the catheter itself or the inflated balloon occludes the pulmonary artery proximal to the tip of the catheter so that the pressure that is obtained is the "venous" pressure, which is reflected back through the capillary bed from the left atrium. Often it is necessary to deliver or support the floating balloon wedge catheter over a wire (similarly to torque-controlled catheters as described above).

The adequacy of the wedge position and the validity of the wedge pressures are verified by several findings. The recorded pressure should be significantly lower than the pulmonary artery pressure and the pressure tracing should have an "atrial" configuration with distinct "a" and "v" waves. If the configuration of the displayed waveform is not characteristic of an atrial pressure curve, a small "wedge angiogram" is performed. 0.5 ml of contrast is introduced into the catheter and this small bolus of contrast is flushed through the catheter by following it with

3–4 ml of flush solution. This should demonstrate the adequacy of the wedge position, as described in Chapter 11. Withdrawing blood back through the wedged catheter and acquiring fully saturated blood from the pulmonary veins has been advocated as a technique to confirm the wedge position. Usually it is not possible to withdraw the blood and even when possible, it has not proven very satisfactory for documenting the adequacy of the wedge pressure. If withdrawal of blood is possible, it must be done *extremely* slowly and even then, a partial vacuum may be created which draws air bubbles into the sample. Once blood has been withdrawn, it is often difficult to clear the catheter of the blood to obtain a satisfactory pressure tracing without forcing the tip of the catheter out of the wedge position.

Pulmonary capillary wedge pressures can be useful when a very accurate wedge position is achieved, however, the accuracy of the wedge pressure at reflecting the actual left atrial pressure *cannot be verified* unequivocally unless a simultaneous left atrial pressure is recorded—nullifying the need for the wedge pressure! The wedge values obtained must correlate with all of the other data and should never be taken as "gospel". Even good wedge pressure waves are damped slightly in amplitude and the appearance and peak times of the various waves are always delayed compared to the actual pressures in the left atrium. This must be taken into account when calculating a mitral valve area from the combined pulmonary capillary and left ventricular pressure waves.

Ventricular pressure waves are generated by ventricular contractility and relaxation, i.e. ventricular emptying and filling. The ventricular systolic wave begins near the end of the QRS complex on the ECG and continues until the end of the "T" wave. Ventricular contraction is normally very rapid and, as a consequence, the upstroke of this ventricular curve is very steep (almost vertical). When the increasing ventricular pressure exceeds the corresponding arterial diastolic pressure, a small "anacrotic notch" occasionally appears on the upstroke of the ventricular (and arterial) pressure curve. This corresponds to the opening of the semilunar valve. The peak of the ventricular pressure corresponds to the end of ventricular contraction. The top of the pressure curve is smooth and rounded but slightly peaked. As ventricular contraction ends, the pressure rapidly begins to drop off. As the pressure curve descends, there is a distinct incisura or "dicrotic notch" in the descending limb of the curve as the ventricular pressure falls below the diastolic pressure in the artery and the semilunar valve closes.

With continued ventricular relaxation, the ventricular pressure drops very steeply to zero and then rebounds to slightly above zero. As the atrioventricular valves open and the ventricle begins to fill during ventricular relaxation, there is a slow, small rise in the ventricular pressure until the end of diastole. The slow gradual rise in pressure is interrupted by a very small positive deflection which is produced by the "a" wave "kick" of the atrial contraction (and pressure), which is reflected in the ventricle, just before the end of diastolic filling of the ventricle. The end-diastolic pressure of the ventricle is measured in the slight negative dip in the ventricular pressure curve *after* the "a" wave and just before the rapid upstroke of the ventricular curve.

The upstroke and downstroke of the normal curves of the right ventricle are slightly less acute (vertical) than the comparable curves in the left ventricle, since the normal peak right ventricular pressure is so much lower while the ejection times of the ventricles are the same. The normal right ventricular pressures are between 15 and 30 mmHg peak systolic and 0 and 7 mmHg end diastolic. The normal left ventricular pressures are between 90 and 110 mmHg peak systolic and 4 and 10 mmHg end diastolic. As with the atrial pressures, the normal ventricular pressure values increase slightly in adulthood.

The arterial pressure curves correspond to the ejection and relaxation times of the ventricles. The arterial pressure curves begin to rise in systole as the ejection pressure of the corresponding ventricle exceeds the diastolic pressure of the arteries and opens the semilunar valves. The arterial pressures peak simultaneously with the end of ventricular contractions. The normal arterial pressure curves have the same peak systolic pressure amplitudes and the same peak systolic configurations as their respective ventricles. At the end of the ventricular ejection time, as the ventricle begins to relax, the arterial pressure, like the ventricular pressure, begins to drop fairly rapidly. As the two pressures drop together, the semilunar valve closes, creating the dicrotic notch on the descending limb of the pressure curves. After the closure of the semilunar valve, the ventricular pressure continues to drop precipitously. The arterial pressure curve continues to decline, but at a much slower rate than the ventricular curve and only slightly further as the blood from the artery runs off slowly into the adjoining vascular bed. This results in a tailing-off or slow decline in the arterial pressure until no further blood runs off and the arterial pressure reaches its diastolic level (Figure 10.6).

The normal systolic pressures in the central great arteries correspond in amplitude and configuration to the corresponding ventricular systolic pressures, with peak pressures of 15–30 mmHg for the pulmonary artery and 90–110 mmHg for the central aorta. The central aortic peak pressure and pressure waveforms are a combination of the forward flow and some reflected or retrograde flow generated from the elastic recoil of the long, elastic vascular walls of the relatively large systemic arterial vascular system. Diastolic pressures in the great arteries are not as consistent from patient to patient, and depend a great deal

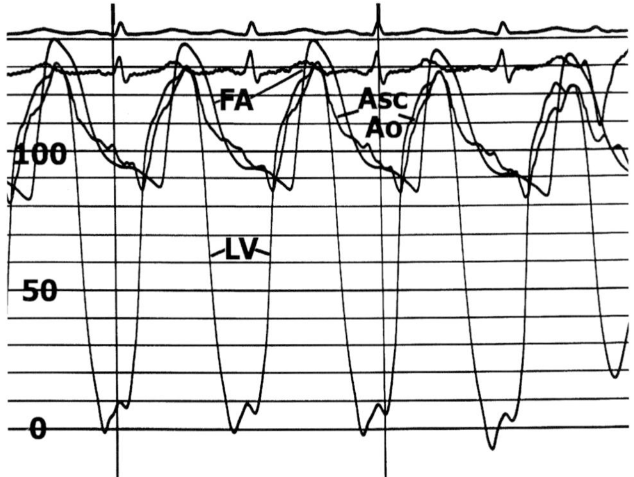

Figure 10.6 Simultaneous left ventricular (LV), ascending aorta (Asc Ao) and femoral arterial (FA) pressure curves.

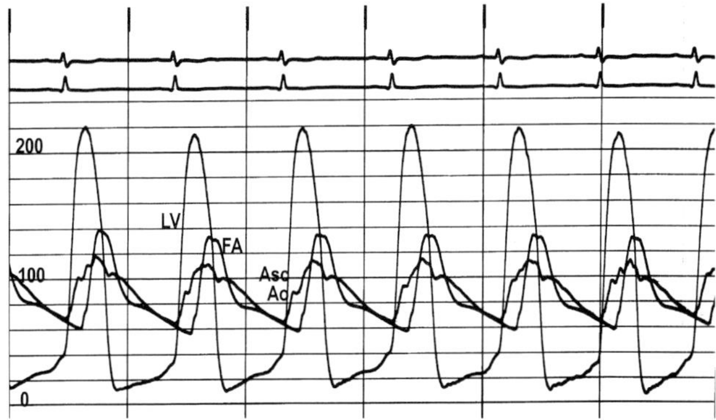

Figure 10.7 Severe aortic stenosis: simultaneous left ventricle (LV), ascending aortic (Asc Ao) and femoral artery (FA) pressure curves showing the left ventricle to aortic gradient and the significant delay and augmentation of the femoral arterial pulse curve compared to the ascending aorta.

on the patient's circulating blood volume and the capacitance of the particular vascular bed. The diastolic pressure in the normal pulmonary artery ranges between 3 and 12 mmHg in the presence of normal pulmonary vascular resistance. The diastolic pressure in the pulmonary artery corresponds closely to the pulmonary capillary wedge pressure. The diastolic pressure in the aorta will range between 50 and 70 mmHg in the presence of normal systemic resistance.

The peripheral systemic arterial pressures have a higher, and a slightly delayed, peak systolic pressure compared to the central aortic pressure. This is a result of pulse wave amplification of the systolic pressure from the central aorta to a peripheral artery (e.g. femoral artery) due to a summation of the reflected arterial waves along the relatively long, elastic, vascular walls. This pulse wave amplification is always present in a normal aorta and arterial system and can be as much as 15–20 mmHg. The delay in the build-up time and the peak systolic pressure in the more peripheral artery is a manifestation of the time and augmentation of the propagation of the pressure wave front through the fluid column (aorta) to the more peripheral arterial site (Figure 10.7).

Occasionally, in complex congenital lesions with pulmonary valve/artery atresia, the pulmonary artery or one or more of its branches cannot be entered, yet pressure information from the particular pulmonary artery is necessary to make a therapeutic decision. Inferential information about the pulmonary *arterial* pressure can be obtained from a pulmonary *venous* capillary wedge pressure. Analogous to the pulmonary artery wedge pressures, a torque-controlled, end-hole (only!) catheter is advanced from the left atrium and into a pulmonary vein. The catheter tip is advanced as far as possible into the pulmonary vein and the tip wedged forcefully into the pulmonary parenchyma in order to record a *pulmonary arterial* pressure. The circumference of the shaft of the catheter in the vein occludes any pressure transmission from the vein while the pulmonary arterial pressure is transmitted through the pulmonary capillary bed to the tip of the catheter. In order to force the catheter tip into the wedge position, it is often necessary to provide extra stiffness to the shaft of the catheter. Similarly to the pulmonary arterial wedge position, this is accomplished with a straight 0.017″ or 0.020″ (depending on the size of the catheter) Mullins Deflector Wire™ (Argon Medical Inc., Athens, TX) introduced through a Tuohy™ wire backbleed/flush device and advanced to a position just proximal to the tip of the catheter.

A proper pulmonary vein wedge position and resultant pressure curve are suggested by the appearance of a higher peak pressure than recorded in the pulmonary vein and the presence of an arterial configuration to the waveform. The pulmonary vein wedge pressure is less reliable even than the pulmonary artery wedge pressure, but may give some idea about the pressure in that segment of the lung. Even a "good" pulmonary vein wedge pressure is usually somewhat damped compared to the actual pulmonary arterial pressure. Pulmonary vein wedge pressures are more reliable when there are low pressures in the pulmonary arteries. A pulmonary vein wedge pressure that is less than 15 mmHg with a good arterial configuration is almost always consistent with a pulmonary arterial pressure of less than 20 mmHg. The contrary reliability in accurately determining higher pressures does not hold true in the presence of high pulmonary vein wedge pressures.

Pulmonary vein wedge angiograms provide some additional direct and some indirect information about the adequacy of the wedge position and about the pulmonary arterial pressure and anatomy. The angiographic appearances of the capillary and arterial beds are reflective of the pulmonary arteriolar pressure. In the presence of low pulmonary artery pressure with little or no competing prograde pulmonary flow, the entire pulmonary arterial tree can be identified from a pulmonary vein wedge angiogram. However, with very high pulmonary arteriolar pressures, the arterioles often do not fill at all, but instead, contrast extravasates into the bronchi when a pulmonary venous wedge angiogram is attempted.

Abnormal pressure curves

Abnormalities of the pressure curves within the heart and vascular system can be a consequence of hemodynamic or "electrical" abnormalities in the cardiovascular system. The pressures may be abnormal only in the context of the surrounding pressures and blood flow. Pressure curves may be abnormal in configuration, in absolute amplitude, in amplitude relative to an adjacent pressure or in any combination of these abnormalities. The normal pressures waveforms and amplitudes for each chamber and vessel in patients of all ages are well established. The pressures observed at various sites within the heart and great vessels during a cardiac catheterization mentally and continuously are compared with the expected normal configurations of the pressure waves and the absolute, as well as relative, amplitudes of the pressures for that area. When there is a deviation from the expected normal pressure waveform or amplitude, the source of the abnormal pressure is investigated and documented at that time during the catheterization procedure.

Configuration of pressure curves

A large amount of hemodynamic information can be obtained from the *configuration* of the pressure waveforms alone. For the configurations of pressure waves to be useful diagnostically, it is imperative that all of the "plumbing" and physiologic artifacts that can occur in the pressure tracings are eliminated. For isolated pressure curves, changes in pressures and any gradients to have any meaning, it is obvious that the *exact location* of the opening(s) at the catheter tip or the exact location of the catheter tip transducer is known. The position of the catheter tip is usually documented radiographically from its position within the cardiac silhouette in relation to the usual cardiac radiographic anatomy, from adjacent "fixed landmarks" which are relatively radio-opaque within the thorax, or by a small angiogram through the catheter.

A wide arterial pulse pressure can be indicative of several abnormalities. A wide pulse pressure occurs in the presence of a slow heart rate as a consequence of the increased stroke volume of the heart and the prolonged diastolic run-off into the peripheral capillaries during the prolonged relaxation time. The source of a wide pulse pressure is obvious from the heart rate and electrocardiogram. On the other hand, a wide arterial pulse pressure with a *normal* heart rate suggests the presence of either significant semilunar valve regurgitation, a large abnormal "run-off" due to a vascular communication such as a shunt or fistula into a lower-pressure vascular system, or a high cardiac output. In the case of a wide pulse pressure with regurgitation or a run-off communication, the stroke volume of the ventricle and the systolic pressure are increased to compensate for the regurgitant (or "run-off") volume. At the same time, diastolic pressure in the artery is decreased by the blood that "escapes" from the systemic arterial system during diastole. The excessive diastolic run-off is flowing into a lower-pressure vascular bed or back into the ventricle. This phenomenon occurs in both the pulmonary and the systemic arterial systems (Figure 10.8).

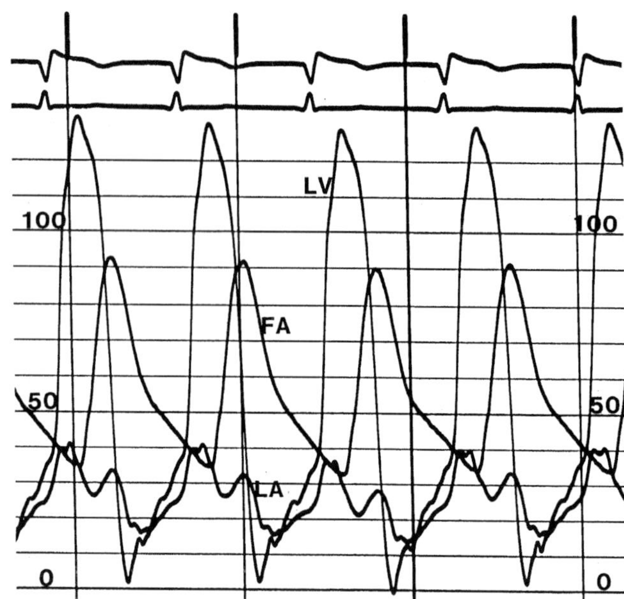

Figure 10.8 Wide femoral arterial pulse pressure and elevation of left ventricular end-diastolic and left atrial pressures in presence of severe aortic stenosis with aortic regurgitation.

In extreme degrees of semilunar valvular regurgitation, particularly in the pulmonary system, the arterial diastolic pressure drops to levels equal to the ventricular end-diastolic pressure. In wide-open semilunar valve regurgitation, the only differential feature between the ventricular and arterial pressure curves is the presence of the characteristic ventricular "end-systolic/diastolic" pressure configuration in the ventricle as opposed to a very low dicrotic notch in the arterial pressure curve. Aortic valve regurgitation widens the pulse pressure, but seldom as wide proportionately, as in pulmonary regurgitation. Patients cannot tolerate as much aortic valve regurgitation for very long without total pump failure and cardiovascular collapse.

A run-off from a systemic to pulmonary artery shunt or a systemic or pulmonary arteriovenous fistula also widens the arterial pulse pressure. The degree of widening of the pulse pressure does not necessarily reflect the size of the abnormal communication and in this respect may be misleading. In addition to the size of the communication, the amplitude of the pulse pressure in the presence of a fistula or shunt is dependent on the resistance and the overall capacitance of the vascular bed receiving the run-off. For example, even a moderate sized patent ductus emptying into a pulmonary vascular bed with normal pulmonary resistance has a very wide pulse pressure, while a very large patent ductus emptying into a pulmonary bed with significantly elevated pulmonary vascular resistance may have a normal pulse pressure.

The increased pulse pressure that is associated with an increased cardiac output is widened because of the increased stroke volume and elevation of systolic pressure, and is not associated with any unusual run-off from the particular vascular bed and, as a consequence, is usually associated with a normal arterial diastolic pressure.

At the other extreme from the wide pulse pressure, a narrow arterial pulse pressure is an indicator of an underlying hemodynamic problem. A very rapid tachycardia, even without any associated anatomic defect, produces a narrow pulse pressure from the low stroke volume of each cardiac beat. However, the tachycardia is often associated with other problems. Patients with either low cardiac output or with a proximal obstruction in the arterial "circuit" have a low amplitude arterial pulse and a narrow pulse pressure. For example, patients with poor left ventricular function and patients with significant aortic valve obstruction have lower than normal (expected) systolic arterial pressure, but, of more significance, they have an associated narrow pulse pressure.

In addition to the pulse pressure, the actual configuration of the arterial pulse wave is revealing. In patients with significant systemic volume depletion, the amplitude of their systemic blood pressure can remain normal as a result of compensation from a catecholamine response, however, the pulse wave has a very narrow pulse width and a wide pulse pressure. The configuration of the pulse wave can become so narrow that it has more of the appearance of a QRS complex of an ECG with a bundle branch block than that of an arterial pulse wave! If the volume is not replaced in the presence of this very narrow pulse waveform, the overall arterial pressure will soon drop.

The configuration of the ventricular pressure curve provides additional information about the hemodynamics in addition to the data from the peak systolic ventricular pressures and the gradients generated across the semilunar valves. In the presence of significant semilunar valve stenosis and in spite of the ejection time being lengthened, the ventricular pressure curve often develops a characteristic, narrower and more pointed shape at the peak systolic pressure. This characteristic curve is suggestive of a significant gradient across the valve (Figure 10.9).

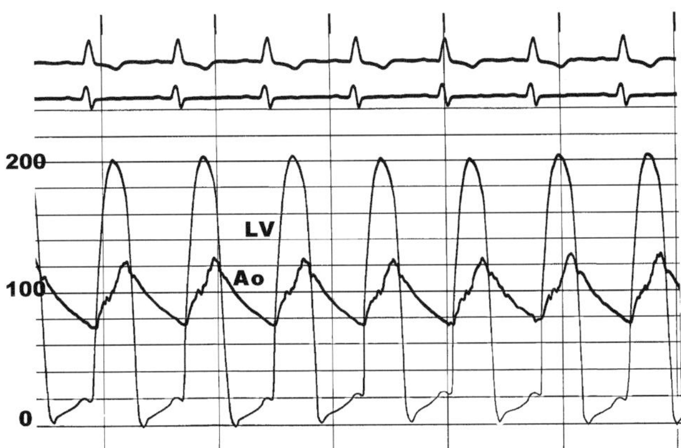

Figure 10.9 Peaked left ventricular pressure curve in the presence of severe aortic stenosis.

The end-systolic/diastolic ventricular pressure provides very valuable information about the hemodynamics (and anatomy). Very low end-diastolic pressures along with end-systolic pressures, which extend below the base line, usually indicates an incorrect (too high) level of the zero level of the transducers. Once a "height artifact" of the transducer is excluded, very low end-diastolic pressures indicate that the patient has significant volume depletion. High end-diastolic pressures can be a manifestation of multiple different real or artifactual problems with the recording. As with low end-diastolic pressures, the first consideration should be the zero level of a transducer, which may be set too low. Once this artifact is excluded, the presence of a true high end-diastolic pressure usually represents compromised ventricular function. This is suspected from the associated clinical findings of the patient and correlated with the subsequent findings during the catheterization.

There are several other causes of high ventricular end-diastolic pressure. The end-diastolic pressure is often elevated to a significant degree from the volume load in the ventricle during diastole in the presence of severe semilunar valvular regurgitation. Similarly, the added ventricular volume of severe atrioventricular valve regurgitation elevates the ventricular end-diastolic pressure (Figure 10.8). Both the semilunar and atrioventricular regurgitation become very evident with the other findings during the catheterization.

Both restrictive and constrictive cardiac problems cause elevation of the atrial pressures along with the ventricular end-diastolic pressure. With a pericardial constriction, the right atrial, right ventricular end-diastolic and pulmonary capillary pressures rise equivalent to the intrapericardial pressure. Eventually with progressive increase in pericardial pressure, the elevation of the end-diastolic pressures

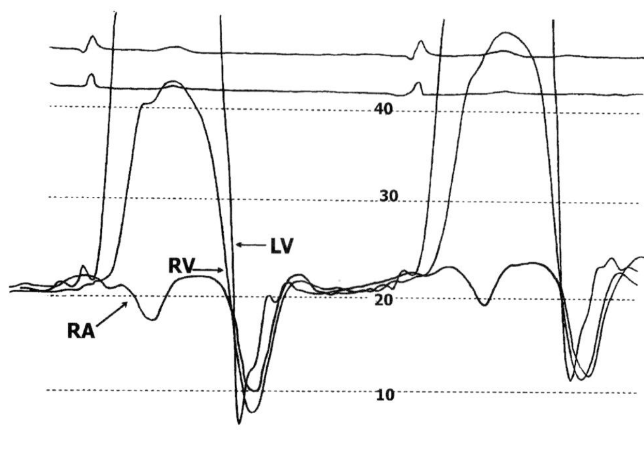

Figure 10.10 "Equal" elevation along with a plateau of the right atrial, right ventricular end-diastolic and left ventricular end-diastolic pressure curves with constrictive/restrictive physiology.

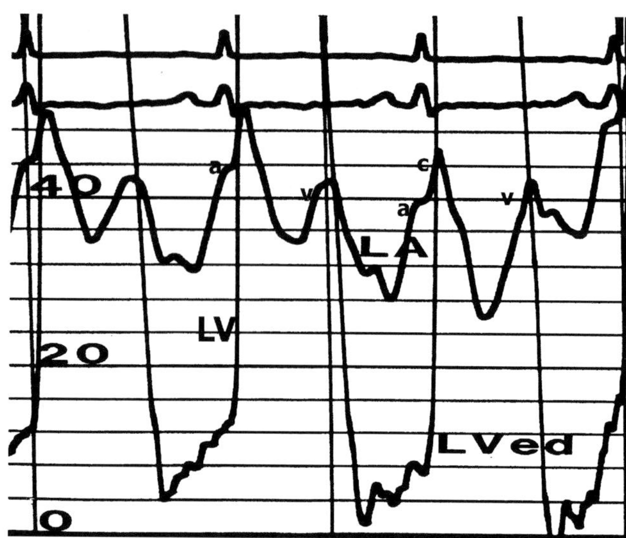

Figure 10.11 Simultaneous pressure tracings in mitral stenosis demonstrating the gradient between the high "a" waves in a left atrial pressure tracing simultaneous with the normal left ventricular end-diastolic pressures.

occurs comparably in *both ventricles* along with an equal rise in the atrial pressures (Figure 10.10). The restrictive/constrictive phenomena produce a fairly characteristic "square wave" or "plateau" configuration to the ventricular diastolic pressure curves and an "equalization" of the peak atrial and ventricular diastolic pressures. In a patient who is volume depleted, particularly from intensive diuretic therapy, the intracardiac pressure changes may not be as characteristic.

With the increase in left ventricular end-diastolic pressure associated with tamponade, there is a concomitant decrease in ventricular filling, which results in a decrease in cardiac output, particularly during inspiration, and the associated development of the characteristic marked decrease in arterial systolic pressure with each inspiratory effort of the patient—the so called pulses paradoxus. An arterial systolic pressure drop of 12 mmHg or more with an inspiratory effort is diagnostic of pericardial constriction restrictive physiology.

Pulses alternans is another pathologic variation that is seen in the arterial pulse. Pulses alternans is, as the name implies, a palpable (and visible, if an arterial catheter/line is in place) consistent alternation in the amplitude of successive cardiac beats, which is not due to an arrhythmia or respiratory variation. Pulses alternans is usually a sign of severe myocardial dysfunction or disease, and the alternating ventricular waveforms actually differ from each other in configuration as well as in amplitude.

Abnormal atrial pressure curves provide valuable hemodynamic information in many cardiac abnormalities. Abnormalities occur in both amplitude and configuration of the atrial waves. A consistently high "a" wave in an atrial pressure tracing, particularly compared to the amplitude of the "v" wave in the same chamber, indicates obstruction to the outflow from that atrium. The obstruction to outflow can be due to obstruction of the orifice of the adjacent atrioventricular valve, poor compliance of the receiving ventricular chamber, or marked asynchrony between the atrial contraction and valve opening (arrhythmia). With an otherwise normally functioning ventricle in communication with the atrium and a sinus rhythm, a high "a" wave indicates atrioventricular valve stenosis and results in a pressure gradient between the atrial chamber and a normal diastolic pressure in the adjoining ventricle (Figure 10.11).

While a very high "a" wave suggests significant stenosis, a normal or only slightly increased "a" wave does not rule out even severe stenosis, nor does it document that the stenosis that is present is only mild. The compliance/capacitance of the atrial chamber or any associated "run-off" openings or vessels from the involved atrium can decrease the amplitude of the "a" wave significantly and, although this does not decrease the significance of the obstruction, it definitely decreases the measured gradient across the particular atrioventricular valve. For example, a very large and compliant right atrium or an associated very compliant venous vascular bed can abolish (mask) the gradient across even a very severe tricuspid valve stenosis. A large atrial septal defect can minimize the gradient across either severe mitral or tricuspid valve stenosis by allowing run-off away from the atrium that is immediately proximal to the stenotic valve. Intermittent high "a" waves with irregular amplitudes, some of which can be very high, are found with electrical atrioventricular dissociation. These very high waves are generated when the atria contract against a completely closed atrioventricular valve.

Atrial "v" waves can be equally revealing. High atrial "v" waves are usually indicative of a large shunt or of significant atrioventricular valvular regurgitation into the atrial chamber. With a large shunt into the atrium, the physical shunting into the atrium tends to extend throughout the entire relaxation phase of the atrial pressure wave, and produces a broad "v" wave. Moderate atrioventricular valve regurgitation tends to generate a later, high "v" wave, which occurs nearer the end of ventricular systole. Greater degrees of atrioventricular valvular insufficiency produce an atrial "v" wave that is broader and begins earlier. An elevation of ventricular end-diastolic pressure will obviously elevate the atrial "v" and "a" waves.

Cardiac arrhythmias interfere with the precise synchronization between the atrial and ventricular contractions. The normal atrial contraction occurs simultaneously with the opening of the atrioventricular valve. With the slight delay in ventricular contraction that occurs with a fairly common first degree atrioventricular block, the atrium begins to contract before the atrioventricular valve begins to open. This, in turn, creates a regularly occurring earlier, but not significantly higher, "a" wave. Complete heart block introduces the effect of an irregularly occurring, total dissociation between the atrial and the ventricular contractions and, in turn, a total dissociation between the atrial and ventricular pulse waves, with the atrial contractions being totally random in relation to the ventricular contractions and to the opening of the atrioventricular valves. As a consequence, when the atrium contracts against a closed atrioventricular valve, it generates a huge pressure and high "a" wave (or "cannon" wave in the jugular venous pulse) while, when the atrium accidentally synchronizes and contracts with the valve opening, the "a" wave amplitude is normal. This same type of atrioventricular asynchrony occurs with atrial flutter with variable block and produces giant "a" waves when the atrium contracts against the closed atrioventricular valve.

Atrial fibrillation completely abolishes the effective atrial contraction and essentially eliminates the "a" waves. The irregularity of the ventricular response also eliminates an effective or recognizable atrial "v" wave so that the atrial pulse wave ends up as an "irregularly irregular", almost undulation of the atrial pressure curve. Fast, even though synchronized, atrial tachycardia increases the "a" wave amplitude, but, more importantly, decrease the systemic arterial pressure by not allowing a sufficient ventricular filling time.

Pressure gradients

The most frequently utilized pressure data from the heart and vascular system are the amplitudes of the measured pressures themselves and the pressure differences (gradients) between two adjacent areas. Gradients or differences in pressure between adjacent chambers or areas result from restriction or obstruction within, or between, chambers or vessels, across stenotic valves, or within stenotic vessels, and the magnitude of the gradient generally reflects the severity of the obstruction. The accuracy and specificity of the measured pressures or gradients are often the determining factor in the subsequent management of the patient, and must be obtained as accurately as possible.

Gradients measured across *isolated* valvar stenosis are the most straightforward pressure gradients encountered in the cardiac catheterization laboratory. In the absence of additional defects, the entire cardiac output passes through each valve and, as a consequence, the measured gradient generally accurately reflects the degree of stenosis of the particular valve. The significance of the gradient across each of the four cardiac valves and the implications of each of those gradients for therapeutic decisions are discussed in detail in the subsequent chapters covering the valvuloplasty of each of the individual valves, and are not discussed in any more detail in this section.

The configuration of the pressure curve immediately adjacent to the pressure gradient is essential for establishing the precise level of obstruction in the arterial system. A peak systolic gradient indicates the severity of the obstruction but, by itself, provides no information about the location of the obstruction. For example, when the obstruction is within the ventricular outflow tract, below the semilunar valve (either subaortic or subpulmonic obstruction), there will be a systolic gradient between the inflow area of the ventricle and the adjacent great artery, but this does not localize the area of obstruction. Only pressure recordings obtained immediately adjacent to the precise area of obstruction will document the area of obstruction. With a subvalvular obstruction, only the maximum systolic pressure of the two curves will differ while the diastolic pressure and the configuration of the pressure tracings (except for amplitude) remain the same above and below the level of obstruction (Figure 10.12).

When there is obstruction in the vessel distal to the semilunar valve (supravalvular, coarctation) there is again a systolic gradient between the ventricle and a more distal arterial site (femoral artery), but this does not establish the level of obstruction. There will be persistence of an arterial pressure curve above and below the obstruction, but with different configurations and peak systolic pressures. Only by recording precisely across the level of the obstruction can the exact area of obstruction be demonstrated by the pressures. The arterial curve immediately proximal to the obstruction has a higher systolic pressure and a wider pulse pressure, while the pressure curve distal to the obstruction is damped compared to the more proximal pressure curve as demonstrated by simultaneous ascending

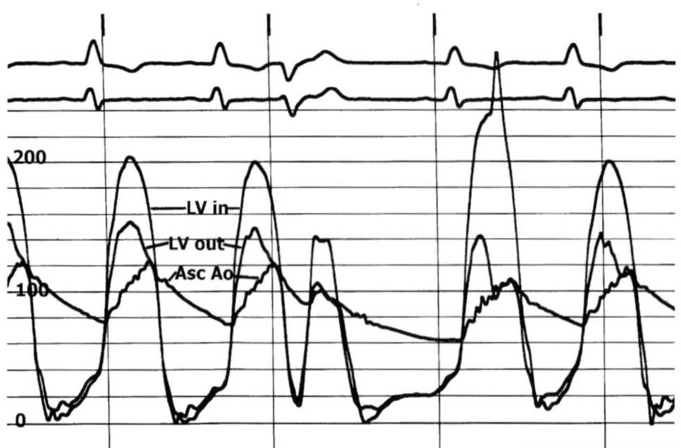

Figure 10.12 Simultaneous left ventricular inflow, left ventricular outflow and ascending aorta pressure curves in the presence of valve and subvalvular aortic obstruction.

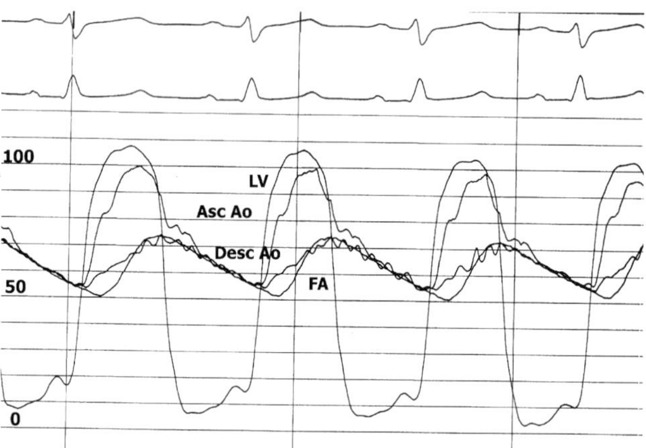

Figure 10.13 Mild aortic stenosis with severe coarctation of the aorta; pressure tracings from: LV, left ventricle; Asc Ao, ascending aorta; Desc Ao, descending thoracic aorta, distal to coarctation; and FA, femoral artery.

aorta, descending thoracic, and femoral arterial pressure tracings (Figure 10.13).

In the presence of multiple area (levels) of obstruction in an arterial circuit, the precise area of change in the amplitude of the pulse wave is even more definitive in determining the level of obstruction. For example, in the presence of subvalvular and semilunar valvular obstruction, a systolic gradient occurs at the subvalvular level, but still with a "ventricular" pressure on both sides of the obstruction. As a catheter is withdrawn across an additional valvular obstruction, an additional systolic gradient would appear at precisely the same time as the pressure curve becomes an arterial tracing with its typical higher diastolic pressure.

There are some notable exceptions where the gradient, including the gradient across a valve, does *not* reflect the degree of stenosis accurately. The measured gradient across a valve or any other obstruction is diminished by a decreased cardiac output. The sedation or anesthesia of a patient during cardiac catheterization decreases their cardiac output compared to what it is when the patient is awake and at a normal level of activity. Decreased contractility of the heart associated with "pump" or heart failure can decreases the cardiac output very markedly and, in turn, diminish the measured gradient across an obstruction. A measured gradient, particularly when it appears only marginally significant, must be correlated with a cardiac output to assure that there is adequate "pump" function.

In complex intracardiac and intravascular lesions where there are associated intracavitary or intravascular communications, the measured gradients have little, or no, significance in the determination of the *severity* of the obstruction. In the presence of an intravascular communication proximal to the obstruction, blood flow can be diverted away from the obstructed valve through the communication, which decreases the gradient across the valve compared to when all of the cardiac output is being forced through the obstructed valve. The gradient across the obstruction would be decreased proportionally to the residual flow across the obstruction. This phenomenon is commonly found in semilunar valve obstruction associated with ventricular septal defects and atrioventricular valve obstruction associated with interatrial communications.

Pressure gradients measured across areas of stenosis in isolated vessels or vascular channels—either in the systemic or the pulmonary arterial bed—similarly have little significance in the determination of the severity of the stenosis. The magnitude of the gradient across a vessel stenosis depends entirely on the vascular anatomy in the surrounding (adjacent) vascular bed. Exactly as with valvular obstructions, the gradient generated across a vessel obstruction is proportionate to the volume of blood forced through the specific area of obstruction. In obstructions of individual vessels, the flow to, and across, the obstruction, and in turn the measured gradient, are reduced (or abolished!) by run-off of the blood flow away from the area of obstruction into branching vessels or collateral channels which arise proximal to the obstruction.

This lack of significance of the gradient is illustrated clearly in several common obstructive congenital vascular lesions. In severe, unilateral, proximal branch pulmonary artery stenosis, the unilateral branch stenosis may obstruct a vessel almost totally, yet only a very small gradient is generated across the obstruction! In this circumstance, all of the blood flow is diverted to the opposite, non-obstructed pulmonary artery and no gradient is generated across the very severe obstruction. Similarly, in the case of coarctation of the aorta where there are extensive collaterals, anatomically (angiographically) there may be a thread-like opening with near total obstruction of the descending aorta, while only a small and insignificant pressure gradient is generated across the obstruction. The extensive, brachiocephalic or thoracic wall collateral vessels divert the majority of the flow away from (around) the area of obstruction in the aorta and diminish the gradient.

An increased volume capacity and compliance of the vascular bed proximal to a stenotic atrioventricular valve, decreases, or even eliminates, any measured gradient across the valve similarly to the diversion of proximal flow through a shunt or collateral. This occurs only with the atrioventricular valves, and particularly with the tricuspid valve because of its relationship to the systemic venous bed. The capacitance/compliance of the systemic venous vascular bed combined with any branching or collateral vessels proximal to areas of venous obstruction, frequently minimizes, or even totally eliminates, gradients across very severe degrees of anatomic (angiographic) obstruction of the venous system. The capacitance of the systemic venous bed is almost "infinite". Very significant degrees of nearly total systemic venous obstruction result in massive dilation of the systemic venous bed (and liver) and cause pooling and very sluggish flow, yet only elevate the venous pressure proximal to the obstruction by a few millimeters of mercury, if at all. In addition, if there is a localized area of peripheral or central systemic venous obstruction, the human body has a remarkable capability of developing collateral channels around the obstruction. These collaterals divert flow away from any obstruction to areas of even minimally lower pressure and mask any gradients.

The absence of significant pressure gradients in the presence of severe anatomic obstruction occurs very commonly in patients following the various permutations and combinations of the "Fontan"/cavo-pulmonary connections or "circuits". The gradients are reduced or even eliminated as a result of the combined systemic venous capacitance and the venovenous collateral run-off channels. It is common to encounter a discrete, anatomic (angiographic) narrowing of as much as 90% of a proximal right or left pulmonary artery (compared to the more distal vessel) while at the same time there is no measurable gradient, or, at most, an insignificant (1–2 mmHg) pressure gradient across the area of narrowing. The management of a severe anatomic obstruction of this degree is obvious regardless of the gradient, however, when the anatomic narrowing is less severe angiographically, the lack of gradient can lead to important true obstructions being considered insignificant and ignored. This represents a very serious error in those patients where every milliliter of pulmonary flow to both lungs is important for survival.

An equally important example of the ability of collateral channels to minimize pressure gradients, even in the presence of severe venous obstruction, occurs in peripheral vein stenosis or even total occlusion of peripheral veins. The entire iliac venous system can be obstructed with no outward physical signs, symptoms or other evidence of the obstruction apparent until a repeat cardiac catheterization through the femoral venous system is attempted! No significant pressure gradient is measured between the peripheral and central venous systems; however, angiography, with the injection proximal in the direction of flow to the area of venous obstruction, demonstrates total obstruction of the vein along with an extensive network of collaterals in the pelvis and abdominal paravertebral areas. Likewise, even total occlusions of the superior vena cava can go unrecognized and produce a minimal gradient at rest when there are sufficient azygos, hemiazygos and other intrathoracic, mediastinal and paravertebral vein collaterals.

The absolute pressure values and the gradients measured from the pressures provide most of the necessary information on which to make therapeutic decisions. Occasionally, however, in addition to the absolute pressure measurements, information about the total resistance of a particular vascular bed or the actual measured or calculated area of a valve orifice or a vessel is very useful, or even essential, for making a clinical decision about a particular patient. These values are not determined from the pressures alone and require additional information about the precise blood flow to the area or the actual total cardiac output in order to calculate them. The measurement of flow and cardiac output along with these calculations is covered later under "Calculations" in this chapter.

Flow, cardiac output and intravascular shunt determination

The detection and quantitating of shunts as well as the quantitative determination of flow in the cardiac catheterization laboratory, are based on the principals of indicator dilution techniques[2]. Indicator dilution techniques depend upon the detection and quantification of indicator substances that have been introduced into flowing fluids. Indicator dilution techniques have been used and validated for the quantitative determination of flow in the fields of hydraulic engineering and physiologic fluid dynamics for over a century. When using an indicator dilution technique for quantitative determinations of flow, a specific amount of an indicator substance is introduced into an inflow or "upstream" location in a constantly flowing fluid within a closed system. Assuming that the substance is uniformly distributed within the constantly flowing fluid, the rate of total flow is determined by measuring the difference in the concentrations of the indicator between the inflow and outflow samples. The change in concentration of the substance in the mixed fluid sampled from a "downstream" or outflow location and measured over time provides the same information. Thus:

$$\text{Flow (Q)} = \frac{\text{Specific amount of indicator introduced per unit of time}}{\text{[Inflow conc. of indicator]} - \text{[Outflow conc. of indicator]}}$$

Indicators are used for the qualitative detection and quantitative measurements of leaks or shunts. The mere presence of even a minute amount of a very sensitive indicator substance in an abnormal location confirms the presence of very tiny leaks or abnormal communications. In addition to merely detecting leaks or shunts in the circulation, shunts are quantitated by measuring the exact amount of indicator that appears in the abnormal location over a specific period of time.

In spite of the general validity of indicator dilution techniques, there are several theoretical and practical problems when applying indicator dilution principals to the human heart. The validity of indicator dilution techniques for quantifying flow in the human circulation depends upon several very general assumptions:

- For quantitating flow there must be a *constant, net flow* into and out of the particular system or circuit during the period of measurement. This premise is fulfilled in the normal human circulation by the fact that, although the heart is actually two separate pumps, the two pumps are in series, and *in the absence of connections or leaks (shunts) between the two sides (pumps)* within the heart, there is a constant and equal flow of blood into and out of each side of the heart. Thus the flow into and out of either side of the heart is equivalent to the net flow into and out of the entire heart.
- There must be complete and uniform distribution within the flowing blood of any indicator substance that is introduced into the bloodstream at the proximal site in the circulation. With the velocity and turbulence of flow within the heart, it is presumed that this occurs when samples are taken at least one chamber distal to the site of introduction of the indicator.
- For the determination of accurate flow there must be no loss of the indicator from the circulating fluid as a consequence of leakage out of the circuit or absorption or retention into the tissues during the period of sampling.
- Not only must the indicator be detectable, but its concentration must be accurately measurable from a site distal to the introduction site in the circulation.

Various indicator substances are used for the determination of flow and the detection and quantification of shunts in the human circulation. The indicators utilized in the catheterization laboratory are chosen specifically to fulfill all of the criteria for the indicator dilution technique to be valid in the human heart. For the quantification of flow or shunts, the exact amount of indicator that is introduced into the proximal area of the circulation must be known, and the amount of indicator leaving the heart or area of shunt must be measurable. On the other hand, for the mere detection of the presence of a leak or shunt, the presence of even a small amount of a very sensitive indicator substance in an abnormal location is sufficient to document the presence of the shunt.

Oxygen content (saturation) in the circulating blood and several exogenous indicators—including cold solutions, indigo-cyanine (Cardio-Green) dye and hydrogen ions—are used for the detection and/or quantification of total flow and shunts. Oxygen, measured as oxygen content of the blood, is the principal indicator used in the determination of flow and the calculation of the magnitude of shunts in the cardiac catheterization laboratory; exogenous indicators are discussed later in this chapter.

Oxygen as the indicator

In the decision-making process for congenital heart patients, a great deal of significance is placed on oxygen saturation determinations. As with the situation with pressures, where the appearance alone of the pressure waves often has significance, certain isolated oxygen saturations can provide important clinical information about a patient early during the catheterization procedure. The presence of desaturation of the systemic arterial blood immediately indicates either right to left shunting or a significant ventilation–perfusion problem with the patient. A systemic venous saturation of less than 50% indicates a very low cardiac output, and an even lower systemic venous saturation of 30–40% or lower indicates a critically low cardiac output which is potentially life threatening to the patient. A high systemic venous saturation that is not due to a left to right shunt, on the other hand, indicates a high cardiac output state.

The calculation of outputs, shunts and resistances are all dependent upon the accurate determination of oxygen saturations in the blood. The several assumptions that are necessary for utilizing any indicator dilution technique in the determination of flow in the human heart have already been listed; when using oxygen as the indicator for the calculation of flow and shunts, additional assumptions are made specifically relating to oxygen. In addition to the assumptions, there also are some practical difficulties in obtaining blood samples as well as significant potential errors in the handling and analysis of the samples for oxygen saturation determinations. In spite of the importance of blood oxygen saturation data obtained during a cardiac catheterization for decision making, as a consequence of the assumptions necessary and the problems with sampling and analyzing the saturations, even under optimal circumstances, oxygen saturations are the *least sensitive* and *most prone to error* of all of the physiologic data obtained during a cardiac catheterization.

When quantifying flow and shunts using oxygen, the *exact* amount of oxygen extracted from the air which the patient is breathing is the indicator. The amount of extracted indicator is measured accurately per unit of time as the oxygen consumption of the patient; the details of measuring oxygen consumption are discussed in a separate section later in this chapter. The oxygen that is introduced into the unsaturated venous blood as it passes through the pulmonary bed, is the volume of oxygen that is extracted from the air as it passes through the lungs. The amount of oxygen introduced into the flowing blood is determined from the difference in oxygen saturation between the mixed systemic venous blood (pulmonary artery blood) entering the pulmonary circuit and the mixed pulmonary venous blood (left ventricular blood) leaving the pulmonary circuit. When using oxygen as the indicator for flow determinations in the absence of intracardiac shunts, either the pulmonary blood flow or systemic blood flow can be measured. In the absence of intracardiac shunts, the pulmonary flow will be equal to the systemic flow and to the *total cardiac output*.

The absolute quantity of blood flow (cardiac output) is determined by dividing the amount of oxygen consumed (in ml O_2/min) by the difference between the inflow and outflow saturations (in ml O_2/100 ml) of the blood across the pulmonary bed. In pediatric and congenital patients this value is "indexed to" (multiplied by) the patient's body surface area and the denominator is multiplied by 10 in order to express the result as liters/min/m^2. The formulas and calculations used in the determination of flow, shunts and resistances when oxygen is used as the indicator are discussed in more detail at the end of this section.

Assumptions necessary using oxygen as the indicator

Possibly the most important assumption necessary when oxygen (percent saturation) is used as the indicator, is that all of the measurements are made with an *absolutely steady blood flow*, i.e. with the patient in an absolutely "steady state". In order for the values to be valid, there can be absolutely no changes in the physical activity, respiratory rate, cardiac rate or level of consciousness of the patient during the sampling. It is desirable (necessary!) to obtain two or more samples from at least *three sites*, which often, in a complex heart, are remote from each other. In order for *cardiac output and/or resistance determinations* to be valid, the samples must be obtained not only while the patient remains absolutely stable, but while the oxygen consumption is being measured. This steady state is often a difficult condition to maintain in infants and children (or any patient) "secured" on a catheterization table, particularly under a "hood" undergoing an oxygen consumption analysis. There is no measure for the degree of the patient's steady state. It is *assumed* that if there is no obvious movement of the patient, no change in the patient's state of consciousness, no change in the heart rate, and if all of the samples are acquired within one to two minutes of each other, then a steady state has been achieved. Even this level of steady state is often difficult to achieve in a patient undergoing a cardiac catheterization. To add to the problem, these same patients are often very ill, the multiple sampling takes a considerable period of time or the patient requires supplemental oxygen to breathe.

Indicator dilution techniques were validated in continuously flowing fluids, while the human circulation has a pulsatile, not continuous, flow. Withdrawing the blood samples for oxygen determinations over at least several seconds is assumed to compensate adequately for this discrepancy.

There is not a single or uniform source of venous inflow on either side of the heart. The normal mixed systemic venous saturation in the right atrium has *three major variable sources* of inflow—the inferior vena cava, the superior vena cava, and the coronary sinus. The superior vena cava and the inferior vena cava receive multiple sources of blood, each with a different saturation!

The superior vena cava receives blood from the jugular veins, the subclavian veins and the azygos system, each of which often has markedly different saturations and flow. Usually the jugular veins have a lower saturation while the subclavian veins contain higher saturated blood from the axillary (peripheral extremity) veins. The saturation from the azygos system is usually slightly higher, reflecting the infrarenal inferior vena caval saturation. The superior vena caval blood normally varies as much as 10% from one area to another just within the lumen of the vein because of its multiple sources of blood.

The inferior vena cava also has sources of both high and low saturation. Inferior vena caval blood, even more than superior vena caval, can vary as much as 10–20% from one adjacent area to another, all within the main channel of the vein. The higher saturated blood in the inferior cava arises from the renal veins while the lower saturated blood is attributed to the gastrocolic and hepatic veins. Because of the contribution of the renal veins, the "net mixed" inferior vena caval blood is generally 5–10% higher than the superior vena caval blood, but even this percentage is not consistent from patient to patient nor even within the same patient.

The coronary venous system contributes significantly to the "pool" of mixed systemic venous blood entering the right atrium from the coronary sinus. Although the coronary sinus and anterior cardiac vein blood makes up only 5–7% of the systemic venous return, the extremely low saturations from the coronary system (25–45%) have a significant impact on the total mixed systemic venous saturation.

With the separate, and different, contributions to the "mixed venous" sample from the superior vena cava, inferior vena cava and the coronary sinus, there is no possible way to measure accurately all of the separate saturations and to compensate for the different volumes of flow from each of these sources. No individual sample from even the right atrium necessarily is representative of the fully mixed venous saturation from all of the venous sources because of the separate streaming of flow into, and even completely through, the right atrial chamber. In the absence of any left to right shunt, a sample further downstream in the flow distal to the right atrium (right ventricle or, preferably, the pulmonary artery) does provide a thoroughly mixed systemic venous sample.

In the presence of intracardiac shunts, which one or combination of the "mixed" saturations from the various systemic venous blood sources is used in the calculation of intracardiac shunts is chosen more or less arbitrarily. Fortunately for the validity of this assumption on the systemic venous side of the circulation, all of the blood from the superior vena cava, inferior vena cava and coronary veins/sinus is mixed together thoroughly in the atrial and ventricular chambers, and in the absence of a left to right shunt this creates a uniform saturation by the time the blood reaches the pulmonary artery. Also, fortuitously and in the absence of any intracardiac shunting, this mixture of all sources of the systemic venous blood in the pulmonary artery results in a mixed venous saturation that is equal to, or very close to, the saturation of the superior vena caval blood alone[3]. Consequently, the saturation in the superior vena cava is assumed to represent the total mixed systemic venous saturation in the calculations of both left to right and right to left shunts when the more distal, mixed samples (e.g. pulmonary artery) cannot be used. At the same time, and even in the absence of intracardiac shunting, this value can easily differ significantly from the true "mixed venous" value. A significant error in this value can alter the calculation of a left to right shunt by 50% or more so several samples that are close or equal in value to each other should be obtained from the superior vena cava before that value is used in the calculations.

Similarly, the mixed pulmonary venous saturation is a combination of the oxygen saturations from somewhere between three and five separate pulmonary veins, each draining different areas of the lungs. Each of these areas of the lungs has a markedly different volume and each area may have markedly different ventilation or perfusion with resultant markedly different saturations from each pulmonary vein. In the presence of a pulmonary parenchymal abnormality or a ventilation–perfusion missmatch, the mixed pulmonary venous saturation measured from a single pulmonary vein can be off by as much as 50–100% from a truly representative mixed sample from all of the pulmonary veins. Owing to the selective streaming into the left atrium from the separate veins, even a sample from any single site in the left atrium has little chance of being representative.

As a consequence, the representative mixed pulmonary venous saturation cannot be measured precisely from any isolated pulmonary vein or even the left atrium. In the absence of any right to left shunting within the heart, a downstream sample from, for example, the left ventricle or the aorta, is preferable to *assuming* that any of the saturation values from a single pulmonary vein or even from the left atrium are correct. In the presence of a right to left shunt, more precarious assumptions must be made. In the absence of known pulmonary disease, it is assumed that all of the pulmonary venous blood coming from the pulmonary veins is fully saturated, or at least that the flows from all of the pulmonary veins have the same or very similar saturations. Similar values that are obtained from several pulmonary veins are usually *assumed* to be representative of the "mixed pulmonary venous" saturation. When the right to left shunt is more distal at either the ventricular or great artery level, samples from the body of the left atrium near the mitral valve are assumed to be representative of mixed pulmonary venous blood. Errors in the samples or the assumptions with the values for mixed pulmonary venous saturation can change the calculation of cardiac output or either a left to right or right to left shunt by 100%!

In addition to the assumptions that are made with the samples and in the calculations, there are also multiple pragmatic or practical problems in both acquiring accurate blood samples and in the analysis of the concentration of the oxygen content in those samples, all of which provide additional potential opportunities for errors, even under optimal circumstances.

Special techniques in blood sampling for oxygen saturation determinations—precautions and errors

There are precise techniques for obtaining *proper* samples and, in the process, techniques for circumventing the innumerable pitfalls that are always present in obtaining these samples. In order to acquire the proper blood samples in the catheterization laboratory, the operator must be very familiar with the principals of, and the calculations for, cardiac output and shunt determinations using oxygen as the indicator.

Sampling site errors

When blood samples are being drawn to determine the magnitude of a shunt, they must be drawn from the proper locations, both well proximal to, as well as distal to any area of shunting. There is significant selective "streaming" of blood flow from the veins as well as into and from the chambers and great vessels of the heart. As a consequence, to ensure complete mixing and no preponderance of input from any one source or contamination from the shunt, ideally the representative sampling for shunt determinations are made at least one chamber removed, or separated both proximally and distally, from the site of shunting. For example, in the detection of shunting through an atrial septal defect, the mixed venous blood samples from the superior vena cava are obtained in the superior vena cava but well proximal to the entrance of the superior vena cava into the right atrium in order to avoid contamination by back flow from the right atrium. The post-shunt mixed blood samples are drawn from the ventricle, or preferably the pulmonary artery, in order to ensure complete mixing of the blood downstream from the shunt at the atrial level.

In order to assure a steady state for the patient, blood samples for oxygen determinations used in the calculation of flow or shunts must be drawn in very rapid sequence over a very short period of time. More than one minute, or at the very most, two minutes between the most proximal and the most distal oxygen saturation values during a right-sided "sweep" potentially invalidates the data because of variations in the steady state of the patient and in the analyzed samples. When the oxygen saturation data are critical and unless there are locations that are very difficult to enter, it is better to obtain the blood samples that will be used to obtain the data during a rapid "oxygen sweep" that is separate from the pressure recordings from these same locations. When more than a few minutes is taken in obtaining samples during an "oxygen sweep" and even in a patient who is in an apparently absolute steady state, at least one blood sample should be repeated from both a proximal and a distal representative area on both sides of the location of shunting. These duplicate samples should be obtained at both the beginning and at the end of the oxygen sweep. The repeat determinations of the oxygen saturations serve as a double check of the patient's steady state and of the consistency of the oxygen analyzing apparatus over the period of time.

In addition to obtaining blood samples for saturation determination in rapid sequence, each blood sample that is to be used in the calculations should be duplicated (or "bracketed") on both sides of the area(s) of shunting for accurate shunt calculations, i.e., at least two samples are obtained in rapid sequence both proximal and distal to the area of shunting. A difference as little as 5% in oxygen saturations can represent a significant difference in oxygen saturation for documenting the presence of a shunt, but only when all of the blood samples for the "oxygen sweep" are obtained in duplicate, the samples from the same location are "identical" to each other, and all of the samples are obtained within *one minute* of each other.

The demonstration of a shunt with an even smaller difference in the saturations is possible in a patient with a low cardiac output and low mixed venous saturations, but still requires careful documentation with duplicate or triplicate values obtained even more rapidly on both sides of the shunt. With a low mixed venous saturation, even a small amount of fully saturated blood added to the mixed venous blood produces a significant "step-up" in the downstream saturation. On the other hand, in patients with a high cardiac output and, in turn, high mixed venous saturations, a small amount of additional fully saturated blood does not create a measurable step-up in the downstream mixture of venous blood (*see* "shunt calculations" subsequently—examples with low and high saturations).

When there are multiple levels of shunting, the selective streaming of blood within the vessels or chambers of the vascular system totally precludes the validity of trying to quantitate the exact amount of shunting at each level from the oxygen saturations alone. The selective streaming of the blood containing different saturations from each different source area while flowing through a particular chamber produces almost discrete, separate columns or channels of blood within the chamber or vessel. When the particular blood sample is obtained from any one of these separate streams of blood, very misleading and erroneous values are produced. The most significant level or location of shunting when multiple levels of shunting are present, is documented better with other data (pressures, angiograms, indicator curves, etc.) and is *not* based on changes in oxygen saturation values at the particular location.

In using the superior vena caval (SVC) blood saturation as the mixed venous sample, at least two separate samples are obtained from slightly different locations (side to side or up and down), with each sample still withdrawn from within the true SVC. The separate saturations obtained from the two adjacent locations should be very close in value to each other. When the saturations of the two separate samples are *not* within one or two percent of each other, a third sample (at least!) is drawn from the SVC in order to determine which of the original samples is more representative. The blood samples from the SVC are drawn from the mid superior vena caval level. Sampling too high in the SVC preferentially samples one of the separate input veins and gives an erroneous value that is not representative of the mixed venous sample from all of the cephalad venous sources. A location that is too high may provide a sample from the axillary (peripheral arm) vein and give an erroneously high O_2 saturation and a sample from the internal jugular vein can give an erroneously low saturation. A sample obtained too low in the SVC (at, or close to, the superior vena cava–right atrial junction) may actually include some blood refluxing into the SVC from the right atrium. Unless there is left to right shunting into the SVC (or more proximally), oxygen saturations in the SVC are usually 5–10% lower than saturations obtained from the inferior vena cava at the same time. If the SVC saturations repeatedly do not agree with each other or continually higher saturations are obtained, the SVC must be investigated with other modalities for lesions such as anomalous pulmonary veins or A–V fistulae entering into the more proximal veins as sources of the higher saturated blood.

Separate samples drawn from the same location can vary in saturation from each other by one to two percent, but should differ by no more than one to two percent. Always recheck any oxygen values that are discrepant from each other and oxygen values that are unexpectedly high or low by obtaining repeated samples from the same site at the same time. Even in the absence of any shunt, saturations during an "oxygen sweep" vary from each other by a few percent. On the other hand, saturations that are *absolutely the same* throughout an entire "sweep" should arouse suspicion about the measuring apparatus and should also be double-checked. Although identical saturations throughout the entire systemic venous system are possible, absolutely consistent values are an indication that the analyzing equipment is malfunctioning. Any discrepancies noted in the saturations, must be rechecked while the catheter is still in the same location or certainly during the catheterization procedure. Once the catheter is removed, there is no means of checking unusual saturations which could result in all of the oxygen data being invalid.

In the absence of any right to left shunting from intracardiac or intravascular communications, left-sided samples throughout the heart and into the aorta are fully saturated. The etiology of any systemic desaturation must be investigated when detected and while the patient is in the catheterization laboratory. Lower than normal oxygen values are frequently encountered in the absence of any central shunting owing to general hypoventilation, isolated areas of hypoventilated lung, or even small but severely hypoperfused lungs or lung segments. Blood gas determinations on room air and while breathing 100% oxygen distinguish between a pulmonary parenchymal disease and a central right to left shunt. If a right to left shunt is suspected, its exact location is determined at that time using indicator dilution curves or angiograms. The injections for the indicator dilution curves or angiograms are carried out in the right heart chamber or vessel that is immediately proximal to the suspected area of right to left shunt. Any central right to left shunting must be consistent with the anatomic and other hemodynamic findings.

Errors in sampling techniques

The catheter, the tubing, the connectors and the stopcocks between the catheter and sampling site represent common, additional sources of sampling error. When a sample is drawn, the entire length of the catheter and the length of tubing between the proximal end of the catheter and the sampling site must be completely cleared of flush solution and blood from a previous sample. Once the catheter and tubing are cleared completely by the withdrawal of fluid or blood, they must be filled with the "sample blood" by further withdrawal of blood through them before the actual sample to be analyzed is withdrawn from the system. When using a 4- or 5-French catheter, a 5 ml syringe is filled during the withdrawal, and when using a 6-French or larger catheter, a 10 ml syringe is filled during the withdrawal. Each withdrawal syringe is filled with fluid or blood from the catheter/tubing before the actual sample is withdrawn from the catheter. If the flush solution (or "old" blood) is not drawn out of the lumen of the catheter completely before the blood for the oxygen determination is withdrawn into the sampling syringe, the sample will obviously be diluted (contaminated) with flush solution or old blood from the previous area, which creates an erroneous reading. This is particularly true when large diameter or very long catheters, which can hold an unexpectedly large amount of fluid, are used.

If too much negative pressure is applied to the sampling syringe or there is not a tight seal between the tip of the syringe and the hub of the catheter/stopcock/side port, micro air bubbles are drawn into the sample and aerate (and oxygenate) the sample. When there is a small bubble of air in the sampling syringe which sits there for any length of time, again, the blood is oxygenated. With rapid sampling and analyzing of the samples, an anticoagulant does not have to be added to the sampling syringe. If heparin is used in the oxygen sampling syringe, even a small amount can contaminate the sample.

The stopcock through which the blood is being withdrawn from the system is another source of fluid contamination of the sample. If the stopcock is switched from the 90°, side port, withdrawing position back to the straight-through, pressure position while the withdrawal syringe is being changed to the syringe for the sample, a very short but definite column of fluid, which is contained within the channel of the stopcock, is reintroduced into the blood column (Figure 10.14). As the stopcock is turned back to the 90° withdrawal position, that small but definite amount of fluid in the lumen of the stopcock mixes with and contaminates the blood sample. This is an equally important source of error when blood gas or ACT samples are being withdrawn. Once the stopcock has been turned to the withdrawal position for sampling, it should remain in that position and the side port should be allowed to bleed during the exchange of syringes until after the actual sample has been withdrawn from the catheter. This potentially results in the loss of a few drops of blood while changing between the aspirating syringe and the sampling syringe, but the amount of blood loss is infinitesimal when the sampling is performed dexterously, even when sampling from a high-pressure system. Even the hub of the catheter, the stopcock or the tubing can trap a bubble of air as

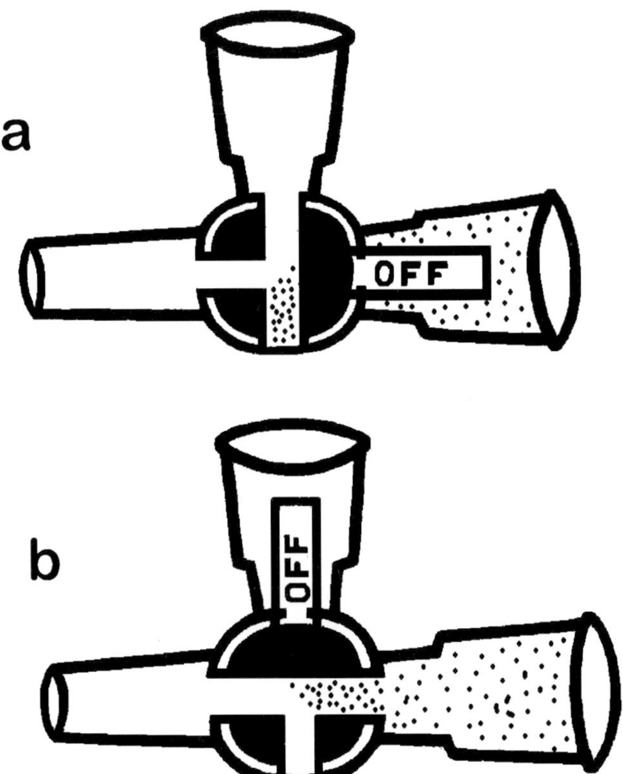

Figure 10.14 Cut-away drawing of three-way stopcock. (a) Stop-cock open to side port with 90° channel open to dead space off through channel (speckled area); (b) stop-cock open to through channel where dead space becomes refilled (speckled area and hub).

a syringe is removed and another one attached if the stopcock is turned back to the straight-through, pressure position. Blood is allowed to drip out of the hub before the sampling syringe is attached.

Samples for oxygen determination should never be withdrawn from the side port of a back-bleed valve/flush apparatus. All back-bleed valves have an internal chamber or dead space between the actual valve and where the sheath or catheter is attached at the opposite end of the apparatus (Figure 10.15). When blood is drawn out of the side port of a back bleed valve, contaminated blood or flush solution, which is always trapped in the valve chamber, is drawn into the sample, ***and/or*** air is withdrawn through the valve leaflets and mixed into the blood sample. In either case, the sample will be contaminated.

The catheterizing physician should never blame an unexpected or unusual saturation on a sampling or technical error without proving it at that time. It is simple and safe enough to redraw a sample and recheck the saturation while the catheter is still in or close to the same location. However, it is absolutely impossible to validate an abnormal oxygen value once the catheters have been removed from the patient! Regardless of the techniques

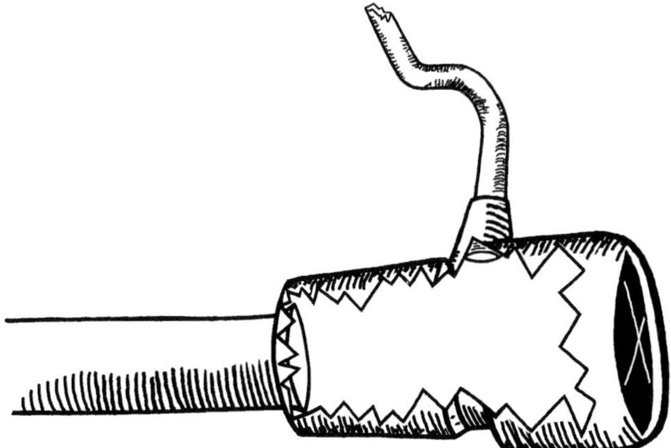

Figure 10.15 Cut-away drawing of the dead space or chamber of a back-bleed valve/flush port.

and type of equipment used, the physician performing the catheterization is totally responsible for the adequacy of the saturation data, making sure that:

- samples are obtained from the proper locations;
- enough separate samples and an adequate quantity of blood are obtained in each sample from each location;
- the samples are not contaminated with air or blood from the previous sample;
- there are no artifactual values overlooked during sampling; and
- samples are obtained in rapid enough sequence to be able to presume that the patient is in a steady state.

Measurement of oxygen saturation/content in blood

Once adequate and accurate blood samples are obtained from a specific site, the oxygen (O_2) saturations or contents in the blood sample are measured using one of several different techniques or machines. In most catheterization laboratories where oxygen saturations are used as the indicator for quantitating flow and shunts, separate blood samples are withdrawn through a catheter or an indwelling line from specific sites within the heart or great arteries. Each separate blood sample is analyzed for the concentration, content or total oxygen in one of several types of oxygen analyzer, which is usually in the catheterization room, close to but physically separated from the sterile catheterization field. All of the oxygen analyzers are very accurate and probably the most reliable part in the "chain of events" required for the determination of oxygen saturation or content of the blood.

The original gold standard for the determination of the oxygen content of blood was with a manometric, "Van Slyke" apparatus, in which both the dissolved oxygen and the oxygen combined with the hemoglobin were extracted physically from the blood and were measured volumetrically[4]. This required a large blood sample, it was a very cumbersome, time-consuming technique, and the procedure required specialized and usually full-time personnel. In the catheterization laboratory environment, the Van Slyke apparatus and technique, fortunately, have faded into historic oblivion and have been replaced by simpler, yet very sophisticated and automated, electronic oxygen analyzers, which are based on indirect spectrophotometric techniques and are equally as accurate or more accurate.

Spectrophotometric analysis—oxygen combined with hemoglobin

Spectrophotometric analyzers determine the percent saturation of the oxygen that is *combined with hemoglobin* in a very small sample of blood. Some of the spectrophotometric analyzers also determine the amount of hemoglobin. From those values, the oxygen content of the hemoglobin is calculated. None of the spectrophotometric analyzers measure the total oxygen content of the blood and plasma since they do not measure the additional dissolved oxygen in the plasma of the blood sample. When the patient is breathing room air the dissolved oxygen is only 0.3 ml O_2/100ml of blood/100 mmHg pO_2. This amount of dissolved oxygen adds less than 2% to the total oxygen content of any sample and, when a patient is breathing room air, is totally insignificant in the calculations of output, resistances and shunts. The significance of the dissolved oxygen when patients are breathing high concentrations of oxygen is addressed later in this chapter in the discussions on blood gas determinations.

The spectrophotometric analyzers currently used include "co-oximeters", whole blood oximeters, and fiberoptic catheter oximeters. The spectrophotometric techniques all depend upon the different absorptions of oxyhemoglobin and reduced hemoglobin in the red, infra-red and even green wavelengths of light between 500 and 930 nanometers. The amount of light transmitted in the red range at approximately 600 nanometers wavelength is a function of the oxyhemoglobin concentration, while at a wavelength of 506.5 nanometers, the light transmission is a function of reduced hemoglobin. Using these and, usually, several additional different wavelengths of light, the light absorbed by the sample is calculated using Beer's equation and reflects the percentage of oxygen bound in the hemoglobin in an essentially linear fashion. Each type of spectrophotometric analyzer uses slightly different combinations of light wavelengths, however, when used and maintained properly, all have a high degree of accuracy for percent saturation of oxyhemoglobin.

A co-oximeter analyzes only the hemoglobin from the cells. In a co-oximeter, the red cells are first hemolyzed in order to eliminate the light scattering due to the intact red cells themselves. The co-oximeter then performs the spectrophotometric analysis on the free hemoglobin alone. Co-oximeters measure total hemoglobin, oxy-hemoglobin, deoxy-hemoglobin, carboxy-hemoglobin and methemoglobin. However, the various co-oximeter apparatuses are expensive and they require special hemolyzing and cleaning solutions and a considerable amount of maintenance to maintain their accuracy. As a consequence, co-oximeters are now used very infrequently in clinical cardiac catheterization laboratories.

The oxygen analyzers used most commonly in the current clinical cardiac catheterization laboratory are "whole-blood" oximeters. These analyzers, as the name indicates, analyze whole-blood samples for percentage of oxygen in the hemoglobin without any processing of the sample. This is done by creating a very thin, uniform, film of the whole blood in special calibrated cuvettes. The transparent walls of each cuvette are machined and calibrated precisely for each particular analyzer so that differences in light absorption between samples are due only to the differences in oxygen saturation. All whole-blood oximeters still depend upon the amount of light transmitted near the 600 nanometers wavelength as a function of the oxyhemoglobin concentration and near a wavelength of 506.5 nanometers as a function of reduced hemoglobin. In addition to the percent saturation of hemoglobin in the sample, some of the wholeblood analyzers also determine the hemoglobin content of the sample. The AVOX oximeter™ (A-VOX Systems Inc., San Antonio, TX), used in our catheterization laboratory, utilizes five different wavelengths of light. Using a multi-spectral analysis, the percent saturation of oxygen in the hemoglobin and the hemoglobin content are measured rapidly, easily, and very accurately, on a very small (0.2 ml) sample of blood and over a full range of saturations and hemoglobin concentrations. With the multiple bandwidths of light in the AVOX oximeter™ analyzer, there is no interference from methoxy or carboxy hemoglobin.

In modern cardiac catheterization laboratories, in order to perform oxygen saturation determinations using whole-blood oximeters, a very small sample of blood (0.2–0.5 ml) is withdrawn from the tip of the catheter or indwelling line positioned in a specific location in the circulation. The sample is withdrawn into a small syringe, which is transferred (handed!) from the sterile field to a "circulating" nurse or technician. The circulating nurse or technician injects the blood sample into the special cuvette for the particular oxygen analyzer, and the cuvette containing the sample is inserted into the whole-blood oxygen analyzer. The oxygen analysis apparatus is separated from the sterile catheterization field; however, it should be in the proximity of the catheterization table and at least in the catheterization laboratory so that the results of the oxygen analysis are available to the operating cardiologist both immediately and conveniently.

A fiberoptic "oximeter" catheter represents a unique alternative technique for analyzing whole blood without having to withdraw a blood sample[5,6]. Fiberoptic catheters still use spectrophotometric principals for the actual analysis. With the fiberoptic catheter, a light source of several specific wavelengths similar to those of the other oximeters is transmitted through the fiberoptic "bundles" of the catheter to its tip, which is positioned at a specific site in the circulating blood. Any differences in the saturation of the blood at the catheter tip change the absorption and reflection of the transmitted light. These changes in the reflected light at the site in the circulation are transmitted back through separate fiber bundles in the catheter to an attached spectrophotometer. The changes in saturation are analyzed similarly to other whole-blood, spectrophotometric analysis.

The fiberoptic catheter was designed to provide a continuous reading of the changes in the saturation occurring at a fixed site in the circulation without any movement of the catheter. The output signal from the fiberoptic catheter is displayed as a continuous graph of the percent saturation. The graph or "saturation curve" is calibrated from 0 to 100 to correspond to the percent oxygen saturation in the blood. This curve, in turn, provides a continuous "read-out" of the instantaneous changes in the saturation at the particular location corresponding to the changes in the patient's condition (and output).

The fiberoptic catheter also function very well at continuously detecting and recording instantaneous changes in the saturations from different locations as the catheter is moved from one location to another. As the fiberoptic tip is withdrawn past the immediate site of a left to right shunt, there is a distinct increase in the height of the curve on the graph, which corresponds linearly to the increase in saturation. There would be an equally distinct drop in the height of the curve as the tip of the catheter is moved to a position proximal to the shunt. With the fiberoptic catheter, a defect resulting in a shunt can be localized very accurately and rapidly. In fact the instantaneous saturation display can be used to guide the catheter toward or through a defect.

However, there are several major disadvantages to the routine use of fiberoptic catheters in the catheterization laboratory. When the fiberoptic catheter tip is positioned *against* a vascular wall, particularly during the movement of the catheter, a sudden loss of the signal occurs. This artifact becomes obvious from the abruptness of the change which occurs in the plotted saturation curve, and is easily corrected by minimal repositioning of the tip of the catheter.

The greatest problem with fiberoptic catheters is the catheters themselves. Unfortunately, although the fiberoptic system functions very well in a single location, the catheters themselves are not suitable for easy or even reasonable manipulation within the heart. Current fiberoptic oximetry catheters are designed to remain in one position and to record changes occurring in the oxygen content at that one location in the circulation. The pediatric/congenital market is not large enough to make it profitable for manufacturers to manufacture fiberoptic catheters that can be manipulated more satisfactorily, and through which pressures can be recorded in addition to their oxygen content sampling capabilities. As a consequence, fiberoptic catheters for oxygen sampling during a cardiac catheterization have never achieved practicality or gained popularity.

Analysis of samples for oxygen saturation determination

As discussed earlier, the actual analysis of the sample for oxygen saturation is usually very accurate. The various problems in acquiring the proper samples have already been discussed. Whichever oxygen-analyzing device is used in the cardiac catheterization laboratory, it should be calibrated at least daily against a control calibration sample with a known, repeatable value. It is also advisable to check the spectrophotometric analyzer against a second, preferably different type of, oxygen analyzer at least once a day, and any time there is even the slightest hint of an irregularity in the values being obtained or expected.

In the current scheme for the determination of oxygen saturations, there are significant potential errors that can occur during the handling of the samples as well as during the displaying and recording of the results from the oxygen analyzer.

Handling, display and recording of oxygen saturation data in the catheterization laboratory

The absolutely "primitive" way in which each blood sample is handled between the drawing of the sample from the patient and the final recording of the oxygen saturation represents another monumental and common source of error in the modern cardiac catheterization laboratory. As alluded to earlier in the discussion of whole-blood oximeters, a potential problem begins with the sample in the syringe on the catheterization table. The physician draws the sample from a particular site through the catheter and into a small syringe on the catheterization table. The syringe containing the blood sample is handed off the sterile field to a circulating nurse or technician who is informed of the (precise!) location from which the sample was obtained. The nurse/technician makes a mental (and possibly written) note of the site of the sample, injects the blood sample into a special cuvette, and inserts the cuvette into the oxygen-analyzing apparatus.

Simultaneous with making a note of the site of the sample or inserting the sample into the oxygen analyzer, the circulating nurse transmits the information concerning the site of this sample by shouting the site to the recording nurse or technician, who is usually in an adjacent, but completely separate, room. The recording nurse/technician manually types the location (only) from which the sample was withdrawn (or whatever site they heard!) at that time, into the timed computer record in the physiologic monitor/recorder. Once the sample is analyzed (in 7–30 seconds) there is an automatic digital read-out of the saturation on the small oxygen analyzer screen within the catheterization room. The value from the analyzer and the site of the sample are again noted mentally or manually (usually by a hand-written note on a temporary flow sheet or small diagram) by the circulating nurse/technician in the room while the analyzer re-calibrates itself (5–10 more seconds) and before another sample can be inserted. The numerical value from the analyzer along with a repetition of the site where that value was obtained and often along with the site of the next sample are "transmitted" by another *shout* to the recording nurse/technician, who is still in a separate room, and as time permits between samples! The recording nurse or technician, in turn, *manually types* the result of the oxygen saturation (*or whatever they heard!*) into the time and previously mentioned site location in the official, timed record on the computer flow sheet. The value for the saturation can be placed into the previously recorded notation for the time and location of the sample. The flow-sheet created by the recording nurse/technician is usually typed into a computer program, which officially times each typed entry of events from the laboratory.

This system of handling the blood samples and getting the data to a recorded source requires a minimum of ***six separate human steps*** by laboratory personnel. The potential sources for error are obviously myriad from this sequence of human steps! Often the samples are drawn from the patient and handed to the circulation nurse/technician faster than the machine can analyze them or faster than the particular nurse/technician (who often has other more urgent duties) is able to put them into the oxygen analyzer or even make a mental (and then written) note of the site and value. As a consequence, the samples are lined up where they can easily be mixed from their proper order or location or even lost altogether. In the noise and occasionally frantic activity of the catheterization laboratory or the control/recording room, the values transmitted verbally to the adjacent control room can very easily be misunderstood. Even when the recording nurse hears the "transmitted" value properly, there is still a further potential for error while entering the value and location during the manual typing into the official flow sheet by the recording nurse, who is simultaneously recording other events that are occurring and items being used in the laboratory!

During this series of events, the oxygen analyzer and, particularly, the display of its read-out often are not immediately adjacent to or visible from the catheterization table. Even when the analyzer is near to the catheterization table, the display of the read-out on the analyzer is very small and not convenient for the catheterizing physician to see. At no time is the read-out from the analyzer prominently displayed, or displayed for the operator to see the values easily and sequentially exactly when they are obtained or in the order in which they were obtained. For the operator to double-check the values for accuracy or consistency and against the previous values takes some extra time and effort away from performing the catheterization.

Similarly, the written notation of the read-out from the oxygen analyzer by the circulating nurse/technician is usually placed on a temporary, small note or small heart diagram which certainly is not timed, not a display which is clearly visible to the operator, and in no way can it act as a valid, or prominent, "prompter". These hand notes of the values from the oxygen analyzer, the actual values from the screen and print-out of the analyzer or the saturations that were transmitted and posted on the official flow-sheet (which, may or may not, have made it to the computer properly) can be reviewed by the operator only when specifically requested. If a spurious sample or recording is obtained and quietly noted or recorded on the flow-chart or there is even a transient distraction due to other activity in the laboratory, the operator can be totally unaware of an unusual but critical result from the "saturation run" until the data are reviewed after the completion of the case. At that time there is no opportunity to verify or disprove the value!

When sampling oxygen saturation data in the catheterization laboratory, there can now be an easily and prominently visible running display of the oxygen findings available to the operator as they are obtained (as is done with pressure data). Most cardiac catheterization laboratories have an electronic *running display* of the ***pressures*** as they are being recorded along with a "running table" of those recorded pressures with different conditions as part of the pressure/recording display on the CRT screen. But most cardiac catheterization laboratories do *not have a prominent and/or even usable* "running display" of the *saturations* that includes the exact time and location of each sample analyzed along with the different conditions when they were obtained.

Usually, at best, the *electronic* running display of the *saturations* is a table of the most recent saturations obtained off the electronic flow-sheet of the computer, which is then displayed on the CRT display of data as a very small table. The display screen in the catheterization room can occasionally display the times and locations from the saturation tables obtained from the computer record, but the values are displayed only intermittently and certainly do not appear instantaneously or live as the saturations are being acquired. In addition, the computer can only display the values that were eventually transmitted to it. As noted, these values are often spurious because of the primitive sequence of "human" steps including the several "verbal transmission links". Obviously, this system of transmitting, recording and displaying oxygen saturations, which requires such a significant personnel involvement, allows the opportunity for numerous human errors. The system for recording and displaying oxygen saturations is absolutely archaic compared to the remaining catheterization laboratory procedures/equipment.

One common alternative that is used in many pediatric/congenital catheterization laboratories for an on-going display of the saturations, is a large, outline diagram of a heart (the particular patient's heart!), which is printed on a chalkboard or erasable display. The diagram is displayed prominently *in the laboratory* and the saturations are written on the diagram as the case progresses. The oxygen saturations are posted manually by a "circulating" nurse or technician. They are recorded accurately, immediately and clearly on the diagram as they are obtained from the read-out of the oxygen analyzer. The large diagram provides a running display of the saturations that is visible to the operator. However, this type of display still does *not* include the time or "condition" of the sample and still involves the very labor intensive steps of retrieving the output from the small screen of the oxygen analyzer, transmitting the value *verbally* within the busy (and sometimes noisy) catheterization room to the recording technician and manually (and accurately) writing the value on the display board—often while many other things are going on in the laboratory.

Fortunately, there now is available one new electronic solution, which provides a large and timed display of the saturations instantaneously on a CRT screen in the laboratory while at the same time requiring minimal human interface. This system utilizes an AVOX oximeter^ETM 1,000 oxygen analyzer (A-VOX Systems Inc., San Antonio, TX) along with a computer program developed by Scientific Software Solutions™ (Scientific Software Solutions, Charlottesville, VA) for a standard PC. The blood sample is taken from the catheterizing physician, injected into the A-VOX™ cuvette and inserted into the analyzer by the circulating nurse/technician. The location of the sample is entered into a built-in electronic table either in the AVOX oximeter™ or into a separate table in the computer program as it is inserted into the analyzer and before the result is displayed on the computer. The saturation values are automatically timed by the oximeter when the sample is inserted into the AVOX oximeter™ for analysis. The timed value for the oxygen saturation is displayed on the small AVOX oximeter™ screen and simultaneously the timed result of the oxygen saturation from the AVOX oximeter™ is transmitted as a digital signal to the computer. The software program acquires the saturation determination, the location of the sample and the time of sampling all as the digital signal from the analyzer and lists the data in a continuously updated, timed, and tabular form on a large computer CRT screen. The displayed table on the computer is timed and up-dated continuously, instantaneously and automatically from the AVOX oximeter™ signal with the only human interface being the designation of the location of each sample as it is placed in the analyzer. A change in the steady state condition of the patient can be designated in the program, and is displayed with a change in the background shading on the computer display. The running table of values is displayed clearly *in the catheterization laboratory* on a prominent "slave" CRT screen, which can be as large as desired and which can be positioned in any desired location in the laboratory. The handling and displaying of the oxygen saturations with this system requires, at most, two human steps, no verbal communications and essentially eliminates errors from the transmission and transcribing of the oxygen data.

As of this writing and primarily because of manufacturer interface problems, the final table of oxygen values with the accurate values, locations, times and conditions is printed out separately and is not electronically integrated into the official computer flow-sheet. It allows absolute verification of all oxygen data that are transmitted verbally to the official record as the case progresses. Ideally (eventually) there will be a large electronic display on an individualized diagram on a CRT screen in the catheterization laboratory of the particular heart for each patient. The computer could then automatically insert both the pressures and saturations into the appropriate locations on the electronic diagram display as well as the official flow-sheet as they are obtained. The electronic display could even be programmed to signal alerts for significant deviations from the expected normal or from the expected sequence of values. This unfortunately will require a major change in the financial priorities of the major manufacturers of cardiac catheterization laboratory computer/monitoring equipment, but in the interim, the separate computer tabulation/display from A-VOX™ and Scientific Software Solutions™ eliminates many of the errors from the human steps in the acquisition of oxygen saturation data.

Dissolved oxygen—oxygen tension analysis

As described previously, *none* of the spectrophotometric methods measure the oxygen that is dissolved in the plasma. The dissolved oxygen in plasma is determined from the oxygen tension (pO_2) of the blood. The oxygen tension is measured with a polarographic electrode in a "blood gas" machine and expressed as mm of mercury (Hg) O_2 tension (or torr). The normal oxygen tension in room air is, at most, 100 mmHg and when a patient is breathing room air, the amount of oxygen dissolved in the plasma is approximately 0.3 ml of oxygen per 100 ml of blood (or 3 ml of oxygen per liter of blood). Compared to the roughly 20 ml of oxygen bound to a "normal" level of hemoglobin, this amounts to less than 1.5 % of the oxygen content of the whole blood. As a consequence, when a patient is breathing room air, the dissolved oxygen is inconsequential and is not considered in the calculations of output, resistances or shunts.

Often, however, oxygen concentrations as high as 100% of the inspired air are used in the catheterization laboratory. High concentrations of oxygen are used diagnostically, particularly when dealing with high pulmonary resistances. Even more frequently, very high concentrations of inhaled oxygen are used for the treatment of ill patients who are hypoxic or in respiratory distress during the cardiac catheterization. When a patient is breathing high concentrations of oxygen, the pO_2 in the pulmonary veins and systemic arterial system can rise as high as 600 mmHg. When the pO_2 is that high, the dissolved oxygen in the plasma becomes a significant fraction of the total oxygen content of the whole blood and must be included in the calculations. The amount of dissolved oxygen in a sample of plasma in ml O_2/100 ml of blood is determined by multiplying the pO_2 of the sample by 0.003. For example, at a pO_2 of 600 mmHg, the dissolved oxygen in the whole blood will be 1.8 ml O_2/100 ml of blood. In blood with a "normal" hemoglobin value, this can represent 10 % of the whole blood oxygen content.

Dissolved oxygen has an even greater significance in the presence of anemia where the amount of hemoglobin, and the oxygen carrying capacity of the hemoglobin in the blood are much lower. In that circumstance, the dissolved oxygen in the plasma becomes a higher fraction of the total oxygen carrying capacity of the whole blood. For example, in a patient with 8 g of hemoglobin, the oxygen content of the hemoglobin in 100% saturated blood would be 10.7 ml O_2/100 ml of blood. The dissolved oxygen at a pO_2 of 600 mm Hg is 1.8 ml O_2/100 ml of blood, or 16.8% of the whole blood oxygen content!

When a patient is breathing oxygen, the pO_2 of *each* of the samples used in the calculation of flow, shunts and resistances is measured and added to the value of the oxygen content of the hemoglobin in the calculations. This includes, for example, the pO_2 of the SVC, PA, LA and systemic arterial samples. When flows are calculated *without* including the dissolved oxygen in patients breathing high concentrations of oxygen, the magnitude of the flow and of shunts are overestimated and resistances are underestimated (since the flow appears in the denominator of the formulas used to calculate resistance). This is illustrated in "Calculations of Shunts" discussion later in this chapter.

At the other extreme, because of the flat oxygen dissociation curve at levels above 65–70%, pO_2 is more sensitive than oxygen saturation in detecting a small right to left shunt or pulmonary hypoventilation in a pulmonary venous or systemic arterial sample of blood. With either of these conditions, the pO_2 of the "saturated" blood is below the usual 80–90 pO_2. When there is a question of the cause of the low pO_2, the patient is administered 100% oxygen. A low pO_2 due to lung disease rises to above 300–500 mmHg with oxygen administration, while a low pO_2 due to a right to left shunt does not rise above 100 mmHg with the same amount of oxygen administration. Low pO_2 is useful in detecting a right to left shunt but, since the value is not linear in relation to the amount of shunting, pO_2 alone cannot be used to quantitate the shunting.

The oxygen saturation of blood can be, and usually is, automatically calculated from the oxygen tension of the blood gas value by blood gas machines. The calculation of oxygen saturation from oxygen tension, particularly at lower saturations, is totally invalid. The steep oxygen dissociation curve from blood at lower saturations does not allow a linear relationship between saturation and pO_2. At the other extreme, because of the flat oxygen dissociation curve at high levels, essentially all oxygen tensions greater than 70 mmHg result in 95% or greater saturation of hemoglobin. The calculations of flow, shunt and resistance, which are dependent upon oxygen saturations, cannot be performed when the oxygen saturations are calculated from oxygen tension in the blood. In the range of very high saturations, the calculated oxygen saturation serves as a valuable check against the saturation value from the spectrophotometric method.

Determination of oxygen consumption

For the precise determination of flow or cardiac output using oxygen saturations, the continuous oxygen consumption must be measured. In infants and children and, now, in older patients in the congenital catheterization laboratory, the expired air is drawn from a hood with a "high-flow" system and is measured for oxygen content with a polarographic oxygen sensor[7]. The polarographic sensor constantly measures the oxygen content of the air drawn past it. The hood is made of a clear plastic material and fits comfortably over the patients without constraining them. In infants, the head and upper chest, and in older patients, only the head is enclosed in the acrylic hood. All openings between the hood, the table and around the chest and neck are sealed loosely with plastic wrap and tape. The seal is tight enough to secure the hood over the patient and to not allow air to flow freely into it, but it is not totally air-tight. The withdrawal pump must be able to draw air through the seal and into the hood at a rate faster than the patient's oxygen consumption utilizes the air. All of the expired "air" from the patient is collected from a hood using a high-flow withdrawal pump.

The withdrawal pump is attached to the polarographic sensor for the oxygen content analysis. The concentration of oxygen in the room air is measured and the apparatus calibrated by drawing room air through the polarographic oxygen analyzer with the withdrawal pump at the same rate that is to be used when the pump is attached to the hood. After the calibration, the hood is attached to the sensor for the oxygen content analysis. The high-flow pump then draws the expired air from the patient out of the hood and through the sensor. The suction from the pump creates a mild partial vacuum in the hood so that ambient air is drawn into the hood (through the loose seals between the hood and the neck or trunk of the patient) and to the polarographic sensor at a rate approximately ten times the patient's estimated respiratory volume. The rate of flow is adjusted according to the patient's size and minute ventilation. The flow into and through the hood is sufficient to prevent any escape of exhaled air but at the same time not so rapid that the expired air is too diluted for accurate analysis. The rate of flow from the hood through the analyzer is kept constant for at least five minutes while the concentration of oxygen in the withdrawn, expired air is measured and samples are drawn from the blood for oxygen saturation determinations.

The difference in the concentration of oxygen in room air and the difference in the concentration of oxygen in the expired air times the volume of gas flow through the hood (and the analyzer) in milliliters per minute measures the oxygen consumed in milliliters per minute (ml/min) by the patient. When divided by the body surface area of the patient in square meters (m^2), the absolute oxygen consumption value is indexed to ml/min/m^2. This value is plugged into the formulas for cardiac output or flow that are discussed subsequently in this chapter. Reliable apparatuses for measuring oxygen consumption based on flow through the hood and the polarographic oxygen analyzer are available commercially in the MRM-2 Oxygen Consumption Monitor (Waters Instruments Inc., Rochester, MN), and no longer need to be assembled by each individual laboratory.

Even with a commercially available apparatus, the measurement of oxygen consumption is difficult. The apparatus and the procedure are cumbersome, require a regular, consistent experience with the apparatus for accurate determinations and cannot be performed with a patient breathing greater concentrations of oxygen than room air or when a patient is intubated. Establishing the proper flow rate through the hood for the required five minutes takes practice and continued experience of a trained individual. During an oxygen consumption determination, one person devotes their full, undivided time and attention to performing the test. Even with an experienced person performing the oxygen consumption, the results are often inconsistent with the other findings and other output determinations. Additionally, it is very difficult to maintain the patient in a steady state for the duration of time required for simultaneously obtaining the oxygen consumption and the necessary blood samples.

Of even greater practical importance, in congenital heart lesions the oxygen consumption value is unnecessary in most of the calculations that are used for the large majority of clinical decisions made utilizing the catheterization data. When oxygen consumption values are used in the calculation of *relative* shunts, they cancel out in the various formulas for the calculations. Often, an assumed oxygen consumption is used in the calculation of cardiac output and shunt determinations when using oxygen as the indicator for dilution studies. The average values for oxygen consumption according to the patient's age, sex, weight and body surface area are available in tables of standard values[8]. The *assumed* oxygen consumption can also be calculated equally as "accurately" by multiplying the patient's body surface area by 150 ml/min. The assumed value and possible errors that might be incurred in these particular calculations, are acceptable in the determinations in congenital heart defects unless there is concern about high pulmonary resistance.

When maximum accuracy in the determination of the cardiac output is necessary for the calculation of absolute flow, resistances and valve areas, either the oxygen consumption is measured in order to calculate the flow and, in turn, the cardiac output or, more often now, cardiac output is measured directly using thermodilution indicator curves. These are easier to perform and just as accurate. For these reasons, oxygen consumption measurements are now used very infrequently in the active, clinical, pediatric/congenital catheterization laboratory.

The calculation of cardiac output and shunts using oxygen saturation

Most calculations in the cardiac catheterization laboratory are now performed by a computer that is on-line in the laboratory. As a consequence, the results are frequently undisputed and taken for granted as "gospel". This could not be further from the truth. The automation of the computations does not remove the obligation of the operator from having a complete understanding of each of the formulas and the importance of each of the numbers used in these formulas. The validity of the specific calculations for the quantification of flows, cardiac outputs, shunts and resistances is dependent upon the validity of each assumption and the *absolute accuracy of every individual number* used in the calculations. The lack of applicability of a necessary assumption or a single, small error in the sampling or in the analysis of a sample results in totally erroneous conclusions no matter how accurate and efficient the computer calculations may seem.

The calculation of total systemic flow (Qs) or cardiac output (CO) using oxygen as the indicator is based on Fick's law of diffusion, which states "a substance will diffuse through an area at a rate that is dependent upon the difference in concentration of the substance at two given points"[2]. An accurate determination of cardiac output using the Fick principal for Qs requires the determination of the oxygen content of the mixed systemic venous (MV) blood and the systemic arterial (SA) blood. Calculation of the pulmonary blood flow (Qp) requires the determination of the oxygen contents of the mixed pulmonary venous (PV) blood and the pulmonary artery (PA) blood. To compensate for the separate and different sources of venous blood contributing to the mixed venous blood on both sides of the circulation and to ensure total mixing of the sample, the mixed venous blood samples are collected as far as possible downstream in the respective circuits (in the corresponding ventricle or great artery). This, of course, assumes that there is no intracardiac shunting. In the presence of an intracardiac shunt, the mixed venous sample must be obtained significantly proximal to the shunt. Often a venous sample from *one* of the sources of the venous inflow is *assumed* to be representative of all of the mixed venous sources on that side of the circulation, whether this is valid or not.

During the same period of time that the blood samples for oxygen content are being obtained, the patient's oxygen consumption (VO_2) is measured. All of these values must be obtained while the patient is in an absolutely steady physiologic state for the Fick principal to be valid. This includes a steady state of consciousness, heart rate, blood pressure and respiratory rate. As mentioned previously, in order for the values to be comparable in pediatric and congenital patients, the absolute values for oxygen consumption and, in turn, for the calculations, are "indexed to" the patient's body surface area. The blood flow per square meter is calculated:

$$\text{Flow (l/min/m}^2) = \frac{\text{Oxygen consumption (ml/min/m}^2)}{(\text{Pul vein O}_2 - \text{Mixed system vein O}_2) \times 10} = \text{CI l/min/m}^2$$

or, in the presence of no intracardiac shunt, calculating for either pulmonary or systemic flow:

$$Q_P = \frac{V\,O_2\ (\text{ml/min/m}^2)}{(PV\,O_2 - PA\,O_2) \times 10} = \text{CI (l/min/m}^2)$$

or:

$$Q_S = \frac{V\,O_2\ (\text{ml/min/m}^2)}{(SA\,O_2 - MV\,O_2) \times 10} = \text{CI (l/min/m}^2)$$

If the oxygen consumption that is used in the formula is not indexed to body surface area (BSA), then the final flow (CO) is multiplied by the body surface area in order to index the CO to BSA.

In these calculations Flow (Q) = Cardiac Index (CI) in liters/minute/square meter; oxygen consumption ($V\,O_2$) is measured in ml/minute/square meter; and the pulmonary artery (PA) pulmonary venous (PV), mixed systemic venous (MV) and systemic arterial (SA) oxygen content (O_2) are in ml of oxygen/100 ml of blood. The denominator is multiplied by 10 to convert the oxygen content of the blood from g/100 ml to g/l of blood, allowing the flow or cardiac output to be expressed in liters/minute. By referencing the measured oxygen consumption to the patient's body surface area, the values for flow are, in turn, indexed per square meter.

By combining the identical multipliers in the denominator the formulas for systemic and pulmonary flow can be simplified so that the direct saturations from the analyzer can be plugged into the calculations:

$$Q_S = \frac{V\,O_2/\text{m}^2}{(SA\ \%\ Sat - MV\ \%\ Sat) \times 1.34 \times Hgb \times 10}$$

And:

$$Q_P = \frac{V\,O_2/\text{M}^2}{(PV\ \%\ Sat - PA\ \%\ Sat) \times 1.34 \times Hgb \times 10}$$

where Hgb = hemoglobin content in g/100 ml.

The *true* oxygen content of a whole blood sample includes the oxygen combined with hemoglobin plus the oxygen dissolved in the plasma. In a patient breathing room air, the oxygen dissolved in plasma is only 0.003 ml of oxygen per ml of blood at 100 mmHg (100 torr) oxygen tension (pO_2). This amount of dissolved oxygen is negligible when determining the oxygen content of the blood, and only the oxygen combined with the hemoglobin is considered as the "oxygen content" when calculations are made on a patient who is breathing room air.

The capacity of hemoglobin (ml O_2/g Hgb) to hold oxygen is determined by multiplying the hemoglobin (g/100 ml) by the Hufner factor, which is a constant corresponding to the capacity of each gram of hemoglobin to hold oxygen. The Hufner factor is variously reported at values between 1.34 and 1.39. A value of 1.34 is currently accepted. The oxygen capacity of the hemoglobin in the blood equals:

O_2 Capacity Hgb (ml O_2/g Hgb) = Hgb (g/100 ml blood) × 1.34 (ml O_2/g Hgb)

The oxygen content of the hemoglobin is the percent saturation of the sample multiplied by the hemoglobin capacity. In patients breathing room air, the oxygen content of the hemoglobin, *not* the oxygen content of whole blood, is used in all of the calculations for flow and shunts. The value for oxygen content of hemoglobin is usually referred to as the "oxygen content".

O_2 content of Hgb (ml O_2/100 ml) =
% saturation of sample × Hgb (g/100 ml) × 1.34 ml O_2/g

This calculation is illustrated by a hypothetical patient who is breathing room air, has an oxygen consumption of 150 ml/min/m^2 and a hemoglobin of 15 g. For consistency in illustrating the calculations, this same hypothetical patient, with necessary variations in the numbers to correspond to the different anatomy or physiology, will be used throughout the subsequent discussions of the various calculations. In this example, the saturations are: 65% in the superior vena cava (SVC), 95% in the systemic artery (SA), 95% in the pulmonary vein (PV) and 65% in the pulmonary artery (PA). In this patient, the oxygen capacity of the hemoglobin is:

15 g/dl × 1.34 ml O_2/g Hgb = 20.1 ml O_2/g Hgb

And the cardiac output in this patient is:

$$Q_S = \frac{V\,O_2(\text{ml/min/m}^2)}{(\text{SA } O_2 \times 15 \times 1.34 - \text{MV } O_2 \times 15 \times 1.34) \times 10} = \text{CI}$$

$$= \frac{150}{(19.1 - 13.1) \times 10} = \frac{150}{6 \times 10} = 2.5\,\text{l/min/m}^2$$

Or, combining denominators:

$$Q_S = \frac{V\,O_2/\text{m}^2}{(\text{SA } O_2 - \text{MV } O_2) \times 1.34 \times 15 \times 10}$$

$$= \frac{150}{(0.95 - 0.65) \times (20.1 \times 10)} = \frac{150}{0.3 \times 201} = 2.5\,\text{l/min/m}^2$$

The same basic formula is used to calculate the absolute pulmonary flow except the pulmonary venous (PV) content is substituted for the SA content and the pulmonary artery (PA) oxygen content is substituted for the SVC content in the denominator.

$$Q_P = \frac{V\,O_2/\text{m}^2}{(\text{PV \% Sat} - \text{PA \% Sat}) \times 1.34 \times \text{Hgb} \times 10}$$

In the absence of any intracardiac or intravascular shunting, PA O_2 and MV O_2 as well as the PV O_2 and the SA O_2 (the only differences in the denominators in either of the formulas) are the same so that the pulmonary flow (Q_P) equals the systemic flow (Q_S) which, in turn, equals the cardiac output (CO).

Effect of oxygen inhalation (dissolved oxygen) on absolute flow

When a patient is breathing higher concentrations of oxygen than room air, the oxygen tension (pO_2) of each sample is determined and used in the calculations. The dissolved oxygen in ml/liter of blood in the sample is calculated by multiplying the pO_2 (in mmHg) by 0.003:

0.003 × pO_2 of sample (in mmHg or torr)
= dissolved O_2 (ml/l of blood)

Example 1: If the pO_2 of a sample in a patient breathing room air is 90 mmHg, then the dissolved oxygen is:

0.003 × 90 = 0.27 ml/l of blood.

Example 2: If, on the other hand, the pO_2 of a sample is 600 mmHg, then the dissolved oxygen is:

0.003 × 600 = 1.8 ml/l of blood.

Dissolved oxygen can be included in the calculations of cardiac output, e.g. using the same hypothetical patient described above, but now breathing 100% O_2 and still with an oxygen consumption of 150 ml/min/m^2 and a hemoglobin of 15 g. The saturations of oxygen in the samples are increased slightly to 70% in the SVC and 98% in the SA. The oxygen capacity of the hemoglobin is still 20.1, while the SA pO_2 is 500 and the SVC pO_2 is 40.

$$Q_S = \frac{V\,O_2/\text{m}^2}{[(\text{SA cont}) + (0.003 \times \text{SA } pO_2)] - [(\text{SVC cont}) + (0.003 \times \text{SVC } pO_2)] \times 10}$$

$$= \frac{150}{[(20.1 \times 0.98) + (0.003 \times 500) - (20.1 \times 0.70) + (0.003 \times 40)] \times 10}$$

$$= \frac{150}{[(19.7 + 1.5) - (14.1 + 0.12)] \times 10} = 2.14\,\text{l/min/m}^2$$

Thus, with the same theoretical patient as above, but who is now breathing 100% oxygen instead of room air, the dissolved oxygen in the plasma changes the cardiac output from 2.5 l/min/m^2 on room air to 2.14 l/min/m^2. This same holds true in the calculation of pulmonary flow, shunt and resistance calculations.

Shunt calculations

When oxygen saturation or content is used as the indicator for quantifying shunts, a volume of blood containing a higher (or lower) percent of oxygen is the indicator. Blood with a specified oxygen saturation is introduced into the venous system on one side of the circulation (a). Blood with a different saturation from the opposite side (b) of the circulation leaks through the communication (shunt) into the original (a) blood. The change in saturation of the blood exiting on the original (a) side of the circulation is measured after it has mixed with the blood which passed through the shunt (a & b). By measuring the exact increase in the oxygen saturation (left to right) or exact decrease in saturation (right to left) in the blood of a previously known (mixed venous) saturation, the amount of abnormal shunt flow is quantitated. In this way, changes in saturations used as the indicator are capable of detecting and quantitating small degrees of shunting.

The problems in obtaining true mixed venous samples on either side of the circulation for the calculation of absolute flows have been discussed. These problems are compounded in the presence of intracardiac shunts where the blood on one side of the circulation begins mixing with the shunted blood from the other side at the level of the shunt. Any downstream locations in adjacent chambers will very likely be at or beyond the area of the shunt, in which case the mixed venous blood has already mixed with the blood that has crossed the shunt. When a more downstream site of completely mixed venous blood cannot be sampled, it is ***assumed*** that *one* (or several) of the multiple inflow veins (upstream) is representative of all of the veins, and the value for that source is used for the mixed venous saturation in the calculations[3].

When intracardiac or intravascular shunts are present, the same formulas with the same oxygen consumption are used for the calculation of the flow in each of the separate circuits. The only variables are the oxygen contents from the different locations in the denominator of the formulas. The actual volume of a shunt can be quantitated using the difference in the total flow in the two separate circuits. As with the determinations of absolute cardiac output, the calculation of the *actual* volume of flow and the volume of the shunt requires a simultaneous determination of the oxygen consumption.

In the detection and calculation of left to right shunts using oxygen saturations, the indicator is the amount of "fully" saturated pulmonary venous blood (coming from the lungs and left side of the circulation) that is introduced through the shunt into, and mixed with, the less saturated systemic venous (right sided) blood. The "fully" saturated and the unsaturated bloods mix in the right heart circulation to produce the saturation of the final mixture downstream. The final mixture distal to the left to right shunt is obtained from the most distal possible site in the right heart blood flow—usually a pulmonary artery. When dealing with only a left to right shunt, the calculation for the systemic flow remains the same as when there is no shunt. The SA O_2 and the MV O_2 in the systemic veins remain the same:

$$Q_S\,(\mathrm{l/min/m^2}) = \frac{\mathrm{V\,O_2\,(l/min/m^2)}}{(\mathrm{SA\ \%\ Sat} - \mathrm{MV\ \%\ Sat}) \times \mathrm{Hgb} \times 1.34 \times 10}$$

In the formula for Q_P, on the other hand, the PA % Saturation is increased as a result of the quantity of the pulmonary venous (PV) blood which crosses the defect mixing with the total systemic venous (MV) blood to result in the final pulmonary artery (PA) blood saturation and volume. The PA % Saturation varies proportionately, according to the magnitude of the shunt:

$$Q_P\,(\mathrm{l/min/m^2}) = \frac{\mathrm{V\,O_2(l/min/m^2)}}{(\mathrm{PV\ \%\ Sat} - \mathrm{PA\ \%\ Sat}) \times \mathrm{Hgb} \times 1.34 \times 10}$$

To illustrate the effect of a large step-up in oxygen as a result of an intracardiac shunt and using the same patient example as used previously, breathing room air with an oxygen consumption of 150 ml/min/m^2, 15 g hemoglobin, a mixed systemic venous saturation of 65%, an arterial saturation of 95%, but now a pulmonary vein saturation of 95% and a pulmonary artery saturation of 85%:

$$Q_P = \frac{150}{(0.95 - 0.85) \times 1.34 \times 15 \times 10} = 7.5\,\mathrm{l/min/m^2}$$

The larger the shunt, the more oxygenated blood is introduced into and mixed with the systemic venous blood, and proportionally the higher the oxygen saturation in the PA becomes. This in turn *decreases* the denominator in the formula and, in turn, increases the Q_P. In the same patient, assuming no concomitant right to left flow, the systemic flow is still 2.5 l/min/m^2, so the ratio of pulmonary to systemic flow is now 3:1.

The *systemic flow* (Q_S) is the total blood that actually flows through the systemic capillaries, while the *pulmonary flow* (Q_P) is the total blood actually flowing through the pulmonary capillaries. The *effective flow* (Q_{EP}) is the volume of desaturated systemic venous blood from the systemic venous system that flows through the lungs and is actually oxygenated in the lungs. The *effective pulmonary blood flow* is equal to the *effective systemic flow* (Q_{ES}), which is the total amount of pulmonary venous blood which is carried to the tissues, and which has oxygen extracted from it in capillaries of the tissues of the body. In the absence of intracardiac shunting the Q_{EP} is equal to the Q_S and to the Q_P. Using the oxygen content (O_2) of the hemoglobin of each sample, the Q_{EP} is calculated:

$$Q_{EP}\,(\mathrm{l/min/m^2}) = \frac{\mathrm{V\,O_2/m^2}}{(\mathrm{PV\,O_2} - \mathrm{MV\,O_2}) \times 10}$$

Using the percent saturation of the separate samples directly in the denominator, the Q_{EP} is calculated:

$$Q_{EP}\,(\mathrm{l/min/m^2}) = \frac{\mathrm{V\,O_2/m^2}}{(\mathrm{PV\ \%\ Sat} - \mathrm{MV\ \%\ Sat}) \times \mathrm{Hgb} \times 1.34 \times 10}$$

In the presence of a left to right shunt, the Q_P equals the Q_{EP} plus the volume of the left to right shunt and the volume of the left to right shunt equals $Q_P - Q_{EP}$. In the presence of a right to left shunt, the Q_S equals the Q_{EP} plus the volume of the right to left shunt and the volume of the right to left shunt equals $Q_S - Q_{EP}$. In order to compare the volume of flow in the pulmonary and systemic circuits and, in turn, calculate the volume of the shunt, the individual flows are calculated separately from the formulas for Q_S and Q_P and then the values compared. Fortunately, and thanks to algebraic rules, the separate formulas can be mathematically merged. In doing so, all of the repeated or duplicated numbers in the two original formulas cancel each other, resulting in a simplified and rapid method for the calculation of relative flows.

Relative flows and pulmonary to systemic flow ratios

The difficulties and inaccuracies encountered in the measurement of oxygen consumption in congenital heart patients makes the determination of *absolute* pulmonary and systemic flows very complicated. The results obtained from the measured oxygen consumption often are not accurate and do not agree with the clinical or other hemodynamic findings. The alternative of using an estimated, or an oxygen consumption calculated arbitrarily, is even less accurate. However, the use of pulmonary to systemic flow *ratios* and the *relative flow* in the two circuits provide sufficient information for the *majority of therapeutic decisions* related to the hemodynamics in clinical pediatric and congenital cardiology. The calculation of pulmonary to systemic flow ratios is as accurate as the blood sampling, considerably easier, and quicker than calculating the absolute flows of the systemic and pulmonary circuits separately and then comparing the results. The relative flow or ratio is customarily expressed as the pulmonary to systemic or $Q_P : Q_S$ ratio, with the Q_S arbitrarily being expressed as unity. The major exceptions where the relative pulmonary to systemic flow ratio does not provide sufficient information are in the presence of suspected high pulmonary vascular resistance, particularly in the presence of left to right shunts of borderline magnitude.

The values for oxygen consumption, hemoglobin concentration, and the Hufner value, which are present in each of the oxygen content values in the separate formulas for absolute flow, all mathematically cancel out in the equations for the calculation of the relative flow between the pulmonary and systemic circulations. As a consequence the *measured saturations alone* are used for relative flow/shunt calculations.

Using the same hypothetical patient as previously described: the patient still has an oxygen consumption of 150 ml/min/m^2, Hgb of 15 g, a mixed systemic venous (MV) saturation of 65%, an arterial saturation (SA) of 95%, and a pulmonary vein (PV) saturation of 95%, but now has a pulmonary artery (PA) saturation of 85%. Using the calculations for flow in the separate circuits in order to determine their relative values:

$$Q_P = \frac{V\,O_2/m^2}{(\text{PV Sat} \times 1.34 \times \text{Hbg} - \text{PA Sat} \times 1.34 \times \text{Hgb}) \times 10}$$

$$Q_S = \frac{V\,O_2/M^2}{(\text{SA Sat} \times 1.34 \times \text{Hbg} - \text{MV Sat} \times 1.34 \times \text{Hgb}) \times 10}$$

Substituting the numbers from the hypothetical patient:

$$Q_P = \frac{150}{(0.95 \times 1.34 \times 15 - 0.85 \times 1.34 \times 15) \times 10}$$

$$= \frac{150}{(19.1 - 17.1) \times 10}$$

$$= 7.5$$

$$Q_S = \frac{150}{(0.95 \times 1.34 \times 15 - 0.65 \times 1.34 \times 15) \times 10}$$

$$= \frac{150}{(19.1 - 13.1) \times 10}$$

$$= 2.5$$

$$\therefore Q_P/Q_S = 7.5/2.5 = 3$$

Or, far more simply using the original saturation values and calculating directly for relative flows:

$$\frac{Q_P}{Q_S} = \frac{\text{SA } O_2 \text{ Sat} - \text{MV } O_2 \text{ Sat}}{\text{PV } O_2 \text{ Sat} - \text{PA } O_2 \text{ Sat}} = \frac{95 - 65}{95 - 85} = \frac{30}{10} = \frac{3}{1}$$

Effect of small errors in oxygen samples

The flow ratios clearly demonstrate how very small errors in sampling for saturations make very large differences in the calculated flows or shunts. Using the same hypothetical patient with an O_2 consumption of 150 ml/min/m^2 and 15 g of Hgb, but now with the saturations ***very slightly different*** from the previous "patient", consider a case in which none of the individual "new" saturations are more than 2% different from the original values (2% being a not uncommon difference between samples even when the two samples are drawn in rapid succession from the same location!). The SA is now 94%, the MV is 67%, the PV is 96% and the PA is 83%. Now the flow ratio is:

$$\frac{Q_P}{Q_S} = \frac{94 - 67}{96 - 83} = \frac{27}{13} = \frac{2.08}{1}$$

The calculated shunt ratio has been reduced by one third by almost inconsequential differences in the saturations of the blood samples. This example is presented in order to re-emphasize with a simple illustration, the importance of paying meticulous attention to all aspects of blood sampling and the handling and recording of oxygen saturation determinations.

Multiple levels of shunting

Often there is a question of the significance of a particular level of shunting when there are several defects and multiple levels of shunting within the heart. There are chapters written in many texts on the calculation of the separate volumes of shunting at different levels through multiple defects—e.g. the separate shunting through an atrial septal defect and a ventricular septal defect. For these calculations, the absolute flow to the body and at each level of shunting is calculated. Basically, the pulmonary flow at each level is calculated separately, using the highest saturation in each chamber receiving part of the shunt as the PA O_2 in separate Q_P calculations for each level of shunting ($Q_{P,A}$, $Q_{P,B}$, etc.). The systemic flow (Q_S) is determined in the normal fashion. The total flow into the most proximal chamber receiving the shunt ($Q_{P,A}$) is determined. The absolute systemic flow (Q_S) is subtracted from the total flow into the most proximal chamber ($Q_{P,A}$) to give the shunt volume at that level. The total volume of flow at the next more distal level of shunt ($Q_{P,B}$) is determined, again using the highest saturation in that chamber/vessel as the PA saturation. The volume of flow into the more proximal chamber ($Q_{P,A}$) is subtracted from the volume of flow at the more downstream chamber ($Q_{P,B}$) to provide the *amount shunted* at the second (more distal) level only. This same process is repeated if there are subsequent levels of shunting. The total flow at the most distal level equals the sum of all levels of shunting and the total Q_P.

Because of the selective streaming of the blood flow within all the chambers, there is *no way* of obtaining the samples in the adjoining chambers either consistently or at all accurately. As a consequence, these calculations of amount of shunt at different levels represent an exercise in mathematical futility and are used only as mental exercises. Other modalities, in particular cine angiography, are far more accurate at separating the relative magnitude and significance of shunts at separate levels when there is multiple-level shunting.

Effect of breathing oxygen on shunt calculations

When the patient is breathing increased quantities of oxygen in the inspired air, the dissolved oxygen becomes important in the determinations of flow and is included in the calculations of shunts. The dissolved oxygen is different for each sample and is added separately to the oxygen content of the hemoglobin of each sample. As a consequence the basic formulas for determining the oxygen content of each separate sample must be used.

Again using the same hypothetical patient as in the previous examples: the oxygen consumption is still 150 ml/min/m^2, the Hgb is 15, but now with the patient breathing 100% oxygen, the mixed venous (MV) saturation is 70%, the systemic arterial (SA) saturation is 98%, but the pulmonary vein (PV) saturation is 100% and the pulmonary artery (PA) saturation is 95%. The oxygen tensions (pO_2 in mmHg) for these same sites are MV, 40; SA, 500; PV, 600; and PA, 80:

$$Q_P = \frac{V\,O_2/m^2}{[(\text{PV cont}) + (0.003 \times \text{PVpO}_2)] - [(\text{PA cont}) + (0.003 \times \text{PApO}_2)] \times 10}$$

Adding the numbers from the hypothetical patient:

$$Q_P = \frac{150}{[(20.1 \times 1.0) + (0.003 \times 600)] - [(20.1 \times 0.95) + (0.003 \times 80)] \times 10}$$

$$= \frac{150}{[(20.1 + 1.8) - (19.1 + 0.24)] \times 10}$$

$$= \frac{150}{(21.9 - 19.34) \times 10}$$

$$= 5.86\ \text{l/min/m}^2$$

The calculated Q_S in the same example with the patient breathing oxygen is 2.14 l/min/m^2 so the ratio of pulmonary to systemic flow is now 5.86 : 2.14 and the Q_P/Q_S is reduced to 2.72 : 1. These small changes in absolute flow become even more important in the calculation of resistances and valve areas.

As long as the separate dissolved oxygen of each sample is added to each separate hemoglobin oxygen content, relative flows and the Q_P/Q_S ratio can still be calculated without determining the oxygen consumption and cardiac output. Using the same hypothetical patient but who is now breathing 100% oxygen, and substituting the appropriate numbers in the formulae:

$$\frac{Q_P}{Q_S} = \frac{\{[(\text{SA cont}) + (0.003 \times \text{SApO}_2)] - [(\text{MV cont}) + (0.003 \times \text{MVpO}_2)]\} \times 10}{\{[(\text{PV cont}) + (0.003 \times \text{PVpO}_2)] - [(\text{PA cont}) + (0.003 \times \text{PApO}_2)]\} \times 10}$$

$$= \frac{\{[(20.1 \times 0.98) + (0.003 \times 500) - (20.1 \times 0.70) + (0.003 \times 40)]\} \times 10}{\{[(20.1 \times 1.0) + (0.003 \times 600)] - [(20.1 \times 0.95) + (0.003 \times 80)]\} \times 10}$$

$$= \frac{[(19.7 + 1.5) - (14.1 + 0.12)] \times 10}{[(20.1 + 1.8) - (19.1 + 0.24)] \times 10}$$

$$= \frac{(21.2 - 14.2) \times 10}{(21.9 - 19.34) \times 10}$$

$$= \frac{70}{25.6} = \frac{2.7}{1}$$

Right to left shunting

In the detection and calculation of right to left shunts, the desaturated mixed systemic venous (MV O_2) blood is the indicator. A quantity of the mixed systemic venous desaturated (MV O_2) blood is introduced (through the shunt) into the fully saturated mixed pulmonary venous (PV O_2) blood. The amount of shunting is determined from the combined saturation of the mixture of systemic venous (MV O_2) and pulmonary venous (PV O_2) blood sampled at a distal arterial (SA O_2) sensing site. The amount of desaturation at the arterial site is a combination of the precise proportions of desaturated systemic venous (MV O_2) and the fully saturated pulmonary venous blood (PV O_2). From the mixed arterial saturation (SA O_2) the amount of systemic venous blood (MV O_2) that was introduced is calculated to quantitate the shunt. The calculation of the absolute flow of each circuit is performed in the same fashion.

In the example patient used previously but back to breathing room air, with an oxygen consumption of 150 ml/min/m², a hemoglobin of 15 and PA = 65%, PV = 95% and MV = 65%. However, now the patient is desaturated and the systemic saturation (SA) only is 85%. The calculations for the absolute flows are:

$$Q_P = \frac{V\,O_2/m^2}{(PV\,O_2 - PA\,O_2) \times 1.34 \times Hgb \times 10}$$

$$Q_S = \frac{V\,O_2/m^2}{(SA\,O_2 - MV\,O_2) \times 1.34 \times Hgb \times 10}$$

And substituting the numbers from the patient into the formulas:

$$Q_P = \frac{150}{(0.95 - 0.65) \times 1.34 \times 15 \times 10} = \frac{150}{0.3 \times 200} = 2.5$$

$$Q_S = \frac{150}{(0.85 - 0.65) \times 1.34 \times 15 \times 10} = \frac{150}{0.2 \times 200} = 3.75$$

From these calculations, the ratio of pulmonary to systemic flow is:

$Q_P/Q_S = 2.5/3.75 = 0.67{:}1$

In this circumstance, the Q_P is equal to the Q_{EP} and with the calculation of the actual amounts of flow in both circuits, the actual volume of the right to left shunt is easily determined by subtracting the Q_P from the Q_S:

Right to left shunt = $Q_S - Q_P$. or $3.75 - 2.5 = 1.25$ l/min/m²

The $Q_P{:}Q_S$ ratio can be calculated directly and more easily in the same patient:

$$\frac{Q_P}{Q_S} = \frac{(SA\,O_2 - MV\,O_2) \times 1.34 \times Hgb \times 10}{(PV\,O_2 - PA\,O_2) \times 1.34 \times Hgb \times 10}$$

Adding the numbers from the hypothetical patient:

$$\frac{Q_P}{Q_S} = \frac{(0.85 - 0.65) \times 1.34 \times 15 \times 10}{(0.95 - 0.65) \times 1.34 \times 15 \times 10} = \frac{40}{60} = \frac{0.67}{1}$$

Bidirectional shunting

In the presence of bidirectional shunting, in order to determine the amount of shunting (flow) in each direction, the absolute flow in the systemic circuit, the pulmonary circuits and the effective pulmonary flow must all be calculated separately. The absolute systemic and the pulmonary flows are compared with the effective pulmonary flow to determine the actual amount of shunting in each direction. The amount of left to right shunt equals the total pulmonary flow minus the effective pulmonary flow ($Q_P - Q_{EP}$) and the amount of right to left shunt equals the total systemic flow minus the effective pulmonary flow ($Q_S - Q_{EP}$). The relative flow or Q_P/Q_S ratio is calculated using only the pulmonary and systemic flows but this value has little meaning in determining the volume of flow to either circuit. Using the same hypothetical patient breathing room air, an oxygen consumption of 150 ml/min/m² and with a hemoglobin of 15 g, but now with a bidirectional shunt so that the MV Sat is 65%, the PA Sat is 85%, the PV Sat is 95% and the SA Sat is 85%:

$$Q_P = \frac{V\,O_2/m^2}{(PV\,Sat - PA\,Sat) \times 1.34 \times Hgb \times 10}$$

$$Q_S = \frac{V\,O_2/m^2}{(SA\,Sat - MV\,Sat) \times 1.34 \times Hgb \times 10}$$

$$Q_{EP} = \frac{V\,O_2/m^2}{(PV\,Sat - MV\,Sat) \times 1.34 \times Hgb \times 10}$$

Substituting the numbers from the hypothetical patient:

$$Q_P = \frac{150}{(0.95 - 0.85) \times 1.34 \times 15 \times 10} = \frac{150}{0.1 \times 200} = 7.5$$

$$Q_S = \frac{150}{(0.85 - 0.65) \times 1.34 \times 15 \times 10} = \frac{150}{0.2 \times 200} = 3.75$$

$$Q_{EP} = \frac{150}{(0.95 - 0.65) \times 1.34 \times 15 \times 10} = \frac{150}{0.3 \times 200} = 2.5$$

From this, the absolute volume of the shunts are determined:

The volume of the left to right shunt = $Q_P - Q_{EP} = 7.5 - 2.5 = 5$ l/min/m²

The volume of the right to left shunt = $Q_S - Q_{EP} = 3.75 - 2.5 = 1.25$ l/min/m²

The pulmonary to systemic flow ratio from these numbers is **Q_P/Q_S = 7.5/3.75 or 2:1**. In this case, the ratio, by itself, suggests a relatively small pulmonary flow compared to the actual 7.5 l/min/m² of measured pulmonary flow. This suggestion or assumption could be catastrophic in determining pulmonary artery resistances and, in turn, operability! This is even more apparent in patients with transposition physiology where the two circuits are in parallel. The shunt that is the only source of mixing may be very small while the absolute flow in both the pulmonary and the systemic circuits is actually very large.

Using a new hypothetical patient example, now with transposition of the great arteries and an atrial septal defect but still with an oxygen consumption of 150 ml/min/m² but now with a hemoglobin of 19 and the following saturations: SA, 80%; MV, 60%; PA, 85% and PV, 98%:

$$Q_S = \frac{V\,O_2/m^2}{(\text{SA Sat} - \text{MV Sat}) \times 1.34 \times \text{Hgb} \times 10}$$

$$= \frac{150}{(0.80 - 0.60) \times 1.34 \times 19 \times 10} = \frac{150}{0.20 \times 255} = 3$$

$$Q_P = \frac{V\,O_2/m^2}{(\text{PV Sat} - \text{PA Sat}) \times 1.34 \times \text{Hgb} \times 10}$$

$$= \frac{150}{(0.98 - 0.85) \times 1.34 \times 19 \times 10} = \frac{150}{0.13 \times 255} = 4.52$$

$$Q_{EP} = \frac{V\,O_2/m^2}{(\text{PV Sat} - \text{MV Sat}) \times 1.34 \times \text{Hgb} \times 10}$$

$$= \frac{150}{(0.95 - 0.60) \times 1.34 \times 19 \times 10} = \frac{150}{0.35 \times 255} = 1.68$$

Here again the $Q_P{:}Q_S$ is only 1.51:1, while the absolute pulmonary flow is *three times* that (4.52).

Vascular resistance

The calculation of vascular resistance is made using Poiseuille's formula. This formula is based on the resistance of a *homogeneous* fluid flowing *constantly* through *rigid* tubing of a *uniform* diameter. The actual formula also takes the length of the tubing and the viscosity of the fluid into account. The viscosity is assumed to be constant, which of course is not true. Blood with higher hematocrits has an exponential increase in viscosity. The diameter and length of the vascular system is not uniform throughout any part of the circulation. The blood flow is pulsatile not constant and, in the elastic vessels, the vessel diameters in any single location are continually changing. In addition, the muscular walls of many of the vessels tend to contract against increased flow, reducing the luminal diameter and increasing the resistance through them with increasing flow. For this formula to be used for the calculation of vascular resistances in the human circulation, like the calculations for flow and shunt quantification, multiple assumptions must be taken for granted. Although absolute resistance cannot be calculated accurately in the human circulation, the formula for resistance has proven useful for comparing measured values against previously calculated "normal values".

The calculation of the absolute resistance of either the pulmonary or the systemic vascular bed requires the determination of the absolute flow across the areas as well as the mean pressure differences across the areas. The flow across the area is determined using blood oxygen saturations and oxygen consumption as previously described. When the flow is indexed to body surface area, the resistance is, in turn, indexed, and is more meaningful in the pediatric and congenital populations. Once flow across a vascular bed has been determined, the calculation of the resistance, already indexed for body surface area, across that vascular bed is fairly straightforward, as follows:

$$R = \frac{P\ (\text{mmHg})}{Q\ (\text{l/min/m}^2)} = \text{mmHg/l/min/m}^2$$

Or:

$$\text{Resistance (mmHg/l/min/m}^2) = \frac{\text{mean pressure drop across vascular bed (mmHg)}}{\text{blood flow (Q) (l/min/m}^2)}$$

Or:

$$\text{Systemic Vascular Resistance } (R_S) = \frac{\text{mean arterial pressure (mmHg)} - \text{mean right atrial pressure (mmHg)}}{\text{systemic blood flow } (Q_S)\ (\text{l/min/m}^2)}$$

i.e. $$R_S = \frac{m\,P_{AO}\ (\text{mmHg}) - m\,P_{RA}\ (\text{mmHg})}{Q_S\ (\text{l/min/m}^2)}$$

And:

$$\text{Pulmonary Vascular Resistance } (R_P) = \frac{\text{mean pul. artery pressure (mmHg)} - \text{mean left atrial pressure (mmHg)}}{\text{Pulmonary blood flow } (Q_P)\ (\text{l/min/m}^2)}$$

i.e. $$R_P = \frac{m\,P_{PA}\ (\text{mmHg}) - m\,P_{LA}\ (\text{mmHg})}{Q_P\ (\text{l/min/m}^2)}$$

Example:
Using our same hypothetical patient with normally related great arteries, no shunt, breathing room air, a measured oxygen consumption of 150 ml/min/m², Hgb of 15 g and saturations: PA, 65%; SA, 95%; PV, 95% and MV, 65% and with pressures: PA, 30/10, mean 15; SA, 100/65, mean 75; LA, a = 8, v = 10, m = 8; and RA, a = 4, v = 3, m = 3. The previously calculated Q_S and Q_P were 2.5 and 2.5 respectively:

$$R_S = \frac{75 - 3}{2.5} = 29$$

$$R_P = \frac{15 - 8}{2.5} = 2.8$$

Or a ratio $R_P{:}R_S$ of 2.8/29 or ~1:10.

When the left atrium is not entered or it is desired to compare the pulmonary arteriolar resistance to the total pulmonary resistance, the pulmonary artery capillary wedge pressure is used in the formula for calculating pulmonary vascular resistance instead of the true left atrial pressure. As long as the pulmonary artery capillary wedge pressure is an accurate reflection of the left atrial pressure, this gives an accurate calculation of the *total* pulmonary resistance. Otherwise it represents the pulmonary *vascular* resistance. The normal total pulmonary resistance is 1–2 mmHg/l/min/m^2, while the normal systemic vascular resistance is 20–30 mmHg/l/min/m^2 and the normal R_P:R_S is ~1:10. These values of resistances in mmHg/l/min/m^2 are also referred to as hybrid units or Woods units. By multiplying the hybrid or Woods units by 80 the value is converted into dynes/sec/cm or absolute resistance units (ARU).

With the accurate measurement of oxygen consumption and cardiac output, and using the values of actual flow across the pulmonary and the systemic circulations in conjunction with these formulas, the differences in flow between the systemic and pulmonary circuits are automatically included in the calculations of the specific resistances in the separate circuits even in the presence of intracardiac shunts.

As an example, using the same hypothetical patient with normally related great arteries, but now breathing room air, in the presence of a left to right shunt, an oxygen consumption of 150 ml/min/m^2, Hgb of 15 g and with saturations of: PA, 85%; SA, 95%; PV, 95% and MV, 65% and now with pressures of: PA, 60/20, mean 33; SA, 100/65, mean 75; LA, a = 10, v = 12, m = 10, and RA, a = 4, v = 3, m = 3. The oxygen consumption is already indexed per meter squared so the results are automatically indexed. The calculated Q_S and Q_P are still 2.5 and 7.5, respectively:

$$R_S = \frac{75 - 3}{2.5} = 29 \text{ mmHg/min/l/m}^2$$

$$R_P = \frac{33 - 10}{7.5} = 3.1 \text{ mmHg/min/l/m}^2$$

Or a ratio R_P:R_S of 3.1/29 or ~1:9.4.

Because of the difficulties encountered in the accurate measurement of oxygen consumption and in determining absolute flows in congenital heart patients, the relative resistances between the pulmonary and systemic circuits are often used in making decisions for therapy in clinical cardiology. The use of the relative (or comparative) resistances eliminates the need for the determination of oxygen consumption since oxygen consumption values of the two parallel circuits in the human circulation mathematically cancel out in the calculation of the relative resistances. The use of these relative resistances is valid in congenital heart patients where the measurement and calculation of oxygen consumption are flawed so easily and, in addition, where the systemic resistance is a significant variable only extremely rarely. To calculate the relative resistance when only the flow *ratios* are known, the drop in pressure across the pulmonary circuit is divided by the *relative* pulmonary flow to the systemic flow. This pulmonary resistance number is divided by the drop in pressure across the systemic circuit which, in turn, is divided by the *relative* systemic flow (Q_S), which is 1.

$$\frac{R_P}{R_S} = \frac{[PA_P \text{ mean} - LA_P \text{ mean}]/Q_P}{[SA_P \text{ mean} - RA_P \text{ mean}]/Q_S}$$

$$= \frac{[PA_P \text{ mean} - LA_P \text{ mean}] \times Q_S}{[SA_P \text{ mean} - RA_P \text{ mean}] \times Q_P}$$

Using our hypothetical patient with normally related great arteries and breathing room air with a 3:1 left to right shunt and the numbers given above:

$$\frac{R_P}{R_S} = \frac{[33 - 10]/3}{[75 - 3]/1} = \frac{7.7}{72} = \frac{1}{9.4} \text{ or } 1:9.4$$

Or:

$$\frac{R_P}{R_S} = \frac{[PA_P \text{ mean} - LA_P \text{ mean}] \times Q_S}{[SA_P \text{ mean} - RA_P \text{ mean}] \times Q_P} = \frac{[33 - 10] \times 1}{[75 - 3] \times 3} = \frac{1}{9.4}$$

Thus, the values calculated from the relative flows are essentially identical to the relative resistance values calculated using the absolute flows in each circuit.

When using any of the resistance calculations, the values obtained must be used in conjunction with the other clinical and hemodynamic findings. The numbers obtained are an *adjunct* to the therapeutic decision and should never be the sole determinant.

Valve area calculation

The gradient across a discrete area such as a valve or narrowed vessel generally reflects the severity of the obstruction quite accurately in patients with congenital heart disease. There are, however, other variables that need to be considered in every case. The gradient is inversely proportional to the area being traversed but directly proportional to the flow across the area. Thus if the flow across the obstruction is reduced, the gradient underestimates the severity of the lesion and vice versa.

Gorlin and Gorlin, over half a century ago, using the laws of hydraulics, derived formulas for calculating the area of a particular obstructed valve or vessel using the combination of the measured flow through the area of the heart or vessel per unit of time along with the measured pressure gradients across that same area[9]. Like the other hydraulic formulas used in hemodynamic calculations, the formulas for the calculation of orifice areas are derived from mechanical models, which had continuous flow of uniform fluids, through rigid tubing of fixed lengths, fixed diameters and with obstructions of fixed diameters. As a consequence, multiple assumptions are required for the use of the formulas for valve areas in the human, with the pulsatile flow of viscous, changing fluid, in vessels that have irregular length and variable diameter and are intrinsically elastic, and passing through valves with variable diameters! In spite of the discrepancies between the human and the mechanical model, the calculated valve areas from these formulas do correlate fairly well with the measured areas in anatomic specimens. The simplified formula is:

$$\text{Area} = \frac{\text{Flow through the valve}}{C \times 44.5 \times [\text{sq. root of } (P_1 - P_2)]}$$

And:

$$\text{Flow} = \frac{\text{Cardiac output (ml/min)}}{\text{DFP (sec/min) or SEP (sec/min)}}$$

Where flow = total flow /min during either systole (SEP) or diastole (DFP); SEP = systolic ejection period (per minute), or the duration in seconds that the semilunar valve is open per minute; DFP = diastolic flow period (per minute), or the duration in seconds that the atrioventricular valve is open per minute; 44.5 = a constant that is related to gravitational acceleration of fluids; and $(P_1 - P_2)$ = the mean pressure gradient across the obstruction; C is an empirical constant to correct for the properties of blood and the geometry of the particular valves. C = 0.85 for the mitral valve and 1.0 for the aortic, pulmonary and tricuspid valves. (C = 0.85 for the mitral valve is more accurate and utilizes the measured diastolic filling time, whereas Gorlin's original C = 0.7 only estimated the diastolic filling time[10].) When the cardiac output is indexed to the BSA, the valve area is indexed to BSA and is more meaningful in the pediatric group of patients.

Since forward flow across a particular valve only occurs during that part of the cardiac cycle when the particular valve is open, the duration of that portion of the flow must be determined. Blood flows through the semilunar valves during systole and through the atrioventricular valves during diastole. The duration of either the systolic flow or the diastolic flow during a single beat is measured from the *crossing points of the simultaneous* pressure curves from the two immediately adjacent areas (chambers or chamber and vessel) on each side of the obstruction. Usually, at least three consecutive sinus beats are measured and averaged to obtain the particular value.

When the pressure curves are recorded during a pullback tracing and not simultaneously from the two areas immediately adjacent to the obstruction, the pressure tracings must be adjusted to correct for the time differences of different heart rates or respiratory variations. If one pressure is recorded remotely from the other, such as a left ventricle and femoral artery pressure, the pressure tracings must be corrected for time and amplitude. The two pressure curves are recorded separately. Then the printed tracings are aligned over each other manually and one pressure traced over the other so that the two curves correspond exactly in time. Once the pressure curves on both sides of the obstruction are aligned properly, the duration of the systolic or diastolic opening period during an individual cardiac cycle can be measured. This duration of the particular valve opening, in seconds, is multiplied by the patient's heart rate to arrive at the SEP or DFP.

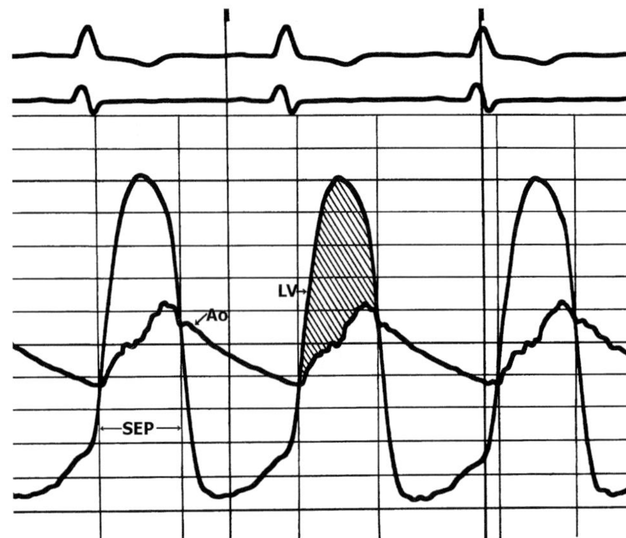

Figure 10.16 Crossing points of the ventricular and arterial pressure curves, which are used in the calculation of systolic ejection period (SEP)—the crossings are designated by vertical lines through the curves.

For the semilunar valves, the systolic ejection time per heart beat is measured from the point where the upstroke of the ventricular pressure curve crosses the arterial pressure curve to the point where the down stroke of the ventricular pressure curve again crosses the arterial pressure curve (Figure 10.16). This value is measured in three consecutive sinus beats, averaged, and the result multiplied by the heart rate to provide the duration of the systolic ejection period (SEP) for the formula for valve area.

For the atrioventricular valve, the atrial and the corresponding ventricular pressure curves are used to measure the diastolic flow period per heart beat. The DFP per beat is measured from the point where the descending slope of the ventricular pressure curve crosses the simultaneously recorded atrial pressure curve to the point where the ascending slope of the ventricular pressure curve again crosses the simultaneously recorded atrial pressure curve (Figure 10.17).

Since the flow through the valves is not constant, but rather accelerates and decelerates, the maximum pressure difference (gradient), *per se*, cannot be used in the Gorlin

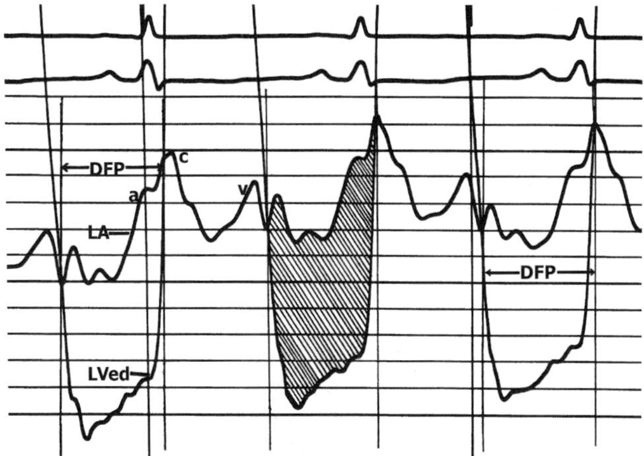

Figure 10.17 Crossing points of the ventricular and atrial pressure curves, which are used in the calculation of diastolic flow period (DFP)—the crossings are designated by vertical lines through the curves.

formulas. To compensate for the accelerating and decelerating phasic flow, the square root of the mean gradient is used along with two empirical constants that theoretically compensate for the characteristics of the blood and the valve. The mean gradient is not a common, nor a simple measurement in the cardiac catheterization laboratory.

The precise way of measuring the "mean gradient" across a valve is to planimeter the area of the differences between the *exactly superimposed*, relevant pressure curves during the particular ejection/filling time for that valve. The number derived by planimetry (in mm^2) is divided by the length of the base of the curve (ejection/filling time) expressed in millimeters to provide the mean gradient. The area between the ventricular and arterial pressure curves during the systolic ejection time is used to calculate the mean pressure across the semilunar valves (*see* Figure 10.16, shaded area). The area between the atrial pressure curve and ventricular end-diastolic pressure curve is used to calculate the mean pressure across the atrioventricular valves (*see* Figure 10.17, shaded area).

Another means of calculating the mean pressure difference is to draw seven, equidistant vertical lines along the maximum horizontal axis from curve to curve between the two curves. The height of each of these lines is measured in mm and the seven values are added together. The sum of these seven measurements, then is divided by seven and this number provides an approximation of the mean gradient in millimeters of mercury. This value corresponds very closely to the mean gradient across the valve as determined by planimetry.

Both of these methods are time consuming and far out of proportion to their accuracy or clinical usefulness in the pediatric and congenital heart catheterization laboratory. Bache *et al.*[11] devised a simplified calculation of the aortic valve area mathematically using the peak systolic gradient and a different constant instead of the mean gradient.

$$\text{AVA} = \frac{\text{CO/SEP}}{37.8 \times (\text{square root of peak systolic gradient} + 10)}$$

$$= \frac{\text{CO}}{37.8 \times \text{SEP} \times (\text{square root of peak systolic gradient} + 10)}$$

This formula is equally as accurate (or inaccurate) as those using the mean pressure gradients, but it still requires the very precise simultaneous recording or the physical overlying of the ventricular and arterial pressure curves if they are not obtained simultaneously, in order to obtain the accurate systolic ejection time interval.

The valve area formulas, like the other hydraulic fluid dynamics formulas, are based on arbitrary constants and many assumptions in order to be applied to the human circulation. In addition, all of these "precise" valve area calculations still depend upon the ***validity and accuracy of the basic data*** that are acquired in the catheterization laboratory.

The pressure curves on both sides of the obstruction must be recorded simultaneously, accurately and at *identical phases of the respiratory cycle*. Any errors in the recording of the pressure curves will be incorporated into the calculated mean gradients and magnify errors in the valve area calculations. In order for the valve area to be valid, the cardiac output must be measured very accurately and at the same time as the pressure measurements are made. A small error in the flow measurement (or assumption of flow) relative to the gradients results in a logarithmic error in calculation of the valve area. In the presence of valvular regurgitation, these formulas are all invalid, underestimating the valve areas significantly. Making matters worse in the modern catheterization laboratory, the computer in the laboratory now rapidly and essentially automatically calculates the valve areas *to the third decimal place, regardless* of the validity or accuracy of the basic pressure data supplied to it.

As a consequence of the difficulties and inaccuracies of the calculations, the calculated valve area should not be considered as "hard scientific data", nor should it be used as a major determinant for or against a decision as to when to intervene on a particular valve in the pediatric and congenital catheterization laboratory. If the clinical information, the non-invasive data, and all of the available data from the catheterization laboratory, are correlated, then all of the information necessary for making the proper decision is available without the mathematical exercises of calculating valve areas.

All of the "natural history" information concerning the indications for surgery on congenital valvar lesions is based on *valvular gradients* ***in conjunction with*** clinical information and clinical judgment. In the vast majority of cases, measured gradients and clinical findings combined with the other findings from the cardiac catheterization and common sense are sufficient to interpret and explain any discrepancies between the measured gradients or valve areas and the severity of the obstruction as judged clinically.

Indicator dilution curves using exogenous indicators

Although oxygen saturation is the most commonly used indicator, most cardiologists envision indicator dilution curves as those obtained with exogenous indicators when considering indicator dilution studies. Indicator dilution techniques, regardless of the indicator substance, are all based on the Fick principal, which has demonstrated that a diffusable substance that is introduced into the circulation mixes uniformly with the blood after its introduction and—assuming no loss from the circulation—the substance is distributed to *all* parts of the body in exactly equal concentrations[2]. It is much easier to conceptualize an indicator dilution curve when using a finite amount of an exogenous substance as the indicator compared to oxygen as the indicator. Exogenous indicators used in the hemodynamic laboratory include small amounts of indocyanine (Cardio-Green) dye, very cold solutions which cause minute temperature changes in the circulating blood, and small amounts of acidic substances, which create very minute changes in the acidity (pH) of the circulating blood.

Small amounts of indocyanine dye or very minute changes in the pH of the blood are used to detect the mere presence of even the most minute shunt. As qualitative indicators, the mere appearance of the indicator at an abnormal site within the heart or circulation confirms the presence of, and identifies the precise location of, a shunt of even the tiniest magnitude.

When exact, measured amounts of indocyanine dye or cold saline (which causes minute changes in the temperature of the circulating blood) are used as the exogenous indicators, they can be used to *quantitate* the absolute flow or to quantitate the amount of shunting at a certain level within the circulation.

Quantitative indicator dilution curves using exogenous indicators

When a known, exact quantity of indicator is introduced into the circulation and a sample from a downstream location in the circulation is analyzed for the concentration of the indicator in solution at that site, the rate of flow of that fluid can be determined. The downstream source of blood is sampled for the indicator using a variety of sensors according to the indicator substance. The sensor is calibrated with a known quantity of the indicator substance in a known quantity of blood. The known quantity of indicator in the precise quantity of blood produces a specific deflection of the sensor. The exact quantity of blood passing the sensor over time is determined by the exact dilution of the indicator at that site. The techniques for performing quantitative indicator dilution curves must be very precise in order to produce accurate and reproducible results.

A precisely measured amount of the particular indicator is introduced into the flowing blood. The changes the concentrations of the dye or the changes in the temperature of the blood that appear at the sensing site are measured over time in order to calculate the net flow. Very accurate and reproducible cardiac output measurements are obtained using either Cardio-Green dye, which is drawn through a densitometer, or a cooled solution in the blood, which is flowing past special thermal sensing catheters for thermodilution curves. A low cardiac output prolongs the appearance of the indicator and lowers the peak concentration of the indicator curve. In extremely low cardiac outputs, the peak concentration may be so low that it may not be measurable. Similarly, if the indicator is injected too far "upstream" (e.g. in a peripheral vein) the indicator becomes too diluted by the time it reaches the peripheral sensor to record a proper output curve. A large intracardiac shunt will lower the peak concentration of the indicator, while the secondary peak on the downside of the curve from the shunted blood containing the indicator provides some estimation of the amount of shunting.

Thermodilution indicator curves

An exact quantity of cold, normal saline at a known temperature that is significantly lower than the body temperature is the indicator. A thermistor probe at the tip of a catheter detects very minute changes in blood temperature for a thermodilution indicator study. The cold flush solution, in small amounts, has the advantage of being non-toxic and it is rapidly dissipated in the body, so many repeated determinations can be made in succession. A precise, known quantity of a cold solution is introduced into the circulating blood. The cold solution causes a minute drop in the circulating blood temperature, which is proportional to the quantity of cold solution and the rate of blood flow. The thermistor detects the minute change in the temperature of the blood as the chilled blood/saline mixture passes the sensor. The thermodilution amplifier plots a curve of the continuous temperature change past the sensor over a finite period of time identical to the curve inscribed with an indicator dye (Figure 10.18).

Using the exact initial temperature of the blood, the exact temperature and amount of the added solution, and the exact overall decrease in temperature of the blood

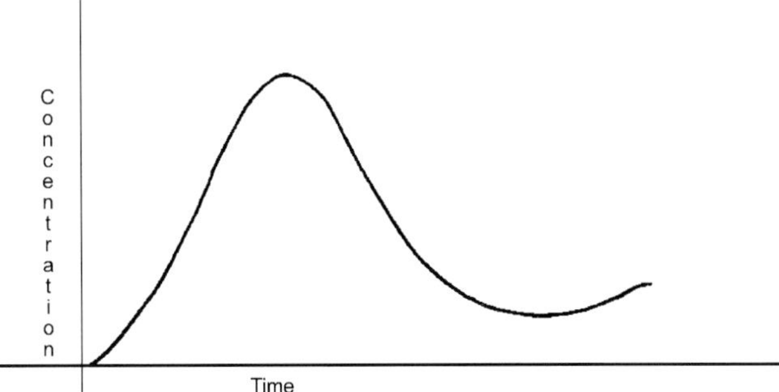

Figure 10.18 A typical inscribed cardiac output curve in the presence of a good cardiac output, showing concentration against time.

downstream as the change in temperature is detected over time, the precise rate of blood flow or "cardiac output" is determined using the following formula and the measured area under the plotted temperature/time curve.

$$CO = \frac{(Tb - Ti) \times (V) \times 60 \times 1.08 \times 0.825}{D6\ (t)\ dt}$$

Where CO = cardiac output (flow); D6 (t) dt = the area under the curve; Tb = the initial temperature of the blood; Ti = the temperature of the injectant; V = the volume of the injectant; 1.08 and 0.825 are two constants which compensate for the ratio of the products of the specific heat of 0.9% saline compared to that of blood, and correct for the loss of heat of the saline during injection, respectively; and 60 converts the result from per second to per minute.

The area under the thermodilution curve can be calculated manually by a "forward triangle" method or by using planimetry. Fortunately, now a simple and accurate analog output computer attached to the thermodilution amplifier plots the curve and calculates the output from the curve automatically, accurately and almost instantaneously. These calculations are more precise than when plotted and calculated manually. The actual curve from the output is plotted and displayed on the screen of the output computer. This graphic plot allows the curve to be inspected visually to ensure that it is at least qualitatively satisfactory in its contour.

The final information from the computer is only as good as the raw data from the samples fed into the computer. As a consequence, performance of thermodilution cardiac output determinations must be very meticulous. Several manufacturers produce thermodilution catheters (e.g. B. Braun Medical Inc., Bethlehem, PA). These different catheters function with several different thermodilution amplifiers, which are also available from several manufacturers (e.g. B. Braun Medical Inc., Bethlehem, PA; Waters Instruments Inc., Rochester, MN). Thermodilution catheters are all flow-directed, floating, balloon catheters. Each thermodilution catheter has three lumens in addition to the thermistor probe, which is positioned at the tip of the catheter. The thermistor is connected by a fine wire that runs within the wall of the catheter to a connector at the hub of the catheter. One lumen of the catheter communicates with the balloon itself for balloon inflation/deflation, the second lumen goes to the tip of the catheter for pressure measurements and withdrawing samples (for blood saturations) and the third lumen is for the injection of the indicator, and exits distally from the side of the catheter approximately 15 cm proximal to its tip.

The thermistor catheter is positioned with the thermistor probe in the main, or a proximal branch pulmonary artery. In most patients, this places the proximal injection port in the right atrium or in the orifice of the adjacent cava. The thermistor connection on the catheter is attached to the amplifier/computer with a reusable, sterilized cable and the computer is calibrated for the specific catheter and patient with the patient's weight and body surface area, and the pulmonary artery and pulmonary arterial capillary wedge pressures.

The greater the difference in temperature between the injectant and the blood, the more sensitive and accurate is the thermodilution output. For the greatest accuracy, the saline for the injectant is cooled in an ice bath. Sterile normal saline is placed in a metal bowl which, in turn, is placed in a larger bowl that is full of iced solution. The saline that is to be used for the injections is allowed to equilibrate with the iced solution for at least 15 minutes. A sterile, electronic thermometer, which comes with the thermodilution set-up, is placed in the solution of sterile injectant and attached to the thermodilution amplifier. This measures the exact temperature of the injectant, which is automatically imported into the formula and calculations in the thermodilution computer.

The body temperature is recorded from the thermistor, which is positioned in the pulmonary artery at the tip of the catheter, and the computer is allowed to stabilize at this base-line body temperature. Once the machine is calibrated with the temperature of the blood and the exact temperature of the cold saline, the exact volume of cold saline that is to be used for the injection is programmed into the thermodilution computer. After beginning the recording on the thermodilution computer, the precise volume of cold saline is quickly drawn into a syringe that has been immersed in the cold saline and *immediately* injected as rapidly as possible through the "injection" lumen of the thermodilution catheter. The rapid withdrawal of the cold solution into the syringe and its *immediate* injection from the syringe prevents the temperature of the injectant from "drifting" before it is injected. The larger the volume of cold saline, the more sensitive is the thermodilution curve, however, the small lumen of the catheter for the injectant limits the amount of fluid that can be injected over a very short period of time. In the pediatric population, the patient's size limits the volume of injectant that can be used even further. 10 ml of cold saline is used for larger children and adults, 5 ml for small children and as little as 2 ml for small infants.

After the injection and the recording of each output curve, the thermodilution computer is allowed to recalibrate to baseline (10–15 seconds). The injection and the output determination are repeated several more times. At least three separate output determinations are performed in order to verify reproducibility of the instrumentation and technique. If performed properly and the equipment is functioning properly, the repeated values will be extremely close. If one or more of the cardiac output values does not agree with the others, several more thermodilution output determinations are performed in fairly rapid succession. By performing many repeat injections, a small scattering of values for the output will be obtained. There should be a group of values that are very close together. Any extreme "outlier" values are discarded, and the values that are close together are averaged as the final cardiac output. If there is a continued wide scatter between the values, the thermodilution catheter is exchanged, the system rechecked and the entire procedure repeated.

Although room temperature flush solution (which is usually significantly cooler than body temperature) is often used as the "cold" injectant, the use of a solution that is any warmer than an iced solution significantly decreases the accuracy of the thermodilution output determination. The less the difference in temperature between the cold indicator solution and the circulating blood, the less sensitive and more scattered the individual thermodilution output determinations will be. An additional error is often incurred when room temperature saline is used for the injectant and the electronic control thermometer for the injectant solution is placed in a separate, non-sterile dish or bag of saline which is situated remotely, off the sterile field. This eliminates the need for using a separate sterile temperature probe for each case, but assumes that there is instantaneous equilibration of the temperature of the various solutions scattered throughout the room. This, of course, is not true unless the room and all of the solutions have been maintained at exactly the same temperature for at least an hour before the output determination. This short cut for measuring the injectant temperature adds additional, potentially monumental error to the determinations. The combination of less accuracy with the lower temperature gradient when using room temperature solutions and the recording of the temperature of the injectant from a remote fluid that is not necessarily at the same temperature, essentially invalidates the thermodilution procedure and certainly explains very discrepant results!

Left-sided thermodilution curves can be used when massive pulmonary or tricuspid regurgitation prevents the recording of a right-sided thermodilution output. The thermodilution catheter is introduced into the left heart by an atrial transseptal puncture technique. The tip of the catheter is manipulated through the left atrium and the left ventricle and into the aorta. Depending on the size of the patient and where the tip of the catheter and the thermistor are placed in the aorta, this positions the proximal, injection port in the left atrium or the left ventricle. Care is taken to ensure that the proximal port of the catheter is at least completely within the left atrium and, in addition, beyond (out of) the tip of the long transseptal sheath, which may still be in the left atrium or left ventricle. The thermodilution curves are obtained exactly as in the right heart.

When performed properly, with properly functioning equipment, the thermodilution cardiac output is extremely accurate and reproducible. It has a very good correlation with the other, established methods for determining cardiac output, including both Fick and Cardio-Green dye output determinations. With the current equipment and techniques, thermodilution is the most satisfactory technique for the determination of cardiac output. It is simpler to perform than a Fick determination, during which oxygen consumption must be measured and during which time the patient must remain in a very steady state. Thermodilution output determinations can be repeated many times and in rapid sequence. No blood samples need to be withdrawn for the thermodilution output. The patient must only be in a steady state during the short duration while the output curve is being obtained. In many catheterization laboratories, the thermodilution technique is the preferred or the only method now used to determine accurate cardiac outputs.

Cardiac output determination with Cardio-Green dye

Indocyanine (Cardio-Green) dye is used as an exogenous indicator for both quantitative and qualitative indicator dilution studies. There have been at least ten different studies over the past half century, all of which demonstrated a close agreement between the values from exogenous indicator dilution studies and the values from the Fick determination for cardiac output/index. Cardio-Green dye is non-toxic and rapidly cleared from the circulation by the liver. Very accurate cardiac output determinations can be performed when an exact quantity of Cardio-Green dye is injected upstream and blood is withdrawn from downstream through a continually reading densitometer at an absolutely steady rate using a constant flow withdrawal pump. The sample can be withdrawn from a peripheral arterial line or catheter positioned in the more downstream location.

If there is intracardiac or other intravascular shunting, an accurate total cardiac output cannot be determined,

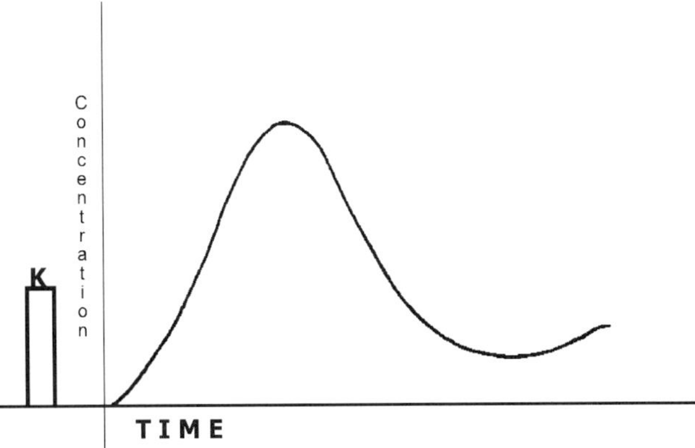

Figure 10.19 Cardio-Green indicator dilution curve with preceding "calibration" deflection.

however, the degree of right to left or left to right shunting can be semi-quantitated using the Cardio-Green dye dilution technique. The Cardio-Green dye curves are extremely sensitive for the *detection* of very minute shunts but the quantification of shunts is less accurate and more cumbersome than utilizing oxygen determinations.

Quantitative indicator dilution studies using Cardio-Green dye require a flow through densitometer connected to a direct current amplifier in the physiologic recorder. The densitometer is calibrated for the concentration of dye in the blood for each use. Exactly 50 mg of the concentrated Cardio-Green dye is dissolved in 10 ml of diluent. As a result, 5 mg of green dye is injected with each 1 ml injection of the diluted solution. Then as a calibrating solution, 0.02 ml of the diluted Cardio-Green solution is introduced into exactly 10 ml of blood. This results in a concentration of 2 ml of the Cardio-Green solution per liter of blood, or 10 mg of Cardio-Green dye per liter of blood.

The densitometer is attached to the recorder, turned on and the tracing from the densitometer on the recorder is adjusted to the zero baseline. With the recorder running, the calibrating solution of Cardio-Green in the blood is drawn through the densitometer at a steady rate using the same constant withdrawal pump that will be used to withdraw the sample for the curve. As the solution containing the dye is drawn through the densitometer, it inscribes a sharp, vertical deflection off the base line and then a straight horizontal line several centimeters above the base line (Figure 10.19).

The height of this deflected line is the calibration factor, K, for that particular batch and concentration of Cardio-Green dye solution. With this particular solution of dye, the height of this calibration deflection represents the height of the deflection that will occur when a concentration of exactly 10 mg/l of dye is drawn through the densitometer. The calibration factor is calculated for various concentrations of dye as follows:

$$\text{K (mg/l/mm)} = \frac{\text{Indicator concentration (mg/l)}}{\text{Deflection of calibration curve (mm)}}$$

Once the solution is prepared and the densitometer calibrated on the recorder, the cardiac output is determined using this same diluted solution of dye as the indicator solution. An arterial line or a catheter positioned in the aorta or in a peripheral artery is attached to a length of sterile tubing, which passes through the densitometer to the constant-flow withdrawal pump. The densitometer, the recorder and the pump are all turned on. The base-line tracing from the densitometer is re-set to zero on the recorder as blood is flowing through the densitometer. One milliliter of the Cardio-Green solution is injected through a catheter positioned in the pulmonary artery. A characteristic time/concentration output curve is inscribed on the recorder (*see* Figure 10.19). The height of the curve corresponds to the concentration of the dye in the blood at that particular instant. The inscribed curve has a relatively sharp upstroke to the peak level, which inscribes a relatively symmetrical peak followed by a down-stroke curve. The down stroke of the curve initially resembles the up-stroke curve, only to begin a very slow tailing off of the lower portion of the down-stroke curve after it has dropped 60% or more toward the baseline. The tailing off or flattening of the curve appears as recirculation of the same dye begins to appear and eventually creates a second, but less significant, peak.

The calculation of the output from the dye dilution curves is dependent upon the total concentration of dye, which "accumulates" beneath a theoretically *symmetrical* curve during a specific period of time. There are two basic methods of determining the concentration of dye beneath the curve manually and, in turn, calculating the cardiac output from the concentration of dye under the curve.

Since the recirculation of the indicator begins before the original curve has fallen to zero, the end of the downward slope of the curve never reaches zero to provide an end point for the curve. Hamilton and associates[12], using principles suggested by Stewart[13], determined that if the time/concentration curve is re-plotted on semilogarithmic paper with the indicator concentration on the logarithmic axis, the descending limb of the curve becomes a straight line until the recirculation curve appears (Figure 10.20).

A continuation of this straight line is plotted (drawn manually) downward on the semilogarithmic paper to the point where the concentration of the dye is 1% of the total concentration. The point where the line crosses the 1% concentration point is arbitrarily chosen as the end of the disappearance time of the initial curve. When the concentration values at the end of the downslope of the original curve are replaced with the extrapolated values obtained from the straight line from the logarithmic curve, the terminal portion of the curve now reaches the baseline on the

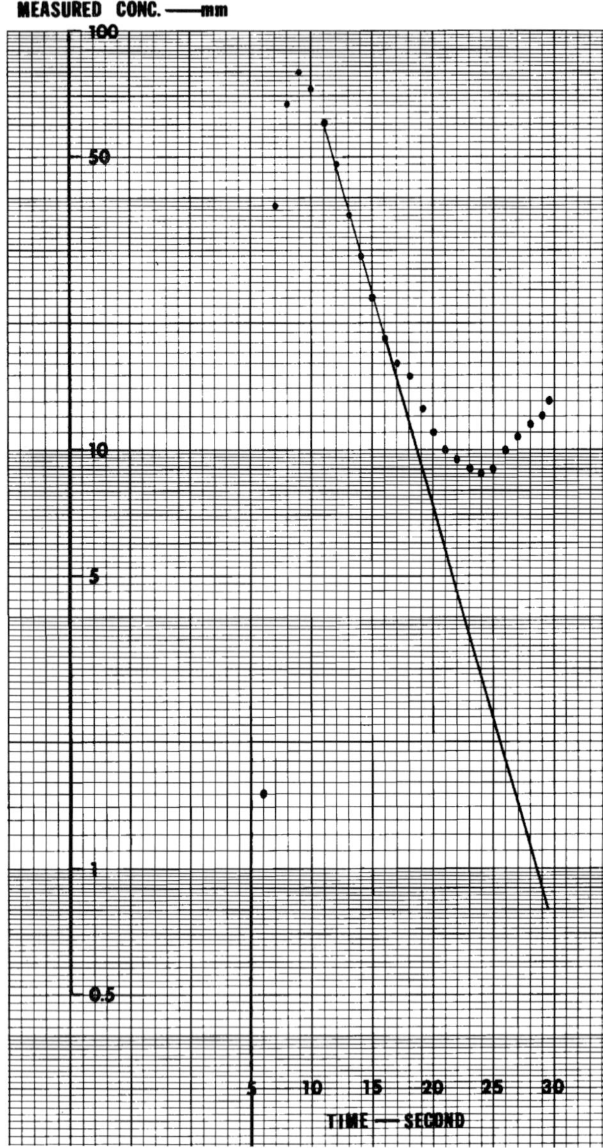

Figure 10.20 Cardio-Green dye curve plotted on semilog paper.

original curve with the recirculation eliminated. This is depicted by the dashed continuation of the downslope line plotted over the original curve, as seen in Figure 10.20. Using this re-plotted descending curve, which now reaches the baseline, the area under the curve, which represents the total concentration of dye, is determined by planimetry. The mean concentration of dye, C_M, is determined by dividing the area, A (in mm^2), obtained from planimetry by the length of the base of the curve, B (in mm).

$$C_M = \frac{A}{B}$$

The cardiac output can be determined using these values in the formula:

$$CO = \frac{I \times 60}{C_M \times K \times t}$$

Where I = the amount of indicator injected (in mg); C_M = the mean concentration of the dye under the curve (in mg); K = the calibration factor for the concentration of dye in solution (mg/l/mm); t (in seconds) = total time of the curve, obtained by multiplying the time lines under the curve by the number of time lines/minute; and the factor of 60 is introduced to give the output per minute.

There is another recognized mathematical method that is an alternative to the use of planimetry to determine the concentration of the dye under the curve, but this alternative method also requires the use of the extrapolated curve of the concentrations transferred from the semilogarithmic paper back to the original curve in order that the curve has an "end" and reaches the baseline. The separate, incremental concentrations of dye under the curve determined from the height of the curve at each one-second interval are added together to calculate the concentration per total time under the curve C_S (in mm–sec). The cardiac output is calculated using these values in the formula:

$$CO\ (\text{in l/min}) = \frac{I \times 60}{C_S \times K}$$

Where I = the amount of indicator injected (in mg); C_S = sum of the one second time concentration values under the curve (in mm–sec); K = the calibration factor for the concentration of dye in solution (mg/l/mm); and the factor of 60 is introduced to give the output per minute.

The "forward triangle" concept provides an even simpler, manual, mathematical method of calculating the cardiac output from an indicator dilution curve. This method is based on the observation that the initial build-up portion of the indicator curve bears a constant relationship to the entire curve[14]. The initial build-up portion of the curve, from the onset to the peak, is considered a triangle. The downslope of the curve bears a constant relationship to the build-up slope, but it obviously is not identical. A constant of 0.34, derived by Benchimol, is used to compensate for the difference in the components of the curve.

Using this concept, the cardiac output is calculated from the original dye curve without the re-plotting on semilogarithmic paper and without the need for planimetry of the area. The only measurements necessary are the build-up time from the onset of the curve to the very peak of the curve and the concentration of the indicator at that highest point in the curve. The formula for cardiac output is:

$$CO\ (\text{in l/min}) = \frac{I \times 60 \times 0.34}{1/2 \times BT \times PC}$$

Where I = the amount of indicator injected (in mg); 0.34 = a constant to correct for the difference from a true triangle; BT = the build-up time from the onset of the curve to the

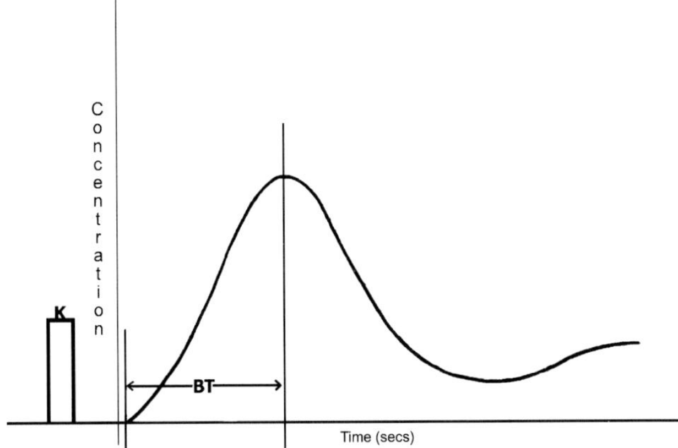

Figure 10.21 Benchimol "forward triangle" calculation of cardiac output from indicator dilution curve. K, calibration concentration; BT, buildup time.

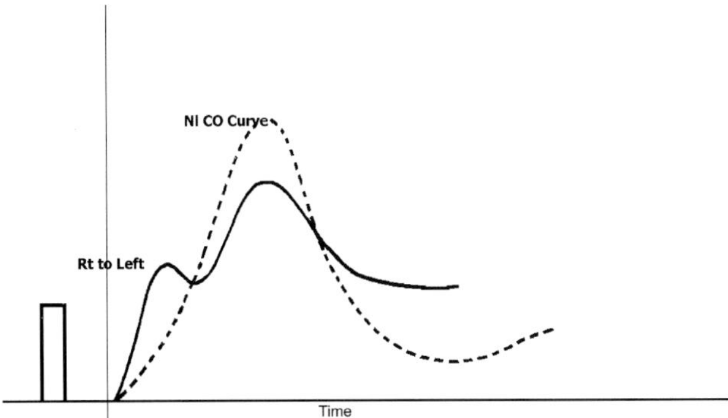

Figure 10.22 Large right to left shunt curve (Rt to Left), superimposed on normal output curve (Nl CO Curve).

highest point in the curve (in sec); PC = the peak concentration of the indicator at the peak of the curve (in mg/l); and the factor of 60 is introduced to give the output per minute (Figure 10.21).

Even using the forward triangle method, the manual calculations are laborious and require tedious measurements of the height of the curve, the various slopes of the curve, the duration of the curve and by one means or another, correlating these values with the concentration of Cardio-Green under the calibration curve. Fortunately, in the few catheterization laboratories where Cardio-Green indicator dilution studies are still used, the densitometer output is connected directly to an analog cardiac output computer, which instantaneously and accurately calculates the cardiac output from this curve.

When used with an output computer, Cardio-Green indicator cardiac outputs are very accurate and fairly simple to perform. They are not dependent upon the patient's being in a steady state and can be performed with the patient breathing any amount of oxygen. Quantitative Cardio-Green output studies do require the withdrawal of a significant amount of blood at a very steady rate from an indwelling line or from a catheter positioned in a systemic artery. Although the blood can be returned to the patient, this requires a special set-up of disposable sterile tubing in the densitometer, and the entire operation of the densitometer must be performed under sterile conditions.

Quantitative shunt determination with Cardio-Green indicator dilution curves

The detection and semi-quantification of both left to right and right to left shunts is possible using Cardio-Green dye curves with an accurate calibration and a constant withdrawal pump. They are easier to obtain and are more sensitive and more accurate for the demonstration of right to left shunts. Any left to right shunt large enough to make a significant change on a peripheral green-dye curve is detected more easily and certainly quantitated more accurately using oxygen saturations and the increase in oxygen saturations through the right heart.

The use of exogenous indicator dilution curves to attempt to quantitate the degree of shunting depends upon the accuracy of the early appearance and the recirculation curves. A right to left shunt using a peripheral sensor to detect green dye demonstrates the very early appearance of a preliminary curve that is caused by the shunted blood before the appearance of the main output curve. This early curve peaks, begins to decline and then blends into the upstroke of the main curve (Figure 10.22). The size of this early curve compared to the size of the main curve provides a general indication of the proportional amount of right to left shunt.

When using an indicator dilution curve to detect (or quantitate) a left to right shunt from peripheral sensing, the beginning of the upstroke of the build up of the main curve is essentially normal in its appearance and in its timing, although its peak amplitude is usually attenuated because of the blood that is shunted away from the central output. However, in the presence of a left to right shunt and shortly after the downslope of the normal output curve begins, there is an abrupt cut-off in the downslope as the curve breaks off horizontally, begins to turn upward and rises to a second peak. The second peak is due to the blood recirculated through the left to right shunt, back through the lungs and arriving early at the peripheral sensor before passing through the systemic venous system (Figure 10.23). As with right to left shunts, the relative sizes of the two curves provide some indication about the magnitude of the shunt.

Tomes have been written on the various mathematical means of using the amplitude and timing of exogenous indicator dilution curves for calculating the exact degree of shunting from the curves. None of the exogenous dye methods are as accurate for quantitating either left to right or right to left shunts as are the quantification of shunts

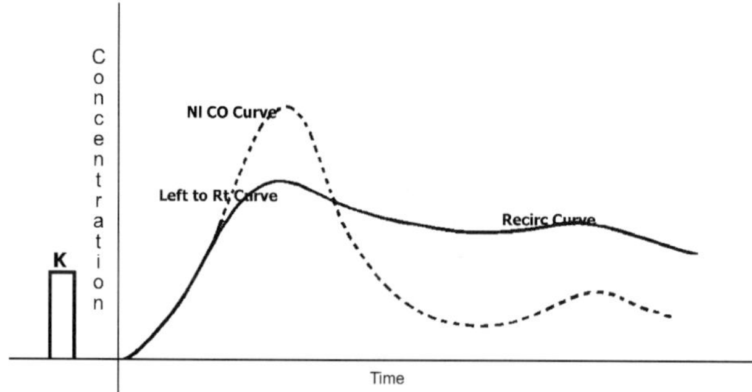

Figure 10.23 Large left to right shunt curve (Left to Rt Curve) superimposed on normal output curve (Nl CO Curve) and followed by recirculation curve (Recirc Curve) of indicator.

using oxygen as the indicator. Owing to the infrequent use of exogenous indicator curves and the generally greater ease and accuracy of oxygen determinations for quantitative data, no further time will be spent on the mathematical exercises of quantitative determinations of shunts using dye dilution curves.

Qualitative indicator dilution curves

Qualitatively, indicator dilution curves are performed rapidly and easily. When used properly, exogenous indicator dilution techniques are the most sensitive techniques available for the detection and localization of the very smallest degree of shunting. Regardless of the material used as an indicator, these techniques are dependent upon the Fick principal of uniform mixing of the indicator within the circulation and the ability of sensors to detect the early appearance of minute quantities of the indicator at some specific point in the circulation.

For the detection *only*, without quantification, of abnormal shunting within the circulation, the distal sensor can be as simple as a densitometer on the skin over a superficial capillary bed through which light can be transmitted (e.g. an ear lobe or fingertip). A sensor that is built onto the tip of a catheter and placed within the circulation can also be used. The catheter tip sensor is positioned within the circulation but blood does not necessarily need to be withdrawn for the detection of the indicator. For the detection only of a shunt, the indicator substance is introduced proximally into the flow on one side of the circulation. The early appearance on the opposite side of the circulation of a minute amount of this indicator indicates the presence of even the very smallest shunt. The amount of indicator introduced does not have to be measured and the amount of indicator arriving at the sensor is only detected and not quantitated.

Indicators used for the detection only of shunts are indocyanine-green dye, ascorbic acid and hydrogen gas. Ascorbic acid and hydrogen gas introduce positive hydrogen ions into the circulating blood, which produces a rapid and very transient lowering of the blood pH, which, in turn, serves as the indictor and can be sensed with an electrode catheter positioned within the circulation.

Qualitative Cardio-Green indicator dilution curves

Right to left shunt detection

When the relative appearance times of indicator curves are utilized only for the detection of a right to left shunt, green dye is an extremely sensitive indicator. For detection only, the amount of indicator injected does not have to be measured and no calculations are required. A qualitative curve that is satisfactory for the detection of a shunt can be recorded without the need for any arterial access and without withdrawing any blood. A special cutaneous earpiece or fingertip densitometer is used as the sensor for Cardio-Green dye. For a better estimation of the amount of shunt, blood can be drawn through a densitometer from an arterial line or the curve from the cutaneous densitometer signal, which is at least qualitatively similar to that obtained by arterial sampling, is amplified and recorded on the catheterization laboratory recorder during a specified period of time.

One to two milliliters of the diluted Cardio-Green dye is injected rapidly through a catheter into a specific location within the right heart circulation. When the location of the injection is proximal to the level of right to left shunting, a discrete, very early deflection of the recorded curve from the peripheral sensor will document even a very minute degree of right to left shunting. This early curve appearing well before the major left-sided output curve is similar to the quantitative curve in Figure 10.22. The dye in the shunted blood passes directly from the systemic venous blood, through the shunt, to the left heart and rapidly to the peripheral arterial sensor, while the dye that is still in the non-shunted blood must pass through the pulmonary circulation to reach the left heart and arrives at the peripheral arterial sensor several seconds later, producing the main output curve. By varying the injection site either proximally or distally within the right heart, the exact site of shunting can be localized. When recorded over time, these inscribed curves are semi-quantitative, with the relative size of the early appearing hump compared to the main curve representing the relative magnitude of the shunting.

Because of streamlining within the heart, green-dye curves cannot differentiate the magnitude of relative degrees of right to left shunting when the shunting occurs at multiple levels within the heart (e.g. with both atrial and ventricular shunting) any better than this can be determined using relative oxygen values. Green-dye curves, however, clearly document the most distal level of shunting. Selective injections in the right or left pulmonary artery can document the presence of unilateral pulmonary arteriovenous fistulae and clearly demonstrate which lung is involved, or if both lungs are involved.

If the sampling is performed through a catheter tip positioned in the left heart and the Cardio-Green is injected through a separate catheter positioned in the right heart, then the Cardio-Green curve can be used for the localization of the most proximal level of the right to left shunt. The reverse of this injection/sampling using two intracardiac catheters can also be used to detect or localize left to right shunts. The injection is performed in the left heart and the sampling is carried out by withdrawing blood from a specific area of the right heart. In general, the qualitative detection of left to right shunting is performed more readily using hydrogen or ascorbic acid dilution curves, which are discussed subsequently in this chapter.

Valvular regurgitation can be detected and even semiquantitated using Cardio-Green dye indicator curves. The indicator is injected into a ventricle or great artery through one catheter, and sensed in the atrium or ventricle immediately proximal in the circulation to the injection site with a second catheter. The amount of regurgitant flow is indicated by the amplitude of the dye curve and by the subsequent rate of disappearance (return to zero) or lack thereof of the dye curve. Normally, no indicator dye should appear in the chamber that is proximal in the blood flow or the valve to the site of the injection immediately after the injection. The early appearance of any dye in the proximal chamber represents regurgitation, and persistence of the dye in the more proximal chamber suggests a more severe degree of regurgitation. The determination of regurgitant flow with indicator dilution curves has the one significant advantage over angiography that the injection of one milliliter of Cardio-Green dye is not likely to result in any ectopy or produce any regurgitation from the injection itself, while a "power" injection of almost any amount of contrast frequently results in ectopy, catheter recoil and induced regurgitation.

Hydrogen gas indicator dilution curves

Hydrogen gas indicator dilution curves are based on the fact that hydrogen gas, when inhaled, passes *instantaneously* through the alveolar wall and is *instantaneously* absorbed into the pulmonary venous blood. The hydrogen that is absorbed into the blood changes the pH of that blood very slightly and very transiently, but significantly enough to be detected. This very slight, transient change is detected by a very sensitive electrocardiographic electrode at the tip of a catheter placed in the right heart. The electrode is actually recording an intracardiac electrocardiogram (ECG) tracing but at a very high gain. The change in the pH does not affect the generation of the electrocardiogram, but rather shifts the baseline stability of the ECG recording such that the appearance of even a minute quantity of this hydrogenated blood produces a sudden, sharp and marked shift in the baseline tracing of the intracardiac ECG. The very early, almost instantaneous, appearance of this shift in the baseline curve of the ECG indicates the presence of a left to right shunt proximal to the location of the sensing electrode.

When the patient inhales hydrogen in the absence of any left-to-right shunt and with the electrode positioned anywhere in the right heart, there is a slow appearance (4–6 seconds) before the occurrence of a somewhat attenuated deflection of the ECG tracing. In the absence of an intracardiac shunt, the "acidified" blood must pass through the systemic arterial system, the systemic capillary bed and the systemic venous system before returning to the right heart. However, in the presence of even a very tiny left to right shunt, the "acidified" blood from the left heart passes immediately into the right heart through the shunt. This results in an immediate, earlier and much larger deflection of the baseline tracing of the ECG recorded in any location in the right heart or pulmonary artery that is downstream from the location of the shunting. Again, this technique does not separate several areas of shunting, but does detect the most proximal level of shunting. By varying the location of the electrode catheter within the right heart, the precise location of an isolated level of shunting or at least the most proximal level of shunting can be identified.

The electrodes on the catheter for hydrogen curves must be new (or "re-platinized") to be sensitive enough to detect the very small changes in the pH of the blood. The baseline intracardiac electrocardiographic tracing from the electrode is adjusted to the middle of the CRT screen. The intracardiac ECG is set at a very high gain and the recorder is turned on at 10 mm/sec. This creates a broad band of tracing across the screen. A control curve is recorded by the inhalation of hydrogen with the catheter tip electrode positioned either on the systemic arterial side of the circulation or in the pulmonary artery wedge position, in order to verify the technique and integrity of the entire system. This control curve should create an instantaneous deflection of the baseline curve, confirming the instantaneous appearance of the indicator at the electrode. To perform the diagnostic hydrogen curve, the electrode catheter is positioned in the desired location in the right heart (systemic venous) circulation in a location that is distal (downstream) to the suspected level of shunting.

Hydrogen is delivered to the patient from an anesthesia bag and mask with an attached three-way rebreathing valve. It takes some practice to release the hydrogen exactly and simultaneously with the patient's inspiration and in doing so not disturb the patient enough for him to interrupt his breathing or even briefly stop breathing, which would delay or prevent the inhalation of the hydrogen into the alveoli and, in turn, into the circulation. The mask with the attached bag, which is filled with hydrogen, is placed gently over the patient's nose and mouth. With the recorder turned on at the slow recording speed, the patient is allowed to breathe room air normally through the side valve of the mask for several minutes in order to become adjusted to the mask. Once the patient is breathing normally, the operator opens the valve in the mask to the hydrogen in the bag precisely with the onset of the patient's normal inspiration. The operator of the mask and valve must indicate the exact instant when the patient inhales the hydrogen (not necessarily when the valve is opened) to the recording nurse/technician. It is better for the person operating the mask to have a foot switch to indicate the moment of inspiration, thus eliminating the verbal transmission time delay to the recording person.

When the electrode is distal to the shunt, there is an immediate and significant deflection of the recorded intracardiac ECG tracing. The sensor on the catheter is positioned forward or backward within the right heart circulation to determine the exact level, or at least the most proximal level, of left to right shunting.

Hydrogen gas is stored in cylinders and transferred to the anesthesia bag for each hydrogen indicator dilution test. Hydrogen gas is explosive, but only when *high concentrations* come in contact with a flame or spark. The concentration of hydrogen exhaled by the patient or escaping from the bag/mask is not sufficient to support an explosion. The combination of the potential danger for explosion of the stored hydrogen gas and the sensitivity of high quality cineangiography for detecting and localizing very small shunts has led to the virtual abandonment of this fairly simple and very useful qualitative indicator dilution technique.

Ascorbic acid indicator dilution curves

A high concentration of injected ascorbic acid can be used as an alternative to inhaled hydrogen as a means of acidifying the blood. The sensor for detecting the change in the blood pH again is an intracavitary ECG electrode catheter, exactly the same as used for hydrogen curves. 500–1,000 mg of ascorbic acid is injected into the pulmonary artery (or actually any position within the right heart) through a venous catheter. The ascorbic acid can be injected through the same venous catheter that is used for the sensing. The ascorbic acid mixes with the venous blood during its passage through the lungs and, as with the hydrogen gas, the acidity of the resultant solution lowers the pH of this blood slightly. As the blood returns to the left heart, any quantity that shunts back into the right heart through a left to right shunt causes a deflection of the ECG curve being recorded from the electrode positioned within the right heart and downstream to the shunting. As with the hydrogen curves, by moving the sensing electrode to different sites within the right heart circulation, the most proximal level of left to right shunting is detected.

Ascorbic acid has several major advantages as an indicator over hydrogen gas. With the availability of the ascorbic acid technique, the problems of the storage and handling of the potentially dangerous hydrogen are obviated. As the ascorbic acid is injected through or adjacent to the sensing catheter, it passes the electrode at the tip of the sensing catheter and produces a marked deflection of the intracardiac ECG at that instant. This very effectively marks the *exact* time of the introduction of the indicator into the system, and makes for very accurate timing of the circulation of the ascorbic acid through the lungs and back to the sensing electrode.

Ascorbic acid dilution curves are uniquely capable of detecting isolated partial anomalous pulmonary venous drainage from a single lung or lung segment. Selective injections and recordings of curves from the right or left lung or even selective branches can be performed. By selectively injecting into the relevant lung or segment, there is rapid reappearance of the acidified blood through the shunt at only the single level or area of shunting, while injections of ascorbic acid into a non-involved segment show no early reappearance of acidified blood.

The only disadvantage of the ascorbic acid indicator technique is that it is more difficult to obtain good curves. In order to perform ascorbic acid curves with most modern recording systems, a special add-on DC amplifier is required. Often the deflection of the recording curve, which occurs as the ascorbic acid is injected past the electrode at the catheter tip, displaces the curve off the scale. The subsequent recirculation from the left to right shunt can occur so rapidly that the baseline curve is not back to baseline (or even on the page) in order to record the second diagnostic deflection. This is obviated by using an electrode catheter with the electrode at least several centimeters proximal to the tip or by injecting through a separate catheter placed several centimeters distal in the circulation to the electrode.

Similar to the situation with hydrogen, the ability to reliably visualize small shunts with cineangiography has essentially eliminated the use of any of the qualitative indicator dilution curves, including ascorbic acid curves. These will probably be relegated to the historical annals of cardiac catheterization.

Data recording and presentation

The cardiac catheterization report should be a summary of all of the procedures performed, events that occurred, equipment used, medications administered, and results obtained during the catheterization. Most catheterization reports contain several components.

All the information is entered on a timed, tabular recording by the recording nurse/technician as the case progresses. In most (all?) current cardiac catheterization laboratories this log is created in a computer program and it is usually printed for a permanent record at the end of the case. The location and time of oxygen samples and pressure recordings along with the numerical results of these samples are entered manually into this timed recording as the case proceeds. This detailed tabular log of the procedure is generated almost automatically by the recording system in most catheterization laboratories. It usually is quite long, yet in fact tells little about the actual procedures or how the data or the hemodynamics were acquired.

The details of the techniques and procedures that were used/performed during the catheterization are presented in a separate, dictated "narrative summary", which must be provided by the catheterizing physician or his designee. A straightforward diagnostic catheterization procedure performed on a simple lesion and with no complications can be summarized in a single short paragraph. However, each pertinent, complex or complicated maneuver or procedure, and particularly any unique components of the procedure, should be described in detail in this summary. Any therapeutic interventions should definitely be described in detail, including the indications and the hemodynamic and anatomic findings before and after the intervention. The details of these complex or unique procedures should include a description of the specific equipment used and how it was used for that particular procedure. This description is usually the only detailed record of such a procedure. The details of this description are particularly important in the event that the same procedure should have to be repeated by a different operator or be part of a review of a particular case.

The narrative description of the procedure includes a listing and a description of the various angiograms that were performed. The description of each angiogram should include the chamber or vessel where the injection was performed, the angles of the X-ray tubes in both planes, the amount of contrast used, the rate and pressure of the injection, and a detailed description of the findings from the angiogram. In complex lesions, these descriptions should contain the details of all of the pertinent anatomic findings of that particular angiogram—both normal and abnormal.

The narrative catheterization summary ***does not*** include, ***necessarily***, a detailed description of the hemodynamic findings but, rather, a tabular summary of the hemodynamics (oxygen saturations and pressures) should accompany the description. When the detailed hemodynamic findings from a very complex pediatric/congenital heart procedure are included in a complex narrative description, this narrative description becomes a tome of words which often leaves the reader very vague or unclear about the exact anatomy or the significant hemodynamics. The differences in terminology that are still used by many different individuals, centers and countries make narrative descriptions even more confusing.

For reporting the data in congenital heart lesions, the adage that "a picture is worth a thousand words"—with the caveat of "an ***accurate*** picture . . ."—could not be truer in attempting to describe the very complex anatomy and associated hemodynamics. Each cardiac catheterization report from the catheterization laboratories at Texas Children's Hospital is accompanied by a "heart diagram", which is *individualized for that particular patient and his particular anatomic and hemodynamic abnormalities*. The narrative summary of the catheterization report usually refers to the individualized diagram of the particular patient for the summary of the findings (e.g. the pressure, oxygen and angiographic data). Each separate diagram is modified in detail and as precisely as possible to illustrate the individual patient's anatomic defects. Chambers or vessels on the diagram are increased, reduced in size or otherwise modified according to the angiographic or anatomic findings. Holes or narrowings are drawn in each separate diagram in proportion to their size angiographically in the patient.

In addition to modifying the anatomic picture, the hemodynamic data on the diagram are "editorialized" to correspond to a single steady state. When oxygen saturations and/or pressures that are obtained during the procedure are different *only* because of different times and/or a different steady state when they were obtained, and which do not actually represent a shunt or obstruction, they are ***not*** reported as differences on the diagrams. When no shunt and/or gradient actually exists, the final, editorialized diagram should not suggest or indicate a shunt or gradient.

This author has previously published a *Diagrammatic Atlas of Congenital Heart Disease*, which contains diagrammatic representations of the basic structures of a large majority of complex congenital heart defects[15]. These diagrams include most of the permutations and combinations of dextro, levo and meso cardia, atrial situs solitus and inversus, atrioventricular concordance and discordance, ventricular–arterial connections, most with either right or left aortic arches and many of the recognized or more common abnormal congenital heart complexes (truncus arteriosus, pulmonary, tricuspid and mitral atresia and anomalous pulmonary venous connections). The basic situs, chamber and vessel abnormalities are difficult to illustrate "from scratch", whereas additional defects (holes) or a narrowing of structures are easy to add to any of the basic diagrams. In addition, the introductory text in the *Atlas* describes in detail a simple way to modify the diagrams in order to make them represent each particular patient's anatomy and hemodynamics absolutely precisely. Almost every heart diagram that is used in a pediatric/congenital cardiac catheterization report undergoes some modification to fit the specific patient.

The modified diagrams can be scanned into a drawing program of a computer, which makes them readily available for the final printed report. The diagrams can be modified on the computer while the report is being generated. Scientific Software Solutions, Charlottesville, VA developed the Pedi-Cath™ computer program that utilizes this collection of heart diagrams and was designed specifically for pediatric/congenital patients. With this program the hemodynamic data (oxygen saturations and pressures) can even be placed into the specific location on an appropriate predetermined basic diagram for the individual patient as the catheterization procedure progresses. The diagrams themselves can be modified and the data editorialized at the conclusion of the procedure.

An accurately created diagram provides a very quick visual image of often very complex anatomy along with a summary of the hemodynamics without having to wade through pages of text. Several representative examples of the heart diagrams without the hemodynamics are included (Figures 10.24–10.27).

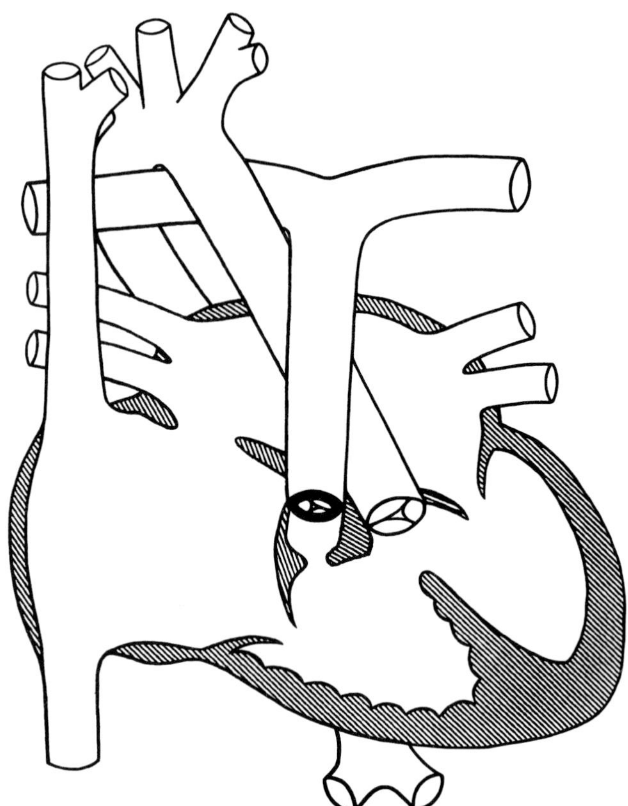

Figure 10.25 Diagram of tetralogy of Fallot with right aortic arch.

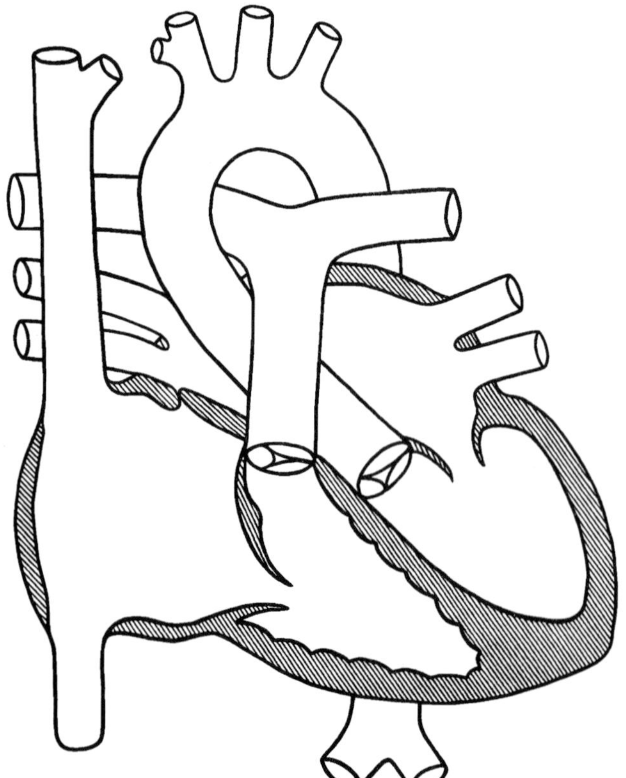

Figure 10.24 Diagram of normal heart with left aortic arch.

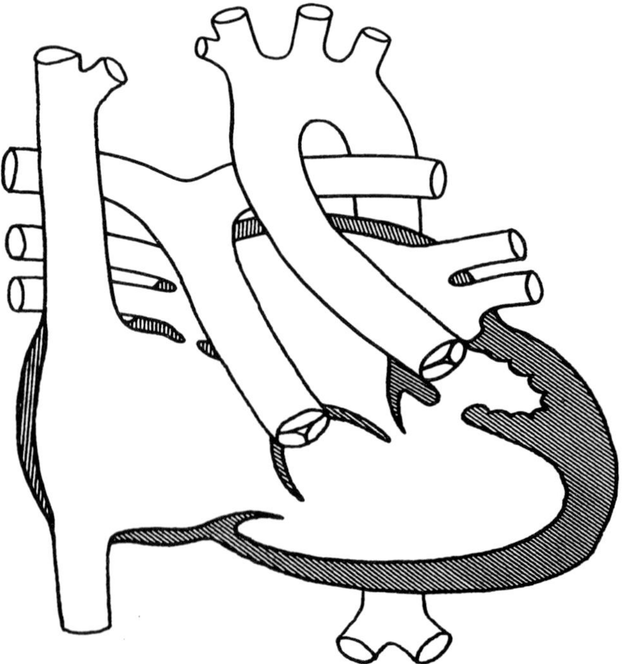

Figure 10.26 Diagram of ventricular inversion, double inlet left ventricle, transposition of the great arteries with an outlet foramen to a hypoplastic subaortic right ventricle.

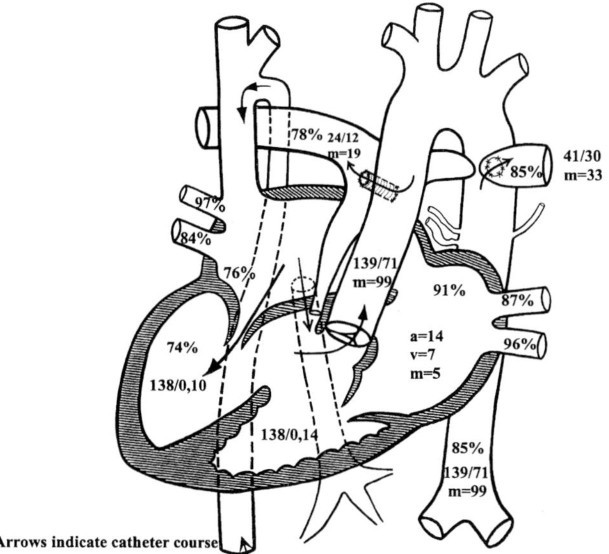

Figure 10.27 Diagram of dextrocardia with situs solitus, ventricular inversion, transposition of the great arteries, pulmonary atresia, ventricular septal defect, interruption of the hepatic portion of the inferior vena cava with azygos continuation to the right superior vena cava, separate hepatic vein drainage into the right atrium, partial anomalous pulmonary venous connection of the entire right lung to the right atrium, atrial septal defect, left aortic arch, systemic to pulmonary artery collaterals to both pulmonary arteries, post operative-direct descending aorta to left pulmonary artery anastomosis (Pott's shunt) with resultant isolation of left pulmonary artery and post operative-5 mm conduit interposition between ascending aorta and main pulmonary artery.

The last heart diagram presented includes representative hemodynamic data as well as very complex anatomy. The simplest and most common of the diagrams is the diagram of a "normal heart" with a left aortic arch (Figure 10.24). This same diagram is available in the book with the atrial and ventricular septa left open; it being much easier to ink in and close openings that are not present clinically than it is to create new openings with white-out. The slightly more complex anatomy of a "straightforward" tetralogy of Fallot with a right aortic arch is illustrated in Figure 10.25. An even more complicated patient with ventricular inversion, double inlet left ventricle, transposition of the great arteries with an outlet foramen to a hypoplastic subaortic right ventricle, is illustrated in Figure 10.26. The final diagram, Figure 10.27, illustrates an actual patient with: dextrocardia with situs solitus, ventricular inversion, transposition of the great arteries, pulmonary atresia, ventricular septal defect, interruption of the hepatic portion of the inferior vena cava with azygos continuation to the right superior vena cava, separate hepatic vein drainage into the right atrium, partial anomalous pulmonary venous connection of the entire right lung to the right atrium, atrial septal defect, left aortic arch, systemic to pulmonary artery collaterals to both pulmonary arteries, postoperative direct descending aorta to left pulmonary artery anastomosis (Pott's shunt) with resultant isolation of left pulmonary artery and postoperative-5 mm conduit interposition between ascending aorta and main pulmonary artery. The diagnoses alone, even without the additional description of the added complex hemodynamic data, fill a descriptive page and still leave the reader confused about the anatomy. At the same time, this complex anatomy, along with the equally complex hemodynamics, are illustrated clearly by the individualized picture. The more complex the anatomy or hemodynamics, the more useful the heart diagrams become.

Near the end of the catheterization report should be included a listing and description of all of the complications of the catheterization and their management. The listed complications should include minor or transient adverse events, as well as major, life- or organ-threatening events, and certainly any events that result in permanent sequelae. The complications listed should include all complications that are related to that particular catheterization either during or after the procedure regardless of the time relationship to the procedure. For example, an infection at the catheterization site or a femoral A–V fistula which does not become apparent until a week after the procedure is still a complication of the catheterization and should be added to the report, if necessary as an addendum.

The catheterization report should conclude with a list of the patient's diagnoses in their order of relative significance to the patient, and with a discussion of the specific recommendations and disposition for the patient. Although ideally the narrative catheterization report is dictated the day of the procedure, this seldom is accomplished. Even when dictated the same day, the final report is not available for at least a week. Even a final completed report can be corrected and edited very easily with the computerized records. This leaves plenty of time to, and no excuse not to, add the details of the final, true disposition, even if it was not decided until a surgical conference a week later.

Responsibility for data

All determinations of flow, shunts, valve or stenotic areas and vascular resistance are only as good as the pressures, flow and oxygen data that are obtained in the catheterization laboratory. Even a small error in the basic data can result in an "exponential" magnification of the error in the calculations. The conclusions drawn from the saturation and pressure data must agree with the other data obtained before and during the catheterization, with the working or final diagnoses, and finally with physiologic principals; e.g. blood does not flow (or shunt) from lower to higher pressure areas nor can there be a measurable step down in saturation in progressing from the systemic veins to the pulmonary artery! Any hemodynamic findings that do not agree or fit with any of the other already available data should be identified *during the procedure* and clarified while the patient is still in the catheterization laboratory. "Second guessing" the day following the procedure never makes up for obtaining accurate data!

References

1. Brown LK *et al*. Anatomic landmarks for use when measuring intracardiac pressure with fluid-filled catheters. *Am J Cardiol* 2000; **86**(1): 121–124.
2. Fick A. *Über die Messung des Blutquantums in der Herventrikeln*. In S. B. phys-med. Ges. 1870: Würzburg. 16.
3. Gutgesell HP and Williams RL. Caval samples as indicators of mixed venous oxygen saturation: implications in atrial septal defect. *Cardiovasc Dis* 1974; **1**(3): 160–164.
4. Van Slyke DD and Neill JM. The determination of gases in blood and other solutions by vacuum extraction and manometric measurements. *J Biol Chem* 1924; **61**: 523–557.
5. Krouskop RW *et al*. Accuracy and clinical utility of an oxygen saturation catheter. *Crit Care Med* 1983; **11**(9): 744–749.
6. Gettinger A, DeTraglia MC, and Glass DD. *In vivo* comparison of two mixed venous saturation catheters. *Anesthesiology* 1987; **66**(3): 373–375.
7. Lister G, Hoffman JI and Rudolph AM. Oxygen uptake in infants and children: a simple method for measurement. *Pediatrics* 1974; **53**(5): 656–662.
8. LaFarge CG and Miettinen OS. The estimation of oxygen consumption. *Cardiovasc Res* 1970; **4**(1): 23–30.
9. Gorlin F and Gorlin S. Hydraulic formula for calculation of the area of the stenotic mitral valve, other cardiac valves and central circulatory shunts. *Am Heart J* 1951; **41**: 1.
10. Cohen M and Gorlin R. Modified orifice equation for the calculation of mitral valve area. *Am Heart J* 1972; **884**: 839–840.
11. Bache RJ, Jorgensen CR, and Wang Y. Simplified estimation of aortic valve area. *Br Heart J* 1972; **34**(4): 408–411.
12. Hamilton W *et al*. Studies on the circulation. IV. Further analysis of the injection method and of changes in hemodynamics under physiological and pathological conditions. *Am J Physiol* 1932; **99**: 534–551.
13. Stewart G. Researches on the circulation time and on the influences which affect it. IV. The output of the heart. *J Physiol* 1897; **22**: 159–183.
14. Hetzel P *et al*. Estimation of cardiac output from first part of arterial dye dilution curves. *J Appl Physiol* 1958; **13**: 92–96.
15. Mullins CE and Mayer DC. *Congenital Heart Disease: A Diagrammatic Atlas*. 1988, New York: Alan R. Liss, Inc.

11 Angiographic techniques

Introduction

In the current era of cardiovascular diagnosis, a large amount of anatomic information is obtained from alternative, non-invasive, imaging modalities such as echocardiography, magnetic resonance imaging (MRI) and computed tomography (CT). However, when precise details of the anatomy are required, angiography still provides the most accurate details plus considerable information about the blood flow that is not available by any other technique. The information acquired from angiograms in patients with complex congenital heart disease usually provides the final, essential data necessary for making the proper therapeutic decision.

In addition to providing very clear and precise images of discrete or specific structures, angiograms provide a great deal of additional information about the actual hemodynamics of the patient. The characteristics of the flow of the contrast within and through structures can be diagnostic of significant functional abnormalities that cannot be demonstrated hemodynamically. The additional angiographic information about flow is useful particularly in the low-flow, low-pressure locations where pressure gradients (or the lack thereof) are often meaningless. With normal blood flow, the blood (and contrast) flow is laminar, appears smooth and uniform and flows in one direction without turbulence through chambers, valves and vessels. In the presence of poor function, the flow of blood (and contrast) becomes stagnated and even pools or reverses direction in isolated locations. This is particularly true on angiograms in the systemic venous circuits of "Fontan" repair patients where often no significant gradients are recorded while the angiogram clearly demonstrates the essentially stagnant flow. Similarly, with obstruction of the tricuspid valve or obstruction to right to left flow across an atrial septal defect, a minimal gradient may be generated, but the angiogram clearly demonstrate a "jet" of restricted flow through the obstruction. In the presence of severe unilateral pulmonary venous obstruction, pulmonary artery pressures or an angiogram in a right or left pulmonary artery may not demonstrate the pulmonary venous lesion specifically, but the reversal of blood (and contrast) flow in that pulmonary artery is almost pathognomonic of the lesion.

This chapter is not intended as a complete text of radiography or angiography of congenital heart disease. There are, in fact, excellent, and very complete, texts devoted to this topic[1,2]. This chapter is intended to provide enough details about the X-ray imaging process to give an interventional cardiologist an understanding of the basic elements of angiography, which are controllable (for the most part) by the catheterizing physician and are essential in the production of quality angiographic images in pediatric and congenital heart patients.

The medical director of the catheterization laboratory must have a major input into the decisions about the specific X-ray equipment that is installed in a pediatric/congenital cardiac catheterization laboratory. The director is also responsible for ensuring that the proper maintenance and functioning of the equipment continue after its installation. The correct installation and calibration and continued proper functioning of the X-ray and image recording equipment are the responsibility of the manufacturer and local biomedical engineers. The major settings of modern X-ray generating and imaging equipment are fixed within the equipment and cannot be altered significantly during any individual catheterization procedure. Any deviation from the optimal performance of the imaging equipment must be recognized and reported by each physician who uses the equipment in order that any problem can be corrected expediently. In addition, there are fine adjustments and specific maneuvers that are necessary to optimize the image obtained during every angiogram. These are the responsibility of each catheterizing physician during each procedure and are the main emphasis of this chapter.

Fixed components of angiographic equipment

All of the current techniques of angiography depend upon images generated by X-rays. In 2001 Bashore published a very nice, short and understandable review of X-ray imaging[3]. X-rays are electromagnetic waves with a very short wavelength and a high penetrating power for tissues. The degree of penetration of tissues by X-rays is inversely proportional to the relative densities of the tissues and proportional to the intensity of the X-rays. The variable penetration of X-rays through the different types of tissue creates images of varying density on the imaging and recording media.

X-ray generators amplify and modulate electrical voltage from a common power line into the very high voltages that are delivered to the X-ray tube[4]. An X-ray tube is a large vacuum tube that contains a (positively-charged) anode and a (negatively-charged) cathode. In the tube a metal filament in the cathode is heated and a high voltage (thousands of volts) is passed to this heated metal filament. This hot metal filament in the cathode discharges (negatively-charged) electrons. The vacuum in the X-ray tube allows the free dispersal of these electrons in all directions. At the same time, an extremely high voltage *positive* charge is applied to the anode of the X-ray tube. The positive charge draws the electrons to the anode with a very high velocity and energy. As these electrons hit a tungsten target on the anode with this high energy, X-ray photons, along with a huge amount of heat, are generated.

The clinical X-ray tube is encased in a very complex and heavily leaded housing. The thick metal (lead) housing around the X-ray tube totally constrains the scattering X-ray photons within the housing except for the very small percentage of photons that are permitted to exit through a small opening, or port, as the X-ray beam. The housing of the angiographic tube also contains an elaborate system for circulating oil to dissipate the heat that is generated.

The X-rays leaving the focal spot and exiting through the single small port are minimally divergent as they travel as beams of photons. These are the usable X-rays which create images on a collecting system as they penetrate structures of variable density. The smaller the focus (focal spot) is on the anode, the less divergence there is of the X-ray beam which exits the tube and, in turn, the sharper the beam of X-rays produced on the eventual optical pick-up (imaging) system. The sharper the focus of the optical image, the greater will be the detail obtained. However, the smaller the focal spot, the greater the electron energy necessary to produce equivalent penetration of the tissues. This produces greater heat and becomes the limiting factor in the production of images with a smaller focal spot.

The intensity and quality of the X-ray beam emitted are controlled by the voltage and amperage of the current delivered to the X-ray tube by the generators. The higher the voltage delivered to the anode, the higher the energy of the electrons, and hence the higher the energy of the photons produced (and the greater the heat produced). The higher their energy, the greater the "force" or penetrating capabilities of the X-ray photons. The separate current that is applied to the cathode filament determines the temperature of the filament which, in turn, determines the number, or quantity, of electrons given off by the filament. The quantity of electrons given off from the cathode determines the current (mA) of the electron stream. The current determines the quantity of X-ray photons produced and is more related to the quality of the X-ray beam and the resolution of the resultant image.

The higher the energy applied to the X-ray tube and anode, the higher the intensity of the X-rays and the greater the heat which is generated by the X-ray tube. Most non-cardiovascular X-ray images involve a single microsecond exposure, which is produced by a single burst of high-voltage energy. In cardiac fluoroscopy, the X-ray beam and the heat are generated continuously for a duration of several seconds. After a very brief pause, the continuous exposure (fluoroscopy) is repeated. During cardiac and vascular cine angiography, an even higher voltage exposure is repeated 30 to 60 times per second for a duration of several seconds. The modern X-ray tube designed for angiography has a high-speed continually spinning anode (a rotating anode) to keep the heat from burning through the focal spot on the anode during these continuous or rapidly repeated exposures. In addition these tubes have extremely elaborate fluid circulating systems for the continuous dissipation of the heat generated. The heat of the X-ray tube is monitored continuously. A limitation of the production and effective dissipation of this heat are critical for the continued function of the X-ray tube.

The focused, almost parallel X-rays are directed to the patient and penetrate the tissues being imaged. The amount of penetration is inversely proportional to the density of the tissues in the various areas of the image. In addition to the photons that penetrate straight through the tissues, many bounce off the tissues in all directions and become non-effective for the production of the image and—of more importance—a danger to the surrounding environment as "scatter radiation". To reduce this scatter, the X-ray system uses filters at the output of the X-ray tube to eliminate some of the more divergent photons which would not be effective for the production of an image. In addition "grids", which are extremely thin parallel strips of metal, are interposed between the imaged structure (the patient) and the receiving screen to align the photons even further. Only the photons that penetrate the body *and* remain as the most parallel beams make it through the grid and are utilized for the final image. In spite of all of these built-in refinements and precautions, there is still a large amount of scatter radiation distributed in all directions from the tissues being imaged.

Originally, before the availability of image intensifiers, the photons emitted from the tissues were captured directly onto a fluorescent screen. The photons reached the screen in proportion to the penetration through the variable densities of the tissues being imaged, and activated the fluorescence of the screen in proportion to the number of photons reaching any particular portion of it. The photons were converted into images by the fluorescent screen where they were visualized directly or recorded on a large sheet of X-ray film. The large film format was ideal for standard X-rays, but created monumental problems (along with some innovative solutions to these problems) for the recording of multiple exposures in the rapid sequence necessary for capturing moving objects during angiography. Once these recording problems had been overcome, the large-film angiograms that were produced were of extremely high resolution. These large-film angiograms had the limitation of, at best, 12, but more often, 6 or even 3 frames per second. These films, at that rate of recording, of course, could not portray structures actually in motion.

On all modern angiographic equipment there is now an automatic brightness control of the image. This is achieved by light detectors in the image pick-up system which capture the photons after they have penetrated the tissues. These sensors sense the intensity of the *light image* produced by the X-rays after they have passed through the tissues of the patient. A reciprocal signal, which depends upon the intensity of the image received, is continuously sent back from these sensors by feedback circuits to the X-ray generators[4]. With the information from the sensors, the X-ray tube delivers more or less energy in order to maintain a constant light intensity for that particular area of the image being sensed.

Depending upon the basic setting of the X-ray system, the X-ray tube converts the electron energy into the correct proportions of photon energy and intensity to produce adequate penetration of the patient and, at the same time, ideal contrast and detail of the image. These basic settings are adjustable according to the size of the patient and the type of study being performed, but are performed almost automatically by modern X-ray equipment. The energy must be pulsed through the patient in a short enough time interval to stop the motion of the heart in order to produce an optimal, clear, X-ray image, and all without excessive X-ray exposure to the patient and operators. All of these variable factors of the X-ray combine together to determine the quality of the image emitted from the object.

Now, in all cardiac catheterization laboratories, the X-ray photons emerging from the tissues pass through an aluminum filter and are captured on an input screen consisting of a thin layer of very sensitive cesium iodide (CsI) phosphor, which converts the absorbed X-ray photons into a very large number of visible light photons. The light photons then generate electrons by either an image intensifier (II) tube or, more recently, a flat-panel detector using an array of transistors in a thin film.

The II takes the light photons from the input screen and generates electrons, which are accelerated and focused through a vacuum tube to impact a small output screen, where they generate very bright light photons that have been amplified to approximately 1,000 times the brightness of the original X-ray source. This results in the visible image on the small output screen. This visible analog light image is captured either by recording directly onto photographic film or by reconversion into a digital image through an analog to digital converter or directly as a digital image with a charge-coupled device (CCD). The marked increase in the intensity of the light image produced by the image intensifier allows for a lower intensity X-ray input into the intensifier along with a much shorter exposure time for each image to be visualized clearly or stored. This allows the X-ray exposure to be performed much more rapidly, which, in turn, allows for moving sequence or "cine" imaging.

The analog light output of the image intensifier is captured by a series of lenses and sent to a video camera or a CCD. In older, but still existing video systems, this light image is then split into two portions. A small portion of this light (15–20%) is diverted to a TV monitor for direct visualization (the fluoroscopy image), and the second and major part of the light beam is diverted to a movie (cine) camera for permanent recording on photographic film. The cine film images are exposed and recorded at a much higher rate than was possible with large-film imaging. When these individual cine images are viewed rapidly and sequentially on movie projectors, the images or structures are seen in motion. Cine angiographic recording replaced large X-ray films as the standard angiographic recording medium. Cine imaging is still used as the primary or back-up recording and archiving medium in some catheterization laboratories.

In the imaging systems in the majority of current X-ray systems in cardiac catheterization laboratories that still use image intensifiers, the analog light image from the video output of the image intensifier is converted into a digital image by an analog to digital converter. The digital image is an array of black and white pixels. The pixels are arranged in variable layers or depths to create different densities or gradations between black and white. The pixels are commonly displayed in a matrix of 512×512, pixels or more recently, $1{,}024 \times 1{,}024$ pixels per mm. The pixels are displayed at depths of 8 bits (which gives 256 different gradations of gray between black and white) and are recorded at speeds up to 60 images per second using biplane imaging. The digital images are visualized directly on a high-resolution cathode-ray screen and are stored on a computer hard drive rather than being reconverted to analog and transferred to film. Direct digital image production, display and recording make up the current standard for the entire imaging chain including visualization in the catheterization laboratory and archiving of the images. In the very latest X-ray systems the output of the image intensifier is picked up by a CCD, which takes the focused light from the input of the intensifier and converts it directly into a digital signal.

Flat-panel detectors are rapidly replacing image intensifiers and CCDs for the conversion of the X-ray energy to usable images. Flat-panel detectors consist of an array of a thin film of micro transistors similar to flat-panel television/computer displays. The separate transistors in flat-panel television/computer screens convert digital numbers into separate light signals, while the transistors in flat-panel *detectors* convert the separate light signals directly into numerical (digital) signals. Current flat-panel detectors do not convert X-ray photons directly, and need the X-ray photons to be converted to light photons using a cesium iodide input phosphor layer. Once the flat-panel detector has converted the light image to a digital signal, this signal is transmitted directly to the display and/or the digital storage system with no degradation of the signal or image.

Obviously, there are many integral or fixed components that form part of this complex X-ray imaging chain, all of which can significantly affect the final image quality[5]. All of the components can, *and do*, change or even fail completely during use. The operator or individual catheterizing physician has little or no immediate control over most of these factors, but should be able to recognize the subtle changes in images that represent changes in the functional status of the equipment.

X-ray generators themselves and the high-tension cables/connections to the X-ray tube can fail. Usually, when these fail, it is sudden, complete and not at all subtle. X-ray tubes can also fail suddenly, however, more often they deteriorate slowly with an insidious degradation of the image quality. Since a gradual deterioration in the X-ray tube does not result in a sudden change in the image quality nor does it shut down the equipment acutely, X-ray tubes are monitored regularly by specific measurements of the X-ray output and by changes in the quality of the image produced. The photon output of the X-ray tubes can be measured directly. The quality of the image is checked for even minimal changes by comparison with previously recorded quality control "ideal" images. In the chain of equipment, the X-ray tubes undergo the most stress, particularly during prolonged use, and are always suspect when there is deterioration in the image quality!

The image intensifier (II) is the next variable in the X-ray imaging chain which is suspect when there is a change in the quality of the images that are produced by the system. The minimum standard image intensifier tube has a cesium iodide input phosphor with high resolution and good brightness. There is some latitude in the quality and contrast of each image intensifier image even in a new system. No two image intensifiers have the same output, even from the moment they are manufactured. Although new image intensifier tubes vary somewhat in the quality of the images they produce, they can still fall within the manufacturing and advertised specifications or standards for the particular tube. Some image intensifiers are more suitable for producing high-contrast images while others produce images with less contrast and better detail.

Of most significance, image intensifier tubes usually do not stop working suddenly, but rather, degrade slowly, insidiously, and steadily with time, and even more so than X-ray tubes. Each image intensifier has its own rate of degradation. The image unequivocally will deteriorate over time because of the inexorable deterioration of the image intensifier tube itself. Major indicators of the deterioration of the image intensifier are from the subjective observations of the users of the system or the need to increase the X-ray energy continually in order to produce comparable images. The images obtained daily must be compared *regularly* to previously obtained, "ideal" images for evidence of even minimal changes in quality. Eventually image intensifiers must be changed for new ones when the quality of the image becomes unacceptable even with a "reasonable" increase in the X-ray dose and even though they are still functioning to produce some images.

From the output image of the image intensifier, a video camera or a CCD picks up the output (the light source) and converts the light output into usable and quality pictures. The video camera, which captures the light from the output of the image intensifier, is the next major variable in the chain. There are many types of video capture system, each with their own particular qualities. The video camera, like the image intensifier, can and will, deteriorate over time. Deterioration in the video camera often results in a striking distortion of the image rather than diffuse or subtle changes in quality. Similarly, changes in the optical system between the video camera and the television screen or film usually result in distortion or "contamination" of the final image with light streaks, shadows or other persistent imperfections on each image.

Flat-panel detectors eliminate many of the components that can fail in the imaging chain. Flat-panel arrays do deteriorate even more subtly than image intensifiers but probably less rapidly and less noticeably. They fail by the failure of individual transistors, which are so small that the absence of an individual sensor will not be noticed; failure will only be noticed if a large cluster of transistors that are adjacent to each other fail. The digital system beyond the flat panel detector has all of the potential problems of any computer system.

For cine angiographic film recording, the light image passes through optical lenses and is split into a small portion for the television monitor image (for direct viewing) and a major portion for the production of the cine image. The cine image is recorded on photographic film in a photographic camera at exposure rates up to 60 frames per second. In addition to the previously mentioned variables in the "X-ray chain", the quality of the cine angiogram depends upon many photographic variables. Cine film is exposed by light at the proper intensity and in the proper proportions, and is developed in a photographic processor using photographic chemicals and techniques. The film type, film speed, the processing chemicals, the temperature of the processor, the exposure time of the film in each of the chemicals, the washing, the drying and the transport of the film in the processor are all major determinants of the quality of the final image. As with all other photographic processes, each variable in the processing is equally important in achieving a quality film.

These photographic variables are often more responsible than the X-ray imaging chain for poor quality angiograms. With the use of cine film, there must be constant screening checks on all of the photographic variables as well as on the X-ray chain. With cine film imaging, even the viewing equipment for the film affects the quality of the visualized image. Dirty or out of focus lenses on the photographic projector blur or distort images which might be perfect on the film itself.

In the film-less, digital system with output from an image intensifier, variations in final image quality still occur as a result of changes in the video pick-up system, in the analog to digital (A to D) conversion system, or in the computer itself. The video pick-up system can deteriorate over time while the A to D converter or the computer itself can undergo "all or nothing" failure. The variables that occurred with the analog video signal and the A to D conversion in the older systems are eliminated by pick-up of the image from the image intensifier with a CCD.

The current minimal standard for a catheterization laboratory for patients with congenital heart disease for both complex diagnostic studies and catheter interventions, is a biplane X-ray system with a biplane angiographic imaging and recording system. Catheterization procedures on pediatric and congenital heart patients in the past were performed using single plane X-ray systems; however, with the type and complexity of the studies and therapeutic procedures being performed now, the use of a single plane system is no longer acceptable, and should not be used for pediatric and congenital cardiac studies, particularly for therapeutic catheter interventions in congenital heart patients.

The use of a single plane X-ray system increases the overall *risk* of any catheterization procedure. A single plane system eliminates the rapid, easy access to "depth perception" or the "third dimension" during catheter manipulation by not permitting the operator to check ***instantaneously*** on the anterior–posterior "depth" of the catheter as viewed in the opposite plane. With a biplane system, the depth relationship of the catheter is available with a one to two *second* glance at the lateral X-ray plane. The single plane X-ray, even with a "C arm" capable of rotation, takes many seconds to rotate to the perpendicular view. Because of this, there is both a reluctance to change and a delay in changing to the opposite view and, as a consequence, many more "blind" probes are performed with the catheter and more prolonged fluoroscopy is used before the X-ray tube is rotated in order to look at the opposite plane. When the X-ray tube is rotated to the opposite or perpendicular plane when using a single plane system, the original plane, obviously, is no longer visible and becomes the blind plane for probing with a catheter. As a consequence, the single plane system very significantly increases the over-all radiation used and increases the time of the procedure because of the prolonged, random probing without this immediate access to the "third" dimension. Finally the use of a single plane system significantly increases the amount of contrast required to obtain the necessary information. A repeat injection with an equivalent amount of additional contrast is required to obtain the comparable second view of any image.

Not only should the standard pediatric and congenital catheterization laboratory have a biplane cine X-ray system, but the system should have the capability of compound angulation of both of the X-ray tubes. Diagnostic imaging and therapeutic procedures performed in the catheterization laboratory require the structure (or structures) to be viewed precisely on edge or in their longest dimension for optimal visualization. To accomplish these optimal views requires either very cumbersome movement of the patients or, preferably, compound angulation of both of the X-ray tubes.

Biplane digital recording is now preferable to biplane cine angiography with video replay. Digital angiography allows instantaneous replay of images of the same quality as the original and of the same quality as the final stored images. The viewed images can be stopped, manipulated to magnify them or enhance contrast and brightness either immediately or once stored on the hard disk. Accurate measurements can be made instantaneously and on-line, during the procedure, with a digital system. Although the actual spatial resolution of a digital angiographic image is slightly less than the resolution of the image on the perfect cine film, the perceived information is superior and far more consistent from frame to frame and from patient to patient with digital images than it ever was on cine angiographic film[6].

Further details of either the X-ray and photographic part of the imaging process are beyond the scope of this monograph. However, the contributions of the "imaging director" interposed between the mechanical components of the system are discussed in detail to follow.

Angiographic technique—individual operator responsibility

It is assumed that all of the truly fixed components of the X-ray equipment are maintained and functioning properly. In addition, there are some adjustments and settings of the X-ray system that are made by the operator during the performance of each catheterization procedure. These settings are changed with each patient in order to produce the optimal visual and angiographic images and, at the same time, use the least radiation. A radiographic technician may make suggestions about these adjustments of the equipment, however the final settings are the responsibility of the individual cardiologist performing the catheterization. During each particular procedure, the catheterizing physician becomes the "director of imaging" in the cardiac catheterization laboratory!

Some aspects for producing quality angiographic images of any type should be intuitive and hold true for any type of image. The subject (patient!) or particular area of the subject should be positioned correctly for the picture, e.g. not inadvertently twisted, rotated or partially out of the field of view! Correct positioning and limiting the size of the image not only produce pictures that are esthetically nicer, but allow the automatic exposure system of the X-ray equipment to provide optimal exposures. The field of the image should be optimized for the precise anatomic area that is being studied. The total area and specific limits of the field of view in both the PA and LAT views are the direct responsibility of the catheterizing physician. If a particular structure within the thorax or even within the cardiac silhouette is the area of interest, the abdomen, neck (or head) and lungs should not be included in the picture! All extraneous areas that are included increase the radiation to the patient (and the operator) and, of equal importance, "confuse" the automatic brightness controls of the system because of the different densities of the tissues that are included in the field. Proper positioning over the area of the structure that is of primary interest keeps the automatic brightness sensors from "seeing" atypically bright or dark adjacent areas and, as a consequence, inappropriately responding to these extraneous areas instead of the main area of interest. For example, if a wedge angiogram in a branch pulmonary artery, which is far distally in the lung parenchyma, is the primary area of interest, but the field that is set on the fluoroscopy image (and recorded image) includes a large portion of the heart shadow, the automatic brightness sensors in the X-ray equipment respond to the dense cardiac image and generate a higher voltage beam. This, in turn, over-penetrates the area of primary interest in the distal pulmonary parenchyma.

There is no longer a place for general and non-selective angiograms in congenital heart patients. Atrial injections are performed only when looking for atrial, atrioventricular valve or atrial septal abnormalities and *not* for looking at abnormalities in the ventricles or great arteries. The exception to using only selective angiography is when the recirculation phase of a right-sided (right heart or pulmonary artery) angiogram is used to obtain information about the general orientation of the left heart structures. The recirculation angiogram should not be used for the purpose of visualizing any details of the left heart or aorta.

In very complex congenital hearts where diagnostic cardiac catheterization is necessary, it is important to obtain information about the general orientation of all of the cardiac structures before highly selective, compound angles are used to visualize the more specific details. For example, the operator must determine the general relationship of the two ventricles to each other before spending time and radiation determining the size and location of a particular ventricular septal defect! In the initial catheterization of a very complex heart, it is advantageous to begin the angiography with ventricular injections in the straight posterior–anterior (PA) and lateral (LAT) projections of the X-ray tubes. Once the general, basic orientation of the heart has been defined by the ventricular angiocardiogram, more specific, special views are used to open up and clarify particular areas within the chambers or vessels. The exact angles of the X-ray tubes necessary to place specific structures "on edge" are determined from the images in the straight PA and LAT views.

The initial angiograms during a procedure are generally performed in the chamber or the area where the most important pathology is suspected. This information is assimilated from the hemodynamic data obtained in the particular case and from other earlier invasive or non-invasive studies. For example, the first injection is performed in the right ventricle (RV) when an obstructive lesion of the RV outflow tract or right to left shunting at the ventricular level is suspected. The initial injections are made in the left ventricle (LV) when looking for LV obstructive lesions or when investigating left to right shunts at the ventricular or great artery level.

Although it may not be in the initial plan for the particular cardiac catheterization procedure, selective angiocardiograms are often performed before all of the hemodynamic data have been acquired. This is particularly true in patients with very complex lesions or where an unexpected or difficult to enter area or an unknown area is entered fortuitously and out of the sequence of the overall planned procedure. The unexpected area is *identified and documented* ***at that time*** with biplane angiography! When the details of the precise anatomy are more important than the specific hemodynamics, the procedure is planned so that details of the anatomy are defined angiographically during the course of acquiring the hemodynamics. The angiograms are interspersed with the hemodynamics as the catheterization procedure progresses. For example, when there are suspected multiple areas of pulmonary branch stenosis, angiograms are performed selectively in the branch pulmonary artery before recording a "pull-back" pressure from the pulmonary artery to the right ventricle.

Contrast media

Another variable in angiography is the particular contrast agent used. Cardiac and vascular angiography depends upon the opacification of the blood by a water-soluble contrast agent, which mixes with the blood and absorbs X-rays as they pass through a particular chamber or vessel. The soluble radiographic contrast agents in use today are iodinated organic compounds, the radiodensity of which depends upon their iodine content. The opacity of the contrast in any particular area is proportional to the iodine content in the contrast material and varies with the relative "thickness" of the contrast material present in any location at any instant in time. Generally speaking, the greater the amount of iodine in the contrast agent, the greater is its osmolarity, the greater is its viscosity and the greater is its toxicity.

There are numerous contrast agents available for cardiac and vascular angiography. Each variation in the formulation of a contrast agent is made in an attempt to increase the amount of iodine (and, in turn, the radio-opacity) while at the same time reducing the toxicity and/or viscosity of the contrast solution. Contrast solutions are divided into ionic media, which dissociate the iodine into ionic particles in solution, and non-ionic media, which do not dissociate into ionic particles but depend upon hydrophilic moieties in their molecules for their solubility. Generally, the ionic media require a much higher osmolality (1,600–2,200 mOsm/kg) to achieve a sufficient iodine content to produce suitable radio-opacity for angiography. The higher osmolality causes more patient discomfort and a slightly higher complication rate, particularly in sicker or more "precarious" patients. The non-ionic media, on the other hand, although they have a lower osmolality are more viscous and far more expensive. All of the large current studies and most current information on the use of different contrast media during cardiac catheterizations have been done in or obtained in adults, and primarily in relation to coronary angiography. The choice of which contrast agent to use represents a compromise between the iodine content, the isotonicity and the osmolality of the individual contrast agents[7].

In addition to the type of contrast used, the total amount of contrast used and the rate at which it is used are also important. A maximum of 4 ml of contrast per kilogram of body weight is the general limit for the amount of contrast used for angiography during any one procedure. This "rule", however, was arbitrarily established decades ago from the clinical finding that the toxicity associated with ionic contrast solutions increased significantly when larger volumes of contrast were used[8]. It is suspected that toxicity is related mostly to the osmolality of the ionic solutions. The 4 ml/kg rule is still accepted, although very different contrast agents are in use today compared to the time when it was established. Although in long complex pediatric/congenital cases much larger quantities of contrast reportedly have been used, there have been no scientific controlled studies performed on the toxic effects and the safe volumes of the ionic and non-ionic contrast agents in pediatric/congenital patients in relation to the duration of the procedure. The complications due to contrast agents during angiography are discussed in detail at the end of this chapter.

Controlable factors—rules for radiography and angiography in the cardiac catheterization laboratory

The adjustable and controllable variables of the radiographic equipment and the variations in technique allow significant control by the catheterizing physician over the quality of the images obtained. Most of these controllable variables add to the safety of the angiograms for the patient and the catheterizing physician. Every angiogram that is recorded should be of a quality that assumes that the particular image is to be used for publication, or that the details and quality of the image may be the operator's defense in a court of law! The operator should pay attention to the precise positioning of the patient, the positioning of the catheter, the overall field which is visualized, the amount, type and rate of contrast and the other radiographic settings which will make each angiographic image a quality, reproducible image.

1 *Collimation.* The smallest possible area of the subject should be visualized in the fluoroscopic and angiographic fields. This is equally important during both catheter manipulations and during angiography. Visualization of the entire chest or even wide areas of the heart are unnecessary during most catheter manipulations. Radiation to the patient (and even more so, scatter radiation to the catheterizing physicians!) increases proportionally to the square of the area exposed to the X-ray beam. This exposure is magnified with the increased doses of X-rays required during angiography. In addition, the greater the differences in the densities of structures that are included in an unnecessarily wide area being viewed, the less accurately the automatic brightness control will function and the poorer the quality of the resultant image will be.

2 *Operator (catheterizing physician) distance*. The catheterizing physician should maintain the maximum distance possible away from the X-ray beam and the patient being X-rayed. The radiation to the catheterizing physician is inversely proportional to the square of the distance from the object (patient). Stepping behind leaded screens and stepping back as far as possible from the patient during angiograms is mandatory in order to reduce radiation exposure to the catheterizing physician(s). However, unless the catheterization laboratory is so small that it prohibits moving at least two meters away from the patient during angiography, it is *not* necessary for the catheterizing physician to actually leave the room (and the patient unattended!) during angiograms.

3 *Image intensifier distance*. The input screens of the poster–anterior (PA) ***and*** *lateral* (*LAT*) image intensifiers should be kept as close to the patient as possible. The greater the distance the input screen of the image intensifier is from the patient, the greater is the magnification of the image, the greater the quantity of X-ray radiation that is required to produce the image, and the greater is the scatter radiation off the patient. The PA image intensifier is usually (and almost automatically) lowered against the patient's chest by the catheterizing physician or the radiographic technicians. The LAT intensifier, on the other hand, is frequently ignored and left far away from the side of the patient! In addition, in order to achieve a really close proximity to the patient with the LAT image intensifier, it takes some extra effort and definite forethought on the part of the nurses and technicians during the initial positioning of the patient for the catheterization. In order for the LAT image intensifier to be positioned against the patient's chest wall, the patient must be positioned at the very edge of the catheterization table at the side of the image intensifier. This has to be done when the patient is being positioned on the table initially before the start of the catheterization procedure and definitely before the patient has been secured to the table with straps or tape. The patient's arms are positioned above their head while at the same time, not forcing the arms into a position that places tension on the brachial plexus. If the LAT intensifier is to be positioned close to the patient, pillows, cushions, pads or other arm supports in the area of the LAT image intensifier *should* ***not*** *extend* beyond the lateral edge of the table on the intensifier side of the catheterization table. Even with maximal preplanning and positioning, the LAT image intensifier almost always remains further from the image isocenter than the PA intensifier. This difference in image intensifier distances from the patient results in higher radiation with the lateral tube and in a different magnification of the images produced between the two monitored views and of the eventual recorded images.

4 *Magnification*. X-ray magnification is used primarily for the visualization of the fine details of individual, small structures or devices and occasionally for the general imaging of very small patients. Each stepwise increase in magnification of the image on the X-ray settings essentially doubles the dose of radiation to the patient (and the scatter to the catheterizing physician). With digital systems, the visualized image can be magnified digitally (with an "acquire image zoom") *without* actually increasing the radiation. This digital magnification results in some degradation of the visualized image, but still allows an image that is usable for catheter manipulations—particularly in a small infant.

5 *Biplane "stored fluoroscopy"*. The ability to save images on "stored fluoroscopy" and particularly with simultaneous biplane imaging, allows the permanent recording of biplane images at a markedly reduced dose of radiation. The image quality with stored fluoroscopy or acquire zoom is not as good as the quality of a biplane angiography image, however for many applications the stored fluoroscopy image is satisfactory. Biplane stored fluoroscopy is useful particularly for test injections, which are used to verify catheter positions as well as for recording balloon inflations or the release of devices from delivery catheters. It is important to have a permanent recording of the balloon inflation or the release of a therapeutic device (particularly when something goes wrong!) but it usually is not necessary to have this information recorded in the fine detail of an actual angiogram.

6 *Image recording rate*. The exposure to radiation of the patient and the personnel in the catheterization laboratory increases in direct proportion to increases in the frame rate of the exposure of the images. The slowest recording rate possible in order to obtain the necessary information should be used for all angiograms. For example, when balloon inflations and release of devices are recorded angiographically, the recording rate could be as low as 7.5 frames per second (fps) (or even 3.25 fps when the equipment allows these low rates). Recording these procedures

at a fast frame rate is like recording grass growing on high-speed film!

7 *Radiation shielding*. "Positionable" transparent leaded glass radiation shields located between the subject and the catheterizing physician(s) should be used whenever possible (at all times!). Most radiation to the catheterizing physician(s) results from scatter off the patient's body above the catheterization table. Radiation is scattered in all directions away from the patient, so a radiation shield between the patient and the operator's chest, neck and head provides very significant protection to the exposed areas of the operator.

8 *Contrast media*. Since most diagnostic catheterizations in pediatric patients and those with congenital heart disease now involve very complex and/or very sick patients, the less discomfort and lower risk of the non-ionic, lower osmotic, contrast agents justifies the greater expense of their use in these cases. Many of the therapeutic interventions in the catheterization laboratory are performed on very sick patients and require multiple injections and, eventually, large volumes of contrast. The necessity for the increased volumes of contrast also justifies the use of the non-ionic, iso-osmotic contrast materials in these patients. The relatively few cardiac catheterizations performed in pediatric and congenital patients that fall outside of these high-risk categories, probably do *not* justify a laboratory's maintaining a separate inventory and separate set-up for a different contrast medium to be used just for the few low-risk cases. A non-ionic, low-osmolar (iso-osmolar!) contrast agent is recommended as the standard contrast agent for a dedicated pediatric and congenital cardiac catheterization laboratory.

9 *Contrast delivery*. For angiograms performed for the purpose of delineating anatomic detail, the bolus of contrast is preferably delivered within one cardiac cycle. When contrast is delivered more slowly, particularly throughout several cardiac cycles, it is diluted by the blood flow and is dissipated away from the area with a resultant poorer image quality. The rapid delivery of more than one or two ml of contrast requires the use of a powered, mechanical, pressure injector. Because of the small lumen of the catheter and the high viscosity of the contrast, more than 2–3 ml of contrast cannot be pushed by hand through a catheter within one cardiac cycle.

There are many varieties of powered, pressure injectors on the market for the rapid delivery of contrast, most of which are electro-mechanical injectors, and most of these have standard features. There is an electrical control unit or console with an "injector head" that contains the drive mechanism for the syringe of the injector. Usually (ideally) the injector head is separate, on a flexible arm or mount, which is detachable and mounted separately from the control console. The control console, which includes adjustments for the volume of contrast and the pressure and rate of the injection, is located away from the patient and can even be in a separate, adjacent room. Ideally, the injector head is supported on an articulated arm which extends from a ceiling mount. An articulated arm and ceiling mount allow the injector head to be moved the entire length of the catheterization table and to any area of the table. The ceiling mount keeps the injector and its connecting cables out of the clutter of equipment on the floor of the catheterization laboratory. The lowest point of the injection syringe when the syringe is in a horizontal position should be 18 to 24 inches above the catheterization table. This height above the table requires that the tip of the injector syringe on the injector head must be tilted *downward* when it is attached directly to a catheter. This makes any air bubbles that might be in the contrast within the injector syringe rise to the top (back) of the syringe away from the attachment to the catheter.

The essential adjustments on commercial pressure injectors include settings for the volume of contrast to be injected, the pressure at which it is injected, and a setting that limits the maximum pressure that can be delivered during the injection. The flow rate at which the contrast is injected is adjustable as long as the combined volume of contrast and the particular chosen flow rate do not cause the pressure limit to be exceeded. The pressure limit provides a safety factor against rupture of the catheter. Most modern commercial injectors also have a setting for "rise time", which is the duration of time for the pressure of the injection to build up from zero to the maximum set pressure. This allows the column of contrast within the catheter to accelerate slowly within the fraction of a second before reaching the peak pressure and flow velocity. This build-up or rise time helps to prevent catheter recoil. A rise time of less than 0.6–0.8 seconds is ineffective at preventing catheter recoil.

10 *Pressure for contrast injections*. The pressure necessary to deliver the contrast in a specified amount of time depends upon the volume of contrast, the viscosity of the contrast material, and the length and internal lumen diameter of the delivery catheter. Most mechanical injectors are capable of generating 1,000–1,200 pounds per square inch pressure! However, the ***lowest*** pressure that will accomplish the delivery of the *desired volume* of contrast within one heart beat is recommended for any injection of contrast within the cardiovascular system. The higher the pressure during the injection, the greater the likelihood of catheter recoil or of intramyocardial injection or extravasation of contrast. Lower-pressure injections of large volumes of contrast are accomplished by the use of shorter length and larger diameter catheters with

relatively large lumens, which are designed specifically for angiography. A rise time of 0.8–1.0 second helps to prevent catheter recoil by allowing the bolus of contrast to "gradually" reach the tip of the catheter before the maximum pressure is reached. This rise time, however, is added to the total delivery time set for the contrast injection. Once the bolus reaches the tightly curved end of a pigtail catheter or the tip of a closed ended angiographic catheter after a slow rise time, the column of contrast pushes the closed catheter tip forward and helps to hold the catheter in place.

11 *Contrast volume*. Although current angiographic contrast media are considered relatively safe, it is recommended that as little contrast is used for each individual injection as is consistent with obtaining good images to obtain the necessary diagnostic information. In addition, as little as possible total contrast medium is used during the entire procedure. Biplane imaging should always be used to conserve the total amount of contrast used. In order to achieve this, there should be a general plan in advance for all of the angiograms that are to be performed during the entire catheterization. In cardiac chambers and in large central vessels, 1 ml of contrast medium per kilogram of body weight per injection is generally used. Significantly less can be used in the presence of non-shunt lesions, in small chambers or unilateral or isolated vessels. Occasionally, in the presence of very large shunt lesions or in very large, dilated chambers, a larger volume of contrast per injection (up to 1.5–2.0 ml/kg) is necessary in order to obtain adequate visualization of the structures.

During a cardiac catheterization procedure of a short duration, a total of no more than 4 ml of contrast/kg should be used during the entire procedure. Although with the newer, and particularly the non-ionic, iso-osmotic contrast materials, far more contrast is frequently used during long and complex catheterization procedures, there have been no clinical, controlled studies to document the safety of this practice. The use of larger volumes of contrast during any one case appears to be safer when the procedure lasts many hours and when the patient is kept well hydrated and diuresing.

Pre-existing renal disease/disfunction contributes to the complications from contrast materials. When there is even the slightest suspicion of renal abnormalities/problems, renal dysfunction should be ruled out before the catheterization or the amount of contrast used must be strictly limited.

12 *Selective injections*. Contrast injections should always be in, or just proximal to, the specific structure of interest and also at the proper location within the chamber or vessel. This selective positioning reduces the amount of contrast necessary during any particular injection and, in turn, the total amount of contrast used during the entire procedure. The injection holes of the angiographic catheter must be positioned free from the walls and intracardiac structures yet centered well within the chamber or vessel. Merely entering a ventricle or other chamber as opposed to making a determined effort to position a catheter in a precise central location or in a specific area of a chamber or ventricle for a contrast injection, represents *poor* and *potentially dangerous* technique. The catheter should be positioned purposefully so that its shaft is supported enough to prevent the tip from recoiling to another area during the injection. At the same time, the tip of the catheter should be free within the cavity of the chamber in order not to produce an intramyocardial injection. A very soft catheter or a catheter where the shaft of the catheter is passing through a long curve to the tip of the catheter, often needs support with a stiffening wire to prevent recoil during a pressure injection. These wires are discussed later in this chapter and in Chapter 6.

13 *Angiographic catheters*. Catheters used for angiographic injections ideally should be the shortest possible length, measuring from the introductory site at the skin to the selective area for the injection. An angiographic catheter should be the largest diameter catheter (French size) as the particular patient can reasonably accommodate and should have the largest luminal diameter possible for the particular French size. The resistance to flow of the contrast material increases proportionally to the length of the catheter, and decreases proportionally to its increasing internal diameter. A catheter with a closed distal tip with multiple side holes that are within one to two centimeters of the distal end of the catheter, is preferable for angiographic injections. The contrast material is delivered more rapidly and uniformly through multiple side holes than through an end hole. Once the maximum pressure of the injection is reached within a closed-tip catheter, the flow of the contrast solution against the closed tip of the catheter pushes the tip of the catheter forward—i.e. the forward pressure holds the catheter in place and reduces catheter recoil. At the other extreme, a high-pressure injection through an end-hole catheter acts like a high pressure fire-hose, with the force through the opening at the tip driving the catheter tip backwards.

There are four basic types of angiographic catheter. The most common of these is the torque-controlled "NIH™-type" catheter. These catheters have a closed distal end with six side holes just proximal to the tip and are manufactured from woven dacron or from various extruded plastics. These angiographic catheters are easy to position selectively and properly within a chamber or vessel, they have the highest flow rates for a particular catheter size, and they tolerate the highest injection pressures.

A variation of the NIH™-type catheter is the side and end hole angiographic "Gensini™ catheter". These have a very tapered distal tip with a relatively small end opening at the tip as well as side holes proximal to the tip. The end hole at the tip allows the catheter to be delivered to a desired location over a wire, but at the same time the opening of the tip is small enough to create some resistance to the flow of contrast through the tip during a pressure injection. These catheters still recoil more than closed-ended catheters during high-pressure injections.

The third type of angiographic catheter is the pigtail type. This is a variation of the end and side hole angiographic catheter, in which 1–2 cm of the distal end of the catheter is looped on itself into a tight 360+° pigtail. Usually the side holes are just proximal to the loop of the pigtail. This configuration helps to keep the catheter from recoiling or burying into the tissues during rapid, high-pressure injections. There are variations of the usual pigtail where the distal loop on the catheter is aligned perpendicular to the long axis of the catheter shaft, giving the catheter a "lariat"-like appearance and allowing contrast to be delivered in a more concentrated area.

The final type of angiographic catheter is the "Berman™ balloon angiographic" catheter. This is a closed distal tip, side hole only, angiographic catheter with a floating balloon that is positioned at the distal end of the catheter just distal to the side angiographic holes. These balloon catheters are manufactured with a softer, extruded plastic shaft to give them some floating characteristics. Balloon angiographic catheters have a second lumen within the catheter shaft for communication with the balloon for balloon inflation/deflation. The space occupied by this second lumen necessarily compromises the diameter of the main, angiographic lumen. The combination of the softer material and the smaller injection lumen results in a catheter that tolerates a lower maximum pressure and has a slower flow rate than comparable sized torque-controlled angiographic catheters.

The inflated balloon provides an extra safety factor against perforation, similar to diagnostic balloon catheters, and when inflated free in a chamber or vessel prevents intramyocardial injections. The distal balloon, when inflated during an injection, allows for partial occlusion of vessels distal to the point of injection for "balloon occlusion angiograms". This prevents any run-off in the vessel distal to the balloon and allows a greater concentration of contrast proximal to the balloon.

14 *Hand injections of contrast.* Angiograms performed with hand injections are invaluable, but primarily only when very small volumes of contrast are necessary—e.g. to test the safety of the location of the tip of a catheter or in very small infants where adequate anatomic detail can be obtained with very small volumes of contrast. Unless extremely large catheters are used, more than 2 ml, or at the most 3 ml, of contrast should be injected with a power injector. A hand injection of more than 2–3 ml of contrast through a 6-French or smaller catheter results in the contrast solution being "dribbled" into the field and the contrast being diluted faster than it can be injected. Such dribbled injections are generally worthless and are a waste of even the small amount of contrast used. Forceful hand injections of 1–2 ml of contrast are used as test injections to determine the safety of the location of the tip of a catheter before a subsequent, large-volume pressure injection is performed through the same catheter. A hand injection of contrast is frequently used to determine the location of the tip of a catheter in an unusual or constrained area and to determine the precise position of dilation balloons or devices before inflation or implant, respectively.

Small hand injections using very slow flow rates are performed purposefully during wedge angiograms or injections into known small or constricted areas. Larger volume, slow, hand injections of contrast are used in areas of the circulation with very slow blood flow—e.g. in the systemic venous circulation of a patient with a cavopulmonary connection.

15 *Pressure hand injections—requirements.* When a hand injection is used to deliver a small amount of contrast rapidly and with good hand pressure, the smallest syringe that will hold the desired amount of contrast is used. The smaller the syringe, the greater the pressure that can be generated in the syringe and delivered to the catheter by a hand injection. Unless an 8-French or larger catheter is being used, a syringe of a maximum of 6 ml is used for hand pressure injections. Additionally, a special syringe with a hard plastic barrel and plunger should be used for hand injection angiograms. The plungers of standard, softer, plastic syringes will bend or break during a truly forceful hand injection. Never use a glass syringe for hand injections. There is always the danger of a glass syringe breaking or shattering during a truly forceful hand injection, with the resulting glass fragments ending up on the operative field (and in the catheterizing physician's hand!).

When performing a pressure injection by hand, the syringe barrel is grasped in a fist of one hand with the barrel of the syringe completely encircled by the hand and fingers while the plunger is pushed forcefully into the barrel with the heel of the other hand—*not* delicately pushed with a finger or thumb and particularly not the thumb of the same hand. Far greater force can be applied to the syringe barrel for a hand injection using this technique.

16 *Hand injections—recording.* Test hand injections that are worth performing, worth the expenditure of contrast, and worth the radiation exposure, should be recorded and saved for review on at least a digital biplane stored fluoroscopy if not as a biplane angiogram.

17 *Biplane.* Essentially all angiograms in pediatric or congenital heart patients are recorded with biplane imaging. Biplane recording conserves the amount of contrast used and prevents the unnecessary hazards of repeated injections in the same location—particularly after moving the patient (or if the patient moves between injections!).

18 *Image measurements—reference calibration.* The *precise* measurement of the diameter of an imaged structure is critical for the successful and safe dilation or device occlusion of that structure. The precise measurement is dependent upon the *precise* measurement of the object along with ***an accurate reference calibration*** for that measurement. Reference calibration is necessary to compensate for the magnification of the image size created by the divergent X-ray beam, the different distances of the objects from the recording apparatus, and the different magnification settings of the X-ray system. The reference calibration is performed with an object with a known, large diameter or length which is imaged and measured accurately in the exact same imaging field (isocenter) as the image of the anatomic structure being measured. This measurement permits compensation for the magnification of the on-screen size of both the reference source and the structure being treated. Only when there is a very accurate calibration factor can the precise diameter of the imaged structure be calculated from the on-screen measurements.

It is common practice, particularly during coronary angiography, to use the diameter of the catheter in the field as the known diameter for the reference calibration. In fact, the X-ray equipment of most digital catheterization laboratories has a built-in edge detection system and built-in reference scale for each French size of catheter. When measuring very small structures (1–4 mm), this technique is relatively accurate, and the visual comparison of structures similar in size to the catheter (e.g. the vessel lumen) prevents gross errors. However, the measured diameter of any catheter is totally unsatisfactory as a calibration reference for measuring the significantly larger structures (valves, central vessels, etc.) being treated in congenital heart lesions. The smaller the diameter (or length) that the reference calibration object is compared to the diameter of the structure being measured, the greater is the potential error from even minute errors in the measurement of the reference image. The larger structures being treated in congenital heart disease (valves, central vessels, intracavitary defects) are almost always measured in centimeters, which creates a marked size discrepancy between the structure being treated and the relatively small diameter of any cardiac catheter used as a reference.

The difference in the diameter between each French size of a catheter is only 1/3 of a millimeter. One third of a millimeter is difficult (impossible!) to measure accurately even when measuring two sharp lines that are magnified on a sheet of paper, with the paper held very steady on a well lit surface! This inaccuracy is compounded when measuring between indistinct pixel lines on a grainy, flickering, computer screen! This inaccuracy in measuring tenths of millimeters is compounded even further when the number obtained from this measurement becomes the reference measurement with which all other measurements must be compared. This grossly inaccurate reference number is then multiplied by or divided into the measurement of the structure on the same grainy moving screen.

The measured diameter of a catheter also varies according to whether there is contrast in the lumen of the catheter or whether the lumen of the catheter is empty. The column of contrast material, or the inner diameter (ID) of the catheter, is measured when the catheter lumen is filled with contrast, while the actual outer wall of the catheter (the outer diameter or OD) is the true catheter diameter that should be used for the reference measurement. The OD of the catheter is not detectable by either the eye or an automatic edge detection system when there is contrast within the lumen of the catheter. The actual difference between the ID and OD of the catheter depends upon the thickness of the catheter wall—which is different for every type of catheter. In addition, particularly when there is no contrast in the catheter, the precise diameter created by the thin external wall of the catheter is indistinct because as the thin circular wall of the catheter is visualized on edge, the visible opacity of the thin wall tapers away from each "side" wall of the catheter.

A numerical example illustrates the potential for error incurred by the use of a catheter as the reference value. A valve annulus (or a vessel) with an actual diameter of 23 mm measures 35 mm on the magnified fluoroscopic screen. If a 7-French reference catheter (2.3 mm OD) measures exactly 3.5 mm on the same magnified screen, the calculated valve diameter will be 23 mm. However, if the measurement of the reference catheter is ***one half millimeter*** too small (either by "automatic edge detection" or attempted actual measurement with cursors) the valve or vessel diameter calculated with the erroneous reference measurement will be 27 mm—a 17% error! If the reference measurement is ***three quarters of a millimeter too small,*** the calculated valve or vessel diameter of the 23 mm structure using this erroneous reference measurement will be 29 mm—a 26% error! Using this calculated measurement, which is 26% over the actual diameter, to determine a balloon diameter for dilation could be catastrophic.

a *Grid or ruler calibration*. An external "grid", "ruler" or "calibrated ball" reference system has been the "gold standard" for accurate calibration of measurements on angiography for several decades. If carried out correctly and precisely, measurements with these techniques are very accurate; however, they are very inconvenient. For accuracy, any such external grid, ruler or ball reference calibration system *must be* filmed in the exact location (isocenter) of the intravascular structure being measured, and the grid or ruler must be exactly perpendicular to the X-ray beam. In order to accomplish this, the isocenter of the image being measured on the X-ray image is determined and recorded, then the patient is physically moved out of the field of the X-ray beam while keeping all of the components (table height and side-to-movement, X-ray tubes, image intensifiers and angles) all in exactly the same positions. The reference calibration system (grid, ruler, ball) is then placed in the field at the exact isocenter of the area being measured, in a plane exactly perpendicular to the plane of the X-ray beam, and is recorded. The reference measurement is taken from this image. All of this calibration requires a major interruption in the procedure in order to move the patient (along with any connecting lines, airways, etc.) completely out from under the image intensifiers.

Ruler or grid lines are usually exactly 1.0 cm apart, providing a relatively large reference distance. With 1 cm marks, no complex calibration factor is necessary after making the actual measurements. When properly aligned, the grid lines are very fine and sharp, which reduces the error in measuring them. With a calibration factor of one centimeter, an error of 0.5 or even 1 mm in measuring the grid lines makes far less difference in the calculated diameter of the measured intracardiac structure. For example, using the same example as above, when the same 23 mm valve or vessel measures 35 mm on the magnified screen and the 10 mm grid measures 15 mm on the same screen, the calculated valve or vessel diameter will be 23.3 mm. If the reference measurement is 0.5 mm too short (or 14.5 mm) the valve or vessel will calculate to be 24.1 mm—only a 3.5% error. Even if the reference measurement is one whole millimeter too short, the valve or vessel will calculate to be 25 mm—still only a 9% error.

b *"Ball" calibration*. In order to avoid the difficulties of aligning the X-ray beam exactly perpendicular to the external reference—particularly when the X-ray tubes are in compound angled views—metal calibration balls of a known, precise diameter are used as the object for the reference measurements. Like the grid or ruler, the ball is not in the field while the angiogram is recorded. The patient is moved out of the X-ray field and the calibration ball placed exactly in the isocenter of the image without moving any of the other elements of the X-ray system. An image of the ball is recorded on the imaging system and the measured dimensions are compensated for with the calibration factor (known vs. the measured diameter of the ball). The ball system has a significant disadvantage compared to a grid or even a radio-opaque ruler. The ball calibration method is very operator dependent. The positioning of the ball in the isocenter must be carried out very accurately. The ball edges are less distinct, and picking the measurement of the maximum diameter of the ball is somewhat subjective. Usually the actual measured diameter of the ball is some odd, fractional number, which makes calculation of the actual diameters cumbersome.

c *Calibration "marker" catheters*. A more convenient reference or calibration system, which is equally as accurate as the grid or ruler, is a catheter which has "calibration marks" built into its wall. The calibration marks are very thin, radio-opaque, metal bands embedded around the wall of the catheter near its distal end, with the bands at a precise, known distance from each other. The bands are exactly one or two centimeters apart (depending upon the manufacturer). The bands on USCI™ NIH™ Marker™ catheters (Medtronic, Minneapolis, MN) are 1 cm apart when measured from top to top or bottom to bottom of adjacent bands, while on Cook™ marker catheters (Bloomington, IN), the bands are 1 or 2 cm apart when measured from inside to inside. These marks can be in the wall of the catheter that is actually being used for the angiography or on another catheter that is positioned precisely in the X-ray field adjacent to or superimposed on the structure being measured. When the calibration marks are aligned exactly perpendicular to the field, they appear as two thin, straight lines or straight bands. If they are not exactly aligned, the bands appear curved or as ovals. The appearance of a curved or an oval band serves as an obvious indicator that the bands are not aligned properly and that, in that alignment, they cannot be used for the reference measurement. When the bands are not aligned exactly, the distance between them is less than one centimeter and the measured distance obviously cannot be used as a reference until the bands are aligned precisely on edge.

When the calibrated marker catheter is used for the contrast injection, the marks on the catheter are usually exactly in the isocenter of the structure being measured during the injection, totally eliminating any errors due to magnification. Usually an angiographic catheter (including its marker bands) moves significantly during a pressure injection and, as the marker bands move, they reorientate through multiple different alignments during the injection. If the bands do not align exactly perpendicular at some stage during the actual injection and angiographic recording, this can be corrected very easily! After the recording of the image has been completed, and without moving the patient, the table or the X-ray tubes at all, the marker catheter is re-maneuvered into the area being measured and manipulated until the calibration marks are in the isocenter of the image and aligned exactly perpendicular to the X-ray beam. The catheter can be moved within the field, but the repeat recording must be made before moving either the structure being measured, the X-ray tubes or the image intensifiers. Once the marks are aligned precisely, a separate, short, slow-frame-rate biplane angiogram or biplane stored fluoroscopy is recorded of the marker catheter with the bands aligned and in the area of the isocenter. If a marker catheter is not used for the injection, a separate marker catheter can be placed either in, or immediately adjacent to, the area being measured. This can be in the same vessel adjacent to the angiographic catheter or in an adjacent or crossing vessel. For example, the marker catheter can be placed in the superior vena cava for measurements in the right pulmonary artery or in the descending aorta for measurements in the left pulmonary artery, or vice versa.

The marker catheter is particularly useful when the structure being measured is at a peculiar angle—for example the left ventricular outflow tract recorded in a long axial view. The marker bands on the angiographic catheter are often aligned along the left ventricular outflow tract and perpendicular to the X-ray beam when the tip of the catheter is positioned either in the left ventricular outflow tract or in the left ventricular apex.

In lesions where exact calibration of the defect is desired, but for one reason or another a marker catheter cannot be used directly for the injection or a second catheter cannot be introduced, the marker catheter can be positioned in the esophagus as an alternative reference object. The esophagus passes directly behind the heart and in very close proximity to most of the intracardiac structures that are being measured. The marker catheter is advanced from the mouth into the esophagus and to a level behind the heart in the area of the intracardiac lesion being measured. To reduce trauma to the esophageus, the small, stiff, 6-French marker catheter can be placed inside of a softer, standard 10-French, naso-gastric tube and the combination passed into the esophagus.

This technique is particularly useful for measurements of coarctation of the aorta, branch pulmonary artery stenosis, and vena caval obstructions, where the calibration bands of the marker catheter in the esophagus lie very close to the actual cardiac lesion, eliminating errors due to magnification. In all of these lesions, the straight PA and Lat projections are often optimal. In these projections, the calibration marks on the marker catheter in the esophagus are lined up properly with minimal, or no, manipulation of the catheter in the esophagus.

The marker catheter and/or any of the other reference calibration systems ***never*** should be placed at any area on the *chest wall* when the object is being used for the reference imaging. Regardless of whether the calibration reference object is on the anterior, posterior or either of the lateral chest walls, it is far from the intrathoracic cardiac image and, in turn, far from the isocenter of the X-ray beam. Since X-ray beams are never exactly parallel and always fan out from the X-ray tube, there is always a significant magnification (or reduction) depending on whether the reference object is on the chest wall in front of, or beyond, the structure being measured, respectively.

d *Calibration systems built into the X-ray imaging system.* An ideal system for the measured reference object in the X-ray field has the calibration reference object and measurement system built into the X-ray imaging system. This requires some extra effort on the part of the manufacturers not only in the production of the system but also to obtain a special "certification of accuracy" of their measuring system before it can be used clinically.

The calibration reference system built into the X-ray system has tiny radio-opaque calibration marks (dots) embedded at precise distances from each other in the input screen of the image intensifier. The ability to use a calibration reference system built into the X-ray system depends upon several critical factors. The intravascular structure being measured must be positioned exactly in the isocenter. The X-ray imaging system has a program in its computer that constantly measures the exact distance from the isocenter of the image to the input screen of the image intensifier, and uses this measurement for its calculations from the measurement of the reference dots.

When the object being measured is positioned *exactly in the isocenter*, the X-ray ***tube*** *to object* (isocenter) *distance* is *fixed* and always is the same in all projections. The only magnification variables are (1) the changing distance from the isocenter to the image intensifiers and (2) the degree of magnification of the X-ray image. The distances, the magnification setting of the image, and the reference marks on the intensifier are controlled precisely or are measured continuously by the internal computer of the X-ray imaging system. These measurements are automatically programmed into the calculations. Assuming a perfectly calibrated and aligned X-ray system and the accuracy of the automatic computer measurement of the distance from the image isocenter to image intensifier screen, this internal calibration system represents the ideal reference calibration system.

There are many advantages to this built-in reference system. Assuming the imaged structure is positioned properly in the field, the reference marks are always in the field and always aligned properly regardless of the angulation of the X-ray tubes. The patient does not have to be moved nor does a special catheter have to be used to have a very accurate reference distance for calibration. The reference marks are usually six centimeters (60 mm!) apart so that even a two mm error in measuring the reference marks on the imaging screen, represents at most a 3% error in the calculated diameter of a valve or vessel!

19 *Catheter positioning for angiocardiograms.* When injecting into chambers during angiocardiograms, the catheter tip must be completely free within the chamber to prevent intramyocardial staining or perforation. By careful observation of the motion of the catheter tip on both the PA and LAT fluoroscopic images, the body of the chamber or vessel can be located and the walls of chambers avoided. Entrapment of the catheter tip is indicated when its motion corresponds exactly to the motion of the wall of the heart. A catheter tip that is completely free has a little extra "dance" during the rest of the heart motion, and often generates occasional premature ventricular contractions.

Finally, a very small but forceful hand test injection is made with angiographic or stored fluoroscopy recording in at least one plane. An injection of 1–2 ml (depending on the size of the patient) is made as forcefully as possible by hand with 2–5 ml "hard" syringe. The idea of the test injection is to detect any abnormal position or entrapment by the location or extravasation of this small amount of contrast at a relatively high pressure, rather than having the full volume of contrast injected into the myocardium at very high pressure! Occasionally, in order to secure a free, non-entrapped position within a chamber, the catheter must be withdrawn from its original position and a new curve formed on it, or a new catheter is used with a different configuration all together.

When positioning a catheter for an angiocardiogram, the last movement of the catheter by the operator should be advancing the catheter forward. By advancing the whole catheter forward, any curve in the course of the more proximal shaft of the catheter is pushed against any "outer circumference curves" along the course of the catheter within the heart or great vessels. The centrifugal force generated during the injection against the curves in the catheter pushes the long curves in the course of the shaft of the catheter against the outer circumference of the cardiac structures. Positioning the catheter shaft against the outer circumference of all the curves prevents, or certainly reduces, recoil of the tip of the catheter during the injection. For example, a retrograde catheter lies along the outside or the outer circumference of the arch immediately after being advanced around the aortic arch into the aortic root (Figure 11.1). If the same catheter is withdrawn several centimeters, the tip initially does not withdraw at all, but, rather, the shaft is drawn away from the outer circumference and against the inner circumference of the arch (Figure 11.2). During a power injection of contrast, the centrifugal force of the contrast flowing rapidly through the curves in the length of the catheter causes all the curves to tend to straighten. If the curve of the catheter is lying against, and supported along, the outer

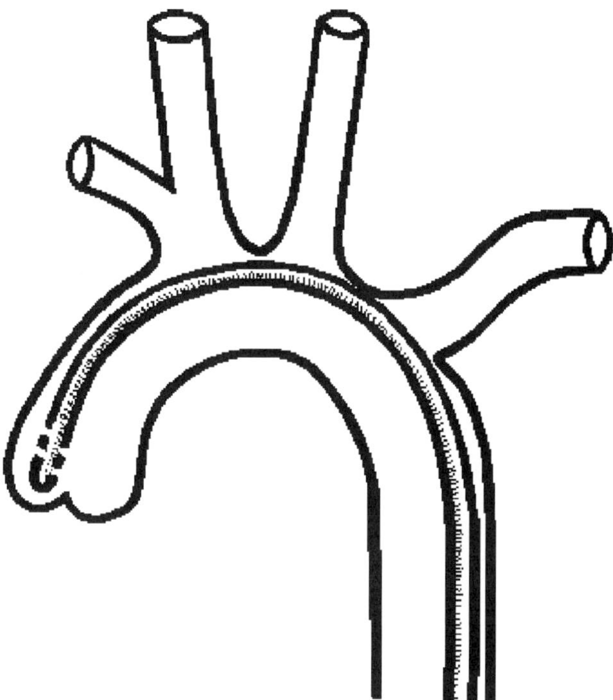

Figure 11.1 The tip of the catheter has been advanced into the aortic root, which forces the entire shaft of the catheter against the outer circumference of the aortic arch. Even with the centrifugal force of the injection, the catheter has nowhere to move away from its position in the aortic root.

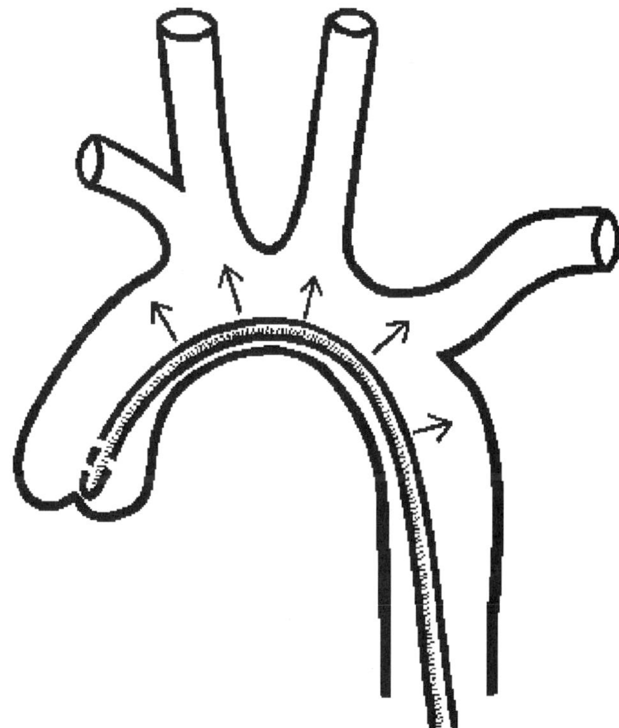

Figure 11.2 Catheter positioned against inner circumference of aortic arch with potential for movement of the entire catheter outward and the tip back (arrows) with the centrifugal force of a power injection.

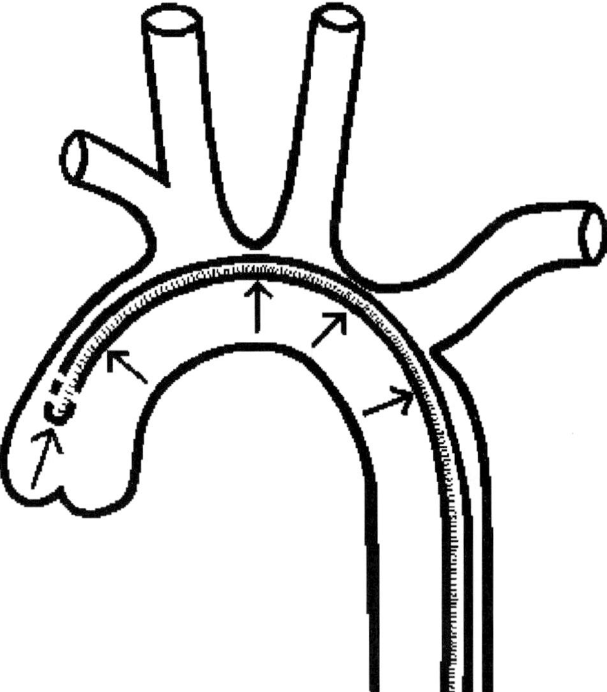

Figure 11.3 Final position of the catheter during a power injection when the catheter has been withdrawn in the aorta and is positioned at the inner circumference of the aortic arch at the beginning of the injection.

circumference of the curves in its course through the vessel or chamber, the catheter remains against the outer curve and the tip is less likely to recoil back and out of the intended site during a high-velocity injection. On the other hand, a catheter that is initially positioned along the inner circumference will tend to straighten and move to the outer circumference, and in doing so withdraw the tip of the catheter (Figure 11.3).

Occasionally, some recoil is unavoidable. This should be considered when positioning the catheter, and may be reduced by a longer rise time, slower overall flow rates, and injecting at lower pressure. The use of a fine, stainless steel, Mullins™ wire within the catheter to stiffen it helps to prevent the recoil of a very floppy catheter. The Mullins™ wire is introduced into the catheter through a high-pressure Tuohy™ valve with a side port in order to allow high-pressure injection. The stiffening wire occupies a very small portion of the catheter lumen but, in catheters which are 6-French or more in diameter, this does not compromise the lumen significantly.

Special angiographic procedures

Balloon occlusion angiograms

A balloon occlusion angiogram is performed with a Berman™-type balloon angiographic catheter with the balloon inflated in and occluding the vessel during the injection[9]. The intention is to increase the concentration of contrast in the vessel proximal to the site of the inflated balloon and to prevent distal run-off of the contrast. During a balloon occlusion angiogram, the balloon is fully inflated for the several seconds' duration of the injection of contrast. This forces contrast into any side or branching vessels proximal to the inflated balloon. This technique is used commonly in both the ascending and the descending aorta and occasionally in the branch pulmonary arteries.

When the balloon is inflated in the ascending aorta in an infant, the purpose of the balloon occlusion is to fill the aortic root and enhance the visualization of the origins and distribution of the coronary arteries. This technique is particularly useful in infants with transposition of the great arteries. In this location, the angiogram is usually performed with an X-ray tube in a steep caudal–LAO position. The balloon catheter is advanced from the ventricle into the ascending aorta, and the injection is performed in the aortic root with the balloon inflated just above the coronary sinuses. To be effective, the occlusion of the aorta must be complete in order to prevent the images of the brachiocephalic vessels from overlapping with the images of the coronary vessel[10]. Obviously in this location, the entire procedure must be performed very expeditiously with absolutely no delays.

Balloon occlusion angiography is also commonly used to visualize branching vessels or collaterals off the descending aorta. In this situation, the balloon angiographic catheter is floated into the ascending aorta, around the aortic arch, and into the descending aorta to a position that is distal to the area to be visualized. The balloon is inflated in the lower thoracic aorta (or just below where the expected side vessels arise) and the injection of contrast performed with the balloon inflated during the entire injection of contrast. This forces contrast backwards against the blood flow and into the side branches.

During the injection the balloon prevents the diastolic filling of the vessels as long as it is inflated. Since the dominant flow into the coronary arteries and collateral vessels is frequently the diastolic flow, balloon occlusion during the angiogram can be counter-productive. As a consequence, often rapid, high-pressure injections, without balloon occlusion, are more effective than balloon occlusion angiograms in these locations.

Balloon occlusion angiography is extremely useful in the pulmonary arteries to fill branching vessels off a more central trunk or, in particular, to visualize a contralateral branch pulmonary artery that is otherwise difficult to enter. In that circumstance the balloon is inflated in the contralateral vessel and just distal to the origin of the vessel that is to be visualized. The inflated balloon in the proximal branch pulmonary artery forces the flow of contrast into the side or contralateral vessel and away from the vessel occluded by the balloon.

Pulmonary arteriolar wedge angiocardiograms

Pulmonary arteriolar wedge angiograms are used to visualize the microvasculature of the pulmonary vascular bed, particularly in patients with pulmonary hypertension. There is enough positive correlation between the vascular images and the degree of pulmonary vascular disease that pulmonary capillary wedge angiograms are now an integral part of the work-up of any patient with pulmonary hypertension or suspected pulmonary vascular disease[11,12]. When wedge angiograms are used for grading pulmonary vascular disease, multiple wedge angiograms are taken with each angiogram in a different segment of the lung. Pulmonary vascular disease is not a uniform disease, so representative pictures must be obtained from as many different areas of each lung field as possible. It is preferable to record the wedge injections using biplane imaging. Often, the capillary bed curves away from the imaging plane and appears "on end" in one plane while it is cut nicely "on edge" in the opposite plane.

Pulmonary wedge angiograms all are performed using hand injections of contrast. There are several techniques for performing pulmonary arteriolar wedge angiograms when looking at the microvasculature. In all cases an end-hole catheter is advanced distally into a branch pulmonary artery and forcefully wedged into the capillary bed. The best wedge pictures are obtained when a standard, relatively stiff, torque-controlled, end-hole catheter is wedged deeply into the capillaries. A balloon wedge catheter can be used, however, even a partially inflated balloon often stops in the more central pulmonary artery proximal to the actual capillary wedge position. In a more proximal "pre-wedge" position, the balloon catheter blocks all of the prograde flow and, in turn, gives a wedge pressure. However an angiogram from this pre-wedge position fills many segments, which often overlap each other and obliterate the details of the individual segments.

1–2 ml of contrast is sufficient for visualization of the capillary architecture. The most effective way of performing a wedge angiogram is with a single-syringe technique. This technique takes advantage of the markedly different densities of the contrast material and a saline flush solution. The difference in density between the contrast and the flush maintains the contrast solution separate from the flush solution when drawn carefully into a single syringe held vertically. Approximately 8 ml of flush solution is drawn into a 10 or 20 ml syringe. Keeping the syringe vertical with its tip pointing down, 2 ml of contrast is drawn *very slowly* into the same syringe. When the syringe is kept in the vertical position and the contrast is drawn into the syringe very slowly, the contrast remains layered at the bottom of the syringe and remains completely separated from the flush solution (Figure 11.4). There will be a distinct interface between the two different density solutions, which can be made even clearer by adding a few drops of blood to color the top layer of flush solution. If the contrast is drawn into the syringe rapidly or with any force, a "jet" of contrast will be created into the column of flush solution as it enters the syringe, and the two solutions will become mixed. The syringe with the separated solutions is maintained in the vertical position as it is attached to the hub of the previously wedged catheter. The attachment procedure must be performed gently so that the two layered solutions in the syringe are not shaken around enough to mix them together.

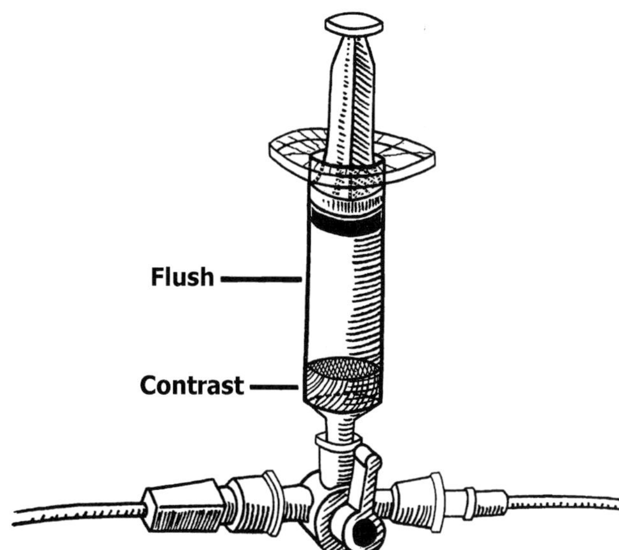

Figurte 11.4 "Layering" of contrast medium and flush solution in a syringe that is held vertically for wedge angiography.

The imaging system is placed on maximum magnification and collimated precisely over the area of distribution of the wedge segment of the lung. The recording frame rate is reduced to 15 or 7.5 frames per second. While observing on fluoroscopy, the catheter is slowly and carefully filled with contrast just to its tip. The angiographic recording is started and while closely observing the area on the screen, the contrast is injected slowly so that the entire capillary bed in the wedge area fills with a fine distribution of contrast. The injection should be fast enough so that the contrast fills the capillaries, but not so fast that the area is obliterated by a diffuse, opaque blush from extravasation into the surrounding tissues. Once the capillaries are filled with contrast, the remainder of the fluid solution in the syringe is forced into the catheter with a slightly greater force (and faster rate) of injection. The flush fluid clears the capillary bed as it "pushes" the contrast through the capillary bed, and the clearing enhances the details of the vasculature. When an operator is just starting to perform wedge angiograms, it usually takes several attempts to develop the correct speed of injection in order to obtain the optimal pictures.

An alternative technique of performing pulmonary capillary wedge injection is to use a two-syringe technique. The two-syringe technique has the one advantage of being able to control or change the exact amount of contrast injected *during* the injection. The contrast is drawn into a 2–3 ml syringe and the flush solution is drawn into a *separate* 10 ml syringe. The two syringes are attached to the catheter through a three-way stopcock. The catheter position and the X-ray field setting are exactly the same as for the single-syringe technique.

With the biplane recording running, the desired amount of contrast is slowly injected into the capillary bed from the smaller syringe, the three-way stopcock is turned to the larger syringe, and the larger volume of flush solution is pushed through with the larger syringe, similarly to fluid injection with the single-syringe technique. This technique has the inherent disadvantage of an obligatory delay of *at least* several seconds during the injection/recording as the stopcock is being switched from one syringe to the other. During this time, the smooth flow of contrast/flush solution into the capillary bed is stopped and, of even more importance, the X-ray is running and continuously exposing the patient and the operator to radiation while no contrast is flowing! There is also a greater chance of small bubbles being trapped within the stopcock between the tips of the two syringes and the hubs within the stopcock. These bubbles are then injected between the bolus of contrast and the flush solution.

Forced "volume" pulmonary arteriolar wedge angiograms

Pulmonary *artery* wedge angiograms are also used for the visualization of pulmonary *venous* structures, particularly when there is obstruction of flow to, or from, a particular pulmonary venous area[13]. With unilateral or segmental pulmonary vein obstruction, contrast that is injected into even the exact pulmonary artery supplying the involved segment, preferentially flows away from the involved segment of the pulmonary artery supplying the obstructed vein and provides no information about the obstructed vein. A pulmonary artery wedge angiogram with injection into the arteriolar supply of the specifically involved venous segment(s) forces contrast through the capillary bed and into the involved pulmonary venous system. This technique provides excellent visualization of the involved pulmonary venous anatomy even in the presence of severely obstructed veins.

The technique for pulmonary arteriolar wedge angiograms used to visualize the *pulmonary veins* is similar to the wedge angiograms used to visualize the capillary bed, except that a greater volume of contrast is used. At least 10 ml of flush solution is drawn into a 20 ml syringe. As the syringe is held vertically, 0.3–0.5 ml/kg of contrast solution is drawn slowly into the syringe. As with the pulmonary arteriolar capillary pictures, the field is set and the image is observed closely and recorded on slow-frame-rate, biplane imaging during the injection. The contrast is injected slowly followed by the flush solution. The larger volumes of contrast with a higher flush rate force the flow through the capillary bed and into the pulmonary veins. The biplane recording is continued until the veins are visualized.

Pulmonary venous wedge angiograms

Another essential type of pulmonary wedge angiogram is the pulmonary venous wedge angiogram. This, as the name implies, is a wedge angiogram performed with an end-hole catheter wedged into the pulmonary venous capillary bed. The pulmonary venous wedge angiogram is used to visualize true pulmonary arteries in which there is low, or no, demonstrable prograde flow[14]. This technique is frequently the only method for visualizing the true pulmonary arteries. Even when areas of the lung are perfused extensively through collaterals, the true pulmonary arteries are frequently not seen adequately. The technique is absolutely essential in identifying the true pulmonary bed in patients with pulmonary atresia or complete isolation of unilateral or segments of pulmonary arteries. The pulmonary vein is accessed from the left atrium either through an existing intra-atrial communication or through an atrial transseptal procedure.

To perform a pulmonary venous wedge angiogram, a torque-controlled, end-hole catheter is advanced from the left atrium into a pulmonary vein and wedged forcefully into the desired distal venous capillary bed. This should produce a pressure tracing through the catheter wedged in the pulmonary vein, which, however, has an arterial contour. The pressure that is recorded is often, but not always, reflective of the true pulmonary artery pressure. Occasionally a transseptal procedure through the atrial septum is necessary to gain access to the left atrium or selectively into a particular pulmonary vein entering the left atrium. Pulmonary vein angiograms in patients with intact atrial septae are one of the absolute essential indications for an atrial transseptal procedure.

For injecting the contrast, the single-syringe technique using a 20 ml syringe is even more desirable for pulmonary vein wedge angiograms, however either the single- or double-syringe technique can be used. If the double-syringe technique is used, extra precautions must be used to eliminate any air in the syringe/stopcock system. Usually 15–17 ml of flush solution and 3–5 ml of contrast are used for these studies. Since the contrast/flush is being forced against the normal direction of blood flow, the contrast is delivered with a significantly greater force and over a longer period of time than are required for a pulmonary arteriolar wedge angiogram.

The X-ray field is set to cover all of the segments of the lung where the true pulmonary vessels have not been visualized from prograde angiograms. As a consequence, the field of view is usually larger than for pulmonary arteriolar wedge angiograms. In order to see as much of the lung field(s) as possible, the field initially is not magnified. A 15 frame per second rate is used for the recording. With the recording started, the bolus of contrast is forced into the pulmonary vein capillary bed. The force and rate of the contrast injection are adjusted by observing the appearance of the contrast entering the pulmonary arteries and the rate of flow in the pulmonary arterial bed. As the injection continues, progressively more force is applied to the contrast injection until the pulmonary arteries are visualized. If the catheter is not wedged sufficiently or insufficient force is applied to the syringe, the contrast merely flows back around the catheter and out of the pulmonary vein. This provides no visualization of the arterioles or pulmonary arteries. As greater force is applied, there is a capillary blush and then the contrast is forced into the distal arterioles, which are distinguished by the direction of flow in the vessels. When the true prograde blood flow into the pulmonary artery is very low, the vein wedge angiogram often fills the entire, true pulmonary arterial tree. On the other hand, when there is significant other flow into the true pulmonary arteries or when too much force is applied to the injecting syringe, the contrast extravasates into the surrounding tissues including the bronchi. When contrast enters a bronchus, the patient usually coughs and produces a small amount of hemoptysis, although a good image of the bronchus is often obtained! The hemoptysis is usually self-limiting and of no clinical consequence.

In addition to the measured pressure from the catheter in the pulmonary vein capillary wedge position, the pulmonary vein wedge angiogram provides indirect information about the pulmonary artery pressure. If the pulmonary arteriolar and arterial vessels are visualized with the pulmonary vein wedge injection, the pulmonary artery pressure can be assumed to be low! The contrast will not fill the true pulmonary arteries satisfactorily or bronchograms are obtained more frequently during attempted vein wedge angiograms in patients who have high pulmonary pressures.

Specific views (angles) for angiocardiograms

When referring to a particular "X-ray angle" or view, the angle refers to the angle or position of the image intensifier in relation to the patient's chest and the tabletop. With an adequate, biplane, X-ray system, both of the X-ray tubes/intensifiers can be rotated around the patient and can be angled both cranially and caudally. Many X-ray systems have different angles or combinations of angles of the two tubes set into an automatic "one-button" control. These settings can be inserted into the X-ray program individually by particular operators.

Most structures of the heart and great vessels are visualized optimally in one specific view. Often, particularly in congenital lesions, a view perpendicular to the optimal view provides significant complementary information about the specific lesion or critical adjacent structures. Although there is a particular angle or view that is superior for the visualization of each separate structure in "known defects", nevertheless there are enough variations in the "typical" anatomy of even very common defects that no single predetermined angle is always optimal, or possibly even satisfactory, in patients with the same diagnosis. Each predetermined angle that is set automatically usually requires some further adjustment in the angles of the X-ray equipment to create the optimal view. Some views are preferable for the "stretching out" or opening up of the particular structures and others are preferable because of the familiarity of the appearance of the particular structure in that particular view[15,16].

Because of the familiarity with the PA and LAT views, and regardless of the anatomy, most catheter manipulations are performed with the X-ray tubes in the straight PA and LAT positions. However, a catheterizing physician should be comfortable with manipulation of the catheter while the X-ray tubes are at unusual angles. Very often, the position of a catheter, a delivery system, or a device will require changing after the X-ray system has been positioned into unusual angles for specific angiography or device implant. It is more expedient if catheters can be re-maneuvered with the X-ray tubes in these unusual angles without returning them to the more familiar and "comfortable" PA and LAT views.

The common angles used for the visualization of particular structures and the particular anatomy or structures for which each angulation is useful are discussed briefly in the following section. In each patient, each of these angles or views requires individual, additional adjustments to the X-ray tube angulation to achieve the optimal visualization of any individual structure. In complex congenital heart lesions, the enlargement or rotation of the heart usually changes the optimal angle for visualization of even the most typical structures. Since, usually, two ideal and complementary angles of the same structure are achieved simultaneously with biplane compound angulation systems, most congenital lesions are studied angiographically with simultaneous biplane imaging.

Common angles and the structures seen in each particular view

Specific structures and lesions are listed under the typical, preliminary or basic X-ray tube angles (positions) that are useful for their visualization. Most of the individual X-ray projections are used with the second X-ray tube in a perpendicular, or nearly perpendicular, complementary projection, whether this is mentioned in the discussion of the structures in that view or not.

Straight posterior–anterior (PA) view

1 The straight PA projection (along with the complementary straight lateral (LAT) projection) provides the best view for a general orientation to the overall anatomy of the whole cardiac structure, particularly in the presence of unknown or very complex anatomy or in the initial study of a complex patient.

2 The entire peripheral systemic venous system throughout the body is visualized optimally in the straight PA view (usually along with a complementary LAT view to provide the anterior–posterior course of the veins).

3 The superior and inferior vena cava.

4 The right atrium (body of the atrium and appendage).

5 The entire right ventricle.

6 The entire length of the right pulmonary artery, the distal right pulmonary arterial tree, and the peripheral left pulmonary arterial tree.

7 The entire pulmonary venous system and the connections of the pulmonary veins to the left atrium.

8 Abnormal pulmonary venous channels—the course of abnormal pulmonary venous channels is usually defined best in the PA view.

9 The cavity of the left atrium and left atrial appendage.

10 The proximal transverse aortic arch with the brachiocephalic vessels and their branches (including surgical shunts off the arch or off the brachiocephalic vessels).

11 The descending aorta, distal to the transverse arch, all of the way to the aortic bifurcation and into the iliofemoral vessels is seen best in the PA view. The PA view is particularly useful for defects, shunts, branches or collateral vessels arising straight off the lateral walls of the descending aorta.

12 The straight PA view provides a good initial view of the coronary arteries-either from an aortic root injection or with selective injections.

13 The PA view gives a good view of the mitral valve in endocardial cushion defects—the so-called "goose-neck" deformity of the valve apparatus. Otherwise there are better views for most mitral valves, normal and abnormal.

14 The straight PA (along with the complementary LAT) view is necessary for the accurate determination of the basic side to side ("D" and "L" relationships of the great arteries) and anterior–posterior relationship of the ventricles and great arteries to each other, particularly in very complex hearts.

15 The straight PA view is best for localizing the mass of the liver. This is particularly important when considering a transhepatic puncture for venous access. The course of the hepatic veins and their entrance into the right atrium during hepatic vein cannulation are seen best in the PA view.

16 In patients with ventricular inversion, with or without a single ventricle, the outlet foramen to the subaortic area and the subaortic area itself are often best seen in the straight PA view.

17 The right and left pulmonary arteries in patients with truncus arteriosus are often best seen in the straight PA view.

Straight lateral (LAT) view

1 The straight lateral view is the usual complementary view to the straight PA view, providing the anterior–posterior relationships of any of the structures mentioned under the PA view. The straight lateral view is usually included when recording an angiogram in the PA view.

2 Type I and type II interventricular septal defects (VSD): high-outflow ventricular defects are often projected better "on edge" in the straight lateral view than in the commonly advocated LAO–cranial view. Because of the spiral course of the septum, the cephalad, subaortic end of the outflow area of the left ventricular outflow tract is aligned perpendicular to the straight lateral view, which usually cuts the perimembranous ventricular defects on edge the best.

3 Most ventricular septal defects (VSD), in the presence of high right ventricular pressure or a dilated right ventricle, with or without right-to-left shunting or with overriding of the aorta, are visualized best in the straight lateral projection when imaged from a right ventricular injection. This is a result of the rotation of the entire septum, which is associated with significant right ventricular hypertrophy or dilation.

4 The precise anterior–posterior relationship of the great arteries in conotruncal abnormalities and true transpositions are established in the straight lateral view.

5 The right ventricular outflow tract (RVOT) is "cut" on edge in the straight lateral view and, as a consequence, this view is particularly good for visualizing obstructions or other abnormalities of the RVOT.

6 The lateral view of the main pulmonary artery "stretches out" the main pulmonary artery maximally and demonstrates the pulmonary valve "on edge" very well.

7 The proximal left pulmonary artery is often cut on edge in the straight lateral view. However, unless contrast is injected selectively into the left pulmonary artery, the images of the main and right pulmonary arteries overlap the image of the proximal left pulmonary.

8 The lateral view separates the origin of the right and left coronary arteries and provides one view of the separated courses of the right, the LAD and the circumflex coronary arteries.
9 The lateral view is particularly good for visualizing the underside of the aortic arch, the high descending aorta and any structures occurring or arising in that area (coarctation of the aorta, PDA and some collateral vessels with a high aortic take-off).
10 The lateral projection provides a side view of the descending aorta and iliopelvic arteries and gives the best visualization of the anterior–posterior course of branches off these trunks.
11 The anterior–posterior course and relationship of normal and collateral iliopelvic veins are visualized only with the lateral view taken simultaneously with the corresponding PA view.
12 The interatrial septum in the presence of right to left shunting: this view is particularly good for visualizing the valve and tunnel of the foramen ovale in the presence of right to left shunting.
13 The entrance of the superior and inferior cava and hepatic veins into the right atrium.
14 The coronary sinus is "stretched" out in the lateral view.
15 The course of the azygos and hemiazygos veins, the lateral course and entrance into the heart of the left superior vena cava to either the coronary sinus or the left atrium.
16 The location of the liver (along with the PA view) for hepatic punctures and the subsequent course of the hepatic veins.
17 The course of the internal mammary arteries behind the sternum along with their branches—particularly into collaterals.

Right anterior oblique (RAO) view

1 Opens up the right ventricular outflow tract along with the main pulmonary artery, and often places the pulmonary valve on edge.
2 Stretches out the junction of the proximal right pulmonary artery with the main pulmonary artery—usually a shallow RAO view.
3 Places the mitral valve more on edge—separates the mitral valve from the subaortic area. (This separation is even better with some associated caudal angulation of the PA intensifier.)
4 Places the tricuspid valve on edge (better with some caudal angulation as well).
5 Places the atrial septum *en-fas*, which is good for visualizing devices placed on the atrial septum.
6 Good second view when selectively injecting coronary arteries.
7 The origin of some arteries, which arise obliquely off the thoracic and abdominal aorta are visualized best in the RAO view (some collaterals, renal arteries).
8 Often the RAO is the best view for an atypically oriented patent ductus off the descending aorta.

Left anterior oblique (LAO) view

1 Opens up the underside of the aortic arch for arch anomalies, (hypoplasia, some coarctations, etc.).
2 Essential for some PDAs with an oblique origin off the aorta.
3 Cuts the mid to high ventricular septum on edge.
4 Cuts some atrial septal defects on edge, particularly the low septum (most of the atrial septum is visualized better with some cranial angulation).
5 Partially opens up and stretches out the proximal left pulmonary artery (even better along with cranial or caudal angulation).
6 Opens up the bifurcation of the left coronary artery.

Straight posterior–anterior with cranial angulation (45° "sitting PA" or straight cranial) view

1 Stretches out the MPA along with the proximal RPA and LPA, i.e. the pulmonary valve and the entire central pulmonary artery tree. Very good view for visualization of the pulmonary valve annulus and valve "hinge points". Straight cranial angulation is the best view for visualizing the central pulmonary arteries when filled by a pulmonary vein wedge angiogram.
2 Opens up the proximal right and left branch pulmonary arteries.
3 Associated slight RAO angulation with the cranial—opens up the right pulmonary artery even better.
4 Associated LAO angulation with the cranial angulation—opens up the proximal left pulmonary artery.
5 The cranial along with a slight LAO is good for stretching out the high RV outflow tract.

Cranial with LAO angulation (45° cranial, 30° LAO [off of horizontal])

1 The posterior and muscular ventricular septum is elongated and cut on edge. This separates type III and type IV ventricular septal defects from each other as well as from type I and II ventricular septal defects.
2 The LV outflow tract is elongated in its longest axis. Gives excellent visualization of the subaortic area (subaortic obstruction and atypical ventricular septal defects are seen well).
3 The left ventricular inflow and the mitral valve are not cut on edge as well unless a very steep cranial angulation can be achieved. Usually the patient's head and shoulders interfere with a cranial angulation that is sufficiently steep to open up these structures.
4 The cranial LAO angle may be the best angle to cut the interatrial septum, or at least part of it, on edge. This angle is particularly useful for visualizing some atrial septal

defects on edge and for the deployment of some atrial septal defect occlusion devices.

"Four chambered" view: cranial with steep LAO angulation (45° cranial and 45° [off of vertical] LAO)

1 Elongates and cuts much of the atrial septum on edge separating posterior (sinus venosus), middle (secundum), and base (primum) parts of septum.

2 Good visualization of the inflow ventricular septum.

3 Puts the endocardial cushion area on edge and is the best demonstration of a common A-V valve overriding the ventricular septum.

4 Clearly distinguishes between mitral insufficiency shunting through an associated ASD versus a pure left ventricular to right atrial shunting.

Cranial–RAO (35° cranial and 45° RAO) angulation

1 Opens up some of the distal RPA branches.

Caudal–RAO (approximately 30° RAO and 30+° caudal)

1 Cuts both A-V valves and the LV outflow tract on edge—creates a perpendicular view to the cranial–LAO view.

2 Mitral valve can be cut precisely on edge. This is an excellent view for the mitral valve and associated subvalve mitral abnormalities.

3 The RAO–caudal cuts both the left ventricular outflow tract and the mitral valve on edge and separates the mitral valve from the left ventricular outflow tract completely.

4 The PA tube in the caudal–RAO allows a simultaneous perpendicular view to the lateral tube in the cranial–LAO, elongating and cutting the LV outflow tract on edge.

5 Places the atrial septum *en fas*—good for visualizing atrial septal defect devices following deployment.

Caudal–LAO (approximately 30° lao and 30+° caudal)

1 Cuts the interatrial septum on edge; good view to use during atrial septal device deployment—moves the image intensifier away from the head of the table while still cutting the septum on edge. Poor view for left atrial angiograms because the left atrial shadow overlies the mitral valve and the left ventricle as contrast empties into the left ventricle.

2 Elongates the proximal left pulmonary artery in the presence of "sea gull" type pulmonary arteries and other late take-offs of the LPA.

3 Very steep caudal with varying degrees of LAO give the "down the barrel" view of the aortic root in order to separate the origin and distribution of the coronary arteries from each other. Usually performed with a balloon occlusion angiogram in the ascending aorta with a balloon angiographic catheter occluding the aorta above the coronaries.

Pre-set angulation

Modern biplane catheterization laboratories often have the capability of programming multiple combinations of pre-set X-ray tube/intensifier angles into "single button" settings. With these pre-settings, the two X-ray tubes rotate simultaneously into the pre-set angles with the touch of one or a set of selected buttons. A combination of angles for the two X-ray tubes is pre-set for each button to correspond to similar angles to those listed above. These pre-set angles are very useful ***to begin*** the positioning of the proper angles for the desired views. Because of the infinite variety of lesions and the different vertical, horizontal and rotational abnormalities within each individual patient, no standard or absolutely fixed set of angles is satisfactory for any particular lesion in every patient. The pre-set angles are used as a starting point for the automatic rotation of the X-ray tubes. Once these pre-set angles are reached, a more precise adjustment of the angulation of each X-ray tube is performed to suit each individual lesion/patient.

Complications of angiography

The most common complication of angiography is an intramyocardial injection with the extravasation of contrast into the wall of a chamber or vessel as a consequence of a high-pressure injection[17]. Usually this results in an intramyocardial "stain" of the contrast with little, or no, identifiable sequelae. When an intramyocardial stain occurs, it is treated according to recognizable changes in the hemodynamics. Usually, observation alone is sufficient. Even when contrast appears in the pericardium, a pericardial tap is rarely necessary. Small intramyocardial pockets or aneurysms have been observed in the area of prior intramyocardial stains, but these are found incidentally and no significant adverse events from them are reported.

A very large or high-pressure extravasation of contrast can extend completely through the myocardium and even into the pericardium with a resultant pericardial effusion or tamponade. The most extreme degree of intramyocardial injection necroses the tissues completely through the myocardium, resulting in a true perforation and massive blood loss. The best treatment, as with all complications, is prevention by meticulous attention to the positioning of the catheter for angiography, pressure test injections with very small amounts of contrast before large injections, and the use of large diameter catheters in conjunction with lower pressures for intracavitary injections. When a large extravasation occurs, it is treated exactly as is any other perforation with tamponade. The tamponade is relieved acutely in the catheterization laboratory and the patient is supported with fluid/blood replacement while being prepared for surgical repair of the perforation.

The injection of air during any contrast injection is always a possibility, but is always preventable. The combination of meticulously clearing every bit of air from both hand-held and power injector syringes before attaching to the catheters, withdrawing a column of blood into the contrast syringe after it is attached to the catheter, and attaching the syringe while advancing a column of contrast forward from the syringe into a back flow of blood from the hub of the catheter, and *always* having the syringe for injection pointing downward during the injection absolutely prevents any air from being injected during an angiogram.

With the earlier ionic and more hyperosmolar contrast agents, many (most) patients experienced discomfort during the contrast injection. The discomfort varied from a sensation of a hot flush passing through the body from cephalad to caudal to actual pain passing first to the head and then to the body. The discomfort was transient but also reproducible with subsequent injections of contrast. There did not seem to be any permanent adverse effects from this sensation. With the newer, non-ionic and iso-osmolar contrast agents this discomfort is seldom encountered.

There are inherent complications due to the contrast agents themselves. The most common of these is a sensitivity or allergy to iodine or to a specific contrast agent. This fortunately is very uncommon in the pediatric and congenital population, but may well become a more frequent problem as congenital heart patients grow into adults. The allergy to contrast or iodine may be known before the procedure, or can occur unexpectedly during the catheterization. Reactions to the contrast range from a minimal skin rash with itching or hives to more extreme reactions including bronchospastic problems, anaphylaxis, shock and potentially even death.

Allergic reactions that occur unexpectedly in the catheterization laboratory are treated with intravenous antihistamines, steroids and, when necessary, epinephrine, and this is usually sufficient to stop the allergic reaction and prevent recurrences if contrast must be used subsequently. Whenever possible, the procedure is completed without the use of more contrast, but if essential anatomic information is still necessary, an additional dose of both steroids and antihistamine is given before any subsequent injection, and both are repeated during the recovery period from the catheterization.

When an angiocardiogram is absolutely necessary in order to obtain critical anatomic information in patients with complex congenital heart disease, it is virtually impossible to obtain the necessary information or perform any therapeutic catheter procedure without the use of contrast. In the presence of a past history of an allergic reaction to contrast or iodine, the vast majority of recurrent allergic reactions in the catheterization laboratory can be prevented or, at least, minimized by appropriate premedication. The risk of a serious allergic reaction is weighed against the risks of not having accurate anatomic information about the lesion. The patient or parent(s) must be counseled accordingly before the procedure.

A patient with a history of allergic reactions to iodine or contrast medium who must undergo a cardiac catheterization is premedicated with intravenous antihistamine and a rapid-acting corticosteroid. Thirty minutes after the premedication and pretreatment with the antihistamine and steroid, a test injection of 0.5 ml of contrast is given intravenously. If no systemic reaction is detected from the initial test, a repeat test injection, using 5.0 ml of contrast, is administered intravenously. If there is no reaction from either of the test injections, the catheterization is carried out normally with contrast injections as necessary. If there is a significant reaction to either test injection, the procedure is either abandoned or, at the very least, performed with only the hemodynamics obtained with no angiograms performed. Fortunately, in the entire experience in the Texas Children's Hospital cardiac catheterization laboratories, no patient has had such a severe reaction to prevent the angiographic procedures after the appropriate premedication. At the end of the procedure, or during the procedure in a very long one, a patient who has a history of an allergic reaction or who has had any reaction to the contrast during the procedure, is given a repeat dose of both antihistamine and steroids. Once the procedure has been completed, any patient who has a history of, or has exhibited, an allergic type of reaction is observed for at least 12 hours after the last dose of antihistamine or steroids.

In addition to allergic reactions to contrast media, all contrast agents have an inherent potential renal toxicity, the manifestations of which vary from patient to patient and between different contrast agents. The majority of the studies and information on contrast nephropathy are on adult patients with significant comorbidity who are undergoing coronary studies[18]. Hematuria or renal failure are reported following cardiac catheterization and angiography. This is usually related to some pre-existing renal problems, the combination of the osmolality of the contrast agents, relative dehydration of the patient, and an excessive, cumulative dose of contrast during the particular procedure. In very long, complex procedures, many pediatric/congenital patients receive large cumulative volumes of contrast agent without apparent adverse effects. These same patients also receive large volumes of intravenous flush solutions and usually diurese generously throughout the long procedure. When the use of a large amount of contrast is anticipated or actually used during a case, the patient is deliberately over-hydrated with extra flush solution administered intermittently during the procedure. An indwelling Foley™ bladder catheter in place during a long procedure, not only makes the patient more comfortable, but also allows constant monitoring of the quantity and the quality of the patient's urinary output. If the extra volume load of fluid in combination with the contrast agent does not result in diuresis of the patient during the catheterization, then the patient is given a dose of an intravenous diuretic along with the extra hydration. Renal failure can occur following the use of contrast agents only, but usually occurs in the presence of pre-existing renal impairment or in association with extremely large doses of contrast used during a catheterization procedure of a very short duration.

The most devastating reactions to contrast agents are damage to the central nervous system (CNS)[19]. CNS reactions may be limited to a severe, persistent headache or to self-limiting seizures, but can include permanent and severe brain dysfunction and even death. These adverse CNS events are probably related to the osmolality of the contrast agents, and occur predominantly when very large doses of contrast are used during very short catheterization procedures.

Both renal and central nervous system complications from contrast appear to be preventable by the judicious control of the amount of contrast used during a catheterization. The original rule of a maximum of 4 ml of contrast per kg of body weight was established with the older ionic and hyperosmolar contrast solutions and *probably* now is too stringent, and no longer applies in the very complex and very long catheterization procedures performed with the non-ionic and iso-osmolar contrast solutions of the current era. Anecdotally, many interventional cardiologists have used doses of contrast up to 8–10 ml/kg during long complex cases without any detectable adverse events. At the same time, there have been no controlled clinical studies in pediatric or older congenital heart patients to document that the "4 ml/kg rule" still does not hold true even using non-ionic or iso-osmolar contrast agents! Until the safety of the higher dosages of the newer contrast agents is documented in a controlled clinical trial, it is judicious to use as little contrast as possible during all procedures, and adhere to the 4 ml/kg rule by very selective injections in precise areas and by using as small a volume of contrast for each injection as is possible to obtain the necessary information. When larger total amounts of contrast are necessary, the patient is given extra hydration, and the larger amounts should be used only in a very prolonged procedure. Usually, when a patient is well hydrated, the contrast itself is an adequate diuretic, however, when large volumes of fluid do not produce diuresis when a patient has received large volumes of contrast and extra fluid, it probably is beneficial to administer an intravenous diuretic.

When small amounts of blood are drawn into a solution of an undiluted, non-ionic contrast agent, irregular aggregates of red cells form in the solution. Initially it was thought that these aggregates were clots and that the non-ionic agents were hypercoagulable[20]. As a consequence, it became common practice to add heparin (3 units/ml) to the solutions of undiluted contrast. It has since been proven that these aggregates were only that, and that they dispersed with any flow of the solution[21]. Nevertheless, many institutions still mix heparin with contrast solution before it is used.

In spite of the potential complications of angiography and from the contrast medium itself, meticulously planned and carefully performed angiography is remarkably safe and produces minimal complications. Even with the more complex catheterizations being performed in the current era, when used in conjunction with other imaging modalities, the number of angiograms that are necessary and the amount of contrast medium used in each study can be reduced. The combination of these adjustments in the way that angiograms are performed improves the safety of these angiographic studies even further.

References

1. Freedom RM *et al. Congenital Heart Disease, Textbook of Angiocardiography*. 1997: Futura.
2. Nihill M. *An Angiographic Atlas of Congenital Cardiovascular Anomalies*. 2001: Blackwell-Futura.
3. Bashore T. Fundamentals of X-ray imaging and radiation safety. *Catheter Cardiovasc Interv* 2001; **54**(1): 126–135.
4. Balter S. X-ray generation and control. *Catheter Cardiovasc Interv* 1999; **46**(1): 92–97.
5. Levin DC, Dunham LR, and Stueve R. Causes of cine image quality deterioration in cardiac catheterization laboratories. *Am J Cardiol* 1983; **52**(7): 881–886.
6. Balter S. Digital images. *Catheter Cardiovasc Interv* 1999; **46**(4): 487–496.
7. Pridjian AK *et al*. Comparison of a low osmolarity nonionic radiographic contrast agent with a standard medium on renal function in cyanotic and normal dogs. *Cathet Cardiovasc Diagn* 1994; **31**(1): 90–93.
8. Stanger P *et al*. Complications of cardiac catheterization of neonates, infants, and children. A three-year study. *Circulation* 1974; **50**(3): 595–608.
9. Keane JF *et al*. Balloon occlusion angiography in infancy: methods, uses and limitations. *Am J Cardiol* 1985; **56**(7): 495–497.
10. Mandell VS *et al*. The "laid-back" aortogram: an improved angiographic view for demonstration of coronary arteries in transposition of the great arteries. *Am J Cardiol* 1990; **65**(20): 1379–1383.
11. Nihill MR and McNamara DG. Magnification pulmonary wedge angiography in the evaluation of children with con-

genital heart disease and pulmonary hypertension. *Circulation* 1978; **58**(6): 1094–1106.

12. Rabinovitch M *et al*. Quantitative analysis of the pulmonary wedge angiogram in congenital heart defects. Correlation with hemodynamic data and morphometric findings in lung biopsy tissue. *Circulation* 1981; **63**(1): 152–164.
13. Bini RM and Bargeron LM Jr. Visualization of pulmonary vein obstruction by pulmonary artery wedge injection. *Pediatr Cardiol* 1982; **2**(2): 161–162.
14. Nihill MR, Mullins CE, and McNamara DG. Visualization of the pulmonary arteries in pseudotruncus by pulmonary vein wedge angiography. *Circulation* 1978; **58**(1): 140–147.
15. Fellows KE, Keane JF, and Freed MD. Angled views in cineangiocardiography of congenital heart disease. *Circulation* 1977; **56**(3): 485–490.
16. Bargeron LM Jr *et al*. Axial cineangiography in congenital heart disease. Section I. Concepts, technical and anatomic considerations. *Circulation* 1977; **56**(6): 1075–1083.
17. Lipton MJ *et al*. Cardiovascular trauma from angiographic jets—validation of a theoretic concept in dogs. *Radiology* 1978; **129**(2): 363–370.
18. Iakovou I *et al*. Impact of gender on the incidence and outcome of contrast-induced nephropathy after percutaneous coronary intervention. *J Invasive Cardiol* 2003; **15**(1): 18–22.
19. Junck L and Marshall WH. Neurotoxicity of radiological contrast agents. *Ann Neurol* 1983; **13**(5): 469–484.
20. Raininko R and Ylinen SL. Effect of ionic and non-ionic contrast media on aggregation of red blood cells *in vitro*. A preliminary report. *Acta Radiol* 1987; **28**(1): 87–92.
21. Grabowski EF. Effects of contrast media on erythrocyte and platelet interactions with endothelial cell monolayers exposed to flowing blood. *Invest Radiol* 1988; **23** (Suppl 2): S351–S358.

12 Foreign body removal

Introduction

With the extensive use of chronic, indwelling, central venous lines for monitoring, hyperalimentation, for chemotherapy and now the numerous interventional catheters, coils and other devices, there are more frequent occasions when iatrogenic foreign bodies become free floating in the circulation. The removal of foreign bodies from the heart and vasculature has shifted from the domain of the radiologist and even the thoracic or vascular surgeon to the interventional cardiologist and, in turn, from the radiographic suite or operating room to the cardiac catheterization laboratory[1,2]. Most of the foreign bodies that are removed from the vascular system are pieces of wire, indwelling, diagnostic or therapeutic catheters, or the therapeutic devices themselves. There are some foreign bodies that are not introduced iatrogenically, but which can be retrieved with a catheter technique[3]. Fortunately all or most of the foreign bodies are radio-opaque, which makes visualization by fluoroscopy and, in turn, catheter retrieval possible. Most of the intravascular foreign bodies end up in the venous circulation, however, when they do end up in the systemic (arterial), circulation, the retrieval materials and "grabbing" techniques are similar. The final extraction from the artery, however, is often more difficult.

There are many catheter devices and techniques that facilitate the removal of intravascular foreign bodies in the cardiac catheterization laboratory. Many of the intravascular retrieval devices have been adapted from urologic instruments. All of the devices that are designed specifically for foreign body retrieval from the vascular system, have the retrieval, or grabbing, mechanism contained in a "carrier catheter". The grabbing (retrieving) mechanism at the distal end of the carrier catheter is activated by a control mechanism that extends out of, or is part of, the proximal end of the catheter. This proximal mechanism moves the distal retrieval mechanism in and out of the carrier catheter and opens and closes the retrieval mechanism. There are several other catheter devices that were designed for other uses, which are helpful in the retrieval of intravascular foreign bodies. The use of all of these devices is included in this chapter.

A prerequisite to attempting the removal of any intravascular foreign material in the cardiac catheterization laboratory is a high-resolution, ***biplane fluoroscopic system***, which includes a quality biplane freeze frame imaging system for "road mapping". Unlike general catheter manipulations in the heart, the maneuvering of a retrieval device to the specific location of a foreign body requires very *precise, controlled* and *purposeful three-dimensional* maneuvers of the retrieval device toward and around the foreign body. Attempting a foreign body retrieval using only a single plane X-ray system relies upon multiple chance or random probes toward the foreign body with the catheter/retrieval device, rather than any skillful, precise, and purposeful catheter maneuvers. Without biplane imaging, the operator can only guess the depth relationships of structures relative to the side-to-side relationships (or vice versa) when manipulating the retrieval device to approach the foreign body. In order to direct the retrieval device purposefully in what is, spatially, a three-dimensional field, the operator must have the capability of reconstructing the position of the errant material in a three-dimensional, spatial orientation. The posterior–anterior (PA) plane of the fluoroscopy provides the side-to-side and cephalad/caudal orientation while the lateral (LAT) plane provides precise and simultaneous anterior–posterior depth orientation. The operator must be able to visualize both planes *simultaneously* or, at the very least, be able to switch back and forth ***instantaneously*** from one plane to the other during every movement of the catheter retrieval device. The capability of displaying a biplane freeze-frame image is necessary to create a three-dimensional "road map" of the location of the foreign body. This is particularly important when attempting to enter one of multiple branching vessels.

Of equal, or even greater, importance, in an attempted catheter retrieval of a foreign body, the use of a single plane X-ray system results in far more and, potentially, excessive radiation exposure to both the patient and the operator. Each unsuccessful, random or chance probing with a catheter in a single plane, which can actually be far away from the foreign body in the opposite plane, uses more fluoroscopy time and radiation exposure than a well-controlled, purposeful maneuver that is directed with simultaneous biplane imaging. The biplane system allows instantaneous visualization of both the depth and side-to-side relationships and prevents repetitive, fruitless manipulations far away from the foreign body.

In addition to a biplane X-ray/fluoroscopic system and the specific catheter retrieval devices, the catheterization laboratory must be equipped with a variety of long sheaths/dilator sets. Long sheaths with radio-opaque bands at their distal tips are very helpful for precise positioning. They should be available in at least 85 cm lengths and in a variety of diameters, up to and including at least 16-French, as part of the standard retrieval equipment. These large sheaths are available from a variety of manufacturers (e.g. Cook Inc., Bloomington, IN, Daig Corp., Minnetonka, MN, Arrow International Inc., Reading, PA, Cordis Corp., Miami Lakes, FL). Super Stiff™ exchange length wires (Boston Scientific, Natick, MA), torque wires, Glidewires™ (Terumo Medical Corp., Somerset, NJ) and various deflector wires (Cook Inc., Bloomington, IN) are also necessary for the precise positioning of the catheters and devices needed for a successful retrieval. Deflector wires should include multiple wire and curve diameters of the Amplatz™ variable curve and deflector wires (Cook Inc., Bloomington, IN) with their deflector handles as well as various sizes of straight stainless steel Mullins™ deflector wires (Argon Medical Inc., Athens, TX), which can be formed into specific "three-dimensional" curves as necessary.

In order to prevent excessive bleeding and to allow frequent (continuous) flushing, which is necessary to prevent clotting within the long sheaths, back-bleed valves with side flushing ports must be available for the sheaths. The back-bleed valves with a flush port are fixed as part of the larger diameter long sheaths, while some of the smaller diameter long sheaths have detachable back-bleed/flush valves. A detachable back-bleed valve has the advantage of allowing even the most irregularly shaped foreign body to be withdrawn completely out of the proximal end of the sheath without having to remove the sheath from the vascular system. Tuohy™ back-bleed valves, which accommodate both the catheters and the wires, are necessary to prevent excessive blood loss and allow continuous sheath/catheter flushing during prolonged manipulation of both wires and retrieval devices. These Tuohy™ back-bleed valves can be used in tandem when a catheter and a wire or when two or more wires are used side-by-side in the sheath with the retrieval catheter.

Access with the retrieval system to the precise location in the vessel or chamber where the foreign body is lodged is often the most difficult part of the procedure. Most errant foreign bodies migrate to a branch pulmonary artery. Preformed, torque-controlled, coronary or peripheral vascular catheters are useful for the purposeful entry into the exact orifice of the major branch vessel where the foreign body is lodged. In addition, torque-controlled wires or curved-tipped Glide wires™ manipulated through a preformed end-hole catheter are essential for selective cannulation into the precise, more peripheral branch vessels. The Amplatz™ variable deflector wires (Cook Inc., Bloomington, IN) are used to tighten the curvature at the tip of a catheter–i.e. to increase its concavity. The preformed (pre-curved) stiff end of a 0.035″ or larger spring guide wire or a preformed Mullins™ deflector wire (Argon Medical Inc., Athens, TX) is used to achieve a "three-dimensional deflection" on the catheter tip or to direct the tip of the catheter away from the concave direction of a more proximal curve on the catheter. With the use of the proper equipment and biplane fluoroscopy, access is possible to all areas or vessels by an experienced pediatric interventionalist.

Technique—general for all retrieval devices

Two separate venous access routes are secured for all types of retrieval procedures in the venous system. One venous access is for the retrieval system itself. The second venous access is used for a separate angiographic catheter, which is used for repeated *small* selective positioning angiograms during the retrieval. When these small, very selective angiograms are performed in the same selective vessel and close to the immediate vicinity of the foreign body or the retrieving catheter/device, then very small amounts of contrast can be used with each injection. Repeated selective angiograms are necessary while approaching the foreign body with the entire retrieval system in order to direct the retrieval device specifically to the foreign body, and repeated selective injections are necessary during the actual retrieval procedure to verify the approximation of the retrieval device to the foreign body. The closer to, and the more directly into the specific vessel where the foreign body is lodged, the less contrast solution will be necessary for each of the selective angiograms.

Injecting the contrast through the long, large diameter, retrieval sheath through which the retrieval device is delivered is occasionally advocated instead of a second catheter for performing the selective, guiding angiograms. Unfortunately this usually does *not* produce satisfactory positioning angiograms. Injections through the retrieval sheath are of little use for the actual positioning of the sheath itself, since the sheath approaching the foreign body must already be in position and in near proximity to the foreign body in order to obtain an effective picture. Secondly, the volume and/or flow rate of injections through the sheath are compromised and frequently insufficient since the injection must be lower pressure through the side arm of a valved back-bleed device and the injection will be restricted around (adjacent to) the retrieval system, which takes up much of the lumen within the same sheath. Finally, contrast medium within the sheath creates "stickiness" between the sheath and the retrieval system, which can compromise subsequent manipulations of the retrieval system.

The angiographic catheter is introduced first. A biplane angiocardiogram is recorded in a more central vessel or chamber, which gives rise to the suspected location of the foreign body. Biplane images identify the exact vessel where the foreign body is lodged and in three dimensions. The angiogram identifies any fixed landmarks in the vicinity of the foreign body and establishes the relationships of other vascular structures to the foreign body. From these pictures, the exact course that will be necessary for a catheter to approach precisely to the foreign body, becomes evident.

A large, long sheath of appropriate length and diameter is chosen for the retrieval. The diameter of the sheath for the retrieval of a device should be two to three French sizes larger than the original sheath that was used to deliver the device. The diameter of the original delivery sheath accommodated the device adequately, but only when it was folded or collapsed purposefully and by hand to its minimal diameter. When the device is grasped as a foreign body loose in the vascular system, it never collapses or folds to that equivalent small diameter. At least a 9- or 10-French long sheath is used for the retrieval of small fragments of indwelling catheter. At least a 15-French sheath is required for the retrieval of a CardioSEAL™, STARFlex™, Amplatzer, other large occluding devices, or other foreign bodies of equivalent size.

The exact location of the foreign material is identified and the course through the vasculature to the foreign body is determined. The long sheath is pre-shaped into a curve that corresponds as closely as possible to the course through the vasculature (and heart) to the foreign body. A curve that is preformed on the sheath will help to maintain the tip of the sheath in position immediately adjacent to the foreign material during the retrieval procedure. The preformed curve is formed "three-dimensionally" in order to conform more precisely to the desired intravascular course and to have the tip of the sheath bend toward the foreign body in all planes of view, once it is in the final position for the retrieval. The curve is formed on both the sheath and dilator together while they are outside of the body.

The specific shaping of the sheath is accomplished by one of several techniques. Straightening of the pre-existing transseptal curve which comes on most long sheaths is accomplished by repeatedly drawing the distal end of the sheath/dilator between a tightly grasped finger and thumb of the opposite hand. The "factory" curve is actually removed completely from the sheath and a partial new curve can be formed using this technique of pulling the sheath/dilator through the clenched finger/thumb while forming a new curve. A more satisfactory curve can be formed by first softening the sheath/dilator by applying external heat to the appropriate area of it. Once softened, the warmed sheath/dilator is reshaped by hand, forming the desired curve. The heat is applied by soaking the exact area of the long sheath/dilator combination in *boiling* sterile water or by placing it in the jet of heat from a heat gun for 30 to 60 seconds. The heat softens the materials of the walls of both the sheath and dilator sufficiently that they can be shaped manually as desired. The warmed segment of the sheath/dilator is removed from the heat source and formed (molded) to correspond to the course through the vasculature (and heart) to the foreign body. The new curve in the sheath/dilator is then fixed with the operator's hands while it is dipped for 5–10 seconds in a bowl of cold sterile water or flush solution. The cold solution fixes this desired new shape. In pre-forming the sheath, each new curve is "over-curved" or tightened slightly more than the curves in the course of the vasculature, since the curves in the sheath/dilator tend to straighten once they are introduced into the warm circulation. The tighter curves in the sheath/dilator help to compensate for this tendency.

Once the large long sheath has been pre-formed, a 6- or 7-French, end-hole catheter is introduced through a standard short sheath. The catheter is maneuvered selectively until the tip of the catheter is positioned *just proximal* to the foreign body using one of the techniques and the equipment described in Chapter 5 on "Catheter Manipulations". A 0.038", Super Stiff™ exchange guide wire with a short floppy tip is passed through this catheter and into the precise vessel in which the foreign body is lodged, or preferably (and very carefully) just *beyond* the foreign body in the same vessel. Once the wire is in place, the catheter and the short sheath are removed over the wire and replaced with the pre-curved, large diameter, long sheath/dilator set. The long sheath/dilator is advanced over the wire to a position where the tip of the dilator is in the exact vessel and just proximal to the most proximal free or loose end of the foreign body. The dilator is fixed securely in place over the wire while the sheath alone is advanced over the dilator until the tip of the sheath is positioned adjacent to the foreign body. The radio-opaque marker band on the distal end of the sheath makes this positioning easier to visualize and maintain.

Once the long sheath is in place, it is maintained in this position while the dilator is removed over the wire leaving the tip of the sheath adjacent to, or even against, the foreign body and supported in the precise area by the stiff wire. The long sheath is drained passively of any entrapped air or blood through the side port of the back-bleed valve and then attached to the flush system. Because of the large dead space within large, long sheaths and the frequent long duration of these procedures, the sheath should be maintained on a slow flush and systemic heparinization is instituted at this time during the procedure.

Sheath positioning and fixation—adjunct techniques

Although the pre-formed sheath can usually be maneuvered into the vessel and to a position immediately adjacent to the foreign body, it is often difficult to keep its tip in the exact position, particularly while the stiff, and often straighter, retrieval catheter is being introduced through the sheath. When the internal diameter of the long sheath is significantly larger than the retrieval catheter being used, the long 0.038″ Super Stiff™ wire over which the long sheath/dilator was delivered and which originally had been passed immediately adjacent to and well beyond the foreign body, is left in place through the sheath, distal to the foreign body after the dilator has been removed. The wire passing through the sheath and adjacent to the foreign body maintains the tip of the sheath directed at the foreign body while the retrieval catheter passes side-by-side with the Super Stiff™ wire within the sheath.

If the long Super Stiff™ wire is removed along with the dilator, there are other alternatives for maintaining the sheath in position adjacent to the foreign body as the retrieval device is being advanced through the sheath. A stainless steel Mullins™ deflector wire, which is precurved to a similar, but somewhat tighter curve to correspond to the course to the foreign body, can be used within the sheath to support and maintain the direction of its tip. The Mullins™ wire is curved in "three dimensions" to correspond to the course of the sheath to the foreign body. As with the initial preforming of the sheath, the curves on the Mullins™ wire are formed tighter than the desired curves in order to maintain the appropriate curves in the large sheath. Mullins™ deflector wires are thinner and smoother and will fit better alongside of the retrieval device within the sheath than the larger Super Stiff™ wire. The smoother surface of the stainless steel wires also allows the smoother passage of the retrieval system next to the wire.

Another way to create a slight change in the direction of the tip of the long sheath is with the use of a 0.038″ or 0.045″, controllable, Amplatz™ deflector wire. The deflector wire is introduced through the sheath adjacent to the carrier catheter of the retrieval device. The active deflector wire is used to redirect the tip of the sheath into the precise vessel branch in which the foreign body is located, and can help to fix the sheath in this position during further manipulations of the retrieval catheter and device. The controllable deflector wire will deflect the tip of the sheath only toward the direction of the concave curve of the sheath in its course through the heart and vesels, and only provides a single plane of deflection.

If a very tight curve is encountered in the approach to the foreign body or the sheath is too stiff to deflect with a single deflector wire, two or even three Mullins™ wires, and even an active Amplatz™ deflector wire, can be used simultaneously, side by side, by using a significantly larger long sheath. Each wire is introduced through a separate Tuohy™ valved back-bleed device, which is added in series to the open port of the previous Tuohy™ "Y" adaptor. Each additional Tuohy™ Y adaptor is attached to the open arm of the previous Tuohy™ while each new wire is introduced through the compression valve of the new Tuohy™ adaptor. With the foreign body lodged in a very difficult or circuitous location, as many as three deflector wires have been used simultaneously alongside of the retrieval catheter in order to maintain the tip of the sheath pointed directly at the foreign body.

When possible, with all retrieval devices it is desirable first to pass the carrier catheter of the retrieval device through a larger, stiffer "guiding" catheter before introducing the retrieval device/carrier catheter into the sheath. This additional guiding catheter must be large enough in its internal diameter to accommodate the retrieval device/carrier catheter and yet small enough in its outside diameter to pass through the sheath with some space between the carrier catheter and the sheath. This extra space within the sheath is desirable to accommodate additional wires. The additional stiffer guiding catheter permits more precise maneuverability and control over the positioning of the carrier catheter/retrieval device. When the stiff guiding catheter is positioned just at the tip of the sheath, it allows the entrapped foreign body to be pulled more forcefully against the combination of the tip of the guiding catheter and the tip of the sheath. The extra guiding catheter helps to prevent the tip of the retrieval catheter or the tip of the sheath from "accordioning" on itself when a very strong force is necessary to pull the foreign body into the sheath. The stiffer guiding catheter within the sheath also helps to prevent the shaft of the sheath from kinking when the route to the foreign body through the vascular system is fairly tortuous.

If there is not a catheter available with a large enough internal diameter to serve as this additional "carrier" catheter, a dilator from a long sheath can be modified and used for this purpose! When the sheath is in position next to the foreign body and the dilator has been removed from the sheath, the tapered distal end of the dilator is cut off one centimeter proximal to the tip. The lumen of the dilator proximal to the tapered tip is very large, yet the wall of the dilator is relatively thick and stiff. This allows the original long dilator to be used as a large diameter, very thick walled guiding catheter. A separate curve can be formed on this modified dilator, in order to increase its maneuverability. The modified dilator within the sheath also serves to "center" the retrieval catheter within the lumen of the sheath, which, in turn, helps to prevent the grasped foreign body from catching on the tip of the sheath as it is being withdrawn into the sheath. When the modified dilator from the same sheath/dilator set is used in this manner, there is obviously no space between the outer wall of the dilator and the inner wall of the sheath for additional support or deflector wires. In this circumstance, however, there usually is enough space between the carrier catheter for the retrieval device and the inner wall of the dilator to accommodate the extra support wires.

Once the tip of the sheath has been secured immediately adjacent to the foreign body, the carrier catheter with the retrieval device is advanced through the sheath/modified dilator. The retrieval device is advanced out of the sheath and, depending upon the characteristics of the foreign body and the exact type of retrieval device being used, placed against or around the foreign body; differences in the devices and grasping techniques are discussed subsequently in this chapter. The retrieval device is activated and the foreign body grasped.

Once a foreign body has been grasped within the vessel, it should be withdrawn *completely* into the long sheath while the tip of the sheath is still in the distal vessel. This is especially important when the foreign body has stiff irregularities or jagged ends or edges that hang out of the end of the sheath (e.g. a Gianturco™ coil or a CardioSEAL™ type atrial septal defect (ASD) occluding device). A foreign body that is positioned in a pulmonary artery ***must be*** pulled completely into the sheath before it is withdrawn through the right ventricle. The use of a much larger diameter sheath from the onset of the retrieval procedure facilitates the withdrawal of the foreign body completely into the long sheath.

If a free leg of an occlusion device or a free loop of coil hangs out of the end of the sheath as the sheath/foreign body is withdrawn through a ventricle, there a very high likelihood of the foreign body's becoming entangled in the atrioventricular valve apparatus. A foreign body entangled in an atrioventricular valve apparatus can require *open-heart* surgery on cardiopulmonary bypass for removal! It would be catastrophic to have an otherwise straightforward transcatheter patent ductus arteriosus (PDA) or ASD occlusion procedure end up as an emergency, open-heart surgical case!

When the foreign body that is lodged in the venous system is retrieved proximal (in the direction of blood flow) to an atrioventricular valve (e.g. from the right atrium, left atrium, or a systemic vein) or distal to the heart in an artery, but cannot be withdrawn entirely into the sheath, an attempt can be made at withdrawing the partially exposed foreign body out of the vasculature and the skin along with the sheath. Often the portion of the foreign body extending out of the sheath is flexible or not too large. The partially collapsed foreign body is held tightly against the distal end of the large sheath/catheter keeping as much of the foreign body as possible within the sheath while the combination sheath/foreign body is withdrawn through the more peripheral vessel. The combination sheath, carrier catheter, retrieval device and foreign body is withdrawn out of the vessel and through subcutaneous tissues and skin as a unit. This certainly is more traumatic to the vessel and the subcutaneous tissues, but usually does not result in any morbidity or permanent damage to the vessel. This procedure for the final removal of an exposed segment of foreign body from the vessel is performed only when there are no stiff or rigid portions of the foreign material projecting at an acute angle beyond of the end of the sheath. Rigid segments that project at acute angles are likely to catch on the vascular structures and can damage them severely.

Before the *sheath* is withdrawn completely from the vessel along with the foreign body, steps should be taken to preserve that particular vascular access. With the tip of the sheath and retrieved device in a more central vein, the stiff end of an exchange length, spring guide wire is introduced into the proximal end of the long sheath and advanced adjacent to the retrieval catheter, through the long sheath, through (or past) the foreign body and into the vessel beyond the tip of the sheath. The stiff end of the wire must be used since, when a foreign body is pulled against the distal end of the long sheath, the soft floppy tip of the guide wire would buckle and fold up against the foreign body, which has been pulled partially within the sheath. As a consequence, the soft tip of the guide wire can seldom be advanced beyond the foreign body at the end of the sheath. Once the stiff end of the guide wire extends into the vessel, *just* beyond the tip of the long sheath, the wire is fixed against the skin outside of the body, which fixes the tip in the vessel in this location. The sheath along with the foreign body is withdrawn out of the vessel over the fixed wire. In this way, the stiff tip of the wire is not advanced within the vessel at all. The wire allows access into the same vein with a new sheath/dilator after the original sheath, along with the foreign body, has been withdrawn from the vessel over the wire. This precaution is particularly important since the foreign body occasionally pulls loose from the retrieval system as it is being withdrawn through the subcutaneous tissues or skin, in which case it will have to be retrieved from that same vessel.

There are several additional steps that help in the withdrawal of larger, stiffer and more difficult foreign bodies into the sheath, or facilitate the withdrawal of the exposed foreign body out through the skin. When the foreign body has been grasped but will not pull completely into the sheath or out of the vessel, it is withdrawn to a position as far distally in the vessel as possible and, particularly, to a position where it cannot embolize centrally and into a worse location in the circulation. Usually larger devices become fixed securely when withdrawn into the smaller, more distal vessels. A second, even larger, long sheath is introduced from a second vessel and a second retrieval device introduced through this larger sheath. If the additional retrieval sheath can be introduced from a different/opposite vessel (e.g. a femoral vein or a jugular vein), this allows the possibility of grabbing the distal end or another portion of the errant balloon, stent or occlusion device.

The distal end of the original guide wire (which may still be through the errant balloon, stent or other foreign body!) is snared, pulled into the new sheath, and exteriorized through the new sheath. A snare is introduced over the distal end of this wire or a basket device is introduced adjacent to this wire into the new larger sheath and maneuvered over or onto the errant device. When the distal end of the errant device cannot be withdrawn into the new sheath alone, a second retrieval system is introduced into the new, larger sheath, but now through the dilator of that larger sheath which has been "modified" as described previously to accommodate the retrieval device. The errant device, still held by the original retrieval system, is grabbed from the different/opposite approach with the new retrieval system through the much larger sheath. Once the embolized device is grasped at a new location with the new retrieval system, it is released from the original retrieval system and an attempt is made at withdrawing the device into the new, larger sheath.

If a second retrieval catheter cannot be introduced, the foreign body is withdrawn forcefully into a smaller, more peripheral vessel, wedged and "secured" in that location in the vessel. When comfortable with the fixation of the errant device in this location, it is cautiously released from the original retrieval device in this "secure" location. The original sheath and retrieval device are withdrawn over the wire and replaced with a new, larger sheath and a new retrieval system over the same wire and into the same vessel. Before its introduction the new sheath/dilator should have a slight, smooth, 15–20° curve preformed at the distal end. This very slight curve allows the side-to-side position of the tip of the new sheath/guiding catheter (with the contained retrieval device) to be changed slightly relative to the foreign body by rotating the retrieval catheter/device slightly while simultaneously moving it very slightly to-and-fro. This ability to reorient the positions of the tip of the sheath and the retrieval catheter allows the foreign body to be grasped from a slightly different angle. The slightly different orientation of the grip on the foreign body is often enough to allow it to collapse better and to be withdrawn completely into the new, larger, long sheath. When the new long sheath is several French sizes larger than the original retrieval sheath, this also helps to allow the foreign body to be pulled completely into the sheath.

Dilating the tip of the long sheath after it has been introduced into the body is another aid to help pull a large foreign body completely into the sheath. This modification is possible only if the sheath used for the retrieval does not have a radio-opaque marker band at the distal tip. The dilation of the sheath tip is performed once the sheath is within the vessel but before the foreign body has been grasped.

If the foreign body has been grasped already and there has been an unsuccessful attempt at pulling it into the even larger sheath, an exchange length Super Stiff™ wire with a long floppy tip is introduced into the sheath. The foreign body, which is still held by the retrieval device, is pushed out of the tip of the sheath to a position several centimeters away from the tip of the sheath. This allows the Super Stiff™ wire that passes through the sheath adjacent to the retrieval catheter to advance beyond the end of the sheath and well past the foreign body to a secure position more distally in the same vessel. The foreign body is released into a "secure" location in the vessel as described above. The carrier catheter and retrieval device are withdrawn completely from the sheath adjacent to the Super Stiff™ exchange wire. A very high-pressure angioplasty balloon with a diameter two to three millimeters larger than the internal diameter of the sheath is introduced into the long sheath over the wire until the center of the balloon is straddling the tip of the sheath. With the center of the balloon secured in a position that is half in and half out of the tip of the sheath, the balloon is inflated to its maximum pressure. If the balloon begins to milk out of the sheath, the inflation is stopped, the balloon is withdrawn into the sheath slightly and the attempted inflation repeated while holding the balloon securely against the end of the sheath. This frequently requires several repeat inflations/deflations and repositioning of the balloon to maintain it exactly in position straddling the tip of the sheath. When inflated in the correct position, the balloon dilates and, in turn, "flares" or even splits the tip of the sheath slightly. When the tip of the sheath has been flared, the balloon is withdrawn out of the sheath over the wire, the retrieval catheter/device is reintroduced adjacent to the wire, and the foreign body re-grasped. The flare and enlarged diameter of the tip of the long sheath facilitates the withdrawal of foreign bodies (particularly disrupted balloons) completely into the sheath.

Pre-positioning of a very large diameter, short, stiff, "recovery sheath" ***over*** the large, long sheath is another technique that helps with the withdrawal of a *foreign body from the vessel and through the skin*. This recovery sheath technique must be planned from the very onset of the procedure, or, at least, before the introduction of a new, larger, long sheath. A very large diameter, short sheath, which is large enough to fit over the large, long sheath, is used as the recovery sheath. The more rigid the material of the wall of this short sheath is, the better it functions as a recovery sheath. In fact, a thin-walled, large diameter, short *metal* cannula serves ideally for this purpose. The long, large diameter, retrieval sheath/dilator is passed through the even larger diameter, short recovery sheath before the long sheath/dilator is introduced into the skin.

The short recovery sheath remains pulled back over the long delivery sheath and positioned against the proximal hub of the long sheath throughout the procedure. The recovery sheath is *not* introduced into the skin unless the endovascular device that is being delivered through the long sheath becomes a loose foreign body, and this grasped foreign body cannot be withdrawn completely into the long sheath when it is withdrawn close to the skin. With the foreign body held firmly in the inferior vena cava or iliac vein and wedged into the tip of the long sheath, the short recovery sheath is introduced into the skin and into the vessel over the long sheath by gently "drilling" it over the long sheath and into the vessel. The grasped foreign body together with the long sheath is then withdrawn into the short recovery sheath. The stiffness of the recovery sheath along with the contained long sheath usually prevents the recovery sheath from "accordioning" on itself. The pull against the rim of the tip of this stiff outer recovery sheath forces the foreign body to fold the remainder of the way into it.

If the foreign body does not pull easily into the recovery sheath, the long sheath with the grasped foreign body is re-advanced out of the short recovery sheath, rotated slightly, and withdrawn again into the short recovery sheath. This slight realignment of the two sheaths to each other allows the foreign body to be pulled into the recovery sheath and, in turn, allows the foreign body along with the original long sheath to be withdrawn out of the vessel. After the withdrawal of the long sheath and foreign body, the short recovery sheath maintains access into the vessel, but without a back-bleed valve. These short recovery sheaths are routinely placed over long sheaths when performing implant procedures with the larger CardioSEAL/STARFlex™ devices. The short recovery sheath is equally effective for retrieving foreign bodies from an artery.

Specific retrieval devices

Snare retrieval devices

Snare retrieval devices are the most versatile and most used foreign body retrieval devices. This type of retrieval device functions like a "western lasso", encircling and then tightening around the object. There are now many different, commercially available, snare retrieval devices, all of which have a retractable loop, or several loops, of flexible wire, which extend(s) beyond the tip of an end-hole (carrier) catheter. When retracted or withdrawn into the carrier catheter the loop(s) constrict(s) on itself/themselves. Any material or foreign body surrounded by a loop of the snare is grasped by the loop as it contracts. These snares are the simplest of the retrieval devices and have a very wide variety of uses. However, they do have limitations to particular types of retrievals and *cannot* be relied upon as the *only* available retrieval device. They can be used only if the foreign body has a "free end", i.e. a piece of an errant catheter or device extending into the lumen of the vessel or chamber, or if a separate wire can be passed and secured through the foreign body and the separate wire grasped with the loop of the snare. There must be an accessible, free portion or end of the object, in order to allow the loop of the snare to encircle it completely. There are many varieties of these snares available. They vary in the material of the wire, the size and the number of loops, the configuration and the angle of the loops off the carrier catheter and in the type of carrier catheter.

"Home-made" snares

Although commercial snares are much more predictable and smoother to operate, before the availability of commercial snares many operators built their own snares for retrieval procedures. The process of building a snare may still occasionally be necessary when, for one reason or another, the precise commercial snare or a particular size of a commercial snare is not available. The materials needed for a "home-made" snare are readily available in every catheterization laboratory.

The main component of a home-made snare is a 240 cm long teflon coated, 0.018″ or 0.021″, spring guide wire. The second component is an end-hole catheter with or without side holes, with a fairly stiff shaft and with an internal diameter large enough to accommodate two strands of the particular spring guide wire side by side within the lumen and still allow some movement of the wires within the catheter. This end-hole catheter becomes the carrier catheter for the snare. Woven dacron catheters are more rigid than most extruded materials and are very effective for this purpose. A long sheath, with a *detachable back-bleed / flush valve*, completes the home-made snare catheter set. The *detachable* back-bleed valve is essential, as it allows the partially opened loop of the snare to be introduced into the sheath without distorting the loop by compressing and squeezing it *through* a back-bleed valve. A detachable valve also allows the grasped foreign body to be withdrawn completely out of the sheath without having to remove the sheath. The sheath must clearly be large enough to accommodate the carrier catheter but, in addition, it must be several French sizes larger than the carrier catheter to allow introduction and passage of the open loop of the snare without compressing it enough to distort it. Also, the larger the diameter of the long retrieval sheath, the more likely will it be to allow the foreign body to be withdrawn completely into the sheath after it has been snared.

Preparation of home-made snares

To build a home-made snare, the end-hole catheter that will serve as the carrier catheter is first passed through a *detachable* back-bleed valve/flush device, which will fit on the long recovery sheath, but before the valve is attached to the sheath. The back-bleed valve will eventually be attached to the long sheath, but only after the partially open snare loop has been introduced into the sheath completely. The two free ends of a long spring guide wire (side by side) are threaded together into the distal end of the end-hole carrier catheter. The two ends of the wire are advanced together completely through the catheter until they appear at the proximal hub of the catheter. Together the ends are drawn out of the proximal hub of the catheter until a loop of the desired diameter of the "snare" is formed by the folded wire at the distal end of the carrier catheter. The loop can be of any diameter and/ or shape.

The two loose ends of the wire are clamped together with a hemostat, which is positioned close to the proximal hub of the catheter and serves as the control handle for the snare. The proximity of the clamp to the proximal hub of the catheter serves as a constant indicator of when, and to what extent, the loop is being extended at the distal end of the catheter. The clamp keeps the loop from being inadvertently extended too far, it keeps the two loose ends of the wires from being pulled completely into the proximal end of the catheter, and it acts as a reminder to keep the loop from being prematurely withdrawn and closed. A slight bend of approximately 30° off the long axis of the catheter is placed on the two wires at the base of the loop at their junction with the tip of the catheter. This bend on the wires creates an offset angle between the long axis of the catheter and the whole loop. This bend allows the loop to extend out of the catheter/sheath at this same angle and facilitates encircling foreign bodies, which may not be aligned exactly perpendicularly to the catheter.

Introducing a home-made snare into a long sheath requires a special procedure in order not to distort (destroy) the loop of the snare and, at the same time, not to exsanguinate the patient. A large diameter, long sheath/ dilator, which does ***not*** have an *attached* back-bleed/flush port, is introduced into the vascular system and positioned adjacent to the foreign body. After the dilator has been removed, the sheath (with no back-bleed valve) is cleared of air and/or clots by passive bleeding directly from the hub of the sheath. When the sheath has been cleared, the flush system is attached directly to the hub of the sheath. When the fabrication of the home-made snare is completed, the shaft of the sheath close to the skin is clamped with a "rubber-shod" Kelly™ clamp to eliminate bleeding from the open end of the sheath after the removal of the flush system and while the loop of the snare is being introduced into the sheath. This clamp on the sheath effectively stops back bleeding and eliminates the "urgency" or rushing of this delicate procedure for the introduction of the loop into the long sheath. The flush tubing is removed from the hub of the sheath and attached to the side port of the detachable back-bleed valve that previously had been positioned on the shaft of the carrier catheter. The open loop of the snare wire is partially compressed between the operator's fingers and, after the flush tubing has been removed from the hub of the sheath, the open loop, along with the carrier catheter is introduced directly into the hub of the previously positioned long sheath. The loop is compressed only enough to allow it to be introduced into the large sheath and not enough to eliminate it between the two strands of the wire. As the open loop of the snare is compressed significantly to fit into the sheath, the operator must use extreme care not to kink, sharply bend or overly compress the loop as it is introduced into the sheath. If the loop is flattened completely, it will not open when extruded from the distal end of the sheath. A sheath diameter significantly larger than that of the carrier catheter allows the loop to be inserted while it is still partially open.

Once the entire open loop of the snare and the tip of the carrier catheter are within the sheath, the clamp on the sheath is released and the system allowed to clear of air by allowing back-bleeding around the carrier catheter. When the sheath has been cleared again, the back-bleed valve that was previously positioned over the carrier catheter is placed on a continuous flush, advanced over the catheter, and attached to the sheath. The clamp on the sheath will compress or even kink the sheath, however, this kink is outside of the body, where it can be reshaped manually before the hand-made loop of the snare is advanced through the area.

Another method of building a home-made snare is to use a long guide wire and the catheter shaft of a balloon angioplasty catheter. The entire balloon is excised from the catheter just proximal to the proximal end of the balloon. The transverse section of the catheter exposes the two lumens of the balloon dilation catheter and provides a unique carrier catheter. The balloon lumen is usually much smaller and eccentric, while the central catheter, or wire lumen is significantly larger. This cut-off balloon catheter is passed through a detachable back-bleed valve, which is positioned back on the shaft of the catheter exactly as was done with the previous home-made snare using an end-hole catheter. A long teflon-coated wire of a diameter that just barely fits into the balloon lumen of the catheter is used to fashion the snare. The floppy end of this wire is jammed tightly into the distal cut-off end of the balloon lumen for at least 4–5 mm. Once the soft end of the wire has been fixed securely in the balloon lumen, the other, stiff end of the wire is introduced into the cut-off opening of the larger central lumen and threaded through the catheter until it appears through the proximal hub of the previous balloon dilation catheter. The stiff end of the wire is withdrawn from the proximal end of the balloon catheter lumen until the other end of the wire, which is jammed into the balloon lumen, forms a loop on itself. This loop forms the snare. This snare is retracted or opened by withdrawing or pushing, respectively, on the single, free end of the wire that extends out of the proximal hub of the catheter. The loop of the snare can be of any size, and shaped or angled just like other home-made snares. This type of snare is introduced into a larger, long sheath without an attached back-bleed valve and with the snare loop open in the same manner as the other home-made snares.

Home-made snares have the advantage that the materials to make them are available at all times in any laboratory. They have the disadvantages of being deformed very easily and of having a very poor "memory" for the preformed loop or for the angle off of the long axis of the catheter. Once the loop of any home-made snare for which spring guide wires were used to make the loop, has been withdrawn into the carrier catheter to tighten the loop, the loop is compressed into a very narrow, slit-like orifice. In order to reuse an individual loop or before it can function as a snare loop again, the carrier catheter is withdrawn from the sheath, the loop extended completely out of the catheter, reformed manually, and then reintroduced into the sheath using the same technique as the original introduction.

As an alternative to a standard spring guide wire and to overcome the problem of the deformation of the withdrawn loops, a 0.021", exchange length, Terumo™ wire can be used to make the home-made snare. The Terumo™ wire looped on itself retains its loop after being withdrawn in and out of the end-hole carrier catheter. However, a side bend cannot be formed on the straight loop and the Terumo™ wire is significantly more difficult to handle.

The technique of retrieval using a home-made snare is different from that used with commercial snares since the home-made loop is delivered in the "open" position and it is already extended out of the end of the carrier catheter. In order to capture the errant foreign body, the sheath must be advanced completely past the foreign body while the loop is still totally within the sheath. Since the snare is already in an open position when it is advanced out of the sheath, the open loop of the snare cannot be forced into, around or over the foreign body. Home-made snares also have variable angles off the long axis of the carrier catheter, and have essentially no memory for the preformed loop once they have been withdrawn into the sheath or the carrier catheter even once. In order to reuse a home-made snare, it must be withdrawn completely out of the body from the sheath, re-formed manually, and reintroduced into the long sheath with each new attempted snaring.

Commercial snares

Curry™ intravascular retrieval sets—guide wire snare

The Curry™ Intravascular Retrieval Set (Cook Inc., Bloomington, IN) is the simplest of the commercially available snare catheters but is a sort of hybrid between home-made and several other more effective commercial snares. The Curry™ Retrieval Set essentially supplies the necessary components for building a home-made snare as a set, which the operator then assembles. These sets consist of an extra long, stainless steel, spring guide wire and a TFE catheter which accommodates two strands of the wire side by side within the catheter and will serve as the carrier catheter. The Curry™ Retrieval Set is available in two different sizes. The CRS 100 set is a 100 cm long, 8-French, TFE catheter with 300 cm long, 0.021" stainless steel spring guide wire. The CRS 200 set is a 100 cm long, 6.3-French, TFE catheter with a 300 cm long, 0.018" stainless steel spring guide wire.

The Curry™ Retrieval Set, although conveniently providing all of the components, still has the significant disadvantages of other home-made snares. The components of the sets are assembled exactly as described for building home-made snares. The formation of the loop, the angling of the loop, and the introduction into the long sheath are exactly the same as with other home-made snares. The lack of memory of the loops is also the same as for the other home-made snares.

In addition to the Curry™ Retrieval Sets, a variety of far more effective commercially manufactured snares are now available. The loops of the other commercially produced snares have a true memory in addition to some unique designs, which makes them far more "user friendly" and effective.

The Amplatz™ Goose-Neck Snare

Amplatz Goose-Neck™ snares (Microvena Corp., White Bear Lake, MN) are wire loops made of Nitinol™ spring wire, which gives them a total memory for return to a specific shape and diameter of the loop. The loop of these snares opens to its fixed diameter and aligns perpendicularly to the shaft of the catheter each time it is advanced out of the tip of the carrier catheter. The loop is very flexible and its angle can be varied slightly by extruding it only partially. Goose-Neck™ snares have an excellent (total) memory for the original loop configuration and size and direction (or angle) off the catheter. This memory persists indefinitely, even after innumerable withdrawals and reopenings in and out of the carrier catheter or long sheath. Even after marked distortion of the loop from manipulations in the vessel, it maintains its original configuration. This "memory" is an indispensable quality in a snare and represents a huge advantage over any home-made snare.

Goose-Neck™ snares are available as sets, which include the snare, a snare introducer, and a specific carrier or snare catheter. The sets are available as standard, petite and micro snare sets. Standard snares are available with loops in diameters between 5 and 35 mm in increments of 5 mm. The 5 and 10 mm loop snares pass through a 4-French catheter, while the larger snares require a 6-French catheter. The "micro snares" are available with loops between 2 and 7 mm in diameter with 3-French delivery catheters, and the "petite snares" are shorter versions of the 10 and 25 mm snare catheters.

The loop of the Goose-Neck™ snare, which is orientated perpendicularly to the shaft of the catheter, has many advantages, particularly when a piece of wire or catheter or the end of a foreign body is aligned parallel to the retrieval catheter in the vascular lumen. On the other hand, this perpendicular orientation of the loop creates a problem during retrieval when the object to be retrieved is oriented across the lumen of the vessel or chamber and perpendicular to the long axis of the retrieval catheter. The perpendicular alignment of the loop to the shaft of the catheter aligns the loop of the snare parallel to an object that is aligned perpendicular to the shaft of the catheter, and makes encircling an object that is perpendicular to the carrier catheter very difficult.

When there is a "mass" of the foreign body (e.g. a balled-up coil or a collapsed occlusion device) the carrier catheter with the snare collapsed within it is advanced *past* the foreign body, the snare is opened and then withdrawn against (over) the foreign body. When firmly against the object, the snare is closed with the intent of grasping either the entire mass or just an edge or end of the foreign body. When the proximal wire of the snare is withdrawn very firmly within the carrier catheter, it creates a very tight grip of the loop on whatever portion of the foreign body is grasped. Because of their memory, relative ease of use, and strength, Goose-Neck™ snares are usually the primary retrieval system in an inventory, and are an essential part of the inventory of every catheterization laboratory.

In addition to foreign body retrievals, these snares are very useful for snaring other catheters or wires during catheter manipulations and positioning. A separate catheter or wire is maneuvered independently either in the same direction or from the opposite direction in the same vessel and snared purposefully in that vessel. The snare for this purpose is pre-positioned so that its loop is aligned across (perpendicular to) the lumen of the vessel or chamber, and the second catheter or wire is maneuvered through the open loop of the snare. This technique is used commonly in both cavae, in the right atrium, in the pulmonary artery and in the aorta when a "through and through" arteriovenous or venovenous long loop of wire/catheter is to be created.

En Snare™

The En Snare™ retrieval and manipulation system (MDTECH [Medical Device Technologies], Gainesville, FL) is a unique snare that is a recent introduction to the armamentarium of the interventional cardiologist. The En Snare™ has three separate interlaced loops of super-elastic Nitinol™ wire, each of which extends approximately 45° off the long axis of the delivery catheter, and each loop is offset circumferentially by approximately 120° from the adjacent loop. Although the loops are separate, they are extended and withdrawn as a single unit. The memory of the loops allows them to be opened and withdrawn repeatedly and innumerable times without distorting or destroying their configuration. There are interwoven strands of very fine platinum wire within each loop, which enhance their visibility during fluoroscopy. The three loops are interlaced with each other along both sides of each extended loop. This provides increased stability of the retrieval loops when they are extended. The snare catheters for all En Snares™ have a radio-opaque band at the tip for extra visualization of it.

The En Snare™ is available in a range of sizes. The size of the snare is determined by the diameter of the loops. There are Mini Snare systems in 2–4 and 4–8 mm diameters. The Mini Snares are delivered through a 3-French, 150 cm long snare catheter. The Standard Snare systems are available in 6–10, 9–15 and 12–20 mm diameters with a 6-French, 100 cm long snare catheter, and in 16–30 and 27–45 mm diameters delivered through a 7-French, 100 cm long catheter.

En Snares™ combine the advantages of most of the other snares put together. The three loops separately flare 45° off the long axis of the end of the catheter, creating essentially a 360° circumferential loop around the end of the catheter, while, at the same time, each forms a separate longitudinal loop almost parallel along the long axis of the catheter. The orientation and arrangement of the loops provide the ability to grasp objects which are orientated parallel to the snare catheter equally as well as those orientated perpendicularly to the long axis of the catheter. As a consequence, the En Snare™ is more versatile than any single-loop snare and can replace several snare catheters in the inventory of a catheterization laboratory. However, the En Snare™ does not create as strong a grip as the Goose-Neck™ snare.

Similar to other foreign body retrieval systems, the En Snare™ is used through a large diameter, long sheath positioned adjacent to the foreign body. The use of this snare is similar to the use of the other snares and depends upon the type and location of the foreign body. The En Snare™ can be advanced forward over the foreign body or withdrawn over the object in order to grasp it. It is used to grasp loose ends or pieces of foreign bodies or to encircle the entire foreign body before grasping it. Positioning and maneuvering the En Snare™ adjacent to the foreign body depend upon the type and location of the foreign body.

Medi-tech™ snare

Medi-tech™ snares (Medi-Tech, Boston Scientific, Natick, MA) are commercially available snares made of memory spring-wire material. The snare loops are an elongated hexagon in shape. The hexagon extends out of the catheter at a slight angle to the long axis of the catheter. The snares come in two sizes—2.0 and 3.5 cms. This snare has a memory for the hexagon loop and the angle after closing and reopening. The Medi-tech™ snare is preferable when the tip of the foreign body extends into the lumen of the vessel or chamber from the side of the vessel—i.e. when the foreign body is more or less perpendicular to the long axis of the vessel and the shaft of the snare catheter. The use of the snare for capturing a foreign body is otherwise similar to that of the other snares.

The Welter™ retrieval loop catheter

The Welter™ Retrieval Loop Catheter (Cook Inc., Bloomington, IN) is a 5-French, braided catheter, which tapers to 4-French, non-braided segment at the distal end. The Welter™ catheter is 100 cm long and has a snare wire uniquely built into the distal 4-French end/side of the catheter. One end of the wire is embedded securely in the wall of the carrier catheter very close to its tip. The wire then wraps 360° around the circumference of the catheter just proximal to the tip and enters a hole in the side of the carrier catheter that is approximately 15 mm proximal to the distal attachment of the wire on the catheter. The wire then extends back through the lumen of the catheter and out of the proximal hub, where it is attached to a control handle. The control handle for the Welter™ loop is similar to the handle of the Amplatz™ deflector wire (Cook Inc., Bloomington, IN), with two fixed side rings and a movable central ring attached to the snare wire.

When the side rings on the control handle are pushed forward (away from the fixed central ring) on the handle, the wire loop extends out of the side of the carrier catheter near its tip. The 360° wrap around the catheter results in the open loop extending in a spiral that is perpendicular to the shaft of the catheter, while the separation of the attachment to the catheter and the entrance into the side of the catheter opens the loop along the long axis as well. The open loop is 15 mm in diameter. When the side rings of the handle are withdrawn toward the fixed central ring (or the central ring is pushed forward) the loop of the snare is retracted. The way the loop of this snare spirals out of the carrier catheter provides a combined perpendicular and parallel orientation of the loop to the shaft of the catheter, which gives it an advantage for the retrieval of foreign materials that have an unusual orientation in the vascular channel, although it provides little or no advantage over the En Snare™ or possibly the Multi-Snare™.

Multi-Snare™ (not approved in US)

The Multi-Snare™ (PFM, [Produkte für die Medizin AG] Cologne, Germany) snare is unique, with a double loop of memory-retention metal. The snare is configured so that the two loops, which are extruded together, cross and align perpendicular to each other. The most distal loop aligns perpendicular to the catheter shaft (and vessel), while the proximal loop aligns parallel to the catheter shaft. The loops cross at the junction between them, but are not attached at that junction, with the result that, as the loops are retracted into the carrier catheter, they "coalesce" into one loop. This allows an object to be grasped by either loop and yet be grasped tightly (similarly to a single loop snare). The two loops are adjustable to approximately 5 mm larger than their stated diameters. Standard Multi-Snares™ are available in 5, 10, 15 and 20 mm diameters and come in a 4-French carrier catheter for the 5 and 10 mm snares, a 5-French catheter for the 15 mm snare and a 6-French catheter for the 20 mm snare. All of the carrier catheters are 125 cm in length.

The two perpendicular loops can be used both for objects that align perpendicular and for objects that align parallel to the vessel and eliminate the need for a "double inventory" of both parallel and perpendicular snares. They also give this snare a great advantage in grasping the end of a foreign body that is mobile and is continuously changing its orientation in the vessel. For example, during the manipulation of the snare adjacent to a foreign body such as the end of a wire or catheter that extends into a large vessel or chamber and moves with each beat of the heart, one of the two loops always remains perpendicular to the end of the foreign body!

There are also micro sets of the Multi-Snare™, which have snare diameters of 2 mm (2–3 mm) and 4 mm (4–6 mm). These are available with 3-French, 175 cm long carrier catheters, which makes them applicable for the retrieval of foreign bodies (e.g. coils!) that have embolized into the very distal pulmonary artery branches, or retrieval from the coronary arteries.

Expro™ Retrieval Microsnare (Not approved in US)

Expro™ Retrieval Microsnares (Radius Medical Technologies, Maynard, MA) are very small diameter snares manufactured of a memory metal wire, which allows the snare to retain its shape after repeated withdrawals/extrusions into and out of the carrier catheter. When the loop is extruded, it angles 45° off the shaft of the catheter. The snare loop is comprised of two strands of fine spring memory wire welded together at their distal tips. The two wires are formed so that they separate when extruded and, in doing so, widen out from each other just proximal to the weld, forming a loop. The weld at the tip of the wires produces a very densely opaque tip of the snare, which is easily seen on fluoroscopy. Together the two wires of the loop are only 0.014″ in thickness creating a very small profile of the collapsed loop and allowing it to pass through catheters with very tiny lumens. The loops of the snare are 2, 4 and 7 mm in width.

Because of the very small size of this snare, it obviously has limited use for the retrieval of errant intracardiac devices. Its small size and the relatively stiff wires of the loop make it particularly useful in very small vessels and very tight vascular locations such as peripheral branch pulmonary arteries. The tip of the Expro™ snare can slide by a tightly embedded foreign body such as an embolized coil. Because of the small size of the wires, it is not particularly strong and, as a consequence, cannot be used to pull larger foreign bodies forcefully into sheaths even if a portion of the foreign body can be grasped. These small snares can be used to loosen a foreign body and withdraw it out of a very small or distal vessel so that the foreign object then can be grasped with a larger, stronger retrieval system.

Techniques of snare retrieval

The snare device is best suited for the removal of a loose or broken piece of catheter or wire where one end (preferably the more proximal end) is lying free in the lumen of a vessel or chamber. The Goose-Neck™ snare has been particularly useful for catching the proximal attaching hub of Amplatzer™ occlusion devices for their retrieval after their release. Snares are also useful for catching the free end of a guide wire which has been purposefully introduced from another vascular entry site in order to create a "through and through" loop or "rail" of wire for the delivery of specific devices.

With both home-made and commercial snares, the retrieving sheath should be significantly larger in diameter than the snare or carrier catheter—at least 2 to 4 French sizes larger. Larger sheaths allow foreign materials to be withdrawn into them more easily once snared, even when the object is folded or pulled against the side of the snare catheter. Extra large sheaths allow home-made snares to be introduced into them without deforming the home-made loops during the introduction into the sheaths or the introduction of the carrier catheter through a stiffening inner sheath/catheter. For the retrieval of pieces of guide wire or small catheters, a large diameter, pre-shaped, commercial guiding catheter can be used instead of a large long sheath. Guiding catheters have the advantages of being more maneuverable and having more rigid walls than long sheaths.

The long sheath or guiding catheter is positioned with the tip just proximal to the foreign body and preferably just proximal to a free end of the foreign body. The activation of the snare to capture the foreign body is completely different for home-made and commercially available snares.

The loop of a home-made snare, which is partially open, is introduced directly into the sheath along with the distal end of the carrier catheter. A detachable back-bleed valve, which the carrier catheter had previously been passed through and which is positioned on the shaft of the carrier catheter, is advanced over the carrier catheter and attached to the sheath as described above under building a home-made snare. With a home-made snare, the exposed, opened, but partially compressed loop of the snare that extends completely beyond the tip of the carrier catheter, is advanced through the long sheath to the tip of the sheath. The sheath, the enclosed partially opened loop of snare, and the carrier catheter are advanced until the entire loop of the snare, which is still within the sheath, is advanced *past* the foreign body. Once the loop is adjacent to or slightly past the foreign body, the sheath is withdrawn, exposing the opened loop of the snare.

A commercially available snare is withdrawn (and collapsed) completely into its carrier catheter, and the carrier catheter is introduced into the long sheath through a previously attached or incorporated back-bleed valve. The tip of the long sheath should already be positioned immediately proximal to the foreign body. The carrier catheter containing the enclosed, collapsed snare is advanced beyond the tip of the sheath and into the vessel immediately adjacent to or just beyond the exposed end of the foreign body. The control mechanism of the commercial snare is advanced (activated), which, in turn, extrudes and opens the loop of the snare.

The angle off the carrier catheter of the various snare loops extends the loop of the snare to a variable degree across the inner circumference of the particular vessel. While carefully observing on biplane fluoroscopy and adjusting the length and location of the carrier catheter or loop, the loop is manipulated around the loose end of the foreign body. This is accomplished by slight to-and-fro motions of the carrier catheter together with the loop of the snare while simultaneously gently torquing the carrier catheter from side to side.

Once the loop is around an end or a piece of the foreign body, the two free ends of the spring guide wire of the home-made snare or the single strand control wire of the commercial snare (at the proximal end of the catheter) are/is fixed in place. The carrier catheter is then carefully advanced over the loop of the snare. This tightens the loop around the loose end/part of the foreign body and pulls the closed loop with the encircled foreign body tightly against the distal end of the carrier catheter. It is important to advance the carrier catheter and not to withdraw the wire(s) of the loop when closing it around the foreign body. Withdrawing the wire(s) into the catheter pulls the loop of the snare off the foreign body before the loop has a chance to constrict around the foreign body. Once the loop has been tightened securely around the foreign body and the proximal end of the loop control mechanism is held or fixed securely with a clamp against the proximal end of the carrier catheter, the carrier catheter and the constricted loop of the snare with the attached piece of foreign body are withdrawn into the sheath.

If the open loop of a snare cannot be advanced around a portion of or over the foreign body from the more proximal end as described above, the commercial memory snares offer several alternative techniques for snaring the foreign body. A small carrier catheter can usually be advanced past the foreign body while the snare is still contained completely within the catheter. Once the tip of the carrier catheter is completely distal to the foreign body, the loop of the snare is opened. The open loop is then withdrawn within the vessel until it is against the foreign body from "behind" the more distal portion of the foreign body. Once the loop of the snare is against/around the foreign body, the snare loop is held in place while the carrier catheter is advanced to close the loop around the foreign body. The grasped foreign body is withdrawn into the sheath in the same fashion as when grasped from "in front".

The use of a separate additional "wire" provides a supplemental technique for grasping a foreign body, when the snare alone cannot grasp any part of it. This is the concept behind the Needle's Eye™ retrieval device (Cook Vascular Inc., Leechburg, PA), which is discussed in detail later in this chapter. A snare that has a perpendicular orientation to the carrier catheter, and a retrieval sheath that is large enough to accommodate a separate guide wire adjacent to the carrier catheter are required for this procedure. A significantly larger recovery sheath is beneficial since the foreign body is often gripped as a "mass" when using this adjunct technique. The carrier catheter with the enclosed snare is advanced out of the long recovery sheath and past the foreign body, and the snare opened just distal to the foreign body as previously described. The large recovery sheath is advanced against the foreign body. Initially, the soft end of a spring guide wire is introduced into the sheath adjacent to the carrier catheter and advanced to the tip of the sheath. From here, the guide wire is maneuvered into and through any opening in the foreign body and then through the open loop of the snare, which is positioned just distal to the foreign body. With the wire through the foreign body and into the loop of the snare, the snare is partially closed, withdrawn back against the foreign body, and then closed tightly.

Once the wire that is passing through the foreign body has been grasped, the combination of the snare, the additional wire and the foreign body is withdrawn into the tip of the recovery sheath. This occasionally requires that the extra wire bends 180° on itself. Occasionally the soft tip of a guide wire cannot be manipulated through a foreign body that is compacted in a small vessel. In that circumstance, either the guide wire is reversed and the stiff end of the guide wire is introduced into the long sheath and used to probe through the foreign body or a Terumo™ (Terumo Medical Corp., Somerset, NJ) wire is used to manipulate through the foreign body. In either case, when the stiff end of a wire is used to pass through the foreign body and is grasped distal to the foreign body, the foreign body along with the still *straight stiff wire* must be withdrawn with the stiff wire remaining straight. The stiff wire is not pulled in a 180° loop on itself before withdrawing it into the sheath, as is done with the soft end of the wire.

Once the foreign body is completely within the sheath, it is withdrawn through the sheath and out of the vessel. The techniques to help get the foreign body into the sheath or the removal from the vessel/skin when the foreign body cannot be drawn completely into the sheath are discussed previously under general retrieval techniques.

Special retrieval devices

Basket retrieval devices

Basket retrieval devices were designed initially for the removal of urinary or biliary stones, but have been adapted by individual cardiologists and have become indispensable for the retrieval of intravascular foreign bodies.

The baskets are comprised of three to five fine strands of stainless steel or other strong wire, which, when extruded out of their carrier catheter, form a helix or "basket" of fine wire strands. Each wire is pre-shaped to form a small, outward bend or curve at its distal end. The wires are welded together at their tips so that they bow away from each other proximally and form the helical basket as the wires are extruded from the tip of the catheter. The basket compresses completely as the catheter is re-advanced over the open wires.

The wires just proximal to the basket are attached together and the combined single strand of wire passes through the catheter and extends out of the hub at the proximal end of the catheter. In most basket devices, the proximal wire is attached to some sort of in/out control mechanism at the proximal hub. Pushing the wire into the proximal hub of the catheter extrudes the basket from the distal end of the catheter, while withdrawing the wire at the proximal hub of the catheter retracts and compresses the basket into the carrier catheter. The baskets come in various shapes, lengths and diameters. Some of them when open have parallel wire strands, but most have a spiral arrangement of the basket wires. These different arrangements of the wires permit slightly different uses. The basket components of retrieval baskets are between 6 and 10 cm in length. Because of the multiple wires of which the baskets are made, the large combined diameter of the compressed wires, and the length of the baskets, basket retrieval catheters/devices are usually larger and stiffer than most other retrieval devices.

All basket retrieval devices—like all other retrieval devices—are used through large diameter, long recovery sheaths, which have a valved, back-bleed device including a side arm flushing port. The long sheath should be at least 3 to 4 French sizes larger than the carrier catheter for the basket device in order to accommodate the foreign body that is being retrieved. The back-bleed device can be built onto the sheath or it can be detachable.

The Medi-tech™ retrieval basket

The Medi-tech™ retrieval basket (Medi-Tech, Boston Scientific, Natick, MA) is available in two sizes. Each basket is comprised of four wires, which form slightly spiraled baskets of 15 mm or 25 mm diameter. Both sizes are available in 5-French carrier catheters of either 120 or 150 cm in length. The control wire at the proximal end of the carrier catheter is attached to a plastic loop that is large enough to accommodate a finger.

The Segura basket™

The Segura™ basket (Medi-Tech, Boston Scientific, Natick, MA) is comprised of four flat wires that do not spiral as they bow out of the carrier catheter. The flat wires prevent torque of the basket when it is rotated and add strength to the wires, permitting them to dilate vessels slightly as they are opened. Segura™ baskets have a locking, slide mechanism to lock them in their open, partially open, or closed position. They are available as 16 and 20 mm diameter baskets, but only with 70 cm carrier catheters, which prevents their use in some more distant or peripheral locations. The 16 mm basket is available in a 4.5-French carrier catheter, while the 20 mm Segura™ basket is only available in a 7-French carrier catheter. The larger 20 mm basket has the advantage of having a 0.038″ lumen through the catheter and through both ends of the basket. This lumen allows the injection of contrast through the catheter/basket as well as the ability to pass a wire through the center of, and out through the tip of the basket. The additional wire passing through the basket adds an additional capability for trapping or holding foreign bodies.

The Dotter™ Intravascular Retriever

The Dotter™ Intravascular Retriever (Cook Inc., Bloomington, IN) was designed specifically for the retrieval of intravascular foreign bodies. This retriever has a large—3 cm diameter by 7 cm long—helical loop basket, which is comprised of 4 stainless steel wires, each of which spirals approximately 90°. The carrier catheter is 8-French, 95 cm long and made of radio-opaque TFE material. The common wire at the proximal hub has an attached torque handle to push and pull the basket in and out of the carrier catheter. This is the sturdiest of the basket devices, but also the largest and most rigid.

Techniques for basket retrieval

The very large diameter long sheath for the retrieval is positioned with the tip of the sheath in the precise vessel where the foreign body is resting and immediately adjacent to the foreign body. The sheath is fixed in this position using the various techniques described previously. The carrier catheter with the enclosed and retracted basket is introduced into the sheath through the back-bleed valve and is advanced through the sheath to its distal end. The carrier catheter with the basket still retracted within it is advanced *very carefully* out of the sheath until the tip of the catheter is beyond the foreign body so that the enclosed and still compressed basket lies side-by-side with the foreign body. The enclosed basket should be centered adjacent to the center of the mass of the foreign object. The maneuver of advancing the tip of the relatively large and stiff basket catheter past the foreign body has the potential for dislodging or pushing the foreign body further into the vessel. This is one of the disadvantages of basket retrieval devices. Occasionally it is necessary to withdraw the basket device completely out of the carrier catheter and to replace the basket with a flexible tipped, torque-controlled wire. The torque wire is manipulated past the foreign body and the carrier catheter for the basket is advanced over the wire. Once the carrier catheter has been advanced well past the foreign body, the guide wire is removed and the basket device is reintroduced into its carrier catheter.

With the basket fixed in position adjacent to the foreign body, the carrier catheter is withdrawn off the basket, allowing the basket to open next to (and around) the foreign body. The inherent "spring" of the wires of the basket in the open configuration forces them against the walls of the vessel or around the foreign body. The expanding wires of the basket necessitate that any loose or free portions of the foreign body will be positioned between the wires of the basket, as they spread out widely. Occasionally the entire foreign body becomes entangled within the wires of the basket. Catching the foreign body is facilitated by rotating the open basket along with a slight to-and-fro manipulation while the basket is adjacent to the foreign body. Once even a single wire of the basket seems to be around a part of the foreign body, the carrier catheter is advanced over the basket. This compresses the basket around the encircled portion of the foreign body and grasps it. Like the snare, if the basket is withdrawn into the carrier catheter when it is positioned over the foreign body, the basket will be pulled away from, rather than grasping, the foreign body.

A second technique with the basket retriever is only effective when using baskets that have spirally arranged wires. The carrier catheter with the basket still within it is advanced entirely past the foreign body so that the entire basket, including its proximal end, is beyond the foreign body. With the proximal end of the basket positioned beyond the foreign body, the carrier catheter is withdrawn while maintaining the basket fixed in position completely distal to the foreign object. This allows the basket to opened fully with it entirely distal to the foreign body. The opened basket and carrier catheter are withdrawn together. This pulls the open basket adjacent to the foreign body. As the basket is withdrawn into the area of the foreign body, its spiral wires encircle and trap any portion of the foreign body that extends into the vessel lumen. Once a portion of the foreign body is between any strands of the basket, the control wire and the basket are held in place or rotated slightly, while the carrier catheter is re-advanced over the basket, closing the basket around the foreign body.

There is a third alternative basket technique that is helpful when the foreign body cannot be grasped with either of the two previous techniques. The carrier catheter tip is positioned immediately proximal to the foreign body. The basket is advanced out of the carrier catheter passing adjacent to, partially through, or past the foreign body. As the basket exits the tip of the carrier catheter, it opens progressively as it is first proximal to, and then adjacent to, the foreign body. The relatively sharp tip of the basket "excavates" partially between the foreign body and the vascular wall. This usually allows at least one strand of the basket to encircle at least part of the foreign body. Again, rotation and to-and-fro motion of the basket as it is maneuvered adjacent to the foreign body facilitate entangling the foreign body with the basket. Once any loose piece or part of the foreign body has been encircled in the basket, the carrier catheter is advanced while the proximal wire of the basket is fixed in position or withdrawn slightly, keeping the relative positions of the basket and foreign material together as visualized on fluoroscopy. One or more of these procedures may have to be repeated many times to catch the foreign material securely enough to withdraw it into the long sheath.

It is usually helpful if the basket can be forced against the side of the foreign material while it is being closed—i.e. the basket is pushed against the foreign body by advancing the entire carrier catheter and basket against the foreign body. Producing this pressure against the foreign body is facilitated if the foreign body is lodged along the convex side of a curve in the chamber or vessel.

Once the foreign material has been caught in the basket, the basket is tightened securely around the foreign material by applying traction to the proximal control wire against the end of the carrier catheter. Once the foreign body has been grasped securely, the basket, catheter, and foreign material are withdrawn into the long sheath and from there out of the body.

The basket device is most useful when there is a loose end of a catheter or a discrete portion of the mass of foreign material protruding at least partially into the vessel or cardiac chamber. It is always helpful if the loose portion of the foreign body is more or less perpendicular to the long axis of the vessel and, therefore, to the basket catheter and device. Occasionally the helix of the basket is used to entrap the side of a loop of a catheter, wire, or larger foreign body when the basket is positioned adjacent to the foreign body with the tip of the basket positioned beyond the loose portion of the foreign body. The basket is also useful in grabbing larger objects such as errant PDA or ASD occlusion devices, which tend to fill the lumen of the vessel. The basket device has the additional advantages of actually compressing the bulk of a foreign body as it is collapsed, and of being much sturdier than most of the other retrieval devices. These features aid in withdrawing a foreign body into the sheath.

Once grasped in the basket, the errant foreign body is withdrawn completely into the sheath before drawing it out of the area where it had embolized. If the foreign body had been lodged in the venous circulation proximal to the heart or in the arterial circulation distal to the heart, an attempt is made at withdrawing it from the vascular system even if the foreign body or carrier catheter cannot be withdrawn completely into the sheath. The foreign body is cautiously drawn tightly up against and as far as possible into the distal end of the large recovery sheath. Once the leading edges of the foreign body (device!) are within the sheath and all acutely angled portions of the foreign body are directed away from the direction in which the sheath is being withdrawn, the entire sheath with the foreign body is withdrawn carefully through the vessels and back to the entrance site of the sheath into the vessel. Usually, if the free portions of the foreign body are angled away from the direction of withdrawal, they are flexible enough to allow withdrawal of the foreign body while it is being pulled against the tip of the sheath and out of the vessel and skin along with the sheath. The final removal of the foreign body out of the vessel and skin is facilitated with the use of a rigid, short retrieval sheath pre-positioned over the long sheath as described previously in this chapter.

At *no* time should a foreign body that is even partially free or open outside of the sheath after it has been grasped with a basket, be withdrawn through *valves* or *intracardiac structures*. Withdrawing *any* partially free foreign body through the right or left ventricle carries a very high potential risk of the irregular portions of the foreign body becoming trapped on or damaging the atrioventricular valve as it is withdrawn through the valve. When a foreign body lodged in a pulmonary artery has been grasped by the basket but cannot be *fully* withdrawn into the sheath, it is better to start the retrieval all over with a different "hold" on the foreign body with the basket. As hard as it is to consider doing, the foreign body is released near its original site. The original sheath is replaced with a much larger long sheath, which will have a better chance of accommodating the grasped foreign body. Then the retrieval procedure is begun all over again! It is obviously better to anticipate the necessary sheath size before introducing the original sheath and starting with an appropriate size or even an unnecessarily large sheath.

The very worst case scenario is to capture a large irregular foreign body in the pulmonary artery with a basket, then not be able to withdraw the foreign body into the sheath and, at the same time, *not be able to release* the foreign body from the retrieval system! This leaves a large irregular device exposed outside of the sheath, but at the same time "permanently" attached to the retrieval catheter. The retrieval system, which then passes from the vein, through the heart to the foreign body, will necessitate an open-heart surgical retrieval. This will most likely occur when the basket device becomes entangled very tightly with a more irregular foreign body such as a CardioSEAL™ type of double umbrella. This potential problem emphasizes the need for using a very large sheath to begin the retrieval procedure and for anticipating the problem. When this possibility is considered before attempting retrieval, it may be more reasonable not to even attempt a catheter retrieval of a large and irregular foreign body from the pulmonary artery.

Basket devices are preferable for the retrieval of larger foreign bodies and those which need some compressing or collapsing before they can be withdrawn. In general, they require a larger vessel or vascular chamber to work in in order to allow the basket to expand around the foreign body. As described earlier, the necessity of having to advance the carrier catheter or the basket past the foreign body in order to grab it, can dislodge the foreign body or push it deeper and more tightly into a smaller vessel. In spite of these shortcomings, basket retrieval devices are another essential instrument in the foreign body removal "arsenal".

Grasping™ or "grabber" forceps

The Grasping™ or grabber forceps (Medi-Tech, Boston Scientific, Natick, MA) is a tiny, four-pronged or legged, wire forceps, which is contained within a small, 5-French carrier catheter. The four metal legs of the forceps are made of fine (0.010″) stainless steel, spring wire. Each leg terminates in a tiny, acute, 90° bend, which faces inward when the spring wires spread apart from each other as they are extruded from the tip of the carrier catheter. As a consequence, these 0.5 mm long, acute, right angle bends at the distal end of each of the tiny legs create tiny hooks, which all face the center of the forceps at the tip of each wire leg. As the legs are extruded from the distal tip of the carrier catheter, they spread apart a maximum of 20 mm away from each other, flaring away from the central lumen into their open position. This flare away from the tip of the catheter creates a wire funnel toward the opening at the tip of the catheter. As the catheter tip is advanced over this wire funnel of the grabber, the distal ends of the four legs of the funnel are compressed progressively together. When completely withdrawn into the carrier catheter, the tiny angled tips of the legs actually overlap each other within the catheter when there is nothing grasped within them. The combination of the compression and the tiny hooks creates a very secure grasp on anything that is positioned between the wire legs before the catheter is advanced over the wires. The opening and closing is controlled by a coaxial wire which extends from the proximal ends of the four legs of the forceps at the distal tip of the catheter, and through the catheter as a bundle to a handle at the proximal end of the carrier catheter. Moving the handle in and out of the proximal hub of the carrier catheter extends and retracts the legs of the forceps at the distal end.

As is the case with the other retrieval devices, the Grasping™ forceps catheter is used through a large, long sheath, which is large enough in diameter (10–15-French) to accommodate the folded or crumpled foreign body once it has been grasped. This long sheath should have a valved back-bleed device (attached or detachable) that can accommodates the carrier catheter system. It is also desirable to pass the small, relatively thin carrier catheter of the Grasping™ forceps through a separate, stiffer and larger end-hole guiding catheter before introducing the carrier catheter into the sheath. The guiding catheter obviously must be slightly longer than the sheath but, at the same time, still shorter than the carrier catheter of the Grasping™ forceps. This stiffer, larger diameter guiding catheter allows the foreign material, once captured, to be drawn tightly against the stiffer guiding catheter, and prevents accordioning of the thin-walled carrier catheter and long sheath. As described earlier with regard to basket devices, the dilator from the long sheath with the tip excised can be used as this inner, stiff, guiding catheter.

Techniques for the use of the Grasping™ forceps retrieval catheter

The tip of the long, large sheath is positioned immediately proximal to the foreign body as previously described. When using the Grasping™ forceps, the tip of the sheath is positioned directly against the foreign body with the sheath aligned in the exact vessel containing the foreign body and as parallel to the long axis of the vessel as possible. The carrier catheter, with the Grasping™ forceps enclosed within it, is introduced through a separate back-bleed valve/flush device into an 8-F end-hole, guiding catheter. The carrier catheter is advanced within the larger catheter until the distal tips of the carrier catheter and the guiding catheter are together. This combination of the 8-French outer and the contained carrier catheter together is introduced through the back-bleed valve at the proximal end of the larger diameter long sheath, and advanced to the distal end of the sheath until the tips of the carrier catheter and the Grasping™ forceps catheter are immediately proximal to the foreign body. Occasionally, during the introduction of the Grasping™ forceps catheter through the sheath, as the combination of the larger, stiffer guiding and carrier catheters approaches the tip of the sheath, it starts to straighten, and dislodges the tip of the sheath away from the foreign body. In that circumstance, the larger 8-French, guiding catheter is fixed in place or even withdrawn slightly within the sheath, while only the smaller, more flexible carrier catheter containing the closed Grasping™ forceps is advanced to the tip of the sheath.

With the tip of the sheath and the tip of the carrier catheter in position adjacent to the foreign body, the sheath, the stiffer catheter, and the carrier catheter are held in place, while the control wire of the Grasping™ forceps is carefully advanced. The legs of the Grasping™ forceps begin to flare out immediately as they extend out of the tip of the catheter (and sheath) and, in turn, open against (and around) the proximal surface of the foreign body. The expanding legs of the Grasping™ forceps usually do not need to extend widely beyond the diameter of the sheath nor completely around the foreign body in order to grasp it. The opening of the Grasping™ forceps is performed very slowly in order not to move or push the foreign body or to open the legs of the Grasping™ forceps too widely.

Once the hooks of the opened legs are at least partially into or slightly around the foreign body, the carrier catheter alone is slowly and carefully advanced over the arms of the Grasping™ forceps while holding the control wire of the forceps at the proximal end of the catheter in a fixed position, keeping the open legs against the foreign body. This closes the legs of the Grasping™ forceps around or into the foreign body and grips it firmly. When grasped tightly with the Grasping™ forceps, the carrier catheter with the foreign body trapped in the forceps is pulled back against the tip of the sheath. If the larger end-hole, guiding catheter was not already at the end of the sheath, it is advanced through the sheath over the carrier catheter of the forceps, until it also is against the foreign body. The carrier catheter/Grasping™ forceps with the foreign body is pulled very tightly against the tip of the stiffer 8-French guiding catheter. While holding the foreign body tightly against the carrier catheter of the Grasping™ forceps and the stiffer guiding catheter, the two catheters with the foreign body are withdrawn completely into the sheath. If a tight enough hold on the foreign body was not achieved with the initial more conservative opening of the legs of the Grasping™ forceps around the foreign body, the legs of the forceps are extended further out of the sheath and further around the foreign body in order to grasp it securely enough to be withdrawn into the sheath.

Once the foreign body is completely within the sheath, it is withdrawn out of the body through the sheath. As with the previously described devices, the foreign body should not be withdrawn through either ventricle of the heart unless it has been withdrawn completely into the sheath. If the device is almost entirely within the sheath with only a tiny portion remaining out of the end of the sheath, then withdrawal through a ventricle vs. starting the retrieval all over requires an on-the-spot decision by the operator. If there is a consideration to withdraw a partially exposed foreign body through a ventricle, none of the protruding foreign body can be angled proximally or even at an acute angle to the long axis of the sheath, and none of the portion of the foreign body hanging out of the sheath can be rigid or stiff. This decision depends upon the nature of the material hanging out, how far it hangs out of the sheath, and what tissues the foreign body is to be withdrawn through.

The Grasping™ forceps catheter has the advantage of being able to grasp the side, end, or almost any part of almost any foreign body. This makes it essential for retrieving foreign bodies that have no loose ends or pieces extending from their surface. The Grasping™ forceps is very useful for retrieving coils that have embolized into a more distal vessel and are wedged as a "ball" with no end of the coil extending off the surface of the "wad" of coil. At least one arm of the Grasping™ forceps will bury into the wadded strands of the coil and grab at least one strand of the coil very securely.

However, there are several disadvantages of the Grasping™ forceps that must be considered before it is used. Once the hook of even a single arm of the Grasping™ forceps has attached onto any part of a foreign body, it tends to stay attached securely to the item and cannot easily be detached from it. This is a huge disadvantage when the foreign body is very large and cannot be withdrawn completely into the sheath and, at the same time, the tight hold on the foreign body prevents its release. The Grasping™ forceps also has a tendency to grab adjacent tissues, especially the walls of the adjacent vessel, along with the foreign body. This, unfortunately, occurs quite commonly, but, although disconcerting, the hook of the Grasping™ forceps usually catches only superficially on the endothelium of the vessel wall and essentially never causes any permanent sequelae. When the Grasping™ forceps does catch on tissues the only way to remove it is to forcibly tear it loose! One way to avoid catching on adjacent tissues is to have the sheath tip tight against the foreign body while opening the forceps. In this way the legs of the Grasping™ forceps do not open as widely, yet are usually able to dig into and grasp the foreign body securely.

If the foreign body is caught in, or even close to, a valve or there are other *intravascular devices* in the immediate area (occluders, stents, etc.), it is better ***not*** to use the Grasping™ forceps. If the forceps inadvertently catches on an adjacent device, the force necessary to pull it free from the device can easily dislodge it and create a new foreign body!

In spite of its shortcomings, the Grasping™ forceps is an indispensable part of the armamentarium of the interventional cardiologist and should be a part of every inventory of devices for foreign body retrieval.

Vascular retrieval forceps—the "Jaw"

The Vascular Retrieval Forceps™ (Cook Inc., Bloomington, IN), which is commonly referred to as the "Jaw", is a 3-French catheter with a tiny 5 mm long stainless steel "jaw" that recesses completely into the shaft of the catheter just proximal to its tip. The tiny jaw has two tiny teeth at its distal end. The jaw opens off one side of a carrier catheter with the opening of the jaw facing the distal end of the catheter. The jaw opens by means of a pivoting mechanism that pivots near the center of a bar similar to a seesaw as the bar crosses the catheter. The proximal end of the "seesaw" opens in the opposite direction on the opposite side of the catheter and is attached to a control wire by a short, hinged segment. The opening and closing of the jaw are controlled by a handle at the proximal end of the catheter, which functions similarly to the control handle of the small, 3-French Cook™ bioptome (Cook Inc., Bloomington, IN). There is a small button on the handle that moves a long, solid, control wire, which is attached to the proximal arm of the jaw, forward and backward as the button slides forward and backward in a groove on the handle. Moving the button forward along the handle opens the jaw and withdrawing the button closes it. To provide some flexibility to the catheter that contains the jaw, and to prevent the jaw from digging into the vessel walls, there is a short—one cm long—segment of flexible spring guide wire attached at the distal tip of the shaft of the catheter just distal to the jaw mechanism. The Retrieval Forceps™ catheters come in catheter lengths of 60, 100 and 135 cm.

Like the other retrieval devices, the Retrieval Forceps™ is used through a long sheath that is large enough in diameter to accommodate the grasped foreign body. The catheter that contains the jaw is the carrier catheter itself and there is no additional carrier catheter, however, as with the other retrieval systems, it is preferable to introduce the Retrieval Forceps™ catheter through a stiffer guiding catheter, which, in turn, is introduced into the large diameter long sheath. The guiding catheter supports the tip of the sheath and helps to prevent the sheath from "accordioning" on itself when a foreign body is being withdrawn into the sheath.

To use the Retrieval Forceps™, the long sheath is positioned with the tip of the sheath just proximal to the foreign body. The Retrieval Forceps™ catheter is advanced to the end of the sheath. As the Retrieval Forceps™ catheter is advanced out of the sheath the jaw is opened. The Retrieval Forceps™ catheter with the jaw opened is advanced into the surface or edge of the foreign body. As the open jaw abuts against the foreign body, the jaw is closed, grasping part of the foreign body with its teeth. When the foreign body has been gripped tightly, the Retrieval Forceps™ is pulled against the guiding catheter and then into the long sheath.

The Retrieval Forceps™ device has the advantages of being able to grasp the side of a wire, strut or catheter and of being able to pass readily into or adjacent to foreign bodies/devices positioned in very small vessels. It also does not tend to grasp adjacent tissues as commonly as the Grasping™ forceps does. The Retrieval Forceps™ is ideal for grasping embolized coils or pieces of wire or catheter that are orientated across, or even filling, a small vessel. This is another retrieval device that should be in the inventory of every interventional cardiologist who performs foreign body retrievals.

The Needle's Eye™ Snare

The Needle's Eye™ Snare (Cook Inc., Bloomington, IN) is a large, complex retrieval device/system manufactured from shape-retentive alloy. The Needle's Eye™ has two separate components, i.e. the "thread" and the "eye of the needle". It is contained within a 12-French carrier catheter and, in turn, is delivered through a 14-French long sheath.

The "eye" portion of the needle is somewhat similar to a standard snare in that the eye opens into a loop as it is extruded from the end of the carrier catheter. The eye is formed from a single strand of fairly thick "memory" metal wire, which in addition to forming a loop, bends back on itself to form a hook comprising the parallel wires and the end of the loop. When inside the carrier catheter, the loop is held more or less straight, but when completely extruded from the carrier catheter and unconstrained by it, the hook curves almost 180° back on itself toward the tip of the carrier catheter, giving it an appearance almost like a cobra head (Figure 12.1a). The space between the two wires forms the eye of the needle.

In addition to the hooked loop of the snare, the Needle's Eye™ device also has a separate wire or "thread" that is an integral part of the device. A single straight strand of relatively stiff memory metal wire (the thread) is extruded separately from the tip of the carrier catheter by advancing a control wire at the proximal end of the catheter. Because of the approximation of the catheter tip to the end, or eye, of the hook, the straight wire passes between the two strands of wire or through the eye, "threading the needle" (Figure 12.1b). The separate wire or thread is extended out of the tip of the carrier catheter after the hook has encircled the foreign body. The needle is threaded through the eye of the snare and the foreign body is totally encircled and grasped very securely. The mechanism of the Needle's Eye™ is similar to the use of a separate guide wire in conjunction with a standard snare.

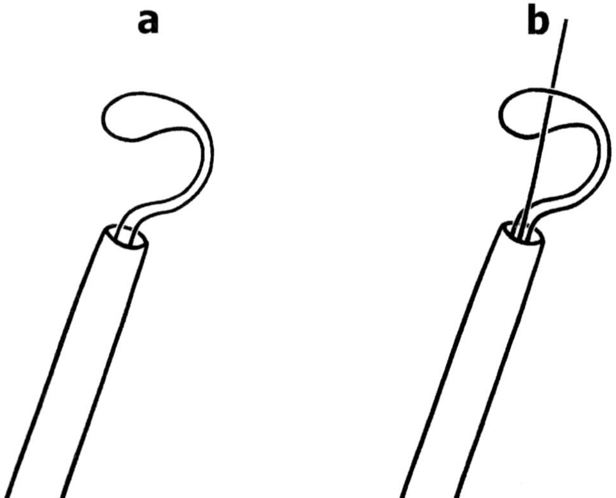

Figure 12.1 Needle's Eye Retrieval device. (a) Loop and hook of eye when extruded from tip of catheter; (b) separate needle advanced out of catheter and through loop of eye.

The hook configuration is formed as the wire loop is extruded out of the carrier catheter, and as the wires are withdrawn into the catheter, the hook straightens and the two side strands of the loop are compressed together. As this stiff, double loop of wire is being extruded out of the end of the catheter and is forming the hook, the stiff, curved loop can actually excavate forcefully under, and encircle, a foreign body that is buried in the tissues. As it completes the 180° loop, the end of the hook approaches the distal open tip of the carrier catheter. The space between the two wires of the curved loop, which is now almost back against the tip of the carrier catheter, forms the eye of the needle. The curved wires of the hook of the device passing behind the foreign body, and the straight thread passing on the opposite side of the foreign body, completely encircle it. The "circle" of the looped wires around the foreign body is tightened against the straight, stiff thread as the curved hook is withdrawn back into the carrier catheter, creating an extremely secure hold on the foreign body.

This system was originally designed for, and is still used primarily as, part of a "lead extraction kit" for the removal of old or non-functioning intracardiac pacemaker leads. The very strong materials and large size of the Needle's Eye™ system make it very effective for grasping and extracting large leads that have become securely embedded in the tissues. Although designed specifically for lead extractions, the Needle's Eye™ device can be used for any other large, securely embedded, foreign body.

The Needle's Eye™ is used through a long 14-French sheath, which comes as part of the lead retrieval set. When used for lead retrieval or other foreign body removal, the large sheath is positioned abutting the lead or other foreign body. The carrier catheter for the Needle's Eye™ is advanced to the tip of the sheath and fixed in a position also abutting the lead or other foreign body. While holding the tip of the carrier catheter against the foreign body, the curved wires of the hook or eye of the needle are extruded somewhat forcefully out of the tip of the catheter. The built-in curvature and the very stiff wire allow the hook to excavate under, and encircle, the foreign body as the wire hook is extruded. Once the hook has successfully encircled the foreign body and the end (or eye) of the hook has been positioned adjacent to the tip of the

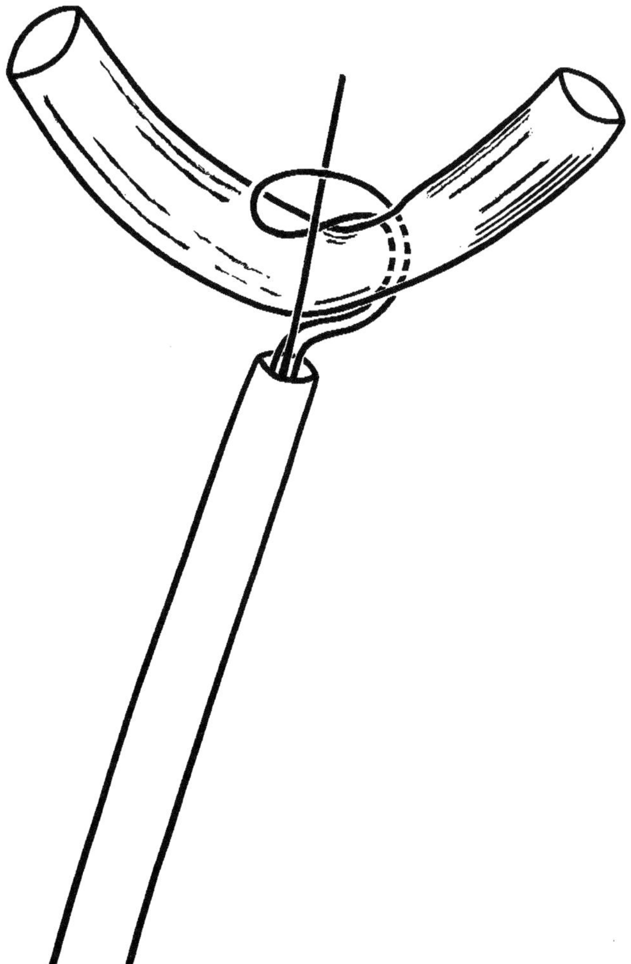

Figure 12.2 Needle and eye encircling a piece of catheter.

carrier catheter, the straight thread wire is advanced out of the carrier catheter and through the eye of the hook. The hook is then withdrawn into the carrier catheter and, in turn, tightens against the thread wire on the opposite side of the foreign body, thus encircling and grasping the foreign body very securely (Figure 12.2).

The Needle's Eye™ snare is the strongest of the retrieval systems and the most likely to be able to dislodge securely embedded foreign bodies. This same characteristic makes this device more dangerous to use. In addition to being very large in diameter, the entire system is very stiff. When the hook is extruded, the wire loop of the hook is capable of digging into the tissues as well as excavating around foreign bodies. As a consequence, perforations are certainly possible both while extruding the hook and when pulling the foreign body loose. The Needle's Eye™ system is very strong, and the grip on a foreign body is very tight and secure. Any tissues around a foreign body that grip it securely will tear before the Needle's Eye™ mechanism releases or gives way, so there is a real danger of tearing vital tissues when extracting a foreign body forcefully with the Needle's Eye™ device. At the same time, the Needle's Eye™ can be released more readily from a grasped foreign body. The hook of the device is re-advanced to loosen it, the thread wire is withdrawn, and then the hook can usually be withdrawn from around the foreign body.

Adjunct devices for foreign body retrieval

There are several other catheter accessories or catheter devices that are designed primarily for other uses which, however, are very useful adjunct devices for the retrieval of foreign bodies. These accessory devices are usually used in conjunction with another specifically designed retrieval device/system. The most commonly used of these adjunct devices are the bioptome forceps and the Amplatz™ controllable deflector wires (Cook Inc., Bloomington, IN).

Bioptome forceps

Relatively large bioptome forceps (6- or 7-French) are used as an adjunct in the retrieval of many foreign bodies. The bioptome is frequently used to loosen, to reorient or to "expose" part of a trapped foreign body so that it can be grasped with another, stronger retrieval device, although occasionally the complete retrieval can be accomplished with the bioptome. The bioptome has the one major advantage of being able to grasp the side or a small portion of a foreign body without the necessity of encircling it completely. Similar to the other retrieval systems, the bioptome is used through a large diameter, long sheath with a back-bleed valve and a side arm flush port. The sheath should be 3–4 French sizes larger than the bioptome catheter in order to accommodate the grasped foreign body.

The long sheath is delivered, as previously described, to a position where the tip of the sheath is pressed against, and abutting a portion of the foreign body. This usually will be against a portion that extends off the surface of the main mass of the foreign body. Keeping the sheath in this position the bioptome is advanced in the sheath until the tip of the bioptome is just within the tip of the sheath. The bioptome jaws are opened as wide as possible *within the tip of the sheath* and maintained in the maximum open configuration as the bioptome catheter is advanced out of the tip of the sheath. As the bioptome extends beyond the end of the sheath, the jaws open further and completely. The opened jaws are now forced against the loose or protruding piece of foreign body, and as the bioptome is advanced, this piece of foreign body becomes forced within the open jaws. If the bioptome jaws are not positioned exactly over the piece of foreign body, the sheath and the bioptome catheter are maneuvered together until the open jaws can be pushed against the desired portion of the foreign body. By continuing to advance the bioptome catheter with some forward force as the jaws are closed, the force is applied against the foreign body and the jaws close around a part of the foreign body. Once the jaws have gripped the loose piece of foreign body tightly, an attempt is made to withdraw the bioptome catheter with the attached foreign body into the sheath and completely out of the body through the sheath. The withdrawal is observed on fluoroscopy to ensure that the foreign material does not become dislodged within the sheath.

Because of the small size of the "mouth" and the smooth but sharp jaws of the bioptome, it is only usable with small diameter pieces of catheters or other foreign bodies of fairly small diameter, such as errant guide wires. When the foreign material is too large or rigid, the bioptome jaws tend to slip off the foreign body. Although the bioptome may not be able to grasp the foreign body securely enough to retrieve it completely, it can often dislodge an edge or part of the foreign body enough for another retrieval device to grasp it more securely. The bioptome is most effective on pieces of foreign material that can be crushed partially by the bioptome jaws such as a piece of catheter, wire or small intravascular plastic tubing. At the same time, the grasped material cannot be too soft. Bioptome blades are designed for cutting rather than grasping, and if the foreign material is too soft, the bioptome cuts through the material creating several pieces instead of the original one piece of foreign material! The bioptome is most useful when the foreign body is wedged very far distally in a small vessel or when only the side of an errant catheter, wire, or tubing is accessible with no free ends protruding into the vessel lumen. The bioptome is particularly useful for retrieving or unwinding coils that have embolized to the distal pulmonary arteries.

The bioptome may not develop a strong enough grip to pull the foreign material completely into the sheath or completely free of the surrounding tissues without cutting it, however, the bioptome is still very useful for dislodging or moving a foreign body from one area to another. It is also useful for dislodging and then holding a piece of foreign material in a fixed position, allowing the foreign material to be grasped with another retrieval device.

For example, a partially opened snare can be introduced over a bioptome catheter that is holding a piece or the edge of a foreign body. The snare loop is advanced into the large long sheath with the partially opened loop of the snare positioned around the bioptome catheter, while the snare catheter passes through the sheath adjacent to the bioptome catheter. As the snare loop is advanced out of the distal end of the sheath, the snare is opened widely and advanced over the piece of foreign material which is already grasped by the jaws of the bioptome. Once past the jaws and now over the foreign body, the loop of the snare is constricted around the foreign body. The foreign body is withdrawn into the sheath while it is grasped by both the bioptome and the snare, or by the snare alone after it has been released from the bioptome.

A bioptome type apparatus with toothed or slightly serrated jaws would be a great adjunct for foreign body retrieval. This would allow a secure grasp directly on the side of the foreign material and diversify the use of a bioptome as a retrieval tool. Even without serrated jaws, a bioptome is a frequent adjunct device in the retrieval of foreign bodies.

Amplatz™ controllable deflector wire

The common Amplatz™ controllable deflector wire (Cook Inc., Bloomington, IN) with a distal curve radius of 10 mm is another very useful device that can be used as an adjunct during foreign body retrieval. Although designed specifically for "bending" or deflecting intravascular catheters, the smaller 0.021″ or 0.025″ deflector wires form a tight curve which creates a 360°, or greater, pigtail type loop when deflected maximally *outside* of a catheter. The deflector wire is most useful for dislodging or moving embedded foreign bodies rather than for actually retrieving them. A deflector wire that is curved around an errant catheter or other foreign body usually does not hold the catheter or foreign body tightly enough to withdraw it completely. Often, however, the deflector wire can be used either to loosen or to fix a free floating foreign body/catheter enough to allow one of the other retrieval devices to grasp the foreign body more securely. The deflector wire is best suited in the situation where neither end of the foreign body is free or only the middle or side portion of an embolized tubing, wire or catheter is accessible to the retrieval system.

The Amplatz™ deflector wire is used through an end-hole carrier catheter that is long enough to pass completely through the long, large diameter retrieval sheath that is being used. A catheter with good torque control and a stiff shaft facilitates the maneuvering of the deflector wire into a position for grasping the foreign body. The deflector wire is introduced through a wire back-bleed valve/flush port on the carrier catheter in order to prevent bleeding around the wire, clots within the catheter, and binding of the wire within the catheter. The distal end of the deflector wire must be able to extend far enough beyond the tip of the carrier catheter (2–4 cm) for the "deflected" portion of the wire to form a complete 360° loop. The long carrier catheter is introduced through a back-bleed valve of a valve/side flush port on the proximal hub of the long retrieval sheath, which must be large enough to accommodate the grasped foreign body and the catheter for the deflector wire as well as another retrieval device/catheter.

The 0.021″ and 0.025″ wires usually form tight 360° loops, however these loops are not very strong, and straighten out if much force is applied to them. The larger diameter deflector wires form stronger loops, but they usually do not form as complete or tight a 360° curve around the foreign body. Because of their minimal strength, deflector wires are used primarily for freeing or reorienting pieces of foreign bodies, wires, catheters or tubing when there is no free end of the foreign body available. Once loosened, a freed end or tip of the foreign body or catheter can be grasped more securely by one of the previously discussed retrieval devices.

When using a deflector wire to grasp a foreign body, the long retrieval sheath is positioned with its tip adjacent to, and *perpendicular to* the piece of catheter, wire, or other foreign material. The catheter that carries the deflector wire is introduced into the sheath and manipulated out of the sheath to a position immediately adjacent to the catheter, wire, or other foreign body that is to be removed. The deflector wire is then introduced through the catheter and advanced out of the tip of the carrier catheter, adjacent to and eventually beyond the errant piece of foreign body. The carrier catheter, deflector wire and deflector handle are rotated so that the concave surface of the carrier catheter (and hopefully the deflector wire) faces the foreign body. When oriented in this direction and the handle of the deflector wire is activated, the concavity of the curve of the deflector wire curves around the piece of foreign body as the wire is advanced further.

When the loose piece of foreign body is definitely within the curve of the deflecting wire, the deflector handle is tightened maximally. With the end of the tip of the deflector wire free outside of the catheter, this allows the wire to create a tight, greater than 360° loop around the loose piece, thus encircling it within the tightened loop. While maintaining a tight grip on the deflector handle, the carrier catheter is advanced against the tip of the deflector wire, which is curved tightly back on itself and holding the piece of foreign body. When the tip of the carrier catheter is forced against the 360° loop of wire, it tends to "lock" the curve on the wire. The combination deflector wire, carrier catheter and foreign body is withdrawn toward and, if possible, into the sheath. If the loop of the deflector wire has a tight grip on the foreign body and the tip of the curve on the deflector wire is entirely within the sheath, the entire unit is withdrawn through and out of the sheath. If, on the other hand, the grip on the foreign body is loose or slipping, once the foreign body is within the sheath, it is better to remove the entire retrieval system, including the long sheath, together as a single unit.

As with all of the other foreign body retrievals, if the foreign body or any portion of it that is grasped by the loop of the deflector wire is still outside of the sheath, it should *not* be withdrawn through a ventricle. If the entire loop of the deflector wire or the loose piece of foreign body cannot be withdrawn completely into the sheath, the combined sheath, catheter, deflector wire and foreign body as a unit is withdrawn very slightly within the distal vessel until one end or a piece of the foreign body is free. Once a part of the foreign body is loosened or the foreign body is in a location where another retrieval device can be used, a second, "true" retrieval device is introduced to grasp the foreign body. The "true" retrieval device can be passed through the same long sheath or through a separate, large diameter, long sheath. When the foreign body is difficult to grasp with the curved deflector wire or is in a precarious location, a separate sheath with the new retrieval device is introduced while the foreign body is held with the deflector wire. A tight enough grip then can be created on the dislodged foreign material with the specific retrieval device to allow its withdrawal into the new sheath.

An Amplatz™ deflector wire can be used adjacent to a true retrieval system or device as part of the planned retrieval system. When a foreign body appears to be tightly embedded, the true retrieval system is introduced simultaneously with the deflector wire with the loop of the snare pre-positioned over the deflector wire before the two are introduced into the long sheath. The snare and the deflector wire are advanced out of the tip of the sheath together. Once the deflector wire is adjacent to, or passes through, the foreign body, a loop is created on the deflector wire and then tightened, as a result of which it partially grabs and loosens the foreign body. Once an end or a loose piece of the foreign body has been freed, the snare is opened completely and advanced around or over the foreign body and the curved deflector wire that is grasping it. Once the foreign body has been grasped securely with the snare, the curve on the deflector wire can be relaxed to straighten and release the deflector from the foreign body. The loosened and now straight deflector wire can be withdrawn from the foreign body, into, and then out of the sheath.

Occasionally, after the foreign body has been held tightly for some time, the deflector becomes entangled with the snare and/or the curve of the deflector wire does not straighten, even after the tension on the deflector handle has been released. When the deflector wire cannot be withdrawn from the foreign body or becomes entrapped within the second retrieval device, the deflector wire and the true retrieval device, along with the foreign body, which is held by both devices, are withdrawn together into the sheath. This does require a slightly larger diameter retrieval sheath.

A third alternative is to release the deflector wire completely once even a part of the foreign body has been freed by the deflector wire and before the true retrieval device is introduced. The loosened foreign body is released from the curve of the deflector wire and the deflector wire is removed from the long sheath. The true retrieval device is introduced through the same long sheath and used to grab the now loosened piece of foreign body.

Combinations of retrieval devices

Each of the various retrieval devices has a unique application for different types and orientations of foreign bodies, as described previously in this chapter. However, the various retrieval devices are frequently used together. This was discussed briefly under "adjunct devices" but holds true for any combination of the "true" retrieval devices. One device may be used to loosen or reorient a foreign body so that a different device can obtain a stronger grip or better orientation on it. The second device may be used in addition to, and simultaneously with, the first one to obtain an even stronger grip on a tightly fixed foreign body.

Pacemaker lead extraction—specialized "foreign body" removal

Pacemaker leads are deliberately implanted very securely in the myocardium. In this sense, they are not an errant or embolized foreign body. However, an intravascular pacemaker lead can be fractured and no longer function to sense or pace the heart. As such, they serve no positive function and at the same time act as a source of thrombi, mechanical irritation to the heart and heart valves, and act as a nidus for bacterial growth and endocarditis. In most cases an attempt is made to remove intravascular pacemaker leads when they are no longer functional. The transvenous pacemaker lead is usually larger than an errant piece of intravenous catheter, wire, or tubing, and it has been fixed very securely into the myocardium of the heart. Pacemaker leads have usually been in place in the vascular system for very long periods of time, which increases their adherence to the surrounding structures throughout their course through the vasculature. All of these peculiarities of pacemaker leads make their retrieval unique and complex, and have resulted in the development of some very specialized equipment for their retrieval.

The removal of intracardiac pacemaker leads is performed only by individuals specifically trained in the use of the specialized equipment and in the techniques of pacemaker lead extraction. This often involves the combined efforts of the electrophysiologist and the interventionist. The tools for freeing up the leads are unique and are designed especially for this procedure. The intravascular leads become tightly encased in dense fibrous tissues (old clot!). This fibrous adherence often extends from the site of entrance of the lead into the more peripheral vein, along the entire course of the lead through the vein, to the attachment within the heart.

The special tools for the "excavation" and freeing-up of the encased lead from the surrounding adherent fibrous tissues include large diameter, thin walled metal sheaths (Cook Inc., Bloomington, IN) and more recently, large diameter, long "Laser™" cutting sheaths (Spectranetics, Colorado Springs, CO)[4]. Laser™ sheaths emit a laser cutting beam from around the entire circumference of the tip of the sheath. They require a very large and expensive Laser™ generator (Spectranetics, Colorado Springs, CO). The Laser™ sheath has the advantage over thin-walled metal sheaths of being more flexible, and it can follow the lead through its curved course in the vein. Also, with the Laser™'s cutting capabilities, somewhat less brute force is required to push it over the encapsulated lead within the vein.

The lead extraction procedure requires a cut-down at the site of the previous, old, scarred cut-down where the lead was originally introduced, and where it enters the vein from the subcutaneous tissues. The entrance site of the lead into the vein is where the lead extraction equipment is introduced. This cut-down is usually in continuity with the surgically formed "pacemaker pocket" and the old pacemaker generator, which is usually removed or replaced. The retrieval sheaths and dilators that are used are larger than much of the comparable equipment used for other transcatheter foreign body retrieval procedures. One piece of large, specialized retrieval equipment developed for lead extraction is the locking stylet and sheath that is now commercially available as the Needle's Eye™ Snare (Cook Vascular Inc., Leechburg, PA), which has already been discussed in this chapter[5,6]. The Needle's Eye™ is particularly useful for "digging" under a lead or catheter that is embedded in the wall of a chamber or large vein.

The first part of the lead extraction procedure is the loosening of the lead from the scarred adhesions along its course from its more peripheral entrance into the vein, centrally through the vein, and to the fixation point in the heart. The cut-down for the lead extraction is usually on the anterior chest wall in the area of the subclavian vein. The lead is freed-up from the subcutaneous tissues outside of the vein and back to the previously implanted pacemaker by blunt and sharp dissection. The lead is disconnected from the pacemaker and the connector is excised from its proximal pacemaker end. The snare end of a special wire snare is introduced from the proximal end of the large extractor sheath and passed completely through the extractor sheath. The extractor sheath can be either a short metal extractor sheath or, preferably, a Laser™ extractor sheath, depending upon the particular circumstances and the preference of the operator.

The freed end of the pacemaker lead is grasped securely with the snare wire and pulled into the distal end of the extractor sheath while still outside of the body. Tension is applied to the snare and, in turn, the freed end of the lead, as the extractor sheath is advanced over the lead and to and into the vein, which is opened with a small incision. While maintaining traction on the snare catheter (and lead), the extractor sheath is forced into the vein and used to cut around the lead, which is encased in scar or old thrombus along its course in the vein. This process requires considerable to-and-fro as well as drilling motion on the extractor sheath, while continually holding tension on the proximal end of the snare wire. As the extractor sheath advances further over the encased lead in the vein and disappears into the vein, eventually the original free end of the lead appears at the proximal end of the extractor sheath. Only the more flexible Laser™ sheath can be used once the subclavian/innominate vein makes its turn caudally into the superior vena cava toward the heart. With the Laser™ sheath, intermittent laser energy is delivered to the tip of the sheath as this pushing/drilling process along the lead is carried out. This procedure is continued along the entire course of the lead through the vein until the lead has been freed all of the way to its attachment in the myocardium.

Once the extractor sheath has reached the "tine" or attachment mechanism of the lead into the myocardium of the heart, the process is continued, but with considerably less force and more cautiously. Ideally, the tip of the extractor sheath will drill just *to* the tip of the lead within the myocardium but no further. Specifically, the tip of the extractor sheath must not drill *through* the myocardium! While holding the long, stiff sheath in this fixed position even more tension is applied to the proximal end of the lead in an attempt to free the lead from the surrounding myocardium. When the lead has been freed from the myocardium, it is withdrawn through the long sheath. If the lead cannot be withdrawn from its attachment in the myocardium and, particularly, if the lead begins to unravel or otherwise come apart, then a secondary technique for withdrawing the lead must be used.

Once the entire course of the lead has been dissected free from the surrounding tissues with the extractor sheath, most of the remaining extraction of the lead is performed from the femoral venous approach. The 14-French sheath of the Needle's Eye™ snare set (Cook Vascular Inc., Leechburg, PA) is introduced from a femoral vein and advanced to a position adjacent to and perpendicular to the side of the loosened lead and as close to the attachment in the myocardium as possible. The tip of the Needle's Eye™ sheath will be in either the right atrium or the right ventricle, depending upon the type of lead being extracted. The Needle's Eye™ snare in its carrier catheter is introduced through this sheath and advanced to the tip of the sheath. The carrier catheter and sheath are maneuvered so that they are touching the side of the lead. The hook of the snare is extruded while simultaneously maneuvering it completely around a free portion of the lead. Once the hook has encircled the lead completely, the thread wire is extruded and advanced through the eye at the tip of the hook (see Figure 12.2). When the eye has been threaded, the hook is withdrawn back into the carrier catheter. This grips the lead very tightly and allows a portion of the grasped lead to be folded on itself and withdrawn into the large sheath. The lead is withdrawn as far as possible into the sheath. By pulling the more proximal lead into the sheath, the tip of the large, long retrieval sheath is pulled against the attachment of the lead in the myocardium. This occurs particularly when the proximal end of the lead has been disrupted or completely withdrawn away from the attachment in the myocardium by the previous manipulations. The side of the lead can still be withdrawn into the sheath, even when the proximal end of the lead is intact and passing out through the superior vena cava and the subclavian vein.

Considerable force with intermittent torsion is applied to the Needle's Eye™ retrieval device that is grasping the embedded lead while counter force is applied by holding or pushing the tip of the sheath over the lead and against the myocardium. This is usually sufficient to pull the lead attachment out of the myocardium. Occasionally, the lead is disrupted further by these forces, leaving a loose segment attached to the myocardium with the free end dangling in the cavities of the right heart. In that circumstance, the Needle's Eye™ retriever is replaced with a basket retrieval device through the same large, long sheath. The basket is manipulated to open around the free end of the lead. The lead is grasped while closing and rotating the basket and, again, as much of the grasped lead as possible is withdrawn into the sheath. Considerable traction and some torque are applied to the basket while the tip of the sheath is pushed against the myocardium to free the lead.

Obviously, there are considerable and sometimes poorly directed forces necessary during this procedure for lead extraction. Also there is no direct control over where the long extractor sheath containing the Needle's Eye™ excavates between the lead and the vessel or chamber wall—only that the lead was originally within the vessel or chamber and hopefully the extractor also remains close to the lead and completely within the channel. All of these factors make the extraction of pacemaker leads a fairly dangerous procedure. In fact, because of the dense adherence of the lead to the vascular wall and the tight, often deep fixation of the tip of the lead in the myocardium, it is not a question of whether there will be a complication from a pacemaker lead extraction, but rather, when. Cardiovascular surgical facilities must be available immediately during the extraction of all transvenous pacemaker leads because of the probability of a major vascular or cardiac perforation.

Special foreign body circumstances

The extensive use of coils and other devices in the PDA, the larger intravascular stents, and the large occlusion devices for both atrial and ventricular septal defects have created a whole new generation of intravascular foreign bodies. When any of these devices become free floating in the circulation, they create an entirely different challenge for foreign body removal. The handling and removal of these devices are covered in the specific chapters dealing with each device, and are not repeated in this section.

Intravascular thrombi and mechanical thrombectomy

Although, strictly speaking, intravascular thrombi/emboli do not represent a foreign body, they do constitute intravascular masses that often need to be dissolved or removed urgently. Intravascular thrombi can be the consequence of vascular stenosis with obstruction, localized vascular trauma, underlying low blood flow situations, the presence of a foreign body in the vasculature, hypercoagulable states, or a combination of any or all of the above causes. As a consequence of a high index of suspicion combined with better imaging modalities, acute thrombosis of large vessels can now be detected early, but unless always considered, will go undetected. Better imaging, the very complex surgical repairs now being performed, particularly in the venous circulation, the more frequent intravenous therapy through indwelling lines that are in place over long periods of time, and the extensive manipulations in the vascular system with large catheters/sheaths, may account for what appears to be an increase in large vessel thrombi/occlusions. When a large vessel thrombus is detected, the earlier definitive management is started, the better the chance of removing the thrombus and maintaining or restoring patency of the vessel.

Thrombolytics are quite effective at "dissolving" thrombi, however, they are less reliable and slower than mechanical removal, which in the presence of "visible" thrombi, is more rapid and more definitive than thrombolytic therapy alone. Thrombolytic therapy can be used as a general systemic infusion, infused directly into the thrombus, or it can be used in conjunction with a mechanical thrombectomy device. When used alone, thrombolytic medications are most effective when infused directly into the thrombus. Thrombolytic therapy is covered in Chapter 2 on medications.

There are a variety of thrombectomy devices which, in one way or another, fragment large thrombi into minute particles. Some of the devices fragment thrombi into particles that are similar in size to, or smaller than, blood cells, which allows the debris to circulate, while some of the devices also (attempt to) extract all (most of) the debris created by the fragmentation. Only one of the current devices that are available for the removal of thrombi from large vessels has a "distal protection" capability of capturing larger fragments that may be dislodged while the thrombus is being fragmented into micro particles or withdrawn.

The original thrombectomy device was the fairly straightforward, Fogarty™ balloon (Edwards Lifesciences, Irvine, CA), which is very effective for extracting thrombi from peripheral vessels. The Fogarty™ device is a small balloon mounted at the distal end of a 4-French catheter similar to a very small Swan™ balloon (Edwards Lifesciences, Irvine, CA). The catheter with the balloon deflated is usually introduced into the thrombosed vessel by means of a cut-down on the vessel. The tip of the catheter with the balloon deflated is advanced past the thrombus. The balloon is inflated and the catheter is withdrawn from the vessel, which pulls the now trapped thrombus, which is adjacent to the catheter and proximal to (in front of) the balloon, back in the vessel. The trapped thrombus is withdrawn through the incision in the vessel or skin and out of the body. This is still an effective procedure for removing thrombi from peripheral vessels, although it has been supplemented by the use of thrombolytics and other more sophisticated thrombectomy devices.

The simplest and one of the earliest and most readily available of the central thrombectomy devices was a catheter with suction applied to it[7]. Using the same principal, but using a long, large diameter (11–16-French) sheath instead of a catheter, makes this technique even more effective and very useful. When a small or fresh thrombus is detected within the vasculature, it can often be withdrawn from the intravascular site by positioning the tip of the large diameter sheath immediately adjacent to the thrombus and then applying a strong vacuum with a large volume (60+ ml) syringe to the proximal end of the sheath. This is frequently sufficient to suck a loose thrombus into the sheath. Large sheaths are readily available and usually require no additional (or expensive) equipment. Occasionally the thrombus must be fragmented or dislodged with a separate catheter, wire, or basket device. A basket retrieval device can be used to try to grasp the thrombus, but usually it tends to slice through the thrombus. Distal embolization is always a potential problem with this type of thrombus retrieval, but if performed expeditiously, can prevent significant further problems from very large thrombi. In addition to these improvised thrombectomy devices there is a variety of commercially manufactured devices.

The Helix Clot Buster™ (ev3, Plymouth, MN) is a pneumatic turbine driven impeller device that has been available for over a decade. The impeller has a rotating helical screw which is contained within a capsule at the distal tip and rotates at 100,000 rpm. The rotating screw creates a very strong vortex of fluid, which macerates the thrombus into particles between 13 and 1000 microns in diameter. The capsule of the Helix Clot Buster™ device is 7-French and it is not introduced over a wire, which makes it more difficult to maneuver into more remote or tortuous locations unless it is introduced through a long pre-positioned sheath. There is no extraction system with the Helix Clot Buster™ with the result that it depends entirely upon all of the resultant fragments being small enough to pass through any distal capillary bed! This makes this device less desirable for use in the systemic arterial circulation.

The Thrombex™ device (Edwards Lifesciences, Irvine, CA) is another rotating helical screw that macerates the thrombus, but it then aspirates the thrombus into an evacuation container. The Thrombex™ is mounted on a 6-French catheter, which makes it usable in smaller patients. Even with built-in aspiration of the debris, there is still a potential for some distal embolization.

The AngioJet™ (Possis Medical, Inc., Minneapolis, MN) macerates the thrombus with multiple, extremely high-velocity jets of saline, which are directed backward from openings adjacent to the tip of the catheter. The high-velocity jets create a partial vacuum by a Bernoulli effect, which sucks the fragments out of the circulation through a separate lumen in the catheter. The extremely high velocity of the jets of saline macerates the thrombus very finely, and the very localized distribution of the jets allows the fragments to be withdrawn effectively from the circulation. AngioJet™ catheters are available in the 4-French XMI™, the 5-French XVG™, and the 6-French Xpeedior™, and they all pass over a wire, which makes them more versatile for entering precise locations and traversing thrombi in smaller vessels. AngioJet™ catheters can be used with a single-use pump set or with a fairly complex, multi-use drive unit. Because of the small size and the over-the-wire use of AngioJet™ catheters, these are the most suitable for smaller pediatric and congenital patients[8]. However, the drive unit, in addition to being fairly complex, is expensive and is usually not available in a purely pediatric/congenital cardiac catheterization laboratory, unless the laboratory has some association with an adult cardiovascular service. The drive unit is mobile, so could be moved between co-operating and near-by laboratories. The AngioJet™ system and catheters can be used to infuse thrombolytics locally into the thrombus as part of the total thrombus removal procedure.

The Oasis™ Thrombectomy Device (Boston Scientific, Natick, MA) has a single small nozzle at the tip of the catheter, which directs a high-velocity jet of saline *back* into the port of a separate lumen in the catheter. The high-velocity jet creates a Venturi effect, which fragments the thrombus while, at the same time, it sucks the fragments back into the catheter. As with the other devices without specific distal protection systems and although the particles are very small, particulate matter that is dislodged can embolize distally.

The Trellis Infusion System™ (Bacchus Vascular Inc., Santa Clara, CA) utilized occlusion balloons in the lumen of the vessel above and below the thrombus to "contain" the debris. A catheter that rotated between the occlusion balloons macerated the clot into fine particulate matter, which, in turn, was evacuated from the area between the occlusion balloons. The rotating catheter tended to denude the endothelium of the vessel where it touched. When the area of the vessel could be isolated with the occlusion balloons, this device had one of the best chances of preventing distal embolization; as of this writing, however, the Trellis™ device has been withdrawn from the market.

The Trerotola Percutaneous Thrombectomy Device™ (PTD) (Arrow International Inc., Reading, PA) is a self-expanding, 9 mm diameter, stainless steel, wire basket, which rotates at 3,000 rpm. The rotating basket fragments the clot into "macro" particles that are as large as 3 mm, but there is *no* evacuation system for these large fragments. The device can be delivered over a wire, which makes it easier to deliver to distal, more circuitous locations such as branch pulmonary arteries. The rotating basket denudes the wall of the adjacent vessel where it touches. The major disadvantage is the potentially larger resultant fragments. As the thrombus is being broken up, the area distal to the thrombectomy must be able to tolerate the embolization of the larger fragments.

Complications of foreign body retrieval/removal

The removal of a foreign body is usually necessitated by an adverse event that can become a complication, but the retrieval procedure itself can create complications. As with all other complications, the best treatment is preventing their occurrence. The retrieval of all foreign bodies requires *extensive manipulation* of often large and stiff catheters and multiple exchanges of wires, sheaths, catheters and the retrieval devices themselves. All of these manipulations and exchanges carry the same, or even higher, risks of the complications that occur from the routine manipulation of any cardiac catheter. Meticulous attention to the details of normal catheterization procedures for the manipulation of catheters, wires and sheaths, and the prevention of air and/or clot embolization are mandatory during every retrieval procedure. Each of the separate foreign body retrieval devices is associated with specific complications, which have been discussed previously in the discussions of each of the devices.

Intravascular structures can be torn or perforated when a foreign body is pulled loose or withdrawn through a vessel. This occurs most frequently during intracardiac lead extractions and is a known, half-anticipated, part of the procedure. It does occur, very rarely, with the forceful extraction of any foreign body that has become embedded in tissue and should always be anticipated. With the unexpected or unexplained deterioration of a patient during any foreign body extraction a tear or perforation is always considered. The treatment is intensive medical support of the patient with the replacement of lost blood until surgical intervention is available to repair the tear.

A foreign body becoming entangled in a ventricle or a cardiac valve is another complication of foreign body retrieval, which for the most part is iatrogenic and should be avoidable. Most dislodged devices (e.g. coils, occlusion devices, stents) in the systemic venous system embolize directly to the pulmonary artery or tumble *through* the ventricles into the pulmonary artery when they become dislodged during or after an implant. They become *lodged in* the ventricle when an attempt is made to withdraw a partially or totally exposed device through the ventricle during a retrieval procedure. Any foreign body that cannot be withdrawn completely into a sheath, *should not be withdrawn through a ventricle.* Avoiding this problem requires a difficult judgment decision before the foreign body is even grasped with a retrieval device. Once a large foreign body is grasped securely with a retrieval device, occasionally neither can it be withdrawn completely into a sheath nor can it be released from the retrieval device!

The probability of this combined problem should always be considered *before* grasping a foreign body with a retrieval device when the foreign body must be withdrawn through a ventricle before its final extraction. When a large, catheter-delivered, intracardiac device becomes trapped in the right ventricle, it usually requires a sternotomy and cardiopulmonary bypass to remove the device, while a direct surgical retrieval from the pulmonary artery requires a thoracotomy, but usually does not require cardiopulmonary bypass. This should be considered before an attempt at grasping or withdrawing an exposed foreign body through a ventricle is even contemplated.

Occasionally, a foreign body is loosened with a retrieval device, but before the foreign body can be withdrawn from the body it becomes released inadvertently or is lost back into the circulation. This results in the embolization of the device to another location. Unless the device embolizes to or through a ventricle, the inadvertent loss of the device usually does not result in any permanent sequelae, but does require a repeat retrieval procedure.

Summary

With the professional expertise which should be present in a well equipped pediatric/congenital catheterization laboratory, and using one or a combination of the retrieval systems described, the removal of virtually all intravascular foreign bodies is possible by a catheter technique. However, even with all of the latest equipment and the best techniques, there are a few circumstances when a foreign body cannot, or *should not* be removed by a transcatheter technique. This applies particularly to large and not easily compressible intracardiac therapeutic devices. Very large devices (large ASD devices, fully expanded intravascular stents) may not compress sufficiently or fold enough to be withdrawn even partially into even the largest, long sheath available. Persistent attempts at the removal of such devices, particularly if the foreign body must be withdrawn through a ventricle, have a high likelihood of causing significant and often permanent intravascular or intracardiac damage. In that circumstance, surgical assistance for the removal of the foreign body is needed.

When a patient in whom a large or difficult-to-remove device has embolized must undergo cardiac surgery to correct the particular defect anyway, or there is some other major defect requiring surgery, there is little wisdom or justification for pursuing an extensive transcatheter removal procedure unless the device is causing an immediate life-threatening problem. Subjecting the patient to the often long, complex, and potentially dangerous transcatheter removal procedure with its large dose of radiation is in no way justified when cardiac surgery is inevitable. This is true particularly when the original defect is not treatable by a similar or larger catheter-delivered device (e.g. an embolized ASD occlusion device in an unusually positioned or large ASD).

It requires more skill, judgment and maturity on the part of the interventional cardiologist to determine when a foreign body is too difficult or dangerous to remove, and then to make the decision *not* to pursue the catheter retrieval any further.

References

1. Dotter CT, Rosch J, and Bilbao MK. Transluminal extraction of catheter and guide fragments from the heart and great vessels; 29 collected cases. *Am J Roentgenol Radium Ther Nucl Med* 1971; **111**(3): 467–472.
2. Lillehei CW, Bonnabeau RC Jr, and Grossling S. Removal of iatrogenic foreign bodies within cardiac chambers and great vessels. *Circulation* 1965; **32**(5): 782–787.
3. Moncada R *et al.* Migratory traumatic cardiovascular foreign bodies. *Circulation* 1978; **57**(1): 186–189.
4. Bracke FA, Meijer A, and Van Gelder B. Learning curve characteristics of pacing lead extraction with a laser sheath. *Pacing Clin Electrophysiol* 1998; **21**(11 Pt 2): 2309–2313.

5. Fearnot NE *et al*. Intravascular lead extraction using locking stylets, sheaths, and other techniques. *Pacing Clin Electrophysiol* 1990; **13**(12 Pt 2): 1864–1870.
6. Byrd CL *et al*. Intravascular lead extraction using locking stylets and sheaths. *Pacing Clin Electrophysiol* 1990; **13**(12 Pt 2): 1871–1875.
7. Greenfield LJ, Kimmell GO, and McCurdy WC 3rd. Transvenous removal of pulmonary emboli by vacuum-cup catheter technique. *J Surg Res* 1969; **9**(6): 347–352.
8. Kirby WC, D'sa R, and Shapiro SR. Mechanical thrombectomy for treatment of postoperative venous obstruction in pediatric patients. *J Invasive Cardiol* 2004; **16**(5/Suppl): S27–S29.

13 Balloon atrial septostomy

Rashkind™ Balloon Atrial Septostomy

The Rashkind™ Balloon Atrial Septostomy (BAS), which was introduced in 1966, was the first intracardiac, non-surgical interventional procedure to be developed and used clinically[1]. The Rashkind™ BAS was not only the first procedure, but it was exceptionally innovative and daring for the time—and even for today. Dr William Rashkind devised the non-surgical technique for the creation of an atrial septal defect as a palliation for newborns with transposition of the great arteries at a time when transposition was one of the most lethal congenital heart defects. The Blalock–Hanlon surgical atrial septectomy was an alternative for the palliative creation of an atrial defect, however, in a critically ill infant, the surgical septectomy was associated with a high morbidity and mortality in most centers at that time. The Rashkind™ BAS procedure, although "crude" by all standards, was *dramatically and instantaneously* successful, and has persisted until today with little change from the original technique as an essential procedure for many congenital heart lesions.

Indications for a balloon atrial septostomy

The need for an atrial septostomy is determined by the underlying cardiac lesion and from the associated clinical findings. Infants or older patients whose clinical signs or symptoms can be improved by better mixing or "venting" of the systemic venous or pulmonary venous blood are candidates for an atrial septostomy. Patients with transposition of the great arteries have parallel systemic and pulmonary circuits and benefit dramatically from mixing of their systemic and pulmonary venous blood at the atrial level. Patients with pulmonary atresia, tricuspid atresia, and other hypoplastic and poorly functioning right ventricles require an adequate interatrial communication to allow systemic venous blood to return back into the systemic arterial circuit. Patients with severe mitral stenosis, mitral atresia or other varieties of hypoplastic left ventricle represent an analogous situation, but for blood to flow in the opposite direction where it is trapped on the left or pulmonary venous side of the circulation. These hypoplastic left heart patients require an atrial septostomy to vent the pulmonary venous blood back into the functional systemic circulation. Patients with total anomalous pulmonary venous connection require an atrial opening to permit both the systemic and pulmonary venous blood to re-enter the systemic arterial circulation.

The BAS is accomplished by forcefully pulling ("jerking") a small spherical balloon through an essentially intact atrial septum, thereby tearing an opening in it. The adequacy of the opening that is created depends upon the toughness of the septum, the size and compliance of the balloon used for the septostomy and the force with which the balloon is pulled through the septum.

Hemodynamics of restrictive atrial septal communications

The necessity for septostomy is suggested by an echocardiogram with the demonstration of a patent foramen ovale or tiny atrial septal defect with restricted flow in a patient with any of the previously mentioned anatomic defects. The restrictive nature of the defect is confirmed in the catheterization laboratory by the pressure difference between the two atria or by angiography demonstrating restrictive flow, or minimal or no mixing at the atrial septal level. The difference in pressure will be very significant when the predominant flow of blood is, or should be, from left to right through the atrial defect. The left atrium is relatively non-compliant, and develops very high pressures when there is restriction to the outflow of the pulmonary venous blood from the left atrium. The right atrium, on the other hand, by itself and along with the hepatic veins and the connected total systemic venous "pool", is very compliant. The right atrium and the systemic venous veins stretch or dilate almost infinitely and in doing so, prevent the development of a gradient from right atrium to left atrium across the atrial septum even with severe restriction of flow and even when the atrial communication is the only outlet of blood from the right atrium! Angiography will confirm the presence or absence of obstruction at the atrial level.

Angiography of the atrial septum

For angiographic confirmation of the atrial obstruction, in lesions with a potential left to right shunt, an angled, cranial–LAO angiogram with an injection at the mouth of the right upper pulmonary vein is used to profile the atrial septum. This angiocardiogram usually demonstrates a bulging of the septum toward the right atrium with a jet of contrast passing through any existing opening in the septum. In lesions with a potential right to left shunt, a straight PA and lateral X-ray view with injection in the right atrium just at the junction of the IVC with the right atrium is used to demonstrate the restrictive flow through the existing atrial defect. The lateral view demonstrates the flow of contrast from right to left most clearly with a vertical jet of contrast passing from the right atrium, through the defect and toward the roof of the left atrium.

Sizing the atrial septal communications in the catheterization laboratory

There are occasions when the existing atrial communication is sized. For larger patients there are static "sizing" balloons that can be passed over a wire and through the defect and used to demonstrate the exact size of the existing atrial opening in questionable cases. These NuMED™ "sausage"-shaped sizing balloons (NuMED Inc. Hopkinton, NY), can be inflated at very low—almost zero—pressure. At this extremely low pressure, the balloon within the defect conforms to the size (and shape) of the defect without stretching or distorting it. The true sizing balloons, however, all are on large catheter shafts, which make them unsatisfactory for use in newborn or small infants. As an alternative, a very small, standard angioplasty balloon, when inflated at very low pressures, can be used in the defect in a similar fashion.

A Swan™ balloon (Edwards Lifesciences, Irvine, CA) or the actual septostomy balloons were used in the past to "calibrate" the atrial communications. The results of this type of sizing can be very misleading, and the technique is no longer recommended. When using a Swan™ or a balloon septostomy catheter to size the defect, the balloon catheter with the balloon deflated is passed through the defect from the right atrium to the left atrium. The balloon is inflated in the left atrium and gently withdrawn against the septum until resistance is first encountered. As the balloon is held gently against the septum, the balloon is deflated in small decrements. The diameter of the balloon when the balloon easily pulls through the septum provides a rough estimate of the size of the opening. This technique is described in detail and illustrated in Chapter 28 ("ASD Occlusion"). There are several major flaws with this type of sizing. The spherical, Swan™ or Rashkind™ type balloons create an acute angle between the edge of the balloon attachment to the catheter and the catheter shaft. As the inflated balloon is withdrawn against the septum this acute, 90° angle—rather than the full diameter of even a partially inflated balloon—catches on the edge of the septal defect, providing resistance to the withdrawal, and gives a false impression of a much smaller defect.

In addition, when the balloon is pulled from the left atrium into the right atrium in the presence of a patent foramen with a sizable "flap valve", the balloon actually pulls the flap of the foramen closed against the septal opening and, in turn, give the impression of a very small opening. When the balloon does pull through the defect after several withdrawals of even the partially inflated balloon through the defect, the defect actually can be stretched and/or dilated significantly during this "sizing" procedure.

The alternative technique for balloon sizing, when using a Swan™ type balloon, is to pass a guide wire from the right atrium through the defect into the left atrium. The Swan™ balloon is advanced over the wire only to the right atrial/inferior vena cava junction where the balloon is inflated maximally. The inflated balloon catheter is advanced over the wire from the right atrium until it pushes against the defect in the atrial septum. The balloon is deflated decrementally while pushing its catheter over the wire against the defect. The size of the balloon as it eventually passes across the defect into the left atrium indicates the size of the defect. Because of the compliance and compressibility of the partially inflated Swan™ type balloons, the gas filled Swan™ balloons are easily compressed, which allows them to "milk" through the defect in an elongated shape. This can also give a false impression of the size of the defect. Of even more importance, none of the sizing techniques provide any information about the functional significance of the defect.

Equipment for a "classic" balloon atrial septostomy

The Miller–Edwards™ (Miller™) balloon septostomy catheter (Edwards Lifesciences, Irvine, CA) is the preferred septostomy balloon for all infants over 3 kg. The Miller™ balloon septostomy catheter has a small latex balloon of 4 ml capacity mounted at the distal end of a

5-French catheter shaft. The balloon material is slightly redundant over the shaft of the catheter and usually requires a 7-French sheath for its introduction. Just at the area where the balloon is attached, the Miller™ balloon catheter has a fixed, slight angulation of the tip of the catheter, which is very helpful for maneuvering the catheter with the balloon deflated from the right atrium to the left atrium across a "closed" patent foramen ovale (PFO). The Miller™ septostomy catheter has only the one lumen, which communicates with the balloon, and no separate catheter lumen, so it cannot be advanced over a wire nor can pressures be recorded or injections performed through the balloon catheter. The Miller™ balloon catheter comes with a very fine, smooth, metal wire stylet, which extends the entire length of the catheter lumen (including through the area of the balloon). The distal end of the stylet can be bent and used like a rigid deflector wire to form a greater or different curve on the tip of the balloon catheter, or it can be used to clear the lumen of the balloon catheter of any obstructions.

The left atrial cavity of an infant who is larger than 3 kg, can safely accommodate the Miller™ balloon inflated with 6 ml of fluid when the balloon is free within the left atrium. Although rated and advertised at 4 ml capacity, these balloons can actually accommodate 10–12 ml before rupturing! When a large diameter septal opening is desired and whenever the left atrium will accommodate it, 6 ml of fluid is used in the Miller™ septostomy balloon. At 6 ml, the balloon not only becomes larger, but the surface of the balloon becomes tense and far less compliant. These are very desirable characteristics for tearing and not just stretching the septum. When the Miller™ balloon is inflated to less than 6 ml, it will be proportionally softer and more compliant. As a consequence Miller™ balloons with lower volumes are smaller and less tense, and "mold" through a smaller defect rather than tearing the edges of it.

There are special circumstances where the Miller™ balloon cannot be inflated to 6 ml. In order to purposefully create a smaller (usually temporary) septostomy or to perform a balloon septostomy in a very small infant, there are smaller balloons available that inflate with a more rigid wall tension at the smaller diameters. The USCI Rashkind™ balloon (United States Catheter, Inc. [USCI] BARD, Glens Falls, NY) was on a 6-French catheter, while the newer and currently available NuMED™ septostomy balloons (NuMED Inc., Hopkinton, NY) are on a 4-French catheter shaft and pass through slightly smaller introducer sheaths.

The more recent USCI Rashkind™ balloon (manufacturer as above) was a latex balloon mounted on and recessed into a 6-French woven dacron shaft. If the balloon deliberately was not fully inflated, when it had been being prepared and cleared of air and bubbles, it passed through a 6-French sheath (as a minimum). Like the Miller™ balloon, this USCI Rashkind™ septostomy balloon did not have a second lumen. The USCI Rashkind™ balloon had the additional major disadvantage of having a much smaller balloon size, with only a 2.5 ml capacity at its maximum inflation volume compared to the 6 ml of the Miller–Edwards™ balloon. Even at its full inflation, the USCI Rashkind™ septostomy balloon was fairly soft and moderately compliant.

The NuMED™ Z-5™ septostomy balloons (NuMED Inc., Hopkinton, NY) are available in two sizes. These balloons are manufactured from a non-compliant thermoplastic elastomer, which results in an essentially fixed diameter, rigid balloon when inflated with the recommended volume. The smaller Z-5™ balloon reaches a diameter of 9.5 mm when inflated with 1 ml of fluid while the larger Z-5™ balloon has a 13.5 mm diameter when inflated with 2 ml of fluid. As a consequence, although they have a volume of only 1 or 2 ml when fully inflated, they produce very rigid balloons with diameters of exactly 9.5 and 13.5 mm. The deflated balloons pass through 5- or 6-French sheaths, respectively.

To facilitate crossing the atrial septum, the distal shafts of the Z-5™ septostomy balloons are angled to approximately 35° just proximal to the location of the balloon. In addition, both of the NuMED™ Z-5™ septostomy balloon catheters have a separate catheter lumen from the balloon lumen. The separate lumen allows the smaller and larger catheters to be introduced over 0.014" and 0.021" wires, respectively. The wire can be positioned securely in the left atrium or a pulmonary vein separately through a more maneuverable end-hole catheter, and then the balloon septostomy catheter is passed over the pre-positioned wire. This is very beneficial in directing the balloon into a very small or malpositioned left atrium and to be absolutely sure that the balloon is in the proper position. The wire through the balloon catheter can be left in place during the rapid balloon withdrawal during the septostomy. The wire remaining in place is helpful in re-entering the left atrium for a repeated balloon withdrawal, and provides a safety mechanism in the event of the balloon separating from the catheter. With the wire removed from the catheter lumen, pressures can be recorded or small contrast injections for angiograms can be performed through this separate lumen to verify the exact location of the balloon.

In patients in whom the shunting is right to left at the atrial level, particularly in those with total anomalous pulmonary venous return, the left atrial chamber is very small. In these very small left atria, the Miller™ balloon conforms to the shape of the small left atrium and begins to stretch and distort the atrium well before it reaches a volume of 6 ml (and its maximum diameter). In that situation, the balloon will be fixed very firmly within the small left atrium and will have no "bounce" or movement. In addition, when the balloon is inflated and either filling the atrium or pulled against the atrial septum, all systemic cardiac output will be stopped totally! Under these circumstances, the balloon inflation must be carried out very cautiously to avoid over distention of the atrium, but at the same time, rapidly to avoid too long a period of hypotension, bradycardia and even cardiac arrest. Once the balloon has assumed the shape of the atrium and stopped moving, inflation is stopped and the withdrawal is performed rapidly with that degree of inflation (usually less than 4 ml). This is the one situation where rapid over-inflation to the full volume of the Miller™ balloon could be disastrous and could cause rupture of the left atrium.

When a very small left atrium is found, particularly in very small infants under 2 kg in weight, in infants where the venous system does not tolerate the 7-French introductory sheath, or in larger patients with right to left shunting, the NuMED™ 2 ml septostomy balloon is used in preference. Neither of these balloons is satisfactory when a large, permanent opening in the atrial septum is desired. The technique and precautions for a balloon septostomy with either of these alternative balloons are similar to those for the Miller–Edwards™ catheter.

Balloon septostomy in the catheterization laboratory

Whenever a balloon atrial septostomy is necessary in neonatal patients, the patient's hemodynamic stability is often dependent upon the atrial communication. As a consequence, the balloon atrial septostomy is performed *at the beginning of the procedure* before any extensive catheter diagnostic studies, whether the septostomy is performed in the catheterization laboratory or the newborn intensive care unit under echocardiography guidance.

The catheterization laboratory has many advantages for the balloon septostomy. All of the ancillary equipment necessary for catheter introduction and the septostomy procedure are available and immediately accessible. Overall visualization of the catheter in relation to the remainder of the anatomy, and the septostomy procedure itself are all visualized clearly using biplane fluoroscopy. With the ancillary equipment in the laboratory and with the use of fluoroscopy, the procedure can be altered to suit any variation in the patient's anatomy. The facilities for cardiopulmonary resuscitation in the event of a problem during the catheterization, and subsequent access to the operating rooms, are usually better in the catheterization laboratory. Performance of the septostomy in the catheterization laboratory does not preclude the use of echocardiography in the catheterization laboratory as an adjunct means of visualizing the septum, the balloon and the results.

Occasionally an umbilical venous line is already present in these infants, and although it is a less desirable approach, it is often used for balloon atrial septostomy out of "expediency"[2]. If the umbilical vein is used, the existing umbilical vein catheter is replaced over a wire with a sheath/dilator set that will accommodate the septostomy balloon. The sheath and dilator are advanced into the umbilical vein until the tip of the sheath is well into the right atrium. The positioning of the sheath with its tip extending centrally past the entrance of the hepatic veins into the inferior vena cava/right atrium assures repeated access to the right atrium and septum with the septostomy catheter. When attempts are made at replacing the umbilical vein catheter directly with the septostomy catheter, often the ductus venosus spasms and the septostomy catheter becomes "detoured" and stuck in the hepatic/portal vein system and cannot be maneuvered to the atrium at all from the umbilical approach. This is a particular problem when using a Miller™ septostomy balloon, which has no separate lumen for a wire.

The femoral vein approach is preferred when a large atrial septostomy is desired, and particularly when it is planned for the atrial septal defect that is created, to last any length of time after the procedure. Although the umbilical vein is patent and even cannulated with an umbilical catheter, the results of the septostomy are less satisfactory from the umbilical vein approach. When the balloon crosses the septum from the umbilical vein, there is a very short distance between the balloon's exit from the small ductus venosus (end of the sheath) to the foramen ovale as compared to the distance from further down in the inferior vena cava to the foramen. This short distance restricts the distance the balloon is able to travel during and after the forceful pull through the septum and, in turn, limits the force that can be applied to pull ("jerk") the balloon through the septum. If the balloon is pulled too far and forcefully against the hepatic veins/ductus venosus, the veins can be disrupted or pulled off the right atrium, and if the balloon is pulled forcefully against the tip of the sheath, it can be ruptured or even totally dislodged from the catheter.

When a smaller opening in the septum is necessary, and it only has to stay open for a few days before proposed surgery, for example in a patient with a simple transposition or a hypoplastic left heart, then the umbilical approach is satisfactory. The smaller NuMED™ balloons can be used and less force (a weaker "jerk") applied via the septostomy catheter. When using one of the NuMED™ septostomy balloons, first an end-hole torque catheter is introduced into the umbilical vein, maneuvered through the septum and into a pulmonary vein, and replaced with a wire that the NuMED™ balloon septostomy catheter will accommodate. When there is a pre-existing umbilical venous catheter, it is replaced with a small spring guide wire that the septostomy catheter will accommodate, and a torque-controlled end-hole catheter is introduced over the wire and maneuvered into the left atrium—and preferably into a left pulmonary vein. The wire is advanced as far as possible and fixed in the pulmonary vein, the catheter is withdrawn over the wire, and the septostomy balloon catheter advanced over the wire and directly into the left atrium. When only a small or temporary septostomy opening is necessary, this is the most expeditious technique for performing a BAS. Without the sheath through the umbilical vein, there is slightly more room for the withdrawal (without hitting against the tip of a sheath), but the withdrawal distance is still limited in order not to pull the balloon into the hepatic veins/ ductus venosus.

During a balloon atrial septostomy procedure performed in the neonatal intensive care unit or the catheterization laboratory, an arterial monitoring line is desirable, and in our laboratory is considered essential. In the newborn infant with congenital heart disease, the arterial line is often present as an umbilical artery line when the infant arrives in the catheterization laboratory. If not, either the umbilical artery is cannulated in the catheterization laboratory with an umbilical artery catheter, or a femoral artery is cannulated with a 20-gauge teflon Quick-cath™ while the sheath is being introduced into the femoral vein.

When a large or persistent opening is desired, the septostomy balloon is introduced from the femoral vein. When a balloon atrial septostomy is the purpose of the procedure or even if it is only a consideration, a sheath that is large enough to accommodate the balloon septostomy catheter to be used is introduced into the femoral vein *at the onset* of the procedure. A standard, short sheath with a back-bleed valve and flush port is used. By starting with the necessarily larger sheath, net trauma to the vein is reduced by eliminating the subsequent exchange to a larger sheath. Starting with the larger sheath also reduces the possibility of not being able to introduce it at all later during the catheterization because of venous spasm of the small femoral vein. A 7-French sheath is required for Miller™ balloons and a 6-French sheath for the larger Z-5™ septostomy balloons. When a balloon septostomy was not planned initially and a smaller sheath was used during the initial part of the catheterization, the existing smaller sheath used for the diagnostic catheterization should be replaced with the larger sheath and dilator as soon as the decision to perform the septostomy has been made. The skin and subcutaneous tissues surrounding the puncture site are re-infiltrated *very liberally* with local anesthesia before exchanging the sheaths.

Once the appropriate sheath for the septostomy balloon has been introduced into the vein, the dilator is removed very slowly, and the indwelling sheath with its side arm and proximal valve chamber is carefully cleared of all air by allowing it to bleed-back as the valve of the side port is opened very cautiously. If the infant is experiencing any respiratory difficulty, particularly with excessive inspiratory effort, no attempt is made to clear the sheath by free or passive back bleeding. With any strong inspiratory effort on the part of the patient, air is easily sucked into an open sheath or an open side port on the back-bleed valve. When there is even minimal inspiratory obstruction, and after the dilator and wire have been removed, the back-bleed valve of the sheath is covered tightly with a gloved finger, a syringe is attached to the side port, and the stopcock on the side port is opened while suction is applied gently to the side port. This allows blood to flow freely from the side port while preventing air from being sucked into the sheath through the valve by the suction on the syringe or the patient's inspiratory effort. Once completely clear of any air, the side arm is attached to a separate flush line and placed on a *slow and continuous* flush.

The septostomy balloon is prepared outside of the body. Normal saline (not dextrose with saline) is used for flushing the balloon and to dilute the contrast to be used in the balloon. Glucose solution, by itself, is sticky and can clog the small lumen of the septostomy catheter. The septostomy balloon is inflated with one, to at most 1.5 ml, of normal saline. This same volume is withdrawn along with any air from the balloon or catheter lumen. The filling with fluid and the withdrawal of the fluid and any air are repeated several times in order to remove as much trapped air from the balloon and catheter lumen as possible. Each time only a very small amount of saline flush is used. The septostomy balloon should *not* be inflated to its full capacity during this preparation. Inflation to the full volume stretches the materials of the balloons, which causes the balloon material to become more redundant around the catheter shaft and, in turn, makes the introduction through the appropriate sized sheath more difficult or even impossible.

The balloon is emptied completely. In a separate syringe, one ml of contrast is diluted with 9 ml of saline to provide exactly 10 ml of a 9:1 dilution of saline to contrast solution. This syringe is attached to the previously flushed and emptied balloon lumen. By starting with exactly 10 ml in the syringe, it is easier and quicker to determine the precise amount of diluted contrast solution that is filling the balloon during the actual septostomy.

The Miller™ septostomy balloon catheter comes with a fine steel stylet within the entire length of the balloon lumen. In preparing the balloon for use, the stylet is removed but is kept on the sterile field. The stylet has several potential critical uses. If the balloon catheter cannot be maneuvered readily from the right atrium into the left atrium through a small or "tight" existing defect, a small, short, smooth 45° curve is formed on the distal end of the stylet. The syringe is removed from the hub of the balloon catheter and the stylet is inserted through the balloon lumen to the tip of the balloon catheter. The stylet within the lumen serves as a rigid deflector wire, creating an additional curve on the distal end of the balloon catheter and stiffening the shaft of the catheter, both of which facilitate advancing the balloon catheter into the left atrium.

The other very important use for the stylet is to assist in the deflation of the balloon after the balloon septostomy procedure has been completed. Even when using very dilute solutions of contrast with saline to fill the balloon, there are occasions when the balloon does not deflate following the septostomy. In this situation, the stylet is reintroduced into the lumen of the balloon septostomy catheter to ream out any dried contrast or other obstructing material within the lumen. This clearing of the lumen usually allows the subsequent deflation of the balloon when the stylet has been withdrawn.

"Classic" balloon septostomy procedure

Regardless of the type of balloon septostomy catheter being used, the surface of the balloon is moistened in the saline flush solution and the rate of flush into the side port of the hemostasis valve on the sheath is increased. Using the syringe attached to the proximal end of the balloon lumen, *mild* negative pressure is applied to the balloon and the balloon is introduced through the valve of the venous sheath. Very slight rotation on the shaft of the balloon catheter often facilitates the passage of the deflated balloon through the back-bleed valve and into the sheath by wrapping the redundant balloon material around the catheter slightly. The balloon is advanced slowly through the sheath while continuing the flush into the side port until the balloon passes beyond the distal tip of the sheath. The redundant material of the deflated balloon advancing within the lumen of the sheath acts as a "plunger" that can create a partial vacuum behind it. The continual flush through the side port fills the sheath behind the balloon as the vacuum develops and, in turn, prevents air from being sucked in through the back-bleed valve by this vacuum as the balloon is advanced through the sheath. Once the balloon has advanced past the end of the sheath, the negative pressure is released from the syringe attached to the balloon lumen and the continual flush on the side port is reduced to a slow drip. The balloon is maneuvered cephalad in the IVC and manipulated through the pre-existing interatrial septal defect and / or PFO into the left atrium.

In the presence of a very tense left atrium or any distortion of the atrial anatomy, maneuvering across the atrial septum can be difficult. With Miller™ septostomy balloons, the solid stylet is introduced into the catheter lumen to help direct the balloon through the atrial communication. When NuMED™ septostomy balloons are being used there are several options to assist in crossing the septum. The stiff end of a small spring guide wire or a Mullins™ wire (Argon Medical Inc., Athens, TX) can be used within the second lumen of the catheter to deflect the tip and support the shaft of the catheter for better maneuverability. A soft-tipped wire can be advanced out of the distal end of the NuMED™ septostomy catheter and the wire maneuvered across the atrial septum and followed by the septostomy catheter. Finally, a separate end-hole, torque-controlled catheter can be maneuvered across the tight atrial communication and into a pulmonary vein and replaced with the fine wire that the NuMED™ septostomy catheter will accommodate, and the septostomy catheter advanced into the proper position over the wire.

The position of the catheter tip within the left atrium is visualized on both the posterior–anterior (PA) and lateral (LAT) fluoroscopy to ensure that the balloon tip is positioned properly in the left atrium, and when available the balloon is visualized simultaneously on echocardiogram. The balloon is initially inflated slowly while its position and motion in the atrium are observed intermittently but frequently on both the PA and LAT fluoroscopy (and echo). The systemic blood pressure and the electrocardiogram (ECG) are monitored continuously and very carefully while the balloon is being inflated. As the balloon begins to inflate, it should move freely within the left atrium and, in fact, begin to "bounce" cephalad to caudally toward the mitral valve or left ventricle with each atrial contraction. The correct balloon bounce is perpendicular to the shaft of the catheter. If this movement of the balloon is not seen, its inflation is stopped immediately. The exact position of the balloon is rechecked carefully on the biplane fluoroscopy and echo. When balloon movement or bounce does not occur or the balloon appears in an abnormal location on echo, there are many dangers and abnormal areas where the balloon may be located. Abnormal positions of the balloon that must be excluded include:

1 *The left atrial appendage.* A balloon in the left atrial appendage appears slightly more anterior in the LAT fluoroscopic view. With the initial balloon inflation, the shape of the balloon begins to distort as the balloon conforms to the shape of the appendage. The balloon in the appendage is seen clearly on echo. Further inflation in the appendage or withdrawal of the balloon when it is trapped in the appendage would tear or totally disrupt it.

2 *A pulmonary vein.* When the balloon is in a pulmonary vein, the tip of the balloon catheter is positioned lateral to (outside of) the outline of the left atrium on the PA fluoroscopic view or posterior to the left atrium on the LAT view. With the initial inflation, the shape of the balloon elongates to conform to the size and shape of the pulmonary vein. It is common that the balloon, or at least its tip, begins to inflate in a pulmonary vein, but with the initial part of the inflation the balloon should "milk" out of the

vein and free into the left atrium. This is probably the safest starting location for the initial inflation as long as the balloon is observed very closely and *does* milk out of the vein on both fluoroscopy and echo. If the balloon does *not* milk out of the vein during inflation, the vein could be split by the full inflation of the septostomy balloon.

3 *In a juxtaposed right atrial appendage*. A balloon positioned abnormally in a juxtaposed right atrial appendage should always be considered a possibility. It is the most difficult abnormal position to recognize and absolutely rule out. The juxtaposed right atrial appendage passes from the right atrium *behind* the great arteries to the left heart boarder and is in very close approximation to the left atrial cavity/left atrial appendage. A juxtaposed right atrial appendage should have been identified by prior echocardiographic or angiographic studies and when present, there should be a high index of suspicion of this area as the balloon is being positioned. A balloon positioned in a juxtaposed right atrial appendage appears in a proper location (in the area of the left atrium) for a septostomy on both PA and LAT fluoroscopy, but not on echo when this is used simultaneously. However, the high index of suspicion, the rigid fixation in the position of the balloon during the initial inflation, the distortion of the shape of the balloon with the early inflation, and the absence of "bounce" toward the mitral valve, will differentiate the position in the juxtaposed appendage from the correct position even without echo. When there is a known juxtaposed right atrial appendage, it is advisable to visualize the balloon with echo as well as fluoroscopy before withdrawing it. Withdrawal from a juxtaposed atrial appendage can totally disrupt the appendage or tear it loose from the right atrium.

4 *In the left ventricle*. As the balloon is inflated in the left atrium and begins to "bounce" properly, it can easily be sucked across the mitral valve and into the left ventricle if there is significant slack on the shaft of the balloon catheter as the balloon is inflated. If the balloon inflation continues with the balloon in the ventricle, the balloon is positioned caudally and laterally in the PA projection and more anteriorly and caudally in the LAT projection. The balloon in the left ventricle becomes relatively fixed in its position on fluoroscopy compared to the bounce when it is in the left atrium. The very caudal location in the ventricle is very apparent unless there are marked distortion and peculiarities in the overall position of the heart and/or the chambers in relation to each other. The balloon in the left ventricle moves and is distorted slightly with each ventricular systole. In the left ventricle, the shaft of the balloon catheter tends to pull away from the operator along the long axis of the catheter in the direction of the apex of the ventricle, rather than the usual bounce perpendicular to the long axis when the catheter is correctly positioned in the left atrium. The balloon in the left ventricle and the catheter passing through the mitral valve are very obvious on echocardiography. A forceful withdrawal of the balloon from the left ventricle would disrupt the left atrioventricular valve.

5 *The right ventricle*. When the septostomy balloon is grossly malpositioned in the right ventricle, the position of the balloon is far anterior on the LAT fluoroscopy and moves (bounces) perpendicular to the long axis of the catheter, but cephalad toward the right ventricular outflow tract during each systole. The abnormal location on lateral fluoroscopy alone should identify this abnormal balloon position and certainly, a simultaneous echo easily confirms this abnormal location. A rapid, forceful withdrawal of the septostomy balloon from the right ventricle results in disruption of the tricuspid valve.

6 *The coronary sinus*. A balloon positioned in the coronary sinus appears very posterior and caudal on LAT fluoroscopy. The otherwise round septostomy balloon assumes a sausage-like shape and becomes very fixed with the initial inflation of the balloon. A septostomy balloon inflated in the coronary sinus usually causes discomfort for the patient, ST changes on the electrocardiogram, or bradycardia. Full inflation of the balloon in, or a forceful withdrawal from, the coronary sinus could tear or split it.

Correct positioning of the septostomy balloon catheter

As the balloon begins to inflate when positioned properly in the left atrium, it begins to "bounce" perpendicularly to the long axis of the catheter shaft and toward the mitral valve. As soon as this motion toward the mitral valve is seen, the balloon is carefully and gently withdrawn toward, and fixed against, the intact interatrial septum during the remainder of the inflation to the desired volume. As the balloon is inflated further, continued care is taken to prevent it from being sucked through the left A-V valve and into the ventricle. This is avoided by maintaining gentle tension on the balloon and careful observation of its motion on fluoroscopy or echo during its initial positioning and *entire* inflation.

The final positioning, the inflation of the balloon in the left atrium, and the withdrawal of the balloon are the times when the adjunct use of the echocardiogram in the catheterization laboratory is extremely useful, and where echo guidance may have a slight advantage over fluoroscopy guidance. The balloon itself and all of the adjacent structures or areas mentioned are seen clearly on the echo. Any abnormal position or motion of the balloon is recognized on the echo image immediately. It is more apparent on the echo image if the balloon is too large for the particular atrium and the left atrium is being distorted extensively during the inflation.

Once confident that the balloon is correctly positioned in the left atrium, and not in any of the danger areas, the balloon is inflated more rapidly to its maximum volume, or at least to the maximum volume and diameter tolerated by the infant's anatomy. For the ***first*** withdrawal ("pull through") and in order to achieve maximum effect from the septostomy, the balloon is filled with the ***maximum volume*** that it is planned to use or that can be tolerated by the infant. The balloon withdrawals should *not* start with a smaller volume and should *not be* performed with graduated and/or gradually increasing diameters of the balloon. Performing balloon withdrawals with gradually increasing volume is more likely to *stretch* the existing opening *temporarily*, rather than actually *tear* a new opening.

As long as the balloon is being inflated, it is observed very frequently or even continuously on biplane fluoroscopy and/or echocardiography. Fluoroscopic observation is predominantly in the PA projection, but it is also intermittently checked in the LAT view to watch for not only the danger areas, but to be sure that the balloon is not exceeding the volume/diameter of the left atrium. If the balloon reaches the maximum *atrial* volume before it reaches the desired maximum *balloon* volume, the balloon becomes distorted as it assumes the shape of the atrium, becomes unusually fixed in the atrium, and usually causes the patient's hemodynamics to "crater". This is more likely to occur in very small infants or in infants with right to left shunt lesions with very small left atria.

The electrocardiogram and systemic blood pressure are observed very carefully during the entire process. As the balloon volume approaches the volume of the atrial chamber, the heart rate slows and the systemic pressure drops. This is a result either of the inflated balloon's occluding all systemic output or of the abnormal stretch on a small left atrium. Such a reaction does not preclude continuation of the septostomy, but is an indication for (1) reassessment of the location of the balloon and its size-relationship to the LA by both biplane fluoroscopy and echocardiogram; (2) pre-treatment with atropine; and (3) a more rapid and dextrous inflation and pull-through of the balloon.

When the balloon is fully inflated to the maximum diameter for the septostomy (up to 6 ml for the Miller™ balloon), the catheter with the balloon is maintained fixed gently against the septum. The shaft of the catheter is grasped with a very firm grip (even to the point of wrapping the shaft of the catheter around a finger several times). A recording with biplane angiography or stored fluoroscopy is started. While recording continuously, the balloon catheter is withdrawn with a very *rapid* and *forceful "jerk"*. At the same time, the withdrawal or jerk from the left atrium back into the right atrium is for a very short distance and must be very controlled. Extreme care is taken to assure that there is no "wind-up" on the catheter just before this rapid withdrawal—i.e. the operator must avoid the almost instinctive tendency to push the shaft of the balloon catheter (and the balloon) forward into the left atrium just before withdrawing it through the septum. Such a "wind-up" allows the balloon to drop away from the septum and potentially through the left atrioventricular valve into the ventricle just before the pull on the balloon starts!

The forceful pull or jerk on the balloon should be performed with the fingers and wrist, ***not*** with the arm and elbow. Withdrawal of the balloon should be so rapid that, when filmed at sixty frames per second, the actual withdrawal is visible on only one frame—i.e. it lasts only 1/60th of a second! The balloon is yanked forcefully back, and completely into, the right atrium during the withdrawal, but it is not withdrawn any further down into the inferior vena cava (or hepatic veins). In the presence of a high-pressure left atrium, the atrial septum bulges to the right, is displaced into the right atrium, and, as a consequence, the foramen is often low and very close to the inferior vena cava. In this situation (and during any septostomy withdrawal) it helps to position the hand that is not pulling the catheter on the infant's leg 5–6 cm caudal to the site where the septostomy catheter is grasped with the other hand or fingers. During the septostomy withdrawal, the second hand serves as a stop to the withdrawal and helps to prevent pulling the balloon too far into the inferior vena cava.

The heart rate and blood pressure drop very significantly immediately following a successful septostomy. While observing the balloon on fluoroscopy, it is immediately pushed back toward (into) the mid right atrium and deflated as rapidly as possible by suction applied to the proximal end of the balloon lumen. When pushed cephalad after a successful pull through the septum, the balloon moves anteriorly on the LAT fluoroscopy while, if the septum was only displaced and the balloon did not pull through it, the balloon moves posteriorly back into the left atrium when pushed cephalad. Following a successful balloon atrial septostomy, the heart rate and blood pressure return rapidly to normal without any extra external effort.

Once the infant stabilizes, the deflated balloon is maneuvered into the left atrium, and the procedure repeated three to six times, or until absolutely no resistance is felt as the balloon is withdrawn rapidly through the defect. Each balloon withdrawal is performed with the balloon inflated to its maximum volume and diameter as determined for that particular patient. Although no increase in balloon size is used during the repeated balloon withdrawals, the repeated withdrawals tend to extend any tears in the septum that were initiated by the initial withdrawal.

Once the operator feels secure that the septum is opened to the maximum possible diameter with the particular balloon, the status of the opening is tested by reintroducing the balloon into the left atrium, inflating it with a slightly smaller volume of the dilute contrast, and performing a slow, gentle withdrawal, allowing the balloon to "float" through the newly created opening. The amount of dilute contrast in the balloon is increased in small amounts until slight resistance to the withdrawal is felt, i.e. starting with 1 ml and working up in approximately 1 ml increments. When an adequate opening has been created, the balloon should float through the defect even with the increasing increments of fluid.

When echocardiography is available in the catheterization laboratory or when it is used for an echo-guided septostomy, the atrial septum and the defect are viewed on the echo. The actual defect is usually defined very clearly and the flow through the defect can be seen on color Doppler.

Once convinced that the opening is adequate, the balloon catheter is withdrawn by applying suction to the proximal end of the balloon lumen while it is being withdrawn through the inferior vena cava, back into the sheath and out of the body. Occasionally, the balloon cannot be withdrawn into the venous sheath. In that case, the balloon is re-advanced several centimeters into the IVC and a 0.025″, soft-tipped, spring guide wire is introduced into the back-bleed valve adjacent to the balloon catheter at the proximal end of the sheath. The guide wire is advanced well into the cardiac silhouette, or even the superior vena cava. The balloon is withdrawn back to the distal end of the sheath and as far into the sheath as possible. The sheath and the balloon catheter are withdrawn together over the wire out of the skin. This allows the removal of the septostomy balloon along with the sheath, but leaves a wire in place for reintroduction of the sheath and a subsequent diagnostic catheter.

An angiographic catheter is introduced and pressure measurements are recorded during a recorded withdrawal from the left to the right atrium. This documents the elimination of the gradient between the atria. The best visual documentation of the atrial communication is with an angiocardiogram. In patients with left atrial to right atrial shunting, an injection is performed in a right upper pulmonary vein with recording in a 45° left anterior–oblique X-ray projection with cephalad angulation (i.e. 4-chambered view). In patients with predominately right to left shunt lesions, the angiocardiogram is performed with an injection into the right atrial–inferior vena cava junction, and recorded in a straight lateral projection.

Echo-guided balloon atrial septostomy

Considerable enthusiasm has been generated for "echo-only-guided" balloon atrial septostomies, which are performed in the neonatal intensive care unit (ICU)[3]. Originally, all balloon atrial septostomies were performed in the cardiac catheterization laboratory during the diagnostic catheterization, when the underlying defect was being diagnosed and evaluated. The majority of infants are now diagnosed definitively by an echocardiogram in the neonatal or nursery ICU, and many balloon atrial septostomies in neonates are performed in the ICU using echocardiographic guidance only. When the septostomy is performed in the neonatal ICU, usually one or more, nurses or technicians from the catheterization laboratory who are familiar with the equipment and the procedure assist with the procedure. The catheterization laboratory personnel provide a special balloon septostomy tray or "cart" containing most of the essential equipment for a routine septostomy. The special tray is brought to the bedside from the catheterization laboratory. The septostomy trays or carts are maintained and restocked in the catheterization laboratory after each use.

The echocardiogram provides an excellent picture of the atrial septum and of the immediately surrounding structures, but not all of the structures can be seen at the same time. Before the septostomy balloon has been inflated and while it is being manipulated, the septostomy catheter is often seen only fleetingly, if at all. Echo views do not provide even two-dimensional perspectives to the structures to aid in catheter manipulations. As a consequence, the maneuvering of the septostomy catheter to the atrium and across the existing defect into the left atrium is semi-blind and more difficult (and occasionally impossible) under echo-only guidance without adjunct fluoroscopy. A very slight inflation of the balloon during these manipulations will help the visualization of the balloon and the tip of the catheter on echo.

Once the septostomy catheter is in the left atrium and the septostomy balloon begins to inflate, the balloon, the septum and the surrounding structures are all seen very well with echocardiography. The exact relationship of the balloon size to the size of the left atrium and the exact location of the balloon against the septum are seen vividly, and their relative sizes are appreciated even better by echo images than by fluoroscopy. The same technique for the actual "ballooning" that is used in the catheterization laboratory is used in the echo-guided procedure in the ICU. Once the balloon pulls through the septum, the hole in the septum and the adequacy of the septostomy are apparent immediately on the echo. At the same time, the balloon disappears completely from the echo field until searched for by readjustment of the position of the echo probe. Even with the balloon out of the field of view, it is still re-advanced from the position of maximum pull until it can be seen in the echo field. After a successful septostomy, the inflated balloon can very easily float from the right atrium into the right ventricle as it is being re-advanced from out of the field. This position must be watched for very carefully on the echo before further maneuvering of the balloon.

Echo-guided septostomy that is performed in the neonatal ICU has the one advantage of not having to transport a sick baby to the catheterization laboratory. Depending upon the availability of staffing, this may be more expedient overall as long as everything goes smoothly. However, in the neonatal ICU there is no option for changes in technique or equipment without incurring a significant delay and disruption of the patient's environment. The size of the sterile field for the procedure in the neonatal ICU is always compromised. Unless the infant already has an indwelling arterial line (umbilical or radial artery) or the catheterization team introduces a separate arterial line, the infant undergoing a septostomy in the neonatal ICU does not always have the benefit of arterial monitoring during the septostomy. In the cyanotic infant the determination of which femoral vessel has been accessed is more difficult by echo where all of the blood is very "blue" and the wire positions in the thorax cannot be checked easily.

Because of the limitations with the totally echo-guided balloon atrial septostomy procedure, it is used mostly for those infants who need a very temporary opening in their septum—i.e. those patients who are expected to have surgery within a few days or weeks and who will be dependent upon their mixing or shunting only until the time of the surgery. Under these circumstances, it is more reasonable to use the umbilical vein for access and to use smaller septostomy balloons for the procedure. In a complex heart where the patient will be dependent on the septal communication for months or years, balloon atrial septostomy is performed preferentially in the catheterization laboratory, where there is in a much more controlled environment and more optimal results can be obtained.

Dilation of the atrial septum (dilation septostomy)

The creation or enlargement of a communication in the atrial septum with a dilation balloon is a balloon dilation procedure that is not exactly a vascular dilation nor is it considered a usual septostomy. Dilation balloons are used for the creation or enlargement of atrial septal defects as an alternative to the fairly crude, and often poorly controlled, rapid withdrawal of inflated, standard atrial septostomy balloons through the septum[4]. A dilation septostomy is used to enlarge a pre-existing opening or, after a transseptal puncture of the septum, to create an entirely new opening. Dilation septostomies are particularly efficacious in the presence of a very thick or tough atrial septum. The shunt created by the atrial septal defect can be right to left or left to right depending upon the underlying hemodynamics and anatomy. When a dilation balloon is used, one or more low-profile angioplasty balloons that are significantly larger than the existing atrial opening, is (are) inflated exactly within the atrial septum. As the balloon(s) expand(s) beyond the diameter of the original opening, it (they) theoretically and hopefully tear(s) a larger opening in the septum. Because of the high degree of control over the rate of inflation and, in turn, the exact diameter of the opening created with dilation balloons, some operators prefer dilation septostomy for all balloon septostomy procedures, particularly in very small and/or very sick infants. At the other end of the spectrum, atrial septostomy performed with a dilation balloon is particularly useful in older, larger patients with very thick or tough interatrial septae, especially when used in conjunction with a blade atrial septostomy. Blade septostomy with dilation septostomy is covered in detail in Chapter 14.

Balloon dilation atrial septostomies are used to enhance both right to left and left to right shunting at the atrial level. A right to left shunt at the atrial level is created in order to vent blood away from the right ventricle while enhancing systemic output by allowing the shunted systemic venous blood to enter directly into the systemic arterial flow. In patients with hypoplastic right ventricles this is the only means of egress of blood from the systemic venous system, and the atrial opening should be as large as possible. The creation of a vent for the right ventricle is also desirable in patients who have a high and fixed pulmonary vascular resistance and have no other intracardiac communication. When an atrial defect is created or enlarged in these patients, the right to left shunting causes the net systemic cardiac output to increase, and the systemic pressure is expected to increase, while there is a concomitant drop in the systemic arterial saturation, and the arterial oxygen saturation is expected to decrease.

In older patients, the goal is to reduce the systemic oxygen saturation by only 8–10%. A sudden decrease of more than 10% in systemic oxygen saturation is usually not tolerated by these patients. The balloon dilation septostomy that is performed in order to enhance right to left shunting is initially performed very conservatively, starting with smaller (6–8 mm) balloons and then gradually increasing the diameter of the balloons as tolerated by the patient. If the systemic arterial oxygen saturation does not drop by at least 6%, the original balloon is replaced with a balloon two millimeters larger in diameter, and the dilation and observation procedure repeated until the desired drop in systemic oxygen saturation and, hopefully, increase in cardiac output, are accomplished. This slow, progressive dilation is necessary to prevent a catastrophic drop in systemic oxygen saturation, particularly in older patients with Eisenmenger syndrome.

When atrial septal dilation is performed to vent a high left atrial pressure, it is often performed to relieve inoperable, obstructive, left heart lesions in order to allow trapped pulmonary venous return to rejoin the general circulation. Infants and children with congenital mitral valve stenosis, mitral atresia and aortic atresia, all with some degree of hypoplastic left heart, are the usual patients undergoing dilation of an interatrial communication for this purpose. In these patients the atrial defect represents the only (or dominant) means of egress of blood from the pulmonary venous circulation, and the defect created should be as large as possible to eliminate all resistance to flow across the septum. The initial balloon (or balloons) used to dilate the septum for this indication should be as large as can be accommodated by the length of the atrial septum. Often these openings are maintained with the implant of an intravascular stent in the atrial septal opening. This is discussed in Chapter 14.

Patients with transposed arterial (TGA) or venous (TAPVC) circulations require an interatrial communication to allow mixing of blood in both directions in order to maintain systemic circulation and oxygenation and to lower the pulmonary venous pressure. The larger these communications can be made, the better are the venting and mixing. In these patients dilation of the atrial septum is performed with the largest diameter balloon(s) that the septum can accommodate.

Procedure for atrial septal dilation

When an atrial septal defect is being created using a dilation balloon alone, the balloon that is used should be considerably larger in diameter than the desired size of the defect. An end-hole catheter is advanced across the septum through either the small existing atrial septal opening or through a transseptal puncture through an intact atrial septum. From the left atrium the catheter is manipulated out into a left upper pulmonary vein and is replaced with a Super Stiff™ (Medi-Tech, Boston Scientific, Natick, MA) exchange length guide wire with a short floppy tip. The wire should be of the largest diameter that the balloon dilation catheter that is proposed for the dilation will accommodate.

A dilation balloon that is approximately twice the diameter of the desired defect is advanced over the wire and positioned precisely straddling the atrial septum. The balloon should be long enough to easily straddle the septum but at the same time must not be long enough to become entrapped in adjacent, narrow vessels. Usually a 2 cm long balloon is used in infants and a 3 or even 4 cm long balloon is used in older patients. All balloons used to dilate the atrial septum should have very short "shoulders" in order for the tip of the balloon not to extend into unwanted, adjacent vessels.

The balloon is inflated slowly while recording each inflation–deflation angiographically in both PA and LAT views. The balloon is observed closely not only for the "waist" near the center of the balloon, but also to ensure that no "second waist" appears on the balloon as a result of the balloon being positioned erroneously in, and/or that it does not move forward into the pulmonary vein or backward into the inferior vena cava during the inflation. When the central waist on the balloon disappear during the inflation or the balloon reaches its maximum pressure, it is deflated. The inflation–deflation is repeated, moving the balloon forward or backward very slightly with each re-inflation.

Often two balloons, positioned side by side across the atrial septum, are used to perform the dilation septostomy. By using two, smaller diameter balloons with their smaller deflated profiles instead of a single very large diameter balloon with a large rough deflated profile, a large diameter atrial septostomy can be accomplished using two much smaller introductory venous sheaths in the peripheral veins as opposed to one very large diameter sheath for the introduction of the large balloon. For example two 12 mm balloons can be introduced through two 6-French sheaths as opposed to the necessity of a large 8- or 9-French sheath for a single 18–20 mm balloon.

When two small balloons are used for dilation of the atrial septum, each balloon individually has an inflated diameter of the desired atrial defect. Ideally, in order to create one large atrial defect, both deflated balloons should pass through the same atrial communication initially. With any pre-existing communication, the second end-hole catheter is maneuvered through the same opening and then into the same or even a separate left pulmonary vein and replaced with a second, identical, Super Stiff™ wire. The two balloons are placed side by side within the defect and the dilation septostomy carried out similarly to the single-balloon technique.

When there is no pre-existing opening in the septum, there are two alternatives for introducing the two wires and then the two balloons through the same initial opening. The simplest procedure is to perform an initial, partial dilation of the septum with the first smaller balloon, which is introduced and positioned across the atrial septum after an initial transseptal puncture. This creates a septal opening through which the second end-hole catheter and eventually the second balloon can be introduced immediately adjacent to the first balloon and in the exact same opening. The second, slightly more complicated alternative is to perform a second transseptal puncture immediately adjacent to (touching) the first transseptal catheter before either balloon is introduced. When performed precisely, using biplane visualization, the second puncture will almost join the first opening, and when dilated with separate balloons the openings will coalesce into one larger hole.

Following the inflation–deflation with either one or two balloons, the angiograms are reviewed for the appearance and then disappearance of the waist(s) with the initial inflation(s) and the absence or reappearance of the waist(s) at the lowest initial pressures during the subsequent inflations. When the septostomy is successful, the waist(s) on the balloon(s) does (do) not reappear at all, or only reappear very late at full inflation during the subsequent balloon inflations. Once satisfied with the inflations, the balloon(s) is (are) withdrawn from the septum over the wire(s). The patient is allowed to stabilize following the septal dilation, the hemodynamics are remeasured, and an angiogram is performed to visualize the atrial defect which has been created. A straight lateral view with injection into the right atrium is usually optimal for visualization of defects that shunt *right to left*, while a left anterior oblique view with cranial angulation and an injection into the right upper pulmonary vein is optimal for visualization of lesions that shunt *left to right*.

When the septum is totally intact before the dilation or it is very tough, a blade septostomy (covered in detail in Chapter 14) is performed initially before any "ballooning" of the septum is attempted. This includes all patients who require an atrial septostomy who are more than three or four weeks old. Although the septum *can* be ballooned at this age, ballooning by itself usually only stretches rather than tears the septum, and only a temporary defect is created. By first making a small incision in the septum with the blade, less wall tension is necessary on the balloon to create a tear and there is more control over the opening created with the balloon. Small incisions in the septum become the beginning of more controlled, linear tears in the specific directions of the cuts as they are split or torn further with the balloon dilation. A controlled tear with the use of less force is accomplished instead of the whole circumference of the opening in the septum being stretched until it forcefully "explodes" in any direction. Once an opening is created in the septum by stretching the hole with a balloon septostomy alone, then a subsequent blade septostomy only stretches and elongates the defect to accommodate the width of the blade as it slides through the opening, and does not incise the septal tissues at all. A dilation septostomy following an initial blade septostomy is very effective when a controlled diameter of the opening is desired.

The hole in the atrial septum formed by dilation, even with preceding blade incisions, as with the other atrial septostomies, often has the same problem of not remaining open. There are now several techniques for stenting the opening in the septum to keep it open. These techniques are described in Chapter 14 on "Special Septostomies". There is also a new fenestrated Amplatzer™ device, which was developed for this problem and for creating atrial septal openings of very specific sizes; this is also discussed in Chapter 14. This device has been used successfully in experimental animals and in a few compassionate cases and appears very promising, but is not available yet for routine clinical use in the United States.

Bioptome septostomy

As an alternative to any type of balloon septostomy for the creation of an atrial defect in a patient with a very small left atrium that cannot accommodate even the smallest septostomy balloon, a biopsy forceps catheter using echo assistance in the positioning of the bioptome jaws has been used successfully for creating a large septal opening[5]. Small pieces of the septum are "chewed" away from the edge of the atrial septal opening with the "jaws" of a 5- or 6-French bioptome catheter. This has been particularly useful in hypoplastic left heart patients, where the left atrium is usually very small and the septum is very tough.

The biopsy forceps is advanced to the right atrium, opened in the right atrium and, using both biplane fluoroscopic and echo guidance, purposefully engaged on the *edge* of the existing atrial septal opening. A simultaneous 2-D echo image of the edge of the atrial septum and the bioptome forceps is essential for the final precise positioning of the open bioptome jaws on the edge of the septal opening before each "bite". Once engaged on the edge of the septal opening, small pieces of the edge of the original septal opening are "nibbled away" by a series of bites with the bioptome. Biopsy forceps septostomy is covered in detail in Chapter 14, on blade and biopsy forceps septostomy.

Complications of balloon atrial septostomy

In spite of the crude and rough nature of the balloon atrial septostomy procedure, there are surprisingly few complications from it when it is properly performed. Virtually all patients have a significant bradycardia and drop in systemic pressure immediately following the forceful withdrawal of the balloon. Almost all of them recover spontaneously and rapidly. For those few who have a sustained, or even progressive bradycardia or hypotension, a dose of atropine and epinephrine appropriate for the patient's weight is given intravenously. In order for this to be administered expeditiously, the appropriate doses of atropine and epinephrine are drawn up and ready to administer before the actual septostomy procedure is even begun for every patient undergoing an atrial septostomy. Unless there is an associated major catastrophic injury during the septostomy, all of the patients recover from the "vagal-like" response with atropine, epinephrine and, rarely, a few external compressions of cardiac massage.

Catastrophic major tears due to gross malpositioning of the balloon before the withdrawal have been discussed.

Abnormal initial balloon positions and how to recognize them and prevent the catastrophe are fairly straightforward. There seldom, if ever, are minor tears during an atrial septostomy. Once a major tear of an appendage, an atrioventricular valve or an atrial wall occurs, the result is a massive blood loss and a rapid demise of the patient. The only real treatment of these tears is prevention. Prevention is possible in almost all cases by meticulous attention to every detail of the procedure no matter how mundane it seems, nor how many septostomies have been performed.

The one major tear that might not be preventable, is a tear at the junction of the right atrium and inferior vena cava from the balloon's being pulled into the inferior vena cava at the end of the forceful jerk, particularly through a bulging or prolapsing septum. Judging the precise distance and controlling the force and distance of the pull on the balloon are often difficult and, unfortunately, are learned only by experience. Fortunately, the inferior vena cava is somewhat compliant or forgiving and "accepts" the inflated balloon for a considerable distance. When a tear occurs at this location, it is in a lower-pressure venous area and often is not as extensive—and therefore not as catastrophic—as a tear within the heart itself. When recognized, the infant is supported with volume replacement and observation while preparing to move them to the operating room. If deterioration continues rapidly, an attempt is made at tamponading the area with a very-low-pressure inflation of the septostomy balloon or an equivalent diameter angioplasty balloon positioned just caudal to or immediately adjacent to the suspected area of tear.

Balloon septostomy, like the many other interventions on the systemic side of the circulation, involves considerable manipulation in the blood that reaches the systemic circulation directly. Most newborns do not receive systemic heparin for a balloon atrial septostomy procedure, so extra attention must be paid to keeping catheters and sheaths flushed and not leaving them in place for long periods of time. The atrial septostomy procedure involves the introduction of balloon catheters into sheaths where air and/or clot easily become trapped, with the ever-present potential for systemic embolization if either the air or thrombi are pushed out of the sheath. Again, the only really effective treatment is recognition of the potential and meticulous attention to the details for prevention.

Several complications are unique to the balloon atrial septostomy procedure. Rupture of the septostomy balloon with or without the loss of the balloon material has occurred in the past, and probably will occur again in the future[6]. This problem is less common with the current universal single use of balloon septostomy catheters and the newer Miller™ and NuMED™ septostomy balloons. When a septostomy balloon that has been properly emptied of air prior to inflation with fluid, ruptures but does not lose part of the balloon, it creates an inconvenience, but does not create a real problem or complication. The ruptured balloon occasionally does not deflate completely and is more difficult to withdraw, but its withdrawal can be accomplished by withdrawing the sheath along with the septostomy catheter. A wire is introduced through the valve in the sheath adjacent to the shaft of the balloon catheter, through the sheath and advanced into the central circulation before the original sheath is withdrawn. This preserves the venous access for the introduction of a new sheath.

When a septostomy balloon ruptures and all or part of the balloon material embolizes, it potentially represents a major catastrophe, but amazingly, usually does not create even a small problem. The balloon material is not radio-opaque. The only indicators of the location of the embolized particle are the signs or symptoms of a vascular occlusion somewhere in the patient, depending upon which organ the piece of balloon lodges in. Any symptoms are treated supportively. Again, prevention by inspection of the balloon and its specifications before using it is the best treatment for balloon rupture. If the balloon catheter is old, past its labeled expiry date, or has been stored in an unfavorable environment, rupture with disruption of the balloon is more likely and the balloon should not be used.

A balloon septostomy catheter shaft can break off and a piece of the catheter embolize with the entire balloon[7]. The piece of catheter is radio-opaque and has a radio-opaque marker that allows the location of the errant piece to be ascertained. In the one reported case of such an incident, the piece lodged in a systemic artery and was retrievable with a catheter retrieval (snare) device. This apparently was an isolated incident and hopefully was a quality assurance problem that will not recur.

Another problem, which is a problem of balloon catheters in general and not unique to septostomy balloons, is the failure of the balloon to deflate after inflation for a septostomy or dilation. Contrast in the balloon catheter lumen which is not diluted sufficiently, or during a prolonged procedure when the contrast remains in the catheter lumen for a long time, both contribute to, but are probably not the only causes of, this problem. Assuming that the balloon is in the right atrium and not lodged in a vital structure or critical orifice, the failure of the septostomy balloon to deflate does not compromise the hemodynamics, but does create a problem of balloon removal. There are several alternative means of overcoming a "non-deflate" problem. The first means of deflating the balloon is to use the stylet that comes with the balloon and try cleaning out the lumen of the catheter by passing the moistened stylet repeatedly in and out of the catheter lumen and all of the way to the balloon. Usually the balloon does deflate very slowly after this reaming out with the stylet.

On the rare occasions that the balloon does not deflate using a stylet, it must be punctured externally. This is accomplished using a second catheter introduced through a second vein. A standard transseptal dilator (alone) as the second catheter and used with a transseptal needle provides the best control as a puncturing device. A small end-hole catheter along with a Mullins™ wire with the safety tip bead cut off, also functions similarly and may allow the use of a smaller second catheter—particularly in small infants. Once the second catheter has been introduced and advanced almost to the right atrium, the non-deflated septostomy balloon is withdrawn into the right atrial–inferior vena caval junction in order to stabilize the balloon in the side-to-side direction. The septostomy balloon is pulled tightly into the inferior vena cava, which fixes it in a fairly stable, non-mobile, position in this location while the second, puncturing catheter approaching from the inferior vena cava is directed at the caudal surface of the balloon. When the catheter tip is against the balloon in both planes of the fluoroscopy, the needle or sharp wire is extruded from the end of the catheter and poked into the balloon. This maneuver is repeated until the balloon has been punctured.

If the fully inflated balloon that will not deflate becomes trapped in a critical location in the course of the blood flow (the tricuspid valve, right ventricular outflow tract or mitral valve), there is usually no time to introduce the second catheter, or the location of the balloon prohibits access for a puncture. The only recourse is to over-inflate the balloon and rupture it deliberately! For Miller™ balloons, this requires 12–13 ml of fluid. This, in itself, is a potential hazard to the infant but when cardiac output is totally blocked by the inflated balloon, there is no alternative. This emphasizes the importance of always knowing the location of the inflated septostomy balloon and the prevention of its moving into critical locations.

Meticulous attention to the details of the septostomy procedure prevents most, if not all, of the previously mentioned complications and remains the best treatment for them.

References

1. Rashkind WJ and Miller WW. Creation of an atrial septal defect without thoracotomy; a palliative approach to complete transposition of the great arteries. *JAMA* 1966; **196**: 991–992.
2. Abinader E, Zeltzer M, and Riss E. Transumbilical atrial septostomy in the newborn. *Am J Dis Child* 1970; **119**(4): 354–355.
3. Perry LW *et al.* Echocardiographically assisted balloon atrial septostomy. *Pediatrics* 1982; **70**(3): 403–408.
4. Mitchell SE *et al.* Atrial septostomy: stationary angioplasty balloon technique—experimental work and preliminary clinical applications. *Pediatr Cardiol* 1994; **15**(1): 1–7.
5. Boucek MM *et al.* Management of the critically restrictive atrial septal defect awaiting infant cardiac transplantation. *Am J Cardiol* 1992; **70**: 559.
6. Vogel JH. Balloon embolization during atrial septostomy. *Circulation* 1970; **42**(1): 155–156.
7. Akagi T *et al.* Torn-off balloon tip of Z-5 atrial septostomy catheter. *Catheter Cardiovasc Interv* 2001; **52**(4): 500–503.

14 Blade/balloon atrial septostomy, special atrial septostomies, atrial "stent septostomy"

Blade atrial septostomy

The blade atrial septostomy catheter and procedure, as the name implies, utilize a blade to incise an opening in the atrial septum. It was designed to create an incision in a resistant or tough atrial septum using the blade to initiate the creation of a larger opening in the septum. The procedure and the unique blade catheter were developed by Dr Sang Park in collaboration with Cook Inc. (Bloomington, IN)[1]. For introduction into the heart, the blade is recessed in a metal housing or "pod" at the distal end of the catheter. Once across the septum, the blade is extended out of the metal housing and withdrawn across the septum to create the incision. A standard Rashkind™ balloon atrial septostomy or a dilation septostomy is used to extend or tear the incision created by the blade.

Indications for a blade atrial septostomy

The indications for a blade atrial septostomy are the same as those for a balloon atrial septostomy, however the blade procedure is used in older patients or in infants with a particularly tough septum. Any patient who has a restriction in the communication between the right and left atria where access of the systemic and/or pulmonary venous blood back into the functional circulation is essential, requires the creation or enlargement of an opening between the two atria. Often such patients do not present clinically until two to three months or even many years of age. There are six general categories of these older congenital heart patients who present from weeks to years after the newborn period, and who are often in desperate need of a new or enlarged atrial communication that usually requires a blade incision to initiate the opening. There is also a growing group of older patients with *acquired* cardiac problems who benefit from the creation of an atrial communication and require a blade incision to initiate catheter atrial septostomy.

1 The first group of patients who require the creation of an interatrial communication are those with transposition of the great arteries, who have insufficient mixing of systemic and pulmonary venous blood with resultant hypoxemia or pulmonary over-circulation/congestion. These patients fall into two subgroups. The first comprises those with an intact ventricular septum without an atrial communication or with an atrial communication that is too small. Patients with an intact ventricular septum or a small or non-existent atrial septal defect have no mixing of systemic and pulmonary blood and usually present very early or are very ill. These infants need an atrial communication created as an emergency regardless of what surgery is planned for them subsequently.

The second subgroup of transposition patients are those with transposition of the great arteries and an associated ventricular septal defect. These patients either have a pre-existing atrial septal defect that is too small or, more often, no atrial communication at all[2]. Patients with transposition of the great arteries, a ventricular septal defect, and an inadequate or absent atrial defect, all need a larger atrial communication for free atrial mixing, but usually not as urgently, and often they do not present for this procedure until several months of age. These patients with only a large ventricular communication "trap" a large percentage of their blood in their pulmonary circulation, develop pulmonary congestion and pulmonary hypertension and, in short order, pulmonary vascular disease unless they have an adequate interatrial communication created.

2 The second major group of patients who require a blade septostomy are those with left atrioventricular valve stenosis/atresia and an associated underdeveloped or hypoplastic left ventricle[2]. Regardless of other intracardiac communications, without an adequate atrial septal opening, the pulmonary venous blood is trapped in the left atrium, creating very high pulmonary venous pressures, preventing adequate systemic oxygenation, and leading to acidosis. Usually the existing atrial communication in hypoplastic left heart patients is very small, making the creation of an opening in the atrial septum an urgent procedure. Even though these patients are very young with very small left atria, they usually have very tough interatrial septae which require some type of blade or other special septostomy.

3 The third group of patients is those with pulmonary valve or tricuspid valve atresia/hypoplasia with hypoplastic right ventricles, in whom the systemic venous return is trapped in the right atrium by the absence of—or a small —atrial communication[3]. In the presence of either a very tiny right ventricular cavity or persistent very high right ventricular end-diastolic and systolic pressures, the right ventricle is not capable of accommodating an adequate volume of systemic venous return with each diastole. In turn, the very small or restrictive right ventricle does not pump an adequate volume through the lungs to the left ventricle to supply an effective systemic output. Without an adequate vent at the atrial level, the systemic venous return remains in the right atrium, the right atrium becomes massively dilated with stasis of systemic venous return, and the cardiac output remains low. Under these extreme circumstances, balloon or blade and balloon atrial septostomy is performed during the initial diagnostic catheterization.

When there is a possibility that the right ventricle will be able to sustain cardiac output once the pulmonary stenosis/atresia has been relieved, the atrial septum is left intact during the initial catheterization. Once the infant has stabilized after the valve perforation/dilation with or without stenting of the ductus or a systemic to pulmonary shunt, then clinical assessment will determine the need for a subsequent atrial septostomy or other intervention.

If the systemic output remains low or the right atrium and liver become distended and enlarged, the atrial septostomy can be performed hours, days or weeks later. If however, the atrial septostomy was performed at the initial catheterization when, in fact, an elevation in right atrial pressure would be essential to augment the right ventricle filling, the potential growth of the right ventricle could be compromised permanently by the adequate atrial communication created by the septostomy. In each individual case of hypoplasia of the right ventricle—and until more data are available on which ventricles will grow with adequate stimulus and with what type of stimulus—the decision as to when to create the septostomy remains an-on-the-spot judgment decision for each individual case in the catheterization laboratory.

4 The fourth group of patients who benefit dramatically from an atrial septostomy are those with total anomalous pulmonary venous connection (TAPVC). In TAPVC both the systemic and pulmonary venous blood returns to the systemic venous circulation and is restricted from returning to the systemic circulation for systemic cardiac output[4]. All of these patients need, or benefit markedly from, a large interatrial communication. Unless these patients have associated, separate obstruction of the pulmonary veins, they present much later in life (weeks, months or even years!) and a blade septostomy is required to initiate the atrial septostomy. When the atrial septum is wide open and the pulmonary veins are non-obstructed, the clinical presentation of patients with TAPVC can be very similar to that of patients with a large atrial septal defect!

5 The fifth group of older congenital heart patients who would benefit from an atrial septostomy are those with pulmonary vascular disease and severe pulmonary hypertension[5]. An atrial septal defect in these patients allows a finite amount of systemic venous blood to shunt from right to left at the atrial level. The right to left shunt vents or decompresses the right heart volume/pressure slightly through the atrial communication and also supplements the blood volume for their systemic cardiac output, as this systemic venous blood is added to the pulmonary venous blood in the left atrium. The admixture of systemic venous blood in the systemic circulation creates some systemic desaturation.

6 The sixth and final group or category of congenital heart patients who benefit from or require the creation of a special atrial communication are those who have undergone a single ventricle cavopulmonary repair and who for one reason or another are "failing", with resultant low systemic cardiac output or refractory protean loosing enteropathy. These patients frequently receive considerable symptomatic relief by the creation of a small restrictive interatrial communication. The tissues are always tough and always require some special procedures both to create and to maintain a septostomy. The interatrial communication usually increases systemic cardiac output, but this is always at the expense of some systemic desaturation. The size of this opening is critical in order to create the optimal balance between increased cardiac output and some desaturation, but without causing symptoms of hypoxia or even resulting in the death of the patient.

As already mentioned, there is also a group of older patients with acquired cardiac problems who would also benefit from an atrial communication. These are the patients with acquired severe progressive right or left heart failure where blood from the failing side of the heart needs to be vented acutely into the better functioning or supported side of the circulation. The creation of an atrial septal communication is required to vent the left heart in patients on extracorporeal membrane oxygenation (ECMO), where left-sided over-circulation and distention can be a significant problem[6,7]. Venting the right heart with an emergent septostomy following acquired acute right heart decompensation has also been done[8,9]. Almost all patients requiring ECMO are older, and in order to create a septal communication that can be relied upon for the period of ECMO and recovery, the opening should be initiated with a blade atrial incision.

When an atrial septostomy is necessary in any patient over one month of age, a blade septostomy procedure is performed as the initial procedure before proceeding with any type of balloon septostomy. Although a standard balloon atrial septostomy or a balloon dilation septostomy (Chapter 13) is usually possible in these older patients, the Rashkind™ type pull-through balloon septostomy is often ineffective against the tougher septum primum tissues of the older patient. The balloon dilation septostomy alone will merely *stretch* the opening of the foramen and not tear a permanent opening in the much tougher septae of the older infant/patient. When the opening in the septum is only stretched and not torn, the beneficial results obtained are very temporary.

If there is a pre-existing septal opening that is over 5 mm in diameter, or if the septal opening has been stretched by any other balloon septostomy procedure that was performed immediately prior to the blade septostomy, a subsequent blade septostomy through this same opening usually only stretches the opening and produces no increase in the septal opening, or at the very best, a very unsatisfactory and still restrictive opening. As the open blade is withdrawn through even a small pre-existing opening, the blade, which is not particularly sharp, distorts (elongates) the pre-existing opening to conform to the linear shape of the blade. The elongation of the septal opening allows the blade to pull through the atrial septal opening by merely stretching the pre-existing opening without incising the septal tissues at all. Whenever there is a question of the septal thickness or when the patient is over one month of age, the septostomy should be started with the blade procedure to reduce the possibility of only stretching rather than cutting and then tearing the atrial opening.

In older patients with a pre-existing small to moderate sized atrial communication but, at the same time, the pre-existing defect is too small for adequate atrial mixing, the blade incision in the septum is performed through a separate transseptal atrial puncture that is at least 5 mm (or more) away from the original opening in the atrial septum. The transseptal perforation is performed with either a standard transseptal needle set or with a radiofrequency perforation catheter[10]. The transseptal puncture is performed 5–10 mm away from the pre-existing opening. In order to create one larger opening, the new opening can be extended into the original opening by angling the blade toward the original opening during the blade pull-through. As an alternative, an entirely separate, second opening can be created with no intention of coalescing the two openings. Trans-thoracic or trans-esophageal echo guidance is helpful for determining the proper distance away from the original opening on the septum for the location of the transseptal puncture.

Equipment for blade/balloon atrial septostomy

For the optimal safety of the patient, the blade septostomy procedure should *always* be performed using a biplane fluoroscopic system and an adjunct echocardiogram. Although the procedure *can* be performed using a single-plane system, single plane X-ray fluoroscopy can only be used when the X-ray tube is capable of rapid rotation to the straight lateral position and, even then, the safety of the procedure is compromised. Patients requiring a blade septostomy are often small patients and often have a very small left atrium. A transseptal perforation to introduce the blade catheter through a very precise area of the septum or just the safe positioning of the blade catheter prior to the incision both require the capability of simultaneous, perpendicular X-ray views in order to "mentally construct" the three-dimensional anatomy. Once the transseptal or the blade catheter is in position, the echocardiographic image provides additional reassurance that the particular catheter is in the proper position.

Park™ blade septostomy catheters (Cook Inc., Bloomington, IN) are available in three sizes—the PBS 100, the PBS 200 and the PBS 300. The cutting surface or blade of the PBS 100 is 0.94 cm in length; that of the PBS 200 is 1.34 cm in length; and that of the PBS 300 is 2.0 cm in length. Although fairly sharp, the blades on the septostomy catheters are *not* finely honed cutting instruments and do not cut on mere contact with tissues, but rather, must have some "slicing" effect to incise tissues. The retracted cutting blade is contained in a tubular metal holder (pod) at the distal end of the catheter. The blade extends to the open position through a slit along one edge in the wall of the pod. Opening and closing of the blade are controlled by a long, stiff, straight, steel wire which extends through the length of the lumen of the catheter from its proximal end to the blade mechanism within the pod at the distal end. At the proximal end of the catheter the stiff wire passes through an adjustable Tuohy™ valve that is attached to the proximal hub of the catheter. The Tuohy™ valve has a "Y" side port that communicates through the catheter lumen to the chamber in the pod containing the blade mechanism, which is used for flushing the catheter lumen and the pod. The proximal, free end of the stiff wire, which extends out of the Tuohy™ valve, has a separate tightening sleeve, which is cinched securely around the wire.

At its distal end, the stiff wire within the catheter attaches to the proximal end of the blade mechanism within the pod. The blade mechanism is tested, adjusted and flushed outside of the body before use. When the stiff wire is pushed into the proximal end of the catheter, the blade mechanism is pushed open and the cutting edge of the blade is extended out of the slit on the pod. When the blade mchanism is opened in the heart, the extended blade mechanism forms a "triangle" in which the apex of the triangle extends away from the shaft of the catheter and perpendicular to the long axis of the body. The blade or sharp cutting edge of the open blade mechanism forms the caudal limb of the triangle. When the blade is extended to the desired 45–60° angle off the shaft (and pod) of the catheter, the loosened tightening sleeve is advanced over the stiff wire until it touches the Tuohy™ valve. The sleeve is cinched tightly on the wire at that position. When fixed at this position on the stiff wire, the tightening sleeve limits the distance the wire can be pushed into the catheter which, in turn, limits the degree of opening of the blade to the desired angle.

The PBS 100 and 200 blades are recessed in catheters with a 6-French shaft, while the PBS 300 is in an 8-French catheter. Because of a bulge at the attachment of the steel housing of the tubular blade container to the shaft of the catheter, blade catheters usually require an introducer sheath one size larger than the advertised diameter of the blade catheter. The PBS 200 (1.34 cm blade) is the blade catheter used routinely for infants, while the PBS 100 (0.94 cm blade) is reserved for very low weight infants or infants with a very tiny left atrium. The PBS 300 (2.0 cm blade) not only has a larger blade but is manufactured from heavier materials and, as a consequence, is a much sturdier device. The PBS 300 is used for all larger infants, older children, and adults. Because of its larger size it can naturally produce a larger incision. Because of the longer length of the blade, withdrawal of the blade through the septum can be performed with the blade extended at a less acute angle off the shaft of the catheter. This less-acute angle off the catheter shaft/carrier pod reduces the diameter of the cut which is made and actually increases the ability of the blade to cut and truly make an incision in the septal tissues. Because of its sturdier construction, the PBS 300 blade is less likely to distort or bend when pulled through a tough septum. The PBS 300 is recommended for *all* patients past infancy.

It is recommended that a long, transseptal type delivery sheath is used to advance the fairly rigid blade catheters from the right atrium into the left atrium even in the presence of a pre-existing opening. The long delivery sheaths now have a radio-opaque band at their distal tip and a back-bleed valve with a side flush port at the proximal end, both of which make their use much safer. The two smaller blade catheters require a 7-French long sheath, while the larger PBS 300 requires a 9-French sheath. These long sheaths must be long enough to reach from the femoral vein to the left atrium, but at the same time cannot be longer than the blade catheter, which is only 80 cm long. Although most patients who require a blade septostomy are infants or young children and a sheath 30–40 cm long would be sufficient (preferable!), most of the available long sheaths are transseptal length sheaths and are considerably longer than necessary for blade septostomy and definitely longer than standard balloon septostomy catheters. When the blade catheter is introduced through any transseptal length sheath, it becomes necessary to exchange this sheath for a shorter venous introductory sheath after the blade procedure, before a Rashkind™ pull-through type balloon septostomy can be performed. Although the distal end of a long transseptal sheath *can* be cut off to accommodate the balloon septostomy catheter, this must be done before its initial introduction. When the distal end is excised, it removes the distal radio-opaque marker on the sheath and results in a very poor fit over the dilator, and a much rougher and more traumatic tip on the sheath.

Transseptal sheaths come from the manufacturer with a 180° curve at the distal end. The curve on the sheath/dilator set is straightened to a gentle 20–30° curve before being used for the blade procedure. All blade septostomy procedures are followed by a balloon atrial septostomy of some type (Chapter 13), and the necessary equipment must be available for this procedure.

Technique of blade atrial septostomy

The usual blade atrial septostomy catheter/sheath is introduced percutaneously through a femoral vein. Although a pre-existing atrial septal defect *can* be crossed from a jugular/superior vena caval approach, the plane of the atrial septum when approached from cephalad is exactly parallel to the course of the catheter coming from the superior vena cava. With this angle of approach, a transseptal puncture with a needle is very difficult, particularly in a small infant. In addition, once the blade catheter has passed through the atrial septum from the superior vena caval approach, a blade incision pulling in this direction will be into the junction of the right atrium–superior vena cava with little intervening septum. A blade pulled forcefully (successfully!) in that direction has a high likelihood of incising the *wall* of the heart at the right atrial–superior vena caval junction or of damaging the sinoatrial node. Because of this, a blade atrial septostomy from the superior vena cava is contraindicated even if technically it could be accomplished.

A blade septostomy catheter can be introduced through the umbilical vein, however, the umbilical vein has usually closed by the time a patient is in need of a blade septostomy procedure. A transhepatic venous access gives a direct access to the atrial septum. The tip of virtually any catheter introduced successfully from the transhepatic approach is directed toward the atrial septum almost as soon as it enters into the right atrium from the hepatic veins. The catheter/needle/blade catheter approach to the atrial septum from a hepatic vein is almost perpendicular to the septum, which makes this approach ideal for crossing a pre-existing defect or for *performing* a transseptal atrial puncture. However, when the blade which has been introduced from the transhepatic route is opened, the open blade aligns exactly parallel to, and lies flat against, the atrial septum when it is withdrawn. As a consequence, the cutting edge of the open blade, which is not particularly sharp, is pulled flat against the surface of the septum. This eliminates any incising effect when the open blade is withdrawn further against or into the septum. Because of this absence of any angle of the blade against the septum, much more force must be used to pull the blade through the septum. Compounding this problem of the angle from the hepatic venous approach, when the blade catheter is introduced from the hepatic veins, there is almost no separation between the atrial septum and the entrance into the hepatic veins where they enter the hepatic parenchyma. This allows much less distance or "free space" for the open blade to "pop into" after it has been pulled forcefully through the septum. The transhepatic route is used for a blade septostomy only after all possibilities of approaching from the femoral veins have been exhausted.

After the hemodynamics have been obtained and the decision has been made to perform a blade atrial septostomy, a biplane angiocardiogram is recorded to visualize the left atrium. This is recorded either from a direct left atrial injection or from a "recirculation left heart" angiocardiogram following an injection into a more proximal location in the pulmonary artery or right ventricle. The biplane left atrial angiocardiogram demonstrates the size and details of the anatomy of the left atrium and provides the fixed radiographic landmarks for the subsequent septostomy. A biplane freeze frame "road map" of the left atrium is saved. Although not always necessary, this angiographic information about the left atrial anatomy contributes significantly to the safety of the procedure. Once this information is available, the diagnostic catheter and original sheath in the femoral vein are removed over a wire.

The catheter and short sheath are replaced with a long transseptal sheath/dilator set which is large enough to accommodate the blade septostomy catheter. Before the standard transseptal sheath/dilator set is used for a septostomy procedure, the original 180° transseptal curve at the distal end of the sheath is straightened into a very gentle, 15–20° curve. This curve is straightened by pulling the sheath/dilator repeatedly through the thumb and forefinger of the opposite hand or by using heat from a water bath, steam or a heat gun to soften the sheath/dilator and then hand straightening them. A 7-French transseptal set is used if a small (PBS 100) or medium (PBS 200) blade catheter is to be used. A 9-French transseptal set is necessary for the large (PBS 300) blade catheter.

If the original diagnostic catheter and a wire were in the left atrium before the diagnostic catheter was removed, the catheter is removed over an exchange length guide wire, which remains in the left atrium. The sheath/dilator set is advanced over this wire and directly into the left atrium. Once the tip of the sheath is well within the left atrium, the wire and the dilator are withdrawn very slowly while maintaining the tip of the long sheath in the left atrium. Once the wire and dilator have been removed, the sheath is cleared meticulously of any air and/or clot by allowing it to bleed back passively through the side port of the sheath whenever possible.

When there is a very small pre-existing atrial opening or a patent foramen ovale, which has not been crossed with a catheter or wire, the long sheath and dilator are advanced over the wire, but only to the area of the right atrium. The wire (only) is withdrawn, the dilator is cleared of any air or clots, attached to a flush/pressure line and flushed. In the presence of even a very small pre-existing atrial communication, the long sheath/dilator combination can often be advanced carefully, using biplane fluoroscopy, directly from the right atrium into the left atrium after the wire has been removed. This manipulation must be very gentle and careful since the tip of the dilator of the transseptal set is sharp and capable of puncturing the atrial wall if any force at all is used. The sheath/dilator is *not* advanced when there is any suggestion of resistance or other difficulty in crossing the original septal defect with it.

When a definite pre-existing opening in the septum cannot be crossed easily with the sheath/dilator combination, the dilator is removed slowly from the sheath, and after the sheath has been cleared carefully of all air or clots, an end-hole catheter of the same French size as the sheath is introduced through the long sheath. The end-hole catheter is advanced beyond the sheath and manipulated into the left atrium through the pre-existing small atrial septal defect or patent foramen. Once the dilator or catheter is within the left atrium, the long sheath is advanced over the dilator or catheter and well into the left atrium. The catheter or dilator is withdrawn slowly out of the sheath and the sheath is again cleared of any air or clots by very carefully allowing the passive free flow of fluid/blood through the side port of the valved back-bleed device on the sheath. Once completely cleared of any air and/or clot, the long sheath is attached to the flush/pressure system and placed on a continuous flush.

When the interatrial septum is intact, or if a second hole adjacent to a small pre-existing atrial septal defect is desired, the long transseptal set is advanced over a wire until the tip of the dilator is in the superior vena cava as the initial position after introduction into the vein. The left atrium is then entered by a standard, long sheath, transseptal needle puncture or, in the very small patient, by a radio-frequency wire transseptal perforation (Chapter 8) using biplane fluoroscopy as well as echocardiographic guidance. Once the tip of the long sheath has been positioned well into the left atrium, the needle and then the dilator are removed slowly and separately. Every time the needle, dilator or catheter is removed from the sheath, the sheath must be cleared meticulously of all air and clots before it is flushed at all. Preferably, the sheath is always allowed to bleed back passively through the side port of the back-bleed valve of the sheath *without* applying any suction to the sheath lumen through the side port. If there is no flow through the side port after the dilator has been removed, the valve at the proximal end of the long sheath is covered tightly with a gloved fingertip and gentle suction is applied with a syringe to the side port of the back-bleed valve. If no blood returns with very gentle suction, the sheath is withdrawn slightly or rotated slightly and mild suction reapplied. It is very important that the withdrawal of blood or air from the sheath is performed *very* gently. The "end-hole only" sheath very easily becomes trapped or totally blocked in a pulmonary vein or against the left atrial wall. When the tip of the sheath is occluded, vigorous suction will preferentially suck air through the back-bleed valve at the proximal end of the sheath! This causes an air-lock within the back-bleed valve chamber and within the lumen of the long sheath, in which case the sheath serves as a direct route into the left atrium *for air* as well as for the blade septostomy catheter! This air will subsequently be flushed into the left atrium and systemic circulation unless prevented or cleared from the sheath! Once the sheath has been cleared of air and clots, it is flushed very carefully, the side arm of the back-bleed device is attached to the pressure/flush system, and the sheath is placed on a slow continuous flush.

In a very small infant, because of the small veins and/or venospasm, occasionally it is not possible to advance a long 7-French sheath all of the way to the heart or the left atrium. In that circumstance, the blade catheter is passed through a short sheath in the femoral vein and very carefully and under continuous direct biplane fluoroscopic visualization it is advanced up the inferior vena cava to the area of the right atrium. Once the tip of the blade catheter is in the right atrium, the patient's shoulders are bent (not twisted) from the mid thorax toward the patient's right side, by sliding his shoulders to the patient's right (without rotating the body). This maneuver is identical to that described previously in Chapter 8 for the transseptal procedure in the presence of a very vertical interatrial septum or when the atrial transseptal puncture is being approached from the left groin. With the patient's trunk bent in this manner, the septum becomes more perpendicular to the long axis of the body (and the inferior vena cava) and allows the straight pod of the blade catheter to pass across the interatrial septum into the left atrium.

Prior to the introduction of the blade catheter into the long or short sheath, all of the fittings on the blade catheter are inspected, tightened and adjusted. The pod actually has a slight convex bow or bend on the surface where the groove is located on the tubular pod. This bend is necessary to assure that the apex of the blade mechanism is pushed out of the groove when the stiff control wire is pushed forward. There should be no leakage at the junctions of the blade catheter with the catheter flush port or around the Tuohy™ valve through which the control wire passes. The blade is tested and should extend easily to the desired angle and retract into the catheter pod without resistance. The degree of extension and the angle of the blade are adjusted and set after all of the other fittings have been tightened. The blade angle is determined by moving the proximal end of the stiff control wire in or out of the proximal Tuohy™ valve. The Tuohy™ valve is part of the flush port, which is attached to the proximal hub of the blade catheter. When the blade has been opened to the desired angle, there is a small plastic cylinder containing a "compression adjuster vice" which fits over the wire. This small vice is advanced over the stiff wire, against the flush port and is tightened on the wire in this position on the proximal end of the wire. With the compression vice tightened at the desired location on the control wire, the blade opens to only the predetermined angle when the distal end of the cylindrical vice on the proximal end of the wire is flush against the proximal hub/valve of the catheter. The control vice and the control wire of the blade must not be twisted or torqued during the adjustments, checking or opening and closing of the blade. Any twist on the control wire can distort or change the angle of the control wire-to-blade attachment and twist the blade in the slot on the catheter, and can cause the blade to jam in either the closed or the open position. The blade should never be withdrawn or retracted *forcefully* back into the recess of the groove in the pod on the catheter. This is particularly true with the two smaller-blade catheters. A forceful retraction into the pod causes the hinge at the tip of the blade (at the apex of the "triangle") to "over-straighten" within the slot of the metal pod. Even with the slight bend on the pod, the forceful withdrawal can "retroflex" the apical hinge point of the blade backward into the groove in the pod. If the angle of this hinge is directed toward the back of the groove, the blade cannot open when the proximal wire mechanism is advanced.

Both the side port on the blade catheter and the side arm of the back-bleed device on the long sheath are attached to the flush system. Once the sheath is in its proper position in the left atrium and the blade mechanism on the table has been checked thoroughly, both the sheath and blade catheter are on a continuous flush, the blade catheter is introduced into the long sheath and passed through the sheath directly into the left atrium. While the blade is introduced into the back-bleed device and once within the sheath, both the side port of the back-bleed device on the sheath and the side port of the blade catheter are maintained on a thorough and continuous flush. If the long sheath does not have a distal radio-opaque marker, the distance from the skin puncture site back to the hub of the sheath is measured accurately on the *sheath* and recorded. This measurement is used as a reference distance in the event that the distal end of a sheath without a marker band cannot be distinguished clearly when the blade catheter is within the sheath and, consequently, the exact position of the tip of the sheath cannot be determined. Once the entire length of the metal pod of the blade mechanism is in the left atrium as visualized on biplane fluoroscopy and echocardiography, the blade catheter is fixed in position and the sheath is withdrawn off the blade catheter and well down into the inferior vena cava (IVC). This leaves the entire exposed but unopened blade mechanism in the left atrium. Both the sheath and the blade catheter are maintained on a flush.

Occasionally, in a very small left atrium, the entire metal pod containing the blade does not fit all of the way into the left atrium and extends partially back through the septum into the right atrium. In this case, the blade and the groove containing the blade also extend partially back through the septum, which, in turn, will not allow the full length of the blade to open in the left atrium. In this circumstance, the blade catheter is advanced with a *mild*, but extra, forward push, which, in turn, indents the tip of the blade catheter into the wall of the left atrium as seen on echo. This "extra push" on the catheter allows more of the groove of the pod and the blade to advance into the left atrium. Once this groove is at least half way into the left atrium, the blade will open entirely in the left atrium as the blade emerges out of the groove. When the blade is retracted, the hinge at the tip of the blade is at the very center of the length of the groove within the metal pod. The hinge at the distal end of the actual blade forms the apex of the triangle of the open blade mechanism. As the blade is opened, this hinge point exits first from the very center of the groove along the metal pod. As long as the *center* of the groove is on the left side of the septum at the onset of opening the blade, the center of the opening blade will open on the left side of the septum and, in turn, hold the entire blade mechanism on the left side of the septum as the blade is opened to its full extent. As the blade opens, the apex of the triangle moves further into the left atrium. In the case of a very small left atrium, the catheter and blade mechanism can actually be advanced slightly into a pulmonary vein or into the left atrial wall to permit the proximal portion of the blade to open within the left atrium. During all of these maneuvers, the blade catheter is observed intermittently with alternate planes of biplane fluoroscopy and continuously with echo imaging. The lumens of both the blade catheter and the sheath are maintained on a continuous flush with heparinized flush solution.

Once the blade has been positioned within the left atrium as determined by comparison of the previously "road-mapped" pictures of the left atrial anatomy on both the PA and LAT angiocardiograms and/or by echocardiogram, the blade mechanism is opened slowly by advancing the control-wire mechanism at the proximal hub of the catheter. The blade mechanism is observed on biplane fluoroscopy and echo to ensure that the blade is not entrapped within a pulmonary vein or the left atrial appendage. To allow a wider opening of the blade in the left atrium, once it is partially opened, the blade catheter is withdrawn very slightly toward the atrial septum to free the tip of the extending blade from the area of the pulmonary veins or left atrial appendage.

Once opened, the blade is angled anteriorly. This angle is determined not only by the angle of the flush port at the proximal end of the blade catheter (which supposedly corresponds to the angle of the blade), but by direct visualization of the tip of the blade within the left atrium as seen on both PA and LAT fluoroscopy. The tip of the blade can be angled either to the right or to the left, but is always at least *slightly toward the anterior chest wall* in order to avoid the possibility of incising the A-V conducting system.

With the blade facing the proper direction, and while manually holding the proximal open/close slide mechanism securely in order to maintain the blade in the open position and at the correct angle, the blade catheter is withdrawn slowly, which draws the *edge* of the blade against the atrial septum. At this point, the hands holding the blade catheter are held against the tabletop to provide stability for the catheter. Withdrawal of the catheter with the open blade is continued slowly, but forcefully toward the IVC until the open blade "pops" through the septum. Prior to this, it is usually necessary to apply considerable force or pull against the septum. The force applied to the blade frequently results in a marked displacement of the atrial septum and the entire cardiac silhouette toward the diaphragm before the blade actually incises and cuts through the septum. If the blade does not cut through the septum, even with a moderate amount of force and in spite of a very significant displacement of the heart, the traction on the blade catheter is relaxed while the catheter with the open blade is re-advanced back into the left atrium. The open angle or cutting angle of the open blade is decreased very slightly by withdrawing the proximal control wire very slightly, which retracts the blade (and decreases the angle of the triangle) slightly into the groove on the catheter. The compression vice is readjusted on the control wire to fix this new angle of the blade when the vice is advanced against the hub. Withdrawal through the septum is reattempted with the reduced angle on the blade until the blade pulls successfully through the septum. If the entire heart is displaced considerably toward the diaphragm without the blade pulling through the septum, the long sheath in the IVC should be withdrawn even further down into the IVC before repeating the withdrawal. Although the blade is withdrawn very slowly and meticulously, when the blade successfully pulls through the septum there is the sensation of the blade "snapping" or "popping" through the septum as the heart "snaps" back in a cephalad direction into the thorax. As soon as the blade pops through the septum, it is immediately retracted back into the catheter by pulling back on the compression vice mechanism on the proximal wire.

After a successful withdrawal of the blade through the septum and with the blade retracted into the pod of the catheter, the blade catheter alone can usually be re-advanced cephalad and back into the right atrium, and from the right atrium, easily back through the newly created septal opening into the left atrium. If the angle of the metal pod of the blade catheter is not sufficient to allow this, the sheath is re-advanced carefully over the tip of the pod of the blade catheter to a position 1–2 mm distal to the tip of the pod. With the sheath in this position, the curvature of the sheath, together with the slight bend in the blade catheter, is usually sufficient to direct the combined blade and sheath into the left atrium with gentle to-and-fro and/or torque motion of the sheath/blade catheter combination. To facilitate the passage back into the left atrium when there is any resistance, it is helpful to bend the patient's thorax to his right similarly to the maneuver when performing a transseptal puncture from the left groin. This tends to position the new opening in the atrial septum more perpendicular to the long axis of the blade catheter.

If the blade catheter cannot be reintroduced into the left atrium very easily, it is withdrawn from the sheath while continually flushing the side port of both the sheath and the catheter. The blade catheter is removed from the long sheath and replaced with a diagnostic catheter, which, in turn, is manipulated back into the left atrium. The sheath is re-advanced over this diagnostic catheter into the left atrium, the catheter removed, the sheath cleared of any air and the blade catheter reintroduced through the sheath. Extreme care must be taken to avoid the introduction of air or clots with the catheter and blade exchanges.

When the blade catheter is out of the sheath, it is very important to inspect the pod which holds the recessed blade to be sure that it is free of any clots or debris, since the entire groove cannot be flushed adequately only by flushing the lumen of the catheter. The lumen of the blade catheter is maintained on a continuous flush while the blade mechanism is inspected and the groove in the pod is cleared of any clot or fibrin. The groove with the distal blade mechanism can be flushed directly by using a needle on a hand-held syringe of flush fluid and forcefully injecting a jet of fluid directly into the groove, over and around the blade.

The reintroduction of the blade catheter into the left atrium and the blade withdrawal are repeated four or five times. With each withdrawal, the angle of the open blade is extended to at least 45° off the shaft of the catheter and the side-to-side angle of the blade within the 180° anterior arc within the heart silhouette is changed with each withdrawal. The blade is always directed anteriorly and either to the right, straight anterior or to the left during subsequent withdrawals. It is to be hoped that at least several small incisions are made at different angles around the anterior 180° circumference of the incised opening in the atrial septum. The posterior 180° is avoided to stay away from the A-V conduction tissues. During the repeated manipulations of the blade, the blade catheter and the sheath are kept under a continuous flush. After four to six blade withdrawals have been performed at different side-to-side angles, or once the blade no longer meets any resistance, it is retracted into the catheter and withdrawn through the introductory sheath.

Following the multiple blade incisions, a balloon atrial septostomy is performed. This can be accomplished with a standard Miller™ septostomy balloon (Edwards Lifesciences, Irvine, CA) or with a static angioplasty balloon. In order to use the Rashkind™ pull-through type of balloon, the long sheath must be replaced with a short 7-French, valved back-bleed sheath. Although the long sheath is of the same French size as the short sheath, a Miller™ septostomy balloon will not pass easily through a long sheath to the left atrium without binding within it. Also unless the long transseptal sheath was shortened before it was introduced initially, it will be too long for both Miller™ and NuMED™ (NuMED Inc., Hopkinton, NY) balloon septostomy catheters.

The side port of the introductory sheath is flushed continuously while the balloon for the septostomy is passing through the sheath into the venous system. The deflated septostomy balloon acts as a plunger within the lumen of the sheath during its introduction into the sheath and creates a significant vacuum behind it. Unless the space in the sheath is filled with flush solution, the vacuum will suck air through the valve on the sheath and into the sheath. Once advanced through the sheath, the septostomy balloon is manipulated across the incised atrial communication and into the left atrium. The balloon is inflated to the maximum volume that can be tolerated by both the balloon and the anatomy of the patient. The fully inflated balloon is jerked very forcefully, but in a controlled fashion, across the septum as with any other Rashkind™ septostomy. The septostomy balloon is pulled through the septum four or five times, each time using the maximum volume that can be tolerated by the size of the left atrium. The goal is to extend the initial incision(s) made by the blade catheter with significant further tear(s) in the septum. In older patients, often the septum is very tough and the maximally inflated balloon cannot be jerked through the septum even after multiple blade incisions.

In these older patients and others with a very thick or tough atrial septum, enlargement of the septum after it has been incised with the blade is performed with angioplasty dilation balloons. A single balloon or, preferably, two balloons side by side are used, depending on the venous access for the balloons and the size of the atrial septal communication that is to be created. Although the femoral approach is preferred, if necessary one or both of the angioplasty balloons can be introduced via an internal jugular or even a subclavian vein approach.

To use an angioplasty balloon following the blade procedure, the blade catheter is replaced with an end-hole catheter which is passed across the newly created defect, into the left atrium and into a left pulmonary vein. The catheter is replaced with a stiff exchange length guide wire and the angioplasty balloon introduced over this wire. The balloon is centered across the septum over this wire and inflated in the defect to its maximum pressure. As with other dilation procedures, a waist appears on the balloon and with full inflation the waist disappears. If two balloons are used for the dilation septostomy, the second balloon is introduced over a wire from a separate venous introductory site. The second balloon is positioned across the atrial septum side by side with the first balloon and the two balloons are inflated simultaneously, observing for the waists on both of them. Using two balloons side by side has the advantage of allowing the use of significantly smaller balloons, which allows venous access from two separate, smaller veins. Double balloons also allow for the creation of much larger openings in a very large patient than is possible with a single balloon. The use of dilation balloons has the advantages of producing a more controlled tear in the septum and allowing access for the septostomy from a greater variety of sites. Furthermore there is far less likelihood of the balloon being disrupted and a piece or all of the balloon material being lost somewhere in the circulation.

The adequacy of the newly created defect is verified by one of several techniques following the balloon septostomy. Measurement of the hemodynamic data including the systemic saturation, right and left atrial pressures, and pulmonary artery pressure gives the best estimate of the functional success of the procedure. The Miller™ septostomy balloon in the left atrium is partially inflated with 1–4 ml of dilute contrast and gently pulled, or allowed to float, through the newly created defect. The "stretched size" of the defect is determined by the diameter of the balloon at that volume of inflation which demonstrates slight resistance at the beginning of the withdrawal. A fairly accurate assessment of the newly created atrial defect at least in one dimension is obtained from an angiographic measurement of the diameter of this balloon as it "milks" through the septum. In the presence of left to right shunting, a left atrial angiocardiogram with the injection in the mouth of the right upper pulmonary vein and filming in the four-chamber (45° LAO–45° cranial angulated) view is performed. This angiocardiogram usually "cuts" the newly created atrial defect on edge and provides a visualization of the new opening. When the shunting through the newly created defect is predominantly right to left, a straight lateral view with injection into the low right atrium/inferior vena caval junction usually provides the optimal angiographic view of the defect. The size and persistence of the newly created atrial defect can also be visualized and the size estimated by echocardiography (especially transesophageal echo).

When performed properly using biplane fluoroscopic and echocardiographic guidance and by always paying meticulous attention to the details of the procedure, the blade septostomy procedure is extremely safe and effective. The actual blade "pull-through" produces a very controlled incision in the septum with the only uncontrolled and unsafe portion of the procedure being the subsequent balloon septostomy enlargement of the defect using a Rashkind™ type, pull-through technique. The greatest hazard of the blade septostomy procedure is not from the blade withdrawal itself or damage produced by the blade incision, but from the potential for the inadvertent introduction of air or clot during the many exchanges of wires, catheters, blades and balloons. Whenever venous access is possible from the femoral approach, the blade/balloon atrial septostomy produces a very effective atrial communication which precludes the need for a surgical atrial septostomy. When femoral venous access is not available or there is a very tough atrial septum with a very small left atrium, alternate routes/procedures are available to create an atrial communication non-surgically.

Cutting balloon septostomy

Often the septum is very tough and resistant to even a dilation balloon, or the opening which is created has been stretched rather than torn and "rebounds" closed very shortly after the dilation. If the patient is a very small infant with a very small or non-existent atrial opening, or the left atrium is too small for even a PBS 100 blade catheter, then a dilation septostomy can be initiated with a cutting balloon catheter (Boston Scientific, Natick, MA).

The maximum diameter of the available cutting balloons is 8 mm. The alternative of using a cutting balloon is only applicable when starting with a very small or, preferably, non-existent opening in the septum. When there is a pre-existing opening which has stretched rather than torn with a dilation balloon and when proceeding to use a cutting balloon, it is better to perform a transseptal puncture with a long sheath set and to start using the cutting balloon in this new, very restrictive opening.

In very small patients, a radio-frequency transseptal perforation as described in Chapter 8 is preferable to a standard needle transseptal puncture because of the size constraints of the patients and their left atria along with better control of the puncture[11]. Once the septum has been crossed with the radio-frequency "burn", either a 0.014" Iron-Man™ (Guidant Corp., Santa Clara, CA) stiff wire or—preferably—a 6-French long sheath/dilator is positioned through the puncture and into the left atrium. The cutting balloon is advanced directly over the wire or, preferably, through the long sheath and positioned across the septum. If a sheath is present, it is withdrawn completely off the balloon and the cutting balloon is inflated to its maximum pressure/diameter in the atrial septum. When inflated, the cutting balloon is moved slightly forward or backward over the wire within the opening to enhance the "incising" effect of its micro blades. The cutting balloon is deflated, rotated slightly within the septal opening and the "inflation–incision" repeated. After at least two separate inflations–incisions with the cutting balloon, it is withdrawn through the long sheath and replaced over the wire with a dilation balloon of a diameter several millimeters larger than the opening that is desired. The dilation is repeated with the larger balloon with the expectation that the incisions made with the cutting balloon will tear further and extend the opening. The size of the dilation balloon is increased incrementally to increase the size of the atrial communication.

Biopsy septostomy

Another alternative to a blade septostomy when the left atrium is extremely small or when there is no access to the septum from the femoral vein is to use a biopsy forceps catheter to "bite away" small segments of the atrial septum in order to create a larger opening in the septum. This procedure was first described by Boucek *et al.* for use in infants with hypoplastic left heart syndrome, intact atrial septum and a very small left atrium[12]. In these patients, it is not possible to open even the very small P 100 blade in the tiny left atrial cavity, and a standard NuMED™ K-5 balloon septostomy catheter (NuMED Inc., Hopkinton, NY) cannot tear the very tough septum.

To perform a bioptome septostomy, a slight curve is formed at the tip of a standard biopsy forceps catheter. The larger the bioptome catheter that can be used, the larger the "bite" and the more effective is the opening that is produced by the bite. A 5- or 6-French biopsy forceps catheter is advanced through a long sheath, which is introduced from the femoral vein and pre-positioned in the right atrium adjacent to the septum. This allows the bioptome catheter to be withdrawn and reintroduced expeditiously without significant manipulation in order to approach the septum between bites. The bioptome is directed using biplane fluoroscopic and echocardiographic guidance, with the fluoroscopy directing the bioptome to the immediate area of the septum and the echo defining exactly where the bioptome bites on the septum. The biopsy forceps is opened in the low right atrium and the jaws are advanced cephalad and posteriorly until a jaw catches on the limbus of the foramen in the atrial septum. If the edge of the septum is not grasped initially, the maneuver is repeated while rotating the biopsy forceps catheter or the long sheath until the edge of the atrial septal opening has been caught by the open jaws of the forceps.

If not successful after several attempts, the bioptome catheter is withdrawn and the curve at the tip of the bioptome is changed slightly to correspond better to the intracardiac anatomy. The rim or edge of the existing foramen is grasped with the jaws of the biopsy forceps and a bite is taken similar to any biopsy. The excised piece is withdrawn and the procedure is repeated until a satisfactory opening has been created in the septum or until a significant slit or cut in the edge of the original septal opening has been created. The long sheath remaining in the right atrium facilitates the repeated bites. Once the edge of the original opening has been incised or "disrupted" with the bioptome, the opening can often be torn further with a dilation balloon septostomy as described in Chapter 13.

The biopsy forceps technique can be used in a patient of any age. It is useful particularly when the septum is extremely tough and resistant to cutting with a blade catheter or when the left atrium is extremely small and cannot tolerate the opening of even a small blade within it.

The biopsy forceps septostomy technique is also useful when there is interruption of the femoral veins/inferior vena cava. When the catheter is introduced from the neck through a superior vena cava approach, the bioptome is directed caudally and the bite with the forceps is on the caudal rim of the original defect. When the bites are taken from this area on the caudal rim of the septum, the procedure *must* have echo guidance to ensure that the atrioventricular valves are not being damaged. When biting on the inferior rim of the atrial septal defect, there is always danger of damage to the atrioventricular conduction system. A more conservative removal of tissue with the bioptome is performed from the superior vena cava approach. The initial opening created with the bioptome bite is expanded further with a dilation balloon.

Stent atrial septostomy

Occasionally it is desirable to maintain the opening in the atrial septum for the temporary, or sometimes even permanent, palliation of complex congenital heart defects. Often the openings or fenestrations created in the atrial septum or atrial baffles by surgery, balloon, or blade and balloon atrial septostomies spontaneously shrink in diameter or even close completely. To prevent this, a standard intravascular stent can be implanted in the atrial opening to maintain its patency. Intravascular stents are used in the interatrial septum or baffles in two different circumstances. In neonates with hypoplastic left hearts, as large an opening as possible is desired in the septum, but the stenting of the septum will usually only be necessary for a matter of months. The other circumstance is in patients who need venting of high right heart or systemic venous pressure, not only to lower the venous pressure but also to enhance systemic cardiac output. These openings may be necessary for an indefinite period of time and usually must be of a specific, much more restricted diameter.

Commonly, rigid P 188 or P 308 stents (Johnson & Johnson, Warren, NJ) are used for stenting the interatrial septum, although recently the "large", pre-mounted Genesis stents (Johnson & Johnson–Cordis Corp., Miami Lakes, FL), which can be dilated to 11 or 12 mm diameter, have been used in newborns where the opening will only be necessary for 3–12 months. The even larger Genesis XD stents (Johnson & Johnson–Cordis Corp., Miami Lakes, FL) are used for the creation of the more permanent larger "fenestrations". Both the initial "dumb-bell" expansion of balloon expandable stents and the overall shrinkage in length as the stents expand, are used to advantage during this particular application in order both to center the stent on the septum and to secure the stent once it has been implanted.

After it has expanded fully and after the shrinkage in length of the stent with expansion, the shorter P 188 stent is almost ideal in length to bridge the usual thickness of the atrial septum. However, this short length is often very difficult to center precisely on the "invisible", moving and relatively thin membrane of the atrial septum. Positioning a shorter stent is made more difficult by the angle that always exists between the delivery wire/balloon/stent and the angle of the septum in small patients. P 308 stents, which are twice as long, provide some margin of error for centering the stent on the septum; however, they have a greater likelihood of extending away from the septum and interfering with access to adjacent areas or to the vital structures themselves—the tricuspid valve in particular. When using the large Genesis™ stent, the choice is between a 19 mm and a 29 mm long one. Since these stents cannot be dilated beyond 12 mm in diameter, the shrinkage in length is less and the 19 mm long large Genesis™ stent is usually sufficient to open the newborn atrial septum completely.

An intravascular stent is particularly useful to splint the atrial septum open in infants with hypoplastic left hearts where there is a restrictive interatrial communication and while the patients are awaiting or have undergone a first stage palliation. In these patients, the left atrium is too small or the interatrial septum is too short and tough to allow the creation of an effective and persistent opening with the usual blade or balloon atrial septostomy. A premounted 19 mm long large Genesis™ or a P _ _ 8 stent, which is mounted as far distally on as short a balloon as possible, is used in these patients. The balloon for the delivery of the stent should have a diameter of only 1–2 mm less than the maximum diameter of the infant's total interatrial septum, and should be significantly larger in diameter than any existing opening in the atrial septum. The forceful over-expansion of these stents into the rim of the existing septal defect is the only mechanism that holds these stents in place in the septum!

The stent placement is controlled using angiography, which is usually performed through a separate catheter. The separate controlling catheter is introduced from a second venous entry site. Transesophageal echo (TEE) or intracardiac echo (ICE) is extremely useful in larger patients, but the large size of the TEE probe or the large sheath necessary for the ICE catheter make both of these modalities in their standard usage too large for use in the newborn infant. The ICE probe has been used successfully as a TEE probe for transesophageal imaging in the newborn infant and may be a viable option to obtain TEE assistance during stent implants. The septum in a small infant is seen very well by trans-thoracic echo. When there is a question about the exact location of the interatrial septum, a small tag of contrast can be placed in the septum with a transseptal needle as described previously in Chapter 8. This is particularly useful in older or larger patients where the opening is being created as well as held open.

An end-hole catheter from one venous access site is maneuvered into a left upper pulmonary vein and is replaced with the largest and stiffest wire which the particular dilation balloon catheter for the selected stent will accept. Whenever possible, it is advisable to introduce an angiographic catheter into the right atrium from a second venous puncture. This catheter will be used for positioning angiograms during the implant of the stent in the septum. For P _ _ 8 stents, a long sheath through which the balloon/stent combination must be delivered is advanced over the wire with its appropriate dilator to the area of the atrial septum, and the sheath alone is advanced off the dilator to the mouth of the pulmonary vein. The dilator is withdrawn from the sheath over the wire and the sheath meticulously cleared passively of any air or clot. The position of the sheath/wire in relation to the pulmonary vein and the atrial septum is visualized with a biplane angiocardiogram (through the sheath or, preferably, the separate venous catheter) and on echocardiogram. A premounted, 19 or 29 mm, large Genesis™ stent can be delivered to the septum directly over the wire without the use of a long sheath, although such a sheath does add some security and additional support.

With the structures adjacent to the septum recorded or committed to memory according to radiographically visible landmarks, the stent/balloon is advanced through the sheath, over the wire or, in the case of the Genesis™ stents, directly over the wire to a position exactly straddling the atrial septum. The sheath is withdrawn off the P _ _ 8 balloon/stent and the position of the stent/balloon in relation to the septum checked angiographically and by echo with either type of stent. In small infants and because of the small size of the atrial structures combined with the stiff delivery wire/balloon/stent combination, the balloon/stent over the wire is always aligned tangentially across the septum, necessitating some delicate manipulations to center the stent on the septum. Once the stent has been centered exactly across the plane of the atrial septum, the balloon catheter and the wire are fixed very firmly and the balloon/stent inflated very slowly. With any movement of the balloon or stent, the inflation is stopped and the position of the stent/balloon is checked with a repeat angiogram and adjusted as necessary. Usually, a considerable simultaneous forward force must be maintained on the balloon dilation catheter and the wire in order to keep the stent in position.

When the stent is in the proper position, it is inflated fully. Usually the stent pushes the rim of any true septal tissue out of the way and no apparent residual waist persists on the stent. When it appears that there is still a significant atrial rim around the fully expanded stent, and if a long sheath was used to deliver the stent, the balloon is inflated to a low pressure within the stent. While the balloon is *being deflated* and while the balloon still is within the stent, the sheath is re-advanced over the balloon and into the stent. The original balloon is withdrawn over the wire and through the sheath, which is now within and through the stent. The original balloon is exchanged for a larger diameter balloon in order to expand the stent to the maximum diameter of the interatrial septum. When a long sheath is not used for the delivery, the replacement with a larger balloon is accomplished over the wire, directly through the stent and *very, very cautiously*! The larger the final diameter of the stent, the better its fixation will be in the thin atrial septal tissues.

Small persistent atrial communications of a fixed, small diameter are desired in patients with pulmonary hypertension and in some patients with intracardiac baffles following single ventricle, "Fontan" surgical repairs. Atrial septal or baffle openings are created to vent the right heart or systemic venous blood while, at the same time, enhancing systemic cardiac output with the additional volume of the added venous blood. The placement of an intravascular stent in the atrial septum in these patients is usually performed only after a balloon or blade and balloon atrial septostomy during previous catheterizations have failed to maintain an atrial communication at least once. Small atrial defects created either surgically or in the catheterization laboratory are particularly prone to spontaneous closure, while slightly larger defects in these particular patients can result in severe and often uncontrollable hypoxemia, which is usually catastrophic. An intravascular stent that is expanded to a very specific diameter at the center of the stent, creates a defect in the atrial septum of a specific size and can maintain the patency of the smaller defect for an extended period of time[13,14].

The stent is prepared ahead of time in order to ensure that the center of the stent expands only to the specific small opening that is desired in these patients, although there now are dumb-bell shaped balloons (NuMED Inc., Hopkinton, NY), which expand the center of the stent only to a specified diameter while expanding the ends of the stent to their full diameter. When using a standard balloon and before the stent is mounted on the balloon, a restraining band or loop of suture of a predetermined fixed diameter is fixed around the center of the stent. The diameter of the loop formed by the restraining band is the same as the diameter of the desired opening in the septum. To create an opening of a very specific diameter which cannot be enlarged further, the restraining band is made from a heavy 1-0 or 2-0, non-resorbable suture or even a fine surgical wire. This creates a very secure band around the stent, but does not allow for any further dilation of the opening even much later in the future. When there is any consideration that in the future the opening in the septum might need to be enlarged, an equally heavy resorbable suture is used to create the band around the stent. A resorbable suture will restrain the lumen of the stent at the diameter which is desired at the time of implant, but it will resorb over several months and allow the stent to be dilated further when desired.

To form the constricting band or loop with either type of suture, the stent is first dilated with an 8–10 mm diameter balloon. Once the stent has been inflated to this diameter, the balloon is deflated and removed from the stent. The partial expansion of the stent separates the struts of the stent by a small amount, creating slight openings between the struts around the circumference of the stent. The openings between the struts allow the suture to be threaded through the adjacent openings at the center of the stent and around the entire circumference of the stent. Once the suture is in place through the struts, a balloon with the precise diameter of the desired opening is placed in the stent and the stent crimped down to that diameter. When the stent has been crimped tightly on the balloon, the suture is tied securely around the stent/balloon to form a loop of the desired diameter. This smaller diameter balloon is deflated and removed. The stent is placed over a deflated balloon that is at least twice, and preferably three to four times, the diameter of the suture loop (and of the desired defect) and recompressed and hand crimped over this larger deflated balloon for delivery.

Two venous introductory routes are secured. An angiographic catheter is advanced into the right atrium and positioned either through a pre-existing small opening in the atrial septum or immediately adjacent to the site where the septum will be punctured. If there is a pre-existing opening in the septum or a small fenestration in a baffle, an end-hole catheter is advanced from the second venous site and through the septal opening until it is secured distally within the pulmonary venous atrium or preferably in a left upper pulmonary vein. The catheter is replaced with a short floppy-tipped, Super Stiff™ wire and the catheter removed over the wire. A slight curve, which conforms to the course from the right atrium through the septum to the left atrium, is formed at the distal end of the long, large diameter transseptal sheath/dilator. The long sheath of the delivery sheath/dilator must be large enough in diameter to accommodate the dilation balloon with the stent mounted on it, including the additional diameter of the suture around (intertwined in) the stent (usually 1–2 French sizes larger). The long transseptal sheath/dilator set is introduced over the prepositioned wire and advanced until the tip of the *sheath* is in the left atrium. In the case of a very small left atrium, the sheath must be advanced off the dilator and into the atrium.

When there is no pre-existing opening in the atrial septum or baffle, the septum or baffle is crossed using a transseptal puncture and a 7- or 8-French transseptal sheath/dilator set. When there is a very tough septal patch/baffle, an original USCI™ Mullins™ transseptal sheath/dilator set (Medtronic Inc., Minneapolis, MN) is used for the puncture. The dilators of these sets have a much finer taper and fit very tightly over the needle and, as a consequence, will penetrate very tough tissues when the other transseptal sets will not! Once the sheath is across the septum or baffle, the needle and dilator are replaced with an end-hole catheter which will accommodate a 0.035″ Super Stiff™ wire. The catheter is maneuvered into a left upper pulmonary vein and replaced with the Super Stiff™ wire. The transseptal sheath is replaced with a larger long sheath/dilator set which is large enough to accommodate the stent/balloon/suture loop. When the created or existing opening in the baffle is very small or very tough, the opening may need to be dilated with a small dilation balloon in order to accommodate the larger sheath/dilator for the stent delivery.

When implanting a stent in the atrial septum or a baffle, either within a small pre-existing opening or through a transseptal puncture, it is very helpful to place a small tag of contrast solution in the tissues of the atrial septum or baffle immediately adjacent to the opening where the stent is to be placed. This tagging of the septum is performed frequently during standard transseptal punctures of the atrial septum (Chapter 8) and the tag is accomplished easily through a transseptal needle just before the transseptal sheath/dilator set is advanced into the left atrium. If the sheath has already passed through a pre-existing opening in the septum, the tag can still be produced using the transseptal needle advanced through a second catheter which is at least 6-French in size and less than 55 cm long, or through a separate transseptal sheath/dilator. The tag on the septal tissues provides a distinct visible marker, which can be seen on fluoroscopy in order to identify the exact position of the septum, which is often very mobile, during the implant. Since the contrast material in a tag tends to dissipate from the tissues fairly rapidly, the tag is placed in the tissues immediately before the stent is to be delivered to the septum.

Once the stent has been prepared completely with the fixed diameter loop of suture around it, it is mounted on the balloon and everything is prepared for the stent delivery, the transseptal needle in the second catheter/dilator is positioned on the atrial septum with the *tip of the dilator* firmly against the septum either immediately adjacent to the small existing opening or in the position where the transseptal puncture will be performed. With the tip of the catheter/dilator, which contains the needle fixed against the septal tissues, the needle is advanced into the atrial septum or the tissue of the baffle just beyond the tip of the dilator or catheter. With the tip of the needle "buried" in the atrial septal tissues and before the needle punctures through the septum, a small (0.3 ml) injection of contrast is forced through the transseptal needle producing an opaque tag or plaque of contrast on the septum.

When there is a pre-existing small, natural atrial opening and/or when a new transseptal puncture is performed in *true atrial septal tissues*, the atrial septum should ***not*** *be pre- or re-dilated* prior to the subsequent implant of the stent. However, when the stent is being implanted in a baffle and even if there is a pre-existing small opening in the baffle, the baffle should first be pre-dilated to the diameter of the desired eventual opening with a balloon *before* the long transseptal sheath *for the stent* delivery is passed through the opening.

Occasionally the pre-existing opening or the newly created puncture cannot be dilated with even a small high-pressure balloon, in which case the opening is incised with a blade septostomy catheter or the dilation is performed with a cutting balloon of the appropriate size. The blade incision in the baffle or the cutting balloon dilation of the baffle is created the same diameter as the eventual desired opening. This is to ensure that the thick, tough, often synthetic baffle material can be dilated at least to the desired restricted diameter of the stent.

Once the sheath of the long sheath/dilator set that is to be used to deliver the stent is in the left atrium over a wire, and the wire is positioned securely on the left side of the baffle, the dilator or end-hole catheter is removed and the sheath meticulously cleared passively of any air and/or clot as previously described in Chapter 8 ("Transseptal Technique"). The tag of contrast in the septal tissues should demarcate the position where the sheath passes through the septum very clearly. The stent, which is mounted on the large balloon with its constraining suture, is introduced over the wire and through the back-bleed valve on the long sheath. The stent/balloon/loop of suture must be covered with a short, protective "sleeve" for their introduction into the sheath through the back-bleed valve. The sleeve is made from a short (5–6 cm long) segment of a sheath of the same diameter as the long delivery sheath. The balloon/sheath/suture combination is introduced into the short sleeve before it is introduced into the back-bleed valve in order to prevent the stent with the encircling suture from being displaced proximally on or even off the balloon as it passes through the tight valve. The stent/balloon with the suture around it is advanced over the wire, out of the short sheath, and into and through the long sheath until the stent/balloon, which is still within the sheath, *straddles* the septum with the center of the stent exactly aligned with the tag on the septum. The long sheath is withdrawn well off the balloon/stent combination leaving the stent straddling the septum. The exact position of the balloon/stent straddling the septum is confirmed with an angiogram after the sheath has been withdrawn by injecting through the second catheter, which is positioned in the right atrium immediately adjacent to the stent/balloon in the defect. A TEE or ICE may be helpful in visualizing the position on a true atrial septum but may not be of any help in visualizing the specific site of puncture in a baffle of synthetic material.

When satisfied that the center of the stent is straddling the defect exactly, the balloon is inflated slowly while recording on biplane angiography or biplane stored fluoroscopy. The "dumbbelling" of the stent as the ends of the balloon expand initially, tends to self-center the stent in the defect within the septum or baffle as the balloon/stent expands. The suture around the center of the stent (or the restriction in the special "dumbbell" balloons) restricts the expansion of the center of the stent to precisely the desired diameter for the opening. The two ends of the much larger diameter balloon expand the two ends of the stent on each side of the septum as the balloon expands completely. Once the balloon and stent are fully expanded at both ends, the balloon is deflated and the security of the stent checked by slight, careful, to-and-fro movements of the balloon catheter.

If the stent seems at all precarious when the technique with the suture securing the central diameter has been used, the balloon is reinflated at a low pressure and then, as the balloon is deflated, the sheath is advanced into and through the stent over the deflating balloon. The original balloon is removed and a larger diameter balloon is introduced over the wire and through the sheath and centered within the stent. The sheath is withdrawn off the balloon and the ends of the stent are expanded even further with the larger balloon. When satisfied with the security of the stent in the septum, the balloon catheter is removed over the wire leaving the stent in place with a new fixed diameter atrial septal opening. This further expansion of the ends is not possible when the stent is delivered over a dumbbell shaped balloon without a central suture tied around the stent unless a very special order balloon with the same central diameter but with larger ends is available.

An alternate technique for fixing a stent in the atrial septum at a specific predetermined central diameter is to use a loop of non-stretchable, radio-opaque, flexible wire fixed at a specific diameter but only around the *balloon under the stent*. The loop of wire remains attached to one long strand of the wire, which will extend out of the body. The wire loop is fixed at the specific diameter by first tying it tightly around a fully inflated, separate, small balloon of the same size as the desired defect which is to be created. The intention is to remove the restraining wire loop along with the balloon after the implant of the stent, which leaves no fixed restraint around the stent even immediately after implant. To accomplish this, the wire loop around the balloon remains attached to one very long strand of wire, which extends off the loop, out from under the proximal end of the stent, along and adjacent to the shaft of the balloon catheter within the delivery sheath, and eventually out of the body adjacent to the proximal shaft of the catheter. The long strand of wire allows the loop of wire to be withdrawn along with the balloon after the stent has been implanted and the balloon deflated.

The loop of wire, which is created to the very specific diameter of the desired opening in the septum, is placed around the *exact center* of a much larger diameter balloon, which is to be used to implant the stent. The stent is expanded partially and then advanced over the partially expanded balloon, which has the wire loop centered loosely on it. It is essential to partially inflate/expand the balloon in order to hold the loop in its precise position on the balloon during the mounting process. This also requires a significant but still partial pre-expansion of the stent in order for the stent to be advanced over the balloon. Once the loop has been positioned properly at the center of the partially expanded balloon and centered under the stent, the stent is crimped progressively over the balloon and wire loop as the balloon is gradually deflated. It is a challenge to maintain the loop, which is relatively loose around the deflated balloon, under the stent and at the exact center of the balloon/stent[15]. When the stent has been mounted securely over the balloon with the loop around it, the balloon/stent/wire loop combination is advanced into and through the long delivery sheath while the long strand of one end of the wire loop trails behind the balloon/stent adjacent to the balloon catheter.

This technique is slightly more cumbersome as it is significantly more difficult to maintain the wire loop in the exact position on the balloon while the stent is being mounted, since the wire loop is larger in diameter than the totally deflated balloon and has *no attachment* to the stent or the balloon. Another disadvantage of this type of loop is that if there is any displacement of the stent on the balloon as the balloon and stent are being delivered or as the balloon is being inflated, the wire loop may not remain exactly at the center of the stent. In addition, once the balloon has been deflated after the initial expansion of the stent, the wire loop will be loose on the balloon, leaving no permanent central band around the stent to maintain the central constriction while the ends are flared further if desired or necessary immediately after implant. However, the absence of the fixed suture around the stent allows the restriction in the stent and, along with it, the opening in the septum to be expanded further immediately after implant as well as at any time in the future.

The central diameter of a stent that has been implanted securely in the atrial septum can be reduced in size with the use of a Goose-Neck™ Snare (ev3, Plymouth, MN). The snare catheter is introduced from the femoral vein and the open loop of the snare is passed over the proximal end of the stent, which extends out into the right atrium. Once maneuvered over the proximal stent, the snare is slowly tightened around the central portion of the stent until the desired diameter is achieved. This does have the disadvantages that the technique cannot be used to reduce the diameter very precisely, and it loosens the stent from its secure fixation within the septum as the narrowest area is decreased further. The precise technique for preparing and delivering a "restricted" stent will depend upon the particular immediate and future needs of each individual patient.

Special devices designed for the creation of a fixed diameter interatrial communication

Small interatrial communications of a specific size are often essential in older patients with pulmonary vascular disease and in patients following "Fontan" types of repair where a specific and small amount of right to left shunting is beneficial, while a larger amount of shunting can be catastrophic.

In order to simplify the process of maintaining the fixed patency of these communications, the AGA™ Company (AGA Medical Corp., Golden Valley, MN) produced a "splint" or "Fenestrated ASD Shunt Device", which has pre-formed holes of specific diameters through its central hub. These devices are manufactured from the same materials and are very similar to the Amplatzer™ ASD occluders (AGA Medical Corp., Golden Valley, MN), except that the splints are manufactured with one or two channels of predetermined size that pass completely through the hub of the device. The hub or central portion of the initial splint prostheses had a diameter of 14 mm and a thickness of approximately 4 mm. The retention disk on each side of the hub varied between 2 and 10 mm depending upon the relation of the hole in the device to the edge of the retention disk. The initial prototype devices had one 10 mm hole or "fenestration" while subsequent clinical models have one or two 5 mm diameter holes.

When these Amplatzer™ fenestrated devices are expanded into the atrial septum, the channel(s) that pass completely through the two end disks and the central hub of the device create one or two small channels between the two atria. When the device is expanded completely and properly in the septum the holes that are created expand to the diameters of the originally manufactured channel(s) in the device[16]. The technique for implanting these "fenestrated" devices is similar to that for implanting Amplatzer™ atrial septal occluders. The channel(s) in the fenestrated device can be expanded a small amount after implant by balloon dilation of the opening with or without the implant of a stent or could be occluded with a separate occlusion device if necessary. Amplatzer™ shunt prostheses require a significantly larger initial opening in the septum than the opening that is usually found or created in patients requiring these small fixed communications, and this opening in the septum must be very close to the diameter of the hub of the device.

Before the fenestrated Amplatzer™ device is implanted, the atrial opening usually requires a blade, and then a balloon dilation, septostomy to a size that will accommodate the hub of the splint device exactly. Since most patients needing this procedure are older and/or have very tough atrial septae or baffles, the sturdier PBS 300 (2 cm) blade is used for the blade incisions. The PBS 300 is delivered to the septum through a 10-F long sheath that has been positioned across the septum/baffle through the pre-existing opening or transseptally through a new area. During each exchange of wires, catheters or devices through the sheath, it is cleared *meticulously* of all air or clot as described previously. The aim of the septostomy preceding the implant of the fenestrated splint device is to create an opening that is large enough to allow the hub of the device to open *completely* and to assume its natural flattened shape when placed in the atrial septum. If the device does not open completely, the retention disks and the hub remain elongated, which compresses the lumen(s) of the channel(s) which extend(s) through the device. The large hole created in the septum before the fenestrated device can be implanted creates another major problem for these particular patients by allowing an excessive amount of right to left shunting, causing marked desaturation and destabilization in some of them, before the fenestrated occluder can be implanted to restrict the opening. The Amplatzer™ fenestrated device along with its precise delivery system must be prepared and ready for immediate implant before any enlargement of the atrial septostomy is begun.

The device is attached to a standard Amplatzer™ delivery cable. Before the device is pulled into the loader, a 0.035″ exchange length wire is advanced *through* the fenestration or channel in the device leaving 4–5 cm of the soft tip of the wire extending distal to the device, and the proximal wire passing through the loader and running parallel with and adjacent to the delivery cable. The wire which is pre-positioned through the device is available in case further dilation of the channel should be necessary acutely after implant of the fenestrated device. Since blade septostomy in these patients is performed using a PBS 300 blade through a 9- or 10-French long sheath, and the device can be delivered through the same sheath, this allows the use of the larger and much sturdier 0.035″ wire, as mentioned above. The proximal ends of the delivery cable and wire are passed through a 9- or 10-French loader or from the distal to the proximal end of a short 10-French sheath, and the cable and extra wire are withdrawn until the attached fenestrated device is against the distal tip of the loader/short sheath and all ready to be loaded.

The fenestrated Amplatzer™ device is delivered using TEE or ICE guidance exactly like the Amplatzer™ ASD occluder (Chapter 28). Since implant of the fenestrated device may be relatively urgent after the septostomy, and echocardiography can be useful during the septostomy, the echo probe which is to be used for the implant is introduced and the intracardiac structures are visualized before the septostomy is begun. Only after the fenestrated device has been prepared for delivery and echo images established, are the blade and then the balloon septostomies performed.

A 10-French long sheath is advanced (with a dilator and over a wire) into the left atrium either through a pre-existing opening or through a transseptal puncture opening. The large, sturdier, PBS 300 blade catheter is advanced through the sheath into the left atrium and the sheath is withdrawn back to the inferior vena cava. In order to provide a good cutting angle and not to create too large an opening initially, the blade is opened to at most 45° off the catheter for the withdrawals of the blade. Following the creation of several incisions at different locations around the circumference with the blade, the blade is replaced in the long sheath with an end-hole catheter, which is advanced into a left upper pulmonary vein. The catheter is replaced with a stiff exchange length wire that the selected dilation balloon will accommodate. The wire passes through the long sheath, which remains positioned at the junction of the right atrium and inferior vena cava. If the patient is not on anticoagulants already, he or she is given 100 mg/kg of heparin at this time. A 14 mm diameter balloon (assuming this is the diameter of the "waist" or "hub" of the fenestrated Amplatzer™ device) is introduced over the wire and advanced through the long sheath, and the septum is dilated. At the end of the dilation there should be no residual waist on the balloon, if the balloon has the same diameter as the hub of the device. Once the opening has been dilated and there is no residual waist, the sheath is advanced over the balloon, into the left atrium and into the mouth of the pulmonary vein. The balloon is slowly withdrawn through the sheath followed by the wire, leaving the sheath in the left atrium or, preferably, in the mouth of the left upper pulmonary vein. During each exchange of wires, catheters, or devices, the sheath is cleared meticulously of all air and/or clot as emphasized earlier. The large sheath through the newly created defect should reduce flow through the defect slightly; however, even with the sheath there the patient may desaturate significantly, and delivery of the fenestrated occluder should proceed as quickly as possible.

The fenestrated Amplatzer™ device is placed in a bowl of flush solution and the device and the wire passing through it are withdrawn into the loader or short sheath. The device is withdrawn to the proximal end of the loader in order to allow the distal tip of the wire that passes through the fenestration to be completely within the tip of the loader. The loader is maintained on a continuous flush while it is introduced through the valve of the long delivery sheath. The device, with the wire passing through it, is advanced into and through the long sheath until the tip of the device reaches the tip of the long sheath. This should allow 4–5 cm of the wire that is passing through the device to extend into the left atrium/pulmonary vein beyond the tip of the sheath. From this point on, with the exception of the wire passing through the device and dangling in the left atrium/pulmonary vein, the delivery of the fenestrated Amplatzer™ device is identical to the delivery of any other Amplatzer™ ASD device (Chapter 28). Once the device has been successfully implanted and the delivery sheath and cable are away from it, the extra wire will still be positioned through the channel in the device, but will be loose within the channel through the device. The wire through the device can be used for the introduction of a balloon dilation catheter for further acute dilation of the channel[16], or even for the implant of a stent within the channel if it does not stay expanded acutely[17]. The device is examined by echocardiography and a right atrial angiogram is performed adjacent to it to define the adequacy of the newly created defect(s). The systemic saturation in patients with either prior "Fontan" type procedures or with pulmonary vascular disease will usually drop to the low 90s or high 80s with a successful, but not too large, atrial communication.

Even these communications can reduce or close completely either acutely or over time as a result of either intimal proliferation, distortion of the fenestrated device if it is not fully expanded, or by acute thrombosis. In each situation, the channel through the device can usually be recrossed (transseptally if necessary) using both echocardiography and biplane fluoroscopic guidance. Once crossed, the channel can be dilated with a balloon or stent[17].

These devices have been used successfully in animals and in several compassionate cases in humans, however, are not yet commercially available in the United States. Because of the size of the opening required for these devices, they are significantly more difficult to implant in the atrial septum than an intravascular stent.

Complications of blade and "special" atrial septostomies

The potential for emboli of air and/or thrombus in the systemic circulation is the greatest danger of a blade or balloon septostomy or any other means for the creation or enlargement of an atrial septal defect. The procedures require the use of a long sheath and many exchanges of wires, catheters, balloon catheters, blade and device catheters through the sheath. The blade mechanism has a very small lumen and a potential "dead space" within the groove in the metal pod containing the blade, which is difficult to flush adequately from the lumen of the catheter. Thromboembolic phenomena for the most part are preventable by meticulous attention to clearing air or clot from the sheath and by specific and repeated flushing of the grooves of blade catheters. This flushing of the groove, as described earlier in the chapter, is performed between each "pull-back incision" with a blade catheter and/or every few minutes when the blade is in the circulation.

An overly successful atrial septostomy in patients where the defect is created to vent the systemic venous blood into the systemic arterial circulation can result in catastrophic desaturation, hypoxemia and even the death of the patient. Prevention by performing these septostomies very conservatively and enlarging the opening incrementally until the desired effect is achieved is the best treatment of this complication. If a patient should decompensate progressively, the defect can be re-occluded acutely using an atrial septal or PFO occluder.

Blade catheters *can* incise the wrong structures if positioned improperly. The use of biplane fluoroscopy *and* echocardiography to guide the procedures and meticulous attention to the details of the technique should prevent blade incisions in any improper location. There have been mechanical problems with the blade mechanism not retracting back into the groove of the pod after the blade has been pulled through the septum. This occurs particularly with the smaller sizes of blade catheters, after a very forceful pull through very tough tissues and/or when the control wire of the blade mechanism is twisted. Prevention by using the sturdier PBS 300 whenever possible is the best treatment. In all of these cases, the blade has retracted *partially* back into the groove and the partial retraction into the groove allows partial withdrawal of the partially exposed blade into a long sheath along with the metal pod. With the cutting edge of the blade withdrawn into the tip of the sheath, the blade can be withdrawn out of the body along with the sheath. This does incur some trauma to the vein and, unless the sheath is much larger than the blade catheter and a wire can be passed through the sheath adjacent to the blade catheter, it results in the loss of immediate access through that sheath/venous site.

Since most blade and special septostomies are followed by a balloon atrial septostomy, all of the complications of the balloon septostomy itself are present and are at least potentially as significant as the complications of the blade procedure alone. A transseptal puncture is necessary to cross the septum for some blade septostomy procedures. The transseptal puncture not only adds the potential complications of a standard atrial transseptal puncture but often the transseptal puncture is in a patient with a very small left atrium or the puncture is performed through an unusual or very tough area of the septum. These complications are discussed in Chapter 8.

Stent septostomies also have potential problems of their own. In small patients, the stents are difficult to position securely on the septum, while at the same time not impinging on other intracardiac structures. When an opening of a precise diameter is desired, the stents must be "hand-prepared" with one of the various central restricting bands. Acute and/or late embolization of these atrial septal stents is always a potential problem. Meticulous attention to the details of the location of the implant and of the implant procedure are most important at preventing this complication. If a stent embolizes acutely while it is still over the wire, the stent should be retrievable enough to withdraw it into the inferior vena cava and implant it there. Distal embolization away from the atrial septum frequently requires surgical retrieval/removal.

Conclusion

Atrial septostomies performed in the cardiac catheterization laboratory for very complex congenital heart patients often represent a "definitive palliation" and are as useful in this era of sophisticated surgical repairs as they were when first conceived over three decades ago. The larger atrial septal defects created with either the blade septostomy or the biopsy forceps septostomy catheters and then extended with a Rashkind™ or dilation balloon atrial septostomy are usually "permanent" and provide a lasting palliation for these patients. The smaller atrial septal openings supported with an implanted stent also appear to represent a relatively permanent palliation. There now are very few indications for a surgical atrial septostomy.

References

1. Park SC *et al.* A new atrial septostomy technique. *Cathet Cardiovasc Diagn* 1975; **1**(2): 195–201.
2. Park SC *et al.* Clinical use of blade atrial septostomy. *Circulation* 1978; **58**(4): 600–606.
3. Park SC *et al.* Blade atrial septostomy: Collaborative study. *Circulation* 1982; **66**: 258–266.
4. Ward KE *et al.* Restrictive interatrial communication in total anomalous pulmonary venous connection. *Am J Cardiol* 1986; **57**(13): 1131–1136.
5. Rich S and Lam W. Atrial septostomy as palliative therapy for refractory primary pulmonary hypertension. *Am J Cardiol* 1983; **51**(9): 1560–1561.
6. Koenig PR *et al.* Balloon atrial septostomy for left ventricular decompression in patients receiving extracorporeal membrane oxygenation for myocardial failure. *J Pediatr* 1993; **122**(6): S95–S99.
7. Ward KE *et al.* Transseptal decompression of the left heart during ECMO for severe myocarditis. *Ann Thorac Surg* 1995; **59**(3): 749–751.
8. Swanson MJ, Fabaz AG, and Jung JY. Successful treatment of right ventricular failure with atrial septostomy. *Chest* 1987; **92**(5): 950–952.
9. Kernis SJ *et al.* Percutaneous atrial septostomy for urgent palliative treatment of severe refractory cardiogenic shock due to right ventricular infarction. *Catheter Cardiovasc Interv* 2003; **59**(1): 44–48.
10. Justino H, Benson LN, and Nykanen DG. Transcatheter creation of an atrial septal defect using radiofrequency perforation. *Catheter Cardiovasc Interv* 2001; **54**(1): 83–87.
11. Du Marchie Sarvaas GJ *et al.* Radiofrequency-assisted atrial septoplasty for an intact atrial septum in complex congenital heart disease. *Catheter Cardiovasc Interv* 2002; **56**(3): 412–415.
12. Boucek MM *et al.* Management of the critically restrictive atrial septal defect awaiting infant cardiac transplantation. *Am J Cardiol* 1992; **70**: 559.
13. Miga DE *et al.* Transcatheter fenestration of hemi-Fontan baffles after completion of Fontan physiology using balloon dilatation and stent placement. *Cathet Cardiovasc Diagn* 1998; **43**(4): 429–432.
14. Pedra CA *et al.* Stent implantation to create interatrial communications in patients with complex congenital heart disease. *Catheter Cardiovasc Interv* 1999; **47**(3): 310–313; discussion 314.
15. Stumper O *et al.* Modified technique of stent fenestration of the atrial septum. *Heart* 2003; **89**(10): 1227–1230.
16. Kong H *et al.* Creation of an intra-atrial communication with a new Amplatzer shunt prosthesis: preliminary results in a swine model. *Catheter Cardiovasc Interv* 2002; **56**(2): 267–271.
17. Chatrath R *et al.* Fenestrated Amplatzer device for percutaneous creation of interatrial communication in patients after Fontan operation. *Catheter Cardiovasc Interv* 2003; **60**(1): 88–93.

15 Balloon dilation procedures—general

History—indications

Transcatheter balloon dilation of *congenital heart lesions* as it is known today began in the early 80s shortly after the reports by Gruentzig on the use of static balloons for the dilation of coronary and peripheral vessels[1], although the concept of dilating stenotic vessels was first conceived by Dotter and Judkins a decade earlier[2]. Since the first use in congenital lesions, there has been a proliferation of dilation procedures for valves and vascular stenosis in congenital heart lesions. Many of these dilation procedures now represent the standard of care for the treatment of the particular defect. Static balloon dilations are often referred to as "angioplasty" or "valvuloplasty" procedures. The specific lesions for which balloon dilation has become an accepted therapy are discussed in separate, subsequent chapters devoted to the specific lesions and to the idiosyncrasies of each particular dilation procedure. The chapters on specific lesions cover the dilation of pulmonary, aortic and mitral valves, coarctation of the aorta and branch pulmonary arteries. Multiple other lesions, which are dilated less routinely, are covered in Chapter 21 on miscellaneous dilations.

During the two decades of the use of balloon dilation procedures for congenital heart lesions, there has been a "learning curve" for the procedures along with continued development and refinement in both the techniques and the equipment. Most developments in the equipment used for congenital heart patients have been coincidental and are a consequence of developments primarily intended for valvuloplasty and/or angioplasty procedures for acquired diseases in adults. As a consequence, the equipment used for balloon dilations in pediatric and congenital patients frequently is not ideally suited for these patients and/or lesions, and almost none of the equipment is "approved" for these specific uses by the FDA, particularly for use in pediatric and congenital heart patients. In spite of this, most of the *developments* in the *techniques* for the dilation of valvular and large vessel lesions have come from pediatric interventionalists treating congenital heart lesions[3].

Equipment for balloon dilation in congenital heart lesions

Balloons

The balloons used for valve and vessel dilations are cylindrical "static" balloons, which expand to a predetermined and "fixed" maximal diameter when inflated to a predetermined maximum pressure. When inflated to their maximum pressure, the balloons develop a very high wall tension and with this become very hard and rigid in their inflated configuration[4]. When the balloon is inflated in a lesion, the wall tension of the expanded balloon is used to split or tear the stenotic tissues.

There currently are dozens of different "angioplasty" balloons in use for dilation of both valves and vessels in congenital heart patients. There are many characteristics of these angioplasty balloons which have different degrees of importance depending upon the particular lesion being dilated and the size of the patient being treated. Balloons with special characteristics used for particular lesions are discussed along with the individual lesions or the specific procedures in subsequent chapters.

The ideal angioplasty balloon is manufactured of a totally *non-compliant* material. The non-compliant balloon reaches its stated, predetermined diameter when it is inflated to its listed maximal pressure, and once it reaches its advertised maximal pressure, the non-compliant balloon does *not* expand further in any area, even with increased pressure. When increasing pressure is applied to the non-compliant balloon, the inflated diameter does not vary from one area to another area over the entire surface of the usable length of the balloon regardless of an external resistance over a particular area of the balloon. While the diameter does not increase, the wall tension of the balloon *does increase* as increasing pressure is delivered to the balloon.

On the other hand, a balloon manufactured from a "compliant" material expands to greater than its stated (advertised) maximal diameter in areas of less external resistance (e.g. areas away from the area of tightest stenosis) at the maximal pressure of the balloon. When increasing pressure is applied to a "compliant" balloon, the less restricted areas on the balloon surface continue to expand even further without adding additional radial force in the area of stenosis. If the "less restrictive" area is in a smaller, but non-stenosed distal vessel, the excess diameter can lead to tears in the adjacent normal vessel.

Ideally, balloons for angioplasty and valvuloplasty in congenital heart patients have a very low and smooth deflated profile. They are mounted on a catheter with a small shaft and the deflated balloon folds tightly over the catheter shaft to create a very small diameter or "profile" of the combined catheter/deflated balloon. This low profile should have a "memory" so that when the balloon is deflated within the patient, it assumes its original smooth fold spontaneously without the assistance of "hand folding" by the operator. The material of the balloon surface is resistant to rupture and tears and has a smooth outer surface. In spite of the desirable "low profile", these balloon catheters must have a central catheter lumen which is large enough to support a relatively large and sturdy guide wire and, at the same time, a balloon lumen which is large enough to allow rapid inflation and deflation of the balloon. When fully inflated, the balloon obstructs all of the forward blood flow through the particular vessel or area during a dilation procedure. In central and common vascular channels, the total cardiac flow is obstructed and the duration of the inflation becomes very critical, so the time of the inflation/deflation must be very rapid.

The "taper" of the ends of a balloon onto the catheter shaft at each end (the balloon "shoulders") for dilation procedures in pediatric and congenital heart patients ideally is smooth and very *short*. The tip of the catheter beyond the distal end of the balloon should also be very short. Any length of the shoulders of a balloon and/or tip of a catheter adds to the *stiff and straight length* of the inflated balloon. The extra rigid and straight length does not contribute to the dilation of the stenotic area but does cause additional trauma to the intravascular structures. The straight, inflated balloon does not conform at all to the natural curvature of the vessels, which frequently is present in vessels being dilated. Any unnecessary extra length of the ends of the balloon makes this discrepancy even worse. As a consequence, the extra, straight length causes balloon displacement and/or vascular trauma.

At the same time, there are occasions when a very smooth taper on the shoulders of a balloon is desirable or even necessary in order to cross very tight valves or stenoses in very small vessels. As a consequence, a few small diameter balloons with relatively long tapered ends are necessary in the inventory of even congenital cardiac catheterization laboratories.

There are balloons designed for specific lesions with characteristics specifically for those lesions. For very resistant stenosis, very high-pressure balloons are necessary. High-pressure balloons are manufactured from tougher (and usually thicker) materials and usually have larger and rougher profiles and require larger introducers. In addition, there are very special, unique balloons, which are available for mitral valve dilation and for the implant of intravascular stents, and the "cutting" balloons. These special balloons are discussed in more detail in subsequent chapters along with the specific lesions and techniques.

Obviously, to accommodate the infinite range in the age and size of patients and the large variety of lesions within pediatric/congenital heart patients, a huge inventory of the full range of balloon diameters and lengths must be available in a congenital cardiac catheterization laboratory. Some of the "ideal" characteristics for dilation balloons are obviously contradictory to each other. As a consequence, most balloon catheters for the dilation of congenital heart lesions represent a significant compromise of several of the ideal characteristics. In any situation, the balloon is chosen which has the fewest or least dangerous undesirable characteristics along with the most essential and favorable characteristics.

Available "static" dilation balloons

Like most of the other materials used in pediatric and congenital heart cardiac catheterizations, the majority of the balloons and the ancillary equipment used for balloon dilations in pediatric/congenital lesions represent an "off-label use" of materials developed and approved for use in the adult patient. The large majority of balloons used in adult cardiac catheterizations are very small coronary angioplasty balloons, which do not have many applications in congenital heart lesions. Fortunately, the adult catheterization "arena" also deals with a wide range of larger balloons which were developed and are used for peripheral vascular lesions. Most of the balloons used in pediatric/congenital lesions are middle and large-sized balloons developed for the biliary, renal, peripheral vascular, large central vessel dilations/implants and a few actually for valvuloplasty. There are innumerable manufacturers of balloons for dilations in adult patients, and there is one manufacturer who actually manufactures balloons specifically for pediatric/congenital use (NuMED Inc., Hopkinton, NY).

Each separate manufacturer produces balloons of different materials, in different sizes and multiple different types of balloon. Each different balloon has some, at least slightly different characteristics from the others, each with some advantages as well as disadvantages. There is no one balloon which is ideal for all lesions of all sizes, with each balloon having some desirable characteristics as well as limitations. New and "better" balloons are developed and introduced so frequently that, often, as soon as they are "inventoried" by a catheterization laboratory, they become obsolete and are replaced with a "new model".

Most of the dilation balloons are available on catheters, which come in several different lengths. Although it might seem ideal to use a specific balloon on a 60 cm long catheter shaft in an infant and the exact same balloon on a 100 cm long catheter shaft in an adolescent, this would require a doubling (or more) of the number of balloons necessary in the inventory of the particular laboratory. For the economy of the inventory and conservation of storage space, only balloons on catheter shafts of at least 100 cm are inventoried, and these balloons are used in all pediatric and congenital patients. A 100 cm balloon catheter can be used in an infant, however a 60 or even 75 cm balloon catheter does not pass completely through the usual long delivery sheath and to a distal branch pulmonary artery in an adolescent or adult-sized patient!

Some of the more common balloons available and used in the United States for congenital patients at the time of this writing are listed. They are listed arbitrarily into several general groups according to a range of diameters of the balloons. Some of the important characteristics and/or uses of each balloon are listed. The "tables" for each type of balloon list the balloon diameters/the catheter shaft sizes in the first column, and the required introductory sheath sizes/wire sizes that the balloon catheter accepts in the second column.

Small diameter dilation balloons

SUB 4™ BALLOON CATHETERS (Medi-Tech, Boston Scientific, Natick, MA)

2–4 mm balloons/3.8-F shaft	4-F sheath/0.018″ wire
4.5–6 mm balloons/3.8-F shaft	5-F sheath/0.018″ wire

These are non-compliant, thin-walled polyethylene balloons, which are available in 2 and 4 cm lengths. They have a very low and smooth profile, a fairly long taper connecting the balloon to the catheter, and a long distal tip. Sub 4™ balloons are covered with a Glidex™ hydrophilic coating. The configuration, size and coating make these balloons excellent for the initial crossing of very small, very tight lesions and for an initial dilation in a staged or sequential dilation of a lesion. They only accept a 0.018″ wire, which offers only marginal support when any "push" on the balloon catheter is required to cross a lesion.

SYMMETRY STIFF SHAFT™ BALLOON CATHETERS (Medi-Tech, Boston Scientific, Natick, MA)

1.5–4 mm balloons/4-F shaft	4-F sheath/0.018″ wire
4.5–6 mm balloons/4-F shaft	5-F sheath/0.018″ wire

The Symmetry™ balloon has a co-extruded, non-compliant balloon material, which makes them smooth, puncture resistant and capable of 15 atms pressure. The extra stiff catheter shaft and a Glidex™ hydrophilic coating enhance the "pushability" over the still relatively small 0.018″ wire. These balloons are excellent for the initial opening of very tight lesions of vessels and valves, particularly for the start of sequential dilations.

TYSHAK MINI™ PTA BALLOONS (NuMED Inc., Hopkinton, NY)

4–8 mm balloons/2.5-F shaft	3-F sheath/0.014″ wire
9–10 mm balloons/2.5-F shaft	4-F sheath/0.014″ wire

These very small balloons are manufactured of a relatively non-compliant thermoplastic elastomer and have maximum inflation pressures of 6 to 3.5 atms for the smaller to the larger diameter balloons respectively. All of these balloons are 2 cm in length. The major use of these balloons is in tiny infants, where their very low profile allows them to be introduced through very small sheaths, yet the relatively "large" balloon diameters for such small sheath sizes makes them applicable for valve dilations. This advantage is almost outweighed by the very small, 0.014″ maximum diameter guide wire which they accept. Currently all available 0.014″ wires support the balloons very poorly during their delivery to the lesion, and are particularly poor at fixing the balloons in place during inflation.

SLALOM™ (Johnson & Johnson–Cordis Corp., Miami Lakes, FL)

3–4 mm balloons/3.7-F shaft	4-F sheath/0.018″ wire
5–6 mm balloons/3.7–4.2-F shaft	5-F sheath/0.018″ wire
7–8 mm balloons/4.2-F shaft	6-F sheath/0.018″ wire

The Slalom™ balloons are low-profile moderately non-compliant balloons of Duralyn™ material, which are available in 2 and 4 cm lengths. They have short shoulders but do have a relatively long tip (6.5 mm) for otherwise short balloons. The 3–5 mm diameter balloons have a burst pressure of 14 atms, the 6–7 mm diameter balloons 12 atms, while the 8 mm diameter balloon has a burst pressure of 8 atms.

Coronary artery dilation balloons

In addition to the four small dilation balloons listed above, there are dozens (hundreds) of additional very tiny balloons manufactured for the dilation of coronary artery lesions. These balloons change "daily" and are too numerous to list, or are obsolete before they can be listed. These balloons reach maximal inflated diameters between 1.5 and 5 mm. They have extremely low profiles, but accept only 0.014″ to 0.018″ wires. In the coronary arteries these balloons are used through "guiding catheters" which help to support the flimsy wires. If a Sub 4™ balloon is not available, a "coronary balloon" of the appropriate diameter can be used as the initial balloon to cross very tight lesions to begin a sequential dilation.

Medium diameter dilation balloons

Balloons between 4 and 12 mm in diameter are far more applicable for the majority of pediatric/congenital valvular and vascular lesions. These "medium" sized balloons are available from many different manufacturers with each balloon type, even from the same manufacturer, having different characteristics.

ULTRA THIN DIAMOND™ AND ULTRA THIN ST™ BALLOON CATHETERS (Medi-Tech, Boston Scientific, Natick, MA)

4–8 mm balloons/5-F shaft	5-F sheath/0.035″ wire
9–12 mm balloons/5-F shaft	6–7-F sheath/0.035″ wire

These polyethylene terephthalate balloons are available in 2 and 4 cm lengths, are non-compliant and are rated at 10 atms burst pressure. They are on a larger catheter shaft than the very small balloons, they are available in larger sizes and they all accept a much larger wire than the very small balloons. Both the standard Ultra Thin™ and the Ultra Thin ST™ balloons are coated with a Glidex™ hydrophilic coating to enhance their passage through sheaths, vessels and stenotic lesions.

The standard Ultra Thin™ balloons have very long, tapering shoulders. The long shoulders make the overall length of the balloon at least twice the actual usable length of the balloon, which can be a problem in a short or curved segment of the vasculature.

The Ultra Thin ST™ balloons are similar to the regular Ultra Thin™ balloons, but have a short stubby taper (shoulder) from the balloon to the catheter. The stubby configuration of the ST™ balloons makes them ideal for both valve and vessel dilation.

SDS™ BALLOONS (Scimed, Boston Scientific, Maple Grove, MN)

4–6 mm balloons/5.2-F shaft	5-F sheath/0.035″ wire
6–8 mm balloons/5.2–5.8-F shaft	6-F sheath/0.035″ wire
9–10 mm balloons/5.8-F shaft	7-F sheath/0.035″ wire

SDS™ balloons have replaced the original Marshall™ balloons. These balloons have very short, stubby tapers or "shoulders" at the ends of the balloons, are available in 1.5, 2, 3, 4, 6 and 8 cm lengths in the 4–8 mm diameter balloons and in all of the same lengths except the 1.5 cm in the 9–10 mm diameter balloons. SDS™ balloons are manufactured of a Rawhide™ co-extruded material with a special Quadra-Fold™ technology, which results in a very low, smooth profile and allows the balloons to return to the same original low profile when deflated. These balloons accept 12 atms of pressure. The slightly "rough" Rawhide™ material, the stubby ends and the multiple lengths of the balloons makes the SDS™ balloon the ideal balloon for the delivery of stents up to a diameter of 10 mm, in addition to their use for routine vessel/valve dilations.

PURSUIT™ BALLOONS (Cook Inc., Bloomington, IN)

4–5 mm balloons/5-F shaft	5-F sheath/0.035″ wire
6–8 mm balloons/5-F shaft	6-F sheath/0.035″ wire
7–10 mm balloons/5-F shaft	7-F sheath/0.035″ wire

Pursuit™ balloons have a very low profile, are non-compliant, and have a rated burst pressure of 15 atms for the 4–6 mm diameter balloons and 14 atms for the 7–10 mm diameter balloons. Most of these balloons are available in 2, 3, 4, 6, 8 and 10 cm lengths although at some diameters the 3 cm length is not available and in the 7–10 mm diameter balloons, the 6, 8 and 10 cm long balloons are not available. In the 4–7 mm diameter balloons, there are alternative balloon lengths, which provides each length of balloon available within one balloon diameter. The balloons larger than 6 mm in diameter refold with a smooth "tri-fold" configuration and all of the balloons have short "shoulders". The balloons are mounted on a stiff Ultra-push™ shaft, which facilitates pushability.

ACCENT™ BALLOONS (Cook Inc., Bloomington, IN)

4–8 mm balloons/ 5-F shaft	6-F sheath/0.035″ wire
9–10 mm balloons/5-F shaft	7-F sheath/0.035″ wire
8–14 mm balloons/6-F shaft	8-F sheath/0.035″ wire
4–10 mm balloons/7-F shaft	8-F sheath/0.038″ wire

These low-profile balloons are available in 2, 3, 4, 6, 8, and 10 cm lengths in balloon sizes up to 8 mm in diameter, in 2, 3, 4 and 6 cm lengths in the 10 & 12 mm diameter balloons, and in 2, 4 and 6 cm lengths in the 14 mm diameter balloons. Accent™ balloons are relatively non-compliant, have short shoulders and will tolerate up to 15 atms in the smallest balloon diameters, with decreasing pressure tolerances down to 5 atms for the 14 mm diameter balloon.

OPTA™ LP BALLOONS (Johnson & Johnson-Cordis Corp., Miami Lakes, FL)

3–7 mm balloons/5-F shaft	5-F sheath/0.035″ wire
8–10 mm balloons/5-F shaft	6-F sheath/0.035″ wire
12 mm balloon/5-F shaft	7-F sheath/0.035″ wire

Opta™ LP balloons are low-profile, relatively non-compliant, balloons with short "shoulders", and are manufactured of Duralyn™. The balloons refold smoothly over the catheter by means of longitudinal folds or "pleats" and track well through the vasculature. Opta™ LP balloons are available in 2, 3 and 4 cm standard lengths with some special 1, 1.5, 3 and 6 cm lengths available. Opta™ LP balloons have a nominal inflation pressure of 6 atms for the 3–10 mm diameter balloons and 4 atms for the 12 mm diameter balloon.

OPTA™ PRO BALLOON DILATION CATHETERS (Johnson & Johnson-Cordis Corp., Miami Lakes, FL)
3–7 mm balloons/5-F shaft 5-F sheath/0.035″ wire
7–8 mm balloons/5-F shaft 6-F sheath/0.035″ wire
8–12 mm balloons/5-F shaft 7-F sheath/0.035″ wire

Opta™ Pro balloons are a newer, low-profile balloon similar to the Opta™ LP balloons of the same Duralyn™ material, although the Opta™ Pro has a nominal pressure of 10 atms for the 3–10 mm diameter balloons and 6 atms for the 12 mm diameter balloons. These balloons are available in 1, 1.5, 2, 3, 4, 6, 8 and 10 cm lengths in the 4–9 mm diameter balloons but only in 4 & 8 cm lengths in the 3 mm diameter balloons and 2, 3, and 4 cm lengths in the 12 mm diameter balloons. These balloons have an abrasion and puncture resistant surface, which makes them advantageous for stent implants.

POWERFLEX™ PLUS BALLOONS (Johnson & Johnson–Cordis Corp., Miami Lakes, FL)
4–5 mm balloons/5-F shaft 5 F sheath/0.035″ wire
6–7 mm balloons/5-F shaft 6 F sheath/0.035″ wire
8–12 mm balloons/5-F shaft 7 F sheath/0.035″ wire

PowerFlex™ Plus balloons are manufactured of Duralyn™ ST balloon material, which makes them moderately noncompliant and reasonably puncture and burst resistant. The nominal burst pressures are 10/14 atms for the 3–10 mm diameter balloons and 6/8 atms for the 12 mm diameter balloon. The PowerFlex™ Plus balloons are available in 2, 3 and 4 cm lengths.

POWERFLEX™ EXTREME BALLOONS (Johnson & Johnson–Cordis Corp., Miami Lakes, FL)
4–5 mm balloons/5-F shaft 5-F sheath/0.035″ wire
6–7 mm balloons/5-F shaft 6-F sheath/0.035″ wire
8–10 mm balloons/5-F shaft 7-F sheath/0.035″ wire

PowerFlex™ Extreme balloons are low profile, significantly higher pressure, balloons which are manufactured from abrasion resistant Duralyn™ and are similar in configuration to the PowerFlex™ Plus balloons. They are available in 2, 4 and 6 cm lengths, with the 8 mm diameter balloon also available in a 3 cm length. The 4–8 mm diameter balloons have a 20 atms burst pressure while the larger 9–10 mm diameter balloons have a 17 atms burst pressure.

Combined medium and large diameter balloon dilation catheters

Some balloons are available in diameters which span both the medium and large diameters. They provide the opportunity of a simpler "inventory" of balloons, however they usually do not have the advantages of balloons manufactured specifically at a narrower range of sizes. The larger the diameter of the balloon, the more important is the catheter material and guide wire size in order to support the delivery of the balloon.

TYSHAK X™ BALLOONS (NuMED Inc., Hopkinton, NY)
8–10 mm balloons/6-F shaft 6-F sheath/0.035″ wire
12 mm balloon/6-F shaft 7-F sheath/0.035″ wire
14–16 mm balloons/7-F shaft 8-F sheath/0.035″ wire
18 mm balloon/8-F shaft 9-F sheath/0.035″ wire
20 mm balloon/8-F shaft 10-F sheath/0.035″ wire
22, 25 mm balloons/9-F shaft 10, 11-F sheath/0.035″ wire

These balloons are manufactured from a micro thin, minimally compliant, thermoplastic elastomer, which gives them an initial, low, deflated profile relative to the balloon diameter. They have short shoulders and are available in a large range of diameters and lengths, which provides a good versatility for balloon dilations in congenital heart lesions. After they have been inflated and then deflated in the body, they collapse to a significantly larger profile with a rough outer surface. The balloons are available in 3, 4, 5, and 6 cm lengths with a 2 cm long balloon available in the 8, 10 and 12 mm diameters only. These balloons have a relatively low, maximum burst pressure ranging from 5 atms for the smallest diameter balloons to 1.5 atms for the largest diameter balloons.

The Tyshak X™ balloon has a new, thicker, braided catheter shaft which accommodates a much larger guide wire (0.035″) without requiring a larger introducer and has far smoother and more satisfactory "pushability" compared to the original Tyshak I & II™ balloons. The Tyshak X™ balloons will probably replace the original Tyshak I and II™ balloons entirely.

Z-MED X™ BALLOON (NuMED Inc., Hopkinton, NY)
8–12 mm balloons/6-F shaft 7-F sheath/0.035″ wire
14–16 mm balloons/7-F shaft 8 & 9- F sheaths/0.035″ wires
18, 20 mm balloons/8-F shaft 10 & 11- F sheaths/0.035″ wire
22–28 mm balloons/9-F shaft 11 & 12-F sheaths/0.035″ wire
30 mm balloon/9-F shaft 13-F sheath/0.035″ wire

Z-Med X™ balloons are manufactured from a slightly thicker, minimally compliant, thermoplastic elastomer material. The thicker material imparts slightly more resistance to puncture and allows a higher pressure for inflation, but because of the thicker material/higher burst pressures, they have thicker, more irregular deflated profiles and require a slightly larger introducer size than the Tyshak X™ balloons of comparable sizes. These balloons have a rated burst pressure of 10 atms for the smaller diameter sizes with the pressure decreasing down to 1.5 atms for the largest diameter (28 & 30 mm) balloons. Z-Med X™ balloons are on the same braided catheter shaft as the Tyshak X™ balloons and accommodate a larger guide wire than the original Z-Med™ balloons.

Z-MED II X™ BALLOONS (NuMED Inc., Hopkinton, NY)

8–10 mm balloons/6-F shaft	7-F sheath/0.035″ wire
12 mm balloon/6-F shaft	8-F sheath/0.035″ wire
14–16 mm balloons/7-F shaft	8, 9-F sheaths/0.035″ wire
18 mm balloon/8-F shaft	10-F sheath/0.035″ wire
20, 22 mm balloons/8, 9-F shaft	12-F sheath/0.035″ wire
23, 25 mm balloons/9-F shaft	13, 14-F sheaths/0.035″ wire
28, 30 mm balloons/11-F shaft	16-F sheath/0.035″ wire

Z-Med II X™ balloons are made from a sturdier, slightly thicker modification of the Z-Med X™ thermoplastic elastomer balloon material, which allows a higher inflation pressure but at the expense of a very rough, bulky, refold configuration. The nominal inflation pressures of these balloons are 6 atms for the smaller (8–10mm) diameter balloons decreasing to 2 atms for the very large (28–30 mm) diameter balloons and the burst pressures for the same balloons range from 15 atms for the smaller diameter balloons to 3 atms for the very large diameter balloons. These balloons require larger introductory sheaths and are often difficult to withdraw through even large sheaths. The Z-Med II X™ balloons have the same braided, more rigid, catheter shaft of all of the other NuMED™ "X" balloons, which makes them easier to push through the vascular system and to control during inflation.

PE-MT™ BALLOON CATHETERS (Medi-Tech, Boston Scientific, Natick, MA)

4–8 mm balloons/7-F shaft	9-F sheath/0.038″ wire
8, 10 mm balloons/8-F shaft	10–11-F sheath/0.038″ wire
12–20 mm balloons/9-F shaft	11–12-F sheath/0.038″ wire

Most of the early valve and vessel dilations in congenital heart lesions were performed using the PE-MT™ balloons. The polyethylene-MT™ material of these balloons is a non-compliant, relatively thick, tough material which refolds fairly smoothly when deflated and the balloons have a medium length taper to the shoulders—a combination of features which is still not available all together on any other large diameter balloon! The PE-MT™ balloons are available in 2 and 4 cm lengths in the 4–6 mm diameter balloons and in 3 (or 4) and 8 mm lengths in the larger diameters, all with a moderate taper of the balloon shoulders. The burst pressure of the balloons varies from 6 atms for the smallest diameter balloons to 3.5 atms for the largest balloons. The size of the catheter shaft and balloon together require a large introductory sheath, which makes these balloons difficult to use in small patients.

Except for the limited available lengths and the large diameter sheaths which were necessary for the combined balloon/mounted stent, the PE-MT balloons were almost ideal for stent delivery. PE-MT™ balloons are still available, but have been displaced for the most part by the newer generation of balloons. For a short while in the US, the PE-MT™ balloons were available on a 5-F shaft as the PE-MT 5™ balloons, which would pass through significantly smaller introducers, however, the market economically was too small for the manufacturer to pursue these balloons for a PMA approval through the FDA.

OWENS™ STANDARD STIFF BALLOON (Scimed, Boston Scientific, Maple Grove, MN)

8–10 mm balloons/8-F shaft	12-F sheath/0.038″ wire
12, 15, 18, 20 mm balloons/9-F shaft	14-F sheath/0.038″ wire

The Owens Standard Stiff™ balloon is a similar (identical?) balloon to the PE-MT™ balloon, but distributed by the SCIMED™ division of Boston Scientific Corporation. The balloon characteristics are the same as the PE-MT™ balloons but these balloons are only available in 3 cm lengths.

Large diameter (only) dilation balloons

In addition to the previously described combined medium and large diameter balloons, several manufacturers provide a separate category of balloons for dilation of intravascular structures which are available only in large diameters.

XXL™ BALLOONS (Medi-Tech, Boston Scientific, Natick, MA)

12, 14 mm balloons/5.8-F shaft	7-F sheath/0.035″ wire
16, 18 mm balloons/5.8-F shaft	8-F sheath/0.035″ wire

XXL™ balloons are manufactured from a co-extruded, non-compliant, polyethylene balloon material. The balloons are mounted on a 5.8-French shaft using a QuadraFold™ technology, which gives them a very low profile for a relatively large balloon. They are available in 2, 4 and 6 cm lengths. These balloons, however, do have horribly long shoulders, which makes the total length of the balloons as much as twice their functional length. These long shoulders contribute to their low profile, but make them difficult, if not actually dangerous, for many vessel and valve dilations, and make them contraindicated for the implant of stents.

OWENS™ LO-PROFILE BALLOON (Scimed, Boston Scientific, Maple Grove, MN)

15, 18, 20 mm balloons/9-F shaft	12-F sheath/0.038″ wire
23 mm balloons/9-F shaft	14-F sheath/0.038″ wire

The balloon material is the same as the Owens Standard Stiff™ balloons, however, these balloons have a unique double lumen to the balloon itself which allows preparation of the balloons without disturbing their folded profile. The 15–20 Owens Lo-Profile™ balloons are only available in a 5.5 cm length while the 23 mm diameter balloon is only available in a 4 cm length. These balloons have relatively low burst pressures of 3.5 to 2.5 atms and have few, or no, advantages over several other lower profile, large balloons. An identical 15, 18 and 20 mm version of this balloon is marketed as an Aortic Valvuloplasty™ balloon.

OMEGA NV™ (Cook Inc., Bloomington, IN)
15, 18, 20 mm balloons/8.5-F shaft 10-F sheath/0.038″ wire
23 mm balloon/10-F shaft 14-F sheath/0.038″ wire

These larger diameter balloons are moderately non-compliant and are available in 3, 5 and 7 cm lengths. Omega NV™ balloons have short shoulders and burst pressure of 4 atms, however, they have no other specific advantages. The Omega NV™ balloon, in fact, is not recommended (by the manufacturer) for valve dilations.

MAXI LD™ (Johnson & Johnson-Cordis Corp., Miami Lakes, FL)
15 mm balloon/7-F shaft 9-F sheath/0.035″ wire

This single diameter, relatively non-compliant, larger balloon is available in 4 and 6 cm lengths. With its compliance, its single available diameter and relatively large deflated profile, the Maxi LD™ has little application in the pediatric/congenital catheterization laboratory.

Special balloon dilation catheters

In addition to the "standard" balloons already listed, there are several other categories of balloons available for very special circumstances and techniques.

High-pressure balloon dilation catheters

The wall of a standard dilation or angioplasty balloon becomes very rigid at a full inflation of even 2–4 atms pressure. The majority of either valvular or vascular lesions in the congenital heart patient do not require balloon pressures higher than this for adequate dilation. There are occasional very resistant lesions—for example scarred, circumferential anastomoses or otherwise densely scarred vessels, which are very resistant to dilation and require significantly more pressure to force open the obstruction. There are several balloons available for these circumstances with very high nominal, and burst pressures; however, most of these balloons sacrifice the profile of the balloon, the length of the balloon and/or introducer size to achieve the higher pressures. These balloons create a potential danger of splitting normal structures and must be used with care and only when using very precise measurements of the structures involved.

ORIGINAL BLUE MAX™ BALLOON DILATION CATHETERS (Medi-Tech, Boston Scientific, Natick, MA)
10 & 12 mm balloons/7-F shaft 10-F sheath /0.038″ wire

These are very high-pressure balloons with a burst pressure of over 20 atms. They are only available in the two diameters and only in 4 cm lengths, which limits their use. These original Blue Max™ balloons were on a 7-French shaft, had very long shoulders and a horrible "refold" profile with very stiff and sharp wings when deflated, particularly when maintained on a negative pressure. These balloons were essential when a very high-pressure dilation was necessary, but are potentially very traumatic to the vessels and intravascular structures and can be very difficult to remove from the vessels after deflation.

"NEW" "BLUE MAX" BALLOON DILATION CATHETERS (Medi-Tech, Boston Scientific, Natick, MA)
4–6 mm balloons/5.8-F shaft 6-F sheath/0.035″ wire
7, 8 mm balloons/5.8-F shaft 7-F sheath/0.035″ wire
9–10 mm balloons/5.8-F shaft 8-F sheath/0.035″ wire

The New Blue Max™ balloon is manufactured from a thin, blended, co-extruded, non-compliant, Poly-5™ material which allows very high inflation pressures, yet has a very smooth, soft and scratch resistant surface which refolds to a very low, smooth profile. The 4–7 mm diameter balloons are available in 2, 4 and 10 cm lengths while the 8–10 mm diameter balloons are available in only 4 and 8 cm lengths. The New Blue Max™ balloons have short shoulders, are on a rigid catheter shaft, and are available with a Glidex™ coating, which allows them to pass easily through tight lesions. All of the New Blue Max™ balloons are rated at 17 atms pressure and are very good for routine as well as high pressure dilations in vascular lesions up to 10 mm in diameter.

CONQUEST BALLOONS (Bard Cardiopulmonary, Tewksbury, MA)
6, 7 & 8 mm balloons/6-F shaft 6-F sheath/0.035″ wire
9 & 10 mm balloons/7-F shaft 7-F sheath/0.035″ wire
12 mm balloon/7-F shaft 8-F sheath/0.035″ wire

These balloons are a composite construction with the outer coating of the balloon made of non-compliant Kevlar™, which makes them very resistant to puncture and allows them to be inflated to extremely high pressures, and at the same time, makes them very non-compliant. The maximum burst pressure of these balloons decreases with increasing diameter and increasing length. The 6 mm diameter balloons can be inflated to 30 atm pressure, the 7 mm diameter balloons to 30–27 atms, while the 12 mm balloons have a burst pressure of 20 atms. They are available in 2, 4 and 8 cm length except in the 9–12 mm diameters, which are only available in 2 and 4 cm lengths. All of these balloons have a relatively smooth "refold" profile and usually can be withdrawn through the original introductory sheath. The extremely long shoulders on these balloons is the one major problem with them. The shoulders make the actual total length of each balloon triple the advertised "working" or usable length. At these high pressures this extreme length of a very rigid, straight balloon straightens all the structures in which the balloon is positioned, which makes them very dangerous when used in an acutely curved vessel or chamber.

ATLAS BALLOONS (Bard Cardiopulmonary, Tewksbury, MA)

12 & 14 mm balloons/7-F shaft	7-F sheath/0.035″ wire
16 & 18 mm balloons/7-F shaft	8-F sheath/0.035″ wire
20 mm balloon/7-F shaft	9-F sheath/0.035″ wire

Like the Conquest™ balloons these balloons are a composite, double layer construction with an outer layer of Kevlar™. Again these balloons are very puncture resistant and have very high burst pressures, particularly for large balloons. The burst pressure of the 12–16 mm diameter balloons is 18 atms while the burst pressure of the 18 & 20 mm diameter balloons is 16 atms. Also, like the Conquest™ balloons, the Atlas™ balloons refold reasonably well back to their original diameters, but they have ridiculously long tapered shoulders, which, again, triples the total length of the balloon compared to its effective length. The long length of such rigid balloons compromises their usefulness in many smaller congenital patients and/or in curved locations.

MULLINS X™ HIGH PRESSURE DILATION BALLOONS (NuMED Inc., Hopkinton, NY)

12 mm balloon/7-F shaft	9-F sheath/0.035″ wire
14 & 15 mm balloons/8-F shaft	10-F sheath/0.035″ wire
16 mm balloon/8-F shaft	11-F sheath/0.035″ wire
18 mm balloon/8-F shaft	12-F sheath/0.035″ wire
20 mm balloon/8 F shaft	13-F sheath/0.035″ wire

Mullins X™ balloons (NuMED Inc., Hopkinton, NY) are a replacement for the original large, Mullins™ high-pressure balloons. They are manufactured from a co-extruded double layer laminate of non-compliant thermoplastic elastomer materials, which allows a very high pressure, yet a relatively low profile, which does, however, result in a rough surface upon refold after inflation. The 12 mm balloons have a rated burst pressure of 14 atms with the maximum burst pressure decreasing with increasing balloon size down to 11 atms for the 20 mm balloon. Each diameter of the Mullins X™ balloon is available in 3 and 4 cm lengths. The balloon catheters, like the other "X" balloons from NuMED™ (NuMED Inc., Hopkinton, NY) are manufactured from stiffer, braided shaft material, which gives them a greater "pushability" and better positional control of the balloon during inflation.

Special purpose balloon dilation catheters

In addition to the "high-pressure" balloons there are several other balloons designed for very special dilation procedures.

BONHOEFFER MULTI-TRACK™ BALLOON DILATION CATHETERS (NuMED Inc., Hopkinton, NY)

14, 16, 18, 20 balloons/7-F shaft	14-F sheath/0.035″ wire

Multi-Track™ balloon catheters have a separate, short, several mm long lumen for a wire ("multitrack lumen") at the very tip of the catheter. This short length of lumen allows a guide wire to pass "in and out" of it just distal to the balloon. With this arrangement, the guide wire of the "multi-track" catheter actually passes adjacent to the balloon and the shaft of the balloon catheter with the wire passing through only the very short segment of the separate "wire lumen". Multi-Track™ balloon catheters were designed to be used simultaneously and side-by-side with a second standard balloon dilation catheter, which can be advanced over the same wire through a standard central catheter lumen. This allows the positioning of the second balloon exactly side by side with the Multi-Track™ balloon[5,6]. With this arrangement a double balloon dilation of a structure can be performed over a single wire. A second Multi-Track™ angiographic catheter can be passed over the wire adjacent to the Multi-Track™ balloon to allow simultaneous pressure recording or angiography while the Multi-Track™ balloon is still in place.

All diameters of the Multi-Track™ balloons are 5 cm in length. They have a burst pressure of 6 atms for the 14 mm diameter balloon, decreasing to 4 atms for the 20 mm diameter balloon.

Because of the wire passing outside of the balloon catheter, these catheters require a significantly larger introductory sheath and a very competent back-bleed valve to prevent massive bleeding at the introductory site. When a second balloon is introduced over the same wire, generally both balloon catheters are introduced directly through the skin/subcutaneous tissues and into the vessel *without an introducer* sheath. This places the two catheter shafts side by side through the same puncture opening in the vessel and results in significant continual bleeding through the site. Multi-Track™ balloon catheters are not available yet for routine use in the United States.

BALLOON IN BALLOON™ (BIB™) BALLOON DILATION CATHETERS (NuMED Inc., Hopkinton, NY)

8–14 mm balloons/8-F shaft	9-F sheath/0.035″ wire
16 mm balloon/9-F shaft	10-F sheath/0.035″ wire
18 & 20 mm balloons/9-F shaft	10-F sheath/0.035″ wire
24 mm balloon/9-F shaft	11-F sheath/0.035″ wire

Balloon In Balloon™ (BIB™) balloons are exactly what the name implies—a separate inner balloon, which inflates within a separate outer balloon. The balloons are designed specifically for sequential dilations and more specifically for the implant of intravascular stents. The sizes of the BIB™ balloons are labeled according to the diameter and length of the *outer* balloon. The inner balloons are 1/2 of the diameter of the outer balloon and 1 cm shorter. The inner balloons all have a burst pressure of 4.5–5 atms while the outer balloons have burst pressures from 10 atms for the 8 mm diameter BIB™ decreasing to 3 atms for the 24 mm diameter BIB™. BIB™ balloons are available in various lengths from 2.5 to 3.5 cm for the smallest balloons and from 3 to 5.5 cm for the largest balloons, all in increments of 0.5 cm. Because of the "two-balloon" construction, these balloons have a significantly larger and somewhat rougher profile and require a significantly larger introductory sheath. In spite of their larger, rougher profile, BIB™ balloons currently are the *optimal balloons* for the implant of stents to the larger initial diameters. They are discussed in more detail in Chapter 22.

CUTTING BALLOONS

2, 2.5, 3, 3.5 & 4 mm balloons/ 3.6-F shaft	5-F sheath/0.014″ wire
5, 6, 7 & 8 mm balloons/ 4.2-F shaft	7-F sheath/0.014″ & 0.018″ wires

Cutting balloons have very small, shallow but sharp steel blades embedded longitudinally on their surface. The 2 & 3 mm diameter balloons have three blades evenly spaced 120° apart over the circumference of the balloon while the 3.5 mm and larger diameter balloons have 4 blades evenly spaced 90° apart around the circumference of the balloon. When deflated, the blades fold against, *and into* the surface of the balloons, but when the balloon is inflated to its full diameter at 10 atms, the blades extend perpendicularly 0.127 mm off the surface of the balloon. The extended blades are very shallow and are intended to incise only the intima and part of the media in a vessel of the same diameter as the balloon. On deflation the balloons refold very smoothly and the blades recess back to their original configuration into the surface of the balloon.

Both the 2–4 mm and the more recently available 5–8 mm diameter balloons are available with blades of 1 or 2 cm length. The blades appear to be very useful in lesions resistant to even high-pressure balloons and in lesions which have demonstrated repeated recoil, but they are not candidates for the implant of intravascular stents.

INOUE BALLOONS (Toray Industries, Inc., Houston, TX)

The Inoue™ balloon is a unique balloon initially designed specifically for dilation of the mitral valve[7]. Inoue™ balloons are manufactured from two layers of latex with a fine layer of nylon mesh sandwiched between them. The latex and nylon mesh are preformed into "dumbbell" shapes and into the different sizes of the available balloons. When used, the distal half of the "dumbbell" inflates initially, then the dilating "waist" of the "dumbbell" and finally the proximal half of the balloon. In this way the distal half of the balloon is inflated, the balloon is pulled back into the valve and the waist and proximal half of the balloon are inflated. This holds the balloon exactly in the valve while the measured waist dilates the valve. Currently Inoue™ balloons are available in four sizes from 20 to 26 mm in 2 mm increments, with each balloon having a 4 mm range in dilating diameter according to the precise volume which is infused into the balloon. This gives the range of balloons a maximum diameter of 24 to 30 mm. These balloon/catheters all have a very large deflated diameter (at least 12-French) and are introduced into the vein and heart without a long sheath. Inoue™ balloons and the details of their use are discussed in Chapter 20, "Mitral Valve Dilation".

Inflation devices—"indeflators"

Although dilation balloons can be inflated with a standard syringe using hand pressure only, this allows no way of *monitoring* or *controlling* the actual pressure applied to the balloon and no way of achieving high pressures in the larger balloon. Precise control of the pressure of the balloon inflation is critical in order to achieve the optimal balloon inflation. The exact recommended maximal pressure is observed in all dilation procedures in order not to exceed the burst pressure of the balloon and cause a pressure rupture of it.

In addition to the absence of any control over the pressure, *pressure applied by hand* to the plunger of a *large standard syringe* cannot produce inflation pressures greater than 1 to 2 atms in a large balloon. Using even a syringe with a capacity of 10 ml to inflate a large balloon and without some locking and screw adjustment mechanism, 3–4 atmospheres (or less!) is the maximum pressure that can be generated in the balloon when the plunger is pushed directly *by hand* into the barrel of the syringe. This pressure limit of "hand inflating" does, however, impose an inadvertent margin of safety during the inflation of *large balloons* with large syringes when pressure monitoring is not used during the balloon inflation!

On the other hand, when small balloons are inflated by hand with *small* (2–5 ml), hard *syringes*, much higher pressures are generated in the balloon and the "rupture pressure" of the balloon is easily exceeded if the balloon inflation pressure is not controlled with a pressure-monitored inflator. This is particularly dangerous in the small, confining vessels in small infants where the smaller balloons are most likely to be used.

The smaller the inflating syringe is, the higher is the pressure that can be generated by hand in the syringe and delivered to the balloon. At the other extreme, the *larger* the syringe is, the greater is the *negative* pressure that can be generated on the balloon lumen during withdrawal of the plunger of the syringe. This becomes important when the inflating syringe is relatively small and when rapid deflation of a balloon is desired. A separate, larger syringe is connected in the system through a three-way stopcock for the deflation.

There are a number of pressure-monitored inflation devices or "indeflators" marketed particularly for the inflation of balloons for the dilation of coronary arteries. These same inflation devices are useful for the very controlled or higher pressure inflations of larger dilation balloons. In general, these indeflators are made of hard plastic materials with a 10–20 ml capacity, an integrated pressure manometer and a screw mechanism between the barrel and the plunger of the syringe for the very precise and controlled emptying and filling of the syringe in very tiny increments. The screw mechanism has a release button, switch or slide which disengages the mechanism to allow rapid filling or emptying of the syringe by direct, hand pushing or pulling on the plunger.

The syringes vary considerably from manufacturer to manufacturer but in general all accomplish the same result. Some of the syringes have a larger volume capacity, sustain higher pressures or even have an electronic pressure monitoring/recording system. The most important criterion for a pressure inflator is that the particular catheterizing physicians who are performing the inflation/deflation are very familiar with the operation and the various idiosyncrasies of the particular inflator they are using. Several common indeflators are listed:

ENCORE™ INFLATION DEVICE (Medi-Tech, Boston Scientific, Natick, MA)
20 ml capacity syringe, 25 atms maximum pressure, push button on barrel of syringe releases screw mechanism of plunger when depressed with the screw mechanism locked automatically when the button is released. Built-in analog manometer for monitoring/control of pressure.

LEVEEN™ INFLATOR (Medi-Tech, Boston Scientific, Natick, MA)
10 ml capacity syringe. The smaller volume is more convenient for use with smaller balloons. A slide mechanism on the handle releases or locks the screw mechanism of the plunger. It has a built in analog manometer.

ANGIOPLASTY INFLATION DEVICE™ (B. Braun Medical Inc., Bethlehem, PA) 25 ml capacity, 30 atms maximum pressure, lever on "wings" attached to the barrel of the syringe releases/locks screw mechanism of plunger.

BARD MAX 30™ Inflation device (C.R. Bard, Inc., Covington, GA)
20 ml capacity syringe, 30 atms maximum pressure, a lever on the center of the "handle" moves from side to side to lock/release the screw mechanism of the plunger.

Technique of balloon dilation—general considerations

The valve or vessel to be dilated is identified angiographically and *measured very accurately* using selective, calibrated angiograms with the contrast injection in, or just proximal to, the lesion. The X-ray tubes are positioned to align the X-ray beams as close to *perpendicular* to the longest dimension of the lesion as possible. This places the area of the stenosis (valve or vessel) "on edge" for the most accurate measurements of the length and diameter of the stenotic area and distances to the adjacent vessels. The diameter of the lesion, the diameter of the vessel/chamber on both sides of the lesion where the lesion is present, and the length of the vessel/chamber on each side of the lesion, are all measured *very accurately* on the angiograms. The measuring system is always calibrated using an *accurate, large diameter,* reference calibration system as described in detail previously in Chapter 11. The balloon(s) that are chosen for the particular dilation procedure depend entirely upon the precise definition of the anatomy and the accuracy of these measurements of the lesion and surrounding structures.

For the balloon dilation of all valves and vessels, the balloon catheter is delivered over a stabilizing very stiff guide wire. Once the lesion and adjacent structures/vessels have been identified and measured, the stenosis is crossed with an end-hole catheter, which is then manipulated as far distal to the lesion as possible. An exchange length, stiff (Super Stiff™ [Medi-Tech, Boston Scientific, Natick, MA]) wire is introduced through a wire back-bleed valve/flush device and advanced through the catheter to a position distal to the tip of the catheter. The balloon catheter that is used must accommodate the guide wire, but the guide wire must be stiff enough to support the delivery of the balloon to the lesion and to *maintain the balloon in its precise position* in the lesion during the balloon inflation. In general, the largest diameter, stiffest wire available, which the lumen of the balloon catheter can accommodate, is used to deliver the balloon catheter. All of the guide wires have a floppy tip and a stiff shaft. The floppy portion at the tip of a guide wire varies in length and is joined to the stiff shaft portion—which also varies in length—by a transition zone (area). When a wire is in a secure position for a dilation procedure, the *stiff portion* of the wire should be *entirely across and significantly beyond* the lesion with both the transition area and all of the floppy portion of the wire positioned well *past* the lesion and secured in a vessel or chamber far distal to the expected balloon position in the lesion. Any portion of the floppy tip or the transition area of the wire positioned in the area where the balloon is sited will compromise the stability of the balloon during the dilation of the lesion.

The choice of the correct wire for the procedure and the placement and maintenance of the wire in the precise position are probably the most important components of the entire dilation procedure. The proper positioning of the wire prior to the introduction of the balloon and the maintenance of that position during the inflation of the dilation balloon often represent the difference between a successful and a failed dilation procedure. The peculiarities of proper, secure wire positioning for each specific lesion are discussed in the separate chapters dealing with each particular lesion.

Balloon preparation

Any potential for air embolization as a result of balloon rupture should be eliminated during the preparation of the balloon before its use. The dilation balloon is "purged" of all air by one of several techniques.

A solution of a 1:5 (or even as dilute as a 1:8) dilution of contrast medium with normal saline is prepared. A separate syringe of an equal capacity to the inflator is filled with the dilute contrast solution and attached to the side, female port of a three-way stopcock. The inflator is attached to the other female port of the three-way stopcock. The pressure/inflation device is cleared of air while it is filled with the dilute contrast solution from the second, side syringe. The dilute contrast is flushed back and forth from the side syringe into the inflator until the inflation device is completely free of air.

During the flushing of the inflation device, it is better to *push* the fluid into the inflator from the second syringe with the tip of the second syringe pointing downward and then to *push* the fluid out of the inflator and back into the second syringe while the tip of the inflation device is pointing upward. This prevents any vacuum from being created while pulling back on either of the syringes, and avoids the introduction of air from outside of the system or from microcavitation as a result of a vacuum that is created by withdrawing with a syringe. Once the syringe of the inflation device has been cleared of all air, the side, "filling" syringe and stopcock are emptied of all air and the balloon is attached, in-line, through the three-way stopcock to the pressure monitoring/inflation apparatus.

There are three different techniques for preparing the balloon and clearing it of all air using this same arrangement of syringes, depending upon the type of dilation to be performed. In the usual balloon preparation, the balloon is inflated, but only *partially*, from either of the syringes attached to the system. In order to avoid stretching or distorting the balloon from its original smooth folds around the balloon catheter, absolutely *no pressure* is applied to the balloon during this filling/flushing. Once the balloon is *partially* filled with fluid, it is positioned vertically (with the balloon tip pointing down and the catheter shaft upward) and the fluid is withdrawn slowly from the balloon as it is tapped gently. This allows any trapped bubbles in the balloon to rise to the "balloon port" on the shaft of the catheter, which communicates with the balloon lumen and is located on the portion of the catheter shaft which is just within the balloon at the *proximal* end of the balloon. The balloon is filled and emptied several times to clear all of the air out of the balloon *and the balloon lumen of the catheter*. As the fluid is withdrawn from the balloon after the final filling, the balloon is refolded manually and smoothly over the shaft of the catheter. While maintaining a vacuum on the balloon/lumen system (with a *gentle* negative pressure) as the balloon empties, the catheter shaft is rotated slowly while holding the balloon between the fingers and "molding" the balloon onto the catheter as the balloon collapses. This rotation is always in the direction of the original "manufactured folds" in the balloon so that the balloon folds naturally and smoothly around the catheter shaft. With balloons that are manufactured with Quadra-fold™ technology (Medi-Tech, Boston Scientific, Natick, MA), the "molding" of the balloon onto the catheter requires no rotation, but rather a straight "smoothing" of the surface of the balloon along its long axis as it collapses. The direction of the folding or characteristic "rotation" of the particular baloon should be committed to memory or even written down for later use during the procedure. With this technique of balloon preparation, the balloon refolds smoothly around the catheter and *all* of the air can definitely be removed from the balloon. This is the type of balloon preparation used for most dilation procedures in the systemic arterial circulation and when mounting stents on dilation balloons.

With some balloon materials, once the balloon has been expanded even slightly and even when inflated at "no pressure", the balloon does not refold smoothly around the catheter or the balloon itself, which results in a relatively rough surface or a profile that is one, or more, French sizes larger than the balloon when it was wrapped in its original manufactured configuration. A "minimal prep" modification of the previously described balloon preparation is used for these balloons. With the "minimal prep", instead of fully inflating the balloon with the diluted contrast, the diluted contrast is introduced only until the fluid is seen to just *enter* the balloon and just begins to form an air–fluid "layer" in the balloon when it is suspended vertically. Not enough fluid is introduced to "unfold" or even partially inflate the balloon. Again, the balloon is held in the vertical position with the tip down so that any air in the balloon rises to the proximal end and is withdrawn before the small amount of fluid that was injected into the balloon is withdrawn. This minimal inflation/deflation is repeated three, four or more times until no more air bubbles are seen in the tubing as negative pressure is applied to the balloon lumen of the balloon catheter. The balloon is refolded manually tightly around the catheter while the last fluid is being withdrawn. This removes all of the air from the balloon, yet leaves the balloon folded smoothly on the catheter shaft. This technique takes more time as only a small amount of the air in the balloon is removed each time the air/fluid is withdrawn.

A special "negative prep" of the balloon is used in cases where there is a very close tolerance of the balloon to a particular sheath, or when there is a very tight stenosis that must be crossed before the dilation. The plastic "retaining" or "shaping" sleeve, which is placed over each balloon in its package by the manufacturer, is left covering the balloon during the entire "negative prep" of the balloon. The balloon lumen is attached *very tightly* to the pressure "indeflator" on the "straight-through" connection of a three-way stopcock. A second syringe, which is of equal capacity to the indeflator, is filled with the diluted contrast solution which will be used in the balloon and is attached, very tightly, to the side port of the three-way stopcock. The syringe of the indeflator is filled with fluid from the attached syringe and then flushed clear of all air and fluid by emptying it into the second syringe through the attached stopcock. The side syringe is detached from the stopcock, any air in the system is emptied from this syringe, and the syringe containing only fluid is reattached tightly to the system. The stopcock is opened to connect the *balloon lumen* with the *inflator device*. The plunger of the indeflator is withdrawn and locked in the withdrawn position. This applies *and maintains* a maximum negative pressure on the indeflator device and creates a high negative pressure in the lumen of the balloon catheter and in the balloon. With the balloon, indeflator, stopcock and side syringe still all attached together, the stopcock is turned to open the side port (and the attached, full syringe) toward the lumen of the balloon. The diluted contrast solution in the side syringe is "sucked into" the lumen of the balloon catheter by the vacuum that was created by the negative pressure generated with the indeflator device. The stopcock is then turned to align the negative pressure in the indeflator device with the catheter lumen once again. This, in turn, sucks more of the remaining air (and some of the dilute contrast solution) from the balloon lumen of the catheter. The balloon itself in its "covering" sleeve is held in a vertical position with the tip facing down and is tapped gently throughout this entire procedure. This same process is repeated many times until no more air is seen streaming from the balloon lumen when it is in communication with the strong negative pressure in the indeflator device.

The stopcock is turned to allow the fluid which remains in the side syringe to enter the inflation device and the air that was previously drawn into the indeflator device is pushed back into the side syringe. The stopcock is turned so that the indeflator is connected to the balloon lumen, which completes the preparation of the balloon. This "negative prep" of the balloon extracts all, or nearly all, of the air from the balloon while not disturbing the original, very tight and smooth "factory fold" of the balloon over the shaft of the catheter.

Balloon introduction

With the exception of the Inoue™ balloon, all dilation balloons are now introduced into the vascular system through indwelling vascular sheaths. Balloon catheter shafts and balloon profiles have decreased dramatically in size over the past two decades so that the sheath size necessary to introduce a balloon is seldom more than one, or at most, two French sizes greater than the shaft of the balloon catheter itself. The exceptions to this are the Mullins X™, the Z-Med™ and the BIB™ balloon from NuMED (NuMED Inc., Hopkinton, NY), all of which require a sheath 2–4 French sizes larger than the shaft of the balloon catheter. These balloons still should be introduced through indwelling sheaths.

An indwelling sheath allows a balloon to pass into a vessel without the rough surface of the balloon causing additional trauma to the vessel. Once the sheath is in place, any additional trauma to the vessel wall at the freshly traumatized entry site as a result of the shaft of the balloon catheter rubbing directly against the vessel wall is eliminated entirely as the balloon catheter is advanced and manipulated within the vascular system. With a sheath in place, there is no gap between the shaft of the balloon catheter and the *hole* in the wall of the vessel, which otherwise would be created owing to the discrepancy between the larger balloon diameter and the diameter of the shaft of the balloon catheter. When no sheath is used, the large hole in the vessel wall around the shaft of the catheter due to this discrepancy results in excessive and continued bleeding. When a much larger sheath than the shaft of the balloon catheter is necessary, it is usually because of a very large balloon with a very large discrepancy between its diameter and the diameter of the shaft of the catheter. The direct introduction of such a balloon into a vessel is far more traumatic to the vessel than the presence of the larger diameter sheath in the vessel.

The direct introduction of balloons over a wire without a sheath was prevalent early in the history of balloon dilations of congenital lesions. The original balloons were on very large *catheter shafts* and they were made of very thick materials so that the deflated profiles of even the small diameter balloons were huge and the balloons often had a very grotesque deflated profile. These earlier balloons usually required sheaths that were three or four French sizes larger than the shaft of the balloon catheter in order to introduce the balloon through them. The consensus then was that a *very* large indwelling sheath would occlude the vessel for a long period of time and would be more traumatic than the rough balloon passing in and out of the opening in the vessel wall. With the current balloons and sheaths, there is little, or no, indication or justification for the introduction of a dilation balloon without a sheath. The indwelling sheath not only protects the vessel from the often very rough balloon surfaces during introduction and withdrawal, but it also isolates the vessel wall from the constant motion of the shaft of the balloon catheter against the vessel at the already traumatized introductory site.

Occasionally, a "negatively prepped" balloon can be introduced into and through a tightly fitting sheath, but, after inflation/deflation in the body, it cannot be withdrawn out of the vessel through the same sheath. In these circumstances, at least the rough, sharp, folds at the proximal shoulder of the balloon can be withdrawn partially into the sheath before the body of the balloon is withdrawn along with the sheath. When the sheath/balloon combination is withdrawn together over the wire from the vessel, it is allowed to rotate in the direction of the still exposed manufacturer's folds in the balloon. When withdrawn together the sheath protects the walls of the vessel and the subcutaneous tissues from the roughest folds and sharper edges of the more proximal shoulder of the balloon. In order to complete the procedure, a new sheath of the same size is reintroduced over the wire that is still in place in the vessel.

Dilation procedure

Once in the vessel, the balloon catheter is advanced over the wire and to the lesion, whether the lesion is a stenosis of a vessel or a valve. Often, while passing through the heart and across the lesion, the stiff guide wire along with the balloon will distort the previously "relaxed" anatomy of the area. The exact position of the balloon in the lesion is verified by a repeat selective angiogram through a separate (additional) angiographic catheter and, after the angiogram, the balloon is positioned exactly in the lesion. Adjustments in the position of the balloon are made with a combination of maneuvers with the stiff guide wire and the balloon catheter. In order to *advance the balloon* further into the lesion, the wire and the balloon are advanced together until they do not advance together any further. If the balloon still needs to be advanced further into the lesion, the wire is held in position and the balloon catheter alone is advanced over the wire. This technique maintains good forward pressure on the wire and the balloon. In order to *withdraw the balloon* in the lesion, *the shaft of the balloon catheter is fixed* at the skin surface while the *wire alone is advanced!* As the wire, which is "buried" and fixed in the distal vessel/capillaries, is advanced against distal resistance, the balloon catheter and balloon will be pushed backward. By using this technique for "withdrawing" the balloon, the wire remains fixed firmly with a forward pressure on it while the wire is wedged in its most distal location. This forward fixation of the wire with no "slack" in its course provides maximum control on the balloon/wire during balloon inflation.

Once the exact position of the balloon, with it centered precisely across the exact center of the lesion, has been confirmed, the lesion is dilated with a controlled inflation of the balloon. The inflation of the balloon should always be performed with a pressure-monitored inflation device. The rate of inflation/deflation depends upon the type and the location of the lesion being dilated. If the inflated balloon is obstructing all of the cardiac output (in a valve or central main vessel) the inflation/deflation must be rapid, while dilations of balloons in isolated branch vessels can be performed more slowly and under better control. The inflation of the balloon(s) during the dilation of a valve or vessel is recorded on either a biplane, slow-frame-rate, angiogram or biplane "stored fluoroscopy" mode. Most congenital lesions, even in small infants, are large in diameter compared to coronary stenoses and as a consequence, very "large" diameter balloons are used which require large volumes for balloon inflation. For the inflation of any balloon over 5 mm in diameter, the screw mechanism of the syringe *is disengaged* and the initial inflation of the balloon is performed with a direct, forceful *hand push* on the plunger of the syringe.

As the balloon begins to inflate, a circumferential indentation or "waist", which is visible on fluoroscopy around the balloon, is created on the balloon's surface by the constriction from the stenosis. To complete the inflation of the balloon with the final few milliliters of fluid and to reach, and maintain, the maximal pressure of the balloon, the *screw mechanism of the syringe is re-engaged* and the remaining inflation fluid is "screwed" into the balloon from the indeflator syringe. The pressure on the syringe manometer is observed carefully in order to reach, but not to exceed, the maximal rated pressure of the balloon. The balloon inflation continues until either the "waist" around the circumference of the balloon disappears or until the maximum rated pressure of the balloon is reached. As soon as the maximum pressure is reached or the "waist" on the balloon disappears, the balloon is deflated rapidly by *disengaging* the screw mechanism and manually and forcefully pulling on the plunger of the syringe of the inflation device. This creates a vacuum in the indeflator, which withdraws the fluid from the balloon as rapidly as possible.

The inflation is reviewed on the angiographic recording of the dilation procedure, looking for the exact position of the balloon in the lesion, the completeness of the expansion of the area of stenosis (disappearance of the "waist"), and the satisfactory diameter of the balloon compared to the diameter of the lesion and the adjacent/surrounding vessel or annulus. Even with all of these factors appearing satisfactory, but certainly when the position of the balloon needs adjusting within the lesion, the inflation of the balloon(s) is repeated several more times. When the dilation of the lesion has been successful and as the balloon is reinflated, there is usually no reappearance of the "waist" on the balloon particularly as the balloon *begins* to be reinflated at a low pressure in the same area. If there is a residual waist or the balloon appears undersized for the lesion, the balloon is replaced with an appropriate larger balloon or a balloon that will accept a higher inflation pressure, and the dilation process is repeated.

Balloon withdrawal

When the balloon is being withdrawn from the lesion and out of the vessel, extra care is necessary to reduce the trauma to the tissues through which the balloon is being withdrawn. Immediately after the deflation of the balloon *but before beginning withdrawal* of the balloon, maximum negative pressure is applied to the lumen of the balloon and the balloon is inspected on fluoroscopy to ensure that it has been emptied completely of all contrast solution. However, this *negative pressure must be* ***released completely*** from the syringe/balloon before the balloon catheter is withdrawn from the lesion. Strong negative pressure applied to the balloon causes the folds and creases on the surface of the deflated balloon to become rigid and to extend out from the balloon surface like sharp "wings" or knife-like blades. These rigid "wings" can catch within small vessels or valve structures as the balloon is withdrawn through them. By releasing the negative pressure, these "wings" become softer and can fold passively more easily against the shaft of the catheter. As the catheter is withdrawn through the heart and vessels with the negative pressure released, the catheter shaft is rotated slowly over the wire in the direction of the natural balloon folds (remembering from when the balloon was being prepared!). The catheter rotation helps to "refold" the balloon over the surface of the catheter shaft and keeps the now looser balloon material from bunching up on the catheter shaft. This creates the lowest possible profile on the balloon as it is withdrawn through the sheath from the vessel.

Extra care is taken as the deflated balloon is withdrawn back through the heart valves. The irregular folds and wings on the deflated balloon can very easily catch on valve chordae as the balloon is pulled through a ventricular chamber. Any resistance must be respected, the balloon re-advanced and rotated and then the withdrawal reattempted. Occasionally either re-advancing the wire alone or just the opposite, withdrawing the wire slightly, changes the course of the balloon/wire through the ventricle and allows an easier withdrawal of the balloon through the ventricular structures.

During the withdrawal of larger balloons in particular, a large amount of resistance is occasionally encountered. When any additional force is required, the entire course of the catheter and wire is examined on fluoroscopy. Twists, kinks or entanglement of the wire or the catheter anywhere within the venous system can occur. When a second right ventricular/pulmonary artery monitoring catheter or a second balloon catheter is used, it is possible for the balloon catheter to become entangled with the second catheter. Assuming none of these problems exists to explain the extra resistance to withdrawal, it is better to re-advance the balloon back into a larger area in a vessel or cavity, reinflate the balloon and, as gentle negative pressure is applied, deflate the balloon again while slowly rotating the balloon catheter as previously described. This process, hopefully, will refold the balloon more smoothly around the catheter. Once the balloon has been deflated and refolded, the negative pressure in the balloon is *released* and the withdrawal back to, and through, the sheath is attempted again. Strong force or pull should never be applied to the catheter with the balloon against the tip of the sheath. A strong pull against the tip of the sheath will buckle or "accordion" the sheath on itself, and actually increases the "mass" being removed. Also, a strong pull on the shaft of the balloon against resistance can actually stretch the *shaft* of the balloon catheter along its length (to the point of breaking!). If the balloon cannot be withdrawn into and through the sheath, the balloon and sheath are withdrawn together over the wire as described previously.

Single versus double-balloon dilation technique

Many vessel and some valve dilations are accomplished with a single dilation balloon inflated in the lesion. The single-balloon technique has the obvious advantage of requiring the introduction of only one supporting/delivery wire and one balloon catheter into the vascular system. With most vessel dilations, the diameter of the balloon used is the same or only slightly larger than the diameter of the vessel being dilated and with the newer, lower profile balloons on smaller catheter shafts, fairly large balloons can now be introduced through relatively small sheaths.

The double-balloon dilation technique has specific uses and several significant advantages, especially for valve dilations[8]. There are circumstances where the combination of two (or three) balloons side by side is essential to achieve a large enough total dilating diameter for an adequate dilation of a valve or a vessel with a very large annulus diameter. Usually a dilation balloon that is 20–50% *larger than the annulus* diameter is required to dilate the stenotic valves adequately when a single balloon is used. Currently, there are no single balloons available with large enough diameters for valves with *very large* diameters of the annulus. Even if available, a single very large balloon that would be necessary to adequately dilate a 30–35 mm diameter valve, would have a very large and horrible deflated "profile" and would require a very large introductory sheath or opening in the vessel. The diameter of the deflated profile of a very large balloon also requires a sheath that is 4–5 French sizes larger than the shaft of the balloon catheter. As a consequence, very large diameter valves make the double-balloon technique obligatory. Two, or even three, smaller balloons can be introduced through separate very small sheaths into separate vessels and placed side by side in the valve, and when expanded simultaneously, achieve a very large effective dilating diameter without damage to any single introductory vessel.

There are many other circumstances where two balloons side by side are not obligatory, but still have significant advantages over a single balloon for certain dilations[8]. A "normal sized" cardiac valve annulus is often very large in diameter compared to the peripheral (entry) vessels of the patient. Even when a balloon that is large enough to dilate such a valve is available, it requires the introduction of a very large balloon or sheath relative to the size of the entry vessel. This is particularly true in small patients. In this situation, two small-profile balloons that are introduced into separate vessels through separate, *small* introducing sheaths, are preferable to a single very large balloon and a single very large sheath. Separate smaller sheaths are less traumatic to the vessels than the one larger sheath, which potentially could occlude the introductory vessel.

When a single balloon is inflated in a valve, it totally obstructs the valve and all forward flow (and cardiac output!). Large balloons, even on the usually larger catheter shafts, take a very long time to inflate and deflate. This slow inflation within a *valve orifice* stops total cardiac output for the duration of the inflation/deflation! Two separate, smaller balloons, even with their smaller catheter shafts, inflate and deflate more rapidly than a single very large balloon. In addition, when two balloons are inflated simultaneously and particularly when inflated fully in a valve or vessel, two separate "lumens" are created adjacent to and between the two balloons. The "lumens" around the two (or more) balloons exist between touching edges of the two circumferences of the two, adjacent, inflated balloons within the single circumference of the valve annulus or vessel (two circles within one larger circle; Figure 15.1). These "lumens" alongside of the two balloons allow significant continued flow through the valve or vessel, especially when the balloons are fully inflated! As a consequence, the drop in the systemic pressure during inflation is less significant and the vagal response is decreased markedly when using side by side balloons compared to a single large balloon, regardless of the size of the valve annulus.

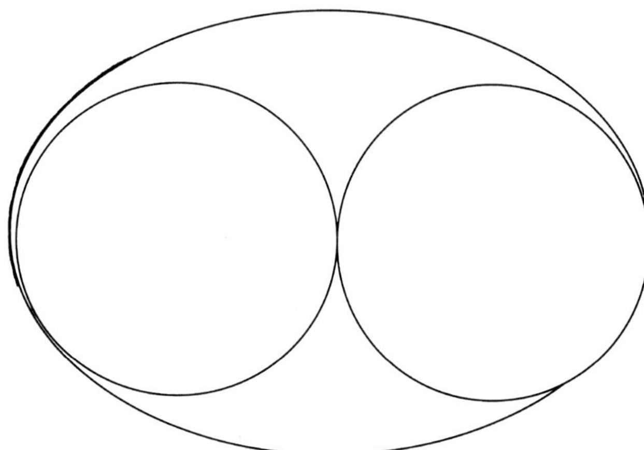

Figure 15.1 Double balloons: circumference of two balloons (circles) within one larger annulus (ellipse) leaves two significant lumens adjacent to the two smaller circles within the larger circle.

Technique of double-balloon dilation

The double-balloon technique essentially is a duplication of the single-balloon technique. The second catheter is introduced through a second vascular puncture. The second puncture is usually into the opposite groin from the first catheter introduction, but can be performed "piggyback" in the same vein immediately adjacent to the site of the first sheath. Once the first end-hole catheter and wire are in place, the course of the first catheter through the heart nicely defines the route to the lesion for the introduction of the second catheter. The second sheath/catheter for the eventual introduction of the second balloon is introduced after the first catheter *and a Super Stiff™ wire* (Medi-Tech, Boston Scientific, Natick, MA) have been positioned securely in the vessel far distal to the lesion to be dilated. The first catheter remains in place *over the wire* to protect intravascular structures from the wire while the second catheter/wire is being positioned. This catheter is placed on a continuous flush over the wire through a wire back-bleed device.

Separate wires, which are introduced through the separate catheters, are secured in place across the obstructed lesion. The second catheter is advanced to a position adjacent to the first catheter/wire. It also is positioned as far as possible distally in the vessel/chamber but not necessarily or desirably into the exact same *distal* branch. A second long Super Stiff™, teflon coated, exchange wire of the maximum size that the balloon catheter that is to be used will accommodate, is passed through this catheter and into the distal vessel with all of the precautions observed for the first wire. While observing on fluoroscopy and also very carefully maintaining the wires in position, the two end-hole catheters are removed one at a time over the wires. If the stiff wires pass through any significant curves in their course to the lesion, unless they are manually fixed in place and held very *purposefully*, the wires tend to straighten and "milk" backwards spontaneously out of their distal locations as they try to assume their straight shape.

When the decision is made to use the double-balloon technique, it is desirable to have a third catheter in place within or adjacent to the involved structure. The third catheter is used for angiograms to confirm balloon positions before and during the inflations, to monitor and verify pressures without having to remove one balloon dilation catheter, and for rapid administration of emergency drugs during the inflation/deflation. When the two balloons are in place through indwelling short sheaths, two "peripheral lines" become available through the side port of the introductory sheath since the balloon catheter shafts are smaller than the sheath sizes necessary for the introduction of the balloon. When these are venous sheaths, these lines are good for the administration of medicine but are of no use for recording central pressures or performing confirmatory angiograms. The third line is introduced "piggy-back" to one of the previously placed femoral vein sheaths or percutaneously into a separate vessel using either the brachial, axillary or internal jugular approach.

The first balloon is inserted and positioned over the first wire as described previously. The second dilation balloon is introduced over the second wire and advanced to a position side by side with the first balloon. The precise positions of the balloons in the lesion are documented with a biplane angiogram with injection through the third catheter. Preferably with separate operators controlling each balloon *and* the wire through each separate balloon, the balloons are inflated simultaneously, similarly to any other inflation of dilation balloons, while the inflations/deflations are recorded on biplane angiography. Both balloons are held in position or manipulated to keep the center of the balloons exactly at the level of the lesion. The inflation/deflation is reviewed on the angiogram. The inflation/deflation is repeated after changing the balloon to lesion position slightly. If possible, it is desirable to change the spacial relationship of the two balloons during subsequent dilations, i.e. if they are lying side by side during the first inflation, an attempt is made to reposition them front to back (or anterior/posterior) to each other during a subsequent dilation.

The success of the dilation is documented by advancing the third (angiographic) catheter across the lesion and recording a "pull-back" pressure with this third catheter as it is withdrawn across the lesion. Although the two deflated balloons, which are still positioned across the lesion, can themselves create some gradient, the gradient from the balloons is minimal and a reasonable estimate of the success of the dilation is obtained even with the balloons in place. If further dilation is necessary, recording the hemodynamics before the balloons are withdrawn facilitates reinflating the same balloons or replacing them over the already secured wires with larger balloons.

If a third monitoring catheter is *not* in place during the double-balloon dilation, then one of the dilation catheters is replaced with an end-hole catheter. The balloon catheter is withdrawn over the wire, keeping the wire securely in place. An end-hole catheter is advanced over the wire, positioned distal to the dilated lesion, and the wire is removed. After clearing and flushing the catheter the distal pressure is measured. Any residual pressure gradient is recorded as this catheter is withdrawn across the lesion. If the lesion has not been relieved sufficiently, the recording catheter is manipulated into a position distal to the lesion, the stiff wire replaced, and the dilation procedure repeated with two new, more appropriately sized balloons.

The final gradient is recorded most accurately with simultaneous pressures recorded through two separate, accurately calibrated, catheter systems. When satisfied from the pull-back pressures that the obstruction has been relieved adequately, both balloons are withdrawn over the wires. The two balloons are removed separately over their wires, in a similar fashion to the removal of a single balloon catheter. Extra care is necessary to prevent catching or entangling one balloon catheter on the other balloon or the third catheter during rotating and removal of the catheters.

An end-hole catheter is advanced over one wire to a position distal to the lesion. The other wire/catheter combination is replaced with an angiographic catheter, which is positioned just proximal to the site of the former lesion. Simultaneous pressures across the area of previous stenosis are recorded and a selective post-dilation angiogram is performed with the angiographic catheter positioned just proximal to the lesion.

In very difficult lesions and where secure positions of the wires are very difficult to obtain, the follow-up distal pressures and angiograms can be obtained without removing the wires by the use of Multi-Track™ catheters (NuMED Inc., Hopkinton, NY) advanced over the wires[9]. The balloon catheters are removed over the wires and, while keeping the wires in their secure distal positions, the Multi-Track™ catheters are advanced over the wires into the distal vessel. Pressures are recorded through the true lumen of a single Multi-Track™ catheter as the catheter is withdrawn along the wire across the previous lesion, or simultaneous pressures can be recorded through the two separate Multi-Track™ catheters with their tips on each side of the lesion. An angiogram is recorded through the Multi-Track™ catheter with the catheter tip positioned just proximal to the dilated lesion. The Multi-Track™ catheters must be two French sizes *smaller* than the *sheath* in order to pass through the sheath *adjacent* to the 0.035″ exchange guide wire. In addition, Multi-Track™ catheters are significantly more difficult to manipulate. For these reasons, Multi-Track™ catheters are only used under very extenuating circumstances.

With the development of some of the newer balloons, the double-balloon technique has become even more appealing for the infant and small child. By utilizing two very low-profile balloons on catheters with small shaft sizes, two balloons of adequate size for very successful dilation of moderately large structures can be introduced and withdrawn through very small sheaths. The sheaths are still at least one size larger than the shaft of the catheters, so there is an automatic solution to an extra line for venous access or arterial monitoring when performing a systemic arterial dilation.

When using a double-balloon technique, the combined diameter of the two balloons is larger than the diameter of the valve or vessel being dilated. How much larger depends critically upon the structure(s) being dilated. Details for each specific lesion are discussed in the following chapters. For example, using "standard pressure" balloons (2.5 to 4.0 atms inflation pressure) for "right-sided" structures, the combined balloon diameters are 1.5 to 1.8 times the diameter of the *pulmonary* annulus or venous stenosis. When *high-pressure balloons* are used, a combined diameter for the two balloons of no more than 1.6 times the annulus diameter should be used.

For the aortic and mitral valve as well as for systemic arterial dilations, the combined diameter of the two balloons, whether low-pressure or high-pressure balloons, should be approximately equal to the annulus or vessel diameter. At the most, the diameter of the two balloons should be no more than 1.2 times the diameter of the aortic valve or the aorta.

Complications of balloon dilation

Most of the complications of balloon dilations are quite specific to the lesion being dilated and are discussed in the chapters on dilations of these separate lesions. There are also complications that are related to the balloons themselves, regardless of which lesion is being dilated.

Occasionally a balloon is punctured during inflation by an adjacent structure such as calcium in the vessel or an intravascular stent. This is an unavoidable "rupture", but also, usually it results in a small discrete "puncture" of the balloon, it occurs at a lower inflation pressure and it is less damaging to adjacent tissues. Punctures of balloons alone are usually more of an inconvenience than they are a "complication" when they occur with a balloon dilation procedure only. Punctures usually result in an incomplete expansion of the balloon at low inflation pressure with a small "dribble" of contrast escaping from the balloon, or difficulty with deflation of the balloon after the attempted inflation, which can usually be treated with patience and time.

Rupture of dilation balloons that are inflated at high pressures within the vascular system, on the other hand, can result in a serious *problem* with the dilation balloons themselves as well as some other unique complications. When a balloon ruptures, it is very obvious as the contrast dissipates out of the balloon, and on the fluoroscopic and/or angiographic imaging, the balloon suddenly "disappears". When dilation balloons rupture, fortunately they usually rupture longitudinally with no loss of balloon material and no permanent sequelae. Following a balloon rupture, the balloon catheter with the ruptured and deflated balloon is withdrawn slowly and gently and the balloon is inspected for the intactness of the balloon material. A dilation balloon can rupture circumferentially and some of the balloon material can be lost. This possibility is covered later in this chapter. A linear tear during a high-pressure inflation causes a localized, extremely high-pressure, linear, knife-like and forceful jet of fluid to be released suddenly through the gap in the balloon. If this forceful jet of fluid is within a *confined* structure, it can damage (lacerate, tear or even rupture) the tissues/structures in its path and can be catastrophic.

Vessel rupture or the possibility of a vessel tear during a balloon dilation alone, with or without the balloon rupturing, should be suspected during *any* dilation when there is deterioration of the patient's hemodynamics during or immediately following the inflation of a balloon! When the inflating balloon results in a rupture/tear of a vessel or a rupture of a cardiac structure, there is usually a rapid deterioration in the hemodynamics of the patient. While supporting the patient medically, the area of the dilation is investigated angiographically. With a unilateral vessel tear, but with the balloon still intact, the dilation balloon is reinflated in the lesion at a low pressure to "tamponade" the lesion and occlude the opening in the vessel or the entire vessel. If balloon rupture is the cause of the tear in the vessel, the original balloon is withdrawn carefully but rapidly over the wire, and replaced with another balloon to tamponade the torn area or whole vessel. This is described in detail in Chapters 17, 18 and 21. When an intracardiac structure tears/ruptures, medical support including the withdrawal of extravasated blood and blood/fluid replacement is continued until the area can be sealed with a device or a covered stent or the patient can be taken to the operating room to repair the tear/rupture.

Balloon rupture during standard angioplasty or valvuloplasty usually occurs when the maximum pressure of the balloon is exceeded. The use of a pressure-controlled inflation device and paying attention to the "advertised" maximal pressure of the particular balloon reduce the likelihood of a rupture to almost zero, and is the best treatment for balloon rupture.

In addition to tissue damage, rupture of a balloon can cause problems with balloon entrapment or the loss of portions of the balloon into the circulation. These problems usually occur when a balloon ruptures circumferentially as opposed to longitudinally. A circumferential tear results in the portion of the balloon distal to the tear acting like a "sail" in the blood flow or like a "scoop" as the balloon is withdrawn through structures. In both circumstances, the distal part of the torn balloon everts over the tip of the balloon catheter either with the flow of blood past the balloon or as the balloon is withdrawn. With any force during the withdrawal, the distal segment of the balloon can be pulled off the catheter as a free-floating piece of balloon. Usually the entire segment of the balloon distal to the circumferential tear comes loose. The material of the balloon itself usually does not contain any radio-opaque material and as a consequence, the loose fragment is "invisible". The fragment can usually be visualized as a "negative shadow" on a selective angiogram in the vessel where the fragment is lodged.

The key to the retrieval of a fragment of balloon is to *maintain the guide wire position* through the balloon and, in turn, through the loose fragment of the balloon which has embolized distally. A *circumferential* piece of balloon remains over the wire even if it pulls loose from the rest of the balloon and the catheter. The balloon catheter with the proximal portion of the balloon usually has been withdrawn over the wire and out of the body before the missing piece of balloon is discovered. The wire is maintained and secured as far distally in the vessel as possible while an angiogram is performed in the same vessel through a second catheter in order to localize the missing piece of balloon as a radiolucent area in the vessel filled with contrast. Once the piece is located, a *10- or 11-French* long sheath dilator set is advanced over the wire to a position *just proximal* to the location of the errant piece of balloon. The wire and sheath are maintained in position while the dilator is removed from the long sheath. When the sheath has been cleared of air, a small repeat angiogram with injection through the sheath is recorded to redetermine the location of the loose piece of balloon. Once the piece is relocated, a 10 mm diameter Microvena™ or Ensnare™ snare is opened slightly and the small open loop of the snare is placed over the proximal end of the wire outside of the long sheath, closed loosely around the wire, and introduced into the long sheath through the back-bleed valve of the sheath. The very slightly opened snare is advanced over the wire to the distal end of the long sheath and the location of the piece of balloon. The snare is opened as widely as possible in the vessel as it exits the long sheath, advanced along the wire and positioned over the area of the loose balloon segment. Repeated small angiograms are performed either through the long sheath or through a second catheter in the same vessel as the open snare is repeatedly advanced over the errant piece of balloon until the snare encircles the segment and the fragment is grasped. Once the fragment has been grasped securely, an attempt is made at withdrawing the fragment over the wire and *into* the long sheath. When the balloon fragment has been grasped tightly over the wire, often the wire must be withdrawn with the fragment in order to retain a tight enough grip on the fragment.

An alternative technique, if the piece of balloon cannot be grasped by the snare *over the wire*, is to introduce a separate, small snare catheter with a small snare loop, through the long sheath and ***adjacent** to*, rather than over, the first wire. The separate snare catheter with the enclosed, closed snare is advanced ***past*** the errant piece of balloon to the distal end of the vessel and to a position immediately next to the tip of the original long guide wire. The original wire should have been maintained in its very distal location and still be passing through and past the errant piece of balloon. The original wire is then withdrawn several *millimeters* while the very small snare is opened as widely as possible and as far distally in the vessel as possible. If the small snare does not open at all, the snare catheter also needs to be withdrawn off the snare very slightly. The open snare needs to be positioned slightly distal to the tip of the original wire in the vessel. With the snare loop open, the original wire is re-advanced, hopefully through the open loop of the tiny snare, which is positioned distal to the tip of the wire in the vessel. Once the wire passes into the loop of the snare, the snare is tightened around the tip of the wire. This usually takes many attempts with both the original wire and the snare withdrawn considerably in the vessel. Once grasped, the tip of the original wire is pulled back on itself, everting the end of the original wire as the tip is pulled back in the vessel. When the original wire is a Super Stiff™ wire, only the flexible tip will turn back on itself, however, the tip of a Super Stiff™ wire with a short floppy tip will make the 180° turn back on itself. The goal is to completely reverse the direction of at least the tip of the original wire and to pull the distal end of this wire into the distal end of the large, long sheath. The piece of balloon is now trapped within the 180° loop of the original guide wire, and as this wire and the snare are withdrawn together into the large, long sheath, the balloon fragment will be pulled into the sheath.

This emphasizes the importance of getting a long sheath to the area of the foreign body, whether a long sheath had been used originally or not. If the snare catheter was delivered separately outside of a sheath and the tip of the original wire was grasped successfully, a *very large loop* of the stiff wire would be formed in the vessel/heart as an attempt is made at withdrawing the grasped wire with the snare. If the separate snare catheter was not advanced through a long sheath which was over the original wire and, in addition, did not pass through the *exact* same course through the heart en route to the foreign body, the large loop in the wire could also encircle valve structures and prevent the loop from being withdrawn or tear intravascular structures during withdrawal! The balloon fragment could also be loose somewhere on the large loop of wire, and if the wire loop became entrapped on a valve or other intracardiac structure, the fragment of balloon would have to be released free in the circulation in order to remove the wire!

Another alternative, if the balloon fragment cannot be grasped with the snare over the wire or the tip of the original wire cannot be snared and pulled back into the sheath with the tiny snare adjacent to it, is to use a "grabber" device (Boston Scientific, Natick, MA) instead of a snare. The large, long sheath is positioned over the original wire with its tip *immediately* adjacent to the piece of balloon. The "grabber" catheter is advanced through the long sheath adjacent to the original wire until the tip of the "grabber" catheter is just proximal to, or preferably against, the loose piece of balloon. The "grabber" device is opened and closed around the balloon fragment. This usually grasps part of the loose balloon material very firmly. The grip on the loose material is tested by several gentle pulls on the "grabber" catheter and a small angiogram is performed through the long sheath to verify what part of the balloon is being held by the "grabber". When comfortable that the foreign material is grasped securely, the original wire along with the grasped piece of balloon held with the "grabber" are withdrawn together into the sheath. The "grabber" almost always grasps the wire along with the foreign material. Occasionally the "grabber" only grasps a small portion, which can tear loose when withdrawn against any resistance such as the end of the sheath, in which case the piece of balloon is grabbed again. The "grabber" also has the tendency to grasp adjacent structures (vessel walls) and "retrieve" small pieces of the adjacent structure along with the foreign material.

A final alternative for retrieving a loose piece of balloon is to use a larger (10 mm) snare through the long sheath next to the original wire. With this technique, the snare catheter is advanced through the long sheath and then past the balloon fragment. The snare is opened in the same vessel distal to the fragment. The original wire is purposefully withdrawn out of the balloon fragment. The fragment of the balloon is then grasped with the snare as the open snare is withdrawn back and, hopefully, around the loose fragment. This, again may take several attempts, but usually is successful. This does require *releasing* the piece of balloon, free in the circulation before re-grasping it!

A very rare occurrence with dilation balloons is the inability to deflate part of the balloon after the inflation. This usually occurs when a balloon punctures/ruptures close to the opening in the catheter where the balloon cavity connects to the catheter balloon lumen within the balloon. This type of rupture allows the proximal balloon to deflate through the tear and to collapse down on the shaft of the catheter over the opening into the "balloon lumen", leaving the distal balloon with no connection to the balloon lumen in the catheter. The inflating fluid is trapped in the non-communicating segment. Usually the combination of time, patience, the pulsation and the pressure of the blood in the vessel around the balloon will deflate the balloon slowly with no other intervention. If this does not occur spontaneously, the partially inflated balloon is probed with a second catheter or a wire passed through a second end-hole catheter. The end of a straight, steel, Mullins™ wire advanced out of the end of an end-hole catheter potentially moves or punctures the partially deflated balloon.

Fracture of the shaft of balloon catheters is an extremely rare, but real occurrence. It occurs with balloon catheters which have expired and/or when the materials of the catheter are damaged from the environment where they are transported or stored. The expiration date of many consumable items relates to the sterility of the packaged material, and some items can be "re-sterilized" and used after their expiration date. However, with most products made of, or containing, "plastics" or rubber materials, the "expiration date" also applies to a deterioration or disintegration of the actual materials with time. This breakdown of the materials is accelerated by adverse environmental conditions, particularly extreme heat and/or dryness. When many "plastic" materials deteriorate, they become brittle. The shafts of catheters, including balloon catheters, become so brittle that they snap like dry spaghetti noodles. If this deterioration is not noted before their use, the shaft of the catheters will snap as they are manipulated around curves within the vasculature. This, of course, is preventable by the proper care of the consumable equipment, paying attention to the expiration dates, and inspecting each balloon catheter before use.

Local vein or artery injury at the introductory site is not unique to, but certainly is more common with, balloon dilation procedures because of the increased diameter of the balloon over the diameter of the shaft of the catheter and the resultant increased diameter of the opening in the vessel that becomes necessary to introduce the balloon into the vessel. It almost always is necessary to use an introducer sheath of one or more French sizes larger than the shaft of the balloon catheter in order to accommodate the balloons, however, as discussed in detail earlier in this chapter, the chance of vessel damage is minimized by always using *sheaths* to introduce and withdraw balloon catheters. Meticulous care of the vessels during the introduction and after the sheaths are removed (as described in Chapter 4), and never using significant force in withdrawing balloons/sheaths out of the vessels, are also critically important at preserving vascular access.

The remaining complications of balloon dilations are discussed in the chapters dealing with the uses of dilation balloons in specific defects, and are not duplicated here.

References

1. Gruentzig A and Hopff H. Perkutane Rekanalisation chronischer arterieller Verschlüsse mit einem neuen Dilationskateter. *Dtsch Med Wochenschr* 1974; **99**: 2502–2510.
2. Dotter CT and Judkins MP. Transluminal treatment of arteriosclerotic obstruction. Description of a new technique and a preliminary report of its application. *Circulation* 1964; **30**: 654–670.
3. Allen HD and Mullins CE. Results of the valvuloplasty and angioplasty of congenital anomalies registry. *Am J Cardiol* 1990; **65**: 772–774.
4. Abele JE. Balloon catheters and transluminal dilatation: technical considerations. *A J R* 1980; **135**: 901.
5. Bonhoeffer P *et al*. Mitral dilatation with the Multi-Track system: an alternative approach. *Cathet Cardiovasc Diagn* 1995; **36**(2): 189–193.
6. Bonhoeffer P *et al*. Percutaneous mitral valve dilatation with the Multi-Track System. *Catheter Cardiovasc Interv* 1999; **48**(2): 178–183.
7. Inoue K *et al*. Clinical application of transvenous mitral commissurotomy by a new balloon catheter. *J Thorac Cardiovasc Surg* 1984; **87**: 394–402.
8. Mullins CE *et al*. Double balloon technique for dilation of valvular or vessel stenosis in congenital and acquired heart disease. *J Am Coll Cardiol* 1987; **10**(1): 107–114.
9. Bonhoeffer P *et al*. The multi-track angiography catheter: a new tool for complex catheterisation in congenital heart disease. *Heart* 1996; **76**(2): 173–177.

16 Pulmonary valve balloon dilation

Introduction

Balloon dilation of valvular pulmonic stenosis in the cardiac catheterization laboratory is now the standard accepted treatment for this lesion in patients of all ages and all sizes. Although a transcatheter treatment of pulmonary valve stenosis was first suggested over 50 years ago[1], balloon dilation of the pulmonary valve was introduced just two decades ago[2]. It has been performed with excellent immediate results since that time and there are now available favorable follow-up data on the patients who underwent balloon dilation of pulmonary valve stenosis as long as 20 years ago. The immediate results for dilation of valvar pulmonic stenosis are as good as those from a surgical pulmonary valvotomy, and the procedure is associated with far less morbidity and mortality[3]. The long-term results are similar to the surgical valvotomies[4].

A very successful pulmonary valvotomy, either by a balloon or a surgical procedure, does result in "significant" pulmonary valve regurgitation as seen on an echocardiogram and often audible to auscultation. In actuality, eighty to eighty-five percent of the ejection fraction of the blood from the right ventricle has "diffused" completely into the distal pulmonary *capillary bed* by the end of systole. Under the usual circumstances, the 15–20% of the systolic ejection fraction which remains in the main and central branch pulmonary arteries at the end of systole and in the presence of otherwise normal heart and lungs, is at a *very* low diastolic pressure. This relatively small amount of blood, which remains in the central pulmonary arteries, represents the total volume of the total regurgitant fraction, which also is at the extremely low diastolic pressure of the pulmonary arteries! This small volume, low-pressure regurgitant fraction has been demonstrated to result in little clinical consequence for patients who have now been followed for more than 35 years following a surgical valvotomy, nor in the follow-up, so far, of patients who underwent *otherwise uncomplicated* balloon pulmonary valvotomies.

When balloon dilation of the pulmonary valve was first introduced into clinical practice, the same indications which were used for a surgical pulmonary valvotomy were used as the indications for balloon dilation of the pulmonary valve. A resting, peak-to-peak *hemodynamic* gradient of 50 mmHg was the general minimum cut-off indication for intervention. The hemodynamic, peak-to-peak pulmonary gradient correlates very well with the echo estimated peak instantaneous pulmonary gradients when these were measured *simultaneously* in the cardiac catheterization laboratory[5]. This provides a reliable, yet accurate and non-invasive means of determining the degree of pulmonary stenosis and selecting patients for pulmonary valvotomy[6,7]. Patients initially were referred to the catheterization laboratory with evidence of right ventricular hypertrophy on examination or electrocardiogram plus an echo *estimated* peak instantaneous *gradient* of 50 mmHg or more in an *awake* patient.

However, in the catheterization laboratory under sedation for catheterization, the same patient often has a peak-to-peak gradient of 35 mmHg or less. Initially those patients with a hemodynamic gradient of less than 45–50 mmHg did not undergo pulmonary valve dilation during that procedure. At the same time, most of these same patients eventually did return for some type of therapy on their pulmonary valves. With the very favorable experience with balloon dilation of the pulmonary valve, the marked improvements in the equipment, and significant changes in the techniques, the dangers of the correctly performed procedure have essentially been eliminated, and the indications for balloon dilation of pulmonary valvar stenosis now are less stringent than they are for surgical valvotomy. The indications for balloon dilation of pulmonary valvar stenosis now are an echo estimated valve gradient of 35 mmHg or more in an awake patient *along with* other objective signs of right ventricular hypertrophy by echo or ECG.

The usual premedications for a cardiac catheterization combined with generous local anesthesia are sufficient for pulmonary valve dilations. General anesthesia is seldom necessary. The patient undergoing pulmonary valve dilation is monitored continuously with a pulse oximeter and an *indwelling arterial pressure line*. The patient in whom a dilation of the pulmonary valve is anticipated, is type- and cross-matched for one unit of whole blood. Having the unit available is good insurance against any major problem and is life-saving in the extremely rare incidence of a disruption of a pulmonary valve annulus.

Patients with very severe pulmonary valve stenosis, particularly infants and patients who are even minimally unstable are placed under general anesthesia and intubated electively. Elective intubation of the "suspect" patient allows total control of the patient's ventilation during the dilation procedure without having to interrupt the procedure with an emergency intubation/resuscitation. In the infant or small child, intubation and controlled ventilation can still be performed with deep sedation and paralysis, usually without general anesthesia being necessary.

Two venous lines (at least) and one arterial line are introduced using standard single-wall puncture percutaneous techniques at the onset of the procedure. A right heart catheterization is carried out from the femoral approach using an angiographic "marker" catheter. The calibrated marks built onto the angiographic catheter validate the accuracy of the calibration and the measurement of the pulmonary valve and annulus from the angiocardiograms. Once significant pulmonary stenosis is confirmed, a right ventricular angiocardiogram is recorded in the posterior–anterior (PA) and lateral (LAT) projections or in a cranial angulated PA view along with the straight LAT projection—whichever view provides the optimal visualization of the valve *on edge* along with the adjacent vascular structures and intrathoracic landmarks. Often the valve structures, and in particular the annulus with the hinge points of the valve, are seen better with a selective main pulmonary artery angiogram in one or more of the same views.

For the accurate measurement of the valve annulus, either a calibrated angiocardiographic "marker" catheter, an external "grid" calibration system, or a "dot" calibration system built into the X-ray system is utilized as the reference calibration system. The diameter or "width" of a catheter is too small, variable and inaccurate to use as the reference measurement for large valvular structures and should *not* be used as the calibration reference for pulmonary annulus measurements. The reference system must be in the same plane and at the same level as the valve being measured with all of the X-ray equipment in exactly the same positions during the angiogram and the calibration. A "dot" calibrated angiographic X-ray system is the preferred reference system in our catheterization laboratory. When the calibration marks on the catheter are used as the reference, a second very brief run of "cine" is occasionally necessary to position and *align* the bands of a calibration "marker" catheter exactly "on edge" in both planes, exactly in the valve orifice (or even just below the valve) and in the same views as the angiogram in order to obtain very accurate calibration. Without moving the patient or either of the X-ray tubes at all, the catheter is repositioned so that the "marker" bands on the catheter are aligned precisely on edge in both planes, placing the marker bands exactly in the plane of the valve in both the PA and LAT projections. The use of the marker bands in this way removes all chances for errors in the measurements because of distortion or magnification and provides assurance by "eying" the relative sizes.

An accurate measurement is made of the pulmonary valve annulus in both the PA and the LAT projections. The valve annulus is measured at the base of the pulmonary valve sinus at the "hinge points" of the valve leaflets and at end systole. The exact diameter of the balloon(s) to be used for the particular pulmonary valve dilation is determined from these measurements.

The straight PA and LAT projections are the most convenient and most frequently used during the actual pulmonary valve dilation procedure. Individual, biplane frames from the angiograms of the valve in the views to be used for the dilation are placed on the CRT monitor as "freeze frame" or "road map" images. Once this angiocardiogram has been recorded and before the patient and/or any X-ray equipment are moved, the exact pulmonary valve location in relation to fixed bony landmarks is noted on the fluoroscope and "freeze frame" screens. If good "freeze framing" for a "road map" of the valve or good fixed landmarks are not available, it is helpful to place small lead markers (#5 lead shot!) on the patient's chest using fluoroscopy to have the "shot" correspond to the location of the valve annulus on the angiograms. The lead markers should be placed so that they are visible in both the PA and LAT projections. The exact angles of the X-ray tubes are recorded with the markers in position.

Single-balloon dilation of the pulmonary valve

Although a double-balloon technique is preferred by this author for most pulmonary valve dilations, a single-balloon technique is used in the newborn and very small infants, and many operators electively still use a single balloon for dilation of pulmonary valvar stenosis in all patients. When a single-balloon technique is to be used for the pulmonary valve dilation, if a second venous line is not already in place, it is introduced once the decision is made to dilate the valve. This sheath/catheter is in addition to the original sheath/catheter used for right heart catheterization. An end-hole catheter is introduced through one of the venous sheaths. The venous sheath through which the end-hole catheter is introduced should be large enough—or is exchanged for a sheath which is large enough—to accommodate the folded balloon of the balloon dilation catheter which is to be used. All balloon dilation procedures are now performed through an indwelling vascular sheath. Even though the sheath may be several French sizes larger than the shaft of the balloon catheter, this extra size, sitting firmly and "immobile" in the vein, is far less traumatic to the vein than the rough profile of *any* of the deflated balloons as they are introduced and withdrawn into and out of the vein before and after a dilation procedure. The end-hole catheter needs to accommodate at least a 0.035″ wire.

The angiographic catheter which is in place through the original venous sheath is maneuvered to a stable position in the right ventricle, preferably in the right ventricular outflow tract. This catheter will be used for continual monitoring of the right ventricular pressure and repeat angiographic injections for balloon positioning, and serves as a rapid access route for medications during the valvuloplasty. The end-hole catheter is advanced through the tricuspid valve and from there into the pulmonary artery. Extra care must be taken when maneuvering this catheter through the tricuspid valve, in order to be sure that the catheter is passing through the *true, central orifice* of the valve and not through any of the chordae or trabeculae in the right ventricle. If there is any question or difficulty in crossing the tricuspid valve with the torque-controlled end-hole catheter, a Swan™ "floating" balloon, end-hole catheter is used to pass from the right atrium into the right ventricle and then to advance into the pulmonary artery. A floating balloon catheter is preferred by many operators for the basic right heart catheterization and, in particular, the entrance into the pulmonary artery for positioning the wire(s) for dilation. However, for those accustomed to, and skilled with using a torque-controlled diagnostic catheter, the balloon catheter seems more difficult.

Occasionally a very tight pulmonary valve is difficult to cross with any catheter. This is particularly true in the presence of very tight, nearly atretic, pulmonary valve stenosis, which is associated with a dilated right ventricle, especially in very small infants. In those circumstances, the pulmonary valve is first crossed with a very *floppy tipped*, spring guide wire, which is followed by the catheter. A pre-shaped Judkins™ right coronary catheter, with the catheter size and the tip curve appropriate for the size of the patient, is used to direct the wire tip toward the pulmonary valve. The right coronary catheter is maneuvered into the right ventricle and then torqued into the right ventricular outflow tract. With these maneuvers, the pre-formed curve at the tip of the catheter is directed almost automatically posteriorly (and pointing at the valve!). A very slow, small, hand-injected angiocardiogram is performed through this catheter to verify that the tip is indeed pointing toward the valve and, of even more importance, to ensure the tip of the catheter is not buried into the muscle of the right ventricular outflow tract.

An exchange length torque-controlled guide wire with a *very* floppy tip is then used to cross the valve. In larger patients, a 0.035″ Magic™ wire (Medi-Tech, Boston Scientific, Natick, MA) is very effective for this, while in smaller patients, the Platinum-Plus™ (Medi-Tech, Boston Scientific, Natick, MA) and the Microvena Ultra-Select™ wire (ev3, Plymouth, MN) are both very useful. Any comparable *very floppy tipped* torque wire can be used. A *curved* tip Terumo glide wire can be use for this probing but, with the understanding that with minimal force, the Terumo wire can *burrow* ***through myocardium*** with no more resistance than passing through the valve! When assured that the tip of the catheter is free, the guide wire with a long floppy tip is advanced through the catheter. The floppy tip is advanced and withdrawn just beyond the catheter tip in very slight increments. Simultaneously, the direction of the *catheter* tip is varied slightly from side to side by torque on the catheter and cephalad–caudad by *slight* to-and-fro motions of the catheter. In this way the very soft floppy tip of the wire is "bounced" softly and repeatedly against the valve leaflets and eventually through the valve orifice. Once through the valve, the wire is advanced as far distally as possible into the right or left pulmonary artery, even to the extent of folding or "balling up" the floppy portion of the wire in the distal vessel.

In most cases, the coronary catheter can be advanced over the wire and far distally into a pulmonary artery. The softer, floppy tipped wire is exchanged through this catheter for the Super Stiff™ wire to be used for the delivery of the balloon dilation catheter. When the preformed coronary catheter will not cross the valve, the coronary catheter is replaced over the fine floppy tipped wire with a tapered tip, end-hole catheter or even a Glide™ catheter, which is *not* preformed to any particular curve. The catheter is advanced over the wire, through the valve and to the distal pulmonary artery. The floppy tipped wire is replaced through this catheter with the Super Stiff™ wire.

In very tight, almost atretic, pulmonary valve stenosis, even a small Glide™ catheter may not follow the floppy tipped wire through the valve, or, on the other hand, when the catheter does pass through the valve, the patient acutely becomes very unstable hemodynamically because of near total obstruction of flow through the tiny orifice. This type of patient should be anticipated from the clinical findings, the right ventricular pressure and/or size and the angiocardiograms of the right ventricle/pulmonary valve. With very tight pulmonary valve stenosis and particularly with an unstable patient, the dilation balloon is prepared even *before* an attempt is made at advancing the wire across the valve, and certainly before a catheter is passed through the valve and positioned across the valve into the distal pulmonary artery.

In the presence of very tight pulmonary stenosis, the valve dilation is performed starting with a very small balloon and using sequentially larger balloons. A very small diameter floppy tipped wire is used to cross the valve initially. A very small wire by itself is usually tolerated across the valve. The initial tiny balloon is introduced over this tiny floppy tipped wire. The dilation of the valve is begun using a very small (2 or 3 mm diameter), finely tapered, low-profile coronary artery balloon dilation catheter. This initial dilation enlarges the orifice slightly in order to stabilize the patient and to allow the introduction of a larger end-hole catheter and, eventually, a larger, stiffer wire. In turn, sequentially larger balloon(s) can be introduced over the stiffer wire and through the enlarged orifice for the final effective dilation[8].

Once a larger end-hole catheter has been advanced through the pulmonary valve and manipulated into the *far distal* right or left pulmonary artery, an exchange length, teflon-coated, Super Stiff™ guidewire with a short floppy tip and of the maximum wire size which the catheter of the prepared balloon will accommodate is passed through the end-hole catheter and advanced into the far distal pulmonary artery. Most balloon catheters currently used for pulmonary valve dilations will accommodate a 0.035″ wire. The teflon-coated wire is used to prevent binding of the wire with the extruded materials of the dilation catheters while the Super Stiff™ wire is used to stabilize the balloon once it is in position for dilation. The short floppy tip on the wire is necessary to ensure that the stiff portion of the wire is well across, and beyond the valve once the wire is in position. The catheter is left in position over the wire while preparing the balloon dilation catheter. The catheter over the wire protects the tissues along the course of the wire from the rough surface of the wire and allows repositioning of the wire should it inadvertently loose its very distal position.

When using a single-balloon technique for dilation of the pulmonary valve, the diameter of the balloon that is chosen for the dilation is 35–50% *larger* than the diameter of the accurately measured pulmonary valve annulus. The length of the balloon depends upon the size of the patient. It is chosen so that the usable length of the balloon (the parallel walls of the balloon) straddles the valve and annulus completely, yet the ends of the balloon do not extend far out into a distal branch pulmonary artery or back into the tricuspid valve. For very tiny infants, the balloon is usually 2 cm in length while for adult-sized patients the balloon is 4 or 5 cm long or even up to 8 cm in length for a very large adult patient.

The preferred technique for balloon preparation is the standard preparation for purging the balloon of all air, as described in Chapter 15. For very tight pulmonary valve stenosis, particularly in small infants and using small, low-profile balloons, a "negative prep" technique is used for the balloon. The solution used for the inflation of the balloon for dilation of a pulmonary valve is a 1:5 dilution of contrast to flush solution. This allows adequate visualization of the balloon, but at the same time facilitates its rapid inflation and deflation.

While holding the guide wire in position and watching this position intermittently on the fluoroscopy screen, the end-hole catheter is withdrawn over the wire and removed from the sheath. With the balloon wrapped smoothly around the shaft of the catheter, the balloon catheter is introduced over the wire into the sheath while maintaining a continuous flush on the sheath and through the catheter through a wire back-bleed device. Once the balloon has passed well into the vein, and to the level of the IVC, the remainder of the passage of the catheter over the fixed wire is observed very carefully (continuously!) on fluoroscopy, watching both the intracardiac course of the wire as well as the tip of the wire. Care is taken to ensure that the balloon does not catch on any intracardiac (tricuspid valve) structures as the balloon catheter is advanced. The balloon catching on the tricuspid apparatus usually indicates that the original end-hole catheter, and in turn, the wire and then the balloon catheter, were passing through the chordae of the tricuspid valve. A course through the chordae not only prevents the balloon's passage, but can lead to disruption of the chordae during the balloon inflation or during the subsequent removal of the balloon.

When there is *any question* of the balloon catching on the tricuspid valve apparatus during its introduction, the balloon catheter is removed and replaced with an end-hole catheter. The *wire*, followed by the catheter, is withdrawn entirely out of the pulmonary artery and the right ventricle. A catheter, preferably this time a floating balloon catheter, is advanced across the tricuspid valve and into the pulmonary artery. Once well out into a distal pulmonary artery, the Super Stiff™ wire is repositioned and the introduction of the balloon dilation catheter is started all over.

As the balloon dilation catheter is advanced, the wire is visualized in its full length within the heart to be sure that the wire does not begin to form a large right atrial or right ventricular loop while the balloon catheter is being advanced. Very often, as the balloon passes from the right atrium to the right ventricle toward the pulmonary artery, the broad "S" course of the wire elongates or widens. As this curve widens the proximal loops in the wire elongate, which, in turn, withdraws the tip of the wire from the distal pulmonary artery if the more proximal wire outside of the body is "fixed" at the skin. The loops in the more proximal chambers can pull the distal tip of the wire completely out of the pulmonary artery. The entire course of the wire from the tip of the wire to the portion of the wire in the inferior vena cava must be watched very closely and *adjusted proportionately* during the balloon's passage through the entire atrium and ventricle. To prevent the wire's withdrawal, the proximal wire is advanced simultaneously as the balloon catheter is advanced to accommodate, exactly, the widening loops in the wire as the balloon catheter is advanced. In a dilated right atrium or right ventricle, even the Super Stiff™ wire can be formed into a complete 360° loop in one of the dilated chambers as the bend in the wire widens into a loop. If the looping of the wire is recognized and is compensated for as it forms by continuing to advance the wire, this 360° loop in the wire can be used to advantage to support the back of the catheter as the balloon is advanced. These maneuvers take considerable time and patience. Even then the wire often does become pulled back from its secure position in the pulmonary artery and has to be repositioned from the very start.

Very careful attention must be paid to the patient's *systemic pressure* and *heart rate* during all of this manipulation. The stretching and/or "bowing" of the stiff wire in the atrium or ventricle can press against intracardiac conduction tissues and cause various degrees of block or ectopic rhythms including even ventricular tachycardia or fibrillation. In the event of an arrhythmia, the manipulations are changed or even stopped until the patient stabilizes. Even the deflated dilation balloon catheter passing through the stenotic valve can occlude, or nearly occlude, the total pulmonary valve orifice and, in turn, all forward blood flow! In such a case, introduction of the balloon catheter and subsequent dilation are carried out very rapidly. If the patient has been at all unstable or if the right ventricular pressure is equal to, or greater than, systemic pressure, atropine is administered before the balloon is advanced across the valve and before the inflation of the balloon, in order to preclude some of the usual vagal response which occurs as a result of the dilation.

Once the balloon catheter has passed through the pulmonary valve, the balloon is positioned with the center of the balloon precisely across the area of the pulmonary valve. The landmarks corresponding to the valve leaflets should be at the center of the balloon. The center of the balloon is the area half way between the metal markers at the proximal and distal ends of the balloon. These marks indicate the "usable" length of the balloon. The position of the balloon in the valve is confirmed by comparing the live fluoroscopic image to the "road map" angiograms. The sternum, vertebral bodies and cardiac silhouette are used as landmarks in the PA view and the sternum, rib cage and the cardiac silhouette as landmarks in the LAT view. If lead markers were previously placed on the chest wall over the position of the valve, these help to identify the exact valve position on the fluoroscopy. As long as the patient is stable and with the separate angiographic catheter already positioned in the right ventricle, a small angiocardiogram is performed to confirm the exact location of the balloon.

A balloon inflation device with a pressure monitor is used for all balloon inflations during dilation of any vascular structures. While observing on fluoroscopy and *recording* on biplane angiography (or stored fluoroscopy), the balloon is inflated with a steady but fairly rapid, "free hand" push on the plunger of the syringe of the inflation device. During the inflation, the "screw mechanism" of the inflation device is initially *disengaged*. Once the balloon is near its full inflation diameter, the "screw mechanism" of the inflation device is engaged and the final volume of fluid is delivered to the balloon by rapid clockwise rotation of the screw mechanism while watching the pressure on the inflator. The balloon is inflated until the "waist" (circumferential indentation) around the balloon disappears ***or*** until the recommended maximum pressure for the particular balloon is reached—whichever comes first. The balloon should not be inflated past its specified maximum pressure.

The "screw mechanism" of the plunger of the syringe is necessary to introduce the last few milliliters of solution into the catheter/balloon and to achieve the maximal pressure of the balloon and/or eliminate the "waist" on the balloon. Direct hand pressure on a syringe which has a capacity greater than 5 ml cannot generate more than 2–3 atmospheres of pressure within the syringe/balloon. As soon as the waist on the balloon is abolished or the maximum pressure of the balloon is reached, the balloon is deflated rapidly by disengaging the "screw" mechanism on the inflator syringe and withdrawing the plunger of the syringe by a direct, maximum pull by hand on the plunger (< 10 to 15 seconds total inflation/deflation time). When the plunger is at the absolute maximal withdrawal from the syringe, the "screw mechanism" is re-engaged to lock the plunger in the withdrawn position, creating a vacuum in the syringe and balloon. The *inflation* of the balloon is observed on fluoroscopy and recorded angiographically, while the deflation needs to be watched but does not necessarily need to be recorded.

During the beginning of the initial inflation, the "waist" caused by the narrow pulmonary valve orifice should appear near the center of the balloon. If the initial "waist" in the balloon is *not* at the center of the balloon during the beginning of the inflation, the balloon is deflated immediately and the patient is allowed to stabilize. The balloon is repositioned according to the location of the initial waist with the previous inflation, and the inflation process restarted. As the balloon is inflated in the correct position, there is frequently a visible "snap" and there is usually a palpable "sensation" as the waist disappears. Once the valve has been successfully dilated, no "waist" should reappear on the balloon as the balloon deflates, nor even at low pressures during subsequent balloon inflations. Because of the curvature of the right ventricular outflow tract, the long straight segment of the balloon bends around this curvature when deflated. As a consequence, there is often a fold or crease on the concave surface of the balloon during the initial inflation before the balloon assumes its straight configuration. It is important to distinguish this from the true waist created by the narrowed valve.

During each inflation of the balloon, the balloon is observed closely for any displacement of the balloon, either forward, further into the pulmonary artery, or backward into the right ventricle. This is a frequent occurrence, which is caused by a combination of the mobility of the valve and by the *tapered portion* of one end of the balloon being positioned erroneously in the narrowed valve. The tight, narrow valve opening "milks" the tapered portion of the balloon forward or backward out of the valve rather than the valve being dilated. The shorter the dilation balloon, the more likely it is to displace during inflations. When any displacement of the balloon is observed, the inflation is stopped immediately and the fluid withdrawn from the balloon. If the inflation continues as the balloon is displaced backward, the tricuspid valve could be damaged. If the balloon displaces distally (forward), it could expand in a smaller branch pulmonary artery and rupture the vessel. After deflating the balloon, it is repositioned and fixed more accurately in the area of the valve.

The Super Stiff™ wire helps to prevent displacement of the balloon during the dilation procedure. During the inflation/deflation procedure, it is imperative that the wire is maintained through the balloon catheter and wedged far out in the branch pulmonary artery in a secure, distal position. When the stiff wire is pushed forward forcefully to maintain its position far distally, it adds stabilization to the balloon within the pulmonary valve by reducing the to-and-fro motion of the catheter. The wire is advanced maximally into the distal pulmonary artery while the balloon is positioned in the valve. During the inflation, forward pressure is applied to both the balloon and the stiff wire together. If the balloon begins to milk *forward* or needs to be withdrawn for any other reason, this is accomplished by advancing the wire forward forcefully, not by withdrawing the balloon. This keeps the maximum forward "push" on the wire and the balloon and, in doing so, maintains the wire with no slack in it in order to keep the balloon in place.

With the stiff portion of the wire maintained entirely through the balloon and well into the distal pulmonary artery, it prevents the sharp tip of the balloon catheter or any sharp kink in the wire from perforating the pulmonary artery distal to the valve. The secure wire position allows a controlled but rapid withdrawal or advance of the deflated balloon in the event of a persistent vagal/hypotensive reaction.

The inflation/deflation of the balloon is repeated four to six, or even more, times depending upon (1) the pressure response in the right ventricle and (2) the adequacy of the disappearance of the "waist" in the balloon at low pressure during subsequent inflations. Repeated inflations of a balloon which is of adequate size to *fill* the annulus and which is positioned correctly across the valve annulus, should produce a successful dilation of a stenotic pulmonary valve.

During the inflation/deflation cycles, the systemic pressure and right ventricular pressures are monitored. There usually is a marked rise in right ventricular pressure and a marked drop in systemic pressure along with a significant bradycardia during the inflation procedure using a single balloon in the pulmonary valve. Preparations to hyperventilate the patient and/or administer atropine are made before the inflation is started. It should also be anticipated that the patient may need several beats of external cardiac massage immediately after the balloon has been deflated. In patients with an associated patent foramen ovale and/or an actual atrial septal defect, there is less of a drop in the systemic pressure and less bradycardia, but a significant drop in systemic saturation does occur during the inflation of the balloon. All of these effects, although occurring to a marked degree during the inflation, tend to be very transient and disappear spontaneously following a successful inflation and deflation of the balloon.

The right ventricular pressure is measured immediately after the dilation through the second indwelling angiographic catheter. Following a successful pulmonary valve dilation, the right ventricular pressure is markedly reduced and the gradient *across the valve* is reduced to near zero. There certainly should be no more than a maximum of 10 to 15 mm residual gradient *across the valve*. In addition to the lowering of the right ventricular pressure following a successful dilation of the pulmonary valve, there usually is an increase in the pulmonary artery pressure and an increase in the systemic arterial pressure.

When there is still an elevated right ventricular pressure, even when the *valve* dilation procedure angiographically appeared satisfactory, it does not necessarily mean that the dilation was unsuccessful. The usual reason for this is the dynamic reactivity of the right ventricular outflow tract muscle following relief of the valvular obstruction that was "distal" to that area of the outflow tract. Prior to opening the valve, the previously very hypertrophied sub-valvular, right ventricular infundibular muscle was held "open" during systole by the high pressure in that area just proximal to the *stenotic* valve.

When the valve is opened successfully, the high pressure in that immediate sub-valve area is eliminated and the very hypertrophied muscle clamps down on itself, creating a new but dynamic obstruction to the right ventricular outflow tract. This same phenomenon was responsible for the "suicide right ventricles" following surgical valvotomies for critical pulmonary valve stenosis. This cause of a residual high right ventricular pressure can be confirmed by three *simultaneous* pressure recordings with end-hole only catheters or catheters with only two side holes very close to the tip, which are positioned in the pulmonary artery, very precisely in the area in the right ventricular outflow tract just below the pulmonary valve and in the body of the right ventricle, or by a very slow, precise, "pull-back" pressure tracing with an end-hole catheter through the same areas. After a successful dilation of the valve, these different pressure recordings demonstrate no pressure gradient *across the valve*!

The hyperdynamic reaction of the infundibulum after the dilation of the valve is seen vividly on a right ventricular angiocardiogram. In spite of a residual right ventricular pressure, sometimes even greater than systemic pressure, there appear to be no adverse consequences of this hyperdynamic obstructive phenomenon. Patients with significant infundibular gradients have been treated variously with infusions of fluid volume, with a beta blocker, and primarily with *time*. The hypertrophy and obstruction resolve over time regardless of which treatment is used.

The other cause of a high residual right ventricular pressure is an unsatisfactory balloon dilation of the valve. This can be due to a technically unsatisfactory dilation procedure or to a truly dysplastic pulmonary valve[9]. The technically unsatisfactory procedure should be apparent with a *critical review* of the *recordings* of the inflation/deflation of the balloon. The measurements of balloon size in relation to the annulus, balloon position during inflation, and the waist on the balloon during inflation are all scrutinized on the recordings of the inflations. When the valve obstruction was not relieved because of poor technique, it should respond to a balloon dilation procedure properly executed.

The "tip-offs" to the presence of a dysplastic valve *often* are the small annulus of the valve and the absence of "post-stenotic" dilation of the main pulmonary artery. These findings are in contrast to the usually large annulus and markedly dilated main pulmonary artery in the "typical" valvular pulmonary stenosis. However, the dysplastic valve may not be obvious anatomically, but is diagnosed definitively by the failure of the valve to respond to a *properly performed* balloon dilation of the pulmonary valve! In a dysplastic valve, the waist on the balloon disappears during dilation when the balloon reaches its maximum inflation pressure, but during deflation of the balloon and with reinflations of the balloon even with the balloon at a low pressure, the waist recurs repeatedly and consistently. Angiography of the "typical" dysplastic valve demonstrates a very thick, immobile mass of valve tissue, which does not change in mobility or appearance after the dilation procedure. These valves require surgical excision of the valve and frequently annular enlargement for relief of the obstruction.

Once satisfied that maximum dilation with the particular balloon has been accomplished, the balloon is removed over the wire. Any "negative pressure" (vacuum) on the balloon is released from the system as the balloon is being withdrawn. The persistent negative pressure on the balloon lumen causes the folds of the deflated balloon to create stiff, very rigid "wings" on the balloon. Releasing the negative pressure causes the folds to soften and allows them to be folded around the catheter. When removing the dilation balloon, the wire is maintained in place in the distal pulmonary artery, the balloon is carefully withdrawn over the wire, out of the pulmonary annulus and through the right ventricle. The balloon catheter and the wire are observed closely on fluoroscopy during the entire withdrawal. It is particularly important to observe the balloon as it is withdrawn through the right ventricle and tricuspid valve as the unwrapped, redundant balloon folds, and the proximal "shoulder" of the balloon can easily "snag" in the tricuspid valve apparatus. Slight rotation of the balloon catheter in the direction of the balloon folds helps to prevent the balloon entrapment.

With the balloon withdrawn into the inferior vena cava, the balloon is refilled very slightly and then, while applying a slow counterclockwise rotation to the shaft of the catheter, a mild negative pressure is applied to the balloon lumen. This maneuver creates a slight vacuum on the balloon and helps to refold the balloon smoothly around the shaft of the catheter. Once the balloon has been "refolded" within the cava, the negative pressure again is released. The balloon is withdrawn over the wire through the sheath.

Following the removal of the balloon, an end-hole catheter is advanced over the wire to the distal pulmonary artery. A follow-up angiocardiogram in the right ventricle or right ventricular outflow tract is performed to anatomically demonstrate the relief of the obstruction, to visualize any secondary infundibular obstruction, and to exclude any intracardiac damage from the procedure. When satisfied with the anatomy and the right ventricular pressures, the wire is withdrawn through the end-hole catheter. It is important to record pressures simultaneously in the pulmonary artery and right ventricular outflow tract as well as simultaneously in the right ventricular inflow and outflow tracts, to establish not only the degree of any residual obstruction but the exact location of the obstruction.

Technique for double-balloon dilation of the pulmonary valve

The double-balloon technique for balloon dilation procedures in general and its overall advantages are discussed in Chapter 15. The double balloon technique is particularly useful in pulmonary valvar stenosis[10]. In the typical pulmonary valve stenosis, the valve annulus is very large in proportion to the patient's size, and because of the compliance of the valve and annulus tissues, a single balloon 35–50% larger than the annulus is necessary to dilate these valves satisfactorily. Because of this combination of factors, when a single balloon is used for pulmonary valve dilation, the single balloon and balloon catheter are disproportionately large compared to the peripheral entry veins. The very large dilation balloons which must be used for single-balloon dilations have very large and horribly rough profiles when refolded. As a consequence, the single balloon requires an inordinately large sheath for entry into the peripheral veins and an even larger opening in the vessel for withdrawal of the deflated balloon. The double-balloon procedure allows the introduction of significantly smaller balloons with much better balloon profiles, particularly for the dilation of pulmonary valve stenosis.

The double-balloon technique allows for better hemodynamic stability during the dilation of severe pulmonary valve stenosis. The two "lumens" created adjacent to the two circumferences of the two smaller inflated balloons within the single larger circumference of the valve annulus (two circles within one larger ellipse) allow some continued flow through the valve even when the balloons are at full inflation. This results in less of a drop in the systemic arterial pressure, less elevation of right ventricular pressure during inflation, and a markedly decreased vagal response with less decrease in heart rate.

The double-balloon technique essentially is a duplication of the single-balloon technique. The second dilation catheter is introduced through a second venous puncture. The sheath for the second dilation catheter is introduced preferably (but not necessarily) into the opposite groin from the first balloon dilation catheter so that the two largest sheaths are not in the same vein.

When using the double-balloon technique for pulmonary valve dilation, a *third* venous sheath/catheter is introduced before the dilation procedure is carried out. The third catheter is used for monitoring pressures in the right ventricle before, during and after the procedure, and to perform selective angiograms during the balloon positioning. This third venous sheath only needs to be large enough to accommodate the angiographic catheter which is used during balloon positioning. In addition, the third line provides a central location for the rapid administration of drugs, particularly when the two balloons are in place. Since the shafts of the balloon catheters are always at least one French size smaller than the deflated diameter of the balloons, the sheaths also provide separate, peripheral venous access "lines" through the side port of the sheaths around the shafts of the balloon catheters. The side ports of these sheaths should be connected to the flush system and the sheaths kept on a slow continuous flush in order to prevent blood stasis and clot formation around the catheters within the sheaths. The third venous sheath and catheter is introduced "piggy-back" under (caudal to) one of the other femoral vein catheters. The third line can also be introduced from an arm or neck vein. This is accomplished percutaneously using either the brachial, axillary or internal jugular vein approach.

The determination of the appropriate size of the two separate balloons for double-balloon pulmonary valve dilation is a controversial issue. There are complex formulas for calculating "equivalent circumferences" for the two circles within one larger circle and for converting the circumference of the circle into the circumference of the "ellipse" created by the two balloons distorting the annulus. These formulas *appear* to give more *credibility* to the sizing but, in actuality, do not help or contribute to the success of pulmonary valve dilations. The numbers now used for choosing the diameters of the two balloons are a result of 20 years' experience with the double-balloon technique. This experience has included some trial and error and some changes along with new developments in the balloons.

Using "standard pressure" dilation balloons (4–6 atms maximum inflation pressure), the combined diameter of the two balloons used for pulmonary valve dilation is 1.6 to 1.8 times the diameter of the pulmonary annulus; e.g., if the valve annulus measures 25 mm, two 20 mm balloons are used simultaneously. (E.g. the annulus of $25 \times 1.7 = 42.5$ is still larger than the combined diameters of the two balloons—$2 \times 20 = 40$). With some of the newer, much higher pressure, lower profile balloons, a more conservative measurement is used for the initial double-balloon inflation (e.g. 1.5 to 1.7 times the annulus diameter for the sum of the two balloon diameters). With either type of balloon, if the result of the dilation with the first two balloons is unsatisfactory, the angiograms of the inflation during the original dilations are reviewed critically to visualize the overall anatomy, the balloon positions during the inflation, the appearance *and disappearance* of the "waists" during the inflation and deflation and, finally, the appropriateness of the diameters of the two balloons in relation to that of the annulus. Assuming the two initial dilation balloons do not appear oversized significantly, they are replaced with two slightly larger diameter balloons and the procedure repeated.

The first catheter/wire is introduced *exactly* as for a dilation using a single balloon. The second catheter for the second wire and balloon is introduced after the first catheter *and wire* have been positioned securely in a distal branch pulmonary artery. The first catheter is left in place over the wire to protect the intracardiac tissues from the rough surface of the wire. The catheter also helps to prevent the first wire from milking back while the second wire is being manipulated through the heart and pulmonary valve, and allows repositioning of the wire if it does become displaced. The second catheter is advanced through the right heart, adhering to the same precautions and techniques for crossing the tricuspid valve. The catheter is advanced through the pulmonary valve and positioned adjacent to the first catheter and wire. The second catheter is maneuvered as far into a distal pulmonary artery as possible, but not necessarily, or desirably, into the same distal branch. A second Super Stiff™, short, floppy tipped, teflon-coated, exchange length wire of the maximal size which the balloon catheter being used will accommodate, is passed through this catheter and again into the distal pulmonary artery. Only a very slight curve is formed on this wire just at the transition area between the soft and stiff segments, prior to its introduction into the catheter. This curve is only formed to help the stiff part of the wire to follow the catheter through the tight curves within the heart. The same precautions which were observed during the positioning of the first wire are used with the second wire. Once the balloons have been prepared, the end-hole catheters are removed over the wires, one at a time, while observing on fluoroscopy and being careful to keep both wires in their very distal positions.

With the "straightness" of the Super Stiff™ wires combined with their tortuous courses through the heart to the distal pulmonary branches, often a conscious effort must be made to hold these wires manually in their distal pulmonary artery locations. The Super Stiff™ wires naturally tend to assume their straight configuration and, in turn, spontaneously work their way out of a curved location in the distal pulmonary artery unless purposefully held in place by a "hands-on" grip, holding and pushing on the proximal wires.

The first balloon is introduced over the wire and positioned precisely in the pulmonary valve exactly as described for a balloon dilation with a single balloon. The second dilation balloon is introduced over the second wire and advanced through the venous system and right heart to a position in the pulmonary valve immediately adjacent to the first balloon. While both balloons are held in position in the valve or manipulated to keep the centers of the balloons exactly at the level of the valve annulus, the two balloons are inflated simultaneously. The inflation equipment and technique are the same as for a dilation with a single balloon, but in duplicate, for a double-balloon dilation. As with a single-balloon pulmonary valve dilation, if there is any displacement of either balloon during the inflation, the inflation is stopped immediately and the fluid is withdrawn rapidly from both balloons. The balloons are repositioned meticulously and the inflation repeated. The repositioning and reinflations are repeated until the "waists" appear appropriately at the centers of the balloons and then disappear at full inflation of the two balloons simultaneously.

Even after an "ideal" inflation, the inflation of the two balloons in the valve annulus is repeated several more times. If possible, the side-by-side/anterior–posterior spacial relationships of the two balloons in relation to each other are changed during subsequent dilations. That is, if the balloons are positioned side by side and next to each other in the PA view during the first inflation, an attempt is made to reposition the two balloon into a front-to-back (or anterior–posterior) relationship to each other during a subsequent inflation.

Following successful dilation, the two balloons are removed over the wires one at a time and in a similar fashion to the removal of a single balloon catheter. With the double-balloon technique, extra care is necessary to prevent catching or entangling one balloon catheter on the other balloon catheter during removal. If it was not possible to have a third, venous, right ventricular, monitoring catheter present during the double-balloon dilation, then at least one of the dilation catheters is replaced with an end-hole catheter and the other with an angiographic catheter. The two catheters are used to measure the resultant pressures in the right ventricle, the right ventricular outflow tract/sub-valve area and the pulmonary artery and to perform post-procedure right ventricular or pulmonary artery angiograms.

With the development of some of the newer balloons, the double-balloon technique for pulmonary valve dilation is even more appealing in the infant and small child. By utilizing two very low-profile balloons on catheters with very small shaft sizes, two balloons of adequate size for very successful dilation of even a large pulmonary valve can be introduced and withdrawn through very small sheaths. This allows the procedure to be performed electively in very small patients without the danger of destroying the venous access sites. With smaller catheter shafts and even with very small sheaths, the sheaths are usually still at least one French size larger than the shafts of the catheters. This provides an extra line for fluid and drug administration even while the balloons are in place. The sheaths in this situation should be on slow continuous flushes to prevent stasis and thrombi around the catheters within the sheaths.

Complications of pulmonary valve dilation

Any of the complications of cardiac catheterizations and of balloon dilations (Chapter 15) in general are obviously possible with any pulmonary valve dilation. In addition, there are complications that are unique to pulmonary valve dilation[11]. These include pulmonary valve and/or annulus disruption, pulmonary artery injury, local trauma from the large stiff wires within the heart or pulmonary arteries, right ventricular/tricuspid valve injury and cardiovascular collapse due to even transient valve obstruction.

Valve and valve annulus disruption usually (always?) is due to balloon over-sizing with a marked discrepancy between the annulus diameter and the balloon diameter or it is due to significant balloon movement during the valve dilation. The best treatment is prevention. The best prevention is by the very *accurate* measurement of the valve and valve annulus using a realistic and accurate reference system, and then *beginning* with a conservative balloon diameter to annulus diameter ratio. When standard inflation pressure balloons and balloon diameter to annulus diameter ratios suggested earlier in this chapter were followed, disruption of the valve or annulus has not occurred in our laboratory and is very unlikely. When a minimal annulus disruption occurs, particularly in a patient who has previously been operated on, usually any extravasation of blood is self-contained in the external perivalvular area. The extravasation may result in a "pseudo-aneurysm" in the area, but probably produces no other sequelae.

On the other hand, a large annulus disruption in a patient who has not had previous thoracic surgery can be catastrophic. There is acute blood loss into the pericardium or pleura with cardiac tamponade and/or massive pleural accumulation of blood. The area where the blood accumulates must be tapped and placed on continuous drainage with a large diameter pericardial or chest drain. Volume replacement with autotransfusion blood can usually be accomplished very rapidly through the existing venous access routes. The type- and cross-matched fresh whole blood is obtained or retrieved as rapidly as possible and more ordered. As soon as the patient with a valve annulus disruption can be stabilized and maintained medically, he or she requires emergent surgical intervention. Unfortunately, in the presence of a large tear/disruption and because of the location, the loss of blood is more rapid than can be kept up with and this complication is usually fatal.

Injuries to the pulmonary arteries are usually due to wire manipulations or wire movement during balloon manipulation. Extra stiff wires are required in order to maintain the balloons in place in the valve during dilations. At the same time, these wires easily perforate distal pulmonary vessels if they are not rigidly controlled during all of the manipulations. The consequences of a vessel perforation depend upon the location of the perforation, the pulmonary artery pressure in the vessel proximal to the perforation, and whether the patient has had any previous thoracic surgery. A small distal perforation in a "wedge" position is usually almost inconsequential, resulting in a small amount of hemoptysis or pleural effusion. If the perforation/tear is in a more central vessel or the patient has significantly elevated pulmonary artery pressures, the consequences and management are similar to those of an annulus tear with a large, rapid bleed.

Large loops or long curves of the Super Stiff™ wires against intracardiac structures produce arrhythmias and hemodynamic instability by holding valves open and "splinting" the contractions of the right ventricle. Complete heart block is a common arrhythmia from these maneuvers, particularly with stiff wires. Although such loops are often necessary to accomplish the delivery of the balloon, the loops must be formed very cautiously. When bradycardia, heart block, or other hemodynamic instability *begins* to occur, the tension or pressure on the loop of wire/catheter is relaxed immediately and the patient is allowed to stabilize. Usually this is sufficient for recovery, although occasionally pharmacologic or mechanical support is transiently necessary.

Tricuspid valve injury can be very insidious but, at the same time, can produce a permanent, debilitating injury. The major cause of tricuspid valve injury is the passage of the catheter, wire and then the balloon through the chordae/papillary muscles of the tricuspid valve[12]. Either during balloon inflation(s) in the pulmonary valve where the proximal end of the balloon extends back into, or milks back into, the right ventricle or, more likely, during withdrawal of the rough, stiff shoulders and folds of the deflated balloon through the tricuspid valve, the chordae are easily disrupted. Once this has occurred, there is no treatment in the catheterization laboratory and if the damage to the valve is severe, the patient eventually requires surgery, hopefully for a repair and not a replacement of the tricuspid valve.

The only real treatment of this complication is prevention. Very careful attention must be paid to the course of the initial catheter passage from the right atrium to the right ventricle. It must pass through the true or central opening of the tricuspid valve and not between chordae. When there is any question (or always!) a floating balloon catheter should be used to pass from right atrium to right ventricle. After the pulmonary valve dilation and regardless of the initial course through the tricuspid valve, the balloons must be withdrawn back through the tricuspid valve very gently and carefully. If there is resistance to the withdrawal of the balloon from the right ventricle, the balloon is pushed back into the ventricle/pulmonary artery, reinflated very slightly, rotated in the direction of the balloon folds, and then withdrawn through the valve gently and carefully once again.

Inflation of the balloon(s) in the pulmonary valve occludes most or all of the forward blood flow through the valve and results in various degrees of hypotension, bradycardia, and occasionally even cardiac arrest. These effects are minimized, but not eliminated, by the use of a double-balloon valve dilation technique. The balloon inflation/deflation in the valve is performed as rapidly as possible while still maintaining control over the position(s) of the balloon(s). Atropine in the appropriate dose for the particular patient is drawn up and available for immediate infusion through an intracardiac catheter before the inflation of the balloon(s) is begun. In more precarious patients, atropine is administered prophylactically immediately before the balloon inflations. Facilities for assisting the patient's breathing and administering external compressions and epinephrine are also available before the dilation is started. Usually with a successful dilation, the heart rate and blood pressure return rapidly, although there have been reported occasions where the resuscitation was not successful.

The presence of an atrial septal defect or even a patent foramen ovale decreases the effects on the heart rate and systemic blood pressure, but at the expense of the systemic oxygen saturation and the constant potential for systemic embolic phenomena. The atrial communication allows a "blow-off" of the right atrial blood through the defect into the systemic circulation during the occlusion of the outflow through the right ventricle. The transient low saturation is usually tolerated very well and certainly better than a severe drop in systemic pressure. The atrial communication permits right to left shunting at any time during the catheterization and, along with this, the continuously present potential for systemic embolization and the consequences of that. Problems from this are avoided by continuous meticulous attention to avoiding the introduction of any air and/or clot into the sheath/catheter systems, heparinization of the patient, and frequent (continuous!) flushing of all catheters, sheaths and lines within the body.

References

1. Rubio-Alvarez V, Limon R and Soni J. Valvulotomias intracardiacas por medio de un cateter. *Arch Inst Cardiol Mex* 1953; **23**: 183–192.
2. Kan JS *et al.* Percutaneous balloon valvuloplasty: a new method for treating congenital pulmonary valve stenosis. *N Engl J Med* 1982; **307**: 540–542.
3. McCrindle BW. Independent predictors of long-term results after balloon pulmonary valvuloplasty. Valvuloplasty and Angioplasty of Congenital Anomalies (VACA) Registry Investigators. *Circulation* 1994; **89**(4): 1751–1759.
4. O'Connor BK *et al.* Intermediate-term effectiveness of balloon valvuloplasty for congenital aortic stenosis. A prospective follow-up study. *Circulation* 1991; **84**(2): 732–738.
5. Mullins CE *et al.* Balloon valvuloplasty for pulmonic valve stenosis—two-year follow-up: hemodynamic and Doppler evaluation. *Cathet Cardiovasc Diagn* 1988; **14**(2): 76–81.
6. Oliveira TC *et al.* Noninvasive prediction of transvalvular pressure gradients in patients with pulmonary stenosis by quantitative two-dimensional echocardiographic Doppler studies. *Circulation* 1983; **67**: 866.
7. Frantz EG and Silverman NH. Doppler ultrasound evaluation of valvar pulmonary stenosis from multiple transducer positions in children requiring pulmonary valvuloplasty. *Am J Cardiol* 1988; **61**(10): 844–849.
8. Ali Khan MA *et al.* Critical pulmonary valve stenosis in patients less than 1 year of age: treatment with percutaneous gradational balloon pulmonary valvuloplasty. *Am Heart J* 1989; **117**(5): 1008–1014.
9. Marantz PM *et al.* Results of balloon valvuloplasty in typical and dysplastic pulmonary valve stenosis: Doppler echocardiographic follow-up. *J Am Coll Cardiol* 1988; **12**(2): 476–479.
10. Mullins CE *et al.* Double balloon technique for dilation of valvular or vessel stenosis in congenital and acquired heart disease. *J Am Coll Cardiol* 1987; **10**(1): 107–114.
11. Stanger P *et al.* Balloon pulmonary valvuloplasty: Results of the Valvuloplasty and Angioplasty of Congenital Anomalies Registry. *Am J Cardiol* 1990; **65**: 775–783.
12. Berger RM *et al.* Tricuspid valve regurgitation as a complication of pulmonary balloon valvuloplasty or transcatheter closure of patent ductus arteriosus in children < or = 4 years of age. *Am J Cardiol* 1993; **72**(12): 976–977.

17 Dilation of branch pulmonary artery stenosis

Introduction

There are several different etiologies and multiple varieties in the type, location and severity of branch pulmonary artery stenosis. Branch pulmonary artery stenosis occurs as congenital ("native") lesions (also occasionally referred to as "coarctation" of the branch pulmonary arteries), as a result of previous surgery on, or in the area of, the involved pulmonary artery or as a combination of these etiologies.

Congenital branch pulmonary artery stenosis occurs either with the stenosis of a single vessel or more commonly with stenosis of multiple branch vessels. Branch pulmonary artery stenosis can occur as the only lesion, in association with other significant cardiac lesions, or as part of a generalized syndrome such as William's, Rubella and Alagille syndromes. In those patients with branch pulmonary artery stenosis associated with generalized syndromes, and in those patients *without* other cardiac anomalies, the involvement of the branch pulmonary arteries usually occurs in multiple areas, bilaterally and throughout the whole pulmonary vascular tree. When the pulmonary branch stenosis involves the distal pulmonary vessels, it involves many or most of the distal branches of the pulmonary vascular tree.

The individual areas of stenosis can be very discrete, or the stenosis can involve a vessel very diffusely. Diffusely narrowed pulmonary arteries, however, usually do have separate, very discrete areas of stenosis within the diffusely involved segments. In addition to the discrete areas of the stenotic lesions themselves, the entire walls of the congenitally stenosed vessels are structurally and histologically grossly abnormal. Patients with "pure" congenital branch pulmonary artery stenoses often have had no previous surgical intervention on or about the pulmonary arteries, and as a consequence have no surrounding "protective" scar tissue. Dilation of the congenital lesions and particularly those in association with systemic syndromes incurs a significantly higher risk for the procedure than dilation of the branch pulmonary stenosis occurring following previous surgery on or around the pulmonary arteries.

Pulmonary artery stenosis is likely to occur in *any* patient who has had surgery on, or even adjacent to, the pulmonary arteries. The walls of otherwise normal pulmonary arteries are very thin and the normally low pulmonary artery perfusion pressures contribute to the acquired pulmonary artery branch stenosis following surgery. The thin walls of the pulmonary arteries are easily distorted or kinked by simple suture lines placed on them. The anastomosis of more rigid materials (patches, conduits) to the pulmonary arteries and the torsion or scarring of suture lines contribute to further stenosis. In addition, the low-pressure, thin-walled, pulmonary arteries are easily and frequently compressed by adjacent intrathoracic structures.

Post-surgical branch pulmonary artery stenosis is common following the creation of surgical systemic artery to pulmonary artery shunts of all types. The direct side to side, aorta to pulmonary artery anastomoses, including the ascending aorta to right pulmonary artery (Cooley/Waterston) shunts and the descending aorta to left pulmonary artery (Potts) shunts are notorious shunts for producing branch pulmonary artery stenoses, and equally notorious for the difficulty in correcting these lesions. At the same time, *all types* of systemic artery to pulmonary artery "shunt" procedures are implicated in causing branch pulmonary artery stenoses from the tension on and distortion of the native pulmonary vessel. Pulmonary artery banding, particularly after a distal migration of a band or the surgical takedown of the bands, commonly creates stenosis of the main or proximal branch pulmonary arteries.

Certain congenital cardiac defects, including tetralogy of Fallot, pulmonary artery atresia with ventricular septal defect and truncus arteriosus, all commonly have separate, congenital, stenotic lesions of the branch pulmonary arteries even before any surgery. Occasionally the congenital branch pulmonary stenosis associated with these lesions is very proximal and just at the take-off of the right and left pulmonary arteries, and does not involve the more distal vessels.

The repair of the *intracardiac lesions* with these complex defects commonly requires surgery on, or about, the pulmonary arteries or the movement or re-implanting of the pulmonary arteries. The surgery itself frequently produces additional acquired branch pulmonary artery stenosis with, or without, the underlying congenital branch pulmonary artery stenosis. Any extensive surgery involving the direct connecting or reconstruction of the branch pulmonary arteries during very complicated repairs of complex intracardiac lesions is likely to result in some areas of stenosis in the pulmonary arteries. The repairs that most often result in some stenosis of the pulmonary arteries include the unifocalization of isolated segments of the pulmonary arteries, patch or conduit insertions from the ventricle to the pulmonary artery, the arterial switch procedures for transposition of the great arteries, the pulmonary artery "conduit" or homograft following the "Ross" procedure, and the various types of caval–pulmonary artery connections. Even the "patch augmentation" of the main or the proximal right or left pulmonary arteries during the repair of intracardiac lesions results in distortion, localized scarring, or constriction of the pulmonary arteries. These stenoses occur at any location along the patch, but they are particularly common at the "ends" of patches where the patches are attached to the native walls of the pulmonary arteries.

Dilation of branch pulmonary arteries was described first experimentally and clinically by Lock *et al.*[1,2]. All varieties of branch pulmonary stenosis appear somewhat "amenable" to balloon dilation with various degrees of disruption of the intima and media of the vessels as a result of the dilation. The degree of clinical success from the dilation of branch pulmonary artery lesions has more to do with the criteria for "success" in each particular institution, than the type of lesion or the exact technique used for the dilation[3,4]. Most branch pulmonary arteries *can* be dilated acutely. In the majority of these vessels, when the dilation balloon is expanded to its full diameter, the area of the original stenosis is doubled, tripled or even quadrupled, and the gradient across the stenosis is reduced acutely and significantly. However, even the acute, immediately post-dilation diameter of the stenotic area seldom remains as large as the diameter of the balloon or the adjacent vessel, the gradient is seldom *abolished*, and very few of these vessels remain at the maximal diameter that is achieved acutely. Many of the pulmonary vessels rebound immediately from the diameter that was achieved acutely with the dilating balloon. Even more of these lesions that were "successfully dilated", re-narrow further with time leaving very few, long-term true, "successes" from branch pulmonary artery dilation alone.

The most satisfactory results from the dilation of branch pulmonary artery stenosis are achieved in pulmonary artery stenosis where the stenosis is a result of previous surgery on, or about the vessel. The scar tissue creating the stenosis is less elastic and the diffuse scar tissue surrounding the vessel allows a safer dilation to a larger diameter. To achieve any "success" with balloon dilation of branch pulmonary artery stenosis, the adjacent native, non-stenosed vessel is often "over-dilated" to as much as 50–100%. The wall of an absolutely "normal" pulmonary artery is very elastic, and tolerates this over-dilation without problems. However, very few (or any) of the stenosed pulmonary arteries, even in the post-surgical stenoses, have "normal" arterial walls. Congenital pulmonary artery stenoses, in particular, have abnormal tissues, which are both hyperelastic following dilation and, at the same time, much more friable. The decision as to which lesions should be dilated and, when dilated, to exactly what diameter and with what type of balloon, is rendered very complicated by all of these variables.

With the availability of intravascular stents for these lesions, the indications for dilation alone of branch pulmonary stenosis have become far fewer. The use of a stent for these lesions allows a predictable dilation of the vessel to its nominal diameter with the elimination of the gradient across any area of stenosis. Using stents, this is accomplished without the need for and associated risk of any *over-dilation* of the adjacent vessel. The stents can be dilated subsequently to accommodate growth and have virtually no "restenosis". The treatment of branch pulmonary stenosis with intravascular stents is covered in detail in Chapter 23.

Even with the availability of stents, there are still definite indications for dilation only of some pulmonary branch stenoses. In *very* small infants, the difficulty and risks are significantly higher for implanting stents that are large enough to eventually be dilated to an adequate diameter to accommodate the vessel's size as an adult. For central branch pulmonary arteries, this requires a stent that can expand to 16–18 mm diameter. Dilation alone of the branch pulmonary arteries is utilized when the only stent that can be implanted is a stent with a small maximum eventual diameter (smaller than the diameter of the same vessel in the adult), which would create a stenosis in the adult's pulmonary artery and which would, itself, necessitate future surgery. Although stents are still occasionally, or *eventually*, placed in these lesions, dilation alone is performed as an initial palliation in small infants. There are also very tight and very resistant branch pulmonary artery stenoses, which do not respond to dilation even with very high-pressure, non-compliant balloons.

The implant of a stent *will not* increase the diameter of these particular lesions and, in fact, a stent in a persistent stenosis produces a more difficult stenosis for eventual surgical repair. These lesions are most suitable for dilation only, using a cutting balloon for the initial procedure. Hopefully the use of a cutting balloon will enhance the result of the dilation of such a lesion. Finally, dilation alone is used for branch pulmonary artery stenosis when it is anticipated that the patient will undergo surgery on the same vessels within a short period of time, in which case a freshly implanted stent could interfere with the planned surgery.

Equipment

The balloons used for dilation of branch pulmonary artery stenoses are described in detail in Chapter 15. It is particularly important that very non-compliant balloons are used in these lesions since branch pulmonary artery stenoses are often very tight (resistant to dilation), while the adjacent vessel is often very similar in diameter to the area of stenosis and this adjacent vessel will not tolerate excessive dilation. A balloon that is even slightly compliant continues to expand *beyond its nominal diameter* in areas of *less resistance* (e.g. in the vessel adjacent to a stenosis) while not expanding to its advertised maximal diameter in the actual area of stenosis[5]. This contributes to tears in the adjacent vessels owing to the over-dilation of the non-stenotic areas. Although there are balloons available from many manufacturers, currently, the Ultra Thin Diamond™ ST balloons (Medi-tech™, Namic, MA) are the most non-compliant and have a very nice low profile for the dilation of vessels of *12 mm or less* in diameter. For vessels larger than 12 mm, Z-Med II balloons (NuMED™, Hopkinton, NY) are available up to 25 mm in diameter, and at their recommended pressures do not expand to more than 10% greater than their advertised diameters. For high-pressure dilations, the New Blue Max™ balloons, (Medi-tech™, Namic, MA) can be inflated to 17–20 atms, pass through 7-F sheaths, and are available in diameters of 4 to 10 mm. For larger diameter, high-pressure and non-compliant balloons, the Mullins X™ balloons (NuMED™, Hopkinton, NY) are available in diameters of 12 to 18 mm and the Atlas™ balloons (Bard Cardiopulmonary, Tewksbury, MA) are available in diameters of 12 to 30 mm. The largest diameter of the Mullins™ balloons has a rated burst pressure of 11 atms, while the largest Atlas™ balloons have a burst pressure of 14 atms. Mullins™ high-pressure balloons have a relatively poor profile and require a 10–12-French introductory sheath, while Atlas™ balloons have a lower profile but have horribly long shoulders, which almost *triple* the length of the balloon.

The fixation of the balloon in a precise location is critically important during the dilation of branch pulmonary arteries, particularly where the distal vessels are often significantly smaller. The balloons are always introduced over stiff wires in order to optimize the fixation of the balloons during the inflation. All of the balloons just mentioned will accommodate a 0.035″ wire, and whenever possible a 0.035″ Super Stiff Amplatz Wire™ (Medi-tech™, Namic, MA) is used for balloon dilations of branch pulmonary arteries.

Technique

The basic technique for the dilation of branch pulmonary artery stenosis is similar regardless of the etiology of the stenosis. The procedure is carried out with deep sedation and local anesthesia or under general anesthesia. In higher risk patients or when long and complex procedures are anticipated, intubation with controlled ventilation under general anesthesia is recommended. If it is suspected that the procedure even *might be* long, an indwelling urinary catheter is placed in the bladder after the patient is positioned on the table and before the patient is scrubbed.

Each patient undergoing dilation of a branch pulmonary artery has at least two venous sheaths introduced and, if a double-balloon or simultaneous balloon dilation is being performed, three venous sheaths are introduced initially. One venous sheath is used for each separate dilation balloon while the additional venous sheath is available for a separate catheter used for selective angiography during the positioning of the balloon(s) for dilation. The additional catheter is invaluable for obtaining pressure measurements and angiograms immediately before, and pressures and angiography after, the dilation without having to remove the balloon dilation catheters or their delivery wires. The additional catheter also serves as a large central line for the rapid administration of medicines or fluids (including blood) during any emergency. All patients undergoing branch pulmonary artery dilations also have an indwelling arterial line placed for the *continual* monitoring of the systemic pressure.

Because of the extensive manipulations in the heart, the often long duration of the procedures, and the frequent total stasis in the vessels distal to the balloons with the resultant propensity to thrombosis, patients undergoing pulmonary artery dilations are administered systemic heparin in a dose of 100 mg/kg. The heparin is administered after all lines and sheaths have been introduced. Because of the risk of vessel tears or rupture, patients undergoing dilation of branch pulmonary arteries are typed and cross-matched and at least one unit of fresh, whole blood is made available immediately in the catheterization laboratory. This is particularly true for those patients with congenital forms of branch pulmonary artery stenosis or patients who are being dilated soon after surgery.

The area of stenosis and adjacent vessels are identified and measured very accurately on *selective* biplane pulmonary artery angiograms. The contrast injections are performed selectively in the involved vessel through the additional catheter. The contrast injections should be performed just proximal to the lesion in order to fill the involved vessel maximally with the contrast while, at the same time, utilizing a smaller volume of contrast and preventing or eliminating most overlapping structures in the recorded images. This permits better quality angiograms and more precise measurements.

There is no single, standard angle or view for any particular branch pulmonary artery or particular stenosis. The X-ray tubes are angled as perpendicular *to the lesion* as possible in order to obtain the *optimal elongation* of the particular vessel and the stenotic lesion. Often a slight cranial and right anterior oblique view will elongate the proximal right pulmonary artery maximally, while a steeper left anterior oblique with either steep cranial or slight caudal angulation will elongate the proximal left pulmonary artery maximally. Often, several repeat angiograms are taken after changing the angle(s) of one, or both, X-ray tubes to obtain better elongation of the particular lesion. A calibrated angiographic "marker" catheter which is actually positioned in the lesion, a calibration grid, or the calibration marks built into the X-ray system are used for *accurate* calibration of the measurements, as described in Chapter 11 on "Angiographic Techniques". As for the reference measurements of all large-diameter structures, the use of the diameter of a catheter is far too inaccurate to serve as an acceptable reference calibration when dilating the larger vessels.

The balloon diameter used for any particular lesion is individualized for that lesion, the particular anatomy, and the etiology of the stenosis in each patient. For dilation of a postoperative branch pulmonary artery stenosis, a balloon diameter is chosen 50–75% larger than the diameter of the *adjacent "normal"* vessel, or alternatively, three to four times the diameter of the narrowest segment of the stenosis, whichever measurement is *smaller*. For "pure" congenital branch pulmonary artery lesions, the diameter of the initial dilating balloon is even more conservative. The diameter of the balloon used for native congenital branch pulmonary artery stenosis should be *no more* than 10–15% larger than the adjacent "normal" vessel or no more than three times the diameter of the narrowing.

Once the lesion has been identified and measured accurately, an end-hole catheter is advanced through the area of stenosis and into the *largest major* distal pulmonary branch beyond the lesion. The major *technical* challenge for the dilation of many branch pulmonary artery lesions often is crossing the very specific lesion with the catheter and *securing* a guide wire across, and *far distal to*, the lesion in order to subsequently support the dilation balloon securely across the lesion. It is critically important that this catheter/wire is in a *large distal continuation* or a very large distal branch of the stenosed vessel to be dilated and not in a small or rapidly tapering extension or side branch. If the catheter and, in turn, the wire (and eventually the distal end of the balloon) are positioned in a very small vessel beyond the stenosis, either the balloon is "milked" backward out of the small vessel *and the lesion*, or the distal vessel is ruptured during the inflation!

When the end-hole catheter has been secured in a far distal position in the vessel, an exchange length, Super Stiff™ guide wire with a short floppy tip and of the largest diameter that can be accommodated by the catheter lumen of the *balloon* dilation catheter, is pre-shaped slightly before introduction. The shaft of the wire is kept in its entirely *straight* configuration with the exception of a short, very slight, 20–30° curve formed just at the transition between the soft tip and stiff shaft of the wire. This curve is formed only to help the stiff wire follow through the curves in the course of the catheter through the central heart. The Super Stiff™ wire is introduced into the prepositioned catheter through a wire back-bleed valve on the hub of the catheter, and advanced through the catheter and into the vessel beyond the tip of the catheter. The short floppy tip on the wire facilitates the fixation of the wire far enough distally in the pulmonary artery to ensure that only the *stiff portion* of the wire remains across the lesion. The catheter is maintained on a slow continuous flush through the back-bleed/flush port.

A short floppy tipped wire carries a slightly higher risk of perforation of a peripheral pulmonary vessel, particularly if the wire is not handled very cautiously. Special care is taken in positioning the wire initially and in *maintaining the wire* far distally in the larger vessel throughout the *entire* dilation procedure. Super Stiff™ guide wires continually tend to resume their *straight* configuration, and when the catheter and wire have traversed a very tortuous course from the introductory site to the lesion, they very readily, and spontaneously, tend to "back out" of their secure distal positions and even out of the lesion. Once a wire is in position in a distal pulmonary artery, a continuous, *conscious effort* must be made to *hold* the wire in position by a manual grip on the wire at the skin's edge even while no other manipulation is being performed with the wire or adjacent wires or catheters. The end-hole catheter remains over the wire until the balloon is ready to be introduced and is kept on a slow, continual flush through the side port of the wire back-bleed valve. The catheter over the wire protects the intracardiac and other intravascular structures from the sharper "cutting" edge of the stiff, bare wire and provides a means of repositioning the wire at the very last minute.

Once the dilation balloon has been prepared, the catheter is removed over the wire and replaced with the balloon catheter. The dilation balloon follows the wire, which is secured distally and, as a consequence, the tip and distal end of the dilation balloon will extend *beyond the lesion* into whichever distal vessel the wire is secured in. In complex or multiple areas of stenosis and in lesions where there is a question about the position of the distal end of the balloon, a static "sizing balloon" or the angioplasty balloon *inflated at very low pressure* is used to define the lesion more precisely prior to the actual therapeutic dilation. This "test" balloon demonstrates the size of the vessel distal to the stenosis very accurately and safely without actually dilating any of the structures at all. Once the wire is in position for the balloon delivery, the "sizing balloon" is advanced into the lesion and inflated at *"zero"* pressure. The very low-pressure balloon exactly conforms to the shapes and diameters of the involved vessel proximally, within the lesion itself, *and in the vessel distal to the lesion* as far as the length of the sizing balloon extends. The expanded, low-pressure, "test" balloon defines the lesion(s) very clearly and establishes the available length and nominal vessel diameters on both sides of the lesion. Once the sizing balloon is inflated in the lesion, the X-ray tube angulation can be changed in order to align the vessel and the area of stenosis optimally in its longest axis perpendicular to the long axis of the balloon and for accurate measurements of all of the areas on the X-ray. When the details of the anatomy have been defined, the X-ray tubes are in the optimal positions, and all measurements completed, the "sizing balloon" is removed and replaced with the dilation balloon. The only disadvantage of this type of sizing, besides the extra effort, is that the smallest, true, very low-pressure sizing balloons (NuMED Inc., Hopkinton, NY) at present require a 9-French introductory sheath.

With the wire secured in the most distal vessel that has been shown to be large enough to accommodate the balloon, the balloon dilation catheter is passed over the wire and the balloon centered across the area of the most severe and/or discrete stenosis. A selective angiogram is performed through the additional catheter to verify the balloon position exactly within the lesion and the size of the vessel in the area of the distal end of the balloon. Particular care is taken to ensure that the distal end of the balloon does not extend into a much smaller diameter branch vessel distal to the lesion. If there is any question about the position or the adequacy of the more distal vessel, the dilation balloon is inflated very slowly and only to a very low pressure similar to the use of the "sizing balloon". Once the wire has been advanced or pushed into its most distal position, the balloon can be repositioned according to the angiogram or "sizing" picture. To move the balloon forward in the vessel, the wire is fixed in position and the balloon catheter advanced over the wire. To withdraw the balloon proximally in the vessel/lesion, the balloon catheter is held in place while the *wire is advanced*. As the wire is advanced, it "pushes" the balloon backwards and, at the same time, maintains the wire (and balloon) securely in place in that area of the vessel.

Balloon inflations in branch pulmonary stenosis are always performed using a pressure-controlled inflation device. Exceeding the balloon pressure often results in balloon rupture, which can be catastrophic in a circumferentially confined vessel. The extremely high-pressure fluid which exits a rupturing balloon through an initial tear or slit has the effect of the edge of a sharp knife blade cutting very forcefully into the vessel wall. In a vessel that has the same diameter as the balloon, the "knife blade" has nowhere to go except *through* the vessel wall. While carefully controlling the wire by maintaining a forward "push" on it and, at the same time, fixing the balloon catheter against the wire with the fingers so that the balloon does not "squirt" forward off the wire into the more distal vessel, the balloon is inflated with a *slow*, controlled, inflation.

Although the balloon occludes the vessel completely, unless the proximal end of the balloon extends completely into the main pulmonary artery or unless the contralateral pulmonary artery is absent or severely stenosed, the balloon is inflated slowly and kept inflated for a period of 15–30 seconds. There usually is sufficient run-off to other areas of the lung and, in turn, little compromise of the overall hemodynamics by the fully inflated balloon in a single branch pulmonary artery. The inflation of the balloon is continued until the "waist" on the balloon disappears or until the maximum pressure of the balloon is reached, which ever comes first. If the balloon begins to move forward or backward during the inflation, the inflation is stopped immediately and the fluid withdrawn from the balloon. The balloon is repositioned, re-secured on the wire and the inflations repeated until the balloon is fixed in the proper location during the inflation.

With the balloon in the ideal location, inflation of the balloon is repeated two or more times, each time repositioning the balloon forward or backward very slightly between inflations, ensuring that the waist does *not* reappear anywhere on the balloon *at the low or initial pressures* as the balloon is reinflated. Many of these lesions have some "recoil", with the waist recurring during each subsequent inflation even though the waist disappeared at full pressure with the prior inflation.

If the "waist" from the stenosis persists on the balloon when a standard dilation balloon reaches its maximum pressure, the dilation of the lesion is reattempted using either a high-pressure dilation balloon or a "cutting balloon". Cutting balloons are only available up to 8 mm in diameter, which limits their use to smaller lesions. The original balloon is withdrawn over the wire, replaced with a high-pressure balloon (or cutting balloon) of the same diameter as the original balloon and the inflations repeated. A much larger introductory sheath is required for the introduction of a larger diameter high-pressure balloon and, in addition, high-pressure balloons have a much "rougher" and larger deflated profile. To use the cutting balloon a long sheath is delivered to the lesion over the original wire and then the larger Super Stiff™ wire must be exchanged for a much smaller and less secure wire to accommodate the cutting balloon. As a consequence, neither high-pressure balloons nor cutting balloons are usually used for the initial dilation of vascular lesions unless the lesion is known to be very resistant to dilation (from a previous attempt at dilation).

When the waist on the balloon has been abolished, an angiogram is recorded through the additional venous catheter before removing the balloon from the body and before withdrawing the wire from its secure position in the distal pulmonary artery. The angiogram is to assure that there is no extravasation from the vessel as a result of a vessel tear. In the case of a tear, and while the balloon is still in the vicinity of the dilation, immediate reinflation of the balloon at a *low pressure* within the lesion can be performed to "tamponade" any bleeding from the vessel. The angiogram also confirms anatomically that there is no return or recoil of the stenosis, which will need even further dilation. Once the operator is satisfied with the dilation and there are no complicating events, the balloon is withdrawn over the wire and out of the lesion.

In most branch pulmonary arteries the balloon can be expanded to its full diameter without a residual waist indicating that the vessels can be dilated acutely. In the majority of these dilated vessels, any remaining stenosis will be at least double the diameter of the original stenosis diameter and the gradient across the stenotic area will be reduced to some degree by balloon dilation alone. Any improvement in the diameter and/or gradient is often considered a successful dilation. However, the dilation alone rarely opens the stenotic area to the full diameter of the adjacent vessel and very few of these vessels remain at the maximal diameter which was achieved acutely. Many of the branch pulmonary artery stenoses rebound immediately from the maximum diameter achieved with the balloon, and most of those vessels which do not rebound acutely or immediately after the dilation, do restenose further with time, resulting in very unsatisfactory net long-term results from balloon dilation of any pulmonary artery.

There has been some enthusiasm for the primary use of high-pressure balloons for the initial dilation of these branch pulmonary artery lesions with reportedly greater success than with standard dilation balloons. Again the "success" represents some immediate percentage "improvement" in the vessel diameter and a "percentage reduction" in the gradient, but, like dilations with standard pressure balloons, high-pressure balloons rarely result in a vessel of *normal* diameter and the *elimination* of the gradient—i.e. they do not *correct* the lesion[6]. High-pressure balloons of an equal diameter to standard balloons often have a much larger initial, deflated balloon diameter (2–3 French sizes larger), have a very rough, even larger, profile after deflation, and generally are significantly more expensive than "standard"-pressure balloons; their advantages for branch pulmonary artery dilations alone are questionable. The indication for the use of high-pressure balloons in our laboratory is only for lesions which are *demonstrated* to be resistant to dilation with standard-pressure balloons.

The very tight areas of stenosis in the very small vessels in congenital branch pulmonary artery stenosis are notoriously very resistant to dilation even with high-pressure balloons. There are increasing numbers of favorable results in these lesions with the primary use of cutting balloons. Cutting balloons are available up to 8 mm in diameter and their use in branch pulmonary artery stenosis has been extended to lesions of almost this diameter.

The catheter lumen of cutting balloons only accepts 0.014″ guide wires, which do not provide particularly good support or control of the balloons. As a consequence, it is preferable to use a pre-positioned, long sheath to deliver the cutting balloon to the distal pulmonary artery branches. The long sheath/dilator is delivered to the area just proximal to or even through the lesion over a larger, stiffer wire and then the wire is exchanged for the finer wire which the cutting balloon will accommodate. The long sheath supports the proximal part of the smaller wire and "constrains" the rigid edges of the blades within the sheath during the delivery of the cutting balloon catheter to the lesion. The long sheath helps to support the cutting balloon catheter/wire during the dilation. Cutting balloons provide a very controlled "incision" in the intima/media of the vessel to allow a satisfactory dilation in an otherwise totally resistant vessel without having to "over-dilate" and potentially rupture the whole vessel. The long sheath also facilitates the removal through any tortuous course of the fairly rigid cutting balloons from distal locations in the branch pulmonary arteries.

Abolishing the gradient in branch pulmonary artery stenosis lesions by dilation alone often requires the disruption of the intima and occasionally even the media and adventitia of the vessel wall[7]. Because of the tendency of these vessels to restenose even with high-pressure dilation, there has even been one report with the recommendation for over-dilating and *purposefully* tearing the pulmonary artery walls by using still larger and high-pressure balloons. Between the creation of a "controlled" intimal/medial tear and the total disruption of a vessel, there is a very delicate balance, which hopefully, cutting balloons will provide in the small vessels. With the ability to use intravascular stents in the larger pulmonary arteries and in doing so, to abolish the gradient and achieve a permanent dilation of the lumen to its normal diameter, all without the dangers of purposefully tearing the vessel, the purposeful tearing of the vessel walls definitely is not recommended, nor even condoned.

Patients who have markedly elevated main or proximal pulmonary artery pressures are very unstable hemodynamically and have the very highest risk of developing adverse events during dilation of the pulmonary arteries. This is particularly true in patients with suprasystemic pulmonary artery pressures in the presence of severe bilateral congenital branch pulmonary stenosis. The risk increases almost proportionally to the elevation of the right ventricular/proximal pulmonary artery pressures. A very high proximal pulmonary artery pressure indicates bilateral involvement. In those cases, occlusion of either the right or left pulmonary artery *alone* during a balloon inflation, compromises the systemic output severely and often results in hypotension, acidemia and a vicious cycle even leading to the death of the patient.

These same patients with the highest pulmonary artery pressures usually have the most severe and most diffuse, multivessel involvement. Patients with the highest pressures are frequently those with generalized syndromes and those who have additional inherent tissue abnormalities of the pulmonary artery wall structure[8]. As an additional risk factor for dilation, these same patients usually have *not* had previous surgery so they have no *protective scar* around the involved vessels. Dilation of these vessels *is* performed, but only with the patient or parents as well as the physician performing the procedure having a full understanding of the higher risks. These same risks in these patients, however, also make them the worst candidates for any surgical intervention.

In addition to the usual precautions for pulmonary artery dilation, elective general anesthesia and intubation are always used in these patients. The intubation not only allows total control over their ventilation, but also provides early information about pulmonary artery bleeding or localized pulmonary edema created by the dilation.

As another precaution in patients with a central pulmonary artery pressures 10 mm or more higher than the systemic pressure, a prophylactic *atrial septostomy* can be performed to temporarily "vent" the high-pressure right ventricle before the balloon dilation of the branch pulmonary artery is attempted. The atrial septostomy or enlargement of an existing atrial defect are performed before any wires or balloons are placed in the pulmonary artery. If there is a totally intact atrial septum, a transseptal puncture is performed and a *dilation* of the transseptal puncture site is performed initially using an 8 mm static dilation balloon in order to create a small atrial communication. Usually no shunting at the atrial level is created immediately or, if there is any, a slight *left to right shunt* occurs immediately after the atrial defect is created. Once even one branch pulmonary artery is obstructed with a catheter or balloon, the right ventricle decompensates and the patient begins to shunt right to left at the newly created atrial defect. The patient has some desaturation, but maintains their systemic cardiac output with the supplemental systemic output from the right to left shunt and, in turn, maintains their blood pressure.

The dilation procedure for the high-risk congenital branch pulmonary artery stenosis is performed much more conservatively and is performed in stages during sequential catheterizations. When high central pulmonary artery pressures are encountered, each pulmonary artery is defined with detailed, *very small*, selective, pulmonary artery angiograms before beginning the dilations. Multiple views are necessary not only to identify, but also to calibrate each of the lesions very accurately. Three venous catheters are used electively in high-risk patients for pulmonary artery dilation. This allows the positioning of *two separate dilation catheters simultaneously in opposite lungs* while still having a separate catheter available for selective angiograms in the precise area of the lesions.

When the patient has significant proximal right and/or left branch pulmonary artery stenosis *plus* additional, multiple distal lesions, the more central lesions are dilated first. It is often considered better *not* to perform further manipulations *through* a recently dilated area in order not to disrupt the recently dilated intima further. However, in the situation of severe combined proximal and distal lesions, the benefits of relieving the more proximal obstruction first, out-weigh the risk of disrupting tissues by manipulating through the proximal area after it has been dilated acutely. By opening the more proximal stenoses first, the high, "head of central pressure" is shifted more distally and to the more distal obstructions in the vessels. If the distal lesions are dilated without first relieving the more proximal obstruction, there will be a low pressure proximal to the distal stenosis, a minimal distal gradient and low flow across the areas *even after the dilation*. As a consequence, there is no way to determine the effect of the distal dilations when performed in the face of significant, more proximal obstruction. Also when the distal lesions are dilated to begin with and when the more proximal obstruction is relieved subsequently, the distal lesions which were dilated earlier are suddenly exposed to the high pressures and become markedly and suddenly over-perfused, resulting in localized pulmonary edema.

Whether or not the more distal lesions are addressed during the same catheterization depends upon the severity of the proximal lesion to begin with and the result from the proximal dilation. When an extremely severe, more central stenosis is relieved even partially, the "head of pressure" is transmitted distally, but also distributed to several vessels and several areas of distal obstructions with a resultant lowering of the more central pressures. In this circumstance, it is better to postpone the dilation of the more distal lesions to a future catheterization. Then, as each distal lesion is dilated, the effect of the dilation of each individual vessel becomes apparent immediately. This reduces the possibility of over-dilating multiple distal lesions and over-perfusing multiple separated segments of lung at the same time.

When multiple bilateral, *peripheral* lesions are present, the one most severe, peripheral lesion in *each* lung is cannulated with a separate end-hole catheter. The catheters are replaced with Super Stiff™ wires across *each* lesion. Balloons are prepared for dilation of each of the lesions. The balloon diameters are chosen to dilate the lesions only *partially*. The balloons should ***not*** be as large in diameter as the "normal" vessel adjacent to the stenosis. The balloons are positioned across both of the separate lesions and *one* of the lesions is dilated. When the first lesion has been dilated, the balloon is withdrawn several centimeters back over the wire while *maintaining the wire securely across the lesion*. The patient is observed for at least 5–10 minutes. During this time, using the additional (third) catheter, the pressure in the vessel just proximal to the lesion is measured and a small, low-pressure, selective, hand angiogram is recorded from the same location. Assuming there is no extravasation of contrast/blood and minimal, if any, hyperperfusion of the area distal to the lesion, the entire procedure is repeated with the balloon already positioned in the opposite lung. In the event of any evidence of bleeding (e.g. hemoptysis, contrast extravasation on the angiogram) or excessive hyperperfusion of the area, the patient is observed for 10–15 minutes. When there is significant hyperperfusion of the lung, the patient is given intravenous furosemide in a dose appropriate for the patient's size. When there is extravasation of blood from the vessel and, particularly if it continues, the angioplasty balloon is re-advanced into the lesion over the wire and inflated at a very low pressure to occlude or markedly reduce further blood flow to the area or to "tamponade" the torn vessel.

When the patient is stable after the initial dilation or after treating a problem and verifying the success of that treatment with an angiogram, the balloon catheter is removed from the wire and replaced with an end-hole catheter. The wire is removed and the end-hole catheter is repositioned into the next most severe stenotic lesion in that lung. The dilation with the balloon already positioned *in the opposite lung* is performed. The entire procedure is repeated in each involved segment, alternating *between lungs* for the next dilation and each time progressing to the next larger vessel or most severe stenosis. The stenoses in the individual vessels are dilated only partially during the initial dilation of each vessel. On the assumption that after multiple vessels have been opened at least a little and there is some drop in the central pulmonary pressure, the dilation procedure is continued with as many of the separate pulmonary branch lesions as possible within a reasonable time for the procedure.

If only a minimal drop in the central pressure occurs and, at the same time, no adverse events were caused during the dilation of the distal lesions, the process is continued, returning to the original vessels which were dilated only partially. They are re-dilated with larger or cutting balloons approaching the desired ultimate diameter for each vessel.

Dilation of bifurcating lesions

Frequently with distal branch pulmonary lesions, the stenosis is present at branch points in the vessels. When these branching lesions are very tight, the intima/media of the vessels are frequently disrupted during a balloon dilation. If the disruption is in a bifurcation or trifurcation area, the intimal disruption can occlude the adjacent branching vessel(s), and any re-access to the occluded branches requires extensive catheter/wire manipulation within the freshly disrupted tissues. This manipulation with wires/catheters can easily re-occlude the original and/or the branch vessels totally. In order to avoid this manipulation, both (or all) branches within the stenotic area are cannulated and have guide wires positioned in them before any one branch is dilated. The pre-positioned wires assure access to all of the branches without any subsequent manipulations of wires/catheters through the area.

Complications of balloon dilation of pulmonary arteries

The balloon dilation of branch pulmonary arteries, even using standard angioplasty balloons, does have potential inherent complications. There are complications associated with the cardiac catheterization of any sick patient and, in addition, complications unique to the dilation of branch pulmonary arteries. The complications from the dilation of branch pulmonary arteries vary in frequency and severity with the etiology of the branch pulmonary artery lesions and have been alluded to previously. Complications are proportionate to the severity of the individual lesions and to the aggressiveness of the treatment of these lesions. They are inversely proportionate to the increasing expertise of the operators and the laboratories where the procedures are performed. The complications can usually be treated in the laboratory but occasionally patients require surgical intervention following dilation procedures. Rarely, patients succumb from branch pulmonary artery dilations even with all emergency therapy available in the catheterization laboratory and immediate surgical intervention.

As is the case with all catheterization procedures, prevention of a complication is the best treatment. A "short cut" or a compromise in the technique or equipment used may be effective in some cases, but inevitably results in avoidable complications. Because of the nature of branch pulmonary stenosis and the severity of some of the lesions, some complications may be unavoidable but, utilizing known, well established procedures and following the known "rules" for each procedure reduces the number of complications encountered.

In the VACA registry of 182 dilations of branch pulmonary arteries in 116 patients there were *five deaths* directly related to the procedure (with two fatal vessel ruptures, one CVA, one sinus arrest and one low cardiac output) and at least eight other life-threatening complications[3]. These data were accumulated during the early experiences with dilation of all congenital heart lesions. Further experience with the procedure has identified some of the risks and has generated some safety factors for the dilation of pulmonary arteries. As a consequence there has been improvement in the results, along with a decrease in the associated complications of balloon therapy for branch pulmonary artery stenosis.

Previous surgery on, or about, the pulmonary arteries, is one of the major causes of branch pulmonary artery stenosis. Fortunately, very old, previous surgery also produces "protective scarring" around the vessel undergoing branch pulmonary artery dilation. Previous surgery which was performed on the vessel, or even in the vicinity of the vessel, at least 6 months (preferably years) prior to the dilation procedure, creates dense scar tissue surrounding the vessel. This scar tissue may be part of, or even the total cause of the stenosis, but of more importance for the safety of the dilation procedure, the scar encases the vessel in a dense "block" of fibrous tissue, which is very resistant to tearing and dissection. Thus, when a vessel is dilated and a tear is created in the intima or even the media of a vessel in a patient where there has been previously surgery, the tear is confined within the scar tissue and does not extend away from the vessel. This allows for a more aggressive dilation with less risk in these older post-surgical lesions.

Previous surgery within the same chest cavity frequently results in pleural adhesions with the pleural space either obliterated or, at the least, very loculated. In the event of a small vessel tear at the location where the vessel is being dilated or the perforation of a tiny distal pulmonary branch (capillary) by the tip of a stiff wire, the pleural adhesions in the chest keep any extravasated blood contained and prevent it from accumulating further.

Recent surgery on a pulmonary vessel, on the other hand, markedly *increases* the risk of a dilation procedure on a vessel. "Healing" of vessels occurs in 6–8 weeks, however, significant scarring does not occur for 6 or even 12 months. The *scarring* protects the vessel from an extended tear or rupture. The sutures and the *healing* acutely hold the vessel wall together under normal circumstances, but the surgery on the vessel itself removes all of the naturally occurring surrounding and supporting tissues. If a vessel needs dilation for residual stenosis shortly after surgery, it is better to perform this within the first few *days* after the surgery while the sutures are still at their strongest. When a vessel must be dilated after there has recently been surgery on it, the dilation should be very conservative, with no attempt to *cure the stenosis* or over-dilate the vessel at that time. The dilation should be only to a diameter *the same or less* than the adjacent "normal-diameter" vessel. If the conservative dilation is not effective, an intravascular stent *of the same diameter* as the adjacent vessel is considered.

The major causes of vessel tears during elective balloon dilation of pulmonary arteries are over-dilation of the adjacent native vessel and balloon rupture during the dilation. When the stenotic area is dilated, it is assumed that there is some *thickened* abnormal tissue causing the stenosis. When dilated, this tissue becomes thin or flattens out as it enlarges in circumference. The normal, adjacent vessel, on the other hand, has only its relatively thin layers of normal intima, media and adventitia with little capability of further "thinning". When the tissues of the normal vessel wall are over-dilated markedly, the tissues can only split (tear) in order to increase their circumference! This, of course, is more likely if the adjacent vessel is smaller than expected or the balloon expands excessively or extends or "milks" into a much smaller branch vessel. Balloon rupture during a high-pressure inflation produces a *very* high-pressure, very discrete, localized, knife-like *jet of escaping fluid* through the narrow slit of the rupture. When the balloon is in the confined space of a small vessel, this knife-like jet has no place to go except through the wall of the vessel.

Disruption of a vessel should be suspected whenever there is the sensation of a sudden "give" in the resistance to the inflation as the balloon is being inflated during the dilation or whenever a dilating balloon ruptures during the dilation. A minor or confined tear can go unnoticed until demonstrated on a follow-up angiogram. A major vessel rupture is suspected when the patient coughs, produces significant hemoptysis and/or becomes unstable hemodynamically very soon after the pulmonary artery dilation. If the patient is intubated, the hemoptysis becomes apparent immediately in the endotracheal tube.

With a massive leak from a pulmonary artery tear, the systemic blood pressure drops along with the onset of the cough. On fluoroscopy, the lung tissues around the area of the dilation become opacified or a pleural effusion appears. Rarely the tear of a pulmonary artery occurs within the pericardium, and along with the other hemodynamic instability the signs of pericardial tamponade occur. The diagnosis of a tear is confirmed with a small selective angiocardiogram injecting into the pulmonary artery just proximal to the area of dilation. When a tear is suspected, the angiogram is performed with a small volume, low-pressure (hand) injection through the additional venous catheter which should be in position in the pulmonary artery already.

When a tear in a branch pulmonary vessel is suspected, the exchange wire must be maintained in place past the lesion. The extent of the tear and the potential for extension of the tear is determined from the angiogram with the wire maintained in place across and distal to the lesion. If a second catheter is not already in place in the pulmonary artery for the angiogram, the second catheter is introduced rapidly through the most accessible venous route. If the patient is deteriorating rapidly and before the precise area has been demonstrated, the balloon dilation catheter arbitrarily is *re-advanced* over the wire, back into the original area of the lesion and reinflated at a low pressure while the second catheter is being introduced. If the balloon had been removed over the wire before the tear/rupture was noted, this is one circumstance where a Multi-Track™ catheter introduced over the same wire is useful to introduce the second catheter rapidly into the area of the pulmonary artery tear. With a large enough introductory sheath, a balloon catheter can be introduced over the same wire, behind the Multi-Track™ catheter in order to "tamponade" the leaking vessel.

When the extravasation is noticed incidentally from a density appearing on the fluoroscopy or when the patient has been very stable for at least 15 minutes, the balloon catheter remains in position proximal to the lesion while the second catheter is introduced. If for some reason, the second catheter cannot be introduced and the patient remains very stable hemodynamically, the wire is maintained in position while the balloon catheter is removed over the wire and replaced with a Multi-Track™ angiographic catheter. The angiogram is recorded with an injection through this catheter without removing the wire, which is still passing through the lesion. The angiogram helps to determine whether, and what type of, further treatment is necessary.

A localized, small tear in an area of the pulmonary artery which has low/normal pressures, usually does not continue to grow and over time, remains confined to the immediate area of the vessel. This is true particularly in those patients whose pulmonary arteries have been previously operated on. On the other hand, a very large tear, even in a low-pressure area or a small tear in a high-pressure area of the pulmonary artery will not be confined to the area of the tear. This is true particularly when there has been no previous surgery in the area of the tear. The extravasation from a non-confined tear continues to increase and extend away from the area of the lesion. The precise treatment of a pulmonary artery tear depends upon the amount of leak from the tear, whether the leak from the tear is confined to the immediate, adjacent area, and on the net hemodynamic consequences to the patient.

In the presence of a non-confined tear associated with extravasation or hyperperfusion of the area, there are several options for treating the lesion as long as the wire is still in place across it. When the deflated balloon over the wire is positioned either in or just proximal to the lesion, the balloon is advanced back over the wire precisely into the lesion and reinflated at a low pressure in order to "tamponade" the tear. The balloon is kept in this position for 10–30 minutes. If the pulmonary artery pressure just proximal to the lesion is not too high, this is usually sufficient to stop the bleeding. If the temporary tamponading of the lesion using the original balloon does not stop the bleeding and control the hyperperfusion, the original balloon catheter is removed over the wire and replaced with a larger diameter balloon and the attempt at tamponading repeated.

When the tear occurs in a small vessel which, however, has very high pressure, balloon occlusion of the tear will usually stop the extravasation temporarily, but it is unlikely that the lesion in the vessel wall will seal with this treatment alone. When the bleeding continues to recur as the balloon is deflated after at least two attempts at "tamponade", the balloon catheter is removed over the guide wire and replaced with a catheter which can be used for the delivery of a coil or some other vascular occlusion device. The wire is removed and the area is occluded by the implant of a coil or other occlusion device. Devices such as an Amplatzer™ patent ductus occluder, an Amplatzer™ Plug or a Gianturco-Grifka™ bag, are considered if the tear is in a moderately large branch pulmonary artery. The occlusion and eventual obliteration of a larger pulmonary vessel is considered only when the occlusion will be life saving or the only alternative is surgical intervention where the vessel and segment of the lung (at least) otherwise would be lost.

Coil occlusion of such a lesion is fairly straightforward *as long as the positions of the wire and the catheter have been maintained* throughout all of the evaluation process. The occlusion procedure, of course, will eliminate all blood flow to the segment of lung distal to the site of the occlusion. In smaller segments of the lung this causes no immediate sequelae, and is exactly what would happen if the patient underwent surgical intervention for the bleeding.

When the area of the tear is controlled successfully by the permanent occlusion of that vessel and the area of lung that was lost was not a major segment (less than 1/4–1/3) of the lung, the dilation of other branches can be continued once the patient is stabilized and while observing the original site after the occlusion.

When the secure position of the wire or catheter across the lesion is lost inadvertently before the bleeding is recognized, this can be catastrophic, particularly if the patient is hemodynamically unstable and requiring resuscitation. An end-hole catheter must be positioned rapidly into the involved lung and preferably into the involved vessel. An attempt is made at re-entering the exact same branch pulmonary artery with the end-hole catheter. If the patient is unstable and the specific vessel cannot be re-entered very expeditiously, the end-hole catheter and then an exchange length wire are secured *anywhere* in the pulmonary artery of the involved lung. An "occlusion" balloon catheter which is large enough to occlude the proximal right or left pulmonary artery is passed over the wire and into the right or left main branch pulmonary artery proximal to the lesion and inflated there. This blocks the flow to the entire involved lung, but allows stabilization of the patient and time to get the patient to the operating room. A Swan™ type balloon is used in smaller patients while a Medi-tech™ occlusion balloon is used in larger patients. These spherical balloons are preferred for this type of "whole lung occlusion" as opposed to a large angioplasty type balloon. A large angioplasty balloon could occlude the vessel effectively, but they are so long as well as large in diameter, that when the *dilating* balloon is occluding a more central right or left pulmonary artery branch, it also extends back into the main pulmonary artery, which is occluded at least partially, and this, in turn, blocks all of the cardiac output.

The larger the tear and the higher the pressure in the involved pulmonary artery, the greater is the extravasation and the less likely the tear is to remain sealed following a temporary "tamponade". Once the involved vessel is occluded proximal to the tear and stabilizes, the patient is observed for at least one hour with the vessel occluded. With no further extravasation during this period of occlusion, the occlusion balloon is deflated *slowly* while observing the patient's vital signs carefully. If the patient remains absolutely stable, a small, low-pressure, hand injection angiogram is performed in the same vessel proximal to the lesion. With no extravasation of contrast from this injection, the patient is observed for at least another hour with the balloon deflated but still in the area.

There is a very high potential for a late recurrence of the bleeding in a high-pressure pulmonary vessel. A decision must then be made for proceeding either with a catheter closure of the involved tear or a total occlusion of the entire vessel while the patient temporarily is stable. The exchange wire should still be in its position *past* the lesion. A coil delivery catheter is introduced separately and advanced adjacent to the wire or, as an alternative, the coil delivery catheter is passed over the original wire to the lesion and the wire is removed gingerly. An occlusion coil which will fill the vessel is advanced to the involved vessel and if possible, the occlusion coil is placed directly over the lesion. It usually is necessary to place several coils in series in the vessel to cover the entire lesion. Covering the entire lesion prevents additional leakage from any *retrograde* flow from the more distal pulmonary artery from reaching the lesion. If the tear is in a very large vessel, an alternative type of vascular occluding device such as an Amplatzer™ PDA or Plug device or an umbrella may be necessary to occlude the vessel.

The availability of "covered stents" in various sizes provides a more appealing alternative therapy for acute pulmonary artery tears, particularly in larger vessels. Ideally, a catheterization laboratory which is performing interventions on vessels, should have an inventory of multiple sizes of covered stents. Unfortunately for pediatric/congenital patients in the United States, the possibility of obtaining these stents ***ahead of time*** to be kept in reserve for emergency compassionate use is still denied/refused by the FDA. Unfortunately, they do not understand that when a pulmonary rupture occurs even Fed Ex™ or UPS™ cannot make the covered stent appear on time! When the appropriate sized covered stent is available, or can be "self manufactured" from available stents and materials, a covered stent is ideal for treating a tear in the wall of a larger vessel. Following the temporary balloon occlusion of the torn vessel, the occlusion balloon in the involved vessel is withdrawn over the wire and replaced with a large long delivery sheath, which will accommodate the specific "covered stent". The covered stent is delivered to the lesion and implanted exactly over the lesion similarly to the delivery of other balloon expandable stents to the pulmonary arteries as discussed in Chapter 23. The entire exchange of the balloon for the sheath for the stent delivery must be completed very expediently since extravasation from the vessel usually continues during all of this maneuvering until the "covered stent" is implanted over the lesion.

Even when the patient stabilizes following the tear and does not require further, immediate interventional treatment, a patient with any extravasation requires at least *several hours* of observation *in the catheterization laboratory* before being moved to 12–24 hour observation in a monitored recovery ward. Definitive treatment can be instituted instantaneously in the catheterization laboratory, but if the extravasation progresses or resumes once the patient is out of the catheterization laboratory, there is an inescapable delay before treatment can be resumed.

Hemoptysis occurs from other causes besides vessel tears. Minor hemoptysis occurring during dilation of branch pulmonary arteries is not uncommon and usually is self-limiting. The most common cause of minor hemoptysis is the perforation of a small distal or "end" pulmonary artery (or capillary?) by the tip of the stiff guide wires. This type of perforation usually presents with a cough, following which the patient produces some blood-tinged sputum, or a small amount of frank blood appears in the airway. In addition to hemoptysis, perforation of an "end" pulmonary artery/capillary by the wire can cause extravasation into the surrounding lung tissues and/or the pleura. The area of the tip of the wire is scrutinized on fluoroscopy for the appearance of an extravasation into the surrounding tissues and/or adjacent pleura, either of which appears as an increasing density.

The best treatment of this complication is, of course, prevention. Very careful, continual attention must be paid to the location of the tip of the wire as well as to the course of the remainder of the wire during the manipulations of the wire and the balloon catheter. When a long curve in the course of a wire passing through the heart straightens during multiple manipulations with the sheath or balloon, the tip of the wire may advance or retract when the proximal end of the wire is *fixed* on the "table top". When the proximal end of the wire is fixed securely outside of the body and the tip advances when it is "buried" very far distally in the distal lung vessel, the only place the tip of the wire can go as the fixed wire straightens, is through the end of the vessel! When a wire perforation of an "end" pulmonary vessel occurs, the magnitude and significance of the extravasation are determined before proceeding any further with the procedure. A small-volume, low-pressure, hand-injected, selective angiogram through the second venous catheter and into the involved vessel demonstrates the amount and rate of leakage. If the perforation occurs in a very low-pressure, distal (capillary) area of the lung, the bleeding will be self-limited and require no treatment. If the perforation is in a very distal vessel, following a successful dilation of a lesion in a vessel with a very high proximal pulmonary artery pressure, the higher pulmonary pressure will then be transmitted to the area of the perforation in the very distal vessel. The higher the pressure is in the involved vessel, the more likely is it that the bleeding will continue, particularly if the pressure is over 40 mmHg. With a high pressure in the area of the perforation, it is likely that some specific interventional therapy will be necessary.

If a perforation of an "end" pulmonary artery by a wire does occur, it is most important, although counter-intuitive, that the wire is ***not withdrawn*** from the involved vessel! The tip of the wire may be withdrawn very slightly so that it is not beyond the end of the vessel into the pleura, but it should *not* be withdrawn any further out of the vessel in which the perforation occurred. *As long as the wire is in place* and the extravasation of blood continues from the perforation of an end artery, the blood flow into the specific small, involved branch vessel can be occluded temporarily and easily with a very small angioplasty, or even a Swan™ balloon catheter advanced over the wire. Whichever balloon is used for this temporary occlusion, it is inflated to the lowest possible pressure necessary to occlude flow past the balloon temporarily.

Temporary balloon occlusion of the vessel involved with the perforation is performed when there is continued extravasation into either the airway, the lung tissues, or the pleura during the few minutes of observation immediately after the distal perforation. The vessel is occluded temporarily for at least 30 minutes and then the occluding balloon is deflated very slowly to check for continued bleeding. If the bleeding reoccurs (continues) after the temporary occlusion balloon has been deflated, the balloon catheter is withdrawn and replaced with a coil delivery catheter. The coil delivery catheter is advanced over the wire in the involved vessel to a location into or just proximal to the perforation. Once the catheter has been positioned in the involved distal branch vessel in, or just proximal to, the perforation, *then and only then*, is the exchange guide wire removed. The location of the tip of the "coil" catheter is verified with a very small hand angiogram through the catheter. The vessel is packed with very small coils as far distally as possible into, and just proximal to, the perforation. Coils are added until the bleeding stops.

When the wire has been withdrawn from the specific, small distal vessel, it often is not possible to re-enter the exact same, very small branch vessel expediently, if at all. A new catheter and then a wire may have to be positioned in a different but adjacent distal vessel arising off the same more proximal trunk vessel. In order to stop the blood flow to the perforated vessel, the more proximal much larger, trunk vessel (and multiple segments of lung) then will have to be occluded with the balloon and then a device to control the bleeding.

When an interatrial communication is created purposefully as a prophylactic "blow-off opening" in an extremely severe branch pulmonary artery stenosis patient, a right to left shunt with the potential problem of systemic embolization is created. The usual meticulous extra precautions are taken to prevent the introduction of air and/or clots into the venous system during all of the subsequent manipulations. These small, catheter-created, atrial openings usually close on their own with time and do not need to be addressed during the initial catheterization when the balloon dilations are performed. If the atrial communication persists and the balloon dilation of the branch pulmonary arteries has been successful, the atrial defect can be closed in the catheterization laboratory later when the patient returns for repeat dilations of the branch pulmonary arteries.

The availability of cutting balloon catheters has introduced a new potential complication. The "blades" on the cutting balloons are very thin and relatively fragile. As a consequence, the blades can be displaced off the balloon surface particularly with any rough handling. Delivery through a long sheath to the site for the dilation reduces the manipulations necessary for cutting balloon catheters and provides a recovery sheath in the vessel for withdrawal of a damaged cutting balloon.

Conclusion

In spite of the temporary or marginal success of balloon dilation of branch pulmonary arteries, and even with a reasonable alternative therapy, balloon dilation of pulmonary artery branch stenosis is still indicated for some lesions. The primary indications for dilation of branch pulmonary artery stenosis are stenoses in very small patients who are symptomatic *owing to the branch pulmonary artery stenosis* or distal branch pulmonary stenosis where there are multiple lesions exactly at the branching points to other distal branches. Balloon dilation of branch pulmonary artery stenosis usually produces some improvement in the vessel diameter and decreases the gradient across the lesion to some degree, but dilation alone is seldom successful at *abolishing* the gradient or opening the vessel to its *normal* or a *persistently* increased diameter. At the same time, there are definite risks unique to balloon dilation of branch pulmonary arteries.

As a consequence, the majority of branch pulmonary artery lesions, particularly in larger patients, are now treated primarily and more definitively with the initial implant of intravascular stents. At the same time, dilation of multiple *distal* branch pulmonary artery stenoses is often performed in conjunction with the implant of intravascular stents in the more central pulmonary arteries. The use of stents in these lesions is covered in detail in Chapter 23.

References

1. Lock JE *et al*. Transvenous angioplasty of experimental branch pulmonary artery stenosis in newborn lambs. *Circulation* 1981; **64**(5): 886–893.
2. Lock JE *et al*. Balloon dilation angioplasty of hypoplastic and stenotic pulmonary arteries. *Circulation* 1983; **67**(5): 962–967.
3. Kan JS *et al*. Balloon angioplasty—branch pulmonary artery stenosis: Results of the Valvuloplasty and Angioplasty of Congenital Anomalies Registry. *Am J Cardiol* 1990; **65**: 798–801.
4. Rothman A *et al*. Balloon dilation of branch pulmonary artery stenosis. *Semin Thorac Cardiovasc Surg* 1990; **2**(1): 46–54.
5. Abele JE. Balloon catheters and transluminal dilatation: technical considerations. *A J R* 1980; **135**: 901.
6. Gentles TL, Lock JE, and Perry SB. High pressure balloon angioplasty for branch pulmonary artery stenosis: early experience. *J Am Coll Cardiol* 1993; **22**(3): 867–872.
7. Edwards BS *et al*. Morphologic changes in the pulmonary arteries after percutaneous balloon angioplasty for pulmonary arterial stenosis. *Circulation* 1985; **71**(2): 195–201.
8. Geggel RL, Gauvreau K, and Lock JE. Balloon dilation angioplasty of peripheral pulmonary stenosis associated with Williams syndrome. *Circulation* 2001; **103**(17): 2165–2170.

18 Dilation of coarctation of the aorta—native and re/residual coarctation

Introduction

During the past two decades, there has been a vast experience with balloon dilation of both re-(residual) coarctation[1] and native coarctation of the aorta[2]. Along with valve pulmonary stenosis, re-coarctation of the aorta was one of the two earliest congenital lesions to be managed by balloon dilation[3,4]. The acute results of dilation of both re-coarctation and native coarctation of the aorta in patients over several months of age are very good, however, they are still not perfect. The criteria for determining the size of the dilation balloon for both native coarctation and re-coarctation are similar, as are the techniques for the two procedures. The results of dilation of both types of coarctation are very similar with the exception that there is a slightly better acute result obtained with the dilation of native coarctation[2].

The complications from the dilation of both re/residual coarctation and native coarctation are rare, but definitely *not* absent, and the complications that do occur often are *not* minor ones. Acute tears in the aortic wall occur, although very rarely, in both groups of patients. Aneurysms of the aorta develop in the area of the dilation in a very few patients who undergo both re/residual coarctation and native coarctation dilation. These aneurysms can occur acutely or they can appear later in the follow-up of a coarctation that was dilated years earlier.

At the same time, surgery for coarctation is not without its problems. There still is the risk of a very major surgical procedure itself, plus the extended recovery following any thoracic surgery. The entire category of "re" or "residual" coarctation patients are a consequence of prior surgical repairs[5]. The acute complications of surgery still occur and can be equally devastating. There still are rare instances of quadriplegia and paraplegia following both native and, particularly, re/residual coarctation surgery[6,7]. Surgery on re-coarctation frequently requires the interposition of an aortic tube graft or prosthetic patch. Significant aneurysms of the aorta are found late after all types of surgical repairs of coarctation of the aorta, but particularly after the "patch augmentation" repair of coarctations[8].

Considering both the results and complications of dilation of coarctation of the aorta and comparing these with the results and complications of surgical repair, most, but not *all* centers and individuals accept dilation of re/residual coarctation and native coarctation as the "standard of care". Some centers and individuals accept dilation of re/residual coarctation, but not dilation of native coarctation, and vice versa. The twenty years of experience with the dilation of both native and re/residual coarctation have provided a much better understanding of both groups of lesions. The development of better equipment has contributed to more refined and safer techniques for the dilation of coarctation. The causes of most acute complications of the dilation of coarctations are now understood better and, as a consequence and to a large extent, most appear to be preventable. The eventual hemodynamic results along with the incidence of complications of the carefully controlled dilation of both native and re/residual coarctation of the aorta appear to be comparable to those obtained with surgical repair, however, only many more years (decades) will provide the real, long-term results and reveal the late complications of balloon dilation of coarctation of the aorta.

Balloon dilation of coarctation of the aorta has benefited significantly from the better understanding of the exact lesions in the native and re/residual coarctations and the effects of balloon dilations on these lesions. This understanding has led to better control of, and a more *conservative* approach to, the dilation procedures. Although the ultimate goal should be the elimination, *totally*, of *any* gradient or anatomic constriction at the site of the coarctation, this does not have to be accomplished at the initial or only procedure. The developments in balloon technology over the past two decades have refined the technique and reduced the local vascular complications[9,10]. The use of intravascular stents in conjunction with balloon dilation for both native and re/residual coarctation in selected *older and larger* patients appears to provide better acute and long-term results for the angioplasty of coarctation. Stents in coarctation of the aorta are discussed in detail in Chapter 25.

Dilation of native coarctation in the newborn or young infant is usually very successful *acutely*. A successful dilation in a sick infant relieves the heart failure and acidosis. However, most of the coarctations that are dilated in neonates and young infants recur within one to six months[9]. When the coarctation does recur, however, the recurrence is without heart failure or any decompensation so that any subsequent treatment of the coarctation becomes totally elective. The infant with a recurrent coarctation can undergo a re-dilation or an elective and less complicated surgery of the recurrent coarctation. Miniaturization of the balloons and meticulous care of the arteries have almost eliminated the acute complications at the local access sites following the dilations of coarctations in infants. In this group of sick newborn and young infants where the surgery represents a much higher risk, there is a significant interest in the dilation of neonatal/infant coarctation in spite of the high incidence of later recurrence of the coarctation. The benefits of the neonatal dilation, even including an obligatory, repeat dilation, still outweigh the risks of surgery on these infant coarctations, which, in itself, is not without the occurrence of re/residual coarctation.

Techniques for coarctation dilation

The techniques used for dilation of coarctation of the aorta are the same for native coarctation and for residual or re-coarctation. Balloon dilation of coarctation of the aorta is usually performed with a single dilation balloon. The balloon used is precisely the same diameter or slightly smaller than the *smallest adjacent* "normal" aortic diameter. The dilation is carried out with a single retrograde balloon dilation catheter, however, in the patient undergoing an elective dilation of a coarctation of the aorta, an adjunct prograde catheter is used in conjunction with the retrograde catheter to assist in balloon positioning, monitor pressures immediately before, during and after the dilation, and for selective aortography. The prograde catheter, which is introduced into the venous system, is then passed into the left heart and eventually is advanced to a position in the proximal descending aorta that is just proximal to the coarctation.

Sedation for the patient undergoing dilation of coarctation of the aorta is similar to sedation for a standard cardiac catheterization. Although some discomfort is created during the actual dilation of the aorta, this is controlled with intravenous analgesics. General anesthesia is usually unnecessary for the otherwise uncomplicated coarctation dilation. A peripheral indwelling intravenous line is secured. A "Foley" urinary bladder catheter is placed in the patient as soon as the patient is sedated. Patients undergoing balloon dilation of a coarctation are type- *and cross-matched* for one unit of whole blood and the blood is made available in the catheterization laboratory.

Both inguinal regions in the areas of catheter introduction are infiltrated *liberally* with 2% xylocaine. Initially a venous sheath is introduced into one femoral vein and small indwelling 20- or 18-gauge cannulae are introduced into one, or often both, femoral arteries. The arterial lines are attached to the pressure monitoring system. A baseline blood gas and an activated clotting time (ACT) are drawn. Patients undergoing coarctation dilation receive 100 mg/kg of intravenous heparin. The exact dose depends somewhat upon their initial ACT. When a prograde arterial catheter is introduced into the left heart by an atrial transseptal puncture technique, the heparin is withheld until just *after* the transseptal puncture. Systemic heparinization is important in these patients particularly because of the long duration of wires/catheters in the central aorta along with the extensive wire manipulation within the left heart and, particularly, in the ascending aorta. The larger sheaths necessary for the introduction of the larger diameter balloon dilation catheters, along with the duration of time the sheaths remain in the arteries, create potential trauma to the femoral arteries. Unless there are other significant intracardiac lesions known or suspected, a brief and "efficient" right heart catheterization is performed once the catheters have been introduced. When associated intracardiac defects are present or suspected, a more thorough diagnostic catheterization is completed before beginning the dilation procedure for the coarctation.

Adjunct prograde catheter technique

The dilation of most coarctations of the aorta are performed using a retrograde arterial approach from the femoral artery, but, at the same time, a prograde venous angiographic catheter is advanced across the atrial septum, into the left heart and from there, into the transverse or descending aorta adjacent to the site of the coarctation. The prograde angiographic catheter along with a long sheath in the left ventricle and a small indwelling femoral arterial line, allow simultaneous pressures from the left ventricle, ascending aorta and femoral artery as well as detailed selective angiography precisely in the area of the coarctation, all to be obtained before a *sheath or catheter* of any size is introduced into an artery. With the prograde catheter remaining just proximal to the coarctation during the dilation, the positioning of the balloon can be checked repeatedly and the hemodynamic and angiographic results of the dilation can be verified immediately without having to remove the balloon from the area.

When there is a pre-existing atrial communication the prograde left heart catheterization is very straightforward. In the presence of an intact atrial septum, the left heart is entered by means of an atrial transseptal puncture, which does not add significantly to the procedure. If there are any peculiarities of the cardiac or thoracic anatomy or if the operator is not entirely comfortable with the atrial transseptal technique, a pulmonary artery angiogram is performed prior to the transseptal puncture specifically to visualize the recirculation phase of the angiogram in order to visualize the anatomy of the left atrium, atrial septum and ascending aorta. This angiogram also provides some information about the coarctation. Once the angiogram has been obtained and unless there is a pre-existing interatrial communication, an atrial transseptal puncture is performed. The transseptal set that is used should be at least one French size larger than the catheter that will be used for the prograde left heart procedure. This allows easier manipulation through the long sheath and, of more importance, allows pressure recordings from the sheath tip (through the side arm of the sheath) and the catheter simultaneously. Even if a pre-existing interatrial communication is present, the use of a long sheath across the septum and into the left heart is still recommended to facilitate catheter manipulation into the aorta and for the purpose of recording pressures from several left heart locations simultaneously.

Once the tip of the long *sheath* is in the left atrium, either the needle or the wire (whichever was used to introduce the sheath/dilator into the left atrium) is removed slowly followed by an equally slow withdrawal of the dilator. The sheath is cleared completely and meticulously of all air and/or clot, the side arm of the sheath is attached to the flush/pressure monitoring system and the sheath is flushed, following which the pressure is displayed from the side port of the sheath. The patient is administered heparin at this time according to the results of the previous ACT. The sheath is positioned with the tip in the mid left atrium being sure that it is not trapped in either a pulmonary vein or the left atrial appendage.

Either a balloon angiographic catheter or a torque-controlled (NIH type) angiographic catheter can be used as the prograde left heart catheter. Whichever catheter is used, it should be at least one French size smaller than the long sheath. The NIH catheter should have calibration or "marker bands" near its tip. A tight 180° curve is formed at the tip of whichever catheter is used while it is still outside of the body by heating or "pulling" and then forming the tip into the desired curve. When a torque-controlled, non-balloon floating catheter is used, the stiff end of a 0.032″ or 0.035″ teflon wire is preformed into a tight 180–270° curve with an additional anterior bend at the tip of the wire (as described in detail in Chapter 6). This wire is introduced into the torque catheter through a wire back-bleed device and advanced to the tip of the catheter *before* the catheter is introduced into the sheath. The catheter lumen of the balloon angiographic catheter or the flush port on a wire back-bleed valve over the wire in the torque-controlled catheter is attached to the pressure/flush system and placed on a slow, continuous flush. The catheter is introduced into the long sheath with both the sheath and the catheter on a continuous flush until the catheter passes beyond the end of the sheath.

As soon as the catheter passes beyond the end of the sheath, the flushes are stopped and pressures are recorded simultaneously from the catheter and the sheath at a 20 or 40 mm maximum gain. These recordings not only provide an initial pressure recording from the left atrium, but also serve as a check for the accuracy of the two transducers. The two pressure curves from the two separate catheters in the same location should generate a *single pressure line* on the monitor and recording! If not, the transducers are checked, re-calibrated and, if necessary, changed until the two curves match exactly.

Once the floating balloon catheter has been advanced beyond the end of the sheath and the pressures have been recorded, the balloon is inflated with carbon dioxide (CO_2). In most cases, the floating balloon catheter with the preformed curve on the catheter and with the balloon inflated will float from the left atrium into the left ventricle with minimal, or no, manipulation. Occasionally it is necessary to use some type of deflector wire to enter the left ventricle from the left atrium even with the balloon catheter. Once the catheter is securely in the left ventricle, simultaneous pressures are recorded from the left atrium (sheath) and left ventricle (catheter) at a low gain and then from the left ventricle (catheter) and femoral artery line at a high gain. These recordings establish or rule out even subtle associated mitral stenosis and provide an indication of the hemodynamic significance of the coarctation. Once the pressures have been recorded, the sheath is advanced over the balloon catheter into the left ventricle. The sheath and catheter pressures are checked against each other again to verify the calibration of the pressure transducers at the higher gain.

If a torque-controlled catheter is used for the prograde left heart procedure, it is advanced through the sheath with the stiff, preformed wire already positioned within the catheter with the tip of the wire all of the way to the tip of the catheter. The catheter is advanced just beyond the tip of the sheath and the simultaneous left atrial pressures are recorded and checked against each other exactly as with the floating balloon catheter. Occasionally, the combination of the wire within the catheter lumen and the compliant tubing of the side port on the back-bleed valve dampens the pressure curve and does not allow a valid recording through the catheter with the wire in place. In that situation, the wire and the back-bleed valve are removed, the catheter cleared of air, flushed and the simultaneous pressures recorded. Once satisfactory pressures are recorded, the back-bleed valve is replaced on the catheter and the wire reintroduced and advanced to the tip of the catheter.

Once the entire curve of the distal end of the catheter is out of the sheath in the left atrium (with the proper preformed wire still within the catheter), the tip of the catheter points almost "automatically" at the mitral valve! If not, very slight torquing or to-and-fro motion of the catheter and wire together redirect the tip toward the mitral valve. Occasionally the sheath must be torqued counterclockwise along with the catheter to direct the combination anteriorly. When pointed at the valve, the *wire* and *sheath* are *held in place* while the catheter is advanced off the wire, out of the sheath and into the left ventricle. The wire is secured to maintain the curve on the wire fixed in the left atrium until the tip of the catheter has advanced well within the left ventricle. The pressures from both the left atrium and left ventricle are recorded through the sheath and the NIH catheter. Once the catheter tip is within the ventricle, the wire is re-advanced to the tip of the catheter to redirect it anteriorly and medially and to support the catheter while the sheath is advanced over it and into the left ventricle.

When the simultaneous left atrial and left ventricle pressures have been recorded, the sheath is advanced over the catheter/wire into the left ventricle. The wire is withdrawn completely out of the catheter, the wire back-bleed valve removed and the catheter thoroughly flushed. The natural direction of a catheter alone coming from the left atrium into the ventricle, particularly through a long sheath, is to point toward the left ventricular apex and exactly away from the aortic valve. A long sheath positioned properly in the left ventricle can facilitate advancing both the floating balloon and the torque catheters into the aorta. When using a floating balloon catheter, merely advancing the balloon catheter, which still should have a slight curve formed at its tip, further out of the sheath within the ventricle with the balloon inflated often "bounces" or deflects the balloon from the apex toward the outflow tract. As the catheter is advanced further through the sheath in the left ventricle, the balloon floats into the ascending aorta and, when the formed curve at the tip of the catheter persists, around to the descending aorta to the area of the coarctation.

When using an NIH or other torque catheter, and occasionally even with a balloon catheter, an active deflector wire is necessary to redirect the catheter tip away from the left ventricular apex to point toward the outflow tract and then into the aorta. A deflector wire with a 5-mm tip curve and of the largest size that will fit into the catheter which is being deflected, is introduced into the catheter through a wire back-bleed valve on the catheter. The back-bleed valve is maintained on a continuous flush. When the deflector wire is at the tip of the catheter and the catheter tip is free and away from the end of the sheath *and away from the wall of the ventricle*, the deflector is activated. The deflection should be slow at first to ensure that the tip of the catheter is free. When the tip bends easily with the initial deflection, then the deflection is formed as vigorously as possible in order to deflect the tip of the catheter the necessary 180°. Once the tip is deflected most of the 180° toward the outflow tract, the catheter is advanced off the wire and toward/into the ascending aorta. Once in the ascending aorta, a pre-curved, torque-controlled catheter often tends to curve around into the descending aorta. If not, the deflector wire is re-advanced to the tip of the catheter and the tip is deflected. The "concavity" of the more proximal curves in the wire in passing from LA to LV and from LV to aorta generally deflects the tip toward the patient's left and, in turn, toward the descending aorta.

An alternative technique for advancing a torque-controlled catheter from the left ventricle to the aorta is to use a curve formed on the stiff end of a rigid wire to deflect the tip of the catheter cephalad from the left ventricle. The tip of the sheath is positioned along the septal surface and approximately half way into the left ventricle. The catheter with the rigid, curved wire at its tip is advanced out of the sheath. The curve on the wire directs the tip of the catheter almost perpendicularly toward the septal wall of the left ventricle. As the tip of the catheter touches the septum, the wire is fixed in position and the catheter is advanced off the wire. This, in turn, bends the catheter tip against the septum and begins to redirect the tip cephalad. As the catheter is advanced further off the wire and, simultaneously, the sheath is advanced further into the ventricle, the catheter bends 180° in the body of the ventricle and points toward the left ventricular outflow tract.

All of the above maneuvering with the prograde catheters may seem complicated and unnecessary. However, with a little experience and expertise these maneuvers are accomplished very quickly. The distinct advantages of the prograde catheter in the aorta compared with the single catheter retrograde technique become very apparent with the first positioning angiogram during a balloon dilation of the coarctation.

With the catheter in the aorta just proximal to the coarctation, the sheath tip in the left ventricle, and with the indwelling femoral line, simultaneous pressures are recorded from these three areas. The coarctation is documented by the pressure differences between the ascending/transverse aorta and femoral artery. The simultaneous left ventricular pressure establishes or rules out any associated left ventricular outflow tract, aortic valve, ascending aorta, or more proximal transverse aorta obstruction.

Coarctation angiography and measurements

The exact type and location of the coarctation is verified by detailed aortograms in the distal transverse aortic arch. The prograde aortic catheter is positioned just proximal to the coarctation site and a selective aortogram is recorded in the PA and LAT projections. If the coarctation is not visualized precisely on edge in these views, the angles of the X-ray tubes are changed appropriately according to these first views, and the aortogram repeated. With the catheter positioned immediately adjacent to the coarctation site, less contrast enters the brachiocephalic vessels (and head!), less contrast is necessary for each injection, and more injections can be performed safely. Accurate measurements with a calibrated measurement system are made of the diameters and lengths of the coarctation site, the aortic diameters both proximal to and distal to the coarctation, and of the locations of and the distances to the brachiocephalic vessels.

If an NIH catheter with calibration marks on it is used for the angiogram, the marks are aligned in their longest axis in both the PA and LAT views so that the calibration marks are aligned exactly perpendicular to the X-ray beam. If the marks are not aligned exactly during the angiogram, without moving the patient or the catheterization table, the *catheter* is repositioned to align the marks properly and a very short biplane angiogram without a contrast injection is performed to record the calibration marks permanently.

When a balloon angiographic catheter is used for the aortogram, another separate system for *accurate calibration* and measurement must be used. A simple alternative to the use of the calibrated "marker" catheter in the aorta during the aortogram is to place a "marker" catheter inside of a nasogastric tube and then advance the nasogastric tube in the esophagus until the marks are positioned immediately adjacent to the area of coarctation as seen on the fluoroscopy. The marks on a catheter in the esophagus can be situated very close to the site of the usual coarctation, and the esophageal catheter can be left in this position as a calibration source for future angiographic measurements of the coarctation area.

If there is a second venous line already in place, a calibration "marker" catheter can be introduced into the superior vena cava through the second venous access. When the marks are at the same cephalad–caudal level as the coarctation, the calibration marks are close enough to the site of the coarctation to eliminate significant magnification effects on either the PA or the LAT images. Another alternative is to introduce the "marker" catheter retrograde into the area of the coarctation just before the angiogram. A built-in calibration system in the X-ray system or a "grid" or "calibrated ball" recorded on an angiogram in the exact same planes as the coarctation after each regular angiogram will provide accurate calibration. Very accurate measurements and, as a consequence, very accurate calibrations of the measuring system are critical for coarctation dilations. The specific calibration devices and procedures are discussed in Chapter 11, "Angiographic Techniques". The width of a catheter does not provide a sufficiently accurate reference system for larger diameter measurements and should never be used as the "calibration factor" for coarctation dilation.

Coarctation dilation

Once the coarctation site has been identified clearly and measured accurately from the aortogram, the lesion is ready for dilation. A balloon is chosen which is the same, or one mm smaller in diameter than the diameter of the ***smallest adjacent aortic segment***. The measured diameter of the coarcted segment itself, the diameter of the aorta at the diaphragm and even the diameter of the thumb have been used to determine the size of the balloon to be used for coarctation dilation. The diameter of the narrowing itself has absolutely no correlation with the diameter of the adjacent aorta! The coarcted segment can be atretic, $1/20^{th}$ or 1/2 the diameter of the adjacent aorta. Certainly no "multiple" of the diameter of the coarctation segment itself can reasonably be used to determine the balloon diameter. If the diameter of a relatively mild narrowing were used, a balloon diameter based on the narrowing could be 2–3 times the diameter of the *adjacent "normal" aorta* and necessarily would tear/rupture this area of the aorta. Although the aorta at the diaphragm (and maybe even the thumb) may have some correlation with the body size of the patient, they have *absolutely no correlation* with, and usually are significantly *larger* than, the diameter of the aorta adjacent to the coarctation. The immediately *adjacent* aorta (not the thumb or the aorta at the diaphragm!) must be able to accommodate the maximum diameter of the fully inflated balloon. The narrowest "normal" aorta that is adjacent to the coarctation is usually the aorta isthmus just proximal to the coarctation. Using a balloon of the same diameter (or smaller) as the adjacent vessel will not over-expand the wall of the adjacent normal vessel at all and, in turn, should not tear normal intima or media, whereas a fully inflated, significantly larger balloon would spit the intima, media and possibly the adventitia when it expands fully. If the maximum diameter of the balloon during the dilation is measured to be small relative to the diameter of the adjacent vessel during the dilation *and* the dilation is not satisfactory, the dilation can always be repeated immediately or at a later date with a slightly larger diameter balloon. However, if the diameter of the balloon is too large for the adjacent vessel and the vessel wall splits, there is no reversing the procedure!

With a native coarctation, where there is a shelf of tissue within the true lumen of the vessel and it is presumed that this shelf will be disrupted with the dilation, a tight narrowing *can* be dilated up to the diameter of the adjacent *narrowest* aorta. With a tight *re or residual coarctation* or a hypoplastic segment of aorta where the narrowing actually is a narrowing of the entire vessel wall, then it is necessary to pay attention to the diameter of the coarctation and *not* to dilate the lesion to more than three times the diameter of the narrowest area.

The length of the balloon should be long enough to cover the area of the coarctation completely, but at the same time, short enough not to extend too far in either direction away from the coarctation. The aorta from the mid transverse aorta just proximal to the coarctation makes a 90° turn to the descending aorta just distal to the coarctation. All dilation balloons become very *straight* and very *rigid* when they are inflated fully. As a dilation balloon expands and straightens, the balloon straightens any structure(s) surrounding it–including the curved aorta. If the curve in the aorta is straightened over a significant distance by a long dilation balloon, the aorta itself can be disrupted and/or torn from the adjoining brachiocephalic vessel.

Once the appropriate balloon has been chosen and prepared for the dilation, the area around the femoral arterial entry site is re-infiltrated liberally with local anesthesia. The small indwelling arterial cannula is replaced with a sheath large enough in diameter to accommodate the balloon chosen for the dilation. An end-hole catheter is introduced into the femoral artery sheath, advanced retrograde across the coarctation, and maneuvered into a location where the wire supporting the balloon can be secured. The location for securing the distal end of the wire for the dilation procedure is determined by the anatomy of the brachiocephalic vessels in relation to the coarctation. Ideally, the wire should be as straight as possible and the distal end should be in a very fixed position so that pushing on the wire does not allow much, if any, to-and-fro movement of the wire in the coarctation area. Either the left or the right subclavian artery is the most satisfactory vessel for stabilizing the wire. The origins of the left subclavian arising directly off the aorta and right subclavian artery arising from the innominate artery are identified from the aortogram.

The left subclavian artery usually arises in the most direct and straightest course off the descending aorta and frequently arises very close to or actually as a part of the coarctation. If the left subclavian artery arises in the coarctation segment and, at the same time, is significantly smaller than the adjacent transverse aortic arch it cannot be used to anchor the distal end of the wire. If the left subclavian artery were used in that circumstance, the distal end of the dilation balloon would be positioned within the base of the much smaller subclavian artery and very likely would rupture the subclavian artery with the full inflation of the balloon. If, on the other hand, the base of the left subclavian artery is either several *centimeters* away from the coarctation or is *as large as the aorta proximal* to the coarctation, it represents the optimal location to secure the wire. If the left subclavian is used, an end-hole catheter is manipulated from the descending aorta far out into the left arm. A long, floppy tipped, Super Stiff™ exchange wire, which the balloon catheter for the dilation will accommodate, is advanced far out into the left arm to secure the wire for the dilation.

If the left subclavian artery is not satisfactory for securing the wire, and unless there is an anomalous right subclavian artery off the descending aorta, the right subclavian artery is the next most satisfactory location for the wire. The right subclavian artery usually arises on the opposite side of the transverse aortic arch from the coarctation and off the right innominate artery. This may present a slightly circuitous course from the descending aorta and require some extensive and very careful catheter manipulation to enter the innominate artery and then the right subclavian artery selectively. Once the right subclavian artery has been cannulated, a long, floppy tipped, Super Stiff™ guide wire is positioned *far out* in the right arm. Once the Super Stiff™ wire is in place in the right subclavian artery, the course from the descending aorta to the right subclavian artery straightens significantly and provides a very secure position for the wire. If the right subclavian artery has an anomalous origin off the descending aorta, it of course, will not be satisfactory to secure the wire for a coarctation dilation.

Early in the experience with dilation of coarctation, the distal end of the wire was positioned in the ascending aorta. The wire positioned in the aortic root actually allows very little control over the wire and, in turn, very little stability for the balloon during the dilation procedure. In addition, the tip of the wire in the ascending aorta can, and does, migrate into the left ventricle, the coronary arteries or even into the carotid arteries. The aortic root position is only used if neither subclavian artery can be accessed or they are not satisfactory for securing the wire.

When it is necessary to position the wire in the aortic root for the dilation of a coarctation, there are several precautions that must be taken. A Super Stiff™ wire with a *long* floppy tip is used. In order to prevent the tip of the wire from entering any of the unwanted and dangerous locations, a tight "J" curve or a "pig-tail" curve is formed at the tip end of the long floppy tip of the Super Stiff™ wire. In addition, a smooth, 180° curve approximately the diameter of the aortic root is formed at the *transition area* between the long floppy tip and the extra stiff portion of the wire. This 180° curve then should "seat" across the aortic root and allow the curled tip of the wire to extend up into the ascending aorta. This still does not overcome the poor control over the wire in this position during the balloon inflation.

Under no circumstances should the wire for dilation of a coarctation be positioned in a carotid or a vertebral artery. Any clot off the wire itself and/or off the arterial wall from irritation by the wire tip goes directly to the brain! During the manipulations of the wire in the area of the coarctation while the balloon is being inflated, the tip of the wire is completely out of the field of view and there can be no control over its movement or the exact location of its tip. The tip of the wire itself, inadvertently and very easily, can be wedged into the tissues of the brain.

When one of the subclavian arteries is used to support the wire for the dilation balloon, the retrograde catheter is maneuvered into the artery and advanced as far distally into the extremity as possible. A long, floppy tipped, Super Stiff™ exchange wire, of the largest diameter which the balloon catheter will accommodate, is introduced through a wire back-bleed valve, passed through the catheter, and positioned as far distally in the extremity as possible. The catheter is left in place over the wire and kept on a slow flush until the balloon dilation catheter is ready to be introduced. With the retrograde wire in place for the dilation, the *prograde* catheter is maintained in position just proximal to the coarctation site while continually flushing the catheter and intermittently monitoring the pressure proximal to the coarctation. The femoral artery pressure is monitored from a second femoral line or through the side arm of the arterial sheath.

The appropriate dilation balloon is prepared so that it is *completely free* of any air. It is advanced over the wire to the area of coarctation. A repeat small aortogram is performed through the prograde catheter positioned adjacent to the coarctation site and any necessary adjustments are made in the position of the balloon. If there is any doubt about the exact position of the balloon, the balloon is inflated very slowly at a low pressure looking for the initial appearance of the indentation or "waist" on the balloon to localize the exact site of the coarctation. Once the balloon is in the exact, desired position, it is inflated rapidly using a pressure-monitored inflation device and while recording the inflation either on biplane angiography or biplane stored fluoroscopy. The inflation is continued until the maximal pressure of the balloon is reached or until the "waist" on the balloon disappears, following which the balloon is deflated rapidly. The total inflation/deflation usually requires less than 10 to 15 seconds. If there is any displacement of the balloon during inflation or an adequate waist does *not* appear at all, the inflation is stopped immediately, the balloon is repositioned, and the inflation is repeated with repeat angiographic recording. Simultaneous pressures are obtained through the previously positioned prograde catheter in the aortic arch and the side arm of the arterial sheath or a cannula in the opposite femoral artery. The prograde arterial catheter thus allows the determination and recording of the pressures across the coarctation site immediately before and after the balloon inflation/deflation without having to move the balloon, and certainly without removing or exchanging any catheters or wires! These recordings alone justify the small extra effort required for the initial placement of the prograde catheter in the aorta for the retrograde coarctation dilation! If there is a question of residual gradient as a result of the deflated balloon still being across the coarctation, the balloon catheter is withdrawn over the wire until it is completely distal to the coarctation area and the pressure recordings are repeated.

An aortogram can be recorded through the prograde catheter (also without the necessity of removing the balloon or advancing catheters or wires past the recently dilated area). The aortogram demonstrates the anatomic result of the dilation and rules out any significant and/or dangerous damage to the aortic wall, before the balloon is removed. When there is no apparent damage to the aorta and there is still a significant residual gradient, or there is a significant anatomic narrowing on the aortogram, the recorded maximum diameter of the balloon during the balloon inflation is compared closely to the diameter of the adjacent aorta on the aortogram. *Precise*, calibrated re-measurements of the diameter of the balloon at its maximum inflation and the diameter of the aorta immediately adjacent to the coarctation site are made. If the maximum diameter of the balloon measured accurately on the angiogram is exactly equal to, or smaller than the diameter of the adjacent aorta, a balloon is used for a repeat dilation that is 1 millimeter larger in diameter than the adjacent aorta in a small patient or 1–2 millimeters larger in diameter in a larger patient. The "advertised" diameter of the new balloon should not exceed the diameter of the adjacent "normal" aorta by more than 10–15%. The original balloon is withdrawn over the wire and the new, larger balloon is introduced over the same, still secured, guide wire and positioned in the exact same manner as the initial balloon. The dilation is repeated while recording the inflation on a biplane angiogram. After achieving the maximal results from the dilation with this balloon, the balloon catheter is withdrawn over the wire from the coarctation site. Repeat, simultaneous pressure measurements are made through the prograde aortic catheter and the indwelling femoral line. A repeat aortogram is recorded with injection through the prograde aortic catheter.

If the waist on the balloon was abolished and the maximally inflated balloon diameter now appears to be slightly larger than the diameter of the normal adjacent aorta, regardless of the residual pressures or the anatomic appearance, the procedure is concluded and the balloon catheter removed. The end-hole catheter is placed on a continuous flush through a wire back-bleed valve and is re-advanced over the wire and very carefully past the just dilated coarctation site. This maneuver through the coarctation site is observed fluoroscopically in order to ensure that the catheter passes through the recently disrupted coarctation site very freely and does not catch on any "roughened" intravascular structures within that area. The guide wire is carefully withdrawn through the catheter and out of the body. While recording pressures the retrograde catheter is carefully withdrawn across the coarctation area into the descending aorta. A post-dilation aortogram is occasionally recorded, injecting through the prograde catheter in the proximal aorta after the balloon, the wire and the catheter have all been removed.

If the adjunct prograde aortic catheter technique is not used, this final procedure of removing the balloon, replacing it with an end-hole catheter, removing the wire completely, performing an angiogram and then measuring the "pull-back" pressure all would have to be performed before *any* results of the initial dilation were known. If the results were not satisfactory, the entire re-manipulation with the catheter, wire and new balloon would have to be repeated, but now across the freshly disrupted coarctation site!

Final simultaneous recordings of pressures from the femoral artery, transverse aorta proximal to the coarctation, and left ventricle are made as the aortic catheter is withdrawn around the arch and into the left ventricle. If there is any question about a mitral valve gradient or if the simultaneous left ventricle and left atrial pressures were not measured as the catheters were being introduced, the left atrial and left ventricular end-diastolic pressures are measured at this time. The sheath tip is withdrawn into the left atrium with the catheter remaining in the left ventricle. The left ventricular end-diastolic and left atrial pressures are recorded simultaneously. The catheters and wires are withdrawn from the sheaths, the sheaths withdrawn from the vessels and skin, and hemostasis achieved by very careful manual compression over the femoral puncture sites, observing the sites and the distal pulses continuously while achieving hemostasis.

By the use of the adjunct prograde technique, the initial hemodynamics, the visualization and measurements of the coarctation are all made with the prograde catheter. The larger arterial *sheath* is not introduced until immediately before the dilation is to be performed so that the time and trauma from any sheath in the artery are reduced markedly. As mentioned earlier, any manipulations with wires and catheters across the *freshly dilated* coarctation essentially are eliminated.

Single-catheter technique

Occasionally with a very sick patient and particularly, a small sick infant, a single *arterial* catheter is used for the entire procedure. Only the artery is punctured. If however the vein is entered while attempting the arterial puncture, at least an indwelling line is kept in that vessel. With the single arterial puncture, a sheath that will accommodate the balloon that is to be used for the dilation of the coarctation is introduced into the artery. A retrograde catheter, which can be used for both the pressure recordings and the aortograms, is introduced through the sheath. An angiographic catheter with calibration marks can be used for the aortogram, the calibration of the images on the aortogram, and the pressure recordings across the coarctation site. An end and side hole, multipurpose catheter can be used for the pressure recordings and the aortogram as well as for positioning the guide wire for the dilation procedure but, currently, these catheters do not provide calibration marks. The retrograde catheter is advanced past the coarctation and a recording of the pressure is performed as the tip of the catheter is pulled across the coarctation. If the catheter does have side holes, care must be taken that all of the side holes are totally on one or the other side of the coarctation during the recording.

After the pressure recording is completed, the retrograde catheter is re-advanced across the coarctation and a biplane aortogram recorded with the injection just proximal to, or actually "in" the coarcted segment. The best "frames" from these angiograms in both PA and lateral views are displayed as a "road map" on a freeze frame system to be used as a reference during the dilation. Since additional aortograms will not be possible once the balloon is in place, special attention is paid to the fixed intrathoracic landmarks or a small lead marker is fastened on the chest wall in a position corresponding to the location of the coarctation on the aortogram. This will serve as an additional reference to use during the balloon positioning and inflation. The calibration measurements are made depending upon which catheter is used for the angiogram and what calibration system is used in the laboratory. The precise measurements of the coarctation and the adjacent aorta are made as previously described.

If the initial catheter for the hemodynamics and aortogram was a closed-end angiographic catheter, it is replaced with an end-hole catheter. The end-hole catheter is advanced retrograde and maneuvered into the desired position (subclavian artery) to secure the wire for the dilation. The proper location and the positioning of this catheter/wire are exactly as described previously. A long, floppy tipped, Super Stiff™, exchange length wire, which the balloon chosen for the dilation will accommodate, is advanced through the catheter as far distally in the extremity as possible and the catheter removed over the wire.

The diameter of the balloon dilation catheter is chosen to correspond to the smallest diameter *of the adjacent aorta* or 1 mm smaller than that diameter for the same reasons described previously. Following the preparation of the appropriate balloon so that it is completely empty of any air, the deflated balloon is introduced into the femoral artery sheath utilizing a gentle rotation in the direction of the folds of the balloon as the balloon passes through the sheath. The dilation balloon catheter is passed retrograde across the site of coarctation until the center of the balloon is positioned exactly at the site of the coarctation as determined by comparison with the "freeze frame" of the coarctation in relation to the bony landmarks in the chest or the lead "marker" on the chest. Usually an adequate femoral arterial pressure can be obtained through the side arm of the sheath around the shaft of the balloon catheter once the actual balloon has passed through the sheath and into the vessel.

A very slow, low-pressure preliminary inflation of the balloon is used initially to determine that the "waist" on the balloon is appearing at the center of the balloon. When satisfied with the balloon position, the balloon is inflated completely with a pressure-monitored indeflator. The inflation is continued until the waist on the balloon disappears or the maximum pressure of the balloon is reached—whichever comes first. The balloon is then rapidly deflated. The inflation–deflation procedure is recorded on slow-speed, biplane angiography or on biplane "stored fluoroscopy". The balloon is inflated at least once more, looking for any evidence of the "waist" at the initial, low inflation pressures as the balloon begins to inflate. The reappearance of no waist at low pressures usually means that the coarctation has been relieved at least anatomically.

Unless a venous catheter is positioned in the left ventricle through a patent atrial septum, the only way of obtaining the definitive results of the dilation is to remove the dilation balloon over the wire and replace it with an end and side hole diagnostic/angiographic catheter. With a prograde venous catheter in the right heart, or even in the left ventricle, vague angiographic information can be obtained about the coarctation site from an injection into the pulmonary artery or left ventricle and observing the diluted contrast as it eventually flows past the area of the coarctation.

There are two possible ways of obtaining direct post-dilation information *without* having to remove the secured wire. By using a diagnostic catheter with a lumen significantly larger than the wire and with a Tuohy™ back-bleed adaptor on the catheter, pressures can be measured through the catheter, around the wire and through the side port of the Tuohy™ adaptor. This technique requires a catheter with a lumen significantly larger than the diameter of the wire. The alternative is to pass a Multi-Track™ (B. Braun Medical Inc.) angiographic catheter over the wire and through the sheath[11]. The Multi-Track™ catheter must be two French sizes smaller than the internal diameter of the sheath in order for the Multi-Track™ catheter to pass *adjacent* to the wire through the sheath. Multi-Track™ catheters are available in sizes as small as 2.5-French, which allows their passage through even a 4-French sheath. The smaller Multi-Tracks™ unfortunately pass over only a maximum of a 0.021″ wire. While the Multi-Track™ is being advanced over the wire, the stiff end of a second wire should be positioned within the Multi-Track™ and advanced to the tip of the true lumen of the catheter to support the very flimsy Multi-Track™ catheter as it is being advanced. There usually is significant blood loss through the back-bleed valve of the sheath with the catheter and wire through the valve side by side.

In smaller patients, only very marginal aortograms can be performed with either of these "over the wire" techniques. When the patient is completely stable after the coarctation dilation and, in addition, when the recorded pressures through the smaller catheter appear satisfactory and the gradient has been abolished, a multipurpose catheter is advanced over the wire, the wire is removed, and a proper aortogram obtained with an injection just proximal to the dilated site. When satisfied with the procedure and the results, the catheter is withdrawn slowly across the coarctation site while the "pull-back" pressure is recorded.

If the results of the dilation are unsatisfactory and it is determined that the diameter of the original dilating balloon as measured on the angiogram of the balloon inflation was small compared to the diameter of the adjacent aorta, the original balloon is replaced with a more appropriately sized, slightly larger diameter balloon before the guide wire is removed. The dilation and all of the post-dilation measurements are repeated. If the relief of the gradient is not 100% successful but does relieve the gradient significantly, the patient can undergo a repeat dilation and/or an intravascular stent implant at a future date.

Dilation of totally "atretic" and/or interrupted coarctation of the aorta

Very rarely a coarctation of the aorta is encountered which is atretic, with absolutely no patent lumen through the site of the coarctation. This abnormality must be differentiated from a classic "interruption" of the aorta, particularly a type A, which can appear similar, but where there is a distinct separation between the proximal ascending and distal descending aorta and no potential or even atretic lumen between the ascending and descending segments. These "atretic coarctations" are assumed to be the extreme degree of narrowing of a coarctation probably due to continued or further constriction of the ductal tissues within the aortic wall with a potential or possibly previous lumen between the two segments. These atretic lesions are all associated with very extensive collateral vessels around the coarctation site. Atretic coarctations are amenable to perforation, dilation, or intravascular stenting depending upon the size of the patient[12].

Excellent biplane angiography, both above and below the atretic area, is absolutely essential in order to visualize the most likely potential area of the lumen and the distance of the two patent vessels from each other. Preferably, the biplane angiograms are performed simultaneously with injections in close proximity to each other in both the proximal and distal vessels. An "atretic coarctation" has a very similar appearance to a "standard" coarctation, with the patent lumens of the proximal and distal areas positioned in very close proximity to each other with what appears to be a membrane or "shelf" between the segments only without even a trace of a tiny communicating lumen between them. Like a true coarctation, there is often a significant discrepancy between the diameters of the two lumens, and the proximal segment is aligned at a fairly sharp angle, anteriorly to the descending segment. If there is a significant tapering toward each other of both the proximal and distal ends along with one or more centimeters of distance between the two ends, the atretic segment is *not* suitable for dilation.

Once the atretic area is defined very clearly and the two segments are in close approximation, a perforation is performed through the area, which corresponds best to the usual site of communication in a standard coarctation, and which hopefully also will be the area of closest approximation of the two patent lumens. The perforation can be performed from above with a catheter introduced separately into a brachial artery or from below with a catheter introduced from the femoral artery. A second catheter remains positioned against the coarctation site in the apposing aortic lumen and is used as both a "target" and for repeated angiograms.

Perforation of the atretic coarctation from above has the advantage that the descending segment is usually larger in diameter, which provides a larger "target". Usually a catheter introduced from a brachial artery and into the proximal area of "coarctation" is easier to align or orient in order to point exactly toward the distal vessel, particularly when the proximal aorta is offset at an angle from the distal or descending aortic segment. The atretic "membrane" can be perforated with the stiff end of a Terumo™ wire or a radio-frequency wire pushed out of the tip of a finely tapered long "transseptal" dilator[12].

The atretic segment can also be perforated from below from the femoral approach. When approached from below, this is a circumstance where a second catheter must be positioned in the proximal segment, and the use of a prograde venous catheter maneuvered to this position is ideal. The tip of the catheter in the proximal segment must be "buried" in the blind end of the segment to provide a fixed "target" as well as to perform angiograms during the puncture from below. The puncture from below usually must be at an angle off the long axis of the descending aorta, which requires some directional control over the puncture. The best directional control is provided by a standard transseptal needle, which is used through a long transseptal set. Often the curve at the tip of the needle must be changed to conform to the angle of puncture into the proximal segment. The puncture from below can also be performed using the stiff end of a wire or, preferably, a radio-frequency wire through a long teflon transseptal dilator. Teflon transseptal dilators are relatively stiff and have enough torque response to provide good directional control over the perforating wire.

Once the atretic area of the coarctation has been perforated successfully, the perforating wire or needle is followed by a fine-tipped, long dilator and exchanged for a stiff exchange length wire. When the wire has been secured across the area, an end-hole catheter is advanced over the wire and positioned in the right subclavian artery.

The next step in the procedure depends upon the size of the patient. The subsequent dilation of the area in all of these atretic patients should be conservative initially. In children and young adolescents, the lesion is dilated to 1/2 to 2/3 the diameter of the proximal adjacent aorta. Regardless of the residual gradient, the recently dilated area is not dilated further at that catheterization, but rather, the operator should plan to further dilate and/or stent the lesion at a later date. In larger patients, even when a stent is placed in the coarctation area primarily, it is not expanded to more than 2/3 the diameter of the adjacent proximal aorta during the initial dilation/stent implant, and then should be re-dilated to re-expand the stent up to the diameter of the adjacent aorta in 6 to 12 months.

Post-coarctation dilation care

There are certain regular precautions that are taken for the vessel(s) at the entry site(s) following a balloon dilation of a coarctation of the aorta. An ACT is obtained at the end of the procedure. Unless the ACT is greater than 300 seconds, the systemic heparin is not reversed. During the procedure with any exchange of sheaths in the artery, the area around the vessel puncture site is re-infiltrated with local anesthesia. Before a sheath is removed from an artery at any time during the procedure, but particularly at the end of the case, the area is re-infiltrated *very liberally* with local anesthesia. Pain causes vessel spasm, which in turn causes decreased flow and results in thrombosis.

The catheter is withdrawn from the sheath first, allowing a small amount of back bleeding through the side arm of the sheath once the catheter is out of the sheath completely. The sheath is withdrawn and pressure applied over the vessel manually. As soon as all the sheaths are out, the drapes over the patient are removed completely so that the lower abdomen and upper thigh areas adjacent to the entire inguinal area are visible. While holding pressure over the arterial puncture site with the fingers of one hand, a pulse distal to the puncture site (dorsalis pedis or posterior tibial) is palpated with the fingers of the other hand. The amount of pressure applied over the arterial puncture site is varied or "titrated" so that just enough pressure is applied to prevent bleeding (or a subcutaneous hematoma formation) while at the same time allowing the palpation of a peripheral pulse continually. In larger or heavier patients, it is better to apply pressure over the arterial site with a firm "roll" of "4 × 4s", since the exact site of arterial puncture deep within thick subcutaneous tissues does not correspond at all to the site of the skin puncture and subsequent pressure. The pressure from the "roll" of bandage covers a wider area deep within the tissues and is more likely to control deep bleeding from the artery. The same technique for monitoring the peripheral pulse is used while pressure is applied with the "roll" of bandage.

In addition to the care of the local puncture sites, these patients are monitored systemically very closely in a recovery area for at least six hours. During this observation period, they should have a secure intravenous line and receive a high maintenance infusion of 1/4 normal saline or Ringer's lactate. The intravenous fluids are continued for twelve hours. A patient following dilation of a coarctation of the aorta usually has diuresed during the procedure from both the contrast agents used and from the increased renal blood flow as a consequence of the relief of the coarctation. Often these patients start out "dry" from being NPO for a prolonged period of time before the procedure begins. The combination of these factors results in a very significant volume depletion, which, in turn, aggravates vagal or other vascular responses caused by the changes in the distribution of arterial blood flow.

Surprisingly, post-dilation patients rarely suffer from the "post-coarctectomy" syndrome that is seen commonly following surgery. Dilation patients rarely have any aggravation of their upper extremity blood pressure, although the systemic pressures may not drop to normal immediately[13]. Post-dilation patients essentially never have abdominal discomfort and usually resume oral intake within 6–12 hours after dilation. There have been reports of serious post-procedure complications following the dilation of coarctations, so no matter how smoothly the procedure went, these patients are observed overnight. Although they may exhibit pain during the actual balloon inflation in the coarctation site, once the balloon is deflated, the pain subsides. Any persistent or recurrent pain should be taken seriously and investigated thoroughly.

Dilation of coarctation neonates and young infants

Coarctation of the aorta in the neonatal patient presents some unique features. These infants frequently present to the cardiologist catastrophically ill with heart failure, in acidosis and in shock. They frequently have additional defects, some of which complicate the catheter management and some of which actually help the catheter management. The identification of any additional defects is made from the clinical examination and the echocardiogram. The echo cannot consistently provide the details about the coarctation size, anatomy and severity, and frequently underestimates the size of the adjacent aortic segments. Decisions about therapeutic intervention for the neonatal coarctation of the aorta should *not* be made entirely on the basis of the echo.

A vigorous, but brief attempt is made at stabilizing infants who are less than three to four weeks old with ventilation, inotropics, volume support and prostaglandin. Stabilization attempts are continued only as long as the infant *improves*. If there is going to be any improvement in the clinical condition, it is noticeable within one to two hours. With, or without, the stabilization after that duration of time, the infant is taken to the catheterization laboratory. If the infant is not responding noticeably to the resuscitative efforts, more time only allows further deterioration. If the infant is responding, the improvement will continue on the way to, and in, the catheterization laboratory. The exact procedure performed depends upon the presence or absence of associated lesions and, when present, which associated lesions are present.

Besides their general hemodynamic instability, the very small femoral arteries with the associated very weak or absent femoral pulses represent the greatest challenge for balloon dilation of coarctation of the aorta in the very small infant. In each individual case, the most expeditious technique possible is utilized to approach and treat the coarctation. Once the coarctation area has been reached with a catheter, the gradient is measured, the selective aortogram(s) performed and accurate measurements of the coarctation and adjacent vessels are made in order to choose the proper balloon.

When the infant responds to the administration of prostaglandins with opening of the ductus arteriosus, the stabilization of the infant is usually rapid and very effective. The presence of the patent ductus indirectly facilitates access to the coarctation by improving perfusion to the lower extremities significantly, and increases the amplitude of the femoral pulses, which facilitates percutaneous arterial access. The presence of a patent ductus, however, compromises the results of balloon dilation of a neonatal coarctation. Without the patent ductus, the balloon is constrained within the aorta and the "path of least resistance" is to crush the abnormal ridge of tissue within the aortic lumen. A wide open ductus arteriosus, on the other hand, allows the dilation balloon to move away from the coarctation "ridge" into the "ampulla" of the ductus rather than crushing or compressing the ridge. In addition, when the ductus does constrict during its normal closure, it probably also constricts some of the adjacent aorta, recreating the coarctation.

Most of the newborns and small infants with coarctation do have at least a potential interatrial communication. In all of these infants, venous access is obtained and an angiographic catheter is introduced into at least the *left ventricle* from the venous approach. At the same time, in a small sick infant, no prolonged effort should be made at advancing this catheter from the left ventricle into the aorta, as is utilized in coarctation dilation in the older patient. The chambers and vessels are very small and the tissues "softer" and prone to puncture. The catheter in the left ventricle provides continual systemic pressure monitoring before, during and immediately after the dilation procedure. The pressure in the left ventricle reflects the severity of the coarctation unless there is associated aortic stenosis or the infant is in terrible heart failure. A left ventricular angiocardiogram is performed which provides some, and possibly, very good information about the coarctation and the overall anatomy.

Infants who do *not* respond to prostaglandins and who have no associated lesions, and those who have associated aortic stenosis, are the most difficult for coarctation dilation. The echocardiogram should diagnose associated aortic stenosis and give an estimate of its severity, although either one of the two lesions can mask the significance of the other. The prograde left ventricular catheter is useful in these patients for monitoring pressures and for the administration of fluid and medication, and is possibly helpful in determining the relative severity of combined lesions.

Percutaneous entry into the *artery* is accomplished with meticulous attention to detail, a very delicate single wall vessel puncture technique, and patience (as described in Chapter 4). The area around the expected arterial puncture site is infiltrated with local anesthesia, being as careful as possible not to puncture the artery with the needle during the infiltration. If the artery is punctured inadvertently, pressure is held over the site for at least 2–4 minutes before beginning the purposeful puncture of the artery. Special 21-gauge percutaneous needles and *extra*-floppy tipped 0.018″ or 0.014″ wires are essential for the percutaneous entry into the artery in these patients. Once the artery has been entered with the guide wire, the area surrounding the puncture site is re-infiltrated liberally with local anesthesia. A 3- or 4-French "fine tipped" sheath/dilator is introduced into the artery. The preliminary diagnostic information about the coarctation is obtained with the retrograde catheter. If the infant is still very unstable, an end and side hole multipurpose catheter is used. This type of catheter allows pressure measurements and quality aortogram(s), and at the same time can be used to position the guide wire for the dilation without the necessity of even one catheter exchange. The second catheter previously positioned in the left ventricle *helps* to confirm the presence of associated aortic stenosis. However, with poor left ventricular function and an associated coarctation of the aorta, even very severe aortic stenosis can be masked.

Once the coarctation has been identified as *the only significant lesion*, it is measured accurately and the dilation of the coarctation is carried out as expediently as possible using the single-catheter, retrograde technique. It is preferable to stabilize the distal end of the guide wire in one of the subclavian arteries, although an excessively long time or effort should not be taken to achieve this location. The balloon for the coarctation dilation is chosen to equal the size of the smallest segment of the aorta adjacent to the coarctation. Once the dilation has been completed and the balloon removed over the wire, the end-hole catheter is re-advanced over the wire and very gently past the coarctation to the aorta proximal to the coarctation. The wire is removed and pressures are recorded simultaneously through the catheter from the ascending aorta and through the side arm of the sheath from the femoral artery. A repeat aortogram is recorded, injecting through the end-hole catheter proximal to the coarctation site.

The catheter should not be withdrawn across the coarctation site until all post-dilation studies or any re-dilation has been accomplished. If the dilation was unsatisfactory and a re-dilation is necessary, the wire is replaced through the catheter which is already across and well beyond the lesion in order that no catheter manipulation back across the freshly dilated area is necessary. When the catheter has been withdrawn across the area, it should not be manipulated back across the area[3].

Co-existent critical aortic stenosis and coarctation in infants

When there is significant aortic stenosis in association with the neonatal coarctation, it is preferable to address the aortic stenosis first. In the presence of the combined lesions, perfusion of the coronary and cerebral circulations is dependent, at least partially, on the increased afterload in the ascending aortic pressure provided by the coarctation. Removing this afterload before opening the aortic valve could compromise the coronary and cerebral circulations even further. In addition, if the coarctation is dilated first, all of the manipulations (sometimes extensive) required for crossing the aortic valve, and the aortic valve dilation, will have to be through the freshly dilated coarctation site with the potential for traumatizing the already damaged aortic intima in the coarctation site even further.

With combined aortic stenosis and coarctation, the diameters of the aortic valve annulus *and* the coarctation with the appropriate adjacent aortic diameters are measured from a left ventricular angiocardiogram or an aortic root injection before an attempt is made to pass a catheter across the stenotic valve. A left ventricular angiocardiogram is obtained with injection through a prograde left ventricular catheter, while the aortic root injection is obtained with the retrograde multipurpose or angiographic catheter that has been manipulated past the coarctation and around the arch to the aortic root. Once the valve and coarctation measurements are obtained, the appropriate dilation balloon for the *aortic valve dilation* is prepared using the "minimal prep" technique but with a prolonged attempt at removing all air. No attempt is made to cross the aortic valve until the balloon for the dilation is prepared and "poised" for introduction. These infants are often so precarious that even a tiny 4-French catheter crossing the stenotic orifice is enough to cause a rapid decompensation in their hemodynamics.

To cross these valves, a 0.018″ or 0.014″, very floppy tipped, exchange length, torque-controlled, coronary artery, guide wire is advanced through a multipurpose or selective right coronary catheter which is already positioned in the aortic root. The wire is advanced out of the catheter and *multiple, rapidly repeated, short probes* are made toward the aortic valve area with the very soft wire tip. Because even a very soft tipped wire exiting the tip of the catheter can be very stiff for the first few millimeters out of the tip, the tip of the catheter is kept a centimeter away from the valve annulus during the probes with the tip of the wire. The tip of the wire is redirected within the aortic root by simultaneously rotating the catheter (to change the anterior to posterior direction) and moving the catheter to and fro (to change the right to left side angle). Unless another wire or catheter is already passing through the valve, the exact location of the orifice really is not known. The more "probes" that are made with the wire along with multiple changes in the angle of the wire, the more likely is the chance of the wire passing through the orifice of the "invisible" valve.

If the wire does not cross the valve after trying for several minutes using the original multipurpose catheter, the multipurpose catheter is replaced with a preformed, either right or left coronary catheter and the "probing" at the valve repeated with similar changes in direction of the catheter tip. The tighter, preformed curves at the tips of coronary catheters allow a greater ability to change the angle of approach toward the small valve orifice.

Once the wire crosses the valve, it is advanced as far as possible into the ventricle, hopefully even looping the soft tip within the left ventricle apex. With the wire passed as far as possible into the ventricle, the catheter is advanced over the wire into the ventricle. If the infant's hemodynamics do *not* remain stable with the catheter across the valve, the wire is fixed in the ventricle and the *catheter* is immediately removed and replaced *rapidly* over the wire with the previously prepared balloon dilation catheter. The dilation of the valve is carried out with as rapid an inflation and deflation as possible and while recording angiographically or on "stored fluoroscopy". After the inflation/deflation, the balloon is immediately withdrawn out of the valve over the wire into at least the ascending aorta.

If the infant remains stable with the end-hole catheter passed through the valve, the wire is removed. A "pig-tail" is formed on the tip of the long floppy tipped, stiffer, exchange guide wire and a 180° curve is formed on the transition zone between the long floppy tip and the stiff shaft of the wire. This individually formed wire is re-advanced through the catheter into the left ventricle. The preformed "pig-tail" on the wire keeps the wire from digging into the myocardium as it is manipulated in the ventricle. The 180° curve at the *transition area* of the wire directs the tip of the wire back toward the left ventricular outflow tract and allows the *stiff portion* of the shaft of the wire to be positioned further across the valve. With the wire maintained in position, the catheter is removed and replaced with the already prepared balloon catheter. The balloon is positioned across the valve and the inflation performed while recording the inflation angiographically or on "stored fluoroscopy". The inflation/deflation is performed as rapidly as possible. During the inflation the left ventricular pressure increases and the infant develops bradycardia. As soon as the deflation of the balloon is complete, the balloon is withdrawn over the wire and out of the aortic annulus. The infant's heart rate should return and the left ventricular pressure will drop to normal levels.

The return of a good heart rate and a good, but lower, left ventricular pressure are immediate indications of the success of the dilation. Ideally, there will be a lower left ventricular pressure, but in the presence of the associated coarctation, the gradient may be "moved downstream" to the coarctation site with little lowering of the left ventricular pressure. The radiographic recording of the inflation/deflation is reviewed. If a "waist" appeared on the balloon and then disappeared during the inflation, some true dilation of the valve orifice is assumed. The balloon is withdrawn back to the area of the coarctation. If the diameter of this balloon is smaller, or, at least, no more than a millimeter larger, than the measurement of the smallest diameter of the aorta adjacent to the coarctation, the coarctation site is dilated with the same balloon. If the balloon is two or more millimeters larger than the adjacent aorta in the area of the coarctation, the balloon is replaced with an appropriate diameter balloon and the coarctation dilated.

After both the aortic valve and the coarctation have been dilated the balloon is removed and replaced with a catheter to re-evaluate the hemodynamics. If there is a left ventricular catheter in place, the "net" results of the combined dilation are determined by measuring the left ventricular and femoral artery pressures simultaneously using the side arm of the sheath for the femoral artery. If the net left ventricular to femoral artery gradient is low, it is assumed that both procedures were successful and the procedure can be concluded. A left ventricular angiocardiogram through the prograde catheter provides visualization of both the aortic valve and the coarctation area. An end-hole catheter is passed over the wire to the left ventricle and the retrograde wire removed. Pressures are recorded on withdrawal of the retrograde catheter from the left ventricle, to the aorta and across the coarctation site to quantitate the residual gradients at each area.

If the net gradient is still significant, the culprit lesion(s) is/are identified from the pressures and angiograms. If there is no prograde catheter in the left ventricle, the results of the dilations must still be determined. A Multi-Track™ catheter provides the most "secure" way of identifying the major residual problem without having to remove the wire from the left ventricle. Pressures are recorded and angiograms are performed through the Multi-Track™ catheter anywhere along the course from the left ventricle to the descending aorta and all *without* having to remove the wire, which can be maintained positioned in the left ventricle. A small, stiff wire is placed in the *true catheter lumen* of the Multi-Track™ catheter to stiffen and support the catheter shaft as Multi-Track™ is being advanced over the exchange wire. Once the Multi-Track™ catheter is in the left ventricle, the wire within the *true lumen* is removed. Angiograms are performed where appropriate and pressures are recorded as the Multi-Track™ is withdrawn over the exchange wire. When a significant area of residual obstruction is identified, the decision is made whether this should or can be treated from the pressures, the review of the balloon dilations and the current angiograms performed through the Multi-Track™ catheter. If a lesion is to be re-dilated, the Multi-Track™ is removed over the wire and the appropriate balloon dilation catheter reintroduced to the culprit lesion.

If a Multi-Track™ catheter is not available or cannot be used with the particular system, then an end-hole, multipurpose catheter is advanced over the wire to the left ventricle and the exchange wire removed. Pressures are recorded and sequential angiograms are obtained through this catheter as it is withdrawn from the left ventricle to the ascending aorta and from the ascending aorta to the descending aorta. This, of course, removes the previously secure wire access back into the ventricle! If the significant or predominant gradient is at the aortic valve, the catheter withdrawal is stopped in the aortic root and a decision is made as to whether further catheter therapy is possible. If the aortic valve is to be re-dilated, the soft floppy tipped wire is reintroduced through the catheter and manipulated across the aortic valve into the left ventricle. The dilation procedure is repeated with a more appropriate diameter balloon.

If there is a significant net left ventricle to femoral artery gradient, but little or no gradient at the aortic valve, the coarctation is still the culprit. The previous coarctation dilation is reviewed. If a larger balloon can be used, the wire is reinserted into the catheter and positioned in the aortic root before the catheter is withdrawn across the coarctation. The end-hole catheter is removed over the wire, the appropriate diameter balloon is passed over the wire and the coarctation re-dilated. Reassessment of the result depends upon which catheters are available, as described above.

Whenever an infant is found to have coarctation of the aorta with aortic stenosis, associated mitral stenosis of some type and degree should be suspected. The Shone's complex of multiple left heart obstructive lesions includes various types of mitral valve stenosis along with the coarctation and aortic stenosis, and frequently results in an even sicker infant. Any one, or all, of the levels of obstructive lesions can be severe and require intervention, however usually the coarctation and aortic lesions are the most pressing and are the only ones that can be addressed reasonably in the newborn period. Congenital mitral stenosis can be treated by balloon dilation in the slightly older child, and is addressed separately in Chapter 20.

The most favorable associated lesions in an infant with coarctation that need dilation are a ventricular septal defect (VSD) and transposition of the great arteries. A VSD provides access to the aorta from the right heart and in turn from the *venous* access. Although access to the coarctation through the VSD is anticipated, these infants should have an indwelling arterial line for systemic pressure monitoring. In these patients, a curved tipped, end-hole or multipurpose catheter introduced through a short sheath from a percutaneous venous introduction is used for the "right heart" procedure. In infants, when manipulating a venous catheter from the right ventricle toward the outflow tract, as the catheter is torqued clockwise, it frequently and, even preferentially, passes dorsally through the ventricular defect and, from there, into the ascending aorta. Otherwise, with purposeful manipulation of the catheter dorsally and cephalad from the right ventricle, entering the aorta almost always is accomplished in infants with a significant VSD. From there, approaching the coarctation around the arch is a straightforward procedure with a wire and curved tip catheter. A selective aortogram is performed and the lesion and adjacent vessels measured accurately. The coarctation is crossed with a prograde end-hole catheter and the catheter is exchanged for the exchange length, stiff, guide wire. The balloon is introduced from the vein and advanced through the right ventricle, through the VSD and to the coarctation. The dilation is accomplished all prograde from the venous entry site without the need for even a 3-French sheath in a femoral artery. The post-procedure measurements are carried out with an end-hole catheter replacing the balloon catheter in the aorta before the "prograde" guide wire is removed.

The same ability to perform a dilation of a coarctation from a venous access holds true for infants with coarctation of the aorta in association with transposition of the great arteries (with or without a ventricular septal defect or aortic or pulmonary override). This is a particularly common association in patients with the so-called Taussig–Bing complex of transposition of the great arteries, ventricular septal defect and pulmonary artery override. A standard end-hole or a balloon "wedge" catheter passes easily from the right ventricle and out into the aorta. With minimal manipulation the catheter is maneuvered into the descending aorta to the coarctation. The diagnosis and dilation are performed similarly to that in the infant with an associated VSD.

Intravascular stents in coarctation of the aorta

The use of intravascular stents for the treatment of coarctation of the aorta has become the primary approach for coarctation in the larger adolescent and adult. The use and advantages of intravascular stents in both native and re/residual coarctation are covered in detail in Chapter 25. Their use in conjunction with dilation of coarctation of the aorta has changed the approach to these lesions dramatically. Intravascular stents not only support the vessels at the maximal dilated diameter of the balloon, but also, in doing so, eliminate the need for *any* over-dilation of the vessel.

However, the basic rules for the implant of intravascular stents in pediatric and congenital lesions apply even more stringently to their use in coarctations. In particular, no stent should be implanted in the aorta if it cannot be dilated up to the *ultimate adult diameter* of the aorta in that particular patient. This "rule" so far has precluded the reasonable and/or sensible use of stents in coarctation of the aorta in infants and small children. The implant of a stent that cannot be dilated to the diameter of the adult aorta, creates a new, very fixed diameter coarctation as the patient grows. A coarctation with a stent in place, which is too small for the aorta and which cannot be dilated further, must be managed surgically. There is a much higher risk for surgery on a coarctation with a stent in place than for the surgical repair of native coarctation, even in an infant. The narrow segment of aorta that contains the stent, at the very least, must be "filleted" open and then patched, if not totally resected or bypassed with a prosthetic graft. At the same time, this same patient who requires such extensive surgery on the aorta, no longer has the extensive collaterals to protect the spinal cord and the lower half of his body. Hopefully, the further development of "open ring" stents or some type of resorbable stent, will eventually make it possible to use stents in the initial treatment of coarctation in infants and children.

In the interim, balloon dilation of coarctation is very effective in infants and children. Even if the obstruction of the coarctation is not eliminated totally with an initial dilation, or even with several balloon dilations, if the aorta is not over-dilated and torn or ruptured, a successful balloon dilation with a stent implant can be accomplished when the patient reaches adolescence or adulthood. For the infant and child, a "conservative" dilation of both native and re/residual coarctation should be the primary approach to these lesions.

Complications specific to coarctation dilation

The majority of the early dilations reported in the Valvuloplasty and Angioplasty of Congenital Anomalies (VACA) registry were for re-coarctation of the aorta and, as a consequence, the majority of the acute complications were in these re-coarctation dilations. In the VACA series of re-coarctation dilations there were five deaths (two vagal, one aortic rupture, one CNS death and one death due to shock)[1].

A better understanding of the effect of the post-dilation vasodilation and the exaggerated physiologic vasovagal response to the pressure drop associated with dilations has helped to eliminate the extreme vasovagal response to the procedure. The patients are maintained on a high maintenance volume of intravenous fluids during the dilation and this fluid infusion is maintained for six to twelve hours after the dilation. The intravenous access is left in place until after the patient is ambulated. With these precautions, the vasovagal type reactions have been eliminated.

Significant central nervous system (CNS) injuries and at least one death attributed to CNS injury have been reported following dilation of coarctation of the aorta. The *exact etiology* of all of the CNS injuries has never been determined unequivocally. Fortunately, with more attention to the position of the distal end of the guide wire for support of the dilation balloon and extremely stringent precautions concerning emboli from the materials and/or the procedure, the central nervous system complications essentially have been eliminated. It is critical that the distal end of the support wire is not positioned in a carotid or vertebral artery or possibly even in the ascending aorta. Catheters passed over wires are maintained on a continual flush in order to eliminate any accumulation of blood and clot around the wire within the catheter or at the wire–catheter interface. Flushing over the wire is accomplished by introducing the wire through a wire back-bleed valve with a flush side port, which is attached to the hub of the catheter. The side port of the wire back-bleed valve is maintained on continual flush from the pressure/flush system. In spite of the theoretical potential for an aortic tear, patients undergoing coarctation dilation are heparinized fully with the hope of eliminating clot formation on the wires or catheters.

Although possible, acute, through and through tears in the aortic wall from the dilation of coarctations have been exceedingly rare. One report early in the history of dilation of coarctation of the aorta was in a patient with re-coarctation of the aorta who had remarkably little or no reaction or scar formation from the prior surgery and apparently little or no reaction to the acute local injury. The patient had a through and through tear in the aortic wall and eventually succumbed to the lesion. Possibly, aortic tears cannot be avoided unequivocally, however it appears likely that aortic tears can be prevented by less aggressive initial dilation of aortic coarctations and not *over-dilating* any segment of the aorta adjacent to the area of the coarctation by measuring that area of the aorta and using that measured diameter to determine the diameter of the balloon for the dilation. Dilation of a typical "native" coarctation presumably tears a "membrane" that lies across the lumen of the aorta and does not extend the tear significantly into the wall of the aorta. Dilation of an equally tight "re or residual" coarctation probably involves dilation of the actual wall of the aorta which has constricted down in the area of the previous therapy and, as a consequence, these should be dilated more conservatively.

Most patients exhibit pain acutely during the process of inflating a balloon in the aorta, however the pain subsides when the balloon is deflated. If a patient has *persistent* pain *after* acute dilation of the coarctation, the area of the coarctation should be investigated carefully with selective aortography or intravascular ultrasound in the area of the dilation. Even without identifying a tear, the patient should be observed in the catheterization laboratory until the pain subsides or for one or more hours if the pain persists. If a through and through tear with progressive extravasation is detected, the balloon is reinflated *at a low pressure* in the area of the tear. The inflation is just enough to "tamponade" the vessel and allow the patient to be taken to the operating room for a repair. Such a surgical aortic repair certainly will require relatively prolonged cross clamping of the aorta and in turn, may require femoral vein to femoral artery bypass.

There has been one report of paraplegia following a balloon dilation of a re/residual coarctation of the aorta in a small infant with associated complex congenital heart disease[14]. The prior surgery on the aorta had involved an uncomplicated end-to-end anastomosis. There was no prolonged ischemia, no evidence of aortic tear nor any evidence for embolic phenomena to explain the paraplegia.

In the early reported series of coarctation dilation, there was an 8.5% incidence of significant enough injury to the arterial introductory site to require intervention or have permanent sequelae at the entrance site into the vessel. In those early years of balloon dilation, the balloon dilation catheters were very large and the balloons themselves were large and grotesque by today's standards. All of the balloons greater than 6 mm in diameter were on 9-French catheter shafts, the balloons were relatively thick walled and they did not fold well around the catheter so that the balloon "mass" had a very large profile. In order to be introduced through a sheath these balloons required an 11- or 12-French sheath! As a consequence to "reduce the size" of the entry hole into the vessel most of these early balloons were introduced into the vessels directly over a wire without a sheath in the vessel. This in fact probably did not reduce the diameter of the "hole" in the vessel wall and certainly contributed to significantly *more* local trauma to the vessel walls. Considering the balloon catheters used at that time, the incidence of arterial injury actually was remarkably low!

Many refinements in the balloons with marked reduction in the size of the catheter shafts and decrease in the balloon profiles have not only allowed a smaller "hole" for introduction into the vessel, but have also allowed dilation balloons routinely to be introduced through indwelling sheaths. With the combination of smaller balloon profiles, routine use of indwelling sheaths, very meticulous care of the introductory sites into the arteries, liberal, repeated use of local anesthesia, heparinization (perhaps?), and personal attention to the site during hemostasis after the balloon/sheath is removed, local vessel injury is now very rare.

When an acute arterial injury does occur, it is treated aggressively at the time of the catheterization. With an absent pulse, the patient is continued on heparin therapy for one or two hours or until the pulse returns. If there is no return of a pulse within 1–2 hours the patient is either begun on thrombolytic therapy with continued heparin or is taken back to the catheterization laboratory for a mechanical recanalization of the vessel, as described in Chapter 34 on purposeful perforations.

With only a 20-year history of balloon dilation of coarctation of the aorta, any long-term adverse sequelae from the procedure are as yet unknown. The "longer-term" adverse sequelae that have occurred so far, seem to occur more with the dilation of "native" coarctation of the aorta where the aorta is not "protected" by a surrounding area of scar tissue, as is found around the re-coarctations. The most bothersome finding after coarctation dilation is the creation of an "aneurysm" at the site of the coarctation dilation. The incidence of these aneurysms has varied markedly in different series, but in general they are rare. The "aneurysms" are usually a small out-pouching in the aortic wall in the area of the balloon dilation. This out-pouching is usually apparent immediately after the dilation. In most cases the out-pouching does not enlarge and in fact seems to remodel into the aortic wall along with the overall remodeling of the aorta. The out-pouching of the aorta is considered an aneurysm when the area "remodels" into a persistent, discrete out-pouching. There are no reported long-term adverse consequences of the aneurysms, however, in at least one series, several of the patients with an aneurysm did undergo surgery for it. The indication for the surgery was not because of any clinical problem due to the aneurysm, but because of the fear of what might happen to the aneurysm over time. The pathology of those aneurysms that were operated upon showed tears through the intima and media of the vessel wall. Some aneurysms have been followed for as long as 18 years with no increase in their size and no sequelae.

Aneurysms of the aorta following surgical repair are not uncommon. These aneurysms are more frequent when there is a persistent narrowing of the aorta proximal to the coarctation repair site or when the surgical repair was carried out with a patch angioplasty. These post-surgical aneurysms are large saccular dilations of the entire area of the coarctation/aorta distal to the more proximal "obstruction". Most of these aneurysms continue to grow with time and most have been referred for surgical revision.

The total incidence of aneurysms following coarctation dilation initially was small and actually seems to be decreasing and, possibly, not occurring at all in more recent series. In the earlier days of coarctation dilation, the measurements of the coarctation and *the adjacent vessels* were less accurate, and less attention was paid to the narrow adjacent structures. Often, marked over-dilation of these areas was carried out with balloons significantly larger in diameter than the adjacent vessel, either because of the inaccuracies in measurement or purposefully in an attempt to achieve a more lasting result. Perhaps the more conservative dilations done with the knowledge that the aorta can be dilated further later or can be held open with an intravascular stent without the need for any over-dilation will totally eliminate the aneurysms associated with coarctation dilations. When a discrete aneurysm does occur, it should be followed closely, probably at least every one or two years with repeated CT, MRI, or angiographic imaging.

A discrete aneurysm can be excluded by a stent graft (large covered stent) or covered with a standard intravascular stent to support the aortic wall in the area and then to have coils packed into the aneurysm behind the intravascular stent.

Conclusion

Balloon dilation is an accepted standard treatment for both native and re/residual coarctation of the aorta in patients of all ages in many major cardiovascular centers dealing with congenital heart disease. The safety of the acute procedure now appears to be very good, perhaps because of a better understanding of the lesions and a more conservative approach to the dilation procedure. A patient who undergoes a conservative dilation of coarctation of the aorta and who has a less than optimal result, but at the same time has no complications, can always have the dilation of the coarctation repeated with, or without, the implant of an intravascular stent to "complete" the procedure.

The success of dilation of coarctation of the aorta over the years and the reduction in the complications and the difficulties with repeat surgery on patients with re/residual coarctation have made dilation of native and re/residual coarctation the procedure of choice in most centers. Most centers stipulate that all patients who have dilation of any type of coarctation of the aorta should be followed indefinitely. In patients who are, or are at least near to, full-grown many centers now regularly perform primary intravascular stent implants along with dilation of coarctation of the aorta. The use of stents in coarctation of the aorta is covered in detail in Chapter 25.

References

1. Hellenbrand WE *et al.* Balloon angioplasty for aortic recoarctation: Results of the Valvuloplasty and Angioplasty of Congenital Anomalies Registry. *Am J Cardiol* 1990; **65**: 793–797.
2. Tynan M *et al.* Balloon angioplasty for the treatment of native coarctation: Results of the Valvuloplasty and Angioplasty of Congenital Anomalies Registry. *Am J Cardiol* 1990; **65**: 790–792.
3. Finley JP *et al.* Balloon catheter dilatation of coarctation of the aorta in young infants. *Br Heart J* 1983; **50**: 411–415.
4. Lock JE *et al.* Balloon dilation angioplasty of aortic coarctations in infants and children. *Circulation* 1983; **68**(1): 109–116.
5. Kappetein AP *et al.* More than thirty-five years of coarctation repair. An unexpected high relapse rate. *J Thorac Cardiovasc Surg* 1994; **107**(1): 87–95.
6. Wada T *et al.* Prevention and detection of spinal cord injury during thoracic and thoracoabdominal aortic repairs. *Ann Thorac Surg* 2001; **72**(1): 80–84; discussion 85.

7. Kalita J *et al*. Evoked potential changes in ischaemic myelopathy. *Electromyogr Clin Neurophysiol* 2003; **43**(4): 211–215.
8. John CN *et al*. Report of four cases of aneurysm complicating patch aortoplasty for repair of coarctation of the aorta. *Aust NZ J Surg* 1989; **59**(9): 748–750.
9. Fletcher SE *et al*. Balloon angioplasty of native coarctation of the aorta: midterm follow-up and prognostic factors. *J Am Coll Cardiol* 1995; **25**(3): 730–734.
10. Anjos R *et al*. Determinants of hemodynamic results of balloon dilation of aortic recoarctation. *Am J Cardiol* 1992; **69**(6): 665–671.
11. Bonhoeffer P *et al*. The multi-track angiography catheter: a new tool for complex catheterisation in congenital heart disease. *Heart* 1996; **76**(2): 173–177.
12. Joseph G, Mandalay A, and Rajendiran G. Percutaneous recanalization and balloon angioplasty of congenital isolated local atresia of the aortic isthmus in adults. *Catheter Cardiovasc Interv* 2001; **53**(4): 535–541.
13. Choy M *et al*. Paradoxical hypertension after repair of coarctation of the aorta in children: balloon angioplasty versus surgical repair. *Circulation* 1987; **75**(6): 1186–1191.
14. Ussia GP, Marasini M, and Pongiglione G. Paraplegia following percutaneous balloon angioplasty of aortic coarctation: a case report. *Catheter Cardiovasc Interv* 2001; **54**(4): 510–513.

19 Aortic valve dilation

Introduction

In most major pediatric centers balloon dilation of the aortic valve in the cardiac catheterization laboratory is the accepted standard for the primary treatment of aortic valve stenosis. Balloon dilation of aortic valve stenosis to treat valvar aortic stenosis was first published in 1984[1]. Balloon dilation of the aortic valve provides palliation that is comparable to the palliation for similar aortic valve stenosis achieved by a surgical aortic valvotomy, but without the risks and morbidity of surgery[2,3]. Significant improvements in the dilation balloons, guide wires and techniques over the past 15 years have improved the success rate and decreased, *but not eliminated*, the morbidity and mortality of the aortic dilation procedure for infants, children and adolescents. The indications for dilation of the aortic valve are similar to the indications for surgical aortic valvotomy and, as with the indications for surgery, the indications for balloon dilation vary with the age of the patient.

In the newborn the diagnosis of aortic valve stenosis comprises a very heterogeneous spectrum of anatomy, including everything from a nearly atretic aortic valve with a small aortic annulus and/or an associated very small, hypoplastic left ventricle, to an equally stenotic valve, but with a large, dilated poorly functioning left ventricle. The exact anatomy and the resultant left ventricular function determine the indications for balloon dilation in this group. The echocardiographic demonstration of aortic valve stenosis with associated poor left ventricular function or low cardiac output, particularly with an otherwise "normal" sized left ventricle, is a major indication for intervention in a newborn regardless of the measured gradient by either echo or catheterization[4].

After the clinical evaluation along with a quality echocardiogram, the definitive diagnosis of valvular aortic stenosis is established by the hemodynamics obtained in the catheterization laboratory. In the older infant and young child with clinical findings of aortic valve stenosis, the indication for valvotomy is determined from the peak to peak hemodynamic gradient measured across the valve in the catheterization laboratory. In the absence of any signs of "poor ventricular function", aortic valve dilation is performed arbitrarily in very young children for a peak to peak gradient greater than 65 mmHg across the valve. Very young children do not participate in organized, severely strenuous, or sustained physical activities and do not create much additional gradient with their level of activity. In adolescent and adult patients, who are more likely to participate in severely strenuous or sustained physical activity, symptoms referable to the heart or a measured peak to peak gradient across the valve of over 50 mmHg is the arbitrary indication for valve dilation. These criteria were established for a *surgical* aortic valvotomy on the basis of "natural history" studies, and probably are too conservative for balloon dilation of the aortic valve.

Technique—general

General anesthesia with intubation and controlled ventilation is used in newborns, in critically ill patients with aortic stenosis, and in any patient in whom the carotid artery approach is being used. The same general procedure is used for the "diagnostic" cardiac catheterization of the patient who is *not critically ill* but who is undergoing aortic dilation, as is used for the catheterization of any other patient. The catheterization is performed under deep sedation and local xylocaine anesthesia with supplemental sedation given intravenously periodically throughout the procedure. A secure peripheral intravenous and an arterial line are established and an indwelling "Foley" catheter placed in the bladder in all patients past infancy who are undergoing a balloon dilation of the aortic valve.

There are several different approaches and techniques utilized to accomplish balloon dilation of a stenotic aortic valve. The specific technique used depends upon the particular circumstances of each individual patient and also on the individual preferences of the operator and/or the catheterization laboratory. The aortic valve can be approached retrograde from the femoral, brachial, umbilical, or carotid arteries. The aortic valve can also be approached prograde from the right heart after passing into the left heart through either a patent foramen ovale or by crossing through the intact atrial septum with a transseptal puncture. The atrial transseptal approach to the left atrium is the preferred technique to acquire the left heart hemodynamics and angiography when the atrial septum is intact, while the retrograde approach through the femoral arteries is the most commonly used approach for the actual balloon dilation of the aortic valve. A double-balloon dilation of the valve using a retrograde approach from both femoral arteries is preferred for most aortic valve dilations[5].

Technique

For the combined prograde and retrograde approach to the aortic valve dilation procedure, a short venous sheath is introduced into one femoral vein and two very small indwelling arterial cannulae are introduced into both the right and left femoral arteries. The right heart catheterization is performed using an angiographic "marker" catheter introduced through the short venous sheath. When a transseptal procedure is to be performed and there are any concerns about or a peculiarity of any part of the anatomy of the left heart, an angiocardiogram is performed with injection into the pulmonary artery before the transseptal puncture. The recirculation of the contrast through the left atrium and left ventricle clearly demonstrates the exact positions and any peculiarities of the left heart anatomy.

The left heart hemodynamics are obtained by means of a prograde left heart catheterization either through a pre-existing interatrial communication or through a transseptal atrial puncture. Using the prograde approach to the left heart, all of the hemodynamics, as well as quality, selective left ventricular or aortic angiograms, are obtained before any "time" is incurred in the arteries with the larger indwelling arterial sheaths. When the necessary right heart information has been obtained, the prograde venous catheter is advanced into the left atrium and from there into the left ventricle. Pressures are recorded from the left ventricle and the femoral arteries, and the left ventricular angiography is obtained to determine the severity and type of the aortic stenosis.

In the absence of a pre-existing atrial communication, the right heart catheter and short venous sheath are replaced with a transseptal set of the largest French size the patient can accommodate comfortably and safely. The long sheath of the transseptal set should have an attached back-bleed valve with a side arm/flush port. A transseptal left atrial puncture is performed using the long sheath/dilator transseptal set as described in detail in Chapter 8. Once the long sheath is positioned in the left atrium and the sheath and its back-bleed valve apparatus are cleared meticulously of all air and clots, the side port of the sheath is attached to the pressure/flush system. At this time in the procedure, the patient is given 100 mg/kg of heparin through the long sheath. An angiographic catheter *one French size smaller than the sheath* is advanced through the sheath and manipulated from the left atrium into the left ventricle. Simultaneous pressures are recorded from the left atrium, left ventricle and a femoral artery. With the knowledge that the femoral artery pressure can be as much as 20 millimeters higher than the aortic root pressure as a result of the elastic recoil of the systemic vasculature, this measured difference in pressures between the left ventricle and femoral artery gives an *estimate*, but does *not* give an accurate measurement of the true transvalvular aortic gradient.

Following the transseptal puncture and when the initial pressures have been recorded, a selective biplane angiocardiogram is performed with an injection into the left ventricle. The angiocardiogram defines the precise anatomy of the aortic root and the aortic valve stenosis, and demonstrates any associated left ventricular outflow track abnormalities. At least one view of the angiocardiograms should be as close to perpendicular to the valve annulus as possible. The lateral (LAT) X-ray tube is placed in a 60° left anterior oblique position with between 30° and 60° cranial angulation. The amount of cranial angulation is determined by how horizontally the heart is situated in the chest–the more horizontally the heart lies in the thorax, the greater the cranial angulation. The posterior–anterior (PA) X-ray tube is placed in a 30°, right anterior oblique position with 30+° of *caudal* angulation. The PA tube should be almost perpendicular to the LAT tube in both planes. If the valve is not cut precisely on edge with the initial picture, the X-ray tubes are rotated appropriately and the angiocardiogram repeated. Very accurate *angiographic* measurements are made of the *diameter* of the valve annulus at the base of the aortic sinuses where the valve leaflets attach or "hinge" in the annulus. The measurements are obtained from a systolic frame where the leaflets are open and the annulus is at its largest diameter during the cardiac cycle. The measurements must be calibrated against a valid reference measurement system.

Depending upon the measurement system in the particular laboratory, an *exact* determination of the *actual diameter* of the valve annulus is made or calculated utilizing an *accurate* reference system for calibration of the measurements. As discussed earlier in Chapter 11, the use of the diameter of a catheter as the reference measurement is not satisfactory, and, in fact, creates dangerous errors when measuring large structures such as valves and large vessels. A calibrated "marker" catheter, which is positioned exactly in the angiographic field, is frequently used and represents a very accurate reference system for calibration. The measuring "bands" on the calibrated catheter are placed in the plane of the valve and aligned *exactly* perpendicular to the left ventricular outflow tract during the injection for the valve measurement. The catheter tip can be either in the aortic root, left ventricular outflow tract, or even in the left ventricular apex. Often the catheter moves during a pressure injection and as a consequence of this movement, the "marker bands" on the catheter will usually align precisely on edge for the calibration measurements during at least several frames of the angiogram. If not, the catheter is repositioned to align the marks on edge before either the X-ray tubes, the table or the patient are moved and a very brief "cine" of the *exactly aligned* marks is recorded with the new catheter position.

As an alternative, a "marker" catheter can be positioned in the superior vena cava immediately adjacent to the aortic root, and in this position it serves as a precise calibration reference in the same reference plane as the aortic valve. The separate marker catheter in the superior vena cava, simultaneously with the use of the transseptal technique, necessitates the use of an additional venous line for the marker catheter. Similarly, a marker catheter can be introduced into the esophagus with the "marks" positioned in a location immediately behind the cardiac silhouette and adjacent to the aortic valve and, in that position, used as an accurate reference system for calibration. Some X-ray systems have calibration marks embedded in the image intensifier screen. The changes in the distance of these marks to the "isocenter" of the image are computed constantly and accurately by the sophisticated computer system, which allows the use of these marks for a very accurate calibration reference regardless of the position and distance of the intensifier. When such a built-in calibration reference system is available and it is verified against a grid or marker catheter reference system, it is the most convenient and accurate calibration system available.

An external grid or a metal "sphere" of a known, precise diameter *placed in the exact plane of the valve* as described in Chapter 11 (Angiography) can also be used as the *accurate* calibration reference. The external grid or sphere is a very accurate but very inconvenient reference system.

Once the measurements of the valve annulus have been completed, the X-ray tubes are placed in the positions that will be utilized during the valve dilation. Biplane records of the best images of the valve from both planes of the biplane angiograms in this same angulation are stored in a "freeze frame" to be used as a "road map" during the valve dilation. If there is not a good "freeze frame" replay capability available, it is useful to place tiny lead markers on the chest wall exactly over the area of the aortic valve annulus on the fluoroscopic image. Fluoroscopy is used to align the "lead" marks on the chest wall according to the location of the valve as seen on the previous angiocardiograms in the same X-ray views.

The long transseptal sheath is advanced over the catheter and into the left ventricle. An "active deflector wire" is introduced through a wire back-bleed/flush valve into the original angiographic catheter and the catheter is deflected 180° toward the aortic valve. While holding the curve on the deflector wire and fixing the wire in place, the catheter is advanced *off the wire*, through the left ventricular outflow tract, and into the aorta. This is accomplished readily when an end-hole or angiographic *woven dacron* catheter is used. These catheters become very soft and flexible after only a few minutes in the circulation at body temperature, and as a consequence are relatively atraumatic and easily deflected.

An alternative technique for advancing a catheter from the left ventricle into the aorta is to use a floating balloon catheter through the long sheath, which is positioned in the left ventricle. The original angiographic catheter is removed from the long sheath while the long sheath is maintained in position in the left ventricle. The long sheath is cleared thoroughly of all air and/or clot. The distal end of a floating balloon angiographic catheter, which is at least *one French size smaller than the sheath*, is "pulled" or softened in heat and then formed into at least a 180° curve at the distal end. The balloon angiographic catheter is introduced into the long sheath and advanced through the sheath and into the left ventricle. During the introduction and the entire time the balloon catheter is being advanced within the sheath, both the sheath and the catheter are maintained on a *constant* flush. Once the balloon tip is beyond the sheath in the left ventricle, the balloon catheter and sheath are switched to pressure monitoring, the balloon is inflated with CO_2, and usually, using minimal manipulations, the balloon catheter floats out of the left ventricle, across the stenotic valve, and into the ascending aorta. In the presence of a very tight stenosis, the balloon must often be deflated partially, or even completely, just beneath the valve in order for the catheter to pass through the stenotic orifice. Occasionally the "active deflector wire" is used along with the floating balloon catheter in order to redirect the catheter tip 180° away from the apex and toward the valve.

Once a catheter has passed into the aorta, simultaneous left ventricular, aortic root, and femoral artery pressures are recorded, with the left ventricle pressure recorded from the side arm of the sheath, the ascending aortic pressure from the catheter, and the femoral pressure from the femoral line. These pressures provide the true peak-to-peak hemodynamic gradient across the *valve* and a comparison with the original left ventricle to femoral artery pressures. In order to obtain even better visualization of the valve leaflets, an aortic root aortogram is recorded through this prograde catheter. The soft catheter alone passing through the valve does not produce significant artifactual aortic regurgitation. When the aortic root angiogram has been recorded, the prograde catheter is advanced further out of the ventricle and the tip advanced around the arch and into the descending aorta (at least beyond the brachiocephalic trunk!). When the hemodynamics have been recorded, both the catheter and the transseptal sheath are placed on a slow continuous flush. The transseptal sheath remains in the left ventricle and the catheter in the descending aorta before, during and after the dilation procedure. This allows simultaneous aortic and left ventricular pressure monitoring and recording during and *immediately after* the dilation procedure. In addition, both the catheter in the aorta and the transseptal sheath in the left ventricle serve as routes for rapid infusions of intracardiac fluids or medications. Of equal importance, the shaft of the catheter that is passing through the stenotic orifice of the aortic valve serves as a visible and definitive "guide" for the subsequent introduction of the retrograde wires/catheters across the valve.

With the prograde catheters in place and the measurements of the valve completed, the balloons for the dilation are chosen and prepared. Extra long balloons are used for balloon dilation of the aortic valve. For smaller patients (and usually smaller 10 and 12 mm diameter balloons), a 4 cm balloon length is used, and for larger patients (and usually larger balloon diameters), 6–8 cm long balloons are used when available. The combination of the double-balloon technique, the use of super stiff wires, and the use of longer balloons, virtually eliminates the problem of the balloons squirting or bouncing in and out of the valve and further damaging the valve during the balloon inflations.

The combined inflated diameters of the *two balloons* for a double-balloon dilation is equal to a maximum of 1.2 to 1.3 times the maximum accurately measured diameter of the aortic annulus. If a single-balloon technique is used, the single balloon diameter to start with is no more than 0.9 to 1 times the diameter of the accurately measured annulus.

For the usual balloon dilation of the aortic valve, the balloons undergo a standard preparation in order to clear them *completely* of any air before introduction into the systemic circulation. A "minimal balloon preparation" similar to the balloon preparation in very small and/or critically ill infants is used when there is concern that the standard balloon prep would increase the deflated balloon profile enough to necessitate a larger arterial sheath. The "minimal balloon preparation" is intended to clear a balloon of air *completely*, but at the same time not to "unfold" it from its "factory wrap" around the catheter.

With the prograde aortic catheter in place across the valve and the dilation balloon(s) prepared, the inguinal areas around the arterial puncture sites are re-infiltrated liberally with 2% xylocaine. The indwelling arterial cannulae are replaced with sheath/dilator sets that will accommodate the balloons chosen for the dilation. An end-hole catheter that accommodates a 0.035" guide wire is passed retrograde around the arch and into the aortic root from one of the arterial sheaths.

Crossing the stenotic aortic valve with the wire(s) and then positioning the catheter(s)/wire(s) securely and safely in the left ventricle is often the most difficult part of the aortic valve dilation procedure. The aortic root is often very dilated and distorted, with the stenotic orifice of the valve located very eccentrically.

The course of the prograde catheter passing through the stenotic valve from the left ventricle into the aorta provides the most reliable technique for identifying the exact position and "direction" of the stenotic orifice, and is a valuable asset for crossing the stenotic aortic valve from the retrograde approach. The course of the catheter passing through the valve orifice provides a visible "guide" to the actual course from the left ventricle, through the narrow and otherwise invisible orifice, and into the aorta.

In the absence of a prograde catheter through the valve, the valve leaflets themselves and the valve orifice are "invisible" on the fluoroscopy and are only identified by comparing the fluoroscopic image to the "jet" of contrast passing through the orifice on the previous angiographic recording. The "freeze frame" of that recording is used as a guide in "finding" the valve orifice during the retrograde approach.

A torque-control catheter with a preformed, slightly curved tip, together with a steerable wire with a slightly curved soft tip, are used to maneuver across the valve. A preformed right or left coronary catheter is most useful for directing the tip of the wire toward the aortic valve orifice. Occasionally the preformed retrograde catheter itself can be directed purposefully and precisely along the course of the prograde catheter and through the valve orifice. Usually crossing the stenotic orifice requires the use of the combination of several catheters and wires, even with a prograde catheter serving as a guide. Rotating the shaft of a catheter clockwise or counterclockwise with the preformed tip positioned in the aortic root, moves the catheter tip (and wire) *anteriorly or posteriorly*. Moving the shaft of the catheter forward and backward moves the curved tip of the catheter (and, in turn, the wire tip) from *side to side* in the aortic root.

The prograde catheter passing through the valve orifice provides the exact "route" through the valve orifice, which is visualized simultaneously as the wire is manipulated through the retrograde catheter. The combination of the known location of the orifice, which is delineated precisely by the course of the prograde catheter through the orifice, and the precise control over the direction of the wire tip, allows the operator to maneuver the tip of the wire purposefully, precisely along and immediately adjacent to the prograde catheter. In contrast to the rapid, repeated maneuvers used during a "blind" probing with a wire at a stenotic aortic valve, the maneuvers with the catheter and the wire when "following along the prograde catheter" are carried out slowly and purposefully. The tip of the wire is observed frequently on both PA and lateral fluoroscopy as the wire is "tracked along" the prograde catheter. This maneuvering of the wire into the ventricle is still not "automatic" and may take several attempts, each with a readjustment of the angle of approach of the wire to the valve. Occasionally, when the angle of the valve orifice is very distorted, it is necessary to change to a catheter with a completely different preformed curve at the tip in order to angle the wire properly at the orifice. A very soft tipped wire can create a problem with this technique. With a very tight stenosis, the high velocity of the jet of blood through the orifice, literally, blows the tip of a very soft tipped wire away from the orifice. When this problem occurs repeatedly, a wire with a slightly stiffer tip is used to accomplish the retrograde crossing of the valve. The technique of tracking along the "adjunct" prograde catheter to guide the retrograde wire through the valve represents the most definitive technique available for crossing the stenotic aortic valve from a retrograde approach.

Some operators prefer not to go through the extra maneuvering for the adjunct prograde catheter technique, and occasionally the prograde catheter from the left ventricle into the aorta cannot be used or accomplished, especially in very small, very sick infants. Various other "tricks" are described for crossing the stenotic aortic valves from the retrograde approach without the adjunct prograde catheter. Most of the techniques first involve the positioning of a precurved, end-hole catheter retrograde into the aortic root. An attempt is often made using the retrograde catheter itself to probe at the "invisible" orifice. A soft tipped catheter is "bounced" gently, rapidly and repeatedly off the valve and occasionally even "backs" through a tight orifice with a 180° loop formed on the catheter. A catheter with a *stiff* tip should *never* be used with this technique. A stiff catheter tip repeatedly bounced off of a stenotic valve can easily *create an orifice* by perforating a leaflet!

When there is no prograde catheter through the valve, a very *soft tip*, small diameter, spring guide wire is maneuvered toward the valve through a precurved, end-hole, retrograde catheter, somewhat similar to the catheter/wire maneuvers just described. The main difference is that the wire is advanced rapidly and repeatedly, in and out of the catheter tip while the angle of the catheter tip is changed repeatedly. This, in turn, bounces, or backs the wire tip in and out of the aortic sinuses until the tip or a loop of the wire eventually falls (somewhat accidentally) through the valve opening. Since the valve leaflets and the orifice are *not visible at all*, this requires rapid, but patient, repetitions rather than any particular skill. The more repetitive "probes" at the valve—each with a change in the direction of the wire by changing the catheter tip position —the more likely is the *chance* of crossing the valve. This is the opposite of tracking along a known course of a prograde catheter through the valve and is an instance where slow, meticulous catheter and/or wire manipulations definitely are *not* indicated. Slow maneuvers in this situation increase the radiation used and, at the same time, decrease the "chances" of hitting the valve orifice per unit time of fluoroscopy used. If one particular wire/catheter combination does not accomplish crossing the valve after several minutes of rapid "probing", the wire and/or the catheter is/are exchanged. A similar "probing" at the valve with the new catheter/wire combination is used.

Although a very soft tipped wire is unlikely to perforate a valve cusp, there *are* potential problems associated with the rapid probing technique. With the rapid in and out movements of the wire, occasionally the wire drops through the valve, but is pulled back and out of the ventricle before the position is recognized because of the rapidity of the maneuvering. This is even more likely in the presence of a markedly distorted aortic root/valve or an unusual course into the ventricle. A more serious problem is the inadvertent and unrecognized cannulation of a coronary artery with the wire/catheter. As the aortic root is probed, the wire passes from the coronary sinus into a coronary artery often more easily than through the stenotic valve. In the presence of a markedly distorted aortic root, the abnormal wire position in the coronary artery can go unnoticed. When the soft tipped wire only is advanced into the coronary artery, it usually does not create a problem, but if the wire is advanced far into the coronary, particularly if the catheter is advanced over the wire deep into the coronary thinking it is in the ventricle, the coronary artery can be damaged. The treatment for this potential problem is awareness and prevention.

Perforation of an aortic valve leaflet during the retrograde probing of an aortic valve is a constant potential problem. When the tip of the retrograde *catheter* is deep into, or actually becomes *buried* in the aortic sinus and then a wire is advanced out of the catheter tip, the wire does not have room to "buckle" or bend and the wire is then more likely to perforate directly through the valve tissue in front of it—particularly the tissue of a thin valve leaflet. If a valve leaflet is perforated by the wire and then a dilation balloon is passed over the wire through the perforation, the valve will be destroyed rather than dilated! The stiffer the wire and/or the catheter that is used for the retrograde probing of the aortic valve, the less ability the wire and/or catheter has of "buckling away" from the aortic sinuses and the greater the potential for this type of leaflet perforation. Even the "soft" tip of a "standard" 0.025″ spring guide wire is *very stiff* for the first few millimeters as it extends out of the tip of a catheter.

A Terumo™ (or Glide™) wire creates an equal or probably greater problem of perforation of the aortic leaflets when it is used to pass retrograde across an aortic valve. Terumo™ wires become much stiffer and much sharper when they have no room to "buckle" between the tip of the catheter and the structure/tissue it is attempting to cross. The Terumo™ wire also "glides" *through* the tissues easily once it does perforate, and as a consequence an abnormal course of the wire within tissues can go unrecognized.

The "blind" retrograde probing technique for crossing the valve usually and eventually is successful, however, it has obvious drawbacks. Crossing the valve depends more on chance and multiple repeated attempts than on any skill. The use of biplane imaging to help "identify" the location of the orifice in "three dimensions" is essential to the success of this as well as all of the other techniques for crossing the aortic valve. Even when the valve, and particularly the orifice of the valve, are not visible, the second plane of fluoroscopy allows the operator to know when the catheter/wire is repeatedly probing in a totally inappropriate or non-productive area of a valve sinus.

Once the left ventricle has been entered with the retrograde catheter and/or wire using whatever combination of retrograde wires, special catheters or special curves happen to work most effectively in the particular patient, a soft, curved tipped, spring guide wire is advanced retrograde as far as possible into the ventricle. When this wire has been secured in the ventricle, an angled, end-hole catheter is advanced over the wire into the ventricle. With a combination of pushing and backing maneuvers of both the wire and the catheter, the tip of the retrograde *catheter* in the ventricle is deflected and directed 180° back toward the aortic valve. When the angled end-hole catheter cannot be directed fairly expeditiously back toward the aortic valve, the original angled catheter is exchanged for a pig-tail catheter over the original wire positioned in the left ventricle. Once the pig-tail catheter passes over the wire and the pig-tail curve is positioned securely in the left ventricular apex, the original wire is removed and replaced with the larger, long floppy tipped, preformed, stiff, exchange length wire, which should almost automatically point toward the left ventricular outflow tract when it is advanced out of the catheter tip.

The largest diameter exchange wire that the balloon catheters chosen for the dilation will accommodate is introduced at this time. In larger patients, the exchange wire is a 0.035″, Super Stiff™ exchange length wire with a long floppy tip. This wire should have a "J" or, even, a >360° pig-tail curve formed manually at its distal floppy tip and a second more proximal, smooth, but short 180° curve formed at the "transition area" between the rigid part and the floppy portion of the wire. The preformed 180° curve at the transition area of the wire will allow the *stiff* portion of the wire to be completely across the valve when the 180° curve at the transition area is seated in the apex of the ventricle. Either the original retrograde, angled, end-hole catheter looping 180° toward the outflow tract or the pig-tail catheter in the apex of the left ventricle directs the tip of the Super Stiff™ wire back toward the left ventricular outflow tract and allows the 180° curve on the stiff portion of the wire to "seat" in the apex of the left ventricle. The tip of the wire is then directed back toward the LV outflow tract or even back across the aortic valve.

When the double-balloon aortic dilation technique is used, the catheter is left in position over the first wire and a slow flush is maintained around the wire while the second wire/catheter is positioned[5]. Once the first stiff wire is in a stable position, the opposite groin is infiltrated liberally with xylocaine. A second sheath/dilator set is introduced into the opposite femoral artery. An angled, end-hole catheter, identical to the catheter which was initially used to cross the valve, is introduced into the second arterial sheath and passed retrograde around the arch. The second catheter is maneuvered retrograde through the orifice and into the left ventricle "following" the first catheter/wire precisely while using the course of the first wire/catheter through the valve orifice to serve as a visible guide for introducing the second wire even if an adjunct prograde catheter was not used. Once the second wire has passed into the ventricle, the angled end-hole catheter is advanced into the ventricle and curved back toward the outflow tract similar to the positioning of the first catheter. When an 180° curve cannot be formed in the ventricle with the angled end-hole retrograde catheter, it is replaced with a pig-tail catheter, which is positioned in the left ventricular apex adjacent to the first wire. A second teflon-coated stiff exchange wire is pre-shaped, identical to the first exchange wire, passed through the second catheter, and positioned in the left ventricle adjacent to and in a similar position to the first wire.

Once the two stiff wires are in a satisfactory, stable position within the ventricle, the end-hole catheters are removed over the wires and the previously prepared balloons are introduced over the wires. It is important that the wires are observed continuously and maintained precisely and securely in their positions during the introduction of the balloons through the sheath and during the process of advancing the balloon catheters retrograde around the arch. The portions of the wires that are outside of the body are maintained straight and are fixed against a firm structure on the table (or against the patient's leg) while the wires and the balloon catheters within the body are observed frequently with fluoroscopy. The wires outside of the body are adjusted in or out slightly in order to keep the left ventricular wire loops from being withdrawn from, or pushed further into (through!) the ventricle during the various manipulations of the balloon catheters. This is important particularly when the balloon catheters are being maneuvered next to each other. The balloons are maneuvered over the wires to a position just above the aortic valve. The two wires are advanced toward the apex of the ventricle until all "slack" is out of the wires and the wires are pushed against the outer circumference of the course from the descending aorta, around the aortic arch, and into the ascending aorta.

Once *all* of the preparations are ready for the *controlled pressure inflation* of the two balloons, the two wires are fixed in position and the balloons are advanced one at a time over the wires and across the aortic valve. The position of the balloons in the aortic valve is compared with the "freeze frame" image of the valve. With the balloons in their proper position, the area of the valve leaflets should be exactly in the center of the two markers at the end of each balloon. This positions the center of the parallel surfaces of the balloons at the narrowest portion of the valve. If the balloons are unstable in the initial position across the valve, they are advanced further over the wires toward the apex of the ventricle while maintaining the parallel walls of the balloons in the narrow portion of the valve and keeping the curved wires in the apex of the left ventricle. This readjustment is easier and safer when using longer dilation balloons. If a balloon is too far within the ventricle, the *wire* is advanced gently in order to push the balloon back rather than withdrawing the balloon. This maneuver maintains the wires at the "outer circumference" of the course around the arch and maintains better control over the wires.

In very severe valve obstruction, the passage of the first deflated balloon across the narrow orifice can cause a sudden and dramatic deterioration in the patient's hemodynamics. In this circumstance, the first balloon is positioned rapidly in the valve, inflated, deflated and withdrawn back into the aortic root. The patient is allowed to stabilize (or is resuscitated) before attempting to position the second balloon. The subsequent positioning of the two balloons is accomplished as rapidly as possible and followed immediately by simultaneous *rapid* inflation/deflation of the two balloons. All inflations/deflations of the balloons during a dilation procedure are recorded on either biplane angiography or "stored fluoroscopy".

During the dilation, the balloons are inflated until the indentations or "waists" in the balloons caused by the stenotic valve disappear or until the balloons reach their maximum advertised pressure, whichever comes first. As soon as the balloons reach this full inflation, they are deflated *as rapidly as possible*. During the balloon inflation in the aortic valve, almost total obstruction of all cardiac output is created by the fully inflated balloon(s). The heart rate slows, the systemic arterial pressure (monitored through the prograde arterial catheter still passing through the valve or through the side arm of one of the arterial sheaths) drops, and the left ventricular pressure (monitored through the transseptal sheath still positioned in the ventricle) increases markedly. With *a successful dilation of the valve*, these hemodynamic parameters rapidly return to "normal" once the balloons are deflated, however, the balloons should be withdrawn rapidly over the wires and back into the aortic root to be sure of, and to facilitate, this recovery.

The inflation/deflation of the balloons is repeated several times, changing the positions of the balloons before each subsequent inflation by moving them in and out of the valve slightly and, if possible, changing their relative anterior/posterior/lateral relationships in the process. With the pressures available through the long sheath in the left ventricle and through the prograde catheter positioned in the aorta, the hemodynamic results of the dilation are known as soon as the balloons have been deflated and without moving the balloon catheters. The end point of the dilation is the absence of any "waist" on the balloons *during the initial phase* of subsequent inflations *and* a reduction of the gradient across the valve to less than 25 mmHg. The left ventricular pressure should approach normal or near normal as monitored by the indwelling transseptal sheath(s).

Occasionally, the heart rate and blood pressures do not return to normal very rapidly after the inflation/deflation. When this return of heart rate/blood pressure is slow, or appears non-existent, if not already accomplished, the balloons are withdrawn over the wires, out of, and away from, the valve. The patient is given atropine through the left ventricle sheath and if necessary given several external manual compressions to stimulate cardiac function. With even partial relief of the aortic obstruction the heart rate and pressure do return.

Before making the *final* post-dilation hemodynamic measurements, both balloons are withdrawn back over the wires into at least the descending aorta so that the only "equipment" passing through the valve is the two retrograde wires and the prograde balloon catheter, which is positioned in the aorta. The residual gradient across the valve is recorded from the pressure in the left ventricle (through the sheath) and the pressure in the aorta (through the prograde catheter) and/or one of the femoral artery pressures through the side arm of the femoral artery sheath. The pressure gradient and the contour of the pulse curves give an excellent immediate indication of the results of the procedure before the removal of any catheters or wires. With a very successful relief of the obstruction, the left ventricular systolic pressure approximates the aortic systolic pressure, the left ventricular end-diastolic pressure is less than 15 mmHg, the gradient across the aortic valve is abolished or reduced to less than 20 mmHg and there is little or no aortic valve regurgitation.

When mild, or no aortic regurgitation is produced, the pulse pressure is 25–30 mmHg even with the prograde catheter and the wires still across the valve. An aortic root angiocardiogram to assess aortic regurgitation is recorded with injection through the prograde catheter. This injection *helps* to assess the aortic regurgitation, particularly if there is a wide pulse pressure. If there is significant aortic regurgitation but good relief of the obstruction, nothing further therapeutic is performed in the catheterization laboratory at this time. If there is a *significant residual gradient and significant aortic regurgitation* as demonstrated by the post-dilation pulse pressure or the aortogram, the wires are removed from across the aortic valve in order to assess the aortic regurgitation more accurately. Occasionally, a stiff wire is forced against one side of the annulus and "holds the valve open", creating false aortic valve regurgitation. Once the wires across the annulus have been withdrawn, the aortic regurgitation is reassessed with repeat pressure measurements and a repeat aortic root aortogram. The prograde catheter passing through the valve alone does not, or very rarely, produce *significant* aortic regurgitation. However, if significant aortic valve regurgitation is demonstrated from the injection through the prograde catheter, the prograde catheter is withdrawn into the ventricle and a repeat aortic root angiocardiogram performed with an injection in the aortic root through a retrograde catheter. If there is still significant aortic regurgitation, regardless of any residual gradient, no further dilation is performed.

If dilation with the original balloons did not produce sufficient relief of the obstruction, but also did *not* produce significant aortic valve regurgitation, the angiographic images of the balloon inflations and the post-dilation angiograms are reviewed. The diameters of the inflated balloon(s) and valve annulus are re-measured accurately on these angiograms of the inflations. If angiographically the balloon diameters are the same or smaller than the diameter of the annulus, the combined balloon diameters are increased up to 1.2 times the annulus diameter and the dilation repeated. If the balloon diameters are 1.2 times (or more) larger than the aortic annulus on the angiographic images of the balloon inflation, no further dilation is attempted. If a single balloon is used for the dilation and the balloon is exactly the same diameter as the annulus on the inflation images, the balloon diameter is increased by at most 10% and the dilation is repeated.

When the transseptal sheath and prograde catheter were not used during the procedure, there are several alternative techniques to record the postdilation pressures *before* the wires are removed. A separate, new transseptal procedure can be performed to enter the left heart and left ventricle. The left ventricular pressure through the transseptal catheter is compared with the femoral artery pressure measured through the side arm of one of the femoral artery sheaths. Another alternative technique is to remove one balloon dilation catheter over the wire. The wire is maintained in the left ventricle and the balloon dilation catheter is replaced over this wire with a Multi-Track™ catheter. The Multi-Track™ catheter is advanced retrograde over the wire all the way to the left ventricle. Pressures from the Multi-Track™ catheter can be recorded from any location along the course of the wire during either the introduction or the withdrawal of the Multi-Track™ catheter and with the wire remaining in place. Angiograms can also be recorded at any location through an angiographic Multi-Track™ catheter. By using the Multi-Track™ catheter, the retrograde wire is still in place in the ventricle without any further manipulations of the wire if a new balloon dilation catheter must be introduced for a repeat dilation.

The third, and least attractive alternative to either of these previous techniques for reassessment of the hemodynamics post-dilation is to withdraw one of the retrograde balloon dilation catheters over the wire and completely out of the body while leaving the wire in the left ventricle. The balloon catheter is replaced with an end-hole diagnostic catheter, which is passed over the wire, retrograde, all of the way to the left ventricle. The wire is then removed completely. The left ventricular pressure is measured through this catheter and compared with the femoral arterial pressure measured through the side arm of the other arterial sheath. If the simultaneous pressures following the dilation demonstrate an unsatisfactory relief of the obstruction, an aortic root aortogram to assess aortic regurgitation *cannot* be obtained without withdrawing this catheter out of its position in the ventricle. Once the catheter is withdrawn and if the dilation *does* need to be repeated, one retrograde wire still is passing through the valve and into the ventricle. This wire serves as a "guide" along which the wire/catheter is directed during the reintroduction of the retrograde catheter back into the ventricle. Once the catheter is positioned back in the ventricle, the stiff exchange wire is re-advanced through this catheter and repositioned *in the ventricle* for introduction of the new balloons.

Once it is determined that a satisfactory relief of the aortic obstruction has been obtained, the balloon catheters are withdrawn slowly over the wires and out of the vessels. As they are withdrawn, the balloon catheters are rotated in the direction of the balloon folds and the *negative pressure* to the balloons is ***released*** during the withdrawal through the aorta and out through the sheaths.

Occasionally the retrograde wires, with their preformed loops and curves, become entangled in the ventricular structures. Once the balloon catheters have been withdrawn out of the sheaths, end-hole catheters are advanced over the wires and into the ventricle. While observing on fluoroscopy, the wires are removed *through these catheters*. Withdrawing them through catheters prevents the wires from damaging or disrupting chordae or papillary muscles around which they may have been entrapped.

There is an additional technique for the guaranteed introduction of a balloon dilation catheter retrograde across even the most stenotic aortic valve. This technique is used only when the aortic valve is particularly difficult or impossible to cross with any of the previous retrograde catheter/wire techniques. This technique is most suitable for a single-balloon dilation technique but can be used for a dilation using double balloons. The technique is a variation of the use of the prograde catheter along with the retrograde technique, but does add some additional complex maneuvering to the procedure. An *end-hole*, floating balloon catheter is introduced prograde into the left ventricle through a long transseptal sheath. The end-hole balloon catheter is advanced (floated) prograde across the aortic valve and into the descending aorta. An extra long (400 cm), exchange length, spring guide wire is passed through the prograde catheter and into the descending aorta. A snare catheter is introduced retrograde from a femoral artery and the distal end of the prograde wire, which was advanced through the prograde catheter, is snared with the retrograde snare and withdrawn out through the femoral artery sheath. This produces a "through and through" wire from the femoral vein to the right atrium, left atrium, left ventricle, through the aortic valve, into the aorta, and out through the femoral artery. The desired balloon dilation catheter is introduced over the *arterial end* of the wire, through an arterial sheath, advanced retrograde over the through and through wire and through the aortic valve. For a double-balloon technique this procedure is repeated from the other femoral artery and a second femoral vein. The position(s) of the balloon(s) in the aortic valve is/are adjusted with the catheters and wires and the dilation of the valve carried out similarly to any other balloon dilation of the aortic valve.

This technique guarantees that the balloon dilation catheters cross the aortic valve *orifice* and provides the maximum control over the position and movement of the balloons during the inflation/deflation. At the same time it does add some complexity to the procedure. The femoral artery and left ventricular pressures can be measured simultaneously before, during and immediately after the dilation through a side arm of the transseptal sheath and a side arm of the arterial introductory sheath since, in order to accommodate the passage of even the deflated dilation balloon, the sheath lumen is always larger than the *shaft* of the balloon dilation catheter.

With the through and through wires in place, the balloon dilation catheters are easily exchanged or removed. Once the dilation of the aortic valve is completed successfully, the balloon dilation catheters are withdrawn over the wires and replaced with end-hole catheters, which are advanced retrograde over the wires and into the left ventricular apex. Once the catheters are *in place over the wires* the wires are withdrawn through the long sheaths from the venous end. The retrograde catheters prevent the stiff wires from cutting intracardiac structures when they "tighten" as they are withdrawn.

When the catheters and wires have been withdrawn out of the sheaths, more local anesthesia is administered liberally around the sheaths at the arterial puncture sites, and the sheaths are withdrawn. Direct manual pressure is applied over the arterial puncture sites to stop local bleeding. Either the dorsalis pedis or the posterior tibial pulse in the same extremity as the puncture is palpated simultaneously while holding pressure on the artery, being sure that the peripheral pulse is not obliterated by the pressure applied to obtain the hemostasis. Pressure is maintained balancing the control of bleeding vs. the peripheral pulse until hemostasis is achieved. The systemic heparin is not usually reversed, so achieving hemostasis safely after the removal of a large sheath can take up to an hour or more.

After hemostasis is achieved, a *very light* bandage just to cover the puncture site is applied. The bleeding should be controlled before the bandage is applied. A tight compression pressure bandage is ***not*** used over the artery. The bandage is left in place for 4–6 hours. The patient is observed in a monitored recovery bed for a minimum of four hours and until they are fully awake. Particular attention is paid to the puncture site and the pulses in the extremity *peripheral* to the puncture site. The "Foley" catheter is left in place until males are awake and until females are moved out of the recovery ward. Patients who undergo aortic valve dilation are observed in the hospital overnight. On the assumption that all of the adrenergic stress and any volume load from the catheterization are dissipated by the following morning, these patients usually undergo an echocardiogram before discharge on the day following the catheterization. This echo information serves as the baseline, non-invasive value for subsequent follow-up evaluations. The patient is discharged with no imposed limitations *because of the catheterization*.

Infant and/or critical aortic stenosis dilation

The diagnosis of aortic stenosis is made from the clinical findings and is based more on the appearance of the valve by echocardiogram and the associated poor left ventricular function rather than on a "gradient"[4]. Dilation of aortic stenosis in the newborn or small infant is one of, if not the most difficult and dangerous procedures performed by pediatric interventional cardiologists. The dilation of infant aortic stenosis is not just a "small version" of any other aortic valve dilation. The newborn or small infant requiring treatment of aortic stenosis is usually very sick, often is on prostaglandin and requires inotropic support before and during the valve dilation procedure. The vascular access is small, particularly in proportion to the sheaths, catheters, wires and balloons that are available for small infants.

These patients usually do have a patent interatrial communication allowing the introduction of a prograde venous catheter into the left ventricle. A left ventricular catheter remaining in place throughout the procedure is invaluable for pressure monitoring and, occasionally, for a left ventricular angiocardiogram. In the *very sick* and small infant, once the left ventricle is entered with the prograde catheter, this catheter is not advanced further into the aorta at this time unless a prograde approach for the dilation is anticipated. When there is no naturally occurring atrial communication, the decision is made at the onset of the procedure as to whether acquiring the hemodynamic information from the left ventricle before it is entered retrograde is worth the extra effort and slightly increased risk of a transseptal puncture in a very small infant.

With meticulous attention to detail, patience, very delicate technique, and some special instrumentation, percutaneous entry into a femoral artery essentially always is accomplished, even in small infants. Small, sick infants are the patients in whom the special 21-gauge percutaneous needles and the *extra* floppy tipped 0.018″ wires are invaluable for entering the artery (Chapter 4). A "single-wall" puncture technique is always attempted. Once the artery is cannulated with the guide wire, the surrounding area to the puncture site is re-infiltrated liberally with local anesthesia. A 3- or 4-French (depending upon the balloon to be used), fine or "feathered" tipped sheath/dilator set is introduced into the artery. Once the sheath is secured in the artery and cleared of any air, an end-hole, pre-curved right coronary catheter is introduced through the sheath and advanced retrograde to the aortic root.

The aortic pressures and aortic root angiocardiograms are performed with the retrograde catheter. This catheter allows baseline pressure measurements, and satisfactory aortic root aortogram(s) can be obtained with end-hole catheters in these small infants. At the same time, an angled, end-hole catheter is the most useful for manipulation of the guide wire across the stenotic valve for the subsequent dilation, all without an unnecessary exchange of catheters. Only one arterial catheter is necessary since a single-balloon, retrograde approach is used for dilation of the aortic valve in small infants. However, if the other femoral artery is entered inadvertently during the puncture of the vessels, it is cannulated with a 20-Gauge, teflon Quick-Cath™ for continual arterial monitoring throughout the procedure.

The "venous" catheter previously positioned in the left ventricle along with the arterial line allows recording of simultaneous left ventricular and aortic pressures. This *helps* to confirm the severity of the aortic stenosis, however, in these infants with poor left ventricular function, the gradient, particularly in very severe aortic stenosis, is often minimal. A left ventriculogram is not usually necessary and potentially is dangerous in a critically ill infant. If a ventriculogram is desired, it is recorded with injection in the left ventricle through the prograde catheter. When the left ventriculogram is accomplished before the valve is crossed, it helps to localize the area of the valve *orifice*.

The diameter of the aortic valve annulus is measured very accurately from the aortic root injection or the left ventricular angiocardiogram. Once the valve measurements are obtained, the appropriate dilation balloon for the aortic valve dilation is chosen and prepared *before* an attempt is made at crossing the valve. The balloon chosen is equal in diameter to the aortic annulus measured at the valve hinge points. The preferred balloons for very small infant and neonatal aortic valve dilations currently are the very small Tyshak Mini™ (NuMED Inc., Hopkinton, NY) balloons. The Tyshak Mini™ balloons up to 8 mm in diameter pass through a 3-French sheath while the 9 and 10 mm Mini™ balloons require a 4-French sheath. The Mini™ balloons, however, accept only a 0.014″ wire. The Hi-Torque Iron Man™ wire (Guidant Corp, Santa Clara, CA) is as effective a wire as any available for supporting these balloons. The dilation balloon is prepared using a "minimal prep" technique. The stenotic aortic valve is crossed only after the balloon has been prepared and is ready to be introduced. These infants are so precarious that the 3- or 4-French catheter alone crossing the stenotic orifice is enough to occlude the orifice and cause the infants to decompensate acutely and occasionally irreversibly.

A 3- or 4-French, pre-curved right or left Judkins™ coronary catheter or a 3- or 4-French curve-tipped multipurpose catheter is advanced retrograde into the aortic root from the femoral artery. To cross the aortic valves in a neonate, a 0.014″ or a 0.018″ very *floppy* tipped exchange length, torque-controlled guide wire is used. The wire used depends upon what the balloon chosen for the dilation will accommodate. When a 0.018″ wire can be used, a Platinum Plus™ (Boston Scientific, Natick, MA) or a V-18 Control™ (Boston Scientific, Natick, MA) wire is very useful both for crossing the valve and for supporting the dilation balloon across the valve. A very slight curve is formed at the tip of the wire to allow changes in direction when torquing the wire. The wire is advanced through the pre-curved catheter positioned in the aortic root.

Crossing the aortic valve in the neonate is similar to the "blind" crossing in an older patient except that all structures are much smaller and, in turn, all catheter manipulations are much finer. Occasionally, the pre-curved catheter will pass through the stenotic orifice when maneuvered directly at the valve. Crossing with the catheter is attempted several times while simultaneously rotating and moving the catheter in and out in the aortic root. When the catheter does not cross the valve, the catheter tip is positioned at least one centimeter above the valve and the very soft tip of a fine guide wire is manipulated out of the catheter. The wire is directed toward the aortic valve orifice by almost continuously rotating the catheter while simultaneously moving both the catheter and the wire to and fro. Multiple, rapidly repeated, short probes are made with the wire toward the aortic valve orifice rather than any slow, methodical maneuvers. The exact location of this orifice really is not known unless another wire or catheter is already passing through the valve. The more "probes" that are made with the wire during the simultaneous, multiple changes in the angle/direction of the wire, the more likely is the tip of the wire to cross the valve. If the wire does not cross the valve after several minutes of trying with the first angled catheter and wire, the catheter and/or the wire are replaced with either the right or left coronary catheter or the multipurpose catheter—whichever was not used initially—and the "probing" with the wire is repeated during continual changes in the direction of the catheter tip. Eventually, more by chance than skill, the wire crosses the valve into the ventricle.

Once the wire crosses the valve, it is advanced as far as possible into the ventricle, hopefully even looping the soft tip of the wire within the apex of the left ventricle. With the wire advanced as far as possible into the ventricle, the catheter is advanced over the wire to the ventricular apex. If the infant remains stable with the *end-hole catheter* passed through the valve, the catheter is fixed in the ventricle and the wire is removed. Preferably, the original fine, soft tipped wire is replaced through the catheter positioned in the left ventricle with a stiffer, exchange length wire of the largest diameter that the prepared balloon will accommodate. The stiffer wire should be pre-shaped before introduction into the catheter/ventricle. A "pig-tail" curve is formed on the long floppy tip of the new guide wire and a 180° curve, which conforms to the cavity size at the ventricular apex, is formed at the transition zone of the wire between the long floppy tip and the stiff shaft of the wire. This specifically formed wire is advanced through the catheter into the left ventricle. The pre-formed "pig-tail" keeps the wire from digging into the myocardium as it is manipulated within the ventricle. The 180° curve at the transition area of the wire prevents the stiffer wire from perforating the left ventricle and, at the same time, directs the tip of the wire 180° back toward the left ventricular outflow tract. This position allows the *stiff portion* of the wire proximal to the curve at the transition area to be positioned completely across the valve and deeper within the ventricle. With the wire maintained in position, the catheter is removed and replaced with the already prepared balloon catheter. The balloon is positioned precisely across the valve and an inflation/deflation is performed as rapidly as possible. The inflation/deflation is recorded on biplane angiography or on biplane "stored fluoroscopy".

During the inflation of the balloon, the left ventricular pressure increases, the systemic arterial pressure drops, and the infant develops bradycardia. As soon as the deflation of the balloon is complete, the balloon is withdrawn over the wire and out of the aortic valve. On relief of the obstruction, the infant's heart rate returns and the left ventricular pressure decreases toward normal. The rapidity of the stabilization of the infant is a partial indication of the success of the dilation. The infant's heart rate should return to a rate faster than the baseline rate and the left ventricular pressure should be lower than predilation. A very sick infant may require some medical or mechanical assistance for return of the cardiac output.

When the infant does *not* remain stable with even the small end-hole *catheter* across the valve, the original wire used to cross the valve is stabilized rapidly and the catheter is *immediately* withdrawn over the wire and out of the valve orifice while leaving the wire in place. The end-hole catheter is *rapidly* replaced with the *previously prepared* balloon dilation catheter, which is passed over the wire and positioned across the valve as expeditiously, but at the same time as accurately, as possible. Dilation of the valve is carried out with as rapid an inflation/deflation of the balloon as is possible. The balloon inflation/deflation is recorded on biplane, stored fluoroscopy or angiographically. After the inflation/deflation, the balloon is immediately withdrawn out of the valve, over the wire and into at least the ascending aorta to allow the infant to stabilize. The wire is kept securely in place in the ventricle whenever possible.

Once vascular access is obtained and the aortic valve is crossed with a retrograde catheter, aortic valve dilation from the femoral route usually is very successful. However, femoral arterial access is the most difficult and the most hazardous part of the procedure in the neonate and small infant. The vessels are very small relative to even the smallest catheters/dilating balloons available for aortic valve dilation. As a consequence, arterial complications are relatively common in this group of patients. Although extreme occlusive problems with necrotic ischemia of a limb are extremely rare, cool extremities with poor perfusion of the extremity immediately after a retrograde catheterization are common and usually represent compromise, if not total loss of the deep femoral artery of the involved limb. These patients usually acutely regain perfusion and warmth of the extremity but often on subsequent attempts at access, the deep femoral artery is totally occluded or occasionally the patient has a relative growth failure of that extremity. As a consequence of the femoral access problems several other routes for aortic valve dilation have evolved.

Carotid artery introduction for the retrograde approach

Transapical balloon dilation of the aortic valve in neonates set a precedent for direct collaboration between the cardiovascular surgeon and the interventional cardiologist for performing aortic valvotomies in critically ill infants. Because of the difficulties with arterial access and then entering the ventricle from the femoral approach, particularly with the earlier balloons, several centers performed balloon dilation of the neonatal aortic valve in the operating room through a thoracotomy and a controlled, apical, left ventricular puncture, but without the necessity of cardiopulmonary bypass. Although this approach avoided cardiopulmonary bypass, it did not avoid deep general anesthesia, the thoracotomy, the ventricular perforation, and all of the inherent problems of these particular procedures. The improvement in balloons and balloon techniques soon put this particular collaborative technique to rest.

An alternative, unique and, initially, seemingly radical collaborative approach for aortic valve dilation was developed as a consequence of the ongoing technical problems with balloon dilation of the infant aortic valve and, at the same time, other vascular technology which had been developing concurrently. The continuing difficulties with the arterial access site when using the femoral artery approach in neonates and the persistent difficulties with the catheter manipulation around the arch and across the aortic valve from both the femoral artery and the umbilical artery approaches made these approaches less than ideal. At the same time the expanded use of extracorporeal membrane oxygenation (ECMO) led to almost "routine" cut-downs *and repairs* of the carotid artery by pediatric vascular surgeons.

The combination of the persistent problems with the femoral/umbilical catheter approaches and the proficiency of the surgeons with the carotid cut-downs resulted in the consideration of a carotid artery approach to the balloon dilation of the aortic valve[6]. The carotid artery itself has considerable appeal as an approach to the aortic valve. Of most importance the approach to the aortic valve from the entrance into the carotid artery is a very short, very straight shot! With this "straight line" from the right carotid artery to the left ventricle, minimal catheter manipulation is required to cross even a severely stenotic aortic valve and to enter the left ventricle with a wire or catheter. The carotid artery is approached and entered by a cut-down procedure performed and repaired by a vascular/cardiovascular surgeon. The carotid approach combined with essentially no vascular or central nervous system sequelae when a skilled vascular surgeon exposes and repairs the artery, makes the carotid approach seem like the ultimate solution to a major problem.

Patients undergoing a carotid cut-down approach for aortic valve dilations are anesthetized with general anesthesia to ensure that they are maintained absolutely still throughout the procedure. They undergo endotracheal intubation for control of their respiration and to keep the head and face out of the "operating" field in the neck. The carotid approach for the dilation is usually used in conjunction with a prograde catheter from a systemic vein and a separate indwelling femoral arterial monitoring line. The majority of the hemodynamic and anatomic information is obtained through these lines before the carotid cut-down is initiated. The venous catheter is advanced through the patent foramen ovale (PFO) and into the left ventricle in almost all of these infants. The venous catheter and femoral arterial line are introduced simultaneously while the surgeon is introducing the sheath into the carotid artery and usually the prograde catheterization and femoral lines do not add any overall time to the procedure. The prograde catheter and indwelling arterial line actually simplify and add to the safety of the procedure. The venous prograde catheter in the left ventricle and the separate indwelling femoral arterial line provide continuous left ventricular and systemic arterial pressure monitoring before, during and after the dilation without having to cross the aortic valve repeatedly with a retrograde catheter.

A vascular surgeon performs a cut-down on the neck over the mid portion of the right carotid artery and isolates the right common carotid artery. A floppy tipped wire that will accommodate the balloon dilation catheter is introduced into the artery either through a small incision performed by the surgeon or through a needle introduced by the pediatric cardiologist.

The surgeon introduces a short 4-French sheath/dilator with an attached back-bleed valve/flush port into the carotid artery over the soft tipped wire, and advances it just to the base of the carotid artery as observed on fluoroscopy. All further introduction and positioning of the sheath tip are performed by the pediatric cardiologist and are visualized continuously on fluoroscopy. If even a short sheath is introduced to its hub in the carotid artery in a small infant, the tip of the sheath extends to (or past) the area of the aortic valve. If the tip of the sheath does not pass *through* the orifice of the valve, it potentially produces catastrophic damage to the aortic valve. Rarely, the sheath/dilator/wire passes into the descending aorta from the right carotid artery cut-down and has to be withdrawn and maneuvered specifically back into the aortic root. Alternatively, the wire may pass directly into the left ventricle during its initial introduction. When the sheath is in the proper position in the ascending aorta, the dilator and wire are removed and the sheath is cleared meticulously of any air or clots before flushing. The sheath is secured in the artery by means of a purse string and subcutaneous sutures so that the tip of the sheath is fixed at least 1–1.5 cm above the aortic valve. An aortic root aortogram is performed with an injection directly through the sheath or through a catheter introduced into the sheath. Accurate measurements of the valve annulus are carried out using one of the reference calibration techniques described in Chapter 11, "Angiography". The appropriate balloon for the valve dilation is chosen from these measurements exactly as it is chosen for the femoral approach. The balloon is prepared with a "minimal prep" in order to eliminate all air from the balloon.

A soft tip exchange wire, with a *very slight* curve at the tip, which will accommodate the prepared balloon dilation catheter is introduced through the sheath. The wire is introduced either directly through the sheath or through an end-hole catheter introduced into the sheath first. A catheter within the sheath provides more control over the tip of the wire and allows this catheter to be advanced over the wire into the ventricle as soon as the wire enters the ventricle. At the same time, the catheter adds considerable "length" outside of the introductory site into the carotid artery, and it extends well above the infant's head for the manipulations. The wire is manipulated through the aortic valve into the left ventricle. This is usually accomplished with only a few "probes" and minimal readjustment in the direction of the wire tip. Once through the valve, the wire is advanced deep into the ventricle until the *stiff portion* of the guide wire is entirely across the valve. The wire is fixed in position in the ventricle while the catheter is removed over the wire from the sheath.

The balloon catheter is advanced over the wire, into the sheath, and to the area of the valve. The balloon is centered precisely across the valve annulus as previously identified by angiography or as visualized on a transesophageal, or even a transthoracic, echocardiogram, and a rapid balloon inflation/deflation is performed. The inflation/deflation is recorded on a biplane angiogram or on "stored fluoroscopy". The balloon is withdrawn over the wire and back into the sheath immediately after it is deflated. As with any other aortic valve dilation, the infant's hemodynamics deteriorate during the balloon inflation in the valve, but usually return rapidly to "normal" (or better) with the deflation of the balloon and its withdrawal from the valve. When the prograde left ventricular and indwelling femoral arterial lines are in place, the hemodynamic results of the dilation are available immediately. The patient is allowed to stabilize while the recording of the inflation/deflation is reviewed particularly for the balloon position and the appearance/disappearance of a waist on the balloon. When the infant's hemodynamics have stabilized, the balloon is reintroduced across the valve and the inflation/deflation is repeated at least one more time. Before each reinflation, the balloon is repositioned forward or backward in the valve slightly. The balloon is observed for any persistent "waist" on it during subsequent inflations, particularly during the very initial phase of the inflation. After a successful dilation, no residual waist should appear on the balloon, even during the early phases of subsequent inflations.

When satisfied with the appearance of the inflations and the resultant hemodynamics, the balloon is withdrawn over the wire and out of the sheath, and the sheath is *passively* cleared very carefully of any air or clot. The balloon dilation catheter is replaced with an end-hole catheter, which is advanced into the ventricle over the wire that is still positioned in the left ventricle. The wire is removed slowly through the catheter, the catheter cleared of air/clot and the simultaneous left ventricle and femoral artery pressures are recorded. If a femoral line was not in place or there was no prograde catheter in the ventricle, the pressures are obtained following the dilation by either a pull-back of the end-hole catheter across the valve or, preferentially, with the left ventricular pressures obtained through the catheter still positioned in the ventricle and the arterial pressure obtained simultaneously from the side port of the carotid artery sheath. In this case, the sheath which is in the carotid artery/aorta must be at least one French size larger than the catheter. When the stenosis is not relieved by the initial dilation *and* aortic insufficiency is not significant, a wire is repositioned in the ventricle (either through the catheter still in the ventricle or by manipulating a wire/catheter back through a valve), and the dilation repeated with a larger balloon or with repositioning of the balloon. If a very wide pulse pressure is recorded or massive aortic regurgitation is visualized by echocardiogram, either the procedure is concluded or the catheter is withdrawn into the aorta and an aortic root angiogram is performed to verify the presence and amount of aortic regurgitation.

When the prograde catheter is already in the ventricle, the pressures are recorded simultaneously from this catheter, the femoral arterial line, and the sheath in the aortic root. When there is no prograde catheter in the ventricle, an end-hole catheter is advanced over the wire into the left ventricle, the wire is removed, and the pressure from the left ventricle is recorded through the catheter with a simultaneous femoral artery pressure from the femoral arterial line. If the resultant pressure in the left ventricle appears satisfactory compared to the femoral arterial pressure, a "pull-back" pressure is recorded as the catheter is withdrawn from the left ventricle into the aorta. A follow-up aortic root aortogram is recorded with injection through the "retrograde" carotid catheter. The decision for any further ballooning of the valve is made exactly as for other aortic valve dilations. When satisfied with the results of the dilation, or if significant aortic regurgitation was created regardless of the residual gradient, the sheath is withdrawn from the artery and the artery repaired meticulously by the vascular surgeon.

There are growing data indicating that the retrograde approach to the aortic valve from the carotid artery may be the safest and, in turn, the preferred approach for balloon dilation of the aortic valve in very small infants. Once the sheath is secured in the carotid artery, the carotid approach represents the most expedient way of crossing and dilating a severely stenotic aortic valve in an infant. The results of the dilation are comparable to other dilation techniques and there are no reported acute complications from the properly performed carotid approach. The repaired carotid arteries have good Doppler flow immediately following the dilation and on short-term follow-up of the carotid repairs. Whether this technique is used routinely in any particular center depends upon the availability and co-operation of the surgeon, the surgeon's skill at vascular access and repair, and the working relationship between the surgeon and the interventional cardiologist. When all of these "elements" fall into place, this is the preferred approach to the dilation of critical aortic valve stenosis in the newborn and small infant.

Umbilical artery introduction for the retrograde approach

In the newborn infant, at least one of the umbilical arteries is potentially patent for up to a week (or more) after birth. In a newborn infant with severe aortic stenosis who requires aortic valve dilation, an umbilical artery approach for the retrograde catheter provides a potential arterial access without compromise of a femoral or the carotid artery[7,8]. The newborn with severe aortic stenosis should have a venous catheterization with a prograde left heart cardiac catheterization. After the first few days of life, the umbilical vein often is not accessible, in which case the usual femoral vein approach is used for the venous catheterization.

The infant with severe aortic stenosis usually is critically ill and frequently already has an end-hole polyethylene "umbilical artery" catheter positioned by the neonatologist in the abdominal aorta from one of the umbilical arteries! In that situation, a fine, very small diameter, but, preferably, relatively stiff, exchange length, teflon-coated wire is passed through the umbilical catheter and as far as possible into the thoracic aorta, ascending aorta and, with the ultimate *luck*, even into the left ventricle. Unless the wire ends up in the left ventricle, the polyethylene umbilical artery catheter is replaced over this wire with a 4-French angled tipped (right coronary) catheter.

When there is no pre-existing umbilical artery line, the umbilical cord stump is scrubbed *very thoroughly* and then "amputated" parallel with and close to the abdominal wall. This exposes the stumps of the two umbilical arteries and the umbilical vein. The two arteries are smaller in diameter, rounder and thicker walled than the single, larger diameter and irregular vein. Usually, all three of these umbilical vessels are obliterated with thrombi, however, patency of the arteries can often be restored by "probing" the arterial lumen with a small diameter, smooth and blunt tipped metal probe. One edge of the exposed wall of the end of one of the arteries is grasped with a small forceps and the occluded lumen of the artery is probed with a very small, blunt, metal, vessel probe a few millimeters at a time until the probe passes several centimeters into the lumen. The probe usually stays within the walls of the vessel as it dissects through the thrombus. With the stump of the vessel opened in this manner, an end-hole "umbilical artery catheter" is introduced into the channel that was created with the probe, and advanced into the newly opened vessel lumen while placing some "counter tension" on the exposed edge of the vessel with the forceps. As the catheter is introduced into the lumen, it is directed posteriorly and *caudally* toward the posterior pelvis. Once the catheter has advanced several centimeters into the artery, it is visualized on fluoroscopy to determine whether the catheter is being directed to the right or the left inguinal area. With that information, the catheter is pushed in that direction toward that groin and the "counter traction" on the "stump" is pulled away from that direction.

Once the catheter has advanced one to two centimeters within the artery, the vessel often seems to "open up" and allow the catheter to move more freely through the umbilical artery. Simultaneously, there may be blood return into the catheter. Usually resistance is encountered in maneuvering the catheter around the sharp 90–130° curve at the junction of the umbilical artery and the iliac artery. Occasionally, advancing the umbilical catheter is facilitated by advancing a fine, floppy tipped, torque wire or a fine, *curved* Terumo™ wire through, and slightly in advance of, the umbilical catheter. Once the umbilical catheter has advanced into the descending aorta, an exchange length wire is advanced further into the thoracic aorta, the ascending aorta and, as before, with considerable luck, into the left ventricle. If the wire does not advance all of the way to the ventricle, the soft umbilical catheter is removed over the wire and replaced with a 4-French right Judkins™ coronary catheter.

From the descending aorta, the combination of the wire and right coronary catheter is advanced/manipulated around the aortic arch into the aortic root. This maneuver is often very difficult and requires several exchanges of different wires and/or catheters. Once the catheter has reached the aortic root, the wire is removed, the aortic pressure recorded, and a biplane aortogram is recorded with the X-ray tubes angled to "cut the valve on edge" (some degree of LAO–Cranial and RAO–Caudal) with the two planes. Accurate measurements of the valve annulus are made using one of the various *accurate* X-ray calibration techniques. A "marker catheter" can be placed in the superior vena cava adjacent to the aorta or even the left ventricle when there is prograde venous access. If there is no venous line, a calibration marker catheter can be inserted gently into the infant's *esophagus* and advanced to the area behind the cardiac silhouette as the reference for the angiographic calibration system. When positioned just behind the center of the heart shadow, the calibration marks on the catheter in the esophagus are in the plane of, and very close to, the aortic valve.

Once the measurements are complete, a very soft tipped, fine torque wire is inserted into the catheter and the stenotic aortic valve is probed with the catheter/wire combination. The technique is exactly as with any other isolated retrograde approach to the aortic valve with the exception that it is far more difficult from the umbilical artery. By the time the catheter/wire has been advanced into the aortic root, the combination catheter/wire has made two fairly acute and nearly 180° curves (passing from the umbilical to the iliac artery and from the descending to the ascending aorta). As a consequence, torque control and to-and-fro control over the catheter are restricted markedly. In addition, the "push" on the proximal shaft of the catheter entering the umbilical artery must be toward the groin and, counter-intuitively, "away" from the direction of the aortic root. Finally, there frequently is significant arterial spasm along the course of the catheter, which restricts catheter manipulation even further.

If the wire can be manipulated across the valve and well into the ventricle, and depending on which wire is used to cross the valve, an attempt is made at passing the catheter into the ventricle. If the shaft of the original wire is relatively soft, and depending upon the lumen diameter of the dilation balloon catheter that is to be used, the initial wire usually must be replaced with a wire which the dilation balloon catheter can accommodate and which is stiffer in order to support the delivery of a balloon/catheter through the circuitous course. Once the proper wire is in place, the catheter that is over the wire is placed on a continuous flush through a wire back-bleed valve and the appropriate balloon is prepared.

When the dilation balloon is ready, the original catheter is withdrawn over the wire leaving the wire positioned securely in the left ventricle. The balloon dilation catheter is advanced over the wire into the umbilical artery and through the circuitous course to the aortic valve. This frequently cannot be accomplished or is only accomplished with one or more exchanges of wires. When the balloon is positioned accurately across the valve, a rapid inflation/deflation is performed while recording the procedure on biplane angiography or stored fluoroscopy. When the infant stabilizes after the balloon deflation, if possible, the balloon is left in place across the valve until the angiograms of the inflation are reviewed. The inflation/deflation is repeated at least one more time. The reinflation/deflation verifies that the "waist" on the balloon does not reappear with the initial reinflation of the balloon. If the infant does not stabilize rapidly after the deflation with the balloon still across the valve, the balloon is withdrawn into the ascending (or descending!) aorta while simultaneously advancing the wire to maintain the wire's position in the ventricle—if at all possible. Once stabilized, an attempt is made at re-advancing the dilation balloon across the valve for at least one more inflation/deflation.

When the dilations have been completed, the balloon is withdrawn over the wire, still leaving the wire in the ventricle. The balloon catheter is replaced with an end-hole catheter, which is advanced over the wire into the ventricle. If there is no prograde catheter in the left ventricle, the wire is withdrawn from the catheter, pressures are recorded from the ventricle, and a biplane left ventricular angiogram is performed through this catheter. Even though the retrograde umbilical catheter is an end-hole catheter, satisfactory left ventricular angiograms can be obtained through these catheters in a neonate. A withdrawal pressure tracing from the left ventricle to the ascending aorta is recorded, following which an aortogram is performed in the aortic root to assess the movement of the valve leaflets and the degree of aortic regurgitation. The catheter is removed and the umbilical artery stump is oversewn. When there is a prograde venous catheter positioned in the left ventricle during the procedure, the pre- and post-left ventricular pressures and any left ventricular angiograms are obtained through this catheter. The prograde catheter obviates the necessity of multiple recrossing of the valve with the umbilical/retrograde catheter.

Because of the difficulties in maneuvering the catheters, wires and balloons from the umbilical artery approach and now with the much smaller balloon dilation catheters that can be introduced into the femoral arteries through very small (3- or 4-French) sheaths, the umbilical artery approach is no longer attempted in our center, although it is still used as the preferred approach in some centers.

Prograde approach to aortic valve dilation

There still are difficulties, particularly in smaller patients, in using any arterial approach for aortic valve dilation. The various potential problems from the different arterial approaches led to the development of techniques for the venous approach for the *prograde* delivery of the dilation balloon(s) to the aortic valve for aortic valve dilation. The usual prograde approach to the left heart is with catheters introduced from the femoral veins, although the umbilical veins have been used in neonates and the jugular/brachial veins have been used in the presence of a pre-existing interatrial communication. These approaches obviate virtually all of the particular problems with the arteries that occur with the arterial approaches, but they do have some significant difficulties of their own[9,10].

Prograde catheterization of the left ventricle and the aorta through a pre-existing intracardiac communication or by means of a transseptal atrial puncture are techniques that are used very commonly. The use of a diagnostic catheter which is advanced prograde into the aorta after it has been introduced into the left heart through a transseptal atrial puncture is part of the routine procedure for dilation of the aortic valve in the older patient as described earlier in this chapter. When a prograde dilation of the aortic valve *is anticipated*, two additional measures are necessary. First, when the transseptal puncture is performed, the transseptal sheath (set) that is used must be large enough in diameter to accommodate the *largest* dilation balloon catheter that is to be used for the prograde aortic valve dilation. Secondly, the passage of the catheter from the *left atrium to the left ventricle* initially is accomplished using a "floating" balloon catheter. The inflated balloon of a floating balloon catheter is more likely to float preferentially *through* the *true, central orifice of the mitral valve*, cleanly between the papillary muscles, and away from any chordae. This is essential in order to avoid the eventual passage or expansion of the relatively large dilation balloons through narrow channels in, or entangled with, these valve structures.

The hemodynamic data are recorded and angiography performed in both the left ventricle and the aorta through the prograde catheters as described earlier in this chapter. Once the hemodynamics and angiography are completed and it is established that aortic valve dilation is indicated, a long transseptal sheath is advanced over the floating balloon catheter and positioned securely in the *left ventricle* as near to the *apex* as possible. If a double-balloon technique is to be used, a second, appropriately sized, long transseptal sheath is introduced into the left atrium and the left ventricle in a similar fashion to the first long sheath. Either an end-hole, floating balloon or torque-controlled catheter is advanced through each long transseptal sheath. As the catheter tip reaches the tip of the sheath, the sheath is withdrawn very slightly to allow the tip of the catheter to exit the sheath without digging into the ventricular myocardium. The catheter(s) is(are) manipulated from the left ventricle, 180° into the aorta, around the arch and well into the descending aorta using the techniques described earlier. The end-hole catheter used for this can be either a soft, torque-controlled catheter or an end-hole, floating balloon Swan™ type catheter. A floating balloon catheter is usually easier and safer to use for this manipulation, although the smaller floating balloon catheters do not accommodate a 0.035" guide wire.

When the end-hole catheter(s) has/have been advanced well into the descending aorta, an exchange length guide wire is introduced into each catheter *through a wire back bleed valve*. With the catheter on a slow continuous flush, the wire is advanced through the catheter and positioned securely in the descending aorta. The exact wires used depend a great deal on the size of the patient and the type and size of balloons to be used. Whenever possible, a relatively stiff wire is desirable in order to provide support for the passage of a balloon catheter around the two 180° curves en route to the aortic valve and to hold the balloon(s) in place during the dilation. At the same time, the wire cannot be so stiff that it holds the mitral valve open and that it "straightens" the normal 360° course from the right atrium to the aorta into a straight line! Occasionally the stiff wire will not traverse around the curves through the original prograde catheter to the aorta or, even if the wire can be positioned in the aorta, it is so stiff that it holds the mitral and/or aortic valves open or "splints" the ventricular walls apart. Any of these difficulties with the wire interferes with the ventricular function to such a degree that it cannot be left in place for even a few minutes. The wires in their course from the left atrium, through the ventricle, to the aorta must have a long loop, deep into the *apex* of the left ventricle and must *not* pass *across* the ventricular cavity. The wires must be maintained in that position throughout the dilation procedure in order to prevent damage to the mitral valve.

Once the appropriate wires are in satisfactory, stable positions and the patient still remains stable, the catheter(s) remain(s) over the wire(s) while all of the catheter(s) and/or the long sheath(s) in the left ventricle are maintained on a slow continuous flush while the dilation balloon(s) are prepared. The dilation balloon for the prograde approach should be shorter than those used for a retrograde aortic valve dilation. The shorter balloons facilitate the delivery of the relatively stiff "balloon segment" of the balloon dilation catheter through the tight curves in the circuitous prograde course to a position across the aortic valve. The shorter balloons also help to ensure that the *proximal* ends of the balloons are positioned entirely in the left ventricular outflow tract and well away from the mitral apparatus when they are inflated. After a balloon is prepared, the original catheter is removed over the wire while maintaining the wire in its position well into the descending aorta and *through the long sheath* and, at the same time, the tip of the sheath is maintained near the left ventricular apex.

Each balloon dilation catheter is introduced over the wire into the long sheath in the femoral vein and advanced to the aortic valve, all of the time maintaining the sheath and the catheter lumen on a continuous flush. This circuitous route through two 180° curves within the heart usually takes considerable and meticulous manipulation of both the catheters and wires while maintaining the sheath in position securely within the left ventricle. Care must be taken that the wire loops neither tighten nor elongate excessively on themselves. When the wires begin to tighten, they pull against, and cut into, the valvular structures and begin to pull the tips of the wires back out of the aorta. When the loops of wire elongate excessively they "stent" the valvular structures open or cut into the valves along the "outer circumference" of the loops. The long sheath maintained in position deep within the left ventricular apex makes the balloon passage from the left ventricle to the aorta slightly more difficult, but this position of the sheath is essential to help prevent mitral valve damage.

When a wire repeatedly pulls back from the aorta and cannot be maintained in the descending aorta as the balloon dilation catheter is advanced over it, a snare introduced retrograde is used to hold the wire in place. A Micro Vena™ snare catheter is introduced into a femoral artery through a 4-French sheath. The distal end of the prograde wire in the descending aorta is grasped with a 10 mm Micro Vena™ snare introduced retrograde. The wire is held securely with the snare in this position, which secures the distal end of the prograde wire in the descending aorta. Alternatively, the distal end of the prograde, exchange length wire is withdrawn through the descending aorta and "exteriorized" through the femoral arterial sheath. Either the snare catheter holding the prograde wire or the exteriorized distal end of the wire is secured on the table outside of the artery. When a prograde, double-balloon dilation is being performed, the second wire also is grasped with a retrograde snare. This can be performed through the same femoral artery with the same snare grasping the two wires simultaneously or with a second snare through the opposite femoral artery. When a single snare catheter is used, unless the first wire or both wires is/are "exteriorized", the exact tension on the separate wires cannot be controlled separately.

If a retrograde sheath/catheter cannot be introduced into a femoral artery for the snare catheter, or the introduction is contraindicated, an attempt is made at manipulating the prograde wire all the way around the arch, to the descending aorta and into one of the femoral arteries, advancing the tip of the wire to a position well beyond the inguinal ligament. The prograde wire can often be fixed in this position by firm, manual, finger pressure directly over the artery, compressing the artery and, in turn, securing the wire in the inguinal area. This fixes the wire but does not allow any "counter traction" or other change in position or tension on the wire from the distal end.

The through and through control on the wire with the retrograde snare keeps the wire from being pulled out of the aorta and back into the left ventricle as the balloon is being advanced. At the same time, the loops in the wire passing through the heart with traction at both ends of the wire, can "tighten" the loops dangerously about the structures in the heart. For many reasons, significant tightening of the wires must be avoided. If the bare wires tighten, they cut into the structures "within" the loops—in particular the medial leaflet of the mitral valve, the mitral chordae, the left ventricular outflow tract and/or the aortic valve itself. As the loops of the wires tighten, the wires pull ***across*** the sub-valve apparatus of the mitral valve. If the wires remain *across* the sub-valve apparatus of the valve as the balloon is advanced, the larger diameter, rougher surfaced, balloon also passes through or is expanded in the sub-valve mitral apparatus causing disruption of the apparatus. The long sheath across the mitral valve helps to protect the mitral valve but does not guarantee that the mitral valve cannot be severely damaged.

Even when the tightening loops do not cause injury, the "tightening" and, therefore, narrower loops in the wire create *more* resistance to the movement of the balloon catheter over the entire course of the wire. The tighter the course of the wire loops, the more difficult the passage of the balloon becomes. The most extreme and dangerous degree of "tightening" of the loops of the wire results in the wire starting from its previous 360° course while passing from the inferior vena cava, to the right atrium, left atrium, left ventricle and out into the aorta, actually *straightening* into an *entirely* straight course through the same structures! This occurs with a sudden "flip" of the wire and unequivocally will damage intracardiac structures. This very dangerous phenomenon is prevented by the continual observation of the course of the wires and never allowing the "loops" in the wires to begin to tighten.

The significant difficulties with the passage of a balloon dilation catheter over the wire require an exchange of the original wire for a smaller diameter wire or a wire with entirely different characteristics. The prograde delivering of the balloon on the balloon dilation catheter to the valve is the most difficult part of this procedure.

Once the balloon is positioned across the aortic valve, any wire loops or curves that were tightened excessively, are "loosened" by advancing the wire very carefully. The *proximal end* of the prograde balloon across the aortic valve must be positioned cephalad in the left ventricular outflow tract and away from the mitral valve apparatus. A long smooth loop of the wire is formed proximal to the balloon in the left ventricular apex so that the wire will be positioned well away from the mitral valve. Initially the balloon is inflated *very slowly* and only partially to be sure that there are no unexpected or unwanted, additional "waists" appearing from entrapment in part of the mitral valve apparatus. When the partial inflation appears "clear" of abnormally located indentations, the balloon is inflated and deflated rapidly as with any other aortic valve dilation.

In addition to the difficulty in delivering the balloon to the aortic valve, there are some additional disadvantages to the prograde technique for the dilation of the aortic valve. The smaller the patient or the smaller the heart, the tighter the 180° curves or loops of wire/catheter become and the more difficult it is to advance the balloons around the multiple curves. When the patient is hemodynamically unstable to begin with, all of the balloon/wire manipulation is not tolerated. These problems are compounded in critically ill infants and particularly in small infants with a *relatively small left ventricular cavity* where it is most appealing to avoid the arterial approach. If the patient does not tolerate the balloon inflation or the balloon across the valve *per se*, it is more difficult to withdraw the balloon quickly from the valve and into a stable location than it is from the retrograde approach. In addition to the risk of damage of the mitral valve and/or valve apparatus from the wire/balloon catheter alone, and during the balloon inflation, there also is a higher incidence of left bundle branch block or complete heart block created during the prograde procedure.

Considering both the technical challenges and the added risks of the prograde approach, the benefits of the prograde approach for the dilation of the aortic valve must be weighed heavily against the disadvantages before embarking on this approach for aortic valve dilation.

Complications of aortic valve dilation

The inability to complete an adequate dilation of the aortic valve is not a "complication", but is a failure of the procedure. The failure of the procedure is not, in itself, an adverse event for the patient unless there is an additional separate complication from the procedure. The underlying disease and not the failure of the procedure itself, creates the necessity for further intervention. At the same time, complications specifically related to aortic valve dilation are more common than with most, if not all, of the other therapeutic catheter procedures.

One of the most common complications specifically associated with aortic valve dilation is injury to a peripheral artery. Although the incidence of arterial injury has decreased as a result of improvements in both the techniques and in the available equipment for the procedure, arterial spasm, clots, tears and disruptions of the artery still occur. Prevention using meticulous technique and the use of the least traumatic equipment possible prevents most arterial injuries (Chapter 4). Early recognition of an arterial problem with early intervention can prevent permanent sequelae. The availability and use of specific catheter interventions and of more effective thrombolytics for arterial thrombi are discussed in Chapters 2 & 35. It is now extremely rare for a patient to require a surgical arterial repair or have any permanent sequelae as a consequence of a retrograde arterial procedure even in a small infant.

The most serious complications from aortic valve dilations are injuries to the central nervous system. As with any procedure on the "systemic side" of the circulation, the potential for embolic events to systemic organs, particularly the head, is always present during aortic valve dilations. There are innumerable opportunities for the introduction of air and/or clots into the circulation proximal to the head vessels during the multiple manipulations in the aortic root, left ventricle, and left atrium. Air embolization absolutely should be preventable by the use of meticulous technique.

Solid particle embolization is a different story. Thrombi easily form on guide wires, on and within catheters and sheaths and specifically on balloon dilation catheters within the folds of collapsed balloons. Patients undergoing these procedures are always anticoagulated with heparin during the procedure. Unfortunately, even this is not sufficient to prevent thrombus formation unequivocally. The best that can be done to prevent thrombi is to keep the patient's ACT level above 300 seconds, to be as expedient as possible with manipulations in the systemic circulation, and to keep all catheters and wires through catheters on a continuous flush. "Parking" catheters and, particularly, balloon catheters in the descending aorta as opposed to the ascending aorta when they are not being used for recordings/procedures specifically in the aortic root, reduces the likelihood of a "head" event.

The most unpredictable, frustrating and probably, the most common complication of aortic valve dilation is the creation of *significant* aortic valve regurgitation. It is the most frustrating complication because the specific cause of the regurgitation in any one patient is still not known although it *is* a potential risk, as a consequence of *every* balloon dilation of the aortic valve. Significant aortic regurgitation occurs in approximately 10% of all balloon dilations of the aortic valve. This number is comparable to its occurrence following surgical aortic valvotomy, but whether it is a problem in the same patients whether they undergo surgery or catheterization is not known. It appears that over-sizing of the balloon for the aortic valve annulus is one predictor for the creation of aortic regurgitation, however aortic regurgitation certainly is created even when using a precisely measured balloon to annulus ratio of less than one. Unquestionably, the wire and then the balloon passage through a valve leaflet rather than through the commissures/orifice of the valve results in significant regurgitation. This problem may not be recognized until after the fact. This particular cause of regurgitation is avoided by gentle retrograde probing of the valve with very *soft, floppy tipped wires* and by directing the retrograde wire along the precise course of a previously positioned catheter that is passing prograde *through the valve orifice*.

Once even a moderate amount of aortic regurgitation is created during a balloon dilation procedure, no further dilation of the aortic valve is attempted regardless of the residual obstruction. Fortunately, patients with very significant aortic stenosis and, particularly, those with significant chronic aortic stenosis tolerate even moderate to severe degrees of acutely created aortic regurgitation without the immediate need for valve repair or replacement. Massive aortic regurgitation with acute left ventricular decompensation does occur, particularly in patients who have only moderate aortic stenosis with no ventricular hypertrophy before the dilation, and whose ventricles are "unprepared" for the sudden volume load. This is the major contraindication to dilation of mild or moderately severe aortic valve stenosis. Facilities must be available for urgent surgery and acute valve replacement in the case of such an occurrence in any patient undergoing aortic valve dilation.

Mitral valve damage during the prograde approach for aortic valve dilation has been discussed previously. Avoiding the prograde approach for dilation of the aortic valve is the best method of preventing this complication. However, the mitral valve apparatus can be disrupted even during a retrograde dilation of the aortic valve. It is possible for the retrograde wire and then the balloon to pass through and become entrapped in the mitral valve chordae. If this is not recognized, the mitral valve can be damaged. An indicator of this potential problem is a *very posterior* and "less mobile" position of the retrograde wire/balloon in the ventricle. A left ventricular angiocardiogram or a transesophageal echocardiogram demonstrates the errant wire/balloon position in the mitral apparatus.

Perforation of the left ventricle is possible during dilation of the aortic valve. A straight wire, particularly with a shorter, straight "floppy" tip is more likely to perforate the myocardium as it is extruded out of the tip of a catheter, although even a wire with a long floppy tip can perforate if enough forward force is placed on the wire when the tip of the catheter is "buried" in the myocardium and cannot bow or bend away from the tip of the catheter. If there is a very sharp kink or angle on the stiff portion of the wire when a "curve" on the stiff or transition zone of the wire is positioned in the apex of the left ventricle *and* the balloon "milks" into the ventricle during inflation, the balloon pushes the acute, sharp angle on the wire further into the ventricle. A straight wire with *no curve* on the transition zone can kink acutely and be driven through the ventricular wall by a rapid forward force on the wire caused by a "squirting" balloon. This is true particularly with small sick infants.

A problem that is more likely to occur in, but is not totally limited to, sicker patients is the inability of the heart to recover and the patient to stabilize after the total obstruction of cardiac output by the balloon inflation/deflation in the aortic valve. Usually, the relief of the obstruction by the dilation is sufficient to allow the rapid return of the heart rate, blood pressure and, in turn, a better cardiac output with rapid stabilization of the patient immediately after the balloon(s) is/are deflated. On rare occasions, the myocardium initially is so damaged and is "stunned" even further by the acute and total obstruction of coronary flow during the balloon inflation that when the balloon is deflated, there is no return of cardiac function in spite of all resuscitative efforts. This may not be entirely preventable. It is less likely to happen if the patient was pretreated adequately and heart failure, shock and acidosis were corrected before the dilation procedure. The double-balloon technique allows some forward flow through the valve when the balloons are at full inflation, which reduces the adverse heart rate and blood pressure effects.

The so-called "hooded coronary" orifice can result in a catastrophic outcome in association with balloon dilation of the aortic valve. With this lesion the orifice of a coronary artery lies low or deep in the coronary sinus. While the valve is stenotic, the "tethering" or doming of the leaflets holds the leaflets away from the abnormally located orifice, but when the valve is dilated successfully, particularly if one leaflet becomes partially flail, the leaflet then folds completely against the wall of the sinus and, in turn, over the orifice of the coronary artery, acutely obstructing flow into the coronary. The best indicator of this abnormality is a very low position of the coronary orifice and the closeness of the aortic leaflet to the coronary orifice before the valve undergoes dilation. Recognition and immediate surgical intervention are the only management for this rare abnormality.

Rupture of the aortic valve annulus is another catastrophic event that can occur during aortic valve dilation, but probably is preventable. This complication is unlikely to occur unless the balloon(s) is/are oversized markedly for the annulus size or the patient has underlying aortic wall disease such as the medial necrosis as seen in Marfan's syndrome. As a consequence, this problem theoretically should be avoidable by meticulous attention to the measurements of the annulus, using *valid reference* calibration measurements, and by thorough knowledge of the patient's history.

In spite of the numerous potentially serious complications of balloon dilation of the aortic valve, the benefits of dilation of the aortic valve still outweigh the risks of the catheter procedure and the risks of the alternative management/therapy as long as meticulous attention is given to the details of the performance of the procedure.

References

1. Lababidi Z, Wu JR, and Walls TJ. Percutaneous balloon aortic valvuloplasty results in 23 patients. *Am J Cardiol* 1984; **53**: 194–197.
2. Rocchini AP *et al.* Balloon aortic valvuloplasty: Results of the Valvuloplasty and Angioplasty of Congenital Anomalies Registry. *Am J Cardiol* 1990; **65**: 784–789.
3. Justo RN *et al.* Aortic valve regurgitation after surgical versus percutaneous balloon valvotomy for congenital aortic valve stenosis. *Am J Cardiol* 1996; **77**(15): 1332–1338.
4. Zeevi B *et al.* Neonatal critical valvar aortic stenosis. A comparison of surgical and balloon dilation therapy. *Circulation* 1989; **80**(4): 831–839.
5. Mullins CE *et al.* Double balloon technique for dilation of valvular or vessel stenosis in congenital and acquired heart disease. *J Am Coll Cardiol* 1987; **10**(1): 107–114.
6. Fischer DR *et al.* Carotid artery approach for balloon dilation of aortic valve stenosis in the neonate: a preliminary report. *J Am Coll Cardiol* 1990; **15**(7): 1633–1636.
7. Beekman RH, Rocchini AP, and Andes A. Balloon valvuloplasty for critical aortic stenosis in the newborn: influence of new catheter technology. *J Am Coll Cardiol* 1991; **17**(5): 1172–1176.
8. Pass RH *et al.* Umbilical arterial cardiac catheterization in infancy: diagnostic and interventional applications. *Cathet Cardiovasc Diagn* 2001; **51**: 551.
9. Magee AG *et al.* Balloon dilation of severe aortic stenosis in the neonate: comparison of anterograde and retrograde catheter approaches. *J Am Coll Cardiol* 1997; **30**(4): 1061–1066.
10. Peuster M *et al.* Anterograde balloon valvuloplasty for the treatment of neonatal critical valvar aortic stenosis. *Catheter Cardiovasc Interv* 2002; **56**(4): 516–520; discussion 521.

20 Mitral valvuloplasty

Introduction

In the more developed countries of the world, mitral stenosis in children is predominately congenital in origin and, fortunately, is a relatively rare abnormality[1]. The stenosis in the congenitally malformed mitral valve has multiple variations and involves all parts of the mitral valve apparatus. The "characteristic" congenital mitral stenosis has a single papillary muscle, the valve leaflets are fused into a funnel-like or "parachute" deformity, and there are no real commissures of the valve. The leaflets alone can be fused without the fusion of the papillary muscles or vice versa. There also often is a "supra-valve" obstructive membrane within the left atrium just above the mitral valve annulus with or without the other abnormalities of the mitral valve apparatus. In spite of the complexity of these lesions, some of these valves are amenable to balloon dilation[2,3].

The success of either balloon dilation or reconstructive surgery for congenital mitral valve stenosis depends a great deal upon the initial anatomy of the stenosis. A successful balloon or surgical dilation opens the stenosis and relieves the obstruction, but still only represents palliative therapy. This palliation hopefully delays the almost inevitable mitral valve replacement. Dilation of congenital mitral valve stenosis by any technique is likely to produce some mitral regurgitation. Fortunately, the degree of insufficiency usually is not great, is tolerated moderately well and certainly is tolerated better than a very tight stenosis. Because of the relative difficulty and the risks and the lack of predictability of the results of dilation of congenital mitral stenosis, the criteria for performing balloon dilation of congenital mitral stenosis are more stringent than for most other therapeutic procedures in the congenital cardiac catheterization laboratory. Even moderate mitral stenosis symptomatically is tolerated quite well and the presence of the stenosis *per se* is *not* an indication for intervention. Patients with congenital mitral stenosis are considered for intervention only when symptoms become significant or when secondary pulmonary hypertension develops. When balloon dilation of a congenital mitral valve stenosis is anticipated, the definite possibility of creating significant mitral regurgitation, which will require a mitral valve replacement, must always be included in the decision for and the discussions about the balloon valvotomy.

In the developing countries of the world where acute rheumatic fever is still rampant, rheumatic mitral valve stenosis is very common and does occur in young children. Because the rheumatic stenosis represents the fusion of what were previously normal, bicuspid, mitral valve leaflets, the dilation of the acquired fusion is far more successful than the dilation of the congenitally deformed valves. As a consequence, the indications for catheter intervention for rheumatic mitral stenosis are much more lenient than for the congenital mitral lesions. The presence of rheumatic mitral stenosis with any symptoms or with even the suggestion of an increase in right ventricular and pulmonary artery pressures is an indication for intervention for rheumatic mitral stenosis in children, adolescents and adults[4].

Balloon dilation is considered the standard primary therapy of rheumatic mitral stenosis at virtually any age, however, in the older patient with mitral stenosis, the decision for valve dilation is weighed against the amount of acquired degenerative changes in the valve[5]. In the child or adolescent with rheumatic mitral stenosis, the degenerative changes in the valve that produce the contraindications to balloon therapy are usually not present. In the younger age group the mitral valve stenosis must be distinguished from congenital mitral stenosis, which may represent a contraindication to balloon dilation of the valve.

The applicability of a stenotic rheumatic mitral valve for a transcatheter mitral valvuloplasty is determined on the basis of a combined echocardiographic and X-ray grading system. The thickness of the leaflets, the restriction in the valve motion, the sub-valvular thickening due to the fusion of the chordae or the papillary muscles and the amount of calcium in the valve on X-ray are all determinates in the "mitral valve score". Each of these factors is graded 1 through 4 according to the worsening degree of severity, and when the numerical grades are added together, give the "score". The higher the score, the less likely the procedure is to succeed and the greater the chances of complications[6]. Thrombi or masses within the left atrium are relative contraindications to balloon dilation of the valve regardless of the other findings.

The balloon types and sizes used for mitral valve dilation vary according to the size of the mitral valve annulus, whether the dilation is with a single "standard" balloon, a double-balloon technique or with the Inoue™ balloon. The dilation technique and type of balloon(s) used are mostly chosen according to the preference of the particular operator and the availability of the particular necessary equipment in the catheterization laboratory. There is a great variability in how the mitral annulus diameter is measured and, in turn, how the balloon sizes are determined for balloon dilation of the mitral valve. The mitral annulus is not actually measured in some adult series, but, instead, the balloon diameter is chosen arbitrarily according to the patient's body size. Other series utilize a formula or a graph according to the patient's measured height and / or body surface area to "calculate" the balloon size to be used.

The size of the Inoue™ balloon is frequently determined according to the patient's height using the formula:

Inoue™ balloon size = patient's height (in cms) ÷ 10 + 10.

This diameter is the maximum diameter of the particular balloon. With the variability in the diameter of the Inoue™ balloon possible during the dilation, this allows the operator to begin the dilation using a diameter 4 mm smaller than the maximum for that balloon and then sequentially increasing the diameter up to the calculated end or maximal diameter of that balloon, all without having to exchange balloons.

For the double-balloon techniques it is better to measure the various diameters of the mitral valve annulus angiographically using several angled views or by echocardiography in several different planes. When actually measured, the dimension of the mitral annulus in the lateral projection usually is 25–30% longer than the posterior–anterior dimension. The *longest* annulus diameter is used in choosing the two balloons. The combined diameter of the two balloons used is usually equal to, or up to, 1.3 times the longest measured diameter of the mitral annulus. Occasionally, when there is very gross malformation of a congenitally stenotic mitral valve, the balloon dilation is started with smaller diameter balloons. If the annulus diameter is not adequately measured by either modality, then a graph of normal valve diameters according to body surface area is used to determine the balloon sizes[7].

Techniques for balloon dilation of the mitral valve

With the exception of one of several retrograde approaches for balloon dilation of the mitral valve and the extremely rare incidence of either transhepatic or transjugular access to the atrial septum, *most* balloon dilation procedures of the mitral valve are performed from the femoral venous approach. The usual, as well as the alternative approaches, to transcatheter dilation of the mitral valve are discussed in this chapter.

The mitral valve can be dilated using a single, large, "standard" angioplasty balloon, with one of several different double-balloon techniques or, in larger patients, dilation with the Inoue Balloon™, which is designed specially for mitral valve dilation. All of these procedures have advantages and disadvantages. Each procedure has its advocates. The double-puncture, double-balloon technique and the Inoue Balloon™ procedure are discussed in detail. The single-balloon technique using a large "standard" balloon and the double-balloon using a single transseptal puncture are mentioned only in comparison to the other two, more preferred techniques.

The safest technique (and the standard of care in developed countries) is to use biplane fluoroscopic guidance for control of the transseptal procedure(s) as well as the actual mitral valve dilation procedure. The actual dilation of the valve also is supported with echocardiographic guidance control. Transthoracic echo (TTE) can be used particularly in the smaller patient, but now the trend is to use transesophageal echo (TEE) or intracardiac echo (ICE) for guidance of the procedure. In addition to the more reliable images of the valve, both TEE and ICE have the advantage that the transducer and the echocardiographer's hands are out of the fluoroscopy field during the dilation procedure. The TEE procedure has the disadvantage that it requires general anesthesia for most patients to tolerate the TEE probe, and at the same time to hold still for the duration of the procedure. The experience with ICE is still limited, and it still requires the presence of an *additional* large venous sheath.

The catheterization and dilation of the mitral valve can be performed with deep sedation and local anesthesia when *transesophageal* echocardiography is *not* used to guide the procedure. If transesophageal echocardiographic monitoring is used during the dilation procedure, then general anesthesia is used for the whole procedure.

Double-balloon, double transseptal puncture technique

A separate venous sheath is introduced percutaneously into both the right and left femoral veins, and a small indwelling arterial cannula placed percutaneously into one femoral artery. As mentioned in the description of the transseptal technique in Chapter 8, it is imperative that the catheter course from the femoral puncture passes through the true femoral vein and not through pelvic collateral veins, which pass deep into the posterior pelvic and perirectal venous system. Right heart pressures and cardiac output determinations are obtained with a right heart catheterization. Pulmonary artery and pulmonary arterial wedge pressures obtained during this part of the procedure *help* to substantiate the severity of the mitral stenosis. Following the acquisition of the "right heart" data, the transseptal left heart catheterization is performed. When the double-balloon, *double transseptal* technique is used, separate transseptal punctures are performed with an approach from both inguinal areas. The *exact* severity of the stenosis and the anatomy of the valve and valve apparatus are determined after the left heart is entered transseptally.

A double-balloon technique through two separate transseptal punctures introduced from separate groins is preferred for children as well as for smaller adults. This allows the introduction of two smaller balloons into smaller peripheral veins and the passage across the intra-atrial septum through two smaller *and widely separated* holes in the atrial septum. With the current balloon technology, both balloon catheters are introduced through long sheaths. The two punctures in the atrial septum are separated from each other by at least a centimeter to prevent the two openings from coalescing and creating one large and permanent hole in the septum! In a large patient with a large mitral annulus, the double-balloon technique allows the use of two balloons of adequate combined diameter without the necessity of using one *very large, very* bulky, and irregular, single, mitral "angioplasty" balloon with its very rough and traumatic deflated profile.

The two transseptal punctures are performed from catheters introduced from the separate right and left femoral veins. (The transseptal technique is described in detail in Chapter 8.) In the adult and in the moderate, or large sized child or adolescent, both transseptal sheath/dilator sets *can be* introduced through *separate punctures* into the *same* femoral vein in either inguinal area when there is an access problem from one side. When using bilateral femoral veins, it is preferable to perform the first transseptal puncture with the catheter that is introduced into the *left* groin. The transseptal procedure from the left groin usually requires bending the patient's thorax to the right in order for the needle to align more perpendicular to the septum and to engage or impinge on the septum during the actual puncture. Performing the first puncture from the left femoral vein allows freer bending and movement of the patient during the first transseptal puncture without fear of dislodging a previously positioned transseptal sheath by the movement of the patient during the second puncture.

Although certainly not essential (or maybe even desirable!), the use of TEE guidance is popular for needle guidance during the transseptal puncture. It is complementary to the fluoroscopy, but should *not* replace the use of *biplane* fluoroscopy as the primary means of visualizing the punctures. Once the tip of the needle and the transseptal set is impinged on the septum, TEE, then, is helpful for localizing the site of the puncture on the septal surface and helps to ensure that the two puncture sites are separated from each other by at least a centimeter. The TEE image of the needle on the septum also provides a security check in avoiding the aortic root and the atrial septum–posterior wall junction during the puncture, particularly when there is a small left atrium.

When the right heart catheterization is performed from the left inguinal area or if sheaths are in both femoral veins, the *left* venous catheter and sheath are replaced over a wire with a 7- or 8-French transseptal set. The transseptal set has a sheath with a back-bleed valve with a flush port and a radio-opaque marker band at the distal tip of the sheath. The transseptal set is advanced over the wire into the superior vena cava and, preferably, into the left innominate vein. The wire is withdrawn from the transseptal set, the dilator cleared of air and flushed, the transseptal needle is introduced into the dilator, advanced to just within the tip of the dilator and *then* attached to the pressure/flush system. The patient's thorax is angled (bent, not twisted!) to the patient's right. This bending creates a more perpendicular angle between the tip of the transseptal needle and the atrial septum once the tip of the needle has been withdrawn into the right atrium. With the pressure from the needle displayed on a 20 or 40 mmHg scale, the sheath/dilator/needle is withdrawn/rotated from the superior vena cava and along the right atrial surface of the interatrial septum, as described in detail in Chapter 8 ("Transseptal Technique").

The transseptal puncture is performed as low on the atrial septum as is possible. For these low positions for puncture through the septum, TEE *is* useful to ensure that the needle tip and, in turn, the puncture is not originating from within the coronary sinus. After the needle tip passes through the septum into the left atrium, visualization of the posterior wall of the left atrium by TEE *helps*, but usually is unnecessary, in avoiding puncture through the posterior wall into the pericardium. While observing pressure continuously through the needle, the needle/dilator/sheath are advanced through the septum and into the left atrium until the tip of the *sheath* is well within the atrium. With any loss of pressure, advancing the needle/long sheath/dilator is stopped, the tip of the needle is rotated horizontally slightly and the location of the needle tip is determined precisely with a small injection of contrast through the needle.

Once the tip of the *sheath* is well into the left atrium, the needle first and then, separately, the dilator are removed slowly from the sheath. The dilator is allowed to bleed back and drip fluid/blood out of the end of its hub as it is withdrawn. The sheath is then cleared meticulously of any air and clots by allowing passive *free flow* of blood out of the side arm of the back-bleed device while tapping and rotating the back-bleed valve chamber. The long sheath in the left atrium along with the wire/dilator/catheter exchanges through the sheath positioned in the left heart represent the greatest potential hazards of the procedure. The wire/catheter manipulations through the long sheath with the sheath tip positioned within the left atrium create a huge potential for the introduction of air or clot into the left heart. Meticulous attention must be taken in clearing the sheath to avoid this. Once the sheath, including the hub/chamber of its back-bleed valve, *unequivocally* is cleared of any air or clot, the side arm of the sheath is attached to the pressure/flush system. At this point in the procedure the patient is given 100 mg/kg of heparin intravenously through the long sheath. When pressures are not being recorded through the sheath, the sheath is maintained on a slow flush of heparinized flush solution.

Once the first transseptal sheath has been secured in the left atrium, the hemodynamics and anatomy of the mitral stenosis are confirmed. An accurate left atrial pressure is recorded through the side arm of the sheath or through a catheter introduced through the sheath into the left atrium. When the catheter is at least one French size smaller than the sheath, pressures can be recorded through both the catheter and the sheath simultaneously. The two simultaneous pressures from the left atrium serve as an extremely reliable method of documenting the accuracy of the two transducers (Chapter 10). The two pressure tracings should produce a *single line* on the monitoring screen. Once the pressure in the left atrium is recorded, angiocardiograms can be performed in the left atrium to define the valve anatomically and to localize various left heart structures. An angiographic catheter is advanced into the left atrium through the long sheath. In order to obtain the most useful anatomic information about the valve, the X-ray tubes are positioned at angles that are as perpendicular to the *annulus* of the valve as possible. The mitral valve usually is "cut on edge" with a right anterior oblique/*caudal* (RAO/caudal) angulation of the posterior–anterior (PA) X-ray tube. A very steep left anterior oblique/cranial (LAO/cranial or "four chambered") angulation of the lateral tube provides the closest to perpendicular view of the valve from the lateral X-ray plane. However, it often is impossible to obtain a steep enough cranial angulation with the lateral X-ray system to cut the valve absolutely "on edge" from the LAO/cranial angle. Even though the entire valve may not be "on edge" with the LAO/cranial view, this view does give a second dimension for measurement of the diameter of the valve *annulus* and the sub-valve apparatus. Since no two patients and valves are the same, frequently several left atrial angiocardiograms with changes in the X-ray tube angulations are needed to position the mitral valve optimally "on edge".

From the left atrial angiocardiograms, the exact size, anatomy and position of the orifice of the mitral valve are determined. During the angiocardiograms, either a calibrated marker catheter, some type of external reference grid, or large diameter calibration system built into the X-ray system is used *in each plane* of the angiocardiograms for accurate measurements of the valve annulus. The measurements should be recorded in as many views as possible including specifically where the valve attachments are visualized within the ventricle. The maximum measured diameter of the valve annulus is used to determine the combined balloon diameters for the dilation. TEE/ICE is used along with the angiocardiogram to define the valvular anatomy and for a corroborative measurement of the annulus.

A frame of the angiocardiogram from both planes of the X-ray is placed in a "freeze frame" image to be used as a "road map" during the dilation. If quality "freeze frame" or image storage capabilities are not available, an external radio-opaque marker can be placed on the skin surface corresponding to the location of the valve as visualized on the angiogram. This marker is used to identify the level of the valve orifice during the dilation. A lead shot (#5!) or a lead number 1 from a radiographic film "labeling set", taped onto the chest wall in both planes, serves as an excellent reference marker.

With the left atrial pressure recorded and the mitral anatomy defined and measured accurately angiographically, an angiographic catheter at least one French size smaller than the long transseptal sheath is manipulated from the left atrium into the left ventricle. With the angiographic catheter positioned in a stable location in the left ventricle and the tip of the larger French sized sheath still within the left atrium, very accurate, *simultaneous* pressure tracings of the left atrial and left ventricular pressures are recorded from the side arm of the sheath and the catheter, respectively. These pressures provide the exact gradient across the stenotic mitral valve. The valve area can be calculated using this gradient along with the cardiac output determinations obtained during the right heart catheterization.

Once accurate and simultaneous left atrial and left ventricular pressures are recorded, the X-ray tubes again are positioned into the angles that are the most perpendicular to the valve annulus and a biplane *left ventricular* angiocardiogram is performed. Often the *negative shadow* of the mitral valve in a densely opacified left ventricular image gives more information about the exact location of the opening, size and excursion of the mitral valve leaflets than the left atrial angiocardiogram. If so, a frame of the left ventricular angiocardiogram in the exact position that will be utilized during the valve dilation procedure is stored on the "freeze frame" to serve as a reference for positioning the dilating balloons once they are exactly within the lesion.

After accurate measurements have been made of the mitral annulus, the balloons are chosen for the dilation. The combined balloon diameters should be equal to or 1.2–1.3 times greater than the measured largest diameter of the mitral valve annulus. Relatively long balloons are used, but, at the same time, balloons with short "shoulders" and short tips are necessary. Some balloons are available with a "pig-tail" curve at the tip rather than a short stubby tip. The "pig-tail" is designed to keep the balloon tip from driving into or through the ventricular wall if the balloon is displaced into the ventricle during inflation. The longer balloons are necessary to span the entire "depth" of the mitral valve and the valve apparatus, and to help keep the dilating surface of the balloons from moving in and out of the valve during the inflation.

Once the angiocardiograms are completed, the measurements obtained, and the size of the balloons chosen, the angiographic catheter is withdrawn from the left ventricle and from the body through the sheath. Preparations are made for the second transseptal puncture. The two balloons will be delivered through the septum through two *separate* long transseptal sheaths. If a larger sized sheath than the one already in the left atrium is necessary to accommodate one or both of the balloons that are to be used for the dilation, the initial transseptal sheath is exchanged for the appropriate larger sized sheath/dilator at this time. The exchange is made over a wire passed through the first sheath into the left atrium or pulmonary vein. Once the new, larger sheath is secure in the left atrium, the second transseptal puncture from the opposite femoral vein is carried out using a second larger transseptal sheath/dilator set that will accommodate the dilation balloon.

The exact location on the septum of the second puncture will depend upon where on the septum the earlier puncture was made. The second puncture should be at least a centimeter away from the first puncture and can be above, below, in front or behind the first puncture—wherever there is the most room and distance from the first puncture. The location of the second puncture on the septum in relation to the first puncture site and the rest of the septum is identified from the earlier left atrial angiograms and by TEE/ICE interrogation. The second transseptal puncture is carried out identically to the first transseptal procedure except that when approaching from the right inguinal area, the patient's body usually does not have to be bent to align the septum better.

After both transseptal sheaths are secured in the left atrium and cleared of air/clot, the side arms of both sheaths are attached to the pressure/flush system and placed on a slow continuous flush. When the two long sheaths are placed on their separate pressure recordings, the two simultaneous pressures from the left atrium again serve to document the accuracy of the two transducers and, in turn, the reliability of the previous hemodynamics. The two pressure tracings should produce a *single line* on the screen.

In order to position the guide wires across the mitral valve for the dilation, an end-hole catheter is advanced through one of the sheaths that are positioned in the left atrium, and maneuvered through the mitral valve and into the left ventricle. It is safer, usually easier and always better to "float" an end-hole, floating balloon catheter through the mitral valve than to maneuver a standard end-hole catheter from the left atrium to the left ventricle. The inflated balloon has a better chance of passing through the "center" and/or the largest orifice of the mitral valve apparatus and not through a narrow slit in a leaflet and/or fused chordae of the valve. TEE/ICE, as well, is very helpful in determining the exact course of the catheter through the valve apparatus.

When the opening in the mitral orifice tolerates it, the sheath is advanced over the catheter and into the left ventricle. Once the sheath and the end-hole catheter are in the left ventricle and well past the mitral valve apparatus, the tip of the catheter is advanced out of the sheath and maneuvered toward the left ventricular outflow tract. The exact mechanism of this maneuver depends upon the stability of the patient, the type of catheter in the left ventricle and the preference of the operator. The sheath over the catheter and through the mitral valve into the left ventricle helps to support the more proximal shaft of a floating balloon catheter in this maneuver. As the balloon catheter is pushed forward through the sheath, the sheath holds the shaft of the catheter in the left ventricle and keeps it from backing up while the tip of the balloon catheter generally is forced to turn or deflect cephalad more or less, toward the LV outflow tract.

When the long sheath cannot be maintained across the mitral valve or the tip of the balloon catheter does not deflect toward the outflow tract on its own in the small left ventricular cavity, a controllable deflector wire is used to deflect the catheter tip toward the outflow tract. The active deflector wire also provides an effective technique for deflecting a standard, "non-floating" end-hole catheter or a floating balloon catheter that is not passing through a sheath, toward the outflow tract. The deflector wire, or any other wire introduced through the catheters in the left heart, are introduced into the catheters *through a wire back-bleed valve* and the catheters are maintained on a slow continuous flush around the wire. The tip of the catheter in the apex of the left ventricle is deflected into a 180° curve with the deflector wire. The *catheter* is advanced *off the wire* toward, and well into, the left ventricular outflow tract (LVOT) or even out through the aortic valve. If the catheter tip deflects in the direction of the aortic valve, but the catheter cannot be advanced into the outflow tract, the deflector wire is removed and replaced with a torque-controlled, exchange length, guide wire with a slightly curved, very floppy tip. While keeping the catheter tip directed *toward* the outflow tract, the curved floppy tipped wire is passed through the catheter and maneuvered out of the catheter and into the ascending aorta using the torque mechanism on the wire to direct the tip. Once the wire has been secured in the aorta, the catheter is advanced over the wire.

In a small patient or in a patient with a small left ventricular cavity, the catheter passage into the left ventricular outflow tract/aorta often cannot be accomplished with a catheter large enough to accommodate the larger Super Stiff™ wire (Boston Scientific, Natick, MA) that is to be used for the balloon dilation of the mitral valve. In that circumstance, the deflection into the outflow tract is performed with a smaller catheter, using a smaller deflector wire, and then is exchanged for a smaller diameter exchange length wire. The smaller exchange length wire, however, will not support the balloon dilation catheters adequately for the dilation procedure. The smaller gauge wire is advanced through the smaller catheter and into the aorta. Once the smaller exchange wire is well into the aorta, the original catheter is withdrawn over the smaller exchange wire and replaced with a 6- or 7-French, end-hole, either woven dacron, extruded polyethylene, or even a Toray™ "Glide" catheter. These catheters are large enough to accommodate a 0.035" wire, but at the same time are malleable enough to follow the smaller wire into the aorta. These larger catheters positioned in the aorta are rigid enough to guide a larger, pre-curved, Super Stiff™ wire through the circuitous route from the venous entry site to the apex of the left ventricle. Once the larger catheter has been advanced over the smaller gauge, exchange length wire and into the ascending aorta, the smaller wire is withdrawn, the catheter cleared of all debris and placed on a slow continuous flush through a wire back-bleed/flush port.

Alternatively, a 6- or 7-French "pig-tail" catheter can be used to position the larger Super Stiff™ wire in the left ventricle. The "pig-tail" catheter is introduced into the left atrium directly through the long sheath and then deflected from the left atrium into the left ventricle. The *loop* of the "pig-tail" passing through the mitral apparatus has the same effect as a floating balloon catheter, as the diameter of the "loop" of the "pig-tail" "backing" through the valve obligates the catheter to pass through the *largest orifice* of the stenotic mitral valve. If a small exchange wire already had been introduced into the aorta or left ventricular outflow tract, the pig-tail catheter is advanced over the smaller wire, through the long sheath and into the left atrium. The pig-tail catheter is advanced through the mitral valve and the curved tip or "loop" is pushed into the *apex* of the left ventricle. When the pig-tail is passed over the small wire, once the curve of the pig-tail is fixed in the apex, the smaller wire is withdrawn completely from the catheter. The pig-tail curve seated in the left ventricular apex will usually deflect the long tip of a Super Stiff™ wire 180° when it is advanced into, and through, the loop and, in turn, directs the floppy tip of the wire toward the left ventricular outflow tract. This allows the transition zone and curved stiffer portion of the wire to "seat" in the apex of the ventricle.

Once the first larger end-hole catheter is positioned securely across the mitral valve with the tip directed into the LVOT, the procedure is repeated through the second long transseptal sheath. The second long transseptal sheath already is positioned in the left atrium. The mitral valve is crossed with a second floating balloon catheter passed through the second long sheath. The catheter is maneuvered into the LVOT or aorta using a technique similar to that used for the first catheter as described above. The patient usually tolerates the two *catheters* across the mitral valve and into the LVOT better than even one of the Super Stiff™ wires within those catheters across the valve.

With the prograde catheters in place and ready for the insertion of the Super Stiff™ wires, the indwelling femoral artery line is replaced with a small arterial sheath. An angiographic catheter is introduced through the femoral artery sheath and advanced retrograde into the left ventricle. This retrograde catheter in the left ventricle was not an absolutely essential part of the procedure up to this point, but during the rest of the procedure, the retrograde catheter facilitates the assessment of the results of the balloon dilation immediately after the mitral dilation without the need for removing or exchanging either balloons or wires.

Once all of the catheters are in place, two Super Stiff™ exchange length wires with long floppy tips (7 cm) (Boston Scientific, Natick, MA) are *pre-shaped* specifically for the mitral dilation and specifically for the particular patient. The wires used must be able to pass through the balloon dilation catheters that have been chosen for the dilation. An exchange length, teflon-coated, 0.035" Super Stiff™ wire with a *long floppy tip* is used to support *each* of the balloons during a double-balloon mitral valve dilation. Preferably, the long floppy tip should have a tight "J" or "pig-tail" curve formed at the very end of the floppy tip. If only straight, long, floppy tipped Super Stiff™ wires are available, a J or tight pig-tail curve is formed on the entire floppy portion of the wire. The J or pig-tail curve at the tip of the wire keeps the wire from digging into the myocardium during the manipulations within the left ventricle. An *additional* fairly tight but smooth 180° curve is formed just at the *"transition" zone between the stiff and floppy portions* of the Super Stiff™ wire. Regardless of the other curves in the wire, this curve at the transition between the *end* of the *rigid* portion of the wire and the beginning of the "floppy" portion is essential to keep the wire from kinking and becoming a "perforating" weapon when "seated" in the apex of the left ventricle outside of a catheter. The diameter of the curve formed at the "transition zone" should correspond to the transverse diameter of the particular patient's left ventricular cavity distal to the mitral valve. During the dilation, this curve in the transition/stiff area of the catheter will "seat" in the apex of the left ventricle. The 180° smooth curve helps to fix the wire in the left ventricular apex while at the same time preventing the wire (and the balloon tip, which is over the wire) from perforating the left ventricle. This 180° curve is particularly important if a balloon "milks" forward during the inflation of the balloons. The straight portion of the wire, which is proximal to the transition curve, *should* direct the dilation balloon toward the apex rather than across the ventricle and/or into the outflow tract of the left ventricle. The floppy portion of the wire distal to the transition curve is directed 180° away from the inflow of the ventricle and toward the left ventricular outflow tract/aorta.

An alternative curve and position for the support wire is to form a 360+° "circular" loop or coil on the *entire* long floppy tip of the wire, beginning with the transition zone of the wire. The wire still should have the 180° curve at the *transition zone* just proximal to this 360+° looping of the long floppy portion. The "coil" of floppy wire remains looped in the body of the ventricle as opposed to extending toward/into the left ventricular outflow tract. This positioning of the wire is simpler than directing the wire specifically into the outflow tract, and gives just as much stability, control and safety for the wires during the inflation. It is slightly harder to keep track of the separate wires/balloons when two wires are looped around in the ventricular apex.

The first pre-curved Super Stiff™ wire is advanced through one of the pre-positioned catheters and fixed with the "transition zone" curve of the stiff wire *seated in the left ventricular apex* and with the tip of the wire heading toward the LVOT or aorta. When the pig-tail *catheter* is used to place the Super Stiff™ exchange wire, the pig-tail loop of the *catheter* first is seated securely into the apex of the left ventricle. The Super Stiff™ wire is introduced into the pig-tail catheter and advanced into the left ventricle. As the wire tip passes through the catheter, ideally, the stiff "pig-tail curve" at the tip of the *catheter* "uncoils" partially and deflects the soft tip of the wire 180° and toward the direction of the LVOT as the wire passes through the loop of the catheter. The Super Stiff™ wire is advanced further into the pig-tail catheter until the preformed *curve* at the *transition zone* of the *wire* reaches the pig-tail curve at the distal end of the *catheter*. This results in the transition curve of the stiff wire "seating" in the apex of the left ventricle still within the pig-tail catheter.

It is imperative to have the straight and stiff portion of the Super Stiff™ wire extending entirely through the mitral valve and to the *apex* of the ventricle. At the same time, the distal "end" of this stiff portion of the wire must be protected by the bend or curve at the transition area of the wire, which directs the stiff straight wire away from the apex. The placement and positioning of this wire may take a variety of maneuvers with the sheath and/or catheters and often is time consuming but, like most other wire positioning for balloon dilation procedures, this particular position of the wire is critical for the successful and safe balloon dilation of the mitral valve. Although it is not absolutely necessary to have the tip of the wire in the aorta, it is desirable to have the soft portion of the wire, which is distal to the "transition" curve, heading at least toward the left ventricular outflow tract. This position helps to stabilize the balloons in the correct area of the valve and reduces ventricular ectopy due to the wires.

The first catheter remains in place over the wire that was positioned first and maintained on a slow flush through a wire back-bleed valve, while the second Super Stiff™ wire is maneuvered into position in the apex of the left ventricle through the second catheter, which is already positioned across the mitral valve and into the apex of the left ventricle. The wires passing through the valve can be visualized with TEE and/or ICE. TEE/ICE will show the position of the wires relative to the valve orifice and verify that they are passing through the center of the orifice of the valve, and ensure that they are not passing through some unwanted structure in the valve or valve apparatus. Once the second wire is in position through the catheter, the patient is ready for the introduction of the balloons and for the dilation of the valve.

If not already across the mitral valve, the two long sheaths are advanced over the catheters and wires and into the left ventricle. The patient's blood pressures and heart rate are observed closely for several minutes for any compromise due to the increased diameters of the sheaths crossing the valve. When the hemodynamic status of the patient tolerates the two sheaths across the valve, the sheaths are maintained across the valve for the delivery of the dilation balloons. If the patient does not tolerate the two sheaths positioned across the mitral valve, the sheaths are withdrawn back into the *left atrium* and maintained in the left atrium. The *catheters* that were used for the introduction of the wires are withdrawn over the wires, through the sheaths and out of the body from each groin while the wires are maintained fixed in place and visualized continuously on fluoroscopy. Extra care must be taken to maintain the wires in their exact positions with the 180° "transition" curve *seated in the left ventricular apex* during the withdrawals of the catheters off the wires. With both wires positioned securely across the septum and preferably, if tolerated, through the long sheaths passing through the mitral valve, with the "transition" curves of the wires in the left ventricular apex and the tips directed into the left ventricular outflow tract, the introduction of the balloons is accomplished.

A double-balloon mitral dilation requires *at least three experienced* personnel to be scrubbed while all of the personnel in the catheterization laboratory assisting with the dilation procedure prepare for the balloon inflations. Recording of the monitored pressures from the left ventricle and left atrium are started on a continuously running, slow-speed, permanent recording. The first balloon is passed over the wire, through the long sheath and across the area of the mitral valve. In very severe mitral stenosis, particularly if the long sheaths could not be maintained across the mitral valve and were withdrawn into the left atrium, the first balloon is "parked" over the wire in the left atrium just proximal to the mitral valve. The second balloon catheter is introduced into the second long sheath and advanced to the left atrium or the mitral valve depending upon where the sheaths are positioned. When the sheaths are across the mitral valve, both balloons are advanced across the valve still within the sheaths. The two balloons are positioned side by side exactly within the valve as compared to the earlier "freeze frame" of the left atrial or left ventricular angiograms of the valve and as visualized on TEE and/or ICE. The sheaths are withdrawn off the balloons and back into the left atrium. The positions of the balloons in the valve again are compared to the earlier "freeze frame" image and/or to a hand injection angiocardiogram through one of the long sheaths and/or a left ventriculogram through the retrograde catheter. TEE or ICE gives a good image of the balloons across the valve and helps verify their proper position in the valve.

If the sheaths had to be withdrawn into the left atrium from the mitral orifice before the balloons were introduced, the two balloons are advanced one at a time from the left atrium, over the two separate wires, into the mitral valve orifice. The first balloon is advanced into position across the mitral valve. If the patient tolerates this balloon across the valve at all, the second balloon is advanced quickly over the other wire and immediately adjacent to the first balloon. The introduction of the two balloons across the valve is performed smoothly, but as rapidly as possible since as soon as even the deflated balloons reach their appropriate positions across the mitral valve, the deflated balloons themselves produce significant obstruction. The centers of each balloon (between the marks at the ends of the balloon) are positioned at the stenotic area of the valve orifice. As described above, the positioning can be verified with TEE and/or ICE when utilized. The balloon positions can be documented further by a hand injection through one of the two long sheaths in the left atrium and compared to the earlier "freeze frame" angiogram of the valve, or the positions of the two balloons relative to the valve and the structures within the *left ventricle* are visualized on a left ventriculogram performed by injection through the retrograde catheter. This angiocardiogram is also important for assessing the amount of mitral regurgitation that is present with the stiff wires (and balloons) across the valve *prior to dilation* of the valve with the balloons.

Not only should the balloons be across the mitral valve, but the proximal ends of the balloons must be well away from the atrial septum while the opposite ends are directed toward the apex of the left ventricle. Neither balloon should be bent or turning across the ventricular cavity either posteriorly toward the mitral apparatus or anteriorly, "across" the ventricle and toward the outflow tract. If the balloons are inflated in either of these abnormal positions, disruption of the mitral apparatus is likely to occur.

When both balloons are in their proper positions across the valve, the two balloons are inflated simultaneously using pressure-monitored and controlled indeflators. Unless the patient is very unstable with the deflated balloons across the valve, the balloon inflations are relatively slow and very controlled. The balloon inflations are visualized continuously fluoroscopically and *recorded* on either slow-frame-rate biplane angiograms or biplane "stored fluoroscopy". The inflation of the two balloons is continued until the recommended maximum inflation pressure of each balloon is reached or the "waist" in the balloons created by the stenosis disappears—whichever comes first. The balloons should not move in their positions within the valve during the inflations and a single, discrete "waist" should appear around the two balloons at the level of the stenotic valve. The appearance of the "waist" on the balloons and then the opening of the valve with the disappearance of the waist are also visible and can be observed on TEE or ICE performed during the balloon inflation. If either of the balloons begins to move either further into, or out of, the ventricle or if an unusual or second "waist" appears on either balloon, especially deep within the ventricle, the inflation is stopped instantly, the balloons are deflated immediately and rapidly and, once they are fully deflated, withdrawn out of the valve.

A very forceful displacement of the balloons *into* the ventricle during the pressure inflation could continue to push the balloon tip, along with the stiff wire, even with the curve at its transition zone, into, and actually *through* the ventricular wall!! If a balloon that is displaced into the ventricle does not push the wire with it, but follows the stiff curve on the "transition" zone of the wire, it "turns" toward the outflow tract and tracks perpendicularly *across* the mitral apparatus. Further inflation in this position could disrupt the mitral apparatus. An "abnormal waist" on a balloon is created by a balloon that is positioned abnormally through a chorda or in a fused papillary muscle in the left ventricle. The presence of any abnormal waist should result in the immediate stopping of the inflation of the balloon. Further inflation of the balloon in such abnormal positions very likely will disrupt the mitral apparatus. Displacement of the balloons backwards into the left atrium pushes the balloons actually *into* the interatrial septum. Continued inflation with the balloon pushed backwards dilates a large and possibly permanent opening in the atrial septum.

If the inflation is interrupted, the inflation angiogram and the TEE/ICE during the inflation are reviewed and the balloons and/or the wires are repositioned to more stable locations. When comfortable with the new positions of the balloons and wires, the inflation is repeated. The inflation again is slow, is recorded on biplane angiography and observed on TEE/ICE following the same precautions concerning abnormal positioning and/or movement during each subsequent inflation of the balloons. Once the maximum pressures of the balloons are reached or the "waists" on the balloons disappear, the balloons are deflated as rapidly as possible and the patient's hemodynamics (vital signs) are allowed to stabilize.

During the inflation of the balloons, the systemic blood pressure drops dramatically as a result of the almost complete obstruction of the forward flow of blood through the mitral valve even when using the double-balloon technique. If the systemic pressure does not *begin* to return *immediately* with just the deflation of the balloons, the balloons are withdrawn over the wires, which remain fixed in place, and out of the valve orifice in order to allow freer prograde flow through the valve. Once the patient has stabilized either with the balloons still across the valve or after reinserting the balloons across the valve, the inflation/deflation cycle is repeated two to four more times. By either advancing the balloons further into the ventricle over the wire or withdrawing them slightly back toward the left atrium by pushing the wires forward, the position of the balloons is changed slightly during each repeat inflation of the balloons. This maneuver is to ensure that the maximum parallel surfaces of the balloons are inflated simultaneously and exactly in the narrowest portion of the stenotic valve. The positioning is verified with TEE or ICE during each change of the balloons' position.

In very severe mitral valve stenosis when even one sheath positioned across the valve cannot be tolerated or even the first deflated balloon crossing the valve causes a significant drop in systemic pressure, preparations are made for an initial, rapid, *single-balloon* dilation in order to open the valve partially before the double-balloon dilation. The partial opening of the valve created by the single-balloon inflation allows the patient to tolerate the two deflated balloons across the valve for a subsequent, double-balloon dilation. The wire(s) is (are) already in place across the valve. With the previous "freeze frame" images aligned with the bony landmarks of the thorax and one of the two balloons ready for immediate inflation, the balloon is advanced across the mitral valve and a rapid, but controlled inflation with biplane angiographic and TEE or ICE recording is started. Exactly as with the *controlled* double-balloon inflation, if there is any displacement of the balloon or the "waist" does not appear in its proper (expected) location as seen on angiography or TEE/ICE, the inflation is stopped and the balloon is deflated rapidly and withdrawn out of the valve. The patient is allowed to stabilize and the procedure repeated when the balloon/wire position and inflation appears correct and stable. Very rarely, a single-balloon dilation must be accomplished before even the second *wire* can be positioned for the double-balloon dilation. When a "good waist" appears on the single balloon and the "waist" is successfully abolished with the balloon inflation, usually the procedure can be continued with a double-balloon dilation as described above.

How the results of the dilation are assessed immediately after the dilation depends upon the placement of the various catheters prior to the actual *dilation* procedure and on whether TEE or ICE imaging is utilized. With the retrograde catheter already positioned in the left ventricle, simultaneous left ventricular and left atrial pressures are obtained immediately through the retrograde catheter and the side arm of one of the long sheaths that are in the left atrium. The estimate of any residual gradient and of the diameter of the valve orifice is also available from the TEE or ICE. If the gradient across the mitral valve is abolished or minimized, then the dilation procedure has accomplished the opening of the valve. The various catheters are removed regardless of the other findings. If there still is a significant gradient across the valve, the decision must be made whether further dilation of the valve can and should be accomplished. An estimate of the degree of mitral regurgitation is made with the TEE or ICE imaging. A left ventricular angiocardiogram is performed to "quantitate" any mitral valve regurgitation very roughly. If significant mitral regurgitation was produced by the dilation, regardless of any residual gradient, no further dilation is performed. If there is no, or minimal, mitral regurgitation and still a residual gradient, the angiograms of the balloon inflations and the TEE information are analyzed to determine if further dilation is possible. The diameter of the valve annulus and the combined diameters of the fully inflated balloons in the annulus are remeasured accurately and together in the same angiographic sequence and by TEE or ICE. If the combined diameter of the two balloons is less than 1.6 times the diameter of the mitral annulus in its largest diameter and the dilation did *not* produce *significant mitral regurgitation*, then larger diameter balloons are used for further dilation.

The larger diameter balloons are introduced with the same technique used for the initial balloons. Occasionally when a larger diameter balloon is used, the diameter of the long sheath will also have to be increased. In that situation the original sheath is withdrawn over the supporting exchange wire, which is maintained in place across the mitral valve and in its position in the left ventricular apex. The new, larger French sized sheath with its dilator is advanced over the wire, into the left atrium and, if tolerated, across the mitral valve. This is repeated with the other sheath if two larger balloons are to be used. The larger diameter balloons are introduced through the new larger sheaths. The dilation procedure is carried out with the larger balloons exactly as with the initial dilation balloons. Usually when the valve is being dilated further during the same catheterization procedure, the patient remains more stable with the sheaths across the valve and during the subsequent balloon inflations.

Reassessment of the results of the dilation is repeated exactly as after the initial dilation. Once the gradient has been eliminated or the waists on the larger balloons no longer reappear during early balloon inflation, the dilation procedure is completed and the dilation balloons are removed. When there is a residual gradient or there is the possibility of further dilation of the valve, the presence of mitral regurgitation is assessed with a repeat left ventricular angiocardiogram and TEE/ICE *before* the wires and balloons are removed from the valve. TEE or ICE is more sensitive at detecting tears and other disruption of the valve leaflets and valve apparatus than angiograms. If there is significant mitral regurgitation and no valve disruption, but with the wires and balloons still across the mitral valve, the balloons are withdrawn back into the sheaths in the left atrium. The TEE and the left ventricular angiocardiogram are repeated. If there still is significant mitral regurgitation, the dilation balloons are removed from the sheaths and replaced with end-hole catheters, which are advanced into the left ventricle over the wires, and the wires are withdrawn carefully through these catheters. The wires with their preformed curves readily catch on the mitral valve apparatus, and must be withdrawn *through catheters* that are fixed in the *ventricle*. Once the wires are removed, the catheters are withdrawn back into the left atrium/sheaths. TEE/ICE and the angiocardiogram are repeated once all balloons, wires and catheters are out of the mitral valve.

TEE or ICE interrogation of the valve and the left ventricular angiocardiogram are repeated with *nothing across the mitral valve*. The presence of mitral regurgitation with nothing crossing the valve represents real mitral valve insufficiency! No further dilation of the valve is considered in the presence of significant mitral regurgitation. If, however, the mitral regurgitation disappears, or even is reduced markedly when the wires are removed from the valve, then the decision is made on the basis of the residual gradient and the valve anatomy seen on TEE or ICE whether the dilation needs to be repeated. If the dilation is to be repeated, it means almost starting from scratch, except that the transseptal sheaths are still in place across the atrial septum. The catheters and then the wires are replaced across the mitral valve, larger balloons inserted, and the dilations repeated as described above.

Once the final dilation is completed, pressure measurements are recorded, a left ventricular angiocardiogram, preferably in the same view as utilized for the original left ventriculogram, and a repeat TEE or ICE analysis of the valve are performed. ICE imaging of the valve can now provide a direct image of the valve orifice facing it from the left atrial side through one of the large long sheaths that are still in the left atrium. A repeat left atrial angiocardiogram, again in comparable views to the pre-dilation left atrial angiogram, is recorded to demonstrate the change in the diameter of the valve orifice, the change in valve motion, changes in the emptying of the left atrium, and the size and amount of leak across the interatrial septum as a result of the transseptal approach.

Occasionally and although it is not advocated, when very large balloons and, in turn, large sheaths must be used to accommodate the balloons, some operators utilize a double-balloon technique for dilation of the mitral valve *without* the long sheaths remaining in the left atrium. In that circumstance, the two venous punctures and two separate transseptal punctures are performed with 7- or 8-French transseptal sets. It still is important that the two transseptal punctures are *at least* one centimeter away from each other so that the two holes do not "coalesce" into one. Once the transseptal puncture is completed, the end-hole catheters and wires are positioned exactly as for a double-balloon dilation through long sheaths. Once the wires are in position, the original transseptal sheaths are removed over the wires and the dilation balloons introduced directly through the skin over the wires. When very large "profile" balloons are necessary for the dilation, the holes in the atrial septum often first must be dilated with a smaller, 6–8 mm diameter angioplasty balloon before the deflated, large dilating balloons will pass through the septum. Once through the septum, the dilation is carried out exactly as with two balloons delivered through two long sheaths.

The only "advantages" of not introducing the two balloons through long sheaths are of not having the long sheaths in the "left heart" for as long and that the "factory" folded balloons introduced directly over the wires *initially* are smaller in outside diameter than the outside diameter of the sheaths which they otherwise would be passing through. However, once the balloons are inflated and deflated in the body their deflated "profiles" and diameters are much larger than the comparable sheaths.

There are multiple disadvantages of *not* using long sheaths, no matter how much larger they might be. The large dilation balloons have horrible deflated profiles, and when withdrawn through the atrial septum they make excellent "septostomy" devices, which are very likely to tear and extend the openings in the septum—resulting in very large communications or tearing the two puncture sites so that they coalesce into a single very large opening in the septum. The deflated large balloons are equally traumatic to the smaller more peripheral venous structures and often disrupt the introductory veins as the balloons are withdrawn, resulting in later total occlusion of the vein.

When the balloons are delivered directly over the wires, there is no way of measuring left atrial pressure immediately after the dilation for assessment of the results of the dilation while still keeping the two wires in position across the mitral valve and while still keeping the two balloons in the left atrium. Either one balloon must be removed over a wire, replaced with an end-hole catheter, and then the wire completely removed, or a *third transseptal puncture* must be performed to introduce a third catheter into the left atrium for the measurements. The third transseptal is possible with an additional long transseptal sheath/dilator introduced "piggy-back" adjacent to one of the other femoral venous punctures. This third transseptal system can be as small as a 6-French, since it will only be used for pressures and possibly angiography.

With the major disadvantages and much greater potential for long-term complications when the balloons are not delivered through long sheaths, it is now standard practice to use the long transseptal sheath technique for double-balloon dilation of the mitral valve. Regardless of how large the diameters of the long sheaths are, they always are less traumatic to the atrial septum and venous structures than "bare" deflated balloons.

Single standard balloon dilation of mitral valve

The single "standard" balloon dilation of the mitral valve is still advocated by some operators for mitral dilations. The single standard balloon technique certainly is useful for the very rare mitral valve dilation when the approach is not from the femoral veins, and particularly the hepatic and jugular vein approaches, which involve significantly different transseptal and dilation procedures. A single balloon also is used in *very small* infants where the mitral annulus is less than 10 mm in diameter. The technique for the transseptal puncture, the acquisition of the hemodynamics, performance of the angiography and the positioning of a single stiff support wire for the procedure, all are the same for a single balloon dilation approached from the femoral vein as described for the first wire of the double-balloon technique.

For a mitral valve dilation using a single, standard angioplasty balloon, the diameter of the balloon used should be the same as the diameter as the mitral annulus. Because of the relatively large diameter of the mitral annulus, this of course necessitates a *very large* balloon relative to the patient's body size. Because of the necessary long "taper" of the ends of these very large balloons, they are also *extremely* long compared to the *usable*, parallel walled sections of the balloons. When the usable length of these large balloons is "centered" in the valve annulus for the inflation, the two ends of the balloon often extend from the apex of the left ventricle back *into* the atrial septum!

Because of the very large diameter of the balloon that is necessary in the larger child or adult for a single-balloon dilation of the mitral valve, these balloons have very large *deflated* profiles, and there often is not a large enough long sheath available to accommodate the larger balloon even with the initial "factory" fold on the catheter. As a consequence, the balloon dilation catheter is usually passed directly over the wire and *not* through a long transseptal sheath or even a short venous sheath. A separate pre-dilation with a separate smaller balloon of the introductory site into the subcutaneous tissues, into the vein and across the atrial septum, often is necessary before the very large sized mitral dilation balloon can be advanced to the mitral valve. The pre-dilation of the subcutaneous tissues and the vein is accomplished with a separate dilator or dilation balloon that is larger than the deflated diameter of the mitral dilation balloon. The atrial septal opening is dilated with a 6 or 8 mm, low-profile, dilation balloon, which is advanced to the septum over the same wire. After the opening in the septum is enlarged, the large single mitral dilation balloon is advanced over the pre-positioned wire, through the septum and across the mitral valve.

In the very small infant, the single balloon for mitral valve dilation is delivered through a long transseptal sheath. In that specific circumstance, the long sheath remains in the left atrium and is available for immediate hemodynamic measurements after the dilation. The long sheath also protects the intracardiac and venous structures from the rough profile of the deflated balloon during its withdrawal.

Similar techniques and precautions are observed during the inflation of the single balloon as are used in the double-balloon technique. The single balloon has to be inflated and deflated as rapidly as possible and carefully but rapidly withdrawn from the valve back into the left atrium over the wire immediately after its deflation to allow the return of the systemic cardiac output. The large single balloon inflates and deflates much slower than two separate balloons used for the same dilation so that the obstruction of cardiac output is much longer during the dilation procedure. As a consequence there usually is a very significant drop in heart rate and blood pressure, and a more prolonged recovery period or even a transient "resuscitation" of the patient is required after the single balloon is deflated.

The single, standard balloon technique superficially appears simpler than any of the other mitral valve dilation techniques. It does avoid the second venous puncture, the second transseptal puncture, and the positioning of two wires across the valve and in the left ventricular outflow tract. This appears as an advantage to very inexperienced operators, however, to gain this small advantage, there are many and significant disadvantages, which have already been described. The slower inflation/deflation of the larger balloon has already been mentioned. In larger patients, the very large diameter single dilation balloon catheters cannot be delivered or positioned through a long sheath. Reassessment of the hemodynamics *immediately* after the single-balloon dilation can be performed only by echocardiography or by placing a second catheter in the left atrium from a *second venous puncture and second transseptal puncture*! Without the second catheter in the left atrium, the balloon catheter must be removed completely out of the body and replaced with a catheter through which pressures can be recorded. By the use of a Multi-Track™ catheter for this post-dilation assessment, at least the wire does not have to be removed as well! If the results indicate that further dilation is required, an even larger balloon would have to be introduced.

A much greater problem with the single standard balloon dilation technique for the mitral valve is that a much larger hole is purposefully made in both the femoral vein and the atrial septum to introduce the large diameter, large-profile balloon. Even worse, when these very large dilation balloons are deflated, they develop an even larger, horribly irregular and rough profile. This profile is guaranteed to tear the septum further as the deflated balloon is withdrawn directly through the septum, and can be very traumatic to the iliofemoral venous system when withdrawn out of the vein. Because of these disadvantages, this technique is not recommended.

Bifoil balloon dilation of the mitral valve

For a while, with the idea of creating a more linear dilation profile as occurs with a double-balloon dilation, but at the same time, still being able to use a single puncture and single wire system, "bifoil" balloon catheters were developed and used for valve dilations. These bifoil balloon catheters had two balloons side by side attached to the same single catheter shaft and central lumen. The bifoil balloon catheter was passed over a single wire similar to a single standard balloon technique, however once the "balloon" was in position in the orifice of the valve, there actually were two balloons side by side, which were fixed securely in their side-by-side relationship.

Unfortunately, all the advantages of a single puncture and single wire are obviated by the multiple disadvantages of the bifoil balloons. The bifoil balloons could not be introduced through any sheaths of any length. Because of the large and irregular profiles of the bifoil balloons even before they are inflated, it was necessary to pre-dilate *the introductory venous tract, the atrial septum*, and even *the mitral valve itself* with a 10 mm angioplasty balloon before the bifoil system could be introduced. The bifoil balloons had problems with unequal inflation and the inability to deflate one or both balloons. After the dilation, there is no means of measuring left atrial pressure without removing the balloons completely. Even when deflated properly, bifoil balloons had an even worse and more traumatic, deflated profile than even one large, single standard balloon. As a consequence bifoil balloons were almost guaranteed to leave a permanent atrial septal defect and permanently traumatize the introductory vein. Because of the real disadvantages compared to any possible advantages, these balloons faded from use *and production* and fortunately are no longer available.

Double-balloon, double-wire, through *single vein* and *single transseptal puncture*: (Block™) technique of mitral dilation

The double-balloon dilation over two wires introduced through a *single* venous and *single* transseptal puncture was developed to "simplify" and expedite the procedure by eliminating one venous and one transseptal puncture. The special double-lumen Block™ catheter was developed specifically for this procedure to carry the two wires through the single puncture. A single catheter was introduced percutaneously into one femoral vein. The right heart catheterization and cardiac outputs were obtained. A single transseptal procedure using a Mullins transseptal set was performed. The hemodynamics and angiocardiograms were recorded from the left heart using the catheter through the transseptal sheath as described previously in this chapter.

Once the anatomy and hemodynamics were obtained, an end-hole catheter was maneuvered through the mitral valve, into the left ventricle and to the left ventricular outflow tract. A stiff exchange length guide wire was passed through this catheter and, preferably, into the ascending aorta. The original catheter was withdrawn over the wire. A low-profile 6 mm dilation balloon was introduced through the sheath and over the wire and positioned across the atrial septum. The sheath was withdrawn off the balloon and an opening was dilated in the atrial septum. With the opening in the septum accomplished, the smaller balloon was withdrawn out of the sheath and body over the wire. The balloon was removed from the wire and the special Block™ catheter was introduced into the vein either through the long sheath if the long sheath was large enough or directly over the wire with the long sheath removed. The Block™ catheter was advanced over the pre-positioned wire, through the septum, through the mitral valve, and into the left ventricular outflow tract. A similar or stiffer exchange length wire was introduced through the second lumen of the Block™ catheter and positioned adjacent to the first wire in the ascending aorta. If both wires were of sufficient stiffness to support the balloons for the dilation, the Block™ catheter was withdrawn off the *two* wires keeping the two wires fixed in position. If the original long transseptal sheath was still in place, it also was removed over the two wires.

The balloon diameters and lengths for the dilation were determined by the earlier measurements of the valve exactly as for the previous double-balloon technique. With the two wires through the same puncture site in the femoral vein, the balloon dilation catheters to be used were introduced one by one over each of the separate wires which passed into the *same venous puncture site* and through the *same hole* in the atrial septum (Figure 20.1). Once the balloons had passed one by one through the septum and into the left atrium, the two balloons were advanced to a position side by side across the valve. The dilation procedure was carried out as with any other double-balloon dilation. Immediate verification of the results could only be estimated by TEE or ICE unless at least one of the two balloons was removed, replaced with a catheter and then that one wire removed from the catheter. After a successful dilation, the balloon catheters were withdrawn over the wires one by one. Separate end-hole catheters were advanced over the two wires into the left ventricle and the wires were removed separately through the two catheters.

The advantages of a single venous puncture and a single transseptal puncture are far outweighed by the many disadvantages of this procedure. The balloons cannot be introduced through sheaths into the skin nor through the atrial septum under any circumstance. Like the single standard balloon technique, unless a separate venous and transseptal puncture was performed, the only assessment of the results *immediately* after the dilation would be by echocardiographic techniques, and many operators are

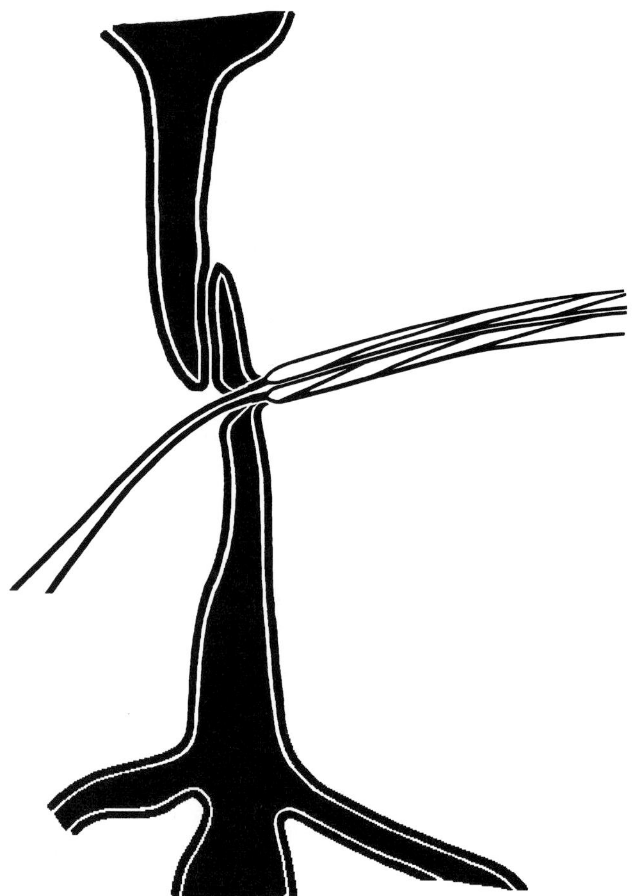

Figure 20.1 Two deflated balloon dilation catheters passing through single small transseptal opening in atrial septum.

comfortable with the echocardiogram assessment only. The two balloon catheters side by side through the same venous puncture hole created a significant, *continual, blood loss* at the venous puncture site, which required constant attention and pressure over the site in order to even minimize the loss let alone prevent an even more significant total blood loss. In addition to the problems with the large puncture hole and bleeding at the venous introductory site, there is an even greater potential problem with the hole created in the atrial septum with the single-puncture, double-balloon technique. Even if one or both balloons did *not* move back into the left atrium/septum during the inflation, the two wires supporting the balloon catheters and passing through the single hole in the septum separated very widely away from each other as the balloons inflated. The distance between the two wires at the maximum balloon inflation becomes equal to the sum of the radii of the two balloons (Figure 20.2). In separating with the inflation, the two stiff wires coming through the one hole in the septum were pushed apart by the expanding balloons and acted like a "reverse scissors" or "blades",

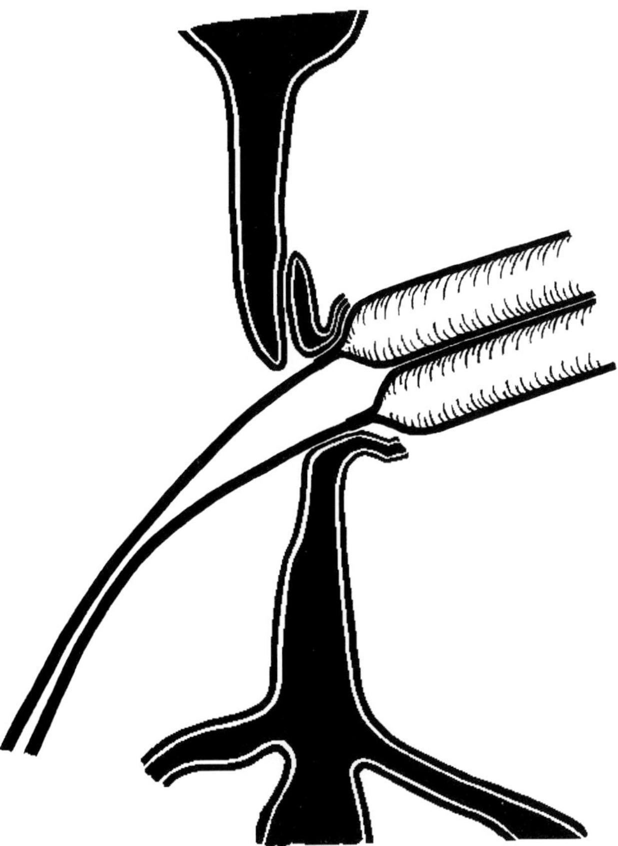

Figure 20.2 The two dilation balloons, which are passing through the same hole in the septum, separate from each other significantly when inflated. The separating balloons separate the *wires* over which the balloons are delivered, which, in turn, tears and enlarges the single opening in the septum.

actually cutting a larger opening in the septum which, in turn, created a permanent atrial septal defect. This phenomenon, of course, was aggravated if the balloons pushed back into the atrium at all during the inflation. When the dilation was completed, the large, deflated, rough profiled balloons had to be pulled back through the already "incised" atrial defect, potentially enlarging it even further. A high percentage of permanent atrial septal defects were created by this procedure, some of them very large.

Double balloons using a Multi-Track™ system over a single wire

The Multi-Track™ balloon dilation catheter (NuMED Inc., Hopkinton, NY) technique is a modification of the double-balloon, single-puncture dilation of the mitral valve[8]. The Multi-Track™ balloon catheter is used along with a "standard" central lumen balloon dilation catheter, and both are introduced over a *single wire*. Multi-Track™ balloons are available as a set. The shafts of both the Multi-Track™ balloon catheter and the "monorail" balloon catheter are reinforced with a steel shaft. After a single venous puncture and a single transseptal puncture the left heart hemodynamics and angiography are acquired through a long transseptal sheath and catheter as described previously. A single stiff support wire with a 6 centimeter floppy "J" tip and a preformed 180° curve at the transition with the floppy segment comes with the Multi-Track™ set, although other 0.035″ Super Stiff™ wires can be individually preformed and used with the Multi-Track™ balloons. The preformed wire is introduced and positioned similarly to the wire positioning with the single wire, standard single-balloon technique. The catheter and the long sheath are withdrawn over the wire. The skin, subcutaneous, venous and septal openings are pre-dilated over this wire with a long, stiff 14-French dilator. The sizes (diameters) of the two individual balloons using the Multi-Track™ technique are determined exactly as for the standard double-balloon techniques.

The Multi-Track™ balloon catheter is introduced into the initial puncture site over the single pre-positioned wire and advanced through the septum into the left atrium. The second standard lumen balloon catheter is introduced over the same wire into the same puncture site. The second balloon catheter passes *adjacent* to the monorail catheter and is advanced over this wire and through the septum to the left atrium. The second standard lumen balloon advances over the wire and into the left atrium better than the monorail balloon and now "covers" the wire within the puncture site and passing through the heart. The tip of the standard lumen balloon catheter advances against the wire loop or holder of the Multi-Track™ balloon so that the two balloons are now aligned exactly side by side. Once both balloons are in the left atrium, they can be advanced into the mitral orifice either individually or both together. When optimally in position across the valve, the two balloons are inflated simultaneously as with any other double-balloon inflation. The separate positions and alignment of the two balloons in the valve with the Multi-Track™ arrangement cannot be adjusted as easily during the inflation as two separate balloons over two separate wires through two separate septal punctures. As a consequence, the two balloons tend to move forward and backward away from each other more during the inflation and must be watched closely for this.

The Multi-Track™ technique eliminates the positioning of a second wire as well as the second venous puncture and the second transseptal puncture. This technique eliminates the separation of the *wires* during the dilation and, although the shafts of the balloons are separate, the shaft of the Multi-Track™ monorail catheter is not as stiff, nor "tethered" proximally as are two side-by-side wires that pass through the same opening. The Multi-Track™ technique, however, does have significant disadvantages. The Multi-Track™ system cannot be used through long sheaths positioned in the left atrium or even through short introductory sheaths into the vein. There still are two catheter shafts through the same venous puncture site resulting in blood loss continuously from the puncture area. Without a completely separate additional venous and transseptal puncture, there is no sheath or catheter in the left atrium during and immediately after the dilation for continuous pressure monitoring and immediate evaluation of the results. The tips of both of the Multi-Track™ balloon catheters should be withdrawn completely into the left atrium before valid left atrial pressures can be recorded after the dilation. As with the single-puncture, double-wire, double-balloon (Block™) technique, the two deflated balloons with their rough profiles must be drawn through the septum and out of the vein directly over the wire with no "protective" sheath over the rough balloon surfaces as the deflated balloons are withdrawn through these structures.

The *double-puncture, double-balloon* mitral valve dilation still is preferred over the double-balloon, single-wire Multi-Track™ technique for this procedure. Because of the disadvantages of all of the single-puncture, double-balloon techniques, a double venous puncture and a double transseptal puncture with introduction of the dilation balloons through long sheaths is recommended for *any* double-balloon dilation of the mitral valve.

Inoue balloon mitral valve dilation

The Inoue™ balloon (Toray Industries Inc., Houston, TX) technique currently is the procedure used most commonly for balloon dilation of the mitral valve in adults[9]. The Inoue™ balloon and technique were developed specifically for the dilation of rheumatic mitral valve stenosis. The Inoue™ technique is also applicable to larger children but because of the overall size (diameter) of the system and the minimum available balloon sizes, it is not applicable to the smaller child or infant.

Each Inoue™ balloon comes as a "kit" which includes the balloon, a special guide wire, a special precurved stylet, a dilator, a metal cannula for "stretching" the balloon, a syringe that is calibrated specifically for each balloon and a ruler/calipers for measuring the inflated balloon diameters very precisely. Each "kit" also includes a detailed, illustrated instruction book about the balloon and the technique. Additional standard catheter equipment is necessary for the basic right heart catheterization, the retrograde catheterization, and the transseptal puncture for the procedure.

Inoue™ balloons are available in multiple sizes varying in 2 mm increments from 20 to 30 mm. The size of the Inoue™ balloon represents the *maximal* dilating diameter of the specific balloon. Each Inoue™ balloon catheter kit contains a syringe, which is specific for the particular balloon, and allows the introduction of precise amounts of fluid into the balloon, which, in turn, produces precise, predetermined and reproducible diameters of the balloon during the dilation procedure. Each of the larger balloons has a range of dilating diameters, which begin at 4 mm less than the listed (maximal) dilating diameter of the balloon. The 20 mm and 22 mm balloons only start with a range of 2 mm smaller than their maximum diameter. For example, a 30 mm Inoue™ balloon has a dilation range of 26 to 30 mm depending upon the exact volume of fluid introduced into the balloon during the dilation.

Inoue™ balloons are uniquely designed, both in the way they inflate and to inflate to a very precise "dilating" diameter when inflated with a very specific amount of fluid. The balloon catheters are equipped with a proximal hub "W connector", which has three "ports" connected to three separate lumens. The two side ports (at the two ends of the "W connector") are connected to the common cavity of the single *balloon* through separate lumens. Each side port connected to a lumen has a two-way stopcock at the proximal end. The *central* hub at the "center" of the "W connector" connects with the lumen passing *completely* through the shaft of the catheter including through the balloon. The central lumen passes through a Lure lock connection at the proximal end of a metal "inner tube" which is built into the catheter shaft. One of the balloon ports acts as a "vent" port, while the other balloon port is a main, or filling port.

While the balloon is still outside of the body, the balloon is cleared of all air (or gas) by flushing fluid into the main *balloon* port and allowing the air to escape from the vent port. Once the balloon is free of all air, the vent port is closed. The syringe, which is specific for the particular balloon, is filled with the *precise* amount of diluted contrast that is required to obtain the maximal diameter of that particular balloon. The filled syringe is attached to the filling port of the balloon catheter. The balloon is *filled* with the *specific amounts* of fluid that each of three diameters of the particular balloon require, while the dilating "waists" on the balloon at each volume are measured precisely with the calipers. The volume in the syringe—and introduced into the balloon—is adjusted so that the waist on the balloon reaches the prescribed measured diameter very precisely. The amount of this volume at each diameter is noted on the scale on the side of the special syringe. The very precise increase in *diameter* by incremental, specific increases in volume in the balloon allows the sequential increase in the diameter of the balloon up to a 4 millimeter larger diameter during the dilation procedure without having to exchange balloons. The diameter of the *balloon* used is chosen to equal the *maximum* diameter to which the valve is to be dilated. The balloon usually is *not* inflated to this maximum diameter initially. This allows the valve to be dilated to less than the maximal measured/calculated diameter initially, yet allows the same balloon to be used for further incremental dilations in 2 mm diameter steps up to 4 mm larger in diameter than the initial inflation when eventually reaching the maximum diameter of the balloon.

During the dilation procedure, the balloon initially inflates in three separate segments, eventually forming a very blunt "dumbbell" configuration with a thick, rigid "waist" at full inflation. First, the *distal* segment of the Inoue™ balloon inflates while it is in the left ventricle, almost as a separate balloon. The inflated "distal balloon" is pulled back against the left ventricular surface of the mitral valve. Next the very *proximal* segment of the balloon inflates on the left atrial surface of the valve, and in doing so leaves a relatively deep "waist" or neck at the level of the valve and between the inflated distal and proximal segments of the balloon. Finally, as the total, specific volume to achieve the particular diameter of the balloon is introduced, the central waist expands exactly in the valve to this predetermined diameter.

As during the other mitral dilations, echocardiography is used to help position and control the balloon during the dilation and to help monitor the effects of the dilation. Although transthoracic echo (TTE) can be used, now usually transesophageal echo (TEE) is used with the Inoue™ balloon as well as with other mitral dilation techniques.

Inoue™ mitral valve dilation technique

A retrograde left heart catheter is maneuvered into the left ventricle from either the right or the left femoral artery. A right heart cardiac catheterization including pulmonary artery wedge pressures is carried out from the right femoral vein. An estimate of the severity of the mitral obstruction is obtained from the gradient between the pulmonary capillary wedge pressure and the end-diastolic left ventricular pressure. The right heart catheter is replaced with a Mullins™ transseptal set appropriate for the size of the patient. A transseptal puncture is performed in the *mid*, or *high* (cephalad) atrial septum. The position of the puncture is controlled using both the PA and lateral projections of the fluoroscopy and comparing the needle position with known, fixed landmarks within the chest. Some operators consider the TEE to be helpful, or even necessary, for positioning the needle properly for this puncture.

Once the tip of the transseptal sheath/dilator set is positioned securely within the left atrium, the needle and then the dilator are removed slowly and the long sheath is cleared meticulously of any air or clot. Accurate left heart hemodynamics and precise angiography of the mitral valve are recorded through the transseptal sheath or a catheter that is introduced through the sheath as described previously. Accurate measurements of both the PA and lateral diameters of the mitral annulus are made from the angled X-ray views of the valve. The proper balloon size for the dilation is determined from these measurements, although in many adult series, the size of the Inoue™ balloon is chosen arbitrarily according to the height and/or the weight of the patient! This arbitrary determination is not applicable in the pediatric population because of the marked variation in size and configuration of congenital mitral valves. The diameter of the Inoue™ balloon is chosen to equal the *largest measured* diameter of the mitral annulus.

Once the hemodynamics and valve diameters have been validated, preparations are made for the introduction of the Inoue™ balloon. The specific balloon chosen for the particular patient is prepared. Each balloon is measured outside of the body at its various inflation volumes/diameters as described above. The diagnostic catheter is withdrawn through the long sheath, which is in the left atrium, and replaced in the left atrium with the specific shaped, Inoue™ exchange length guide wire. This guide wire is fairly stiff and has a large diameter 360+° curve at the distal end. The large loop in the guide wire is looped around in the left atrium. The long sheath is removed over the wire and replaced with the 14-French Inoue™ dilator. The dilator is advanced over the guide wire, through the skin, into the vein and through the atrial septum well into the left atrium. This creates a wide tract from the skin to the left atrium for the subsequent introduction of the Inoue™ balloon catheter. Once the tract is created, the dilator is removed over the special guide wire. The Inoue™ balloon catheter is introduced over the guide wire and advanced just to the introduction site at the skin.

A metal stretching tube, which has a configuration similar to a Ross™ transseptal needle without the sharp tip, is introduced into the inner tube of the balloon catheter only after the catheter has been positioned over the special guide wire. The long metal Inoue™ *stretching tube* is introduced over the wire into the *inner tube* in the shaft of the Inoue™ catheter. The *stretching tube* is advanced into and locked to the Lure™ lock hub of the *inner tube* of the catheter. The *inner tube* with the contained metal stretching tube is advanced into the catheter, and the locking pin on the hub of the inner tube is locked into the slot on the central *hub* of the balloon catheter. The fully inserted and locked *inner* and *stretching tube* elongates the otherwise fairly fat and stubby Inoue™ balloon into an elongated tubular structure. All of these maneuvers and attachments are made with the balloon catheter still outside of the body but over the guide wire that is in the left atrium. When the balloon elongates, the outer *diameter* of the *balloon* shrinks to a diameter approximately the same as the shaft of the Inoue™ catheter.

The "stretched and elongated" Inoue™ balloon catheter with the contained stretching and inner tubes locked in place is advanced over the exchange guide wire directly through the skin and into the femoral vein. The catheter with the still stretched balloon is advanced to, and partially through, the atrial septum. When the *balloon* is 1/2 to 2/3 through the septum and approaching the left atrial posterior lateral wall, the *stretching tube* is released from the hub of the catheter and withdrawn 1–3 cm. The catheter is advanced a few centimeters, which, in turn, advances the remainder of the balloon into the left atrium. The *stretching tube* is withdrawn proportionately as the catheter is advanced. Once the balloon is completely within the left atrium, the *inner tube* is released from the locking pin and withdrawn within the catheter until resistance is met. The withdrawal of the stretching and inner tube causes the balloon to expand slightly and allows it to flex and bend around within the left atrium.

Once the balloon is completely within the left atrium, the *stretching tube and the guide wire* are withdrawn together from the catheter shaft and the balloon catheter lumen is cleared of air by allowing passive back flow until there is only blood return and, once cleared, the lumen is flushed. The special Inoue™ stylet is introduced into the balloon catheter and advanced to the tip of the catheter. The wire of the Inoue™ stylet has a three-dimensional 220° and anterior curve at its distal end and in addition has a polished "blunt" elongated "bead" over its distal tip. The purpose of the stylet is to direct the balloon anteriorly as well as caudally toward the mitral valve, similarly to the use of a precurved, rigid, Mullins™ deflector wire for crossing the mitral valve (Chapter 6). Before its introduction, the Inoue™ stylet can be reshaped manually to conform more precisely to the size and anatomy of the particular patient's left atrium.

The pre-shaped stylet is introduced into the Inoue™ catheter and advanced within the catheter into the left atrium. As the curved tip of the stylet enters the left atrium, the tip of the balloon begins to deflect in the direction of the curve in the wire and, in turn, toward the mitral valve. At this juncture of the procedure, with the "vent" port *closed*, the balloon is inflated with 5–8 ml of carbon dioxide (CO_2) through the "fill" port. This expands only the distal segment of the balloon to 10–15 mm in diameter and allows the partially filled Inoue™ balloon to act like a "floating" balloon to help pull the balloon through the central orifice of the mitral valve. The stylet is advanced further into the catheter until the balloon is pointing directly at the mitral orifice. The balloon catheter is advanced off the stylet. The combination of using the stylet as a "deflector" wire and the floating tendency of the balloon essentially assures passage through the mitral orifice and once through the annulus, through the center of the valve apparatus.

Occasionally, the valve orifice is so small that the inflated balloon in the left atrium not only does not pass into or through the valve, but rather, obstructs all flow through the mitral orifice. In that situation, the balloon is deflated slowly and partially and an attempt made at advancing the smaller diameter balloon through the valve. If the balloon does not pass through the valve when it is inflated at all, the catheter with the deflated balloon is manipulated through the valve using the stylet as a fixed or rigid deflector wire, as described in Chapters 6 & 8. The stylet may have to be withdrawn and reshaped to conform to the particular atrium in order to accomplish a successful deflection through the valve.

Occasionally, in the presence of a very large left atrium, deflection with the stylet, even with the balloon inflated, does not direct the balloon through the mitral valve. In this circumstance the stylet is withdrawn behind the *proximal* end of the balloon on the catheter and the balloon is partially inflated. The catheter, with the balloon, is then rotated clock-wise toward the *rightward-posterior* wall of the left atrium. The stylet is fixed in position while the balloon catheter is advanced. This forces the balloon to loop 360° within the left atrium, which, in turn, directs the balloon tip leftward and anteriorly directly toward the mitral orifice. As it is advanced with continual minimal adjustments in its direction, the balloon advances from this 360° loop through the valve and into the left ventricle.

Once the balloon is into the left ventricle by whichever manipulation, or when the *distal segment* of the balloon was *deflated* completely in order to enter the left ventricle, the balloon is partially reinflated with CO_2. The partially inflated balloon is moved to and fro within the valve apparatus in order to verify that it is not entrapped within the chordae. A TEE or ICE is helpful for identifying the location of the balloon within the valve and ensuring that it is not entrapped within the chordae or not passing through a small secondary valve orifice. A left ventricular angiogram through the separate retrograde catheter also helps identify the correct position of the balloon through the valve. When satisfied with the position across the valve, the *main* input stopcock is *opened* while a diluted contrast solution is flushed *into* the *vent* stopcock and completely through the balloon. This forces the CO_2 out of the balloon and replaces it with dilute contrast while still not inflating the balloon *at all*. When the balloon is empty of CO_2, the *vent* stopcock is closed. The syringe, filled with the predetermined, specific amount of dilute contrast for the *minimal diameter* of the particular balloon, is attached to the *main* stopcock. The precise amount of inflation fluid necessary to reach the *minimal* diameter of the particular balloon was noted previously on the red scale on the side of the special syringe during the trial inflations. The dilation procedure is begun.

The balloon inflation is begun by first filling *only* the *distal* segment of the balloon with fluid. With this segment of the balloon filled, the balloon is withdrawn against the ventricular side of the stenotic area of the valve and into the orifice of the valve. The balloon positioning is visualized on the fluoroscopy while comparing the balloon position with fixed landmarks within the thorax, and the position is verified by TEE or ICE interrogation. While the balloon is held precisely in that position, the remainder of the balloon is inflated sequentially but continuously and rapidly with the predetermined volume to create the minimal central "waist" on the balloon. The second part of the inflation fills only the *proximal* segment of the balloon which, in turn, positions the proximal and distal inflated portions of the balloon on each side of the obstruction and "locks" the whole balloon in place straddling the narrowest area of stenosis. As the inflation of the balloon continues, the center "waist" of the balloon inflates to the pre-set diameter determined by the exact amount of fluid injected into the balloon. The expansion of the central "waist" in the balloon accomplishes the dilation of the valve. The entire inflation process is recorded on biplane angiography and observed on TEE or ICE. As with other mitral valve dilations, if the balloon does not inflate symmetrically or displaces forward or backward out of the valve, the inflation is stopped immediately and the balloon deflated. After repositioning, the inflation is repeated.

Once the dilation is completed, the balloon is withdrawn into the left atrium and the results of the dilation assessed by echo, hemodynamics and angiography. With the balloon withdrawn, there is nothing across the valve to compromise this assessment. The echocardiogram immediately demonstrates any mitral regurgitation qualitatively and provides an estimate of any residual stenosis. An angiocardiogram through the retrograde left ventricular catheter documents any regurgitation and gives some indication of any change in the movement of the valve leaflets. By removing the stylet from the balloon catheter in the left atrium, pressures can be recorded from the left atrium through the balloon catheter, and with the retrograde catheter in the left ventricle the precise post-dilation gradient is measured across the mitral valve. If the gradient persists and there is *not* a significant amount of mitral regurgitation, the balloon catheter is maneuvered across the valve and the inflation repeated to the next larger diameter of the balloon. The entire process with a 2 mm increase in diameter each time can be repeated twice by increasing the inflation volume in increments for a total increase of 4 millimeters in the *diameter* of the balloon "waist", while still using the same Inoue™ balloon. The balloon requires a slightly higher inflation pressure at the full inflation diameter and, in turn, has a slightly greater wall tension, possibly providing a better dilation. If significant mitral regurgitation is produced by the dilation, no further dilation is performed regardless of any residual gradient.

Once the dilation is completed, the balloon catheter is removed by a *very specific* reversal of the introduction procedure for the balloon. The curved guide wire is reintroduced into the left atrium through the balloon catheter. This tends to "straighten" the balloon slightly and eliminate any "kinks" in the lumen of the catheter. The metal elongating tube is reintroduced *over the guide wire* into the catheter and attached onto the inner tube with the Lure™ lock connection. The inner tube and the contained elongating tube are advanced into the catheter and locked on the central catheter hub with the pin lock. The balloon is observed on fluoroscopy during this maneuver to be sure that the balloon does not kink and that the advancing, stiff elongation tube does not perforate through the side of the catheter lumen. The inner tube and elongating tube are *always* introduced over a guide wire within the balloon catheter. The proper reinsertion of the inner and elongating tubes straightens and elongates the balloon, which narrows it back to a diameter similar to the diameter of the catheter. Once the balloon is elongated completely, it is withdrawn through the septum and out of the body over the guide wire. An end-hole catheter or the dilator is advanced over the guide wire and the guide wire removed through this catheter.

Once the operator becomes familiar with the equipment and the technique, the Inoue™ mitral valve dilation in the adult is easier and quicker than the double-balloon technique. The results and complications of the two techniques seem equal in large comparative series[10,11]. Because of the size of the equipment and the limited sizes of the balloons, the Inoue™ balloon and technique are not used in small children. The balloon design is ideal for dilation of the fused rheumatic valve commissures, but may not be satisfactory for some congenital mitral stenoses where the combined valve and the sub-valve apparatus have a long "funnel"-like configuration. For most congenital mitral stenosis, particularly in smaller patients, the double-balloon technique is preferred.

Retrograde mitral dilation—through and through wire "rail" technique

Because of concerns over the creation of permanent interatrial septal defects by all of the double-balloon and the Inoue™ balloon mitral valve dilation techniques, several investigators have developed retrograde procedures for delivering the dilation balloons to the mitral valve from an arterial introduction site. The first of these retrograde techniques involves the use of two balloons introduced retrograde from the two separate femoral arteries over two complex "through and through" venous to arterial wire "rail" systems[12].

A standard right heart catheterization is carried out from a femoral vein. A retrograde catheter is introduced from the femoral artery and the degree of mitral stenosis estimated with simultaneous pulmonary capillary wedge and left ventricular end-diastolic pressures. Once the hemodynamic and angiographic data have been obtained, a transseptal puncture is performed from one femoral vein using a *9-French* Mullins™ transseptal set. The sheath is positioned in the left atrium and cleared of all air and clot. The hemodynamics are confirmed with simultaneous left atrial and left ventricular end-diastolic pressure recordings. A 7-French Swan™ floating balloon catheter (Edwards Lifesciences, Irvine, CA) is passed through the sheath, into the left atrium, the left ventricle, and out into the ascending aorta.

The retrograde catheter is replaced with a Microvena Gooseneck™ snare catheter (Microvena Corp., White Bear Lake, MN) with a 20 mm snare loop. The snare catheter is advanced around the arch and the prograde Swan™ catheter encircled with the loop of the snare. A 400 cm long exchange length wire is passed through the Swan™ catheter into the ascending aorta and grasped with the snare. The snare catheter with the grasped exchange wire is withdrawn and exteriorized from the femoral artery. This "exteriorizes" the arterial end of the exchange wire, which now extends from the femoral artery, retrograde around the arch into the left ventricle, back through the mitral valve to the left atrium, into the long venous sheath, back across the interatrial septum, and finally out of the femoral vein. The Swan™ catheter is withdrawn off the wire and out of the body.

Once the first through and through wire is in place, the 7-French Swan™ catheter is reintroduced into the same long 9-French sheath adjacent to the first exchange wire and advanced through the left heart into the ascending aorta similarly to the introduction of the first floating balloon catheter. The same snare catheter is introduced into the second (opposite) femoral artery and advanced into the aortic root. The entire snare procedure with a second exchange length wire advanced through the Swan™ catheter in the aorta is repeated, creating two through and through venous to arterial "rail" wires, although the two wires exit through the two separate femoral arteries.

An even more satisfactory method of positioning these wires is to introduce the Swan™ catheter through two separate venous and two separate transseptal punctures so that the through and through wires will be entering two separate venous sites and passing through *separate and separated holes* in the atrial septum. In addition to having the separated holes in the septum, the two separate routes through the right heart and septum through two separate long transseptal sheaths permit a Swan™ catheter to remain over each exchange wire as it passes through the mitral and aortic valves. The catheter over the wire protects the intracardiac structures from the "cutting" properties of a spring guide wire that is rubbing continuously against moving tissues.

The diameter and length of the balloons for the dilation are chosen exactly as for any other double-balloon mitral valve dilation technique. Once the two through and through wires are in place, the appropriate dilation balloons are introduced over the two wires separately into each of the femoral *arteries* and advanced *retrograde* into the heart. When the Swan™ catheters are still over the wires, as the tip of each balloon is advanced against the Swan™ catheter, the Swan™ catheter is withdrawn proportionately. The balloon dilation catheters are advanced one at a time over their wire, through the aortic valve, and into the left ventricle, and looped back through the mitral valve. This maneuver takes some careful manipulation of the wire/balloon combinations. The combination wire/catheter must not *form a tight loop* that constricts around the mitral and aortic valves or the wire/catheter must not become *too loose* and, in turn, form such a loose loop within the left ventricle that the balloon will not make the 180° curve in the ventricle in order to pass retrograde through the mitral valve. Once the balloons are retrograde across the mitral valve, the balloons must not extend too far into the left atrium and close to (or into) the atrial septum. When the two balloons are in the proper position as determined from the previous angiograms and by TEE or ICE visualization of the balloons within the valve, the mitral dilation is performed, inflating and deflating both balloons simultaneously while recording the procedure on biplane angiography.

Without very extensive catheter manipulation the *immediate* results can be assessed only by an echocardiogram. The same criteria are used to consider a repeat dilation with larger balloons as are used for the other double-balloon dilations of the mitral valve. Unless an *additional* arterial catheter is introduced into the left ventricle or a separate transseptal procedure is performed through a separate venous puncture, an accurate hemodynamic assessment cannot be made until one (or both) of the balloons is (are) removed entirely. If there is significant mitral regurgitation detected immediately by TEE or ICE, the balloons *and wires* must be removed in order to determine whether the mitral regurgitation is real or artifactual caused by the balloons/wires wrapped tightly through or across the valve. If indeed it is artifactual and there is residual stenosis, the entire procedure for the reintroduction of the wires and balloons must be repeated!

The entire advantage (and purpose) of this technique was to avoid creating a large atrial septal defect. If a single transseptal puncture for the initial positioning of the two wires is used, the danger of splitting the septum when the balloons initially are positioned in, or move into, the left atrium during the inflation is the same as for a prograde, single-puncture, double-balloon technique! The creation of the two "through and through" wire systems and the actual positioning of the balloons in the valve are more complicated than any of the other techniques for the balloon dilation of the mitral valve. The introduction and presence of balloons with very large and rough profiles in the *arteries* has an equal or greater potential for trauma and damage to the arteries similar to the damage to the veins with the prograde techniques. The introduction of these large, retrograde mitral balloons through sheaths in the arteries was not attempted because of the necessarily very large size of the sheaths at the time when this procedure was used. Because of these multiple disadvantages, this retrograde mitral technique never was widely used and for the most part, now is no longer even considered.

Retrograde mitral valve dilation—steerable catheter technique

There is a second, totally retrograde arterial technique available for mitral valve dilation, which does *not* require a complex "through and through rail" wire[13]. Instead of the through and through wire, this technique uses a specially designed 9-French, steerable, guiding catheter to pass a supporting guide wire retrograde from the left ventricle across the mitral valve and into the left atrium. The steerable catheter is an end-hole catheter with a single very large central lumen. The catheter lumen is large enough to accommodate the 0.014" "steering or deflecting" wire *and*, side by side within the lumen, the "support", 0.035" guide wire which the dilation balloon will accommodate. The "steering" wire passes into the central common lumen of the catheter through the proximal hub and exits from the central lumen *through the side of the catheter* approximately two centimeters from the tip of the catheter. The very distal end of the "steering" wire then is attached securely to the *outside* of the very tip of the catheter. When traction is applied to the proximal end of the "steering" wire, the wire pulls against the tip of the wire/catheter where the wire is fixed at the tip of the catheter external to the lumen. This traction creates a tangential force against the tip of the catheter similar to the string at one end of a bow. The force, in turn, generates a curve as much as 160° back on itself at the distal end of the catheter. The catheters are available with three different "tip curves" of 1.7 cm, 2.2 cm, and 3 cm. The difference in the curvature of the distal end of the catheter depends upon how far from the tip of the catheter the steering wire exits the lumen of the catheter on the shaft.

At the proximal end, the catheter lumen is attached to a triple port device with Touhy adaptors on two of the ports for the two wires. The "steering" wire passes through one Touhy valve and has an adjustable wire "lock-nut" on the wire proximal to the Touhy valve. The guide wire for the balloon dilation procedure passes through the second Touhy valve. The third port to the lumen is attached to a flush/pressure system. With the two wires passing through the lumen and the multiple catheter/wire manipulations occurring within the systemic arterial circulation, all three of the lumens are maintained on a continuous flush with only occasional intermittent pressure recordings through the third pressure/flush lumen.

The hemodynamics and anatomy are recorded from a combined right heart catheterization with pulmonary capillary wedge pressures and a retrograde left ventricular catheterization used for both pressure recording and left ventricular angiocardiograms. The X-ray tubes are positioned in an RAO–caudal and LAO–steep cranial angulation for the best "on edge" visualization of the mitral valve. Once this information is available, the angiographic images, which demonstrate the valve apparatus in the best angles, are stored in a "freeze frame" image, which can be displayed simultaneously or repeatedly replayed while the dilation is being performed. The retrograde diagnostic catheter is replaced through the arterial sheath with the special "steerable" catheter. The steerable catheter is advanced, retrograde, far into the ventricle and the tip of the steerable catheter is deflected 160–180° by creating traction on the proximal end of the "steering" wire. The catheter is rotated in the ventricle appropriately while visualized on biplane fluoroscopy in order to turn the deflected tip toward the mitral orifice. The catheter is withdrawn within the ventricle while maintaining the formed loop at the distal end of the catheter. This pulls the tip of the catheter into or close to the mitral valve orifice. If the tip actually enters the orifice, a left atrial pressure is obtained through the pressure lumen of the catheter. With the catheter tip in, or pointed at, the left atrium, a "J" tipped, standard, exchange length 0.035" wire is advanced through the catheter and passed either far out into a pulmonary vein or looped around several times within the left atrium. Often, the deflected curve at the tip of the catheter must be readjusted or the catheter rotated or moved in or out slightly to accomplish the passage of the wire into the left atrium. *When* the catheter tip can be visualized adequately with TEE or ICE, this can be useful at redirecting the catheter tip more specifically toward the mitral orifice.

With the standard stiffness, exchange length guide wire secure in the left atrium/pulmonary vein, the tension is released gradually from the "steering wire" of the steerable catheter and the steerable catheter is withdrawn over the wire and out of the artery. An end-hole Swan-Ganz™ catheter is introduced over the wire, advanced to the left ventricle, and maneuvered retrograde back into the left atrium and to the distal end of the wire in the left atrium/pulmonary vein. The original "J" guide wire is removed through the Swan-Ganz™ catheter and replaced with an exchange length, Super Stiff™ wire (Boston Scientific, Natick, MA) that the balloon catheter(s) to be used for the dilation will accommodate. If the catheter tip is back in a pulmonary vein, a short floppy tipped Super Stiff™ wire is used. If the catheter is looped around in the left atrium, a long floppy tipped Super Stiff™ wire is used. The Super Stiff™ wire is advanced through and out of the tip of the Swan-Ganz™ catheter. Once the Super Stiff™ wire is secured in the left atrium so that the stiff portion of the wire is well across and completely past the valve, the Swan-Ganz™ catheter is withdrawn over the Super Stiff™ wire and back into the left ventricular outflow tract.

In order to ensure that the wire has taken the proper course through the true orifice of the valve apparatus, the Swan-Ganz™ balloon is inflated and pushed over the wire from the outflow tract, back into the ventricle and toward the mitral orifice. The balloon moving freely through this course helps to ensure that the wire is not passing through the side of the valve or through a small chordal attachment. Here, TEE or ICE should be able to follow the balloon and confirm the proper course of the wire.

The diameters and lengths of the balloon(s) for the dilation are chosen as for any other balloon dilation of the mitral valve. If a double-balloon technique is to be used, the retrograde positioning of the second wire is repeated through a steerable catheter introduced from the opposite femoral artery. The procedure is identical, but somewhat easier than positioning the first wire since the first wire delineates the track of the exact course through the valve. The original, smaller short sheaths in the femoral arteries are replaced over the pre-positioned wires with larger diameter short sheaths that will accommodate the deflated balloons of the balloon dilation catheters.

The balloon dilation catheters are introduced through the sheaths and over the wires and maneuvered retrograde around the arch, through the aortic valve, through the left ventricle and back into the mitral valve. The manipulation around the tight 180° curve in the left ventricle is very tricky, particularly after the balloon dilation catheter has already made the previous 180° turn around the aortic arch. The balloon dilation catheters tend to bind on the wires in the tight curves, and as the balloon catheter is advanced, the wires are easily pulled back out of the left atrium. The balloons *must be* aligned with the long axis of the ventricle and *not* across the ventricle when they are in the correct, final position through the mitral valve for the dilation of the valve. Without a through and through wire "rail" as used in the other retrograde technique, there is nothing to "hold" or control the distal ends of the wires in place with this retrograde technique. This part of the procedure takes extreme patience and considerable skill at simultaneous wire/balloon catheter manipulations. As always is the case with the positioning of dilation balloons and wires, the further "forward" the wire can be advanced or pushed, the better the fixation of the wire becomes against the "outer circumferences" of the total course of the wire to the site for dilation and, in turn, the more control is available over the wire/balloon.

The exact position of the balloons across the valve is verified by comparing the fluoroscopic image of the balloons to the original "freeze frames" of the left ventricular angiograms of the mitral valve and by visualizing their positions in the valve on TEE or ICE. When precisely positioned, the balloons are inflated while observing on the TEE/ICE and recording on biplane angiography. With the dilation catheter passing through two 180° curves in order to be positioned in the mitral orifice and with the distal end of the wire completely free, there is very poor control over the balloon(s) during their inflation. The same criteria as for other mitral balloon dilations are applied for stopping the inflation if the balloons begin to move or appear malpositioned during the inflation.

The immediate results of the dilation can be assessed only by TEE/ICE without the introduction of a third arterial or a transseptal catheter. A pulmonary wedge pressure can be obtained through the original right heart catheter, but precise hemodynamic assessment of the gradient and angiographic visualization cannot be performed until one or both of the balloon catheters *and wires* is/are removed and replaced with diagnostic catheter(s).

A modification has been made to the Inoue™ balloon to allow its use with this particular retrograde mitral dilation technique. The balloon shaft is lengthened in order to traverse the distance from the femoral artery retrograde to the mitral valve. Otherwise, the procedure is reportedly the same as the single-balloon retrograde technique. The Inoue™ balloon apparently is no more difficult to deliver retrograde, and achieves similar results to the other retrograde techniques. The Inoue™ balloon requires a 14-French introductory site in the femoral artery!

This "steerable" retrograde mitral valve dilation technique has the one potential real advantage that it could be used for transcatheter balloon dilation of the mitral valve in the presence of true, total, bilateral occlusion of the iliofemoral venous systems and/or interruption of the inferior vena cava. Otherwise this technique, like the "through and through wire" retrograde technique, potentially is very traumatic to the femoral arteries and is more complicated than any of the prograde techniques. In experienced hands, the transseptal procedures are straightforward and safe and allow more direct access to the mitral valve.

The special steerable catheters do have other uses for the retrograde catheterization of the pulmonary venous chambers in the specific complex postoperative anatomy following "Mustard" or "Fontan" types of repair.

"Prograde" balloon dilation of the mitral valve from other than the femoral approach

There are extremely rare occasions when there is no direct access to the interatrial septum from either of the femoral veins, and an alternative route to the mitral valve must be used to perform a prograde, mitral valve dilation. The retrograde arterial approach using a steerable catheter has just been discussed, however, it has many drawbacks in most users' hands, and the retrograde, arterial approach to the mitral valve is unacceptable in pediatric and other small patients. Alternative approaches for the atrial transseptal procedure, including both the transjugular approach and the transhepatic approach, are described in Chapter 8 ("Transseptal Techniques"), and both approaches provide access to the mitral valve for balloon dilation. When either of the "non-femoral vein" approaches to the atrial septum is used, a single-balloon technique for the dilation of the mitral valve is used.

Transjugular approach for balloon dilation of the mitral valve

The transjugular approach to an atrial transseptal puncture is used for access to the left atrium in patients in whom the iliofemoral venous access is obstructed, but the superior vena cava is open. In patients with mitral stenosis, a jugular access is more justified, more straightforward, and safer than the transseptal procedure from the transhepatic approach. The atrial transseptal procedure from the jugular approach is described in detail in Chapter 8 ("Transseptal Techniques").

The atrial septum in patients with significant mitral stenosis invariably bulges from the left into the right atrium (unless there is a pre-existing opening in the septum). This bulge of the atrial septum creates a "shelf" on the cephalad end of the septum protruding into the right atrium just caudal to the entrance of the superior vena cava into the right atrium. This bulge or "shelf" seems to have been "created" for the purpose of a transseptal puncture from the superior vena cava! The course from the right jugular vein to the "bulge" in the septal surface essentially is a straight line, making the impinging on the bulging septum straightforward and seldom a problem in these patients. As a consequence, before beginning the puncture from this approach, the curve at the distal end of the standard Brockenbrough™ needle is straightened to a very slight ~10° curve.

Even when performed for the purpose of the mitral valve dilation where a much larger delivery sheath is necessary, a standard 8- or 9-French MTS™ set is used for the *initial* transseptal puncture from the jugular vein. There are no MTS™ sets or transseptal catheters in a "transseptal length" that are large enough to accommodate either the single standard mitral "angioplasty" balloons or an Inoue™ balloon. In addition, better control of the transseptal puncture is possible with a standard diameter and length MTS™ set, and much less force against the septum is required compared to using a very large sheath/dilator set. Before the standard MTS™ set is introduced into the jugular vein the combined sheath/dilator is straightened, leaving only a 15–20° curve at the tip of the sheath. This straighter curve is more advantageous for both the puncture of the septum and for proceeding directly to the orifice of the mitral valve after the atrial septal puncture.

The transseptal puncture from the right jugular vein is completed as described in Chapter 8. Once the needle and then the sheath/dilator are through the septum, there usually is a long distance and a relatively straight course to the orifice of the mitral valve from the very high puncture site on the septum. After the successful *puncture* into the left atrium, the sheath/dilator combination is advanced *over the tip of the needle*. With the needle still *within* the tip of the sheath/dilator for directional control, the tip of the sheath/dilator is directed towards the patient's left and anteriorly within the atrium. The combined *needle/sheath/dilator* is advanced until the tip of the *sheath* is well within the left atrium. The needle and dilator are removed *separately* and very carefully, as with all transseptal procedures. The sheath is cleared meticulously of any air or clots, attached to the pressure flush system, and placed on a slow flush. The patient is administered 75–100 mg/kg of heparin at this time.

A 7-French, end-hole "floating" balloon catheter is advanced through the sheath and into the left atrium and the inflated balloon catheter is manipulated (floated) through the orifice of the mitral valve and into the left ventricle (LV). The inflated balloon advancing through the stenotic mitral orifice ensures that the catheter passes through the largest central orifice and not through a chordal attachment of the mitral valve. Pressures are recorded simultaneously from the left ventricle through the catheter and from the left atrium through the sheath. Once the hemodynamics have been recorded, angiography is performed in both the left ventricle and the left atrium as described earlier in this chapter for any other mitral valve dilation. When the anatomy has been defined and the valve measured, preparations are made for the dilation.

Even though the jugular vein is as large as a femoral vein, "piggy-back" sheath techniques are not reasonable in a jugular vein, so only a single-balloon mitral dilation technique is possible from this approach. Single-balloon techniques require either a very large diameter MTS™ system for the "angioplasty" balloons or a very large dilator for the Inoue™ technique. Once the hemodynamics and angiography have been obtained, the end-hole balloon catheter is "re-floated" through the valve and manipulated into the left ventricular apex. If possible the transseptal sheath from the jugular/SVC is advanced over the catheter and almost to the LV apex. Using the support of the sheath or with the use of an active deflector wire, the floating balloon catheter is "turned" in the apex of the left ventricle and directed toward or into the left ventricular outflow tract/aorta. Exactly as for the wires for the other prograde mitral dilations, an exchange length 0.035″ Super Stiff™ wire with a long floppy tip is *pre-curved* to form a 180° curve just at the transition zone between the stiff and floppy portions of the wire and a multi-looped "pig-tail" curve is formed on the long floppy segment. The wire is passed through and out of the end-hole balloon catheter. The distal floppy portion of the wire is allowed to pass into the aorta or to curl back into the ventricular cavity while the 180° curve at the transition zone of the wire is "seated" in the apex of the left ventricle.

Once the wire is stable in this position in the left ventricle, the floating balloon catheter is withdrawn out of the sheath, over the wire and replaced with a 6 mm diameter angioplasty balloon. The angioplasty balloon is positioned across the site of the septal puncture and the long sheath is withdrawn completely out of the left atrium and the septum, leaving only the balloon over the wire and across the septum. The septum is dilated with the balloon following which the balloon and long sheath are withdrawn from the jugular vein leaving the Super Stiff™ wire in the jugular vein, through the septum and mitral valve and secure in the apex of the left ventricle.

If available in a large enough size to accommodate the mitral "angioplasty" balloon, an MTS™ is straightened to a gentle 15–20° curve at the distal end. The pre-curved MTS™ is introduced into the jugular vein over the Super Stiff™ wire and advanced through the septum into the left atrium. Once this is accomplished, except for the size of the sheath in the jugular vein, the introduction of the "angioplasty" balloon and the dilation of the mitral valve are straightforward, with the very straight course from the jugular vein to the mitral valve providing excellent control over the balloon.

If an Inoue™ balloon is used from the jugular approach, the stiff portion of the special Inoue™ guide wire is straightened and a tighter 180° curve is formed at the junction of this stiff portion and the floppy tip. This modified Inoue™ wire is positioned in the *LV apex* through the floating balloon catheter similarly to the way the Super Stiff™ wire was positioned for the "angioplasty" balloon. A 6 mm diameter angioplasty balloon is positioned over the Inoue™ guide wire to dilate the jugular venous tract and the septum. The small angioplasty balloon is replaced over this same wire with the large Inoue™ dilator. Once the tract from the skin, through the jugular vein, through the septum and into the left atrium has been enlarged, the dilator is withdrawn, but the same Inoue™ guide wire is left in place in the left ventricle. The Inoue™ balloon is "straightened" with the metal straightening catheter and the inner catheter and is advanced into the left atrium over the Inoue™ guide wire. From the jugular approach and the high septal puncture site, the "straightened" Inoue™ balloon advances straight toward the mitral valve.

When the *balloon* is 1/2 to 2/3 through the septum and approaching the mitral valve, the *stretching tube* is released and withdrawn 1–3 cm. The catheter is advanced a few centimeters, which, in turn, advances the remainder of the balloon into the left atrium. The *stretching tube* is withdrawn proportionately as the catheter is advanced. Once the balloon is entirely within the left atrium, the *inner tube* is released from the locking pin and withdrawn within the catheter until resistance is met. The withdrawal of the stretching and inner tubes causes the balloon to expand slightly as it shortens. Once the balloon is completely within the left atrium, the stretching tube *alone* is withdrawn from the catheter lumen over the guide wire. The balloon catheter is cleared of air and flushed. With the straight course from the neck and with the wire already pre-positioned in the ventricle through a floating balloon catheter, the Inoue™ balloon can usually be advanced directly over the guide wire and easily through the mitral valve without CO_2 inflation, without the special Inoue™ stylet, and without all of the special stylet manipulations that are required from the femoral approach. The "three-stage" dilation with the Inoue™ balloon is carried out otherwise exactly as when the Inoue™ balloon is introduced from the femoral veins.

Transhepatic approach for balloon dilation of the mitral valve

Transhepatic access to the vascular system is described in detail in Chapter 4 ("Vascular Access"). Transhepatic access is used for venous access in congenital heart patients who have obstructed or obliterated iliofemoral *and* obliterated superior vena caval access to the venous system. This route is used for the introduction of a variety of relatively large sheaths to accommodate dilation balloons, stents on balloons for implants, and various intracardiac occlusion devices. It is possible to use this route for very selected mitral valve dilations. Only a single transhepatic puncture has been performed and a single large sheath introduced during any separate transhepatic procedure. In turn, only "single-balloon" dilation techniques of the mitral have been used from this approach. Because of the large sheath and balloons necessary for the dilation of a mitral valve, this route is only considered when no other venous access is possible and when the advantages of the transcatheter dilation far outweigh the surgical risks.

From the transhepatic approach and hepatic veins, catheters enter the right atrium just at the entrance of the inferior vena cava. As a consequence of the rightward and lateral puncture site into the liver and the course through the hepatic veins to the right atrium, a catheter from the transhepatic approach points almost directly at, and perpendicular to, but usually very caudal on, the interatrial septum.

The atrial transseptal puncture is performed using the standard Brockenbrough™ needle and MTS™ sheath/dilator set, however, the distal curves on both the needle and the MTS™ set are modified to better conform to this approach. The distal end of the transseptal needle is straightened to approximately 10° to allow for the straight course to the puncture into the septum, while at the same time still allowing some directional control of the tip by the very slight remaining curve. The 180° curve at the tip of the MTS™ set is reduced to 70–90° to conform to the course from the septal puncture site to the mitral valve. From the transhepatic approach the needle cannot always be positioned at a specific, desired area of the septum. To facilitate entry into the mitral valve, yet leave room away from the septum in the left atrium for the proximal end of a dilation balloon, a mid to even cephalad position on the septum is desired, but not always possible, from the transhepatic approach.

Once the tip of the *sheath* on the needle/sheath/dilator combination has passed through the septum, the needle and the dilator are removed separately with the same meticulous techniques and precautions as with any other atrial transseptal procedure. The sheath is cleared completely of air/clots by allowing it to bleed back passively and then it is attached to the pressure-flush system and placed on a continuous slow flush. Once the sheath is secure in the left atrium the patient is administered 75–100 mg/kg of heparin.

Often, the combination of the minimal angle from the septum to the mitral valve along with the preformed curve on the sheath results in the sheath tip dipping directly into the mitral orifice and left ventricle with little or no special manipulation. Even when this occurs almost automatically, the sheath tip should be withdrawn to the left atrium and the mitral valve crossed with an end-hole, floating balloon catheter, which is advanced through the sheath into the left ventricle to ensure that the valve is crossed through the largest true orifice. Thereafter the positioning of the wire and the dilation balloon as well as the performance of the balloon mitral valve dilation basically is identical to a single-balloon mitral dilation from a femoral vein approach.

Either the standard single "angioplasty" balloon or an Inoue™ balloon is used from the transhepatic approach. Both techniques necessitate some additional extra dilation of the tract through the liver and septum and then the exchange through the hepatic tissues of the original transseptal sheath for either a very large sheath/dilator or a special dilator as described previously in this chapter for single-balloon mitral dilations. Because of the usual low (caudal) puncture site on the septum, when the balloon is across the mitral valve and ready for the dilation, the operator must take special precautions to be certain that the proximal end of the dilation balloon is well within the left atrium and none of the balloon is straddling the atrial septum when the balloon is inflated.

After the dilation of the valve, the withdrawal of the exposed balloon through the septum and the hepatic tissues is the most difficult and hazardous part of the procedure. Whenever possible, the "angioplasty" balloon is withdrawn into the large long delivery sheath positioned in the left atrium in order to protect the septum and hepatic tissues during the withdrawal of the rough, large, deflated balloon. When the balloon cannot be withdrawn into the sheath, the short distance and almost 90° angle from the mitral valve to the septum create sharp angles in the folds (or "wings") of the deflated "angioplasty" balloon material, which, in turn, interfere with the withdrawal of the balloon through the septum. Once through the septum, the rough folds of the deflated balloon offer significant resistance to the withdrawal and create a large tract through the liver. The tract through the liver is always occluded with large coils after a dilation balloon is withdrawn through it.

The withdrawal of an Inoue™ balloon probably is slightly less traumatic to the septum and liver than the usual large "angioplasty" balloons. The "straightened" Inoue™ balloon is larger than most mitral "angioplasty" balloons but when straightened is considerably smoother.

Cribier percutaneous metallic mitral commissurotome (PMMC) for transcatheter dilation of the mitral valve

The most recent addition to the equipment and procedures for transcatheter dilation of the mitral valve is the Cribier™ percutaneous metallic mitral commissurotome (PMMC) (Medicorp, Nancy, France)[14]. This device is a scaled down, metal valve dilator similar to the surgical Tubbs™ mitral dilator, but which is capable of being delivered to the mitral valve by a transcatheter technique. The Cribier™ commissurotome has been used extensively in France, where it was developed, as well as in India[15]. The mechanical dilator has not been introduced into the United States.

The PMMC operates by squeezing an adjustable, proximal control handle ("pliers"), which, in turn, expands a single pair of relatively blunt "blades" 180° away from each other at the distal end of the "catheter" when the proximal "pliers" are squeezed. The blade dilator mechanism and the handle are both manufactured entirely of metal, both are detachable from the "disposable" connecting catheter, and both can be sterilized in an *autoclave* so that they can be reused (up to six times suggested by the manufacturers). The PMMC is delivered to the left atrium through a transseptal technique, positioned across the stenotic mitral valve over a special stylet, and the dilator operated by squeezing the proximal handle, which expands the blades. As the blades of the dilator expand, they tend to align with, and expand along, the "natural" lines of the commissures and are very effective at splitting fused commissures, particularly in the presence of calcification of the valve.

The PMMC has adjustable expansion diameters and can be expanded from 18 mm up to 40 mm by setting the desired diameter on the handle. The present smallest metallic commissurotome collapses down to a 13-French size. The collapsed dilator is passed directly over a special guiding stylet without the use of a sheath. While no sheath passes through the atrial septum, the septum is crossed initially with a transseptal technique. The transseptal puncture is performed fairly low (caudal) on the atrial septum, closer to the mitral valve than the usual transseptal puncture, so that the stylet and, in turn, the PMMC does not form a large curve in the left atrium. After the transseptal procedure, the atrial septum is dilated with an 8 mm diameter angioplasty balloon or a special, solid, 14- or 18-French dilator that is part of the PMMC "set" and is equivalent in diameter to the diameter of the collapsed valvulotome. The stylet is a smooth, stiff, solid, stainless steel wire, which has an attached distal floppy portion. There is a small "ball" or "stop" fixed on the wire, located just proximal to the junction between the stiff portion of the wire and the distal floppy portion. This "stop" prevents the dilator from passing beyond the stiff and supportive portion of the wire. There now is a down-sized, 9-French prototype version of the metal dilator which already has had a preliminary clinical trial and should be available outside of the United States by the time of publication of this book.

The hemodynamic and anatomic information about the mitral valve is gathered as for any other transcatheter mitral valve dilation. The left atrium is entered by a transseptal puncture as low (caudal) on the septum as possible and preferably using the long sheath technique. An exchange wire is positioned in the left atrium or pulmonary vein and the atrial septum is dilated with an 8 mm diameter, low-profile angioplasty balloon or with the 18-French, long dilator that comes with the set. The dilation balloon or dilator is removed over the exchange wire in the left atrium and replaced with, preferably, an end-hole, floating, balloon (Swan™) catheter, although a torque-controlled end-hole catheter could be used. The regular exchange wire is removed and the end-hole catheter is advanced through the stenotic mitral valve and into the left ventricle. The tip of the end-hole catheter is deflected cephalad from the left ventricular apex toward, or into, the left ventricular outflow tract/aorta. The special stylet for the PMMC is passed through this catheter, across the mitral valve, and positioned with the stiff portion completely through and beyond the valve toward the apex while the floppy portion is looped securely within the body of the left ventricle. The "stop" on the stylet is positioned well within the left ventricle beyond the annulus of the valve but it should not be buried into or curving away from the apex of the ventricle. The end-hole catheter is removed over the stylet. The PMMC is advanced directly over the special stylet, through the septum and left atrium until the mechanical dilator is straddling the stenotic mitral valve. The position across the valve is verified by comparison of the fluoroscopic position with fixed landmarks within the thorax, the prior left ventricular and/or left atrial biplane "road map" angiocardiograms, and as visualized on a TEE image. Some operators place a retrograde pig-tail catheter in the aortic root as an added "opaque" reference marker to help localize the position of the mitral valve. The relationship of the mitral valve to the aortic root catheter is established by prior left ventricular angiocardiograms with a retrograde catheter in position in the aortic root.

The desired diameter of the metal commissurotome is set with the adjustments on the handle and the PMMC is expanded to that diameter by squeezing the handle ("pliers"). The dilation procedure is observed on TEE and biplane fluoroscopy and recorded on biplane angiography. As the dilator opens, the dilator and the whole heart are displaced into a very "horizontal" position within the thorax as the dilator straightens significantly as it opens. The squeeze on the handle is released, which retracts the blades of the dilator. The commissurotome is withdrawn over the stiff stylet and out of the mitral valve while the stylet remains in place across the valve. The anatomic and hemodynamic results of the dilation are verified by TEE. When there is a retrograde catheter in the aortic root, it is advanced into the left ventricle and the degree of mitral regurgitation documented by a left ventricular angiocardiogram. If the valve was not opened sufficiently and significant mitral regurgitation was *not* created, the PMMC is adjusted to a larger diameter, re-advanced across the mitral valve, and the dilation repeated. On the other hand, if any increase in mitral regurgitation was produced by the dilation, the procedure is terminated. The commissurotome is withdrawn completely out of the body over the stylet and replaced with an end-hole catheter, and the stylet is removed through the end-hole catheter. Follow-up hemodynamics and/or angiograms are recorded through the end-hole catheter.

In extensive European and other worldwide use outside of the United States, the Cribier™ metallic mitral commissurotome has already been shown to be as effective as balloon dilation for the treatment of rheumatic mitral stenosis[16]. The Cribier™ dilator has a great appeal in countries severely constrained by economics. The metal handle and dilator components of the device can be cleaned, re-sterilized and reused safely at least six times, decreasing the cost per procedure considerably. The 14- and 18-French systems make this device and procedure unacceptable for smaller pediatric cases but the development of the 9-French system should make it applicable for rheumatic mitral stenosis in most pediatric patients.

The large French size of the present devices and the stiffness of the catheter/device as it crosses the septum and mitral valve appear to be real disadvantages of the PMMC. The advantage of creating a very linear dilation in the valve with *rheumatic* stenosis actually may be a disadvantage for congenitally stenotic mitral valves where, often, there are no well-defined commissures. To date there has been no experience with the mechanical dilator with congenital mitral stenosis.

Complications of transcatheter dilation of the mitral valve

Transcatheter dilation of the mitral valve remains one of the most technically challenging and difficult procedures performed in the *pediatric and congenital* cardiac catheterization laboratory. Most of the information and data about percutaneous mitral valve dilations are from the adult experience with the dilation of rheumatic mitral stenosis. The anatomy of rheumatic mitral valve stenosis generally is more suitable for a transcatheter procedure, and rheumatic patients who require intervention are usually larger than patients with congenital mitral stenosis who undergo dilation. In spite of these "advantages" in rheumatic patients, there still are major potential complications from the dilation of these valves[17].

All of the potential complications of manipulations with long sheaths, catheters, wires and "devices" in the systemic arterial circulation are compounded for transcatheter dilation of the mitral valve, where extensive and prolonged manipulations with sheaths, catheters, and wires are required. The long sheaths in the systemic arterial circulation along with the multiple exchanges of wires and catheters through the sheaths create a continual *potential* hazard for the embolization of air or thrombus. These particular complications are avoided by the operator's knowledge of the source and causes of the embolic material along with the use of continuous and meticulous attention to the details of the techniques for avoiding these sources of emboli, as covered in Chapter 8 on transseptal procedures.

The transseptal puncture itself has reported complications. The most commonly reported complication is unrecognized perforation of the cardiac wall or aortic root by the needle and the subsequent enlargement of the abnormal communication by advancing the sheath and dilator through the perforation. The enlarged opening results in cardiac tamponade. By using biplane fluoroscopic guidance, paying meticulous attention to the details of the transseptal technique, and refraining from using "short cuts" to the transseptal technique, complications of the transseptal puncture, *per se*, are decreased significantly, if not completely. Details of the correct techniques for the transseptal procedure are described in Chapter 8.

Dilation of the mitral valve using the transseptal approach can result in the creation of permanent atrial septal defects. The exact incidence and significance of these defects really are not known, but in most reports vary between 20 and 50%[18]. The larger the opening created in the septum during the procedure, probably the greater the likelihood of creating a permanent defect. Larger openings are created by purposefully dilating the septum, by the use of very large or rough "profile" balloons that are advanced through the septum without the protection of a long sheath, or by two or more balloons/wires passing through the same septal opening and separating from each other in the septum as the dilation balloons are expanded. Techniques for performing mitral dilation using the transseptal approach, which, at the same time, minimize the dilation of the septum and reduce the likelihood of creating a permanent opening, have already been described in this chapter. In the present era, if a significant atrial defect is created and persists, it can be occluded readily with one of the ASD occlusion devices.

Complications occur from the dilation of the valve itself. The valve leaflets, the chordae, or the annulus can all be torn during a dilation of the mitral valve[19,20]. Valve or valve apparatus tears result in mitral regurgitation while an annulus tear, in addition to the valve regurgitation, results in a tear externally from the vascular system and massive extracardiac bleeding. The more malformed the valve, the greater the likelihood of damage to the valve or valve apparatus. The chances of damaging the valve/valve apparatus are *minimized* by paying meticulous attention to the positions of the wire(s) and the balloon(s) during the dilation procedure, and the use of appropriately sized balloons. Wires and balloons must not pass through narrow openings in the chordae or small, abnormal (accessory) openings in the valve. As described under proper technique, the wires and balloons should be aligned in the direction of the valve and not across the valve apparatus during dilations.

One of the most serious and dreaded complications of transcatheter dilation of the mitral valve is a tear or perforation of the left ventricle[21,22]. The best treatment is prevention by very careful attention to, and control of, wire and balloon positions during a dilation, although even with maximum precautions, perforations or tears may be unavoidable. Both potentially create massive bleeds into the pericardium.

The wire or the balloon can be pushed through the ventricular wall and cause perforation of the left ventricle. The seriousness of this complication generally depends on the size of the opening and recognition of the problem. An isolated wire passing straight through the ventricular wall often causes a minimal, if any, problem if recognized and if nothing else (a catheter or balloon) follows the wire through the hole. The wire alone perforates because of extrusion out of the tip of a catheter that is buried in the myocardium, or an unusually stiff wire or too vigorous manipulations with the wire. A perforation with a wire *alone* usually is managed by observation or with a pericardiocentesis to drain any accumulation of blood from the pericardium.

More commonly, however, perforation with a wire occurs as the *balloon* over the wire "milks" forward forcefully into the ventricle as the balloon is being inflated and the combined wire and balloon perforate the ventricular wall. This complication has been reported only with balloon or other dilating devices that are passed and secured in the mitral valve/left ventricle over wires. Unless special precautions are taken during the positioning of the wire and balloon and during the subsequent inflation of the balloon, the balloon can be pushed forward into the ventricle very forcefully as it is inflated. The stiff tip of a balloon which is straightened and stiffened with full inflation along with a sharp kink in a wire, can easily perforate the ventricular wall. In this circumstance, a large perforation is created usually with an acute and sudden exsanguination of the patient, similar to a large tear in the ventricle. A smaller perforation due to the same cause may be more controllable by occluding the perforation with a catheter-delivered device[23].

Perforation with a balloon or wire during over-the-wire balloon inflations ironically are prevented by the use of *Super Stiff™ wires* to provide maximum control of the inflating balloon. A 180° smooth *curve* is preformed *on the transition area of the Super Stiff™ wire* between and including the end of the *stiff portion of the wire.* This smooth curve is positioned securely in the apex of the left ventricle. In addition, the balloon that is over the wire must be in the exact proper position in the valve and the balloon's position(s) must be observed very closely and controlled very precisely during the inflation.

A tear in the valve annulus that extends through the ventricular wall is equally as catastrophic as a large ventricular perforation. Tears in the mitral annulus occur when the balloon(s) used for the dilation is/are over-sized significantly for the size of the valve annulus, or when the valve and valve apparatus are particularly malformed, degenerated, sclerotic or calcified. An annulus tear usually creates a sudden, massive hemopericardium or hemothorax, which usually cannot be controlled by any transcatheter means. In any grossly abnormal valve, the diameter of the balloon(s) for the dilation should be more conservative and the diameter of the balloons only increased sequentially and gradually. When an annulus tear occurs and no matter how futile it may seem, an attempt is made at evacuating and replacing the blood from the pericardium while preparing for a surgical thoracotomy.

Unusual routes of access for a mitral valve dilation increase the likelihood of complications. The arterial retrograde approaches to the valve increase the likelihood of arterial injury at the entry site(s). The jugular and hepatic routes make post-procedure hemostasis difficult and increase the likelihood of local hematoma or hemorrhage.

Prevention is the best treatment of all complications. Prevention is accomplished by the use of proper equipment and the meticulous attention to every detail of the procedure. Deficiencies in equipment and "short cuts" in the established procedures increase the likelihood of complications significantly.

References

1. Collins-Nakai RL *et al.* Congenital mitral stenosis. A review of 20 years' experience. *Circulation* 1977; **56**(6): 1039–1047.
2. Grifka RG *et al.* Double transseptal, double balloon valvuloplasty for congenital mitral stenosis. *Circulation* 1992; **85**(1): 123–129.
3. Moore P *et al.* Severe congenital mitral stenosis in infants. *Circulation* 1994; **89**(5): 2099–2106.
4. Shrivastava S *et al.* Percutaneous balloon mitral valvuloplasty in juvenile rheumatic mitral stenosis. *Am J Cardiol* 1991; **67**(9): 892–894.
5. Zaibag AM *et al.* Percutaneous double-balloon mitral valvotomy for rheumatic mitral valve stenosis. Lancet 1986; **1**: 756–761.
6. Wilkins GT *et al.* Percutaneous balloon dilation of the mitral valve: an analysis of echocardiographic variables related to outcome and the mechanism of dilatation. Br Heart J 1988; **60**: 299–308.
7. King DH *et al.* Mitral and tricuspid valve annular diameter in normal children determined by two dimensional echocardiography. *Am J Cardiol* 1985; **55**: 787–789.
8. Bonhoeffer P *et al.* Mitral dilatation with the Multi-Track system: an alternative approach. *Cathet Cardiovasc Diagn* 1995; **36**(2): 189–193.
9. Inoue K *et al.* Clinical application of transvenous mitral commissurotomy by a new balloon catheter. *J Thorac Cardiovasc Surg* 1984; **87**: 394–402.
10. Ruiz CE *et al.* Comparison of Inoue single-balloon versus double-balloon technique for percutaneous mitral valvotomy. *Am Heart J* 1992; **123**(4 Pt 1): 942–947.

11. Park SJ *et al.* Immediate and one-year results of percutaneous mitral balloon valvuloplasty using Inoue and double-balloon techniques. *Am J Cardiol* 1993; **71**(11): 938–943.
12. Babic UU *et al.* Percutaneous transarterial balloon valvuloplasty for mitral valve stenosis. *Am J Cardiol* 1986; **57**: 1101–1104.
13. Stefanadis C *et al.* Retrograde nontransseptal balloon mitral valvuloplasty. Immediate results and long-term follow-up. *Circulation* 1992; **85**(5): 1760–1767.
14. Cribier A, Rath PC, and Letac B. Percutaneous mitral valvotomy with a metal dilator. *Lancet* 1997; **349**(9066): 1667.
15. Eltchaninoff H, Tron C, and Cribier A. Effectiveness of percutaneous mechanical mitral commissurotomy using the metallic commissurotome in patients with restenosis after balloon or previous surgical commissurotomy. *Am J Cardiol* 2003; **91**(4): 425–428.
16. Eltchaninoff H *et al.* Percutaneous mitral commissurotomy by metallic dilator. Multicenter experience with 500 patients. *Arch Mal Coeur Vaiss* 2000; **93**(6): 685–692.
17. NHLBI Registry. Complications and Mortality of Percutaneous Balloon Mitral Commissurotomy: A report from the National Heart, Lung, and Blood Institute Balloon Valvuloplasty Registry. *Circulation* 1992; **85**: 2014–2024.
18. Cequier A *et al.* Left-to-right atrial shunting after percutaneous mitral valvuloplasty. Incidence and long-term hemodynamic follow-up. *Circulation* 1990; **81**(4): 1190–1197.
19. Cequier A *et al.* Massive mitral regurgitation caused by tearing of the anterior leaflet during percutaneous mitral balloon valvuloplasty. *Am J Med* 1988; **85**(1): 100–103.
20. O'Shea JP *et al.* Unusual sequelae after percutaneous mitral valvuloplasty: a Doppler echocardiographic study. *J Am Coll Cardiol* 1992; **19**(1): 186–191.
21. Berland J *et al.* Percutaneous balloon valvuloplasty for mitral stenosis complicated by fatal pericardial tamponade in a patient with extreme pulmonary hypertension. *Cathet Cardiovasc Diagn* 1989; **17**(2): 109–111.
22. Robertson JM *et al.* Fatal left ventricular perforation during mitral balloon valvuloplasty. *Ann Thorac Surg* 1990; **49**(5): 819–821.
23. Ruiz CE and Bansal RC. Percutaneous closure of a left ventricular perforation post balloon mitral valvotomy. *Catheter Cardiovasc Interv* 1999; **48**(1): 78–83.

21 Dilation of tricuspid valve stenosis, systemic vein stenosis and miscellaneous intravascular/intracardiac stenoses

Introduction

Dilation of almost all narrowed structures and orifices that occur in or with congenital cardiac or vascular diseases has been attempted and accomplished with success[1]. Dilation of the pulmonary, aortic and mitral valves, pulmonary branch stenosis, and of both "native" and re/residual coarctation of the aorta are "standards of practice" and have been discussed in previous chapters dealing with each of those specific lesions. The dilation of tricuspid valve stenosis is included in this chapter under "miscellaneous" dilations since it is so rare and so variable, and often occurs in association with other significant congenital cardiac abnormalities. There are numerous other vascular narrowings that occur in patients with congenital heart disease which are neither pure valvar stenosis nor stenotic lesions of great vessels, but which are amenable to balloon dilation. These lesions occur both congenitally and as a consequence of prior surgery, particularly at the site of vascular anastomoses. This chapter deals with the dilation of most of these miscellaneous stenotic lesions within the heart and great vessels. Dilation of many different structures has been attempted, some with reproducible success and others with only occasional or transient success. The exact procedure and its outcome depend upon the nature of the particular lesion as well as upon the technique used for the dilation.

Dilation of tricuspid valve stenosis

Tricuspid valve stenosis rarely occurs as an isolated lesion. Congenitally it occurs with, or as the cause of, various forms of hypoplastic right ventricle and in conjunction with Ebstein's malformation of the tricuspid valve. Tricuspid valve stenosis also occurs as a consequence of rheumatic fever and carcinoid syndrome, and in prosthetic tricuspid valves made of biological materials. Many stenotic tricuspid valves also have significant regurgitation. The most significant hemodynamic component of the tricuspid lesion must be determined before a catheter intervention is undertaken. None of the multiple heterogenous types of stenoses of the tricuspid valve are common, nor are any of them particularly amenable to balloon dilation. At the same time, the alternative of surgical treatment of tricuspid valve stenosis is very tenuous and frequently results in a valve replacement or a "single-ventricle" type of repair, which totally bypasses the tricuspid valve/right ventricle. As a consequence, all varieties of predominantly stenotic tricuspid valves are approached initially with an attempt at balloon dilation in the catheterization laboratory[2].

In the catheterization laboratory, tricuspid valve stenosis is suspected hemodynamically from the presence of a very high "a" wave in the right atrial pressure curve and/or a gradient between the "a" wave and the right ventricular end-diastolic pressure, although because of the massive compliance of the right atrium/systemic venous "pool", neither of these hemodynamic findings may be found even in the presence of significant tricuspid valve stenosis. Angiographically, tricuspid valve stenosis is suggested by the appearance of a small or immobile valve and by the flow characteristics of a "jet" of contrast through the stenotic valve. Tricuspid valve stenosis is documented most satisfactorily by the presence of a definite "a" wave gradient across the valve when demonstrated by the *recording of simultaneous pressure curves* from both the right atrium and the right ventricle from two separate catheters. The "giant a" wave must be distinguished from a high right atrial pressure with a dominant "v" wave, which is a consequence of tricuspid valve regurgitation, or of a large left to right shunt into the atrium. Because of the usual, very marked respiratory variations that occur in the right atrial pressures, "pull-back" recordings across the tricuspid valve using a single catheter usually are not satisfactory for documenting tricuspid valve stenosis.

Simultaneous right atrial and right ventricular pressure curves can be acquired with a single catheter by using a long sheath delivered to the right atrium. A catheter that is at least 4–5 cm longer than and at least one French size smaller than the sheath is manipulated into the right ventricle while the tip of the long sheath remains positioned in the right atrium. Simultaneous pressures then are recorded from the right ventricle through the catheter and from the right atrium through the side arm of the sheath. Since two venous catheters eventually are used for a dilation of the tricuspid valve, the simultaneous right atrial and right ventricular pressures can also be measured from the two separate venous catheters.

The absence of a high "a" wave gradient alone does not rule out significant tricuspid valve stenosis. The right atrium, along with the systemic venous system in general, is very compliant, particularly when there is significant dilation of these structures from a long standing, "sluggish", right heart flow or high right atrial pressures. Because of the compliance of the systemic venous vascular bed, the large capacitance of this vascular bed "absorbs" any high-pressure waves and minimizes the elevation of right atrial pressure.

The presence of an associated atrial septal communication, which is very common with the congenital forms of tricuspid valve stenosis, can eliminate any significant pressure gradient across the tricuspid valve. The associated atrial septal communication results in right to left shunting through the defect which "vents" the right atrial pressure by shunting the blood away from the right atrium and the tricuspid valve and, in turn, diminishes the forward flow across the tricuspid valve, reducing or eliminating any gradient. For an accurate *hemodynamic* assessment of tricuspid valve stenosis in the presence of an atrial septal defect, the atrial septal defect is occluded temporarily while the gradient across the tricuspid valve is measured. This requires the use of one, or more, separate "occluding" or "sizing" balloons. The large, specially designed, very soft, static, "sizing balloons" from NuMED™ (Hopkington, NY) are the most satisfactory for the test occlusion. They are easier to control across the atrial defect and cause less overall compromise of the hemodynamics than the large Medi-tech™ (Namic, MA) "occluding" balloons, which were designed, and used originally, for this purpose. A static sizing balloon larger in diameter than the estimated size of the atrial defect, is introduced through a 9-French venous sheath over a wire which is pre-positioned in a left upper pulmonary vein. The sizing balloon is positioned across the atrial defect and inflated until a "waist" appears on the balloon and the flow through the atrial communication is stopped completely. This is verified by a small, hand angiogram with injection into the right atrium or by a transesophageal echocardiogram (TEE) or intracardiac echocardiogram (ICE) when one of these echo-imaging modalities is being used to guide the dilation procedure. The large, static, sizing balloon, when inflated across the tricuspid valve, can also be used to determine the size of the tricuspid valve orifice very accurately, however, when inflated the balloon totally obstructs forward flow and can lead to a rapid cardiovascular collapse unless the sizing of the valve itself is performed extremely rapidly.

Because of the relatively large annulus of the tricuspid valve, a double-balloon technique is used in order to reduce the profile of each individual balloon at the venous introductory site. A right ventricular angiocardiogram is performed in the right anterior oblique or caudal/right anterior oblique view. The diameter of the valve annulus is measured by angiocardiogram, by TEE or by ICE, when either of these modalities is available and being used. The combined *diameters* of the two balloons for the dilation should be approximately 1.5 times the longest measured diameter of the tricuspid valve annulus. The balloons should have very short and stubby "shoulders" and the balloon catheters must have short distal tips. Depending upon the patient's size, balloons 4–6 cm long are used in order to completely straddle the valve.

Technique

The tricuspid valve is dilated from either the femoral or the internal jugular venous approach. Access to the valve is "straight" and more direct from the internal jugular vein(s), however, two relatively large venous sheaths are required to accommodate the dilation balloons and, as a consequence, usually tricuspid valve dilation is approached from the femoral veins.

Venous lines are established in both femoral veins with standard venous introductory sheaths. These sheaths should be large enough in diameter to accommodate the dilation balloons which are to be used. End-hole, *flow-directed, balloon catheters* are advanced from each vein into the right atrium. The catheter lumen of these floating balloon catheters should be large enough to accommodate the support guide wires that will be used for the dilation. The end-hole floating balloon catheters are used to cross the tricuspid valve when entering the ventricle from the right atrium in order to ensure that the catheters cross through the *central orifice* of the stenotic tricuspid valve. The long "row" of short, widely spaced chordae of the tricuspid valve leaflets allows a standard torque-controlled catheter easily and frequently to pass through the chordal attachments rather than through the true valve orifice, while the larger diameter of the inflated balloon of the floating balloon (flow-directed) catheters prevents the catheters from passing between these small chordal openings and facilitates the catheters "floating" through the true valve orifice as they pass from the right atrium to the right ventricle. Once a catheter has crossed the proper area of the valve, the wires that are introduced through the catheters and, in turn, the balloons for the tricuspid valve dilation will pass through the correct *central area* of the true valve orifice. As a "double check", the valve is interrogated with TEE or ICE for the position of the catheters across the valve, when either of these modalities is being used.

The two wires to support the double balloons can be positioned either in the apex of the right ventricle or, as an alternative, distally, out into a pulmonary artery branch. The wires positioned in the pulmonary artery are more stable, however, the wires and, in turn, the balloons tend to pass tangentially through the tricuspid valve and have the possibility of detaching chordae from the septal wall of the right ventricle during the dilation. Having the wires positioned in the right ventricular apex is preferable because of the resultant angle of the wires/balloons passing through the valve annulus. Wires that are positioned in the apex of the right ventricle will pass perpendicularly through the annulus of the valve; however, this position in the apex provides a more "precarious" stability for the balloon because of the relatively shallow right ventricular cavity and the difficulty in keeping just the *stiff portion* of the wires completely across the valve.

In order to position the wires securely in the right ventricle, the end-hole, floating balloon catheter is passed from the right atrium, through the tricuspid valve and as far as possible into the *apex* of the right ventricle. Securing the tip of the floating balloon catheter in the apex of the right ventricle is facilitated by deflating the balloon as soon as the balloon has passed completely *through* the tricuspid valve. Once the balloon catheter is deep into the apex, an *active* deflector wire is advanced to the tip of the floating balloon catheter and the tip of the catheter is deflected 180° toward the right ventricular outflow tract. A partial, or even complete, inflation of the balloon may help to prevent the tip of the catheter from digging into the trabeculae/myocardium during these deflections. When possible, this area in the right ventricle is interrogated with TEE or ICE for the position of the catheters/wires in the apex. Once deflected, the catheter is advanced off the deflector wire, keeping the curved deflector wire deep in the apex of the ventricle. The balloon catheter is advanced as far as possible toward the right ventricular outflow tract. Once this 180° curve is formed on the catheter, the deflector wire is withdrawn and replaced with a pre-curved Super Stiff™ wire.

A 0.035" Super Stiff™ wire with a *long floppy tip* is used to support each balloon across the tricuspid valve. The wires are pre-shaped before introduction into the catheter. A 360+° "pig-tail" loop is formed on *the entire floppy portion* of each wire and a separate, smooth 180° curve is formed at the *transition portion* of each wire between the stiff and the floppy portions. The wires are introduced into the pre-positioned end-hole balloon catheters, one at a time. As the wire is advanced out of the tip of the catheter, the catheter is moved to and fro very slightly, allowing the floppy portion of the wire to coil freely in the right ventricular cavity or right ventricular outflow tract rather than burrowing into the myocardium. The first wire is advanced until the 180° curve *at the transition portion* of the wire has been advanced into, and is fixed in the apex of, the right ventricle. When the first wire is in place, that catheter is left in place over the wire to help support the wire and protect the tissues while the second wire is being positioned. The same curves are formed on the wire and the same procedure for positioning the wire is used for the second wire.

Once both wires are in place, the end-hole, flow-directed balloon catheters are withdrawn over the wires and replaced with the balloon dilation catheters. The dilation balloons are advanced as far as possible into the right ventricle by pushing both balloons *and wires* forward into the ventricle. The smooth curves on the transition portions of the stiff wires prevent the wires/balloons from pushing *through* the wall of the ventricle. The positions of the balloons across the valve are interrogated with TEE or ICE in order to verify the correct passage through the center of the valve orifice. The balloons are inflated and then rapidly deflated while recording the inflation on a biplane angiogram. The angiograms are reviewed for the appearance of "waists" on the balloons and then the disappearance of the waists with the full inflation of the balloons. The inflation/deflation of the dilation balloons arbitrarily is repeated several times, each time trying to hold/advance the balloons further into the right ventricle. The double balloons allow some flow between the balloons when they are inflated, however, forward flow through the right ventricle is compromised significantly during each inflation of the balloons.

After a presumed successful dilation of the valve, the balloons are withdrawn over the wires back into the right atrium and out of the body and replaced with end-hole catheters. The end-hole catheters are advanced into the right ventricle over the wires and the two wires are withdrawn carefully through the catheters positioned in the right ventricle. The valve is interrogated with TEE or ICE for relief of the stenosis and for any tricuspid regurgitation. One of the catheters is withdrawn into the right atrium and *simultaneous* right atrial and right ventricular pressures are recorded. An angiogram to evaluate tricuspid regurgitation is recorded with a hand injection through the end-hole catheter in the right ventricle, but if the angiogram obtained is not satisfactory, the end-hole catheter in the right ventricle is easily replaced with an angiographic catheter.

If the dilation balloons cannot be maintained far enough into the apex of the right ventricle to remain fixed in position across the tricuspid valve during the inflations, the floating balloon catheters and then the wires are repositioned distally in a pulmonary artery branch and the dilation procedure is repeated. It is very important to use the floating balloon catheters for crossing the tricuspid valve and passing into the pulmonary artery in order to avoid passing through the chordae as the catheters are manipulated from the ventricle and into the pulmonary artery. Once the catheters, and then the wires, have been positioned securely in a distal pulmonary artery, the same size dilation balloons are used. The only difference is that they will be aligned tangentially across the valve during the inflations. Even longer balloons may be necessary when they are positioned tangentially across the valve.

When there is a problem with access from the femoral veins and/or the balloon catheters cannot be fixed securely across the tricuspid valve for the dilation, then the jugular approach is used. Both jugular veins are cannulated with short sheaths that are large enough to accommodate the dilation balloons that are to be used. The two separate flow-directed balloon catheters are advanced from the jugular veins, through the right atrium and into the right ventricle. The catheters are positioned as deeply as possible straight into the apex of the right ventricle, using the same maneuvers with the floating balloon catheter and deflector wires that were described previously for the approach from the femoral veins.

The two Super Stiff™ wires are precurved exactly as when the approach was from the femoral vein to the right ventricle. Once the floating balloon catheters have been positioned securely in the apex of the ventricle, the wires are passed through the catheters and the 180° curve at the *transition zone* of the wires is "seated" in the apex of the right ventricle. The essentially straight course from the jugular vein to the apex of the right ventricle allows a better support of the wire and, in turn, the balloons. When the balloons have been secured across the tricuspid valve, the dilation procedure is identical to when it is performed from the femoral approach.

Dilation of systemic veins and venous channels

A normal vein is very thin walled and compressible, providing very little intrinsic support from the wall or resistance to kinking or external compression. Occasionally there are *congenitally* narrowed areas in the systemic venous system or external compression of a vein by an extrinsic mass or structure. However, most stenoses of systemic veins in children and in older congenital heart patients are acquired as a consequence of other systemic diseases, prior surgical intervention, cardiac catheterizations, or indwelling venous lines or pacing leads[3].

Any surgery on the thin-walled veins themselves, results in narrowed or compressed channels. As the area around the venous channel heals and as the patient grows, further stenosis occurs over time from the combination of the scarring of the venous wall tissues, the constriction of suture lines, or by external compression from surrounding scar tissue or adjacent extrinsic structures. A common type of postoperative "venous" lesion requiring intervention is the stenosis of the superior or inferior limb of the intracardiac baffles following a "Mustard" or "Senning" venous switch repair of transposition of the great arteries[1]. Areas of stenosis in the baffles or venous channels following the "Fontan" cavo-pulmonary repair of single ventricles are appearing more frequently as patients with these surgical repairs return for follow-up. All of the venous stenoses occurring following prior surgery on a venous channel have the "advantage" for the catheter interventionist of the vessel being *surrounded* externally by thick, dense scar tissue.

Stenosis of systemic veins following prior cardiac catheterizations or stenosis as a result of a prior indwelling line usually is a result of "internal" trauma and internal obliteration of the vein. Thrombosis around transvenous pacing leads that are present in otherwise normal hearts also falls into this category. The materials of the indwelling pacing leads, the central lines themselves, or the solutions that are infused through the lines, cause chronic irritation of the intima, thrombosis, and an eventual, obliterating, organized thrombus and scar. Cardiac catheters, guide wires or an intravascular device scraping or banging against the wall of a vein cause(s) acute venous wall trauma which can result in thrombosis. Even venous spasm around a catheter as a result of straightforward catheter manipulations in the vein lead to intimal damage or disruption of the venous wall with subsequent thrombus formation. These lesions usually occur more peripherally and in the smaller veins, but certainly also occur in, or extend into, the larger, more central veins. These "internal" venous stenoses frequently are very long and often result in total obliteration of the particular venous channel. The venous stenosis/obliteration which occurs from internal trauma to the vein also, unfortunately, does not result in *any external scarring* (or external "protection") of the vein against disruption. In addition to all of the acquired venous stenoses, there are also apparent occurrences of congenital stenoses of the veins. These appear as band-like indentations circumferentially around the vessel wall and also have no surrounding supporting scar tissue.

The type and etiology of the stenosis determines if, and what type of, therapy can be used. When a venous stenosis or even a total obstruction can be crossed with a wire, it almost always can be crossed subsequently with a catheter and dilated acutely. The post-surgical and post-catheter stenoses in venous channels expand *acutely* to balloon dilation with at least a temporary opening of the channel. With the combination of the very low intravenous pressures to distend the acutely opened veins and the very thin walls and compressible nature of the veins, there is very little intrinsic wall support or resistance to external compression to maintain the patency of these veins. The stenosed area of the vein must be "over-dilated" to at least *twice* the diameter of the nearest normal vein in order to achieve *any* lasting result from a dilation alone of a systemic vein. Even with the "over-dilation", the stenosis of the vein usually recoils acutely or is re-compressed by any external surrounding structures shortly after an initial, successful expansion. Because of their propensity to restenose, most operators now treat systemic venous stenosis with primary intravascular stent implants at the time of dilation, as described in Chapter 24.

Dilation of central systemic vein stenosis

Since most of the more central venous lesions occur postoperatively, there is usually dense scar tissue surrounding the area of stenosis of the vein. This scar tissue contributes to the stenosis and creates resistance to dilation. At the same time, the surrounding scar tissue also provides a "safety factor" against vein rupture or perforation and prevents wide extravasation around the area when a vein does rupture or split during dilation. Usually, the major challenge to dilation of the stenosis of the systemic veins is crossing the stenotic area at all, even with a wire. Many of the areas of central venous or baffle stenosis following previous surgery on the area are stenosed, "folded" or kinked so severely that they have absolutely no lumen. Each area of venous stenosis is different from any previously encountered, and must be addressed as an individual new and different lesion.

Total occlusions of the *central* venous channels, which occur following the surgical creation of venous baffles, can usually be perforated and crossed using one of the techniques described subsequently in this chapter and in Chapter 31. These areas of total obstruction usually have a patent lumen or channel of a large diameter on each side of the obstruction. The obstruction usually is short and the entire area is encased in dense post-surgical scar tissue. This creates an ideal situation for purposeful *perforation* through the localized area of total obstruction with a transseptal needle or a radio-frequency (RF) perforating system. As examples, a prior "bidirectional Glenn shunt" purposefully creates an "atresia" with total separation of the pulmonary arteries from the right atrium, and, along with this, from the inferior vena caval/hepatic vein blood[4]. An obstruction in the superior limb of a "Mustard" or "Senning" baffle totally occludes the superior vena caval return to the heart. When re-communication of either of these "circulations" is desired, a perforation between the two areas is straightforward.

The venous channels on each side of these obstructions are identified angiographically with *both* PA and lateral angiograms with injections in the open channels/chambers on both sides of the obstruction. From the two complementary views in both the proximal and distal channels/chambers, a "three-dimensional" image of the area is constructed mentally. Whenever possible, a separate catheter is positioned in the channel/vessel on both sides of the obstruction. The catheter on the opposite side from the perforating needle/wire serves as a continuously visible "target" for the needle/wire.

The obstruction is perforated approaching it from either the internal jugular (cephalad) or the femoral (caudal) vein approach. The choice is made according to which approach aligns the *needle* (or other "perforating" tip) in the straightest direction *toward the largest patent venous "target" channel* on the opposite side of the obstruction. The needle or perforating catheter may have more of a curve proximal to the obstruction, but this is of less importance than the tip being directed straight *toward a larger open channel ("target")*. When the angle of approach is comparable from both the jugular and the femoral veins, the femoral approach is used. The femoral route is always preferable since the majority of cardiac catheterization tables are oriented to operate more conveniently from the femoral venous approach.

A transseptal sheath/dilator set is manipulated over a guide wire and positioned so that the tip of the dilator is against the obstruction. If necessary, before it is introduced the distal end of the transseptal needle either is straightened slightly or curved more in order to correspond to the angle of puncture through the obstruction. The needle is introduced into the sheath/dilator set and advanced until the tip of the needle approaches just within the tapered tip of the dilator. A small (2–3 ml), *hard* syringe is filled with contrast material and is attached to the hub of the needle. Pressure monitoring *through the needle* during punctures through a venous obstruction is useless. The pressure through the needle is dampened as soon as the needle exits the tip of the dilator, and remains dampened during the entire, often long, course of a puncture through a venous obstruction, which provides no helpful information for the puncture. Repeated tiny injections of contrast through the needle during the puncture demonstrate the position of the tip of the needle in the "tract".

The needle is advanced out of the tip of the dilator into the obstruction until the needle tip is exposed fully. The needle with the sheath/dilator is advanced into the obstruction, always directing the needle tip toward the "target" chamber. There often is considerable resistance to advancing the needle into the dense tissues and, as a consequence, a significant displacement of all of the tissues in the area as the needle/dilator is pushed. As the needle is advanced in small increments through the dense obstruction, ***very*** small amounts (0.1–0.2 ml) of contrast are pushed very forcefully through the needle into the obstructed tract. The contrast injection produces a very small opacification, or "tag" of contrast medium *in the tissues*. It is important to inject only a *very tiny amount* of contrast through the needle during this particular procedure. A larger amount of contrast injected into the tissues obliterates the visualization of the entire area. If the needle punctures out of the scarred channel into adjacent tissues or spaces, the contrast injection demonstrates this very clearly. The needle alone or the tiny amount of extravasated contrast in an adjacent structure causes no problem when recognized and the needle is *not* followed with the dilator into the abnormal area. If the needle has detoured away from the exact course toward the patent, open channel at the opposite end of the obstruction, the needle is withdrawn, redirected and re-advanced in the proper direction. When the needle enters the patent channel on the opposite end of the obstruction, a sensation of the needle advancing forward more easily or "giving" in the tissues is usually experienced. Another small injection of contrast is performed verifying the proper location. When a chamber/vessel is entered, the contrast flows freely into the chamber/vessel. Once the needle is through the obstruction into the patent channel on the opposite side of the obstruction and the contrast swirls around freely in the desired channel, *then* a pressure line is substituted for the syringe with the contrast, and pressure is observed and/or recorded during the remainder of the puncture.

When the needle is still not through the obstruction or has deviated away from the direction of the patent channel into adjacent tissues or some other undesired vascular space, the small amount of contrast injected into the tissues creates another visible "tag" or the contrast injected into a "space" or erroneous chamber swirls around with the flow in that structure. In either case the contrast injection serves as a landmark to the abnormal location. As long as the dilator and sheath are *not* advanced into the abnormal area over the needle, the needle puncture alone from a venous channel into the abnormal location *will not* cause problems. Using this landmark, the needle is withdrawn, redirected, and the puncture repeated until the true "target" channel is entered. Once the proper location is verified with the tiny contrast injection, the syringe is removed and the needle attached to the flush/pressure system, flushed and a pressure recorded.

Occasionally the needle must be withdrawn completely from the sheath/dilator and the tip of the needle "re-curved" in order to direct the angle of the tip of the needle in the correct direction for the puncture into the desired patent channel. The puncture may take several repeated attempts with several different "tissue tags" and angles on the needle. Once the needle is through the area of stenosis and into the channel on the opposite side of the obstruction, the proximal end of the needle is flushed and attached to the pressure monitoring system. While closely observing and maintaining the pressure obtained through the needle during this part of the puncture, the needle tip is redirected to follow the direction of the patent channel, and the entire needle/dilator/sheath unit is advanced through the obstruction into the patent channel using the extra stiffness of the needle to support the dilator and/or sheath as they are pushed forcefully through the tissues.

Occasionally, only the very tip of the dilator advances into and through the obstruction and the whole dilator and sheath will not follow it into, or through, the dense tissues. In that case, forward pressure is maintained on the sheath/dilator to maintain the tip of the dilator through the obstruction while the needle is withdrawn carefully. Once the needle is out of the dilator, the needle is replaced with a *long floppy tipped*, but otherwise stiff wire of the largest diameter that the tip of the dilator will accommodate. This stiff wire is advanced further into the channel to provide support for the dilator without danger of the wire perforating through the opposite wall of the channel. Once the *stiff portion* of the wire is across the stenosis and secured, the sheath/dilator are withdrawn and replaced with only the dilator or a smaller diameter sheath/dilator set, which is then advanced through the stenosis over the wire. If even the smaller sheath/dilator set or the dilator alone cannot be advanced further through the lesion, there are two alternatives.

When a second catheter coming from the "opposite direction" has already been positioned in the channel/chamber that is being entered (the "target channel"), the catheter in the "target channel/chamber" is replaced with a snare catheter and a 10 mm diameter snare is introduced into the "target" area. The tip of the wire that was advanced through the obstruction is snared in the "target area/channel", pulled through the obstruction, and exteriorized through the introductory sheath of the second catheter. Once the wire is exteriorized, firm traction is applied to both ends of the wire to create a very taught, through and through venous "rail" over which the dilator can be advanced, even through the toughest tissues. Once the dilator is through the lesion, the dilator is exchanged over the through and through wire for a low-profile dilation balloon and the tract dilated. Often only a very small diameter balloon will pass through the stenosis even over the "rail wire". In that circumstance, the lesion is dilated sequentially over the same wire using larger and larger balloons.

If no catheter was in, or could be advanced into the "target channel/chamber", and only the tip of the dilator could be advanced through the obstruction, a small diameter, floppy tipped, but otherwise, stiff wire is advanced through the dilator into the "channel". This wire must be small enough for a low-profile "coronary" balloon dilation catheter to pass over it and stiff enough to support the balloon. While the wire is maintained in position, the dilator is removed and replaced with a very low-profile 2 or 3 mm coronary dilation balloon. The stenotic tract is dilated with the balloon inflated to a high pressure (15–20 atms). Often the balloon only partially enters the tract, in which case the tract is dilated in steps as the balloon is advanced several millimeters after each balloon inflation/deflation. Once this dilation is accomplished, the coronary balloon is replaced with a larger balloon or a cutting balloon and a sequential dilation of the occluded tract is carried out until a balloon that is significantly larger than the "channels" adjacent to the obstructed area can be used.

Once the area is expanded to nearly the diameter of the adjacent vessels, the decision is made on the basis of the etiology and tissue "characteristics" whether to continue with the dilation alone or to proceed with an intravascular stent implant. If dilation is to be the only intervention, the area is dilated to at least *twice* the diameter of the adjacent channels. Even with this degree of over-dilation, dilation alone is not as effective at creating a permanent opening of the channel as an intravascular stent implant, as described in Chapter 24.

Dilation of small peripheral systemic veins

The more peripheral and smaller venous stenoses are usually those secondary to the "internal" vascular trauma. These obstructed veins are usually occluded totally with thrombi and/or scar *within* the vein and the lesions can be very long. Because the "initiating trauma" to the vein was internal, there is usually no external, surrounding, "protective" scar tissue. The obstruction in these veins is usually long, difficult to cross and, in some cases, cannot be traversed at all with the present equipment. Because of the combination of the small diameters of the more peripheral veins, the nature of their obstruction, and the relatively slow venous flow, early *re-occlusion* following *dilation alone* is the *rule* rather than the exception. Once a small vein re-occludes following a dilation, the chances of crossing the obstructed area a second time are even less than originally. As a consequence, dilation with intravascular stent implant is used *primarily* for these lesions whenever the area of stenosis can be crossed. The catheter procedures for crossing these areas of vein stenosis and the details of techniques for dilation with stent implants in these veins are covered in detail in Chapter 24 ("Venous Stents").

There are occasional small vein stenoses which are not necessarily associated with prior surgery or catheterizations and which are very discrete and very resistant areas of stenosis. These lesions are unusual, in that the discrete area of stenosis does not expand even when dilated using a very-high-pressure balloon. There are some anecdotal reports of very favorable results using a "cutting balloon" in this type of lesion. Unfortunately, in the United States, the largest cutting balloon was 4 mm in diameter, so this technique was limited to *very tight* stenosis in relatively small veins. There are 6 and 8 mm diameter cutting balloons available outside of the United States, and good results have been obtained with these balloons in larger vessels in a very small number of selected cases.

When a cutting balloon is considered, it is important to use the cutting balloon initially before any other dilation of the area. The "cutting blades" of cutting balloons are very thin and really not particularly sharp. A preceding dilation will stretch the area of stenosis, and when an attempt is made at further or re-dilation with the cutting balloon, the blades merely push the now stretched and "elastic" tissues aside rather than cutting into them. In the presence of a tight discrete stenosis that does not appear to be the result of prior trauma/thrombosis, the *initial dilation* of the area should be with the cutting balloon when the appropriate sized cutting balloon is available.

Pulmonary vein dilation

One of the first vascular lesions to be dilated clinically in the catheterization laboratory was stenosis of the pulmonary veins[5]. Although these initial pulmonary vein lesions were a result of multiple etiologies, they *appeared* ideal for dilation. The stenoses were often discrete and were localized in the vein to only the area just at the junction of the vein with the left atrium. Experimentally, in both animals and postmortem specimens, the normal pulmonary vein could be dilated to three times its normal diameter without tearing the vein, making dilation a very appealing approach.

Usually a transseptal approach to the left atrium is required to reach the pulmonary veins, but otherwise the positioning of the wires and balloons in the pulmonary veins is not a major challenge. As predicted from the anatomy and the nature of the veins, pulmonary vein stenoses did respond acutely and dramatically to balloon dilation. Unfortunately, after the first few cases, it became apparent that the success with pulmonary vein stenosis was very short lived. Within four to six weeks, the pulmonary veins re-stenosed to as severe, or even worse, a degree of obstruction than before the dilation.

Initially it was thought that intravascular stents would be the answer to re-stenosis in the pulmonary veins.

However, as described in detail in Chapter 24, besides the technical challenges of the implant procedure for pulmonary vein stents, *re-stenosis of the stents* in the pulmonary veins is even more aggressive than the re-stenosis which occurs with dilation alone. There are a few cases of mid term success with stents implanted in pulmonary venous channels where the stenosis was *secondary to prior surgery* on the left atrium, the general area of the pulmonary veins, or the pulmonary veins themselves. These particular stenotic lesions in the pulmonary veins are still considered for the implant of a stent initially in association with the dilation of the veins.

However, for the most part, dilation and intravascular stent implant for native or congenital pulmonary vein stenosis has been abandoned. At the same time, the natural history of pulmonary vein stenosis and the prognosis of surgical therapy for pulmonary vein stenosis are so terrible that when a patient is deteriorating because of pulmonary vein stenosis, dilation, and/or intravascular stent implant almost always is attempted as a "last resort" therapy for these lesions. The procedure is described in detail in Chapter 24 ("Venous Stents") in the section dealing with pulmonary vein stents, and is not repeated here.

Dilation of pulmonary valve in tetralogy of Fallot

Although most of the obstruction of the right ventricular outflow tract in tetralogy of Fallot was considered to be in the infundibular area, there essentially always is a pulmonary valvar component of the total right ventricular outflow tract obstruction. The time-honored therapy for the hypoxemic infant with tetralogy of Fallot has been the creation of a surgical shunt or, more recently, very early "total repair". Neither of these therapeutic options is without its own inherent problems plus the additional general risks of surgery for a small, sick infant. Surgical shunts have a long history of distorting pulmonary arteries, and either decreasing the flow or producing over circulation in one lung. These problems can cause unequal growth of the pulmonary bed, unilateral pulmonary vascular disease, or isolation of a unilateral pulmonary artery. The early "repairs" represent a significantly higher acute surgical risk for the infant and the "final chapter" still is not in concerning the real *long-term* results of these extensive, very early "total repairs". These persistent concerns about surgical therapies, plus the excellent results of pulmonary valvar dilation, led to dilation of the pulmonary valve being considered as an option to surgical palliation for infantile tetralogy of Fallot[6].

Early in the course of pediatric heart catheterization it actually was considered too dangerous, and, even, bad practice to cross the pulmonary valve with a catheter in infants with tetralogy. However, as definitive surgical repairs of tetralogy patients were performed, catheterization of the pulmonary artery became increasingly necessary to obtain definitive information about the complex distal pulmonary artery anatomy prior to this surgery. As the preparation of infants for catheterization and the control of their systemic pressures and circulating volumes during catheterization procedures improved, catheterization of the pulmonary arteries became more routine and much safer. The infants do develop some transient hypoxia, but their systemic pressure is maintained from flow through the ventricular septal defect. This set the stage for attempts at pulmonary valve dilation in infants with tetralogy of Fallot.

The initial results of pulmonary valve dilation in the infant tetralogy patient proved to be even more beneficial than expected[7]. There are minimal adverse events associated with crossing the valve with the guide wire, catheter and even with the dilation balloons, and favorable results were achieved acutely in at least 85% of these patients undergoing dilation of the pulmonary valve/right ventricular outflow tract. Most of these favorable results persist for six months or more, allowing for an elective total surgical correction at a more reasonable age and size. The dilation appears to provide a better and more uniform overall growth of the pulmonary arteries during the period of time prior to surgical correction. As the procedure for dilation of the pulmonary valve in these patients evolved, it appeared possible that much of the infundibular stenosis may be secondary to the valvar component and possibly not part of the primary lesion. However, the infundibular stenosis does seem to respond to the dilation as well! Relief of the infundibular obstruction appears to be even more satisfactory when a cutting balloon is used for the dilation of the infant tetralogy.

Technique of pulmonary valve dilation in infants with tetralogy

Although the pulmonary valve can be crossed in these infants, the crossing and dilation of the valve must be accomplished expediently. Even a small wire across the valve can cause the systemic saturations to drop. These patients are monitored with the pressure from an indwelling arterial line and a reliable, peripheral pulse oximetry sensor in place throughout the procedure. This assures an *instant to instant, accurate* monitoring of the status of the infant during the procedure. The infant who is to undergo right ventricular outflow tract/valve dilation is intubated electively and placed on assisted ventilation using deep systemic sedation or general anesthesia (preferably). The infant is kept on a separate intravenous infusion of approximately 10 ml/kg/hr of 5% dextrose in quarter normal saline or in Ringer's lactate once in the catheterization laboratory.

All preparations for the balloon dilation procedure are made even before an attempt is made at crossing the valve even with a fine wire. A biplane right ventricular angiocardiogram with a steep cranial angulation of the PA X-ray tube is performed to visualize the pulmonary valve, the valve annulus, the right ventricular outflow tract and the proximal branch pulmonary arteries. It is important to document if either the proximal right and/or left pulmonary arteries is/are significantly hypoplastic or separately stenotic. If one pulmonary artery is *very significantly* smaller than the *valve annulus*, that pulmonary artery should *not* be used for the distal position of the wire and, in turn, the balloon placement during the valve dilation. The diameter of the valve annulus is measured on the angiocardiogram in both the PA and lateral views. A "freeze frame" of both views of the angiogram, which includes both the right ventricular outflow tract and the valve, is stored for comparison during the dilation. The position of any fixed intrathoracic landmarks (trachea, manubrium, vertebrae) and their relation to the area of the valve are identified.

A balloon with a diameter 1.5 times the maximal diameter of the valve annulus and 1.5 or 2 cm long is prepared with a negative preparation of the balloon in order to keep the balloon at its very lowest profile. When the valve or infundibulum is very tight initially, a sequential dilation may be necessary, in which case the initial balloon is a very low profile, 2–3 mm "coronary" balloon. If the balloon that is chosen for the final or maximum dilation of the valve will require a larger introductory sheath than the original diagnostic catheter, the sheath is changed to the larger size at this time.

Just before the valve is crossed with even the wire, the patient arbitrarily is given an additional 10 ml/kg bolus of D5/saline and a supplemental dose of sedation/anesthesia. For the very hypoxic and unstable infant, additionally, 0.1 mg/kg of propranolol is given *very slowly* intravenously. A 4- or 5-French, 2.5 or 3.0 right Judkins™ coronary catheter is manipulated into the right ventricle. While comparing the fluoroscopic image with the "freeze frame" image, the catheter tip is directed toward, or even into, the right ventricular outflow tract with careful, gentle to-and-fro probing and torquing of the catheter. A slight (approx. 45°) curve is formed on the tip of a very floppy tipped, torque-controlled, guide wire (Microvena™ or Platinum Plus™), which the balloon that has already been prepared for the dilation will accommodate. This wire is advanced through the catheter that is pre-positioned in the outflow tract, advanced out of the catheter, and manipulated through the stenotic valve. The wire is advanced very gently through the valve with a combination of torque on the wire and/or the catheter as the wire is moved to and fro in the outflow tract until the wire pops through the valve.

Once the wire passes through the valve, it is advanced as far as possible out into a distal pulmonary artery. The left pulmonary artery is preferable but, assuming neither pulmonary artery is disconnected or severely hypoplastic, either vessel will suffice as long as the wire can be advanced far enough distally. All of the floppy portion of the wire must be beyond the valve/main pulmonary artery and, additionally, the *stiff portion* of the wire must extend completely beyond the area of the valve and well out into the branch pulmonary artery. Although it may be gratifying to the catheterizing physician just to accomplish getting the tip of the wire through the valve, the wire must be manipulated much further, and maintained *far into* a distal pulmonary artery branch in order to support the dilation balloon. If the wire by itself cannot be manipulated into a position in the distal pulmonary artery, an attempt is made at advancing the small coronary, guiding catheter over the wire and past the valve. If the catheter passes through, and is tolerated across, the valve, the wire is withdrawn into the tip of the catheter, while the catheter tip is redirected more selectively toward the right or left pulmonary artery. Either the catheter itself is advanced into the distal branch pulmonary artery or the torque wire is re-advanced out of the catheter into the distal branch. With the catheter tip pointed directly at the branch pulmonary artery, the wire often can be advanced further into the far distal pulmonary branch.

Often the selective right "coronary catheter" with the stiff, pre-formed curve at its tip, will not follow the torque wire across the valve, or, if across the valve, will not advance distally into either branch pulmonary artery. In that situation, the wire is fixed as far as possible into the pulmonary artery and the selective coronary catheter in the right ventricle is replaced over the wire with a 4-French, end-hole, multipurpose or curved tipped Terumo Glide™ (Boston Scientific, Namic, MA) catheter. Either one of these two types of catheter usually can be maneuvered over the wire and then into a distal branch pulmonary artery. Either the original floppy tipped guide wire with a stiff shaft, or an extra stiff guide wire that the chosen balloon catheter will accommodate, is advanced through the catheter and positioned as far as possible distally in the right or left pulmonary artery. As soon as the wire is in a satisfactory position, the catheter is withdrawn into the right ventricle over the wire. All of these maneuvers must be performed expediently, often with intermittent pauses between the manipulations to allow the infant to stabilize between the manipulations.

The end-hole catheter is removed over the wire and replaced with the previously prepared balloon dilation catheter. The balloon is advanced into the right ventricle *inflow* area. The "freeze frame" pictures of the valve area are reviewed and displayed on the fluoroscopy screen, while the location of the valve is identified by its relation to the intrathoracic landmarks. With the area of the valve identified and all preparations for the balloon inflation ready, the balloon is advanced over the wire into position across the *infundibulum and the valve*. An attempt is made at having the balloon straddle the infundibulum as well as the valve with the hope that the balloon inflation will dilate any fibrous portion of the infundibular stenosis and "stun" the hyperdynamic infundibular muscle during the valve dilation.

The balloon is inflated rapidly and deflated immediately after full inflation, recording the entire inflation/deflation on biplane angiography. If there is any instability of the infant, the balloon is withdrawn very quickly over the wire and into the body of the right ventricle. As the balloon just crosses the valve and, certainly, during the dilation, the infant's saturation and heart rate usually drop significantly. As soon as the balloon is deflated and withdrawn into the ventricle, the infant should respond with an immediate increase in systemic saturation while the other hemodynamic parameters stabilize over a few more minutes. If the saturation and heart rate do not increase, or if there is any further drop in any of these parameters, the infant is given a further bolus of fluid, a repeat dose of ketamine and, if necessary, 10 microgms/kg of neo-synephrine, intravenously.

Once the infant is stabilized and before removing the balloon or wire from the body, the hemodynamic results of the dilation are reassessed. The systemic pressure and saturation are compared to the pre-dilation values. The angiograms of the balloon inflation(s) are reviewed to ensure proper position of the balloon *and* disappearance of the waist on the balloon during the inflation. If there is any question about the adequacy of the dilation, the same, or when indicated, a larger balloon is advanced over the wire across the outflow tract and the valve, and the inflation repeated. When satisfied with the adequacy of the dilation, the balloon is withdrawn over the wire, out of the body and replaced with the end-hole catheter. The end-hole catheter is advanced over the wire and into the pulmonary artery well beyond the valve.

By using a catheter with an internal diameter considerably larger than the wire diameter and with the wire passing through a Tuohy "Y" back-bleed/flush adaptor, pressures and saturations can be obtained and angiocardiograms performed with the fine wire still in place across the outflow tract and into a distal pulmonary artery. The pressure recording and angiograms also can be accomplished without removing the wire by using a Multi-Track™ (NuMED, Hopkinton, NY) angiographic catheter over the wire. Otherwise, the wire is removed through the catheter and the pressure and the saturation in the pulmonary artery are recorded through the catheter. The pressure is recorded while withdrawing the catheter very slowly across the pulmonary valve and into the right ventricular infundibulum. An angiocardiogram is recorded with injection directly within the right ventricular outflow tract.

If there is persistence of significant infundibular hyperreactivity or the infant is still hypoxemic, the infant is slowly given an additional 0.1 mg/kg of intravenous propanolol and started on 1–2 mg/kg/24 hr of oral propanolol after the procedure. There is no definitive information that the beta blocker will relieve this obstruction in this particular circumstance, however, beta-blocker therapy is useful in the treatment of non-catheter induced infant "tetralogy spells" by slowing the heart rate. When the dose of the beta blocker is adjusted carefully, it does not cause any apparent harm to the infant. Once the infant is stable, the catheter is removed and the infant is allowed to awaken. A good intravenous line is maintained and, in addition to any oral intake, the infant given high maintenance intravenous fluids for the first twenty-four hours after the procedure.

Even with persistent clinical improvement, a repeat cardiac catheterization is recommended within three to four months after the valve dilation. The repeat study is primarily to evaluate the branch pulmonary arteries for any residual unequal pulmonary flow. Occasionally the pulmonary artery into which the dilating balloon was directed during the dilation procedure, is dilated significantly during the valve dilation and, as a consequence, receives most of the prograde pulmonary blood flow. When unequal pulmonary flow is documented, the opposite pulmonary artery is dilated to at least an equal size.

"Cutting balloon" for dilation of tetralogy of Fallot

The availability of "cutting balloons" has created a new option for the catheter dilation of the right ventricular outflow tract in the infant with tetralogy of Fallot. The major argument *against* balloon dilation therapy for infants with tetralogy of Fallot was that the majority of the stenosis was assumed to be dynamic and in the infundibular area or that this type of stenosis theoretically would not respond to dilation. Whether either, or both, of these premises are true or not, the cutting balloon offers a possible solution. Initially, only 4 mm or smaller diameter cutting balloons were available in the United States, so the procedure is limited to smaller infants or very tight stenosis. Cutting balloons come in 1, 1.5 and 2 cm lengths (Boston Scientific, Namic, MA) although only the 1 cm long balloon is applicable in the small infant or when the course to the obstruction is very circuitous. When the decision is made to use a cutting balloon for this lesion, *no* pre-dilation should be performed on the area before the use of the cutting balloon.

The preparation of the patient, the localization of the stenosis angiographically, and the delivery of the guide wire and its positioning in a distal pulmonary artery for the dilation with the cutting balloon are identical to the procedures for dilation with a standard balloon, except that current cutting balloons only accommodate a maximum 0.014″ guide wire. The Iron Man™ wire (Guidant,™ St Paul, MN) appears to be the stiffest and most applicable wire in this size to support the cutting balloon. The major difficulty with the procedure is delivering the cutting balloon to the lesion. Over the bare wire, this often entails forming a large 360° loop in the right atrium to support the "back curves" in the wire as the balloon is pushed over it. An alternative, which requires more initial preparation and manipulations before the cutting balloon is introduced, is to form a small "S" curve at the distal end of a long 5-French sheath and then to advance the long sheath/dilator over the wire from the femoral vein to the right ventricle (outflow tract!). The dilator is removed and the cutting balloon advanced over the wire and through the sheath as far as the right ventricle. To deliver the sheath/dilator to the right ventricular outflow tract usually requires the use of a sturdier wire than the 0.014″ wire, which in turn, means initially placing a larger wire distally through the outflow tract, delivering the sheath/dilator to the right ventricular outflow tract, then replacing the larger wire through a catheter placed distally in the pulmonary artery with the 0.014″ wire when the sheath/dilator are in place.

The cutting balloon is advanced over the wire into the lesion and the dilation carried out using similar techniques to the dilation with a standard balloon, except that the cutting balloon is moved forward and backward very slightly during the inflation. Dilation with the cutting balloon usually is repeated 3 or 4 times, changing the position of the balloon each time during each subsequent inflation, and moving the balloon slightly forward or backward. Usually the dilations with the cutting balloon are followed with one or more further dilations with a larger diameter, standard angioplasty balloon that is more appropriate in diameter for the size of the pulmonary valve annulus or main pulmonary artery. In Europe and much of the rest of the world outside of the US, there are now 6 and 8 mm diameter cutting balloons available. These sizes may extend the applicability of this technique to slightly older/larger patients with tetralogy.

The initial results at Texas Children's Hospital using the cutting balloon for dilation of the right ventricular outflow tract/pulmonary valve in infants with tetralogy of Fallot have been extremely gratifying. There have been no complications and each patient has had a significant and sustained increase in systemic oxygen saturation. No patient has had any complication from the procedure nor required a shunt prior to definitive correction.

There is one report of the successful use of a coronary atherectomy catheter to open the right ventricular outflow tract in an infant with tetralogy of Fallot as the initial palliation, and a report of an experimental "thermal ablation" of the right ventricular outflow tract[8,9]. There have been no further reports following the one successful case using the atherectomy catheter or any reported clinical applications of the "thermal ablation", but both ideas certainly support the concept of directing the initial palliation of these patients primarily at the right ventricular outflow tract obstruction.

Dilation of surgical shunts and collateral arteries

Often, patients whose pulmonary blood flow is dependent entirely on a surgically created systemic to pulmonary artery shunt or on one or more native, systemic to pulmonary artery collateral arteries will develop increasing cyanosis over time or occasionally acutely clot or otherwise close off. These patients are catheterized specifically to look at the adequacy of these systemic to pulmonary artery communications and at the overall pulmonary artery anatomy. If a localized area of stenosis/thrombosis has developed at the anastomosis, within the lumen of the shunt, or within the course of a collateral vessel, and the patient is not considered large enough, or otherwise is unsuitable, for a "definitive repair", dilation of the vessel that is providing the pulmonary blood flow, with or without thrombolysis, is performed[10,11].

The diameter of the shunt or the collateral vessel adjacent to the stenosis is measured accurately. A dilation balloon is chosen *equal* in diameter to the nominal diameter of the *shunt* or up to 1.5 times the diameter of the native vessel adjacent to the stenosis in the collateral vessels. The balloon used is as short as possible and should have very short shoulders. The balloon is prepared with a partial negative prep in order to keep the profile as smooth as possible. An end-hole catheter is introduced into a femoral artery through a sheath that will accommodate the prepared balloon dilation catheter. The catheter is maneuvered into and through the stenosis within the shunt or collateral. A stiff exchange length guide wire, of the largest diameter that the balloon catheter will accommodate, is advanced through the catheter and to a location as far distal to the area of stenosis as possible.

Once the wire is in a secure position with the *stiff portion* of the wire entirely across the lesion, the catheter is withdrawn over the wire and replaced with the prepared balloon. The balloon is advanced to a position straddling the lesion and the inflation and deflation accomplished while recording on biplane angiography. The balloon inflation is repeated several times until the "waist" from the stenosis no longer appears on the balloon surface even at low pressures. Usually this is sufficient to relieve the stenosis at least temporarily.

When an acute thrombosis is present, it usually is recognized angiographically as a filling defect in the vessel. The end-hole catheter is manipulated into the shunt/collateral and advanced adjacent to the location of the thrombus. Local thrombolytic therapy (Chapter 2) is administered through the catheter before attempting to cross the lesion with a wire or a catheter and before performing the balloon dilation.

When the stenosis is very tight and either it was not relieved or when the lesion was known or suspected to be very resistant to dilation to begin with, the use of a cutting balloon for the initial or a repeat dilation should be considered. In the United States, these were limited to very small or tight lesions by the 4 mm maximum diameter of the available cutting balloons. The procedure for delivering the cutting balloon to the lesion is similar to the delivery of a standard angioplasty balloon. However, the actual inflation/dilation is *different* in that the cutting balloon is purposefully moved slightly forward and backward in the lesion while the balloon is inflated at its maximum pressure, with the intention that the very shallow, and not too sharp, blades will have a greater likelihood of cutting with some movement. Hopefully, cutting balloons will become suitable for more lesions with the availability of the 6 and 8 mm diameter balloons in the US.

The implant of intravascular stents in these shunt and collateral lesions usually is *not* considered unless the patient otherwise is inoperable, and the dilation of the particular shunt/collateral represents the only "permanent palliation" available. The implant of stents in these areas, in that circumstance, is covered in Chapter 24.

Dilation of conduits and/or surgical anastomoses

There are increasing numbers of conduits, manufactured from various prosthetic materials, being implanted in congenital heart patients. Conduits are placed in surgically constructed ventricular to pulmonary artery connections, in many systemic venous to pulmonary artery connections, and in some pulmonary artery to pulmonary artery and systemic artery to systemic artery reconstructions. Many of these prosthetic vascular structures eventually become stenotic, and many of the stenoses in these conduits are amenable to balloon dilation when the narrowing is *not* the circumferential diameter of the prosthetic material itself. The tubular conduits themselves cannot be dilated to greater than their manufactured diameter. Many of these conduits are not amenable to intravascular stent implant because of the location of the attachment of the conduit adjacent to contractile tissues. The success of the dilation is more dependent upon the characteristics and location of the stenosis than on the technique for dilation.

Some of the conduits are fashioned of homograph or heterograph tissues, while other conduits are tubes constructed from various synthetic materials, including Dacron™ and Gortex™. The conduits may or may not contain a tissue valve. The conduits *usually* are circumferential tubes but occasionally are 1/2 or 3/4 circumferential patches. All of the conduits have the potential for stenosis either at their anastomosis to the native tissues or within the lumen of the conduit itself, particularly at the area of a tissue valve. The luminal stenosis usually is a result of shrinkage of the walls of the tissue conduits, sclerosis and shrinking of the tissue valves within the conduits, intimal proliferation, which can create "peals" within conduits, or folding or kinking of the prosthetic conduits. The anastomotic stenoses occur with scarring of the areas or angulation and torsion of the anastomosis with the native tissues.

Unlike native vessels, none of the circumferential conduits, regardless of materials, can be dilated beyond their original diameters. Both the tissue conduits and the synthetic conduits have very little initial elasticity and all types of conduit materials become very stiff, rigid, even calcified and totally non-elastic after being in place in the body for any length of time. Any attempts at *over*-dilation with very high-pressure balloons result in a significant risk of through and through splitting of the conduit and/or its anastomoses to the native tissues, regardless of the material from which the conduit was made. Although a through and through split in these conduits *usually* is contained within the surrounding scar tissue, the "scar tissue" itself can become so rigid that the split extends through the scar and can result in a massive extravasation.

The technique for conduit dilation is similar to the technique for any other vessel dilation except that the balloon diameter of a single balloon should *not* exceed the diameter of the conduit. If a double-balloon dilation is used, the combined diameters of the two balloons can be up to 20% greater than the diameter of the conduit. The dilation procedure is the same whether the obstruction is at the anastomosis or within the lumen and regardless of whether the intraluminal obstruction is due to the conduit shrinking, intimal proliferation, conduit kinking, or tissue valve sclerosis/constriction within the conduit.

Similar to other "vessel" dilations, a Super Stiff™ wire is positioned across and well beyond the area of stenosis. The dilation balloon is advanced over the wire until the balloon straddles the area of stenosis. If the "waist" on the dilation balloon created by the stenosis is not abolished using a standard pressure dilation balloon, the standard pressure balloon can be replaced with a high-pressure balloon of the same diameter, however the risk of "cracking" the conduit and creating a through and through tear of the conduit is increased significantly when the tissues are this tough. Even if the "waist" does not disappear or the waist returns as the balloon is deflated, a larger balloon is *not* used.

When the "waist" is abolished by the full inflation of a standard or high-pressure balloon, but then recurs as the balloon is deflated to lower pressures, the use of an intravascular stent is considered only when the conduit stenosis is away from actively contracting muscular tissues. Stent fracture is likely to occur when the stent is placed in an area where the stent will be compressed or at the anastomosis of the conduit with the contracting ventricle—which, unfortunately, is a common site of stenosis. The stents crush and then fracture, usually within a short period of time. Frequently fragments of the stent embolize away from the area of implant. In these locations, dilation alone is attempted as a palliation of the obstruction without the adjunct use of a stent.

The presence of calcium in the walls of a conduit of any material or in a valve within a conduit is a danger sign for dilation and particularly for stent implant. The calcium indicates a very rigid obstruction and a conduit which is likely to fracture or split rather than dilate. The calcium within the conduit also frequently has small, sharp spicules ("teeth"), which puncture or rupture dilation balloons. With dilation alone a balloon puncture/rupture usually is an inconvenience and requires some extra effort at removing the balloon; however, a balloon rupture during a stent implant is a disaster, often resulting in balloon entrapment within an incompletely expanded stent.

Subaortic stenosis

There is some interest, even enthusiasm, and there have been a *few* favorable *reports* on the dilation of "discrete, membranous" sub-valve aortic stenosis[12]. Unfortunately, the large majority of sub-valve aortic stenosis is *not* a discrete membrane and usually is associated with significant fibromuscular and/or pure muscular tunnel stenosis. The "membranous" subaortic stenosis also frequently has attachments to and involvement of the aortic valve leaflets even before balloon dilation. Although there may be a transient relief of a gradient across the area during a dilation procedure, neither the fibromuscular nor the tunnel obstructions respond to dilation with *any* persistence of the relief and there is no effect upon the aortic valve involvement. When in the very rare instances where the subaortic obstruction does appear to be a thin, membranous, very discrete stenosis without any associated fibromuscular obstruction, and has no significant aortic valve involvement both by echocardiographic interrogation and by angiography, an attempt at balloon dilation of the lesion is warranted as a first-stage *palliation*.

Sub-valve aortic membranous stenosis is dilated using the retrograde approach. The aortic valve and the subaortic obstruction are crossed with a retrograde, end-hole catheter using the same techniques and equipment used for aortic valve dilation (Chapter 19). A Super Stiff™ wire is preformed and positioned in the apex of the left ventricle similarly to aortic valve dilations. A dilation balloon, *equal in diameter* to the *aortic valve annulus*, is prepared with a standard preparation to eliminate all air within the balloon. Although the obstruction is not at the valve, the limiting factor for the *maximum diameter* of the balloon still is the aortic annulus. The dilation balloon is passed retrograde over the pre-positioned, Super Stiff™ wire and positioned to straddle the area of sub-valve obstruction. The balloon is inflated/deflated very rapidly while maintaining its position fixed within the sub-valve area. As occurs during the dilation of the aortic valve, the blood pressure drops precipitously during the balloon inflation but usually returns immediately upon deflation of the balloon. Although the sub-valve area adjacent to the obstruction may appear larger in diameter, or the obstruction is not relieved with the original balloon, a balloon with a larger diameter than the aortic annulus is *not* considered for a repeat dilation. The balloon dilating the subaortic membrane, out of necessity because of the proximity of the valve to the sub-valve membrane, also extends back across the aortic valve/annulus and, as a consequence, a larger diameter balloon would dilate the aortic annulus excessively at the same time.

Even though the subaortic gradient decreases, or even disappears during the procedure, it usually recurs, often as soon as 24 hours after the dilation, because of the usual, associated, fibromuscular stenosis! Dilation of sub-valve aortic obstructions also has a high incidence of creating left bundle branch block and, rarely, even complete heart block. As a consequence of the minimal permanent effect on the gradient and the potential for bundle or complete "electrical" heart blocks, dilation of sub-valve obstructions is only recommended in the very rare instance when *all* data suggest a pure, *thin, discrete, membranous* sub-valve obstruction.

Dilation of supravalve aortic stenosis

Dilation of supravalvar aortic stenosis is not recommended. In spite of the apparent appealing appearance of some of these lesions for dilation, the tissues of the supravalvar aortic stenosis are very abnormal, thickened, histologically disarrayed and do not respond at all permanently to dilation. The elasticity of these tissues allows stretching of the lesion, but only with immediate recoil.

Intravascular stents have been considered for supravalvar aortic stenosis, however, because of the location of the lesions exactly at the position where the aortic valve leaflets open, its usual actual involvement of the origins of the coronary arteries, and the location of the obstruction immediately proximal to the carotid vessels, stent therapy for this lesion is not considered seriously as a reasonable approach.

Dilation of aortic obstruction secondary to aortitis and/or vasculitis

Diffuse obstructive lesions of the descending aorta *therapeutically* often are grouped with coarctation of the aorta, or more specifically as abdominal coarctation. However, these lesions all are associated with a generalized systemic disease or are presumed to be acquired lesions. These associated conditions include neurofibromatosis, rubella, Williams Syndrome and Takayasu's aortitis. As a consequence of the very heterogenous underlying pathology, the response to balloon dilation is very unpredictable. At the same time, surgical "repair" of these aortic lesions in smaller patients is not entirely satisfactory, and balloon dilation without the implant of intravascular stents is the preferred initial approach.

The largest experience in balloon dilation of these lesions has been in patients with lower thoracic/abdominal aortic obstructions presumably due to Takayasu's type of arteritis, and most of this experience with dilation alone was before the introduction and common use of intravascular stents[13–15]. In these particular aortic lesions, balloon dilation alone was very effective. The dilation of these lesions appeared to be conservative in terms of balloon to vessel diameters, and minimal acute complications were reported. Most of the lesions did have some residual gradient and there were some recurrences, both of which were amenable to re-dilation. In a later series of patients, the same authors utilized intravascular stents to treat both intimal dissections and/or residual stenosis following initial balloon dilation[16].

Most aortic obstructions are now treated with primary intravascular stent implants (Chapter 25), except in smaller patients, where stents that eventually can be dilated to the diameter of the adult vessel cannot be implanted because of the patient's size. In smaller patients, a very conservative balloon dilation of the obstruction, which knowingly leaves some residual obstruction or gradient, probably is the best palliative therapy until the patient is large enough for the implant of a potentially adult diameter stent. The balloons used for the dilation of these "mid-aortic" obstructions should be no larger in diameter than the diameter of the smallest *adjacent* "normal" vessel—even with the realization that the "adjacent normal" vessel also probably is involved with the disease process and will be smaller than the "expected" normal for the patient's size. Residual or re-obstruction of these lesions can be re-dilated later, while an acute dissection as a result of a balloon that is too large for the vessel may require the emergent implant of a stent, which eventually will be too small for the patient, and/or emergency surgical intervention.

Dilation of systemic arteries

Similarly to obstructions in the aorta, smaller systemic arteries in younger or congenital heart patients have, or develop, obstructions as a consequence of multiple different etiologies[17]. These etiologies include diffuse systemic diseases, inflammatory arteritis, fibromuscular hyperplasia, local trauma to the vessel, and prior surgical/catheter intervention. Any multiple vessels, including the carotid, vertebral, subclavian, renal, mesenteric and iliofemoral arteries, can be involved. These lesions, regardless of etiology, potentially are amenable to balloon dilation, and most of these lesions now are treated with balloon dilation with or without primary intravascular stent implant.

The results of balloon dilation alone depend upon both the etiology and the location of the obstruction. Each lesion individually must be investigated for etiology and degree of involvement. Unlike an atrial septostomy, where an initial large or maximal dilation usually will produce the best results, these arterial lesions are treated conservatively and if necessary, with the use of sequentially larger balloons to achieve a successful dilation without over-stretching or tearing the involved vessel. There is a large number of balloons available for the dilation of even the smallest systemic arterial lesions, although none are designed or manufactured for that purpose. From the innumerable balloons manufactured for coronary and adult peripheral artery dilations, there is a wide variety of balloons that are ideally suited for the dilation of pediatric and congenital peripheral arterial lesions. The specific balloon diameter, length and profile are chosen to match the size and location of the involved vessel. Those arterial lesions that occur acutely and are associated with thrombus, usually are treated concomitantly with thrombolytics[18–20].

Dilation of the atrial septum

The creation or enlargement of a communication in the atrial septum with a dilation balloon represents a balloon dilation procedure that is not exactly a "vascular" dilation nor is it considered as a usual "septostomy". Dilation of an atrial septal communication is performed to enlarge a pre-existing opening or, after a transseptal puncture of the septum, to create an entirely new opening in order to create palliative shunting at the atrial level. Balloon dilation of the atrial septum is covered in detail in Chapter 13, "Balloon Atrial Septostomy", and is not repeated in this chapter.

Dilation of miscellaneous structures—general

Balloon dilation of almost any stenotic intravascular lesion is possible. Most of the miscellaneous, non-valve and non-great vessel lesions are covered in this chapter. Other areas of intravascular stenosis may occur and should be amenable to balloon dilation. The risks of dilation of a still-undefined miscellaneous lesion depend upon the location, the etiology of the lesion, and the technique utilized. There already is enough prior experience with the dilation of a large variety of lesions to devise a safe and effective dilation technique for any new or different vascular lesion that may arise.

Properly performed balloon dilation of stenotic lesions usually is effective and generally is safe. Even if the dilation of the lesion does not result in a permanent "cure", balloon dilation alone usually provides at least some temporary palliation. Balloon dilation frequently is the initial procedure for the treatment of many intravascular stenoses in pediatric and congenital heart patients, and particularly those who are too small to tolerate an adult sized stent.

Complications of balloon dilation of the tricuspid valve, systemic and pulmonary veins, tetralogy of Fallot, and miscellaneous vascular lesions

The complications of balloon dilation in general are covered in detail in Chapter 15, and the complications of atrial septostomies are covered in Chapters 13 and 14, and none of these are repeated here.

The complications related to tricuspid valve dilation are a result of the anatomy of the valve and the specific lesions involving the valve rather than the dilation procedure. None of the heterogenous lesions of the tricuspid valve are very common, and the characteristics of the tricuspid valve stenosis may not be particularly suitable for balloon dilation. Unlike the other three valves of the heart, even the normal tricuspid valve does not have a nice, discrete annulus, which clearly separates two large or well defined chambers or vessels. The normal tricuspid valve has a large and somewhat ill-defined annulus and support structures with the chordae of the valve, in essence, "blending into", and partially obliterating any real, discrete cavity of the right ventricle. As a consequence, there is little or no space in the cavity of even the normal right ventricle to position the "ventricular half" of a cylindrical dilation balloon that is positioned across the valve for a dilation procedure. This problem is compounded with stenosis of the tricuspid valve, which often involves hypoplasia of the valve and/or ventricle or displacement of the valve even further into the ventricular cavity.

During dilation of the tricuspid valve, the balloon/wire combination is pushed forcefully and continuously toward/into the right ventricular apex. Even with a strong, continuous push on the balloon/wire, the resulting dilation of the tricuspid valve frequently is less than satisfactory because of balloon movement out of the valve. The risk of ventricular perforation or rupture from the wires and tips of the balloons being forced into the ventricular wall is significant and, if perforation does occur, it essentially is not treatable. This risk must always be considered when a dilation of the tricuspid valve is attempted.

As with the dilation of any valve, disruption of the valve leaflets and/or valve apparatus resulting in significant tricuspid valve regurgitation is a significant possibility because of the basic anatomy of the valve. Fortunately, because of the usual low pressure of the right ventricle, the acute hemodynamic and symptomatic consequences of even significant tricuspid valve regurgitation usually are minimal and tolerated, often for years and certainly tolerated better than significant tricuspid valve stenosis.

Complications of the dilation of systemic veins are rare or go unrecognized. The veins are very compliant and resistant to tearing and rupture. Because of the relatively low venous pressure and the confined spaces where most of the veins are located, when a vein is perforated during attempted crossing of an obstruction, or even tears during a dilation, the puncture/tear usually results in the extravasation of very little blood into the surrounding tissues and, even then, the extravasated blood self "tamponades". The major problem with the dilation of venous structures is the almost universal restenosis/reocclusion after dilation alone. Because of this, most venous lesions now are supported with the implant of intravascular stents at the time of the initial dilation procedure.

Balloon dilation of the right ventricular outflow tract/pulmonary valve in infants with tetralogy of Fallot carries the possibility of not only not succeeding, but at the same time actually "aggravating" the infundibular obstruction and precipitating a hypoxemic spell. Each patient must be individualized and the procedure performed as expediently as possible. The use of a cutting balloon appears to optimize the results and minimize the risk of the dilation not being effective. Measures to prevent, and preparations for the acute treatment of, hypoxemic spells must be made before the dilation is started, and surgical support must be available within the institution. In addition to the risk of the procedure not working, as with any dilation, the risks of tearing or disrupting structures are always present. The best treatment of this complication is prevention by rigidly adhering to established, safe, techniques during the dilation procedure. If a major vascular disruption occurs, only extremely proficient, massive resuscitative efforts with huge volume replacement and the immediate availability of cardiovascular surgical intervention are likely to salvage the patient.

Dilation of arterial shunts and collateral vessels carries only a very small risk of vascular disruption, particularly in the younger group of pediatric and congenital heart patients, where the vessels are usually more elastic and pliable than in the adult atherosclerotic population. With a disruption of a shunt or a significant collateral vessel, a major intrathoracic extravasation of blood results, but possibly of more importance, a significant (or only!) source of the pulmonary blood flow can be disrupted, with resultant acute hypoxia. The bleeding usually can be managed acutely with evacuation from the thorax and replacement of any lost volume. If bleeding from a tear continues and if the torn vessel is one of several sources of pulmonary blood flow, the vessel can be occluded in the catheterization laboratory or the patient is taken to surgery urgently. When the vascular tear/disruption interrupts the major source of blood flow to the lungs, emergent surgery to re-establish some flow to the pulmonary circuit is the only potential for salvage.

When shunts or conduits made of synthetic fabrics are dilated, there is always the possibility of disrupting an intimal lining within the synthetic tube and, in doing so, creating a "peal" of tissue which can occlude the lumen. This possibility should always be considered if a patient deteriorates acutely immediately after the dilation of a shunt or conduit made of synthetic material. The obstructive "peal" can be identified angiographically as a radiolucent area within the lumen of the recently dilated shunt or conduit. Such a "peal" can lead to total obstruction of the shunt or conduit and, in turn, create a very acute, catastrophic emergency which requires instantaneous treatment.

The most definitive and rapidly available management of this "peal" is to immediately "re-tack" and/or compress the "peal" against the wall of the shunt or conduit with an intravascular stent. The pre-mounted Genesis™ or Express™ stents are applicable for small shunts, however, one of the hand-mounted, larger stents would be required for a "peal" within a larger conduit. An alternative, faster but less definitive, treatment is to try to move or partially compress the "peal" using repeated dilations with the original angioplasty balloon, which is usually still in the body and over the wire when the peal becomes apparent. This often is partially effective and can be used to palliate the patient while the stent is being prepared. Surgical intervention is a third and definitive alternative, but in the case of a total obstruction of a major conduit, probably could not be performed rapidly enough to salvage the patient.

Although the potential for complications as a result of the dilation of this heterogenous group of lesions is present, fortunately, the actual incidence of complications is very small, most of the complications are not life threatening, and the incidence in this group of lesions should remain rare by the adherence to established and safe techniques in performing the various dilation procedures.

References

1. Mullins CE *et al*. Balloon dilation of miscellaneous lesions: results of valvuloplasty and angioplasty of congenital anomalies registry. *Am J Cardiol* 1990; **65**(11): 802–803.
2. Khalilullah M *et al*. Double-balloon valvuloplasty of tricuspid stenosis. *Am Heart J* 1987; **114**(5): 1232–1233.
3. Kimura C *et al*. Membranous obliteration of the inferior vena cava in the hepatic portion. (Review of 6 cases with 3 autopsies.) *J Cardiovasc Surg* (Torino) 1963; **4**: 87–98.
4. Ward CJ *et al*. Use of intravascular stents in systemic venous and systemic venous baffle obstructions. Short-term follow-up results. *Circulation* 1995; **91**(12): 2948–2954.
5. Driscoll DJ, Hesslein PS, and Mullins CE. Congenital stenosis of individual pulmonary veins: clinical spectrum and unsuccessful treatment by transvenous balloon dilation. *Am J Cardiol* 1982; **49**(7): 1767–1772.
6. Qureshi SA *et al*. Balloon dilatation of the pulmonary valve in the first year of life in patients with tetralogy of Fallot: a preliminary study. *Br Heart J* 1988; **60**(3): 232–235.
7. Sluysmans T *et al*. Early balloon dilatation of the pulmonary valve in infants with tetralogy of Fallot. Risks and benefits. *Circulation* 1995; **91**(5): 1506–1511.
8. Qureshi SA, Parsons JM, and Tynan M. Percutaneous transcatheter myectomy of subvalvar pulmonary stenosis in tetralogy of Fallot: a new palliative technique with an atherectomy catheter. *Br Heart J* 1990; **64**(2): 163–165.
9. Neya K *et al*. Experimental ablation of outflow tract muscle with a thermal balloon catheter. *Circulation* 1995; **91**(9): 2445–2453.
10. Marx GR *et al*. Balloon dilation angioplasty of Blalock–Taussig shunts. *Am J Cardiol* 1988; **62**(10 pt 1): 824–827.
11. Marasini M *et al*. Balloon dilatation of critically obstructed modified (polytetrafluoroethylene) Blalock–Taussig shunts. *Am J Cardiol* 1994; **73**(5): 405–407.
12. Lababidi Z *et al*. Transluminal balloon dilatation for discrete subaortic stenosis. *Am J Cardiol* 1987; **59**(5): 423–425.
13. Khalilullah M and Tyagi S. Percutaneous transluminal angioplasty in Takayasu arteritis. *Heart Vessels Suppl* 1992; **7**: 146–153.

14. Tyagi S *et al.* Balloon angioplasty of the aorta in Takayasu's arteritis: initial and long-term results. *Am Heart J* 1992; **124**(4): 876–882.
15. Tyagi S *et al.* Percutaneous transluminal angioplasty for stenosis of the aorta due to aortic arteritis in children. *Pediatr Cardiol* 1999; **20**(6): 404–410.
16. Tyagi S, Kaul UA, and Arora R. Endovascular stenting for unsuccessful angioplasty of the aorta in aortoarteritis. *Cardiovasc Intervent Radiol* 1999; **22**(6): 452–456.
17. Schmidt B and Andrew M. Neonatal thrombosis: report of a prospective Canadian and international registry. *Pediatrics* 1995; **96**(5 pt 1): 939–943.
18. Smith PK *et al.* Urokinase treatment of neonatal aortoiliac thrombosis caused by umbilical artery catheterization: a case report. *J Vasc Surg* 1991; **14**(5): 684–687.
19. Silva JA *et al.* Rheolytic thrombectomy in the treatment of acute limb-threatening ischemia: immediate results and six-month follow-up of the multicenter angiojet registry. Possis Peripheral Angiojet Study-Angiojet Investigators. *Cathet Cardiovasc Diagn* 1998; **45**(4): 386–393.
20. Weiner GM *et al.* Successful treatment of neonatal arterial thromboses with recombinant tissue plasminogen activator. *J Pediatr* 1998; **133**(1): 133–136.

22 Intravascular stents in congenital heart disease—general considerations, equipment

Introduction

In 1986–8 the (J & J) P 308 and P 204 intravascular stents (Johnson & Johnson, Warren, NJ) underwent a two-year animal study of implantation into pulmonary arteries and systemic veins at Texas Children's Hospital[1]. The animal study included two-year follow-up examinations of the anatomic and histologic characteristics of the vessels in the locations with the implanted stents. In 1989, as a result of the excellent results that were demonstrated in the animal study for these stents in large arteries and veins, these same stents were introduced into an FDA, investigational device exemption (IDE) protocol, human clinical trial for similar lesions in congenital heart patients.

In 1994, while the clinical trial for congenital lesions still was in progress, these same stents received FDA approval for clinical use *in biliary and vascular lesions* in *adult human patients*. As a consequence of this approval for *human use* and, although not specifically approved for the lesions being studied in the congenital heart trial or for pediatric patients (although they are human!), the stents became commercially "available" for use in humans and consequently for use in any lesion, to physicians in the United States as well as the rest of the world. The commercial availability of the stents combined with the very favorable data up to that time in the one US trial and several other trials outside of the US, led to the acceptance of these stents by most centers involved with the care of congenital heart patients throughout the United States and the rest of the world for the routine treatment of branch pulmonary artery stenosis and systemic venous stenosis in congenital heart patients[2]. At Texas Children's Hospital, over 900 intravascular stents have been implanted in more than 500 congenital heart patients for various forms of vascular stenosis over the 15 years since the beginning of the IDE trial.

It has now been established that the implanted intravascular stent represents a mechanism that safely maintains a vessel at the same diameter to which the stent/vessel is dilated. Even with the well-documented and very favorable data which were available from the trial, the manufacturer of the P 308 stents (Johnson & Johnson, Warren, NJ) never considered pediatric/congenital heart disease commercially important enough to pursue a final FDA, IDE approval for this particular limited use. Although intravascular stents still do not have "FDA approval" (or recognition) for use in congenital lesions and pediatric patients, since 1996 the use of intravascular stents for these congenital vascular lesions has been accepted *as the standard of care* by all centers and all professional medical societies associated with the care of pediatric and congenital heart disease throughout the world, including the United States.

There still are many stenotic vascular lesions in pediatric and adult congenital heart patients that are not amenable to surgical correction, and for which balloon dilation alone does not maintain the full patency of the vessel. This is particularly true for branch pulmonary artery stenosis and stenosis of systemic and pulmonary veins. Whether the stenosis of these vessels is congenital in origin, is a consequence of previous surgery, or is a combination of both etiologies, these lesions, in fact, are frequently made worse by attempts at surgical repair. The dismal surgical outcomes are a result of a combination of the delicate or abnormal nature of the vessels themselves, the inaccessible locations of the lesions in these vessels, and the scarring that occurs in the vessels following the surgery. The normal branch pulmonary arteries and both the systemic and pulmonary veins are very thin-walled, normally very low-pressure vessels and, as a consequence, are easily compressed or distorted by adjacent structures. The more proximal branch pulmonary arteries and systemic veins are surrounded by or crossed by higher-pressure, more ridged structures. In their "natural" or native (non-operated) state, there is some mobility of these vessels, which allows them to "fit" between or move away from the more ridged and higher-pressured structures that might compress them. However, with the scarring and adhesions in the area of these vessels following surgery, this "mobility" of the individual vessels is lost. The more distal pulmonary arteries and the pulmonary veins are small and lie deep within the pulmonary parenchyma. As a consequence, these distal pulmonary vessels are essentially inaccessible for surgical repair because of their location.

The thin, delicate vessel walls of pulmonary arteries and systemic veins, even under the best of circumstances, do not permit surgical reconstruction of the vessels, which persist as *tubular* structures. Unless ridged, artificial materials are used in the reconstruction, even the optimally repaired branch pulmonary artery or systemic vein is easily compressed by surrounding structures. At the same time, any ridged material used in such reconstructions distorts and constricts the thin-walled, native vessels at the anastomotic sites. The materials and the suture lines connecting them to the natural tissues cannot grow or stretch with the future growth of pediatric patients, which results in even further distortion and stenosis. Once operated, the scarring around these thin-walled vessels both constricts the vessels and prevents their natural mobility and movement away from compression by adjacent structures.

Balloon dilation of all types of stenotic vessels is and has been performed with mixed reports of success. Dilation of any type of stenosis of pulmonary veins, unequivocally has been unsuccessful at maintaining patency over any length of time. Although the pulmonary veins can be dilated acutely with instantaneous relief of obstruction, this obstruction almost universally returns over weeks to at most several months, and when it returns, it does so to a worse degree than originally[3]. This experience has been repeated in many centers over the past decade and a half. For the most part, dilation alone of stenotic pulmonary veins is attempted only as a "stop-gap" to other therapy.

Balloon dilation of systemic vein stenosis has had mixed results regardless of the etiology of the stenosis. There certainly are individual cases which are improved acutely both hemodynamically and symptomatically. Unfortunately, many, if not most of the patients who have acute success from the dilation of systemic venous stenosis, do have re-stenosis within months. The re-stenosis recurs even after several repeat dilations of the same vessel. There are no reported *series* of *sustained* successful dilations of systemic vein stenosis *to normal vessel diameters* and *without residual gradients* following dilation alone in even a majority of the patients in any series.

The "success" of balloon dilation of branch pulmonary artery stenosis is related more to the criteria of each individual institution for a "successful dilation" as opposed to the actual *correction* of the lesion[4]. For example, a *statistically significant*, acute increase in vessel diameter or acute "percentage decrease" in the gradient is an improvement and is considered an acute success by some. This improvement may be only a 50% increase in diameter and/or a 50% decrease in the gradient, and may not be permanent, but still is an acute "improvement" and is considered a success[4,5]. The ultimate goal of a dilation procedure is a *permanent* increase in vessel diameter to the *normal size* for that particular patient and vessel, and/or a permanent *elimination* of *any gradient* across the lesion. Utilizing the establishment of *lasting, normal* hemodynamics and the "normalization" of the vessel diameter angiographically as the criteria for the successful dilation of a vessel, the success of balloon dilation alone for branch pulmonary stenosis is *very* low.

These less than optimal results from dilations in all types of vessel in congenital heart patients led to the adoption of intravascular stents as the standard of care in the treatment of congenital vascular obstructions. A large experience with the use of J & J™ Palmaz™ intravascular stents (Johnson & Johnson, Warren, NJ) in these lesions in the United States as well as throughout the rest of the world, has now provided extensive data on the mid to long-term results of intravascular stents in all of these lesions. This very extensive worldwide (including the US) clinical experience with stents demonstrated between good and spectacularly good results for the treatment of these lesions[6]. These results are equally good in growing patients. The most favorable results in congenital lesions are in the vascular stenosis acquired following surgery on, or about, the vessels, that occurs in congenital heart lesions postoperatively. The success of stent implants in all lesions varies directly with the equipment used and with the skill and experience of the catheterizing physicians who implant the stents.

One factor that always must be considered with the implant of all existing intravascular stents, is that these are *permanent* implants. These stent implants will remain in the patients for their entire life, and the *maximal potential* expanded diameter of the *implanted* ***stent*** determines the ***eventual, final diameter*** of the vessel. Animal studies, and now extensive human experience, demonstrated that when the stent initially is expanded purposefully to less than its maximal diameter at the time of implant, the same stent can be expanded further, and/or re-expanded, up to the *maximal diameter of the* ***stent*** at a much later time[7,8]. This is critically important in smaller pediatric patients in order to be able to accommodate their subsequent growth. The subsequent expansion of the stent can be up to the *potential maximal diameter* of the *specific* ***stent***, even when the stent has been in place for years.

When a stent with a maximum diameter that is smaller than the maximum *eventual* diameter of the vessel is implanted in such a vessel, it represents the *purposeful creation of a future, very fixed stenosis* in that vessel. As a consequence, except in extremely extenuating, life-threatening circumstances, stents with small maximum diameters are *not used* in a vessel that eventually will be larger than the maximum diameter of that particular stent. There are several basic "rules" that have evolved for the implant of stents in congenital heart lesions.

Rules of stent implant in congenital heart lesions

The implanted stent itself must not create a present or future stenosis! A stent should not be implanted purposefully, which knowingly, and *by itself will necessitate* future *surgery* on the same lesion because of stenosis created by the stent itself either because of future growth of the patient or because of known aggressive re-stenosis caused by the particular stent. Small stents that cannot be dilated to the full, potential adult diameter of the particular vessel, should not be implanted in that vessel. The only exception to this "rule" would be under extreme, life-threatening circumstances where there are *no* alternatives to the particular therapy.

A stent with a small maximal diameter implanted in a potentially large central vessel of a patient means, unequivocally, that the patient will require subsequent surgery to correct the "iatrogenic stenosis" regardless of the need for any other surgery. The subsequent surgery is complicated further by the ingrowth of the implanted stent into (or through!) the vessel walls. Once intravascular stents have been in place for several years, they become completely incorporated into the wall of the vessel and they cannot be *removed* without removing the segment of vessel containing them!

Rule number two is not to "jail" major branch vessels, or vessels to major areas, which may require later catheter access. Whenever possible, major branch vessels arising from, or adjacent to, the area of stenosis to be stented *are not crossed or covered* with the present J & J™ stents (Johnson & Johnson, Warren, NJ). Even with full dilation of any of the Palmaz™ J & J™ stents, catheters of any significant diameter and certainly *therapeutic* catheters cannot be passed or manipulated between or through the open side "mesh" or "cells" of the stent. Even when a small catheter passes through these openings, the side openings of the P _ _ 8 or P _ _ 10 stents (Johnson & Johnson–Cordis Corp., Miami Lakes, FL) cannot be dilated enough to allow the passage of a larger catheter for an intervention in the side branch. When an important side branch (or bifurcation) is present in the area to be stented with a Palmaz™ stent, both the major vessel and the side branch are stented simultaneously with a "bifurcating" stent technique in order to secure access to both vessels for future therapy.

The availability of the Double Strut Stent™ IntraStent™ (Intra Therapeutics Inc., St. Paul, MN) (ITI) and the Mega™ and Maxi™ stents (ev3, Plymouth, MN) with their "open cell" designs may obviate the problem of "jailed" side vessels. A catheter can readily be manipulated through the side "cells" of these stents, and the individual "cell" can be dilated to as large as 12 mm in diameter. More data about these stents are necessary before recommendations can be made about their use as a total substitution for the already extensively used and "proven" J & J™, Palmaz™ stents. The Genesis XD™ stent (Johnson & Johnson–Cordis Corp., Miami Lakes, FL) allows passage through the side cells, which are attached by the "omega" connections, and probably these cells can be dilated with higher pressure balloons in order to overcome "jailing". This is still being investigated.

Rule number three is not to implant a stent that knowingly results in aggressive tissue reaction/proliferation and, in turn, causes a more severe degree of stenosis. To date, only balloon expandable stents appear satisfactory for growing patients, while the self-expanding stents, so far, have been disastrous for these same growing patients[9]. When a self-expanding stent with a small *maximum* expanded diameter, is used in a correspondingly small vessel, it has the same effect of creating a future stenosis as implanting any other small stent. At the other extreme, when a self-expanding stent with an eventual large diameter that is significantly larger than the vessel in which it is implanted at the time, is implanted in a smaller vessel, it generates a continual force to expand further in an attempt to reach its "built-in" maximum diameter. This continual force against the walls of a smaller vessel creates a continual, *stress/irritation* against the intima of the vessel, which results in an extremely aggressive intimal proliferation. This intimal proliferation has been demonstrated to even obliterate the involved vessel completely. This reaction occurs regardless of the materials of the self-expanding stent. There is still no detailed information concerning the use of self-expanding stents in the particular stenotic vascular lesions that are present in fully grown, adult, congenital patients.

General equipment necessary for the implant of intravascular stents in congenital lesions

1 A biplane catheterization laboratory with capabilities for compound angulation of both tubes and very high resolution X-ray imaging is essential. Although a single stent can be implanted safely in a distal pulmonary artery with a single-plane system, in congenital patients it is often necessary to implant several stents simultaneously, each with a very different orientation, because multiple or bilateral lesions are present. Without biplane imaging and compound angulation, the precise, simultaneous implant in different planes is very difficult if not impossible and certainly more dangerous. The absence of this capability certainly compromises the accuracy of an implant, the overall success of the procedure, and the safety of the patient.

2 Biplane "freeze-frame" imaging capabilities are essential. It is imperative to be able to "road-map" the lesions during implant with an identical reference frame from the earlier angiogram of the area. If the "road mapped" images of the lesions are of marginal quality or cannot be utilized during the very critical positioning of the stent, multiple and possibly otherwise unnecessary, repeat angiocardiograms will become necessary during the implant.

3 The specific stent(s) must be available for the *particular lesion* and, along with the stents, the particular balloons, long sheaths, and long Super Stiff™ wires (Boston Scientific, Natick, MA) that are required for the implant of each particular stent.

4 In addition to the specific materials for the stent delivery, a large inventory of miscellaneous diagnostic catheters, general spring guide wires as well as special torque and deflector wires is necessary for the stent implant procedures. Often the stenoses are in very inaccessible locations and require every piece of equipment in addition to all of the physician's skill and experience to position the stiff wires and delivery sheaths securely in these very difficult areas.

It is inexcusable to fail and/or abandon the necessary implant of a stent because of the lack of a specific, known and required item of equipment.

Specific equipment for stent implants

Stents, general

The "ideal" stent for congenital lesions still probably is not available, and perhaps is only a dream for such a "small" commercial market; no pun intended. Ironically, most of the stents used in pediatric and congenital lesions are very large in diameter compared to the small coronary and even the peripheral stents used in acquired lesions in larger adult patients. The ideal stent for congenital use has a low profile when collapsed yet expands to the ultimate *adult diameter* of the vessel in which it is placed. At its fully expanded diameter, the stent must have sufficient wall strength to support the vessel at its maximally expanded diameter and to prevent any rebound or collapse of the stent/vessel over time. Obviously, the stent cannot be irritative to the tissues where it is implanted and should not cause an excessive tissue response or abnormal intimal proliferation. Ideally a stent for congenital use should be flexible in its compressed state in order to bend or "flex" as it is being advanced around tight curves en route to the site of stenosis. The stent also should be somewhat flexible in its expanded state in order to conform to "curved" locations in the vessel once it is implanted. The ideal stent should have ***no*** sharp ends or tips that can perforate the delivery balloon or the walls of the vessel where it is implanted. An added desirable quality is the capability for the side openings in the "wall" of the stent to "stretch" or be opened further. This would allow subsequent entrance into any side vessels which were crossed by the stent and, in turn, would eliminate the "jailing" by the stent crossing its orifice. Finally, having the stents pre-mounted securely on appropriate balloons and balloon catheters for delivery to the complicated congenital locations would simplify the procedures significantly as well as add consistency and safety to the procedures.

Unfortunately, in the absence of an "ideal stent" that is manufactured specifically for use in congenital lesions, the stents and delivery equipment that are available for adult vascular interventions in acquired (atherosclerotic) disease are used and modified to suit the delivery and implant of stents in congenital lesions. Because of the lack of "official" recognition for pediatric/congenital patients, all of the manufacturers of stents test and "label" their stents with the "maximum" diameters for use in the "approved" smaller diameter biliary system and peripheral vessels rather than their true potential maximum diameters. This creates some confusion in their use in the larger vessels that are encountered specifically in pediatric/congenital lesions. For example, the "Large" Genesis™ stent (Johnson & Johnson–Cordis Corp., Miami Lakes, FL), with a maximum diameter of only 11–12 mm, is not a true *large diameter* stent, and only represents a 1–2 mm increase in maximum diameter compared to the Medium Genesis™ stent (Johnson & Johnson–Cordis Corp., Miami Lakes, FL). The Mega LD™ and Maxi LD™ stents (ev3, Plymouth, MN) are both labeled for a maximum expansion diameter of 12 mm with no distinction between the two, whereas in reality the Mega LD™ expands to 18 mm and the Maxi LD™ expands to 26 mm! Other examples of this are the labeling of the Palmaz™ P _ _ 8 stents and Genesis PG _ _ 10 XD™ stents (Johnson & Johnson–Cordis Corp., Miami Lakes, FL). The last numbers of the label (8 and 10, respectively) represent the maximum "legitimate" diameters of the stents for these adult lesions while, in reality, these exact stents are capable of expansion to 18 mm diameter, and they have been tested to be safe, as well as having adequate wall strength at the larger diameters[1]. The Palmaz™ P _ _ 8 stents have been used successfully and safely in pediatric/congenital lesions at diameters up to 18 mm for over a decade and a half.

The stent that is most appropriate for the individual lesion must be available in the inventory of stents in the particular catheterization laboratory. The specific stent usually cannot be chosen until during the actual procedure to implant the stent. As a consequence, a cardiac catheterization laboratory performing interventions including intravascular stent implants on pediatric/congenital heart patients is required to have in its inventory a large variety of types and sizes of stents and all of the appropriate balloons and necessary expendable equipment for their delivery. Cases that require the implant of a particular or a special stent must be planned in advance and the necessary special stents for the particular case are ordered in advance on the basis of previous catheterization data and non-invasive studies in anticipation of the type and size of lesions. This unfortunately does not account for new or different findings encountered unexpectedly during the catheterization for the implant of the stent.

Specific stents applicable for use in *major central* vessels

Genesis Extra Diameter™ (XD™) stents

The Genesis XD™ stent (Johnson & Johnson–Cordis Corp., Miami Lakes, FL) which is marketed as the Cordis™ PG _ _ 10B series of stents, has become the standard stent for most congenital vascular stenosis in large vessels that will not exceed 18 mm at their adult diameters. The Genesis XD™ is available in 19, 25, 29, 39 and 59 mm lengths. The Genesis XD™ stents expand to the same diameters and shrink in length when expanded, comparable to the original P _ _ 8, Palmaz™ series stents (Johnson & Johnson, Warren, NJ). Like the earlier Palmaz™ stents, the Genesis XD™ stent is laser cut from stainless steel tubing and is a "closed cell" design. The laser cut in the Genesis™ stents, however, is more complex and produces small "S" or "Omega" hinges between each circular row of "diamond" cells. These "hinges" provide some flexibility during delivery and allow the stent to conform to slight curves in the vessels once implanted, while the circumferential rows of "diamond" cells create a very strong cell configuration and wall strength. The "Omega" hinges may allow dilation of the side cells with "separation" of those hinges to allow access through the side of the stents in order to overcome "jailing" of side vessels. The end "cells" of the Genesis XD™ stents are closed, producing rounder ends without the sharp "points" of the earlier P _ _ 8 stents. The Genesis XD™ is comparable to the J & J, Palmaz™ P _ _ 8 series stent both in size and strength while at the same time having some flexibility and closed cells at the ends. Genesis XD™ stents are available in 19 mm (PG1910B), 25 mm (PG2520B), 29 mm (PG2910B), 39 mm (PG3910B) and 59 mm (PG5910B) lengths and are *advertised* to expand to 10–12 mm in diameter. *In vitro*, and in clinical use, this stent expands successfully to 18 mm in diameter, and at that large diameter the Genesis XD™ stent still retains its wall strength.

There have been reports after implant of the entire rows of adjacent cells separating from each other at the "Omega" hinges, but there are no reported adverse effects or clinical consequences from these separations. When expanded to 15–18 mm in diameter with a single inflation on a single large balloon, the shrinkage of the expanded stent in overall length is similar to that of the P _ _ 8 stents. The closed cells at the end of the stent and, in turn, the smoother, rounder ends presumably are less likely to puncture the delivery balloon, any adjacent balloon, or the adjacent vessels. The Genesis XD™ series of stents has replaced the P _ _ 8 stents for most central vessels in congenital heart lesions.

Unlike the standard Medium and "Large" sizes of the Genesis™ stents, the PG _ _ 10B Genesis XD™ stents, for some inexplicable reason, are ***not*** pre-mounted on balloons for delivery. The versions of the Genesis XD™ stents that were tested *in vivo* in animals were pre-mounted on various sizes of balloons. With the special manufacturer's pre-mounting of the other Genesis™ stents, the stents essentially are incorporated into the balloon surface and, in turn, the stents are fixed very firmly on the balloons. In the animal trials, the pre-mounted Genesis XD™ stents were delivered through very circuitous vascular channels without the use of a long sheath and without displacement of the stents. Although the smaller Genesis™ stents are all available pre-mounted, the current commercially available Genesis XD™ stents require individual hand mounting and, as a consequence, they are delivered through long sheaths and, of more importance, have the significant potential problem of the stents moving or slipping on the balloons during delivery to the lesion!

If pre-mounted versions of the Genesis XD™ stent and the larger "aortic" sizes ever do make it past the corporate decisions and come to market, they will reduce, if not solve, most of the current problems during the implant of intravascular stents in pediatric and congenital heart patients, and certainly will make the procedures infinitely safer. Pre-mounting, along with the already present flexibility and smoother ends of the Genesis XD™ stents, would create an easier and safer delivery. Pre-mounting would allow the stents to be introduced through smaller diameter, short sheaths and potentially allow the stents to be advanced to the lesions in all cases without the absolute necessity of a long sheath. At the very least, pre-mounting would prevent all dislodgement of the stents from the balloons during a standard delivery through a long sheath.

The "rounded" smoother ends combined with the flexibility of these stents allow passage around tighter curves within the vascular system during delivery "en route" to the target lesion. The flexibility in turn allows the use of the "braided", more flexible sheaths, which do not kink at all when bent, for delivery of the stents. Pre-mounting of the stents would enhance this capability for stent delivery very significantly. The smoother, non-sharp ends do not tend to puncture the implanting balloons, adjacent balloons, or vessels, and the flexibility allows a single stent to conform better to the curvature of a vessel after its implant than a series of shorter stents.

Although there still is no stent commercially available which fulfills *all* of the optimal criteria for use in congenital lesions, the "Genesis XD™ Series" of stents is getting closer to that nebulous "ideal" stent. The "Genesis™ type" stent still is *not* available in the *very large* diameters and lengths comparable to the P _ _ 10™ series stents (Johnson & Johnson, Warren, NJ) and, as a consequence, still is not suitable for central aortic, central common venous channel, or main pulmonary artery use.

Mega LD™ stents

The Mega LD™ stent (ev3, Plymouth, MN) is another stent that can be dilated to 18 mm diameter. The Mega LD™ is laser cut from stainless steel tubing in a very elaborate, "undulating" pattern, which creates an irregular but repeating configuration of openings between the adjacent rows of struts, which pass entirely around the circumference of the stent. These openings produce the "open-cell" design. The configuration of the "cells" is similar to that of the earlier Double Strut LD™ stents (Intra Therapeutics Inc., St. Paul, MN), but the "single struts" are cut from a tubing of an initially thicker material, which makes each strut thicker and stronger than the double struts of the Double Strut LD™ stents. The Mega LD™ stents are available in 16, 26 and 36 mm lengths and expand to a maximum diameter of 18 mm, which makes them applicable for the same size lesions and vessels as the Genesis XD™ and the original Palmaz™ P _ _ 8 stents.

The "open-cell" configuration provides flexibility to these stents in both the unexpanded and expanded states and, when the stents are *expanded sequentially*, allows the stents to be expanded to their full diameter without shrinking significantly in length. If, on the other hand, these stents are expanded with a single large balloon and expanded from their collapsed state directly to 15 or 18 mm in diameter, the ends are "compressed" toward each other by the "dumbbelling" of the balloon, which results in a significant shrinkage in the overall length of the stent. The characteristic end expansion ("dumbbelling") of a large balloon as it is inflated with a Mega LD™ stent mounted on it, actually *compresses* the cells of the Mega LD™ stent lengthwise *and holds this longitudinal compression*, while the center of the stent is expanding to its full diameter! This does not occur if these stents are expanded sequentially—i.e. first on a 10–12 mm diameter balloon and then to their full 15–18 mm diameter with a second balloon inflation. When the final *length* of the stent at the larger diameters is critical, the delivery of these stents requires either the use of separate, sequential balloons starting first with a small balloon followed by the second, larger balloon, or a sequential inflation using a BIB™ balloon (NuMED Inc., Hopkinton, NY).

The "open cells" allow access through the sides of the stent for catheters, balloons or even devices. The side "open cells" can be dilated up to 12 mm in diameter. Like their predecessors, the Double Strut LD™ stents, the end cells are closed and smooth, decreasing the likelihood of puncture of the implanting balloon or adjacent structures.

The "open cells" of the Mega LD create an irregular surface when mounted over the delivery balloon and, as a consequence, can catch on any structures that they pass through, including the back-bleed valves on sheaths. Because of this, Mega LD™ stents are always introduced into a short "loading sleeve" (Figure 22.1a) before being introduced through the back-bleed valve on the long delivery sheath (Figure 22.1b). If the Mega LD™ stent is introduced directly through a back-bleed valve, the individual rows of cells tend to be lifted off of the surface of the balloon, which distorts the stent or prevents its introduction.

While the Mega LD™ stents have the advantage of having *no* sharp ends that can dig into and damage the balloon or the vessel wall, at the same time, because the ends do not dig into the vessel wall the stents can be moved to and fro easily within the vessel during and immediately after implant, particularly with any subsequent catheter or balloon manipulations immediately after the implant!

a

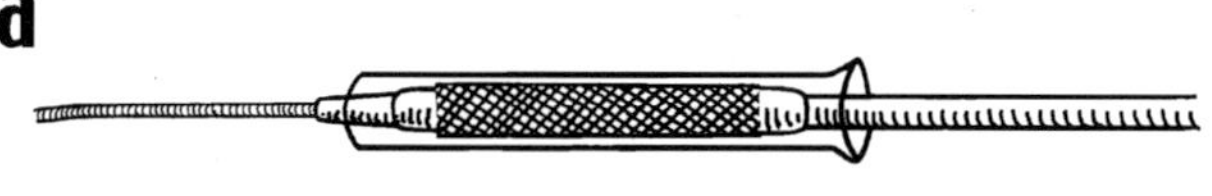

b

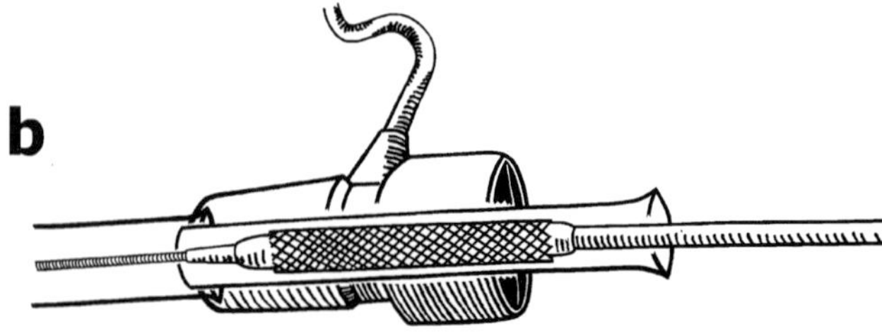

Figure 22.1 Stent on balloon and "loading sleeve". (a) Stent mounted on balloon and placed within a short "loading sleeve"; (b) "loading sleeve" with enclosed balloon/stent introduced through back-bleed valve of long sheath and seated on "flange" (or flare) at the proximal end of the sheath within the chamber of the back-bleed valve.

The wider, "looser" side cells not only can be crossed purposefully with a catheter or dilator, but during manipulations immediately after implant, the individual cells can be pushed out of shape by the tip of a catheter which, in turn, distorts the geometry of the entire stent. Significant longitudinal distortion of the cells elongates and narrows the implanted stent, which in turn can result in the freshly implanted stent being displaced. As a consequence, a vigorous effort is made to implant the Mega LD™ stents to their "final" configuration with the initial delivery balloon so that *no* subsequent manipulations within the stent are necessary during the initial implant catheterization. When the Mega LD™ stent has been implanted "successfully", and even if it is not in an *exactly* perfect position, it is *not* manipulated at all immediately after implant. Remanipulation or re-dilation is reserved for a subsequent catheterization after the stent has been allowed to fix into the tissues for several months.

The thicker struts of the Mega LD™ stents make these stents more resistant to compression and eliminate *most* of the recoil of the stent/vessel at the larger diameters. In *in-vitro* tests of Mega LD™ stents which were dilated sequentially to 15 and 18 mm diameters, the wall strength appears similar to that of the J & J, P 308 stents at the same diameters. The stiffer material reduces, but does not eliminate, the flexibility of the unexpanded or the expanded Mega LD™ stent. Mega LD™ stents have replaced the original Double Strut LD™ stents for most uses in congenital lesions. The Maxi LD™ stent, which is discussed later in this chapter, is larger and has similar but even sturdier characteristics. Although it can be dilated to significantly larger diameters for use in very large vessels, the Maxi LD™ can be used in place of the Mega LD™.

Palmaz™ P 308 stents

Although the J & J™ Palmaz™ P 308 stents (Johnson & Johnson, Warren, NJ) are not ideal, for over the first decade of use in congenital heart patients they were the only balloon expandable stents available for intravascular use in pediatric/congenital patients in the United States. The P _ _ 8 stents have passed the test of time and still are used in some of these patients. These stents fulfill the minimal criteria for use in the *large* central vessels and they meet most of the *minimal* acceptable criteria for stents in congenital lesions. *Once* these stents had been delivered successfully to the particular sites, they performed admirably for the treatment of congenital heart lesions for over a decade and a half of use, and have demonstrated no long-term adverse events from the stents themselves.

The P 308 "Iliac" stent is laser cut from a small stainless steel tube which is 30 mm long and 3.4 mm in diameter. The laser cuts produce multiple rows of interrupted, longitudinal slits, which encircle the "tube" and run the entire length the "tube". The opening of each slit is approximately 5 mm long and alternate rows of slits are staggered 50% so that when the tube is expanded, the slits along the walls of the stent create small diamond-shaped openings. At full expansion of the stent, these "diamonds" become very narrow and the resultant "diamond openings" are very resistant to compression circumferentially. As the slits expand into the "diamonds" the overall length of the stent shrinks proportionally to the expansion of the stent. The "diamonds" have very strong radial strength but, at the same time, are so small that there is no possibility of a *catheter* being *manipulated* through even the fully opened, side "diamond" openings of the stent once the stent is implanted. The slits at each end of the stents are "open" and, as a consequence, become rings of very sharp points when the stent is expanded.

Palmaz™ P 188 and P 108 stents

The Palmaz™ P 188 and P 108 stents (Johnson & Johnson, Warren, NJ) are 18 and 10 mm long versions, respectively, of the P 308 stainless steel, "expanded slot" design stents. The shorter J & J™, P _ _ 8 series stents are manufactured from the same diameter tubing with an initial 3.4 mm non-expanded diameter. The only difference is the overall length of the initial segment of tubing and, in turn, the length of the eventual stent.

All of the P _ _ 8 stents can be expanded up to 18–20 mm in diameter (advertised maximal diameter is 8 mm), and at the 18–20 mm diameter they still maintain their wall strength. When expanded to 18 mm diameter, the P 308 stents shorten to approximately 55% of their original length. At 18–20 mm expansion, the shorter P _ _ 8 stents also shorten to 50% of their original length, which in the P 108 stent, in particular, creates a very short and narrow circular "band". All of the P _ _ 8 series stents are rigid in both their collapsed and expanded state, which allows no "bend" or flexibility during delivery or after implant. If expanded to a large diameter with a single, continuous inflation with a large balloon, the longer P 308 stents tend to kink permanently at the center as the two ends of the balloon/stent expand away from the center with the initial inflation. This "kink" often remains as a residual "waist" at the center of the stent/vessel at full expansion. All of the adverse characteristics of these stents affect the delivery techniques and the potential complications of these stents.

The shorter stents are useful in central vessels in *very* small infants where the initial inflation diameter is no more than 7–8 mm, but where the eventual, anticipated diameter of the vessel is 15–18 mm. The shorter length P _ _ 8 stents are compressed or "crimped" to a slightly smaller collapsed diameter (on smaller balloons) and pass around tight curves within the vasculature more easily during delivery than the longer P-308 stents. Both of these features make delivery of the P-108 stent easier in small infants. The extremely short length at 15–18 mm expansion becomes of no consequence when these stents are used for the *initial implant* in vessels with a small diameter at the time of implant. When further dilation and greater support of the vessel are necessary when the patient and the vessel are larger, a longer, large-diameter stent can be implanted *within* the original short stent.

Multiple, shorter, P 188 stents placed in tandem within curves or bends in vessels are preferable to a single, longer, straight and rigid P 308 stent. In curved lesions, multiple, tandem and overlapping expanded P 188 stents can conform to the curvature of the vessel, in contrast to the single straight, rigid and longer expanded P 308 stent.

Double Strut LD™ stents

Double Strut LD™ stents (Intra Therapeutics Inc., St. Paul, MN) were the original open-cell stent from this manufacturer. They are cut by laser energy from very thin stainless steel tubing in an irregular and repeating "open-cell" configuration but with *double rows* of relatively fine parallel struts, which pass around the circumference of the stent. The thinner material of the struts and the open-cell configuration provide *very* significant flexibility to these stents in both the unexpanded and expanded states, while the double struts of each row provide wall strength that is equivalent to a single strut of thicker material.

The Double Strut LD™ stents are advertised as expandable to a maximum diameter of 12 mm, and *at diameters up to 12 mm* reportedly have the same tested wall strength and "crush resistance" as the J & J™ P _ _ 8 stents. Like the J & J™ P _ _ 8 stents, Double Strut LD™ stents can be dilated to 18–20 mm in diameter; however, when expanded to diameters greater than 12 mm, Double Strut LD™ stents definitely do *not* have the wall strength of the comparably sized J & J™ stents at these larger diameters. Since Double Strut™ stents do not shrink, there is less metal per unit of wall length than in any stents that shrink significantly with expansion. Implanted in larger diameter vessels with resistant stenosis, Double Strut LD™ stents tends to recoil immediately after implant or collapse under persistent high wall stress.

There is only a single row (or a single strut) at each end of the stent and each end cell is closed. The single row of closed struts at each end creates "rounded", smoother and "softer" ends on each stent. Like the Mega LD™ stents, the open-cell wall design allows access through the side of the stent for catheters and balloons, which allows the side "cells" to be dilated up to 12 mm in diameter. This has been documented in animal work in our laboratory. This decreases, or possibly even eliminates, the problem of "jailing" side branches.

The open-cell design of the Double Strut LD™ stent obviated many of the problems with the original J & J™ Palmaz™ stents, as well as the need for some of the more specialized implant procedures. The rounded, softer ends of the Double Strut LD™ stents do *not* puncture the inflating or any adjacent balloons during simultaneous implants. The thinner material and open-cell design of the Double Strut LD™ stents make them very flexible in both their compressed (crimped) and in their expanded configurations. The flexibility in their compressed configuration and the ability to bend when mounted on a balloon allows them to pass very easily around tighter curves and, in combination with the smoother, "rounded" ends, permits tracking around much tighter curves during delivery through long sheaths.

The flexibility of the Double Strut LD™ stents after implant allows them to conform to the shape of a curved vessel after implant and, as a consequence, a single, "longer" stent can be used in a curved vessel as opposed to a series of multiple, short, overlapping, rigid stents. Double Strut LD™ stents are available in a variety of lengths including a 76 mm long stent, which allows the use of one long stent instead of multiple overlapping stents in some special circumstances. When Double Strut LD™ stents are overlapped, the "open cells" of the overlapping stents tend to interlock and hold them together securely.

Like the Mega LD™ stent, when a Double Strut LD™ stent is *expanded sequentially* to the larger diameters it shrinks less than 10% in total length, but when expanded with a single large balloon expansion from its collapsed state directly to 15 or 18 mm in diameter, the characteristic end expansion ("dumbbelling") of a large balloon as it is inflated with a Double Strut LD™ stent mounted on it, actually *compresses* the cells of the Double Strut LD™ stent lengthwise toward the center *and holds this longitudinal compression*, while the center of the stent is expanding to its full diameter at the shortened length! This does *not* occur if these stents are expanded sequentially—i.e. first on a 10–12 mm diameter balloon and then to their full 15–18 mm diameter with a second balloon inflation. When the final length of the stent at the larger diameters is critical, the delivery of these stents requires either the use of separate, sequential balloons, starting first with a small balloon followed by the second, larger balloon, or a sequential inflation using a BIB™ balloon (NuMED Inc., Hopkinton, NY).

Because of the somewhat irregular shape to the cell design, the Double Strut LD™ stents, like the Mega LD™ stents, do not compress or crimp as smoothly or tightly over the dilation balloons when mounted on the balloons using hand crimping. The "wires" of each strut must be compressed almost *individually* along the length and circumference of the stent and, even then, the surface of the mounted stent often is rough. Because of the irregularity and "looseness" of the cells on the surface, Double Strut LD™ stents, like Mega LD™ stents, are always introduced into a short "loading sleeve" before being introduced through the back-bleed valve on the long delivery sheath (*see* Figure 22.1).

Like Mega LD™ stents, Double Strut LD™ stents have the advantage of having *no* sharp ends to dig into and damage the balloon or the vessel wall. Because of their smooth ends that do not dig into the vessel wall and their overall "softer" construction, they can be moved to and fro or distorted within the vessel even more readily than Mega LD™ stents during or immediately after implant. As a consequence, the Double Strut LD™ stent should always be implanted to its "final" diameter and configuration with the initial delivery balloon so that *no* subsequent manipulation within the stent is necessary during the initial implant catheterization. Like the Mega LD™ stents, when the Double Strut LD™ stent is implanted "successfully" and even if it is not in an *exactly* perfect position, it is *not* manipulated at all immediately after implant.

The clinical use of these stents in congenital lesions has been limited. The results were encouraging, although the lack of strength of these stents at the larger diameters prevents their more universal use. They are very good for lesions in very curved vessels and in thinner walled vessels where the wall strength of the stent is not as critical. The Mega LD™ stents (ev3, Plymouth, MN) are sturdier versions of the Double Strut LD™ stent, which were discussed earlier in this chapter and now are available commercially. The Mega LD™ stents have almost replaced the Double Strut LD™ stents in congenital use. Certainly, the rounder ends of the Double Strut LD™ stents eliminated many of the problems and complications that resulted from the sharp, rigid ends of the J & J™ Palmaz™ stents. The final decision on their use for any of the multiple varieties of congenital lesions requires at least several more years of experience and follow-up data.

Cheatham-Platimum™ (C-P™) stents

Cheatham-Platinum™ (C-P™) stents (NuMED Inc., Hopkinton, NY) were available on special order for emergency or special compassionate use in the US, and are available for routine use outside of the US. These are balloon expandable stents manufactured from strands of platinum wire, which are welded together to form a "zigzag" tube of a wire mesh. This configuration results in a closed-cell, tubular stent, but the larger "zigs" allow the passage of a catheter/balloon through the opening in the "zigs" in the side-wall of the larger stents. The size of each "zig" and number of rows of "zigs" determine the diameter of the stent, while the number of "zigs" in a row determines the length of the stent. C-P™ stents are available in a very wide range of lengths (from 15 to 90+ mm!) and in diameters (up to 30+ mm) by special or custom order. These stents have "rounded" smooth ends and are slightly flexible. The platinum material makes them highly visible on fluoroscopy and X-ray. The wall strength is reportedly equal to or greater than that of the comparable J & J™ stents expanded to the same diameters.

The larger sizes of the C-P™ stents allow access to side vessels/branches through the individual "cells" of the stent. These stents are in routine use throughout most of the world *except* in the United States. The design of the C-P™ stents gives them some of the favorable characteristics of the ev3™ stents. They have rounded smoother ends as well as some flexibility in both their non-expanded and expanded configurations. They have side cells that can be traversed and at the same time the stents are very stable after implant. There was some question about the persistent strength or integrity of the welds of these stents under the continued stresses of repeated compressions. This concern resulted in a design/materials change from the original C-P™ stent to obviate this problem.

The C-P™ stents had been available in the US for selected cases by special order, only for compassionate and/or individual humanitarian emergency use as covered stents and when no other comparable stent was available. However, even that life-saving availability has been curtailed in the US by the US FDA. C-P™ stents are available outside of the United States and, there, have had a very wide and very satisfactory use with an excellent safety record. The ability to order "custom sizes" allows the use of C-P™ stents in extremely versatile and often unique circumstances, which are not possible with any other stent.

Outside of the US, a covered version of the C-P™ stent is available and can be ordered in almost an infinite variety of custom sizes. The results with the extensive use of C-P™ stents throughout the rest of the world and in a large variety of congenital lesions, particularly in some unique situations, have been very encouraging. Hopefully, the regressive trend in the US will eventually be reversed, and these stents will become more available routinely in the US within the foreseeable future.

Stents available for *very large* central vessels (aorta, central pulmonary artery/conduits or central venous channels and conduits)

P 3010, P 4010 and P 5010 (P 3015, P 4015 and P 5015 outside of the US)

P _ _ 10 stents (Johnson & Johnson–Cordis Corp., Miami Lakes, FL) are larger versions of the Palmaz™ P _ _ 8 series stents. They are manufactured from slightly thicker and larger diameter stainless steel tubing and each laser cut is slightly larger and longer than in the P _ _ 8 stents. The

P _ _ 10 stents are available in 3, 4 and 5 cm lengths and expand up to 28 mm in diameter. These stents maintain their wall strength at their full, expanded diameters. Like the Palmaz™ P _ _ 8 stents, the P _ _ 10 stents are absolutely rigid in both their unexpanded and expanded configurations. The rigidity of these stents and their sharp ends are even more apparent than in the P _ _ 8 series stents, and when inflated in one stage on a very large balloon, the flaring of the sharp ends and kinking at the center represent an even greater problem than with the P _ _ 8 stents.

The P _ _ 10 series stents can be expanded to a large enough diameter to accommodate the central aorta, main pulmonary artery or central systemic vein or pulmonary venous channels in even the largest adult patient and have already had a fairly extensive use in these areas.

Maxi LD™ stents

Maxi LD™ stents (ev3, Plymouth, MN) are a slightly thicker and larger version of the single strut Mega LD™ stent (ev3, Plymouth, MN). Similar to the other ev3™ stents, Maxi LD™ stents have an "open-cell" design and have smoother "rounded" ends. These stents are available in 16, 26 and 36 mm lengths and can be expanded to 24–26 mm in diameter. Like the other ev3™ stents, Maxi LD™ stents, when *expanded sequentially* to their full diameter, do not shrink in length significantly. However, when compressed (crimped) tightly on a large diameter BIB™ balloon for such a sequential dilation, there is considerable resistance to the start of the initial expansion of the inner balloon. Usually the inner balloon must be inflated with pressures 3 to 4 atmospheres greater than the rated burst pressure of the inner balloon, or inflation of the outer balloon must be started before the inner balloon begins to inflate.

Up to 24 mm diameter these stents have a wall strength similar to that of the J & J, P _ _ 8™ stents, however, when placed within a significant curve in a vessel, Maxi LD™ stents do tend to kink along the concave surface of the curve after their implant. In very limited usage these stents have been very successful in coarctations of the aorta and in very large central branch pulmonary arteries in large patients.

Cheatham-Platinum™ (C-P™) stents

The Platinum wire C-P™ stents (NuMED Inc., Hopkinton, NY) used to be available in much larger diameters (up to 30+ mm) by special order for unique, compassionate/emergency use even in the US, but this emergency availability has been suspended in the US. The larger stents are available outside of the US with a CE mark of approval. The large C-P™ stents are manufactured of thicker wires, with more rows of cells and in longer lengths. The size and number of rows of "zigs" in each stent determine its size and strength. As with the other "standard sized" C-P™ stents, these larger C-P™ stents are available outside of the US as "covered stents". The covered stents all are available only by special order but now cannot be used for even compassionate and/or humanitarian use in the United States.

Stents available for small vessel use (*peripheral* branch pulmonary arteries and small, very *pheripheral* systemic veins)

There are multiple stents available which *cannot* be dilated to diameters large enough to be used for *central* vessels in any patient, but which do have a definite use in the smaller peripheral pulmonary arteries, very peripheral systemic veins, and selective, small systemic arteries or shunts where a restricted diameter actually is desired and there *never will be a need* for a larger diameter than the maximum diameter of the stent as a consequence of the growth of the patient. Many of these smaller diameter stents are available commercially pre-mounted very securely on delivery balloons. Because of their smaller sizes and the pre-mounting, these stents are introduced and delivered through much smaller diameter sheaths and are easier to deliver through tortuous courses through the vascular system. In spite of the temptation to use these stents in potentially large vessels in small infants because of their small collapsed size and easier use, these stents should ***not be used*** in ***any vessel*** that is expected to grow to a diameter larger than the maximum diameter of the stent. When a small stent is used in these potentially larger vessels, the maximum diameter of the *stent itself* produces a fixed diameter stenosis which cannot be dilated further and unequivocally will require a very difficult, and otherwise unnecessary, surgical repair in the future to correct the iatrogenic stenosis created by the small diameter stent.

Medium Genesis™ and "Large" Genesis™ stents

The "standard" Genesis™ stents (Johnson & Johnson–Cordis Corp., Miami Lakes, FL) replaced the earlier J & J™ P _ _ 4 and the Cordis™ Corinthian™ line (Johnson & Johnson–Cordis Corp., Miami Lakes, FL) of stents and are a smaller version of the previously described, significantly larger, Genesis XD™ stent. The *"Large"* Genesis™ stents are misrepresented as "large" stents since their maximum diameter is only very slightly larger than the maximum diameter of the Medium Genesis™ stents. The "Large" Genesis™ stents definitely *cannot* be expanded to the required large diameters of the adult central pulmonary arteries, central systemic veins, and the aorta, and *should never be used* in these locations.

Like the Genesis XD™, the Genesis™ Medium and "Large" stents are laser cut from stainless steel tubing with a complex cut which produces a closed-cell design, but with each ring of the "diamond" cells attached to the adjacent ring of cells with an "Omega hinge" similar to the larger Genesis XD™ stents. The "hinge" gives the stents flexibility in both their non-expanded and their expanded configurations. This flexibility markedly improves their ability to "track" around tight curves during delivery and allows them to conform somewhat to the "curved" configuration when implanted in a curved vessel. The "end cells" are closed, which gives the ends of the stents a much smoother configuration. These smoother ends should reduce, or even eliminate, the problems of balloon/vessel puncture during delivery of the stents.

The advertised maximum diameters of the Medium Genesis™ is 7 mm and of the "Large" Genesis™ is 9 mm but, like the P _ _ 4 predecessors, the Medium and the "Large" Genesis™ stents can be expanded up to 10 and 11 or 12 mm in diameter respectively. Medium Genesis™ stents are available in lengths of 12, 15, 18 and 24 mm, while the "Large" Genesis™ stents are available in lengths of 19, 29, 39, 59 and 79 mm.

The Medium and "Large" Genesis™ stents are available pre-mounted on a variety of Cordis™ balloons (Cordis Corp., Miami Lakes, FL). The pre-mounting represents a unique "incorporation" of the stent *into* the wall of the balloon. This incorporation with the wall of the balloon fixes the stent very securely on the balloon and allows delivery of the stents to very circuitous locations without the use of a long sheath and with no displacement of the stent on the balloon when delivered through a long sheath. The balloon on which the particular stent is premounted depends upon the length of the stent, the desired implant diameter of the stent, the introductory sheath diameter, and the guide wire diameter.

The Medium Genesis™ stents are mounted on 4–7 mm diameter Cordis™ Aviator™ balloons, 3–7 mm diameter Cordis™ Slalom™ balloons and 4–7 mm diameter Cordis™ Opta Pro™ balloons (Cordis Corp., Miami Lakes, FL). The "Large" Genesis™ stents are mounted on 5–9 mm diameter Cordis™ Opta Pro™ balloons. All of the balloon catheters are advertised as being available in 135 cm as well as shorter lengths. The Opta Pro™ balloon catheters pass over a 0.035″ wire while the Slalom™ balloon catheters only accept a 0.018″ wire and the Aviator™ balloon catheters accept only a 0.014″ wire.

All lengths of both the Medium and "Large" Genesis™ stents are also available independently and not premounted. These individual stents can be hand-mounted on any other desired balloon for delivery. As yet, neither the non-mounted nor the pre-mounted Medium and "Large" Genesis™ stents have had extensive use in congenital lesions, so the final indications and advantages/disadvantages are yet to be determined. In all likelihood, these stents will replace all of the other "smaller" stents in the Cordis™/J & J™ line of stents which are discussed later.

Express™ Biliary LD stents

Express™ Biliary LD stents (Medi-Tech, Boston Scientific, Natick, MA) are similar in *size* to the standard Medium and "Large" Genesis stents (Johnson & Johnson–Cordis Corp., Miami Lakes, FL). These stents have a "tandem" construction of alternating large ("macro") and small ("micro") rings of struts, which provide maximum flexibility during delivery and after implant and at the same time, provide considerable wall strength when expanded. The alternate rings of struts are attached to each other by lengthwise metal bands which connect only every third loop of the larger rings to every forth loop of the smaller rings. This arrangement provides a very "open-ring" configuration when expanded, which allows catheter/balloon access through the side "cells" in the wall of the implanted stent.

These stents are pre-mounted on Ultrathin™ SDS balloons (Medi-Tech, Boston Scientific, Natick, MA) and are available in 6 through 10 mm diameters and in 17, 37 and 57 mm lengths on the 6–8 mm balloons and in 25, 37, and 57 mm lengths on the 9 and 10 mm diameter balloons. All of these balloon catheters pass over a 0.035″ wire, so they can be delivered over Super Stiff™ wires (Medi-Tech, Boston Scientific, Natick, MA). The stents mounted on 6–8 mm balloons are introduced through a 6-French sheath while the 8 mm diameter, 57 mm long balloons and all of the 9 and 10 mm diameter stent/balloons require a 7-French sheath. The non-compliant Ultrathin™ SDS balloons can be inflated to 12 atmospheres, and at that pressure have a very uniform inflation diameter regardless of the resistance in any particular area around the balloon. Like the other smaller stents, these stents can be expanded to only 11–12 mm maximum diameters and, as a consequence, are useful *only* in *distal* branch pulmonary lesions or in *very peripheral* systemic arterial or venous lesions and *never* should be used in central, potentially large vessels.

Intrastent Double Strut ParaMount stents

ParaMount™ stents (ev3, Plymouth, MN) are a premounted version of the Double Strut™ stents with an advertised diameter up to 8 mm, but like the other Double Strut™ stents, they presumably can be dilated to even larger diameters. They are pre-mounted very securely on 5–8 mm diameter, Bard Opti-Plast XT™ balloons (Bard Cardiopulmonary, Tewksbury, MA), and are available in lengths of 16 and 36 mm. At these small diameters, like the other ev3 balloons, these balloons have little longitudinal shrinkage and have similar wall strength to the other pre-mounted smaller stents. There is very little reported use in pediatric patients and congenital lesions.

Palmaz™ P-204, P-154 and P-104 stents

The smaller Palmaz™ P _ _ 4 or "Renal" stents (Johnson & Johnson, Warren, NJ) are part of the original "line" of J & J™ intravascular stents that have been in use for one and a half decades. They are made from smaller stainless steel tubing and cut with a similar "expanded slot" design by the same manufacturing process as the larger P _ _ 8 stents. The *non-articulated* P-204 stent is 20 mm long and 2.4 mm in its non-expanded diameter. The P-154 and P-104 stents are 15 and 10 mm long, respectively. All of the P _ _ 4 stents are expandable to a maximum of 11 mm in diameter (advertised maximal diameter is 4 mm). Similar to the larger J & J™ stents, the P _ _ 4 stents are rigid and have very sharp ends when expanded.

The P-204 stent also is available with an "articulation" (open gap at the center with the two 1 cm long halves attached by a single strand of stainless steel). This "articulation" provides some flexibility for the longer stent during delivery, but leaves a narrow gap between the two ends and allows asynchronous motion between the opposing ends of the two halves, which results in excessive tissue reaction and rapid re-stenosis between the two segments after implant. The articulated versions are contraindicated in pediatric/congenital lesions.

The P _ _ 4 stents have been supplanted by the Medium and "Large" Genesis™ stents, and will probably disappear from availability and clinical use.

Double Strut™ stents

The Double Strut™ stent (Intra Therapeutics Inc., St Paul, MN) is a similar stent to the Double Strut LD™ (Intra Therapeutics Inc., St Paul, MN), which is used in large vessels. These stents are stainless steel, of an "open-cell" design, and are available in 10, 16, 26, 36, 56, and 76 mm lengths. These stents can be expanded to a minimum of 5 mm in diameter at implant yet eventually can be dilated to 18 mm (advertised maximal diameter of 10 mm). These stents are very flexible, have rounded smoother ends and, with their open-cell design, provide access to side vessels/branches through the "cells" in the sides of the stents. When expanded to less than 10 mm in diameter, these stents have a wall strength that reportedly is comparable to the J & J™, P _ _ 8 stents. The ITI Double Strut™ stent is ideal for the small vessel in the growing child where the eventual end diameter of the particular vessel is unknown.

Balloons for stent delivery: general

The specifications of the balloons used for *stent delivery* in congenital heart patients are much more stringent than the specifications for the balloons used in the balloon angioplasty of valves and vessels in the same patients. All of the specifications of the balloons for stent implant are very important, not only for an adequate dilation of the vessel/stent, but for the "interaction" and compatibility with the particular size and design of the stent. The *ideal* balloon for the delivery of all stents in pediatric/congenital lesions is not available. The specifications of the "ideal" balloon are as follows:

The surface of balloons for stent delivery *should be* scratch- and puncture-resistant and should allow "fixation" of the collapsed stent to the balloon surface. The *usable length* of the balloon for stent delivery, which is the length of the *parallel walls* of the balloon, should be 1–2 mm ***shorter*** than the length of the non-expanded or collapsed stent. The balloon material should be *totally non-compliant* in order to provide uniform expansion of the stent to exactly the same diameter *throughout the length* of the balloon/stent when inflated at the maximum pressure of the balloon regardless of external resistances. The uniform expansion is particularly important in the area of the tightest stenosis, which usually has the most resistance to dilation. At the same time the areas of the balloon which are not covered by the stent and where resistance is the least, should not be expanded more than the advertised diameter of the balloon and/or the diameter of the balloon in the restricted confines of the stent.

While the balloons should be non-compliant and made of tough materials, the balloons for the *delivery and initial implant* of the stent do ***not*** have to be high-pressure balloons. The maximum pressure of the balloon required for implant only has to be enough to expand the stent out to the walls of the *non-stenosed* vessel, but not necessarily enough to expand the area of stenosis completely! Ideally, the balloon for stent delivery and implant is on a relatively small catheter shaft and has a low and *smooth deflated profile*. The balloon should refold to the same low profile with a *smooth surface* and *very even contour* when deflated in the body—without the aid of external or manual hand "folding". Because of the long skin to lesion distances necessary to reach many of the locations for intravascular stent implants in congenital heart patients, the *shaft* of balloon catheters for stent delivery should be at least 100 centimeters in length.

The "ideal balloon" for the delivery of intravascular stents should have *all* of the above characteristics *and, in addition,* would have the stent *pre-mounted securely* on a separate balloon by the manufacturer. A pre-mounted stent significantly simplifies the procedure for the catheterizing physician by allowing delivery without the use of a long sheath and entirely eliminating the problems of the stent dislodging from the balloon during delivery to the lesion even with the use of a long sheath. The smaller diameter, "biliary" stents are available pre-mounted. These pre-mounted smaller stents are usable in the *very distal pulmonary arteries and the peripheral systemic veins* in congenital patients but are *not* satisfactory for any of the more common central, vascular stenoses.

Unfortunately, the commercial market (profit capability) for balloons for the delivery of large diameter stents specifically for congenital lesions is very small. The small potential market, combined with the regulatory restrictions imposed by the US FDA on the development of new balloons/stents, imposes prohibitory costs and hurdles for the manufacture of such balloons specifically for a very limited, pediatric/congenital use. As a consequence, "ideal" balloons, and especially ideal large balloons with stents pre-mounted on them, do not exist for the delivery of stents to the large central vessels in congenital lesions.

The large majority of balloons currently used for stent deployment still are adapted from the adult peripheral vascular angioplasty and "biliary" applications. Of all of the many balloons used currently for stent delivery and implant for congenital lesions, only the BIB™ balloons (NuMED Inc., Hopkinton, NY) are designed specifically for stent delivery in the pediatric/congenital population, and particularly for stent delivery to lesions greater than 12 mm in diameter. Even these balloons cannot be considered "ideal" because of their large deflated diameters and their very rough deflated profiles. As a consequence, the "ideal" balloon/stent for the delivery of truly large stents in pediatric/congenital lesions is not available. For the *initial implant* of the truly larger stents to an initial diameter of less than 12 mm, several of the peripheral angioplasty balloons do fulfill most of the ideal criteria. However, the particular balloons used currently for each stent implant in pediatric/congenital patients still represent a compromise of one or more of the most important characteristics of each balloon.

When balloons that *do not* have all of the ideal characteristics are used for stent delivery, they often result in less satisfactory stent implants *and* in a much higher incidence of complications. These complications include, but are not limited to, the necessary use of *very* large delivery sheaths/systems, stent displacement, rupture of the balloons, and balloon entrapment within the stents during stent implant. When a balloon is chosen for stent delivery for any particular lesion, the balloon is chosen primarily for the specifications of that particular balloon that are *least likely to cause a major complication* during the stent delivery. Occasionally, the balloon is chosen according to those specifications which, it is anticipated, *will* result in the complication, but which is the *least serious* of those complications, which inevitably are going to occur! The advertised length of a dilation balloon is the "effective" length of the balloon or the length of the *parallel surfaces* of the balloon when the balloon is expanded. The balloon length for stent delivery ideally should be several millimeters *shorter* than the length of the stent and certainly, *no longer* than the stent. As the balloon with the stent mounted on it is expanded, the stent mounted over the surface of the balloon compresses and constricts the balloon, which increases the resistance to expansion and restricts it from expanding *under the entire length* of the stent. If the ends of a balloon extend beyond the ends of the stent, they do not have this constraint and always expand first (and almost completely) before the balloon under the stent even *begins* to expand. When the balloon is *significantly longer* than the stent, the ends of the balloon expand initially *beyond* each end of the stent in a "dumbbell" like configuration (Figure 22.2). The "dumbbell" ends are separated by the non-expanded stent and expand in areas proximally and/or distally away from the specific area of stenosis. As the "dumbbell" expands further, the ends of the stent begin to follow at a very acute angle off the rest of the stent as a circumferential ring of sharp points (Figure 22.3). For the same reason, even the "shoulders" of the balloon beyond its usable length should be very short or "blunt" and should extend a minimal distance beyond the ends of the mounted and non-expanded stent.

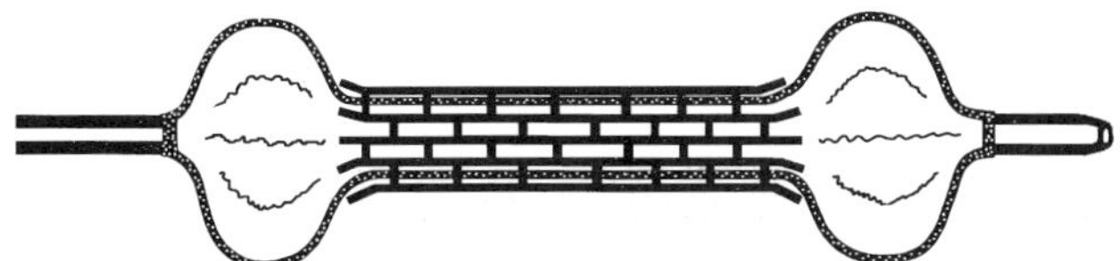

Figure 22.2 Beginning expansion of only the ends of the balloon beyond ends of stent.

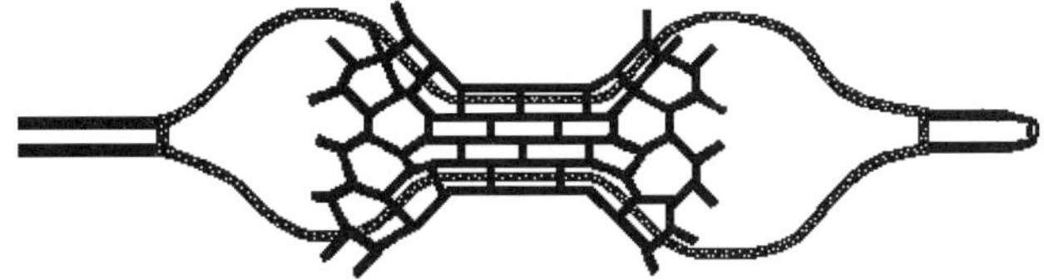

Figure 22.3 With the further expansion of the ends of the balloon and beginning expansion of the stent, the "dumbbelling" of the balloon is exaggerated. The circumferential rows of "spikes" at the ends of the stents are raised off the surface of the balloon.

When a hand-mounted stent is advanced within a sheath through a very tortuous course within the heart, the stent frequently tends to slide proximally on the balloon. In a very acute bend in the course, the stent can even slide completely off the balloon and onto the more proximal shaft of the catheter. In this circumstance, a slight extra length and extension of the balloon material beyond the *proximal end* of the stent will be desirable or necessary to keep the stent from sliding proximally on the balloon —or even completely off the balloon! When the stent repeatedly slides backward on the balloon during delivery, it becomes necessary to compromise and use a balloon slightly longer than the stent in order that the balloon

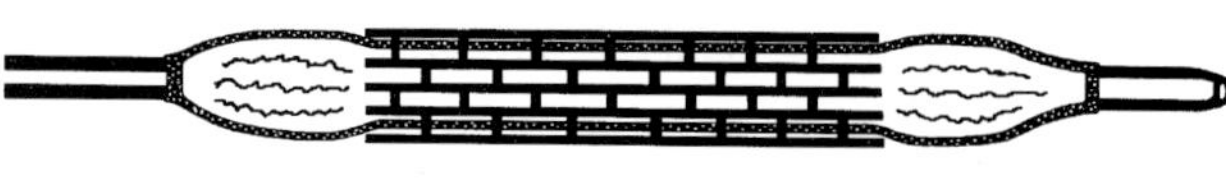

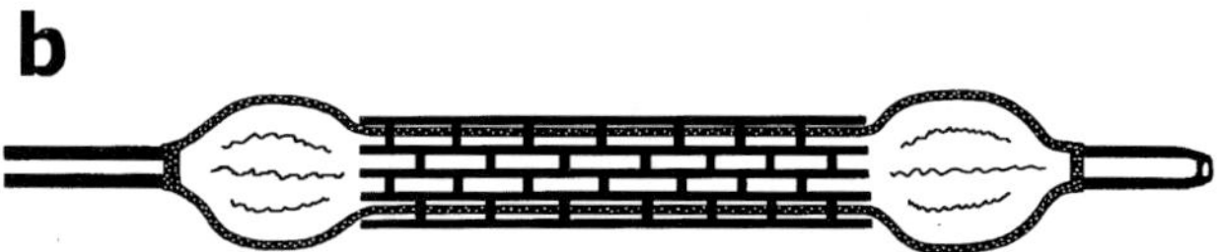

Figure 22.4 Stent mounted on balloon for delivery: (a) stent crimped on balloon with "shoulders" extending beyond end of stent; (b) "shoulders" of stent expanded *slightly* (while in sheath) to keep stent from sliding off balloon.

can deliberately extend 1–2 mm beyond each end of the mounted stent (Figure 22.4a). Once the stent with the slightly longer balloon is introduced completely into the delivery sheath through a protective sleeve, the balloon is partially expanded within the sheath at a very low (1 atm) pressure (Figure 22.4b). With the stent/balloon "confined" within the delivery sheath, this "partial expansion" creates small "shoulders" on the balloon beyond each end of the non-expanded stent. The shoulders, in turn, help to keep the hand-mounted stent from sliding off the balloon during delivery. This, of course, represents a compromise from the "ideal" balloon for the *delivery and ideal eventual expansion* of the stent, and also increases the possibility of balloon puncture as the balloon expands further and more acutely at both ends during the stent implant. In the absence of a pre-mounted stent that is very secure on the balloon, the operator *chooses his complication*!

For the implant of the short Genesis XD™ stents (Johnson & Johnson–Cordis Corp., Miami Lakes, FL), the shorter P-188, P-204 (Johnson & Johnson, Warren, NJ), and the 19 mm long Mega LD™ stents to *initial implant* diameters of *less than 12 mm*, a 2 cm long, 4, 6, 8, or 10 mm diameter balloon with very stubby "shoulders", on either a 5- or 6-French, 100 cm long catheter, is used. For the initial implant of the 36 and 39 mm long Genesis XD™ stents, the P-308 stents and the longer Mega LD™ stents to diameters *less than 12 mm*, a 3 cm long, 6 or 8 mm diameter or occasionally even a 2 cm long 10 or 12 mm diameter balloon with very stubby shoulders, and on a 5-, 6- or 7-French, 100 cm long catheter is used. For the longer Mega LD™, Maxi LD™ and C-P™ stents when initially implanted to *less than 12 mm* diameter, balloons *equal to, or as close to*, the exact length of the stents are used for their implant. The diameter of the balloon used for the stent implant is chosen according to the planned or expected diameter of the stent and vessel *at the time of the initial implant*. The implant diameter can be the *minimal* expanded diameter of the stent that *will fix the stent* securely into the lesion. With a tight stenosis, the stent does ***not*** have to be expanded to the nominal diameter of the adjacent vessel during the *initial* expansion during implant. Many standard angioplasty balloons are available for the delivery of even the potentially largest stents, when they are implanted at initial diameters of *less than 12 mm*. These balloons are available in diameters from 4 to 12 millimeters, in lengths several millimeters shorter than the stents being delivered, and have as many of the other ideal characteristics of balloons for the delivery of stents as possible.

All balloons that are even minimally longer than the stents which are mounted on them, and even balloons that are "the same length" as the stent, expand initially at *both ends* during the initial inflation of the balloon/stent (*see* Figure 22.2). This expansion at each end of the balloon (and the stent) often is to the full diameter of the balloon before the central portion of the stent even *begins* to expand! As a consequence, the stent flares away from the parallel surfaces of the stent at both ends (*see* Figure 22.3). The angle of this flaring is proportionate to the diameter of the balloon and relative to the length of the stent and the balloon. At balloon diameters of less than 10–12 mm, the angle of the flaring at the ends of the stent off the long axis of the stent will not be as acute. For the implant of stents *up to 12 mm* in diameter, a single balloon of the desired diameter, shorter than the stent and with as many of the other ideal characteristics as possible is used.

Balloons used for stent implants to *initial diameters* greater than 12 mm have separate requirements. For the implant of stents to *an initial diameter of over 12 mm*, the Balloon in Balloon™ (BIB™) balloons (NuMED Inc., Hopkinton, NY) are recommended and used routinely. As the name indicates, the BIB™ balloon has a smaller diameter inner balloon within an outer, larger diameter balloon. The inner balloon is one half the diameter and one centimeter shorter than the outer balloon. During stent implants, the inner balloon is inflated first, expanding the stent *uniformly* to half of its final diameter. Once the stent has been expanded uniformly on the inner balloon, then the outer balloon in inflated. This expands the stent to the full diameter of the outer balloon without the marked flaring of the ends of the stent as the stent expands initially.

These balloons have three distinct and important advantages for the expansion and implant of stents to the larger diameters. As a stent is expanded initially *on a single, large diameter balloon* to an initial diameter of more than 12 mm, the angles of the flaring ends of the stent become even more acute and align almost perpendicularly to the long axis of the stent and the vessel wall before the center of the stent begins to expand. With the current J & J™ P _ _ 8 and P _ _ 10 stents, this initial expansion at the ends of the stent results in a circumferential ring of sharp points at each end of the stent (*see* Figure 22.3)! These sharp points align perpendicularly to, and can actually penetrate, the vessel wall as the stent expands to its larger diameter. This initial flaring of the ends of the stents is minimized by the initial *uniform expansion* to one half of the maximum diameter by the shorter, inner balloon of the BIB™ balloons. The uniform diameter of the "half-expanded" stent throughout its length, also allows the stent to be repositioned within the lesion before the full expansion of the stent with the outer balloon is begun.

The final, and possibly most important advantage of the BIB™ balloons, is during the implant of a stent to an initial diameter of 15 mm or larger. When a stent is expanded initially and directly to these larger diameters with a standard, *single*, large diameter balloon, the angle of the expanding ends and the flaring of the two ends of the stent are even more acute. As the two flaring ends "meet" at the center, non-expanded, area of the stent, the struts of the stent wall can develop an acute angle, or kink, in the struts toward the central lumen and at the center of the stent (Figure 22.5). As the remainder of the stent expands to its full diameter, this acute, central "kink" often cannot be forced out of the stent and remains as a permanent, non-expanded "waist" or stenosis in the stent (and vessel) (Figure 22.6). The initial, partial and more uniform expansion with the inner balloon of the BIB™ balloons eliminates this problem.

Even with the very important advantages of the BIB™ balloons for expanding large diameter stents, the BIB™ balloons also have some disadvantages. The balloons themselves have a very large deflated profile, and with a stent mounted on them they require a very large sheath

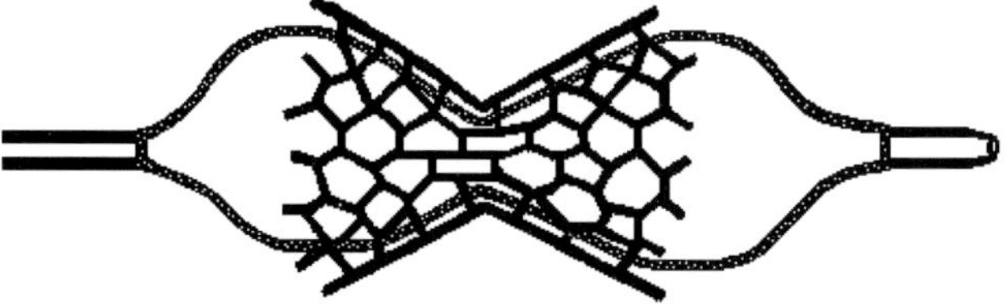

Figure 22. 5 Mid non-expansion of a stent on a large diameter balloon creates a fold or angle in the wall at the center of the stent.

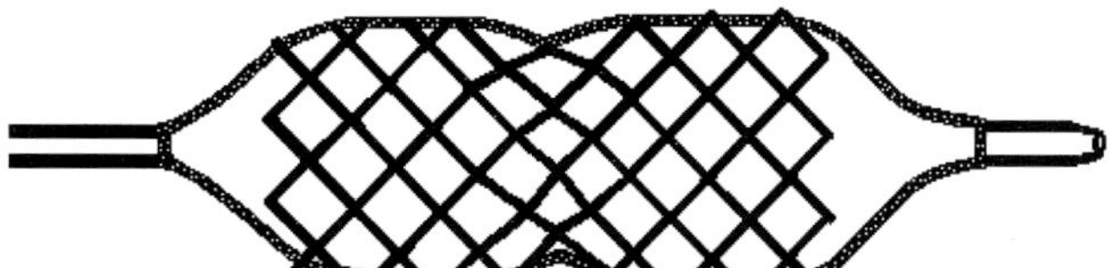

Figure 22.6 Residual kink created at the center of a stent after direct inflation to a large diameter with a single total inflation of a large diameter balloon.

for the introduction (10–14-French). In addition deflated BIB™ balloons have a very large, rough profile, which makes their withdrawal out of a recently implanted stent, very precarious and often difficult. The profile of the deflated BIB™ balloon often is *larger* than the initial diameter of the balloon/stent combination and, as a consequence, the deflated BIB™ balloon often cannot be withdrawn back into the long, large diameter, delivery sheath.

In addition to the balloons described for the delivery and implant of stents, a variety of high-pressure balloons in multiple diameters is frequently required for the final expansion of the stents in congenital vascular lesions. High-pressure balloons are necessary to complete the expansion of an implanted stent which has a residual stenosis in the stent/vessel due to a very resistant lesion, and to further expand stents which were implanted with a lower pressure balloon. Unfortunately, the "high" pressure balloons in the larger sizes, either are extremely long with very long shoulders or have a large deflated diameter and have horrible, rough, deflated profiles after their initial inflation. Because of these features, the larger high-pressure balloons are *not* used for the initial delivery and implant of the stents. The long shoulders of the Atlas™ high-pressure balloons result in displacement of the stents during implant and the rough, poorly refolded profiles of the Mullins X™ high-pressure balloons result in difficulty in removing the balloons, particularly from within a freshly implanted stent. For these same reasons, high-pressure balloons are used very cautiously even to further expand *freshly implanted* stents.

Specific balloons currently available

All of the balloons for stent delivery are listed in detail and discussed in Chapter 15 ("Balloon Dilations—General"). Their specific characteristics that provide particular advantages and disadvantages for the delivery of intravascular stents are discussed here.

Balloons for delivery of potentially *large diameter* stents to *initial* diameters up to 10 mm

Many of the smaller, standard, angioplasty balloons are satisfactory for the delivery and implant of stents up to an initial diameter of 10 mm. Although some stents are pre-mounted on balloons of these smaller sizes for delivery, the *pre-mounted* stents, to date, only expand to a maximum of 11–12 mm diameter and *are only used* in small peripheral pulmonary arteries and very peripheral systemic veins. The major problems that still occur with the balloons for the delivery of the majority of stents, occur when the *stents* eventually must be dilated to diameters much greater than 10 mm and, in turn, must be individually hand-mounted on the balloons.

Ultrathin SDS™ balloons

SDS™ balloons (Scimed, Boston Scientific, Maple Grove, MN) are an upgraded version of the previous Marshall™ balloons (Scimed, Boston Scientific, Maple Grove, MN) and are designed particularly for stent delivery. The SDS™ balloons are *non-compliant* balloons with a composite wall construction. This construction gives them a smooth refold profile after inflation/deflation while, at the same time, they are very tough and puncture resistant. In addition the balloons have a non-slippery, almost "rough" (Rawhide™) surface, which grips the stents better than an absolutely smooth or "hydrophilic" surface. SDS™ balloons have very short stubby shoulders, can be inflated to a maximum pressure of 12 atmospheres, and are available in diameters of 4–10 mm and in 1.5, 2.0, 3.0, 4.0, 6.0, and 8.0 cm lengths, which makes them *ideal* for the implant of all varieties of stents when the stent only needs to be inflated to these small *initial* diameters. While the balloon surface purposefully is "rough" and non-slippery, the shaft of the catheter has a Glidex™ Silicon™ (Boston Scientific, Natick, MA) coating making the catheter shaft slippery. All of the SDS™ balloons pass over a 0.035″ wire and, *with a stent mounted* on them very tightly, the 10 mm balloons require only an 8-French long sheath for delivery. This combination of features makes these balloons the most satisfactory of all of the balloons for the delivery of the larger diameter, non-pre-mounted stents *to initial implant diameters of 10 mm or less.*

Pursuit™ balloon angioplasty catheters

Pursuit™ balloons (Cook Inc., Bloomington, IN) are available in diameters from 4 to 10 mm and in lengths of 2.0, 3.0, 4.0, 6.0, 8.0 and 10.0 cm—although all lengths of the balloons are *not* available in each diameter. These are low profile and relatively non-compliant balloons, which pass over a 0.035″ wire and, with a stent mounted, pass through a 7–9-French sheath. These balloons have had a limited but reportedly successful use for stent delivery.

Accent™ AXM7 balloons

Accent™ balloons (Cook Inc., Bloomington, IN) are very thin walled, slightly compliant balloons. The AXM7 balloons (Cook Inc., Bloomington, IN) are on a 7-French catheter shaft and accommodate a 0.038″ wire. The balloons are available in diameters of 4–10 mm in 1 mm increments and in 2.0, 4.0, 6.0 and 10.0 cm lengths in all diameters. Although they have been used in selected circumstances, because of their thin-walled construction, these balloons generally are not recommended for the deployment of the large J & J™ Palmaz™ P _ _ 8 stents, even to small initial diameters and particularly not into tortuous or curved areas. The longer length Accent™ balloons are appropriate for the delivery of very long stents into peripheral venous locations.

Balloons for delivery of large diameter stents to *initial* diameters up to 12 mm

Ultra-thin™ Diamond™ balloons

Diamond™ balloons (Medi-Tech, Boston Scientific, Natick, MA) are non-compliant balloons with very short shoulders which refold very smoothly after inflation/deflation. The balloons are available only with a Glidex™ Silicon™ coating (Boston Scientific, Natick, MA), which makes the surface of the balloon very slippery. This slippery surface is beneficial for passing through tight lesions during standard angioplasty procedures, however, it is detrimental for stent delivery as the slippery coating makes it even more difficult for the stent to adhere to the balloon during delivery. Before a stent is mounted on an Ultra-thin Diamond™ balloon, the Glidex™ coating must be wiped completely off the balloon surface by vigorously rubbing the balloon surface with a 4 × 4 swab. Ultra-thin Diamond™ balloons are available in diameters of 5–12 mm and all except the 12 mm diameter balloon inflate to a maximum pressure of 12 atmospheres. The 12 mm diameter balloon has a maximum inflation pressure of 10 atmospheres. They are available only in 2.0 and 4.0 cm lengths with a 3.0 cm length (best for the more common P 308 stents) available only in the 8 mm diameter balloons. All of these balloon catheters have a 5.8-French shaft and accommodate a 0.035″ wire. A stent mounted on a 10 mm diameter Ultra-thin Diamond™ balloon requires only an 8-French sheath for delivery. This balloon is satisfactory for the *initial implant* of larger stents up to an initial diameter of 12 mm or less. The Diamond™ balloon is not quite as resistant to puncture as the SDS™ balloon.

PowerFlex™ P3 balloons

PowerFlex P3™ balloons (Cordis Corp., Miami Lakes, FL) are non-compliant balloons manufactured of Duralyn™ ST material (Cordis Corp., Miami Lakes, FL) which is quite resistant to puncture. They are available in diameters of 4–12 mm with a maximum pressure of 15 atmospheres for all sizes except the 10 and 12 mm diameters. The 10 mm balloon withstands 14 atmospheres while the 12 mm balloon has a burst pressure of 8 atmospheres. These balloons are available in 1.0, 2.0, 3.0, 4.0, 5.0, 6.0, 8.0 and 10.0 cm lengths in the 4–8 mm diameter balloons, with no 10.0 cm lengths in the 10.0 mm balloon and only 2.0, 3.0 and 4.0 cm lengths in the 12 mm balloon. All of these balloon catheters pass over a 0.035″ wire. A 12 mm diameter PowerFlex P3 balloon with a stent mounted on it passes through an 8-French sheath. PowerFlex P3™ balloons are very satisfactory for the delivery of larger stents to initial diameters of 12 mm or less and provide a wide range of lengths to accommodate the exact length of the stent.

Opta™ Pro balloons

Opta™ Pro balloons (Cordis Corp., Miami Lakes, FL) are slightly compliant, lower profile balloons, and are available in diameters from 8 to 12 mm and withstand a maximum pressure of 8 atmospheres. These balloons are available in 1.0, 1.5, 2.0, 3.0, 4.0, 6.0, 8.0 and 10.0 cm lengths, except in the 10 mm balloon where there are no 1.0 or 1.5 cm lengths, and in the 12 mm balloon, which is only available in 2.0, 3.0 and 4.0 cm lengths. These balloon catheters accommodate a 0.035″ wire and, with a stent mounted, pass through 7–9-French sheaths. The Opta™ Pro balloons have had widespread, reportedly successful use for stent implants to less than 12 mm in diameter. The shorter balloons are ideal for delivery of very short stents.

Accent™ AXM5 balloons

AXM5 balloons (Cook Inc., Bloomington, IN) are very thin walled, slightly compliant balloons, which are available on a 5-French catheter shaft with balloon diameters from 4 to 8 mm with balloon lengths of 2.0, 3.0, 4.0, 6.0, 8.0 and 10.0 cm, and in 10 and 12 mm diameters with balloon lengths of 2.0, 3.0, 4.0 and 6.0 cm. These balloons do have slightly longer shoulders and a distal tip which is longer than any of the previously described balloons. The smaller diameter balloons have a maximum pressure of 12 atmospheres while the 8, 10 and 12 mm balloons have a maximum pressure of 6 atmospheres. The balloon catheters pass over a 0.035″ wire and, *with a stent mounted* on the balloon, pass through 8- or 9-French sheaths.

Although they have been used to deliver stents in selected circumstances, because of their thin-walled construction, these balloons are not recommended for the deployment of the large J & J™ P _ _ 8 stents even to small initial diameters, and particularly into tortuous or complex areas because of the sharp spikes which develop at the ends of the expanding stents. The longer length Accent™ AXM5 balloons are appropriate for the delivery of any of the very long stents into peripheral venous locations.

Accent™ AXM6 balloons

AXM6 balloons (Cook Inc., Bloomington, IN) are also very thin walled, moderately compliant balloons, which are on a 6-French catheter with balloon diameters from 8 to 14 mm, in balloon lengths of 2.0, 4.0 and 6.0 cm. The 8 mm diameter balloon inflates to a maximum pressure of 12 atmospheres, the 10 mm to 9 atmospheres, the 12 m to 7 atmospheres and the 14 mm diameter only to 5 atmospheres.

Like the other Accent™ balloons, these balloons are not recommended for the deployment of the large J & J™ P _ _ 8 stents with their sharp ends, even to small initial diameters, and particularly into tortuous or complex areas. The longer length Accent™ balloons are appropriate for the delivery of very long stents into peripheral venous locations.

Small *maximum* diameter balloons with *pre-mounted small maximum diameter stents* for use *only* in *smaller peripheral vessels* and *not* suitable for use in potentially large, central vessels

The smaller "Medium" and "Large" Genesis™ stents (Johnson & Johnson–Cordis Corp., Miami Lakes, FL) and the Express™ stents (Boston Scientific, Natick, MA) are available pre-mounted on several different balloons from their respective manufacturers. These stents and balloons are suitable for use *only* in *distal branch pulmonary arteries* and *small peripheral systemic arteries and veins* that are not expected to grow to more than 8–10 mm in diameter.

Aviator™ balloons

The 12, 15, 18 and 24 mm long Medium Genesis™ stents are mounted on 4–7 mm diameter Aviator™ balloons (Cordis Corp., Miami Lakes, FL). The balloons accept only a 0.014″ guide wire, but with the mounted stent pass through 4–6-French sheaths. These balloons inflate to 10 atmospheres. The balloons/stents are available on 75 and 135 cm length catheters. These balloons/stents are suitable *only* for use in peripheral branch pulmonary artery stenosis or very peripheral veins.

Slalom™ balloons

The 12, 15, 18 and 24 mm long Medium Genesis™ stents are available mounted on 3–7 mm diameter Slalom™ balloons (Cordis Corp., Miami Lakes, FL). The balloons accept a 0.018″ guide wire, and with the mounted stent pass through 5- or 6-French sheaths. These balloons inflate to 10–12 atmospheres. The balloons are available on 80 and 135 cm length catheters, and like the stents on the Aviator™ balloons, these stents/balloons are suitable *only* for use in distal branch pulmonary artery stenosis or very peripheral veins.

Opta Pro™ balloons

The 12, 15, 18 and 24 mm long Medium Genesis™ stents are available mounted on 4–7 mm diameter Opta Pro™ balloons (Cordis Corp., Miami Lakes, FL). The 19, 29, 39, 59 and 79 mm long "Large" Genesis™ stents are available mounted on 5–9 mm diameter Opta Pro™ balloons (Cordis Corp., Miami Lakes, FL). Opta Pro™ balloons accept a 0.035″ guide wire, and with the pre-mounted stent pass through 6- or 7-French sheaths. These balloons inflate to 8 atmospheres. The balloons are available on 80 and 135 cm length catheters but, like the same stents on the Aviator™ and Slalom™ balloons, these stents/balloons are suitable *only* for use in distal branch pulmonary artery stenosis or very peripheral small veins.

Ultra-Thin SDS™ balloons

Express™ stents are available pre-mounted on Ultra-Thin™ SDS balloons (Medi-Tech, Boston Scientific, Natick, MA). They are available in 6 through 10 mm diameters and in lengths according to the length of the stent. These balloon catheters all pass over a 0.035″ wire and through a 6- or 7-French sheath with the stent mounted. These balloons have ideal characteristics for stent delivery. Like the other pre-mounted stents, these stents are only suitable for use in peripheral branch pulmonary arteries and peripheral systemic veins and arteries.

Balloons for delivery of stents to initial diameters over 12 mm

Balloon In Balloon™ (BIB™) balloons

The general characteristics of Balloon in Balloon™ (BIB™) balloons (NuMED Inc., Hopkinton, NY) have been discussed earlier in this chapter. BIB™ balloons are slightly compliant balloons and are available with an outer balloon diameter of 8 to 24 mm. The outer balloons are available in lengths of 2.5 to 5.5 cm (with other lengths available to special order). The inner balloon of the BIB™ is one half the diameter and is 1.0 cm shorter than the outer balloon. Both the inner and outer balloons have maximum inflation pressures of 6–4 atmospheres, the maximum pressure of the balloons decreasing with their increasing diameter.

Sequential inflation of the BIB™ concept balloons provides the most uniform and safest expansion of a stent when the stent requires expansion to larger diameters at the time of the initial implant. With a stent mounted on the BIB™ balloons, the combination stent/balloon requires a 10–14-French sheath for the delivery of the stent. BIB™ balloons have a large, very rough profile when deflated and the deflated balloons by themselves require the same, or even a larger diameter sheath for withdrawal, even after the stent is implanted and is no longer on the balloon.

In spite of their several disadvantages, BIB™ balloons are the best balloon and possibly should be the *only* balloon for the implant of stents expanded to diameters greater than 12 mm *at the initial* implant. The large sheaths that are necessary with BIB™ balloons usually are not a significant problem in the larger diameter lesions, since patients who require an implant to the initial large diameters are usually larger patients.

Z-Med™ II X high-pressure dilation balloons

Z-Med™ II X balloons (B. Braun Medical Inc., Bethlehem, PA) are relatively non-compliant, thick walled peripheral angioplasty balloons with relatively short shoulders. The Z-Med II X™ balloons are available in diameters from 5 to 10 mm in 1 mm increments, and in additional larger diameters of 12, 14, 15, 16, 18, 20, 22, 23 and 25 mm. The smaller sizes are available in lengths of 2.0, 3.0 and 4.0 cm while the balloons larger than 12 mm diameter are available in 3.0, 4.0 and 6.0 cm lengths. Multiple other combinations of diameter and length are available by special order from NuMED™ (NuMED Inc., Hopkinton, NY). The five smallest diameter Z-Med™ II X balloons have a maximum inflation pressure of 15 atmospheres. Thereafter, the larger the balloon diameter, the lower the maximum pressure, with the 22, 23 and 25 mm balloons having a maximum pressure of only 4 atmospheres. All of the Z-Med™ II X balloons accept a 0.035″ wire.

Z-Med™ II X balloons have fairly thick walls and are fairly puncture resistant. The "X" balloons have a braided catheter shaft, which gives them a good "pushability". With a stent mounted on them, these balloons require an 8-French sheath for the smallest diameter balloons and up to 15- or 16-French sheaths for the largest balloons. These balloons also have a very rough profile after deflation. As a consequence these balloons offer little advantage for the delivery of stents to large initial diameters compared to the more desirable BIB™ balloons.

Maxi LD™ balloons

Maxi LD™ balloons (Cordis Corp., Miami Lakes, FL) are moderately compliant balloons that have a diameter of 15 mm at their advertised inflation pressure of 4 atmospheres. When inflated with the maximum inflation pressure of 6 atmospheres, these same "15 mm" balloons reach 15.9 mm in diameter. They have short shoulders and are available only in 4.0 and 6.0 cm lengths. These relatively large balloons do have a slight size advantage with a stent mounted on them. The 15 mm balloon with a stent mounted on it passes through a 9- or 10-French sheath. With the initial inflation these balloons produce maximal flaring of the ends of the Palmaz™ P 308 and Genesis XD™ stents, and are less resistant to puncture than the old PE-MT™ balloons (Medi-Tech, Boston Scientific, Natick, MA) of comparable size. The initial inflation to 15 mm is almost guaranteed to flare the ends of the stent acutely.

Tyshak™ II X balloons

Tyshak™ II X balloons (B. Braun Medical Inc., Bethlehem, PA) are a thinner walled (earlier) version of the Z-Med II balloons (B. Braun Medical Inc., Bethlehem, PA). These *balloons* are available in the same sizes as the Z-Med™ II X balloons, however they are mounted on catheter shafts which are one French size smaller than the comparable Z-Med™ II X balloon. The new "X" balloons, even in the smaller sizes (4–8 mm) now pass over a 0.035″ wire. As a consequence of the thinner balloon material and the smaller diameter catheter shaft, these balloons with a mounted stent can be introduced through a slightly smaller sheath. However, the thin walls of the balloon and the small catheter shaft make these balloons generally more prone to puncture and, as a result, particularly unsatisfactory for the delivery of stents with exposed, sharp ends. When stents are inflated to large diameters initially with these thin-walled balloons, the problems of puncture are compounded.

PE-MT™ balloons

PE-MT™ balloons (Medi-Tech, Boston Scientific, Natick, MA) are large, and at the same time, very non-compliant balloons. In addition to being non-compliant, the PE-MT™ balloon material is very puncture resistant. PE-MT™ balloons are available in 12, 15 and 18 mm diameters, but currently only in 3.0 and 5.0 cm lengths, and only on 9-French catheter shafts. These balloons have a maximum pressure of only 3–5 atmospheres and have moderately long shoulders. The long shoulders at each end of the stent flare maximally and unnecessarily before the center of the stent even begins to expand. The catheter shaft of these balloons accepts a 0.038″ wire, but because of regulatory idiosyncrasies, the same balloons on 7- or 8-French catheter shafts, which were used to implant the first thousand plus P-308 stents in pediatric and congenital heart lesions, are no longer available. With a stent mounted on the current PE-MT™ balloons on the 9-French catheter shafts, the stent/balloon combination requires an 11–13-French sheath for the delivery of a stent. As a consequence of the *9-French* catheter shafts and in spite of their other advantages, the PE-MT™ balloons are rarely used now for stent delivery.

Omega NV™ balloon angioplasty catheters

Omega NV™ balloons (Cook Inc., Bloomington, IN) are large diameter, moderately compliant, angioplasty balloons that can be used for stent delivery. The balloons are available in diameters of 15, 18, 20 and 23 mm, and all of these sizes in lengths of 3.0, 5.0 and 7.0 cm. All of the Omega NV™ balloons have a rated burst pressure of 4 atmospheres. These balloons accommodate a 0.038″ wire; however, with a mounted stent, they require a 12- to 16-French sheath for stent/balloon introduction. The balloon material is not as resistant to puncture as either the PE-MT™ material (Medi-Tech, Boston Scientific, Natick, MA) or the BIB™ balloon material (NuMED Inc., Hopkinton, NY). As a consequence, Omega™ balloons are not as satisfactory as either of those two balloons for the implant of stents at larger initial diameters.

Balloons for the re-dilation of resistant stenoses within implanted stents

There are several additional "high-pressure" balloons that are not particularly useful for the delivery of intravascular stents, but which are very useful for the re-dilation of resistant stenoses that persist after the implant with a standard delivery balloon. The details of all of these balloons are covered in Chapter 15, but they will be mentioned here.

For stents which still have a residual stenosis in them and are less than 10 mm in their implanted diameter, the New Blue Max™ balloons (Medi-Tech, Boston Scientific, Natick, MA) are available in diameters of 4–10 mm and can be inflated to 20 atms. These balloons have an excellent profile for stent/vessel dilation. Conquest™ balloons (Bard Cardiopulmonary, Tewksbury, MA) are available in diameters of 6–12 mm, with burst pressures up to 30 atms for the 6 mm balloon decreasing to 20 atms for the 12 mm balloon. Unfortunately, these balloons have horribly long shoulders and can only be used when there are long straight areas of the vessel adjacent to the stent.

For larger stents with residual stenosis, the Mullins X™ balloons (NuMED Inc., Hopkinton, NY) are available in diameters between 12 and 20 mm with a burst pressure of at least 11 atms for the largest balloons. These balloons have a large initial deflated profile as well as a very rough surface and large profile when deflated. These balloons can only be used safely when the stent is fixed very securely in place in the vessel. Atlas™ balloons (Bard Cardiopulmonary, Tewksbury, MA) are a larger version of the Conquest™ balloons, and are available in diameters of 12–20 mm. These balloons have a burst pressure of 18 atms for the smaller and 16 atms for the larger balloons. Like the Conquest™ balloons, the Atlas™ balloons have horribly long shoulders. The total length of the balloon is triple the usable length of the balloon so they should be used only when there is a sufficient length of straight vessel beyond each end of the implanted stent.

Sheaths for stent delivery

General criteria

All of the stents that are "hand-mounted" on the delivery balloon, as well as some of the "pre-mounted" stents, are delivered to the lesion through long sheaths. The sheath/dilator sets for stent delivery are extra long "transseptal" type sets with an attached back-bleed valve/flush port. For stent delivery, the sheaths in these sets must be extra long (75 to 85 cm) in order to reach the distal branch pulmonary arteries in larger (taller) patients. In a very tall patient, even an 85 cm long sheath passing through significant curves within the heart may not reach the distal branch pulmonary arteries, and if the implant of a branch pulmonary artery stent in such a patient is necessary, even longer sheaths should be specially ordered ahead of time and/or one of the pre-mounted smaller maximum diameter stents can be used in the smaller *peripheral pulmonary vessels*. For a hand-mounted stent, the *sheath* length must be sufficient to reach *beyond* the desired location for implant and should be available in 8- through 14-French sizes. Additionally, the sheath for stent delivery *must be* resistant to kinking. The course of the sheath through the bends and curves within the heart and great vessels often is very tortuous, with occasional, additional acute turns. A kink occurring in a long sheath creates a transverse ridge within the sheath, which prevents a stent mounted on a balloon from passing the area even after the sheath is straightened within the body. The larger the diameter of the sheath, the greater the tendency of the sheath to kink when positioned across fairly tight curves.

The sheaths should be radio-opaque throughout their length or should have a very distinct radio-opaque marker band at their distal tip. When a sheath without a distal radio-opaque band is in position over the stent/balloon combination, the exact tip of the *sheath* often is very difficult to visualize. As a consequence, a radio-opaque marker at the distal end of the sheath allows more *exact* placement of the stent and significantly reduces the radiation necessary for visualizing the sheath.

Specific sheaths for stent delivery

The Check-Flo II Mullins™ teflon long sheath with RF bands

Check-Flo™ RB-MTS™ sheaths (Cook Inc., Bloomington, IN) currently are the most suitable non-braided sheaths for the delivery of *rigid* stents to vascular lesions in patients with complex anatomy. Check-Flo™ sheaths are available in sizes 6- through 14-French with sheath lengths up to 85 cm. These long sheaths are moderately kink resistant. Generally, if this sheath kinks when it is otherwise handled properly, the curvature in the course to the lesion where the sheath kinks will be too tight to allow the passage of a 3 cm long *rigid* stent. The Cook™ sheath/dilator sets are labeled according to: the presence of a marker band or not; the type of back-bleed valve; the "internal diameter" of the tip of the sheath; the internal diameter of the dilator tip; the length of the sheath; and the type of sheath. For example, an RCF-11-38-85-MTS™ is an 11-French, 85 cm long Check-Flo™ sheath with a radio-opaque tip band and with a dilator which accepts a 0.038″ wire. Most of the large, long sheaths have a significantly *larger internal diameter* than the stated size *and the dilator*, except at the very tip of the sheath, where the sheaths taper to fit fairly tightly over the dilator.

When desired, a specific curve can be formed on the tip of the sheath or dilator by either cold-shaping by repeatedly pulling the *combination* between the fingers and thumb as a curve is "molded", or by heating the *combination* in boiling water or in the hot air jet of a heat gun and then hand forming the desired curve and "fixing" the curve by dipping it in cold flush solution while still holding the formed curve by hand. A specific curve is useful to help the tip of the sheath/dilator advance around a tight curve or to "seat" the sheath in an area with a complex curvature without the curvature of the body causing constant tension on the sheath.

Super Arrow-Flex™ sheaths

Arrow-Flex™ sheaths (Arrow International Inc., Reading, PA) have a tightly wound spiral of coil wire sealed between ultra-thin outer and inner layers of the flexible polymer walls of the sheath. This "metal framework" makes the sheaths very kink resistant even when the sheath is tied into a knot! These sheaths are available in diameters of 5–11-French, but only in maximum lengths of 80 cm in the largest diameters. All of the Arrow™ introducer sets come with an integral, color-coded, side port/hemostasis valve. All of the 35 cm and longer Super Arrow-Flex™ sheaths have a radio-opaque marker band at the distal tip of the sheath. Because of the reinforcement within the wall of the sheath, the outer diameter of the sheath is at least one French size larger than the outside diameter of a non-reinforced sheath of comparable internal diameter.

The great advantage of these sheaths in forming very tight curves without kinking also is a disadvantage during the delivery of *rigid stents*. The sheath forms such tight curves in the course through the heart that when a *rigid stent*, which will not bend on the balloon, is advanced within the sheath, the balloon/stent combination cannot be advanced through the tight curve in the sheath. As a consequence, either the stent/balloon stops at the tight curve or the stent "milks" off the balloon onto the proximal catheter shaft while the more flexible balloon passes through the tight curve. These sheaths are very useful for the delivery of truly flexible stents. The new generation of stents may obviate the problem of stent displacement in tight curves completely.

Flexor™ introducer sheaths

The Flexor™ sheath (Cook Inc., Bloomington, IN) has a metal wire winding reinforcing the wall of the sheath with very similar kink-resistant characteristics to the Super Arrow-Flex™ sheath. Flexor™ sheaths are available in 6–10-French diameters and lengths up to 80 cm, with the tip of the dilators accepting a 0.038″ guide wire. Flexor™ sheaths are available with and without an integral Check-Flo™ side port/hemostasis valve and a radio-opaque band, which is located one mm proximal to the tip of the sheath. Flexor™ Check-Flo™ introducer sets are available in multiple lengths and with a large variety of preformed tip configurations. Flexor™ sheaths are very kink resistant and, like the Super Arrow-Flex™ sheaths, may form curves without kinking that are too tight to allow a *rigid* balloon/stent combination to pass through. Flexor™ sheaths can be manually formed into specific distal curved shapes.

Brite Tip™ sheaths

The long Brite Tip™ sheaths (Cordis Corp., Miami Lakes, FL) are a long version of the standard Brite Tip™ line of short sheath/dilator introducer sets (Cordis Corp., Miami Lakes, FL). These sheaths are co-extruded of two separate layers, which give the sheaths extra strength and flexibility without kinking when they are bent into fairly tight curves. All of the sheaths come with color-coded side port/hemostasis valves and have a distal tip that incorporates an extra radio-opaque band for excellent visibility. The tip of the dilator accepts a 0.035″ guide wire. The sheaths are available from 5- to 11-French, and by special order in lengths up to 90 cm. Like the Cook™ MTS™ sets (Cook Inc., Bloomington, IN), the Brite Tip™ introducers can be formed into specific tip shapes with cold shaping by pulling the combination between the fingers and thumb or by heating the sheath/dilator and then hand molding the sheath/dilator into the desired curve. These sheaths do not appear to have any great advantages over the Cook™ RB-MTS sheaths for stent delivery and are not as readily available.

Special purpose sheaths

Cook™ Inc. makes large long Check-Flo™ Introducer sets in 16- and 18-French diameters in 70 and 85 cm lengths respectively (Cook Inc., Bloomington, IN). These very large sheaths are for the delivery of very large balloon/stent combinations in addition to their use for the retrieval of particularly large or "non-collapsible" foreign bodies. In addition Cook™ manufactures extra large Check-Flo™ Introducers in 18-, 20-, 22- and 24-French sizes (Cook Inc., Bloomington, IN). The sheaths in all of these sets are 65 cm long but in the past could be specially ordered in longer lengths. All of these introducer sets require 6 to 12 weeks for delivery on "routine order" and, as a consequence, several of each size should be in stock in interventional laboratories dealing with congenital heart lesions for the purpose of retrieving large foreign bodies.

Wires for sheath/dilator and stent delivery—general

The ideal wire for the delivery of a stent is a *very* stiff exchange length wire. In addition to the delivery of the stent/balloon combination through the long sheath, the guide wire first must support the introduction and delivery of the long, large diameter, stiff sheath/dilator sets through which the stents are delivered. In addition to a very stiff shaft the wire should have a very short "transition zone" between the "floppy" distal portion and the stiff support portion of the wire and should be available with a very short, distal "floppy" tip. When the wire is in position for sheath/dilator delivery or stent implant, the *stiff* portion of the wire *must* extend *entirely beyond* the area of stenosis in the vessel where the stent is to be implanted. The very stiff wire is necessary to direct and support the large sheath/dilator set through the tortuous course and tight bends through the heart to the site of obstruction. Once the dilator is removed, the stiff wire helps to support the large, long sheath and prevent its kinking. The stiff wire then supports the stent/balloon combination and "straightens its course" as it is advanced through the sheath to the site. Finally, and probably of most importance, the wire must be stiff enough to maintain the stent/balloon in a precise position and keep the balloon catheter from moving forward or backward as the balloon/stent is being inflated. The one disadvantage of very stiff wires is that they tend to straighten *everything* in their path and, in turn, often prop open the tricuspid and/or the pulmonary valve(s) when the long sheath is positioned in the pulmonary artery. In the smaller patient, this decreases forward flow significantly and, in turn, decreases cardiac output and drops systemic blood pressure while the wire is in place.

The most satisfactory wires available for stent delivery at the present time are the Amplatz Super-Stiff™ (Medi-Tech, Boston Scientific, Natick, MA) exchange length guide wires. These wires are available in both 0.035″ and 0.038″ diameters and both diameter wires are available with the standard long (7 cm) floppy tips and the special short (1 cm) "floppy" tips. While the 0.038″ wire is only 0.003″ thicker than the 0.035″ wire, it is more than twice as stiff. This extra stiffness of the 0.038″wire often is necessary in order to deliver very stiff, *very large* diameter sheath/dilator sets through the tortuous course to the pulmonary arteries. Unfortunately, none of the balloon catheters that are satisfactory and are now available for stent delivery, will accommodate the 0.038″ wire. When the 0.038″ Super Stiff™ wire must be used to deliver the long, large sheath/dilator, and after the sheath is delivered to the exact position, the heavier wire is exchanged through the dilator or through a separate end-hole catheter for a 0.035″ Super Stiff™ (or smaller diameter) wire in order to accommodate the particular balloon/stent being used. The original dilator is replaced over the 0.038″ wire for the separate end-hole catheter when the dilator cannot be advanced to the very tip of the 0.038″ wire. Then the 0.038″ wire is exchanged through the catheter for the 0.035″ or smaller wire for the delivery of the stent.

If a long, floppy tipped, Super Stiff™ wire is used for pulmonary artery stent implants, all of the long floppy portion of the wire must be "balled" or "wadded-up" in the distal pulmonary artery *beyond the area of stenosis* in order to have only the stiff wire in the stenotic area with the transition portion *and part of the stiff portion* of the wire completely through and well beyond the area of the lesion. Whichever wire is used, once the stiff wire has been positioned through a tortuous course in the heart to a distal position in the lung, the wire must be held manually in order to maintain it in this location. Otherwise the straight, stiff wire will attempt to resume its straight configuration and "back" itself out of the distal location.

The very short (1.0 cm) floppy tipped, Super Stiff™ wire is used for stent implants only into the pulmonary arteries. The short floppy tip is wedged distally in a pulmonary *capillary* in the peripheral lung field. The advantage of the short floppy tipped wire is that it allows more of the true stiff portion of the wire as well as all of the "transition" portion of the wire to be positioned well past the lesion so that only the *stiff* portion of the wire remains positioned *across* and also *well past the lesion.* The disadvantage is that the short floppy tip, itself, can be quite stiff and minimally flexible, and can easily penetrate through the pulmonary capillaries into the lung parenchyma. Even when observed very carefully and controlled very precisely and with even very slight to-and-fro movement, the tip of the wire can perforate the vessels in the capillary bed leading to hemoptysis and/or hemothorax. The *short floppy tipped* Super Stiff™ wire is ***not*** used for stent delivery to *any* other location. When the tip of a Super Stiff™ wire is to be located in a central or peripheral vein, in any systemic artery, or in any cardiac chamber, the 7 cm *long* (standard), floppy tipped Super Stiff™ wire is used to avoid excoriation or perforation of the walls of either vessels or chambers by the short floppy tip of the wire.

The Lunderquist™ wires (Cook Inc., Bloomington, IN) are very stiff "guide wires" in which the proximal shaft of the wire is a solid stainless steel mandril, which has an attached flexible tip of coil wire. These wires are available as exchange length, 0.035″ wires, which have either a 3 cm or 7 cm coil (floppy) tip. These wires are even stiffer than the 0.038″ Super Stiff™ wires (Medi-Tech, Boston Scientific, Natick, MA) and certainly have a greater tendency to "straighten" themselves and everything in their path. As a consequence, when the proximal wire passes through any significant curves en route to the lesion, it must be held manually, purposefully, continuously, and very securely in its distal position in order to prevent the wire from spontaneously "backing-out" of its position.

Other wires such as the Amplatz Extra Stiff™ (Cook Inc., Bloomington, IN) and the Road Runner™ wires (Cook Inc., Bloomington, IN) are not as stiff as either the Medi-tech™ Super Stiff™ or Lunderquist™ wires. When these other wires are used, even if the sheath is delivered to the area of stenosis successfully, these wires always represent a compromise in the *control* of the position of the stent/balloon during the inflation/implant of the balloon/stent.

Very rarely in very small infants, stents must be delivered on balloon catheters that do not accommodate even the 0.035″ wires, and it becomes necessary to use a smaller diameter, but non Super Stiff™ wire. Smaller diameter 0.014″, 0.016″ and 0.018″ Road Runner™ extra support wires (Cook Inc., Bloomington, IN), 0.014″, 0.016″ and 0.018″ HyTek™ wires (Microvena Corp., White Bear Lake, MN), 0.014″, 0.016″, 0.018″, 0.025″ and 0.035″ Ultra-Select™ wires (Microvena Corp., White Bear Lake, MN), 0.014″, 0.018″ and 0.035″ FlexFinder™ wires (Microvena Corp., White Bear Lake, MN) and 0.018″ and 0.025″ Platinum Plus™ wires (Medi-Tech, Boston Scientific, Natick, MA) have all been used with success in selected cases, but again, always with some compromise in the control of the balloon/stent combination during the implant procedure.

Manometer balloon inflation devices

A pressure-monitored inflation device with a capacity of 20 ml or greater and capable of generating and holding at least 20 atmospheres of pressure is used for the balloon inflation for the delivery of *all* stents. Pressure against the plunger of a small standard syringe can exceed the burst pressure of a smaller balloon if not monitored. At the other extreme, manual pressure by itself against the plunger of a large (20 ml or more), standard syringe often *does not* produce the necessary pressure to reliably expand a large balloon with a stent mounted on it, and certainly not in the presence of a severely stenotic area. In addition, a syringe without a manometer does not allow *any control* over what inflation pressure is achieved. The mechanical inflation device is necessary to achieve the higher balloon pressures, while the manometer is necessary to control the *exact* balloon pressure for the expansion of the stent. Exceeding the maximum inflation pressure of the balloon leads to balloon rupture and the potentially serious consequences of a ruptured balloon in a partially inflated stent.

A large variety of these inflation devices are available from most of the balloon and some independent manufactures. The inflation devices, in addition to a ratcheted or screw inflation/deflation mechanism, must have a non-ratcheted, "free or rapid" inflate/deflate, sliding mechanism for large balloon inflations/deflations. The "free" sliding inflation/deflation mechanism is used for the initial, rapid volume inflation of the balloon and the rapid deflation of the balloon after the implant. The ratchet mechanism is used for the final, precise high-pressure inflation and fine adjustments in the volume/pressure at the end of the inflation/implant. The inflation device must be accurate for both volume and pressure and it should be capable of generating and maintaining relatively high pressures. The inflation device must hold a volume that is greater than the volume capacity of the balloon that is being inflated. Each different device has its own specific idiosyncrasies for its operation.

Encore™ indeflator device

The Encore™ device (Medi-Tech, Boston Scientific, Natick, MA) has a clear polycarbonate syringe barrel encased in a covering that holds an analog manometer. The manometer is attached to the syringe lumen and has a maximum pressure of 26 atms. The syringe has a capacity of 20 ml. The ratchet mechanism on the syringe plunger is engaged all of the time unless deliberately released by compressing a squeeze/release button on the side of the barrel.

B. Braun™ angioplasty inflation device

The B. Braun™ angioplasty inflation device (B. Braun Medical Inc., Bethlehem, PA) has a 25 ml clear polycarbonate syringe barrel with an analog pressure gauge, which reaches and holds 30 atms pressure. The syringe has a rapid action "winged" locking mechanism, which locks very quickly, adjusts very accurately and holds at high pressures.

Merit Medical™ inflation devices

Merit Medical (Merit Medical Systems, Salt Lake City, UT) has four different inflation devices, all with a clear 20 ml polycarbonate barrel. The syringe has a squeeze "bar" on a "T" handle to release the ratchet mechanism. The difference in the four inflation devices is in the type of manometer gauge. All of the gauges are electronic, but are available in analog or digital and in local or remote configurations and with, or without, built in timers.

Bard Max 30™ inflation device

The Max 30™ (C.R. Bard, Inc., Covington, GA) has a "T" shaped handle over the polycarbonate barrel of a 20 ml capacity syringe. A lever which moves from side to side across the "T" locks or releases the ratchet mechanism of the syringe. The Max 30™ inflation devices can deliver 30 atmospheres of pressure.

The only additional criterion for the use of any of these inflation devices is that the *operator* must be very familiar with the operation of the specific device that is being used.

Technique for the implant of intravascular stents

The technique for the delivery and implant of the J & J™, Palmaz™ stents (Johnson & Johnson, Warren, NJ) has been developed and modified extensively during the fifteen years of the clinical use of these stents in congenital and pediatric cardiac patients. Unfortunately, the stent and balloon technology for this "non-approved" use has not kept pace adequately with the complex congenital lesions for which stent therapy now is routinely utilized. Relative to the developments in stents and stent techniques for coronary arteries, the stents and delivery equipment for congenital lesions are a decade behind in development and in their introduction for clinical use in the United States. There have been some improvements in the stents which are approved for use in adult peripheral vascular disease and which have filtered down to the pediatric/congenital population. At the same time, the changes/improvements in the delivery/implant techniques for congenital heart patients were developed predominately in pediatric/congenital catheterization laboratories during the decade and a half of the use of stents in these patients.

All "self-mounted" or "hand-mounted" stents are currently delivered through or with the use of a long sheath advanced to and past the lesion where the stent is to be implanted. To date, there are no satisfactory ways of hand-mounting stents and securing them tightly enough on the balloons to allow *confident and safe* delivery of a stent without the use of a long sheath. Even if secured to the balloon, without the use of a long sheath, the stiff, sharp exposed ends of a rigid stent that is hand-mounted on a balloon, easily extend off the balloon, catch on intravascular structures, and are displaced off the balloon during its passage through the vascular channels to the lesion. If the stent catches on structures as the stent/balloon is being advanced, the stent is displaced proximally on the balloon catheter. This prevents delivery to the lesion and creates a problem in getting the stent out of the vessel and body, but usually does not result in an errant, free-floating stent. If the stent catches on structures during the withdrawal of the balloon/stent/catheter, the stent is displaced onto the wire distal to the balloon. Without sophisticated and difficult retrieval techniques, this results in a stent potentially free floating in the circulation! At present, a long-sheath technique is recommended and is always used for the delivery of hand-mounted stents.

The equipment and techniques for the delivery of all of the available large diameter, hand-mounted stents to the proximal pulmonary arteries, to the central systemic veins, and to the large systemic arteries are almost identical, although the delivery to the pulmonary arteries is usually more complex and difficult. The similarities in the equipment, and the general techniques for the delivery and implant used for all of the stents currently available for the larger vessels are described in this chapter. The delivery and implant of the rigid Palmaz™ P _ _ 8 and P _ _ 10 stents are the most difficult and dangerous. Familiarity with the techniques for delivering those stents should make the delivery of most other stents relatively straightforward. The availability of pre-mounted large stents on appropriate sized balloons may change these techniques dramatically within the next few years.

The peculiarities and particular difficulties with the delivery of stents to specific locations in specific vessels are discussed in Chapters 23, 24 and 25, which cover the use of intravascular stents in pulmonary arteries, systemic veins and systemic arteries, respectively. Peculiarities in the general delivery of the newer, more recently available stents are discussed at the end of this section on technique.

General technique for stent delivery

Most intravascular stent implants in congenital heart patients can be performed with well controlled, deep sedation and liberal local anesthesia. However, since the procedures can be very long, which becomes uncomfortable for the patient, general anesthesia often is used electively. General anesthesia becomes essential when the implant of a stent or even part of the procedure is performed from the neck, when it is known that the procedure definitely will be of a very long duration, or when the patient needs endotracheal intubation for some other reason. General anesthesia has the advantage of another physician besides the catheterizing physician monitoring the patient and having some responsibility for the patient's degree of sedation and the control of the patient's airway.

With the use of either sedation alone, or when general anesthesia is used, the patient requires a secure intravenous line for the administration of supplemental sedation and other medications during the procedure. Often, *just before* the actual expansion of the stent for implant and even though the patient appears sound asleep, the patient is given a supplemental dose of sedation/anesthesia in order to ensure that the patient remains absolutely still at the moment of implant.

All patients undergoing stent implant have an *indwelling* arterial line in place during the entire procedure. This line allows *instantaneous and continuous* monitoring of systemic blood pressure and the obtaining of necessary blood gases throughout the procedure. It always is better to anticipate and, in turn, to prevent problems with the patient than to try to compensate for a catastrophe once it has occurred. A subtle change in the continuously displayed intravascular blood pressure which is on a monitor provides an *early* indicator of impending trouble, while the periodically displayed pressure from a "cycling" arm blood pressure cuff recorder may well appear long after the adverse event begins.

Every patient undergoing a stent implant has an indwelling bladder catheter (Foley™) placed at the beginning of the procedure. No amount of sedation or analgesia compensates for the discomfort of an over-distended urinary bladder during a long procedure—particularly if it is unexpectedly long!

In a patient undergoing stent implant in the pulmonary arteries or systemic venous systems, one *extra* venous *catheter* is introduced into the venous system *in addition to* the venous line(s) which will be necessary for the delivery of the stent(s), in order to have an *extra* catheter in the venous system *in addition to* the number of catheters through which stents will be delivered. Thus, in a patient in whom two stents are to be implanted simultaneously, *three* venous catheters are introduced. A separate line is used for each individual stent delivery, while *the additional venous line* is used to perform *precise selective* angiograms pre, during, and immediately after the expansion of and implant of the stent. The additional, angiographic catheter is positioned in the same vessel, close in proximity and proximally in the flow of blood to the stenosis/stent implant area.

Some operators advocate performing the "placement" angiograms during the stent implant through the long delivery sheath after the sheath has been withdrawn off the stent/balloon combination and back into the more proximal vessel. This technique is of no use during the positioning of the stent/balloon combination before it is completely out of the delivery sheath (and no longer retrievable). Often the details of the anatomy from angiograms with injections through the sheath are *not* suitable. The shaft of the balloon catheter fills and compromises most of the lumen of the sheath and the pressure of the injection through the side port of the sheath is limited by the loose "seal" of the back-bleed valve of the sheath over the shaft of the catheter. As a consequence, a sufficient amount of contrast cannot be delivered rapidly enough with a high enough pressure to visualize the stenosis–stent relationships *accurately*.

In addition, in order to perform the angiogram through the sheath during the stent implant, the sheath must be withdrawn *completely off* the *balloon* and not just off the stent. Once the sheath is completely off the balloon/stent, further readjustment of the stent/balloon position is more difficult. In addition, this places the distal tip of the sheath very proximal to both the stent *and the area of stenosis* in the vessel. As the contrast is injected relatively slowly through the sheath and into the more proximal vessel, the contrast is diluted by adjacent, rapidly flowing blood, preventing an adequate visualization of the area of interest. Also when the sheath tip is far proximal to the area of stenosis, the tip is often proximal to a bifurcation or a large branching vessel, in which case, the majority of the small quantity of slowly injected contrast is diverted into the branch vessel and away from the stenotic area. Poor angiographic imaging is more "the rule" than the exception with the "through-the-sheath" technique and, as a consequence, this technique is not recommended. Inadequate angiograms compromise the precise positioning of the balloon/stent.

The implant of stents into smaller, more peripheral veins is the one exception where through-the-sheath angiograms can be useful. In this circumstance the vessel is small, the sheath is "upstream" in the flow of blood, the blood (and contrast) flow is slow and the injection is into a very confined channel that is being stented. Occasionally, however, when the implant of a venous stent is "retrograde" in the vein (e.g. a stent delivered into a femoral vein from the jugular approach) the end of the sheath is "downstream" in the *flow* from the lesion, with the result that the contrast injected through the sheath flows *away* from the lesion/stent and is of no value.

The area(s) to be stented is(are) identified and quantitated both hemodynamically from the pressure measurements and angiographically with *selective* angiograms *into the precise vessel/area* to be stented. The techniques for *accurate*, quantitative measurement are described in detail in Chapter 11 and definitely should be adhered to for the implant of intravascular stents. After identifying and measuring the stenosed area(s) of the involved vessel(s) very accurately, an end-hole catheter is advanced from the access site, across *and well beyond* the area of obstruction. It is extremely important that the vessel that is entered *distal* to the obstruction is of a large diameter *and* is the longest distal branch or tributary beyond the stenosis. This vessel must be *long enough* to allow the very distal placement of the tip of the supporting guide wire and of a *large enough diameter* to accommodate the distal end of the *fully* inflated balloon which will be used to deliver and implant the stent. When the balloon and stent are centered on the stenotic lesion during the stent expansion, the distal end of the implanting balloon will always extend well beyond the lesion and into the distal vessel. Considerable extra time is often required to enter this largest, distal vessel. The extra time spent in locating and achieving a good position in this largest vessel with the end-hole catheter is essential.

Once the catheter has been manipulated far into the largest distal vessel, it is replaced with a Super Stiff™ exchange length guide wire. If a long "floppy-tipped" Super Stiff™ wire is used, the vessel must be very long (and large enough in diameter) to accommodate the entire curled up ("balled-up") long floppy portion of the wire. It is imperative that the *entire*, long floppy tip, *along with the transition zone* of the wire and a significant portion of the extra stiff portion of the wire all extend a significant distance beyond the lesion. The balloon and stent are supported only by the very stiff portion of the wire and by a wire that is in a very secure distal position without the capability of any to-and-fro movement. The precise wire position contributes significantly to the ultimate success and safety of the procedure. All the extra time required in positioning the wire securely and very distally adds to the likely success of the procedure, while any compromised location of the wire is inviting a catastrophe.

Over-dilation and tearing of a smaller branch vessel that is just distal to the stenosis, is one of the greatest hazards during the implant of intravascular stents. It usually is a consequence of the wire and tip of the balloon being malpositioned prior to the stent implant. When the balloon tip is positioned and fixed in, and then inflated in, an erroneous and unusually small vessel that is just distal to the lesion, either it will rupture the vessel or the balloon will be "milked" back out of the vessel during the inflation and, in turn, the stent will be displaced proximally.

When there is a question about the size and configuration of the particular anatomy in the area of the stenosis and, in particular, a question about the adequacy of the vessel distal to the stenosis, the anatomy is defined precisely with a low-pressure, "sizing" balloon. This is ***not*** a pre-dilation of the area but rather, a "zero-pressure" inflation with a very low-pressure *sizing* balloon in the area to determine the *contour* of the entire area! The most satisfactory balloon for this sizing is the NuMED™ low-pressure "angioplasty" ("sizing") balloon (NuMED Inc., Hopkinton, NY), although any angioplasty type balloon can be used for the sizing if it is inflated only at very low pressure. The sizing balloon is advanced over the pre-positioned stiff guide wire and positioned exactly in the area of stenosis where the balloon/stent is to be inflated. The sizing balloon is inflated at a *very low (zero!)* pressure. The balloon at this "zero" inflation pressure fills, and *conforms to*, the exact anatomy of the stenosis and vessel(s) both proximal and distal to the lesion without dilating the area at all. This technique is useful particularly to determine if there is sufficient diameter distal to the stenosis to accommodate the distal tip of the balloon during inflation of the balloon for the stent implant. If the vessel distally is too small, the zero pressure "sizing" balloon either does not inflate in the area or it gently "milks" back out of the vessel. The only disadvantage of this particular low-pressure sizing balloon is that it requires a 9-French introductory sheath, but at least this size will usually be required for the delivery of the stent.

As long as the stenosis is more than 3 to 4 mm in diameter, pre-dilation of stenotic lesions before implanting a stent is ***not*** performed. Only very tight stenoses, which are too tight to allow a large, long delivery sheath for the delivery of the stent to pass through the lesion, are pre-dilated routinely. When pre-dilation is performed, the stenosis is pre-dilated *only* enough to allow the particular delivery sheath to pass through the stenotic area. When the vessel adjacent to the stenosis (either proximal or distal to the obstruction) is significantly larger than the proposed initial delivery balloon for the stent, pre-dilation *unequivocally should* ***not*** be performed. A "successful" pre-dilation of a stenotic area temporarily will dilate the area *acutely*, but it also temporarily makes the area of the stenosis very compliant and even "patulous". When a stent is implanted in this patulous or "softened" area, the stent does not fix securely to the now elastic walls, even when it is fully expanded and is in the proper position. As a consequence, the stent/balloon can be displaced very easily either during the balloon inflation or, even more likely, during the attempted removal of the balloon from within the lumen of the stent after the implant. Any movement of the stent immediately after implant usually results in migration of the stent to a non-stenosed area of the vessel or, even worse, results in a stent "free floating" in a vessel/chamber.

The main argument *in favor of* pre-dilation of a lesion in which a stent is going to be implanted, is to ensure that the balloon/stent combination *can* open the lesion sufficiently during the implant/expansion of the stent to allow removal of the balloon from the stent after implant. The inability to dilate the lesion during the implant of the balloon/stent combination can leave not only the original vessel stenosis, but also a stent with the same stenosis in it. The presence of the stent on the balloon does ***not*** add any *additional dilating* force or dilating capability in addition to that of the balloon alone. The expanded intravascular stent only *maintains* the degree of dilation that is achieved acutely by the particular *balloon*. When a significant residual stenosis persists in the stent/vessel after a stent is implanted with a usual "standard-pressure" balloon, the original implanting balloon is replaced with a high-pressure balloon and the dilation of the stent/vessel repeated. Very few (no!) residual stenoses do not respond to a balloon dilation when a *non-compliant*, high-pressure balloon is used for the reinflation and the balloon is inflated to 20 to 25 atmospheres within a stent! This is true particularly when the attempt at re-dilation is six, or more, months after the original stent implant.

Pre-dilation of the area and the diameter of the pre-dilation constitute a judgment decision during each stent implant procedure. The decision is individualized in the catheterization laboratory as the anatomy is visualized and sized. When pre-dilation of the vessel *is* performed before a stent implant, there is one major "*rule*" for the pre-dilation. The pre-dilation of any stenotic lesion which precedes the implant of an intravascular stent should be only to a diameter that will accommodate the delivery sheath and which is *significantly smaller in diameter* (at least 3 mm smaller in diameter) than the diameter of the adjacent vessel or to the diameter to which the *stent* is to be expanded at its *initial* implant. In order to ensure fixation of the stent into some residual, more rigid tissues in the vessel wall, pre-dilation with a minimal diameter balloon ensures that the balloon that is used for the delivery of the stent can be larger and can expand the *stent* to a diameter which is definitely *larger* than the pre-dilated ("softened") stenotic area.

The pre-dilation is performed over the same Super-Stiff™ wire over which the long sheath/dilator eventually will be delivered. Once the wire is securely in place, a *standard* pressure dilation balloon is advanced over the wire to the obstruction. The pre-dilation balloon used is only 2–3 mm larger in diameter than the diameter of the *stenosis* in the vessel and is at least 3 mm *smaller* than the *adjacent* vessel, which should be the anticipated *implant diameter* of the stent. The pre-dilation documents at least some "give" to the stenosis in the vessel as well as opening the vessel to accommodate the large sheath for the stent delivery. After a pre-dilation is performed, the Super Stiff™ wire is maintained in its secure distal location, while the separate balloon used for the pre-dilation is withdrawn, leaving the wire in place across, and well beyond, the stenosis.

If a very tight area of stenosis cannot be pre-dilated *at all* with a *standard-pressure* balloon, a high-pressure balloon which is similar in *size* to the standard-pressure balloon is used over the same wire in a repeat attempt to pre-dilate the stenosis to the *minimal diameter* that will accommodate the delivery sheath. Pre-dilation with the high-pressure, but smaller, balloon ensures that if the standard, lower-pressure balloon for the delivery of the stent does not fully expand the area of stenosis, the area of stenosis will be expanded to at least the diameter of the high-pressure, pre-dilation balloon. This newly permitted increase in the diameter provides sufficient evidence to be certain that the implanting balloon can be *removed* from a partially expanded (but secured) stent without displacing the stent.

Long indwelling sheath stent delivery technique

A long sheath/dilator set which will accommodate the particular balloon/stent combination is advanced over the pre-positioned Super Stiff™ wire and past the area of stenosis which usually has *not* been pre-dilated. The tip of the *sheath* is positioned at least several *centimeters* distal to the area of obstruction in the vessel. The delivery of the sheath to the lesion and securing the sheath in position without creating kinks in the sheath, particularly to branch pulmonary artery lesions, often is the most difficult and challenging part of the entire procedure for the implant of an intravascular stent. Once the sheath and dilator are in position with the tip of the *sheath* well beyond the lesion, the Super Stiff™ wire in the distal vessel and the long sheath are fixed in place while the dilator is slowly and carefully withdrawn over the wire and out of the sheath. The sheath is allowed to *bleed back* from the side port on the back-bleed valve until it is clear of all air and possible clots—remembering that the large, long sheaths hold 10–15 ml of fluid (or air and/or clot!). Once *cleared* by "passive drainage", the sheath is flushed thoroughly by hand and then is attached to a *continuous* slow flush to prevent the development of clots in the large potential dead space within the sheath and around the wire. After any pre-dilation is accomplished and as soon as the delivery sheath is in position, if not administered earlier, the patient is administered systemic heparin in a dose of 100 mg/kilogram of body weight.

If a long sheath with an attached back-bleed valve/flush port or a separate back-bleed valve/flush port that which will accommodate the delivery catheter and fit on the long sheath is not available in the particular catheterization laboratory, the massive bleeding which would occur from the open sheath can be prevented with a "make-shift" solution. The bleeding through a non-valved sheath with a wire within it is stopped effectively (and temporarily) with a "rubber-shod" Kelly™ clamp placed across the sheath (containing the wire) just outside of the body where the sheath exits the skin. This prevents the massive blood loss around the wire and through the sheath after the dilator is removed from the sheath. Of equal importance, it prevents air from being sucked into the sheath during a deep inspiratory effort by the patient. The clamp on the sheath does not allow any acute or continuous flush of the sheath, and the clamp indents the sheath, but only in an area *outside of the body* where the clamp is applied. This indentation in the sheath does not interfere with the passage through that segment of the sheath that is outside of the body and can be straightened manually, nor with the eventual delivery of the stent. Of most importance, the "external" indentation does not involve any areas that are in tight curves or bends in the sheath in the course of the sheath to the target site.

When a separate, detachable back-bleed valve, which is not built onto the sheath, is used for a stent delivery on a large sheath with no built-in back-bleed valve, the balloon alone is passed through the detached, separate back-bleed valve and is slid back onto the shaft of the *balloon dilation catheter before* the stent is mounted on the balloon. In this way the stent mounted on the balloon does not have to be forced through the smaller diameter lumen of the removable, back-bleed valve. After the stent has been mounted on the balloon, the stent/balloon unit is introduced completely into the *non*-valved sheath, the pre-mounted back-bleed valve is advanced forward on the shaft of the catheter onto the proximal hub of the sheath, and attached to the hub. The clamp on the sheath is released, the sheath is allowed to bleed back thoroughly through the side port of the attached back-bleed valve, and then the side port is attached to the flush system.

The exact stent and balloon that are used depend upon the current, desired and eventual adult size of the vessel and the location of the lesion in the vessel. For ***all*** vessels, a stent *always* is used which eventually can be dilated to the ***eventual adult diameter*** of the particular area of the vessel. The length of the stent depends upon the length of the actual lesion, the expected shrinkage in the length of the stent with full expansion, the curvature of the vessel, and the distances within the vessel before any branching or bifurcations. The exact anatomy is defined angiographically or, when there is any question, by inflating the "sizing" angioplasty balloon in the precise area at a very low pressure.

In choosing the appropriate stent for a particular lesion, the operator must always consider the amount of shrinkage in the length of the stents with each increase in diameter of the stents. This is particularly important with the J & J™ Palmaz™ (Cordis Corp., Miami Lakes, FL) and Genesis XD™ stents (Johnson & Johnson–Cordis Corp., Miami Lakes, FL), which shrink as much as 50% when inflated to their largest diameters. Shrinkage in length to some degree must be considered with almost all stents. When a stent is to be expanded to 15 mm or larger in diameter, in order to account for the shrinkage, the stent used often must be longer in its collapsed state than the length of the vessel where it is to be implanted. This shrinkage in length makes it extremely important that the balloon and stent are positioned precisely over the exact lesion at the beginning of, and maintained in that position throughout, the expansion of the stent during its implant. With a stent properly and precisely placed on the delivery balloon, the shrinkage usually, *but not necessarily*, is symmetrical from both ends of the stent. As a consequence, most balloon/stent inflations should be slow and observed very carefully so that any asymmetric expansion or movement in the position of the stent relative to the anatomy can be adjusted before the stent is fully expanded and fixed securely in an abnormal position. The expected shrinkage of a stent occasionally is used to the operator's advantage, utilizing the further decrease in length with further expansion of a stent to move the ends of the stent away from crossing or branching vessels. The use of a BIB™ balloon (NuMED Inc., Hopkinton, NY) is helpful in order to allow some purposeful adjustment for an asymmetrical inflation or shrinkage after the stent has been expanded to only half of its final diameter.

The balloon is chosen specifically for the stent that is being used and the diameters adjacent to the area of implant while the exact *stent is chosen* for the particular anatomy of the lesion as well as the diameters of the immediately adjacent vessels. To prepare the balloon for the stent, the balloon lumen is attached to the inflation device and the balloon is inflated partially, but not to a high pressure. The balloon is cleared of air by repeated partial inflations/deflations while holding the balloon in a vertical position with the *tip of the balloon facing down*. Once the balloon is cleared of air, the balloon is deflated slowly while simultaneously refolding the balloon manually around the shaft of the catheter. Once the balloon is refolded as smoothly as possible, the balloon is maintained on "negative pressure" by withdrawing the plunger of the inflation device and locking it in the fully withdrawn position. The appearance of a continual stream of tiny bubbles after applying negative pressure to the balloon with an inflation device indicates a leak in the balloon or the inflation system. The source of any leak is identified and eliminated before proceeding, even if it requires replacing the balloon or the inflation device.

There are some special preparations for the BIB™ balloons. Each BIB™ balloon catheter has three lumens: one lumen (with a blue hub) to the inner balloon, one lumen (with a white hub) to the outer balloon, and a central catheter lumen of the catheter itself (with a green hub). In the original BIB™ balloons, where the central lumen passed through the area of the balloons and before it passed out through the tip of the catheter, the tubing of the central lumen was very narrow and thin walled. This narrow tubing allowed the collapsed balloons to compress to a diameter only slightly larger than the diameter of the catheter shaft, but did not provide much longitudinal support in that area when there was no wire in this lumen. To compensate for this during the preparation of the balloons, each balloon catheter comes with a blunt, solid metal, 0.035″ stylus. This metal stylus is inserted into the distal end of the catheter lumen during balloon preparation and while the stent is being crimped on the balloon. The stylus passes through the area of the balloon(s) and back into the shaft of the catheter well proximal to the balloons and, in this position, keeps that area of the catheter and the balloons very straight and elongated.

For preparation of BIB™ balloons, both balloon lumens are connected to manometered inflation devices. The inner balloon is inflated and cleared of air and then the outer balloon is inflated and cleared separately. Once the balloons have been prepared, cleared of all air and rewrapped around the catheter, the balloon lumens are opened to *neutral* pressure and the stylus is removed. The stent is passed over the refolded balloons, the stylus is reinserted, and both balloons are again placed on negative pressure. Since the stent over the balloons covers the radio-opaque "markers" on the catheter within the balloons, the BIB balloons with the stent mounted are viewed under fluoroscopy in order to align the stent precisely and evenly within the marks within the balloons. The stent then is compressed (crimped) over the balloons by hand exactly as with any other stent–balloon combination. The stylus remains in the catheter during the "crimping" and until just before introduction over the delivery wire.

Any balloons that have a Silicon™ or other "slippery" coating also require "pre-preparation" before a stent is mounted on them. The balloon is inflated until it is tense and then the "slippery" coating is rubbed off the balloon surface very vigorously with a dampened, 4 × 4 gauze sponge. Once it is "rubbed clean" the balloon is manually rewrapped over the catheter as it is deflated. When the balloon has been cleared of air, the balloon is placed on negative pressure and simultaneously is rotated and "refolded" onto the shaft of the catheter in order to collapse the balloon maximally onto the catheter shaft. Some slight "irregularities" on the surface of refolded balloons actually are desirable when using balloons for the delivery of stents. The irregular surface of the balloon helps to keep the stent, which is hand-crimped on the balloon, from sliding on the balloon during its passage through the sheath. Before the stent is advanced over any balloon for mounting on the balloon, the stent and surface of the balloon are both coated with undiluted contrast solution. As the contrast dries, it becomes very sticky and serves as a "glue" that will help to hold the stent on the balloon.

To prepare the stent for mounting on the delivery balloon, the entire length of the stent is dilated sufficiently to allow the stent to pass easily over the balloon, and one end of the stent is flared even wider by inserting the tip of a large dilator (the dilator from the delivery sheath) into one end of, and advancing it through the length of, the stent. As the dilator is withdrawn from the end of the stent, the dilator is angled slightly and rotated around within the proximal tip of the stent, which, in turn, "flares" or makes a "funnel-like" opening in one end of the stent. When much larger delivery balloons are used, the entire stent is dilated even further before introducing the stent by gently advancing an even larger dilator into, and through, the stent. The dilation and flaring of the stent facilitate advancing the stent over the balloon and help to prevent the ends of the stent from catching on the folds of the balloon. With the Palmaz™ J & J™ stents, this is essential to prevent the puncture of the balloon by a sharp tip at the end of the stent.

With negative pressure applied to the balloon lumen, the tip of the balloon catheter is introduced carefully into the flared end of the stent and while the stent is *allowed to rotate* slowly and very slightly (less than 360°) to correspond to the direction of the folds of the balloon, the balloon is advanced very gently into the stent. The catheter and balloon always should slide *freely* into the stent. The introduction of the stent over the balloon is performed very gently and slowly to prevent a sharp tip at the end of a stent from digging into, and puncturing, the balloon during the mounting process. Particular care is necessary with the J & J™ Palmaz™ stents (Johnson & Johnson, Warren, NJ) which all have multiple sharp tips at each end. If the stent catches on the balloon at all, the stent is withdrawn, the balloon is re-formed or the stent dilated/flared further. The stent is advanced over the balloon until it is positioned over the *exact center* of the length of the balloon. The stent is centered lengthwise as precisely as possible by aligning the ends of the stent with, or equally between, the metal markers on the shaft of the catheter beneath the balloon material. When there is any question about the exact positioning of the stent on the balloon, the stent/balloon should be visualized under fluoroscopy.

Once the stent is centered exactly on the balloon, the metal stylet of the BIB™ balloons is introduced into the distal end of the catheter lumen of the balloon catheter and pushed far enough into the distal end of the catheter lumen of the balloon catheter to be entirely proximal to the balloon. This stylet within the lumen supports the lumen of the catheter during the subsequent forceful compression of the stent over the balloon. Strong negative pressure is maintained on the balloon lumen while the connecting tubing and the inflator are inspected carefully for any balloon leaks. A new puncture or leak is indicated by a continual stream of small bubbles flowing into the tubing or the inflator as the negative pressure is applied.

Once assured that there are no leaks, the stent is compressed (crimped) uniformly on the balloon by manual finger compression. There are no "crimping tools" available that are applicable universally for the large variety of stents, balloon sizes, and balloon types or for the different diameters of the catheter shafts of the different large balloon dilation catheters used for the large variety of congenital lesions. As a consequence, the crimping of all non-pre-mounted stents is performed by hand. Several more drops of contrast are placed on the surface of the stent before the manual crimping on the balloon is started.

Starting with *light* finger pressure, finger pressure is gradually increased while moving the fingers over the entire length and around the circumference of the stent. The circumference of the stent is squeezed onto the balloon as the stent/balloon is rolled between the fingers. Once the stent is relatively smooth and secure on the balloon, then the fingers are squeezed *as tightly as possible* and *repeatedly* over the entire surface of the stent/balloon as the combination is rotated between the fingers. The process is repeated using the tips of the fingernails to compress the individual longitudinal struts forcefully between the circumferential "bands" of the stent. This fingernail compression creates a slightly irregular surface on the mounted stent, which, in turn, helps to secure the stent on the balloon, but does not affect the eventual stent expansion or strength.

The short length of plastic tubing which is present over the balloon in its sterile package is occasionally used as a "smoothing" tool over the stent once it is mounted on the balloon. When the stent has been compressed over the balloon, the plastic tube is advanced over the combination of the balloon/stent. The tube over the stent/balloon is compressed manually between the fingers as tightly as possible while the tube, stent, and balloon are rotated between the fingers. However, this step usually is not necessary and does not crimp the stent as tightly as direct finger compression on the stent.

Once the stent is compressed securely on the balloon, several more drops of undiluted contrast solution or albumin solution are spread on the surface of the balloon–stent combination. The additional contrast is allowed to dry briefly on the surface of the balloon–stent. This serves as additional "glue" to help retain the stent on the balloon and keep it from "sliding" on the balloon during delivery through the sheath. The contrast "glue" works most effectively if it is allowed to dry for 15–20 minutes.

Stent delivery over a wire and through a pre-positioned sheath

The delivery of the stent/balloon combination to the lesion, over a pre-positioned stiff wire and through a pre-positioned long sheath, is the original and established technique for the delivery of stents to the various congenital lesions. This technique is the most tested and reliable technique available for the delivery of the current stents. With the sheath and wire fixed in their position beyond the area of obstruction, the balloon catheter with the mounted stent is introduced over the proximal end of the wire and advanced to the valve of the sheath. The introduction of the balloon with the mounted stent into and through the valved sheath depends on the length and type of stent. The J & J™ Palmaz™ stents, which are longer than 3 cm, can be pushed directly through the back-bleed valve by gripping the most *proximal* end of the stent very tightly with the tips of the fingers. As the proximal tip of the stent is squeezed tightly and continuously in order to maintain the stent in *its exact* position on the balloon, the entire length of the stent is advanced through the valve of the sheath, and the combination stent/balloon is advanced into, and all of the way through, the attached back-bleed valve chamber and into the sheath. There is a small "flare" at the proximal end of the sheath within the distal end of the back-bleed valve housing (chamber) where the back-bleed apparatus is attached to the sheath (Figure 22.7). This flare of the sheath creates a flange or "ridge" within the back-bleed valve chamber between the distal end of the valve housing and the proximal end of the sheath within the valve "chamber". This ridge is not visible from outside of the back-bleed housing, but can catch the distal end of the stent and block the passage of the mounted stent from passing into the lumen of the sheath from the back-bleed valve chamber. Longer stents can be held securely at the *proximal* end of the stent with the tips of the fingers and supported on the balloon as the stent is advanced *all of the way through* the "valve" and *past* this ridge.

The shorter P 108, 188, and 204 stents are too short to maintain a grip with the fingers on the proximal end of the stent as it is advanced *all* of the way through the back-bleed valve and *past the flange*. When introducing the shorter stents is attempted by just holding the stent with the fingers, the stent is easily displaced proximally off of the balloon as the proximal end of the stent passes

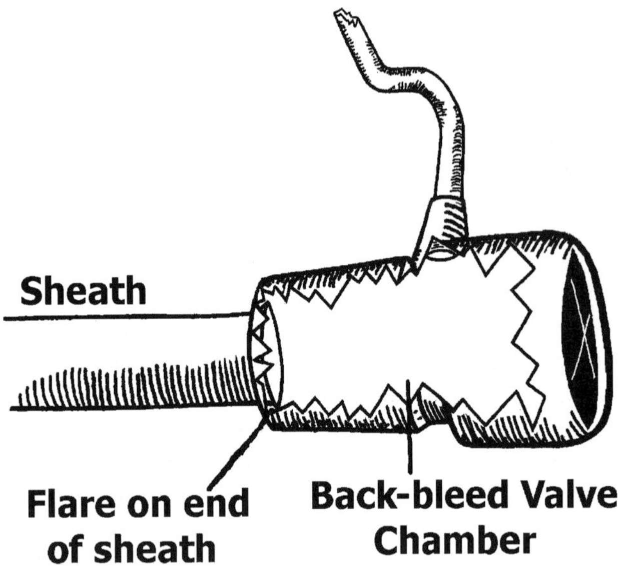

Figure 22.7 Flange (or flare) on proximal end of sheath within the back-bleed valve chamber.

through the valve beyond the grasp of the fingers. This is overcome by using the short "metal introducing tube" supplied by J & J™ (Johnson & Johnson, Warren, NJ), or a short, cut-off length of sheath as an introducing sleeve (*see* Figure 22.1). The short length of "introducer" sheath should be the same diameter as the delivery sheath, made from a fairly stiff sheath material and approximately five centimeters long. The *proximal*, cut, end of the short segment of sheath can be dilated with a forceps to flare the end slightly. The balloon with the mounted stent is introduced very carefully into the flared end of this sleeve until the stent is completely within the sleeve. The sleeve along with the contained balloon/stent are all held together and are passed through the back-bleed valve and into the long sheath until the *sleeve* seats on the flange between the valve apparatus and the proximal end of the sheath (*see* Figure 22.1). The balloon, stent, and catheter are advanced out of the sleeve and into the shaft of the long sheath. The sleeve is withdrawn out of the valve and back to the hub on the shaft of the balloon catheter. The introduction of the stent/balloon through the short sleeve can be used for the P 308 stents, and may make their introduction through the valve more secure. The short sleeve should definitely be used with all of the open-cell stents (ev3, Plymouth, MN). The pattern and the "looseness" of the cells of the open-cell stents cause them to catch on the back-bleed valve itself and cause the cells to pull apart if they are pushed directly through a back-bleed valve.

When a long sheath *with a separate and non-attached* back-bleed valve/flush port is the only long sheath available, the *balloon* and the balloon catheter are passed through the removable back-bleed valve/flush port separately before the stent is mounted as described previously. The balloon with the mounted stent is introduced into the open end of the stent and the back-bleed valve, which is on the more proximal shaft of the catheter, is pushed forward on the shaft of the catheter and attached to the large sheath with a continuous flush delivered to the pre-mounted back-bleed valve. The remainder of the stent delivery then becomes identical to the delivery through a long sheath with a built-in attached back-bleed valve.

Once the *proximal* end of the stent/balloon combination has been introduced and advanced several centimeters beyond the valve and hub of the sheath, the balloon is inflated very gently (~1 atmosphere) with the inflator and the inflator is locked to maintain this pressure in the balloon. This minimal pressure to the balloon expands the exposed shoulders of the balloon, which extend beyond each end of the stent, very slightly, without expanding the stent at all. This is particularly useful when the balloon is the same length or slightly longer than the stent. The slightly expanded balloon and the "exposed" shoulders of the balloon help to keep the stent from sliding proximally on the balloon as it is advanced through the sheath. Unless the balloon is inflated too vigorously, this still allows the balloon to pass easily through the sheath. If the balloon/stent does not move easily within the straight area of the sheath, the balloon has been inflated with too much pressure, and some of the pressure on the inflator should be released. This slight inflation of the ends of the balloon is important, particularly where there is a very tortuous course of the delivery sheath through tight bends in the vascular system.

While frequently observing the balloon/stent combination within the sheath as well as the position of the tip of the wire and sheath and the course of the wire and sheath on fluoroscopy, the balloon catheter with the mounted stent is advanced over the wire within the sheath to the involved narrowing in the vessel. As long as the wire and sheath are maintained securely in place, advancing the balloon and stent is usually accomplished quite easily. It is important to repeatedly observe the *entire course of the sheath* as well as the tip of the sheath and wire while the catheter and the balloon/stent are being advanced within the sheath. Occasionally, the "circumference" of a long curve *in the course of the sheath/wire* as it passes through the heart is *widened* as the balloon, stent, and catheter are pushed against the outer circumference of any curve in the sheath while it is passing through a dilated chamber or vessel within the heart. As the balloon, stent, and catheter push on and increase the curvature of the sheath, the *distance* along the wire from the skin entry site to the lesion lengthens. If the increasing circumference of this curve in the sheath/wire and, in turn, the actual length of the distance to the lesion are not noticed and not *compensated for* by advancing the *sheath and wire* along with the catheter at the skin, the *tip* of the sheath and the wire will be withdrawn out of their secure positions distal to the lesion. As soon as this "widening of the circumference" of the curve begins to occur, instead of the sheath and wire remaining firmly fixed outside of the body, the sheath and wire outside of the body are advanced along with the balloon/stent/catheter just enough to compensate for the increased length being caused by the large curvature within the heart.

Once the stent and balloon have been advanced through the sheath to the area of the lesion, the *stent* (on the balloon) is centered exactly at the area of maximal narrowing. The slight pressure in the balloon lumen is released and the balloon deflated completely *before* the sheath is withdrawn off the stent/balloon. With the stent/balloon still within the sheath and with the guide wire still buried far out into the lung parenchyma, the *wire, catheter, and balloon/stent* are fixed in this location while the sheath alone is carefully withdrawn off the balloon/stent/catheter/wire combination. This uncovers the stent on the balloon over the wire centered in the proper location in the area of narrowing.

After withdrawing the sheath, it is important to repeat a selective angiogram through the separate venous catheter either within, or *just* proximal to, the lesion in order to verify the exact positioning of the stent in the stenosis. Because of the stiffness of the wire, the catheter and the sheath, often there is distortion of the vessel and a change in the curvature and position of the wire/balloon/stent combination relative to the stenosis or to relatively fixed landmarks in the thorax after the sheath has been withdrawn. This can displace the stent/balloon away from the exact central area of stenosis compared to the location before the wire was introduced. The repeat selective angiocardiogram identifies any changes in relative positions and allows the stent/balloon to be readjusted into the precise area of narrowing. Repositioning of the stent/balloon/catheter in the area is similar to the repositioning of a balloon/catheter for angioplasty. The stent, balloon, and catheter are advanced over the fixed wire to advance the stent further into the lesion, but in order *to withdraw the stent/balloon/catheter*, the *wire alone* is pushed forward forcefully. As the wire advances, it pushes the stent/balloon/catheter backwards while, at the same time, keeping the wire forced forward into the distal location in a very secure position.

During the passage of the balloon/stent/catheter through the sheath, occasionally the stent slips on the balloon and is displaced proximally on the balloon. If this displacement is less than 1–2 mm and the stent is still *completely over the balloon*, it usually is of little or no consequence. However, the balloon and stent positions should be inspected *very carefully* while the balloon and stent are *still within the sheath* and *before the sheath is withdrawn*. If the *stent* is displaced more proximally *on the balloon*, the stent still may be in its proper position within the lesion, but the distal end of the *balloon*, off of which the stent is displaced, will be positioned further into the distal vessel and away from the narrowing. A distal positioning of the balloon usually results in the balloon/stent combination milking backwards before the stent even begins to expand during the initial balloon inflation. This results in the stent's being displaced and implanted in an improper location. If the "extra distal balloon" extends into a small distal vessel and the distally displaced balloon does not milk back out of the vessel, the expansion of the balloon can result in rupture of the small vessel.

If the stent is displaced more than 1–2 mm on the balloon, and certainly if the stent extends completely off the balloon at all while the stent and balloon are still within the sheath, the implant procedure is abandoned temporarily and the sheath is ***not*** withdrawn off the balloon/stent combination. With the balloon/stent still within the sheath and with the stent now positioned over only the proximal end of the balloon, the balloon again is inflated very slightly. This inflates only the distal end of the balloon and creates a larger "shoulder" of balloon *distal* to the stent. The entire catheter/balloon/stent is withdrawn through the sheath, over the wire, and out of the body. The larger "shoulder" of the balloon, which is now completely distal to the displaced stent, helps to keep the stent from sliding distally off the balloon as the combination is withdrawn through, and out of, the sheath. Even with the "distal shoulder" on the balloon the stent often catches at the valve of the sheath and is retained in the valve chamber of the sheath after the balloon has been withdrawn. Usually, the very end of the stent is visible just within the valve and still over the wire. When the end of the stent is visible just within the valve, a tip of the visible end of the stent is grasped with a small forceps and pulled out through the valve.

If the stent cannot be retrieved from within the sheath/valve, the entire sheath must be withdrawn over the wire. Once the sheath is completely out of the body and off the wire, the stent is pushed forward, through and out of the distal end of the sheath with a dilator or balloon catheter. Once the stent is retrieved from the withdrawn sheath, the dilator is replaced in the sheath and the sheath/dilator is re-advanced over the wire into the vessel and to the lesion. If the sheath is damaged *at all*, a new sheath/dilator set is used.

Unless it was damaged in the removal process, the retrieved stent is re-mounted on the same or a new balloon. When re-mounted, the stent is positioned 1–2 mm *forward* (distally) of the center of the balloon. This leaves the stent mounted slightly more *distally on the* balloon with more "shoulder" exposed "behind" and more proximal to the stent toward the shaft of the catheter. The balloon catheter with the re-mounted stent is reintroduced over the wire, into and through the back-bleed valve of the sheath, and advanced several centimeters into the sheath. The balloon is again inflated minimally (with approximately one atmosphere of pressure). The "forward" positioning of the stent on the balloon allows more of the proximal "shoulder" of the balloon to *expand slightly* behind the stent, which, in turn, helps to prevent the stent from sliding backward as the balloon/stent is advanced through the sheath. Once the balloon/stent has been advanced to the proper position as verified fluoroscopically, the balloon again is deflated before the sheath is withdrawn off the balloon/stent.

Very rarely, as the sheath is being withdrawn off of the stent/balloon, the stent again slides backward (proximally) on the balloon along with the sheath or, inadvertently, the stent/balloon is exposed with the stent already displaced proximally on the balloon. In this circumstance, after the sheath is completely off the *stent* but still partially over the proximal balloon, the sheath is gently readvanced over the balloon. Usually, the edge of the distal end of the sheath catches on the proximal end of the stent and does not allow the stent to be withdrawn back into the sheath. By continuing to advance the sheath forward *very gently*, the stent can be pushed forward, and often can be positioned back onto the proper location on the balloon! This maneuver must be performed very gently and carefully with no excessive force. If the stent does not move forward easily, it suggests that the sharp distal ends of the stent struts are caught on the balloon. Any excessive force applied to the sheath can push one of the sharp tips of the end of the stent *into* the wall of the balloon and puncture the balloon. This is a particular problem with the J & J™ Palmaz™ stents with the very sharp tips at both ends. Fortunately, even the Palmaz™ stents and all of the other stents can usually be re-advanced over the balloon quite safely by using this maneuver with the tip of the sheath.

The sheath is withdrawn off the proximal end of the balloon but no further. The sheath positioned in close proximity to the balloon helps to support the shaft of the balloon catheter during the implant. Once the stent is in the exact, proper position in the stenosis and its correct position on the balloon has been verified, the balloon is inflated slowly to its maximum advertised pressure and hopefully to the maximum diameter of the balloon. During the inflation the stent is observed continuously *and recorded* on biplane angiography or biplane stored fluoroscopy. The inflation of the balloon expands the stent into the stenosed area of the vessel to the diameter of the implanting balloon. If there is even the suggestion of stent displacement during the initial slow inflation, the inflation is stopped and the stent/balloon repositioned correctly within the stenosis using manipulations of the catheter, wire or sheath. Once the stent is expanded fully or the balloon has reached its maximum pressure, the balloon is deflated rapidly. Often, there is some waist or incomplete expansion of the stent with the first inflation of the balloon; however, with accurate prior sizing and positioning, the stent will be centered on the lesion and fixed securely in the vessel. The deflated balloon is repositioned over the wire very slightly forward or backward and the inflation is repeated several times to achieve maximal expansion of the entire length of the stent with the particular balloon.

After implanting the stent securely in the area of stenosis and while the balloon is still within the stent, the stent position and fixation are confirmed with a repeat angiogram through the adjacent catheter. With the balloon still positioned within the stent, the balloon is reinflated at a low pressure. Then, simultaneously, as the balloon is being deflated slowly and with the balloon still within the stent, the long delivery sheath is re-advanced gently and gradually over the balloon and into the stent as the balloon deflates within the stent[10]. The inflated balloon within the stent *centers* the proximal shaft of the balloon catheter *and the advancing edges of the tip of the sheath* within the lumen of the stent. This "centering" keeps the edge of the distal end of the sheath from catching on the proximal end of the stent as the sheath is reintroduced into and through the stent. Often, as the sheath tip is pushed against the balloon and as the balloon is deflating, the balloon and the following tip of the sheath slide forward together and through the stent before the balloon deflates completely. This still accomplishes the goal of the sheath advancing completely through the stent without catching on, or dislodging, the stent.

Once the sheath is in or completely through the stent, the balloon is deflated completely by applying negative pressure to the balloon lumen. When the balloon has been deflated completely, the negative pressure *is released* from the inflating syringe. The balloon is withdrawn over the wire and into the sheath with the balloon lumen on "neutral" pressure while the balloon catheter is rotated very slightly in the direction of the balloon folds (determined earlier while preparing the balloon), and it is withdrawn into the sheath. The release of the strong negative pressure "softens" the folds or "wings" on the deflated balloon. When the sheath can be repositioned and maintained in its position *through* the stent, the sheath allows the balloon to be withdrawn through the stent while the stent walls are "protected" completely by the sheath from any rough folds or "wings" on the deflated balloon as the balloon is withdrawn. With the long sheath through the stent, a catheter or a new, larger or different balloon can easily be advanced reliably and safely through, or into, the newly implanted stent without danger of dislodging the stent.

This balloon-assisted procedure for re-entering the stent is extremely valuable in even the most straightforward stent implant procedures but it is particularly important when there are any curves in the vessel immediately proximal to the area of the stent[10]. The greater the angle or curvature of the vessel entering the stent, the more essential the balloon-assisted re-entry technique becomes. The stiff guide wire through the stent tends to "remain straight" and to orient itself tangentially across a curved vessel (and stent). This consistently forces the wire, catheter, and sheath against one edge of the proximal end of the stent, which, in turn, prevents even a finely tapered dilator or catheter from entering the stent after its implant. The balloon-assisted procedure for re-entering the stent with the sheath is now the standard technique used after essentially every stent implant.

Once the deflated balloon has been withdrawn from the stent, preferably through the sheath with the wire and sheath remaining through the stent, the balloon catheter is withdrawn from the vessel and out of the body through the sheath. The necessity for further dilation or for placing additional stents is determined from pressure measurements and repeat angiography while the sheath is still passing through the stent. With the sheath in place within the stent, any subsequent steps in the procedure are far more straightforward. If a partially inflated stent is fixed in the vessel and the vessel and stent are still stenotic, the initial implanting balloon is replaced with a high-pressure balloon to further expand the stent and vessel together.

Occasionally the sheath cannot be re-advanced into the stent even over the actively "deflating" balloon, and on withdrawal of the balloon through the stent, the balloon catches on, and begins to dislodge, the stent. In this situation the sheath is re-advanced until the edge of the *distal end of the sheath* purposefully is pushed *against* the *proximal end of the stent* and purposefully caught against the stent. The sheath that could not be advanced *into* the stent is now caught on the end of the stent and is used to "buttress" the stent in its position in the vessel. With the sheath fixed in this position against the stent, the stent is held in place as the balloon is carefully withdrawn. Simultaneous *rotation of the balloon catheter* facilitates the withdrawal of the balloon out of the stent and into the sheath. It can be helpful to advance the balloon *beyond* the stent, reinflate the balloon at least partially, and then deflate the balloon while rotating the balloon catheter to help "refold" the balloon. Once refolded, the strong negative pressure is released from the balloon before attempting to withdraw the balloon from the stent.

If the sheath cannot be re-advanced into the stent while the balloon is deflating within the stent, but the balloon *can be* withdrawn out of the stent, the balloon is withdrawn out of the stent, through the sheath and out of the body. The long dilator is reintroduced into the sheath and an attempt can be made at reintroducing the combined sheath/dilator into and through the stent. Unfortunately, even with an apparent tight and smooth fit of the tip of the dilator over the wire and the tip of the sheath over the dilator, the tip of the dilator or sheath often catches on the proximal end of the stent and cannot be reintroduced into the stent without dislodging the freshly implanted stent. Occasionally the use of a new dilator, which is one size *larger* than the sheath (particularly the 11- and 12-French sheaths) and with a different curve formed on the tip of the dilator, will facilitate the sheath and dilator re-entering the stent. Advancing or slightly withdrawing the wire separately while simultaneously advancing the sheath/dilator, occasionally changes the angle of the wire as it enters the stent enough to allow the tip of the dilator and subsequently the sheath to enter the stent. However, remarkably, the very tiny interspace *between the wire and dilator or sheath and dilator* frequently is very effective at catching on the sharp, exposed end of the stent and totally prevents reintroduction of the sheath into the stent. This problem provides the rationale behind the reintroduction of the sheath into the stent *over the initial balloon* as it is being deflated within the stent whenever it is possible.

When the balloon cannot be withdrawn into the sheath once it has been withdrawn out of the stent, both the balloon and sheath are withdrawn from the body over the wire *with the wire still fixed securely through the stent into the vessel far distal to the lesion*. Even when the balloon cannot be completely withdrawn into the sheath, at least the partially refolded, proximal "shoulder" of the balloon usually can be withdrawn into the distal end of the sheath, which, in turn, "covers" the rough folds in the shoulder at the proximal end of the balloon and partially protects the vein and tissues as the combination sheath and balloon are withdrawn. This partial covering of the shoulder of the balloon allows the partially folded balloon to be withdrawn through the vein puncture site, subcutaneous tissues, and skin without causing significant vessel/tissue damage. Again, it is important to *release any negative pressure* from the collapsed balloon in order to "soften" the exposed folded edges or "wings" on the balloon.

Once the balloon and large sheath are out of the body and off the exchange wire, either a *new* long sheath or a *new* short sheath/dilator of the same diameter as the previous long sheath is introduced over the wire, into the vein. The *new, large* sheath prevents bleeding and is less traumatic to the vein for any subsequent catheter or balloon introductions. In the past, large balloons for subsequent or further dilations were introduced into the vein directly over the stiff exchange wire without a sheath. However, this is no longer recommended. The rough walls of a large "folded balloon" passing directly into the tissues and particularly on withdrawal from the vessel/tissues are significantly more traumatic to the vessel than a larger diameter, but fixed, indwelling and immobile sheath.

The larger balloons used for re-dilation of a stent, particularly the 15 and 18 mm balloons, are prepped "negatively" or at most, minimally inflated during their preparation before their introduction in order to prevent the development of the large "wings" or rough irregular shoulders from a previously fully inflated/deflated balloon. When introduced through a short sheath and advanced over the wire without a long sheath passing through the stent, the balloon must be advanced very carefully into and through the stent. Even though the proximal end of the stent is wide open, because of the tendency of the Super Stiff™ exchange wire to "straighten", the wire usually presses against one edge at the end of the stent and the tip of the balloon, or the folds of the balloon almost always catch on the ends of the proximal wires of the stent. Again, slight, alternating traction with pushing or advancing the wire as the balloon is advanced, often changes the angle and relative positions of the wire/balloon/catheter as the tip of the balloon enters the stent. In particular, as traction is applied to the wire, the wire often is pulled away from the wall of the stent. This allows the tip of the balloon to enter the stent first and then the entire balloon to pass into and through the stent. This traction on the wire must be performed very cautiously since any traction on the wire *also* can withdraw the tip of the wire from its secure position in the distal pulmonary artery!

As a last alternative, partial inflation of the balloon with the balloon tip positioned just proximal to the stent may be enough to move the wire away from the edge of the stent and "center" the tip of the balloon catheter in the vessel/stent. As the balloon is deflated slowly, the tip of the balloon catheter and, hopefully, the balloon itself can be advanced into the stent over the "centered" wire. This inflation of the balloon is used as a last resort since the inflation eliminates the original smoother "factory fold" of the balloon and may make the introduction of the rest of the balloon into the stent impossible.

Occasionally, no maneuver allows the reintroduction of a sheath, catheter, or balloon back into a *freshly* implanted stent without some movement of the stent. If a stent moves at all in its freshly implanted state, it can easily be displaced! Even if the position of the implanted stent does not "look or measure" perfectly, if the freshly implanted stent moves *even slightly* with subsequent manipulations, reintroduction of anything back into it should be *abandoned* at that time. When the stent has been in place for three to six months, it becomes fixed very securely into the vessel wall and can safely be re-entered and re-dilated during a subsequent catheterization.

Once the re-dilation balloon has been introduced into the stent by whichever method is successful, the larger or high-pressure balloon is centered exactly within the stent and inflated to its maximum pressure or diameter to expand the stent to its final diameter. The inflation/deflation is repeated several times to ensure maximum expansion of the stent in the previously stenosed area. After maximum inflation of the balloon within the stent, the balloon is deflated completely with maximum negative pressure. The negative pressure is released from the balloon lumen before withdrawing the balloon from the stent. If a long sheath was used with the re-dilation balloon, if possible the sheath is re-advanced into and through the stent as the balloon is deflating, as described previously.

With all dilation and stent implant procedures, the follow-up pressure measurements and selective angiograms in the proximal vessel are performed before the deflated balloon is withdrawn from the stent. This allows further reinflation to correct for residual hemodynamic problems or abnormalities seen on the angiogram or for the reintroduction of the sheath into the stent. Once satisfied with the repeat hemodynamics and the anatomic appearance, the balloon is withdrawn carefully out of the stent and into the sheath or more proximal vessel and from there, out of the body. When the balloon has been removed from the body, an end-hole catheter is passed over the wire, and, if possible, to a position distal to the stent. If it is not possible to get it through the stent, the catheter is positioned just proximal to the stent. The Super Stiff™ exchange wire is withdrawn carefully through the catheter, out of the stent, and out of the body.

"Front-loading" stent delivery

The "front-loading" stent delivery technique was developed because of repeated problems with hand-mounted stents sliding proximally off the balloons while they were being advanced through long delivery sheaths[11]. Front-loading of the stent eliminates this problem. In addition, with the "front-loading" technique, a delivery sheath one, or even two, French sizes smaller can often be used for the delivery of a comparably sized stent/balloon. For the front-loading technique, an end-hole catheter and then a Super Stiff™ guide wire are positioned exactly as for the standard long sheath stent delivery. The same extra effort is used to position the catheter tip and, subsequently, the distal end of the wire, as securely and as far distally to the stenosis in the vessel to be stented as possible.

Technique for front-loading

The stent and balloon are prepared very differently for the "front-loaded" delivery. The long sheath that is used for front-loaded stent delivery is chosen so that the balloon with the stent mounted can just barely be *accommodated* within the sheath. This permits the use of a long sheath that is *at least* one, if not two, French sizes smaller than the long sheath that is used for a standard, through-the-sheath delivery of the same balloon/stent. While outside of the body, the delivery balloon is passed from the proximal to the distal end and completely through the long sheath until the balloon is exposed entirely beyond the distal end of the sheath. The stent is mounted on the balloon while the balloon extends out of the distal end of the sheath, but otherwise, the stent is mounted exactly as for the standard, through-the-sheath delivery technique.

Once the stent is mounted and tightly crimped on the balloon, the balloon catheter *with the mounted stent* is *withdrawn* into the *distal end* of the sheath. The withdrawal into a tight fitting sheath requires considerable "finger compression" of the tip of each individual exposed strut at the proximal end of the stent as each strut is withdrawn into the sheath. The balloon, stent, and catheter are withdrawn into the distal end of the sheath until the entire *stent* (on the balloon) is within the distal tip of the sheath, but at the same time, the tip and the "shoulder" of the balloon, which are distal to the stent, extend just beyond the distal tip of the sheath. The balloon is inflated very slightly. Since most of the balloon and all of the stent are within the very tight fitting sheath, the inflation only expands the exposed distal "shoulder" of the balloon, which extends just outside of the tip of the sheath. In this position, the inflated distal tip of the balloon extending out of the tip of the sheath forms a "dilator tip" for the sheath while the "inflated" portion of the balloon, which is within the sheath, helps to "fix" the relative positions of the balloon and stent tightly against the inner diameter of the sheath.

While religiously maintaining the distal position of the previously positioned long wire, the original short sheath used for the diagnostic catheterization and the positioning of the delivery wire is removed over the wire. The tract into the vein is dilated to at least the diameter of the long sheath containing the balloon/stent. While the balloon catheter and the long sheath are *fixed together very tightly* by finger compression over the balloon/stent at the distal end of the sheath and the balloon catheter and stent at the proximal end of the sheath, the combination of the balloon catheter with the stent mounted on the balloon, which is positioned just within the tip of the long sheath, and the long sheath all are advanced as one unit, over the wire, and introduced through the skin subcutaneous tissues and into the vessel. The partially inflated balloon extending beyond the tip of the sheath acts as the "dilator tip", although it does not have as smooth an interface with the sheath or as stiff a "dilating" tip as a regular dilator. The balloon catheter within the sheath does not provide as rigid support for the shaft of the sheath as the standard long dilator provides. Once through the skin and into the vessel, the combination balloon/catheter/sheath is advanced *together* as one unit over the wire, through the heart and to the lesion. Very careful attention and a very tight grip on the sheath along with the enclosed shaft of the catheter are necessary to keep the balloon/stent/sheath combination all *fixed together* in precisely the same relationship while the combination is advanced through the vascular system and heart. The introduction and advancing of this combination requires at least two *pairs* of "knowledgeable" hands! It is impossible for a single catheterizing physician to advance the sheath while at the same time keeping the catheter and sheath fixed together as one unit and maintaining the wire securely in place. The hands of the additional *and knowledgeable* operator or assistant maintain the wire in position and the sheath and catheter fixed together while the primary operator advances the sheath/catheter combination. This is the most difficult part of a "front-loaded" stent delivery.

In addition to the difficulties in introducing the combination sheath/balloon/catheter/stent over the wire and through the skin and subcutaneous tissues, the front-loading delivery technique has several other very significant problems, which occur while the combination is being advanced *through the heart* to the lesion. These problems are significant enough to prevent the technique from being used more regularly. The inflated tip of the balloon extending out of the tip of the sheath does *not* create a smooth "dilator" tip nor a smooth interface between the surface of the balloon and the "lip" of the distal end of the sheath. Often, when there are any curves in the course to the lesion, a wide gap is created in this interface. As the sheath/catheter/stent combination is advanced, the gap or "lip" at the leading edge of the tip of the sheath may catch on intravascular or intracardiac structures and prevent the sheath from advancing further.

The inflated balloon within the distal end of the sheath does not *fix* the balloon–sheath relationship together very *securely* and, as a consequence, the balloon/stent/sheath combination functions very poorly as a "single unit". As the combination balloon/stent/sheath is advanced over the wire and through the heart, the balloon with the mounted stent is very easily pushed *out of the sheath.* Inadvertent displacement of the balloon/stent *out* of the sheath opens the stent partially and precludes any further advancing of the sheath or stent. If the stent on the balloon advances out of the sheath completely, it easily becomes entrapped in the intracardiac structures. Conversely, the *sheath* can be *pushed forward* over the stent/balloon, which, effectively, pushes the stent/balloon *back into the* sheath. When the stent/balloon/catheter is further back in the sheath and the tip of the balloon is away from the tip of the sheath, the balloon tip no longer extends beyond the tip of the sheath as the "dilator", and the open tip of the sheath without any "dilator" creates a very blunt and sharp "leading edge", which prohibits the sheath from being advanced any further.

When the balloon is inflated to a significantly higher pressure in order to prevent balloon/stent movement within the sheath, the lumen of the balloon catheter as it passes *through the balloon* is compressed by the pressure in the balloon and, in turn, prohibits the movement of the combined balloon/stent/sheath over the wire.

Finally, the *shaft* of the balloon catheter within the sheath does not provide the stiffness and support for "pushing" the sheath compared to the true long dilator. As a consequence, this lack of "shaft" support of the sheath results in kinks in the sheath, buckling of the sheath, or even "accordioning" of the sheath on itself when the sheath is advanced against any resistance. This precludes advancing the sheath any further and can result in the stent/balloon being extruded out of the sheath prematurely as the catheter alone is advanced beyond a stuck sheath which "shrinks" in length as it accordions. The multiple *disadvantages* of the front-loading technique outweigh most advantages over the standard long sheath delivery technique. The front-loading technique is used only when the standard delivery technique through a pre-positioned long sheath has failed several times.

When a front-loaded stent can be advanced all of the way to the stenotic area, and as soon as the stent is centered in the lesion, the balloon, which is partially inflated within the sheath, is *deflated completely*. After the balloon is deflated, this "loosens" the balloon/stent within the sheath and removes any inflating pressure from the balloon. With the balloon deflated, the sheath is withdrawn off the balloon/stent. The remainder of the implant of the stent is exactly as with the delivery technique through a pre-positioned long sheath.

"Ing" technique of front-loading

To overcome the "interface" problems between the tip of the partially inflated balloon and the tip of the sheath, Dr Frank Ing further refined the front-loading technique so that a *tip* segment of the long dilator which came with the long delivery sheath that is used to deliver the stent/balloon, is used as the "dilator" during the sheath delivery[12].

This modification of the front-loading technique and equipment eliminates the problems of the discrepancy of the "balloon shoulder/tip of sheath" interface. This modification also allows P 108 or P 188 stents to be mounted on even smaller balloons and delivered through sheaths as small as 6- or 7-French! This, in turn, allows the implant of stents which eventually can be *expanded to* the *final large adult diameters* into the central vessels of infants and small children. The smaller sheaths used with this modified technique follow the stiff wire to the lesion without kinking better than the larger diameter sheaths. The shaft of the balloon catheter still does not create as much support for the sheath as does the long dilator which comes with the sheath and, as a consequence, extreme care must be used in order not to bend or kink the sheath as the combination smaller sheath/balloon catheter is advanced through curves or bends within the cardiac structures.

The "Ing" modified, front-loaded device is advanced to the lesion over a pre-positioned Super Stiff™ wire which must still be positioned far distal to the lesion with the same care and attention used for the standard long sheath delivery technique. The stent mounting and the preparation of the balloon catheter and sheath require more individual preparation by the operator than the more "standard" front-loading technique.

The long dilator is removed from the long sheath that is to be used for the front-loaded delivery of the stent. Like the "standard" front-loading procedure, the balloon catheter first is advanced from the proximal to the distal end and through the long sheath so that the entire balloon is outside of the distal end of the sheath. The distal end of the *long dilator* is *amputated 2–3 cm* proximal to the tip of the dilator. The lumen of the dilator at the proximal end of this cut-off segment of the dilator is significantly larger than the "wire" lumen, which is at the very distal tip of the dilator. By rotating the *proximal end* of the shaft of this cut-off segment of dilator in the "jet" of heat from an electric "heat gun", the proximal end of the cut-off segment of dilator is softened. While the proximal end of the segment of dilator is still soft, the lumen of the softened proximal end of the segment of dilator is forced over the distal tip of the balloon catheter that is to be used for the delivery of the stent. As the lumen of the amputated tip of the dilator is forced over the tip of the balloon catheter, it is twisted or "screwed" slightly onto the tip of the catheter distal to the balloon. While the portion of the dilator is still "soft", an umbilical tape is tied tightly around the *proximal portion* of the cut-off tip of the dilator, which is now positioned over the very distal tip of the balloon *catheter*. As the segment of dilator cools with the tie around it, the wall of the cut-off segment of dilator shrinks with a circumferential "groove" in it created by the tie around it. The combination of the shrinking as it cools and the groove within the segment of dilator which is over the tip of the balloon catheter, forms a tight bond between the amputated dilator tip and the tip of the balloon catheter. This process fixes the proximal end of the cut-off tip of the dilator against the distal shoulder of the *balloon*. The dilator tip now, essentially is a part of the balloon catheter.

The stent is mounted on the balloon similarly to the previously described "front-loading". The stent is centered on the balloon, making sure that the distal end of the stent is behind the proximal end of the attached segment of the cut-off tip of the dilator. The balloon, stent, and catheter, with the attached tip of the dilator, are withdrawn into the sheath until the *proximal, straight portion* of the newly attached segment of the tip of the dilator is withdrawn just within the tip of the sheath. The withdrawal of the balloon/stent into the sheath requires the same individual crimping maneuvers over the tips of the struts of the stent as it is withdrawn into the distal tip of the small sheath. Only the tip of the dilator, which is attached to the tip of the balloon catheter, should extend out of the sheath. This tip of the original dilator for the long sheath re-creates the original, smooth interface between the sheath and the "dilator". The balloon is inflated partially within the sheath to help secure the balloon/stent/catheter within the sheath at that position. With the balloon and stent front-loaded they are delivered over the pre-positioned stiff delivery wire exactly as with the previously described front-load technique.

Even with the "Ing" modification, it still is somewhat difficult to maintain the front-loaded balloon/stent precisely together with the sheath as the combination is advanced through the heart, and the shaft of the balloon catheter still does not provide as strong support for the advancing sheath as the true long dilator. The biggest disadvantage to this technique, however, is that the "special tips" for the balloon catheters must be "hand-made" and "hand-mounted", which requires some talent and considerable additional time on the part of the operator during each case.

"Sheath-within-a-sheath" technique for the delivery of stents—combined front-loading and pre-positioned long sheath delivery technique

The final sheath technique for stent delivery is a combination of the standard pre-positioned long sheath delivery and a front-loading delivery technique. It is used in very extenuating circumstances where a large stent must be delivered through an extremely dilated heart or a very tortuous course within the heart, and particularly to lesions in the pulmonary arteries. The "sheath-within-a-sheath" technique usually is not used unless one or all of the previous long sheath techniques have failed. The sheath-within-a-sheath technique is particularly useful when there is a recurrent problem of the stent being displaced off the delivery balloon as it is advanced to the lesion through a long sheath. An end-hole catheter and a Super Stiff™ exchange guide wire (Medi-Tech, Boston Scientific, Natick, MA) are pre-positioned across the lesion and well into the vessel distal to the lesion as is accomplished with all of the other stent delivery techniques.

With the sheath-within-a-sheath technique, the stent is *front-loaded* into the smallest diameter long sheath that will accommodate the desired stent when it is mounted on the delivery balloon. The front-loaded stent, balloon, and sheath, in turn, are delivered to the lesion through another, still larger diameter, pre-positioned, long sheath. This second, larger diameter sheath/dilator set must be *six to seven centimeters* ***shorter*** than the smaller long sheath into which the stent/balloon is front loaded and must be *large enough* in its *internal diameter to accommodate* the outer diameter of the smaller diameter long sheath in which the balloon/stent is front-loaded. The outer extra-large long sheath is usually two French sizes larger than the long inner sheath. The second, larger diameter, long sheath/dilator set is advanced over the pre-positioned Super Stiff™ wire and well past the lesion in the vessel. The dilator is removed from the extra-large sheath while maintaining the Super Stiff™ wire in its secure distal location. With this extra-large sheath in place, the dilator removed over the wire, and the sheath cleared of all air and clot, the smaller diameter long sheath with the previously front-loaded balloon/stent/catheter is introduced into the proximal end of the pre-positioned, larger diameter long sheath. The front-loaded balloon/stent/catheter/sheath is advanced to the lesion *through the larger long sheath*. The front-loaded inner sheath/catheter prevents the stent from sliding on the balloon while it is being advanced through the outer sheath, while the outer larger sheath provides a smooth course through the heart for the front-loaded balloon/sheath tip interface and obviates most of the problems of the pure front-loaded delivery. The inner sheath/balloon catheter combination provides some additional support for the outer sheath to prevent kinking of either sheath. This technique has always been successful when the other techniques have failed. The major disadvantages of the sheath-within-a-sheath technique are the extra equipment necessary and the necessity of using the even larger diameter outer sheath.

Non-sheath delivery of stents

The delivery of stents *which are* currently available *and suitable for central vessels* in congenital heart lesions has been attempted without a long covering sheath, but without consistent or *reliable* results. Stents that are not premounted on balloons by the manufacturers cannot be fixed securely on the balloons. In addition, the J & J Palmaz™ stents (Johnson & Johnson, Warren, NJ) have exposed, rigid ends, which protrude off the surface of the balloon when the balloon/stent passes through any curve. These tips of these stents frequently catch on intracardiac structures and can easily be pushed off the balloons as the stent/balloon combination is advanced through any curves in the vascular course to the lesion, especially through the intracardiac structures. Once the stent has slipped off the balloon, the loose stent on the catheter shaft has sharp exposed ends. When the catheter/balloon with the loose hand-mounted stent is moved either forward or backward, the stent can catch on intravascular structures and make removal difficult and dangerous to the patient.

The Medium and "Large" Genesis™ stents (Johnson & Johnson–Cordis Corp., Miami Lakes, FL) are pre-mounted commercially and *can* be delivered safely without a sheath. The walls of the balloons actually are "incorporated" into the mesh of the stents and fix the balloon on the stent very securely until the balloon is expanded. Unfortunately, these pre-mounted Genesis™ stents are only available on balloons up to 9 mm in diameter, and the stents can be expanded further *only* to a *maximum diameter* of 10–11 mm. Although they are commercially available in the United States as well as the rest of the world, they ***are not applicable*** for use in ***any central vessels*** in humans except possibly under very extenuating, life-threatening situations. Although these stents are much easier to deliver, the stents themselves *create* a future iatrogenic stenosis in any vessel which eventually and normally will grow to a diameter greater than 11–12 mm! The stenosis created by a *limited diameter* of a stent unequivocally will require surgery on the stent/vessel for relief of the iatrogenic stenosis.

Larger, prototype Genesis XD™ stents (Johnson & Johnson–Cordis Corp., Miami Lakes, FL) applicable for use in central vessels were developed and produced *pre-mounted* for experimental *in vivo* studies, and were tested successfully in animals[13]. These prototype stents are flexible and have closed cells at the ends producing a smoother end to the stent. Like the smaller diameter versions, these larger Genesis XD™ stents were "embedded" very firmly on the balloons and could be delivered through all varieties of tortuous vasculature without a sheath and without dislodging the stent. Unfortunately, these pre-mounted, larger stents would be primarily for congenital heart patients and, as a consequence, the "small market" for these apparently does not "justify" the commercial investment to produce them. If the larger Genesis XD™ stents (Johnson & Johnson–Cordis Corp., Miami Lakes, FL) were made available pre-mounted, these stents would obviate almost all of the difficulties of stent delivery and make the implant of intravascular stents in pediatric and congenital heart patients easier for the operators and infinitely safer for the patients.

Special circumstances for stents

Dilation of rigid stents to large diameters

As discussed earlier in this chapter—in the discussions of large balloons—when balloon expandable intravascular stents are expanded on standard dilation balloons, the ends of the balloons inflate first causing the ends of the stents to flare out before the center of the stents even begins to expand. With large rigid stents, the flared ends of the stent create an acute angle off the long axis of the stent and vessel (*see* Figure 22.3). The ends of the stent, in turn, project toward and into the walls of the vessel. The flaring of both ends of the rigid stent also creates an angle at the center of the stent between the two flaring ends. With an initial expansion up to 10–12 mm in diameter, neither the angle of the distal tips against the walls of the vessel at the end of the stent nor the central angle appears to be of any consequence. However, with *initial expansion* to larger diameters than 12 mm, the flared, distal ends of the stent become almost perpendicular to the walls of the vessel. When the ends of the stent are sharp, they dig into, and create a ring of small, punctate circumferential "perforations" in, the vessel walls before the center of the stent begins to expand. As the center of the stent begins to expand, these embedded tips of the stent are pushed linearly along the vessel wall creating small linear tears at each puncture site. In vessels surrounded by dense scar tissue this probably is of no consequence, but in a "native" vessel these tears can be through the media and even through the adventitia.

With the initial expansion of rigid stents to diameters greater than 12 mm, the angle created at the *center of the stent* also becomes significant (*see* Figure 22.5). When the angle at the center of the stent becomes more acute than 90°, it very likely *cannot be* "re-straightened" as the stent is expanded to its full diameter and, in turn, leaves a "kink" or "waist" in the expanded stent as further pressure against that area pushes against a perpendicular ridge of struts at the center of the stent (*see* Figure 22.5).

Because of this phenomenon, when rigid stents are implanted with initial diameters greater than 12 mm, they are expanded sequentially, starting with a balloon less than 10 mm in diameter. This is achieved in the case of smaller vessels or very tight stenoses by beginning the implant with a single, smaller, delivery balloon. In the larger diameter vessels/stenoses, the initial implant is performed using a Balloon In Balloon™ (BIB™) balloon (NuMED Inc., Hopkinton, NY), which allows sequential expansion and still allows fixation in a large vessel with a larger diameter stenosis.

When a stent initially implanted at a very small diameter, or when a residual small central "waist" is being re-dilated to a larger diameter, the re-dilation is performed incrementally with separate balloons which are increased sequentially in diameter. If there is a central waist in a stent which is 10 mm or less in diameter, a full, further expansion up to 15 or 18 mm expands the ends of the stent first and aggravates the central "waist", possibly creating a kink in the center of the stent and making it impossible to dilate it completely.

Bifurcating stents

The primary indication for bifurcating stents is the presence of stenosis at, or very close to, the branch point or bifurcation of two or more significant vessels. If a single Palmaz™ P _ _ 8 or P _ _ 10 series stent (Johnson & Johnson, Warren, NJ) is placed across the bifurcation or branch, the *flow* to the vessel usually is not blocked, but the *physical access* to the branching vessel will be blocked ("jailed") by the initial stent crossing the non-stented branch, which, in turn, will eliminate any subsequent access to that branch with a catheter. Branch or bifurcating vessels of any significance are stented with the branching or bifurcating stents implanted simultaneously with the stent in the main vessel. Occasionally the *orifice* of the bifurcating or adjacent branch vessel is wide open, but the distal branches in that same vessel have significant stenosis which will need intervention either immediately or in the future. In that situation, the proximal, non-stenosed branch must be protected with a stent implanted simultaneously and "bifurcating" with the primarily stented vessel to "protect" the *access* into the non-stenosed more proximal branch vessel.

The implant of large stents in areas of bifurcation or at the origin of large branch vessels, particularly in the pulmonary arteries, is technically the most challenging procedure performed by the pediatric interventional cardiologist. First, it involves the implant of two (or more) stents simultaneously along with the use of three (or more) simultaneous venous catheters. The *exact* location of the stenosis *and* the relation of the stenosis to the branch or bifurcation must be defined *very precisely*. The two (or more) stents must be implanted simultaneously and very precisely into their exact locations. Unless very precise implant techniques are used, the simultaneously implanted and bifurcating stents can easily create a catastrophic situation. When simultaneous stents are to be implanted, both branches are analyzed very carefully for the degree of stenosis, the distance from the bifurcation to the stenosis, and the distance to any additional branch points.

When implanting bifurcating stents simultaneously, it is even more important to use *balloons* slightly ***shorter*** than the stents which are being implanted. Longer balloons flare ("dumbbell") the ends of each stent during early inflations much more than balloons that are slightly shorter than the stent. Flaring of the ends of the stents creates the perpendicular radius of sharp tips of the struts at the ends of the stents, particularly with the rigid, J & J™ Palmaz™ stents. When adjacent stents are implanted simultaneously, these exposed extended sharp ends of the struts very likely will puncture the adjacent balloon, which is expanding the second expanding stent.

When crossing stents are implanted, both stents should be at least 3 cm long and the crossing points of the two stents should be at, or as close to, the center of each of the stents as possible. At the same time, the proximal open ends of both stents must be proximal enough in the more proximal vessel to allow access and not be obstructed by the side of the adjacent (crossing) stent (Figure 22.8). If there is a relatively long area of stenosis in either of the vessels, the more proximal areas which include the *crossing points* of the stents, are addressed with the initial implant of the stents. Although two stents implanted simultaneously tend to support and fix each other in place, each separate stent should be appropriate for the size of the separate branch vessel in which it is implanted and be capable of fixing securely into the walls of that vessel on its own.

Occasionally, one of the stents in a bifurcating or crossing situation can be implanted without inflating and expanding the second balloon and stent *simultaneously*. However, *access* to the branching vessel, in which the stent is *not* being implanted (expanded) initially and simultaneously, must be "protected" before and during the implant of the first stent in the other branch. This "protection" of the branch is achieved by delivering the wire *and the sheath/dilator* to the other branch vessel before the first stent is implanted. The sheath/dilator is left in place in the side branch vessel during the entire implant of the initial stent in the first vessel.

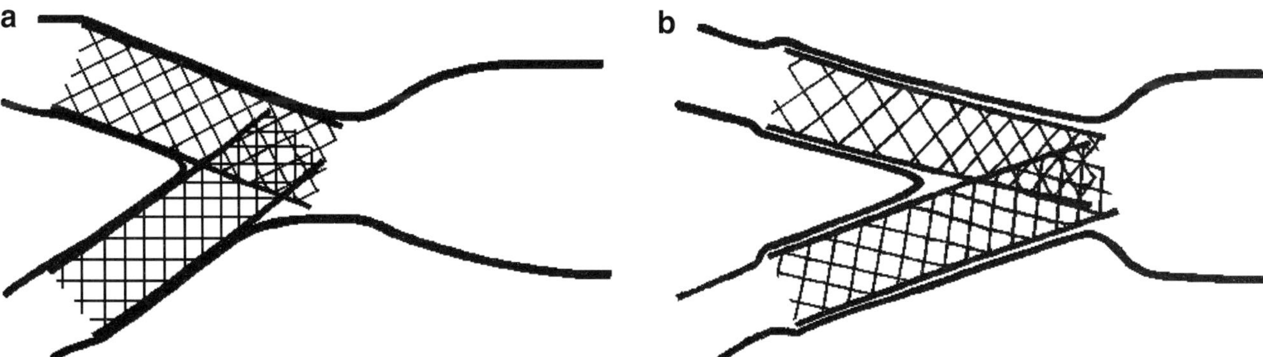

Figure 22.8 Crossing stents implanted in a bifurcating lesion: (a) stents implanted too far distally—proximal ends of implanted stents overlap each other, obstructing subsequent access into at least one of the bifurcating/branch vessels; (b) bifurcating stents implanted more proximally with stents "crossing" each other nearer their centers. Proximal ends of stents extend into more central vessel and provide subsequent access to both branches.

This separate implant of the stents has the advantage that there is no simultaneously inflated stent to puncture the adjacent balloon during the inflation for the implant of at least the first stent. At the same time, when the second stent is implanted in a position crossing or next to the previously implanted stent, the *balloon* in the *first* stent *must be inflated along with and* during the expansion of the balloon in the second vessel/stent in order to prevent the initial stent from being crushed. The expanded balloon within the stent which is already implanted and expanded, helps to "protect" the second balloon from the sharp ends of the struts of the original stent and helps to prevent puncture of the adjacent (second) balloon by these sharp tips of the original stent. The technique of implanting crossing or bifurcating stents one at a time has the disadvantage of not creating the support against the tissues provided by the two expanded stents adjacent to (crossing) each other when they are implanted into large vessels. This is particularly true when one of the adjacent, more proximal *orifices* is not stenotic.

When there is a bifurcation stenosis occurring distally in association with an *additional and contiguous more proximal single stenosis* in the main, feeding vessel (Figure 22.9), management of the combined lesions with the implant of intravascular stents becomes more complex. Although it is counterintuitive to implant a stent in the more proximal vessel and then have to work through the freshly implanted stent to implant more distal stents, the single *more proximal stenosis*, in fact, must be addressed first *before* the additional bifurcating stents are placed in the more distal branching areas of stenosis!

To overcome these problems, the larger single stent, which will be in the more central stenosis that is proximal to the bifurcating stenosis, is implanted first (Figure 22.10). Once the more central stent is secured, the more distal branching stenotic vessels are cannulated simultaneously *through* the more proximal stent with two (or more) catheters and wires passed separately but adjacent to each other through the proximal stent. The two or more stents in the branching vessel are implanted with the *proximal ends* of the bifurcating stents both implanted and overlapping *within* the distal end of the more proximal single stent (Figure 22.11).

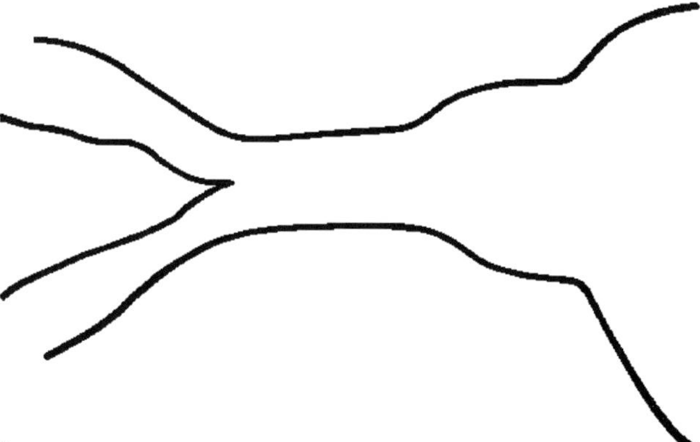

Figure 22.9 Diagram of combined central proximal right pulmonary artery stenosis along with distal bifurcating right branch pulmonary artery stenosis.

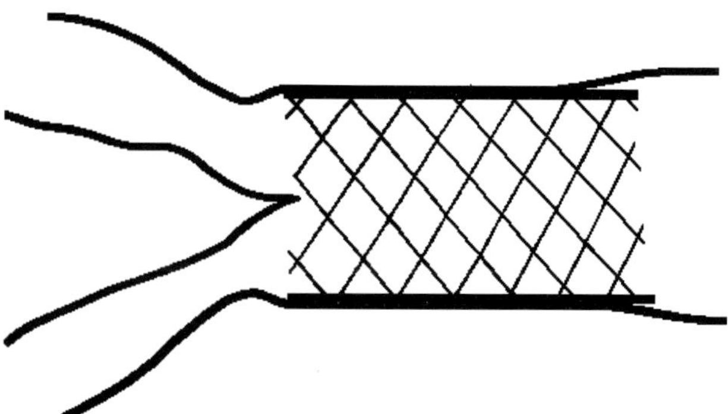

Figure 22.10 Single large stent implanted first in the single, more central stenosis, which is proximal to the bifurcating stenosis in the same vessel.

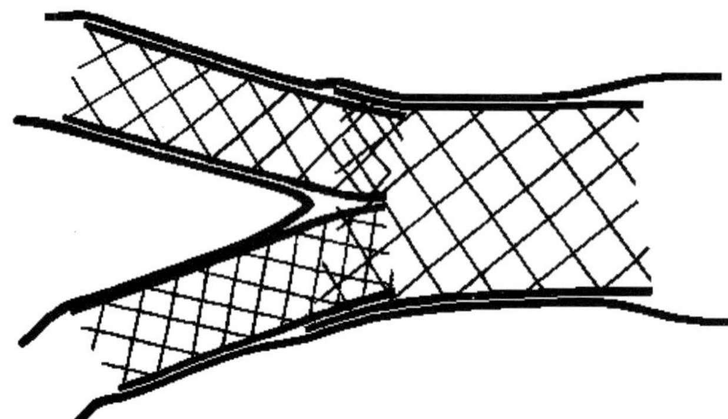

Figure 22.11 Distal bifurcating stents implanted *through (out of) and in tandem with* the single more proximal stent.

When the more proximal stent is very secure, the distal bifurcation stenoses can be addressed immediately after the more proximal stent is implanted. However, if there is a question about the stability of the first stent, the distal branch stenoses are addressed at a subsequent catheterization. Once the bifurcating stents are in place, *any* subsequent dilation, of the single more proximal stent and/or *either one* or both of the distal stents, must be performed with the number of balloons equal to the number of the more peripheral, distal stents. These balloons are always inflated simultaneously with the proximal ends extending back into the single proximal stent and the distal ends extending out of the proximal stent into each of the branching stents/vessels.

If two (or more), distal side-by-side or bifurcating stents are implanted first, in order to dilate and also support the more proximal single vessel stenosis with "a stent" after the two distal stents have already been implanted, ***two*** *side-by-side* stents would have to be implanted in the more proximal *single* vessel stenosis in order not to crush one of

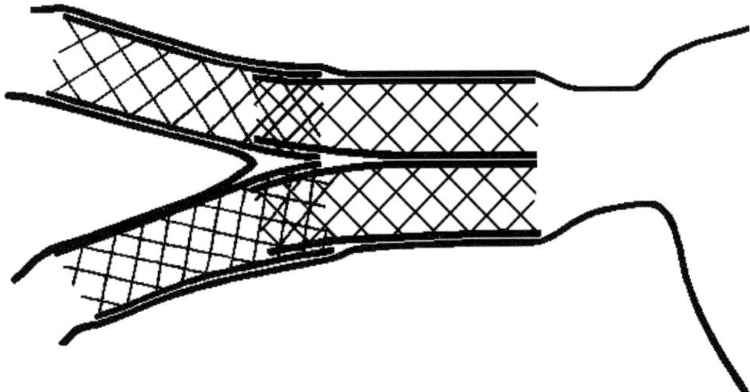

Figure 22.12 Parallel tandem stents extended back into single proximal channel.

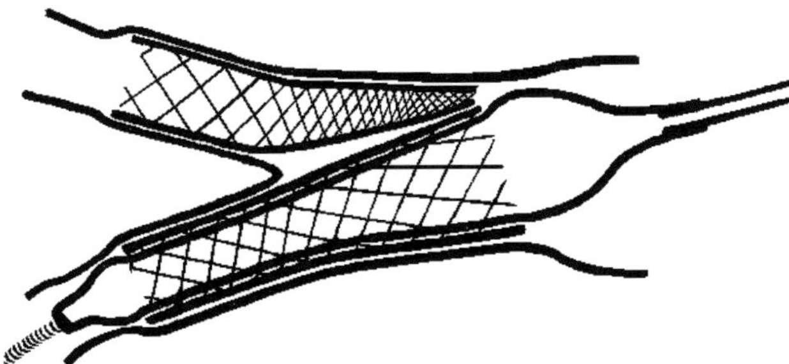

Figure 22.13 "Unprotected" stent in an adjacent vessel crushed by balloon expanded in adjacent vessel.

the more distal stents! This would create (and necessitates) a *dual channel* in the *single* vessel. The dual channel would have to extend as far proximally as any more proximal stenosis in order to treat the stenosis with implanted stents (Figure 22.12).

When there are dual stents and/or two stent orifices adjacent to each other anywhere in a vessel which requires dilating and/or the implant of an additional stent, separate balloons must be inflated *simultaneously in* ***each*** of the adjacent stents during any subsequent dilation of *either* of these stents. This of course holds true as well if there are more than two adjacent stents (e.g. in a trifurcating branch stenosis!). Any dilation more proximal (with or without stents) made with a single balloon that is adjacent to and outside of a stent which is not being supported by a second balloon in that stent, will crush the adjacent stent that is *not* supported with an inflated balloon in it at the bifurcation or where the stents are next to each other (Figure 22.13). Any balloon and/or catheter in the adjacent but unprotected stent/vessel could be trapped *outside* of the expanding new stent!

When a single, more central stent is implanted in a lesion that is very short and immediately proximal to the bifurcation stenoses, occasionally a "skirt technique"—which was originally described for coronary lesions—is used to implant the initial, proximal stent[14]. In order to ensure dilation and support with a stent of the short more proximal stenosis as well as to guarantee access to both branches of the distal bifurcation, and in order not to overdilate either of the distal branches while implanting the single, much larger, more proximal stent, the proximal stent is mounted on, delivered over, and implanted on *two separate, adjacent balloons within the single proximal stent*. A stent is chosen that will expand the proximal vessel/stenosis to the desired diameter. Then, the two smaller balloons, which together will expand the single stent enough to fill and open the proximal pulmonary artery to the desired diameter, are chosen and "negatively prepped". The two balloons are placed side by side within the single stent and the stent is compressed and crimped tightly *over the two balloons*. A single, *larger diameter* long sheath is used that will accommodate the combined diameter of the two balloons together with the single stent mounted over them. The large, long, sheath/dilator set is introduced and advanced over a Super Stiff™ wire which is positioned as far distally as possible into one of the stenotic branches. The tip of the long sheath is positioned distally in the stenosis in the proximal vessel where this initial stent, which will be delivered on the two balloons, will be implanted. The large, long *sheath* is advanced as far distally as possible over the dilator/wire within the single proximal vessel and just to the area of the bifurcation stenosis off the central vessel. The long dilator and Super Stiff™ wire are removed, leaving the sheath in place.

A small torque-controlled end-hole catheter, through which the wire which will be used in *one* of the balloon catheters on which the stent is mounted will pass, is introduced into and advanced through the large, long sheath. From the tip of the long sheath, the catheter is manipulated into and far distally in one of the stenotic bifurcation branches off the more central artery. Once the first catheter is securely in place, a second similar catheter is advanced through the long sheath adjacent to the first catheter, manipulated and advanced distally into the *other* stenotic branch of the bifurcation. Two separate exchange length wires, which the two balloons on which the stent is mounted will accommodate, are advanced through the separate catheters and wedged into the respective separate distal pulmonary artery branches. The two catheters are withdrawn over the separate wires and the two balloons which are compressed within the single stent are introduced *over the two side-by-side wires*, into the large long sheath and advanced as a single unit over the two wires and through the long sheath to the stenotic area of the more proximal pulmonary artery.

It is imperative that the two separate end-hole catheters and, in turn, the two separate wires are advanced initially to the separate stenotic pulmonary artery bifurcating branches through the *single long sheath* which was positioned initially in the more proximal pulmonary artery. This ensures that the two catheters, and in turn, the two wires are passing through the *exact same course* through the heart and do not deviate separately around even a single chorda!

As the stent and two balloons are advanced distally from the tip of the sheath, which is positioned in the proximal pulmonary artery, the tips of the two balloons, which extend out of the single stent, follow the separate wires into the separate bifurcating branches off the more central single pulmonary artery. By pushing the balloons/stent forward as far as possible, the single stent becomes positioned immediately adjacent to the bifurcation, while at the same time buttressed against, and straddling the two branches equally. The sheath is withdrawn proximally off the two balloons/single stent, and with the wires and balloon catheters pushed forward as firmly as possible, the two balloons are inflated simultaneously. This expands the single stent into the proximal vessel with the distal end of the stent "flared" like a "bi-legged skirt" toward the two distal stenotic branches. Any subsequent dilations or stent implants in the proximal vessel or the branches are performed with separately delivered, but simultaneously inflated, balloons.

Tandem stents

Tandem stents are frequently necessary in vessel stenoses that are longer than the available stents or in curved lesions in order to have the straight rigid stents conform better to the contour of the vessel. The use of tandem stents is particularly important with the limited available lengths and the lack of flexibility of the J & J™ Palmaz™ stents (Johnson & Johnson, Warren, NJ).

In the deployment of tandem stents, it is important that no gap is left (or allowed to occur later) between adjacent stents. Alternatively, the adjacent ends of two stents that are within the same vessel, should have a wide separation between the approximated ends of the abutting stents at the time of implant. The exposed, rigid and sharp end of a *single stent*, by itself, creates an irritation, which results in a build-up of the intima. The irritation of the vessel wall between the apposing *ends of two stents* that are in close approximation to each other, is aggravated by the movement or bending of the vessel that occurs in the gap between the two stents. The vessel movement causes the two apposing, sharp ends to "grind" the tissues between them, resulting in very aggressive, localized, intimal proliferation. Intimal proliferation in these "gap" areas is one of the few documented causes of significant re-stenosis in the many pediatric/congenital lesions that have been stented.

At implant, the adjacent tandem stents are overlapped by a *minimum* of 35 to 70%. The degree of overlap depends upon the type of stent, the expected implant diameter of the stents, which effects the shrinkage in length of the stents, and the *age* and *expected growth* of the patient and, in turn, the future growth in *length* of the vessel. When P _ _ 8 stents are implanted in *potentially large* (15–18 mm diameter) vessels, which, however, are small in diameter at the time of implant, they are overlapped *at least 60–70%*. This degree of overlap is necessary to prevent separation of the stents as the stents shrink in length as they expand *and* to allow for subsequent growth of the vessel in *length*. P _ _ 8 stents shrink ~50% in length with expansion to their largest diameters. The newer ITI™ stents (ev3, Plymouth, MN) shrink minimally in length when expanded *sequentially* and do not require as much overlap to allow for the initial shrinkage or for shrinkage later with further dilation.

When tandem stents *of all types* are implanted in small, but *growing patients*, the potential growth of the patient and *length of the vessel* must be taken into account and an even greater overlap of the stents created at the time of implant. None of the stents "elongate" after implant, and, in fact, when stents are dilated further in diameter to accommodate the growth of a vessel, most stents shrink even further in length with re-dilation! At the same time, the tissues elongate as well as increase in diameter with growth, which results in the adjacent, tandem stents, which have a fixed length and are fixed in the tissues of the wall of the vessel, separating from each other, even when there was a significant overlap at the time of implant. When there is insufficient overlap of the adjacent stents, the ends actually separate and create an area of extreme irritation and intimal proliferation between the ends of the stents. As a consequence, when sufficient overlap of adjacent tandem stents cannot be provided to allow for the patient's growth, it is better to leave a large gap of *at least 5–6 mm* between the ends of the adjacent stents at the time of the initial implant. An additional stent can be implanted between the original stents after several years, when the patient is re-catheterized and the original stents are re-dilated.

When the area of stenosis to be stented is in a curved vessel, two, or more, overlapping, short rigid stents should be implanted in tandem around the curve, rather than one long, straight, rigid stent. This is particularly important with the J & J™ Palmaz™ stents. A shorter stent on a short balloon is easier to deliver and implant in a curved vessel and a series of overlapping, tandem, short stents conforms better to the curvature of the vessel than a single long stent. A longer straight, rigid stent implanted in a curved vessel not only does *not* conform to the curvature of the vessel, but leaves the long, sharp ends of a rigid stent digging into the outer circumference of the curvature of the vessel wall at an acute angle. The sharp ends of the stents implanted at an acute angle to the wall of a vessel are another *demonstrated* cause of excessive intimal proliferation and re-stenosis following stent implant in congenital lesions with the longer J & J™ stents (Johnson & Johnson, Warren, NJ).

If multiple tandem stents are anticipated, at the initial implant of each of the earlier stents, the earlier stents implanted are not expanded to their final maximum diameter with their implant, but with their initial expansion are expanded only enough to fix the stents in place. This smaller initial diameter of the earlier stents allows several more millimeters of expansion with the implant of *each* subsequent stent. This, in turn, allows subsequent stents to be implanted at a slightly larger diameter than the original stents in order to ensure the fixation of each additional stent as it is expanded into the same vessel. The stents which were implanted earlier and initially, are expanded further and incrementally with the implant of each additional stent. Eventually the full diameter of that particular vessel can be achieved after the entire length of the tandem stents has been implanted, yet without significant over-dilation of the particular vessel when the initial stents have been implanted at smaller than final diameters. If, on the other hand, the first or earlier stents are expanded to the full diameter of the vessel with their implant, in order to "over-expand" the subsequent stents, they must be expanded to a diameter slightly *larger than the vessel* to secure the additional stent(s) in the vessel and within the initial stents.

When tandem stents are implanted in veins, the most distal (*in the direction of blood flow*) stent is implanted first. If the proximal (in the direction of blood flow) stent is implanted first, stasis of blood flow occurs in the newly created lumen within the stent (proximal in the flow to the more distal stenosis). This blood, which is not flowing, tends to clot before the more distal stents are implanted and more adequate flow can be established through them. In the pulmonary arteries with pulsatile, more vigorous flow, the opposite occurs. The more proximal stent is implanted first. If the more distal area is opened with *no* blood flow coming from the more proximal, still stenotic vessel, the blood in the dilated pulmonary bed distal to the obstruction stops and will thrombose.

Recent developments in stents

There are some improvements in the stents and in the delivery systems for peripheral vascular use, which somewhat inadvertently have "trickled down" or been modified for the pediatric and congenital arena. Of the hundreds of new stent designs and stent materials that have been introduced in the past decade for use in adult vascular diseases, several have applicability, although not "approval", for the pediatric and congenital population. The three "groups" of relatively new or "pending" stents which already have promise for congenital lesions are the Cheatham-Platinum™ (C-P™) stents (NuMED Inc., Hopkinton, NY), the Mega™ and Maxi™ stents (Intra Therapeutics Inc., St Paul, MN) and the Genesis XD™ stents (Johnson & Johnson–Cordis Corp., Miami Lakes, FL). All of these have been discussed in some detail earlier in this chapter.

The Cheatham-Platinum (C-P™) stent (NuMED Inc., Hopkinton, NY) has had extensive use world wide (except in the United States) for the standard congenital lesions. It is not available *routinely* in the United States. It was the first stent available in the much larger diameters, which also had some flexibility and had rounded ends for safe use in larger lesions. Because of its unique characteristics and wide range of "available" and "custom" sizes, and its availability with an expandable "covering", the C-P™ stent has had some unique investigational and compassionate use applications throughout the world, including even in the US. The most innovative of these uses is the "re-building" or "creation" of "internal venous tunnels" with very large, long and covered C-P™ stents for the "completion of the Fontan" in the catheterization laboratory. This catheterization procedure, if perfected, could replace two major cardiac surgical procedures.

The Double Strut™ stent (Intra Therapeutics Inc., St Paul, MN) was the first stent approved for "human use" in the US which had both flexibility and a truly open-cell design, which have considerable appeal for use in congenital lesions. Several newer stents from ITI™ are now approved for human use in the US and appear to be even more suitable for pediatric and congenital lesions. The Mega™ and Maxi™ stents (ev3, Plymouth, MN) still have the favorable open-cell design as the Double Strut™ stent but are stronger and/or larger.

The Genesis XD™ stent (Johnson & Johnson–Cordis Corp., Miami Lakes, FL) is an apparent replacement (successor) for the Palmaz™ P _ _ 8 series of stents (Johnson & Johnson–Cordis Corp., Miami Lakes, FL). The Genesis XD™ has some flexibility, smoother ends and a partially flexible design, all of which improves the ease and safety of its use. Even with the improvements in its design, the Genesis XD™ *appears* to have retained the strength of the P _ _ 8 stents. The Genesis XD™ stent appears to fulfill most of the criteria of an ideal stent for many of the central congenital heart vascular stenoses, although more clinical experience with it is necessary before too much complacency develops about the delivery of stents!

Stenting of the atrial septum

Standard intravascular stents are occasionally used to maintain an opening in the atrial septum for the temporary, or sometimes even permanent, *palliation* of complex congenital heart defects. Often the septal openings created by a balloon atrial septostomy (Chapters 13) or a blade and balloon atrial septostomy (Chapter 14) spontaneously shrink in diameter or even close completely. Standard intravascular stents can be placed in the atrial openings to maintain their patency. Stents with a restricted central diameter are used to create openings, but with a restricted flow in atrial baffles in "failed Fontan" patients. These uses of intravascular stents are covered in detail in Chapter 14.

"Future" developments in intravascular stents

Large flexible stents without sharp tips at the ends

It should be possible with a few adjustments of the laser cutter to produce an even larger version of the Genesis XD™ stent comparable in size and strength to the Palmaz P 4010 and P 5010 stents (Johnson & Johnson–Cordis Corp., Miami Lakes, FL). A larger stent with the smoother ends and with the slight flexibility of the Genesis XD™ would improve the safety of the stents for use in the aorta or any other very large vessel. The smoother ends alone probably would eliminate the aneurysms that develop during the implant of stents in the aorta as a result of the sharp tips of the rigid J & J™ stents. Whether the pediatric/congenital "market" is large or important enough for the manufacturers to make this happen, still remains to be seen. Hopefully, the already available Maxi™ stent (ev3, Plymouth, MN) will fulfill the same criteria or the large C-P™ stents (NuMED Inc., Hopkinton, NY) will become available in the US to provide this added safety for these patients.

Pre-mounted, flexible stents

A prototype, pre-mounted version of the Genesis XD™ stent (Johnson & Johnson–Cordis Corp., Miami Lakes, FL) was mentioned earlier. This pre-mounted stent underwent *in vivo* animal tests in early 2001[13]. The pre-mounting of these stents, like the other Genesis™ stents, is unique, with the stent almost "incorporated" into the surface of the balloon. This pre-mounting along with the "smoother" ends of these stents allowed the Genesis XD™ stents to be delivered safely *without* the protection of a long sheath, even when passing through the right heart and through very tortuous vessels, and without the stent catching on intravascular structures or being dislodged from the balloon. This very secure type of pre-mounting requires a great deal of collaboration between the manufacturers of both balloons and stents.

The commercial availability of the larger pre-mounted intravascular stents would make the implant of stents for all of the pediatric and congenital heart patients easier and infinitely safer. At the same time, pre-mounted stents initially would increase the cost of the procedure significantly. When stents that are *not* pre-mounted are used, a single stent is suitable for use in many different lesions and vessels with many different diameters. The separate stent merely is mounted on the particular diameter balloon, which is applicable to the particular lesion. For the most part, the *balloons* that are used to implant the intravascular stents are already in the inventory of the catheterization laboratory for the balloon dilation of vessels and valves. However, when using *pre-mounted* stents, an inventory of a full range of each size of the pre-mounted stent/balloon combination would be necessary and the balloons with the pre-mounted stents would not be useable for other angioplasties without stent implant. Eventually, the costs of the procedures would "even out", with less time required for the preparation and delivery procedure for the stents, less loss of balloons and stents from stent slippage or balloon rupture/entrapment, and certainly less time used as a consequence of the significantly worse complications now encountered with some of the "hand-mounted" stents.

Unfortunately, the major (and almost only!) applications for the larger pre-mounted stents are for *pediatric/congenital heart lesions*. As such and in the environment of the US FDA, which does not recognize *any* stent for pediatric or congenital heart use, this population does not represent a market, much less a profitable market, and certainly not an area for future development, for Johnson & Johnson–Cordis™ or, so far, for any other stent manufacturers to pursue specifically for this use.

Covered stents

There is considerable interest and ongoing development of "covered stents" for the exclusion of aortic aneurysms in atherosclerotic adults. Covered stents have been used occasionally on a compassionate basis for emergency "bail-out" in a few unique pediatric/congenital patients. The early covered stents that were used in congenital patients were hand-made by wrapping a "sleeve" of fabric or freshly harvested vein over or around a non-expanded stent. The sleeve of covering material had the same diameter as the desired *final* diameter of the vessel that was being stented. The sleeve of fabric or tissue was attached to the stent by several sutures and the stent with the covering sleeve was mounted on a balloon. The combination was compressed and delivered through a sheath similar to the delivery of other balloon-expandable stents. These hand-made stents required a significantly larger introductory sheath than the stent/balloon alone. When the stent expands, the covering sleeve expands and/or unravels and creates an "impervious" channel in the area which is "covered" by the sleeve. Hand fabrication of these covered stents was tedious and very time consuming and, of equal or more importance, the end product was very unpredictable and imprecise.

Eventually, new modifications with the covering material built into, or onto, the stents were developed and a variety of covered stents now are manufactured and are available commercially for the adult market. (Manufacturers include: WALLGRAFT-Medi-Tech, Boston Scientific, Natick, MA; JoStent-Jomed Implantate, GMH, Rangendingen, Germany; Zenith-Cook Inc., Bloomington, IN and Excluder-W. L. Gore & Associates, Flagstaff, AZ). These covered stents are for adult vascular use and for use predominantly outside of the US. Simultaneously, more needs are arising for covered stents in congenital heart lesions.

Covered stents for use in congenital patients have even more stringent limitations than standard stents. Besides the lack of availability for congenital use, the major problem for the use of covered stents in many congenital patients is the subsequent growth of the patients and vessels. There is one oral communication which suggests that some expandable polytetrafluoroethylene (ePTFE) covered stents can be dilated further in order to accommodate the growth of a patient even several years after their implant. Until the single observation can be duplicated and demonstrated to be reproducible in further animal or human trials, this observation cannot be taken for granted for all patients and types of stents/coverings. Certainly, a non-stretchable "covering" or fabric material over a stent, which is similar to a circumferential prosthetic conduit, cannot expand beyond the manufactured maximum diameter of the material, particularly after there has been tissue ingrowth into the covering/fabric. This type of covered stent, in turn, would create a *fixed maximum diameter* for that vessel, which is fixed by the diameter of the covering of the stent at the time of implant. Until new materials/designs are available that can definitely be dilated further once the covered stent has been in place for many months, covered stents should be used only in patients who have reached adult size, or in extremely extenuating, life-threatening, circumstances.

The covered stents which have been or currently are being used in pediatric/congenital lesions, are those which are available for adult peripheral vascular lesions and, for the most part, have been used in isolated, "emergency bail-out" situations. The first uses of covered stents were for the control of acute tears in vessels. Originally, these were tears in smaller vessels (coronary arteries), and usually the tears were iatrogenic following balloon dilations. Subsequently, the same concept was used for the occlusion of degenerative tears and aneurysms of the aorta. There are at present extensive developments and multiple clinical trials for the treatment of aortic aneurysms in adults with covered stents. With favorable outcome of these trials and newer developments in the covered stents, covered stents eventually will be more applicable to, and more readily available for, congenital lesions.

There already has been a sporadic use of covered stents in pediatric/congenital heart lesions for the repair of acute tears in vessels, which occurred during balloon dilation procedures. This currently involves the problem of the necessary individual, "hand" preparation of the covered stent during such an emergency—which is time-consuming and somewhat inconsistent. The humanitarian approval or off-label availability of a commercially manufactured, more sophisticated covered stent in multiple sizes would make this application more effective, more consistent and, again, much safer and even life-saving in acute catastrophic emergencies. Covered stents also have an application for the occlusion of "window type" systemic to pulmonary communications, particularly those arising from the ascending aorta or entering into difficult to reach locations in the more distal pulmonary arteries (e.g. unusual ductus and/or Potts descending aorta to left pulmonary artery shunts)[15,16]. However, if a covered stent is used for this purpose in much smaller patients, the covered stent must be capable of further dilation to accommodate for the patient's growth! A few hand-made covered stents have been used under extenuating or emergency circumstances in congenital patients for the purposeful occlusion for managing iatrogenic tears in vessels following balloon dilation of branch pulmonary arteries.

Covered stents have been used for the treatment of aortic tears that occur during the dilation of coarctations of the aorta, or even are suggested for use in the routine stenting of coarctation of the aorta[17]. A long covered stent potentially obliterates the vasa-vasorum, intercostals and/or the *spinal artery* in the areas which can be included under the stent and covered by the stent, with the possibility of causing tissue ischemia or even paraplegia. In the adult atherosclerotic, dissected aorta, where covered stents are being used extensively, these critical side/branch vessels in general have not created a problem. Additionally, there is a real incidence of stent displacement during stent implants for coarctations of the aorta. Usually the errant stent is "re-implanted" in a smaller distal area of the aorta, and with a non-covered stent and the knowledge that flow is preserved *through the side of the open stent*, there is little concern when the stent crosses side branches. However, a covered stent which becomes displaced in the aorta, potentially would occlude critical side branches which it crossed! In addition, there is the necessity of very large introductory sheaths for hand-made and commercially available covered stents which are currently available for the aorta.

In spite of the lack of prospective or planned commercial development in this area, the most innovative uses of covered stents to date have been in congenital heart lesions. Covered stents were used to "rebuild" intra-atrial, venous channels which were disrupted and leaking significantly in several complex patients with single ventricles who had undergone "Fontan" cavopulmonary type single ventricle repairs[18]. There now are proposed, surgical/interventionist ("hybrid") collaborative trials for the use of covered stents to "complete a Fontan" procedures prospectively. These developmental uses of covered stents are described in more detail in Chapter 32.

"Open-ring" stents

The use of intravascular stents in the central and *potentially* large vessels still represents a problem in *very* young or *very* small patients who have a very significant potential for further growth. *Small diameter*, pre-mounted stents, which can be delivered easily to the pulmonary arteries or to other sites in very small infants, are readily available, however, these small diameter stents *cannot be dilated* subsequently to a size adequate to the diameter of even a *small* adult central vessel. Any stent with a small or limited diameter, which *cannot eventually be dilated to the adult diameter of the vessel*, represents an *iatrogenic stenosis* and should *not be used* in these vessels. This problem has been overcome partially by the "Ing" modified, front-loading delivery technique, which was described earlier in this chapter and which allows the delivery of the current, shorter, P 108 and P 188 stents through as small as 7-French sheaths. These particular shorter stents can be dilated to adult diameters; however, this is not the perfect solution. Even these stents and the necessary sheaths/dilators are large and rigid relative to the size of a *very small* infant. Another area of potential future stent development is a small stent, which either dissolves or can be opened later to allow dilation to a diameter ***beyond*** *the nominal diameter of the original stent* in order to allow dilation of the particular vessel to the eventual diameter of the adult vessel.

Dr Ing developed a simple but very innovative "open-ring" stent and validated its usefulness in one animal study[19]. With his technique, one or two longitudinal cuts were made along the entire length of standard P 154 or P 204 stents (Johnson & Johnson, Warren, NJ), which have a maximal diameter of 10–11 mm. This created a small stent, which was split and "opened" longitudinally, completely along one side, or with two longitudinal cuts on the opposite sides of the stent, a "bi-valved" stent. The incised halves of the stent were reattached to each other with two or three 6-0 *resorbable* sutures, which were placed along each cut edge. These "reattached" small diameter stents were mounted on a balloon, delivered and implanted easily through a *6-French sheath* exactly as any other very small stent. These small, potentially "open" stents were then dilated acutely up to 11 mm in diameter during their implant *without* disruption of the sutures holding the two halves together. The resorbable sutures fixed the two longitudinal halves of the stent together securely enough to allow dilation to the full diameter of the particular stents. The expanded, sutured stent, when implanted, supported the dilated vessels at the widest diameter of the implanted stents, while the sutures maintained the edges of the stents together securely and long enough to allow secure fixation of the stents into the tissues and to provide adequate support of the dilated vessel. The sutures resorbed over 8 to 12 weeks. Any time thereafter, further dilation of the vessel in the area of the stents separated the previously incised and sutured, longitudinal cut(s) in the stents, allowing further dilation well beyond the nominal limits of the original standard, smaller diameter stents. This unrestricted dilation of the "opened" stents in the vessel is sufficient to compensate for *any* subsequent growth of the vessel. The "open-ring" stent allows the delivery of a very small stent to very small central vessels in young infants as small as 3–4 kilograms, while the "opened" stent subsequently allows the *vessel* to be dilated eventually to an adult diameter as the small stent splits.

The stents which were utilized in the animal investigation were prepared specifically for the study by the manufacturer (Johnson & Johnson, Warren, NJ). The manufacturer performed the longitudinal cuts in the stents and polished and coated the cut edges in order to resist corrosion similar to the surfaces and ends of all stents. Unfortunately, the very small number of patients who would require these stents prohibits a prospective human study which could reach enough statistical significance to satisfy the FDA, even if it lasted a century. As a consequence, these professionally cut and polished stents are no longer produced for any use. The only current alternative for the "Ing" open-ring stent is to "hand-cut" the stents, which would leave the edges rough and not coated and, in turn, create some added unknowns for a clinical trial. Hand cutting in order to individually produce the "open-ring" stents also increases the difficulty and consistency of preparing each stent, and certainly would decreases the safety of their use in these precarious positions in these already critically ill infants.

Recently, the "open-ring" concept has reappeared in Europe as the "Growth Stent"[20]. The growth stent is laser cut and electro polished as a "bi-valved" stent with specific, facing, "tongue and grove" areas where the two longitudinal halves fit together in order to maintain the edges together more securely (QualiMed, Winsen/Luhe, Germany). The edges are held together with the same resorbable sutures used by Dr Ing and are completely reabsorbed after 8 weeks. In addition to its small size, this stent has the advantages of having some open side cells and "Omega" hinges between adjacent rows of cells, which together give the stents considerable flexibility. The greatest advantage is that it is professionally manufactured and commercially available at least outside of the US.

Hopefully, with some enlightenment of the FDA toward the humanitarian use of "congenital" devices in adult patients, the precedence might extend to the very small, unique and otherwise untreatable populations of neonatal congenital heart patients. Without resistance from the FDA, it might be possible to import these unique but rarely used stents or to persuade one or more of the US stent manufacturers to make these or similar "open-ring" stents available even for this commercially non-profitable group of patients.

Future stents

New intravascular stents continue to be developed and improved for acquired vascular diseases in the adult population. Secondarily, but presently only fortuitously and certainly not "officially", these new stents become available for congenital and pediatric heart patients. With some enlightenment of the FDA, hopefully some Objective Performance Criteria (OPCs) can be agreed upon between the professionals caring for these patients, industry and the FDA which would allow not only the approval of existing stents for congenital lesions, but would permit and even encourage the *development* of stents *specifically* for the pediatric/congenital population.

An alternative to the small open-ring stent might be a small, but at the same time, a totally biodegradable stent. Biodegradable stents have been developed primarily with the goal of preventing re-stenosis, but up until now, have not proven satisfactory. Such a small resorbable/degradable stent, which is developed for larger coronary arteries, could be ideal in order to "buy time" for severe stenosis of major vessels in very small infants.

Complications of stent implants

With the exception of the inappropriate use of a stent in a particular location, the complications of intravascular stents in the pediatric and congenital populations, are almost all related to the *implant procedures*, and not to the stents themselves. Once successfully and accurately implanted, and unlike the stents used in acquired adult vascular diseases, there are very few late complications of the stents themselves in pediatric/congenital patients. This is particularly true for the currently available, new generation of stents. Those late complications which have occurred, are usually related more to specific peculiarities of the underlying congenital lesions than to the stents themselves. Complications can occur during implants into any location in congenital lesions; however, implants into the pulmonary arteries (Chapter 23) are technically more challenging and result in more complications.

The most significant complication of the stents themselves is iatrogenic and occurs when an inappropriate stent is implanted in a particular vessel. This occurs most commonly when a small stent, which *cannot* be dilated to the eventual adult diameter of the vessel, is implanted in a growing patient. This, in turn, will eventually result in stenosis of the vessel that will be of equal or greater significance to the stenosis caused by the initial lesion. A stenosis in a vessel due to a stent that is too small and cannot be dilated any further, will require *complex* surgical intervention to correct it. To relieve the stenosis due to a small stent, the entire segment of the vessel must be excised or the entire length of the stent/vessel must be divided and patched, whether any other surgery is required for that particular patient. The use of a stent that knowingly will eventually be too small for the vessel, is justified only in life-threatening situations, and/or when the patient will require surgery in the area of the stent for some other reason—for example a "conduit" exchange necessitated for growth.

With the continued necessity of having to "make do" with the materials available rather than having the specific stents and/or specific equipment designed for stent delivery in pediatric and congenital lesions, the physician implanting stents in pediatric/congenital patients with complex lesions must anticipate a variety of problems with stent deployment and implant. In turn, the operator must be prepared to handle these so they remain "adverse events" and do not result in permanent adverse sequelae for the patient.

The most important "treatment" of the complications of stent implants, like all complications, is prevention! Tried, true and established delivery equipment and techniques are used as often as possible. Very careful attention must be paid to all of the details of the procedures that have been demonstrated to be successful as well as safe for the implant of the stents. Very careful observation of the catheter, wire, sheath/dilator, balloon/stent, and finally, the position of the stent, is essential at *all* stages of the procedure. Taking "one step backward" and "regrouping" in order to correct an erroneous position of any of the components of the system at any time during the implant procedure helps to prevent complications or, at the very least, prevents repetition of most of the preceding procedure. "Short-cuts" in the techniques and changing to different, not previously tested equipment or techniques, frequently result in problems with delivery or implant of the stent. New materials (wires, sheaths, balloons and even stents) and new techniques using unproven materials or new materials should be tested on animal models and then have extensive, totally successful, human use with adequate follow-up, before being advocated and published as "successful" or certainly "routine".

With all complications that occur during stent implant, it is extremely important (critical) to maintain the secure position of the delivery wire through the stent in order to facilitate a recovery from the misadventure.

Specific complications of stent implants

Local vessel injury can and does occur at the introductory sites in the vessels where the stents are introduced. Because of the usual large diameter of a stent mounted on a dilation balloon, the introductory sheaths for the delivery of stents are necessarily large even in smaller patients. In spite of this, both arterial and venous complications following the implant of intravascular stents in pediatric and congenital patients have been extremely rare. Venous damage at the location where the large sheath was introduced can lead to total obstruction of the vein, but this may go unnoticed until a subsequent cardiac catheterization is attempted through the same vein.

In spite of the very large sheaths required for the balloon/stent combinations, particularly during the first five years of the original stent implant protocol in congenital heart patients, there were remarkably few venous occlusions found during the required routine follow-up catheterizations of these patients. This lack of venous occlusions is attributed to the routine heparinization of these patients during the procedure and to the meticulous care of the entry sites during the sheath introduction, during the procedure, and following the removal of the large sheaths. All of these patients were placed on aspirin for six months following the procedure, which also may have contributed to the paucity of venous occlusive problems!

The experience with intravascular stents in systemic arteries is relatively limited, but like the venous stents, requires a large introductory sheath. Like the venous entry sites, the complications from the even larger sheaths that are necessary for implanting stents in coarctation of the aorta, have been very rare and probably also are infrequent because of the close, personal attention and care of the arteries during the introduction of the sheath, during the procedure, and after the removal of the sheath from the artery.

Although the majority of the central complications of intravascular stents occur during stent implants, there are a few problems which occur in or around previously implanted stents during catheter manipulation or additional interventional procedures in vessels that were stented previously. Stents implanted even years earlier, can cause problems during subsequent catheter manipulations.

It is quite easy to trap a catheter or wire in an exposed, side "cell" of a J & J™ Palmaz™ P _ _ 8 stent. Catheters as large as 8-French easily pass into and through the *side, fully "expanded diamond"* opening of an expanded J & J™ Palmaz™ P _ _ 8 stent, but at the same time, even a very small catheter or wire can be difficult to withdraw from these same "diamond" spaces. Because of the diamond configuration of the spaces, a catheter that is perpendicular to the wall of the stent passes easily *into and through* the *center* of the diamond space (Figure 22.14a) but, when attempting to withdraw the catheter out of the diamond of the cell and if the catheter assumes even the slightest angle to the stent, the catheter is pulled to the side of the cell and wedged into a corner of the diamond and, in turn, becomes entrapped in the acute, sharp corner by the acute angles of the diamond (Figure 22.14b). The more forcefully the catheter is pulled, the tighter the catheter is pulled into the acute angle in the diamond and the tighter the catheter becomes entrapped. This same mechanism of trapping occurs with smaller catheters and/or wires, which pass into the side cells of the stents more easily. Prevention of this problem is the most important treatment. As a consequence, great care should be taken in the manipulation of *any* catheter or wire *in the area of*, or back through, a previously implanted stent.

When a catheter becomes trapped in the side of a stent, however, recovery is possible. A relatively stiff, curved wire is used within the trapped catheter to free the catheter. A 3–4 cm long, 60–90° curve is formed on the stiff end of a standard 0.035″ or 0.038″ teflon-coated guide wire. The curve on the stiff end of the teflon wire is formed outside of the body and outside of the catheter. The curved, stiff end of the wire is introduced into the proximal end of the entrapped catheter and advanced to the area where the catheter is trapped through the side hole of the stent. The preformed curve of the wire within the catheter, in turn, creates a new curve in the shaft of the *catheter* at the location where it enters the side of the stent and, in doing so, *changes the angle* of entrance of the catheter through the side, diamond shaped opening in the stent to a more perpendicular orientation to the side of the stent. The more perpendicular the catheter becomes relative to the long axis of the stent, the more likely the catheter will be to move to the center of the "diamond" and spring free of the stent. The new curve formed on the *catheter* by the wire eventually will be sufficient to change the direction of the catheter as it passes into the side of the stent enough to loosen the catheter from the corner of the "diamond" in the stent wall. While holding the wire in this location, the catheter is withdrawn in very small increments while gently "jiggling" it out of the stent. If this does not accomplish the release, the position of the wire within the catheter or the curve in the wire is changed until the catheter eventually becomes aligned perpendicularly and springs free.

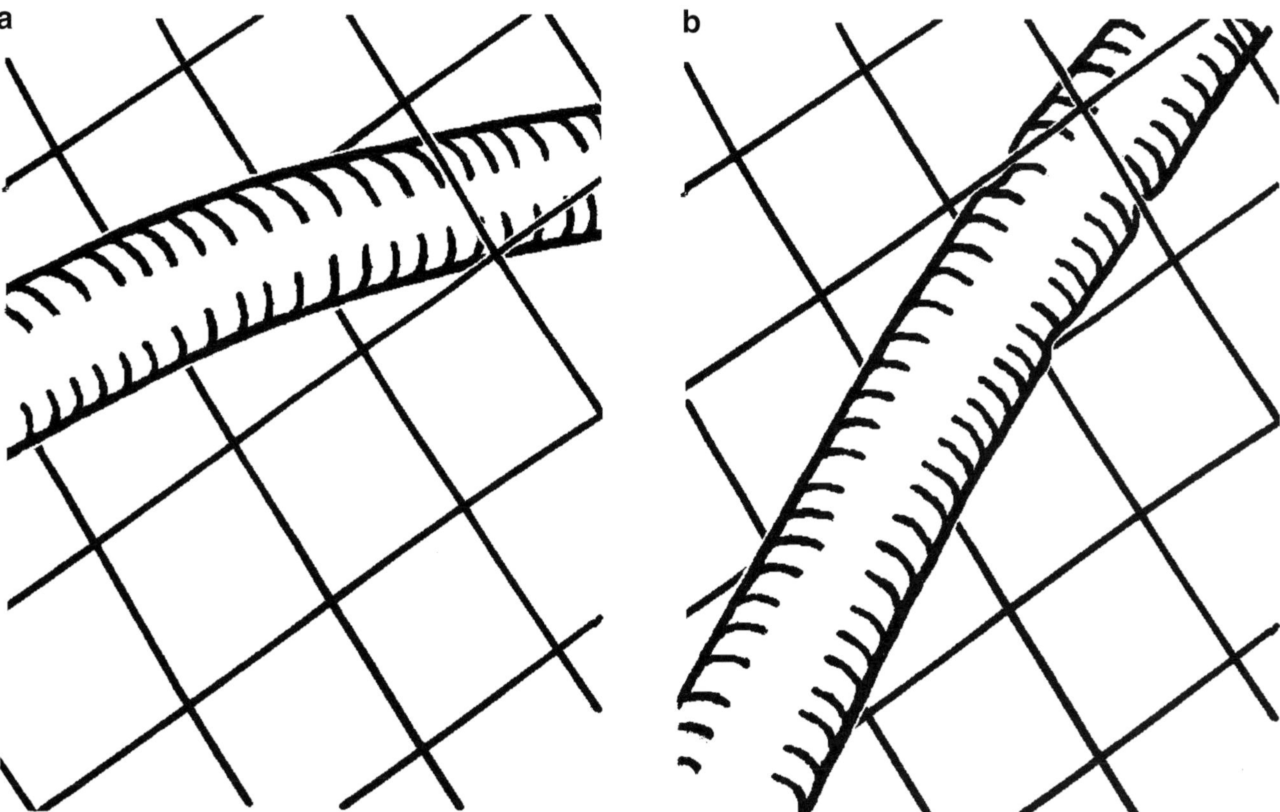

Figure 22.14 (a) Catheter passing straight (perpendicular) through side cells of stent; (b) catheter passing through side cell on an angle and trapped in side cell of stent.

The same "change in the curve" of the catheter can be accomplished using a 0.035″ or 0.038″ "active deflector wire" within the trapped catheter. The active deflector wire is introduced into the trapped catheter as a straight wire and advanced to the area where the catheter enters the stent. A "deflection" curve is formed gradually on the tip of the wire (and, in turn, the catheter). As the catheter curve changes, gentle traction along with slight "jiggling" is applied to the catheter. When there still is resistance to withdrawal of the catheter, the amount of, and location of, the curve are altered until eventually the catheter becomes perpendicular to the "diamond", loosens, and can be withdrawn from the side of the stent.

When a wire is entrapped in the side of a stent, any attempt at a forceful withdrawal will unravel the spring guide wire. A torque-controlled, end-hole catheter *with a fairly rigid preformed curve* on the tip is advanced over the wire to the stent. The change in the angle at which the catheter/wire enters the stent, is usually enough to allow withdrawal of the wire with minimal subsequent manipulations *and no force*.

Even years after implant, any tip at the ends of the struts of a J & J™ Palmaz™ stent, which continue to protrude into the vessel, remain very sharp. These sharp tips can easily puncture balloons that are within or adjacent to the implanted stent. Occasionally a sharp tip of a strut of a previously implanted stent bends and protrudes inward toward the lumen of the vessel/stent and, as a consequence, the sharp tip pointing toward the lumen will puncture any subsequent balloon that is inflated within the same stent. This problem of potential balloon puncture should always be anticipated in the presence of a previously implanted stent. An attempt is made to avoid the area of protrusion when balloons are expanded adjacent to the area where the stent protrudes. When recognized, a protruding tip occasionally can be pushed "flatter" against the wall of the stent/vessel with a large catheter or sheath, which is stiffened with a heavy, stiff wire within it or with one of the kevlar covered balloons, which is less likely to puncture.

When the *tip* of a strut is protruding at the *end* of a previously implanted stent, the protruding tips are "protected" at least partially from *adjacent* balloons being inflated, by the balloon that is being inflated within the original stent with the protruding tip(s) in order to keep the original stent from being distorted/crushed by the adjacent balloon. This is particularly important when new stents are being implanted in the area of, or within, a previous stent.

Puncture of the implanting balloon during the expansion of a stent results in the balloon being trapped within a partially expanded stent, in which case, the balloon cannot be inflated further nor deflated. When a new stent is to be implanted and there is even *the possibility* of a protruding portion of a previous stent in the area, a "test" inflation with only the balloon is performed. The balloon only is inflated in the precise area where the new stent will be implanted but without the new stent. A punctured balloon alone which is adjacent to a stent is an inconvenience, while a punctured balloon within an unexpanded stent can be a catastrophe.

Previously implanted stents can be compressed, or even crushed, by external pressures which occur in an area/vessel adjacent to the vessel where the stent is implanted. Often this is unavoidable. Compression of stents occasionally occurs with stents that are positioned adjacent to the aorta or the sternum in patients who have had previous surgery. The surgical scarring eliminates the "mobility" of the adjacent vessels in relation to each other. These stents usually were placed in these particular locations to treat stenosis caused by the very same external compression of the vessel. When stents are used in these areas, compression is expected or unavoidable. Some of the Double Strut LD™ stents (Intra Therapeutics Inc., St Paul, MN), which were implanted at diameters of 16 mm or greater, rebounded or shrank from their implant diameters acutely or collapsed partially over time *without* being in areas known to be particularly vulnerable for collapse from external pressure. These particular stents are no longer used in large-diameter vessels. Stents which do shrink or collapse can be treated with re-dilation along with the implant of a second, but stronger, stent within the collapsed stent.

Stents can also be crushed from external, iatrogenic forces. This occurs in the operating room, when a vessel containing the stent is "retracted". The iatrogenic compression of a stent in the operating room can be prevented when the surgeon is aware of the potential problem with the stent, the problem is anticipated, and any external force on the stent is avoided. In the catheterization laboratory, previously implanted stents can be compressed when a vessel is being dilated or an additional stent is being implanted in a vessel which is immediately adjacent to the original vessel with a previously implanted stent. In order to prevent collapse of the original stent, a second balloon should always be positioned in and inflated within the original stent in order to "protect" the original stent and prevent its compression by an expanding balloon in an adjacent vessel. Most stents which are compressed only partially and remain in place, can be treated by re-expansion with a balloon and the implant of an additional stent within the original stent.

The most significant potential late complication from an *implanted stent* has been the erosion *through* the wall of an adjacent structure. In spite of the large number of stents that have been implanted in positions adjacent to the aorta, fortunately, this is an extremely rare occurrence and seems to occur when a stent is implanted adjacent to, and compressed by, a large and markedly dilated aorta and only when there has been previous surgery on one or both of the adjacent vessels. The causes of the erosion in particular patients are unexplained and this problem must be considered in the face of a sudden deterioration of a patient who has a stent implanted adjacent to a large dilated aorta.

Surprisingly, even with the extensive manipulation required in very sick patients and the use of often very large, stiff catheters, wires and sheaths/dilators, there have been very few reported adverse events or permanent sequelae from the *wire/catheter/sheath manipulations* during the delivery and implant of intravascular stents in pediatric/congenital heart patients. This probably is due to the overall extensive experience and the established techniques used by the majority of operators who are performing intravascular stent implants in these patients.

There are, at the same time, numerous, relatively common problems which occur during the delivery and implant of the stents themselves. Displacement of the stents, at least to some degree, during their implant is common in congenital lesions even when the *current* optimal equipment and techniques are utilized. When a stent is displaced significantly, it becomes a complication. Displacement of a stent often is the result of not utilizing the best techniques/equipment available and, in turn, is best treated by prevention. Inaccurate centering of the stent on the balloon or displacement of the stent off the center of the balloon during delivery causes the balloon to inflate asymmetrically and, in turn, "milks" the stent forward or backward during the balloon inflation. Expanding a stent on a balloon which is too large in diameter or too long for the vessel that is immediately *adjacent* to the stenosis, can cause the balloon to be squeezed out of the narrower vessel and away from the area of stenosis. Any unusually narrowed area should be identified angiographically or with sizing balloons before the implant is started and, in turn, avoided by starting with a smaller initial balloon for the implant.

Not using an *extra stiff wire* or poor positioning of the wires during the delivery of stents, will compromise the control over the position of the stent during implant. Inadequate distal wire position, either from softer wires, poor initial position or by loss of position during sheath and/or balloon/stent delivery is a major cause of stent displacement. During the stent expansion, the *stiff portion* of a Super Stiff™ (Medi-Tech, Boston Scientific, Natick, MA) wire must be positioned *entirely* across the lesion and *fixed securely* across the precise area being stented with the floppy tip *and the transition zone* of the wire advanced *well distal to and beyond* the area of stenosis. Also, the Super

Stiff™ wire is pushed forcefully into an "advanced" position into the distal tissues beyond the balloon/stent so that there is no "slack" in the course of the wire or balloon catheter, and no to-and-fro movement of the wire or balloon catheter is possible. When the wire and balloon catheter are maintained in this position, advancing the *wire alone*, even minimally, pushes the balloon catheter and the stent/balloon *backwards* over the wire! With the wire so positioned, the position of the stent can be controlled very precisely—a minimal push on the balloon catheter alone advances the balloon/stent further into the vessel/lesion, while a minimal push on the wire "withdraws" (pushes) the balloon/stent slightly backward in the vessel/lesion, and a forward push on both the balloon catheter and the wire fixes the stent/balloon securely in position. Finally, the balloon/stent is inflated *slowly* so that the balloon/stent position can be adjusted or the inflation can be stopped with any movement of the balloon/stent relative to the lesion.

Once the stent has been implanted with the initial inflation, the stent still can be moved or displaced accidentally by manipulations with a deflated balloon. The relatively rough surface of the deflated balloon can easily become caught within open spaces (cells) of a freshly implanted stent. When any slight rotation or to-and-fro movement of the balloon results in comparable movement of the freshly implanted stent, the likelihood of dislodging the stent becomes very high. This occurs more frequently when a balloon ruptures, but can also occur with any of the deflated "angioplasty" balloons, which have very rough, deflated profiles even when not ruptured. Entrapments of the balloon in a stent owing to balloon ruptures are more serious and are covered in detail in subsequent paragraphs. Entrapment of a rough but still intact balloon for the most part is preventable or treatable. First, the choice of a balloon with a *smoother profile* for the implant of the stent helps to prevent this. Secondly, always reintroducing the sheath into the stent over the ***deflating*** balloon *as the implanting balloon is being deflated* separates the rough surface of the balloon from the inner surface of the stent and prevents the balloon from becoming entrapped within the stent.

In the situation where the sheath cannot be re-advanced over the deflating balloon and the freshly implanted stent moves every time the balloon is moved, the additional angiographic catheter, which is already adjacent to the stent, is used to "buttress" the stent while an attempt is made at withdrawing the balloon from the stent. A gentle (25–30°) curve, which corresponds to the curve in the vessel *proximal to the stent*, is formed at the transition portion of a *short floppy tipped*, 0.035" Super Stiff™ wire. This wire is introduced into the adjacent angiographic catheter and advanced to the tip of the catheter. The now "stiffened" catheter is advanced against the exposed proximal end of the stent. As the catheter is pushed against the end of the stent, the balloon is "jiggled" gently and withdrawn carefully out of the stent. Occasionally the rounded end of the angiographic catheter will pass preferentially into the stent (when *not* desired!) and will not catch securely against the end of the stent. In this situation, the angiographic catheter is replaced with an end-hole catheter. The same stiff wire is introduced into, and advanced to *just within the tip* of the end-hole catheter to be used to stiffen the end-hole catheter. The "squared" hollow tip and the distal opening of the end-hole catheter definitely will catch on, and, in turn, will tend to "buttress" against the end of the freshly implanted stent, supporting the stent enough to withdraw the balloon out of the stent.

Balloon punctures, leaks or disruptions during stent implants produce even more serious "events" and often result in major or even permanent sequelae. These problems occur primarily (only?) with the J & J™ Palmaz™ stents. Balloon leaks and disruptions are a result of several different problems. Both punctures and balloon ruptures/disruptions are more common with thin-walled dilation balloons and during stent implants into the pulmonary arteries. The punctures can be very tiny with miniscule leaks or, at the other extreme, can be massive as a result of a total disruption of the balloon. Both small leaks in balloons and disruptions of balloons create significant problems during stent implants.

The most common causes of balloon *puncture* are the sharp points that occur as the distal ends of the struts of the J & J™ Palmaz™ stents. The effects of the sharp tips are accentuated by the "flare" created at the ends of the stents when each end of the *balloon* expands significantly before any of the stent itself begins to expand (described and illustrated previously in this chapter). The likelihood of this type of puncture is increased when the balloon which is used for the implant is *longer* than the particular stent and, in turn, extends significantly beyond the ends of the stent, or when the implanting balloon/stent is expanded to a very large initial diameter with a single expansion of a large balloon. This combination results in the distal ends of the balloon expanding almost completely before the ends of the stent even begin to expand (*see* Figure 22.2). As the balloon continues to expand ahead of the ends of the stent, the sharp tips of the struts of the stent are directed *into the expanding wall* of the balloon. These punctures occur during the initial expansion of the ends of the stent and can result in the majority of the stent *not expanding* at all. The incidence of this particular type of puncture is decreased by using balloons that are *shorter* than the length of the stent for the delivery of the stents, using balloons that do not have long shoulders, and by using stents that do not have sharp tips at the ends.

Another potential reason for the puncture of a balloon is when J & J™ Palmaz™ stents are implanted in *curved* lesions. This cause of puncture is somewhat similar to the condition which occurs when the balloon for delivery of the stent is too long for the stent. When a balloon begins to inflate in a curved location, the balloon expands very asymmetrically and the concave surface of the balloon, which extends beyond the end of the stent, is "folded" over, and initially expands acutely against the end of the straight stent. This places the surface of the balloon perpendicularly against the pointed tips at the end of the struts of the stent. Again the problem is avoided, or at least lessened, by using balloons shorter than the stent and by using stents with "rounded" ends.

When "bifurcating" J & J™ stents are implanted simultaneously, the flaring sharp tips of one of the stents can easily puncture the balloon which is being inflated in the adjacent stent. This is particularly true as the balloons inflate to large diameters and the flaring, sharp struts at the ends of the stents develop a very acute angle off the inflating balloon. The remedy for this is to minimize or prevent the flaring by using shorter balloons or to expand each stent *sequentially* using separate, sequential balloons or BIB™ balloons (NuMED Inc., Hopkinton, NY) for the delivery of larger stents. Using stents without sharp tips at the ends of the struts probably will help to prevent this problem.

Occasionally a balloon is punctured while the stent is being mounted onto the balloon or during any lengthwise repositioning of the stent on the balloon. These punctures in the surface of the balloon are very minute openings, which cannot be seen and can easily go unnoticed until an attempt is made to expand the balloon/stent. This type of puncture is avoided by "opening" the stent slightly and "flaring" one end of the stent with a dilator, before introducing the balloon into the stent during the mounting of the stent and by very precise, meticulous, and gentle introduction of the stent into the balloon. If at all possible, "repositioning" of the stent on the balloon is avoided by the proper centering of the stent on the balloon initially and before the stent is crimped on the balloon. A tiny puncture that cannot be seen, becomes apparent when the balloon with the mounted stent is placed on strong negative pressure while the stent is being mounted/crimped on the balloon. With strong negative pressure, a tiny, continuous stream of bubbles appears in the fluid within the syringe of the inflator. A strong vacuum should always be placed on a mounted stent/balloon to test for tiny leaks before the stent/balloon is introduced into the patient.

A *small* leak in the balloon during the implant of a stent is indicated by the stent not expanding properly, if at all, as fluid is delivered to the balloon as pressure is applied slowly with the inflator. Simultaneously, as the balloon inflation is attempted, a faint "whiff" of contrast will appear distally in the vessel where the stent is being implanted. This "free" contrast is very subtle and may not be seen at all when there is a tiny leak. These leaks in balloons can be the beginning of a major crisis or, at the very least, a significant problem. The management of this "crisis" depends upon at which stage in the expansion of the stent the leak occurs, when it is noted and, of course, the magnitude of the leak. If there is a large leak due to a large tear in the balloon, the leak is more obvious, the problem usually is much more serious and there are fewer alternatives for recovery.

If the balloon is noted to have a tiny leak before the stent even *begins* to expand, there occasionally can be an effective fairly simple remedy. Stop the balloon inflation immediately and apply negative pressure to the balloon. An attempt is made at withdrawing the balloon/stent carefully back into the sheath. Even when the stent does not expand at all, this usually is *not* possible and an alternative recovery technique is used. When the leak is first noticed after the ends of the stent have started to expand and the ends are expanded to a diameter just larger than the sheath, there are several choices for recovery. The alternatives again depend upon the degree of expansion of the stent and the magnitude of the leak in the balloon. In the presence of a very tiny "pin hole" or "puncture" leak in the balloon where the ends of the stent have expanded very slightly while the center stays collapsed and the stent otherwise stays in position, an attempt is made to further inflate and implant the stent in spite of the small leak.

The further expansion of the stent is attempted by inflating the balloon/stent combination faster than the injected fluid can leak from the tiny hole! A *hard syringe* with a capacity the *same as the balloon* is filled with *normal saline*. The saline has a much lower viscosity than the diluted contrast and flows faster through the balloon lumen of the catheter. The saline is injected into the balloon as rapidly, and with as much hand force, as possible. Usually, this expands the balloon with the stent at least a little further. An even more rapid inflation of the leaking dilation balloon can be accomplished by using a pressure (power) injector, which is used for the contrast injections for angiograms, for the rapid inflation of the balloon! The syringe of the power injector is filled with a volume of normal saline 1.5–2 times the capacity of the balloon. This volume is delivered into the balloon at 600 psi with the power injector. The very rapid injection usually dilates the stent further. The increased dilation often is sufficient to fix the stent at least loosely in place within the vessel and allows the removal of the punctured and now torn balloon. The rapid inflation with the injector *usually ruptures* the balloon, necessitating some further tricks for removing the balloon after the stent has been expanded. *Usually* the rupture in the balloon is longitudinal and the balloon material remains intact except for the tear.

After the "power inflation" and slight further expansion of the stent, the balloon, which now definitely is ruptured, is deflated as much as possible. First an attempt is made at advancing the sheath into the stent over the ruptured balloon and withdrawing the balloon out of the stent through the sheath. This usually is not possible, in which case, the long sheath and/or the adjacent catheter is/are advanced against the proximal end of the stent to "buttress" and help hold the stent in position while the balloon catheter is withdrawn very carefully out of the stent. This often requires a relatively forceful withdrawal to pull the balloon out of the stent and back into the delivery sheath. If the ruptured balloon can be withdrawn out of the stent but not into the sheath, the wire is maintained in position and the balloon and sheath are withdrawn completely out of the body. All of this maneuvering is observed almost continuously on fluoroscopy. During the withdrawal of the balloon, the balloon catheter is rotated very slowly to try to "refold" the torn "wings" of the balloon around the catheter. This maneuver is very delicate and can easily dislodge the stent in spite of the buttressing with the sheath/catheter.

If the original ruptured balloon cannot be withdrawn out of a minimally expanded stent without dislodging the stent, an attempt is made to expand the stent further starting with a new, much smaller, low-profile balloon, which is advanced within the stent adjacent to the ruptured balloon over a separate wire through a separate introducer! This obviously is a major undertaking. The original, additional angiographic catheter is replaced with an end-hole catheter, or if the second catheter was not in place, a small end-hole catheter, which will accommodate a 0.035″ wire, is introduced from a separate venous puncture and manipulated into the involved pulmonary artery. Using torque-controlled wires, skill and patience, a wire and then the second catheter is maneuvered into the partially expanded stent, adjacent to the trapped, ruptured balloon and completely *through* the stent into the more distal vessel. Once the catheter is distal to the stent, the end-hole catheter is replaced with as stiff a wire as possible, which will accommodate a new, small, *very low-profile* balloon dilation catheter. The diameter of the balloon must be sufficient to expand the stent further but the deflated balloon must be able to pass adjacent to the original balloon. The very low-profile balloon is advanced/manipulated over the wire and into the stent, next to the ruptured balloon. The new balloon is expanded within the stent (and adjacent to the trapped, ruptured, original balloon). This expands the stent further and helps to fix the stent more securely in place in the vessel. This first expansion/fixation with the low-profile balloon usually is sufficient to allow the withdrawal of the ruptured balloon. Occasionally, however, a second, even larger balloon may have to be used in sequence and adjacent to the ruptured balloon to expand the stent enough before the ruptured balloon can be withdrawn safely and completely. Using sequentially larger balloons, the stent is expanded until the ruptured balloon can be removed, and eventually the desired diameter of the stent is achieved. Once the original, torn balloon has been removed, a new balloon of the size necessary to expand the stent fully is introduced over the original wire and into the stent to complete the expansion of the stent to the desired diameter.

During all of these manipulations, there is nothing to prevent the stent from being displaced forward if pushed by the balloon or a catheter entering it! When a stent does displace distally, the wire still should be maintained through the stent and in a very distal, secured position. If the stent is displaced forward (distal to the stenosis) and off the original balloon during these maneuvers, a balloon that is slightly larger than the diameter of the partially inflated stent is advanced over the wire, into and completely *through* the stent until at least the *distal* end of the balloon extends beyond the distal end of the stent. The *proximal* end of the balloon will be positioned *within* the distal end of the stent or rarely the entire balloon will be *totally distal* to the stent. The balloon is inflated slowly and at low pressure, hopefully expanding the part of the *balloon* that is distal and outside of the stent, and expanding the balloon (only) to a diameter equal to the diameter of the stent *without expanding the stent at all*. In this way, the stent becomes "trapped" on the proximal catheter *shaft* or actually on the proximal end of the balloon. The catheter, balloon, and stent are withdrawn over the wire back into the area of stenosis until the stent is against the "buttressing" edge of the long sheath or the second catheter. The original delivery wire should remain fixed in its position as far distally as possible during all of the maneuvers with the balloon/stent/catheter. With the stent maintained in place by the tip of the long sheath or the tip of a second catheter, the balloon is slowly deflated partially while simultaneously withdrawing the balloon very carefully further *into* the stent until it is centered within the stent. This balloon/stent is then inflated in the lesion, in order to secure the stent within the lesion at least partially. While still "buttressing" the proximal edge of the stent with the long sheath, this balloon, which is smaller than the lesion, is withdrawn carefully over the wire and replaced with a larger balloon that is sufficient to secure the stent firmly in the lesion.

Occasionally during some of these maneuvers, the *sheath* actually passes over the *balloon* and enters, or even passes completely through, the loose *stent*. The *sheath within* a loose stent is a "double-edged sword". The ruptured balloon certainly can be withdrawn more easily through and out of the stent with the stent "protected" from the balloon by the sheath. However, the sheath *within* or through the stent provides no support for holding (buttressing) the stent in its desired position. If the partially inflated diameter of the stent is not enough to hold the stent against the wall of the stenosis, the stent can easily move forward *or backward* in the vessel *over* the sheath within the stent. When the sheath passes into the stent in this circumstance, the *second catheter* positioned against the proximal end of the stent is absolutely *essential* in order to buttress the stent and keep it from being pulled *back* out of the lesion into a larger more central vessel! With the stent maintained in this position with the second catheter, a new, larger diameter balloon is advanced through the sheath (and stent) and centered within the stent. While "buttressing" the stent in this location with the second catheter, the *sheath* is withdrawn out of the stent and off of the balloon. The balloon is inflated to expand and fix the stent in its proper location.

If the stent moves forward (distally), and cannot be "trapped" and withdrawn by a balloon passed completely through it as just described, the stent is expanded and fixed in the more distal location in the involved vessel. Even though this is not the originally desired position, there is little, or no, consequence from implanting the stent in a distal, normal vessel. The major potential problem is that the distally displaced/implanted stent may cross a significant, side or branching vessel when expanded. This usually can be avoided but, if it does occur, is of little or no consequence in the more distal vessels.

When the stent, which is not fixed in the vessel, does move backward (proximally) from the lesion and over the sheath which has passed *within the stent*, the situation becomes more precarious. Attempts at withdrawing the sheath from within the stent usually aggravate the situation by withdrawing and displacing the stent still further proximally along with the sheath. This is another situation where the second (or third) additional catheter(s), which *already are present* in the vessel being stented, is/are essential! If the additional catheter is not in place or is *not* an end-hole catheter, the manipulations with the long sheath and loose stent are *stopped* immediately. A separate, preferably large French size, *end-hole*, catheter is introduced into a vein and advanced to a position just proximal to the stent in the involved vessel. A slight (25–30°) curve is placed on the *stiff end* of a standard 0.038″ teflon guide wire. The wire is advanced to just within the tip of the end-hole catheter, which is positioned proximal to the stent in the involved vessel. The stiff end of the wire is used to stiffen and provide more control over the "extra" catheter.

The catheter, which is "reinforced" with the wire, is advanced and manipulated until the tip of the catheter "catches" against one of the ends of a strut at the proximal end of the stent. Because of its rounded distal tip, the separate *angiographic* catheter, which may have been in place already, usually will *not* catch on, or allow a significant push against, the end of the stent. When the only *additional* catheter is an angiographic catheter, it is replaced with an end-hole catheter. The "squared" end, along with the opening of the end-hole catheter, usually catches the end of the stent with minimal manipulations of the catheter. Occasionally the angle of the wire *within the catheter* must be modified several times in order to accomplish this. The "stiffened" catheter against the end of the stent is used to stabilize the stent in position while the sheath is manipulated. When there is any proximal displacement of the stent out of the lesion, the reinforced catheter is used to attempt to "push" the stent forward (distally) over the sheath and back into the precise lesion. The catheter with the stiff end of the wire within the catheter and both pushing against the stent usually are sufficient to hold the stent in place during further manipulations of the sheath. During all of these maneuvers, extra care is taken to maintain the position of the *original delivery wire* through, and well distal to, the stent and balloon.

Once the stent is supported, the original ruptured balloon is withdrawn through the sheath and replaced with a new, larger diameter balloon and preferably a balloon shorter than the original balloon initially used to implant the stent. The new balloon is centered within the stent while the sheath still is within the stent. While "holding" the stent with the additional venous catheter(s) and holding the balloon in position over the wire within the stent, the sheath is withdrawn slowly and gently from within the stent and completely off the balloon until the sheath tip is just proximal to the balloon. The stent may need to be pushed purposefully distally by the "holding" catheter as the sheath is being withdrawn. Once the sheath is removed, the balloon is expanded at low pressure and just enough to approximate the inside of the partially expanded stent. With the larger balloon expanded at low pressure within the stent and before expanding the stent further, the balloon catheter can be used to help reposition the stent. An angiogram is performed to confirm the exact position. The stent is expanded in this position with the new balloon.

When a high-pressure, rapid inflation of a *punctured* balloon in the stent does not expand the stent sufficiently to fix the stent or to allow the removal of the balloon, the original balloon must be extracted from the very minimally expanded stent by alternative means. The sheath is advanced forward against the proximal end of the stent and used to "buttress" the stent as the balloon is withdrawn forcefully (hopefully intact!). If the sheath alone is not rigid enough to hold the stent in place, the tip of an additional end-hole catheter supported by a stiff wire, as described above, is advanced against the end of the stent adjacent to the tip of the sheath. During all of these manipulations, extra attention must be paid to maintaining the delivery wire through the stent and in its very secure distal location. By utilizing both the tip of the sheath *and* the tip of a stiffened, extra catheter together against the proximal end of the stent, the stent is held in place while the balloon is rotated and forcefully withdrawn from the stent. This maneuver usually is successful in removing the balloon although it may distort the stent significantly or further disrupt the balloon in the process. If the stent is distorted, the proximal end of the stent is reopened with a very low-profile, very small, dilation balloon passed over the wire and into the proximal end of the distorted stent. The low-profile balloon is *advanced* sequentially through the stent and reinflated until the entire stent is expanded to the diameter of the balloon.

Once the original, ruptured balloon has been removed from the non-expanded stent and the stent has been opened even slightly, but is still held in place only by the end of the sheath or the tip of the extra catheter, the smaller balloon is replaced with a slightly larger diameter, still low-profile, dilation balloon. If possible, the balloons that are used for the sequential dilations are made of a thicker walled, tougher material even at the expense of the low profile. Eventually a large enough balloon is introduced into the stent to fix the stent in place in the original lesion.

Large tears or total disruptions of balloons occur during stent implant. They occur as an extension of a small puncture or leak, but more commonly, are a consequence of excessive pressure applied locally to the balloon or the use of balloons which basically are unsatisfactory for stent implant. The management of longitudinal tears generally is similar to the management of large punctures. Circumferential tears in the balloon can lead to displacement of the distal part of the balloon and are more likely to dislodge the stent during attempted removal of the balloon.

All of the problems of balloon rupture and entrapment during a stent implant are more common and are far more serious when the involved stent is in a pulmonary artery. A bare, partially opened stent, particularly with expanded ends, should *never* be withdrawn through the right ventricle. When the stent is displaced *distally* into a branch pulmonary artery and cannot be withdrawn and secured back into the original stenotic lesion, it is expanded and fixed in the distal branch pulmonary artery distal to the original stenosis as described above.

If the stent, now with the new balloon within it, is displaced proximally into the larger more proximal branch pulmonary artery or even into the main pulmonary artery, the first attempt is to re-advance the stent/balloon combination over the wire and back into the original stenotic site. When the partially expanded stent cannot be maneuvered back to the stenosed area, the next alternative is to reposition the proximally displaced stent into the contralateral pulmonary artery, which in the presence of unilateral branch pulmonary artery stenosis, usually is larger. The balloon/stent combination is withdrawn over the wire, completely into the main pulmonary artery, and the balloon is partially deflated but kept within the stent. It is imperative to maintain a secure wire position through the errant stent to maintain at least partial control on the alignment of the stent in the pulmonary artery. If the wire is inadvertently withdrawn from within the stent, the stent will become free floating and tumble around in the main pulmonary artery or even back into the right ventricle (particularly in the presence of significant pulmonary regurgitation). This makes recapture of the stent difficult, time consuming, or even impossible. The deflated balloon remains partially reinflated in order to help fix and align the stent in the main pulmonary artery.

In order to move the displaced stent from the main into the contralateral pulmonary artery, a new, additional wire must be passed *through the stent* and then positioned securely in the contralateral pulmonary artery. An additional end-hole catheter is introduced into another vein. This additional catheter is manipulated adjacent to the original delivery wire and the partially deflated balloon and *through* the central lumen of the loose stent. After it has passed *completely through* the true lumen of the errant stent, the *new catheter* is manipulated into the contralateral pulmonary artery, far distally and into a large branch of that pulmonary artery with the use of torque-controlled wires or deflector wires. A new Super Stiff™ wire is advanced through the catheter and fixed in the contralateral pulmonary artery. Once the new Super Stiff™ wire is in a secure position through the stent and *into the contralateral pulmonary artery*, the original balloon is deflated fully and withdrawn from the stent and then the *original* Super Stiff™ delivery wire is withdrawn from the original lesion, out of the stent and out of the body.

Once the new stiff wire is secured through the stent in the contralateral vessel and the original wire is withdrawn, a new balloon, which is slightly larger than the partially expanded, loose stent, is introduced over the new wire and into the stent. The balloon is inflated *at a low pressure* with the balloon centered or slightly distally within the stent in order to fix the previously loose stent on the balloon, but not to expand the stent further. With the stent fixed on the balloon, the balloon/stent is advanced into the larger contralateral pulmonary artery over the wire. The rounded tip of the balloon extending distally to the stent facilitates this maneuver. When successfully maneuvered into the contralateral vessel, the balloon and stent are "wedged" into the most distal possible part of the vessel and the balloon is expanded to its maximum diameter/pressure to fix the stent in place. In order to fix the stent more securely in this vessel, it may be necessary to replace this balloon with a slightly larger balloon and repeat the inflation. It usually is necessary, and certainly is advisable, to secure the stent in this position by "buttressing" the stent with the tip of the additional end-hole catheter during the exchange to a larger balloon. Once the original stent is fixed in this location, the balloon and wire are withdrawn and the implant of a stent into the original lesion is restarted with the positioning of a new wire through the lesion!

If the balloon/stent cannot be advanced into the contralateral vessel, then significantly more serious alternatives must be considered. One possible solution is to dilate and fix the balloon/stent in the main pulmonary artery. This usually is not possible because of the very large diameters of the central pulmonary artery. Only if all of these maneuvers and positions for the stent have been considered/tried and are not possible, is the withdrawal of the stent over a balloon and out of the pulmonary artery, through the right ventricle and back into the inferior vena cava even considered. There is *absolutely* ***no totally safe*** way to withdraw an exposed, even minimally expanded, stent/balloon through the right ventricle and tricuspid valve. If any parts of the ends of the struts of the stent are elevated off the surface of the balloon when the balloon is inflated within a stent, withdrawal should never be considered.

The withdrawal of a displaced, partially expanded balloon/stent from the pulmonary to a more proximal systemic vein may be considered in only two circumstances. The first is when the *proximal end* of the incompletely expanded stent either still is within, or can be withdrawn back into, the tip of the sheath, or at the very least, the proximal end is not expanded ***at all*** on the balloon. In that circumstance, the proximal end of the stent forms a tight fit and a "tapered trailing funnel" extending distally over the ruptured balloon. With this rare situation, an attempt at withdrawing the combination stent, balloon and sheath through the right ventricle is considered. At the same time, the consequences of the partially expanded balloon/stent becoming entrapped in the right ventricle/tricuspid valve apparatus must always be considered very seriously and surgical support must be available immediately.

The other circumstance when a withdrawal of the exposed, partially expanded balloon/stent through the right ventricle is attempted, is when the partially inflated balloon fills the entire, partially expanded stent very "snugly" with the stent fitting *tightly* on, and expanded *smoothly* over the surface of the balloon. There must be no free or flared ends or struts of the stent extending off the surface of the balloon proximally, and the balloon ends should be expanded slightly *larger* in diameter than the ends of the stent. It is *not* advisable to consider withdrawing a partially opened stent through the tricuspid valve if there is ***even one*** sharp end of a strut or edge of the stent extending away from the surface of the balloon.

Even with a balloon expanded smoothly within a stent, there is still a chance of a tip of the exposed stent becoming "elevated" off the balloon and catching on the valve apparatus! The combination of the inflated balloon filling the partially expanded stent along with the sheath, is carefully withdrawn all together over the Super Stiff™ wire which is still fixed across the lesion and into the far distal pulmonary artery. Once the partially inflated balloon/stent combination is through the right ventricle (and tricuspid valve!), the combination is withdrawn until the stent can be fixed in a benign location more proximally in the venous system (e.g. the inferior vena cava or iliac vein). When the original stent has been fixed securely in a peripheral venous location, the implant of an additional stent into the original location is reconsidered.

If, before the original balloon ruptured, the stent was expanded too much for the stent to be withdrawn back into the sheath but, at the same time, the balloon did not expand the stent enough to allow removal of the balloon by any of the previously described techniques, then the choices depend more upon the location of the stent. Usually, in this circumstance, the ends of the stent are flared and the flared ends are the only part of the stent which expanded! Repeated attempts are made at introducing the sheath into and through the stent over the ruptured balloon or withdrawing the balloon forcefully from the stent supported against the end of the sheath and extra support catheter. The risks of further attempts at catheter recovery are significantly higher when the ruptured balloon cannot be withdrawn from the stent at all and, at the same time, the stent is expanded partially off the surface of the balloon.

When a non-expanded stent with the entrapped balloon is secure in the *pulmonary artery* and while the patient is still in the catheterization laboratory, surgery can be scheduled and performed, on a less than "urgent" basis on that same day, and the removal of the stent/balloon from the pulmonary artery can usually be performed without cardiopulmonary bypass. If, on the other hand, the stent/balloon combination becomes entangled in the right ventricle/tricuspid valve during an attempt at withdrawal, the valve is both propped open and partially obstructed or there may be damage to the valve. If the stent *over the balloon* does become trapped within the right ventricle, an attempt is made at withdrawing the deflated balloon over the wire and out of the stent, leaving the stent in the right ventricle. The stent alone does not cause obstruction to flow and occasionally the stent can be grasped and gently teased out of the ventricle[21]. If not, with the patient remaining stable, the patient can be scheduled for relatively elective surgery. When the stent with the balloon becomes trapped in the right ventricle and the balloon cannot be withdrawn from the stent, the patient requires emergency surgery, which now must be performed on cardiopulmonary bypass. The alternative of a referral for elective surgical removal of a partially expanded stent on a ruptured balloon, which is positioned securely in a pulmonary artery and cannot be manipulated to a benign position in either pulmonary artery, is prudent and *always* should be considered.

When a partially expanded stent on a ruptured balloon is present in, or is withdrawn to, a position *in the right atrium or in either vena cava*, and the balloon catheter is still over the wire, the preferable approach is to implant the stent securely in the inferior vena cava in a position away from significant branching/side veins. The wire within the stent/balloon is maneuvered through the stent/balloon, across the right atrium and into the opposite vena cava. This provides a guarantee that a stent that could become totally free from the balloon, cannot embolize into the right ventricle. The original balloon is withdrawn from the stent and a balloon large enough to expand and fix the stent in the caudal inferior vena cava is advanced over the wire and into the loose, partially expanded stent. The balloon is expanded at a very low pressure and just enough to fill and "trap" the partially expanded stent. This usually results in the ends of the balloon expanding slightly larger than the stent and, in turn, "covering" or extending over the ends of the loose stent. The balloon/stent combination is withdrawn into the appropriate location in the inferior vena cava and the balloon is inflated fully, hopefully fixing the stent in that location in the cava.

The alternative for a loose stent that is in the right atrium or either cava, is to attempt removal of the combination stent/balloon from the vascular system by a catheter technique. If a wire is *not* present through the balloon catheter, an exchange length wire is advanced through the balloon catheter, out of the tip of the catheter and maneuvered as far as possible into the opposite vena cava. The partially expanded stent, which is stuck over the balloon, potentially can be "re-compressed" over the balloon with a snare and then withdrawn, at least to a superficial vein, and partially if not completely into a large sheath and out of the body. A 20 mm Microvena™ snare in a snare catheter is introduced through a separate very large sheath. The separate introductory site preferably is into the same vessel and immediately adjacent to the original long sheath. An alternative introductory site is through the internal jugular vein when the original balloon/stent was introduced from the femoral vein or, just the opposite, from the femoral vein when the original balloon/stent was introduced from the jugular approach.

The snare catheter, which is introduced from the separate puncture site, is advanced with the enclosed snare to a position immediately adjacent to the *distal end* of the wire, which is in the opposite vena cava. The snare is opened in the opposite cava and maneuvered next to the *distal end* of the wire, which more proximally is passing through the balloon catheter/stent. The guide wire within the balloon catheter, which is still passing out of the tip of the balloon catheter and across the atrium, is withdrawn slowly until the tip of the wire is withdrawn just *proximal* to the open snare. This allows the open snare to be maneuvered over the tip of the wire and eventually maneuvered/withdrawn over the balloon catheter and around the balloon/stent combination. The wire is re-advanced out of the balloon catheter so that it again is secure in the opposite vena cava. The wire passing completely across the atrium provides a control or "safety net" to ensure that a "dislodged" stent cannot embolize into the right ventricle. With the wire in this position, the snare, which is over the stent, is tightened around the balloon/stent until the stent begins to collapse *slightly*. The snare is loosened and moved several millimeters up or down the stent and the tightening is repeated. The entire process is repeated until the entire length of the stent has been re-compressed slightly over the balloon. The "squeezing" of the stent is performed in small increments, moving along the length of the stent. A very strong compression in any one area can indent and distort the stent, which would prevent further uniform compression.

This repeated "squeezing" process along the entire length of the stent with the snare compresses the stent close to its original, non-expanded diameter. Even if this compression still does not allow the stent to be withdrawn into the original delivery sheath, it does allow the stent to be withdrawn into a very peripheral vein near the introductory site into the vessel. The snare is positioned around the *most proximal part* of the stent, and while compressing the proximal end of the stent along with the disrupted balloon with the snare, the combination of the balloon/stent, the original long sheath, the encircling snare and the adjacent snare catheter are withdrawn as far into the introductory vein as possible, while all of the time keeping the guide wire across the right atrium and into the opposite vena cava. The stent can usually be withdrawn to within a few millimeters of the introductory site into the vessel, where the balloon/stent should be palpable beneath the skin just cephalad to the puncture site. The snare is released and an attempt is made at withdrawing the catheter/balloon/stent through the puncture site. When significant resistance is encountered, the balloon/stent on the catheter is removed through a small cut-down over the vessel.

In addition to the previously discussed complications of stent implants, all of the complications of balloon dilation alone also occur during the implant of stents, but the usual complications associated with the balloons alone occur far less frequently. Rupture of vessels is a complication of balloon dilation but rarely occurs during stent implant. With stent implants that are performed properly, the vessels are dilated only to the diameter of the adjacent normal vessel and *not* over-dilated. Dilation to the nominal vessel diameter seldom ruptures a vessel.

Hyperperfusion of dilated segments of the lung occurs with stent implants, and probably to a greater degree than with balloon dilation alone. Once a vessel is opened to a certain diameter with a stent, no "recoil" or spasm of the stented vessel can occur to reduce the flow to the vessel distal to the *dilated and stented* area as opposed to a vessel which undergoes dilation only. Treatment of the complications that are common to both balloon dilation alone and balloon dilation with stents is the same for both etiologies and is covered in Chapter 15 on "Balloon Dilation—General" and Chapter 17 on "Balloon Dilation of Branch Pulmonary Arteries".

Once implanted, intravascular stents have had remarkably few late complications in congenital heart patients. There usually is a less than one half to one mm of a normal layer of protective neo-intima build-up within the lumen of the stent. This thin layer is present between the metal struts as well as over the surface of the struts and does not narrow the lumen of the larger vessels significantly. This usually occurs within three months, is smooth, and has not been shown to accumulate further even over very extended lengths of time for as long as a decade or more.

A greater intimal build-up does occur in stents/vessels when significant discrepancies remain in the diameters of the lumens within the vessel and stent. This atypical, selective, intimal build-up does *not* narrow the vessel to a diameter which is less than the narrowest *adjacent* non-stented lumen or the narrowest area within the stent which is present at the time of implant. The selective neo-intimal reaction is thought to be a consequence of the excessive turbulence in the blood flow caused by the variable diameters at the involved areas within the vessel. The turbulence results in an exaggeration of the normal stimulus to neo-intima formation caused by the implanted stent itself. The extra build-up of intima tends to "streamline" the vessel, narrowing the overall vessel to the narrowest diameter that exists immediately postimplant, rather than actually narrowing the vessel or stent lumen further. This neo-intima tends to create a vessel of uniform, smoother diameter, which is equal in diameter throughout its length to the *narrowest* contiguous area of the vessel/stent at the time of implant.

When a residual "waist" or narrowing persists within a stent immediately after implant, the neo-intima within the stent fills in the adjacent, wider area of the stent over time. This, again, "streamlines" or "smoothes" the entire lumen to correspond to the narrowest residual diameter within the stent immediately after implant. This build-up of intima has been interpreted as "re-stenosis", but it does *not* narrow, or re-stenose the vessel to a *narrower* diameter than the narrowest diameter that was present at the time of implant.

Similarly, when a stent is *over-expanded* to a diameter larger than the adjacent normal vessel during the initial implant, the stent, over time, tends to work its way into, or even *through, the wall* of the vessel. As the stent migrates into and through the wall of the vessel, the vessel wall "heals behind" the expanding stent and grows back within the stent to a diameter equal to that of the *normal adjacent* vessel. The over-expanded stent eventually appears to rest on the outside of the vessel, and creates a measurable distance from the lumen of the vessel to the stent. Even though the stent appears to be outside of the vessel lumen, there have been no consequences of this phenomenon. This thickness of wall within the stent also has been misinterpreted as "re-stenosis" whereas, in fact, the vessel again is "streamlining" and does *not* narrow to a diameter that is less than that of the adjacent vessels. This phenomenon appears to have no consequence, but can be avoided for the most part by not over-expanding a stent beyond the diameter of the *adjacent, non-stenosed* vessel.

There are very rare, true "re-stenoses" in stents implanted in pediatric and congenital vascular lesions. In essentially all cases, however, when re-stenosis is seen, there is some unusual circumstance about the particular implant or it is in a very unusual vessel or with some peculiarity of the tissues of the vessels themselves. Re-stenosis due to malpositioning of a stent or as a result of malalignment in the vessel is avoided by carefully positioning the stent so that the stent aligns exactly *in line with the lumen* of the vessel during implant. In curved or angled vessels, this requires the use of multiple overlapping, shorter, rigid stents or the use of a "flexible" stent in order for the implanted stent to conform to the curvature of the vessels. A long rigid stent placed in a curved vessel results in the sharp ends of the stent digging into the outer curvature of the vessel at an acute angle. In this circumstance, there is continual irritation of the vessel by the sharp tips, and an excessive intimal build-up will occur in those areas.

There are several areas or vessels in congenital heart patients where re-stenosis of the stented vessel occurs almost predictably. The most frustrating of these "vessels" are the pulmonary veins. Regardless of the type, the etiology or the location of stenosis in the pulmonary veins, re-stenosis recurs even after an apparently very successful dilation with a concomitant stent implant, and the re-stenosis recurs within a short period of time. As of this writing there is no satisfactory definitive solution to this particular problem.

The branch pulmonary arteries in patients after an arterial switch procedure for transposition of the great arteries represent another area after stent implant of more frequent re-stenosis. Re-stenosis of these vessels after dilation with stent implants only appears to occur when the particular pulmonary arteries are "stretched" longitudinally and excessively without sufficient freeing up of each pulmonary vessel at each hilus as the pulmonary arteries are pulled anterior to the aorta during a "Le Comp" maneuver. When re-stenosis has occurred in these unique pulmonary arteries after stent implants, it has been treated successfully in all of the cases with re-dilation and further stent implants in any of the re-stenotic areas.

Stents placed in tandem, which do not overlap when implanted or which separate a short distance from each other later during longitudinal growth of the vessel, create a "grinding" area between the ends of the two stents. When the ends of two stents are within one mm of each other, very aggressive intimal build-up and stenosis occurs between the stents. This is avoided by creating sufficient overlap at implant to prevent separation and to allow for the growth of the vessel in length as well as diameter. The alternative is to leave a distance of *at least 5–6 mm* between the ends of the adjacent tandem stents when they are implanted—e.g. when trying to avoid a significant branch vessel which arises between or within an area of stenosis.

Stents implanted adjacent to strong external compressing forces can be compressed or can even collapse. For example, a stent placed in a pulmonary artery directly behind a large dilated aorta occasionally is compressed into an ovoid cross sectional shape or even fractured longitudinally and collapsed. The compression of the pulmonary vessel often was at least part of the indication for the stent to begin with and, in this circumstance, is hard to avoid. A compressed stent is treated by re-dilation with the implant of additional stent(s) within the original compressed stent.

Stents within right ventricular to pulmonary artery conduits, which are situated between the sternum and the muscular beating heart, frequently collapse or actually fracture. This almost is the expected outcome of stents in this location. The collapsed stent may remain in the outflow tract or pieces of these stents break off and embolize to the pulmonary arteries. The distal pieces appear to have no consequences even when left in place in the distal pulmonary arteries. With this knowledge about stents in this location, the decision to implant a stent in this location is made after weighing the temporary relief of the obstruction, which can be achieved by the stent, versus the known, relatively frequent and early adverse events from the collapse of stents there.

There are several reports of "aneurysms" of the aorta appearing acutely *after* the implant of large stents in coarctations of the aorta. In the reported cases, the stents presumably were implanted to their maximum diameters on a single large balloon with a single inflation where a circumferential ring of the sharp ends of the stents could protrude perpendicularly toward (into!) the vessel wall during the initial balloon expansion and before the center of the stent even began to inflate. These aneurysms are not reported with stents implanted in the aorta with gradual or sequential dilation of the stents. The use of BIB™ balloons for sequential enlargement of these large implants, and the availability of large stents with rounder (smoother) ends, should obviate this complication completely. The reported cases were addressed surgically without further information about them but with no other reported sequelae.

Conclusion

The use of intravascular stents actually has reduced the complications of balloon dilation in all vessels. The adverse events and complications during delivery are minimized by close attention to the details of proven delivery techniques. Hopefully many of the delivery problems have been or will be eliminated by improvements in the stents, balloon technology and delivery techniques. Currently, even with the existing technology, intravascular stents are considered as the primary therapy for vascular stenosis occurring in most congenital heart patients.

References

1. Mullins CE *et al.* Implantation of balloon-expandable intravascular grafts by catheterization in pulmonary arteries and systemic veins. *Circulation* 1988; **77**(1): 188–199.
2. O'Laughlin MP *et al.* Use of endovascular stents in congenital heart disease. *Circulation* 1991; **83**(6): 1923–1939.
3. Driscoll DJ, Hesslein PS, and Mullins CE. Congenital stenosis of individual pulmonary veins: clinical spectrum and unsuccessful treatment by transvenous balloon dilation. *Am J Cardiol* 1982; **49**(7): 1767–1772.
4. Rothman A *et al.* Early results and follow-up of balloon angioplasty for branch pulmonary artery stenoses. *J Am Coll Cardiol* 1990; **15**(5): 1109–1117.
5. Zeevi B, Berant M, and Blieden LC. Midterm clinical impact versus procedural success of balloon angioplasty for pulmonary artery stenosis. *Pediatr Cardiol* 1997; **18**(2): 101–106.
6. Shaffer KM *et al.* Intravascular stents in congenital heart disease: short- and long-term results from a large single-center experience. *J Am Coll Cardiol* 1998; **31**(3): 661–667.
7. Morrow WR *et al.* Re-expansion of balloon-expandable stents after growth. *J Am Coll Cardiol* 1993; **22**(7): 2007–2013.
8. McMahon CJ *et al.* Redilation of endovascular stents in congenital heart disease: factors implicated in the development of restenosis and neointimal proliferation. *J Am Coll Cardiol* 2001; **38**(2): 521–526.
9. Cheung YF *et al.* Early and intermediate-term complications of self-expanding stents limit their potential application in children with congenital heart disease. *J Am Coll Cardiol* 2000; **35**(4): 1007–1015.
10. Recto MR *et al.* A technique to prevent newly implanted stent displacement during subsequent catheter and sheath manipulation. *Catheter Cardiovasc Interv* 2000; **49**(3): 297–300.
11. Salazar OH *et al.* Feasibility of a technique for branch pulmonary artery stent implantation. *J Vasc Interv Radiol* 1996; **7**(1): 41–46.
12. Ing F *et al.* A new delivery system for implantation of large stents through small sheaths in infants and children with

branch pulmonary artery stenoses (Abstract). *Cardiol Young* 2000; **10** (Suppl): 152.

13. Forbes TJ *et al*. The Genesis stent: A new low-profile stent for use in infants, children, and adults with congenital heart disease. *Catheter Cardiovasc Interv* 2003; **59**(3): 406–414.
14. Kobayashi Y *et al*. The skirt technique: A stenting technique to treat a lesion immediately proximal to the bifurcation (pseudobifurcation). *Catheter Cardiovasc Interv* 2000; **51**(3): 347–351.
15. Preminger TJ, Lock JE, and Perry SB. Traumatic aortopulmonary window as a complication of pulmonary artery balloon angioplasty: transcatheter occlusion with a covered stent. A case report. *Cathet Cardiovasc Diagn* 1994; **31**(4): 286–289.
16. Sadiq M, Malick NH, and Qureshi SA. Simultaneous treatment of native coarctation of the aorta combined with patent ductus arteriosus using a covered stent. *Catheter Cardiovasc Interv* 2003; **59**(3): 387–390.
17. Khan MS and Moore JW. Treatment of abdominal aortic pseudoaneurysm with covered stents in a pediatric patient. *Catheter Cardiovasc Interv* 2000; **50**(4): 445–448.
18. Richens T *et al*. Interventional treatment of lateral tunnel dehiscence in a total cavopulmonary connection using a balloon expandable covered stent. *Catheter Cardiovasc Interv* 2000; **50**(4): 449–451.
19. Ing F *et al*. The new "open-ring" stent; evaluation in a swine model. *Catheter Cardiovasc Interv* 1998; **44**: 109.
20. Ewert P *et al*. Novel growth stent for the permanent treatment of vessel stenosis in growing children: An experimental study. *Catheter Cardiovasc Interv* 2004; **62**(4): 506–510.
21. Hoyer MH *et al*. Transcatheter retrieval of an embolized Palmaz stent from the right ventricle of a child. *Cathet Cardiovasc Diagn* 1996; **39**(3): 277–280.

23 Intravascular stent implant—pulmonary branch stenosis

Introduction

The use of intravascular stents is accepted by most centers as the safest, most effective and most definitive means of treating branch pulmonary artery stenosis. Surgical repair of these lesions can relieve the stenosis, but surgery on branch pulmonary lesions also directly or indirectly is a major *cause* of branch pulmonary artery stenosis[1]. Balloon dilation (angioplasty) of branch pulmonary stenosis alone, at best, partially or temporarily relieves the obstructions[2–4], while properly placed intravascular stents open the lesions to the nominal diameter of the adjacent vessel, totally relieve the gradient across the area of obstruction and, in addition, appear to be the most cost effective treatment[5,6].

The delivery of intravascular stents to the branch pulmonary arteries in complex pediatric and congenital heart patients probably is the most difficult and challenging procedure encountered by the pediatric or congenital interventional cardiologist. This results from the combination of the complex nature of the lesions along with the "stagnation" in the development of the equipment necessary for these procedures. The delivery of almost all stents to the pulmonary arteries first involves advancing the large and stiff stents, which are hand-mounted on the delivery balloons, through major, often acute turns in the course through the heart to the pulmonary arteries before the target lesion even is reached. Branch pulmonary artery stenoses often have peculiar and acute angles of origin, multiple areas of stenosis, large dilated or displaced main pulmonary artery/right ventricular outflow tracts and large dilated right atria and ventricles—all of which complicates the delivery of stents. Most of the significant branch pulmonary artery lesions are located in the larger, more proximal areas of the pulmonary arteries and require large, rigid stents with very strong walls which ***must be capable*** of dilation to the eventual large diameters of the adult central pulmonary arteries of that particular patient. All of these factors require the use of very large, often stiff and complicated delivery systems. The problems with the anatomy are compounded by the relatively crude, and unnecessarily "antiquated", expendable equipment, which is still the only equipment available for the implant of stents in the larger or potentially larger branch pulmonary arteries in pediatric and congenital heart patients.

The delivery and implant techniques described in this chapter are the techniques that are used for the delivery of the Palmaz™ P-308, P-188 and P-128 balloon expandable "iliac" stents (Johnson & Johnson, Warren, NJ) to the major branch pulmonary arteries[7]. These particular stents were the original stents used for the central and branch pulmonary arteries and were the only stents available for this use in large vessels for the first decade of stent implants in pediatric/congenital heart patients. There now are several new stents with more favorable characteristics for delivery, which can be dilated to satisfactory diameters of the adult central pulmonary arteries *and*, at the same time, have sufficient wall strength to support these large vessels when they are dilated to diameters over 12 mm. The characteristics, advantages and disadvantages of these newer stents are discussed in detail in Chapter 22.

So far, all of the larger diameter stents which should be used in central vessels must be hand-mounted on the delivery balloons, and most of the delivery and implant techniques used for the original J & J,™ P _ _ 8 stents are still used for the newer generation large stents. Once the delivery and implant of the original J & J™ P _ _ 8 stents are mastered, the delivery of any of the new or improved larger stents is far easier and more straightforward. The smaller, J & J™ P-204 "renal" stents (Johnson & Johnson, Warren, NJ) as well as the newer "Medium" and "Large" Genesis™ stents (Johnson & Johnson–Cordis Corp., Miami Lakes, FL) of similar diameters are currently available and can be *delivered* far more easily using smaller delivery sheaths and wires. However, these smaller diameter stents are ***only*** suitable for the *smaller more peripheral* branch pulmonary arteries and ***not** acceptable* for any of the *central* pulmonary arteries or major, central pulmonary artery branches.

Pulmonary artery stent equipment and delineation of the lesions

A biplane X-ray system with capabilities for compound angulation of the X-ray tube is absolutely essential for the implant of all but the simplest of pulmonary artery stents. In most cases, multiple branch pulmonary arteries are involved, the lesions are in curved vessels, and the separate lesions occur in different vessels which arise at markedly different angles from each other. Multiple simultaneous views are necessary, not only for the implant of several stents at the same time, but during the implant of each individual stent in order to visualize the entire stent as well as the vessels adjacent to the target lesion. In addition to a biplane system, a high-quality, biplane "freeze frame" replay system is required to perform pulmonary artery stent implants. The number of small "positioning" angiograms can be reduced by the appropriate use of a good system to "road map" lesions from a prior image.

Currently, all stents are delivered to the pulmonary arteries over Super Stiff™ wires and through long sheaths. Although it occasionally is possible to deliver the stents that are currently available over a standard strength wire, the softer wires provide much less control over the stent/balloon and result in a much greater likelihood of the stent being displaced away from a fixed location, which, in turn, results in failure of the stent delivery/ implant. Similarly, *none* of the current stents that are suitable for central branch pulmonary arteries are premounted. Although these larger stents occasionally have been delivered without a long sheath, there is a very high likelihood of stent entrapment on right heart structures or displacement off the balloon during the delivery to the lesion. Both the use of "standard" guide wires and the delivery of stents without a long sheath increase the risks of the procedure and decrease the likelihood of success of delivering stents to the pulmonary arteries, and are not recommended.

For the delivery of a *single* stent to a branch pulmonary artery, at least *two* veins are accessed at the beginning of the procedure. One venous access is used for the wire and the sheath for the delivery of the stent and the second venous access is for a separate catheter, which is used for monitoring angiography. When two stents are being delivered simultaneously, a *third* venous line is accessed for the additional angiographic catheter. The best access veins for delivery of stents to the pulmonary arteries are the two separate femoral veins. In larger children, adolescents, and young adults when one femoral access site is obstructed and simultaneous stent implants are necessary, two venous lines can be "piggy-backed" into a single femoral vein. When "piggy-backing" sheaths in a single vein, it is preferable, when at all possible, not to place the two (or more) very large sheaths for stent delivery in the same vein! As an alternative, a femoral vein and an internal jugular vein are used for the introduction of the large delivery sheaths for the stent implants with the third, smaller, "monitor/angiographic" catheter introduced "piggy-back" into the femoral vein. A final alternative venous access for stent delivery to the pulmonary artery is through the transhepatic approach, which is described in detail in Chapter 4. This certainly provides a "straight shot" to the right ventricle and right ventricular outflow tract, and is preferable to any of the more circuitous more peripheral veins. The transhepatic route is not a "standard" access route, but has been used successfully for the introduction of large diameter sheaths.

In the absence of access from either femoral vein, access is obtained from the combination of an internal jugular vein and a hepatic vein for large sheath access while a brachial, axillary or subclavian vein can be used for the introduction of the extra diagnostic/angiographic catheter. The more peripheral veins in the upper extremities usually are *not* suitable for *stent delivery* to the pulmonary arteries. The size of these peripheral veins usually is too small and, of more importance, the tortuous curves encountered through the upper extremity venous channels prevent the delivery of the rigid stents to the pulmonary arteries.

The area of branch stenosis is identified and quantitated accurately from the pressure gradients and from the measurements on selective biplane pulmonary artery angiography. There is no one universal or specific angle or position which demonstrates any one particular area of pulmonary branch stenosis the best. The particular angles of the X-ray tubes for each area of stenosis vary from patient to patient and from lesion to lesion within the same patient. The view utilized for the primary "operating" X-ray plane is the view in which the area of stenosis is displayed maximally in its *longest axis*. The second X-ray plane is positioned to obtain the optimal view of any crossing or branch vessels that arise off the target vessel. Frequently, several small *selective* angiograms into the involved vessel, each time changing the angulation of the X-ray tubes slightly, are necessary to obtain the optimal views. These angles can be anywhere from straight AP, lateral, RAO and LAO projections, to any combination of these angles along with cranial or caudal angulation.

When the two X-ray tubes are in the optimal positions for the dilation and subsequent stent implant, a *selective* biplane angiogram is recorded *in the area* of the stenosis by injecting *into the vessel* being treated through the "extra" angiographic catheter. The angiographic catheter is introduced from an additional available venous access, but preferably, not the vein(s) where the delivery sheath(s) is(are) introduced in order not to have too many sheath/catheters in the immediate area of the delivery sheath. "Freeze frame" views of the stenosis in both planes of the selective pulmonary angiogram are saved and are used for "road maps" of the area during implant of the stent. If a record of the angles of the X-ray tubes is not automated in the X-ray equipment, it is important to make a separate notation of the X-ray tube angles for future reference.

When either suboptimal fluoroscopic images or only poor quality "road-mapping" is available, an alternative radiographic "positioner" is established on the *skin* of the patient to identify the specific site of the lesion. Once the X-ray tubes are placed in their final, optimal positions, this "identification" of the lesion is accomplished by using fluoroscopy to place small lead marker(s) on the chest wall, which will correspond with the area(s) of stenosis as seen on the fluoroscope or angiogram. These markers on the chest wall, combined with the known X-ray tube angles, provide a relatively consistent reference for the area(s) of stenosis during stent implant. The positions of the markers on the chest wall should be verified and, if necessary, readjusted immediately before proceeding with the stent delivery to compensate for any changes in the patient's position between the original positioning of the markers and the final stent delivery.

In order to acquire the optimal, *selective* picture of the lesion to be stented, the angiographic catheter is positioned just proximal to, or actually in, the area of stenosis. A calibrated NIH type angiographic "marker" catheter (Medtronic Inc., Minneapolis, MN) is ideal for these angiocardiograms. "Pig-tail" angiographic catheters, with or without "marker bands", should *not* be used for these injections in the pulmonary arteries. The holes in the pig-tail catheters are on the straight shaft of the catheter proximal to the looped end of the catheter. As a consequence, for an adequate angiogram, the loop of the pig-tail must be positioned within, or even distal to, the lesion. This loop of the pig-tail positioned in the precise area during the stent implant interferes with subsequent sheath and stent positioning and must be removed during stent deployment. Also it is difficult to perform precise and very selective injections with a pig-tail catheter.

When the NIH type marker catheter is aligned exactly perpendicular to the X-ray beam, the marker bands on the catheter will be positioned exactly on edge and appear as narrow straight lines with no blurring or "rounding" of the edges of the marks. When these marks are aligned accurately in the lesion, the marks also help to determine the alignment of the vessel in its longest axis on the X-ray. The marks, which are separated exactly one centimeter when the catheter is aligned properly, provide *accurate* "reference" calibrations for the *precise* measurement of both the length and diameter of the area of stenosis as well as the diameters of the adjacent vessels. The measurements acquired include the diameters and lengths of the vessel adjacent to the stenosis and should include the distances both proximally and distally to the nearest branching vessels from the area of stenosis. These measurements determine the length of the stent that can be used and the diameter and length of the balloon which will be used to deliver the stent.

Stent delivery into the pulmonary arteries

When the lesion has been delineated precisely angiographically and hemodynamically, a second 7- or 8-French, end-hole catheter, which will accommodate at least a 0.038″ guide wire, is introduced into the venous access that is the most suitable for the *large sheath* introduction and the access to the particular pulmonary artery. This catheter is maneuvered through the area of branch stenosis to a position as far distally in the involved branch pulmonary artery as is possible. The tip of the catheter should be maneuvered into the vessel that has the largest diameter distal to the lesion and should be advanced as far distal to the obstruction in that vessel as possible. The catheter should be in a peripheral capillary wedge position at the extreme periphery of the particular lung field. It is preferable that the tip of the catheter actually overlies the stomach or liver at the base of the lung fields!

This very distal position of the catheter in the pulmonary artery is essential in order to secure a Super Stiff™ guide wire (Medi-Tech, Boston Scientific, Natick, MA) as far distal to the obstruction as is possible and to ensure that the *stiff portion* of the wire, *only*, is not only across, but well past, the stenotic lesion. Any extra time and effort necessary to obtain this very distal, peripheral position for the tip of the catheter is time well spent. The extra time at this stage of the procedure not only saves time in the long run, but may very well make the difference between a successful and a failed implant procedure for a pulmonary artery stent. *The placement and securing of the stiff wire is one of the most important parts of the implant of pulmonary artery stents*. Displacement of the stiff wire during stent delivery or implant is one of the major causes of stent displacement and malposition.

Once the end-hole catheter is wedged in the proper distal vessel, a 0.035″ Super Stiff™ exchange guide wire (or the largest wire which the balloon catheter to be used will accommodate) with a 1 cm "short", floppy tip (Medi-Tech, Boston Scientific, Natick, MA) is advanced through and beyond the tip of the end-hole catheter and embedded in the lung parenchyma. It is desirable to form a slight, short curve just and only at the *transition zone* between the stiff and floppy portion of the Super Stiff™ wire in order to allow the stiff part of the wire to follow the catheter around tight curves. This is particularly true if the catheter is very soft or if the course to the distal vessel is very tortuous and associated with any acute bends.

At the same time, *long curves* are ***not*** preformed on the more proximal, stiff shaft of the Super Stiff™ wire even though they might appear to correspond to the potential course of the wire within the heart. Except for the small curve at the transition between the stiff wire and the floppy tip, an essentially "straight" super stiff exchange wire is necessary. Long curves on the more proximal shaft of the wire prevent all rotation of the wire and, in turn, interfere with the passage of the stiff wire to the tip of the catheter. If the stiff wire has a curve in the more proximal part and with the curve positioned within the heart, as the straight tip of the stiff sheath/dilator set approaches the curve, the sheath/dilator tends to proceed in a *straight* direction. As the tip of the stiff sheath/dilator advances, the tip pushes against the concavity of the preformed long curve, which is positioned within the heart. As a consequence, the *curve* in the wire is increased as the sheath/dilator pushes perpendicularly against the curve as the "circumference" of the preformed bend (curve) elongates. With the proximal end of the wire fixed and the curve in the wire lengthening, if the increase in the length of the curve is not compensated for, the *tip* of the wire will be withdrawn out of its distal location. This tendency to widen the curve on the wire within the heart is aggravated by *the pre-existing, preformed curve on the wire* where it passes through the curves within the heart.

When there is any question about the exact area of stenosis from either the angiocardiograms or the site of the gradient, a low-pressure "sizing balloon" (NuMED Inc., Hopkinton, NY) or even a standard angioplasty balloon inflated to a low pressure is used to size and exactly define the stenosis. The "sizing balloon" is advanced over the wire that is already in place for the stent delivery. A sizing or angioplasty balloon, which is inflated to a very low pressure, is used to define the area of stenosis and the surrounding structures more precisely. The specifically designed low-pressure, "sizing balloons" (NuMED Inc., Hopkinton, NY) are preferable for this purpose. These balloons are manufactured from a very thin walled material, which is much softer and more pliable than the walls of balloons that are designed for angioplasty. The NuMED™ sizing balloons do have the one disadvantage that they require a 9-French sheath for introduction into the vein, but at the same time, most sheaths for delivery of stents to the pulmonary arteries are larger than this. Once the wire is in place, the end-hole catheter is removed over the wire and replaced with the low-pressure sizing balloon. When this balloon is inflated *at a very low pressure* in the area of the stenosis, the area (or areas) of indentation ("waists") in the partially inflated balloon identify the exact diameter, the length of the stenosis, and if there are multiple areas of stenosis all very precisely. The sizing balloon will also demonstrate any unusual configuration of the vessel itself, which might contribute to stent displacement during the inflation of the delivery balloon.

Once the straight Super Stiff™ wire is secured in an optimal position, the original catheter or the sizing balloon catheter is kept over the wire until just before the sheath/dilator set is introduced. Either the end-hole or the balloon catheter should be maintained on a slow flush through a wire back-bleed device. A separate operator or an assistant *manually, purposefully and very attentively* should hold the catheter and wire in this position while the sheath/dilator and balloon/stent are being prepared. Super Stiff™ wires tend to assume their "straight" configuration and in doing so, unless *purposefully and attentively* held in place, they spontaneously tend to work their way back out of their secure distal position.

In a small heart and/or where there are very tight curves into the pulmonary arteries, the 0.035″ Super Stiff ™ wire may not be sufficient to support the passage of the large diameter, long and stiff sheath/dilator sets necessary for stent delivery. The much stiffer, 0.038″ Super Stiff™ guide wire (Medi-Tech, Boston Scientific, Natick, MA) must then be used to deliver the long, large and stiff delivery sheath/dilator set. However, *none* of the current balloon catheters used for stent delivery will accommodate a 0.038″ wire. In that circumstance, the 0.038″ Super Stiff™ wire is used to deliver the long sheath/dilator set to, and well beyond, the lesion. The larger 0.038″ wire is then exchanged through the sheath/dilator for the smaller diameter 0.035″ wire once the sheath and dilator are in place and before the dilator is removed.

When the large sheath/dilator cannot be advanced far out into the distal pulmonary artery over the 0.038″ wire, and once the *sheath* is well past the area of stenosis following the delivery of the sheath/dilator over the wire, the dilator alone is removed over the 0.038″ wire leaving the wire and sheath in position. A smaller French sized end-hole catheter is passed through the sheath over the 0.038″ Super Stiff ™ wire and wedged as far as possible, deep into the lung parenchyma. The 0.038″ wire is removed and replaced with the 0.035″ short tipped, Super Stiff™ wire (or the largest gauge Super Stiff ™ that which will accommodate the balloon catheter that is to be used for stent delivery). The 0.035″ wire is passed through the catheter and as far as possible beyond the tip of the catheter into the lung parenchyma. The catheter is left in place and on a flush over the Super Stiff™ wire, and again the catheter, wire, and sheath are purposefully held in place, manually maintaining a "push" on the catheter/

wire/sheath until the stent and balloon are prepared and ready for introduction.

If a Super Stiff™ wire with a standard *long* (7 cm) floppy tip (Medi-Tech, Boston Scientific, Natick, MA) is used for pulmonary artery stent implants, the long floppy portion must be "wadded" or "balled" up in the pulmonary artery distal to the stenosis in order to have all of the floppy and transition (between the soft tip and the stiff shaft) portions of the wire *entirely beyond* the area of stenosis with only the *stiff portion* of the wire across the stenosis. It is important that none of the *flexible* distal *or transition* portions of the wire are in, or even near to, the area to be stented. This "wadding" of a long floppy tip far into the distal pulmonary artery often requires considerable manipulation and multiple exchanges of wires and catheters—and extra trauma to the vessels!

Regardless of the time and effort necessary, the proper wire positioning is an absolutely essential step before any attempt at sheath/dilator or balloon/stent delivery in order to ensure that the wire position is not lost during the stent deployment. During the delivery of the stent/balloon over the wire, the wire must be continually advanced or "pushed" forcefully into the vessel in order to maintain the wire in a forward, rigid position with absolutely no slack on the wire. When the floppy portion or even the transition zone of the Super Stiff™ wire remains in the area of stenosis, as the large sheath and dilator are advanced over the wire around the bends within the heart, the wire tip can be pulled out of the more distal branch vessel. Even if the sheath/dilator can be positioned over the wire with the wire in an unstable distal position, any of the softer portion of the wire within the area of stenosis results in very poor control over the stent/balloon combination during balloon inflation.

When the balloon and stent are inflated, the balloon/stent combination straightens to the *maximum length of the balloon*. This straightening tends to push the distal end of the balloon out of, and away from, any even slight curve in the distal vessel. If a soft portion of the wire is in the area of stenosis or if the wire is "loose" in the area, no control can be maintained over the balloon/stent during the inflation. The balloon/stent will push any slack in a wire back out of the lesion or allow the balloon to "milk" proximally over the wire, resulting in an abnormally proximal deployment of the stent. In this circumstance, particularly if the stent is being expanded in a vessel with a larger proximal diameter than the diameter of the delivery balloon, the stent will not be secured in the vessel by the expanded balloon when the balloon has been displaced, and the stent ends up floating freely on the delivery wire in the larger, more proximal pulmonary artery!

Rarely, when there is an *extremely short*, acute or circuitous course of the pulmonary artery immediately distal to the stenosis, it is necessary to place the *stiff end* of a Super Stiff™ wire distally in the pulmonary artery in order to obtain the necessary fixation of the wire for the secure delivery of the stent. Before the stiff end of the wire can be delivered to the distal pulmonary artery, a relatively stiff end-hole catheter first must be delivered to the distal location in the pulmonary artery. The edge of the very stiff tip of the stiff end of the Super Stiff™ wire can catch on the inner walls of the catheter during the attempted delivery of the wire and, in turn, will not allow the wire to pass through the catheter. A small, short, approximately 45° curve formed at the very tip of the stiff end of the wire may help in advancing the wire through the curves in the catheter in this circumstance.

If the stiff end of the Super Stiff™ wire still cannot be advanced through the pre-positioned catheter, an alternative technique is possible for positioning the stiff end of the wire in the distal branch pulmonary artery. The stiff end of the Super Stiff™ wire with the slight curve at the tip is passed through a 6- or 7-French end-hole catheter that will accommodate the wire, while the catheter is still *outside of the body*. The stiff wire is advanced in the catheter until the tip of the stiff end of the wire is positioned just within the tip of the catheter. A second end-hole catheter of the *same French size* as the first catheter is maneuvered to the desired position in the pulmonary artery and wedged distally to the stenosis in the vessel. This second end-hole catheter is replaced with the "soft end" of a 0.035" short tipped, Super Stiff™ exchange guide wire. The second end-hole catheter is removed over the wire leaving the wire embedded in place. While maintaining the wire in position, this same catheter, once outside of the patient, is placed through a *long sheath* of the same French size. This combination of the *catheter and the long sheath* (6- or 7-French) is advanced over the previously positioned 0.035" Super Stiff™ exchange guide wire to a position as far distal to the stenosis in the pulmonary artery as possible. The *sheath* is advanced over the catheter/wire to, and then past, the tip of the catheter. A continuous flush is maintained through the catheter through a wire back-bleed/flush system as the *catheter* and the *stiff wire* are withdrawn very slowly, leaving only the *long sheath* in place in the distal pulmonary artery site.

The catheter with the curved, *stiff end* of the Super Stiff™ wire pre-positioned at its tip is introduced into the long sheath and advanced through the right heart within the sheath to the desired position well beyond the area of stenosis. When the catheter reaches the end of the sheath, the stiff end of the Super Stiff™ wire is advanced out of the tip of the catheter as far as possible beyond the distal end of the catheter into the desired distal pulmonary artery position. Once the stiff end of the wire is in position, the catheter and smaller, long sheath are removed very cautiously over the wire while observing the wire continuously on fluoroscopy. This leaves the stiff end of the Super Stiff™ wire in place in the distal pulmonary artery.

The large and stiffer, 11- or 12-French delivery sheath/dilators can usually be advanced over this wire to the desired location distal to the stenosis. At the same time, the stiff end of the wire is even more likely to be displaced or to perforate the distal pulmonary capillary bed than the short floppy tip on a Super Stiff™ wire. As a consequence, this technique does require extra precaution and meticulous attention to the position of the tip of the wire. Close observation and extreme care must be taken *not* to allow the tip of the wire to move to and fro in the distal pulmonary bed during further sheath or catheter manipulations. Even with maximum precautions, the stiff end of a wire in the lung creates an extra hazard for perforation.

In the majority of circumstances, it is recommended that the stenosis in a pulmonary artery that is to have a stent implanted, should ***not be*** pre-dilated prior to the delivery of the stent. When a stent is to be implanted, the stenosis in the vessel will be expanded along with the initial expansion of the stent. The area of stenosis ensures that the stent will be fixed tightly in the stenosis as the stent expands into the stenosis with the expansion of the stent/balloon. The tighter the fixation of the stent in the stenosis of the vessel, the less likely is it that the stent will be dislodged with further balloon or catheter manipulations. Pre-dilation does guarantee that the particular area *can* be opened acutely, but at the same time, pre-dilation produces a temporary expansion and a "softening" of the wall of the vessel. This "patulous" area of the vessel at the site of stenosis prevents the stent from fixing *securely* in the lesion. Unless the balloon for stent *implant* is *significantly larger in diameter* than the balloon used for pre-dilation, the stent will not be fixed securely in the lesion after a pre-dilation of the area.

There are only two circumstances when pre-dilation of the stenosis in a pulmonary artery is recommended. The first circumstance is a stenosis of a pulmonary artery that did ***not*** respond at all to *prior dilation* during a *previous catheterization*. Such an area of the vessel, which cannot be dilated at all, will not expand with a stent on a balloon of the same pressure. When the stent does not expand at all in the stenosis, it can trap the delivery balloon in the minimally or incompletely expanded stent within the segment of the vessel. The second indication for pre-dilation is when the diameter of the area of stenosis is so tight that the delivery sheath/dilator set cannot be advanced through the stenosis without some prior dilation of the area. This degree of stenosis would be less than 2–3 mm in diameter!

In either of the circumstances where a pre-dilation of the stenosis is performed, the pre-dilation is performed with a balloon that is *significantly smaller* in diameter than the diameter of the balloon which will be used for the delivery and implant of the stent. In small diameter pulmonary arteries, the balloon used for the pre-dilation should be 2–3 mm *smaller* than the diameter of the balloon that will be used for the implant of the stent. In larger vessels, the balloon used for the pre-dilation should be 3–5 mm *smaller* in diameter than the diameter of the balloon intended for the implant of the stent. The exact balloon length and diameter depend upon the anatomy and diameters of the adjacent vessels.

When pre-dilation is necessary, the smaller dilation balloon is advanced over the previously positioned Super Stiff™ wire and positioned so that the balloon is centered in the area of stenosis. The balloon in the pulmonary artery should be inflated only to the manufacturer's maximal recommended pressure to avoid balloon rupture. Balloon rupture in a small, constrained pulmonary artery likely will lead to vessel rupture from the violent "cutting pressure" which occurs through the slit-like opening as a balloon ruptures.

During the positioning and inflation of any balloon in a branch pulmonary artery for the delivery of a stent or for pre-dilation with a balloon only, it is imperative that the *tip* of the balloon is *not* wedged in a very narrow or short distal branch segment of the involved pulmonary artery. It also is imperative not to let the balloon "milk" *forward or distally* into a narrower portion of the distal artery during the balloon inflation. If a balloon is positioned in or milks forward into a very small distal vessel which cannot accommodate the maximum diameter of the balloon, the distal branch pulmonary vessel is very likely to rupture!

The "waist" which is visible around the inflating balloon on the fluoroscopic image may reappear during the deflation of the balloon or during the *early, low-pressure* reinflation of the balloon during a pre-dilation. This reappearing "waist" at low pressures in the balloon is a result of the elastic recoil of the stenosis in the vessel, and disappears with minimal further inflation. The transient "waist" which appears only *at low pressures* is of no consequence for the subsequent stent implant. The balloon inflation for pre-dilation is repeated several times to the maximum advertised pressure of the balloon in order to verify the elimination of any "waist" or area of persistent stenosis on the balloon at the maximum pressure of the balloon. If there is a persistent waist on the balloon during inflation at the *maximum* recommended balloon pressure, this waist is measured accurately using the calibrations of the marker catheter. It is *unlikely* that during the subsequent stent delivery, a stent that is mounted on a standard or similar pressure balloon will expand a narrowing that persisted with a pre-dilation balloon, any further than the expansion by the pre-dilation balloon. If a *very significant*, narrow residual indentation remains persistently during the pre-dilation with a standard-pressure balloon dilation catheter, then an additional *pre-dilation* is performed of the area with a higher pressure (Ultra-thin™ or Blue-Max™) balloon (Medi-Tech, Boston Scientific, Natick, MA) of the same size as the original pre-dilation balloon. The high-pressure pre-dilation balloon should be of a diameter 2–3 mm *smaller* than the balloon which will be used for the implant of the stent.

If there is still a persistent and significant residual waist when the high-pressure balloon used for the pre-dilation is inflated to its maximum pressure, then the decision to implant a stent becomes far more complicated. A stenotic lesion which cannot be dilated at all with a high-pressure balloon also will *not* dilate any further initially with the addition of a stent over the balloon! In *most* cases, however, once a stent has been in place in a vessel for at least several months, the stenotic areas which previously were resistant to dilation, "soften" and can be dilated with a balloon that is inflated to the identical high pressure some months later. After completion of the pre-dilation, the balloon dilation catheter is withdrawn over the wire while keeping the wire fixed securely in place in the distal pulmonary artery.

All of the large balloon-mounted stents that currently are suitable for use in large or central pulmonary arteries, are delivered to the pulmonary arteries over a wire and *through special, extra-long sheaths*. Although some operators who have had difficulties in advancing or positioning long sheaths in the branch pulmonary arteries have advocated and gotten by with the delivery of hand-mounted stents to these locations without the use of a long sheath, this is not recommended. Without the long sheath, hand-mounted stents and particularly the more rigid, larger stents, which are exposed on the surface of the balloons, can (and will!) become caught on intravascular structures or dislodged from the balloon during delivery to the pulmonary artery. In addition to the protection of the stent that the long sheath provides during its delivery to the pulmonary artery site, the long sheath adds additional support to the shaft of the delivery balloon and permits some "readjusting" in the position of the exposed stent in the lesion before the final expansion of the stent. The long sheath *absolutely is indispensable* in the recovery of an implanting balloon in the event of puncture or rupture of a balloon during the implant of a stent. Possibly, newer stents *and* the secure pre-mounting of these stents on the balloons by the manufacturers will eventually obviate the need for a long sheath for delivery to the pulmonary arteries, but with the currently available large stents, the long sheath delivery technique still provides the only *safe* and *reliable* means of delivering large, hand-mounted stents to the pulmonary arteries.

The sheath used for the stent delivery must be long enough to reach several centimeters *beyond* the area of pulmonary branch stenosis. In a tall or older child, and certainly in adult sized patients, this requires a sheath that is 75 or even 85 cm long. The sheath must be kink resistant, should have a back-bleed valve with a flush port at the proximal end, and should be very radio-opaque or have a radio-opaque marker band at the tip. The valved/flush system is essential for this stent delivery technique, both to avoid excessive blood loss and to keep the sheath continually flushed and free of clots during the implant. The most suitable sheaths for the delivery of hand-mounted stents to the pulmonary arteries currently are the 75 or 85 cm long "transseptal" type RB-MTS sheaths (Cook Inc., Bloomington, IN), which were described in Chapter 22. The diameter of the long sheath depends upon the stent and the type and diameter of the balloon which is used to deliver the stent. An 11–12-French sheath is necessary to accommodate the delivery of the larger diameter balloon/stent combinations (on 15–18 mm "standard" balloons and on BIB™ balloons [NuMED Inc., Hopkinton, NY]), while P 188 and P 308 stents, which are mounted on 10 mm (or smaller) diameter balloons can be delivered to the branch pulmonary arteries through 8- or 9-French sheaths.

Since a large sheath, once in position to deliver the stent, obstructs distal flow in the particular vessel significantly and results in blood stasis in the pulmonary artery beyond the stenosis, systemic heparinization with 100 mg/kg of heparin is given just before the introduction of the long delivery sheath.

The *sheath* is pre-shaped before introduction to conform to the anatomy of each particular patient's right ventricle and pulmonary arteries. All reshaping of the sheath is performed with the dilator within the sheath to prevent kinking of the sheath. Most long sheaths come from the manufacturer with a 180° "factory transseptal" curve, which usually is very unsatisfactory for stent delivery to the pulmonary arteries. The distal end of the *sheath* needs to be specifically re-curved to conform to the curvature of the course of the vessel *just proximal* to the area of the pulmonary artery branch where the stent is being implanted. A new curve can be formed on the sheath by pulling the distal portion of the sheath/dilator set repeatedly between the tightly gripped thumb and forefinger of the opposite hand. This "softens" the sheath/dilator slightly and straightens the original curve. The pulling between the thumb and finger is continued until the desired, new curve is formed on the sheath/dilator. Alternatively, the sheath and dilator can be "softened" by heating the *sheath/dilator* set *together* in boiling water or in the "jet" of a "heat gun" for 30–60 seconds. After the sheath/dilator material has "softened" for 30–60 seconds, the sheath/dilator together are pulled gently and smoothly between the fingers and thumbs in order to "hand-form" the sheath/dilator combination into the curve which is desired for the sheath. When heating the sheath/dilator together, the very *tip* of the *sheath* is protected from the heat (held between the fingers!) to keep it from softening and "flaring" in the heat. After forming the new curve on the sheath by either technique, the combination sheath and dilator is cooled in a cold flush solution to "fix" the desired curvature on the sheath.

Once the proper curve has been formed on the *sheath*, the dilator is removed from the sheath and the *dilator alone* is reheated and reshaped to form a more acute 70–90° smooth curve just at the very *tip* of the dilator. After heating the dilator alone, the more proximal curve (which was created on the dilator while forming the curve on the sheath) is straightened and a tight, *smooth* 90° curve is formed at the very tip of the dilator alone. This curve at the tip of the dilator facilitates the passage of the stiff sheath/dilator through the sharp curves of the right ventricle and out into the pulmonary arteries.

When the dilator is reinserted into the sheath, the tip of the sheath/dilator combination assumes the curve of the stiffer dilator, however, once the sheath is in place in the pulmonary artery and after the dilator has been removed, the sheath "remembers" the curve formed on it earlier. When the sheath and dilator have been prepared, the catheter which remained over the previously positioned wire is withdrawn carefully over the Super Stiff™ wire while observing the wire very carefully and maintaining its tip as far distally in the pulmonary artery branch as possible. With a #11 blade the skin puncture site is enlarged to accommodate the larger, long sheath/dilator. The pre-curved long sheath and dilator set is introduced into the venous system over the previously positioned Super Stiff™ wire and is advanced over the wire to the area of the right atrium. While very carefully observing both the course of the wire within the cardiac silhouette *and the tip of the wire* in the distal pulmonary artery on fluoroscopy, the long sheath/dilator set is maneuvered/pushed carefully over the wire, through the right heart and into the main pulmonary artery. As the curved tip of the sheath/dilator set advances into and through the right ventricle, the sheath/dilator is rotated or "torqued" smoothly in a clockwise direction similar to the maneuvering of any torque catheter being advanced through the right ventricle. Once securely into the pulmonary artery, the sheath/dilator is advanced further into the branch pulmonary artery until the tip of *the sheath* is well beyond the area of stenosis where the stent is to be implanted.

During the introduction of the sheath/dilator, the tip of the stiff sheath/dilator initially tends to "straighten" the curves on the wire as it passes from the inferior vena cava to the right atrium, to the right ventricle, and into the pulmonary artery. This "straightening" first tends to push the most proximal curve toward the superior vena cava and, in doing so, "elongates" the entire complex curve, which will withdraw the tip of the wire unless the "elongation" is compensated for by advancing the wire at the introductory site. Once the tip of the sheath/dilator has made the initial turn into the right atrium, the sheath/dilator follows the initial curve, passing from the right atrium to the right ventricle, and tends to pass straight toward the right ventricular free wall. As a consequence, the curved course of the wire through the right ventricle to the pulmonary artery now is pushed laterally and "bowed outward" toward the right ventricular free wall, again elongating this curve in the wire. The larger the right atrium and/or right ventricle, the more exaggerated the elongation in the course of the wire becomes. Unless carefully watched and compensated for, this straightening and then extra bowing of the wire curves within the heart lengthen the circumference of the curves in the wire, and when the wire is *fixed* at the skin surface, the lengthening of the curves in the wire within the right heart, necessarily withdraws the wire tip from its distal position! In order to avoid this, the wire not only is given extra slack, but also is advanced slightly along with the sheath/dilator proportionately as these curves are created and widened, and then retracted as the curves straighten. During all of this maneuvering with the sheath/dilator and wire, the *tip* as well as the course of the wire must be watched very closely in order to maintain the tip in its most distal position.

The wire bowing or displacement is particularly common when a smaller, 0.035″ Super Stiff™ wire, is used to deliver a larger, long 11- or 12-French sheath/dilator combination in large dilated right hearts. When a 0.035″ Super Stiff™ wire absolutely cannot support the delivery of the 11- or 12-French sheath/dilator set which is necessary for the stent delivery, the regular end-hole catheter is passed over the 0.035″ wire to the very tip of the wire and the 0.035″ wire is replaced with a 0.038″ Super Stiff™ wire as described previously. Although a 0.038″ wire is only 0.003″ thicker than a 0.038″ wire, it is $2\frac{1}{2}$ times stiffer! After the large sheath/dilator has been delivered to the branch pulmonary artery over the 0.038″ wire and the dilator removed, the 0.038″ wire is replaced with the 0.035″ wire by using an end-hole catheter through the sheath.

Very rarely, even when using a 0.038″ super stiff wire, the large 11- or 12-French sheath/dilator combination cannot be advanced into the pulmonary artery or, particularly, to one of its branches. Even if the sheath/dilator is advanced, in doing so, the tip of the wire becomes displaced so far proximally that it cannot support the subsequent delivery of the balloon/stent combination. This happens more frequently in the presence of either a very large dilated right atrium or a very large dilated right ventricle. If the relatively stiff *sheath/dilator* combination cannot be advanced through the right heart and into the pulmonary artery over a 0.038″ Super Stiff™ wire by any of the above maneuvers, alternative supportive techniques are used to deliver the sheath/dilator to the difficult distal location.

In the presence of a very large right atrium or ventricle, even the heavier and stiffer 0.038″ Super Stiff™ wire is pushed and displaced far laterally toward the lateral wall of the right ventricle as the stiff 12-French sheath/dilator combination is advanced into the ventricle. This displacement of the wire, in turn, aims the tip of the sheath/dilator set toward the lateral wall of the right ventricle and perpendicularly to the desired course toward the pulmonary artery. In this circumstance as more wire is introduced at the skin to compensate for the elongating curve, the more proximal portion of the wire in the *right atrium* will bow toward the *superior vena cava* and eventually loop 360° on itself in the right atrium. Unless the wire is purposefully advanced significantly at the introductory site while the wire is going through this looping, the tip of the wire definitely will be withdrawn from its distal location and probably even completely out of the pulmonary artery! However, if this looping is recognized and *totally compensated for* by advancing the wire proportionately, the loop formed can often be used to redirect the forward direction of the tip of the sheath/dilator toward and into the pulmonary artery. While the tip of the Super Stiff™ wire is maintained in its secure distal pulmonary artery location, a large, *smooth* 360° loop of the Super Stiff™ wire is formed in the very large right atrium as both the sheath/dilator and the wire are advanced together. The full, outer "circumference" of the large wire loop conforms to the maximum outer diameter of the right atrial cavity. Once this loop is formed with the wire, the wire is maneuvered slightly to *maintain the loop in the right atrium and the tip of the wire in the distal pulmonary artery* while the sheath/dilator set is advanced over the wire and around the loop in the right atrium. After passing through the 360° loop in the atrium, the pre-formed curve at the tip of the sheath/dilator now will be directed cephalad in the right ventricle and toward the pulmonary artery. The extra support provided to the proximal portion of the wire/sheath/dilator set pressing against the outer circumference of the right atrial lateral wall allows the tip of the sheath/dilator to advance into the main and then the branch pulmonary artery. This maneuver requires extremely careful observation of the entire course of the wire/sheath/dilator, skill, and at the same time caution, observing for *persistent* bradycardia or other arrhythmias. With this maneuver, there always will be some ectopy and/or bradycardia, especially when the "loops" are formed initially and as the sheath/dilator is being advanced with a "push" on the circumference of the loops of the stiff wire. These arrhythmias should be allowed to subside by relaxing the loops or pausing in the forceful or extreme maneuvers. Usually the arrhythmia/instability resolves spontaneously and the maneuvering of the sheath/dilator can be resumed.

An alternative technique, which at first may seem somewhat more extreme, is to use a second (and even third!) Super Stiff™ wire *together* with the initial Super Stiff™ wire *within the dilator* of the sheath/dilator set. Usually the difficult part in the delivery of the long sheath/dilator is to advance the tip of the sheath/dilator from its position in a very dilated right ventricle into the main or right or left pulmonary artery. In that circumstance, the tip of the sheath/dilator is displaced far laterally in the right ventricle, and as the relatively "straight" sheath/dilator combination is advanced over the wire further into a dilated right ventricle, the tip of the sheath/dilator pushes perpendicularly *against the broad curve* and the course of the more distal wire, which is passing from the ventricle to the pulmonary artery. Instead of the tip turning and advancing into the pulmonary artery, the more proximal wire bows or loops in the right atrium, which begins to create the previously described back curve or loop in the right atrium. This back curve, in turn, directs the tip of the sheath dilator more laterally and *caudally*. When the previously mentioned 360° right atrial loop with one 0.038″ wire does not permit successful delivery to the pulmonary artery, additional 0.038″ Super Stiff™ wires are used side by side within the 11-French dilator to add support to the original Super Stiff™ wire!

The sheath/dilator set is advanced as far as possible into the right ventricle and toward the outflow tract over the original 0.038″ wire until *just before* the curve on the more proximal wire begins to bow or bend more within the right atrium. If possible, the sheath/dilator is torqued to direct its "curved" tip cephalad. A short (2–3 cm), smooth 30–40° curve corresponding to the curve from the cavity of the right ventricle into the right pulmonary artery is formed on the ***stiff end*** of a second 0.038″ Super Stiff™ wire. This curved, *stiff end* of the second Super Stiff™ wire is introduced *adjacent to the original Super Stiff™ wire* through the wire back-bleed valve on the dilator and into the proximal end of the long dilator. The second wire is advanced through the dilator *to the tip of the dilator*. The lumen of the shaft of an 11-French dilator will accommodate up to *three* 0.038″ Super Stiff™ wires side by side while the tip of the dilator only allows the passage of one of the 0.038″ wires! The curve on the stiff end of the second wire will rotate cephalad and help to direct the tip of the dilator in that direction as the wire reaches the tip of the dilator. While fixing the original 0.038″ (guiding) Super Stiff™ wire in position, the sheath/dilator *and the second Super Stiff™ wire* are advanced together over the original wire. The shaft of the sheath/dilator now is supported by the additional Super Stiff™ wire, which is positioned within the dilator. This support is particularly important proximally and prevents the back of the sheath/dilator from bowing within the right atrium or right ventricle and allows the forward force on the proximal sheath/dilator/wire to be transmitted forward and cephalad to the tip of the sheath/dilator. This advances the tip into the pulmonary artery by the forward motion of the combination. Occasionally, even a second Super Stiff™ wire will not provide sufficient support to allow the combination sheath/dilator/extra wire to be advanced through a very dilated or distorted right ventricle. In that circumstance, a similar curve is formed on the stiff end of a *third* Super Stiff™ wire and it is introduced into the proximal end of the dilator alongside of the *other two* Super Stiff™ wires. The third wire is used in conjunction with, and exactly the same as, the second wire. This seemingly extreme technique has provided sufficient support to deliver the sheath/dilator to the branch pulmonary artery in every case in which it has been attempted. Once the tip of the dilator has advanced into the desired proximal branch pulmonary artery, the "extra" super stiff wires along with the "guiding" Super Stiff™ wire all are held in place while the sheath and dilator alone are advanced further into and past the lesion. Once the sheath and dilator have been advanced to a position where the *sheath* is well beyond the area of stenosis, the original Super Stiff™ wire and sheath are fixed in position while the "extra" wires are withdrawn slowly.

Regardless of which means was used to accomplish the sheath position, once the *tip of the delivery sheath* is well distal to the area of stenosis, the guiding Super Stiff™ wire and sheath are fixed in position and the dilator alone is withdrawn slowly over the wire, out of the sheath, and out of the body. The slow withdrawal of the dilator allows blood from the pulmonary artery to flow into the tip of the sheath and follow the dilator tip as it is withdrawn through the entire sheath. A rapid withdrawal of the dilator creates a vacuum within the sheath, which causes air to be sucked into the dilator and sheath around the wire. Once the dilator has been withdrawn completely, the sheath is allowed to *bleed back* passively from the side port until it is completely free of air or clots, remembering that these large sheaths accommodate a volume of as much as 12 ml. When there is a wire passing through the back-bleed valve of the sheath, withdrawal from the side arm of the sheath with a syringe should ***not*** be attempted. Suction applied to the side arm invariably causes air to be drawn *into the sheath* through the back-bleed valve around the wire before blood is withdrawn through the shaft of the sheath from the distal tip! This suction will fill the hub and proximal sheath with air rather than clearing it! Once the sheath bleeds passively until it is free of air and clots, it is flushed thoroughly with a syringe and then placed on a slow continuous flush. The slow flush can be stopped intermittently when pressures are to be recorded through the side port of the sheath. If it has not been administered earlier during the procedure, the patient is given 100 mg/kg of heparin at this stage of the procedure.

If the sheath/dilator was advanced to the pulmonary artery over a 0.038′ wire, the wire must be exchanged through the dilator, the sheath, or a new catheer for a wire that will accommodate a delivery balloon catheter for the stent. If the tip of the dilator is positioned *very far* distally in the pulmonary artery branch, the wire can be exchanged for a smaller diameter wire through the dilator before the dilator is withdrawn. Otherwise (and more frequently) the wire is exchanged through an end-hole catheter after the large dilator has been withdrawn. A 6- or 7-French end-hole catheter is passed through the sheath and over the 0.038″ wire to the most distal position of the wire in the branch pulmonary artery. The catheter is fixed in this position and the 0.038″ wire is withdrawn and replaced with a 0.035″ Super Stiff™ wire (or largest diameter wire which the proposed balloon for the stent will accommodate). The catheter is removed slowly and the sheath cleared of air passively and re-flushed.

The exact balloon to be used depends upon the diameter of the stenosis, the diameter of the vessel being treated, the length (and type!) of stent being used, the difficulty of entering the particular area, and what types of balloons are available at that particular time. All of these factors must be considered initially during the procedure before determining the diameter of the sheath for the stent delivery. The balloon for stent delivery is chosen according to the length of the stent and the diameter to which the stent is to be dilated at *implant*. Generally, a balloon is used which is the diameter of the "normal" non-stenotic area of the vessel adjacent to the stenosis. In the presence of a very tight stenosis, a balloon can be used which is smaller than the anticipated final diameter for the stent/vessel at implant and can be considerably smaller than the adjacent "normal" vessel. As long as the *lesion* is tight enough to secure the stent very firmly in the location at this smaller diameter, the ability to use a smaller balloon often allows the use of a more desirable balloon for stent delivery or a smaller delivery sheath. After a successful implant, the smaller diameter stent can be expanded during the same procedure (or at a later procedure) with a larger balloon, which might not have been as satisfactory for the delivery of the stent. If the lesion was pre-dilated and, in particular, if there was no residual waist on the balloon used to pre-dilate the area of stenosis, then a balloon *at least* 2–3 mm larger in diameter than the measured waist or 2–3 mm larger than the balloon that was used to pre-dilate the lesion, is used as the initial diameter of the balloon which is used to deliver the stent.

The ideal balloon for delivery of stents to the pulmonary arteries should have as many of the optimal balloon characteristics as possible because of the tortuous course in the approach to the lesions and the complexity of the lesions themselves. The ideal characteristics of balloons for stent delivery are discussed in Chapter 22. Because there is no *ideal* balloon available for the delivery of stents that need to be dilated initially to large diameters, often there is a compromise between one or more of these ideal characteristics of the balloons. When there are specific characteristics that are more likely to reduce serious complications, these are the characteristics that have the highest priority in the choice of the particular balloon being used.

The lengths of dilation balloons are "labeled" by the manufacturers according to the "usable" dilating length—i.e. the length of the *parallel walls* of the balloon when the balloon is fully inflated. Usually there are radio-opaque markers on the shaft of the catheter beneath the balloon to correspond to the "usable" balloon length, although in some rare instances the radio-opaque marks are at the actual tips of the balloon. Unfortunately, the "advertised length" is not very precise and not consistent between manufacturers or even on different balloons from the same manufacturer. There always is a taper from the expanded parallel surfaces of the balloon to the attachment onto the catheter shaft at each end of the balloon. The taper varies according to the manufacturer and the type of balloon. It can be very long (even centimeters) or, *preferably*, relatively short, "squared off" or even "blunt". The taper can begin several millimeters distal to the advertised length of the "parallel" surfaces or occasionally exactly at the precise end of the advertised length (and the end of the parallel surfaces). The taper produces the "shoulders" which extend beyond the parallel surfaces on both the deflated and inflated balloons.

It is important that the taper or "shoulders" of the balloons for the delivery of the P 308 J & J "Iliac" stents to the pulmonary arteries are blunt and short. The length of the parallel surface of the balloon ("advertised length") should be shorter (definitely no longer) than the 3 cm length of the non-expanded P 308 stent. When a longer balloon is used, the extra length represents exposed balloon both proximally and distally to the ends of the stent, which expands before the stent. When a balloon with a mounted stent is inflated, the portions of the balloon extending beyond the ends of the mounted stent represent the areas of least resistance to inflation and expand significantly (completely!) before the center of the balloon and stent itself, which causes the "dumbbell" appearance of the balloon (and stent). Asymmetrical and/or premature inflation of *one end* of a balloon that is positioned beyond one end of a stent, can result in forward or backward displacement of the stent on the balloon and/or of the balloon/stent combination before the *stent* begins to inflate. In either case, the displacement results in an improper location for the stent implant.

Of equal importance, the premature expansion of an end of the balloon causes an initial expansion and marked flaring of the *end(s)* of the stent before the center of the stent even begins to dilate. The expanding "flared" end(s) of P _ _ 8 stents result(s) in radial rings of sharp *points* extending perpendicularly toward the vessel wall at the end(s) of the expanding stent. The larger the balloon, the more acutely these "points" are angled toward the vessel wall. In addition, when the balloon is significantly longer than the stent, these points occur within the ends of the incompletely expanded balloon and can puncture the balloon itself during inflation—particularly when the expanding balloon is positioned around the curves in the pulmonary arteries.

A balloon *slightly* shorter (1–1.5 mm) than the stent is ideal for the expansion and implant of stents. A balloon that is shorter than the stent expands the center of the stent first with the expansion of the ends of the stent actually following during the inflation of the balloon. The expanded center fixes the stent exactly in the stenosis without any forward or backward displacement by the balloon/stent. The ends of the stent are expanded by the "shoulders" of the balloon, but only after the center of the stent is fully inflated and fixed in place and, in turn, will not puncture the balloon. The very ends of the stent, in fact, often are expanded using a shorter balloon. This is remedied easily after the stent is fixed in place. The balloon is deflated and first advanced slightly (distally) within the stent. The balloon is inflated, opening the distal end of the stent. The procedure is repeated with the balloon withdrawn proximally within the stent to fully open the proximal end of the stent. Because of the taper of the ends of the balloons and even with short "shoulders", and as long as the balloon is only *slightly* shorter than the stent, the stent ends will expand slightly so the balloon, which is shorter than the stent, does not become trapped within the "partially expanded" stent when the balloon is deflated.

The one disadvantage of using a balloon that is shorter than the stent, occurs during the delivery of the stent/balloon through a tortuous course to a stenosis in the pulmonary arteries. When such a balloon is used, there are minimal or no portions of the folded "shoulders" extending beyond the ends of the collapsed stent on the balloon. Even short folded shoulders, which extend very slightly beyond the end of the stent, create small "bulges" on the balloon just beyond each end of the stent, and these bulges help to maintain the stent in place on the balloon as the stent/balloon is advanced through the long sheath. As a consequence, when a balloon is used that is shorter than the stent, proximal displacement of the stent on the balloon is more common as the stent/balloon is advanced through the sheath.

The solution for the severe "dumbbelling" of balloons and stents when expanded on larger balloons is the use of a stepwise inflation of the balloon/stent combination using separate, sequentially larger balloons for the inflation. In very tight stenoses or small vessels, sequential inflations are accomplished by the use of a smaller balloon for implant, followed by a separate larger balloon for the final inflation. This, of course, cannot be used in larger diameter vessels/stenosis, in which case balloon in balloon (BIB™) balloons (NuMED Inc., Hopkinton, NY) are used.

The development of the BIB™ balloons represents a solution for the implant of stents with sequential expansion in larger vessels, but using one balloon catheter. BIB™ balloons are exactly what their name implies–there is a smaller diameter balloon within a larger diameter balloon. The inner balloon is one half the diameter of the outer balloon and usually 0.5–1.0 cm shorter than the outer balloon. The diameter of the outer balloon of the BIB™ balloon determines the final diameter of the stent implant. The stent is mounted on the BIB™ balloon and delivered to the lesion through a long sheath exactly as with other balloons. However, in the lesion, the inner balloon alone is expanded initially and completely. This smaller balloon eliminates the severe "dumbbelling" and often allows some repositioning of the partially, but uniformly expanded stent. When the stent position is satisfactory, the outer balloon is inflated to finish the implant. The major disadvantages of BIB™ balloons are their deflated size and their deflated profile. Because they actually are one balloon within another, they are considerably larger in deflated diameter than a "single" balloon of comparable diameter. With their larger deflated diameter, they also have a fairly rough profile. In spite of their disadvantages, BIB™ balloons are recommended for implant of all stents in the pulmonary arteries that require an initial implant diameter of 12 mm (or more).

The appropriate balloon is chosen according to the lesion and the stent to be used. To prepare any balloon for the mounting of a stent on it, the balloon is partially inflated with a solution of diluted contrast (1:5 dilution of contrast solution to normal saline) and then cleared of all air. The balloon is *not* inflated at any pressure and no attempt is made to "test" its maximum pressure. Full or high-pressure inflation totally unfolds the folded balloon and makes refolding the surface of the balloon smoothly difficult. Before the balloon is pre-inflated, it is inspected (and if necessary measured) for the location of the metal radio-opaque bands within the balloon and for the direction in which the balloon is folded (wrapped) around the catheter. The balloon is alternately inflated partially and deflated using the 1:5 dilution of contrast solution and normal saline. The balloon is tipped so that the "port" within it is positioned at the "up" end of the balloon and all air is sucked out of the balloon as it is deflated. With most balloons this is with the *tip* of the balloon pointing *down*.

Once the balloon has been cleared of air, as it is emptied of fluid for the last time the balloon is re-wrapped carefully around the catheter in the direction of the balloon's natural folds as the flush solution is withdrawn. This usually entails a smooth, slow counterclockwise rotation of the shaft of the catheter while "molding" the balloon with the fingers around the catheter shaft in a clockwise direction (as the tip of the balloon is pointing away from the operator). This refolding varies with different types of balloon and depends upon in which direction the initial inspection determined the "wrapping" of the balloon to be. When refolding the balloon before mounting a stent, slight irregularities on the balloon's surface or slight protrusions of the balloon's "shoulders" may appear that actually become beneficial during the *delivery* of the stent. The irregularities help to keep the stent from slipping on the balloon as the combination stent/balloon catheter is advanced through the long sheath.

The appropriate stent for the vessel and stenosis is opened and inspected. Until recently, the only stents available for central pulmonary arteries and their major branches in the United States were the J & J P308, P188 and P108 stents (Johnson & Johnson, Warren, NJ). All of the P _ _ 8 stents are expandable to 18 to 20 mm in diameter. This diameter is suitable for the adult, central, branch pulmonary artery in most patients. In the last several years, several new Intra Stent™ (ev3, Plymouth, MN) and the Genesis XD™ stents (Johnson & Johnson–Cordis Corp., Miami Lakes, FL) have been approved for human use and are in increasing use for stent implants in the large pulmonary arteries. None of the P _ _ 8 series of stents, nor any of the other larger stents suitable for central pulmonary arteries, are pre-mounted on delivery balloons commercially and, as a consequence, all of the stents applicable for use in the central branch pulmonary arteries are hand-mounted and delivered to the lesions through long sheaths. The P _ _ 8 stents represent the majority of stents that have been implanted in pulmonary arteries, and most of the discussion about the "techniques" for pulmonary stent delivery is based on experience with these stents. At the same time, the techniques for delivery and implant of the P _ _ 8 stents are applicable to all of the hand-mounted stents that currently are appropriate for implant into the larger proximal branch pulmonary arteries.

The smaller diameter P 104, P 154 and P 204 stents (Cordis Corp., Miami Lakes, FL), and more recently, the "Medium" and "Large" Genesis™ Stents (Johnson & Johnson–Cordis Corp., Miami Lakes, FL), are available on smaller balloons and are *easier* to *deliver* to the pulmonary arteries. The "Medium" and "Large" Genesis™ stents, in particular, are pre-mounted very securely on the delivery balloons, which eliminates many of the delivery problems. Unfortunately, all of these smaller stents are suitable ***only*** for the *smaller, more* ***distal pulmonary artery branches*** and should ***never be used*** in central pulmonary or proximal branch pulmonary arteries in any patient who otherwise will not need the particular segment of artery *removed surgically*. These smaller stents *are* suitable for the treatment of stenosis in *small* right ventricle to pulmonary artery conduits that unequivocally will require subsequent surgical replacement. The stent in this circumstance is used to buy time before the inevitable surgical replacement.

These smaller stents certainly *are easier to* deliver, they *are easier* and safer to implant, particularly for the less experienced operator, and they *appear* appropriate, or even large in size for the pulmonary artery in an ***infant** at the time of implant*. However, these stents *cannot* be dilated or re-dilated to diameters greater than 11 mm, which represents a very significant iatrogenic stenosis in a grown patient's central pulmonary artery! The stenosis created by a small stent which has been implanted in a pulmonary artery for as little as several years, unequivocally obligates the patient to a very complex surgical procedure which, possibly, would otherwise have been unnecessary, and during which the stented segment of pulmonary artery must be resected, or at the very least, will require "filleting" of the stent with a surgical patch over the stented segment! These small stents have been advocated for use in the *central* pulmonary arteries in small infants by a few operators who are not comfortable with the more difficult techniques for delivering the larger short stents to the pulmonary arteries. The rationale for the use of the smaller stents is that the *creation of a significant later and permanent obstruction* will not be important, relative to the immediate, but temporary, clinical gain. There are anecdotal reports of small stents being surgically "pealed" out of the lumen of a pulmonary artery, however, only after being in place for a matter of months. Once a stent has been in place in a pulmonary artery for more than a few months, it becomes incorporated into the structure of the vessel wall and often extends "through the wall" into adjacent structures. After any period of time, the stent is not "removable" from the vessel without removing that segment of vessel!

To mount the J & J™ P _ _ 8 stents or any of the available larger diameter stents on a balloon for delivery and implant, one end of the stent is flared open and the entire length of the stent is dilated slightly with a rigid dilator before the balloon is introduced into the stent. The dilation of the stent is accomplished by passing the tip of a large dilator (from the long delivery sheath) into and through the stent. As the dilator is withdrawn from the stent, it is angled slightly and rotated circumferentially around within the very end of the stent to accomplish the flaring of the end. Flaring of the P _ _ 8 stents, in particular, prevents the sharp ends of the struts of these stents from puncturing the surface of the balloon, while the slight dilation of all of the various stents prevents the folds and irregularities on the balloon from catching on the sides of any of the stents as the stent is advanced over the balloon for hand mounting.

With negative pressure maintained on the balloon and the balloon wound tightly around the catheter, the outside surface of the balloon is moistened with undiluted contrast material and the tip of the balloon catheter is carefully introduced into the flared end of the stent. A *slow, slight*, and smooth rotation is applied to the balloon/balloon catheter together so that the spiral of the wrapped balloon "screws" smoothly into the stent in the direction of the balloon, "wrapping" around the catheter as the balloon on the catheter is advanced very carefully and slowly into the stent. Once introduced into the end of the stent, the balloon should slide easily into the stent. With larger balloons, the stent may expand (dilate) slightly further as the stent advances over the large diameter balloon and catheter. The balloon is advanced into the stent until the stent is positioned over the *exact center* of the balloon. The exact position of the stent on the balloon varies with the length and type of balloon and stent used, and is determined by the metal markers within the ends of the balloon. The positioning of the stent slightly forward or backward on the balloon varies according to any anticipated difficulties in passing the balloon/stent combination through the long sheath. Once the stent is in position over the balloon, a few more drops of undiluted contrast are spread over the surface of the stent and balloon. As the contrast dries, this contrast becomes very sticky and serves as a transient "glue" that helps to hold the stent on the balloon.

After moistening the stent/balloon with the contrast, the stent is compressed ("crimped") onto the balloon using manual finger pressure. Negative pressure is maintained on the lumen of the balloon all of the time during the "crimping". Manual finger compression is used over the stent for "crimping" the stent onto a delivery balloon rather than using one of the "crimping tools". Each combination of the balloon/catheter-shaft/stent is a little different from any other, so that no single "crimping tool" is satisfactory for the wide variety of combinations of balloon catheters and stents necessary for pediatric and congenital lesions. When a crimping tool is used, it must be of the exact size for the balloon/catheter-shaft/stent combination; otherwise there is a danger of the crimping tool distorting or damaging the balloon or stent owing to unequal compression of the stent over the balloon.

For the manual "crimping" of all of the larger stents, *initially*, gentle finger compression is applied circumferentially and sequentially over the entire surface of the stent. As the stent/balloon combination is rotated slowly between the fingers, the force of the fingers applying compression as they move over the entire surface of the stent is increased. Finally, the finger compression on the stent/balloon is as forceful as the operator can apply. It is helpful to use the fingernails circumferentially into the rows of slots or "cells" around the P _ _ 8 stents during this final, very firm compression. Although this last maneuver during the manual compressing of the stent over the balloon appears to distort and indent these "slots" in the stent, it does *not* affect the eventual diameter nor the eventual wall strength of the stent. The plastic sleeve which comes with the stent is occasionally used to assist in the initial "crimping" of the stent on the balloon. The sleeve is advanced over the balloon/stent after the stent has been mounted loosely over the balloon. The stent is compressed tightly onto the balloon through this sleeve by very firm finger compression while "rolling" the fingers over the entire surface of the sleeve and over the stent/balloon within the sleeve. This smoothes the stent over the balloon but does not compress the stent as firmly as direct finger/fingernail compression over the stent itself. This combination of maneuvers and techniques secures the stent on the balloon as tightly as possible. Additional contrast is applied over the surface of the mounted stent. The longer the contrast is allowed to dry, the tighter the bond becomes between the stent and the balloon.

The hand-mounted stent is now ready for introduction into the sheath. The previously positioned Super Stiff™ wire and sheath are held securely in position and the side arm of the long sheath is maintained on a slow flush. The negative pressure is released from the lumen port on the balloon. The longer P 308 stents are introduced directly through the back-bleed valve of the sheath without a protective sleeve over the balloon/stent. The *proximal* end of the P 308 stent on the balloon is gripped firmly, with the fingers squeezing the proximal end of the stent against the balloon. The finger grip on the stent is maintained until the stent has passed completely through the valve *and through the junction of the valve chamber with the sheath.* There often is a small ridge or "shelf" where the sheath is attached to the back-bleed valve chamber. The distal tip of the stent can catch on this ridge as it is being advanced into the sheath, and if the stent is not held tightly in place, this ridge can displace the stent proximally on the balloon. The P 308 stent is long enough that the operator can hold the very proximal end of the stent during all of the distance as the *distal end* of the stent is passing through the back-bleed valve and valve/sheath junction. P 308 stents are rigid and straight enough to be pushed through the back-bleed valve mechanism without distorting them.

The P 188 and P 108 stents are too short to maintain a grip on the stent as it advances all of the way through the valve chamber to the sheath, and the ITI™ and hand-mounted Genesis™ stents are not rigid enough to be pushed through the back-bleed valve apparatus itself without protecting the stent from the valve. In order to introduce a P 188, P 108, ITI™ or Genesis™ stent through the back-bleed valve on a long sheath, the stent/balloon combination is first introduced into either a metal "introducing tube" (Johnson & Johnson, Warren, NJ) or a short segment (4–5 cm long) of introducer sheath of the same, or one French smaller, diameter than the long delivery sheath. The introducing tube or short segment of sheath serves as a protective cover completely over the length of the stent/balloon. The introducing tube or short segment of sheath is advanced over the stent/balloon combination to form a sleeve over the stent. The sleeve, now containing the balloon/stent, is introduced through the back-bleed valve of the long delivery sheath and advanced to the junction of the proximal end of the sheath and the back-bleed valve chamber. The sleeve or short segment of sheath is fixed or "seated" in the junction of the valve chamber, with the sheath within the back-bleed valve, as the stent/balloon combination is advanced through the sleeve and into the lumen of the long sheath. Once the balloon/stent is well within the lumen of the long sheath, the sleeve is withdrawn onto the proximal shaft of the balloon catheter. This short sheath or metal introducer can be used with the P 308 stents, but usually it is not necessary with this particular stent.

The balloon catheter with the hand-mounted stent on the balloon is advanced several centimeters into the straight shaft of the sheath, just beyond the hub of the back-bleed valve. When the balloon and stent are completely past the chamber of the back-bleed valve on the sheath, a small amount of positive pressure (approximately one atmosphere) is applied to the lumen of the balloon. This inflates the "exposed" shoulders of the balloon very slightly where they extend beyond the ends of the stent. The *slight* inflation/expansion of these shoulders, in turn, helps to keep the hand-mounted stent from sliding along, or, even, all of the way off, the balloon as the combination is advanced through the sheath, particularly around tight curves. After *slight* pressure is applied to the balloon, the catheter/balloon/stent still should move freely within the sheath. If there is resistance to movement, the pressure is released *partially* from the lumen of the balloon.

The catheter/balloon/stent is advanced over the wire, through the long sheath, through the right heart and to the area of obstruction. This manipulation is performed very carefully and smoothly while observing the balloon/stent combination within the sheath continuously on fluoroscopy in order to ensure that the stent does not slide backward on the balloon at all while the stent/balloon is being advanced through the sheath. This movement on the balloon can be a problem, particularly as any hand-mounted stent on a balloon is advanced around very tight bends in the sheath. If the stent moves on the balloon more than 1 or 2 mm, the catheter/balloon/stent should be withdrawn over the wire and completely out of the sheath, and the entire mounting and delivery process started over. If expansion of the stent for implant is attempted with the stent not centered appropriately on the balloon, the balloon will expand eccentrically and is very likely to "milk" the stent off the balloon or move the stent out of its proper location, either of which can result in balloon entrapment in the stent, an improper position of the stent, or embolization of the stent.

After removal from the body, the stent is repositioned on the balloon very carefully and re-crimped on the balloon. An attempt is made to identify the cause of the stent sliding on the balloon. A kink in the wall of the sheath, a kink in the wire, or an unusual or very tight curve in the course of the sheath through the right heart, all are obvious causes for displacement of the stent. Very tight curves or true kinks in the sheath often are not apparent until the dilator is removed from the sheath. The *catheter* lumen of the balloon catheter, particularly within the balloon area, may be too *thin walled* and not allow the stent to be compressed tightly enough on the balloon without compressing the *catheter* lumen of the catheter. Compression of the catheter lumen results in resistance or stoppage of the movement of the balloon catheter, particularly as it passes around curves. When the cause of the stent displacement has been identified, the problem is corrected before reintroducing the stent/balloon. When there is a kink in the sheath or wire, either one or both is/are replaced. Occasionally, mounting the stent 1 mm forward on the balloon will allow a slightly larger shoulder to expand behind (or proximal on the balloon) the stent when the balloon is inflated slightly within the sheath. This slight increase in the proximal shoulder is usually enough to keep the stent from sliding proximally on the balloon during delivery, but should not be enough to interfere with a proper expansion of the stent. When no obvious cause of stent displacement is found, or the cause cannot be corrected, with the result that the hand-mounted stent repeatedly slides proximally on the balloon as the balloon and stent are advanced through the sheath, an alternative technique must be used for the balloon/stent delivery.

The standard "front-loading" technique described in detail in Chapter 22 is one alternative technique for the delivery of any hand-mounted stent to the pulmonary arteries. The front-loading technique is applicable when the standard sheath delivery technique has been tried and failed on several occasions. The front-loading technique is more difficult and often is less successful than the *standard through-the-sheath* technique. With the front-loading technique, the sheath is withdrawn from the patient over the wire and completely out of the body with the wire maintained in its secure position in the distal pulmonary artery. The balloon with the hand-mounted stent is introduced into the sheath while it is outside of the body, and the balloon and stent are advanced just to the distal tip of the sheath. Alternatively, the balloon alone is advanced completely through, and out of the distal end of, the sheath. The stent is hand-mounted on the balloon while the balloon extends completely out of the distal tip of the long sheath. The balloon with the mounted stent is then withdrawn back into the tip of the sheath while manually compressing the proximal end of the stent into the sheath. With either technique of introducing the stent/balloon into the sheath while the sheath is outside of the body, the *stent* is positioned entirely within the distal end of the sheath while the tip of the balloon, which is distal to the mounted stent, *extends out of the end of the sheath.* This exposed tip of the balloon serves as a "dilator" as the sheath/balloon/stent combination is reintroduced.

The balloon is inflated partially to "secure" the balloon and stent precisely in this position just within the distal end of the sheath and to expand the exposed tip of the balloon to form a fairly taut but "smooth tip" just beyond the tip of the sheath. This balloon/stent/sheath combination is introduced over the pre-positioned wire with the tip of the balloon now acting as the dilator for the sheath as it is reintroduced over the wire, through the skin, into the vein and advanced through the right heart to the area of obstruction in the pulmonary artery. Particular care must be taken to maintain the balloon/stent/sheath relationship *exactly* the same at the tip during this introduction. If the balloon/stent slides back into the sheath, a very discordant interface is created between the tip of the balloon and the wider tip of the sheath while, if the balloon/stent advances out of the sheath at all, the distal end of the stent begins to expand. If the balloon/stent/sheath can be advanced to the lesion with the stent/balloon properly within the sheath, the positive pressure on the balloon lumen is released before the sheath is withdrawn from the balloon/stent combination.

This technique has several inherent disadvantages. The tip of the balloon, which is extending out of the sheath and serving as the dilator, does not create a smooth dilator/sheath interface. The rough and inconsistent interface between the tip of the balloon and the tip of the sheath often catches on the tight curves within the intracardiac right heart structures and prevents the combination from advancing to the pulmonary artery. Also it is very difficult to maintain the balloon/stent/sheath in their exact positions in relation to each other. If the balloon is inflated very tightly within the sheath, the *wire lumen* within the balloon becomes compressed and limits the movement of the catheter over the wire. If the balloon advances out of the sheath even slightly prematurely, the distal end of the stent is exposed and begins to expand. The partially expanded stent will catch on every intracardiac structure. If the sheath is advanced forward off the balloon/stent, an even more discordant interface is created at the tip of the sheath. Delivery of the long, large sheath to the pulmonary arteries often is difficult even with a tight and smooth fitting dilator, the support of a stiff dilator, and over the extra support of a 0.038″ Super Stiff™ wire. The current delivery balloons only accommodate the much floppier 0.035″ Super Stiff™ wire. The combination of the softer wire, softer, smaller shaft of the catheter within the sheath, and the poor interface between the tips of the sheath and balloon, frequently prohibits the delivery of any hand-mounted stent to the pulmonary artery by the "front-loading" technique.

A "front-loaded" delivery technique for the stent is more successful when the stent can be mounted on a much smaller delivery balloon and, in turn, introduced through a sheath of a significantly smaller diameter. When a smaller delivery balloon and sheath can be used, a *sheath-within-a-sheath* modification of the "front-loading" technique can be used for the delivery of hand-mounted stents that could not be advanced through a standard long sheath. A large—11- or 12-French—long delivery sheath is positioned over the Super Stiff™ wire and across the area of stenosis as previously described for a standard, through the sheath, delivery. The stent is mounted and crimped very tightly onto a smaller profile balloon on a balloon catheter with a smaller catheter shaft. The smaller balloon/stent combination is "front-loaded" (as described above) outside of the body into a separate, *smaller diameter*, long delivery sheath. The separate, smaller, "front-loaded" sheath must be at least two French sizes *smaller* in diameter and at least 3–4 cm ***longer*** than the original, outer, large, long sheath which is already positioned across the lesion in the pulmonary artery. The smaller diameter, long sheath with the "front-loaded" balloon/stent is introduced over the wire and into the larger, pre-positioned long sheath. The stent/balloon, which is front-loaded in the smaller sheath, passes very smoothly to the lesion in the branch pulmonary artery through the larger sheath.

All of the disadvantages of the standard front-loading technique are overcome by passing the front-loaded stent/balloon/sheath through the larger long sheath. The "sheath-within-a-sheath" front-loading technique requires the positioning of the larger long sheath across the lesion, and can be used reasonably only when the stent can be deployed at a smaller initial diameter. Deployment of the stent in the lesion is similar except that both sheaths must be withdrawn off the balloon/stent before the balloon/stent inflation. All pressure that had been applied previously to the lumen of the balloon is released before the sheaths are withdrawn. If the smaller sheath is withdrawn off the balloon/stent first and while the stent/balloon is still within the larger sheath, the entire delivery system is retrievable through the large sheath in the event of any stent displacement at the last minute.

The "Ing" modification of the front-loading technique represents a third alternative for delivery of large stents to lesions in small pulmonary arteries. This technique is described in detail in Chapter 22. The Ing technique utilizes the amputated tip of the dilator that comes with the long sheath, as an extension on the tip of the delivery balloon. The amputated *tip of the dilator* is attached to the tip of the *balloon dilation catheter*. When the stent has been mounted on the balloon and the balloon/stent front-loaded into the sheath, the attached dilator tip extends out of the tip of the long sheath for a "front-loaded" delivery. The dilator tip on the balloon eliminates the "interface" problems of a partially inflated balloon serving as the "leading tip". Standard diameter, but short P _ _ 8 stents can be mounted on small balloons and introduced with small diameter (6- or 7-French) long sheaths. Unfortunately, the dilator tip and balloon modifications are not available commercially and all have to be hand-made for each individual case. As a consequence, this technique adds a great deal of complexity to the procedure and is not widely used.

By one or a combination of these delivery techniques, hand-mounted stents essentially can always be delivered to a pulmonary lesion that can be crossed with a wire. Once the balloon/stent combination is advanced successfully to the lesion, the center of the stent (and balloon!) is positioned exactly at the area of tightest stenosis. The exact relationship of the stent to the delivery balloon and to the stenosis is verified with a repeat, selective angiogram performed through the "extra" angiographic catheter, which was positioned immediately adjacent to, or actually in, the area of stenosis. Repeat angiograms are necessary to re-establish the exact location of the stenosis in relation to the balloon/stent position and alignment when the stent/balloon is in place in the lesion. The stiff wire, the large sheath with the balloon catheter and, particularly, the straight stent, passing through the curves to the pulmonary artery all distort the original "relaxed" pulmonary artery anatomy very significantly and, in particular, any relationship to relatively fixed anatomic landmarks within the thorax.

The Super Stiff™ guide wire is pushed forward to maintain it as rigid and as far distally in the pulmonary artery as is possible. Major adjustments in the position of the balloon/stent in the lesion are performed *before* the sheath is withdrawn off the balloon/stent. To move the balloon/stent more distally, the balloon catheter is advanced over the wire or both the wire and the balloon catheter are advanced together. To adjust the balloon/stent proximally (backwards), the balloon catheter is held in place while the ***wire*** alone is advanced—this "pushes" the balloon catheter backwards with the balloon/stent while maintaining the wire "buried" in its most distal and very secure location. This maneuver maintains the forward tension on the wire against the "outer circumference" of all the curves in the course to the stenosis. This "forward tension" provides the most control of the wire/balloon catheter. If, on the other hand, the balloon is withdrawn over or with the wire, this forward tension and control on the wire are lost.

Between each of the adjustments in the balloon/stent position in relation to the stenosis, repeat, very small, selective, biplane pulmonary angiograms through the additional angiocardiographic catheter are performed to verify the positioning of the stent. When there is any choice or decision about the exact stent position in the lesion, the balloon/stent is centered slightly *on the distal side* of the obstruction, but *at no time* even slightly *proximal* to the stenosis. If the stent is delivered too distally, it may not cover the area of stenosis satisfactorily, but the stent will be fixed in a smaller vessel, and does not become free floating. If necessary, the lesion can be covered by the placement of a second stent slightly more proximally within the first stent. The first stent, in fact, will provide a very precise "landmark" for the positioning of the additional stent.

However, if the stent begins expanding proximal to the stenosis, and particularly if during inflation the balloon/stent "milks" backward (proximally) at all, the stent very likely will be inflated in a vessel which is too large to allow the stent to be fixed in place with the particular balloon being used. This results in the stent floating freely (over the wire!) in the proximal pulmonary artery or right ventricle once the balloon is deflated!

When the desired position of the stent/balloon has been achieved, the balloon catheter, the attached stent, and the guide wire are fixed securely in place. Any pressure that had been applied to the balloon lumen is released and the sheath is withdrawn carefully off the enclosed balloon/stent. The sheath is withdrawn completely off the proximal junction of the balloon/catheter where the balloon is attached to the catheter, but should not be withdrawn much further proximally on the catheter. The sheath in proximity to the balloon helps to support the balloon/stent in the correct position during balloon inflation. A repeat small selective pulmonary angiogram is performed after the sheath is withdrawn to verify that the balloon/stent did not shift in relation to the stenosis as the sheath was withdrawn. If there was any movement of the stent/balloon as the sheath was withdrawn, the balloon/stent *again* is readjusted slightly forward or backward (as described above) before the balloon/stent is inflated.

With the stent and its delivery balloon centered at the narrowest area of the stenosis, the balloon/stent is inflated slowly to its maximum recommended pressure. The balloon inflation with the stent expansion is *recorded* on biplane "stored fluoroscopy" or on a slow frame-rate, biplane angiogram. As the balloon inflates, the stent expands along with the balloon. Initially the ends of the balloon, both proximally and distally to the stent, begin to expand, then the center of the balloon along with the entire stent expands. Once the balloon and stent are at full inflation/expansion within the limits of the balloon pressure, the balloon is deflated, leaving the stent expanded and fixed in place across the area of narrowing. To ensure a uniform and maximum expansion of the stent throughout its length with the particular balloon, the inflation of the balloon is repeated several more times, each time with a slight forward or backward repositioning of the balloon within the expanded stent.

Following successful fixation of the stent in the area of narrowing, the exchange guide wire is maintained in its secure position as far distally beyond the stent as possible. The balloon, still within the stent, is re-inflated but at a low pressure. While slowly deflating the balloon, the sheath is re-advanced over the balloon catheter/balloon and advanced back into or through the stent[8]. The inflated balloon within the stent "centers" the tip of the sheath within the lumen of the stent and keeps the edges of the tip of the sheath from catching on the struts at the ends of the stent. Occasionally, as the sheath is advanced onto the deflating balloon, the tip of the sheath pushes the balloon distally and completely through the stent. In either case, the balloon "centers" the tip of the sheath within the stent and allows the sheath to pass into and through the stent without catching on the stent. With the tip of the sheath beyond the stent, the balloon is deflated completely and the balloon catheter is withdrawn carefully into the sheath and through the stent. The reintroduction of the sheath through the freshly implanted stent using this technique is now performed in all cases of stent implants, particularly in the pulmonary arteries, where the stents often align at an angle to the approach from the more proximal artery. When the sheath is re-advanced within the stent, it protects the freshly implanted stent from the rough deflated balloon as the balloon is withdrawn and allows the safe and easy introduction of additional balloons or catheters through the freshly implanted stent.

In the rare instance when the sheath cannot be re-advanced into the stent, the balloon is withdrawn out of the stent over the wire without the sheath protecting the stent from the rough balloon. The balloon after the initial stent expansion is deflated with maximum negative pressure. Once the balloon is completely empty of contrast, the ***negative pressure is released*** from the balloon *before* attempting to withdraw the balloon. Strong negative pressure on a deflated balloon causes the folds of the balloon to extend out from the surface of the balloon as rigid, sharp "wings". These "wings" can prohibit the withdrawal of the balloon from the stent or displace the stent as the balloon is withdrawn. While fixing the wire in its position and with the negative pressure in the balloon released, the shaft of the balloon catheter is rotated slightly as the balloon is withdrawn very gently out of the stent. This often takes some persistent, gentle, to-and-fro manipulation or rotation of the balloon catheter to free it from within the stent. During all of these manipulations while the balloon is still within the stent, special care is taken to maintain the secure, very distal wire position through the stent.

If the stent begins to move as the balloon catheter is withdrawn, the *sheath* is advanced over the balloon catheter until the tip of the sheath touches the proximal edge (end) of the struts of the stent. The edge of the sheath pushing against the end of the stent helps to hold the stent in place as the balloon alone is withdrawn out of the stent, again using some gentle to-and-fro manipulation or rotation of the balloon catheter. Extreme care is necessary during this maneuver to avoid withdrawing the wire while concentrating on the balloon and stent or dislodging the stent into the more proximal larger pulmonary artery.

Once the initial delivery balloon has been withdrawn carefully over the wire and completely out of the *stent*, the wire is fixed in place and the balloon catheter is withdrawn over the wire, through the sheath (if possible) and out of the body. If the balloon cannot be withdrawn completely back into and through the long delivery sheath, the sheath is withdrawn with the balloon over the wire and they are both withdrawn together out of the body. Even if the balloon cannot be withdrawn completely into the sheath and is withdrawn only partially back into the tip of the sheath, the very rough and angular proximal end/shoulder of the balloon is covered by the distal end of the sheath, which protects the vein from the worst trauma from the ragged, deflated balloon surface exiting the vein. Again, continued attention and care are taken to ensure that the *wire* is not withdrawn from its very distal position through and beyond the stent while the operator is concentrating on the entrance site of the wire at the skin.

If the sheath was withdrawn from the body along with the balloon, the balloon is withdrawn through and out of the sheath when they are outside of the body. Outside of the body, the partially expanded balloon is molded by manual compression with the fingers of the operator back into the tip of the sheath. If the sheath tip is *not* distorted when the balloon is withdrawn, the dilator is reinserted into the long sheath and the sheath reinserted into the vein. If the tip of the original sheath is distorted even slightly, a new sheath/dilator set is prepared and introduced into the vein over the existing wire. If possible, the sheath/dilator is advanced over the wire and carefully back to, into, and through, the stent without moving the stent. The smooth interface of the new sheath/dilator facilitates, but does not guarantee, the passage into and through the freshly implanted stent. Even the finely tapered tip of a long *dilator* passing over the wire has a tendency to catch on the end of the stent! If a long sheath can be positioned through the stent, it makes all subsequent maneuvers much easier.

When the balloon used for the initial implant of the stent was smaller in diameter than the ultimate desired diameter of the vessel, the initial balloon is replaced with a dilation balloon of the desired maximum diameter to which the stenotic vessel is to be dilated at this time. If there was a residual and persistent stenosis or a waist on the stent after the original expansion with the initial, standard-pressure balloon, and in order to completely expand the stent, a high-pressure balloon is used for the repeat dilation.

With the sheath in place through the stent and while observing carefully on fluoroscopy, the new balloon is passed over the wire and through the sheath until the new balloon is in position at the center of the stent. The sheath is withdrawn off the balloon. The balloon is inflated very carefully, observing the further expansion of the stent. This inflation is repeated several times, again with slight forward or backward changes in the balloon's position between inflations. The balloon is inflated to its maximum pressure, care being taken to avoid exceeding this. Exceeding the maximum pressure is very likely to rupture the balloon during the inflation. If there is still a significant residual waist in the stent after the reinflation sequence or after inflation with a new larger balloon, a high-pressure polyester Blue-Max™ (Medi-Tech, Boston Scientific, Natick, MA) or Mullins™ balloon (NuMED Inc., Hopkinton, NY) of the same or even slightly smaller diameter is used for the subsequent inflations. The same technique is used for the exchange of the high-pressure balloons as any other balloon. However, when *preparing* the Blue Max™ or Mullins™ balloon, it is inflated and deflated repeatedly using a "negative prep technique". With the protective sleeve over the balloon and a strong negative pressure maintained on the inflator, a minimal amount of the inflation fluid is sucked into and out of the balloon during the prep of the balloon. With such a minimal inflation during preparation, the air is removed from the balloon without actually "unfolding" the balloon, so that the balloon does not lose the manufacturer's smoother fold on the catheter.

High-pressure balloons usually require a larger sheath than even a balloon with a stent mounted on it. If the original or larger sheath cannot be re-advanced through the partially expanded stent at some point after the stent implant, the new larger or higher-pressure balloon is introduced over the wire into the vein through a short sheath and advanced "bare" over the pre-positioned wire to the stent. This is only attempted with a new balloon that has undergone a "negative prep" and has not been inflated previously, so that it retains the smoothest possible profile on the catheter. It is uncanny how even the tapered tip of a balloon catheter that fits very tightly over the guide wire, will catch repeatedly on the tip of a proximal strut of the stent! Usually with patience, careful maneuvering of the wire and the balloon catheter, the balloon eventually can be advanced into the implanted stent without displacing the stent as long as the secure wire position is maintained. This often requires significant to-and-fro motion of the wire and balloon catheter together as the balloon approaches the stent. Once the balloon is within the stent, the reinflation is the same as when the balloon was delivered through the long sheath.

Occasionally, the balloon catheter tip, even with a very tight fit over the wire, catches repeatedly on one of the proximal ends of the stent and prevents the balloon from re-entering the stent. In that situation, re- or further dilation of the freshly implanted stent is abandoned at that time. It is always better to leave a stent that is securely implanted, even if it is not expanded "ideally", than to dislodge the freshly implanted stent with subsequent catheter or balloon manipulations. The stent can be re-entered more easily and re-dilated very safely at a later, subsequent catheterization after it has healed and fixed very securely in place.

Once the final re-expansion of the stent has been achieved, and assuming that the long sheath is in the proximity of the stent, the balloon is reinflated within the stent and the sheath is re-advanced into the stent as described following the original expansion of the stent. The deflated balloon is withdrawn carefully over the guide wire, into the sheath, and completely out of the body. While carefully maintaining the wire and sheath in their positions, an end-hole catheter is introduced over the wire and into the sheath, and advanced through the sheath beyond the implanted stent. The sheath is withdrawn out of the stent and into the pulmonary artery just proximal to the stent. The wire is withdrawn through the catheter and out of the body, the catheter is cleared of all air and debris and attached to a flush/pressure system through a wire back-bleed/flush valve. This last maneuver facilitates the removal of the sheath and the wire and keeps either of them from becoming caught on, or entangled with, the stent. Withdrawing the wire through a catheter prevents the rough surface of the wire or the relatively stiff, sometimes curled, end of the wire from dragging through the stent and the entire heart on its way out of the body. Once the wire is removed, with the catheter tip positioned *distal* to the stent and the sheath tip just proximal to the stent, simultaneous pressures are recorded from the side arm of the sheath and the hub of the catheter. This permits accurate, simultaneous, postimplant proximal and distal pressure measurements without the necessity of any further catheter manipulation or probing in the area of the newly implanted stent.

If the sheath cannot be reintroduced over the balloon and back into and through the stent after the final balloon inflation, the balloon is withdrawn from within the stent over the wire and out of the body through the sheath. An end-hole catheter is advanced over the wire, through the long sheath, through the right heart and into the pulmonary artery. If it is *possible* with minimal effort, the catheter is advanced over the wire *through* the stent. This allows the wire to be removed through the catheter and positions the catheter distal to the stent for accurate pressure recording. Again, it is remarkable how the tip of the catheter, which fits tightly over the wire, can repeatedly catch on one strut of the stent during this attempt. If the catheter cannot be passed over the wire through the stent with minimal effort and without disturbing the stent, the Super Stiff™ wire is withdrawn from the distal location and into the catheter that is positioned in the pulmonary artery adjacent to the proximal end of the stent. When the wire has been removed from the catheter and out of the body, the catheter tip itself, without the stiff wire pushing it against one side of the stent, occasionally can be maneuvered through the stent more easily. Extra care is used in maneuvering catheters or wires through freshly implanted stents in the pulmonary arteries. Because of the turns and angles within the pulmonary arteries, the catheter or wire easily crosses inadvertently into the now open side "diamond cells" of the stent, becoming entrapped in the stent. A catheter as large as an 8- or even 9-French can pass through the side "diamond" of a fully expanded P 308 stent!

While carefully recording pressures, the catheter is withdrawn back through the stent to the proximal pulmonary artery. The angiographic catheter, which already is in the vicinity of the branch pulmonary artery, is utilized to obtain a final, post-stent implant, pulmonary artery angiogram. The pulmonary artery angiogram is performed with the X-ray tubes angled appropriately to position the stent in its longest axis. With this information satisfactorily recorded, the catheter and sheath are withdrawn and hemostasis achieved by pressure over the puncture site.

Distal branch pulmonary artery stenosis

Although distal branch pulmonary artery stenoses are usually multiple and represent more complex lesions, developments in new stents have made it easier and safer to implant stents in these lesions. The smaller, pre-mounted "Medium" and "Large" Genesis™ stents (Johnson & Johnson–Cordis Corp., Miami Lakes, FL) and Express™ stents (Medi-Tech, Boston Scientific, Natick, MA), although ***not suitable*** for the more *central or proximal* branch pulmonary arteries, are very suitable for use in most of the distal branch pulmonary artery stenoses, which occur at or beyond the first branching of the right or left pulmonary artery.

These stents, which are pre-mounted on and almost embedded in the surface of the smaller delivery balloons, can be introduced and advanced to the lesions through much smaller sheaths. The mounting on the balloons is secure enough that the stents can be delivered to the peripheral locations without the use of a long sheath when desired. The smaller diameters of these pre-mounted balloon/stent combinations or their required delivery sheaths allow two or even three stents to be delivered simultaneously and reasonably, side-by-side to distal bifurcating or even trifurcating lesions. The same "rules" apply to the implant of small distal bifurcating/trifurcating stents, as are necessary in the more proximal pulmonary arteries for the larger stents and which are discussed in the next section of this chapter.

Special circumstances (also discussed in detail in Chapter 22)

Bifurcating or branching pulmonary arteries

Stenotic lesions located exactly at branch points or bifurcations of pulmonary arteries add a significant additional challenge to placing stents in the pulmonary arteries. When the stenosis is very proximal or just at the take-off of either the right, left or both pulmonary arteries, or when bifurcating, adjacent, branch vessels both need to be dilated with stent implants, it is necessary at least to protect the access to the contralateral or adjacent pulmonary artery during the inflation of the first stent, or to implant stents simultaneously into the two adjacent branching vessels. To protect the access for simultaneous implants, a second long, large delivery sheath is delivered to the second vessel *before* the first stent is deployed. This guarantees access to the second vessel for the delivery of a second stent even if the first stent crosses or encroaches on the origin of the second vessel. Even when the take-off of the contralateral or branch pulmonary artery is *not* stenotic, but is located in very close proximity to the area of the vessel to be stented, it is necessary to stent the contralateral or branching vessel simultaneously in order to preserve *any* later access to that branch.

During the implant of simultaneous, crossing stents in the pulmonary arteries, each stent is delivered and deployed similarly to the previously described implant of a pulmonary artery stent, but with several special precautions. When the proximal ends of the two simultaneously implanted stents extend into the more proximal common vessel:

- Long stents should be used.
- The proximal ends of the stents should overlap the maximal possible distance to preserve future access.
- Both stents must be inflated simultaneously to keep the balloon in one stent from crushing the other stent or to keep a protruding strut at the end of a stent from puncturing the balloon of the second stent.

The use of either the Mega™ (ev3, Plymouth, MN) or the Genesis™ XD stents (Johnson & Johnson–Cordis Corp., Miami Lakes, FL) is recommended for crossing lesions with the hope of preventing balloon puncture problems. With either simultaneous implants or with the "protected" implant of a stent, a third venous line is absolutely essential in order to obtain repeated angiograms for verification of the exact positions of the other two catheters/stents.

Tandem stents

In very long pulmonary artery lesions, tandem stents are often necessary to "cover" the entire area of stenosis. Tandem stents are frequently used in conjunction with bifurcating stents. Often multiple, short rigid stents have been used in tandem along a curvature in a pulmonary artery in preference to a single long straight stent. The multiple shorter stents conform better to the curvature of the vessel than a single, long, straight stent.

Tandem stents in the pulmonary arteries are implanted with 50–75% overlap of the adjacent stents! This marked degree of overlapping is necessary to accommodate for both the marked acute shortening of the current stents (approximately 50%) when they are expanded to full adult diameters or for the growth *in length* of the particular vessels after the stents have been implanted. With longitudinal growth over any duration of time, stents that are fixed within the tissues of the vessel walls pull away from each other in proportion to the longitudinal growth of the vessel. When tandem stents are implanted in the pulmonary arteries, it is preferable to implant the most distal stent (in the direction of blood flow) first. This prevents over-dilation of the distal area prior to the stent implant, allows the more proximal stent to "catch" on the distal stent, and reduces the manipulation through a freshly implanted stent. The exception to this is when the more distal area is in a bifurcation and requires bifurcating stents.

Bifurcating lesions off a stenotic, more proximal, central vessel

Bifurcating stenotic branch pulmonary arteries arising from a more proximal, long segment of pulmonary artery stenosis, is the one exception where the *more proximal stent* in tandem implants is implanted first. When there is a long proximal stenotic segment of a vessel leading to a more distal vessel with bifurcating or branch stenosis off the same vessel, the *most proximal stenosis* is approached *first* when it is anticipated that both the proximal vessel and the distal bifurcation will require stents! Although intuition would suggest that the more distal vessels should be treated first in order not to require extensive manipulations through the recently implanted, more proximal stent, this is not true. Once bifurcating or side-by-side stents have been implanted distally, any additional more proximal stents, which extend proximally out of the side-by-side stents, must be implanted with additional side-by-side stents implanted simultaneously even if the more proximal area is a single vessel! Occasionally when the two distal branches are very small, the "skirt technique", which was originally described for coronary arteries, is used to position the first more proximal stent properly in the bifurcation[9]. These techniques are described in detail in Chapter 22.

Stents extending back into the lumen of major or central pulmonary arteries

When the open end of a stent extends back out of a branch pulmonary artery and more than a few millimeters back into the larger more proximal, or even the main, pulmonary artery, the stent partially "jails" the orifice of the vessel. This produces one of the more difficult situations for re-entering the stent and the branch vessels distal to the stent. This is particularly true when the proximal end of a left pulmonary artery stent extends significantly into the main pulmonary artery. Although the normal left pulmonary artery arises as an almost "straight" extension off the main pulmonary artery, in most congenital heart lesions the left pulmonary artery has a sharper angle off the main pulmonary artery. The proximal end of the stent extending back into the main pulmonary artery creates a "wire fence" around the orifice of the left pulmonary artery, which prevents a catheter from "sliding" straight off the main pulmonary artery into the left pulmonary artery. The greater the angle of the branch pulmonary artery off the main, the greater the problem this creates.

The best management of this, like most other problems in the catheterization laboratory, is prevention. It is better to place a stent slightly distal and within an obstruction which is located just at the orifice of the branch than to allow a significant amount of a stent to hang out into the more central vessel. This more accurate positioning is accomplished more satisfactorily with the shorter P 108 and P 118 stents. A shorter stent on a shorter balloon is positioned more easily with the proximal edge of the stent positioned just at the stenosis of the branch vessel. If the shorter stent moves significantly distal to the obstruction and leaves a significant residual stenosis, a second (or third) short stent can be implanted within the first stent during the same, or at a later procedure. Initially, when the shorter stents were not available, extension of the stent proximally into the central vessel was more frequent, and was almost impossible to prevent during the implant of the longer stents into very proximal lesions in either the right or left pulmonary artery. With the use of longer stents, simultaneous, large, long crossing stents can be placed in the bifurcation of the main pulmonary artery in order to protect both orifices.

When a single stent hanging out significantly into the proximal or more central vessel cannot be avoided, there are several techniques that help in entering the overhanging end of the stent and providing access to the branch vessel beyond it. A biplane fluoroscopic system is absolutely essential to accomplish these very complex maneuvers. A large diameter, long sheath is advanced into the main *pulmonary artery*. The tip of the sheath is positioned anterior in the main pulmonary artery and, as a consequence, anterior to the open end of the stent extending from the right or the left pulmonary artery into the main pulmonary artery. A very slight (~30°) curve is formed at the tip of the long sheath before it is introduced. This slight curve at the tip of the sheath allows the direction or position of the tip of the sheath to be changed by slight to-and-fro motions and rotations of the shaft of the sheath.

An end-hole catheter with *an angled tip* is advanced through the long sheath and out of the sheath into the main pulmonary artery, also adjacent to the open end of the stent. The end-hole catheter is manipulated toward the open end of the stent and if possible advanced into the stent. An active tip deflector (Cook Inc., Bloomington, IN) is used within the catheter to deflect the tip of the catheter toward the opening at the end of the stent as visualized on *biplane* fluoroscopy. The long sheath maintains the shaft of the catheter anteriorly and away from the posterior (back) wall of the central pulmonary artery and the sides of the stent where the stent actually enters the branch pulmonary artery. This helps to keep the tip of the *catheter* away from and out of the *sides* of the stent as it is maneuvered out into the central pulmonary artery.

If the catheter itself cannot be advanced into the open end of the stent, a torque-controlled, *exchange length*, spring guide wire with a tight "J" curve at the tip is advanced through the angled tip, end-hole catheter. This usually requires the use of a catheter with a *fixed, stiff and more rigid* angle at the tip. The wire is advanced through the catheter and with the aid of the angled tip of the catheter and the curve on the sheath the "J" curved wire is manipulated toward the open orifice of the stent. The tight "J" curve at the tip of the wire helps to preferentially "back" the curve on the wire through the central *lumen* of the stent rather than "threading" or "weaving" a straight tip of the wire into and through the side cells of the stent. Once the wire has passed into the true lumen of the stent, the wire is advanced (and maneuvered) as far distally in the branch pulmonary artery as possible before attempting to follow the wire with the catheter. Often the catheter with the rigid angle at the tip, which was necessary to direct the wire into the stent, will not follow the wire into the distal vessel. In that case the original catheter is replaced with a Terumo Glide™ catheter (Boston Scientific, Natick, MA), which is advanced into the distal pulmonary artery.

When entering the open end of the stent cannot be accomplished after a *few attempts* with one particular wire or catheter, the wire or catheter or both is/are changed for a different wire or catheter, each with a different curve or tip configuration. Twenty or thirty attempts using exactly the same equipment/technique are no more likely to accomplish the maneuver than the first three or four attempts!

Another alternative for entering a partially "jailed" vessel off the main pulmonary artery is to use a Swan™ floating-balloon catheter, still through the long sheath positioned in the proximal main pulmonary artery "in front of" the "orifice" in the stent. The Swan™ catheter, on its own, more than likely, will "float" toward the *contralateral* pulmonary artery. An active tip deflector (Cook Inc., Bloomington, IN) used within the Swan™ catheter while the balloon is still deflated directs the tip toward the open end of the stent, and then partial inflation of the balloon allows the balloon to be "pulled" into and through the stent as the balloon catheter is advanced off the deflector wire. An additional alternative, still using the Swan™ catheter through the long sheath, is to place a large occlusion balloon in the contralateral branch pulmonary artery. Transient inflation of the occlusion balloon in the contralateral vessel forces all of the pulmonary blood flow into the stented vessel and often helps to "push" the Swan™ balloon into the stent.

A third alternative is to attempt to grasp and pull the open end of the stent toward the catheter with an additional catheter/device while the original catheter is being manipulated into the stent (from the long sheath). An additional end-hole catheter is positioned in the pulmonary artery, *adjacent to the long sheath* and with the tip of the end-hole catheter adjacent to the *side* of the exposed stent. A 0.025", 5 mm curve, active deflector wire is advanced through the second end-hole catheter, the tip of the deflector wire is advanced out of the tip of the catheter, and purposefully passed through the most proximal *side* of the stent. The deflector handle is activated and, in turn, the curving tip of the deflector wire encircles a side strut of a "cell" of the stent, which extends into the proximal pulmonary artery. Once the deflector has been tightened around the strut of the stent, the deflector wire with the tightly curved tip grasping the stent is used to pull the free end of the stent to one side of the central pulmonary artery. This slight change in direction of the stent is often enough to allow one of the other catheters or wires to enter the true central lumen of the stent.

Once a wire or catheter has passed through the lumen of the stent to the distal pulmonary artery beyond the stent, a stiff wire is exchanged for the original wire/catheter and an appropriate long sheath/dilator set is maneuvered through the stent into the distal pulmonary artery. This occasionally is not possible because of the acute angle of the original stent off the main pulmonary artery.

Stent implants in conduits to the pulmonary artery

Stenosis frequently occurs or develops in conduits that have been implanted between a ventricle and the main pulmonary artery. Conduits that are formed from a tube of synthetic material have a fixed diameter. The stenosis in the conduits develops as a result of kinks in the conduit materials, from intimal proliferation within the conduit, from stenosis of prosthetic valvular tissues within the conduits, and from scarring at the anastomoses between the conduit material and either the right ventricle or the pulmonary artery. Although the conduit itself cannot be dilated to a diameter larger than its initial diameter, the stenoses within the conduit are usually amenable to dilation and the implant of stents. Similarly to other intravascular stenoses in pediatric/congenital heart patients, dilation alone of the stenosis in a conduit seldom produces a lasting result. At the same time, pre-dilation with a balloon slightly *smaller* than the desired eventual diameter, is usually performed in order to verify that the stenosis can be opened with a balloon (and stent) at all.

The diameter of the balloon for the delivery of a stent to a conduit is determined from the known original diameter of the conduit tubing or from the measured largest diameter of the pulmonary artery distal to the conduit. A balloon that is larger than the known diameter of the conduit can be used when the pulmonary artery adjacent to the distal end of the conduit widens markedly, but in that situation, the balloon should not be inflated at extremely high pressures. A stent successfully implanted across the area of the valve within the pulmonary conduit, usually will relieve the stenosis, but at the same time will produce wide-open pulmonic regurgitation. The implant of a stent should be questioned when the stenosis is at the proximal end of the conduit in the area of contracting myocardium. Stents subjected to repetitive compressive forces usually fracture fairly quickly or even fragment, with embolization of pieces to the distal pulmonary arteries.

Even with a successful total relief of the stenosis by dilation with an implant of a stent in a pulmonary artery conduit, the stent implant will represent only palliation of the problem. Even if the stent is large enough for the flow in an adult pulmonary artery, pulmonary valve regurgitation develops in the conduits whether a stent is compressing the valve and holding it open or not. Although stenoses occur in conduits in small patients and these can be opened with dilation and a stent implant, the small diameter of the conduits which must be implanted in smaller patients is outgrown and eventually require replacement to compensate for the growth of the patient. When the conduit itself is small, a smaller diameter stent, which will be limited by the diameter of the conduit, can be used in this situation for temporary *palliation*. The stent, which otherwise would have created a stenosis, eventually will be removed along with the small conduit when the conduit is replaced.

Complications of pulmonary artery stents

All of the problems and complication associated with stent delivery and implant to any other location are certainly possible, and actually are even more likely, during the implant of stents in the pulmonary arteries. The general complications of stent implant are discussed in detail in Chapter 22 and are not repeated here. There are particular problems that occur with stent implants into the pulmonary arteries and that are more or less unique to the implant of stents in these locations. Some of the problems that are common with the delivery of all stents occur far more often in the pulmonary arteries. These complications are discussed in this section.

Because of the tight curves encountered in advancing stents to the pulmonary arteries and the curved locations where the stents are implanted, the displacement of any or all of the hand-mounted stents during delivery and implant is more common in pulmonary stent implants than stent implants in any other area. Meticulous attention to the use of the proper equipment, the details of mounting the stents on the delivery balloons, the delivery of the stents through long sheaths, the maintenance of wire position during stent deployment, and the final positioning of the stents/balloons in the lesions all help to prevent stent displacement.

With any of the individually hand-mounted stents, it is quite common to have a stent slide proximally off the balloon and partially or all of the way onto the shaft of the catheter as the balloon/stent is advanced through a tortuous course to a branch pulmonary artery. This *event* is easily recognized on fluoroscopy and can be managed *before* it becomes a *complication*. The balloon catheter is withdrawn through the sheath while the sheath and delivery wire are maintained in their precise positions. The proximal end of the balloon usually catches and pulls the dislodged stent back with the balloon at least to the valve of the long sheath. Occasionally, the dislodged stent will slide back onto the balloon as the balloon catheter is withdrawn. This is *not* necessarily a good thing! If this *even starts* to occur, the balloon is inflated slightly within the sheath to prevent the stent from sliding back over, on, or even off the distal end of the balloon. No attempt is made to deliver the stent at this time even if it appears to reposition itself on the balloon as the combination is being withdrawn. The original cause of the displacement is still present and the stent almost certainly will displace from the balloon again during any attempt at re-advancing the balloon/stent.

Usually the end of a strut of the proximal end of the dislodged stent will catch on the valve mechanism of the sheath as the balloon with the trapped stent is withdrawn to the hub of the sheath. The end of the caught stent, however, usually can be visualized through the valve and grasped with a fine forceps in order to withdraw the stent completely out of the long sheath. Rarely, the stent cannot be grasped through the valve, in which case, the balloon catheter, the stent and the long sheath all must be withdrawn outside of the body over the delivery wire in order to remove the stent from the sheath. In that situation, the delivery process, beginning with the placement of the long sheath across the lesion, is started all over. Once the loose stent and the balloon catheter have been removed from the sheath, an attempt is made to determine what caused the stent to dislodge off the balloon. The stent can dislodge owing to an inappropriate balloon, the stent catching on a flattening surface or kink at a curve in the sheath, an inappropriate positioning of the stent on the balloon initially, or insufficient inflation of the balloon as the balloon/stent is being advanced through the sheath. Once the cause has been determined, the stent is remounted on the same, or a more appropriate balloon and the delivery repeated. If, after several attempts, the cause of the stent dislodgement cannot be corrected, one of the alternative stent delivery techniques must be utilized.

Very rarely and particularly during an implant location in an acutely curved artery *and* when not observing the stent/balloon closely, a hand-mounted stent will slide proximally on the balloon just as the balloon/stent is advanced *out of the sheath*. If this movement is significant and is noticed *before* the stent is completely out of the sheath, the balloon/stent combination is withdrawn over the wire, completely back into the sheath, out of the body, and the stent remounted on the balloon. If the stent moves proximally on the balloon after the sheath is withdrawn completely off of the stent/balloon, the tip of the sheath is used against the proximal end of the stent to "push" the stent back to the center of the balloon. This "pushing" of the stent is performed very cautiously and *gently*, as there always is the danger of a sharp strut at the distal end of particularly the J & J™ P _ _ 8 stents puncturing the balloon as it is pushed back over the balloon. This is more of a problem in a sharply curved vessel. Even a tiny puncture results in an incomplete or no expansion of the stent when the attempt is made at inflating the balloon. The techniques for removing a balloon from a partially expanded stent are covered in detail in Chapter 22.

A very rare and probably preventable problem is the occurrence of a free-floating stent which is still over the guide wire, but totally *distal* to the balloon. This can occur with any of the hand-mounted stents when the stent/balloon combination is withdrawn forcefully against a fixed resistance, for example, against a tight curve within the long sheath, when the stent/balloon which is exposed outside of the sheath is pulled back into the lesion, or during an attempt to pull the stent/balloon combination back into the sheath after the stent on the balloon has been exposed completely out of the sheath. When a stent is free floating and still over the wire distal to the balloon, there are several options. The best option is to replace the original balloon with a smaller balloon, which then can be manipulated back into the unexpanded stent and inflated very slightly—just enough to secure the stent on the balloon. The stent/balloon combination with the partially inflated balloon is then withdrawn very cautiously back into the lesion and the balloon inflated there with the goal of implanting the stent initially with the smaller balloon. If the smaller balloon cannot be introduced completely into the stent, the balloon then is used to push the stent into a far distal branch pulmonary artery. The balloon is pushed into the stent as far as possible in the distal location and the balloon/stent inflated. The balloon is deflated, advanced further into the stent, and the inflation repeated. The entire process is repeated sequentially until the stent is secure in the distal, albeit not the target, location.

Free-floating, fully expanded, stents have ended up in the main pulmonary artery. These usually are a result of a stent/balloon milking proximally during balloon/stent inflation or the stent being pulled back into the larger, more proximal vessel as a balloon is being withdrawn from the stent. With proper technique and control of the wire, the expanded, free-floating stent should still be over the wire as described above. No attempt should be made at withdrawing the expanded stent back through the right ventricle and tricuspid valve, but an attempt can be made at re-advancing the original balloon or an even larger balloon into the stent, "trapping" the stent loosely on the balloon and then pushing the balloon/stent back into the lesion. If the stent was already expanded to a diameter too large to re-enter the original, intended stenotic site, an alternative is to place the "loose" expanded stent in the contralateral pulmonary artery, assuming that the contralateral artery is neither stenotic nor inherently smaller than the "target" vessel.

A stent that is "free-floating" in the main pulmonary artery, but is still over the original wire, is re-cannulated with a separate, additional, end-hole catheter, which is introduced from a separate venous puncture site. The new catheter is maneuvered into and through the "free-floating" stent and then into the contralateral pulmonary artery. This may require the introduction of a third catheter or long sheath with a deflector wire or bioptome, which can be used to grasp the free-floating stent securely in order to control and withdraw the loose stent to a more proximal location in the main pulmonary artery while the other catheter is being manipulated into the contralateral pulmonary artery. Once the new catheter has been manipulated into the contralateral vessel, an exchange length Super Stiff™ wire is advanced through the new catheter and fixed far distally in the contralateral pulmonary artery. The end-hole catheter is removed and a *larger* dilating balloon is advanced over the new Super Stiff™ wire and into the stent. Until this time the original wire passing through the stent and the original lesion serves to secure the "free-floating" stent in the main pulmonary artery and may help to stabilize it while the new catheter, wire and balloon are advanced into and through it.

Once the new wire and/or the new balloon is/are in position in the stent, the original wire is withdrawn completely out of the free-floating stent. The expanded, free-floating stent is "trapped" by expanding the new balloon within the stent enough to secure the stent on the surface of the balloon, but not enough to expand the stent any further. The combination balloon/stent is advanced carefully over the new wire as far as possible into the contralateral pulmonary artery and there the balloon is expanded to its full diameter. If the errant stent is not fixed securely in the contralateral vessel, additional stents can be used over the same wire and placed in tandem through the original stent to fix an unstable stent in the more proximal vessel by the creation of a "very long stent" of multiple overlapping standard stents.

Balloon puncture during stent deployment is more common with P _ _ 8 stents delivered to the pulmonary arteries. This results from the stents necessarily and frequently being delivered to stenotic sites that are present within tight curves in the pulmonary arteries or associated with the implant of "crossing stents" in the pulmonary arteries. In any curved location or against the surface of an adjacent balloon, the very sharp tips of the exposed and extended struts at the ends of the P _ _ 8 stents very readily puncture balloons. Balloon rupture occasionally is due to inflation of the balloons with excessive pressure but, most often, it is at least partially associated with an initial *puncture* of the balloon. The use of the ITI™ Double Strut LD™ and Mega™ stents and the Genesis™ XD stents in these locations should reduce and hopefully even eliminate the problems of balloon puncture and possible balloon rupture during stent implants. Further experience with these stents is necessary in order to determine the effect of the new stents on these serious complications. The unfavorable consequences of balloon puncture/rupture during stent implants, including partial or no stent expansion, balloon rupture and entanglement within the stent, or even balloon separation from the catheter within the stent, all are discussed in detail in Chapter 22 along with their prevention and treatment.

In addition to the problems with balloon displacement and balloon rupture being more common with stents implanted in pulmonary arteries, when they do occur the problems are compounded by their location, which is "downstream" from the right ventricle and, in particular, distal to the tricuspid valve. This always makes access to, and management of, the problems with stents more difficult. The withdrawal of an exposed stent from a pulmonary artery through the right ventricle is very likely to result in the stent/balloon becoming entrapped in the ventricle. This creates an extremely hazardous situation, which in most cases should not even be considered, since it usually requires emergency open-heart surgery to rectify.

Probably the most common "adverse event" that is unique to pulmonary artery stent implants is bleeding into the lung (chest) due to a distal pulmonary vessel (capillary) *puncture* by the tip of the stiff guide wires that are used to deliver and support stent implants. The fairly rigid tip of a stiff delivery guide wire can easily puncture through the *end* of the distal pulmonary artery into (or through) the pulmonary capillary bed. These perforations occur at any time and with even minimal wire manipulation; however, the more manipulations are required with the wire, the sheath/dilator, the catheters, and the balloons over the wire, the greater is the likelihood of such perforations. Since most branch pulmonary artery stents are placed in patients who have had previous intrathoracic surgery, the bleeding from these perforations usually, but not necessarily, is self-limited. Rarely, in the case of such punctures, a thoracocentesis is necessary to evacuate blood from the pleura or the bleeding vessel requires a localized coil occlusion just proximal to the puncture to stop the bleeding. When a puncture from the wire with bleeding does occur and is recognized, the wire ***should not be removed/withdrawn*** until an end-hole *only* catheter can be advanced over the wire to the very far distal location of the wire in the pulmonary parenchyma. Extremely rarely, surgical intervention will be required because of uncontrollable bleeding. When surgery is required, it usually requires at least a pulmonary lobectomy.

Localized, segmental, pulmonary edema distal to an implanted stent is more common following stent implants than following balloon angioplasty of the pulmonary arteries without a stent implant. The implanted stent produces a wider, more effective and permanent opening of the vessel/stenosis with no capability of recoil of the artery compared to balloon dilation alone. Localized pulmonary edema results in a cough, slightly increased respiratory effort, or even frothy sputum along with an increased X-ray density of the pulmonary parenchyma in the involved area. The localized edema *usually* responds to the administration of an intravenous diuretic and results in no real consequence. At the same time, in situations where there are extremely high (systemic or greater) proximal pulmonary artery pressures, the localized pulmonary edema is progressive and can even be life-threatening.

When a stent is being implanted in a branch pulmonary artery in the presence of a high proximal pulmonary artery pressure, the area of narrowing initially should always be opened *only partially* with the implant of the stent. The stenosis eventually can be relieved totally with very small incremental enlargements of the stent during subsequent repeat cardiac catheterizations. However, if in the presence of very high pressures, the stenotic area initially is opened widely and all at once, the maximum high pressure and flow are delivered suddenly to the distal, previously "protected" and "unprepared" pulmonary capillary bed. Since the resistance is so much lower in such an area, a disproportionately large flow is delivered to the area and causes massive, localized, hemorrhagic pulmonary edema. The most drastic, but definitive treatment in the catheterization laboratory of this type of extreme overperfusion is the occlusion of the involved vessel(s) with some type of occlusion device delivered selectively to the involved branch(es) of the pulmonary artery. The alternative treatment is even more drastic and would be a surgical lobectomy or even a pneumonectomy!

Pulmonary artery rupture/disruption probably is the most serious adverse event that occurs during the implant of pulmonary artery stents. Because stents do not need to be and normally are *not* overexpanded purposefully to diameters larger than the adjacent vessels, this complication is less common during stent implants in the pulmonary arteries than during balloon dilation alone of these vessels. The exception to this is in patients with very tight, multiple, stenoses in congenitally narrowed pulmonary arteries, where the proximal pulmonary artery pressures are extremely high, the "narrowed" area is less than one millimeter in diameter, and the "good" adjacent vessel is 3–4 mm or less in diameter. The tissues themselves of the pulmonary arterial walls in these diffuse congenital pulmonary artery stenoses are abnormal. The vessel walls of these pulmonary arteries are thicker, but are less elastic than in normal pulmonary arteries. The stenotic areas in particular, but also the adjacent vessels in these branch pulmonary arteries, are so narrow initially that they necessarily must be dilated to at least three or four times their initial diameter just to accommodate even a pre-mounted stent/balloon. The smaller pre-mounted stents allow delivery without a long sheath and, in turn, allow stent implants to smaller initial diameters. This should reduce the problem of vessel rupture in the distal arteries in these patients. The problem is exaggerated in very tight more proximal vessels, where hand-mounted larger stents must be delivered through large diameter sheaths. These multiple factors result in vessel disruption with even the *very slight* further dilation required as the stent is being implanted. The very tight proximal vessels may not be amenable to treatment with the hand-mounted intravascular stents, however, there is no alternative treatment for most of the multiple branch pulmonary arteries, which are most likely to have vessel rupture, so dilation with stent implant is attempted even in these late stage patients.

Vessel rupture due to distal movement of the balloon during balloon expansion with or without the implant of a stent is not unique to pulmonary artery stents. This occurs when the distal end of the balloon inadvertently is placed in, or "milks" into, a distal vessel that is too small to accommodate the diameter of the expanded balloon. If the balloon does not "milk" back proximally and remains in that small vessel during the balloon inflation, the vessel can tear. Very careful delineation of the size of the target lesion as well as the vessel immediately distal to the lesion is always performed before the stent and delivery balloon are chosen for a lesion. With the properly sized stent and delivery balloon, paying meticulous attention to the positioning of the stent, and controlling the sent during implant, this complication is avoidable. Stent displacement as described previously is a far more common consequence of balloon–vessel size discrepancies and seldom produces as serious a consequence as vessel rupture.

Another group of patients where pulmonary artery stents are used and where the implants are particularly dangerous is the patients who have had *very recent* surgery on their pulmonary arteries (within days to 2 months) and who require emergency "bail-out" for residual critical branch pulmonary artery stenosis or total obstruction. Recent suture lines themselves are not as strong as native vessels, and most of the surrounding adventitia and other supporting tissues, which *were* present around the pulmonary arteries, have been dissected away from the involved arteries during the surgery. At the same time, the fresh sutures in the first few days in the vessels are probably stronger than the "healing" vessels will be for next three to six months. "Healing" occurs in six weeks but "good scarring" of the surrounding tissues takes six or more months. As a consequence, if pulmonary dilation is considered necessary in these patients, dilation with a stent implant should be performed earlier in the post-operative period, and in every case the expansion/implants must be extremely conservative. The implant of a stent in these circumstances eliminates the need for "over-dilation" of the area in order to achieve a result.

In spite of the potential for many or very serious complications during the implant of stents in the pulmonary arteries, with the use of proven techniques, paying meticulous attention to the details of the procedure and (hopefully) with the use of the newer stents, these complications can be minimized, if not totally prevented.

References

1. O'Laughlin MP *et al.* Use of endovascular stents in congenital heart disease. *Circulation* 1991; **83**(6): 1923–1939.
2. Rothman A *et al.* Balloon dilation of branch pulmonary artery stenosis. *Semin Thorac Cardiovasc Surg* 1990; **2**(1): 46–54.
3. Zeevi B, Berant M, and Blieden LC. Midterm clinical impact versus procedural success of balloon angioplasty for pulmonary artery stenosis. *Pediatr Cardiol* 1997; **18**(2): 101–106.
4. Formigari R *et al.* Treatment of pulmonary artery stenosis after arterial switch operation: stent implantation vs. balloon angioplasty. *Catheter Cardiovasc Interv* 2000; **50**(2): 207–211.
5. O'Laughlin MP *et al.* Implantation and intermediate-term follow-up of stents in congenital heart disease. *Circulation* 1993; **88**(2): 605–614.
6. Trant CA Jr *et al.* Cost-effectiveness analysis of stents, balloon angioplasty, and surgery for the treatment of branch pulmonary artery stenosis. *Pediatr Cardiol* 1997; **18**(5): 339–344.
7. Mullins CE *et al.* Implantation of balloon-expandable intravascular grafts by catheterization in pulmonary arteries and systemic veins. *Circulation* 1988; **77**(1): 188–199.
8. Recto MR *et al.* A technique to prevent newly implanted stent displacement during subsequent catheter and sheath manipulation. *Catheter Cardiovasc Interv* 2000; **49**(3): 297–300.
9. Kobayashi Y *et al.* The skirt technique: A stenting technique to treat a lesion immediately proximal to the bifurcation (pseudobifurcation). Catheter Cardiovasc Interv 2000; **51**(3): 347–351.

24 Intravascular stents in venous stenosis

Introduction

Prior to the use of intravascular stents, the treatment of essentially all types of systemic venous stenosis/occlusions was *unsuccessful*. Attempts at surgical repair of venous *stenosis* almost universally resulted in total venous *obstruction*, or, at the very least, a more severe degree of obstruction. There were a few "successful" results from balloon dilation of systemic venous obstruction, however, only the acute or immediate results were reported and even these acute results were very inconsistent and none were long lasting[1].

Intravascular stents have been used to treat venous obstructions for over three decades. Small polyethylene tubes were used more than 35 years ago to "stent" a tract from the protal to the hepatic veins[2]. More than a decade later, metallic, self-expanding and balloon expandable stents were used clinically in systemic veins and to create portacaval shunts[3,4].

During the animal trials of the Palmaz™ P 308 stents (Johnson & Johnson, Warren, NJ), which led to their use in the more common pediatric/congenital lesions, these stents were placed in large central pulmonary arteries and in central systemic arteries as well as in multiple different systemic venous channels of various sizes[5]. The results of the systemic venous stent implants were equally satisfactory to those in the central pulmonary and systemic arteries. There were no thromboses, no re-stenosis, and no unusual intimal proliferation in the veins as a consequence of the stents in the vessels for as long as 24 months as long as the stent/vein had flow through it immediately after implant. As a result of the very favorable animal results in systemic veins, the use of the J & J™ Palmaz™ stents in systemic venous obstruction was included in the original IDE clinical protocol trial for the use of intravascular stents in pediatric and congenital heart lesions[6]. During the sixteen years since the onset of that trial, there has been an extensive use of intravascular stents in a wide variety of systemic venous obstructive lesions in pediatric and congenital heart patients with extremely favorable results in all types of systemic venous obstruction[7]. The venous obstructions that are treated most frequently are obstructions that are secondary to prior interventions including prior surgery on, or even adjacent to, the vein or the venous channel, and following trauma to the intima of the veins from catheter manipulations or indwelling lines. There are rare congenital venous obstructions, venous obstructions secondary to external compression by adjacent structures, and acquired obstructions due to inflammatory changes and neoplasms all of which respond to treatment with intravascular stents.

Equipment

Similarly to the use of stents in other locations, *only stents that can be dilated up to the potential eventual adult diameter of the particular vein are used in the venous channels in any patient*. The very peripheral venous channels, like the peripheral pulmonary arteries, with their significantly smaller diameter of the lumen, even in adult patients, allow the use of some of the smaller diameter stents which, because they are now available pre-mounted, represents a very significant advantage for their delivery and implant. The same stents and the same criteria for the usage of those stents in a vessel of a particular size are used in the systemic veins as are used in the pulmonary arteries.

The newer generations of Genesis™ XD stents (Johnson & Johnson–Cordis Corp., Miami Lakes, FL) along with the Double Strut LD™, Mega™ and Maxi™ stents (ev3, Plymouth, MN) are the predominant stents used in systemic veins at this time. These newer stents have replaced the various sizes of the J & J™ Palmaz™ stents (Johnson & Johnson, Warren, NJ), which were used almost exclusively during the first decade of venous stenting, and for which most of the "longevity" history of stents in these venous structures has been developed.

Genesis™ stents

There are several "lines" of the Genesis™ stents (Johnson & Johnson–Cordis Corp., Miami Lakes, FL), all of which are described in detail in Chapter 22. The "Medium" and so-called "Large" Genesis™ are available very securely pre-mounted on various sized balloons, which makes them easier and safer to deliver. However, both the "Medium" and the "Large" Genesis™ stents can only be expanded to a *maximum* diameter of 11–12 mm and, as a consequence, they are applicable only for implant in the smaller, peripheral veins. The larger Genesis XD™ (or PG _ _ 10B) series of stents (Johnson & Johnson–Cordis Corp., Miami Lakes, FL) are comparable in size to the original Palmaz™ P _ _ 8 series stents and are suitable for all but the very large "common" central systemic venous channels and veins and now are used in most large venous locations because of their relative flexibility and smoother ends.

Intrastents™ in venous stenosis

Like the Genesis™ stents, there are several varieties or "lines" of Intrastent™ (ITI, ev3, Plymouth, MN), all of which are described in detail in Chapter 22. The initial stents from ITI, which were used in pediatric/congenital lesions, were the Double Strut LD™ stents, which are manufactured with an elaborate and complex laser cut, which gives the stents an "open-cell" configuration with considerable flexibility and smoother ends. These stents are available in 16, 26, 36, 56 and 76 millimeter lengths and have an *in vitro* tested wall strength, *up to their advertised diameter of 12 mm*, that is comparable to the J & J™ Palmaz™ P_ _8 series of stents. The particular cell design creates an interlock with adjacent stents when they are overlapped in tandem. This combination of characteristics makes Double Strut LD™ stents very appealing for implants at smaller diameters, and especially in longer, peripheral venous lesions. They can be dilated up to 18–20 mm in diameter if necessitated by the growth of a patient.

At diameters greater than 12 mm, the Double Strut LD™ stents definitely have less wall strength compared to the P _ _ 8 stents, and, as a consequence, have been replaced by the Mega™ and Maxi™ stents (ev3, Plymouth, MN) for primary use in the larger veins. The Mega™ stents can be dilated to diameters comparable to the Palmaz™ P _ _ 8 stents, and at the larger diameters they appear to have comparable wall strengths. The Maxi™ stents are comparable in size and wall strength to the even larger, J & J™ P _ _ 10 stents (Johnson & Johnson, Warren, NJ) and are used in the very large, "common" central venous channels.

As in the pulmonary arteries and any other area, all of the ITI™ stents are easily distorted or dislodged by any catheter or balloon manipulations within the stent immediately after they are implanted. As a consequence, once implanted, they are not manipulated *during the same catheterization* procedure. The wires, sheaths and delivery balloons are the same as those used for pulmonary artery stents (Chapters 22 & 23).

Technique—stent implants in central venous and baffle obstructions

Usually, superior vena caval and other central vein obstruction in the more cephalad venous system is manifest by varying degrees of a "superior vena caval syndrome", with general swelling and edema of the head, upper trunk and upper extremities, headaches and eventually even hydrocephalus. Occasionally, however, significant central obstructions of the superior vena cava or the superior baffle of a venous switch repair will have remarkably few signs and symptoms because of the large and extensive collaterals around the area of obstruction. The obstructions may only become apparent when venous access to the heart is attempted from an upper extremity or jugular vein. This occurs frequently in patients who have undergone "venous switch" repairs of transposition of the great arteries, and who often require access from the superior vena cava for the implant of a transvenous pacemaker.

Inferior vena cava and inferior baffle limb obstruction can be even more subtle, but eventually presents with hepatomegaly, lower extremity edema and/or ascites. The treatment of these lesions with dilation and concomitant intravascular stent implants is very successful and is recommended at the earliest detection of even mild to moderate degrees of obstruction even before any significant signs or symptoms appear. Some of the consequences of central venous obstruction (hydrocephalus and liver damage in particular) are irreversible. It is better to prevent these complications than to treat them after they occur, and dilation with the implant of intravascular stents now offers a safe and effective therapy.

The implant of most venous stents can be performed using deep sedation with liberal local anesthesia at the site of catheter introduction. General anesthesia, however, is recommended when long, extensive recanalizations or other manipulations are necessary from any approach, if any of the procedure is to be carried out through the internal jugular vein approach, or if multiple superior venous (brachial, axillary, subclavian, or jugular) access sites are necessary. "Transseptal" type punctures through venous obstructions in the cephalic venous channels, which are performed from the neck, and the delivery of stents from the superior vena caval approach, both are definite indications for the use of general anesthesia.

As with all therapeutic catheterizations, an indwelling arterial line is utilized for continuous arterial pressure monitoring and/or arterial blood gas sampling. Since these procedures can be very long, an indwelling urinary catheter in the bladder is placed in all of these patients. This is particularly important when stents are being implanted in veins in the iliofemoral area. A bladder full of contrast, in addition to making the patient very uncomfortable, completely obliterates the lateral view of the pelvic area of the iliofemoral veins! Because of the generally sluggish flow in the venous system and the potential for total obstruction to this flow by the catheters and sheaths during the dilation and stent implant procedures, heparin is administered intravenously once all of the lines for the procedure have been introduced. The patients are given 100 units/kilogram of heparin and in long cases supplemental doses are given to maintain the ACT in the 300–350 second range.

The areas of venous stenosis are identified by *biplane* angiograms either in the combined PA and lateral views or in biplane angled views, depending on the site of the obstruction. The degree of stenosis is determined primarily from the angiographic appearance of the lesion, comparing the diameter of the obstructed area to the diameters of the adjacent "normal" venous channels. The X-ray views used to visualize the stenosis during the procedure are the X-ray angles that place the area of stenosis in its longest possible axis, which, in turn, place the X-ray tubes perpendicular to the obstruction. Contrast is injected into the vein in a location proximal to (in the direction of the flow of blood), and as close to the obstruction as possible. The angiograms are performed using a *large-scale calibration system* such as a calibrated 1 or 2 cm "marker" catheter, a separate grid calibration system, or a *centimeter* calibration system which is built into the X-ray system in order to obtain very accurate measurements of the diameters and lengths of both the stenosis and the adjacent vessel(s).

Low or absent pressure gradients across venous lesions have essentially *no* meaning in relation to the degree of stenosis. Because of the generally low pressures in the venous channels, the frequently extensive and often multiple collateral channels around any area of obstruction and, of even more importance, the high compliance of the entire systemic venous system, *usually* no "significant" pressure gradient is generated across even very severe (or even total) obstructions in systemic venous channels. The pressures and gradients across the areas often are not even recorded in the evaluation and treatment of venous stenosis, although when any pressure gradient *is present* across an area of stenosis, it represents very significant obstruction.

The major challenge for the implant of stents into systemic venous channels often is entering the channel initially and then traversing the severely stenotic or *often totally obstructed* venous channels. Once the obstructed venous channel is entered and its entire length traversed with even a wire, it can be dilated with stents implanted to open the channel completely. In general, the "routes" to venous obstructions are straighter and there is a shorter distance from the venous introductory site to the stenosis than for other intravascular stent implant procedures.

There are four common areas of significant venous obstruction commonly encountered in pediatric and congenital heart patients. These are:

1 Baffle obstructions in the superior and inferior limbs of the systemic venous return following venous switch repairs ("Mustard" or "Senning") for transposition of the great arteries;

2 Superior vena caval obstruction secondary to prior surgery on or in the vicinity of the superior vena cava or indwelling venous lines in the internal jugular veins and/or superior vena cava;

3 Femoral vein or iliofemoral vein obstruction secondary to indwelling venous lines or previous cardiac catheterizations through those veins; and

4 Obstructions in the systemic venous/pulmonary artery circuits following all types of cavopulmonary ("Fontan") surgical repairs.

The introduction of the venous lines and the approach to the catheter/stent recanalization is different for each of these areas and for the different obstructions within each type of lesion.

A total venous obstruction is identified angiographically with an injection of contrast solution proximal to, or "upstream" to the obstruction. Often, even a total venous obstruction creates relatively few, if any, signs or symptoms and is discovered incidentally during an attempted cardiac catheterization. Although localized, total venous obstruction causes no obvious signs or symptoms in the child or young adult, venous obstructions do generate long-term problems of venous stasis with aging, and venous obstruction often prevents the necessary access for trans-catheter diagnostic or therapeutic procedures.

For obstructions in the superior baffle limb or the superior vena cava itself, a catheter is introduced into an upper extremity or the right internal jugular vein and advanced until the tip of the catheter is positioned immediately adjacent to the site or area of obstruction. A selective angiogram is performed through this catheter for the visualization and quantification of the precise area of the superior venous obstruction and to visualize all adjacent structures. The vessels/channels are calibrated usually using a "marker" angiographic catheter or the centimeter calibration system built into the X-ray system. A separate venous catheter is introduced from the inguinal/femoral area and advanced to a position in the vein that is adjacent to the distal end of the venous obstruction, which is, in turn, "downstream" from the lesion. A separate or simultaneous angiogram is performed with an injection through this second catheter and/or both catheters at the same time. The angiograms from "both ends" of the obstruction demonstrate the exact area and extent of the venous obstruction.

Occasionally there is a tiny residual "string like" channel extending through a venous obstruction. In that situation, an attempt is made at cannulating this channel with a fine tipped, *exchange length*, torque-controlled or a Terumo™ Glide™ wire (Terumo Medical Corp., Somerset, NJ). The exact wire used depends upon the course of the channel. The 0.021″ curved tip or straight Glide Wire™ or the 0.018″ Platinum Plus™ (Medi-Tech, Boston Scientific, Natick, MA) are both effective for precise, controlled manipulations through very narrow residual channels. If one of these wires can be passed entirely through the obstruction from either direction, an attempt is made at passing a small, fine tipped ("feather tipped"), long dilator through the channel over the wire. The 6-French, 52 cm long dilator from a Mullins™ Pediatric Transseptal set (Medtronic Inc., Minneapolis, MN) has a very fine, smooth taper over a 0.025″ wire and makes an excellent instrument for "drilling" through obstructions over a fine, long wire.

When there is too much resistance in the scarred tissues to allow the dilator to be advanced (pushed) over the wire alone, the angiographic catheter at the opposite end of the obstructed area is replaced with a snare catheter. The free, distal end of the wire that had passed through the obstruction is grasped with the snare and is pulled taut with the snare. This traction on both ends of the wire pulls the wire very taut and provides support to the wire while the dilator is "drilled" through the channel from the opposite end. Rarely, only a very fine 3- or 4-French dilator can initially be advanced through the channel using this technique. Once any dilator has been pushed/pulled through the channel, it is replaced over the through-and-through wire with successively larger dilators with larger openings in their tips until a larger, stiffer exchange length guide wire can be passed through the dilator. Once a large stiff wire has passed through the obstruction, a long sheath/dilator set is advanced through it. Thereafter, larger stiffer wires, dilators or dilation balloons are sequentially advanced through the area, gradually dilating it. Eventually a long sheath that is large enough to accommodate the delivery of the desired stent is passed through the obstructed area.

If a small, fine-tipped dilator cannot be pushed over the wire and through the stenotic tract through the obstruction even when using the tension from the snare catheter pulling from the other end, the dilator is replaced over the wire with a 2 or 3 mm diameter very low-profile "coronary artery" balloon with a very finely tapered tip. The coronary balloon is advanced into the stenotic venous channel over the snare-supported wire and sequentially inflated and deflated as it is pushed/pulled further into, and eventually through, the channel. Once the very small dilation balloon has been advanced through the stenotic channel completely, it is replaced with a 5-French sheath/dilator set. The original fine wire is replaced through the sheath with an appropriately larger, stiffer exchange wire for the delivery of further balloons and the stent.

Traversing totally obstructed venous channels

If there is no residual channel through the obstruction or if the channel cannot be cannulated with a wire and dilated, then the totally obstructed area often can be crossed with a *transseptal needle* and a transseptal sheath/dilator set (Medtronic Inc., Minneapolis, MN). The use of a transseptal needle provides precise directional control to the puncture through the obstructed area, as opposed to probing with the stiff end of a wire that has no directional control. Puncture through a totally occluded area *absolutely requires* biplane fluoroscopic and good "freeze frame" imaging. By paying precise attention to the anatomy and to the details of the procedure, obstructed areas as long as 3–4 cm can be crossed safely with the directional control provided by the needle. Venous obstructions that occur in areas where there has been previous surgery are surrounded by dense scar tissue, which is difficult to puncture but does provide a solid mass of "supporting" tissue around the obstructed vein. Angiograms are recorded in any adjacent chambers or vessels as well as at both ends of the obstruction of the venous channel in order to visualize all of the important landmarks. As long as the tip of the needle is maintained in the precise, desired, directions as observed on *biplane* fluoroscopy, no other vital structures or vessels adjacent to the area surrounding the superior vena caval obstruction (or the course of the needle puncture!) will be in the path of the needle. The needle should not be advanced, rotated or otherwise moved unless the needle tip is being visualized fluoroscopically.

The "transseptal" puncture can be approached from either the right internal jugular vein or from either femoral vein. Because of the arrangement of most catheterization laboratories and tables, the femoral approach generally is more "convenient". The approach used, however, is determined by the anatomy of the visible *patent venous channels* at *both ends* of the obstruction. Intuitively, the approach that gives the "straightest shot" directly at the obstructed area would be chosen. However, the size and location of the venous channel *at the opposite end of the obstruction* which represents the "target" of the puncture is of far *more importance* in determining from which direction to perform the puncture. The approach used is that from which the tip of the particular transseptal needle used during the puncture can be directed precisely toward the center of the lumen of the ***venous "target" channel*** at the opposite end of the obstruction. "Engaging" the proximal end of the obstructed venous channel with the needle is not a problem when approaching from either direction; however, keeping the needle tip directed at a small, patent, venous "target" channel at the opposite end of a long obstruction, is often very difficult or impossible when using the femoral approach and, in particular, when a very forceful "push" must be applied to the needle in order to cross the obstruction. A catheter is positioned and maintained in the venous channel which represents the "target" at the *opposite end* of the obstruction from the "puncture side". The catheter in the "target" channel provides a persistent landmark for the direction of the puncture regardless of any distortion caused by the force on the needle.

An end-hole catheter is positioned adjacent to the obstruction at the end where the puncture is to be performed and a guide wire with a short, floppy tip is passed through this catheter to the site of the obstruction. The catheter and the original venous sheath are removed over this wire and replaced with a 6-French transseptal sheath/dilator set. The tip of the dilator of the transseptal set is positioned as close to the area for puncture as possible. The "original" USCI™ Transseptal Set™ (Medtronic Inc., Minneapolis, MN) has the tightest, smoothest and finest taper over the needle of any of the transseptal dilators. As a consequence, this represents the best transseptal *dilator* for this particular procedure. The curve at the tip of the transseptal needle often must be changed slightly to conform to the course and direction from the initial puncture, into the obstruction, and toward the open "channel" at the opposite side of the obstruction as determined from the previous angiograms. This may require straightening or, just the opposite, increasing the bend at the distal end of the needle according to the particular anatomy. Once the proper curve has been created on the needle, the guide wire is removed from the dilator, the needle is introduced into the sheath/dilator set and advanced to the tip of the dilator. With the tip of the needle still within the tip of the dilator, the combination needle/sheath/dilator is rotated and moved gently in order to point the tip toward the "target channel" at the opposite end of the obstruction.

With this type of puncture, the pressures obtained through the needle during the puncture procedure have absolutely no meaning or value, so continuous pressure monitoring is *not* used during punctures through totally obstructed venous channels. Instead, a small (2–3 ml), hard syringe is filled with contrast and attached to the hub of the needle.

The needle is advanced into the tissues toward the "target" venous channel while observing the direction of the needle continuously in both planes of the fluoroscopy. As long as the needle remains directed precisely at the "target" area, the needle/sheath/dilator all are advanced together into the obstruction. Biplane imaging is accomplished either by rapidly alternating between the PA and the LAT fluoroscopy planes or by observing the two planes simultaneously (available with some systems). A single plane X-ray system is *totally unsatisfactory* for this procedure. Even with a rapidly rotating X-ray suspension C-arm, the changes in direction and position of the needle during these punctures are too rapid and too frequent to be controlled with a single-plane system.

When the needle is advanced into areas that are not well identified, *very tiny* (0.1 ml) injections of contrast are made through the needle and into the tissues along the tract while recording on biplane angiography. The tiny "tag" of contrast in the tissues verifies that the needle tip is still moving in the correct direction or that the needle tip is no longer within the surrounding scar tissues. Only a *very tiny amount* of contrast should be injected through the needle. If a larger volume of contrast is used for this "tag", the entire area is obliterated by the opacity of the contrast extravasating into the tissues. The extravasated contrast can take up to several hours to clear from the tissues so larger volumes are avoided at all costs.

When, even with various rotations of the needle/dilator/sheath, the needle tip no longer can be directed precisely at the "target" area as it is being advanced into the obstruction, the needle is withdrawn from the sheath/dilator set leaving the sheath/dilator in the obstructed tract, while the needle is reshaped to form a more appropriate curve on it. The needle is reintroduced into the sheath/dilator and the advancing of the needle/dilator/sheath is resumed.

When the needle reaches the previously positioned catheter in the "target" venous channel at the opposite end of the obstruction or while advancing the needle, any sensation of "give" is felt, a small injection of contrast is made through the *second catheter* positioned in the "target channel" to verify the relative position of the needle tip in relation to the "target" channel. The relationship of the needle to the "target" channel can distort the tissues in the area from the pressure and torsion of the needle pushing into the tissues. As a consequence, the needle tip can appear to be "touching" the second catheter, while it actually still can be separated by several millimeters of tissue. When, from the first angiogram, the tip of the needle appears to be in the proper position in the distal "chamber", a repeat *0.1 ml* of contrast is injected *through the needle*. When the needle has entered the "target" venous channel, the contrast swirls freely away from the needle. When the tip of the needle still is in the tissues, another small "tag" of contrast is created in the tissues at the tip of the needle. The "tag" of contrast demonstrates any distortion of the tissues by the needle and provides a definitive relationship of the tip of the needle to the potential "target". The angle of the needle is adjusted to compensate for any distortion and the puncture is continued in the corrected direction until the "target" channel is entered.

Once the tip of the needle is *in* the channel of the "target" vessel, the tip of the needle is directed to follow the course of the most open channel, and the entire transseptal set is advanced through the obstruction. Occasionally, only the tip of the needle and just the tip of the dilator can be advanced through the dense scar around the obstruction and into the open channel. In this circumstance, the transseptal needle and dilator are fixed in this position while the angiographic catheter in the lumen of the "target" channel is replaced with a snare catheter. The snare is opened and positioned around the tip of the needle/dilator in the target channel. The dilator is held in place very securely in the tract by maintaining a slight "push" on it while the needle alone is carefully withdrawn from the sheath/dilator. An exchange length guide wire that can pass through the tip of the dilator is advanced through the dilator, into the open "target" channel and grasped with the snare. The exchange guide wire is pulled taut with the snare and the sheath/dilator set "drilled" through the obstruction by pushing and "spinning" the set over the *taut* wire. If the sheath still cannot be advanced through the scarred tissues, the sheath/dilator set is exchanged over the *snared exchange wire* for a long dilator of a smaller French size and with a very fine tipped orifice, or for a low-profile, 3–4 mm diameter, high-pressure coronary angioplasty balloon.

The tract is dilated by sequentially advancing either the dilator or the dilation balloon over the taut wire. Once the dilator or balloon has passed completely through the obstruction, the dilator or balloon is exchanged over the still grasped, small wire for a new dilator with a larger lumen at the *tip*, which will accommodate at least a 0.035″ wire. The original small wire is exchanged for a Super Stiff 0.035″ wire and either a slightly larger angioplasty balloon or the dilator with the sheath for the delivery of the stent is introduced. Even the larger wire may have to be grasped with a snare from the opposite end to keep it taut in order to "pull" the larger dilator through the tract. The tract usually is pre-dilated only enough so that the long sheath for the delivery of the desired stent can pass through it.

If a very tight and resistant stenosis is encountered when the stenosis is being traversed initially, the tract is pre-dilated to a slightly larger diameter to ensure that it can be expanded at all when dilated during the stent implant. The tract is pre-dilated to no more than approximately 75% of the ultimate desired diameter. Often, a high-pressure balloon is necessary for the predilation in this area or for the final dilation of the stent after implant.

A stent is chosen that can be dilated to the eventual *adult diameter* of the vein/venous channel and in a length that covers the lesion but, at the same time, does not extend into adjacent chambers or veins. The length of the stent is particularly important in the reconstruction of "venous switch" ("Mustard" or "Senning") baffles in order not to cross the channel of the opposite baffle or to be too close to the left atrioventricular valve. The obstruction of the superior limb of these baffles often occurs just at the cardiac end of the baffle and usually is on a curve, which can be as acute as a 90° angle, off the more proximal portion of the channel. In the presence of a sharp curve, either multiple shorter stents, which are implanted in tandem and overlapping, or a very flexible stent should be used to conform to the curvature. When the J & J™, Palmaz™ P _ _ 8 or P _ _ 10 stents are used in these curved central venous locations, it is better to place two or more shorter stents in tandem in order to create a final "curved stent" that will conform to the vessel, than to use one long stent which would "straighten out" (and distort) the area or impinge on adjacent structures.

In smaller patients, a single, long, ITI™ Double Strut LD™ stent (ev3, Plymouth, MN) can be used in these superior baffles. These stents conform to the curves in the venous channels very well and they will support even fairly dense, resistant stenoses and hold the vessels open as well as a J & J™ P _ _ 8 stent (Johnson & Johnson, Warren, NJ), but only *up to 12 mm in diameter.* A single, ITI™ Double Strut™ stent definitely will *not be* strong enough to hold a very constrictive stenosis open at a diameter over 12 mm. However, Double Strut LD™ stents can eventually be dilated up to 20 mm and maintained at these diameters by implanting an additional stent within the original Double Strut™ at the time of redilation. In smaller patients, Double Strut LD™ stents have the advantage that they can be delivered to the smaller diameter vessels on smaller balloons and, in turn, through smaller sheaths.

The Cordis™ Genesis XD™ stents (Johnson & Johnson–Cordis Corp., Miami Lakes, FL) and the ITI™ Mega™ and Maxi™ stents (ev3, Plymouth, MN), all expand to the necessary diameters of adult "central" veins, they all are available in multiple lengths, they all have some flexibility, and *none* have the sharp ends of the earlier J & J™ Palmaz™ stents. As a consequence, the Genesis XD™, the Mega™ and the Maxi™ stents currently are the preferred stents for use in these central venous areas. The Maxi™ is the only stent available which is both "flexible" and can be dilated to *over* 18 mm diameter. All of these larger diameter stents still must be "hand-mounted" and delivered to larger vessels (diameters) through relatively large, long sheaths. These newer generation stents are replacing the J & J™ Palmaz™ stents completely in these areas.

Once the stenotic central venous area has been traversed and a long delivery sheath has been passed through the area of obstruction, the stent delivery is relatively straightforward. The course of the sheath to the area of obstruction usually is relatively straight, which decreases the likelihood of stent displacement during the delivery of the stent to the site. Similar to stent implants in other areas, venous stents are expanded to the diameter of the nearest normal vessel. When tandem stents are required, each additional stent is implanted at a diameter at least 2 mm larger than the previous stent in order to secure it in place.

Stent implant in peripheral vein obstruction

Iliofemoral vein obstruction is the most common venous obstruction encountered in the pediatric/congenital catheterization laboratory. When femoral vein or iliofemoral vein obstruction is present, it is usually discovered incidentally during attempts at percutaneous entry into the femoral vessel. Obstruction of these veins rarely produces signs or symptoms in children or young adults, although a barely noticeable "Medusa" of superficial veins over the involved inguinal area and lower abdominal wall frequently represents an indicator of potential obstruction of the deeper veins. Although obstructions of these veins are not associated with symptoms, at least not during childhood, they do frequently produce a major problem for venous access in patients where repeated or multiple venous access is essential for subsequent management. It is important to address venous obstruction therapeutically and aggressively in the catheterization laboratory whenever it is discovered, but particularly when it is found early in the course of a staged repair of a complex cardiac defect or in patients who, it is anticipated, will require frequent, subsequent cardiac catheterizations[8]. Patients in these categories include cardiac transplant patients, hypoplastic left heart and other patients who will require "single ventricle" repairs, patients with more than a single isolated branch pulmonary artery stenosis as a result of either congenital defects or post-unifocalization, and any other complex anatomy where multiple or staged repairs are necessary.

The long-term patency of "rebuilt" peripheral veins depends upon establishing adequate flow through the vein which has been freshly opened with the implant of a stent. Even when a vein is opened widely with one or more stents, but, at the same time, there is no flow through the vein/stents, the venous channel will thrombose and re-occlude almost unequivocally. This creates a real and frequent problem when attempting to establish flow in stenosed or occluded veins where the stenosis/obstruction extends close to the inguinal area. If the most proximal end of the stent (in the direction of flow) cannot be positioned within a lumen of the vein where there is adequate flow, the stent very likely will re-occlude up to an area where good venous flow has been established. Unfortunately, in the inguinal area, stents cannot be extended back into the skin puncture site! At the same time, when the vein is totally obstructed but has been traversed with a wire, an attempt *should be* made to rebuild the vein with intravascular stents. If the vein does re-occlude totally, there will be *no less* blood going through the vessel! As a consequence, nothing except the time and effort of the implant procedure is lost by the attempt at rebuilding the occluded vein! In addition, the easily visualized course of the previously implanted stents in the iliofemoral area creates a very visible "target" during subsequent catheterizations for the puncture into, and subsequent recanalization of, the same venous tract, which is now within the stent. This type of recanalization of a tract *within* an iliofemoral venous stent that has become totally obstructed, has proved successful and extremely useful on multiple occasions, and has allowed repeat catheterizations through the same route in very complex patients.

Technique for peripheral vein stent implant

The diagnosis of vein obstruction is suspected when the percutaneous needle enters the vein with a good blood return and the wire ***easily*** advances, but only a *short distance* (1–2 cm) beyond the tip of the needle before it stops advancing. The puncture area is visualized on fluoroscopy *in both planes* to confirm the positions of the wire and the needle. The course of the wire *must be* viewed in the lateral (LAT) as well as the posterior–anterior (PA) projection to be sure it is not passing deep, posteriorly into the pelvis even when, in the PA projection, it appears to be passing in the direction of the normal femoral vein. If the wire is passing roughly parallel to the skin surface in the LAT view and in the typical course for the femoral vein, the *wire* is fixed securely in this position while the puncture needle is withdrawn over the wire and replaced with the plastic cannula of a Medi-cut™. Blood should return through the cannula of the Medi-cut™ *around the wire* as the Medi-cut™ is introduced into the vein. The Medi-cut™ is advanced over the wire into the tissues as far as possible. If there is still blood return through the cannula of the Medi-cut™, the wire is slowly removed and a small gentle hand injection of contrast is performed through the cannula of the Medi-cut™ while *recording* in *both the PA and LAT* projections. A very fine, slightly irregular tract of contrast often is seen following the *usual* course of the femoral vein. This tract *is* what is left of the original vein. The tract usually has a blind end before it actually empties into any other vein. A 0.021″ Terumo™ wire (Terumo Medical Corp., Somerset, NJ) is introduced into the Medi-cut™ and advanced as far as possible into this tract.

An alternative scenario is that the needle enters the vein and blood return is obtained, but a wire cannot be introduced beyond the needle at all. When this is repeated several times and blood is still flowing freely from the hub of the puncture needle, a *biplane* angiogram of the area is performed with a ***small, slow and gentle*** hand injection of 1–2 ml of contrast *through the needle*. A large or forceful injection through this needle will extravasate contrast into the surrounding tissues and obliterate everything in the area for many minutes. Usually the contrast flow from the needle following a gentle injection will track forward in a straight direction for at least several millimeters and then detour through numerous very circuitous collateral venous channels which course predominantly posteriorly and into the pelvis. Very often, however, a fine, *straight*, thread-like tract of contrast does appear and continues anteriorly, parallel to the surface of the skin in the LAT view following the course of what *was* the femoral vein! Because of the multiple overlapping collateral veins in the PA view, this tract often is a tiny, straight, anterior tract, which is apparent only on the *lateral view* of the angiogram. When this tract is present, a soft tipped wire is introduced under direct fluoroscopic visualization and advanced as far as possible past the tip of the needle. With careful, gentle manipulation the wire often enters the fine tract. In any case the puncture needle is replaced over this wire with the plastic cannula of the Medi-cut™. The soft tipped wire is replaced with a 0.021″ straight Terumo™ wire (Terumo Medical Corp., Somerset, NJ) and the straight tract is cannulated as far as possible with the Terumo™ wire.

In either scenario for entering the scarred "tract of the femoral vein", once the Terumo™ wire is 2 or more cm into this tract, the Medicut™ is withdrawn over the Terumo™ wire and replaced with a 5- or 6-French *fine tipped, long,* stiff dilator. The long dilators from the original USCI™ transseptal sets have the best tips for this vein dilation. The long dilator is straightened so that there is only a *very slight* curve formed at the tip of the dilator before it is introduced. The straightened dilator allows for more "forward" push on it while the slight curve permits some directional changes in its course as it is advanced. The dilator is advanced to the tip of the Terumo™ wire. With the tip of the dilator pointed in the direction of the course of the venous "tract", the Terumo™ wire is pushed several millimeters forward out of the dilator. The dilator again is advanced to the tip of the wire. The wire and fine dilator frequently follow the course of the original vein, in all likelihood dilating through old thrombus as they advance. This procedure is repeated in very small increments, continually observing the course with biplane fluoroscopy, until the wire has either "popped into" a patent venous channel connecting with the inferior vena cava (IVC) (rarely) or reached the site of the usual bifurcation of the IVC into the iliac vein.

If the wire does not enter the patent venous channel, an end-hole venous catheter is introduced from a vein on the upper trunk (arm, jugular, etc.) and is manipulated through the right atrium and as far as possible caudally into the portion of the more proximal IVC, which is still patent. In order to reach the most caudal limits of the patent IVC/iliofemoral veins, this often requires the use of a combination of a torque-controlled, end-hole catheter along with a torque-controlled wire and multiple small angiograms in the veins along the way. Once the most caudal limit of the patent inferior vena cava is reached with this catheter, a biplane angiogram is recorded with an injection through this catheter from above. The PA and LAT angiograms demonstrate the caudal-most limits of any still patent venous channel/IVC from above and the relationship of this channel to the tip of the wire/dilator coming from below.

The end-hole catheter from above is "pushed" into the most caudal end or "stump" of the patent cephalic venous channel and maintained in that position. The dilator/wire from below is directed toward the tip of the catheter coming from above. The tip of the catheter that was introduced from above should be positioned in the area of the *true*, patent venous channel closest to the wire/dilator that is coming from below. The Terumo™ wire is advanced out of the dilator toward the tip of the end-hole catheter. The wire is withdrawn and advanced many times, each time "inching" the dilator forward until the wire enters the patent cephalad vein *or* until it becomes obvious that it is not going to traverse the intervening tissues. When the wire does enter the patent channel, it is followed with the dilator using one or more of the assist maneuvers described previously for traversing obstructions in the venous channel from above.

When the wire does not enter the patent channel on its own and the patent area is within 0.5–1 cm of the tip of the dilator, the Terumo™ wire in the dilator is replaced with a transseptal needle. This may require first replacing the original dilator over the wire with a dilator that will accommodate the transseptal needle; however, the 21-gauge tip and the "pediatric" transseptal needle will advance through a 5-French "feather tipped" dilator. The needle is pre-curved outside of the body to correspond to the angle necessary to traverse the "gap" between the tip of the dilator and the patent, more central, venous channel. The needle is introduced into the dilator and the same procedure is utilized for puncture through an obstruction as described previously in this chapter for puncturing through an obstructed area of a superior caval baffle. Biplane fluoroscopic control of this puncture is absolutely necessary. Once the needle enters the patent channel, the same procedures for switching to a wire, then to the dilation balloon or to a sheath for stent delivery is used as described previously.

There is one, very significant difference in the nature of these peripheral obstructions compared to the central, large venous obstructions. In obstructions in the central venous channels, there almost always has been previous surgery in the area of the venous channel, and the obstruction is surrounded by dense scar tissue. This usually is *not* the situation in peripheral obstructions, where the obstruction is a consequence of internal "trauma" to the vein and there is little or no surrounding scar tissue. As a consequence, any puncture outside of these peripheral veins is into the free tissue spaces around the veins or into *adjacent structures.* In the case of the pelvic and abdominal veins this is into the retroperitoneal space. When a small injection of contrast is performed outside of the vessel channel into the retroperitoneal tissues, the contrast moves away from the area very slowly and gradually dissipates in the tissues without further accumulation of blood in the area. Because of the very small puncture hole from the needle alone, the low venous pressures, and the confined space of the retroperitoneal space, these punctures do not result in significant extravasation of blood nor result in any lasting problems. When a puncture between the blind end of the occluded venous channel and the open more central channel is performed, it often is through this "open retroperitoneal space" with no surrounding scar tissue. Even when this "open space" is stented *for a short distance* and good flow is established through the stent, there is surprisingly little extravasation of blood!

The exception to this lack of scar tissue surrounding the peripheral veins is in the circumstance when the obstruction is secondary to a previous puncture or tear of the vein which resulted in a significant retroperitoneal bleed. In that circumstance, the entire retroperitoneal space is filled with scar tissue and puncture through the area is safer.

Once the peripheral venous obstruction has been identified, calibrated, and, if necessary, re-cannulated as just described, the angiographic or dilating catheter is removed over the through-and-through wire and replaced with an end-hole catheter that will accommodate a 0.035" guide wire. Usually the catheter is advanced, and the venous stents are introduced and implanted, *in the direction of the venous flow*. The end-hole catheter is maneuvered through the area of venous stenosis into the patent, more central vein to a position far from the obstruction. A Super Stiff™ 0.035" guide wire with a long flexible tip is passed through the catheter to a position well beyond the obstruction and into the patent more central vein. A long sheath/dilator set that will accommodate the proposed stent is introduced over the Super Stiff™ wire. The Super Stiff™ wire is important, particularly in cases where there is a bend or circuitous course between the puncture site into the venous system and in or through the site of venous obstruction.

If the area of stenosis is large enough to accommodate the diameter of the intended delivery sheath, it is not pre-dilated. If the area of stenosis is less than 4 mm in diameter or was very difficult to traverse initially, a 5 or 6 mm diameter dilation balloon is advanced over the 0.035" wire, positioned so that the balloon is centered in the area of the stenosis, and a pre-dilation of the area is performed. The size of the pre-dilating balloon should be no more than 50% of the diameter of the nearest normal vein that is adjacent to the area of stenosis and no more than 50% of the anticipated implant diameter of the stent. The balloon is inflated to the maximum recommended pressure or until the waist on the balloon is eliminated as visualized on fluoroscopy. This pre-dilation is necessary to allow the larger delivery sheaths to pass through the area of stenosis and to ensure that the stent will open to a large enough diameter to allow removal of the initial, lower-pressure, stent delivery balloon. After successful pre-dilation, the balloon is withdrawn over the wire leaving the 0.035" wire in place across the stenosis in the vein and with the tip of the wire as far distal to the stenosis as possible. The appropriate diameter, long transseptal sheath/dilator set is straightened to correspond to the wire course to the particular area of stenosis that is to be stented.

A smaller (8- or 9-French) long sheath is chosen when the area to be dilated with a stent is very tight and it is anticipated that a stent expansion to 10 mm or less in diameter initially will match the size of the adjacent vessel *and* fix the stent tightly in the area of stenosis. If the adjacent vessel is much larger in diameter or the stenosis dilates easily to at least 12 mm in diameter, then an 11- or 12-French sheath/dilator system is used in order to allow the delivery of the stent on a BIB™ balloon (NuMED Inc., Hopkinton, NY). Whenever possible, the largest diameter, long, delivery sheath/dilator set which, it is anticipated, will be necessary for the balloon/stent or subsequent dilation, is introduced initially. The specifically preformed, long sheath/dilator set is introduced over the previously positioned wire. When pre-dilation was performed, the balloon catheter used for pre-dilation is replaced with the long sheath/dilator set over the wire. The long sheath must be long enough to reach beyond the area of stenosis. The combined sheath/dilator set is advanced over the wire until the *tip of the sheath* is beyond the area of stenosis.

The wire and the sheath are fixed in their respective positions while the dilator is withdrawn from the sheath over the wire. Blood is allowed to bleed back passively from the side arm of the sheath until the sheath is free of air and then the sheath is thoroughly flushed, remembering that an 11- or 12-French, 75 or 85 cm long sheath holds 11–15 ml of blood or solution. At no time when there is a wire passing through the back-bleed valve should suction be applied to the side arm of the long sheath to "help" or "speed up" the clearing of air. The path of least resistance to the vacuum created by suction on the side arm of a back-bleed valve will be for air to enter through the back-bleed valve around the wire passing through it rather than blood returning from the tip of the sheath! Once the sheath has been cleared passively of all air and flushed by hand, the sheath is attached to a slow continual flush. The patient is given 100 mg/kg of heparin systemically at this time.

The stent that is used should be capable of dilation to the potential *adult diameter* of the particular vein where it is implanted. The size of the balloon to deliver and implant the stent is chosen by the diameter of the nearest and *largest* adjacent vein *at the time of implant*. The implanted stent should be slightly larger than the largest adjacent vein, particularly the vein that is more central (distal) in the direction of venous flow. The stent is hand-mounted and "crimped" onto the appropriate balloon as described in Chapter 22. The stent, which is now mounted on the balloon, is advanced over the previously positioned wire and into the long sheath. As the stent passes through the back-bleed valve, the proximal end of the stent is held firmly on the balloon until the stent "disappears" into the valve and into the shaft of the catheter. Shorter stents will have to be introduced through the valve through a short "sleeve" as described in Chapter 22.

The wire and sheath are fixed in their positions through the stenosis and the balloon/stent combination advanced and centered at the area of stenosis. Generally, the course through the sheath to areas of venous stenosis is straighter than the course to other areas of intravascular stenosis and, as a consequence, there is less chance of the stent being displaced off the balloon, even without having to partially inflate the balloon/stent within the sheath. While the balloon catheter with the mounted stent and the guide wire are fixed securely in place, the sheath is withdrawn carefully off of the contained balloon and stent. The sheath is withdrawn completely off the balloon, but to a position just at the proximal end of the balloon. The sheath adjacent to the balloon helps support the balloon/stent in its position and allows a final small, low-pressure, angiogram through the sheath to verify the exact position of the balloon/stent in the stenosis. After the stent has been implanted, the short distance between the balloon and sheath also facilitates re-advancing the sheath over the balloon and into the stent.

With the balloon/stent combination fixed in a position centered over the maximal area of obstruction, the balloon is inflated to its maximum recommended pressure or until the stent is fully expanded. The balloon is deflated, leaving the stent fixed in the vein. In order to ensure a uniform expansion of the stent, the inflation of the balloon is repeated several times, each time with slight forward or backward repositioning of the balloon within the stent. With the sheath over the shaft of the balloon catheter with its tip proximal (in the direction of flow) to the stent, a small hand injection of contrast is performed through the sheath. This demonstrates the fixation of the stent within the vessel and, of equal importance, will show if there is any residual obstruction in the vein proximal to the stent. Following successful fixation of the stent in the area of narrowing, the exchange guide wire is secured as far distally beyond the stent as possible and the balloon is inflated at a low pressure within the stent. As slight negative pressure is applied to the balloon and as the balloon deflates, the sheath is advanced over the *deflating* balloon and *into* the stent. With the sheath and wire fixed in place, the balloon catheter is withdrawn carefully over the wire, into the sheath and out of the stent. The sheath positioned over the wire and within the stent facilitates the introduction of additional balloons or stents if further dilation/stents are necessary.

If the sheath cannot be advanced back into the stent, or if, as the balloon catheter is withdrawn from the stent, the stent begins to move, the tip of the *sheath* can be used to support the stent in its position in the vein. The sheath is re-advanced over the balloon catheter until the tip of the sheath contacts the proximal edge of the stent. The distal end of the *sheath* against the proximal end of the stent will help to fix the stent in place as the balloon is withdrawn back into the sheath. This may take some gentle to-and-fro manipulation along with simultaneous "torquing" of the balloon catheter. Occasionally, even the sheath must be rotated slightly to facilitate the balloon's re-entering the sheath. Extreme care is necessary in these maneuvers to avoid withdrawing the wire out of the stent, or even worse, pushing and dislodging the stent further distally into the more "downstream" (and larger diameter!) venous system. Once the initial balloon is successfully withdrawn out of the stent over the wire, it usually is quite easy to withdraw the balloon through, or with, the sheath over the wire and out of the body.

If the balloon used to deliver the original stent was smaller than the nominal diameter of the vessel adjacent to the stenosis, or there is a residual "waist" or stenosis in the expanded stent, the stent is dilated further, but only when no more stents are to be implanted during the same catheterization. When the sheath can be re-advanced over the original balloon into, and through, the stent after the stent implant, the original balloon easily can be replaced with a larger diameter balloon, a higher-pressure balloon, or the same balloon with an additional stent. If the new balloon that is necessary for the further dilation is too large for the original sheath, the original sheath must be withdrawn out of the stent and out of the body over the wire and replaced with a larger sheath/dilator set that will accommodate the larger balloon.

The larger sheath/dilator is advanced to and, if possible without distorting or pushing the stent, into and through the stent before the new balloon is advanced through it and into the freshly implanted stent. If the larger sheath and dilator do not advance easily into the stent, the tip of the sheath is positioned several millimeters proximal to the stent when only a re-dilation is to be performed. The new, deflated and smoothly folded balloon is advanced over the wire, through the sheath and, very gently, completely into the stent. In each case the balloon should undergo a "negative prep" to maintain the lowest and most "streamlined" delivery profile as is possible. With very close observation on the fluoroscope, the new balloon for the re-dilation is advanced slowly and delicately into the stent until the balloon is precisely positioned exactly in the center of the stent. The larger balloon is inflated while observing the further expansion of the stent. This inflation is repeated several times until the maximum pressure of the particular balloon is reached, and each time between inflations with slight forward or backward changes in the balloon's position within the stent. After the final inflation for expansion of the stent, the balloon is reinflated in the stent at a low pressure. Again, as the balloon is deflating slowly, the sheath is advanced over the balloon and into the stent. After the sheath is advanced completely within the stent as the balloon deflated, the negative pressure is *released* from the deflated balloon and the balloon is withdrawn very carefully into the sheath, out of the stent and out of the body over the guide wire.

When the area of venous stenosis is long and requires more than one stent, the most *distal* stent (in the direction of blood flow and closest to the heart!) should be the first stent to be implanted! In the more sluggish venous circulation, when the first stent(s) is/are implanted in the more proximal (in the direction of blood flow) areas of the stenosis, because of the persistent stenosis further "downstream", there is insufficient run-off from the freshly dilated and stented vessel, and intrastent thrombosis is likely to occur!

After each subsequent, more proximal stent has been implanted, a small contrast injection is performed through the sheath in order to visualize the implanted stents and adjacent vessels on a biplane angiogram. When satisfied with the stent fixation and position, the balloon still within the stent is inflated, the *sheath* is re-advanced very gingerly into the just implanted stent as the balloon is being deflated, and the balloon is withdrawn through the sheath as previously described. When additional stents are necessary, the next stent is mounted on the *same* balloon. Each additional stent is implanted overlapping the previous stent by 25–50% depending upon the anticipated shrinkage of the stents at their full expansion and the potential future growth of the patient. This procedure is repeated until the entire area of stenosis is "lined" with stents. The progress of the stent implants is monitored very accurately with repeated small biplane angiograms. These injections are made directly through the long sheath and can be made around the balloon catheter when the area proximal to the last stent implanted is to be visualized or after the balloon catheter is removed when the area within the stents is to be visualized.

After the final stent implant, the dilation balloon and the long sheath are removed over the wire from the venous site, a short sheath/dilator set is introduced over the wire into the venous system, and the wire and dilator are removed. An angiographic catheter is introduced into the venous system and advanced to a position just proximal (in the direction of blood flow) to the most proximal of the newly implanted stent(s). The X-ray tubes are angled appropriately to view the stents in their longest axis. A final angiogram of the implanted stents is recorded with injection through this catheter. No attempt is made to maneuver a catheter through the freshly implanted stents to a position distal to them. Since the hemodynamics of venous obstructions are so meaningless, the extra manipulation is of little benefit and could very easily dislodge the recently implanted stents.

Occasionally, venous stents are implanted "against the flow" of the venous blood. For example, stents are implanted in the superior vena cava through a sheath introduced from the femoral vein or, just the opposite, stents in the iliofemoral vein are implanted from the internal jugular vein approach. In the case of tandem stents implanted "against the flow", the most distal stent in the *direction of the flow of the blood* (and closest to the heart) still is the first stent implanted. Angiography performed during the "against the flow of blood" implant of venous stents must be performed through a separate catheter that is introduced into a separate vein at the opposite end of the obstruction, or through a second catheter introduced "parallel" to the stent delivery system. If the second catheter is introduced parallel to the stent delivery sheath, the angiograms are recorded with the second catheter passing through the lesion and alongside the delivery sheath. This catheter ***must be*** withdrawn from the area before each stent is expanded or the catheter will be trapped *outside of the stent* in the area of obstruction! If post-implant angiograms are desired, the second catheter is manipulated very cautiously back through the newly implanted stent(s) in order to inject "upstream" to the stent/obstruction.

Post-implant care of venous stents

Assuming there are no other extenuating circumstances, stents implanted in venous channels are treated the same as in any other lesion undergoing stent implants. Heparin is not reversed at the end of the procedure, but no additional heparin is given. Patients are observed in the recovery room environment for several hours and during this time are continued on maintenance intravenous fluids. When awake, they are transferred to a cardiology ward and usually observed over night, primarily for bleeding at the introductory sites. Unless the patients are tolerating, and taking, a liberal oral intake, they are maintained on the intravenous fluids overnight. When they are awake fully and taking oral fluids liberally (usually the next morning) they are started on 82 mg of aspirin a day, which is continued for the next six months. They otherwise have no imposed limitations or restrictions because of the stents.

Stent implants in the Fontan circuit

Stent implants anywhere in the systemic venous "Fontan" circuits are treated as all other "venous" stent implants. At the same time, some of these stent implants are in the *pulmonary arteries*. When in the pulmonary arteries, the implants still are in very low-pressure, non-pulsatile, low-flow areas. Even more so than the other venous obstructions, the absence of pressure gradients across areas of obstruction in these patients has very little, if any, meaning. The systemic venous system is very compliant, dilating almost infinitely to accommodate all possible increase in pressure. There usually are several alternative, major systemic venous, "inflow channels" into the heart and the central pulmonary arteries in "Fontan" patients. As a consequence, venous flow preferentially is diverted away from any area of localized systemic venous or unilateral pulmonary arterial obstruction so that *no gradients* are generated. Because of the multiple sources of blood "inflow" into the pulmonary bed, it is impossible to quantitate any unequal distribution of pulmonary flow by current nuclear perfusion studies. As a consequence of these multiple factors, obstruction in the "Fontan circuit" is determined entirely from the angiographic anatomy.

Obstruction can occur within both or either caval channel(s), at the anastomotic sites to the pulmonary arteries, or in the branch pulmonary arteries themselves. With the relatively precarious nature of the pulmonary perfusion in these patients, *any* minimal obstruction of flow is significant. A narrowing in the diameter of the lumen of a vessel to two-thirds or less of its nominal diameter represents a significant luminal stenosis. A diameter of a right or a left pulmonary artery that is less than two-thirds of the diameter of the comparable, contralateral vessel *is stenotic* and will have significantly decreased flow.

These lesions are treated when discovered. Most of these channels are treated effectively by dilation along with intravascular stent implants. The implant of stents into these vessels is relatively straightforward except that most of these channels are very large in diameter and have very compliant vessel walls adjacent to the stenotic area. These characteristics require that the stents are implanted at very large diameters at the time of implant. Otherwise the stents used, and the procedures for implant of the stents, are the same as in other large central vessels.

By the time most of these patients come to treatment of these stenoses, they have reached twenty or more kilograms in weight and readily accept large sheaths for stent delivery. The one problem for transcatheter therapy in the "Fontan" patient is that all of these patients have had at least several prior surgeries with indwelling venous lines and multiple prior cardiac catheterizations. Venous access to the central channels can be problematic and may require peripheral venous reconstruction with stent implants even to approach the central vessels.

When stents are *implanted* at diameters over 12 mm, Balloon In Balloon™ (BIB™) balloons (NuMED Inc., Hopkinton, NY) are recommended for the implant. These balloons allow the initial implant with a large (15 or 18 mm or even larger) diameter balloon but at the same time allow for the stepwise or sequential expansion of the stent using the one balloon. The initial smaller expansion of the stent on the inner balloon eliminates the marked initial "dumbbell" expansion of the balloon and stent that occurs when a stent is expanded with a single larger balloon with one continuous expansion of the balloon/stent from deflated to a full large diameter. The sequential inflation of the stent avoids most of the problems of the balloon/stent shifting forward or backward during the inflation. The radial rings of sharp tips at each end of the early "dumbbell" shape of the expanding stent are eliminated. This reduces vessel trauma and the possibility of balloon puncture by the stent. With the stent partially expanded on the inner balloon of the BIB™, the stent can be repositioned forward or backward within the area of stenosis before the final full inflation of the outer balloon.

Pulmonary venous stents

Pulmonary vein dilation was one of the first "angioplasty" procedures attempted in congenital heart defects. The dilation of the pulmonary veins was very successful *acutely* but pulmonary vein stenosis universally recurred, and recurred with a vengeance, within a relatively short time[9]. The use of stents to treat pulmonary vein stenosis seemed a natural evolution after the success of intravascular stents in the treatment of stenosis of the other congenital venous lesions. The major problem *envisioned* was the slightly more difficult access to the pulmonary veins. Unfortunately the results of stents implanted in congenital pulmonary vein stenosis are even less satisfactory than the dilation of these same lesions. Stenosis of the pulmonary veins not only recurred following stent implants, but recurred to a more severe degree. Stenosis developed within the stents, but of equal or even greater significance, the more proximal areas of the pulmonary veins *within the lung parenchyma* became severely stenotic from a very aggressive intimal proliferation. The results usually are ultimately fatal.

The procedure for the implant of stents in pulmonary veins is technically very challenging. The approach to the pulmonary veins usually requires a transseptal procedure. The transseptal procedure is straightforward, however, following a standard atrial transseptal procedure, the subsequent approach within the left atrium to all except the left upper pulmonary veins is compromised, particularly in smaller patients. The course of the long delivery sheath, which is coming from the inferior vena cava through the fixed, small opening in the atrial septum, is *fixed* in a fairly rigid direction/course in the left atrium, which in turn compromises maneuvering into the separate pulmonary veins.

Of even greater significance, the pulmonary veins themselves are very *short*. This leaves little distance between the orifice of the pulmonary vein at the left atrium and the proximal pulmonary capillary bed with *no* length for the stent and the distal end of the implanting balloon to extend into the lung parenchyma proximal to the obstruction. Any displacement of a stent during its implant into a pulmonary vein will be back into the left atrium with no possible area to secure the stent. Displaced pulmonary vein stents frequently embolize systemically.

The use of stents in some *post-surgical* pulmonary vein stenoses is one exception to the almost universal failure of stents in pulmonary veins. There have been a few examples of stenosis of pulmonary venous anastomoses following anomalous pulmonary venous return repairs, which have maintained their response to intravascular stent therapy. These patients are different from those with congenital stenoses in several respects. The stenosis is in scar tissue, which is not always associated with the aggressive abnormal intimal proliferation seen in congenital pulmonary vein stenosis, and there usually is a dilated and long vessel proximal (upstream) to the stenosis. This length of the vessel allows the implanting balloon to be positioned far enough into the vein, but at the same time, the balloon does not encroach on or damage the more proximal lung parenchyma. The length of the vein proximally allows some distance within the vein for the stent to be implanted in a secure position. As a consequence of these features, there are some pulmonary vein stents that have been implanted in post-operative stenosis that have remained open for several years.

The implant of stents into native stenosis of pulmonary veins is challenging. The involved vein and the area of stenosis must be measured very accurately to determine the exact size of stent and balloon to be used. This is a most critical measurement because the vein *normally widens* as it courses the short distance from the lung parenchyma to the left atrium. As a consequence, the *wall* of the pulmonary vein not only does *not* grip or hold the stent but tends *to extrude* the stent toward the cavity of the left atrium! In *no case* should pulmonary vein stenosis *ever* be pre-dilated. Ideally, there is a discrete area of the pulmonary vein stenosis just at the entrance (orifice) into the left atrium with a more proximal (within the lung) area of dilation of the vein.

In most cases of pulmonary vein stenosis, a transseptal procedure is necessary just to gain access to the left atrium. After gaining access into the left atrium an end-hole catheter must be manipulated selectively into the involved pulmonary vein(s) from the long sheath, which is in a very fixed location within the atrial septum. The tip of a Super Stiff™ wire then is secured well into the vein (or lung parenchyma) through this catheter. The long, relatively stiff delivery sheath/dilator for the delivery of the balloon/stent is advanced over the stiff wire into the vein and the sheath "secured" within the stenotic vein over the wire.

The difficulty of these manipulations is compounded by several factors. When the stenotic vein enters into the right side of the left atrium, the angle into the stenotic vein is very difficult (if not impossible) to manipulate into from the fixed area of the puncture on the atrial septum and the resultant "leftward" direction of the relatively stiff sheath. To facilitate entry into the right upper pulmonary veins, the transseptal puncture must be performed in an "abnormal", but more favorable location on the septum, which is caudal and toward the patient's left on the septum relative to the usual puncture site. Similarly, access to the left lower pulmonary vein creates a very acute angle from the usual puncture site and the direction of a standard transseptal puncture. Often access to the left lower pulmonary veins can only be accomplished from a transseptal puncture performed with an approach from the superior vena cava. When the *puncture* can be accomplished from this approach, the route through the interatrial septum from the superior vena cava provides a direct approach to the left lower pulmonary veins and a better approach to the right lower pulmonary veins.

Another complicating anatomic feature is that the stenotic orifices of the pulmonary veins often are immediately adjacent to each other. This side-by-side relationship of the veins requires the simultaneous implant of side-by-side stents, both through separate venous access and separate transseptal punctures.

For stent implants into pulmonary vein stenosis, the stents must be mounted on *very* short balloons with *very* stubby shoulders. The initial wire position and the maintenance of this position are extremely critical. The size of the stent and balloon also is extremely critical and no attempt should be made to implant a pulmonary venous stent without the optimal balloon and stent. Any extra length of the implanting balloon almost guarantees that the balloon/stent will milk out of the vein during the inflation of the balloon. In order to prevent or reduce the possibility of the stent's "milking" out of the vein by the expanding balloon, the balloon catheter is pushed forward over the wire continuously and forcefully by the operator as the balloon with the stent is inflated. Mounting the stent distally on the balloon results in the proximal balloon inflating first and actually aggravates the problem of the stent milking out of the pulmonary vein!

If a stent does milk out of the vein, it becomes free floating in the left atrium, hopefully still over the wire! In that situation, the wire is maintained fixed well into the pulmonary vein and the tip of the sheath is kept within the left atrium adjacent to the "free stent". With the stent still over the wire, the sheath and the wire are fixed very securely in the pulmonary vein and the balloon is removed from within the stent and out through the sheath. If the original delivery sheath was an 8-French or smaller, the original long sheath is withdrawn over the wire and replaced with a 10-French long sheath dilator set, all of the time meticulously maintaining the distal end of the wire buried in the pulmonary vein. Once the tip of the new larger long sheath is well within the left atrium, the larger dilator is removed over the wire. An opened 15 or 20 mm snare (depending upon the diameter of the expanded stent) is placed around the proximal end of the wire and then closed loosely over the wire. The snare catheter with the closed snare loop over the wire is introduced into the valve of the sheath with the catheter adjacent to the wire. The snare is advanced through the sheath over the wire into the left atrium. When the snare passes beyond the tip of the sheath, the snare loop is opened and manipulated over the expanded stent, which is "floating" over the wire. The wire is maintained in the pulmonary vein while the snare is manipulated around the proximal end of the stent. Once the snare is around the stent, the snare is closed tightly, compressing (collapsing) the stent. While holding the stent with the snare, the sheath is pushed against the proximal end of the stent while the wire is maintained securely in the pulmonary vein. This should push the stent, which is over the wire and held by the snare, firmly against the wall of the left atrium. Once the stent is in a fairly rigid position, the snare is relaxed, moved slightly proximally or distally along the stent, and re-compressed as tightly as possible. This sequence of tightening the snare over the stent is repeated, moving the snare along the entire length of the stent until the proximal end of the stent can be withdrawn at least partially into the sheath. Once the proximal end of the stent is into the end of the sheath and while tightening the snare as much as possible around the exposed stent, the entire "unit" (sheath, snare catheter and collapsed stent) is withdrawn over the wire, through the septum and out of the body. If possible, this "unit" is withdrawn over the wire leaving the wire in place, however, once the stent is pulled into the sheath, the wire may be gripped so tightly by the closed snare that it will have to be withdrawn with the sheath, snare and stent.

If, after a reasonable try, the stent cannot be snared, or if snared, it cannot be withdrawn even partially into the sheath, the wire is withdrawn from the vein and the stent. This allows the stent to be totally free floating. The stent tumbles around within the left atrium and eventually will embolize to the left ventricle and out into the aorta. The even partially dilated stent *usually* does pass through all of these chambers and eventually to the descending aorta. Usually the stent tumbles within the course of the predominant blood flow (in the central aorta). The stent itself is too large in diameter to enter, or at least, pass far into any critical side branch. Once the stent has reached its final destination during the embolization, then a decision is made whether to try to retrieve it from the artery or to dilate the stent further in order to fix it permanently in its errant arterial location.

Because of the dismal overall, even short-term results with the use of stents in pulmonary veins, their use in these locations is recommended only when the patient is unequivocally and progressively deteriorating because of the pulmonary vein obstruction. When pulmonary venous obstruction is progressing, most patients have a very grim and ultimately fatal prognosis. As a consequence, in the face of this alternative, treatment with pulmonary venous stents is tried in many patients as a "last-ditch" effort. Hopefully, future developments in stent technology, stent coatings, and direct treatment of the tissues of the area will improve the outcome in these patients.

Pulmonary venous baffle obstructions

Obstructed, post-surgical, large, pulmonary venous channels in intra-atrial baffles, like other post-operative stenoses of large systemic venous channels, respond favorably to intravascular stent implants. These lesions occur predominantly in the pulmonary venous baffle channel in patients who have undergone "venous switch" ("Mustard" or "Senning") repairs of transposition of the great arteries[10,11]. The pulmonary venous baffle channel has several unique characteristics. The pulmonary venous baffle channel is the *only channel* for the *entire* pulmonary venous blood flow. As a consequence, it must be a *very* large diameter channel, and any stent used in this area also must be very large and able to be dilated sufficiently to accommodate the *total cardiac output* during the venous flow. In addition, these patients often are very precarious hemodynamically by the time they appear for management of this problem. They often have very high pulmonary venous pressure proximal to the obstruction and, as a consequence, significant elevation of pulmonary arterial pressure. Any catheter or the large sheath passing through the stenotic area results in further, possibly critical, obstruction of this compromised channel. The expanded dilating balloon during the inflation for the implant of a stent obstructs the already precarious flow totally and unequivocally, which in turn, stops the entire cardiac output while the balloon is inflated! Transcatheter treatment of these lesions not only is technically challenging and must be performed very expeditiously, but also is potentially very hazardous for the patient.

The approach for transcatheter treatment of an obstructed pulmonary venous baffle requires a "transseptal" puncture and passage of a very large, long delivery sheath through the wall, usually, of the inferior limb of the surgically placed intracardiac venous baffle. A "recirculation" phase of a left ventricular or pulmonary artery angiogram is necessary to visualize the obstructed pulmonary venous channel as well as both the "proximal" and the "distal" pulmonary venous atrial "chambers", which are positioned on each side of the obstruction. Usually, the "recirculation" phase of a large volume, biplane, main pulmonary artery angiogram provides a sufficient "pulmonary venous" angiogram to roughly define this anatomy. When very high pulmonary artery pressures are present, selective, very distal pulmonary artery or even pulmonary artery capillary wedge injections are performed to obtain the "recirculation" pictures of the pulmonary venous chambers without a large bolus pulmonary artery angiogram. It is imperative to visualize the anterior and lateral limits of the "distal pulmonary venous" chamber (original right atrium), which is adjacent to the tricuspid valve. This part of the atrial chamber is the "target" area for the trans-baffle, "transseptal" puncture.

The "transseptal" puncture of the inferior baffle is performed far *caudally* within the inferior limb of the baffle in order to allow sufficient space for the eventual positioning of the stent within this "distal" pulmonary venous channel. If the puncture is too far cephalad, the stent and/or balloon can remain partially in the baffle during or after the implant! Before the introduction of the needle, it is helpful to bend the patient's thorax toward the patient's *left* in order to position the inferior baffle more perpendicular to the needle approach. (This "bend" of the thorax is in the opposite direction to the "bend" in the patient for a standard transseptal puncture!) The needle itself is "straightened" prior to introduction into the long sheath/dilator so that it has only the very slightest curve at its tip. The straighter needle delivers more "forward" force to the tip of the needle during the puncture. The sheath of the delivery sheath/dilator set used must be large enough to accommodate the very large stent when it is mounted on the large dilation balloon. The dilation balloon must be large enough to fix the stent securely in this location during the initial inflation of the balloon/stent. This will require a 12- or 14-French sheath. None of the "transseptal sets" are available in these very large sizes, so the initial "transseptal" procedure through the baffle is performed with a standard 7- or 8-French transseptal set. The transseptal set is introduced over a wire and positioned at the cephalic end of the *inferior baffle*. The introductory wire is withdrawn and the dilator cleared of any air. The needle is introduced into the dilator, advanced just to the tip of the dilator within the transseptal "set", and the needle is attached to the pressure system. The combination needle/dilator/sheath is withdrawn together caudally within the inferior limb of the baffle while directing the tip of the needle *anteriorly* and *laterally*. When the desired, caudal location is reached for the puncture within the channel of the inferior limb of the baffle, the needle is advanced out of the tip of the dilator, into the baffle and the "transseptal" puncture through the baffle is performed. The needle tip is observed continuously on both planes of the fluoroscopy and the pressure transmitted through the needle is watched closely as the needle is advanced. The baffles often are very tough or even "hardened" over time and as a consequence, usually are very difficult to puncture. It often requires multiple adjustments in the exact location and/or the direction of the needle tip before the puncture is accomplished successfully. Often successful puncture can only be accomplished at the very edge of the baffle where the baffle is anastomosed with the native tissues. Regardless of the site of puncture, the transseptal set and needle must be pushed very forcefully, and when the needle does traverse the baffle, it usually crosses suddenly and with a forward lurch of the tip of the needle.

Once the needle has punctured and crossed through the baffle successfully, the pressure from the distal pulmonary venous chamber appears on the pressure curve observed from the needle. If no pressure is visualized after the needle has advanced forward noticeably, a *tiny* (< 0.1 ml) injection of contrast is performed through the needle. As with other "transseptal" punctures when the needle is in the proper position, the contrast "swirls" away from the tip of the needle. When the needle is buried within the tissues of the baffle, the injection of the tiny amount of contrast will be very difficult, and when accomplished, a "tag" of contrast appears in the tissues and identifies the errant location. Once the needle is in the distal chamber, the dilator and sheath are advanced with the needle into the distal pulmonary venous chamber. Occasionally, even a 7-French sheath/dilator cannot be advanced successfully through the baffle and only a smaller diameter transseptal set or even just the dilator will follow the needle through a thick, tough, baffle after the initial puncture. In that situation the initial small opening created through the baffle with the smaller diameter sheath/dilator set or dilator alone is dilated open with a small, high-pressure dilation balloon in order to widen the "tract" enough to allow the introduction of the large sheath. Rarely, sequential dilations of the baffle are necessary to enlarge the opening to allow the passage of the very large, long sheath/dilator.

Once the long sheath is within the "distal pulmonary venous" chamber, the needle and dilator are removed slowly and carefully and the sheath is cleared passively of all air and any possible clots. The first catheter used through the long sheath will depend upon the estimate of the degree of stenosis and the difficulty of the puncture through the baffle. When the patient is very stable and the position of the tip of the long sheath is optimal for entering (pointing at!) the obstructed venous channel, an angiographic "marker" catheter is introduced into the distal pulmonary venous chamber through the long sheath. With a catheter even one size smaller than the sheath, simultaneous, separate pressures can be obtained through the catheter and the side arm of the long sheath. The pressures are recorded from both the catheter tip and the sheath while they are adjacent to each other in the distal pulmonary venous chamber. The simultaneous pressures will verify the accuracy of the pressure recording systems. The angiographic catheter then is manipulated through the obstruction and into the "proximal" pulmonary venous chamber while simultaneous pressures are recorded from the proximal and distal pulmonary venous chambers through the catheter and the sheath, respectively.

The X-ray tubes are angled in order to align the portion of the catheter passing through the obstruction (and hopefully the obstruction as well) in its longest axis, and a biplane angiogram is recorded with injection into the "proximal" pulmonary venous chamber. This angiogram demonstrates the anatomy precisely and allows accurate measurements of the diameter of the stenosis, the length of the stenosis, and the dimensions of the pulmonary venous chambers at both ends of the obstruction. Once the angiograms are recorded and the stenotic area measured accurately, the angiographic catheter is withdrawn into the long sheath. The angiographic catheter is replaced with an end-hole catheter.

The end-hole catheter is attached to the flush/pressure system through a wire back-bleed valve with a side port and is introduced into the long sheath. The catheter is maneuvered through the pulmonary venous obstruction, into the more proximal "pulmonary venous chamber", and as far into a *left* pulmonary vein as possible. The left pulmonary vein provides the "straightest" course from the baffle puncture, through the obstructed venous channel and into a vein. This maneuvering is accomplished with a combination of a torque-controlled catheter, deflector wires, and torque-controlled or floppy tipped wires. Once the catheter is well into the pulmonary vein, a short tipped Super Stiff™ wire is passed through the catheter and wedged out in the pulmonary vein. As long as the patient tolerates the small diameter of the catheter through the stenosis without hemodynamic deterioration due to obstruction of the total pulmonary venus flow, the catheter is left in place over the wire. No attempt is made at advancing the large sheath across the lesion at this time. A continuous flush is maintained around the wire through the catheter and through the sheath.

If the stenosis is so severe that the diagnostic catheter passing over the wire through the stenosis compromised the patient's hemodynamics, then there is no way that the patient can tolerate the larger delivery sheath and/or balloon/stent through the area long enough to allow the deployment of a stent. In this circumstance the area is "pre-dilated" partially before proceeding with the stent implant. If the long sheath that is in the distal pulmonary venous chamber is large enough to accommodate the large stent/balloon combination, the balloon dilation catheter can be advanced easily through this sheath. If the sheath in the distal pulmonary venous atrium is the smaller diameter sheath used for the "transseptal" puncture, this smaller long sheath is exchanged over the wire for the very large, long sheath/dilator which will accommodate the delivery of the large stent/balloon combination. The larger sheath/dilator is advanced into the distal pulmonary venous chamber and the dilator is removed over the wire. The sheath is allowed to clear passively of all air and clot and then placed on a continuous flush.

The balloon that is used for the pre-dilation should have a diameter that is no more than 70% of the anticipated diameter of the stent at *implant*. Once all the preparations for the inflation of the balloon have been completed, the angioplasty balloon is advanced through the large sheath, over the pre-positioned wire and into the lesion, and the stenotic area is dilated with a very rapid inflation and deflation of the balloon. The balloon inflation/deflation is recorded on biplane angiography. In the hemodynamically precarious patient, the balloon immediately is withdrawn out of the lesion after the deflation of the balloon and then the results of the balloon inflation are reviewed on the angiograms. The patient is allowed to stabilize and the dilation repeated at least one more time.

After the lesion has been dilated several times and particularly after any residual "waist" on the dilation balloon has been eliminated, the balloon dilation catheter is withdrawn over the wire and an angiographic catheter is introduced into the sheath adjacent to the wire and advanced *adjacent to the wire*, through the very large sheath, and manipulated back into the proximal pulmonary venous chamber. The angiogram in the "proximal" chamber is repeated and all areas/structures are remeasured. Along with these measurements any fixed thoracic landmarks in the area of the stenosis along with the particular angles of the X-ray tubes are noted and "freeze frame" images of the lesion are stored as a "road map". When satisfied that the stenosis is open at least slightly, the angiographic catheter is withdrawn from the long sheath.

With the Super Stiff™ wire still in place across the pulmonary venous baffle, a second venous catheter is introduced and maneuvered into the channel on the *systemic* venous side of the baffle and into the *superior* limb of the baffle (the catheter can be introduced from above or below!). An angiogram is recorded in the channel of the *superior* limb. This provides an indication of the proximity of the area of the pulmonary venous obstruction to the channel through the superior limb of the baffle and, in particular, if there is any associated narrowing of the superior limb of the baffle. If there is narrowing of both the superior limb of the systemic venous channel and the common pulmonary venous channel, and particularly if the two narrowed areas are in close proximity to each other, "protection" of the access of the channel through the systemic venous limb is necessary before, and while, the pulmonary venous stent is being implanted. An end-hole catheter is positioned and maintained across the superior baffle so that if the superior limb channel is compressed by the pulmonary venous stent, there is guaranteed catheter/wire access back through the superior limb of the systemic channel.

It is desirable to have a second (angiographic) catheter in the distal pulmonary venous chamber. The second catheter is extremely helpful for "positioning angiograms" during the actual stent implant, but it does require a second "transseptal" puncture through the baffle of the inferior limb. Without the second catheter in the pulmonary venous chamber, there is no other good way of obtaining verification/positioning angiograms during the stent deployment. Once the large delivery sheath or the stent/balloon is in place across the obstruction in the common pulmonary venous channel, the hemodynamics frequently deteriorate rapidly, which leaves little time for significant further "decision making" or adding catheters.

The length of the stent used is determined from the previous measurement on the angiograms. The ultimate diameter of the stent used must be capable of dilation to the largest diameters currently available in intravascular stents. Regardless of the current size of the patient, the stent used in a common pulmonary venous channel must be capable of dilation to a diameter that will allow the *entire blood volume* to pass through the stent at low venous pressures and eventually at the patient's maximal, adult size. In virtually all patients, this requires a J & J™ P _ _ 10 or an ITI™ Maxi™ stent, either of which can be dilated to diameters of 25–30 mm. A balloon is chosen with a diameter that unequivocally will expand the stent enough *to fix the stent securely in place* and, at the same time, allow the most rapid expansion of the stent. During the *initial* implant, the stent does *not* have to be opened to the maximal diameter anticipated eventually, but it does have to be expanded enough *to fix the stent* securely in place. In the critically narrowed channel, even after pre-dilation, the large sheath or the balloon/stent combination alone, even before inflation, can occlude the entire channel and, in turn, stop systemic cardiac output. The goal of the initial stent expansion in these lesions is to fix the stent securely in place and then deflate the implanting balloon as rapidly as possible. Once the channel is opened and fixed open even partially, further dilation of the stent is accomplished safely with sequentially larger balloons, each with a rapid inflation/deflation. This is one circumstance where a BIB is not usable for the delivery of the stent to larger than 10–12 mm diameter. The extra time required for the separate inflation and then deflation of both balloons of the BIB system usually cannot be tolerated in this particular lesion. The problems of the stent "dumbbelling" and kinking in the center during a single large balloon expansion are tolerated better in this particular location. The ends of the stent usually are expanding into large dilated "chambers" as opposed to the more usual constrained, linear walls of a vessel. When a *very large* stent is used, the residual central "kink" or waist does not result in a significant narrowing of the channel.

The stent is mounted on the appropriate balloon and *all* preparations for the implant are made before introducing the balloon/stent into the sheath. The X-ray tubes are placed in their optimal positions, the "road map" images of the lesion and surrounding tissues are displayed, the injector is attached to the second catheter in the distal venous chamber (when available) and this catheter is positioned as close as possible to (or through!) the obstruction. The injector is filled with a sufficient volume of contrast for several injections, is set for the appropriate volume and pressure for each separate injection, *and is armed*! Once all preparations are completed, the large sheath/dilator is advanced through the lesion over the wire. If the patient remains reasonably stable with the large sheath across the lesion, the subsequent implant of the stent is fairly straightforward and similar to any other stent implant through a long sheath. However, if the patient's clinical signs deteriorate immediately when the sheath/dilator is advanced across the lesion, the sheath/dilator immediately is withdrawn over the wire back into the distal pulmonary venous chamber and an alternative stent delivery technique must be used.

An attempt is made at a semi "front-loaded" delivery of the stent with the stent/balloon acting as the dilator, as the stent, balloon, and sheath are advanced through the *lesion* together. The large delivery sheath/dilator is advanced over the wire until the tip of the dilator is positioned in the distal pulmonary chamber immediately *distal and adjacent to* the obstruction. The dilator is withdrawn over the wire and out of the sheath while the tip of the *sheath* is *advanced* as close as possible to the distal outlet of the obstruction. The stent/balloon catheter is introduced over the wire until the distal end of the *stent* is positioned *just within the end of the sheath,* which leaves the tip of the balloon extending just beyond the tip of the sheath. The balloon (within the sheath) is inflated slightly to expand the distal, exposed tip of the balloon outside of the tip of the sheath, which in turn, creates a "dilator" for the large sheath. The combination sheath/balloon/stent is advanced expediently over the wire until the *stent* is centered within the obstruction while, simultaneously, its location is being compared to the location on the "road map" images of the area. Without pausing in the movements, the sheath is withdrawn off the balloon/stent. If the patient remains stable with the deflated balloon/stent across the lesion, a verifying angiogram is obtained, injecting through the second catheter (already attached to the injector which is set and armed!) before the stent/balloon is inflated. The injector immediately is rearmed. Any necessary adjustments in the stent or second catheter position are performed and verified with an additional angiogram if absolutely necessary.

If the patient begins to deteriorate with only the balloon/stent across the lesion, once the stent/balloon appears to be in the proper location within the stenosis as compared to the "road map" images, the balloon/stent is inflated and the balloon deflated, both as rapidly as possible. Using this last technique, there is a greater chance of the stent being malpositioned slightly, but the total combined time of obstruction by first the large diameter sheath alone followed then by the time of the deployment of the stent is less than 15–20 seconds. The patient should stabilize immediately with the deflation of the balloon, now with the channel held open significantly by the expanded stent.

Occasionally the large sheath with the "front-loaded" balloon/stent catheter will not follow even a Super Stiff™ wire through a tight obstruction. After several failed attempts at that maneuver, the stent/balloon catheter is withdrawn over the wire, and out of the sheath. The stent/balloon catheter is replaced over the wire with a balloon dilation catheter only. If the area was pre-dilated earlier, a slightly larger or higher-pressure dilation balloon than was used with the initial pre-dilation is used, and the area of stenosis is re-dilated with the new balloon. If the area had not been pre-dilated previously, a balloon is used that is 60–70% of the expected diameter of the stent when it is implanted or 3–4 times the diameter of the stenosis itself—whichever is *smaller.* After the area is expanded by the pre-dilation, as demonstrated by the disappearance of the waist on the dilation balloon or by angiography, the balloon dilation catheter is removed over the wire and withdrawn through the long sheath. The balloon dilation catheter is replaced over the wire with the dilator that came with the large sheath. The sheath/dilator is advanced over the wire and through the obstruction, again observing the patient for any deterioration. If the patient now remains reasonably stable, the dilator is removed immediately and rapidly from the sheath over the wire and replaced with the balloon dilation catheter with the stent mounted on the balloon.

As with the front-loaded delivery, when the sheath is positioned across the obstruction even after pre-dilation, the patient frequently begins to deteriorate and the stent must be delivered very expediently. The stent/balloon is reintroduced rapidly into the sheath and the balloon/stent advanced into the lesion, keeping the sheath on a continuous flush. The sheath is withdrawn off the stent/balloon. If the patient does not remain stable with either the sheath or even just the deflated stent/balloon alone across the lesion, the balloon is rapidly inflated and deflated to deploy the stent in the lesion by comparing the position to the "road map" image and without any confirmatory angiograms.

An alternative when, even after pre-dilation, the patient becomes unstable with the sheath only across the lesion, is to reattempt the "front-load" crossing of the lesion for the stent implant. Although this still involves the same size sheath and balloon/stent combination, when the front-loaded stent/balloon can be advanced through the lesion, the "front load" saves more than a *minute* of the time to stent expansion compared to the standard balloon/stent delivery through a sheath that was pre-positioned over a dilator.

The deterioration in the hemodynamics caused by the sheath or balloon/stent occlusion of the lesion begins to reverse immediately and rapidly once the stent is expanded in the lesion and the balloon is deflated, even with the deflated balloon still across the lesion. Once the patient stabilizes, the balloon is reinflated gently and, while the balloon is deflating, the sheath is advanced into the stent over the deflating balloon and wire. The initial balloon is withdrawn and replaced with the larger final diameter balloon for further expansion of the stent.

Complications of venous stents

The implant of pulmonary venous stents is very complicated, very risky and usually is an exercise in futility. Intravascular stents *very seldom, if ever, benefit* pulmonary vein obstructions and are no longer recommended for these lesions unless the patient is on a fulminant progressive fatal course because of the pulmonary vein stenosis.

Although the *potential* for complications during the implant of systemic venous and baffle stents is the same as for the implant of other vascular stents, the actual complications from the implant of systemic venous stent are less than with any other type of stent implant. With the rebuilding of the peripheral venous channels, there has been extravasation of blood into the retroperitoneal tissues. In each case this has been self-limited, requiring minimal if any specific therapy and resulting in no permanent sequelae. Small persistent perivascular leaks into the retroperitoneal space following the implant of stents into the systemic veins have been occluded with the deposit of several coils into the area through the wall of the stent.

There have been several re-occlusions of small, reconstructed, systemic peripheral veins. These re-stenoses either have been associated with the subsequent immediate use of the recently stented veins for infusions through indwelling lines in the stented veins, or have been in stented veins where flow was never established through the vein by the stent implants. On several occasions, the totally occluded veins that had been previously stented were reopened by re-cannulation with wires, re-dilating, and re-stenting the area. When flow was established through the reopened stented veins, the veins then remained open.

Displacement of stents during the implant of "venous" stents rarely occurs. In each case where it has occurred, the stent was "trapped" with a balloon and re-implanted in the same, or in a non-involved vessel with no serious consequences or permanent sequelae. As long as flow is established through the stented vein, there has been no *in situ* clotting in the central venous system in spite of the inherently often sluggish venous blood flow. Probably as a consequence of the more straightforward route for the implant of most venous stents, there have been no major vein ruptures or tears during the implant of venous stents.

Systemic venous stents, particularly in totally occluded veins, appear to be a "win–win" situation. The implant procedure for venous stents is safe and the stents generally remain open; however, if a totally occluded vein re-occludes after a stent implant, the patient is no worse off.

References

1. Mullins CE *et al.* Balloon dilation of miscellaneous lesions: results of Valvuloplasty and Angioplasty of Congenital Anomalies Registry. *Am J Cardiol* 1990; **65**(11): 802–803.
2. Rosch J, Hanafee WN, and Snow H. Transjugular portal venography and radiologic portacaval shunt: an experimental study. *Radiology* 1969; **92**(5): 1112–1114.
3. Wright KC *et al.* Percutaneous endovascular stents: an experimental evaluation. *Radiology* 1985; **156**(1): 69–72.
4. Palmaz JC *et al.* Expandable intraheptaic portacaval shunt stents: early experience in the dog. *Am J Radiol* 1985; **145**: 821–825.
5. Mullins CE *et al.* Implantation of balloon-expandable intravascular grafts by catheterization in pulmonary arteries and systemic veins. *Circulation* 1988; **77**(1): 188–199.
6. O'Laughlin MP *et al.* Use of endovascular stents in congenital heart disease. *Circulation* 1991; **83**(6): 1923–1939.
7. Ward CJ *et al.* Use of intravascular stents in systemic venous and systemic venous baffle obstructions. Short-term follow-up results. *Circulation* 1995; **91**(12): 2948–2954.
8. Ing FF *et al.* Reconstruction of stenotic or occluded iliofemoral veins and inferior vena cava using intravascular stents: re-establishing access for future cardiac catheterization and cardiac surgery. *J Am Coll Cardiol* 2001; **37**(1): 251–257.
9. Driscoll DJ, Hesslein PS, and Mullins CE. Congenital stenosis of individual pulmonary veins: clinical spectrum and unsuccessful treatment by transvenous balloon dilation. *Am J Cardiol* 1982; **49**(7): 1767–1772.
10. Hosking MC, Murdison KA, and Duncan WJ. Transcatheter stent implantation for recurrent pulmonary venous pathway obstruction after the Mustard procedure. *Br Heart J* 1994; **72**(1): 85–88.
11. Abdulhamed JM, Alyousef SA, and Mullins C. Endovascular stent placement for pulmonary venous obstruction after Mustard operation for transposition of the great arteries. *Heart* 1996; **75**(2): 210–212.

25 Coarctation of the aorta and miscellaneous arterial stents

Introduction

The initial investigations for the use of intravascular stents were for use in the peripheral arteries[1,2]. There was an almost simultaneous and explosive development in the use of stents for the treatment of stenosis of coronary arteries, which established a new era in the management of coronary artery disease and stimulated the development of these stents for use in other vascular areas. Although no stent has "FDA approval" for use in any pediatric/congenital lesion, by 1997 intravascular stent treatment had become the accepted, *standard therapy* for pulmonary artery branch stenosis and systemic venous stenosis in congenital heart patients[3]. The extensive use of the larger J & J™, P 308, "iliac" stents (Johnson & Johnson, Warren, NJ) in the pulmonary arteries and systemic veins in pediatric and congenital heart patients as well as in multiple adult systemic arterial lesions, led to a natural extension of the use of these stents to the treatment of coarctation of the aorta and other arterial lesions in pediatric/congenital heart patients.

When implanted in experimentally produced coarctations in animals, the P 308, "iliac" stents provided a sustained relief of the obstruction[4]. The ability to re-dilate at a later time the P 308 stents, which had been in the descending aorta chronically, in order to accommodate for the growth of the animal was also demonstrated in these studies[4,5]. However, for most adult human aortas, the 18 mm *maximum* diameter of the commercially available Palmaz™ P _ _ 8 stents represented a major limitation in the use of the "iliac" stents in the central aorta of humans. A lumen with an absolute maximum diameter of 18 mm, by itself, creates a stenosis in the proximal descending aorta of most moderate and large sized adults.

In spite of this major drawback, there were a few sporadic uses of the P 308 stents in the central aorta and other systemic arteries in various pediatric and "congenital" patients in the United States and the rest of the world[6–8]. The early cases included several acquired "abdominal coarctations" which were in the more distal, smaller descending aorta as well as some re-stenosis of classical congenital coarctation of the aorta. The acute results in these cases were very favorable, although the stents still could not be expanded beyond 18 mm in diameter. In the meantime, the larger diameter, thicker, and sturdier P 4015 and P 5015 stents (Johnson & Johnson–Cordis Corp., Miami Lakes, FL) became available for clinical trials in Europe. These larger stents, which except for size were identical to the P _ _ 8 stents, logically and quickly received CE approval for clinical use in large vessels in Europe and much of the rest of the world including the rest of the Americas *outside of the United States*. These larger P _ _ 15 stents can be dilated to 26+ mm in diameter, which makes them suitable for implant in the central aorta, even in very large (or potentially large) patients, in which location they now have had extensive use outside of the US. In addition to the P _ _ 15 stents, the larger diameter, Cheatham-Platinum™ (C-P™) stents (NuMED Inc., Hopkinton, NY) also became available commercially for use in larger vascular lesions outside of the US. Special C-P™ stents can be dilated to as large as 30 mm in diameter. The C-P™ stents have had very successful use in Europe, and a rare compassionate use in the United States.

With the introduction of the larger stents, intravascular stent therapy was rapidly expanded for use in native coarctation as well as re-coarctation of the aorta in all countries where the larger stents were available. Similar to all other vessels, when intravascular stents are implanted during a dilation of a systemic artery, the artery and the stent can be expanded to the exact, desired diameter of the artery and no larger. Unlike dilation angioplasty alone of vessels, the artery does *not* have to be over-dilated at all in order to compensate for the rebound or recoil of the vessel after dilation. This makes dilation with the simultaneous implant of a stent, inherently safer than a balloon dilation alone.

The limited use of the P 308 stent along with an occasional "compassionate" use of the larger J & J™ stents and the C-P™ stents continued in the United States with satisfactory results until eventually, in 1999, the larger J & J™ P 4010 and P 5010 stents (Johnson & Johnson–Cordis Corp., Miami Lakes, FL) were finally approved by the FDA for "arterial use" in the United States. In the meantime, several "aneurysms" in association with the implant of P _ _ 8 stents in coarctation of the aorta were reported. These cases were very rare and sporadic, but their occurrence did dampen the initial enthusiasm for the routine use of stents in coarctation of the aorta. The exact etiology of these aneurysms still has not been documented, however, the appearance of the aneurysms and the particular technique of implant suggest that the mechanism of the aneurysms is related to the particular stents that were used and the technique of delivery of those stents.

When either the P _ _ 8 or the P _ _ 10 stents are expanded by a single, initial inflation on a single large balloon with a diameter of 15 mm or more, and are expanded directly to the maximum diameter of the balloon, the balloon, along with the stent, expands initially and completely at both ends before the center of the balloon and stent itself even begin to expand. In doing so, the balloon assumes a "dumbbell" configuration which, in turn, flares both ends of the stent almost perpendicularly off the surface of the balloon and toward or into the vessel wall. The expanding, open, "end-struts" of the J & J™ P _ _ 8 and P _ _ 10 stents create a radial ring of *sharp points* at each end of the struts of the stent. These rings of sharp tips at the end of each strut with the initial inflation of the balloon/stent align almost *perpendicular* to, and pointing directly at, the wall of the vessel. As the ends of the stent expand further along with the remainder of the stent, these sharp tips dig into the vessel wall creating multiple circumferential tiny intimal (and medial! and adventitial!) perforations in the arterial wall. As the center of the stent expands, the circumferential ring of points that are imbedded in the vessel wall moves away from the center of the stent, creating short longitudinal tears/lacerations in the wall before the center of the stent eventually aligns parallel to the wall! These circumferential rings of perforations or tears probably are implicated in the creation of the aneurysms. It appears that a change in the type of stent or the technique for the expansion of the P _ _ 10 stents eliminates, or markedly reduces, the development of these aneurysms.

Until 2002, the P 4010 and P 5010 stents, with their distal sharp ends, were the only stents *commercially* available for the very large (or potentially very large) aorta. In 2002 FDA approval of the ITI™ Maxi™ stent (ev3, Plymouth, MN) provided an additional stent in the US which can be expanded to at least 25 mm in diameter for use in the central aorta, and which does not have sharp tips at the ends of the stent.

Equipment for arterial stent implants

Stents

The evolution of the stents that are available for use in the central aorta is discussed earlier in this chapter. Obviously, only stents that *eventually* can be expanded to the expected *adult diameter* of the aorta (or other artery) of the particular patient, should be used in the systemic arteries, regardless of the patient's size at the time of the implant.

J & J™ P 4010 & P 5010 stents

The J & J™ P 4010 and the P 5010 stents (Johnson & Johnson–Cordis Corp., Miami Lakes, FL) were the first stents suitable for use in the central aorta of large sized patients and, eventually, that were available commercially in the United States. These stents are laser cut from a slightly larger and thicker stainless steel tubing than the P _ _ 8 stents, in 4 & 5 cm lengths, respectively, and are balloon expandable to 25+ mm in diameter. When expanded above 15 mm these stents shrink in length similarly to the P _ _ 8 stents, and at 25+ mm diameter they shrink by > 40% in length. In addition to their larger diameters, the thicker stainless steel of these stents provides a wall strength that is significantly greater than that of the P _ _ 8 stents. Like the P _ _ 8 series stents, the laser cuts of the P _ _ 10 stents are straight, longitudinal, interrupted slits. This cutting pattern of the alternate rows of "slits" results in a very strong, "diamond" configuration of each "cell" when the stent is expanded. The open slots at each end of the stents result in radial rings of the very sharp tips of each strut.

J & J™, P 308, P 188 & P 108 stents

The characteristics of the J & J™ P _ _ 8 series stents (Johnson & Johnson–Cordis Corp., Miami Lakes, FL) are described under the "General Characteristics of Stents" (Chapter 22). These stents are expandable to a maximum of 18 mm (advertised to 8 mm maximum) diameter and are available in lengths of 30, 18 and 10 millimeters. When these stents are expanded to 18 mm in diameter, they shorten to approximately 55% of their original length. They are suitable for the central aorta *only in small sized adults*. They are suitable for use in the more peripheral systemic arteries and arterial branches.

Genesis XD™ stents

The Genesis XD™ stents (Johnson & Johnson–Cordis Corp., Miami Lakes, FL) are comparable to the J & &™ P _ _ 8 stents in size and apparent strength. These are balloon-expandable and must be hand-mounted on the desired balloon for implant. The Genesis XD™ stent is laser cut with alternating rows of slots; however, the alternate rows have an "s" cut so that after expansion, each ring of "diamond" shaped cells ends up connected to the adjacent ring of "diamonds" by a slightly flexible "omega" shaped hinge or joint. The end cells are "closed" so that they do not produce sharp tips when expanded. The Genesis XD™ stents are used in comparable locations to the P _ _ 8 stents, and are not suitable for use in the central aorta of most normal or large sized patients.

Double Strut™, Maxi™ and Mega™ stents (ev3, Plymouth, MN)

Double Strut™ Stents

The ITI™ Double Strut™ stents (ev3, Plymouth, MN) are available for use in the same lesions where the J & J™ P _ _ 8 series stents are used. These stents also are laser cut from stainless steel tubing. The laser cutting of these stents, however, is more elaborate and somewhat serpentine, resulting in an "open-cell" wall configuration. This wall configuration gives the stents flexibility in the non-expanded state, allowing them to bend on the balloon as they are delivered around curves. The flexibility persists in the expanded state, permitting the Double Strut™ stents to conform to curvature in the arterial walls after they are expanded and implanted. The "cutting" of the cells of the Double Strut™ stent results in closed cells at the *ends* of the stent, which gives these stents smoother ends than the comparable J & J™ stents, and may provide additional protection against aneurysm formation in the aorta. The "open cells" of the side of the stent allow access through the side of the implanted stent and these openings in the sides can be expanded up to 12 mm in diameter.

Double Strut™ stents are balloon-expandable up to *only* 18–20 mm diameter (advertised to 12 mm maximum) and are available in lengths of 16, 26, 36, 56 and 76 millimeters. When expanded *sequentially*, the Double Strut™ stents do *not* shrink appreciably in length even at their maximum diameter. However, when expanded above 12 mm in diameter with a single, large diameter balloon inflation, these stents not only shrink, but are compressed in length by the expanding ends of the balloon. The Double Strut™ stent does ***not*** have as much radial strength as the J & J™ P _ _ 8 stents when expanded to diameters greater than 12 mm, and the radial strength often is not sufficient to maintain an acutely dilated large vessel. With it maximum diameter of 18 mm, the Double Strut™ stent is not suitable for use in the central aorta, except in very small adult patients.

The Mega™ stent

The ITI™ Mega™ stent (ev3, Plymouth, MN) is a recently approved single-strut, thicker metal, but still open-cell design stent. Its laser-cut construction is similar to that of the Double Strut™, but with thicker metal and only single struts. The resulting single-strut, open-cell stent, is comparable in size to the Double Strut™ and P _ _ 8 stents, but with a wall strength of the expanded stent which, reportedly, is comparable to that of the P _ _ 8 stents. This stent has only recently entered clinical use. Hopefully, it will overcome some of the problems of the rigid configuration and the sharp ends of the P _ _ 8 stents. Like the P _ _ 8 and the Double Strut™ stents, the Mega™ stent is usable only in the *distal* aorta and peripheral arteries, and does *not* expand to a large enough diameter to make it usable in the central aorta of most patients.

The Maxi™ stent

The ITI™ Maxi™ stent (ev3, Plymouth, MN) has been approved for use in humans in the United States. This is a larger diameter, thicker walled, single-strut stent, but still with an open-cell design similar to the original ITI™ Double Strut™ stents. The open-cell design allows some flexibility. Maxi™ stents can be expanded to 25 mm in diameter and reportedly have the same wall strength as the J & J™ P _ _ 8 stents. As such this stent should be a viable option for central aortic stenting; however, the open-cell design of the Maxi™ allows the stent to kink when placed in sharp curves and allows the cells of the stent to be distorted during subsequent catheter manipulations within the freshly implanted stent. This distortion of the "cells" allows catheters or balloons to pass through the side cells. There is not sufficient documentation of the use of the Maxi™ stents as yet to recommend it over the P _ _ 10 stents.

NuMED Cheatham-Platinum™ (C-P™) stents

C-P™ stents (NuMED Inc., Hopkinton, NY) are manufactured from platinum wire. The wire is welded in rows in a particular "zig-zag" pattern. The particular design of the welded rows results in a closed cell configuration, which however, is slightly flexible. The number of rows of "zigs" determines the eventual diameter of the stents, so these stents can be manufactured in very large diameters and any particular length desired. These stents have CE approval and are in very wide clinical use throughout the world except in the United States—although they have had occasional emergency or compassionate use in the United States. Extensive data comparable to the other large diameter stents are not yet available in the United States.

Balloons for the delivery of arterial stents

The same or even more critical requirements for the balloons that are used for the delivery of any other stents, are necessary for the balloons that are used for the delivery of arterial/aortic stents. As is the case with the balloons for the delivery of stents to the other congenital locations, the "ideal" balloon is not available for the delivery of a stent into a central arterial/aortic location. When the systemic arterial stenosis is very tight and the artery immediately distal to the stenosis is not significantly larger than the artery proximal to the lesion, a balloon that is smaller than the expected, final diameter of the artery is used for the *initial implant* of the stent. However, if the arterial narrowing is not tight or the artery progressively enlarges immediately distal to the stenosis, then a larger diameter balloon must be used for the initial implant. The balloon for the final dilation and fixation of a stent in a systemic artery should be the same diameter or, at most, 10% larger than the smallest diameter of the "normal" artery immediately adjacent to the stenosis. The balloon used to implant the stent initially does *not* need to be a high-pressure balloon and, because of the very rough deflated surfaces of all of the available high-pressure balloons, these balloons usually are contraindicated for the *implant of* stents. High-pressure balloons can be used to further expand stents when they are already fixed securely in the artery.

In small patients where an initial stent expansion to a diameter of 10 mm or less is acceptable, the Ultrathin SDS™ balloons (Boston Scientific, Natick, MA) are the preferred balloons for the implant of the stent. These balloons are discussed in Chapter 22, and their use for the delivery of stents to the smaller diameter pulmonary arteries is described in Chapter 23. Even when implanted initially at these small diameters, the particular *stent* that is implanted in the aorta, *ultimately must be capable* of expansion to the eventual, full *adult diameter* of the patient's aorta!

The Balloon In Balloon™ (BIB™) balloons (NuMED Inc., Hopkinton, NY) are recommended for stent delivery when the *initial* diameter for implanting the stent is greater than 12 mm. Arteries that require these larger sizes of balloons for the initial implants, represent the majority of arterial/aortic stents. Although BIB™ balloons require a significantly larger sheath for the delivery of a stent, the step-wise expansion of the stents which these balloons allow has many advantages which far outweigh the disadvantage of the larger sheath. The outer balloon of the BIB™ balloon used for stent implant is the same length as the stent, and the inner balloon is 1 cm shorter than the stent. The smaller and shorter inner balloon expands the stent uniformly throughout the length of the inner balloon without flaring the ends of the stent. If anything, both ends of the stent remain slightly under-expanded, which eliminates the circumferential, radial row of sharp tips that otherwise extend out from each end of the expanding stent. With the step-wise expansion of the stents, there essentially is no "dumbbell" effect of the balloon within the stent. The initial expansion of the stent to the smaller inner balloon diameter of the BIB™ balloon, also allows repositioning of the partially expanded stent before final maximal expansion and fixation with the outer balloon.

When the Double Strut,™ Mega™ or Maxi™ stents are expanded to an initial large diameter with a single expansion of a single, large diameter balloon, the expanding "dumbbell" of the expanding balloon compresses the stents from both ends and actually "shrinks" the stents in length by as much as 50%. However, when ITI™ stents are expanded stepwise or sequentially expanded with BIB™ balloons, this eliminates any lengthwise shrinking of these stents. None of the ITI™ stents have sharp points extending from either end during or after expansion and, as a consequence, are less likely to puncture the balloons or arterial/aortic wall. At the same time, the smoother ends do not "fix" into the vessel wall as securely as the sharp, rigid tips of the Palmaz™ P _ _ 8 or P _ _ 10 stents (Johnson & Johnson–Cordis Corp., Miami Lakes, FL), and unless fixed in place by a very tight initial lesion, do tend to move in the artery during any subsequent balloon/catheter manipulations within the freshly implanted stent.

Stents and balloons for implant into arteries which normally and ultimately will be smaller than 18 mm

There is now a large variety of smaller stents that are pre-mounted on balloons and that are ideal for implant in arteries that *ultimately will be small* in their diameter at their full adult size. Examples of this type of artery include the systemic to pulmonary artery collaterals, systemic to pulmonary artery surgical shunts, peripheral or branch systemic arteries, and the patent ductus arteriosus. The most suitable stents for use in the smaller systemic arteries at the time of this writing are the pre-mounted, balloon-expandable, "Medium" and "Large" Genesis™ stents (Johnson & Johnson–Cordis Corp., Miami Lakes, FL) and the Express™ stents (Boston Scientific, Natick, MA). Any one of a number of pre-mounted, balloon-expandable, coronary artery stents appear to be suitable for implant in the ductus of a newborn infant with a ductus dependent pulmonary artery circuit. These smaller balloons/stents are discussed subsequently in this chapter under the discussions of stenting the specific arteries.

Sheaths for arterial stent delivery

All of the stents currently used in central arterial/aortic lesions must be hand-mounted and, as a consequence, are delivered to the lesions through long sheaths similar to the delivery of hand-mounted stents to other sites. The delivery sheath must be long enough to extend from the entry site in the artery to a location several centimeters past the lesion. For the implant of arterial stents, a back-bleed/flush port on the sheaths is essential to prevent massive blood loss during the procedure. Ideally, the sheaths are kink-resistant and are themselves very radio-opaque or have a radio-opaque marker band at the distal end for easy visualization. When mounted on 10 mm or smaller balloons for their initial implant, even the larger diameter stents can be delivered through 8- or 9-French sheaths, while the stents delivered on the BIB™ balloons require 11–13-French sheaths. Currently, the long RB-MTS™ sheaths (Cook Inc., Bloomington, IN) are the most satisfactory for stent delivery to the central aorta.

The smaller diameter, pre-mounted stents often can be introduced through a short peripheral introductory sheath and delivered to the lesion "bare" over the wire.

Wires for arterial stent delivery

Exchange length, Super Stiff™ wires (Medi-Tech, Boston Scientific, Natick, MA) are used for the delivery of all large arterial/aortic stents. Because of the force of the arterial blood flow and the fact that the stents usually are being implanted against this flow of blood, there is a greater tendency for the balloon/stent to be pushed by the force of the blood flow as the balloon is inflated and displaced distally. The stiffer the support wire and the more securely the wire can be positioned, the less the problem of stent displacement due to the force of the blood flow. As opposed to the short floppy tip on the wires that are used in pulmonary artery implants, a minimally traumatic, *long floppy tipped*, Super Stiff™ wire is used for arterial implants. From the femoral approach, the distal end of the wire is positioned far out into an artery in an upper extremity. With arterial/aortic stent implants, there seldom is a problem of getting the stiff portion of the wire completely across the lesion being stented even using the wires with long floppy tips. Only when access to an artery in either upper extremity is not possible with the retrograde catheter, is the long, soft end of the Super Stiff™ wire looped in the central ascending aorta during a stent implant. The *stiff portion* of the wire must be entirely across the lesion, around the arch and into the aortic root. The balloons that are available and used currently for the delivery of large systemic arterial/aortic stents, will accommodate only a maximum of a 0.035" inch wire. The Amplatz™ Super Stiff Wire™ (Medi-Tech, Boston Scientific, Natick, MA) currently is the most satisfactory wire available.

Technique for coarctation (central arterial) stent delivery

Intravascular stent implants currently are used routinely to dilate and support both native and re-coarctations[9]. Although the use of stents eliminates the need for any "over-dilation" of the aorta in the area and results in a more persistent lumen, the use of stents does not eliminate, or possibly even reduce, the potential complications which occur from balloon dilation of coarctation of the aorta[10–12]. All precautions used for a balloon dilation of a coarctation of the aorta are observed for stent implants in both the native and re-coarctations. *Very accurate* measurements of the area of stenosis and the adjacent artery are mandatory. For balloon dilation and stent implants in coarctation of the aorta, specific, consistently reliable, separate X-ray calibration systems are used for these measurements. Stents (or balloons) are not expanded more than 10% larger than the adjacent "normal" aorta. Very tight coarctations of the aorta are expanded sequentially with a staged expansion of the lesion during sequential catheterizations. Very special precautions are utilized during the expansion of stents to large diameters and are discussed in detail in this section.

The implant procedures for arterial stents are performed using general anesthesia or very heavy analgesia/sedation. A balloon expanding in a systemic artery produces pain at the dilation site, so general anesthesia or deep sedation with heavy analgesia is *necessary* for this procedure[13]. Chlorpromazine (thorazine) is an excellent adjunct to the premedication or sedation of these patients. The vasodilation effect of chlorpromazine helps to reduce the extreme elevations of proximal systemic pressure encountered during the transient total aortic obstruction that occurs during balloon inflations, and to counteract the "rebound" hypertension encountered following the dilation of a coarctation of the aorta. In addition to either heavy sedation or general anesthesia, 2% local anesthesia is infiltrated around the arterial puncture/entry site. The local anesthesia is administrated *very liberally* initially and *repeated frequently* during and again at the very end of the procedure.

For the implant of most stents in coarctation of the aorta and other central aortic locations, one venous and one or two arterial lines are secured at the beginning of the case. Initially, only a small, "Quick-Cath" cannula or a 5-French dilator is placed in the artery. Once lines are secured, blood is obtained for a measurement of a baseline activated clotting time (ACT), but heparin is not administered at this stage of the procedure. Once the initial dose of heparin is administered later in the case, the ACT is monitored periodically throughout a long case and maintained at 275–350 seconds with the administration of additional heparin.

The majority of "arterial/aortic stents" are delivered retrograde and usually there is a fairly direct "route" and an essentially straight course to the involved arterial stenosis. The major problem with the delivery of stents to systemic arteries is the necessity of introducing a large delivery sheath into the artery and the potential problems of local arterial damage from these large sheaths. Arterial lines initially are secured in the femoral artery with a small arterial cannula or small vessel dilator. Although the actual delivery of the stent will be retrograde, a predominantly prograde approach is used for the diagnostic catheterization, angiograms, and measurements of the coarctation of the aorta and, particularly, during the implant of a stent into the coarctation. By using the combined prograde and retrograde approach, the duration of "time" in the artery with a large sheath or catheter and manipulations with large sheaths/catheters within the artery are reduced, which markedly reduces the incidence of arterial complications.

A right heart catheterization is performed from a femoral venous approach. After the completion of the right heart catheterization, and from the same venous entry site, the left heart is entered through the atrium. When there is no pre-existing atrial communication, a transseptal left atrial puncture is performed and a long sheath/dilator set is advanced from the femoral vein into the left atrium. The sheath/dilator or the sheath with a catheter within it are maneuvered into the left ventricle from the left atrium. Once the tip *of the sheath* is in the left ventricle, the dilator or catheter is removed and the sheath is allowed to bleed back passively through the side port of the sheath. Once cleared of all air and clot, the side port of the sheath is attached to the flush/pressure system, flushed vigorously, and then placed on a slow continuous flush. When the transseptal puncture is completed, the patient is given 100 mg/kg of intravenous heparin.

Using a "heat gun" or boiling, sterile water, a 360° loop is "pre-formed" on the end of a Berman™ balloon angiographic catheter (Arrow International Inc., Reading, PA), as described in Chapter 7. The balloon angiographic catheter that is used, is *one French size smaller* in diameter than the French size of the transseptal sheath. With both the sheath and the balloon catheter on a *continuous* flush, the balloon catheter is introduced into the sheath and advanced to the left ventricle. Just as the balloon exits the tip of the sheath the Berman™ balloon is inflated. Usually with the support of the sheath, which is positioned in the left ventricle, and with the "pre-formed" curve on the catheter, minimal manipulation of the balloon catheter is required in order to "float" the balloon into the ascending aorta and, from there, again with the help of the preformed curve, *around to the descending aorta*. Occasionally it is necessary to redirect the tip of the balloon catheter positioned in the left ventricular apex to a more cephalad direction with a deflector wire that can be used within the balloon catheter.

These same type of maneuvers can be accomplished with a tip deflector wire in a soft, but "non-floating" angiographic catheter in order to manipulate a catheter other than a floating balloon catheter, prograde from the ventricle into the aorta. The current woven dacron catheters (Medtronic Inc., Minneapolis, MN) very rapidly become very soft at body temperature, which makes them quite safe for deflection in the left ventricle and subsequently for manipulation out into the aorta. Whichever catheter is used, it should be at least one French size smaller than the long sheath that is maintained in the left ventricle. This size discrepancy allows intermittent monitoring of pressure through the sheath simultaneously with pressures from the catheter.

Once around the arch and into the descending aorta, the balloon is deflated and the tip of the catheter is positioned just proximal to the obstruction in the aorta. Simultaneous pressures are recorded from the left ventricle (through the side arm of the sheath), from the aorta proximal to the stenosis (through the catheter) and distal to the obstruction (through the indwelling arterial line[s]). A biplane aortogram with the injection through the prograde catheter positioned just proximal to the lesion is recorded in the PA and lateral views. The ideal angulation of the X-ray tubes in order to elongate the lesion into its longest axis is determined from these angiograms, and the X-ray tubes adjusted accordingly.

For precise measurements of the coarctation and both the adjacent proximal and distal aorta, a calibrated "marker catheter", a calibrated, centimeter, reference "grid" system, or the "centimeter distance" calibration "dots" built into the X-ray system are used. The built-in calibration using the width of a catheter as the reference is not reliable when measuring large vessels. In order to use a marker catheter as the calibration system (unless the catheter which was deflected from the left ventricle into the aorta was an angiographic "marker" catheter), the "marks" of the marker catheter must be positioned exactly *in the field* of the coarctation and aligned properly just before the aortogram is recorded. This is accomplished most expeditiously by replacing one of the indwelling arterial lines with a 6-French sheath and then introducing a 6-French marker catheter retrograde exactly into the area of the lesion *just before* the aortogram is recorded.

As long as the patient, the catheterization table, the X-ray tubes, and the image intensifiers are *not moved at all* between the recording of the marks on the "marker catheter" and the performance of the aortogram, the marker catheter can be positioned before, during or after the actual aortographic injection. Once the "bands" are lined up exactly in the plane of the lesion, a separate very short run angiographic recording is performed without any contrast injection in order to record the calibration bands again without moving the patient or the X-ray equipment. Similarly, the calibration "marks" can be recorded from a venous catheter before or after the prograde catheter is introduced into the aorta or even using a separate venous "marker" catheter placed in the field as long as neither the patient nor any element of the imaging system is moved between the recording of the properly aligned "marks" and the actual aortogram.

The exact type, length and diameter of *stent that will be used* are determined from the anatomy and these angiographic measurements. The stent used also depends upon the expected *eventual adult* diameter of the stented area as a result of any future growth, the position of adjacent branch vessels, and the contour of the aorta in the area where the stent is to be implanted. Once the exact *stent* and its diameter for implant have been chosen, then the decisions are made concerning which balloon and, in turn, which sheath will be used to deliver the particular stent. The diameter of the balloon that will be used to implant the stent depends upon the *smallest* "normal" vessel diameter *adjacent* to the coarctation.

For an aorta with a current or expected diameter of 20 mm or more in the particular area, only the J & J™ P 4010 or P 5010 stents or the ITI™ Maxi™ stents are suitable (in the US) for implant into the central aorta. The current Palmaz™ P _ _ 8 series of stents, the Genesis™ XD and the other ITI™ stents cannot be dilated to greater than 18 mm and should not be used in arteries larger, or expected to be larger, than 18 mm. Both the ITI™ Mega,™ the Palmaz™ P _ _ 8 and the Genesis™ XD series stents, however, could be used in a patient who, it is anticipated, will be very small ***and** consistently* has fallen in the lower percentiles on their growth curve—i.e. those patients who are very unlikely to become even average sized adults and definitely not large adults.

By using a step-wise or sequential expansion even to large diameters, the *perpendicular* radius of sharp tips at the ends of the J & J™ Palmaz™ type stent, which occur as the stents are expanded, are minimized. However, even after a stepwise expansion, all of the J & J™ Palmaz™ family of stents *at full expansion* are very straight and rigid, and end up with sharp ends that flare *slightly* radially around the circumference of the stent and into the arterial wall. This potentially is a problem, particularly in locations in the aorta that have a significant curvature such as the proximal descending aorta. ITI™ stents conform better to curves in the arteries and have "rounded" ends that are less traumatic to the arterial walls. At the same time, the ITI™ stents do tend to move forward or backward in the artery spontaneously, particularly during any manipulation of balloons or even catheters within them immediately after implant—possibly because they *do not* have sharp tips at the ends to "dig" into the vessel wall! The choice between the Maxi™ and the Palmaz™ P _ _ 10 stents in suitable patients is a decision of the operator, and currently depends upon each individual operator's experience.

The Super Stiff™ delivery wire that is used for the sheath/dilator and stent delivery is positioned securely in one of the *subclavian* arteries for the implant of a stent in a coarctation of the aorta. The use of a subclavian artery to secure the delivery wire is preferred over the earlier technique of looping the long floppy tip of the stiff wire in the ascending aorta. When the distal end of the wire is positioned in the ascending aorta, the entire soft portion of the distal end of the wire becomes looped loosely in the ascending aorta. This results in a long, free, 180° curve of the stiff portion of the wire extended around the arch from the descending into the ascending aorta. With the floppy tip of the wire free in the ascending aorta, this long, floppy tip of the wire cannot be pushed or "fixed" against anything and, in turn, precise control is lost over the to-and-fro motion of the wire/balloon/stent in the area of stenosis. In addition, a long floppy tip that is looped in the ascending aorta easily drops into the left ventricle or, even worse, works its way into a coronary artery.

To position the wire in the subclavian artery, if a marker catheter had been used retrograde through the arterial sheath, it is replaced with a long end-hole catheter. The end-hole catheter is maneuvered retrograde across the coarctation and as far out into either the right or left subclavian artery as is possible. In most cases, the *right* subclavian artery is used to secure the Super Stiff™ wire for a balloon/stent delivery in a coarctation of the aorta. Once the retrograde, end-hole catheter has been advanced through the obstruction, it is maneuvered across the transverse aortic arch and far out into the right subclavian artery. The right subclavian artery allows the wire that is coming from the descending aorta to make a gradual, slight curve through the lesion and across the transverse aortic arch. This position allows a very secure "fixation" of the distal end of the wire.

The left subclavian artery can be used when it *arises off, and courses relatively parallel* to, the *descending* aorta *and*, at the same time, the origin of the subclavian artery is far enough *proximal* to the obstruction, so that the implanted stent will not encroach upon this orifice of the left subclavian artery. At the other extreme, when the origin of the subclavian artery actually is involved at the site of obstruction of the coarctation, it may be desirable to implant the stent purposefully extending partially into the origin of the left subclavian artery.

Whichever subclavian artery is used, the end-hole catheter is manipulated into the artery and maneuvered as far distally into the respective extremity as possible. In order to maneuver the catheter very far distally in the artery and far out into the arm, it usually requires the use of a torque-controlled, floppy tipped wire in advance of the tip of the catheter in order to maneuver through the course of the distal artery. The 0.035″ Magic™ wire (Medi-Tech, Boston Scientific, Natick, MA) has been very effective and safe for this maneuvering. Once the tip of the *catheter* is positioned far distally in the extremity, the torque wire is replaced through the catheter with a 0.035″

Amplatz, Super Stiff Wire™ with a long floppy tip (Medi-Tech, Boston Scientific, Natick, MA). The Super Stiff™ wire is advanced as far as it will go in the artery. The retrograde arterial catheter is maintained in its position over the wire and maintained on a slow flush until the sheath/dilator is ready for introduction. During all of the positioning of the *retrograde* catheter/wire, the prograde catheter is maintained with the tip of the catheter just proximal to the lesion and maintained on a constant flush.

The appropriate stent is mounted on the appropriate balloon before the delivery sheath is introduced. Once the stent is mounted on the balloon and ready for delivery, the area around the femoral arterial sheath through which the catheter and wire are passing, is re-infiltrated very liberally with local anesthesia. The re-infiltration should be down to and around the artery. With the stiff wire fixed in place, the catheter over the wire and the short sheath are replaced with the large, long sheath/dilator set that is to be used for the stent delivery. A sheath is used which accommodates the *largest possible* balloon/stent that *might* be used in the particular case. It is better to start with a sheath that is one to two French sizes larger than it is to have to exchange large sheaths in and out of an artery even once or twice. The long sheath/dilator set is advanced retrograde until the tip of the *sheath* is several centimeters past (proximal to) the lesion. While keeping the wire in its secure position well distally in the upper extremity, the dilator is removed over the wire and out of the sheath. The sheath is allowed to bleed back passively in order to clear it of any air or clot and then placed on a continuous flush.

The stent, which is mounted on the appropriate balloon, is introduced over the wire, into the long sheath. The walls of the J & J™ stents are rigid enough to be introduced through the back-bleed valve of the long delivery sheath without distorting the stent, however, a short protective sleeve should be placed over ITI™ stents while they are being introduced through the back-bleed valve of the large, long sheath. The protective sleeve can be made from a short, cut-off segment of sheath of the same French size as the long delivery sheath. The stent/balloon is positioned within this short segment of sheath as the combination is advanced through the back-bleed valve of the long sheath. Once the balloon/stent is well into the long sheath, the short "sleeve" is withdrawn back onto the shaft of the balloon catheter. With both the sheath and the balloon catheter maintained on a continuous flush, the stent and balloon are advanced through the long sheath to the lesion. A selective aortogram with the injection through the prograde catheter is performed precisely in the area of the stenosis, and any adjustments that are necessary to center the stent exactly in the lesion are made in the balloon/stent position.

When the stent is in the precise position across the stenosis, the sheath is withdrawn off the stent and completely off the proximal end of the balloon, but at the same time, not far away from the balloon. The wire is advanced to be sure it is positioned securely with no "slack". A "forward push" is maintained on the wire *and* balloon/stent/catheter combination to secure the balloon/stent in position. When the position of the wire and the balloon/stent are correct, or once they have been adjusted to correct the position, a selective aortogram is repeated and a "road map" image of the angiogram saved. The prograde catheter is withdrawn just enough to be entirely away from the cephalad end of the stent in order that the prograde balloon does not become trapped by the stent when the stent expands.

When the stent is in the optimal position, the balloon is inflated. With large diameter lesions, the inner balloon of the BIB™ balloon is inflated and the position of the "half way" inflated stent rechecked against the "road map" or with another aortogram. If necessary the balloon/stent or wire is/are adjusted to reposition the stent precisely in the center of the stenosis. The outer balloon then is inflated, which expands the stent and fixes it in position. Often, with maximum balloon/stent expansion in the aorta, the patient experiences significant discomfort while the balloon is being inflated. Even when they are sedated adequately, they may move slightly or groan. Although the patient does not remember the event the next day, any movement of the patient can move the relative position of the stent in the coarctation. The pain decreases, but may not disappear, with the deflation of the balloon.

Various maneuvers including the administration of adenosine or the institution of very rapid ventricular pacing in order to stop the effective cardiac contractility just before the balloon inflation are utilized to keep the balloon with the stent from moving during the balloon inflation. With the use of Super Stiff™ wires and with the wire positioned properly and securely in one of the subclavian arteries, these adjunct measures have not been necessary in our experience.

With a long segment of stenosis or a stenosis extending around a curve in the artery, two or more stents placed in tandem are preferable to cover the entire area *or* to conform better to the curvature of the artery. When any stents that potentially will be dilated to a large diameter are implanted in tandem, the adjoining stents should overlap the adjacent stent by at least 50%. When several stents are being implanted in tandem in the aorta, there is a critical decision that must be made concerning which of the stents should be implanted first. This depends predominantly upon the particular anatomy of the area.

When there is a relatively uniform diameter of the entire area involved, the stent that will be more "downstream" (in the direction of blood flow) and further from the heart is implanted first. During the implant of the first stent, whenever possible, the stent is expanded to *less* than the *eventual* desired diameter of the stent/vessel but, at the same time, to a large enough diameter to fix the stent securely in the vessel/stenosis. Implanting the first stent at a slightly smaller initial diameter allows the second stent to be expanded within the first stent at a slightly *larger* diameter than the first stent, but not having to over-dilate the adjacent vessel. The larger diameter of the second stent fixes the second stent securely in the aorta and flares the proximal end of the first, and more distal, stent slightly. This flaring traps the second stent within the first stent, while the slightly larger balloon expands both stents further for a more secure hold in the artery.

When there is progressive widening of the artery/aorta distally, as is often encountered with "post-stenotic dilation" of the aorta beyond a coarctation, the more proximal (or "upstream or cephalad") stent is implanted first. This implant is more precarious. The more distal area widens to a diameter that is significantly larger than the aorta proximal to the coarctation and often is larger in diameter than the more proximal area possibly can be dilated to. This creates the perfect situation for the more proximal stent to migrate distally! The balloon for the more proximal stent implant should be slightly larger in diameter than the proximal *vessel* and the first, more proximal stent is implanted as far proximally in the vessel as is possible while still including the area of stenosis/coarctation. The more proximal location usually is at a significant angle to the wider descending aorta, which helps to keep the stent from moving distally. This positioning of the proximal stent also leaves the distal end of the proximal stent "hanging free" in the larger diameter, more distal segment of the aorta! The sheath, very cautiously, is reintroduced into the freshly implanted stent while the implanting balloon gradually is being deflated. The original balloon is withdrawn through the sheath, which is now positioned through the stent. The second (more distal) stent is mounted on a balloon that is at least 10% larger in diameter than *the distal portion of the area* being stented, and at least as large as the aorta distal to the obstruction. The balloon/stent is advanced within the sheath and the first stent until there is at least 33–50% overlap of the stents. The sheath is withdrawn very cautiously off the stent/balloon. The position is checked with a repeat, selective aortogram, injecting through the prograde catheter. The balloon/stent is expanded while continually holding the stent/balloon in place by pushing the stent/balloon/catheter toward the original stent. The original stent flares further to oppose the vessel wall while the second (distal) stent expands wider at the free, distal end, opposing the arterial wall at its distal end and, hopefully, creating a significant angle from the first stent which, in turn, helps to hold the combined stents in place. This very precarious implant is one situation where rapid ventricular pacing during the actual implant is considered in order to stop cardiac output temporarily.

Once the stenosis is expanded and completely "covered" with one or more stents, the balloon again is inflated and the sheath re-advanced into the stent *as the balloon is deflating*. The sheath within the stent provides a "protective separation" of the "rough" walls of the deflated balloon from the freshly implanted stent, which, in turn, allows the withdrawal of the balloon from the stent or the easy introduction of additional larger or higher-pressure balloons for further expansion of the stents. Stents in the aorta occasionally are "flared" in order to conform better to the contour of the aorta by further dilation of *just the ends of the stents* with larger balloons. Generally, this flaring of the ends of the stents into the arterial wall probably is not necessary. Usually, smoother large balloons, which are less likely to dislodge the stent, but which otherwise would not have been satisfactory for stent *implant*, can be used for this "flaring", however, any "re-moulding" or flaring of the stent is performed much more safely, months later at a subsequent catheterization, when the stents have become fixed firmly into the wall of the aorta. Once satisfied with the fixation of the stents a final aortogram is performed and simultaneous pressures proximal and distal to the stent(s) are recorded through the already positioned combination of catheters.

Pressures also are recorded through the prograde catheter as it is withdrawn from the ascending aorta, the left ventricle, the left atrium and finally, the right atrium. An ACT is checked and the heparin is reversed with protamine only when the ACT is greater than 300 seconds. The areas of the arterial punctures *again* are infiltrated liberally with local anesthesia. The large arterial sheath is withdrawn and bleeding controlled with finger (hand) pressure manually over the site until the bleeding has stopped completely. While pressure is held over the puncture site with one hand, the posterior tibial or dorsalis pedis pulse in the same extremity is palpated with the other hand. Enough pressure is applied over the puncture site to prevent bleeding or hematoma formation, but at the same time not so much pressure as to eliminate the pulse peripherally. The amount of pressure over the puncture is "titrated" in this manner until the bleeding stops. Control of the bleeding from these large puncture sites often takes considerable time and even more patience. Surgical repair or any of the available "vascular seals" has not been necessary in our experience in order to achieve hemostasis and yet maintain good peripheral perfusion.

Abdominal aorta stents

In addition to the classical "coarctation", more distal areas in the aorta ("middle aortic syndrome") are amenable to treatment with intravascular stents[14,15]. These distal aortic lesions usually (always!) are acquired lesions and secondary to some type of prior arteritis. The involved area in the aorta usually is a long segment, fairly tight and irregularly narrowing, and very frequently involves major side branches off the aorta. The tissues of the arterial wall usually are very abnormal with a thickened vessel wall, which, at the same time is very "friable". Most of these lesions are amenable to dilation with stent implants.

Because the involved area of the aorta is more distal and normally much smaller in diameter than the area of the arch and proximal descending aorta, the P _ _ 8, or comparable sized Genesis™ or Intrastent™ stents usually are sufficient for these lesions. In addition, since these areas of stenosis usually are very narrow, the stents can usually be implanted on relatively small balloons and through smaller sheaths compared to stents in the "classic coarctation". The exact lesion, the adjacent branching vessels, and the nearest "normal" aorta that is adjacent to the lesion, are visualized by selective biplane aortography and accurately measured using an accurate angiographic calibration system as described earlier in this chapter. This aortography usually is performed through a retrograde catheter, although a prograde approach following a transseptal puncture can be used to position an additional catheter just proximal to the lesion(s) and even as far distally in the aorta as the distal bifurcation of the aorta at the origin of the iliac arteries. A catheter that is introduced prograde and advanced to the descending aorta is preferable when very precise positioning of stents adjacent to or above and below branching vessels is required. The prograde catheter, which is in position in the descending aorta, allows small selective angiograms to be performed just proximal to the lesion while the stent actually is being implanted from the retrograde approach.

Once the anatomy of the entire lesion has been visualized and measured accurately, the appropriate stent(s) is (are) chosen. These acquired aortic lesions are expanded very conservatively at the time of the implant of the stent. The actual narrowing in the artery is not expanded to more than two and a half times the diameter of the most severe ***stenosis*** during the initial implant procedure, even if the final expanded diameter of the stent is not as large as the diameter of the adjacent "normal" aorta. An acute dilation of the lesion to a larger diameter has a significant chance of tearing these very abnormal tissues of the arterial wall. Once the patient has recovered from the initial stent implant and the aorta has had a chance to "heal" for at least several months following the initial implant of the stent, the patient is re-catheterized and the stent(s) can be dilated further.

At the present time, if the stenosis extends across a significant branching vessel, separate stents are implanted above and below the side/branch vessel covering as much of the lesions in the adjacent aorta as possible without crossing these branches. With a little more experience using stents with "open-cell" designs, stents will be placed across these side or branching vessels and yet still allow access to the side branches.

Stents in arterial shunts/collateral vessels

Rarely, enlargement of or preservation of a systemic artery to pulmonary artery surgical shunt or a systemic artery to pulmonary artery collaterals is desirable for symptomatic improvement in congenital heart patients[16,17]. As with most of the other vascular lesions, dilation alone of theses arteries usually does not produce persistent results. The patency of these lesions can be maintained very well with the implant of one or more intravascular stents.

There are many technical *advantages* when implanting stents in these arteries, compared to placing stents in the larger central arteries in pediatric/congenital heart patients. The maximum desired or eventual diameter of any of these vessels is significantly smaller than the central aorta so that "smaller" stents, smaller delivery balloons and, in turn, smaller diameter introductory/delivery sheaths can be used. Because of the similarity of these stenoses to acquired lesions in the adult patient, there is a much larger variety of balloons, stents and delivery systems available for these lesions. Lesions in the branch systemic arteries or collaterals are ideal in size for the pre-mounted "Medium" and "Large" Genesis™ stents (Johnson & Johnson–Cordis Corp., Miami Lakes, FL) and the Express™ Biliary LD stents (Boston Scientific, Natick, MA). Both of these types of stents are available pre-mounted very securely on balloons in multiple sizes of the balloon delivery catheters.

"Medium" Genesis™ stents are mounted on balloons between 3 mm and 7 mm in diameter, and are available in lengths of 12, 15, 18 and 24 mm. Depending upon the particular balloon, the balloon delivery catheters for the "Medium" Genesis™ stent are delivered over a 0.014" or 0.018" wire and all have small catheter shafts. As a consequence, these stents can be introduced through a 4–6-French sheath (or 6–7-French guide catheter). The "Large" Genesis™ stents are mounted on balloons between 5 mm and 9 mm in diameter and are available in lengths of 19, 29, 39 and 59 mm. The balloon catheters for the delivery of the "Large" Genesis™ stents accept a 0.035" wire and require a 6- or 7-French introductory sheath (or an 8- or 9-French guide catheter). All of the pre-mounted stents can be introduced through a short sheath and usually can be delivered "naked" to the lesion without the use of a long sheath or guiding catheter. When there is a very tortuous course or sharp curves in the course to the site of implant, a long sheath is recommended to prevent the stents from catching on the angles or edges in the vessel. The slight flexibility and smoother ends of these stents allow the stents mounted on the balloons to pass smoothly through the long sheath. The use of a long sheath also allows repeated "positioning" angiograms to be performed in the vessel just proximal to the stent/implant area during the delivery without the necessity of a second catheter.

The architecture of the Express Biliary LD™ stents has alternating micro and macro circumferential elements attached together in "tandem" to provide an open-cell design. This design provides optimal flexibility and superior wall strength. Express™ stents are pre-mounted on Ultrathin™ SDS balloons in diameters of 6–10 mm and are available in stent lengths of 17, 37 and 57 mm. A pre-mounted 25 mm length is available only on the 9 and 10 mm diameter balloons. All of these balloon delivery catheters accommodate a 0.035″ wire. The stents mounted on the 6–8 mm balloons pass through a 6-French sheath while the 9 and 10 mm balloons require a 7-French sheath. If there is any tortuosity or sharp angles in the approach to the lesions, these stents are delivered through a long sheath or a guiding catheter.

The delivery of stents to the systemic arterial lesions is similar to the delivery of stents to the distal pulmonary artery branches. The involved vessels frequently are difficult to enter initially and difficult to cannulate further with a catheter or with a stiff delivery wire that is adequate to support the balloon/stent combination. The lesion is identified and quantitated on the basis of selective biplane angiograms with injections into the proximal "feeding" vessels. Freeze-frame, "road map" images of the lesion are stored with special notations made about adjacent radiographically visible tissue and structures that are in the vicinity of the lesion and that can be used as reference structures at the time of implant. A stent/balloon is chosen that is 1 mm larger in diameter than the adjacent "normal" vessel (the nominal diameter of the surgical "shunt" or the adjacent larger segments of the particular collateral) and long enough to cover the stenotic lesion. The lesion is crossed with an end-hole catheter, which is advanced as far distal to the lesion in the vessel as possible using the combination of the catheter and torque wires. The torque wire is replaced with a stiff exchange length guide wire of the largest diameter that the balloon catheter that is to be used to deliver the stent will accommodate.

In most circumstances, the pre-mounted balloon/stent is introduced directly over the wire, through a short arterial sheath, and advanced "bare" over the wire to the lesion. Unless there is an additional arterial catheter for another angiogram, the "freeze-frame" reference pictures are used to position the stent. Occasionally, and particularly when there is a difficult tortuous course to reach the lesion, a long sheath/dilator is first delivered over the wire and past the lesion. The dilator is removed over the wire and the balloon/stent is delivered over the wire through the long sheath similar to the delivery of most of the non pre-mounted stents. When the sheath is withdrawn off the balloon/stent in the lesion, small hand injection of contrast through the sheath into these confined arteries provide very adequate angiograms for the final positioning of the stent. The balloon/stent inflation is usually very straightforward, with very little movement of the stent/balloon during implant in these locations.

Ductus arteriosus stents

Growing experience in patients with hypoplastic left hearts, hypoplastic right hearts, and other patients with ductal-dependent pulmonary blood flow has demonstrated that intravascular stents implanted in the newborn ductus for the purpose of keeping the ductus open represent a very effective palliation for many of these patients.

Ductus arteriosus stents in "ductus-dependent" pulmonary artery circulations where there is no prograde access to the ductus

In neonatal patients with pulmonary valve atresia or other ductus-dependent pulmonary artery circulation, including infants with hypoplastic right hearts, a "permanent" patency of the ductus provides an adequate substitute for a surgically created systemic to pulmonary shunt for maintaining pulmonary blood flow. Temporary patency of the neonatal ductus initially is achieved by a continuous intravenous infusion of prostaglandin. Subsequent, persistent patency of the ductus arteriosis which, in many newborn patients, provides adequate systemic to pulmonary blood flow can now be achieved by maintaining the patency of the ductus with a catheter-implanted, intravascular stent[18].

Many newborn patients with a ductal-dependent pulmonary artery circulation do not have a prograde route to the pulmonary artery and, in turn, to the ductus. These patients require an arterial, retrograde approach to the ductus and include most patients with pulmonary atresia and a ventricular septal defect, some patients with severe tetralogy of Fallot, some patients with tricuspid atresia, and even some patients with pulmonary atresia with an intact ventricular septum. In most of these patients, the ductus arteriosus has been maintained open with prostaglandin by the time the patient is first seen by a pediatric cardiologist/interventionalist. The patent ductus in many of these patients is long and tortuous and arises from an unusual location/angle off the aorta and, as a consequence, *not all* patents will be candidates for stenting of the patent ductus arteriosus.

Experience with surgical shunts has demonstrated that the ideal diameter of a systemic to pulmonary shunt in an average sized newborn is 3–4.5 mm in diameter. These same diameters have proven satisfactory for adequate pulmonary blood flow through a ductus that is maintained open with a stent in a newborn. The original stents that were available, even in these small diameters, were rigid and were delivered on balloon catheters with large diameter catheter shafts. The difficulties in the delivery of these early stents through the arterial system in very small infants created many complications in the initial attempts to use stents to maintain ductal patency[18]. However, as a result of the extensive developments in stents that are available for the treatment of coronary artery stenosis, fortuitously, there now is a very large variety of very low-profile, flexible, pre-mounted, stents that can be delivered "bare" over a wire and through very small arterial introductory sheaths—all of which makes them very suitable for stenting of the PDA and/or systemic to pulmonary shunts in newborn infants[19]. Although a flexible stent is desirable, a stent with *small* wall "cells" also appears essential because of the propensity of the ductal tissue to prolapse or contract through any open or uncovered spaces in the wall of the stent.

Medium Genesis™ stents (Johnson & Johnson–Cordis Corp., Miami Lakes, FL) are small stents with a maximum diameter of 10 mm and a closed, relatively small, cell design. They are available premounted on 3–7 mm diameter balloons and in lengths of 12, 15, 18 and 24 mm. These stents can be delivered "bare" over a wire and through a short sheath as small as 5- or 6-French. In addition to the Medium Genesis™ stents, there are innumerable pre-mounted coronary stents that can be dilated up to 4 to 5 mm in diameter, in a variety of lengths, and that are available from many different manufacturers including Cordis–J & J™, Boston Scientific™, Guidant™, Medtronic™, and Cook™. These stents are too numerable to list and the specific characteristics of the coronary stents change almost weekly. The local, adult interventional laboratory will have the most up to the moment information on these stents, their characteristics and, in all likelihood, will have a large inventory of multiple varieties. The Express™ stents (Boston Scientific, Natick, MA) have a relatively large, open-cell design, but the smallest diameter pre-mounted Express™ stent is 6 mm. The large open-cell design and the minimal pre-mounted diameter of the Express™ stents make these stents unsatisfactory for stenting the neonatal ductus.

When a newborn infant has a ductus-dependent pulmonary circulation and the use of a stent is *considered* in the management of the patient, the infant requires a cardiac catheterization with high-quality angiography in order to demonstrate the exact location, course, anatomy and precise measurements of the ductus. This information is *suggested* by echo/MRI studies, but the absolutely necessary, precise information, so far, can only be obtained by selective angiography.

The infant is maintained on the intravenous prostaglandin infusion. A biplane aortogram is performed in the straight PA and lateral views with the injection of contrast in the proximal *descending* aorta. This angiogram preferably is performed through a venous catheter advanced prograde through the left heart either through a patent foramen ovale, left atrium and left ventricle or, more directly, from the right ventricle, through a ventricular septal defect and into the ascending aorta. The prograde angiographic catheter positioned in the descending aorta allows repeat angiograms during the actual implant of the stent, which will be delivered through a separate retrograde catheter. When a prograde catheter cannot be positioned in the descending aorta, the angiogram is performed through a 4-French, end and side-hole catheter introduced retrograde from the femoral artery. The angiogram demonstrates the location, course and size of the ductus and, in turn, its potential applicability for the implant of a stent. The angles of the X-ray tubes frequently have to be altered and the aortogram repeated in order to elongate the ductus maximally and to visualize both ends of the ductus adequately. The patent ductus must be capable of being entered reasonably easily, traversed completely by a wire, and then with the balloon/stent catheter from the particular aortic approach. This implies a reasonable angle of the aortic end of the ductus off the aorta when approached from the introductory site in the artery, and a patent ductus that is not *too* tortuous throughout its course, although significant curves/tortuosity will be straightened by a catheter/wire and eventually a balloon/stent positioned in a ductus.

Once the ductus is visualized and appears reasonable to enter and stent, an angled, end-hole catheter is introduced into the femoral artery and advanced to the area of the ductus. A very floppy tipped, torque-controlled, guide wire is advanced through this catheter and manipulated through the ductus and into a distal pulmonary artery branch. The ductus, which has usually been maintained on prostaglandin, is very friable and the wire or catheter should never be forced *at all* into or through it. A repeat aortogram is recorded once the wire is positioned through the ductus in order to demonstrate any changes in the ductus length, contour or diameter caused by spasm of the ductus or tension/straightening from the wire. This angiogram preferably is performed through the separate prograde catheter in the aorta, although an adequate angiogram usually can be recorded through the original catheter and over the wire with the use of a Tuohy™ high-pressure "Y" adaptor attached to the hub of the catheter over the wire. If an adequate angiogram cannot be obtained by either of these techniques, a second, small retrograde catheter should be introduced. A freeze-frame "road map" of this angiogram of the ductus is stored for reference use.

After the angiogram has been obtained, an end-hole catheter with a smooth tip is advanced over the wire very *gently*, through the ductus and into the distal branch pulmonary artery. Once the catheter is in the distal pulmonary artery, the original floppy, torque-controlled, guide wire that was used to manipulate across the ductus is replaced with the stiffest possible exchange length guide wire that the delivery balloon/stent that will be used to deliver the stent to the ductus, will accommodate.

The exact length of the stent used in the PDA is determined from the angiogram of each particular ductus. Ideally the stent must cover, and extend slightly *past both ends* of the ductus but, at the same time, should not extend too far into the lumen of either the pulmonary artery or the aorta. Once the delivery wire is secure through the ductus and well into a distal pulmonary branch, the second angiographic catheter is positioned adjacent to the aortic end of the ductus. The correct stent/balloon is chosen and prepared on the catheterization table and the prostaglandin infusion is stopped. The patient is observed closely for at least 30 minutes, and assuming no acute or severe deterioration of the patient during that time, the aortogram is repeated. Usually the ductus constricts and changes in configuration rapidly once the infusion of prostaglandin is stopped. Occasionally the rebound constriction of the ductus is very severe and very rapid which, in turn, necessitates either the reinstitution of the prostaglandin infusion or the rapid introduction of, and the implant of, the stent. The ductus tissues are friable, so the balloon/stent introduction must be very gentle and very precise, and the stent must pass easily through the ductus. Because of these factors, some operators prefer to prepare the balloon stent and position the stent/balloon across the ductus before stopping the prostaglandin infusion and then wait for the prostaglandin to wear off with the deflated balloon/stent already in place across the ductus. The second catheter adjacent to the aortic end of the ductus is essential at this stage of the procedure in order to allow very rapid and precise final positioning of the stent within the ductus just before deployment.

With any deterioration of the patient, or after 30 minutes, the angiogram is repeated, the stent/balloon position adjusted, and the balloon/stent is inflated to its advertised pressure or until all indentations in the balloon/stent have disappeared—whichever comes first. The balloon is deflated immediately and rapidly. With a properly implanted stent, the patient immediately will oxygenate better and stabilize as soon as the balloon is deflated. The balloon is withdrawn carefully out of the stent/ductus and with the wire still through the stent and ductus, the aortogram is repeated to visualize the adequacy of the coverage of the stent in the ductus and the new flow to the pulmonary arteries. If there are *any areas* of the ductus, particularly at either end of the ductus, which are not covered by the stent, a second (or more) stent(s) is/are implanted during the same catheterization. The additional stent(s) is/are placed overlapping the first stent and covering *all* of the ductal tissues entirely. Any "exposed" ductus tissue is notorious for constricting and closing completely, even with a stent in the remainder of the ductus. For the implant of an additional stent immediately after the implant of the first stent, all of the catheters and wires are already in place and minimal further manipulation or time in the catheterization laboratory is necessary for the implant of an additional stent. Once the ductus is covered adequately and the patient is stable, the delivery wire is withdrawn from the stent and the catheter withdrawn. The infants are maintained on 21 mg aspirin per day.

Stenting of the ductus in patients with pulmonary atresia with intact ventricular septum

In infants with pulmonary atresia and intact ventricular septum, along with the opening of the pulmonary valve, a systemic to pulmonary "shunt" can be performed in the catheterization laboratory by implanting a stent in the ductus arteriosus. The stenting of the ductus is addressed after the pulmonary valve has been perforated and dilated successfully. This allows the delivery and implant of the stent into the ductus arteriosus through a venous route and the use of a smaller catheter system in the artery. When a stent is to be implanted in the ductus during the catheterization, before any intervention on the ductus and if not administered earlier when the lines were established, the patient is administered heparin systemically. After the pulmonary valve has been perforated and dilated, the final balloon dilation catheter for the pulmonary valvotomy is removed over the guide wire. Following the perforation and balloon dilation of an atretic pulmonary valve, a long guide wire usually has already been advanced through the ductus creating a "through-and-through" route from a femoral vein, through the right heart and ductus, down the descending aorta and out through a femoral artery sheath/catheter.

If the through-and-through "rail" wire was not established during the valve perforation/dilation, the "rail" is established at this time with an exchange length wire which the proposed balloon catheter for stent delivery will accommodate. The balloon dilation catheter used for the pulmonary valve is replaced with a long 4- or 5-French end-hole catheter, which is advanced through the venous sheath, over the original guide wire and into the pulmonary artery or ductus (wherever the end of the wire is positioned). If the tip of the prograde venous catheter is in the pulmonary artery, it is manipulated through the ductus into the descending aorta and maneuvered through and out of the femoral artery sheath with the help of a torque-controlled wire. Occasionally the prograde catheter in the pulmonary artery cannot cross the ductus easily into the descending aorta. In that circumstance a floppy tipped wire and then a snare catheter is maneuvered *from the aorta*, through the ductus and into the pulmonary artery. A soft tipped wire is advanced through the venous catheter prograde into the main pulmonary artery and is snared with a Microvena™ snare (ev3, Plymouth, MN), which has been passed through the retrograde catheter into the main pulmonary artery. The snared prograde wire and the prograde venous catheter are withdrawn through the ductus and out through the femoral arterial sheath with the retrograde snare. Once both ends of the *catheter* are available outside of the body, the original floppy tipped exchange wire is removed and replaced with a stiff exchange wire of the maximum wire diameter that the particular coronary stent/balloon catheter or other pre-mounted stent/balloon that will be used for implanting the stent in the ductus, requires. This wire is secured outside of the body at both the arterial and venous ends.

An equally effective alternative is to advance the floppy tipped wire from the retrograde catheter through the ductus and into the main pulmonary artery and to introduce the snare catheter into the pulmonary artery from the venous route. The retrograde wire then is withdrawn through the right heart and out through the venous sheath to complete the through-and-through wire.

Even when previously visualized very adequately, a *repeat* aortogram with the injection adjacent to the ductus is performed either through a Tuohy™ adapter attached to the hub of the catheter over the through-and-through wire or through a separate prograde or retrograde catheter positioned in the descending aorta adjacent to the ductus. This angiogram of the ductus is imperative because of spasm or distortion of the ductus caused by the various wire/catheter manipulations through it. The diameter and length of the ductus are remeasured very accurately. As with the implant of a stent in any other ductus, the goal is to "line" the entire lumen of the ductus, including covering both ends of the ductus with the stent. Similarly to the patients with pure ductus-dependent pulmonary circulations, a 4 mm diameter stent is used in these patients. Once the through-and-through wire is established and the appropriate balloon/stent for the particular ductus is chosen *and prepared for delivery*, the prostaglandin infusion is discontinued. Assuming no acute or sudden deterioration in the infant's saturation/hemodynamics, the infant is observed for at least 30 minutes while off the prostaglandin infusion and the aortogram repeated. Often the combination of the irritation of the through-and-through wire/catheter, the preceding manipulations during the balloon dilations of the valve, and the discontinued prostaglandin infusion distorts the ductal anatomy significantly. The ductus anatomy is re-examined carefully and the measurements repeated.

If the ductus acutely goes into spasm or the infant deteriorates significantly when the prostaglandin infusion is stopped, the prostaglandin infusion is restarted and the stent is delivered to the ductus before re-stopping the prostaglandin as described previously.

The pre-mounted stent on a 4 mm balloon dilation catheter is introduced over the *venous end* of the through-and-through wire and advanced over the wire, through the right ventricle, pulmonary valve and into the ductus arteriosus. Although small stents notoriously are poorly visible, or even invisible in large adult patients, in small infants they are seen clearly in both the collapsed and the expanded states. Once the balloon/stent combination is in position in the ductus, and before the stent is expanded in the ductus, the anatomy of the whole ductus and, in particular, the exact location and diameter of the areas of minimal ductal diameter are re-imaged angiographically. If there is not a second catheter in the aorta, the aortogram is accomplished by advancing a 4- or, preferably, a 5-French, end and side-hole catheter retrograde over the arterial end of the through-and-through wire. The catheter is advanced just to the aortic end of the ductus and a pressure, Tuohy™ "Y" adaptor is attached over the wire at the proximal end of the retrograde catheter. An angiogram is performed over the wire through this retrograde catheter, the tip of which should be adjacent to the ductus and the stent/balloon catheter coming from the other end of the wire. With the anatomy precisely identified and recorded, the retrograde catheter is withdrawn back into the descending aorta as the stent/balloon catheter is positioned exactly in the ductus.

The *stent* should cover *both ends* of the ductus completely including, in particular, the area of the narrowest portion of the ductus, which usually is at the pulmonary end of a long tortuous ductus. When satisfied with the stent length and location, the stent is expanded by inflation of the balloon to its full diameter or to the recommended maximum pressure of the balloon—whichever comes first—followed by a rapid deflation. A repeat angiogram is recorded with injection through the aortic catheter *before* the deflated balloon is withdrawn from the stent positioned in the ductus. When satisfied that the stent is fully inflated and fixed in the ductus, the deflated balloon is withdrawn cautiously out of the stent, over the wire and out of the body. The retrograde catheter is re-advanced to the aortic end of the stent and a final repeat angiocardiogram is recorded through this catheter before the wire is withdrawn. Similarly to the other stents in the neonatal ductus, if there is an area of the ductus which is not covered completely, a second, overlapping stent should be implanted at that time.

When satisfied with the position, the adequacy of expansion of the stent and the "lining" of the entire ductus by the stent(s), an end-hole catheter is introduced over the venous end of the wire and advanced into the pulmonary artery. The wire is carefully withdrawn out of the stent through the venous catheter.

The hemodynamics and anatomy are carefully reassessed and a decision is made whether an atrial septostomy is to be performed. Hemodynamically, an atrial communication in the presence of some elevation of the right atrial pressure enhances *left* ventricular filling and systemic output, albeit with some systemic desaturation and at the expense of some forward flow through the right ventricle/pulmonary arteries. On the other hand, with at least a moderate sized right ventricle, the right ventricular pressure near normal, and even in the presence of significant tricuspid valve regurgitation, a *restrictive* atrial communication and the associated elevated right atrial pressure *should enhance* right ventricular filling and, in turn, encourage forward blood flow through the right ventricle, pulmonary artery, and lungs. Until more definitive data are available on which ventricles will grow with adequate flow, and with what type of stimulus, this remains an on the spot judgment decision, which must be made in the catheterization laboratory, during each individual case.

Stenting of the ductus in the hypoplastic left heart syndrome

The patent ductus is essential for the systemic output in the infant with severe left heart obstructive lesions and, particularly, an associated "hypoplastic left heart" syndrome. In most cases, the open ductus is maintained with prostaglandins until the infant undergoes the first stage "Norwood" surgical palliation. In that surgery, the entire ductal tissue is excised purposefully and widely when the distal pulmonary artery is anastomosed to the aorta and *no catheter intervention* on the patent ductus should be considered when a "Norwood" surgical palliation is considered.

An alternative approach to the "Norwood" and "single ventricle" approach to the patient with a hypoplastic left heart is an orthotopic cardiac transplant. However, when the infant is "listed" and awaiting the transplant, the ductal patentcy must be maintained until the transplant is performed—often for weeks or months. To maintain the patency of the ductus medically requires a continuous, precisely controlled, intravenous (IV) infusion of prostaglandin. The maintenance of the IV and the precise control of the rate of the prostaglandin in a neonate require a 24/7 neonatal intensive care environment. Even in this environment the infant is in a very precarious situation. An alternative technique is to maintain the ductal patency with an intravascular stent[20,21].

Once the decision is made to "list" the patient for a transplant, then the implant of a stent in the ductus should be considered immediately. The longer the patient waits, the lower the pulmonary resistance becomes and the sicker the infant becomes. The longer the patient remains on prostaglandin, the greater the likelihood of systemic infection and the more friable the ductal tissues become.

The infant with a "hypoplastic left heart" who is to undergo the implant of a stent in the ductus is taken to the catheterization laboratory with the ductus patency maintained with the prostaglandin infusion. The infant is intubated and ventilated on 17–18% oxygen. If the patient does not have an indwelling arterial line, a femoral artery is cannulated with a 20-gauge Quick-Cath™, and a multipurpose, end and side-hole catheter is introduced through a sheath in the femoral vein. This catheter is manipulated through the right ventricle to the pulmonary artery and to the ductus arteriosus. A biplane angiogram is recorded in the PA and lateral views with the injection directly into the ductus. This angiogram is to visualize the exact diameter, length and configuration of the ductus. If necessary, the X-ray tubes are re-angled to "cut the ductus on edge" more precisely and the angiogram repeated. Precise measurements are made of the length and diameter of the ductus from the views that elongate the ductus optimally. Freeze-frame images of the desired views are stored for use as "road maps" during the implant of a stent into the ductus.

The end and side-hole catheter is advanced through the ductus into the distal descending aorta. A 0.018″ or 0.035″ exchange length guide wire (depending upon which stent and which balloon catheter is to be used), is advanced far into the distal aorta, the tip of the wire is fixed in the ilio-femoral artery, and the catheter is removed over the wire. If there appears to be any distortion of the pulmonary artery–ductus–descending aorta anatomy by the wire, a repeat angiogram is recorded over the wire and through the catheter in the ductus before the catheter is removed. This angiogram performed with the catheter over the wire is accomplished by injecting the contrast through a Tuohy™ high-pressure "Y" adaptor attached to the hub of the catheter while the catheter is still positioned over the wire.

A stent is chosen that is as large in diameter as the ductus/descending aorta can accommodate and long enough to extend completely through the ductus. The expanded stent must extend from well within the pulmonary artery, through the ductus, to well into the descending aorta.

Unlike the stents in the ductus for pulmonary atresia patients, where a very controlled flow using a small stent (3–4 mm) is desired, in patients with hypoplastic left heart, the stent must be large enough to accommodate all of the cardiac output and not create any resistance to this flow because of restriction from a limited diameter of the stent. Depending upon the patient's size, this usually requires an 8–12 mm diameter stent. The pre-mounted standard "Large" Genesis™ stents (Johnson & Johnson–Cordis Corp., Miami Lakes, FL) are satisfactory for this use up to 10 mm in diameter. The Genesis™ stents are available pre-mounted in diameters up to 9 mm and in lengths of 19, 29 and 39 mm. These stents can be introduced through a short, 6-French sheath and advanced over a 0.035″ guide wire without the necessity of prepositioning a long sheath across the lesion. "Large" Genesis™ stents are very flexible and conform to the curvature of the ductus. None of the coronary artery stents are suitable for this use because of the maximum diameter of 4 to 5 mm. The Express™ Biliary LD stents (Medi-Tech, Boston Scientific, Natick, MA) are available pre-mounted in similar sizes, but have larger side "cells" as a consequence of their open-cell design, which may be a problem for any use in the *ductus* because of the propensity for rapid ingrowth of the ductal tissues through any space.

Once the wire is in place and the stent is ready for delivery, the prostaglandin infusion is stopped. The stent is advanced over the wire and positioned across the ductus. The balloon/stent is maintained in this position while monitoring the patient's distal arterial pressure and systemic saturation for 30 minutes or until the patient's hemodynamics begin to deteriorate. The idea is to allow the large diameter, often patulous, ductus to constrict enough after the prostaglandin is stopped to hold the stent in place. The blood pressure and systemic saturation decrease as the prostaglandin wears off and the ductus begins to close. Unless a second venous catheter has been introduced into the pulmonary artery or the stent/balloon was delivered to the ductus through a long sheath, an angiogram in the pulmonary artery to verify the status of the ductus and the stent position is not possible at this time.

After the 30 minutes or with any deterioration of the patient, the stent's position is compared to the freeze-frame "road map" images of the ductus, and when in the appropriate position, the balloon is inflated slowly to deploy the stent precisely in the ductus. Once fully inflated, the balloon is deflated rapidly. The large diameter stent should fix very securely in place in the ductus. The inflation/deflation is repeated one, or more, times and then the balloon is removed from the body over the wire.

An end- and side-hole catheter is advanced over the wire and into the stent. An angiogram is recorded within the ductus (stent), injecting over the wire with the use of a Tuohy™ "Y" connector on the catheter. If the stent is not fully expanded, if it is at all unstable, or if there are areas of ductal tissue that are "exposed" or "uncovered" by the stent, a further dilation of the stent or the implant of an additional stent will be necessary to cover the ductal tissue completely. If a second stent is necessary and the wire still is in place, the additional stent can be implanted during this same procedure without any significant further or repeated manipulations through the freshly implanted stent.

Once satisfied with the location and expansion of the stent(s), the wire is removed from the catheter and the catheter withdrawn. The infant is maintained *off* the prostaglandin infusion. Depending upon the status of the pulmonary vascular resistance, the infant usually can be discharged and observed as an outpatient until a donor heart becomes available. Even with a very satisfactory stent in the ductus, the infant still needs very close follow-up. As the pulmonary vascular resistance falls significantly, the infant's lungs can become flooded, with a proportionate decrease in the effective systemic cardiac output through the ductus.

The presence of the stent in the ductus does not interfere with a cardiac transplant procedure since the stented ductus and the adjacent tissues are removed at the time of the transplant. The main *disadvantage* to stenting the ductus in an infant with hypoplastic left heart syndrome is when a donor heart does *not* become available of for some other reason, the decision for the course of treatment is reversed and a "Norwood" procedure is required. A large stent in the ductus arteriosus complicates, or even possibly renders impossible, the usual "Norwood" surgery.

Complications of arterial stents

Complications of systemic arterial stents include exaggeration or extension of any of the complications of balloon dilation of any vessel including, particularly, coarctation of the aorta or dilation of other arterial lesions. At the same time, since the implant of a stent requires *no over-dilation* of the artery, complications related to dilation with the balloons are very rare.

Iatrogenic obstructions caused by the implant of stents that have a maximum diameter that will be too small for the *eventual size* of the adult aorta, should be a totally avoidable "complication" of stents used in the treatment of coarctation of the aorta and other arteries. There now are stents available that can be dilated to 25+ mm, which makes these stents large enough in diameter for any adult proximal descending aorta. These potentially larger diameter stents should be used in any growing patient with even the potential of having the aorta in the area of coarctation grow to larger than 16–18 mm in diameter. A stent with a limited diameter, which creates an obstruction because it is too small for the aorta, creates an obstruction that is much more difficult to repair than the usual native or "residual" post-operative obstruction. When the patient is too small to implant a stent that can be dilated to the anticipated diameter of the adult aorta, it is preferable to treat the patient with balloon dilation without a stent or with surgical repair initially. A stent can be implanted later to "finalize" the correction of any residual lesion following prior dilation or surgery.

A very serious complication of the catheter treatment of coarctation of the aorta using balloon dilation with or without stent implant is injury to the central nervous system (CNS) during the catheterization procedure. CNS injury most likely occurs from air and/or clot embolization coming from catheters, sheaths or wires that are present in the systemic circulation proximal to the carotid and vertebral vessels. Meticulous attention to clearing fluid lines, catheters and sheaths of any air and/or clot, keeping guide wires in the circulation "covered" with a catheter that is maintained on a continual flush for as long as possible, the continual flushing of *all* catheters and sheaths that are positioned in the heart, and the routine use of systemic heparin, particularly during "left heart" procedures, should reduce or eliminate CNS problems. Direct injury from the tip of a wire positioned in a cranial artery has been implicated in central nervous system injury. Never positioning a wire tip in either a carotid or a vertebral artery eliminates this particular possibility.

Probably the most common complication of the use of stents in the arteries is injury to the local artery at the site of catheter/stent introduction with subsequent compromise of arterial blood flow in the involved extremity. These injuries occasionally are unavoidable because of the necessarily very large sized balloon catheters/sheaths that are used to deliver stents to the aorta. Meticulous care of the arteries, which was discussed earlier in this chapter and in Chapter 4, is the best prevention and, in turn, best treatment of this problem. Local anesthesia is used liberally and repeatedly around the artery and surrounding tissues before, during, and at the end of the procedure. Local anesthesia is administered even if the patient is receiving general anesthesia. A precise, single-wall puncture is utilized for the entrance into the artery. Although an indwelling sheath often is as much as 2–3 French sizes larger than the dilation *balloon* or balloon catheter that is used for the stent delivery, an indwelling sheath, which is relatively fixed in the artery, is always less traumatic to the artery than a constantly moving catheter or a bare, rough, "folded" balloon/stent being introduced into and withdrawn out of the artery. When the sheath is removed from the artery, the puncture site is compressed manually and *personally* while continually monitoring the puncture site for bleeding and, *at the same time*, the artery distal to the puncture for a pulse. This hemostasis can take 30, 60, or more minutes, but should be accomplished *before* the patient leaves the observation and care of the catheterizing physician!

Stent displacement is relatively common during the implant of stents in coarctation of the aorta. There often is a large discrepancy in diameter between the aorta proximal to the coarctation and the aorta distal to the coarctation. A stent that is expanded to a diameter that is calculated to fix the stent in the aorta proximal to the coarctation, can easily become free-floating in the much larger distal aorta. At the same time, expanding the stent to a diameter satisfactory for the diameter of the aorta distal to the coarctation would split the smaller-diameter aorta that is proximal to the obstruction. In order to avoid displacement, the stent is implanted with the majority of the stent positioned in the aorta proximal to the narrowing and *no* attempt is made at "approximating" the distal end of the stent to the larger distal aorta during the initial implant procedure. If a stent dislodges and moves further distally in the aorta, the stent is purposefully repositioned in the distal aorta so that it does not compromise vital side branches, and then it is expanded and fixed in the more distal location.

Tears in the arterial wall or flaps off the intima/media are less common, or at least, less recognized, during stent implants in systemic arteries, including congenital coarctation of the aorta, than with balloon dilation alone of these same lesions. When the proper sized stents are used after the artery is measured properly and very accurately, the adjacent aorta should not be "over-dilated" at all and, at the same time, any slight disruption of the intima/medial tissue within the area of the stent is compressed back against the wall of the aorta by the stent. As the endothelium and neointima develop over and around the stent, the combination of the wall "thickening" by the "new endothelial tissues", the scarring as a consequence of any tears that did occur, and the "metal scaffolding" of the stent within the area, all together create a very solid arterial wall. The artery in the precise area of the stent is very non-compliant, but no more so than a surgical scar involving the same area!

Aneurysms have occurred acutely during the implant of stents in coarctations of the aorta. These occurred more commonly with the use of the larger Palmaz™ stents (Johnson & Johnson, Warren, NJ) and occurred predominantly (only?) when the stents were dilated acutely to their final large diameters with a single inflation of a large diameter balloon. Acute aneurysms are not reported with the sequential dilation of stents to their precise, eventual large diameters, or with the use of stents that do not develop sharp tips at their ends as they expand. Aneurysms following the implant of stents in coarctation of the aorta are still being studied, and should be looked for in every patient who undergoes a stent implant in the aorta.

Tears or ruptures of the aorta occur with dilation of native coarctation, re-coarctation of the aorta, and middle aortic syndrome, but should not occur with the *conservative* implant of the correct size stent in coarctations. Meticulous, accurate measurements of the lesion itself and the adjacent vessels, and avoiding oversized dilations/stents compared to the size of the lesion itself and the adjacent vessel, presumably should prevent this complication during stent implant. In cases of very severe stenosis of classic coarctation or middle aortic stenosis, a staged dilation/implant during several sequential catheterizations is utilized to avoid splitting very narrowed vessels by a single dilation to a very large diameter. A stent that is still narrowed within a vessel can always be dilated further at a later date. Once the artery/aorta is split or torn, there is little or no "turning back", although several operators have reported on the successful use of a covered stent as an emergency "bail-out" therapy in the catheterization laboratory[22,23].

Stents implanted in coarctation of the aorta have been reported to fracture or kink[24]. This probably is a result of the type of stent used in the area. There have been no adverse events from these findings and a recurrent narrowing as a result of a fracture or kink can be treated with the implant of an additional stent within the original stent.

The implant of stents into the patent ductus of newborn infants has its own specific complications. These complications are in addition to the inherent complications of extensive catheter manipulations in very sick newborn or small infants. As with all complications, the best treatment is prevention by paying meticulous attention to the details of the procedure and the use of known, established techniques until newer/better techniques are proven. Irritation and spasm of the ductus is a potential problem with any manipulation around or through the ductus. This spasm is not always responsive to prostaglandin infusion or re-infusion. Should intractable ductal spasm occur, having the equipment ready for immediate deployment of a stent is the best treatment. This, however, is not a guarantee of successful recovery since the "mass" of even the "tiny" stent/balloon occasionally cannot be advanced through the ductus once it begins to spasm. Disruption/tears of the ductal tissues is another potential with stent implant into the patent ductus, particularly when the stent delivery is rushed. The tissue is inherently very friable and cannot tolerate rough handling. When disruption of the ductus does occur, it usually is catastrophic.

Stent displacement during implant into the "patulous" ductal tissue in an infant is a real problem. Prevention, by the use of a slow meticulous positioning and by waiting for the prostaglandin to wear off before deploying the stent, is the best treatment. When a stent displaces from the ductus, an attempt is made to capture the stent on a balloon and reposition it back into the ductus. A new balloon which is at least 1 mm larger than the maximum diameter of the stent is more effective for "capturing" an errant coronary stent. When a *coronary* stent becomes displaced from the *ductus* and is positioned or implanted in *any other artery* (even *very* peripherally), the coronary stent, unequivocally, eventually will produce a very significant stenosis in that vessel because of its very small maximum diameter. If a displaced stent cannot be captured and reimplanted successfully in the ductus or removed from the patient with a catheter, the stent should be removed surgically from the errant vessel within a few days after the attempted implant procedure, unless the errant vessel is considered "expendable".

The majority of the complications of stent implants in arterial locations are eliminated by the use of extremely accurate measurements, a conservative diameter at the initial implant, and by paying meticulous attention to the details of *every step* of the procedure. The morbidity and complications of dilation with intravascular stent implant for systemic arteries appear to be comparable to or even less than surgical therapy of these same lesions. Dilation with stent implants in coarctation and other congenital systemic arterial lesions still represents a "new" treatment, which requires decades of follow-up to determine its real efficacy and safety.

References

1. Dotter CT *et al.* Transluminal expandable nitinol coil stent grafting: preliminary report. *Radiology* 1983; **147**(1): 259–260.
2. Palmaz JC *et al.* Atherosclerotic rabbit aortas: expandable intraluminal grafting. *Radiology* 1986; **160**: 723–726.
3. Shaffer KM *et al.* Intravascular stents in congenital heart disease: short- and long-term results from a large single-center experience. *J Am Coll Cardiol* 1998; **31**(3): 661–667.
4. Morrow WR *et al.* Balloon angioplasty with stent implantation in experimental coarctation of the aorta. *Circulation* 1994; **89**(6): 2677–2683.
5. Grifka RG *et al.* Balloon expandable intravascular stents: aortic implantation and late further dilation in growing minipigs. *Am Heart J* 1993; **126**(4): 979–984.
6. Suarez de Lezo J *et al.* Balloon-expandable stent repair of severe coarctation of the aorta. *Am Heart J* 1995; **129**(5): 1002–1008.
7. Rosenthal E, Qureshi SA, and Tynan M. Stent implantation for aortic recoarctation. *Am Heart J* 1995; **129**(6): 1220–1221.
8. Bulbul ZR *et al.* Implantation of balloon-expandable stents for coarctation of the aorta: implantation data and short-term results. *Cathet Cardiovasc Diagn* 1996; **39**(1): 36–42.
9. Cheatham JP. Stenting of coarctation of the aorta. *Catheter Cardiovasc Interv* 2001; **54**(1): 112–125.

10. Mendelsohn AM *et al.* Stent redilation in canine models of congenital heart disease: pulmonary artery stenosis and coarctation of the aorta. *Cathet Cardiovasc Diagn* 1996; **38**(4): 430–440.
11. Cheatham J *et al.* Early experience using endovascular stents in children with coarctation of the aorta: promising results . . . but proceed with caution (abstr). *Cardiol Young* 1998; **9**(Suppl 1:11): (abstr).
12. Suarez de Lezo J *et al.* Immediate and follow-up findings after stent treatment for severe coarctation of the aorta. *Am J Cardiol* 1999; **83**(3): 400–406.
13. Sapin SO, Rosengart RM, and Salem MM. Chest pain during stenting of a native aortic coarctation: a case for acute intercostal muscle ischemia and rhabdomyolysis. *Catheter Cardiovasc Interv* 2002; **57**(2): 217–220.
14. Thanopoulos BV *et al.* Long segment coarctation of the thoracic aorta: treatment with multiple balloon-expandable stent implantation. *Am Heart J* 1997; **133**(4): 470–473.
15. Tyagi S *et al.* Percutaneous transluminal angioplasty for stenosis of the aorta due to aortic arteritis in children. *Pediatr Cardiol* 1999; **20**(6): 404–410.
16. Redington AN and Somerville J. Stenting of aortopulmonary collaterals in complex pulmonary atresia. *Circulation* 1996; **94**(10): 2479–2484.
17. El-Said HG *et al.* Stenting of stenosed aortopulmonary collaterals and shunts for palliation of pulmonary atresia/ventricular septal defect. *Catheter Cardiovasc Interv* 2000; **49**(4): 430–436.
18. Gibbs JL *et al.* Stenting of the arterial duct: a new approach to palliation for pulmonary atresia. *Br Heart J* 1992; **67**(3): 240–245.
19. Michel-Behnke I *et al.* Stent implantation in the ductus arteriosus for pulmonary blood supply in congenital heart disease. *Catheter Cardiovasc Interv* 2004; **61**(2): 242–252.
20. Ruiz CE *et al.* Brief report: stenting of the ductus arteriosus as a bridge to cardiac transplantation in infants with the hypoplastic left-heart syndrome. *N Engl J Med* 1993; **328**(22): 1605–1608.
21. Slack MC *et al.* Stenting of the ductus arteriosus in hypoplastic left heart syndrome as an ambulatory bridge to cardiac transplantation. *Am J Cardiol* 1994; **74**(6): 636–637.
22. Khan MS and Moore JW. Treatment of abdominal aortic pseudoaneurysm with covered stents in a pediatric patient. *Catheter Cardiovasc Interv* 2000; **50**(4): 445–448.
23. Tyagi S, Rangesetty UC, and Kaul UA. Endovascular treatment of aortic rupture during angioplasty for aortic in-stent restenosis in aortoarteritis. *Catheter Cardiovasc Interv* 2003; **58**(1): 103–106.
24. Ledesma M *et al.* Stent fracture after stent therapy for aortic coarctation. *J Invasive Cardiol* 2003; **15**(12): 719–721.

26 Occlusion of abnormal small vessels, persistent shunts, vascular fistulae including perivalvular leaks

Introduction

Occlusion of abnormal or persistent arterial or arteriovenous structures or vessels feeding vascular leaks or tumors by catheter embolization techniques has been utilized for over thirty years[1]. The embolization techniques were developed and perfected primarily by the vascular radiologists working in the abdominal viscera, gastrointestinal areas and the central nervous system, particularly in "end artery" vessels. Many materials and devices, including the patient's own clotted blood, Gelfoam™, colloidal plugs, "glues", detachable balloons and coil occlusion devices have been used for these peripheral occlusions[1–6].

In the pediatric and congenital heart population there are numerous abnormal congenital and acquired vascular communications and intravascular "leaks" which require or, at least, can be benefited by transcatheter occlusion. The occlusion of these vascular lesions in pediatric and congenital heart patients has been performed in the catheterization laboratory for over two decades. The abnormal flow through these communications usually results in significant abnormalities of the underlying hemodynamics and compromises the patient's symptomatic and hemodynamic status. The abnormal vascular communications which are encountered in pediatric and congenital heart patients include traumatic fistulae, systemic to pulmonary artery collaterals, systemic arteriovenous fistulae, pulmonary arteriovenous fistulae, coronary arterial-cameral fistulae, perivalvular leaks and a variety of residual, surgically created systemic to pulmonary artery communications including Blalock–Taussig, modified Blalock–Taussig, Potts, and Waterston/Cooley shunts.

There are numerous different catheter-delivered devices and techniques available for the occlusion of these abnormal vascular structures. There is no single device applicable for every lesion and multiple devices may be suitable, and used, for any one lesion. These devices/materials are used either by themselves or (frequently) in combination with one or more of the other devices. The specific occlusion device used depends upon the type, size and location of the communication/leak as well as the availability of a particular device either locally or as approved, in the particular country. Some of these devices are designed specifically for a particular lesion and are discussed in detail in other chapters in the description of the occlusion of the specific intracardiac defect. These same descriptions are not repeated in this chapter.

Since most of the devices can be utilized for the occlusion of multiple different structures and many of the abnormal vascular communications can be occluded with several different devices, each of these miscellaneous vascular lesions and the separate vascular occlusion devices that are used for that lesion are included in the discussion of the particular lesions in this chapter. The multiple devices themselves that are available for these occlusions are discussed initially in this chapter, before the details of their use in the various lesions for which they can be used.

Devices/equipment for vascular occlusions

Occlusion coils

Stainless steel occlusion coils are the most widely used of the catheter-delivered occlusion devices and have had the longest continued use in pediatric and congenital heart lesions. They are particularly useful for small or tortuous vessels and have gained enormous popularity and use for the catheter occlusion of the patent ductus arteriosus (PDA). The specific coils used for PDA occlusion and the modifications of the delivery system/techniques specifically for the PDA are discussed separately and in detail in Chapter 27 ("PDA Occlusion"). Many of these modifications, which were developed specifically for PDA occlusions, are useful for the occlusion of general vascular structures.

Occlusion coils are available as specific lengths of various sizes (gauges) of stainless steel, spring guide wire. The "guide" wires are pre-formed during manufacturing so that they will coil into a cylindrical tube of a specific diameter of the wire in their "resting" state. The number of loops of coil and the length of the "tube" of coils depends upon the original length of the straightened wire. Most of the "occlusion coils" have multiple tiny threads or filaments of nylon fabric intertwined within the windings of the spring wires to promote better thrombosis within a vessel.

Occlusion coils are best suited for the occlusion of long and/or tortuous vessels with irregular internal diameters, and especially those which have a significant narrowing somewhere along the course of the vessel. Since a successful occlusion is expected to cut off *all* blood flow through the vessel, the vessels being occluded should not be the sole blood supply to a particular area of tissue unless necrosis of the tissues that are supplied by the vessel is desired.

Gianturco™ coils and 0.052″ stainless steel coils

The coil occluder with the most extensive use in pediatric and congenital heart patients is the standard Gianturco™ coil. The Gianturco™ coil is a length of special stainless steel spring guide wire in which the stiffening "core" wire is pre-formed to curl into a "coil" or "wire cylinder" of a specific diameter in its "free" or "resting" state. These coils are available in multiple sizes of the spring wire, multiple diameters of the coil ("cylinder") and multiple lengths of the coil wire. The Gianturco™ coil has multiple fine nylon fiber segments embedded within the windings of the spring wire in order to increase the thrombogenicity of the implanted coil. Gianturco™ coils are available in *spring wire diameters* of 0.025″, 0.035″, 0.038″ and now, an additional coil of 0.052″ wire diameter, in lengths between 1.2 and 15 cm and in *coil diameters* from as small as 2 mm to as large as 20 mm in diameter. The very smallest diameter, short coils are available only in the 0.025″ diameter wires while very large diameter coils are available only in the more recently available 0.052″ wires. The total length of the straightened segment of coil wire in conjunction with the particular diameter of the preformed loops of the coils, determine the number of loops which are formed by any particular length of coil. Each Gianturco™ coil comes from the manufacturer in a straight metal introducer tube. The internal lumen and the length of the introducer tube are specific for the diameter of each wire and the straightened length of the wire.

The mass of the wire of the coil itself creates a mechanical occlusion and the embedded nylon fibers add to the thromboses in the area where the coil is deposited and, in turn, occlude the vessel or communication. The coils are best suited for deposit into tubular vessels that have some length and vessels that have an area of narrowing somewhere within the channel of the vessel or the abnormal communication. A stenosis distally in the channel of the vessel prevents even coils that are undersized from migrating out of the target vessel and embolizing to an area or vital organ distally beyond the vessel.

The coils are delivered through polyethylene, end-hole *only*, catheters, which have an internal diameter which is just *slightly greater* than the diameter of the *wire* of the spring coil. Other *end-hole only* catheters manufactured from materials that impart a smooth or slick inner surface and that are slightly larger in their internal diameters than the wire of the coil can be used for coil delivery. The catheter for coil delivery must ***not*** have side holes. Side holes allow the potentially curved tip of the coil to catch in, or pass into, a side hole of the catheter as the tip of the coil crosses the side hole. The tip of a coil catching in a side hole of the catheter will prevent the coil from being delivered through the tip of the catheter. Since the standard Gianturco™ coils have no attachment to the delivery wire, the coil catching in a side hole also prevents any retrieval of the coil without totally removing the delivery catheter. Both the material of the catheter and the internal diameter of the catheter are critically important in order to prevent the coil from "binding" within the lumen of the catheter during the delivery through the catheter.

A catheter that is smaller in internal diameter than the coil wire obviously does not allow the coil with its imbedded fibers to be introduced into, or advanced through, the catheter. A catheter with an internal diameter significantly larger than the diameter of the wire of the coil allows the coil to bend and partially "coil" within the catheter or allows the pusher wire to push past the coil instead of actually "pushing" the coil through the catheter. Either occurrence will cause the coil to bind within the catheter. The delivery catheters are available with many preformed tip configurations in order to facilitate entry into specific areas. Straight delivery catheters, which the operator can pre-shape to suit his particular needs, are also used to deliver coils. End-hole, only, floating balloon catheters can be used to deliver the coils to certain locations or in particular circumstances. The inflated balloon helps to fix the tip of the catheter in place and/or prevents portions of the coil from extending *back* into a more proximal main vascular channel. The catheter lumen of the floating balloon catheter obviously must be of a slightly larger internal diameter than the diameter of the coil *wire* that is being delivered through the balloon catheter.

The coil is introduced into the proximal hub of the delivery catheter through the straight metal "loader" as a straight length of wire. The straightened coil is pushed out of the loader, into the delivery catheter and through the delivery catheter with a teflon-coated, spring guide wire of the same or similar wire size as the coil wire. The coil is delivered by pushing it completely through and out of the distal end of the delivery catheter. As the coil is extruded out of the delivery catheter, it *immediately* begins to form the small loop of its predetermined "coil" diameter as it opens into its coiled configuration. Once the extrusion from the catheter *starts* with the standard Gianturco™ or the 0.052" coils, there is *no way* of withdrawing the coil back into the catheter or stopping or reversing the delivery. Even if the coil is noted to be in an unsatisfactory position as it starts to extrude from the catheter, it can only be extruded completely and then retrieved with a separate retrieval catheter and system.

When choosing the appropriate occlusion coil, the diameter, the length and the general configuration of the vessel to be occluded are imaged angiographically. The length and diameters of the vessel are measured very accurately on the angiograms. The Gianturco™ coil occludes the vessel by the creation of an irregular mass of the coil wire and the nylon fiber strands that are incorporated within the wire in which a thrombus forms. The *coil* used should be 1–2 mm larger in diameter than the vessel that is to be occluded. The slightly larger diameter results in the coil unraveling in an *irregular configuration* within and across the vessel lumen rather than into a neat "donut" like cylinder or smoothly coiled configuration. If the diameter of the coil is far larger than the diameter of the vessel, the coil does not "coil" at all, but rather tends to align straight within the vessel lumen and, in turn, does not form an effective occlusive mass in the vessel. When the coil is extruded from the catheter, it not only must have the appropriate diameter and length to fix to the walls of the vessel, but also must not be excessively long. When the coil is too long, it can extend proximally out of the target vessel and into the more central feeder vessel, which potentially can be back into the normal circulation and interfere with vital structures. If, at the other extreme, the diameter of the formed coil is too small for the vessel, the coil rolls up into a tight "donut", does not occlude the entire vessel, and is likely to tumble distally or even out of the desired vessel. Once one coil is secured within a vessel, additional coils of different sizes and/or diameters can, and frequently are, intertwined within or deposited proximal to the original coil to complete the occlusion. Even when used in tandem, but without a distal narrowing or some other type of device for fixation, the standard Gianturco™ coil generally is only usable in tubular structures of no more than 7–8 mm in their distended diameter. For larger vessels and vessels without an area of discrete stenosis, either the standard Gianturco™ coils are used in conjunction with other intravascular occlusion devices or the 0.052" coils are used initially to begin the occlusion of the vessel.

Occlusion coils can be deposited into long vessels that have a discrete distal narrowing, where the coil then lodges in place at the narrowing, although it is not "fixed" against the wall. In that circumstance, coils can be "floated" into the vessel, one after another to create a mass of coils, proximal to the stenosis in the vessel. When this technique is used, the final coil in the vessel should be of a slightly *larger* diameter then the diameter of the vessel in order to wedge the last coil against the walls of the vessel. The one "fixed" coil assures that the "loose" coils packed within the vessel do not "float" back out of the vessel into the vital circulation.

Currently, by far the most common use of the Gianturco™ coil in congenital heart lesions is for the closure of the patent ductus arteriosus. This is an entirely separate subject and is discussed in detail in Chapter 27 and is not covered in this chapter at all. There are many abnormal vessels, collaterals and persistent surgically created systemic to pulmonary artery shunts, which frequently are associated with more complex lesions. These vessels require occlusion when the additional systemic flow competes with normal pulmonary flow, particularly when the abnormal communication persists after the major intracardiac defect has been corrected. These communications traditionally required surgical division during the corrective procedure or as a separate, later, surgical procedure. When the occlusion of these defects is performed surgically during the intracardiac repair, it significantly prolongs or complicates the surgery. Most of these abnormal communications now are occluded with Gianturco™ coils either before or shortly after the major surgery[7]. With the use of coils, further extensive extra surgery or repeat surgery is unnecessary for the elimination of persistent systemic to pulmonary artery collaterals or for any surgically created systemic to pulmonary artery shunts that are present at the time of, or following, the "total" correction.

Other lesions in which the coils are useful are arteriovenous fistulae, including systemic coronary-cameral, peripheral arteriovenous fistulae as well as pulmonary arteriovenous fistulae. These lesions can produce either left to right or right to left shunts. In these lesions it is critical to identify a stenotic or "end" vessel into which the device can be fixed very securely in order to reduce the dangers of embolization to an essential more distal vessel or vital structure in the systemic circulation.

The 0.052 inch stainless steel coil

In order to provide a more robust coil, a more occlusive coil and a coil particularly for use in the patent ductus arteriosus, the 0.052" stainless steel coil was developed. The 0.052" coil is a larger, stiffer version of the standard Gianturco™ coil with the wire of the coil being the heavier gauge 0.052″ diameter. The 0.052″ coil provides a much sturdier occluding device for the miscellaneous vessels and is particularly useful for the occlusion of much larger vessels with higher pressures and higher flows[8]. The use of the 0.052″ coils for the occlusion of the patent ductus arteriosus for which they were developed, is discussed in detail in Chapter 27.

In an end vessel or in a vessel with definite distal stenosis, the 0.052″ coils are delivered with a "free release" technique exactly like the standard, smaller sized, Gianturco™ coils. However, when choosing the diameter of the 0.052″ coil for a particular *constrained* vessel, the diameter of the *coil* used should be no more than 1–1.5 mm larger than the stretched diameter of the vessel being occluded. The 0.052″ coils are very rigid and have a much greater tendency to form into a symmetrical "donut" shape after they are extruded, and they have very little tendency to form into irregular or elongated shapes. In a vessel that is significantly small in diameter for the coil and non-elastic, the 0.052″ coil is likely to elongate into an almost straight wire rather than to bunch up into an irregular coil.

Because of the larger wire size alone, the 0.052″ coil requires a delivery "catheter" of a larger internal diameter for implant than the standard Gianturco™ coils. The necessity of using the larger delivery catheters can prohibit the use of the 0.052″ coils in infants and very small children. This becomes an even greater problem when the 0.052″ coil embolizes away from the implant location and must be retrieved. To overcome the necessity of using the larger French sized delivery *catheters*, the 0.052″ coil is usually delivered through a 4- or 5-French, long, transseptal type *sheath* with a radio-opaque band at the tip rather than through a separate delivery catheter. This allows the delivery of the larger diameter coil wire without an overall increase in *outside* diameter of the delivery system. The long sheaths have the disadvantages of having less flexibility, less ability to bend at acute angles and, as a consequence, a greater tendency to kink than most "delivery catheters". This tendency to kink compromises the access to vessels or lesions arising at acute angles off the major vessel (aorta). When the long 4- or 5-French sheath is used to deliver the 0.052″ coil, it is advisable to introduce the long sheath into the peripheral entry vessel through a *short*, 6- or 7-F sheath. Then, if the totally extruded coil needs to be withdrawn, it can be withdrawn into the larger, short 6- or 7-French sheath, which is already in the vessel. In the larger patient, the 0.052″ coil, of course, can be delivered through a 6- or 7-French guiding catheter.

The "bioptome controlled" delivery technique is preferable to the "free release" technique for the delivery of the 0.052″ coils to all locations, but particularly when there are *any* concerns about the proper "seating" or possible distal embolization of this coil. Bioptome-controlled delivery is described in detail, later in this chapter and in Chapter 27 on "PDA Occlusion".

Delivery techniques for the Gianturco™ and the 0.052″ stainless steel coils

"Free-release" technique for coil delivery

An end-hole only delivery catheter is chosen with a shape of the tip of the catheter that will facilitate entry into the specific area to be occluded and of an internal diameter to match the diameter of the coil *wire* being used. The delivery catheter/sheath is manipulated and advanced as far as possible into the vessel to be occluded. The tip of the delivery catheter/sheath is fixed securely in the vessel at, or distal to the site for, implant of the occlusion device. Extra effort should always be made to ensure that the delivery catheter/sheath is positioned very deep into the vessel that is to be occluded. Often during the process of advancing the coil through the catheter or extruding the coil wire out of the tip of the delivery catheter/sheath, the tip of the delivery catheter/sheath can be pushed backward in the vessel. The catheter/sheath must be far enough into the vessel initially to allow for this.

Once the catheter is positioned properly, the thin tubular end of the coil introducer is introduced into the proximal hub of the pre-positioned delivery catheter or sheath. The coil introducer should be introduced through a wire back-bleed/flush device that previously was attached to the proximal hub of the coil delivery catheter/sheath. The back-bleed/flush device allows a continual flush of the delivery catheter or sheath during the introduction of the coil and during any exchange of pusher wires, which, in turn, "lubricates" the lumen of the catheter. The stiff end of a straight teflon-coated spring guide wire (of the same size as the internal diameter of the delivery catheter/sheath and the same size or slightly larger [if possible] than the *wire* of the coil itself) is introduced into the proximal end of the straight tubular coil introducer. As the straight spring guide wire is introduced into the proximal end of the coil introducer, the coil is pushed through and out of the distal end of the introducer tube and into the delivery catheter/sheath by the "pusher" spring guide wire. The coil wire has *no* attachment or connection to the pusher wire so that once the introduction of the coil into the catheter has begun, the coil can be *advanced only* within the catheter. Standard Gianturco™ or 0.052″ coils cannot be withdrawn at all! Once the coil is completely within the proximal end of the delivery catheter/sheath, the coil introducer is withdrawn from the catheter over the "pusher" wire and pulled back to the proximal end of, or off, the pusher wire. The teflon-coated spring pusher wire is reversed and the soft end of the wire is advanced within the catheter, which, in turn, pushes the coil (still as a straight segment of wire) through the length of the delivery catheter/sheath. Once the wire and coil are well within the catheter, the catheter, pusher wire and enclosed coil wire are observed carefully on fluoroscopy as the coil is advanced within the catheter or long sheath. The coil is distinguishable from the pusher wire by its slightly "undulating" configuration and the different density of the wire of the coil compared to the pusher wire. As a check of the two wires, a small radiolucent "interspace" can be created between the proximal end of the coil and the distal end of the pusher wire by withdrawing the pusher wire several millimeters while observing under fluoroscopy.

Once the distal end of the coil has reached the tip of the catheter/long sheath, the coil begins to extrude from the tip of the catheter/sheath by continuing to advance the "pusher" wire. As the coil is extruded from the tip of the catheter or sheath, the "coil wire" immediately begins to curl into its pre-formed coiled configuration and/or push the tip of the delivery catheter/sheath away from the site. Exactly how the coil positions itself within the vessel depends upon the size relationship of the diameter of the pre-formed coil and the internal diameter of the vessel at that particular location.

It is important to choose a *coil* diameter of the standard Gianturco™ coil that is 15–20% larger than the stretched or expanded internal diameter of the vessel at the area where the coil is to be implanted. If the coil diameter is smaller than the vessel diameter, the coil wire "coils" into a tight, smooth circular coil with the appearance of a small "donut" and is likely to embolize further along in the vessel. When it tumbles and if it does become lodged in the more distal vessel, the lumen within the "donut" of the coiled wire can line up with the vessel lumen and prevent effective occlusion. On the other hand, when the diameter of the coil is much larger than the diameter of the vessel lumen, then the coil cannot "coil" on itself at all and stretches out longitudinally in the lumen of the vessel and again, probably will not occlude the vessel. When the coil diameter is so large that the coil cannot "coil" at all, as the pusher wire and coil wire are advanced through the catheter or sheath and as the coil wire is pushed out of the tip of the delivery catheter or sheath, the coil wire remains straight and actually pushes the tip of the delivery catheter/sheath back in the vessel. The catheter or sheath tip can be pushed completely back out of the vessel into which the coil is being delivered. This leaves some, or all, of the coil extending proximally out of the target vessel. The ideal coil/vessel size relationship allows the coil to partially coil on itself yet partially stretch out into a very irregular shape or mass. When the coil is to be delivered into a very critical and short segment of vessel, the "distensibility" of the particular vessel can be tested precisely at that location by a low-pressure inflation of a small angioplasty balloon that is slightly larger in diameter than the vessel at that area.

After the successful implant of a coil, a small injection of contrast is performed through the delivery catheter or sheath to verify the degree of occlusion. Often, it is necessary to deposit more than one coil, and often even multiple coils of different sizes, in any single vessel to complete the occlusion. As long as there is room in the vessel, additional coils are deposited at the same location, through the same delivery catheter or sheath, and during the same procedure until the vessel is occluded completely.

In most cases of the occlusions of discrete vessels, standard coils are extruded into a confined segment of the vessel and are released automatically by the "free-release" technique as they exit the delivery catheter. The majority of vessels that are occluded (except the PDA), have some distal tortuosity or narrowing on which the extruded coil becomes trapped. The very accurate "teetering" across the narrowest segment of a vessel that is required for coil occlusion of the PDA, seldom is encountered in the majority of other vascular/small vessel occlusions. With accurate information about the size of the vessel to be occluded and when the proper size and type of coil is used for the occlusion of discrete vessels, there is full expectation that the coil will "fold up" into a compacted, irregular shape, reorient and move (usually distally) after its release and then lodge securely in the vessel. When there is a high likelihood of this type of seating in an appropriate vessel there is little need for the more complicated and expensive detachable/retractable coils. Although unnecessary for the majority of coil deliveries for vascular occlusions, control of the release and retrievability of the coil, however, does become essential in some circumstances.

Special techniques for the delivery or modification of the Gianturco™ and 0.052″ coils to improve the safety of their delivery

When the coil must be delivered in a *very specific site* in order not to occlude adjacent or branching vessels that are critical for the supply of essential viable tissues (e.g. coronary branches adjacent to a coronary-cameral fistula), then a controlled release/retrievable system must be used. When the vessel more proximal to the area being occluded is significantly wider than the area of the vessel where the coils are being implanted or when the coils are delivered near to the aortic entrance of the vessel and as the vessel becomes full of coils, then a retractable or controlled release coil is desirable or even essential. Similarly, if the vessel has only minimal length or the coil is at all large in diameter relative to the vessel diameter, there is a high probability that the coil will elongate too much during delivery and will extend back into the central vessel (aorta!) as it is extruded from the delivery catheter, and a control of the release of the coil is essential. Even when multiple coils are being "wadded" into a long vessel, easy and immediate retrievability of the last and most proximal coil always is desirable.

When the free-release coil is too small in diameter for the vessel, it "balls-up" into its "donut" configuration, "bounces around" in the vessel, which is too large, and easily can embolize *backward* and out of the vessel into the central, critical vessel. With standard free-release Gianturco™ coils, there is absolutely no control over this tumbling, once the extrusion of the coil has started. "Retrieval" of a free-release Gianturco™ coil after the extrusion of the coil has started, thereafter, represents a "foreign body" retrieval of a coil which has embolized to a distal location from the site of implant!

Special techniques to achieve control over standard Gianturco™ and 0.052" stainless steel coils

In order to overcome the non-retrievability, "all or nothing" delivery of standard Gianturco™ and 0.052" coils, multiple modifications of the delivery system/technique have been developed. With a *controlled* attach/release coil, the fit and fixation of the completely extruded coil can be tested once the coil is extruded completely into the vessel before the coil is released from the attached delivery wire/cable. If the position/fixation is not satisfactory, the coil can be withdrawn back into the delivery catheter and repositioned before it is released, or the coil can be withdrawn totally out of the body and the procedure restarted with a more appropriately sized coil. When there is a residual leak through the coils and even when the vessel proximal to the coils is short or otherwise not ideal, by using a controlled-release coil system, an additional coil can be extruded safely into earlier coils in the vessel and tested for both occlusion and fixation before release. If either fixation or occlusion is not satisfactory, the additional coil can still be withdrawn from the original coil(s), although care must be taken because each successive coil tends to become entangled with any previous coil(s).

The various commercially available and the self-made techniques for controlled release of the coil, all are effective to some degree at accomplishing retrievability of the coil during delivery. The minute details of all of these modifications are described in detail in Chapter 27 on "PDA Occlusion", where these coil "control" systems are more of a necessity. The specific uses of the various "controlled-release" systems for general vascular occlusions are discussed here.

Because of the problem of a "no-return" delivery once the extrusion of standard Gianturco™ and 0.052" coils is started and, in the long absence of a commercially available and viable "detachable coil" in the United States, there have been several very innovative techniques developed in order to overcome this shortcoming and make the Gianturco™ and 0.052" coils safer and more reliable.

Latson *catheter* modification for Gianturco™ coil delivery

The Latson™ modification of the *delivery catheter* provides some degree of control and retrievability for the standard Gianturco™ coil[9]. The tip of the delivery catheter is heated and then pulled into a tapered tip over a short, solid, smooth wire or "mandril" of *exactly* the diameter of the *bare coil spring wire* of the particular coil. The mandril is removed and the pulled tip of the catheter is cut off at the narrowest area of the "pulled taper" on the catheter. This creates an opening in the tapered tip of the catheter, which is tight around the bare spring wire of the coil and *very* tight around the coil wire when the nylon fabric is embedded in the wire of the coil. This modified tip configuration is now available commercially as the Latson™ multipurpose catheter: #248498 (Cook Inc., Bloomington, IN) and as the modified Vertebral catheter: #WN27750 (Mallinckrodt Inc., St. Louis, MO).

As a result of the narrowed orifice of the tip of the catheter, the coil now is gripped very tightly as it passes through the *narrowed* orifice of the tightened, modified tip of the catheter. As a consequence of the tight grip on the wire, it is necessary to apply considerable force to the delivery/pusher wire to extrude the standard Gianturco™ coil through the tip of the Latson™ catheter. Because of this tight grip on the coil created by the modified tip of the catheter, and unless the coil has become entrapped on something in the vessel (a previous coil!), the now "dangling" coil, which has been extruded *almost* entirely but is now gripped tightly by the tip of the modified catheter, can be withdrawn from a vessel and out of the body along with the catheter when the delivery catheter is withdrawn through a peripheral introductory sheath.

During the withdrawal of the Latson™ catheter, the coil cannot be withdrawn back into the Latson™ catheter but rather the coil, which is now mostly extruded, will be "dangling" at the tip of the catheter, exposed in the circulation and *not* "protected" as it is being withdrawn within the circulation. The coil cannot be repositioned or reused with this catheter while it still is within the circulation. To start over, the coil and delivery catheter are withdrawn completely out of the body through the peripheral introductory sheath, and a new coil is introduced through the same delivery catheter.

The technique for the delivery of a Gianturco™ coil to a vessel using the Latson™ modification is almost identical to the delivery of the "free-release" coils. Usually, but not necessarily, the retrograde approach is used with the Latson™ catheter. Once in position the coil is pushed out of the catheter with the pusher wire, but now with the necessary considerable additional force on the pusher wire. Because of the force required, more attention must be paid to the extrusion process in order to extrude the coil in small, *controlled* increments in order to deliver the coil to the precise location. The *grip* on the coil by the tip of the catheter is dependent completely on the *very accurate* "tolerances" of the internal diameter of the tip of the catheter whether the catheter is built by hand or by commercial manufacturers. The Latson™ catheter tip is not as strong or dependable as any of the other attach/release mechanisms and does not allow the reuse of the coil during the same procedure without first withdrawing the coil out of the body completely. Although the Latson™ catheter does provide some extra safety in the delivery of a standard Gianturco™ coil, the necessary tolerances and the inability to withdraw the coil into the catheter are disadvantages to this catheter modification for coil delivery.

Balloon-assisted coil delivery to branch vessels

Floating end-hole balloon catheters occasionally are used to deliver any 0.035″ or smaller Gianturco™ coils to abnormal branch vessels. Balloon catheters are used with several different techniques for the delivery of the coils. The end-hole, floating balloon catheter may be the only catheter that can be manipulated into the vessel by the particular operator. In that circumstance, usually, once in the vessel, the balloon is deflated within the vessel and the end-hole balloon catheter is used like any other end-hole catheter for the delivery of the coil. Because of the "ragged" surface of the deflated balloon over the tip of the catheter, extra attention is necessary during the withdrawal of the catheter after the coil has been delivered to prevent the balloon from snagging on the fabric strands that are dangling from the freshly implanted Gianturco™ coil.

The end-hole floating balloon catheter is also used with the balloon *inflated* securely in the vessel in order to wedge coils forcibly into distal locations or to keep the coils from extruding back out of the target vessel. For these purposes, the balloon catheter is manipulated into the vessel to be occluded and *then* the balloon is inflated tightly against the walls within the particular vessel. With the balloon catheter fixed tightly within the vessel, the "free-release" Gianturco™ coil is extruded into the vessel distal to the balloon. When the inflated balloon is fixed tightly enough in the vessel, the coils can be pushed into the vessel with some force to "pack" them more tightly in the vessel. This usually represents a delicate balance between the fixation of the balloon in the vessel and the force used against the pusher wire. If too much force is applied, the inflated balloon can be pushed out of the vessel along with the coils that are being packed into the vessel. If the entrance of the vessel being occluded is close to the entrance of a vital branch vessel, some of the coils can extend into the adjacent vessel or the entire coil can embolize distally into the more central circulation!

Bioptome-assisted coil delivery

The bioptome-assisted delivery of coils for PDA occlusion, and in particular the 0.052″ coils, is discussed in detail in Chapter 27 ("PDA Occlusion")[8]. The bioptome-assisted technique is effective for the precise control of the delivery of any Gianturco™ coil to locations other than the PDA where the exact localization of the coil is extremely critical. Bioptome-assisted delivery is equally as effective when using the more frequently used 0.038″ coils as it is with the 0.052″ coils. Bioptome-controlled delivery is offered an alternative to the commercially manufactured, detachable coils, which in their *more robust form* are only available outside of the USA. The bioptome technique allows complete retrievability of the coil at any time until the purposeful release of the grasp with the bioptome. The bioptome technique is used as an adjunct technique to the "free-release" technique in the placement of the coils into very specific locations or the "final" coils in more critical or precarious locations.

The bioptome attachment to the coil requires the *lumen* or internal diameter (ID) of the delivery system to be at least 1.3 mm (4-French *ID*). A 4-French long sheath with a back-bleed valve and distal radio-opaque marker is used as the *minimum* sized delivery system for bioptome-controlled delivery. However, a 5-French sheath allows a "more comfortable" delivery and more reliable withdrawal of the coil/bioptome back into the delivery system when necessary particularly with the 0.052″ coils. As a consequence, a 5-French sheath with distal radio-opaque marker is usually used with bioptome-controlled coils except in the very smallest infants.

An end-hole catheter is introduced through a 6- or 7-French short sheath and advanced well into the vessel to be occluded. The end-hole catheter is replaced with a stiff, exchange length wire. The 4- or 5-French long sheath/dilator that is to be used to deliver the coil/bioptome is introduced over the wire and through the short introductory sheath and advanced until the tip of *the sheath* is significantly past the "target" area within the vessel to be occluded. Because of the use of a sheath for the delivery and the stiffness of the bioptome itself, bioptome-controlled delivery does have some limitations as to which vessels it can be used in. Often, if there is significant tortuosity of the vessel proximal to the implant site, the bioptome-controlled technique cannot be used.

The bioptome technique requires a special preparation of the occlusion coil, which is used in order for the coil to be grasped with the bioptome. All Gianturco™ and 0.052″ coils consist of a very fine stainless steel wire tightly wound to form the larger "spring guide" type wire of the advertised coil "*wire*" diameter. One end of the "spring" wire is sealed and polished with a small "weld", while the opposite end is open with a very tiny hollow tube created by the fine wires. The coils, including the 0.052″ coils, come loaded in a metal "loading tube" with the welded end of the coil at the distal end of the loader.

The stiff end of a separate 0.038″ spring guide wire is introduced into the proximal end of the coil holder/loader and advanced until just *1–2 mm* of the *distal*, closed (welded) end of the coil is exposed exiting the distal end of the metal loading tube. This exposes the tiny welded tip, which seals the end of the fine coiled "wire tube" of which the "spring coil" is made. While holding the short more proximal and exposed portion of the coil tightly between the fingers, the small welded tip (only) is grasped tightly with a forceps and pulled 0.25 to 0.5 mm away from the remainder of the spring coil which is held by the fingers of the other hand. This maneuver separates the small welded ball approximately 0.5 mm away from the windings of the coiled portion of the "spring wire", but still attached by a single, stretched-out, strand of the fine, very stiff wire. This separation of the welded "ball" allows the bioptome to grasp the "ball" firmly while at the same time allowing the bioptome jaws to close *almost* completely over the stretched out strand of fine wire. This allows the outside diameter of the combination of the closed, 3-French bioptome jaws, over and holding the welded "ball" of even the 0.052″ coil, still to be less than 4-French in outside diameter.

The closed bioptome jaws over the tip of the coil, however, do not fit back within the original metal loader. The combination must be withdrawn into a separate slightly larger "loader" in order to be *front-loaded* into the delivery sheath. Before the coil is grasped with the bioptome, the bioptome is passed through the *separate* slightly larger metal loading tube (which comes with the 0.052″ coils) or through a segment of a 4-French short sheath which can be used as a loader equally as well as the new, larger metal loading tube which is provided only with the 0.052″ coils. The 4-French sheath must be long enough to contain the entire straightened length of whichever coil is being used. After the bioptome is passed through the separate metal loading tube or the 4-French sheath and during the attachment to the "prepared coil", the metal loading tube or length of sheath is withdrawn on the bioptome shaft back to its proximal control handle. Once the new "loading tube" is back on the shaft of the bioptome catheter, the bioptome jaws are opened and then closed tightly around the "prepared" separated, welded ball at the end of the coil.

With one operator/assistant holding the bioptome jaws closed tightly over the "ball" at the tip of the coil, the "new", larger diameter "loading tube" through which the bioptome was previously passed, is advanced over the bioptome jaws which now have the tip of the coil grasped within them. The entire coil is drawn out of the original metal loading tube directly into the new larger "loading tube" or segment of short sheath. The coil is withdrawn completely into this new tube until the now distal (originally proximal) end of the coil is *just within* the tip of the new loading tube. The bioptome-controlled coil is now ready to be delivered from the new loading tube into the pre-positioned delivery sheath. The distal end of the loading tube is introduced into the back-bleed valve at the hub of the pre-positioned delivery sheath and the bioptome catheter (with the attached coil) is advanced into the loader/sheath and the shaft of the delivery sheath.

The bioptome jaws are held closed very tightly while the coil is advanced to the end of the delivery sheath. The entire delivery is observed closely on fluoroscopy. The coil and the bioptome jaws can be visualized very clearly on fluoroscopy. The sheath is withdrawn slightly until the tip of the sheath is exactly in position for implanting the coil. The bioptome catheter and coil are advanced together, extruding the coil out of the tip of the sheath. The combination bioptome/coil is advanced together with the sheath held in position until the bioptome jaws with the grasped coil are just *1–2 mm within* the tip of the sheath. At this point the security of the extruded coil is tested by very slight, gentle, to-and-fro movement of the sheath and bioptome catheter together. The degree of occlusion can be tested by a contrast injection into the involved vessel through a second catheter. This obviously can only be accomplished if such a catheter is in place. If not satisfied with the fixation of the coil in the vessel or the degree of occlusion, the coil can easily be withdrawn into (and, if desired, out of) the sheath, and the procedure restarted in a new location of the delivery sheath or with a different coil. When satisfied with the fixation in the vessel and the degree of occlusion, the bioptome catheter is advanced until the jaws have advanced completely out of the tip of the sheath. The bioptome jaws are opened, releasing the coil.

The advantages of the bioptome-controlled delivery of coils are the obvious complete control over the actual release of the coil and the complete retrievability of the coil until the moment of its *purposeful* release. The major disadvantages to this technique are the requirement for a slightly larger delivery system, the lower flexibility of the long sheath delivery system for entering more tortuous locations or vessels arising at acute angles off the major feeding vessel (aorta), and the added expense of the bioptome.

Special commercial modifications of the delivery system or the coil to *control* the delivery of the Gianturco™ type coil

Detachable™ coils: Jackson™ coils, Cook detachable and Flipper™ coils

Outside the United States–i.e. in countries not under US FDA jurisdiction–the Jackson™ (or Detachable™) coil is available commercially from Cook™ Inc., Europe. This is a safe, detachable or controlled-release variation of the standard Gianturco™ coil. The Detachable™ coil is in widespread, standard, use for PDA occlusion as well as all other types of vascular occlusions, particularly in Europe[10]. The European Detachable™ coil is not available in the United States. The Detachable™ coil is slightly less robust than the standard Gianturco™ coil, however, for the occlusion of most vascular lesions other than the PDA, this relative flimsiness is of little consequence. The relatively simple attach/release mechanism of the Detachable™ coil gives complete control over the release and retractability of the coil, making vascular occlusions in even the most precarious vessels a safer and more effective procedure. The Detachable™ coil, with its specific pusher/delivery wire is, however, slightly more expensive than the standard "free-release" Gianturco™ coil.

The Detachable™ coil essentially is a standard Gianturco™ coil that has been fitted with a screw mechanism for the purposeful attachment and release from the delivery or "pusher" wire. The European Detachable™ coil comes from the manufacturer as a "set" containing the coil, a special clear loader, a special delivery/pusher wire and a fine movable mandril, which passes through the delivery wire *and* the coil. The clear loader has a slight funnel at the proximal end where the "female" screw mechanism in the coil is located. The Detachable™ coil itself outwardly has the same appearance as a standard Gianturco™ coil, with the distal end of the occlusion coil sealed with a rounded, smooth and polished "weld" while the proximal end of the coil is hollow. The open, proximal end of the straightened occluder coil is "squared off", hollow and appears slightly irregular on very close inspection. The fine wire windings within the proximal, hollow end of the coil form a "female screw thread" for the attachment of the "pusher" wire. The special attach/release delivery or "pusher" wire consists of a spring guide wire of the same diameter as the coil to be used. The pusher wire has a long, tapered "male" screw mechanism as an integral part of its *distal* end and comes with a removable "torquing" device for purposeful rotation of the wire/screw tip. The coil attaches to the delivery/pusher wire with this very simple screw mechanism.

In addition, the special delivery/pusher wire has no fixed "core" wire, but is *hollow throughout* its entire length, *including* through the fine screw at the distal end. The small lumen throughout the wire allows a very fine, smooth, steel "mandril" or stiffening wire to pass completely through, out of the end of the pusher wire and through the coil. The fine, totally removable "mandril" wire, which is approximately 10 cm longer than the combined pusher wire and the straight coil wire, comes packaged within each pusher wire. The mandril passing within the delivery/pusher wire and the coil acts as a stiffening "core" wire. The mandril has a short segment of "spring" wire attached at its proximal end to serve to identify the proximal end and as a "hub" for moving and torquing the mandril. Detachable™ coils commercially come stretched out as a straight spring wire positioned within a thin, *clear*, straight loading tube of approximately the same ID as the OD of the coil.

Once the delivery catheter is positioned properly and secured in place, the coil is attached to the pusher wire. The clear loader containing the occluder coil is inspected very carefully. Each end of the occluder coil is positioned slightly more than one centimeter within the ends of the loader. The proximal and distal ends of the occluder coil/loader are identified. The screw end of the delivery/pusher wire is introduced into the proximal (funneled) end of the loader. The mandril wire is advanced through the delivery/pusher wire and 8–10 mm beyond the distal tip of the "screw" mechanism of the delivery/pusher. Very carefully and without pushing the coil forward in the loader, the mandril is introduced into the proximal end of the coil by gentle trial and error probing and then advanced 8–10 mm *into* the hollow coil. The delivery/pusher wire is advanced over the mandril until the screw at the tip of the delivery/pusher wire enters into the proximal end of the coil. When the screw tip has engaged in the proximal end of the coil, the coil and pusher wire are attached by two and a half clockwise turns on the pusher wire or on the coil loader when it is gripped facing the pusher wire. The screw at the tip of the pusher wire enters and engages with the proximal end of the coil. Once the screw has tightened within the coil, the delivery/pusher wire is turned *counter*-clockwise *one half* turn to slightly loosen the attachment. *Gentle*, and *very slight* to-and-fro motion of the pusher wire within the loader is used to test the attachment of the coil to the pusher wire. Holding the pusher wire, the core/mandril wire is advanced the remainder of the way into the coil until the mandril reaches the distal, closed tip of the straightened coil within the loader.

The distal end of the clear coil loader is introduced through a wire back-bleed/flush device into the hub of the previously positioned delivery catheter. The delivery/pusher wire with the enclosed mandril is advanced into the loader, which, in turn, pushes the attached, straightened Detachable™ coil out of the loader and into the delivery catheter. The mandril remains in the delivery/pusher wire as the pusher wire is advanced. The distal end of the catheter is observed continually on fluoroscopy as the coil advances through the catheter to the tip of the catheter and as the coil is advanced out of the tip of the catheter into the desired location for implant by advancing the delivery/pusher wire further. The mandril is maintained within the delivery wire *and coil* until the coil is at least partially out of the delivery catheter and the tip of the coil is in or slightly *distal* to the correct position for implant. The mandril still within the coil keeps the coil straight and allows easy adjustments in the position of the coil. Once the coil is partially out of the catheter and in proper position for implant, the mandril is withdrawn slowly, allowing the coil to curl into its "coiled" configuration in the vessel/lesion. The pusher catheter and coil are advanced further while the mandril is withdrawn to just within the *proximal end* of the coil and until the coil is totally extruded from the catheter and formed into its full coil configuration. At this point the coil is tested for its proper location and its fixation in the vessel by slight to-and-fro motion of the pusher wire or with an angiogram. When satisfied with the fixation of the coil and the occlusion of the vessel, the small "vise" is attached to the proximal end of the delivery/pusher wire and the vise with the pusher wire/mandril is rotated counter-clockwise until the coil detaches from the pusher wire. The release of the coil as the coil is being detached is observed very closely under fluoroscopy to ensure a smooth "unscrewing", and that there is no binding or twisting of the still-attached coil.

If the Detachable™ coil is not in the exact, desired position, at any time before it is purposefully "unscrewed", it can easily be withdrawn back into the delivery catheter. As the coil is withdrawn into the catheter, the mandril remains positioned proximal to and *outside* of the coil. If the same coil is to be repositioned using the same catheter, the mandril is re-advanced into the coil (which now is straightened within the catheter) before the coil is re-extruded into the vessel. This retrievability during delivery adds total control and a significant degree of safety to the occlusion of any vascular structure. The total European Detachable™ coil systems are slightly more complicated and significantly more expensive than the standard Gianturco™ coils by themselves.

Flipper™ coils

The Flipper™ coil (Cook Inc., Bloomington, IN) is an attempt in the US at a version of the European Detachable™ coil. The earlier US version of a detachable stainless steel coil of a size considered reasonable to use in PDA occlusions was a catastrophe. The original "larger" detachable coil which became available in the US was made from a smaller, less robust spring wire, had far fewer incorporated "thrombotic" fibers, and had a bizarre, unnecessarily complicated attach/release mechanism. As a consequence this coil had very little use. The Flipper™ coil is a revised version of the Cook, Inc., US detachable coil, which became available in 2001 with an attach/release mechanism similar to the European Detachable™ coils. The Flipper™ coil wires are 0.035″ wires and still do not have comparable robustness nor the occlusive capabilities of the 0.038″ standard Gianturco™ coils. Flipper™ coils are available in 3–12 cm lengths and with coil diameters between 3 and 8 mm. Current Flipper™ coils have more fiber strands embedded in the coil wire than the original US version of the detachable coil, and for a 0.035″coil do seem to have comparable occlusive properties to the smaller 0.035″ standard Gianturco™ coils. Flipper™ coils require a delivery catheter with a 0.041″ inner diameter, which generally is a 5-French catheter.

The lack of robustness of the 0.035″ coil compared to the 0.038″ coil is a limitation of this coil for its use for primarily closing a patent ductus arteriosus, but the controllability and retrievability of the Flipper™ coil make it very appealing for most other vascular occlusions or for the implant of additional coils for the "final and total" occlusion of a patent ductus which already has a larger, secure coil in place.

The packaging, attaching, loading, delivery and release of the Flipper™ coils are all similar to the European Detachable™ coils described above.

Alternative occlusion coils including "Micro" coils

In addition to the standard and large sized Gianturco™ *type* coils, there is a large variety of other small coils available for *small vessel occlusion*. The alternative coils are delivered through significantly smaller and more flexible catheters, and as a consequence can be placed in more circuitous and distal locations. None of the smaller alternative coils are as robust as the stainless steel Gianturco™ coils.

Target™ platinum coils and their delivery technique

Target™ Coils (Target Therapeutics, Fremont, CA) are similar in concept to the Gianturco™ coils. They are segments of very fine spring guidewire-like wires with thrombogenic fibers intertwined in the spaces between the wire coils of the spring wire. There, the similarity ends. Target™ coil wires are made of very small diameter 0.014″ and 0.018″ platinum wires. In spite of their very small diameters, and because of the platinum material, these coils are very radio-opaque and easily visible under fluoroscopy in the catheterization laboratory. Because of the material and tiny size of these coils, they are more flexible and pass through tortuous catheters/vessels easier than Gianturco™ coils. Target™ coils do not open into a cylindrical "coil" in their relaxed state but rather, into complex "helix" configurations which vary between 4 and 7 mm in diameter. Because of their size and less "fiber material", these coils are more compressible in a particular vessel and, in turn, not as occlusive as the larger stainless steel Gianturco™ coils.

Target™ coils are delivered through specific, *very small (3-French), very flexible* Tracker™ delivery catheters (Target Therapeutics, Fremont, CA). The Tracker™ catheters are small and "trackable" but are *non*-radio-opaque throughout their entire length except for a tiny radio-opaque marker at the very tip of the catheter. This tip marker identifies the most distal location of the tip but, once the delivery/pusher wire is removed from the Tracker™ catheter, the course of the catheter proximal to the tip is *invisible*! Tracker™ catheters are advanced to the *orifice* of the vessel to be occluded through a larger torque-controlled 5-French, guiding catheter. From the guiding catheter, the Tracker™ catheter is advanced through the vessel over a special, very fine, Dasher™ guide wire (Target Therapeutics, Fremont, CA). The Dasher™ guide wire is pre-positioned in the target vessel. Because of its torque control, its very floppy tip and its very small size, this wire can be manipulated very readily to very distal locations and through very tortuous and long vessels.

To deliver the Target™ coils, a pre-formed, torque-controlled, 5-French guiding catheter which accommodates the Tracker™ catheter is positioned *in* the orifice of the vessel to be occluded or, alternatively, into a trunk vessel off of which the target vessel arises. The special Dasher™ tracking wire, which is 0.014" in diameter and 175 cm long with a very flexible tip, is passed through the guiding catheter and into the target vessel. The specifically curved floppy tip of the Dasher™ wires can be manipulated selectively through very tortuous and very circuitous, distal vessels using a "torquer vice" on the stiff shaft of the wire to help to direct the tip of the wire to the specific location. An appropriately sized Tracker™ ("Tracker™-18", 150 cm) catheter (Target Therapeutics, Fremont, CA) is then advanced over the Dasher™ wire and through the guiding catheter to the orifice of the target vessel. As the Tracker™ catheter is being advanced over the wire a *continual flush* is maintained through the guide catheter *and* the Tracker™ catheter through the special double "Y" adaptors attached to the proximal ends of *both* the Tracker™ and the guiding catheters.

When the Tracker™ catheter is being advanced over the wire beyond the tip of the guiding catheter and through the more tortuous areas of the vessel, the Tracker™ catheter is advanced several centimeters at a time while alternately withdrawing or tightening the Dasher™ wire very slightly. In this way the Tracker™ catheter is "inched" along the Dasher™ wire without displacing the wire. All of this time, *only the tip* of the Tracker™ catheter is visible over the wire. Occasionally the Tracker™ catheter does not follow over the Dasher™ wire and the wire is pulled out of position. In that circumstance, often the very flimsy Tracker™ catheter with just the tip of the exposed, very floppy Dasher™ wire maintained just beyond the tip of the catheter can be advanced (manipulated) together as a unit back to the appropriate location. Once the Tracker™ catheter has reached the desired location, the Dasher™ wire is withdrawn very carefully and very slowly from the Tracker™ catheter. The Tracker™ catheter is maintained on a slow constant flush while the opaque tip of the catheter is observed continuously on fluoroscopy to be sure that the tip is not being displaced during the removal of the wire. Once the wire is removed, *again*, only the opaque marker at the tip of the Tracker™ catheter will be visible. A small, ***slow*** hand injection of contrast is performed through the Tracker™ catheter and recorded on biplane angiography or stored fluoroscopy in order to "road map" the actual "course" of the Tracker™ catheter for future reference. After the "road map" is recorded, the Tracker™ catheter is flushed *very slowly* but very thoroughly to clear it of all contrast material. A rapid or forceful flush of the Tracker™ catheter can easily "blow" the tip of the Tracker™ catheter back out of the vessel.

Each Target™ coil comes straightened in a separate, tiny, metal tubular holder/introducer. The introducer tube is flushed gently and the end, which does not have a hub, is fitted into the straight segment of the "Y" connector at the proximal end of the Tracker™ catheter. The coil is pushed out of the introducer and into the proximal end of the Tracker catheter with the short "plunger tool" which comes with the coil. Once the plunger tool has been advanced to the "hilt", the coil is completely within the Tracker™ catheter as a short, straight, *free* segment of wire. Target™ coils fortunately are very radio-opaque. The plunger tool and the introducer tube are removed. The *stiff end* of the special "coil pusher wire" is introduced into the proximal end of the Tracker™ catheter and advanced approximately *30 cms*. This "pre-advances" the coil that distance within the Tracker™ catheter. The stiff end of the coil pusher is withdrawn, the pusher wire reversed, and the soft nylon distal end of the pusher "wire" introduced into the Tracker™ catheter. All of this time the Tracker™ catheter and guiding catheter are *maintained on a slow continuous flush*. As the coil pusher (soft nylon end first) is advanced in the Tracker™ catheter, the coil is advanced proportionately through the catheter. This part of the delivery is observed particularly carefully on the fluoroscopy. Extreme care is taken as the coil is advanced within the Tracker™ catheter to ensure that the tip of the Tracker™ catheter is not withdrawn even slightly by inadvertent traction applied to it. When the advancing coil and coil pusher wire begin to enter curves and bends in the course of the Tracker™ catheter, the advancing coil and coil pusher wire tend to "straighten" the Tracker™ which, if not compensated for by advancing the proximal end of the Tracker™ catheter, can pull the tip of the Tracker™ catheter back out of the desired position. The course of the coil, which now is visible through the "invisible" catheter, is compared to the previously obtained angiographic "road map" of the catheter course. This is to help ensure that the coil and pusher are not displacing the "invisible" catheter during the introduction of the coil.

When the coil reaches the tip of the Tracker™ catheter, by further advancing the coil pusher, the coil is extruded from the distal end of the catheter and is free in the vessel to be occluded. Like the standard Gianturco™ coils, the Target™ coils have no attachment to the pusher wire and once extrusion begins, the coil cannot be withdrawn. Also like the Gianturco™ coils, the way the coils unwind and coil in the vessel depends upon the relative size of the coil compared to the vessel size. In order to accomplish complete occlusion of a vessel, usually many coils or multiple sizes of the coils are used. As with other occlusions and whenever possible, the total occlusion of the vessel should be accomplished completely before the procedure is abandoned.

Controlled release micro coils

There are two varieties of controlled release systems for the "micro" coils, which do provide retrievability of the coils even after they have started to be extruded. The two mechanisms are entirely different, but both are manufactured by Target™ Therapeutics (Target Therapeutics, Fremont, CA). Although the primary use of these coils is by neuroradiologists, they are equally suitable for small vessel occlusions in the pediatric/congenital population.

The first of these controlled release micro coils is the Guglielmi™ electrolytically detachable coil (GDC) (Target Therapeutics, Fremont, CA). These are, as the name implies, released from the delivery wire by a micro current delivered through the wire, which, in effect, melts a connection between the delivery/pusher wire and the coil. The second type of controlled release coil is the Interlocking Target™ coil (Target Therapeutics, Fremont, CA). These coils have a unique system of micro machined, overlapping pins or "couplers" which are compressed within a tiny delivery catheter until the final millimeter of the coil is extruded from the tip of the catheter. Both of these controlled release micro coils otherwise are used in similar circumstances to the other micro coils.

Tornado™ coils

The Cook Tornado™ coils (Cook Inc., Bloomington, IN) functionally are almost a cross between the standard Gianturco™ coils and the Target™ coils. As their name implies, these coils are shaped like a tiny tornado "funnel" which along with their size and material gives them more compressibility and, supposedly, more coil "exposure" to the lumen of the vessel. These coils are constructed of platinum wire, which is more radio-opaque than stainless steel wire of comparable size. The coil wires are available in both 0.018" and 0.025" spring wire sizes, which, in turn, are less robust than the standard Gianturco™ coils. Each coil has multiple strands of tiny synthetic fibers embedded along the coil wire to facilitate thrombosis. The Tornado™ coil sizes are labeled corresponding to the largest and the smallest diameters at the ends of the "funnel". For example, a 6/2 coil has a 6 mm diameter large end, which tapers down to a 2 mm diameter small end. The 0.018" Tornado™ coils are available in sizes from 3/2 to 10/4 with lengths of the straightened coil varying from 2 to 14 cm, while the 0.025" Tornado™ coils come in sizes from 5/3 to 10/5, with lengths of the straightened coil from 4 to 12 cm. From the standard packaging of the Tornado™ coils, the small end of the "funnel" is delivered first from the "coil" holder and loads first. By special order the Tornado™ coils can be packaged so the large end is delivered first. Tornado™ coils are delivered through catheters with internal diameters of 0.025" or 0.032", which allow the use of very small, trackable catheters.

The 3-French Slip-Cath™ (Cook Inc., Bloomington, IN) is ideal for the delivery of these coils. The Slip-Cath™ is very flexible and has a very slick hydrophilic coating, which allows it to track through very circuitous and small vessels. Its small outer diameter allows it to be advanced to the orifice of the vessel that is to be occluded through a torque-controlled, 5- or 6-French guiding catheter. The nylon 3-French infusion catheter (Cook Inc., Bloomington, IN) with a radio-opaque tip is less flexible than the Slip-Cath™ but also makes a good delivery catheter for delivery to more proximal areas in small, but less tortuous vessels.

The technique for loading and delivering the Tornado™ coil is similar to the delivery of a "free-release" Gianturco™ coil. There is no attach/release mechanism. The coils are introduced into the pre-positioned delivery catheter from their loader and advanced through the catheter with a 0.025" pusher wire. When there is a very tortuous vessel proximal to the site of delivery, a very soft tipped pusher wire is used. A concomitant slow, continuous flush through the delivery catheter assists in advancing the coil through the catheter. The smaller Tornado™ coils occasionally can be advanced through the delivery catheter by a strong flush on the catheter alone. The strong flush, however, may cause the tip of the catheter to recoil out of position, making the "flush" delivery much less reliable and less precise. As with other micro coil occlusions, usually more than one coil essentially is always required to complete the occlusion. After one or more coils are delivered, a small hand angiogram is performed through the delivery catheter to check the degree of occlusion. If there still is any residual leak, additional coils are delivered until the vessel is occluded or there is no more space in the vessel for additional coils.

Nester™ coils

The Nester™ coils (Cook Inc., Bloomington, IN) are still another variety of coil for vascular occlusions. These are 0.035″ platinum coils with synthetic fibers entwined in the coil wire. In their relaxed, free shape, the coils have a cylindrical configuration. Nester™ coils are all 14 cm in length and available in 4–12 mm diameter "cylinders". These coils are softer than even the comparable diameter Tornado™ coils. The Nester™ coils are designed to occlude by bunching up and packing into a relatively large (1–2 cm) mass within the vessel.

The Nester™ coils are delivered through a catheter with a 0.035″ or 0.038″ inner diameter and advanced through the delivery catheter with a 0.035″ teflon-coated spring guide "pusher" wire identically to the delivery of the Gianturco™ free-release coils. The standard Nestor™ coils have no attach/release mechanism so, like the Gianturco™ coils, once extrusion of the coil begins, there is no turning back. Because they are so soft and flimsy, these coils are used mostly as additional or supplemental "stuffing" coils rather than primary occlusion devices. They are added as "packing" to complete the occlusion within a previous, stiffer coil or other device already placed in a vessel.

Particulate materials and non-coil intravascular devices available for vascular occlusions

There are several materials and intravascular devices in addition to the intravascular coils that are available and occasionally used for the occlusion of abnormal vascular communications.

Particulate materials

Vascular radiologists use particulate materials extensively for the acute occlusion of vessels and abnormal communications. These materials usually are used to control bleeding from a specific vessel and/or to totally occlude vessels with the intent of necrosing the tissues "downstream" from the occlusion (tumors, neoplasms). The particulate materials are useful mostly for very diffuse, but, at the same time, "end artery" lesions. The materials used include autologous blood clots, pieces of Gelfoam™ and pieces of Polyvinyl Alcohol (Ivalon™). The autologous blood clots and Gelfoam™ usually only provide a temporary occlusion and for that reason seldom are used in congenital vascular lesions where a more "permanent" occlusion is desired.

The autologous clots are just that–small solid particles of the patient's recently clotted blood, which are injected from a syringe through a catheter that is pre-positioned in the culprit vessel[1]. The "clot particles" that are used should be slightly larger than the vessel that is to be occluded. The already clotted blood acts as a temporary occlusive mass to occlude the small, preferably "end" vessel. The clot usually thrombolyses over a short period of time, however, it usually remains in place long enough to allow acute bleeding from the vessel to stop and occasionally long enough for the vessel to thrombose.

Gelfoam™ is an insoluble material made from dried pork skin gelatin and formed into porous foam sheets. The foam material can absorb many times its own weight in blood and/or other fluids. When left in the tissues it resorbs into the body within 4–6 weeks. Gelfoam™ is approved to enhance coagulation on the *surface* of bleeding tissues but is not "approved" for intravascular use. It comes in sterile sheets, which can be cut to any desired size or shape, and the pieces can be compressed into very small particles.

Very small, cut and compressed pieces of Gelfoam™ are soaked in a dilute solution of contrast and then are forced into the end vessel that is to be occluded through a catheter by a strong flush with a syringe[2]. In the vessel, the "wad" of Gelfoam™ expands and absorbs blood to create an occlusive mass. Gelfoam™ is useful to "complete" or "finalize" the occlusion of a vessel/fistula which has been started with another occlusion device. Obviously, this soft gelatin like material cannot be used to occlude high-flow and/or high-pressure vessels, and like autologous clot, the Gelfoam™ itself may not create a permanent occlusion. The Gelfoam™ particles themselves are not radio-opaque, so embolization to distal locations is only apparent from any contrast solution that might be retained in the particles and/or signs or symptoms that are produced by the embolized particles.

Ivalon™ (Polyvinyl-alcohol or PVA) foam particles are available for a similar use to the autologous clots or Gelfoam™ pieces. The Ivalon™ does provide a more permanent occlusion but, as small soft particles, still is useful only for end vessel and/or "completion" of other vessel occlusions. Ivalon™ particles are available commercially from Cook Inc. (Bloomington, IN) as dried particles in multiple different particle sizes between the smallest 50–100 micron and the largest 2000–2800 micron sizes to accommodate multiple different vessel sizes. The dried Ivalon™ particles are mixed with contrast material to soften them and give them some radio-opacity for injection into the circulation. The particles mixed with dilute contrast are drawn out of their sterile container into a syringe and injected with the same syringe into the desired site through a pre-positioned catheter. Similar to the autologous clots and Gelfoam™, there is little control over the location where the particles are delivered and essentially, no retrievability.

"Intravascular" glues

There was a transient interest by several different investigators for the use of the tissue adhesive isobutyl 2-cyanoacrylate (Bucrylate™) as an occlusive/embolic material to occlude large vessels/vascular communications[4]. The Bucrylate™ polymerizes into a solid mass instantaneously on contact with blood. The area for deposit of the Bucrylate™ must be "isolated" from the surrounding circulating blood and/or the Bucrylate™ must be injected very specifically into the area. Bucrylate™ was very difficult to handle and to control during delivery both during animal testing and during several clinical uses. If injected too fast it embolized distally and/or backward into proximal branches and, in doing so, occluded all areas that it entered. If injected too slowly, it occluded the injecting catheter when only partially extruded. The difficulties with delivery of Bucrylate™ compared to other occlusion materials/devices, and the unknowns about long-term carcinogenic effects of Bucrylate™ in humans, led to it being abandoned for human trials in the United States.

Occlusion devices for large vascular communications

Gianturco-Grifka Vascular Occlusion Device™ (GGVOD™)

Although it does contain spring guide wire and is approved for use in the US as a variation of the Gianturco™ coil, the Gianturco-Grifka Vascular Occlusion Device™ (GGVOD™) (Cook Inc., Bloomington, IN) has little resemblance in either appearance or use to the Gianturco™ coils. The GGVOD™ is a nylon bag or sack of a predetermined fixed diameter into which a specific length of spring wire is wadded to achieve a tense, fixed diameter, mass of spring wire[11]. The wire for the packing of the bag of the GGVOD™ is a spring guide wire with the stiffening core and safety wires removed. The bag only serves to contain the mass of wire within the fixed diameter of the bag. The bags are available in diameters of 3, 5, 7 and 9 mm, each coming with a specific length of "packing" spring guide wire. The bags are somewhat flattened and elongated so that they do not form a circular or spherical configuration in their length or cross section. The stated diameter is the largest measured cross-section of the particular bag and not the actual circumferential diameter of the bag.

The GGVOD™ is usable only in tubular vascular structures that are at least 1.5 times longer than their respective diameters. The GGVOD™ is held in the vessel by the radial force created by the wad of spring wire within the bag and exerted against the surrounding vessel wall. The bag diameter should be at least one millimeter larger than the diameter of the vessel to be occluded. If the particular vessel is very distensible, then a larger diameter bag to vessel ratio is used.

The technique for delivery of the GGVOD™ to most abnormal vascular communication is similar to the delivery of the GGVOD™ to the PDA (as described subsequently in Chapter 27) with one major exception. When delivering the GGVOD™ to a collateral or branch vessel compared to the delivery to the PDA, the delivery sheath initially and, in turn, the bag is delivered exactly to the implant site and *all* of the wire extrusion into the bag is directly into the site where the bag is to be implanted. This is in comparison to the delivery to the usual patent ductus, where the sheath and the bag are advanced *beyond* the implant location and some of the filler wire is extruded into the bag in this distal location before the bag/delivery catheter is withdrawn back into the specific site within the ductus for the implant. The fixation of the bag and/or the ability to push all of the filler wire into the bag depend(s) upon a relatively precise and, at the same time, tight fit of the filled bag into the vessel/channel. As with the delivery of coils to critical locations, the vessel/channel can be "sized" with a small angioplasty balloon that is slightly larger than the vessel/channel and inflated at a low pressure in the vessel/channel.

Because of the complexity of the delivery and release of the GGVOD™ and the critical importance of each individual step, the details of the GGVOD™ delivery to vascular communications other than the PDA are listed here in a tabular, "cook book" form.

Components of the GGVOD™ system

- A long, 8-French, valved outer delivery sheath with a distal marker band.
- The nylon "sack" or "bag": in 3, 5, 7 and 9 mm sizes (diameters).
- An **inner**, stiff walled, pusher catheter to which the bag is attached.
- A long variable length (according to bag size) detachable, coiled spring filler wire within the pusher catheter.
- A stiffer pusher wire (attached to the proximal end of the filler wire and extending out of the proximal end of the pusher catheter).
- A second, stiff, middle, "bag release" catheter which is pre-positioned over the pusher catheter.
- A complex attach/release system which joins all of these components.

• A short length of 8-French "peal away" sheath which comes over the distal ends of the two catheters and the attached "bag".

Six major steps in the implant of a GGVOD to an abnormal vascular communication (except a PDA)

• The long delivery sheath is advanced into the abnormal vascular communication until the sheath tip is just within the area where the "sack" is to be implanted.
• The "sack" is introduced into the long sheath through the "peal away" sheath.
• The "sack" is positioned *precisely in the area* to be occluded and the sheath is withdrawn off the sack.
• The filler wire is pushed into the sack.
• The pusher wire is separated from the filler wire.
• The filled "sack" is separated from the pusher catheter.

Details of the six major steps for the GGVOD delivery to an abnormal vascular communication

Step 1: The long delivery sheath is positioned in vascular communication with the tip of the sheath 1–2 cm beyond the area where the sack is to be implanted

• The abnormal vascular channel is entered with an end-hole catheter which is advanced as far beyond the area to be occluded as possible.
• A second catheter from a second vascular entrance site is placed adjacent to the proximal (in the direction of flow) end of the communication.
• The end-hole catheter is replaced with a 0.035″ stiff exchange wire.
• The special 8-French, valved delivery sheath/dilator set with a marker band at the distal tip of the sheath is advanced over the wire into the abnormal channel until the tip of the *sheath* is just beyond the area of the channel where the GGVOD™ is to be implanted. Unless the delivery sheath tip can be advanced just distal to the location for occlusion, the GGVOD™ cannot be used.
• The dilator and wire are removed, the system is cleared of air and clot and then the sheath is flushed thoroughly.

Step 2: The "sack" and delivery system introduction into the long sheath

• All of the components of the GGVOD system are inspected carefully.
• The "sack", which is attached to the pusher catheter and the wire/delivery/release system, is introduced into the pre-positioned long sheath as a single unit through the short "peal away" sheath.
• The short "peal-away" sheath is removed after the "sack" is completely within the sheath.
• The "sack" is advanced with the attached delivery system to the tip the sheath (but still within the sheath tip) to the exact location where the GGVOD™ is to be implanted.

Step 3: The "sack" is positioned in the vessel/channel

• With the pusher catheter held in place, the sheath is withdrawn off the "sack" which now is in the precise position for implant. The "sack" itself is invisible, but the attaching band on the proximal neck of the "sack" is visible and defines the proximal limit of the "sack".
• While observing on fluoroscopy, several loops of the "filler" wire are advanced very loosely into the "sack" by advancing the stiff pusher *wire* 5–10 cm. The "sack" is not packed tightly with the filler wire at this point.
• The position of the "sack" is checked with a small angiogram through the second catheter positioned in or adjacent to the proximal end of the channel.

Step 4: The filler wire is pushed into the sack

• With the "sack" in the proper position, the remainder of the filler wire is fed *completely* into the "sack". This is checked on fluoroscopy being sure that the connection point of the filler wire with the pusher wire is *within the sack*. This is identified by a difference in X-ray densities at the connection point.
• The exact "sack" position in the vessel and the degree of occlusion are checked by another angiogram through the second catheter.

Step 5: The pusher wire is separated from the filler wire

• When sure the filler wire is completely within the "sack" and while observing on fluoroscopy, the *wire* release mechanism is activated by pushing forward on the two side "loops" of the special attach/release handle. This detaches the pusher wire from the filler wire.
• The *pusher wire* is withdrawn into the pusher catheter —this releases and separates the pusher *wire* from the "sack". This withdrawal of the pusher wire should be very slow—until absolutely sure that the pusher wire is separated from the filler wire.

Step 6: The pusher catheter is separated from the sack

• The stiffer, middle, *release catheter*, which is over the pusher catheter but within the sheath, is advanced snugly against the neck of the "sack".

• With the tip *of the release catheter* held *exactly* in place against the sack, the inner *"pusher" catheter* is withdrawn forcibly from within the neck of the "sack". (If the *release catheter* moves *at all*, the position of the "sack" very likely will move with it!!)
• The forceful withdrawal of the "pusher catheter" releases the "sack" in the channel entirely free from the delivery system.

The advantages of the GGVOD™ for vascular occlusions are the same as its advantages for occlusion of the PDA. The GGVOD™ is excellent for the occlusion of relatively large and/or high flow vascular channels or structures that have any associated length. In this type of lesion, the GGVOD™ usually produces immediate, complete occlusion. Even the largest "sack" is delivered through only an 8-French sheath, which is reasonable in all patients past infancy. Once delivered and before it is released purposefully, if the "filled bag" does not fit in the vessel, is loose in the vessel or otherwise does not occlude the vessel, the wire can be withdrawn and the bag repositioned or even replaced with a bag of a different size. The larger diameter GGVOD™ devices also are applicable to some larger, high flow vessels and channels where coils alone are not sufficient–for example in large abnormal venous channels or large pulmonary arteriovenous malformations. One of the greatest advantages of the GGVOD™ is that it is approved for this use and is available in the United States.

The GGVOD certainly is not a "universal" device, only being applicable to tubular vascular lesions that are somewhat longer than they are in diameter. Another disadvantage of the GGVOD for vascular occlusions relates to the size and stiffness of the delivery sheath. Since most small vessels requiring occlusion arise from the aorta and require arterial access, the 8-French delivery sheath represents a significant disadvantage for use in infants or small children. In addition to its diameter, the GGVOD™ is delivered through a long sheath which is not as flexible as most delivery catheters, so delivery of the device into acutely angled and/or tortuous vessels is difficult, if not impossible. Replacing the delivery sheath that comes with the GGVOD™ with a Flexor™ type sheath overcomes some of this problem. A final disadvantage is that the GGVOD™ is quite complicated to use and when used infrequently, the delivery/release technique must be "relearned" with each use.

There have been rare complications encountered with the use of the GGVOD™ even in the occlusion of vascular structures other than a PDA. On several occasions the filler wire either could not be or was not pushed entirely into the "sack" and/or was pulled partially out of the "sack" as the pusher wire was withdrawn (incompletely released?), resulting in a segment of the filler wire extending into the lumen of the vascular channel after the release of the "sack". In most occlusions other than the PDA, this creates little or no problem since the goal is to occlude the entire channel. If the filler wire extends back into a necessary or vital feeding channel and cannot be "wadded" back into the channel that is being occluded, the wire can be captured with a vascular snare. The wire can be bent back and forth repeatedly against the orifice of the target vessel and, in doing so, broken off from the more distal wire, which is within the target vessel. If the wire cannot be broken, the entire wire can be withdrawn from the sack and out of the body. This, unfortunately, leaves the "sack" empty and often destined to embolize to a more distal location. Under these circumstances and before withdrawing the wire completely out of the "sack", the "sack" should be grasped with a separate retrieval device and/or the vessel distal to the "sack" selectively occluded with a temporary occlusion balloon unless it is determined that the more distal vessel is expendable if permanently occluded with the embolized empty sack.

When undersized and/or in a very compliant vessel, the entire, full "sack" can embolize distally from its desired site in the abnormal channel. Occasionally this merely occludes the desired channel in a different, but still effective location. If, however, the embolized "sack" migrates into the central or other vital areas of the circulation, the embolized sack must be removed, which cannot be accomplished as a full sack. First, the full bag is snared to hold it in position. If the neck of the sack can be snared, it should not be pulled with any force. Unusual tension on the neck can detach the only radio-opaque part of the bag itself!! Once the bag is grasped, a hole is "chewed" in the bag with a bioptome forceps introduced from a separate vessel and through a slightly larger sheath. Once a hole is created in the full "sack", loops of the packed filler wire usually will extrude immediately through the hole, and/or while "chewing" the hole, a loose portion of the filler wire becomes exposed and is grabbed. The grasped wire then is carefully withdrawn with the forceps while the "sack" is held with the snare or other retrieval device. The emptied bag is then withdrawn utilizing the device that is holding the sack.

In spite of the disadvantages and rare complications, the GGVOD™ has some very specific uses and it should be available to any laboratory heavily engaged in therapeutic catheterizations.

Spring wire alone

The steel wire of a spring guide wire itself is thrombogenic. This property of the wire causes unwanted thrombosis on the wires within the blood stream and within sheaths and catheters. Thrombosis on spring guide wires represents a continual potential for embolic complications. This same property of the wire can be used purposefully to promote thrombosis and/or occlusion in very large abnormal chambers (aneurysms) or channels, either alone or packed on top of other occlusion devices. In order for a spring guide wire to be used as a stimulant to thrombosis and vascular *occlusion*, the wire should be capable of being wadded into a fairly compact mass. Flexibility of the wire is accomplished by removing the straight, stiffening safety core wire(s) from inside of a standard stainless steel spring guide wire. Once the safety core is removed from a spring guide wire, the remaining spring wire becomes very soft and can be compacted easily into a tight mass. Once a guide wire has the core wire removed, several *meters* of 0.025–0.038″ spring wire can be delivered into a 2–3 cm diameter space. Once packed within any confined area that has little or no flow within it, such as a pedunculated aneurysm, thrombosis and obliteration of the area occur very effectively.

Like a "free-release" coil, long spring wires used in this fashion cannot be retracted back into the delivery catheter once the extrusion of the wire has started. If part of the wire inadvertently protrudes out of the specific area being "packed", usually the loose end of the wire can be recaptured with a snare catheter and can be withdrawn completely if it cannot be positioned ideally.

Amplatzer™ Vascular Plug

The Amplatzer™ Vascular Plug (AGA Medical Corp., Golden Valley, MN) is the latest addition to the armamentarium for the occlusion of abnormal vascular communications and is available even in the United States. This unique device is still another modification of the Nitinol™ wire weave or "basket-like" occlusion devices already in common use for the occlusion of the patent ductus, atrial septal defects, patent foramen ovale and ventricular septal defects. The Amplatzer™ Vascular Plugs are small, cylindrical, Nitinol™ wire mesh "plugs", which are available in various diameters, but have no flanges or retention disks at either end of the "plug". The plugs are manufactured of 144 strands of a finer, 0.004″ Nitinol™ wire. Unlike most of the other Amplatzer™ occlusion devices, the vascular plugs have no polyester disks within them and, in turn, rely on the fine mesh of the Nitinol™ metal mesh for occlusion of the vascular structure. Similar to the other Amplatzer™ devices, the plugs do have similar metal posts or markers at the center of each end of the plug, with a female micro screw within the post at the proximal end of the device. The female micro screw allows attachment with an identical screw mechanism to a standard Amplatzer™ delivery cable. The plugs achieve their fixation in the particular vessel by the tension against the wall of the vessel by the expansion of the device against the wall of the vessel/structure similarly to the other Amplatzer™ devices.

The plugs are available in diameters from the smallest of 4 mm increasing in 2 mm increments up to a maximum of 16 mm in diameter. The 4–10 mm plugs are 7 mm long while the 12–16 mm plugs are 8 mm in length. The finer metal wires and the lack of polyester disks allow the plugs to be implanted through smaller delivery systems than the comparably sized Amplatzer™ PDA and VSD occlusion devices. The 4–8 mm diameter devices are delivered through a 5-French, 0.056″ internal diameter sheath, the 10 & 12 mm devices through 6-French, 0.067″ internal diameter sheaths and the 14 & 16 mm devices are delivered through 8-French, 0.088″ internal diameter sheaths.

The Amplatzer™ Vascular Plugs are usable for the occlusion of multiple different venous and arterial structures, all of which, however, must have some "tubular" configuration. This includes residual Blalock–Taussig type shunts, the tubular PDA, systemic to pulmonary collaterals, systemic to pulmonary vein communications, pulmonary arteriovenous fistulae, and even some perivalvular leaks. The diameter of the plug that is used should be 2–3 mm larger than the diameter of the lumen that is to be occluded. The Amplatzer™ Plugs, like the other Amplatzer™ devices, have the advantage of being fully retrievable until they are purposefully released, which makes a test occlusion with the device possible before the operator is committed to releasing the plug.

In addition to "the tubular" characteristics of the lesion, the use of the Amplatzer™ Vascular Plug depends upon the ability to maneuver the delivery catheter into (and past) the lesion that is to be occluded. The current delivery sheath along with the relatively stiff delivery cable precludes the use of the plugs distally in very tortuous locations, while, at the same time, the retrievability of the plug allows its placement more proximally in tortuous vessels where other non-controlled release devices would be inappropriate.

PFM Nit-Occlud™ device for occlusion of abnormal vascular channels

Although designed specifically for the occlusion of the PDA, the Nit-Occlud™ device (PFM, Cologne, Germany) is another effective tool for the occlusion of certain abnormal vessels and vascular channels where precise control over the release is an issue. The Nit-Occlud™ device is discussed in detail for its use for PDA occlusion in Chapter 27. Unfortunately, this device is only available *outside* of the United States and in a limited clinical trial in the US. Nit-Occlud™ devices are tightly wound coils of Nitinol™ wire, which are pre-shaped to conform to several different shapes of "typical" conical PDAs. Like its predecessor, the Duct-Occlud™ device, the Nit-Occlud™ devices have no fibers intertwined in their coil windings to help promote thrombosis/occlusion. Nit-Occlud™

devices depend entirely on the tightness of the coil configurations, the mass of Nitinol™ wire, and the thrombogenicity of the metal itself to occlude the vessels. The precise control/release mechanism of the Nit-Occlud™ device makes it useful in situations in vascular channels where a precise and very controlled positioning is essential. Like the bioptome control for the delivery of standard stainless steel coils, the attach/release system for the Nit-Occlud™ makes the delivery system somewhat stiffer than the usual Gianturco™ type coil delivery catheters which, in turn, makes these devices less useful for lesions in more tortuous vessels and/or circuitous locations. Where it is available outside of the US (and hopefully sometime eventually in the US) the Nit-Occlud™ device should be considered for the occlusion of larger and unusual and/or abnormal vessels/vascular communications/leaks where the placement of the occluder is very precarious.

Catheter delivered detachable vascular occlusion balloons

Several types of detachable occlusion balloon were available around the world and even in the United States in the past. Although still available in some locations around the world, none of the detachable occlusion balloons are available any longer in the US market.

B-D Mini-Balloon™

The B-D Mini-Balloon™ occlusion device (Becton Dickson Co.) probably had the widest use in congenital heart defects when it was available[12]. These were very tiny occlusion devices. The balloons were 1 mm in diameter when deflated and up to 5.3 mm in diameter when inflated. They were delivered "hydraulically" by a unique (and complex) delivery system. The deflated balloon came attached to the tip of a very soft, flexible, 1 mm diameter delivery catheter. This catheter, with the attached deflated balloon, was coiled into a spherical "delivery chamber". These delivery chambers were flattened at two opposite ends, giving the chamber the appearance of a toy "rotating top". The delivery chamber had an inlet and outlet port at the opposite flatter ends of the chamber.

A larger, more maneuverable, guiding catheter, which accommodates the 1 mm delivery catheter, is maneuvered *into* the origin of the vessel to be occluded. The outlet port of the delivery chamber which contained the delivery catheter and attached balloon was attached to the proximal end of the guiding catheter with a Lure-lock connection. By a rapid, forceful, hand flush into an inlet port in the chamber, the delivery catheter with the *deflated* balloon attached at the tip was hydraulically forced into and through the guiding catheter, and from there into the vessel. The catheter with the deflated balloon actually floated along with the flow of the fluid and blood in the vessel. With this delivery technique, the tiny deflated balloon and catheter would traverse almost any bend, curve or loop throughout the course of the vessel. Usually the catheter with the deflated balloon traveled completely through the vessel to, or even past, the end of the vessel. There was, however, no way to direct the course of the balloon/catheter purposefully if there was a branch or bifurcation in the vessel. Once delivered, the fine soft, delivery catheter with the attached deflated balloon was withdrawn slowly until the deflated balloon reached a position precisely at the site within the vessel where the occlusion was to occur.

The balloon then was inflated with a predetermined amount of contrast solution, which was diluted to be exactly isotonic. With this inflation and with the balloon still attached, the degree of occlusion and, of more importance, the tightness of the fixation of the balloon within the vessel were tested. If the balloon migrated distally and/or did not fix securely in a suitable position in the vessel, it was deflated and withdrawn to a different more proximal area or withdrawn completely. If the fixation and occlusion seemed satisfactory, then the balloon was further inflated with several tenths of a ml more of the dilute contrast, which, in turn, fixed the balloon in place more securely and occluded the vessel. The delivery catheter was pulled away forcefully from and out of the "neck" of the "fixed" balloon, hopefully leaving the balloon in place. The B-D Mini-Balloon™ had a self-sealing valve in the neck of the balloon, which kept the balloon inflated after the delivery catheter was pulled out of the valve. The isotonic contrast within the balloon would neither leach in nor out of the balloon, once the balloon was inflated in position. Occasionally, even with this technique, the tiny balloons would work loose and migrate (embolize) more distally—usually with no consequences as long as they remained in the same vessel. A 10 mm occlusion balloon on a 2 mm diameter catheter, which was delivered with the same system, was developed at about the time the entire system/concept was abandoned.

The B-D Mini-Balloon™ had the capability of being able to be delivered through very tortuous channels to otherwise inaccessible locations. At the same time, the delivery technique was quite complex and initially was difficult for many operators to master, so most operators would choose an alternative device (coil) unless the location mandated the use of the occlusion balloon. In addition, because of the balloon material, these occlusion balloons had a definite and relatively short (one year) shelf life before the materials of the balloon deteriorated and became unusable. There have been other detachable "mini-balloons" used sporadically and in isolated cases for the occlusion of congenital heart lesions, but like the B-D Mini-Balloon™ they have been withdrawn from the market, not because of complications, but because of the very small overall market, the small demand for the more complicated balloon occlusion techniques, and the availability of alternative devices which are simpler to use.

A second larger Goldvalve™ Detachable Balloon Embolization Device™ (DB™) was, and may still be, available in Japan. The Goldvalve™ balloons are manufactured of latex and are available in multiple sizes varying from a small 6 mm cylindrical to a large 15 mm diameter, 30 mm long balloon. The Goldvalve™ balloons attached to a 2–3-French delivery catheter are delivered through a 9-French catheter. The 9-French delivery catheter is advanced over a long, stiff wire all of the way to the site for the implant/occlusion and the balloon advanced through the delivery catheter to the site. Once in its proper position the balloon is filled with a 2-hydroxy-ethyl methacrylate (HEMA) solidifying solution. Two different liquid components of the HEMA compound are introduced into the balloon, and because of a glucose oxidase in one of the liquids, the liquids within the balloon spontaneously solidified over 40–60 minutes to form a solid occlusive device[13]. Once the material solidifies, the 9-French outer catheter is pushed against the inflated balloon, the attached small delivery catheter is pulled against the 9-French outer catheter to free it from the balloon, and both catheters are removed.

Because of the necessity of delivering the large 9-French delivery catheter to the lesion, these balloons had no advantages in either delivery or occlusion capabilities compared to standard occlusion coils and other occlusion devices. Because of the relative unknowns of the HEMA materials in the human body over long periods of time, these DB™ devices probably will not make it to the United States.

At this time there are no balloon occlusion devices commercially available on the US market for permanent occlusion of vessels and abnormal vascular channels.

Amplatzer™ PDA & VSD devices for the occlusion of abnormal vascular channels

The Amplatzer™ PDA and VSD occlusion devices (AGA Corp., Golden Valley, MN) are better suited for the occlusion of larger vascular channels than many of the previously discussed devices, and are relatively recent additions to the devices available for the occlusion of abnormal and/or unwanted vascular channels—even in the United States. The Amplatzer PDA and VSD devices are described in detail in Chapters 27 and 30, respectively. There also is the Amplatzer™ Plug (AGA Corp., Golden Valley, MN), which is discussed earlier in this chapter and is somewhat similar to the VSD and PDA devices.

The three devices vary only a little from each other in their design. All three are roughly cylindrical, short, closed tubes of a fine weave of Nitinol™ memory metal. The VSD devices have small 2 mm lips or rims at *each end* of a "cylinder" and the cylinder or hub is not tapered. The central "tube" of the PDA device is tapered slightly and has a rim, but only at the more distal end, which has the slightly larger diameter. The "Plug" is a short cylindrical tube with no "rim" at either end and is manufactured of a finer Nitinol™ wire. Which one of the devices is preferable for any particular vascular channel, depends upon the particular anatomy of the lesion and the flow within the particular channel.

The Amplatzer™ PDA and VSD devices as well as the Plug, all occlude by the same mechanism. The Amplatzer™ devices all self expand into their "resting" configurations in a vascular channel when extruded from their delivery sheath. When the channel is smaller in diameter than the particular device that is used, the device applies pressure against the vessel walls outward and all around the lumen to hold the device in place and fill the lumen of the channel. Although none of these devices was designed specifically for other types of vascular lesions or channels, this mechanism of occlusion does make them ideal for the occlusion of larger abnormal vascular channels/leaks, which are broad, not necessarily very long, and which have high flow through them.

As opposed to the delivery to the PDA or VSD, where the Amplatzer™ devices are positioned more or less straddling the lesion, their delivery to vascular channels and/or fistulae usually involves implanting the devices within the body of the channel or vessel or even in a channel which tapers further distally. As a consequence, these devices, when expanded, potentially fix even more securely into the walls of the channel rather than when "teetering" on a specific area of narrowing. Since these devices are designed to fit into a specific sized defect, when used in vascular channels they often cannot open immediately to their designed, fully expanded size and/or shape. In those circumstances, they initially assume unusual configurations within the vessels, but generally occlude the abnormal channel very completely. With the "memory" of the Nitinol™ metal in these devices, the devices eventually will achieve their designed configuration even within a constrained vessel!

Both the Amplatzer™ VSD and ASD devices have been used in a variety of abnormal vascular channels in patients outside of the United States and in a few extenuating, compassionate circumstances in the US. Now the Amplatzer™ muscular VSD device, the Amplatzer™ PDA devices and the Amplatzer™ Plugs are available for use in the United States. This does give physicians around the world including in the US, a better choice of occlusion devices in order to be able to use the most appropriate device for the occlusion of unusual and/or large vascular channels.

Atrial septal occluders for miscellaneous vascular occlusions

Occasionally there are vascular channels that require occlusion that are very large in diameter and relatively short. All of these lesions are large enough in diameter to be hemodynamically significant, yet so short in length that they will not accommodate any of the more common and accepted vascular occlusion devices without compromising the adjacent vital blood channels that are connected by the abnormal communication. These very large diameter channels include but are not limited to the afferent vessels of pulmonary arteriovenous fistulae, anomalous left superior vena cava draining into the left atrium, and persistent azygos/hemiazygos veins following "Glenn" type shunts. In these cases, an Amplatzer™ ASD device (AGA Corp., Golden Valley, MN), an Amplatzer™ PFO device (AGA Corp., Golden Valley, MN), a Rashkind™ PDA device (USCI, Glens Falls, NY) a CardioSEAL™ ASD device (NMT Medical Inc., Boston, MA) and a Sideris Button™ device (Pediatric Cardiology Custom Medical Devices, Athens, Greece) all can be of an appropriate size and configuration to fit into, and all of these devices have been used to occlude, these unusual communications. Some persistent aortic pulmonary communications that were created surgically (Waterston-Cooley or Potts shunts) are very short, they have high flow, and they are present between very large, high-pressure and very essential vessels. As a consequence, they require a very low-profile and sturdy device for occlusion.

These devices and their delivery to their designed lesions are described in detail in Chapters 28 ("ASD Occlusion") and Chapter 29 ("PFO, Fenestration, and Baffle Occlusions"). In the large diameter, short and more or less, "flat" lesions between two large, adjacent "tubes" (great arteries), the positioning and fixation of the device in the vessel are critical in order to prevent "movement" of the device during or after implant. The occlusion of the short aortopulmonary vascular communications often involves a more circuitous route to the lesion in order to deliver a device, and the implant procedure usually requires a very unusual and/or acute angle for the delivery of the device. This makes the delivery to these unusual locations more difficult and the release/implant of the device more precarious. Once the delivery sheath is in position through the lesion while at the same time, *not kinking the sheath*, the particular device extrusion and implant is similar to the device delivery into an atrial septal defect/PFO.

Caval filters or Cook "Spider"

Rarely there are *very* large diameter, abnormal, venous channels and/or communications with very compliant walls that require occlusion. Because these veins distend very easily and extensively, none of the previously described devices can be fixed securely in the vessels. In these vessels, the Spider™ device (Cook Inc., Bloomington, IN) is used as a "scaffold" or framework for the implant of other devices, particularly coils. The Spider™ "springs" into a broad, spread-out configuration as it is pushed out of its delivery catheter and attaches to the walls of the vessel by tiny, very sharp hooks in addition to the spring tension of the arms of the device against the vessel wall. The Spider™ itself is not occlusive, but other devices such as coils are intertwined in the Spider™ to form an occlusive mass.

Stents as a scafold for occlusion devices

Although designed for, and used primarily for, maintaining the patency of vessels, specially prepared intravascular stents are used to assist in the occlusion of very large diameter channels/vessels[14]. The stents are used in a manner similar to the previously described Spider™ as a "scaffold" for coils or other occlusions devices. By fixing the center of the stent at a restricted diameter by means of a circumferential suture tied around the stent when it is mounted on the balloon, a large diameter stent can be expanded purposefully into an "hour-glass" shape. The suture is "woven" into the spaces between the struts of the collapsed stent and tied around the stent in a circumference with a small fixed diameter before the stent is mounted on the delivery balloon. The diameter of the suture around the stent maintains the center of the stent expanded only to the desired restricted diameter of the suture. When the stent is expanded on a large diameter balloon (15+ mm), the ends of the stent flare widely with this "narrowing" at the center of the stent creating an "hour-glass" configuration of the stent. With the center of the stent fixed at the narrow diameter by the suture, the tendency of the ends of the stent to extend and align almost perpendicular to the walls of the particular vessel/channel is exaggerated even more than usual. The very sharp ends of each strut of particularly the J & J P _ _ 8 or P _ _ 10 stents create sharp fixation points into the wall of the vessel. This fixes the stent very securely in the vessel. A stent can be implanted using this technique and using a P _ _ 10 stent, into vessels/channels up to 25 mm in diameter. Once the stent is in place, then coils and/or occlusion devices can be intertwined into or packed into the "afferent end" of the stent/vessel to achieve the occlusion of the vessel.

Covered stents

Another mechanism with which intravascular stents are used to "occlude" vessels is by the use of "covered stents" to purposefully occlude side or branching vessels and/or tears in the wall off a main channel/vessel. The covered stent will cover all areas that are adjacent to the stent and prevent flow into those vessels and other abnormal openings/tears. This is a very selected use and requires the availability of a covered stent of the exact diameter of the torn central or main channel or vessel. The covered stents are available commercially only for adult peripheral vascular use and/or in investigational studies. For use in the isolated congenital patient, commercially manufactured covered stents have been available only for compassionate use in very extenuating circumstances. More frequently the stents are modified extensively from the commercially available covered stents and/or hand fashioned using ultrathin expanded polytetrafluoroethylene (ePTFE, Gore-Tex™) membranes (W. L. Gore & Associates, Flagstaff, AZ) over existing intravascular stents of appropriate size for the involved vessel[15]. The ultrathin ePTFE material has a considerable capability of stretching acutely so that each diameter of ePTFE tubing can be used with several sizes of stents. However, none of the means of acquiring and producing covered stents for congenital heart patients in the United States are rapid enough or satisfactory for emergency use. For such use, the stent should be available immediately from the inventory of the catheterization laboratory for emergency use.

Except in emergencies, the covered stents probably only should be used in fully-grown patients since there is no suggestion or information about the ability to re-dilate the covering materials on the stents even months, much less years, after implant and/or in the presence of significant growth of the vessels. At the same time, in a life-threatening emergency, the use of a covered stent that was rapidly available and of a size to fit even a small vessel would be preferable to massive blood loss and exsanguination from an acute vascular tear.

Occlusion procedures for specific lesions

Systemic to pulmonary collaterals

The systemic to pulmonary collateral vessels originate from the aorta or from major branches off the aorta. They usually are relatively long, tortuous, tubular lesions of varying diameters throughout their course and usually have one or more discrete narrowing as they course distally into the pulmonary parenchyma. Because of this anatomy the occluding device usually does not have to "fix" tightly against the vessel wall and, in fact, almost is expected to move distally a small distance after release. The anatomy of these lesions makes them the ideal lesions for occlusion with "free-release" Gianturco™ coils. The most difficult part of the occlusion of these lesions frequently is the initial access into, and then obtaining a secure position *well within*, the vessel. The cannulation of some of the collaterals often requires a great deal of imagination as well as a large inventory of specific catheters and/or deflector wires. Very often, a more secure access into a collateral off the descending aorta is achieved when the catheter is approaching from the ascending aorta to the descending aorta. This approach to the collateral vessel can be accomplished through a co-existing ventricular septal defect, through a transseptal atrial septal puncture in conjunction with the use of a floating balloon catheter, or by introduction of the catheter into a brachial artery.

The collateral vessels that come directly off the aorta usually are entered directly with the catheter for the delivery of the coil. Those vessels arising more remotely off a brachiocephalic branch of the aorta, those with a very tortuous course, and/or those where the occlusion must be accomplished in a more circuitous and distal location in the vessel, often require the use of a separate "guide catheter" to engage the orifice of the main collateral vessel. Then, a small, very flexible, or even "floating" smaller delivery catheter such as the Target Tracker™ catheter (Target Therapeutics, Fremont, CA) or the Cook Slip-Cath™ (Cook Inc., Bloomington, IN) is passed through the guide catheter to deliver the smaller coils and maneuvered to a more secure distal location into the vessel that is to be occluded.

The exact type and size of coil that is used depend upon the access to the vessel as well as the length and the diameter of the vessel. The "free-release" Gianturco™ and Tornado™ coils usually are ideal for the smaller vessels with sufficient length to accommodate several "compacted" coils placed in series. In the same size but shorter length vessels or in vessels where multiple coils already have been implanted and are filling the vessel back to or near the orifice of the entrance from the main vessel, a controlled release coil or device is desirable. Using a controlled release coil during the extrusion of the final coil, if the entire coil does not fit completely and securely within the vessel to be occluded, the detachable coil can be withdrawn, repositioned, "packed" into the vessel, or even completely and simply withdrawn.

The 0.052" coils (Cook Inc., Bloomington, IN), particularly with a bioptome-controlled release system, are very good for the occlusion of larger diameter collaterals in smaller patients. As long as the vessel that is to be occluded does not arise too acutely off the aorta, these coils can be delivered through as small as a 4-French sheath. The controlled release allows repositioning, or even complete withdrawal of the coil if either the position and/or occlusion are not satisfactory. In the larger patient with a large, longer collateral, the Gianturco-Grifka Vascular Occlusion Device™ (GGVOD™) (Cook Inc., Bloomington, IN) and the Amplatzer™ plug (AGA

Medical Corp., Golden Valley, MN) are excellent choices for these occlusions. The use of the GGVOD™ and the larger diameter plugs is dependent upon being able to use an 8-French delivery sheath safely through an arterial approach and to have the stiff sheath make the acute curve from the aorta into the collateral.

Surgical shunts

Occasionally, systemic to pulmonary shunts persist after "corrective" surgery and require closure following a previous repair of the underlying congenital lesion. Although the "Blalock" and "modified Blalock" shunts are similar to the collateral vessels in that they are tubular "vessels", the remaining characteristics of the shunts are very different. The shunt, which is created surgically, usually arises at a very acute angle off the base of a brachiocephalic vessel, which, in turn, makes access into the shunt from the arterial approach very difficult. The "modern" shunts usually are made of synthetic materials that are very noncompliant, they usually are uniform in diameter with no tortuosity, no narrowing and no distal tapering, which makes the fixation of an occlusion device within a Blalock type shunt depend entirely upon the firm pressure of the occluder against the walls of the shunt.

The "free-release" Gianturco™ coil is still the most commonly used device for transcatheter occlusion of these lesions. The larger, 0.038″ or preferably, 0.052″ coils are used to ensure firm pressure against the walls of the shunt. Ancillary maneuvers frequently are employed to assure the fixation of the coils in these shunts. Occasionally, there is a narrowing of the *pulmonary artery* at the entrance/anastomosis site of the shunt into the pulmonary artery. In this circumstance and when the patient is large enough to accommodate it, an intravascular stent can be implanted in the pulmonary vessel in the area of the stenosis, which will *cross* the exit orifice of the shunt. This effectively "jails" the exit of the shunt and allows coils to be packed into the shunt against the struts of the stent, which are crossing the orifice of the shunt into the pulmonary artery.

When there is no stenosis of the shunt and/or no stenosis of the pulmonary artery (or the patient is not a candidate for a pulmonary artery stent), an angioplasty type balloon can be inflated in the pulmonary artery across the distal end of the shunt for the purpose of temporarily occluding flow through the shunt while the coils are being implanted. The balloon inflation is maintained as coils or other devices are placed in the shunt. The inflated balloon occludes the distal end of the shunt and stops blood flow through the shunt while coils are packed and intertwined with each other within the shunt. Unfortunately, this technique is not foolproof. Unless the coils are packed very tightly against the walls of the shunt and/or when the coils are placed in a shunt with a very uniform diameter and/or no distal narrowing, the implanted coils still can embolize into the pulmonary artery when the balloon is deflated.

A sturdy, 0.038″ or even 0.052″ *controlled release* coil is the preferred device for the residual surgical shunt which has no narrowing within its lumen. The controlled release coil is implanted in the shunt and, before the coil is released, *tension* on the attached delivery wire is relaxed. In this way the coil is allowed to reposition itself within the shunt and usually, if it is not going to hold, the coil will pass through the shunt and to the pulmonary artery while still attached to the delivery, attach/release wire. When this occurs with the coil still attached, the coil can be withdrawn into the delivery catheter.

Another alternative for occluding residual surgical shunts is to deliver a much sturdier device into the shunt from the venous/pulmonary artery approach. A 0.052″ coil, a Gianturco-Grifka Bag™, or even a small Amplatzer™ Vascular Plug can be delivered from the venous approach. The venous and pulmonary artery approach may have a straighter course to the shunt. The venous introduction and straighter course allow the use of a larger and/or stiffer delivery system.

An end-hole catheter introduced into the venous system is manipulated into the pulmonary artery where the shunt enters, into the shunt from the pulmonary artery end of the shunt, through the shunt and into the aorta. The catheter is replaced with an exchange length, long floppy tipped, Super Stiff™ wire. The specific delivery catheter/sheath for the device to be used is advanced over the wire through the venous system and into the shunt. The dilator and wire are removed, the sheath is cleared of all air and/or clot and placed on a slow flush. Once the delivery catheter/sheath is in place *through the shunt*, the device is delivered to the site within the shunt for implant/occlusion. With the device maintained in the precise position, the sheath is withdrawn, which, in turn, deploys the device in the shunt. The degree of occlusion is verified with an angiogram, injecting into the arterial end of the shunt through a separate catheter.

Occasionally, entry with any catheter or wire into the shunt from the pulmonary artery end is very difficult or even impossible. In that circumstance, an exchange length, floppy tipped, 0.035″ wire is advanced through an end-hole catheter, which is passed retrograde from the artery, through the shunt and into the pulmonary artery. The end of the wire is snared in the pulmonary artery with a snare introduced from a vein and advanced through the right heart to the pulmonary artery. Once snared, the wire is withdrawn through the right ventricle, right atrium and out of the venous system, creating a through-and-through wire, which passes through the shunt. The delivery system for the occlusion device can then be advanced over the wire from the venous approach and into the shunt for venous delivery of the desired device.

Short, large-diameter aorto-pulmonary communications

Congenital aorto-pulmonary (A-P) windows and residual, direct aortic to pulmonary artery (Cooley–Waterston or Potts) shunts can be occluded with devices in the catheterization laboratory. Coils are unsatisfactory for these lesions because of the very short, broad, "window" nature of these communications. The most satisfactory device for these "window-like" shunts is one of the "double umbrellas". The double umbrella (Rashkind™ PDA, Clamshell™ and CardioSEAL™ ASD) devices, the Sideris double umbrella modification of the Inverted Button™, and a modified Amplatzer™ ASD device all have been used to occlude this type of lesion[16–18].

A-P window type communications are occluded from either the arterial or venous approach. The choice of approach depends upon the vascular access for the particular approach and which approach gives the best "angle" from the vessel into the lesion for the implant of the device and, in turn, the best control over the particular delivery system. Because these communications essentially are part of, and parallel to, the walls of the adjacent vessels and the vessels have *relatively* small diameters compared to a cardiac chamber, there usually is *no good* angle for the delivery of any one of these devices! The devices initially used for these lesions required an 11-French delivery sheath, however, the Amplatzer™ PFO device potentially can be delivered through a smaller sheath. Because of the sheath size, the venous approach is preferred when all of the other factors in the choice in the approach are otherwise equal.

The congenital or residual surgical A-P communication is identified and measured accurately by echocardiogram and by selective angiograms with injection immediately adjacent to the systemic arterial side of the lesion and/or actually within the communication. The X-ray tubes are angled so that the communication is "cut on edge" at least in one plane. Once identified and measured, the defect is crossed with an end-hole catheter. Preferably, a through-and-through, artery to vein wire "rail" is created with an exchange length wire. The catheter/wire can be introduced from either the arterial or venous approach and then captured with a snare catheter, which is introduced from the opposite vascular access. When there is any question about the size and/or configuration of the defect, the communication can be sized and "shaped" using a NuMED™ sizing balloon (NuMED Inc., Hopkinton, NY) advanced over the wire. It is advantageous, if not essential, to have a second systemic arterial catheter to be used for "positioning" angiograms during the procedure.

For occlusion of the "window type" communication with any of these devices, a long delivery sheath first is positioned *through* the defect with great care taken not to kink the sheath because of the unfavorable angles involved. The through-and-through wire facilitates the delivery considerably of the delivery sheath/dilator through the communication. Once the delivery sheath is through the defect and the wire and dilator are removed, the "umbrella" type devices are delivered exactly as for the occlusion of a PDA with the old Rashkind™ PDA device or the occlusion of a fenestration with a CardioSEAL™ device. The distal umbrella/disk is opened on the "distal" side of the defect. The sheath, the delivery system and the device are withdrawn as a unit, pulling the open umbrella/disk tightly against the defect. The device may have to be pulled very firmly against the defect, in which case, the device becomes markedly distorted, very similar to the delivery of an umbrella/disk during the closure of a fenestration, particularly where there is a long communication. Usually, the vessel walls surrounding and adjacent to A-P communications are fairly rigid and the defects are small, so that a marked distortion of the device from the strong "pull" on the device against the vessel wall is possible during the delivery without pulling the device through the defect. When the center "hinge" or "hub" of the device is within and/or through the defect and the proximal legs/disk still are within the delivery sheath but completely through the defect, the sheath alone is withdrawn, opening the proximal umbrella/disk on the more "proximal" side of the defect. After angiographic confirmation with an injection on the systemic arterial side of the lesion, the device is released. The device often reorients itself markedly after release from the torsion of an acutely angled delivery system.

Coronary cameral fistulae

Closure of most coronary-cameral fistulae with a catheter-delivered device in the cardiac catheterization laboratory now is the standard approach for these lesions. The fistulae arise off either the right, left and/or any branch or combination of branches off the coronary arterial system. They usually have a fairly long and often tortuous course and empty into a right-sided cardiac chamber or the pulmonary artery. They rarely empty into the left atrium or even the left ventricle. The choice of device and delivery technique depends upon the specific anatomy of the fistulae, the length of the fistulous tract and the distance away from the true and essential coronary arteries. Test occlusion of the fistula with a balloon is recommended in all cases to help to define the anatomy and distensibility of the fistulous tract, and to determine if there is any myocardial tissue dependent on the blood supply off the fistula. This is tested by the inflation of a small Swan™ balloon in the fistula tract while observing the electrocardiogram very closely for any ST-T wave changes.

A retrograde, end-hole arterial catheter is introduced into the "feeding" coronary artery and maneuvered into the fistula as far as possible using torque-controlled and/or Glide™ wires as necessary. The fistula is defined angiographically with *selective* coronary angiograms into the feeding coronary artery or, preferably, into the orifice of the fistula itself. Multiple views are obtained to define the course, branchings, narrowing and the site of emptying of the fistula. Often there is a narrowing and/or an acute tortuosity in the fistula tract, which will help to fix an occlusion device.

An exchange guide wire is passed far into, and if possible, completely through the fistula. The original catheter is replaced over the wire with a small Swan™ end-hole, balloon catheter or a very short, small balloon angioplasty catheter, which is to be used for sizing and test occlusion. Several (multiple) *low-pressure* test inflations at different locations along the fistulous tract are performed with the balloon. It is useful to have a second arterial catheter already in position in the aortic root or even in the selective coronary artery in order to perform small selective angiograms in the aortic root and/or in the coronary artery proximal to the fistula and the site of test occlusion. In addition to the degree of occlusion of the fistula, this injection demonstrates additional tracts off the fistula and any significantly under-perfused areas of the myocardium distal to the balloon occlusion.

When the fistula is to be closed from the retrograde arterial approach, the balloon catheter in the fistula is replaced over the exchange wire with an end-hole only, torque-controlled catheter. The end-hole catheter is passed as far distally in the fistula as is possible. A "free-release" type coil is satisfactory for coronary-cameral fistulae *only* when (1) there is no myocardial tissue dependent on the flow from the proximal fistula, (2) there is a long tract of the fistula that is distal to the origin of the fistula off the true coronary system and (3) the delivery catheter can be manipulated reasonably easily and far distally into the fistula. With lesions that fulfill these criteria, the coils usually are delivered from the retrograde approach through a catheter maneuvered selectively into the fistula from the feeding coronary artery.

When delivered retrograde, the occlusion device is implanted as far *distally* in the fistulous tract and as far away from the orifice of the fistula off the true coronary artery as possible. The distal location keeps the coil away from the true coronary vessel and allows the deposit of additional coils more proximally in the fistula. Once the delivery catheter is in position for the coil delivery, a selective angiogram is recorded in the fistula through this catheter to verify the precise location. A coil for occlusion of the fistula is chosen which is 1–2 mm larger in diameter than the "balloon sized" diameter of the lumen of the fistula. The coil must expand against the walls of the fistula in order to fix the coil in place in a non-stenotic location. In a fistula with a significant narrowing and/or an area of acute tortuosity more distally in the fistula, a coil is chosen just larger than the diameter *proximal* to the narrowing or to straddle a specific narrowing similar to the retrograde implant of a coil into the "narrowing" of the PDA. How the coil is delivered into the fistula depends upon the precise anatomy, and is different in each case. At least 2–3 minutes after the first coil is implanted, the degree of occlusion is tested with a repeat selective injection into the fistula through the coil delivery catheter. Frequently there are residual leaks through one, or even several, coils in a coronary-cameral fistula. Leaving a small residual leak through the fistulae, particularly with the coils in place, increases the patient's likelihood of developing endarteritis in the future, and when there is a "jet" of residual leak through the coils, there also is a high chance of creating hemolysis.

Several (or multiple) more coils are deposited in the fistula sequentially until the flow through the fistula is stopped. The choice of the additional coils depends upon the residual anatomy and the remaining proximal length of the fistula. Additional coils are intertwined with the initial (earlier) coils to prevent their movement backward toward the coronary artery. When the most proximal coils will be close to the entrance of the fistula from the coronary artery, a *controlled release coil* and technique are used for the final coil(s).

The prograde venous (retrograde into the fistula) approach for the transcatheter closure of some coronary-cameral fistulae has several distinct advantages over the retrograde arterial approach. Fewer catheter manipulations are required in and/or through the somewhat precarious true coronary arteries and the central arterial system in general. Larger and stiffer (less bendable) delivery systems can be introduced from the venous approach than from the retrograde arterial approach. This extends the options to a larger variety of occlusion devices that can be used to occlude coronary-cameral fistulae. From the venous approach, the delivery sheaths for the large 0.052" coils and Duct-Occlud™ device as well as the larger sheaths for the Gianturco-Grifka™ Bag, the Amplatzer™ Vascular Plug or the Amplatzer™ muscular VSD occluders can be positioned in the fistula without kinking the sheaths and without compromising the systemic arterial entrance site and/or the proximal coronary arteries themselves.

In order to establish the venous access to the fistula, it almost always is necessary first to create an arterial to venous, through-and-through wire. The catheter/wire is introduced from the arterial approach, into the coronary artery, through the fistula and into the venous circulation, where the wire is snared with a catheter introduced from a vein. The introduction site for the venous catheter should be from the peripheral vein (femoral or jugular) that will give the best angle of approach into the distal end of the fistula. An end-hole retrograde catheter is introduced into the feeding coronary artery and from there, manipulated into the origin of the fistula. A torque-controlled, floppy tipped or curved tip Glide™ wire is maneuvered through the fistula and into the "exit chamber" of the fistula within the heart. The distal end of the wire is snared at the "venous" end, where it exits the fistula and is exteriorized through the venous entry site.

The retrograde catheter should remain over the arterial end of the wire while the delivery catheter or sheath/dilator is advanced from the venous end of the through-and-through wire and into the fistula. The arterial catheter over the wire protects the tissues within the coronary artery from damage by the bare wire and allows a continuous flush around the wire to prevent clotting in the coronary system. The tip of the delivery catheter/sheath is positioned according to both the anatomy of the fistula and what type of device is being used. In general, the tip of the delivery catheter/sheath is positioned just proximal (in the direction of blood flow in the fistula) to the location where the device(s) is(are) to be implanted. Once the delivery catheter/sheath is securely in position, the through-and-through wire is withdrawn through the arterial catheter and the catheter is cleared carefully of any air and/or *clot*. The retrograde *arterial* catheter remains positioned in the coronary artery in the end of the fistula or at least in the coronary artery just proximal to the fistula. The retrograde catheter is used to perform sequential selective angiograms during the positioning and delivery of the device(s) and/or to add additional occlusion devices after the implant of the original device.

An occlusion device/coil is chosen which is appropriate for the particular anatomy of the coronary fistula. When delivered from the venous approach the choice of type and size of device is much greater, allowing the delivery of very retrievable devices such as the Amplatzer™ vascular plug and the GGVOD™ devices. When delivered from the venous approach, the device is implanted in the fistula straddling an area of narrowing or *proximal* (in the direction of blood flow) to any areas of narrowing and/or sharp bends in the fistulous tract, but at the same time distal to any true coronary artery branches off the fistula. The one disadvantage to the venous approach is that subsequent devices that are delivered through the same delivery system, must be implanted "downstream" or *distal in the flow* from the original device and often into a larger diameter area of the fistula than the site of the original device. The "downstream" devices, which are predominately coils, may not fix in the vessel as securely, and complete occlusion is less likely. Any subsequent device and, in particular, coils delivered in a "downstream" location must be significantly larger than the diameter of the fistula in that location and must be "intertwined" and attached to the original device.

It always is preferable to implant additional coils/devices proximal to the original device. If additional coils are to be delivered from the *venous side* and are to be placed proximal to the first device, a delivery catheter must be *advanced through and/or past the original device* and into the more proximal fistula without dislodging the original device/coil. This is accomplished using a Terumo Glide™ (Boston Scientific, Natick, MA) wire and a tiny, end-hole-only catheter similar to crossing a freshly implanted coil in a PDA. As the coil is being extruded from the catheter, which has passed through/past the original device/coil, the catheter is withdrawn into, or adjacent to, the original device/coil in order to catch or entwine the additional coil(s) on the original device/coil.

A preferable technique for the implant of additional coils proximal to the original device, which was delivered from the venous approach, and particularly when the first device is implanted distally in the fistula away from the entrance of the fistula off the coronary artery, is to deliver additional coils "upstream" through the *retrograde catheter* that is already positioned in the proximal part of the fistula. Using a *controlled-release system* additional coils are "stacked on top of" the original device to complete the occlusion. Often, with a very large coronary-cameral fistula, this combination of venous and arterial approaches is the planned procedure.

In certain circumstances during the catheter occlusion of coronary-cameral fistulae it is imperative to use a controlled-release device for the delivery of the occlusion device. The presence of a particularly short fistulous tract and particularly one with a wide orifice off the true coronary system necessitates a controlled-release device. A fistula of any length into which multiple coils are implanted and when the next, and most proximal, coil must be implanted near the true coronary artery, is the other definite indication for a controlled-release system. In these circumstances, the coil and/or any other type of device must be retrievable immediately in the event that the device or part of the device extends back into the lumen of the true coronary artery during the delivery of the device. The tip of a coil with its attached filament strands dangling into the lumen of a true coronary artery is very likely to shed thrombotic emboli into the high flow in the coronary artery and can result in infarction of myocardium distal to that area.

Pulmonary arteriovenous fistulae

Pulmonary arteriovenous (AV) fistulae can be congenital or "acquired", they can be isolated or multiple, they can occur in thousands and they can be large or small. These lesions *can be* occluded with catheter-delivered devices. How they are occluded and with what particular device are determined by the exact anatomy of the lesion(s). Each pulmonary AV "fistula" may have several afferent and efferent vessels. The central communicating vessels *usually* are small, tortuous and restrictive, but can be relatively large and even form an almost straight communication from the pulmonary artery to the pulmonary vein.

The rare, isolated, congenital pulmonary AV fistula usually is large, with multiple and usually tortuous afferent pulmonary arterial and efferent pulmonary venous channels. The size(s) of the major central AV communication(s) through the fistula is(are) determined by detailed angiography. An occluding device significantly larger than the major central communicating AV channel must be used initially to prevent the occlusion device from passing through the fistula and into the pulmonary vein/systemic circulation. The goal is to occlude the major afferent channel(s) while, at the same time, occluding no, or as few as possible, normal pulmonary arterial vessels, which supply adjacent normal lung tissue. In the presence of multiple channels, test occlusions of the various afferent channels using a balloon angiographic catheter or a Swan™ balloon catheter is performed to determine the largest and/or most significant feeding vessel(s). In most cases, the actual communication between the artery and vein is relatively small and one or many standard "free-release" Gianturco™ coils can be used for the occlusion. When the communication is large, the large 0.052" coils, the Gianturco-Grifka™ bag, the Amplatzer™ PDA, VSD devices or vascular Plug or even an "umbrella" occluding device all can be used to at least begin the occlusion in these lesions. Once a larger device is in place, standard Gianturco™ coils can be packed proximally to the larger device in the afferent channel to complete the occlusion of that particular vessel/segment.

Biplane fluoroscopic and angiographic systems are absolutely essential for the treatment of these lesions. The branching pulmonary arteries are very "three-dimensional" and arise at multiple angles to, and at different planes from, each other. The branches of the arteries to be occluded must be cannulated selectively, and then subselectively. A single-plane system does not provide the depth relationships for this precise cannulation. Probing with a single-plane system results in exponential increases in the radiation use/exposure and of the amount of contrast used for localizing and cannulating any specific lesion.

It is desirable to have a second venous angiographic catheter, which is positioned selectively in the pulmonary artery and immediately adjacent to the delivery catheter for the occlusion device. Once the precise afferent vessel has been identified, it is cannulated selectively with an end-hole catheter. The catheter is replaced with an exchange length, short tipped, 0.035" Super Stiff™ wire. The delivery dilator/sheath set with a sheath appropriate for the device to be used is advanced over the wire into the major afferent vessel and *as close to the fistulous communication as possible*. Multiple normal pulmonary artery branches, which supply vital normal lung tissue, usually arise off the major afferent pulmonary artery proximal to the fistula. The more proximally the occlusion is performed in the afferent pulmonary artery that feeds the fistula, the greater the number of vital vessels that supply the normal adjacent functional lung parenchyma will be occluded.

The occlusion device is introduced into the precisely positioned sheath and extruded as accurately as is possible into the exact location and released. Before release of the device, an angiogram is performed through the second venous catheter to determine the effectiveness of the first occlusion device and to determine the location(s) of the next most important afferent vessel(s). With residual flow through the fistula from this artery, either a second large device is implanted through the same delivery catheter or a coil delivery catheter is introduced through the delivery sheath and the occlusion is completed with supplemental coils packed proximal to the original device in the afferent vessel of the fistula.

Once the first feeding artery is occluded, the delivery sheath/catheter is repositioned into the next most important feeding vessel and the procedure repeated. Once the initial, larger vessels are occluded, the remaining vessels may be occluded more satisfactorily with a different and/or smaller device. In that case the original delivery sheath/catheter is exchanged for the delivery sheath/catheter for the different device or the new delivery catheter is advanced to the lesion through the original delivery sheath/catheter. The procedure is repeated until the individual fistula is occluded. Each time an occlusion device is implanted, it is important to perform the implant as close to the lesion as possible.

In the presence of multiple pulmonary arteriovenous fistulae, patients often are very cyanotic and very symptomatic. At the same time, there usually are too many separate pulmonary AV fistulae to consider occluding all of them. In the very symptomatic patient, the largest and most important AV lesions are identified with detailed angiography and an attempt is made to occlude as many of the major fistulae as possible without further compromising the remaining normal lung tissue. This, of course, does not cure the patient, but often, enough of the lesions can be occluded to provide a significant, albeit temporary, symptomatic palliation for the patient. The technique is the same for multiple fistulae as for an isolated large fistula. The exact device and the technique used are determined from the selective angiographic anatomy of the individual lesions. With each successful occlusion of one or more *significant* lesions, the patient's systemic arterial saturation rises slightly. If this does not occur after the occlusion of three or four *more significant* fistulae, the patient probably will not receive benefit from further occlusions.

The multiple diffuse (thousands) of tiny pulmonary arteriovenous fistulae seen frequently after isolated superior caval to pulmonary artery anastomoses are not directly amenable to occlusion therapy. The exception is when there are a few separate large fistulae associated with the other multiple diffuse tiny fistulae. These larger systemic to pulmonary fistulae can, and should, be occluded. Even with the multiple small fistulae, occlusion of associated larger pulmonary fistulae provides some symptomatic relief for the patient.

The approach to the multiple tiny pulmonary arteriovenous fistulae is to anticipate their development, and in turn, prevent their occurrence by proceeding with the completion of the connection of the inferior vena cava so that hepatic blood flow *reaches both lungs*. Even after these multiple tiny pulmonary A-V fistulae have appeared, the patient's systemic saturations seem to improve with the completion of the inferior caval connection to both lungs, even though the multiple tiny fistulae do not, objectively, seem to regress.

Systemic artery to pulmonary artery and veno-venous collaterals post "Fontan corrections"

The complete caval-pulmonary repair of single ventricle lesions has created a whole new spectrum of systemic artery to pulmonary artery and systemic vein to pulmonary vein collaterals/fistulae. These are usually small but can be multiple and/or very large, especially some of the hepatic vein to pulmonary venous fistulae. Regardless of the size of an individual fistula, each fistula provides "competition" to the flow to the already precarious, "forward" pulmonary blood flow, produces extra volume on the "single ventricle" and/or creates a "right to left" shunt with systemic desaturation of the patient. These abnormal vascular communications usually are *not* obvious from clinical or noninvasive studies. They are detected only during a cardiac catheterization and then, only when they are looked for specifically with selective angiography. These abnormal fistulae arise from any systemic artery or vein within the thorax, neck or even from the abdomen. The arteries communicate with the pulmonary arteries, the pulmonary veins and/or even the systemic veins. The systemic venous channels communicate with the pulmonary veins and/or with other systemic veins draining to an entirely different systemic venous bed. The arterial communications usually are small tortuous channels but on aortography or systemic venous angiography, the pulmonary arteries and/or veins light up with contrast long before the normal "recirculation" from the pulmonary arteries has time to reach the pulmonary veins. When a catheterization is performed for any reason on any of these single ventricle, "Fontan" type patients, these lesions should be looked for specifically while the patient is in the catheterization laboratory and when found, occluded.

The major challenge in occluding these lesions is locating and then cannulating their origins off the systemic arterial or systemic venous systems. Once located and cannulated, they usually are occluded quite simply with free-release coils or other available occlusion devices. The smaller of these lesions are ideal for the small Tornado™ (Cook Inc., Bloomington, IN) or Target™ (Target Therapeutics, Fremont, CA) coils and delivery systems. The hepatic vein to pulmonary venous fistulae usually are much larger and require one or more of the larger occluding systems. Fortunately, access to these hepatic to pulmonary venous channels is usually directly from the central hepatic veins, allowing introduction of the larger, stiffer delivery systems for the large coils, Gianturco-Grifka™ bags (Cook Inc., Bloomington, IN) or one of the Amplatzer™ occlusion devices (AGA Medical Corp., Golden Valley, MN).

In 2004, most of the abnormal vascular communications were treated in the catheterization laboratory with the available devices even in the United States. With the addition of the devices that are on the horizon in protocol studies in the US and/or routinely available in the rest of the world, even more of these lesions will be amenable to catheter therapy. The catheter management of all abnormal vascular communications will be safer and more widely distributed with the introduction of a wider choice of devices that are more appropriate for specific lesions.

Occlusion of aortic root/coronary sinus to left ventricular tunnels

Congenital tunnels from the aorta to the left ventricle are rare fistulous tracts, which usually present in infancy. The combination of the clinical findings of a nondescript systolic murmur, which is followed immediately by a long diastolic, decrescendo murmur over the base of the heart and in association with a widened pulse pressure are indistinguishable from the findings of aortic valve regurgitation. The diagnosis of an aortic to left ventricular tunnel is made by echocardiogram and confirmed with an aortic root angiocardiogram. A biplane angiogram is necessary to determine the precise origin, the course and the exit of the tunnel and to obtain accurate measurements of the diameter of various areas of the tunnel. Generally, these lesions have a fairly straight origin off the aortic root, are some distance from the aortic valve and coronary arteries and, as a consequence, are very amenable to occlusion with a catheter-delivered device.

Once the tunnel has been identified angiographically, it is cannulated selectively with a floppy tipped spring guide wire and then a catheter over the wire. Selective angiograms are recorded with injections directly into the tunnel in order to define the anatomy of the tunnel more precisely. The X-ray tubes are angled in order to align the tunnel on edge and in its longest dimension. If there is any question about the anatomy and/or diameters of the tunnel, the guide wire is passed through the tunnel into the left ventricle and a Swan™ floating balloon catheter is advanced over the wire into the tunnel. The balloon is inflated very gently and at a low pressure within the tunnel and, if the tunnel has any significant length, in several different locations along the course of the tunnel. The balloon inflation in the tunnel provides information about the distensibility of the fistulous tract and how the patient will tolerate an occlusive device in the tunnel. The combined angiographic and "sizing" information determines the most appropriate device for occlusion of the tunnel. A static sizing balloon would give the same or better information, but would require the use of a 9-French sheath in the artery!

The tunnels usually are large relative to the patient's size and all of the tunnels from aorta to left ventricle have a high-velocity flow through them. This requires the use of a sturdy occlusion device, which will fix securely in the high-pressure, high-flow tract. Because of the usual small size of the patient, usually either a controlled-release, large coil and/or a small Amplatzer™ PDA or Vascular Plug is/are used. A coil with a bioptome-controlled release (in the US) requires a 5-French long sheath for true controllability and the smallest sizes of both the Amplatzer™ PDA and Vascular Plug devices (4 mm) pass through 5-French sheaths. The Detachable™ coils, available in the rest of the world, utilize a 4-French delivery catheter, but these coils often are not robust enough for these lesions. In the rare larger patients, larger devices including the GGVOD™ can be considered for the occlusion of these tunnels.

A wire is maneuvered from the retrograde catheter, through the tunnel and into the left ventricle. The retrograde catheter is replaced over this wire with the delivery sheath/dilator or catheter that is to be used for the device chosen for the particular tunnel. The delivery sheath is advanced through the tunnel, to the left ventricle or, at least, to the distal end of the tunnel. Once the delivery sheath is positioned securely in the tunnel, the wire and the dilator are removed from the delivery sheath. The sheath is cleared passively and meticulously of all air and/or clot as with all other delivery systems particularly in the systemic circulation. The appropriate device is loaded into, and advanced to the end of the sheath within the tunnel. The sheath and occlusion device are withdrawn together until the device, which is still within the sheath, is positioned in the desired location for implant in the tunnel. If the device being used is a coil, the coil is extruded from the sheath into the tunnel until the attach/release mechanism of the coil is just within the tip of the sheath. With the other devices, the delivery catheter/cable and device are fixed in position and the sheath withdrawn off the device until the device is fully deployed in the tunnel.

The fixation of the occlusion device is tested by fairly vigorous to-and-fro motion of the delivery system, and a small, hand injected angiogram is performed with an injection of contrast through the delivery sheath. The delivery sheath still is over the delivery catheter/cable with the tip of the sheath just proximal to the device within the tunnel and even a slow, small injection demonstrates the position of the occlusion device and the degree of occlusion of the tunnel—particularly if the tunnel is occluded satisfactorily. When satisfied with the fixation and the degree of occlusion, the release mechanism of the particular device is activated. By using a device with a controlled-release system, if the fixation of the device and occlusion are not satisfactory, the device readily can be withdrawn into the delivery system and the procedure restarted with a more appropriate size or type of device.

Perivalvular leaks

Perivalvular leaks occur around and adjacent to surgically implanted prosthetic valves. They usually occur adjacent to prosthetic aortic or mitral valves, they often are multiple, and they usually are in very sick patients, all of which makes these lesions difficult and precarious to treat. Fortunately, perivalvular leaks occur around the outside of the "sewing ring" of the prosthetic valve, which usually places the fistulous communication away from the functioning "leaflets" of the prosthetic valve.

The aortic prosthetic perivalvular leak hemodynamically is similar to a coronary sinus to left ventricular fistula (previously in this chapter), although perivalvular leaks frequently are multiple and usually occur in significantly larger and older patients. The diagnosis of, and the number of aortic perivalvular leak(s) are suggested by transthoracic echocardiography and/or from biplane, aortic root aortograms. The treatment of perivalvular leaks is monitored in the catheterization laboratory with *both* selective biplane angiograms, which are performed actually within the perivalvular leak, and by trans-esophageal echo (TEE). The aortic perivalvular leak is accessed with a retrograde catheter from the aorta above the prosthetic valve. The orifice of the perivalvular leak is usually located directly off the ascending aorta adjacent to the "ring" of the prosthetic aortic valve.

The location(s) of the aortic perivalvular leak(s) is(are) identified with TEE.

Once an aortic perivalvular leak is suspected and then identified, the leak is cannulated selectively with a retrograde, end-and-side hole catheter. The *exact location* of the aortic opening of the perivalvular leak in relation to the aortic valve prosthesis, its *shape*, its *maximum and minimal diameters*, its *length* and its exit site into the left ventricle all are defined very accurately with selective biplane angiograms with injection directly into the fistulous tract, with the X-ray tubes angled to elongate the tract maximally. The perivalvular leaks often are short and have an elliptical shape adjacent to the rigid, prosthetic valve "sewing ring". Once the precise anatomy and size are defined angiographically and correlated with the TEE findings, an occlusion device is chosen which will occlude the perivalvular leak, but, at the same time will *not* extend out of the orifice of the fistula and interfere with the function of the adjacent prosthetic valve.

An exchange wire is placed through the retrograde catheter, into and through the tract of the perivalvular leak and into the left ventricle. The original catheter is replaced over the exchange wire with the specific delivery system for the device to be used and the delivery system is advanced deep into the tract of the perivalvular leak. The tract of the perivalvular leak and the delivery system are interrogated continuously with the TEE. It is useful, if not absolutely necessary, to introduce a second, retrograde catheter into the aortic root in order to perform small, repeated, selective angiograms during the actual delivery of the device, which is being performed through the other retrograde catheter/delivery system.

When the fistulous tract has any length and has any constriction within its course, a controlled-release, large coil often is the ideal device for these lesions, but only when the coil can be implanted completely *within* the tract so that none of the attached coil fibers extend out of the tract and into the area of the moving leaflets of the prosthesis.

For the short, broader perivalvular leaks, the smaller diameter Amplatzer™ PDA, the Amplatzer™ muscular VSD occluders or the newer Amplatzer™ Vascular Plug are used. The choice of which of these devices to use depends upon the size of the proximal orifice and the presence of any narrowing along the course of the leak. In spite of the usual elliptical shape of the orifice of these perivalvular leaks, the Amplatzer™ devices, when initially implanted, often conform to the shape of the tract. The Amplatzer™ devices are placed either at the aortic orifice of the leak or within the tract of the leak utilizing the "ridge" created by the valve ring as the "central narrowing" to straddle with the "waist" of the device. The exact location where the occlusion device is implanted within a perivalvular leak depends upon the length, diameter and configuration of the perivalvular leak, the proximity to the prosthetic leaflets and, often, a trial and error deployment of the device. The "lips" or "rims" of the Amplatzer™ PDA and muscular VSD devices usually are short enough that they do not interfere with the leaflets of the prosthesis, even when the "rim" of the device is outside of the orifice of the fistulous tract.

Once a coil or one of the Amplatzer™ occluders has been delivered into the tract, but before its release, a repeat biplane angiogram in, or very close to, the aortic orifice of the leak is performed to visualize the tract, to visualize the degree of occlusion, and to check the position of the coil/device in relation to the movement of the prosthetic valve leaflets. The area is interrogated with the TEE/Doppler™ to identify the distance of the particular coil/device away from the leaflets of the prosthetic valve and to check for residual leak through the tract. When the occlusion is satisfactory and there is no interference with the function of the prosthetic valve as seen on the TEE, the coil/device is released. The angiogram and the TEE are repeated after the release of the coil/device to confirm the degree of occlusion, changes in the position of the coil/device, the freedom from interference with the prosthetic valve apparatus, and/or the presence of any additional perivalvular leaks.

Any residual and/or additional perivalvular leak is addressed during the same catheterization procedure. Residual leaks through devices can result in hemolysis and, if not closed during the initial implant procedure, may have to be closed later as an emergency. In addition, when performing additional occlusions during the same procedure, all of the anatomy is fresh in the operator's mind and the wires and catheters already are in place for the implant of an additional occluder, even though it may be a different type from the original occluder.

Small PDA "double umbrella" occlusion devices, which could be implanted completely within the tract of perivalvular leaks, were used in the past for the occlusion of perivalvular aortic leaks, however, all of the double umbrella devices require a much larger and stiffer delivery system. As a consequence, the double umbrella devices on a rigid frame no longer are used for the occlusion of aortic perivalvular leaks.

Perivalvular leaks around a prosthetic mitral valve represent significantly greater challenges for transcatheter occlusion. Mitral perivalvular leaks frequently are multiple and they are more difficult to image precisely by either echo or angiography. Both prograde access through a transseptal atrial septal puncture to the left atrium and retrograde access from the left ventricle are used for the catheter occlusions of mitral perivalvular leaks. Devices in perivalvular mitral valve leaks are delivered and implanted from the left atrial (outlet) end of the leak, which is against the direction of the flow of the blood through the mitral perivalvular leak. As with the occlusion of the aortic perivalvular leaks, the delivery and the implant of occlusion devices for mitral perivalvular leaks are visualized and controlled by both selective biplane angiography and TEE/Doppler.

Mitral perivalvular leaks initially are identified by transthoracic echocardiography and biplane, left ventricular angiography. Once the perivalvular mitral leak is defined angiographically and a decision is made to perform a transcatheter occlusion, a pre-curved, end-and-side hole, retrograde catheter is positioned in the left ventricle, a prograde, long, transseptal sheath is positioned in the left atrium (usually by transseptal atrial puncture), and a TEE probe is introduced to visualize the mitral annulus. The specific leak(s) is(are) identified, then they are defined more definitively by TEE/Doppler™ interrogation and more selective biplane angiograms with the injections preferably performed directly *into the perivalvular tract* from either a prograde or retrograde approach. Selective views of the angiograms in the left ventricle and/or selective views in the tract of the leak are displayed as "road maps" of the overall anatomy of the area.

A Judkins™ left coronary catheter or another "J" shaped catheter is introduced retrograde into the left ventricle. The 180° curve on the pre-curved, retrograde, left ventricular catheter helps to direct the tip of the catheter toward the mitral annulus or, more specifically, toward the left ventricular (entrance) end or into the left ventricular "entrance" of the perivalvular leak(s) in order to obtain more "selective" injections.

Using the angiographic "road maps" and TEE, from the venous approach, a separate 6- or 7-French, end-and-side hole torque-controlled catheter with a fixed slight angle at the tip is maneuvered, usually along with a torque-controlled guide wire, into the *left atrial (exit) end* of the perivalvular leak. In order to prevent extensive, unnecessary and "blind" maneuvering, *biplane* fluoroscopy is absolutely essential for this maneuvering in order to direct the catheter purposefully both from side to side and from front to back. The catheter is advanced well into, or through, the fistulous tract. The X-ray tubes are angled as perpendicular to the long axis of the catheter (and tract) as possible and to place the catheter, which is positioned in the tract, at one "edge" of the valve ring as seen in at least one view. A high-pressure, Tuohy™ "Y" adaptor is attached over the wire to the hub of the catheter and a biplane angiogram recorded while injecting through this catheter, over the wire and directly into the tract of the perivalvular leak. The biplane angiograms define the diameter, shape and length of the tract and demonstrate the distance of the proximal and distal openings of the tract from the prosthetic valve leaflets. The diameters, lengths and distances are measured very accurately on both the angiogram and on the TEE images. The proper device to occlude the perivalvular leak is chosen on the basis of these angiographic measurements and the corresponding TEE images. The original torque wire, which still is through the catheter, is replaced with a long, preformed, floppy tipped Super Stiff™ (Boston Scientific, Natick, MA) wire, which is looped in the ventricle after passing through the perivalvular tract.

The choice of the device used to occlude a perivalvular mitral valve leak is similar to the choice of device used to occlude perivalvular aortic valve leaks. The available devices include large, *controlled-release* coils, the Amplatzer™ PDA, muscular VSD and Vascular Plug devices, and the Gianturco-Grifka Vascular Occlusion Devices (GGVOD™). In addition to these devices, the larger and stiffer delivery systems that are necessary to accommodate the "double umbrella" devices, can be tolerated from the venous/transseptal approach, allowing the use of virtually any occlusion device that is suited for the particular anatomy. Once the exact device is chosen, the appropriate delivery system/catheter is delivered to the perivalvular leak from the prograde/transseptal/left atrial approach. The specific delivery system/catheter for the occlusion device can be delivered to the perivalvular leak over the Super Stiff™ wire through the *original* transseptal sheath, or the new long delivery sheath/dilator is introduced over the exchange wire after removing the original transseptal sheath. If the original transseptal sheath does not accommodate the delivery system/catheter for the device that is chosen, the original transseptal sheath is replaced with a larger diameter long transseptal sheath which is one or two French sizes larger than the particular delivery system that is to be used for the device delivery. The larger diameter transseptal sheath is pre-curved before it is introduced to conform to the course from the inferior vena cava, through the right atrium and atrial septum and to a position just over the mitral annulus. The large long sheath positioned in the left atrium provides extra support for the delivery catheter, and when the larger sheath is advanced to the left atrial end of the perivalvular leak over the delivery catheter, the large sheath allows "postioning" angiograms to be obtained just at the distal end of the leak during the delivery of the device without the necessity of another catheter in the left atrium. When the device is deployed and flow through the tract is decreased/stopped, the contrast will reflux "backward" into the tract slightly.

The device is delivered into the tract of the perivalvular mitral leak and positioned in the tract similarly to the positioning in perivalvular aortic leaks and according to the type of device being used. Once opened in the tract, the positioning, degree of occlusion and distance away from the leaflets of the prosthetic valve are examined by repeat biplane angiography, injecting through the retrograde catheter or through the long sheath over the delivery catheter, and by TEE/Doppler™ interrogation. When satisfied with the occlusion and the position, the device is released. A large volume left ventricular angiocardiogram is performed through the retrograde catheter to visualize the final occlusion of the perivalvular leak and the function of the prosthetic mitral valve, and to exclude any additional perivalvular leaks. If there is persistent flow through the original perivalvular communication and/or if there are any additional perivalvular leaks detected, these are addressed during this same catheterization for the same reasons as for residual perivalvular aortic leaks.

Complications of vascular occlusions

As with all other therapeutic catheterization procedures, there are potential complications related to the catheterization itself and those more specifically related to the occlusion procedure. Since a majority of the abnormal vessels and/or vascular channels requiring occlusion arise off a systemic artery, most transcatheter occlusion procedures are performed entirely or, at least, partially from an arterial approach. This, alone, increases the likelihood of local arterial injury and of systemic embolic complications. These complications and the steps taken to prevent them are discussed in detail in Chapter 4 ("Vascular Access") and Chapter 9 ("Retrograde Technique").

Embolization of the occlusion device and/or inadvertent occlusion of the blood supply to a vital structure or organ are the major complications unique to intravascular occlusion of systemic vessels, fistulae and perivalvular leaks. Occlusion of unwanted vessels/structures is prevented by test occlusion with a balloon catheter before depositing an occlusion device and by the use of controlled-release/retrievable devices whenever there is any question about compromise of a vital adjacent vessel/structure. This is particularly important in the occlusion of coronary-cameral fistulae, where the extension of even a small part of the occlusion device into a vital coronary artery can obstruct and/or thrombose an essential coronary blood supply.

Remote embolization of a vascular occlusion device is always possible, but almost always is preventable. Certainly, the use of the controllable and retrievable devices adds to the safety and secure positioning of occlusion devices for peripheral vascular occlusions. When "controllable" release devices are not available or cannot be used, extra care is taken in the sizing of the device for the lesion and in choosing the safest location for the implant of the occlusion device. When a vascular occlusion device does embolize to a different unwanted and/or dangerous area or structure, it becomes a foreign body that requires removal. It is imperative that the catheterization laboratory performing vascular occlusion procedures has the equipment and expertise for the removal of all types of foreign bodies.

The migration of a coil or other small occlusion device completely through a large pulmonary arteriovenous fistulous communication into the pulmonary vein and, in turn, embolization into the systemic arterial circulation always is a possibility and potentially, results in very serious consequences. This type of embolization is prevented by the use of a much larger device and/or an "irregular" device, like an umbrella, which becomes trapped securely in the afferent vessel of the fistula.

Whenever there is incomplete occlusion of a vessel or other lesion with a resultant high-velocity residual "jet" leak through or adjacent to an implanted device, any of the vascular occlusion devices can produce hemolysis. Again, treatment is prevention by occluding the lesion completely during the initial catheterization for the occlusion. When a high-velocity lesion does remain and does result in hemolysis, the patient initially is treated medically with extra volume infusions and blood replacement as necessary for symptoms. Often the hemolysis is self-limited after 2–7 days, but when it is unrelenting and/or progressive, re-intervention to eliminate the high-velocity lesion is necessary. Usually additional transcatheter delivered occlusion devices to stop the flow will solve the problem, but rarely surgical removal of the device and closure of the vessel/leak will be necessary.

Complications of catheter occlusions of aorta to left ventricular tunnels and peri-prosthetic valvular leaks

Like all other therapeutic catheterization procedures, and particularly those within the systemic arterial system, all of the basic hazards of the cardiac catheterization procedure are present with these procedures. The occlusion of aortic to left ventricular tunnels and perivalvular leaks of both the aortic and mitral valves with catheter-delivered devices involves very extensive manipulations proximal to the head vessels in the systemic arterial system with wires, catheters and delivery systems, which, in turn, creates a very high potential for cerebrovascular embolic problems. There must be constant vigilance to *prevent* the introduction of air into the system and to keep all wires passing through catheters, catheters and delivery systems on a continuous flush to prevent thrombi from forming. The potential for embolization of the occlusion device itself from the defect to the systemic circulation is always present. The equipment must be available for the immediate capture and retrieval of any embolized device before it results in permanent damage to a vital organ.

The occlusion of perivalvular leaks around mechanical prosthetic valves involves extensive catheter/wire/delivery system manipulations adjacent to the valve orifice and the mechanical leaflets of the involved prosthetic valves with the potential for entrapment in the valve and significant interference with the valve's function. The manipulations in the area of these valves must be directed very precisely and cautiously, and observed continually on *biplane* fluoroscopy to avoid the valves.

Any of the occlusion devices placed in perivalvular leaks can interfere with the function of a mechanical prosthetic valve. Prevention is the optimal management by the use of retrievable devices and the very careful positioning and testing of each device as it is delivered. If the function of a prosthetic valve is compromised significantly, the device must be removed either by retrieval with a catheter technique or surgically.

Summary

Unwanted shunts and/or vascular leaks in virtually all cases can be occluded with a catheter-delivered device. Refinements in the imaging systems, the variety of available devices, and improvements in delivery have made these procedures more effective and far safer. In 2005, trans catheter occlusion of residual and/or unwanted vascular communications and/or leaks should be the primary approach for their management.

References

1. Bookstein JJ *et al.* Transcatheter hemostasis of gastrointestinal bleeding using modified autogenous clot. *Radiology* 1974; **113**(2): 277–285.
2. Gold RE and Grace DM. Gelfoam embolization of the left gastric artery for bleeding ulcer: experimental considerations. *Radiology* 1975; **116**(3): 575–580.
3. Kaufman SL *et al.* Transcatheter embolization with microfibrillar collagen in swine. *Invest Radiol* 1978; **13**(3): 200–204.
4. Zuberbuhler JR *et al.* Tissue adhesive closure of aortic-pulmonary communications. *Am Heart J* 1974; **88**(1): 41–46.
5. Serbinenko FA. [Balloon occlusion of saccular aneurysms of the cerebral arteries]. *Vopr Neirokhir* 1974; **4**: 8–15.
6. Gianturco C, Anderson JH, and Wallace S. Mechanical devices for arterial occlusion. *Am J Roentgenol Radium Ther Nucl Med* 1975; **124**(3): 428–435.
7. Yamamoto S *et al.* Transcatheter embolization of bronchial collateral arteries prior to intracardiac operation for tetralogy of Fallot. *J Thorac Cardiovasc Surg* 1979; **78**(5): 739–743.
8. Grifka MR and Jones TK. Transcatheter closure of large PDA using 0.052″ gianturco coils: controlled delivery using a bioptome catheter through a 4 French sheath. *Catheter Cardiovasc Interv* 2000; **49**(3): 301–306.
9. Kuhn MA and Latson LA. Transcatheter embolization coil closure of patent ductus arteriosus—modified delivery for enhanced control during coil positioning. *Cathet Cardiovasc Diagn* 1995; **36**(3): 288–290.
10. Uzun O *et al.* Transcatheter occlusion of the arterial duct with Cook detachable coils: early experience. *Heart* 1996; **76**(3): 269–273.
11. Grifka RG *et al.* New Gianturco-Grifka vascular occlusion device. Initial studies in a canine model. *Circulation* 1995; **91**(6): 1840–1846.
12. White RI Jr *et al.* Therapeutic embolization with detachable balloons. Physical factors influencing permanent occlusion. *Radiology* 1978; **126**(2): 521–523.
13. Goto K *et al.* Permanent inflation of detachable balloons with a low-viscosity, hydrophilic polymerizing system. *Radiology* 1988; **169**(3): 787–790.
14. Moore JW and Murphy JD. Use of a bow tie stent occluder for transcatheter closure of a large anomalous vein. *Catheter Cardiovasc Interv* 2000; **49**(4): 437–440.
15. Khan MS and Moore JW. Treatment of abdominal aortic pseudoaneurysm with covered stents in a pediatric patient. *Catheter Cardiovasc Interv* 2000; **50**(4): 445–448.
16. Tulloh RM and Rigby ML. Transcatheter umbrella closure of aorto-pulmonary window. *Heart* 1997; **77**(5): 479–480.
17. Jureidini SB, Spadaro JJ, and Rao PS. Successful transcatheter closure with the buttoned device of aortopulmonary window in an adult. *Am J Cardiol* 1998; **81**(3): 371–372.
18. Richens T and Wilson N. Amplatzer device closure of a residual aortopulmonary window. *Catheter Cardiovasc Interv* 2000; **50**(4): 431–433.

27 Transcatheter occlusion of the patent ductus arteriosus (PDA)

Introduction

Transcatheter closure of patent ductus arteriosus (PDA) with one or more of several (many) devices/techniques now represents the established, standard approach for the correction of a PDA throughout the entire world including even the United States (US). There now is one device approved even by the US Food and Drug Administration (FDA) specifically for closure of the PDA.

The patent ductus arteriosus presents in an infinite variety of shapes and each shape appears in an equally wide range of sizes[1]. The most common shape is conical with a large aortic end (ampulla) tapering to a narrower pulmonary end. The persistent ductus however, can be long and "finger-like" with or without an additional tapering at the pulmonary end; it can have several areas of narrowing or even be shaped like a long tube with no tapering at any area. The long tubular ductus usually is relatively straight but can be tortuous. At the other extreme the PDA can be a very short and flat communication or "window", between the aorta and the pulmonary artery. Each shape of the PDA can vary in diameter at its narrowest portion from less than 1 mm to greater than 10 mm. The flow through the ductus and the differential in pressure between the two ends of the ductus depend upon the size of the ductus and the relative resistances of the pulmonary arterial and systemic arterial circulations. Obviously, no single device can be optimal or even applicable for all of the varieties in the size and shape of the PDA, and fortunately over the past three plus decades multiple devices and the procedures for delivering them have been developed for transcatheter closure of the patent ductus arteriosus.

Transcatheter occlusion of the PDA was first introduced by Porstmann in 1967 *et al.*[2], however, PDA occlusion in the catheterization laboratory was not popularized until the early 1980s, when the more practical Rashkind™ PDA occluder was introduced into clinical trials in the US and the rest of the world. Since the introduction of the Rashkind™ PDA device, many different devices and techniques for transcatheter occlusion of the PDA have been introduced and used clinically for almost 25 years with minimal morbidity and no mortality from the *catheter procedures*. The success and complications of the procedures for transcatheter occlusion of the PDA have been variable and are related both to the type and size of the ductus, the particular device used, the delivery procedure utilized, and to the experience and skill of the operators performing the occlusion.

Depending upon where one resides in the world, in 2004 there were between three and ten devices and/or techniques *available* for PDA occlusion in the catheterization laboratory. The availability of devices in any particular area or country depends upon the developmental stage of new devices and the approval for human use by the regulatory agencies of the various countries. Ironically, most of the viable devices and techniques for occlusion of the PDA in the catheterization laboratory were designed, developed and clinically validated in the US. Unfortunately for the pediatric and adult patients with congenital heart lesions in the US, the FDA has been ultra conservative toward children in their review and approval of specific devices. As a consequence, the United States has the fewest devices available and the most restricted "approval" for the use of those devices that are available for specific congenital heart lesions throughout the rest of the world.

There are several devices that are approved by the FDA in the US for the occlusion of "vascular lesions" that have been adapted for transcatheter PDA occlusion and are used for PDA occlusions in the catheterization laboratory in the US. These devices and their special delivery techniques have been demonstrated to be extremely safe and effective and are *accepted as the standard therapy for PDA occlusion* by all knowledgeable medical professionals throughout the world, including in the US. However, in 2004, the Amplatzer™ PDA device was the *only* device approved by the FDA in the US specifically for *"PDA occlusion"*.

Many of the devices and techniques used for PDA occlusion are discussed in Chapter 26 ("Small Vessel Occlusions"), however, the peculiarities of their use and delivery for the occlusion of the PDA are discussed in more detail in this chapter. The patent ductus arteriosus, in essentially all patients over 3 kg in weight, is amenable to one of the transcatheter-delivered, device occlusion techniques.

More than three decades ago Dr Werner Porstmann in what was then East Germany, developed the first device used for the transcatheter occlusion of the PDA. The Porstmann PDA Device™ was an Ivalon™ foam "plug" which was introduced and delivered through a very large arterial sheath. At that time, the procedure required a surgical "cut-down" on a *large* artery and the overall procedure was quite complicated by the use of a "through-and-through" arterial to venous "rail" wire. Because of these multiple factors, although effective at closing the ductus[3], the Porstmann procedure was never used in smaller children, nor used very widely even in larger/older patients. In spite of the size and complexity of its delivery system, the Porstmann PDA Device™ still has a very limited use in larger patients in several areas of the world[4]. Although the Porstmann PDA Device™ no longer is in continued or widespread use, it did demonstrate conclusively and for the first time that a congenital heart lesion could be *corrected* successfully and safely in the cardiac catheterization laboratory.

The original, hooked, Rashkind PDA device was the first catheter-delivered device to be used successfully to close a PDA in an infant or a small child[5]. Although this device was effective at closing the ductus, the hooks on the device created significant problems, which prevented its approval and widespread use. The more practical, and very effective, double umbrella Rashkind™ PDA Occluding Umbrella was first introduced into clinical trials in the US in 1981. The double umbrella concept of the Rashkind™ Double Umbrella PDA device was similar to the original King–Mills ASD devices, which had been introduced several years earlier[6]. The Rashkind PDA devices were comprised of two opposing, tiny umbrellas attached together at their centers. Each of the two umbrellas had a stainless steel wire frame to each of which a thin sheet of *polyurethane* foam was attached. For transcatheter delivery to the ductus, the two umbrellas folded away from each other from the center of each umbrella. The device was available in two sizes. Initially there was only a 12 mm diameter device, which had three relatively fine legs on each umbrella. Eventually a 17 mm diameter device was added which had four legs, which were slightly sturdier, on each umbrella. The smaller device required an 8-French delivery system while the larger device required an 11-French delivery system. Because of the opposing umbrella configuration of the device, the Rashkind PDA Device™ was best suited for the shorter and/or broad, patent ductus and poorly suited for a longer, more tubular ductus.

In the United States, the Rashkind™ Device was available only in a *very extended*, FDA, Investigational Device Exemption (IDE) trial[7]. The Rashkind™ device did receive Pre Market Approval (PMA) from the *professional medical* panel of the Device Division of the US FDA in 1989. However, in spite of this approval by the *professional panel*, the Rashkind™ PDA Device never made it through the final step of the bureaucratic paperwork and, as a consequence, it never reached the commercial market in the US. During this same period of time, the Rashkind™ Device had been accepted and approved as the standard of care for transcatheter occlusion of the PDA throughout most of the rest of the world. Because of the inability to enter the US market and, at the same time, the introduction of other less expensive (while often less effective!) devices, production of the Rashkind™ Device was discontinued and at present the Rashkind™ Device no longer is available commercially anywhere in the world.

The protocol trial of the Rashkind™ PDA Device in the United States and the successful, routine use of the Rashkind™ Device in the rest of the world, did demonstrate conclusively that non-surgical, catheter, closure of the PDA in infants and children, not only was possible, but also, was safe and effective as a *practical, corrective*, transcatheter therapeutic procedure for a congenital heart lesion. The delivery technique using the long sheath, which was developed for the delivery of the Rashkind PDA Device™, is the same technique used today for the delivery of most of the devices used for the closure of the patent ductus arteriosus, atrial septal defects, the patent foramen ovale, and ventricular septal defects.

Following almost a decade of successful transcatheter PDA therapy with the Rashkind™ PDA Device, the device was withdrawn totally from worldwide use. During almost five years *before* it was withdrawn from use in the rest of the world, the Rashkind™ device had not been available in the United States. Having become accustomed to the significantly better standard of care provide by transcatheter closure of the PDA and then suddenly having *no* device available, pediatric cardiologists, particularly in the United States, became almost desperate for another non-surgical technique for occlusion of the PDA. As a consequence, several pediatric cardiologists and other interventionists became very innovative in developing alternative methods for transcatheter PDA occlusion.

The standard Gianturco Occlusion Coil™ had been available and approved worldwide for *"vascular occlusions" (even in the US)* for almost three decades[8]. After the total and abrupt withdrawal of the Rashkind™ Device, the standard Gianturco™ coil was considered for occlusion of the PDA and after successful PDA occlusions in an animal model, PDA occlusion with the Gianturco™ coil in children was attempted clinically in 1992[9]. The coil quickly was demonstrated to be very effective and relatively safe for PDA occlusion in humans[10]. After over a decade of use for the occlusion of the PDA, the Gianturco™ coil still is in widespread use for closure of the PDA, particularly in the United States where, until May 2003, according to FDA criteria, no device officially was "approved" for the occlusion of a PDA.

The Gianturco™ coil is very effective at occluding the ductus arteriosus, but, at the same time, using the standard delivery of a Gianturco™ coil, there is no control over the release of the coil, and once the standard Gianturco™ coil *begins* to extrude from the delivery catheter, the coil must be delivered completely with no retrievability of the coil with the same delivery catheter. In Europe, the manufacturers of the Gianturco™ coils (Cook™, Europe) developed a modification of the coil (the Detachable or Jackson™ Coil) which added an effective attach/release mechanism to the *standard* Gianturco™ coil without altering the other characteristics of the coil[11]. The Detachable Coil™ is available and is in routine use in Europe and in most parts of the world *outside of the US* as the "standard" method of treatment for the PDA.

The manufacturer of the Gianturco™ Coil in the US (Cook™ Inc., Bloomington, IN) developed an attach/release system for the vascular coils (the Flipper™) but, in doing so, decreased the size and "robustness" of the actual coils and decreased the number of embedded thrombogenic fibers, the combination of which made the US version unsatisfactory for routine ductal occlusions.

Because of the lack of controllability and non-retrievability of the standard Gianturco™ coil, some unique, specialized delivery techniques have been developed by individuals in the US to make the use of the coil safer for PDA occlusion. These techniques include the use of a balloon to hold the coil in the ductus during its extrusion[12], a snare catheter to control the coil during and after its release into the ductus[13], a small bioptome to act as a retaining and/or attach/release mechanism for the coil[14] and the use of a "drawn" or tightened catheter tip to hold the coil tightly before it is forcefully extruded from the catheter[15]. All of these modifications and techniques are discussed in detail subsequently in this chapter.

In addition to the Gianturco™ coils there are several other vascular occlusion devices available for PDA occlusion. In the US, the Gianturco-Grifka™ Vascular Occlusion Device (GGVOD™) is approved for occlusion of "vascular lesions" and is very effective for occlusion of the long tubular type of PDA. In Europe, and Germany in particular, the Duct-Occlud™ PDA Occlusion Device was developed specifically for PDA occlusion. The Duct-Occlud™ has had significant use throughout Europe and had a preliminary clinical trial in the US. The Nit-Occlud™ PDA Occlusion Device is an improved version of the Duct-Occlud™ device, and at the time of writing is in use in Europe and in clinical trials in the US. The smaller sizes and/or special modifications of at least four different devices that were designed for the occlusion of atrial septal defects, have been used for PDA occlusion in unique circumstances. The Clamshell™, the CardioSEAL™, the Amplatzer Atrial Septal Occluder™, and the Amplatzer Muscular Ventricular Septal Defect Occluder™ all have been used to close the large patent ductus. Specific modifications of the Sideris Button™ ASD device and the Amplatzer™ ASD device were made particularly for occlusion of the patent ductus, and both of these PDA devices have been available for clinical use in Europe for several years. The Amplatzer™ PDA device completed clinical IDE trials in the US in 2002 and in May 2003 was the first device to receive US FDA approval specifically for PDA occlusion in the US.

One, or more, of these devices or their modifications now provide effective alternatives for the safe catheter occlusion of all PDAs in patients who are past early infancy. The appropriate or "ideal" device and technique for PDA occlusion used in any particular patient depends upon the size of the ductus, the configuration of the ductus and upon what devices are available in any particular country. The catheter size and technique depend upon the device being used and the operator's preference.

PDA occlusion technique

The initial diagnosis of a PDA as well as the exclusion of additional cardiac lesions is made clinically from the physical examination, ECG, X-ray and echocardiogram. In general a cardiac catheterization is only performed when a therapeutic PDA occlusion procedure is to be accomplished. During the catheterization, the definitive diagnosis, the hemodynamics and, in particular, the *exact size and configuration* of the ductus are confirmed during a diagnostic catheterization before the therapeutic procedure to correct the defect. A high-resolution biplane fluoroscopy and angiographic system with a quality recording and freeze frame playback system are essential for the precise visualization and measurements of the ductus and for the visualization of the device and the delivery system during the occlusion procedure. An X-ray system with compound angulation capabilities is desirable for delivery of a PDA device and the biplane fluoroscopy becomes absolutely essential if an occlusion device embolizes away from the PDA and a catheter retrieval of the device becomes necessary.

General anesthesia is not absolutely necessary, but often is used in order to ensure a very quiet, totally immobile patient at the moment of the delivery of a device. Patients are anesthetized and/or sedated through a secure intravenous line and positioned on the catheterization table. Lidocaine is administered around the femoral vessels and the patient is prepped and draped to produce sterile fields around both inguinal areas. A short, 7-French sheath is placed in either the right or left femoral vein, and a short 4-French sheath is placed in a femoral artery; preferably, but not necessarily, in the opposite groin from the venous sheath. Using a 6-French Gensini™ marker catheter (Cordis Corp., Miami, FL) or a 6- or 7-French NIH™ "marker" catheter (Medtronic Corp., Minneapolis, MN), a prograde right heart catheterization is performed to define the hemodynamic effects of the PDA and to rule out other lesions. In spite of the preferential course from the main pulmonary artery into the PDA, an attempt is made *not* to cross the ductus with the prograde catheter during the "right heart" phase of the procedure. Any manipulations with the catheter through the ductus can irritate the ductal tissues and cause the ductus to spasm. After the hemodynamics are obtained, the venous catheter is positioned to align the "calibration marks" on the catheter "perpendicular" to the planes of the two X-ray tubes". This often is achieved optimally by positioning the venous angiographic "marker" catheter straight in the superior vena cava.

An aortogram is performed through a 4-French pigtail catheter or a high-flow NIH™ type catheter, which is introduced retrograde from the femoral artery and positioned in the descending thoracic aorta just *distal* to the aortic end of the ductus. The retrograde aortic catheter, which is positioned adjacent to the ductus and used for the aortogram, will not "irritate" and change the configuration of the ductus, which can happen when the prograde venous catheter is advanced into/through the ductus. By injecting just *distal* to the aortic end of the ductus, the maximum concentration of contrast medium is delivered into the ductus during diastole with little dissemination of the remaining contrast into the head or other extraneous areas. A biplane aortogram is performed in order to determine the shape and direction of the ductus off the aorta and to measure the exact size of the PDA. The straight PA and lateral projections usually provide the best visualization of the ductus anatomy and demonstrate the exact angulation of the ductus off the aorta. The exact size and anatomy of the ductus and the relationships to the adjacent fixed landmarks within the thorax such as the tracheal air shadow and the vertebrae usually are seen best on the straight lateral aortogram. The minimum and maximum diameters, as well as the length, of the PDA are measured very accurately from the aortogram in the lateral or near straight lateral projection using a valid calibration reference system. A still frame "road-map" of the ductus and the surrounding, fixed landmarks is created on the angiographic replay system in the catheterization laboratory.

It is possible to perform the aortogram for visualization of the ductus through the venous catheter that has been advanced from the pulmonary artery, prograde through the ductus and into the descending aorta immediately distal to the aortic end of the ductus. However, any catheter manipulation through the ductus *can* result in spasm or, occasionally, even *dilation* of the ductus. The catheter itself positioned in the ductus also *distorts* the ductus anatomy and changes the apparent angle of the ductus off the aorta. Occasionally, however, in the presence of a very large, high-flow ductus, the best or only way to obtain an adequate visualization of the exact size and anatomy of the ductus is to perform the angiogram with the holes of the angiographic catheter *actually centered within the lumen of the ductus*. With a catheter in the ductus, the side holes of an NIH™ or a pigtail catheter actually straddle the length of the ductus.

In a very small ductus, the measurement of the exact diameter is less critical and the narrowest diameter of the ductus can be *estimated* fairly accurately by comparing the smallest diameter of the ductal lumen to the known diameter of the angiographic catheter that is used for the angiogram. However, for the larger patent ductus, a more accurate technique for the measurement of the ductus must be used. The various techniques available for the calibration of the measurements are discussed in detail in Chapter 11 and include the use of calibrated "marker catheters" aligned and positioned exactly in the area of the ductus, a "dot calibration" system built into the X-ray system, or even an external calibration "grid" or "ball" placed in the exact plane of the ductus after the completion of the angiogram. The external grid or ball is considerably more cumbersome and seldom used any more. The larger the ductus is, the more important the accurate calibration and precise measurement techniques become.

Ideally, the operator should have a choice of any, or at least several of the available, clinically tested varieties of PDA occluders in order to have the best and safest device for the particular ductus size and configuration.

Specific devices for PDA occlusion

Each of the various devices that are available for catheter occlusion of the PDA in at least some parts of the developed world are discussed in detail. The delivery catheters and techniques used for the delivery of each of the available devices are discussed along with the advantages and disadvantages of each.

Gianturco coil

The Gianturco™ coil (Cook Incorporated, Bloomington, IN) has been in clinical use for over three decades with US FDA approval for "vascular occlusions" in humans. In 1992 Cambier and Moore reported the successful use of a standard 0.038″ Gianturco™ occlusion coil for a transcatheter PDA occlusion[9]. Within a very short time thereafter, Gianturco™ coils became used routinely for the occlusions of the PDA in multiple centers in the US and throughout the rest of the world. The Gianturco™ coil proved to be effective, very safe and relatively cheap for the occlusion of the small to moderate diameter PDA. *Physicians* throughout the world (including even the United States) who were caring for patients with a patent ductus soon accepted the Gianturco™ coil occlusion as the *standard treatment* and the standard of care for treatment of the PDA.

When using the previously established techniques for the delivery of Gianturco™ coils into constrained vessels and in spite of its very successful use in the PDA, there still is very limited control and no retrieval of the Gianturco™ coil with the delivery catheter during a coil implant into a ductus. This lack of control complicated the closure of the patent ductus with the Gianturco™ coil and resulted in an unacceptable number of embolizations away from the PDA during attempted implants of the coils. In addition, the standard available sized Gianturco™ coils frequently do not hold well enough in the larger PDA and, as a consequence, are not as effective and safe for the larger PDA. When Gianturco™ coils are used to occlude a ductus that is large and/or unusual in shape, very often multiple coils must be implanted into a single ductus in order to totally occlude the defect[16]. Now, for the closure of the larger PDA, FDA approval and the commercial availability of the Amplatzer™ PDA occluder will probably cause the replacement of the coils completely for this use, at least in the US. At the same time, the coils are far cheaper and very effective at closing the smaller PDA and until an even better, smaller and cheaper device becomes available, the Gianturco™ coil still is the preferred *device* for catheter closure of the small ductus.

Gianturco coil; standard "free-release" ("slinky") technique

Gianturco™ coils are small lengths of special stainless steel spring guide wires that are pre-formed into "coils" or small "cylinders" of specific diameters. The coils come in different coil *wire* diameters, different diameters of the loops of the coils, and different lengths of the "straightened" coil wires, the combination of which determines the "size" of the coil. Each Gianturco™ coil has multiple fine "filaments" or fibers of nylon embedded within the windings of the coil wires to increase the thrombogenicity of the coil. The standard coils are available with 0.025″, 0.032″ and 0.038″ diameter *wires*. The different, pre-formed diameters of the loops of the Gianturco™ coils range between 3 mm and 15 mm. The different straightened lengths of the coil wire along with the diameter of the loops of the specific coil determine the *number* of loops that are formed by each coil. The sequential numbers on the label of the *standard* Gianturco™ coil *in the US* represent (1) the coil *wire* diameter, (2) the total *length of the coil wire* and (3) the *diameter of the coil loops*. From the length and the diameter of the coil loop, the operator *calculates* the number of loops that will be formed as the coil forms. The formula for this calculation is:

Number of loops = coil length in cm $\div \pi \times$ D in mm $\times$ 10.

The Gianturco™ coils that are available *outside of the US*, are labeled more logically according to the number of loops rather than the length of the coil wire! The coils are packaged in a straight metal introducer tube as a straightened wire when they come from the manufacturer.

For the "free-release" technique, the coils are delivered through a polyethylene, *end-hole-only*, catheter with an internal diameter that is only very slightly larger than the diameter of the *wire* of the coil. The coil delivery catheter must *not* have side holes. Side holes in the catheter result in the tip of the coil, which is curving in an attempt to resume its coil configuration, catching in one of the side holes of the catheter and preventing the delivery of the coil out of the distal *end* of the catheter. Both the material and the internal diameter of the catheter are critically important to prevent the coil from "binding" within the catheter during the delivery through the catheter. The internal diameter of the catheter must be sufficiently larger than the diameter of the coil wire to also accommodate the enmeshed fibers in the coil wire. A catheter that is smaller (or even exactly the same) in its internal diameter than the diameter of the coil wire, does not allow the coil even to be introduced into the catheter. A catheter with an internal diameter significantly larger than the diameter of the coil wire allows the coil to bend and begin to partially "coil" on itself while still within the catheter and/or allows the pusher wire to push past the proximal end and the entire coil within the catheter. Either of these occurrences causes the coil to bind within the catheter and prevents its delivery. Catheters for the delivery of coils are available with many pre-formed curves at the tip of the catheter to facilitate entry into different orientations of the ductus, and as straight catheters that the operator can individually pre-shape to suit his particular needs.

The coil for the "free-release" technique is chosen according to the narrowest diameter of the ductus, the shape of the ductus, the length of the ductus and the size (diameter) of the aortic ampulla of the ductus. The heavier

0.038″ coils are preferred for all but the very tiniest ductus. The diameter of the coil loops should be at least two times the diameter of the *accurately measured* narrowest portion of the ductus. The length of the coil is chosen to allow one full loop at the pulmonary end of the ductus and three, or preferably four, loops to form in the aortic ampulla of the ductus. When the ampulla is very short or narrow, occasionally the relative amount of coil on each side of the ductus is altered so that the implanted coil does not extend significantly into the lumen of either the aorta or the pulmonary artery.

The delivery of a Gianturco™ coil to the patent ductus by the "free-release" technique can be either prograde from the pulmonary artery through the ductus from the venous system or retrograde directly into the ductus from the aorta. A delivery catheter is chosen to suit the specific ductus, the route to be used and the size of the coil wire.

The retrograde approach is preferred for the "free-release" delivery of the Gianturco™ coil. After the exact size and anatomy of the ductus have been determined angiographically, a 4-French coil delivery catheter is introduced through an indwelling short sheath in the femoral artery. The catheter can be one of many varieties as long as it has a similar internal diameter to the external diameter of the coil *wire* being used and it is an *end-hole only* catheter. A "road map" of the lateral aortogram of the ductus is displayed on the fluoroscopy screen for reference for the remainder of the procedure. The end-hole delivery catheter is passed retrograde in the aorta, through the ductus and well into the pulmonary artery. This usually is accomplished with minimal manipulation, but occasionally requires passing some type of guide wire through the ductus first and then following it with the catheter.

Once the delivery catheter is well into the pulmonary artery, the appropriate coil is loaded into the proximal end of the catheter through a wire back-bleed/flush port valve. The tubular metal coil container/loader is introduced through the wire back-bleed/valve device on the catheter and advanced deep into the proximal hub of the catheter. The soft end of a teflon-coated spring guide wire that has the same or slightly larger diameter than the coil wire, is introduced into the proximal end of the coil container/loader and advanced through the loader well into the catheter. This pushes the coil out of the loader and into the delivery catheter. Once the coil is completely within the catheter, the coil loader is withdrawn off the proximal end of the wire. While observing the distal end of the catheter on fluoroscopy, the wire is advanced into the catheter. This pushes the coil in advance of the "pusher" wire. The coil, the separate pusher wire and the separation between the two are clearly visible within the catheter on the fluoroscopy as the combination approaches the tip of the catheter.

As the coil approaches the catheter tip, the pusher wire is advanced slowly, allowing *2/3 to one full loop* of the coil to form in the pulmonary artery. With this one loop formed in the pulmonary artery, the catheter with the pusher wire and the partially extruded coil all together are withdrawn very carefully and slowly until the exposed loop of the coil touches the pulmonary end of the ductus. This is determined by comparing the position of the coil loop to the "road map" of the prior lateral aortogram and by the slight straightening and/or distortion of the loop of coil as it touches the pulmonary end of the ductus. If there is any question about this location, an angiocardiogram is recorded through the separate diagnostic venous catheter, which can still be in the pulmonary artery.

An adequate, repeat aortogram to demonstrate the exact position of the coil within the entire ductus cannot be performed without introducing a second catheter into the aorta. A second aortic catheter can be introduced prograde through the left heart and ascending aorta to the descending aorta or, preferably, a second retrograde arterial catheter is introduced from the other femoral artery. In either case, when it is anticipated that a second catheter will be needed in the aorta, it should be introduced before the delivery of the coil is started.

Once the single loop has touched the pulmonary end of the ductus, the proximal end of the pusher guide wire, which is extending out of the proximal hub of the catheter outside of the body, is fixed *in a straight line* against the patient's leg and/or against the catheterization table. With the pusher wire fixed very securely and absolutely straight, the catheter, alone, is withdrawn over the fixed "pusher" guide wire. This maneuver "uncovers" and extrudes the remainder of the coil into the descending aorta as the catheter is withdrawn. The pulmonary loop of coil is observed closely during this maneuver, adjusting the tension on the pusher wire and the position of the catheter to be sure that the single loop of coil in the pulmonary artery remains in the proper location and is not pulled through the ductus or pushed back into the pulmonary artery. As the catheter is withdrawn off the coil, the coil often begins to coil or loop just at the tip of the catheter which, in turn, places tension on the loop in the pulmonary artery. This tension on the coil must be compensated for by advancing the delivery catheter over the wire very slightly. At the other extreme, the coil can be stretched straight as it extrudes out of the delivery catheter and, as it is released completely, the coil springs up and down in the descending aorta several times like a "slinky" before coiling up into the aortic ampulla of the ductus. Some operators rely on this rapid recoil of the coil occurring, and purposefully withdraw the catheter rapidly off the coil wire during delivery.

An alternative technique to fixing the pusher wire outside of the catheter as the catheter is withdrawn off the wire is to advance the pusher wire in small increments as the delivery catheter simultaneously is withdrawn in equally small increments. This allows the loops of coil to form on the aortic side of the ductus without placing tension on the loop on the pulmonary end of the ductus and/or creating the "exciting" springing up and down of the entire coil in the aorta. This slow release may allow the aortic end of the coil to "seat" better in the aortic ampulla end of the ductus but, at the same time, can allow more of the coil loops to be pulled *into* the pulmonary side of the ductus.

With either of these "free-release" techniques from the retrograde approach, there is no real control over the coil itself, and once the extrusion of the coil has started, there is no way of withdrawing the coil or repositioning it. This remains a major drawback to the use of the standard Gianturco™ coils with the "free-release" technique, and has led to many modifications in the delivery of the Gianturco™ coils for PDA occlusions.

When a small portion of the aortic loops of the coil does remain protruding into the aortic lumen, this usually can be "pushed" gently toward, and into, the ampulla with the tip of the retrograde catheter. If a very large portion hangs into the aorta and cannot be repositioned into the ampulla, the entire coil is grasped with a snare loop introduced through the retrograde catheter, and the coil is withdrawn out of the ductus through the artery and out of the body through the arterial sheath. After the first coil is withdrawn, the implant procedure can be started all over with a different, more appropriate coil.

With the coil in its proper position and after waiting approximately 10 minutes, a repeat aortogram is performed in order to verify the position of the coil and the complete closure of the ductus. Occasionally there is a *very tiny* smoke-like swirl of contrast through the ductus between the coils. This very tiny, irregular "smoke" of contrast usually is of no consequence, and a complete closure usually occurs by the following morning. On the other hand, even a small, high-velocity, *jet* of contrast that passes through or adjacent to the loops of coil in the ductus, represents a residual leak, which probably will not close, and more than likely will become larger with time and/or result in hemolysis.

In the event of the persistence of a residual, jet-like leak for 10 minutes or more, additional coils are added sequentially at that time until the ductus is closed angiographically in the catheterization laboratory. The necessity of closing the ductus completely while still in the laboratory is based on the experience that a jet-like lesion seldom closes on its own, and such a residual leak through the implanted coil(s) leaves the patient not only with a small residual PDA but also with a "foreign body" in that PDA. This results in a higher risk of endocarditis and is an even greater indication for closing the defect. Of equal, and often more immediate importance, some of these residual "jet-like" leaks through the coils (or any device in the ductus) result in hemolysis. Hemolysis through the coils often is of a very significant degree and can require transfusions and/or emergency intervention to close the ductus completely and/or remove the device.

In order to add additional coil(s) to the ductus immediately after the initial coil(s) has/have been implanted, the ductus is crossed very carefully from the aorta to the pulmonary artery with a Terumo Glide™ wire. A small, straight or very smoothly curved coil delivery catheter is advanced carefully from the aorta over that wire, through the original ductus coil(s) and into the pulmonary artery. The additional coil is chosen depending on the size and location of the leak. Usually, coils with the loops of the coils several millimeters smaller in diameter, and often smaller sized coil wires than the original coil, are used for the additional coil implants. A similar technique to the original coil implant is carried out with the exception that as the aortic loops of the coil are extruded, an attempt is made to extrude the aortic loops *within* the loops of the original coil—i.e. the aortic loops are pushed out of the catheter more than entirely pulling the catheter off the coil. The aortogram is repeated 10–15 more minutes after the additional coil is implanted. If there still is a residual jet-like leak, additional coils are added using the same retrograde procedure.

When it works, the retrograde Gianturco™ "free-release" technique has the advantages that it is quite quick, simple and inexpensive to perform and *usually* results in complete ductus occlusion. The ductus usually is crossed easily by the retrograde approach. It requires only a small catheter in the artery. It has the major disadvantage that once the coil has begun to be extruded, there is no "turning back"; i.e. the coil cannot be withdrawn nor even retained in the catheter even if it is observed to be malpositioned early during its delivery. As a consequence, there still is an incidence of embolization of the coils away from the ductus to either of the pulmonary arteries or to the aorta with this technique.

The alternative delivery route for the "free-release" coils is from the prograde venous approach. The anatomy and size of the ductus are determined and "road mapped" exactly as with the arterial approach. The coil is chosen in the same manner according to the ductus anatomy and diameters. For delivery from the venous route, the operator must calculate *exactly* how many *loops* of coil are formed from the length of the particular coil that is to be used. The coils that are available outside of the US are labeled more logically and more conveniently according to the number of loops rather than the length of the coil wire! The appropriate coil delivery catheter is manipulated through the right heart, pulmonary artery, through the ductus, and well into the descending aorta distal to the ductus. Because the usual coil catheters are small and often poorly maneuverable, this may require first crossing the ductus with a more maneuverable end-hole catheter, replacing this catheter with an exchange wire and then passing the coil delivery catheter over this wire.

The coil is loaded into the pre-positioned delivery catheter and advanced to the tip of the catheter. One or two loops of coil are extruded into the descending aorta while the tip of the catheter still is a few millimeters distal to the aortic ampulla of the ductus. The catheter tip, together with these exposed aortic loops of coil, is withdrawn into the aortic ampulla of the ductus. With the catheter tip positioned there, the pusher wire is advanced carefully, extruding the additional loop(s) of coil that are to be positioned on the aortic end of the ductus into the ampulla. At this juncture of the delivery, enough of the coil must remain in the delivery catheter to be able to form one full loop of coil on the pulmonary side of the ductus (as determined from the known length of the coil). The pusher wire is fixed on the table outside of the body and the delivery catheter is withdrawn off the last loop of coil as it forms in the pulmonary artery. This should extrude the one last loop of coil into the pulmonary end of the ductus. Similarly to delivery by the retrograde approach, an aortogram is performed through a retrograde catheter for angiographic verification of the position of the device and the degree of closure of the ductus. If there is a residual leak, a repeat coil implant is carried out during the same catheterization procedure, but it is performed more effectively and safely from the retrograde approach, as described earlier in this chapter.

The only advantages that the venous approach has over the retrograde technique while using the "free release" of the standard Gianturco coils, is the ability to intermittently perform small *aortograms* during the delivery of the coil to verify its position during the process while still using only one arterial catheter. Otherwise the control of the delivery is no better, and, perhaps, even worse, and the standard "free release" coil still cannot be withdrawn to reposition it once the extrusion has started. The coil cannot be retained nor retrieved with this delivery catheter.

Occasionally, the venous delivery approach is used simultaneously with a retrograde approach in order to deliver a second coil *simultaneously* from the retrograde approach while using separate prograde and retrograde catheters. There even have been two prograde coils delivered simultaneously with one retrograde coil in a very large ductus. With these multiple coil delivery techniques, the prograde venous and the retrograde delivery *catheters* all are positioned through the ductus exactly as they are when coils are delivered individually. Each coil is delivered exactly as it was individually. The simultaneous delivery of two (or more) coils from two separate approaches does require two (or more) operators. The delivery of the two coils simultaneously reportedly allows the closure of a larger PDA using 0.038" coils. This simultaneous delivery of several or more of the 0.038" coils through separate catheters has been replaced through the availability of larger coils, the various adjunct delivery techniques, and the availability of the Amplatzer™ ductus occlusion devices.

In spite of the shortcomings of the standard Gianturco™ coil, its effectiveness, its low cost, and its widespread availability, along with the modified delivery techniques, have resulted in the Gianturco™ coil becoming an accepted, standard device for transcatheter PDA occlusion in the United States.

Modifications of the Gianturco™ coil and coil delivery technique for controlled delivery

Various adjuncts for the delivery of the standard Gianturco™ coil were developed by individual pediatric cardiologists to provide more control over the *standard* coil during implant. These modifications include:

1 the use of a balloon catheter to hold the coil in place during implant[12];

2 a snare to hold the extruded end of the coil during implant[13];

3 a bioptome to hold the coil in the delivery catheter[14]; and

4 a specific narrowing of the lumen of the tip of the delivery catheter to retain the coil[15].

These techniques increase the safety of the coil delivery but also increase the technical demands of the procedure and the cost to the patient.

In Europe, the manufacturers of the coils added a "screw" attachment/release mechanism to the Gianturco™ coil to create a Detachable™ Coil[11]. This screw mechanism gives total control over the release of the coil even after complete extrusion from the catheter and allows total retrieval of the coil until the coil purposefully is released by "unscrewing" it. The Detachable™ Coil is the standard PDA closure device for the small PDA in Europe and most of the rest of the world. A modification of this mechanism by the same, parent company in the US for use in the US resulted in a "less robust" coil, which is not very useful for PDA occlusion. In Germany, the Redel Duct-Occlud™ Device was developed and introduced into clinical use in Europe. It is a variation of a larger coil, which however, is specifically shaped to fit in the usual conical shape of the ductus. This device has only been used in pre-clinical trials in the United States and now has ben replaced with the Nit-Occlud. Most recently, a larger 0.052" standard non-controlled Gianturco™ type coil was developed and approved in the US for vascular occlusions. This has been very effective for the occlusion of the larger PDA, particularly with the addition of a bioptome-controlled delivery system. The details of the procedures for all of these devices and modifications of the delivery system for PDA occlusion are covered subsequently in this chapter.

Detachable coils

Because of the relatively high incidence and continued potential for embolization of the Gianturco™ coils when they are delivered using the standard "free-release" technique for PDA occlusions, multiple modifications of the coils and the delivery techniques appeared. Probably the most practical and universally accepted of these is the controlled-release, Cook™ Detachable™ coil, often referred to as the "Jackson™" Coil. The Detachable™ coil is manufactured and distributed commercially by Cook Europe, Inc.™, and is available commercially and in *routine use* everywhere in the world *except in the United States*. The Detachable™ coil has a very simple screw attachment mechanism at the proximal end of the coil. Dr Gianturco utilized this same screw mechanism many years ago on the attach/release mechanism of inferior vena caval filters. This simple mechanism has a fine, long, slightly tapered and hollow screw at the distal end of a special, torque-controlled, delivery wire. The standard Gianturco™ coil is hollow within the windings of the fine outer steel wire and, while one end is sealed with a "weld", the other end remains open, with the winding of the wire creating a "female" screw connector. The fine screw at the end of the delivery *wire* is screwed into the open end of the coil. A long, very fine, straight mandril passes through the entire delivery wire, through the screw mechanism of the wire and through the attached coil in order to provide stiffness to the system during attachment and passage of the coil through the delivery catheter. The detachable coil requires the use of a 5-French delivery catheter with a minimal lumen ID of 0.041 inches.

The identification and sizing of the ductus and the positioning of the delivery catheter through the ductus are identical to the delivery of standard "free-release" Gianturco coils. The Detachable™ coils can be delivered from either the prograde approach from a venous introduction or retrograde from the femoral artery, although the retrograde approach is preferred and used predominantly. The Detachable™ coils are only available outside of the US and are labeled differently (and *more logically*) than the standard Gianturco™ coils in the US. The numbers on the labels of the European Detachable™ coils more logically represent (1) the *diameter of the coil loops* and (2) the *number of loops* which are formed by the coil when it is extruded. This information is more *useful* and more sensible to record on the packaging, particularly for use in the PDA. All of the Detachable™ coils in Europe at this time are 0.038″ coils, so that number is not included in the label.

The Detachable™ coil is packaged as a straight wire in a thin, clear, straight plastic, loading cartridge or tube. The mandril, which is already passing through the separate delivery wire and its distal "screw", is advanced further out of the distal (screw) end of the delivery wire, introduced into the proximal end of the loading cartridge, and into and through the coil to the distal end of the coil. The screw tip of the delivery wire is advanced to and into the proximal end of the coil within the clear loading cartridge. Once the screw tip is engaged in the coil, the delivery wire (or the loading cartridge) is rotated gently *clockwise* approximately eight times, which tightens the "screw" to engage the whole length of the threads on the delivery wire into the end of the coil. Once the threads are completely into the coil, the cartridge now is rotated one turn *counterclockwise* to unwind or back the screw threads out of the coil approximately 1 mm in order to loosen the coil slightly.

Once the coil is attached and loosened slightly, the distal end of the loading cartridge is introduced into the proximal end of the delivery catheter through a wire back-bleed/flush device. The coil delivery catheter should be pre-positioned through the ductus from the desired approach. With the mandril through the entire system, including the coil, the coil, which is attached to the pusher/delivery wire, is advanced from the clear loader, into the catheter, carefully through the catheter and *to the tip* of the delivery catheter. The catheter, the delivery wire and the course of the coil advancing through the catheter are observed closely on fluoroscopy. Care is taken not to rotate either the pusher/delivery wire or the catheter in either direction during the passage of the coil through the delivery catheter. Any rotation of the delivery wire and/or catheter could "unscrew" or excessively tighten the attach/release screw mechanism of the coil.

Once at the end of the catheter, the mandril is fixed outside of the hub of the catheter against the table at the proximal end of the catheter as the pusher/delivery wire is advanced within the delivery catheter. This advances the coil off the mandril and out of the catheter tip and allows the still attached coil wire to begin coiling by effectively "withdrawing" the fixed mandril a corresponding distance from within the coil as the coil is advanced out of the catheter. With the exception of also maintaining the mandril position in relation to the *catheter* during the extrusion of the coil, the *delivery of the coil* thereafter is identical to the "free-release" coil regardless of which delivery route is chosen.

The huge advantage of the Detachable™ coil is that at *any* point during the extrusion of the coil, the coil can be withdrawn into the delivery catheter, repositioned and/or redeployed. This can be repeated, essentially, as many times as necessary! The coil can be tested for the security of its position after it is extruded completely and, even after it is completely out of the delivery catheter, it can be withdrawn back into the catheter any time until it is released *purposefully*. Once the operator is satisfied with the position and fixation of the coil, the release is accomplished by turning the delivery wire *counterclockwise* by means of the small "pin vise" on the wire until the coil falls free from the delivery wire. The "unscrewing" takes many (8–10) *complete* turns of the pin vise. All steps after the implant of the coil are the same as with the "free-release" coils, including repeat occlusions as necessary.

This controlled-release feature, obviously, adds a remarkable degree of safety to the closure of the PDA with a "Gianturco™" coil. It is particularly useful for the prograde venous approach for the delivery of the coils, which without the controlled release is more precarious than from the retrograde approach. The controlled release does not eliminate embolization due to inappropriate sizing and/or the changes in the ductus diameters after a coil is implanted, but has essentially eliminated embolization due to changes in the patient's positioning and other placement errors during implant. As a consequence, the controlled-release coils represent the standard of care for PDA occlusion throughout the world *except in the United States*. The major disadvantage of this Detachable™ Coil is the fact that, in spite of its worldwide acceptance as the standard for coil delivery, it is *not available* to patients in the United States. The only other disadvantage of the controlled-release coil is the slightly higher cost of the Detachable™ coils because of their included special delivery wire. This extra cost is easily justified by the simplification and the increased safety of the procedure.

"Flipper" PDA occluding system

For at least three years, there has been considerable speculation and rumor about the availability in the United States of a controlled-release delivery system for the coils from Cook Inc. (Bloomington, IN). The first version of the controlled-release (or detachable) coils available in the US actually were manufactured from a smaller diameter coil wire than the standard "free-release" Gianturco™ coil of the same advertised size. These detachable coils also had fewer nylon fibers embedded in the coil. As a consequence, these coils were not as "robust", were less occlusive, and proved to be very unsatisfactory for primary PDA occlusion. The original "detachable" coils in the US also came with a rather complex attach/release mechanism similar to the mechanism of the Gianturco-Grifka Vascular Occlusion Device™. The major use for this version of the Cook™ detachable coil now is for the delivery of the second (or more) coil(s) when there is residual leak after the implant of an initial standard coil.

More recently, the Flipper™ Detachable Coil PDA Occluding System (Cook Inc., Bloomington, IN) was released in the United States! From the brochures, the specifications of this coil look identical to the Cook, Europe ("Jackson") Detachable™ coil. However, the earliest versions of the Flipper™ Coils appear to be similar in their characteristics to the original "detachable" coils in the US except for the simpler, original European detachable coil "screw release mechanism" which now is present on the Flipper™ coils. In addition, the new Flipper™ coils apparently are available in a non-ferrous material which is compatible with MR scanners. If these newer detachable coils are available with *coil* characteristics that are equivalent to the standard Gianturco™ coils, coil occlusion of the PDA (and other structures) in the United States immediately will become much easier, cheaper and safer. A true detachable coil of comparable sturdiness and occluding capacity to the standard Gianturco™ coil would eliminate the need for many of the adjunct delivery techniques that are described in the following sections of this chapter.

Adjunct techniques and devices to control the delivery of "free-release" coils

In the United States, where the safer, controlled-release coils are not available, multiple and very innovative modifications to improve the safety of the coil delivery have been developed. The preliminary steps to identify the ductus and to measure its exact size and configuration are the same regardless of which of these modifications are used to control the delivery of the coil.

Balloon "fixation" during coil extrusion

One method to control the extrusion of the coil is with the use of the inflated balloon of a floating balloon (Swan™ or Berman™) catheter to fix the pulmonary end of the coil during the retrograde delivery of the occlusion coil to the ductus[12]. There are several techniques for using such a balloon to assist the coil delivery.

Once the ductus size and anatomy have been determined, an end-hole catheter is advanced from the right heart, through the ductus and into the distal descending aorta. This catheter is exchanged for a 0.038", stiff, Terumo™ exchange length Glide™ wire. An 8-French long transseptal type sheath/dilator with an incorporated hemostasis valve is preshaped to conform to the course of the catheter from the right ventricle, through the pulmonary artery to the ductus. The preshaped sheath/dilator set is introduced over this wire from the venous entry site and advanced into the proximal main pulmonary artery. The dilator is removed from the sheath over the wire and, after the sheath is cleared thoroughly of any air and/or clot, a 7-French floating balloon *wedge* (Swan™) catheter is advanced prograde over the wire, through the long sheath and into the pulmonary artery. The balloon is filled with a solution of very dilute contrast and positioned just distal to the end of the sheath. The balloon is inflated so that it is positioned just against the tip of the sheath. The wire through the ductus and the long sheath in the pulmonary artery are used to support the relatively flimsy balloon catheter as it subsequently is used to "hold" the pulmonary loop of the coil, which is delivered from the retrograde approach.

The retrograde angiographic catheter is replaced with a coil delivery catheter. The retrograde coil delivery catheter is passed through the ductus and positioned well into the pulmonary artery. The first "pulmonary" loop of the coil is extruded in the pulmonary artery through the retrograde catheter similarly to any other retrograde Gianturco™ coil delivery. The retrograde delivery catheter along with the extruded loop of coil is withdrawn back to the pulmonary end of the ductus exactly as with the "free-release" coils. As the pulmonary loop of coil reaches the pulmonary end of the ductus, it begins to flex or straighten. The balloon of the "Swan" catheter is inflated and together with the long sheath, is pushed over the Terumo™ wire, which still passes through the ductus and against the single loop of coil, which is against the pulmonary end of the ductus. The wire passing through the ductus ensures that the balloon pushes toward and against the pulmonary end of the ductus while the long sheath over the balloon catheter adds further support to the shaft of the floating balloon catheter. The forward pressure on the balloon catheter/sheath forces the balloon against the pulmonary end of the ductus and fixes the partially extruded coil against the pulmonary end of the ductus. This prevents the pulmonary loop of coil from pulling through the ductus and, of equal importance, prevents additional loops of the coil from working their way back into the pulmonary side of the ductus as the remainder of the coil is extruded into the aortic ampulla. With the pulmonary end of the coil held in this manner, the aortic end of the coil is extruded in small increments. Each time a loop of coil is exposed in the aorta, the retrograde delivery catheter is re-advanced, pushing each individual loop of coil into the ampulla instead of the single "slinky" type release of the aortic loops of the coil.

Once all of the aortic loops are extruded into the ampulla the coil is released from the delivery catheter by the final 1–2 mm extrusion. With the balloon still against the pulmonary loop of coil and while the Terumo™ wire is still passing through the coil/ductus, a descending aorta aortogram is performed through the delivery catheter with the tip of the retrograde catheter positioned immediately adjacent to the aortic ampulla of the ductus. This aortogram is to check the position and fixation of the coil in the ductus.

The balloon fixation technique still does not allow the withdrawal of the coil back into the *delivery* catheter. If the coils appear in an unsatisfactory or unstable position and while it still is held in place by the balloon on the pulmonary side of the ductus pushing firmly against the loop of coil in the pulmonary end of the ductus, the aortic end of the coil is grasped with a retrograde snare or "grabber". Once the coil is grasped with the snare or grabber, the balloon in the pulmonary artery is released from its "forward pressure" and the coil is withdrawn out of the body through the arterial sheath. The wire remains through the ductus and the sheath and "floating" balloon catheter are still in place in the pulmonary artery. The procedure is restarted with a new different sized coil using the same technique for holding the pulmonary loop of coil.

When satisfied with the position of the coil after its complete extrusion from the delivery catheter, the forward pressure (push) on the balloon catheter/long sheath is relaxed very slowly and the combination balloon/long sheath is withdrawn very gingerly *over the wire* that remains through the ductus and coil. Once the sheath and balloon are away from the coil/ductus, the balloon is deflated. A repeat aortogram is performed to recheck for residual leak. If there is a significant residual leak, the ductus and first coil are recrossed with the retrograde delivery catheter and additional coils are delivered retrograde through the original coil(s) while the support Terumo™ wire is still in place through the ductus. With the prograde Terumo™ wire still through the ductus and the initial coil, the pulmonary loop of any additional coils can be fixed against the pulmonary end of the ductus by reinflating the balloon in the pulmonary artery and pushing it forward with the sheath over the wire during the delivery of the additional coil.

Once satisfied with the position of the coil(s) and the degree of occlusion of the ductus, the support wire that is passing through the coils in the ductus is withdrawn. The balloon is reinflated, the balloon catheter and the sheath are pushed gently against the pulmonary end of the ductus and the implanted coils while the long support, Terumo™ wire is withdrawn slowly and carefully out of the ductus and the coils(s). The Terumo™ wire is withdrawn into the end-hole balloon catheter while observing the balloon catheter/sheath, the wire and the coils closely on fluoroscopy. Once the Terumo™ wire is completely out of the ductus (and coils), the balloon catheter and sheath are withdrawn carefully away from the ductus, the balloon deflated and the balloon is withdrawn from the pulmonary artery. The position of the coil(s) and the degree of occlusion are verified with a final descending aortogram adjacent to the ductus. If there still is a residual leak, the ductus can be recrossed with the small retrograde catheter, similarly to the procedure with "free-release" coils, and additional coils are added until there is no residual "jet-like" leak.

The balloon technique has the advantage of securing the otherwise "free-release" coil in position while it is being extruded. One disadvantage of the technique is that the balloon may occlude a residual leak while the balloon is still being pushed against the pulmonary end of the ductus and, in turn, falsely suggest there is no leak. The balloon support technique also has the potential disadvantage of dislodging the implanted coil as the support wire is being withdrawn from the ductus or when the balloon catheter is moved away from the recently implanted coil. It does add to the complexity of the procedure as well as the additional expense of the balloon catheter, long sheath and the Terumo™ wire.

There is an alternative to this technique, which does not require the wire passing through the ductus (and through the freshly implanted coils). The *coil* still is delivered through a retrograde catheter. A Swan™ balloon catheter is introduced through either a standard short introductory sheath or through a long Mullins™ sheath which has been preshaped and positioned in the pulmonary artery as previously described. The balloon catheter is advanced into the main pulmonary artery. The *stiff end* of a very stiff spring guide wire or a 0.021″ Mullins™ wire is *pre-formed* outside of the body to match the contour or course of a catheter through the right ventricle to the main pulmonary artery to the ductus. The pre-formed stiff wire is advanced to the tip of the balloon catheter. The balloon is inflated in the pulmonary artery and pushed forward to be sure that the pre-formed stiff wire will hold the balloon in the proper position and allow the balloon to be pushed directly against the pulmonary end of the ductus. If the balloon catheter was introduced through a long sheath, the sheath adds additional support and directional control of the balloon against the ductus. When the proper curves on the wire and the long sheath have been established, the stiff wire/sheath will push the inflated balloon against the partially extruded coil in the pulmonary artery and hold the pulmonary loop of coil in place, similarly to the previous version of this technique.

This variation in the technique avoids the necessity of the wire passing through the implanted coils and then the need for withdrawing the wire through the freshly implanted coils immediately after their implant in the ductus. This variation of the balloon-assisted delivery has the disadvantage of not fixing the balloon as securely against the pulmonary loop of coil as with the balloon assisted technique with the wire passing through the ductus.

Snare-assisted Gianturco™ coil delivery

Another innovative technique for control of the standard Gianturco™ coil during its delivery is the use of a snare catheter to hold the *distal end* of the coil in place during its extrusion into the ductus from the delivery catheter and to maintain total control over the coil after its extrusion from the delivery catheter[13]. This snare technique is used primarily for the retrograde delivery of coils, however it is also applicable to the prograde delivery of coils.

The ductus configuration and size are established and a retrograde coil delivery catheter is advanced from the aorta and through the ductus as with all other retrograde coil deliveries. A 4- or 5-French snare catheter with a 10 mm diameter snare (Microvena™ Corporation, White Bear Lake, MN) is advanced into the pulmonary artery from the venous approach. In spite of the poor maneuverability of the snare catheters, this usually is accomplished either by maneuvering the snare catheter directly to the pulmonary artery or with the use of a floppy tipped guide wire passed through the snare catheter and advanced first into the pulmonary artery. An alternative, and *preferable* approach, which adds considerable additional safety to the procedure, is to position a 6- or 7-French *long sheath* in the pulmonary artery from the venous approach before introducing the snare catheter. Once the long sheath is in position in the pulmonary artery, the snare catheter is advanced to the pulmonary artery through the long sheath. The long sheath provides immediate and direct access to the pulmonary artery plus some additional support and control over the snare catheter once it is in position in the pulmonary artery. Of even more importance, if a snared coil inadvertently pulls through the ductus into the pulmonary artery, it is essential that the coil is withdrawn *into* a long sheath *before* it is withdrawn through the right ventricle. With the snare already advanced through the long sheath, this becomes automatic.

The 10 mm snare is opened in the pulmonary artery and maneuvered around the tip of the retrograde delivery catheter, which has already passed through the ductus into the pulmonary artery. This "capturing" of the delivery catheter takes some combined, simultaneous manipulations of the snare and the retrograde catheters as well as "three-dimensional" imaging using biplane fluoroscopy. The snare is closed loosely around the distal tip of the retrograde delivery catheter. The snare around the delivery catheter purposefully is allowed to slip distally to within 1–2 millimeters of the tip of the delivery catheter as the delivery catheter is withdrawn toward the ductus. The snare is tightened securely enough around the delivery catheter at this position to hold the snare one to two millimeters from the *tip* of the catheter, however, the snare must *not* be tightened so much that it compresses or indents the coil delivery catheter.

The appropriate coil for the occlusion of the PDA is introduced into and advanced just to the tip of the delivery catheter while the tip of the delivery catheter in the pulmonary artery is held securely with the snare. 1–2 *mm* of the coil wire is extruded cautiously from the tip of the delivery catheter and through the encircling snare. No more than 1–2 mm of the coil is exposed as even this short segment begins to curve away from the long axis of the catheter. Any extra length of coil passing through the snare will curl further and interfere with, or even prevent, the later release of the coil from the snare. Even this very short, 1–2 mm segment of extruded coil extending from the tip of the catheter creates a 45–90° angle off the long axis of the catheter. The snare is loosened very slightly and withdrawn very carefully to the tip of the delivery catheter. With continual slow and very careful withdrawal of the snare catheter, the minimally loosened snare slides just off the tip of the catheter and around the short segment of the exposed coil. The snare is immediately tightened around the small length of the exposed coil. The snare is tightened *just enough* to hold the coil (although instinctively the inclination is to tighten the snare very tightly). The snare *must not* be tightened so much that it indents into the windings of the coil of the coil wire.

With the tip of the coil in the pulmonary artery grasped with the snare, the delivery catheter alone is withdrawn very slightly, exposing 1/4 to 1/2 loop of coil in the pulmonary artery. Once the 1/2 loop of coil is exposed, then as the retrograde delivery catheter is withdrawn toward the ductus along with the minimally extruded coil, the snare catheter is *advanced a comparable distance* along with the delivery catheter and attached partial loop of coil. This allows the delivery catheter to be withdrawn while maintaining the same loop of extruded coil. The delivery catheter with the coil is withdrawn while the snare is advanced until the extruded partial "pulmonary loop" of the coil is against the pulmonary end of the ductus. The exposed loop of coil bends or "flexes" against the pulmonary end of the ductus as it reaches that location. The snare now is held in place along with the "pulmonary loop" of the coil while the delivery catheter is withdrawn into the descending aorta. This obligates the remainder of the coil to extrude into the aorta/aortic ampulla of the ductus while the partial loop is held securely in the pulmonary artery by the snare. While the snare is controlling the position of the coil in the ductus, there is no need for a rapid "slinky" deployment of the aortic end of the coil. With the snare holding the pulmonary end of the coil, the delivery catheter is withdrawn very slowly and in small increments, observing the exact deployment of each loop very carefully. During a slow controlled deployment while controlling the pulmonary loop with the snare, each aortic loop of the coil can be "pushed" into the aortic ampulla by re-advancing the delivery catheter/wire against the extruding aortic loops of coil.

If there is less than 1/4 to 1/2 loops of the coil in the pulmonary artery after the coil is fully deployed and completely freed from the delivery catheter, the snare catheter holding the coil is withdrawn very slightly. This pulls more of the length of the coil from the aortic ampulla into the pulmonary loop of the coil on the pulmonary artery side of the ductus. This must be performed *very* cautiously as the entire coil can easily be pulled through the ductus and into the pulmonary artery. When satisfied with the position of the coil, a confirmatory descending aortogram is performed for verification of the position and degree of closure. If not satisfied with the degree of closure, an additional "free-release" coil can be added using the original delivery catheter while still holding the original coil in place. Alternatively, the original coil is released from the snare and the additional coil delivered using the same snare technique after the retrograde delivery catheter has repassed through the ductus and the first coil, or even a totally "free-release" can be used for the additional coil(s).

Releasing and withdrawing the snare from its grip on the coil can be very tricky and difficult. When satisfied with the position and closure of the ductus or when planning to use the snare for a second coil implant, the snare is opened completely by advancing the snare control wire. Once the snare is open completely, the snare catheter is withdrawn ***very carefully and very slowly*** away from the coil. It is *very common* for the fiber strands of the coil and/or the wire of the coil itself, to hang up on the snare. When the snare does not release freely and completely from the wires of the coil itself, it is obvious *only when this problem is anticipated and looked for*. When the snare is caught on the coil, as the fully opened snare is withdrawn slowly from the coil, the shape of the loop of the snare begins to distort, part of the opened *loop of the snare* does *not* move away from the coil and/or, at the same time, the end of the coil begins to move toward the snare. When the snare remains entangled only in the fibers of the coil, the entrapment is far less obvious, and unless there is a very high index of suspicion it will be missed. The entanglement of just the fibers in the windings of the snare loop can occur by itself and/or after the snare has been released from entanglement with the wires of the coil itself. When the snare catches on only the fibers of the coil, the opened snare can move as much as 1–1.5 *cm away from*, and *appear free* of the coil, even when the snare loop is still *attached tightly* by long strands of the coil fibers. When attached by the fibers only, and when this is not anticipated, as the snare is withdrawn further, the coil is pulled along with the snare and out of the ductus by the fibers only attached to the snare! Although the fibers on the coil seem to be caught securely on the snare, there is not enough real, or persistent, control of the loose coil by this fibrous connection to allow any control over, and the retrieval of, the coil.

The snare hanging up on the coil windings and/or fibers ***always*** *should be anticipated* and always must be managed *patiently*. When persistent attachment to the wire windings of the coil is encountered, the opened snare is rotated very gently in both directions while simultaneously moving it back and forth very slightly. Partially opening and closing the snare during this movement often is helpful. All of the time the *coil* is observed very closely and should not be moved significantly by the manipulations with the snare. Eventually and usually, the snare springs free of the *wire windings* of the coil. Once free from the wire windings, the operator *should assume* that the snare *also is caught on the fibers* of the coil! Further withdrawal of the snare is performed very cautiously and under continual fluoroscopic observation. When caught on the fibers, the coil moves synchronously with the snare movement, but now the snare loop is one or more *centimeters* away from the coil! Again this is treated with patience. First an attempt is made at re-closing the snare and "withdrawing" the snare into the snare catheter by *advancing the snare catheter* over the snare loop—all of the time watching the coil and making sure it is not being pulled along with the snare. If this is not successful the snare is opened and closed into the catheter slowly and repeatedly while at the same time rotating and moving the snare to-and-fro very carefully. Usually one or a combination of these manipulations eventually will free the snare from the fibers. Even when fairly sure that the fibers are free, the snare is withdrawn very slowly and with continual fluoroscopic observation of the coil in order to be certain that there are no additional fibers holding the snare—even as far as 2 cm away from the coil!

The advantage of the snare technique is the controlled retention of the pulmonary loop as the aortic loops are being extruded. Once the aortic loops are extruded completely, the ability exists to readjust the coil position toward the pulmonary artery by pulling more of a loop into the pulmonary artery with the snare. The snare still does not provide any capability for withdrawal of the coil back into the original delivery catheter if too much becomes extruded into the pulmonary artery. If the coil is markedly malpositioned or actually pulls completely through the ductus into the pulmonary artery, the snare then has a hold on the coil for control and retrievability from the pulmonary artery side.

It is recommended that when the snare technique is used, the snare catheter *always* should be delivered to the pulmonary artery through a larger diameter, long sheath, which remains positioned in the pulmonary artery during the coil delivery. The advantage of beginning the procedure with the snare catheter through a long sheath positioned in the pulmonary artery is that a malpositioned or displaced coil in the pulmonary artery can be pulled directly into the long sheath and out of the body.

If the snare catheter initially was not positioned in the pulmonary artery through a long sheath and even though the snare has a hold and control of an errant coil, when a snared coil pulls completely into the pulmonary artery, matters become even more complicated. When an opened and exposed coil is pulled from the pulmonary artery through the right ventricle, there is a very high likelihood that the coil will become entangled tightly in the tricuspid valve apparatus. If a coil that is entangled in the tricuspid valve cannot be untangled easily and without trauma to the valve, then the relatively straightforward transcatheter ductal occlusion procedure or even the alternative "simple" and elective lateral thoracotomy surgical division of a ductus has been converted into a far more complex, urgent and open-heart surgical repair!

When the snare catheter had not been passed through a long sheath initially and a coil that is grasped by the snare is pulled through the ductus into the pulmonary artery, a second venous catheter is introduced and a large, long sheath is introduced into the pulmonary artery utilizing this second catheter. A second snare or a "grabber" retrieval catheter is delivered to the pulmonary artery through the long sheath which is now positioned in the pulmonary artery. The errant coil is re-snared or "grabbed" with the new retrieval device which is passing through the long sheath, released from the first snare, withdrawn into the long sheath and out of the pulmonary artery through the long sheath.

In addition to the disadvantages of only partial controllability and of snagging of the snare on the coil, the snare-assisted technique requires the additional expertise for the use of the snare and incurs the additional expenses of the snare and long sheath.

Latson delivery catheter modification

One of the more unusual, simplest and probably, the more effective of the "modified techniques" for the delivery of coils to the PDA is the Latson modification of the delivery catheter for the delivery of the standard "free-release" Gianturco™ coils[15]. The distal end of a 5-French Mallinckrodt™ vertebral catheter is softened in the dry heat jet of a heat gun or in boiling sterile water. The warmed tip of the catheter is pulled away from the shaft of the catheter until the softened portion stretches, thins and then pulls apart. This leaves the catheter with a very long tapered tip, which also has a *very small*, almost pin point distal opening. A standard 0.035″ spring guide wire is introduced into the proximal end of the catheter and advanced through the catheter until it stops at the newly created taper at the distal tip of the catheter. Starting very distally on the newly tapered and very fine tip of the catheter, the tip is excised (amputated) sequentially in minute (1/2 to 1 mm) increments until the tip of the 0.035″ wire can be *forced* barely through the now shortened but finely tapered tip of the catheter and forced through the tip only by a very firm push from the proximal end of the wire. In order to create a reasonably smooth tip, a very sharp razor blade is used to excise the segments of the tip.

The opening that eventually is created (reached) as the catheter is excised back to the new tip, allows a 0.038″ Gianturco™ occlusion coil (which actually is a 0.035″ spring wire) to be pushed through the tip, but also only with some significant force to overcome the extra resistance of the newly narrowed opening. The slight, added diameter to the coil wire that is created by the enmeshed nylon fibers results in a catheter tip that the occlusion coil must be *forced* through for delivery (extrusion) from the catheter.

The fit over the coil wire (and fibers) is tight enough that when the catheter is withdrawn with even as little as 2–3 mm of the coil still within the catheter, the exposed coil still will be withdrawn along with the catheter rather than being pulled out of the catheter! The catheter with the partially extruded coil actually can be withdrawn carefully out of the body through a sheath without the coil being pulled out of the catheter. Currently there are two commercially available 5-French end-hole catheters with the tip of the catheter appropriately modified for this technique. They are the Latson™ multipurpose catheter: #248498 (Cook Inc., Bloomington, IN) and the modified vertebral catheter: #WN27750 (Mallinckrodt Inc., St. Louis, MO). These commercially available catheters obviate the need for "hand-making" each catheter, however their effectiveness is dependent upon the *very close* tolerances of the manufacturers.

Up until the moment of coil extrusion, the prerequisites of the anatomy of the ductus and techniques for coil delivery using the Latson™ catheter with the modified tip are the same as for the standard "free-release" coils. The occlusion of the ductus using the modified catheter tip technique can be used from either the retrograde or the prograde approach, and depends entirely upon operator preference.

For the retrograde approach, the specially modified delivery catheter is introduced into the femoral artery through an indwelling short sheath, advanced retrograde in the aorta, and manipulated across the ductus and into the pulmonary artery. The coil is introduced into the proximal end of the catheter through a wire back-bleed device, however, the *stiff end* of the spring guide wire is used as the pusher wire to advance the coil through the catheter to the tip. When the catheter is in position across the ductus and adjacent to the pulmonary end of the ductus, the coil is pushed forcefully and in very small increments out of the catheter with the pusher wire. One half to one full loop of the coil is formed on the pulmonary side of the ductus. The catheter with the partially extruded coil is pulled back against the pulmonary end of the ductus. As the delivery catheter is withdrawn into the ductus, the pusher wire is advanced in small, forced increments equivalent to the distance that the catheter is withdrawn and according to how the coils are forming on the aortic side of the ductus. If too much coil is advanced into the pulmonary side of the ductus, the delivery catheter *with the partially extruded coil* is withdrawn back toward the aorta. This straightens part of the coil in the ductus and shortens or decreases the pulmonary loop of coil. As the aortic loops of coil are formed, the delivery catheter is re-advanced intermittently to push the multiple loops of coil into the aortic ampulla while the catheter is still attached and just before the final several millimeters of the coil are forced out of the delivery catheter. If the coil does not seat properly in the ampulla, the delivery catheter in the aorta is withdrawn in order to stretch out and straighten the coil in the aorta slightly. This repositioning of the coil in the ampulla is attempted without "releasing" the coil. This is possible since the final release of the coil requires a purposeful, *forceful* push on the pusher wire to extrude the final several millimeters of coil.

If a satisfactory position of the coil in the ductus cannot be accomplished, the delivery catheter with the attached coil dangling at the end of the delivery catheter is withdrawn from the ductus, down the descending aorta and carefully out of the artery through the femoral artery sheath. The procedure can then be restarted with a different coil. The retrograde approach using this catheter has the advantage over the prograde approach that the fully extruded, but still attached coil can be withdrawn completely from the body without crossing and possibly becoming entangled in vital cardiac structures such as the tricuspid valve, which can occur when the prograde venous approach is used.

When the prograde approach is used with this catheter, it is recommended that the modified coil catheter initially is delivered to the pulmonary artery *through a long 6-French sheath* similar to the introduction of the snare catheter when the "snare-assisted" technique is used. With the prograde delivery catheter already passing through a long sheath, which is positioned in the pulmonary artery, and if the coil inadvertently does pull completely out of the ductus into the pulmonary artery, the extruded coil automatically is pulled into the long sheath *before* it is withdrawn through the right ventricle and tricuspid valve.

Using the prograde approach with the Latson™ modified catheter, the tip of the delivery catheter is advanced through the ductus and positioned in the descending aorta. When, for example, a "four-loop" coil is used, 2 1/2 to 3 loops are extruded into the descending aorta adjacent to the aortic ampulla. The coil, which has the "aortic" loops extruded but is still "attached" to the delivery catheter, is withdrawn into the ductus ampulla. A small aortogram is performed injecting through a separate retrograde catheter, which should be positioned immediately adjacent to, but just distal to the ampulla. With satisfactory seating of the coil in the ampulla (and occlusion of the ductus!), the tip of the delivery catheter is withdrawn across the narrowest portion of the ductus while simultaneously and forcefully pushing the pusher/ delivery wire forward the same distance, which, in turn, extrudes more of the coil. This portion of the coil, which is still attached to the tip of the catheter, begins to loop in the pulmonary artery. The position is rechecked with another aortogram. When the position appears satisfactory, the final 1–2 mm of coil are pushed forcefully out of the catheter, releasing the coil. At any time up until this purposeful release, the coil still is attached securely to the delivery catheter and can be pulled back to reposition more coil on the pulmonary side of the ductus and/or to totally withdraw the extruded coil into the long sheath.

This modified catheter has the distinct advantage of providing significant control over the extrusion of the coil as well as retrievability of the coil until the final 1–2 mm of coil forcibly and purposefully are pushed out of the tip of the catheter. The major disadvantage until recently was that the modified catheters were not commercially available and had to be hand-made for each case. Even with the commercially available modified catheters, the tolerances vary slightly making the "grip" on the coil variable and not totally reliable. When the modified opening is very tight, the extrusion of the coil requires a very hard push to accomplish the extrusion of the coil, which makes it difficult (or impossible) to extrude the coil in fine, precise increments. When the modified opening is not tight enough, the delivery catheter will act like a standard free-release catheter. The coil delivery catheter cannot be withdrawn when the coil is partially extruded without the coil being delivered completely.

Modification of the pusher wire for coil delivery

A unique but very simple modification of the "pusher" wire and a standard Gianturco™ coil provides some retrievability of the coils somewhat similarly the Detachable™ coils. This modification is based on the fact that the coils themselves, except for the very distal tip, are hollow and the proximal end of the coil actually opens into a hollow lumen, which has a "spiral metal" lining formed by the inside of the wire windings. A standard spring guide wire one size smaller than the coil wire can be "inserted" forcefully into the open end of the coil. This technique is limited to use with the larger 0.038″ and 0.052″ coils.

A 4-French, long *sheath* is positioned through the ductus from either the prograde venous or the retrograde arterial approach. This usually requires the passage of an end-hole catheter and then replacing that catheter with the long sheath/dilator over an exchange wire. The coil is chosen according to the size and shape of the ductus.

The tip of a 0.038″ spring guide wire is introduced into the *distal* end of the metal loader containing the 0.038″ coil and is advanced several millimeters until it pushes the *proximal* end of the straight, loaded coil several millimeters *backward* out of the *proximal* end of the metal loader/holder. This exposes several millimeters of the *hollow* proximal end of the 0.038″ coil. A 4-French end-hole coil catheter, which just barely will accommodate a 0.035″ wire, but will *not* accommodate the 0.038″ (or larger) coil wire, is used as the "pusher" catheter. (When a 0.052″ *coil* is being used, a 0.038″ pusher wire and a "pusher" catheter that will just accommodate the 0.038″ wire are substituted for the 0.035″ wire and 4-French catheter.) The 4-French catheter is passed from the proximal to the distal end through a short 4-French sheath. The short, 4-French sheath must be long enough to accommodate the length of the particular occlusion coil when the coil is straightened completely. The short, 4-French sheath is withdrawn back over the shaft of the "pusher" catheter. A 0.035″ spring guide wire, which fits *snugly within the 4-French pusher catheter*, is advanced through the 4-French end-hole "pusher" catheter until the distal tip of this 0.035″ wire extends just beyond the tip of the catheter. The tip of this 0.035″ guide wire is forced a short distance *into* the exposed, hollow, proximal end of the 0.038″ coil that is to be used for the occlusion. When forced into the end of the larger coil wire, this 0.035″ wire creates a reasonably tight connection between the 0.038″ coil and the proximal, open tip of the 0.035″ spring guide wire. The short sheath is advanced over and past the tip of the "pusher" catheter and just over the tip of the guide wire now attached to the coil. The guide "pusher" wire, the "pusher" catheter and the attached coil are withdrawn together and, with this, the straight coil is withdrawn completely out of the metal loader and completely into the short 4-French sheath. This 4-French sheath now serves as the coil loader.

The 4-French sheath containing the coil is introduced through a back-bleed valve on the hub of the long 4-French delivery sheath which has been pre-positioned through the ductus. By advancing the 4-French "pusher" catheter and the guide wire together as a unit, the coil is advanced out of the short ("loader") sheath and completely into the long delivery sheath. The short, 4-French "loader" sheath is withdrawn out of the hub of the long sheath, over the "pusher catheter" and back to the hub of the pusher catheter. The combination coil, guide wire and 4-French "pusher" catheter are advanced as a unit through the long sheath. As the elongated coil passes through the ductus and approaches the end of the long sheath, the guide wire and the 4-French pusher catheter are advanced together, which in turn, advances the coil further and extrudes it out of the tip of the delivery sheath. Under close fluoroscopic observation, the coil is extruded out of the tip of the long delivery sheath exactly as it would be out of a catheter with a "free-release" coil (depending upon whether the prograde or retrograde approach is used). The major difference and advantage of this "attachment system" is that if too much coil is extruded in any location or if the coil generally needs to be repositioned, the coil can be *withdrawn* back into the long sheath by withdrawing the "attached" guide/pusher wire, the pusher catheter and the coil together back into the sheath.

When the coil is positioned correctly, the 4-French covering, "pusher" catheter is advanced over the guide wire until it pushes tightly against the attached, proximal end of the *larger* diameter occlusion coil. The larger coil cannot enter the 4-French "pusher" catheter, so when the spring guide pusher wire is withdrawn forcefully while holding the "pusher" catheter and long sheath in place against the end of the coil, the 0.035" wire pulls out of the end of the larger occlusion coil, releasing the coil in the ductus.

The advantage of this control over the coil is obvious. The disadvantage is that fixation of the tip of the 0.035" spring guide wire within the end of the coil is very inconsistent, with a very limited or no control over the degrees of tightness. If the pusher/delivery wire is not pushed into the coil tightly enough, the coil can come free during any attempt at withdrawal. If the guide wire is pushed into the coil too far and, in turn, too tightly, the coil does not release when the wire is withdrawn or when it does release, it does so violently. The violent withdrawal of the attach/pusher wire from the coil easily can displace the implanted coil. A manufactured version of this presently improvised attach system, but with resultant very tight and consistent tolerances, would make this system much more appealing.

Bioptome-controlled delivery

The most recent, very innovative and very effective modification of the Gianturco™ coil delivery technique is to use a small, 3-French bioptome (Cook Inc., Bloomington, IN) to hold one end of the coil during delivery[14]. The coil is held with the bioptome during implant, repositioning and until the coil is in an ideal position before releasing it purposefully. The technique is usable with both the standard 0.038" and 0.052" Gianturco™ coils. The bioptome control technique for coil delivery became more widely used and almost essential with the introduction of the larger and much stiffer 0.052" coils and their availability for PDA occlusion[17].

Using the bioptome-controlled technique, the patient undergoes a right heart catheterization and an aortogram through a retrograde catheter in the descending aorta exactly as with any other PDA occlusion procedure. The bioptome-controlled modification does not alter the way the ductus is studied and measured nor any other parts of the catheterization prior to the PDA occlusion. Bioptome control of the coil delivery is applicable from either the prograde or the retrograde approach. The prograde venous approach for the bioptome-controlled technique does have the advantage of allowing a larger sheath/delivery system for the large coils without compromising an artery.

The bioptome-controlled coil is delivered to the ductus through a long 4- or 5-French sheath, which is used as the "delivery catheter". The sheaths have an attached back-bleed valve with a flush port on the proximal end and a radio-opaque "marker band" at the distal end of the sheath. The use of a long sheath for the coil delivery rather than a "delivery catheter" allows the use of this technique and the larger coils without a significant increase in the size of the "delivery catheter". The marker band on the long sheath allows easy and definite visualization of the end of the sheath during the critical extrusion of the coil, but at the same time does not allow for any "stretching" or *circumferential* distortion and/or change in the *round* cross-sectional configuration of the tip of the sheath. The fit of the "closed" bioptome while grasping the 0.052" coil is tight within a 4-French sheath, particularly as the bioptome attached to the coil exits the distal end of the sheath in the area of the marker band. Because of the "tightness" of the bioptome when grasping the 0.052" coil in the 4-French sheath, a 5-French long sheath is preferred for the delivery of the 0.052" coils.

Because of a significant problem in withdrawing a fully extruded *0.052" coil* back into either a 4- or 5-French sheath, the 4- or 5-F delivery sheath is advanced to, and positioned in, *the pulmonary artery* through a larger diameter, 6- or 7-French long sheath as an added safety procedure during any *prograde approach* for the bioptome-assisted coil delivery technique. A 6- or 7-French *long sheath* first is positioned in the pulmonary artery and then the smaller diameter, long 4- or 5-French coil delivery sheath is delivered to the pulmonary artery *through the larger, long sheath*. The long, 4- or 5-French coil delivery sheath obviously must be at least several centimeters longer than the outer 6- or 7-French long sheath. The larger, long outer sheath in the pulmonary artery ensures that a coil that is grasped in the pulmonary artery and regardless of any angulation, can be withdrawn into a sheath before the coil is withdrawn through the right ventricle. Since the coil delivery sheaths are introduced into the vein through sheaths of the larger sizes anyway, this does not increase the French size of the introductory system. This is the standard technique used by the author.

Since most of the long sheaths have a built in, 180° "transseptal" curve at the tip, both the longer, 4- or 5-French coil delivery sheath and the outer 6- or 7-French long sheaths are "straightened" to a 40–50° smooth curve at the tip which corresponds to the course from the right ventricle into the pulmonary artery and to the ductus as seen in the lateral fluoroscopic view. The curve is formed slightly tighter for the smaller, longer coil delivery sheath. The sheaths are straightened into the less acute curves by pulling the distal end of the sheath/dilator combination several times between the tightly gripped thumb and forefinger, or by heating the distal end of the combination sheath/dilator in boiling water and manually reshaping them to the desired curve while cooling the combination in a bowl of flush solution.

The ductus is crossed from the pulmonary artery to the aorta with a maneuverable, torque-controlled, end-hole, diagnostic catheter (a Goodale–Lubin or Gensini type catheter), advanced well into the descending aorta, and then replaced with an exchange length spring guide wire. The long "pre-shaped" 6- or 7-French sheath/dilator is advanced to *the pulmonary artery* over the exchange length wire, which remains fixed in position passing through the ductus. The long dilator is removed over the wire leaving the sheath in the pulmonary artery over the wire, which is still passing through the ductus. The larger, long sheath is cleared of air/clot and placed on a slow, constant flush. The "pre-curved" 4- or 5-French coil delivery sheath/dilator is advanced through the long sheath, over the wire, and passed *through* the ductus into the proximal descending aorta several centimeters distal to the aortic end of the ductus. If the additional, larger diameter, long sheath is not used, the 4- and 5-French long sheaths are introduced into the vein through short 6- and 7-French sheaths, respectively, and advanced over the wire and through the ductus until the tip of the long delivery *sheath* is positioned in the descending aorta. The long 4- or 5-F dilator and the exchange wire are removed, leaving the 4- or 5-French long sheath in place across the ductus. The delivery sheath is cleared very carefully of any air or clot by allowing it to bleed back through the side port and then the sheath is flushed.

In order to be used with the bioptome technique, the occlusion coil requires a special preparation to be grasped with the bioptome. All Gianturco™ coils consist of a very fine stainless steel wire wound to form a larger "spring guide" type wire of the advertised "wire" diameter. One end of the "spring" wire is sealed with a small "weld" while the opposite end is a very tiny, open tube of the fine wires. The coils, including the 0.052″ coils, come loaded in a metal "loading tube" with the "welded" end of the coil at the distal end of the loader.

The bioptome jaws when clamped over the tip of the coil will not fit back into the original metal loader. The combination must be withdrawn into a separate slightly larger "loader" in order to be front-loaded into the delivery sheath. Before the coil is grasped with the bioptome, the bioptome is passed through the *separate* slightly larger metal loading tube (which is available with the 0.052″ coils) or in the absence of this specific loading tube, a short length of 4-French sheath is used as the new, larger loading tube. The length of the 4-French sheath must be long enough to contain the entire length of the *straightened* coil. After the bioptome is passed through the separate metal loading tube or the short 4-French sheath, the metal loading tube or length of sheath is withdrawn back onto the shaft of the bioptome catheter toward its control handle, and remains there while the coil is prepared and attached to the bioptome.

The stiff end of a separate 0.038″ or 0.052″ spring guide wire is introduced into the *proximal* end of the coil holder/loader and advanced very slightly until just *1–2 mm* of the *distal* (sealed or welded) end of the coil is extruded out of the distal end of the metal loading tube. This exposes the tiny welded tip, which seals the end of the finely coiled wires of which the "spring coil" is made. While holding the short exposed more proximal portion of the *coil* tightly between the fingers, the small welded tip (only) is grasped tightly with a forceps and pulled 0.25 to 0.5 mm away from the remainder of the spring coil, which is being held by the fingers of the other hand. This maneuver leaves the small welded ball separated approximately 0.5 mm from the windings of the coiled portion of the "spring wire" but still attached by a single, stretched-out strand of the fine, very stiff wire. This separation of the welded "ball" allows the bioptome jaws to grasp the "ball" firmly while at the same time allowing the bioptome jaws to close almost completely over the stretched out single strand of the coil wire. This allows the combination of the closed 3-French bioptome jaws holding the 0.052″ coil wire along with the welded "ball", still to be less than 4-French in diameter.

With the "new" larger loading tube or short sheath positioned on the proximal shaft of the bioptome catheter, the bioptome jaws are opened and then closed tightly around the separated, welded ball at the end of the coil (still within the original loading tube with the "weld" just barely sticking out of it). With one operator holding the bioptome jaws closed tightly over the "ball" at the tip of the coil, the separate "new" loading tube/short sheath through which the bioptome previously was passed is advanced over the bioptome jaws which now have the tip of the coil grasped within them. The entire coil is drawn out of the original metal loading tube directly into the "new" short sheath or "loading tube". The coil is withdrawn into this new tube until the now distal (original proximal) end of the coil is *just within* the tip of the "new loading" tube. The bioptome-controlled coil is now ready to be delivered from the new loading tube into the long delivery sheath.

The distal end of the new "loading" tube is introduced through the hemostasis valve and "seated" in the proximal end of the long 4- or 5-F coil delivery sheath. The straight coil is introduced into the sheath by advancing the shaft of the bioptome into the sheath, all of the time with the second operator holding the bioptome jaws closed tightly over the "ball" of the coil. The coil is advanced to the end of the sheath by advancing the bioptome catheter within the sheath while observing the end of the sheath on fluoroscopy.

With the sheath tip maintained in the descending aorta just distal to the ductus ampulla, two to three loops of coil (depending upon the eventual total number of loops) are extruded slowly from the sheath into the aorta. Once the coil has formed into several coiled *loops* in the aorta, the delivery sheath, along with the bioptome and extruded loops of coil are *withdrawn together* as a unit until the extruded loops are positioned within the aortic ampulla of the ductus. The marker band at the tip of the sheath is now at, or near, the narrowest area of the ductus or even slightly on the pulmonary end of the ductus. The larger long outer sheath tip is maintained in the proximal main pulmonary artery, being sure that it does not advance into the ductus over the smaller diameter long delivery sheath.

The opened loops of the stiff 0.052″ coils prevent the tip of the delivery sheath with the coil extruding from the tip, from pulling too far and through the pulmonary end of the ductus. The remaining, still straight portion of the coil and the bioptome jaws are visible on fluoroscopy extending back through the ductus, but still *within* the sheath. Fixing the sheath in this position, more coil wire is extruded into the ampulla by advancing the bioptome catheter until there is a short, straight length of coil equivalent to only 1/2–2/3 of a *loop* of the coil still remaining in the sheath and attached to the bioptome. The necessary length is calculated from the calculated length of straight coil it takes to make one loop of the particular "coil". An aortogram is repeated in the descending aorta adjacent to the aortic end of the ductus to verify the satisfactory coil position in the ductus. If the coil is not in the correct position and/or does not appear to be creating sufficient occlusion of the ductus, it is withdrawn partially or completely back into the delivery sheath and the implant restarted. Usually, as traction is placed on the coil to begin withdrawing it into the delivery sheath, the sheath can be re-advanced back through the ductus into the descending aorta in order to restart the extrusion without further repositioning of the delivery sheath!

When the coil is in a satisfactory position and while holding the bioptome in its precise position, the sheath is withdrawn off *most* of the remaining coil. This allows the final loop of coil to *begin* looping on the pulmonary side of the ductus. Because of the stiffness of the 0.052″ coil, the sheath/bioptome/coil combination often must be re-advanced intermittently during this last extrusion to allow the coil to form a loop without pulling the "aortic" loops through the ductus. It is preferable *not* to allow the *jaws* of the bioptome holding the very tip of the coil to advance out of the sheath at this point in the delivery process. As the final, pulmonary loop of the stiffer 0.052″ coil along with the jaws of the bioptome are deployed out of the tip of the 4- or 5-French sheath during the delivery of the 0.052″ coil, the coil usually and immediately angles 90° off the long axis of the jaws of the bioptome. This does not interfere with the grip on, and/or the release of, the coil, but does make any withdrawal of the coil back into the 4- or 5-French delivery sheath more difficult, if not impossible. Before the final portion of the coil with the "jaws" is extruded on the pulmonary end of the ductus, a repeat aortogram is performed with the retrograde catheter. The aortogram confirms the exact coil position, orientation and degree of closure, all while the coil is completely and easily retrievable.

If there is not enough of a loop of coil on the pulmonary side of the ductus and the bioptome jaws still are within the tip of the sheath, the entire sheath, bioptome and coil are withdrawn carefully. This pulls a very small additional amount of the coil into the pulmonary end of the ductus. After pulling more of the loop of coil to the pulmonary end of the ductus, the sheath *and* bioptome again are advanced slightly. This allows the coil to re-loop and provides a test for a sufficient loop of coil on the pulmonary end of the ductus. If there are too many loops of coil on the pulmonary side of the ductus, the sheath is advanced over the still grasped coil while withdrawing the bioptome/coil slightly. This allows the sheath to advance over the coil, back into and through the ductus, particularly when using the large 0.052″ coils. Once the sheath is back through the ductus, more loops are extruded on the aortic end and the implant process restarted. Occasionally, as the sheath is advanced over the coil, particularly with the 0.038″ coils, this actually withdraws most of the coil back into the delivery sheath, which is still on the pulmonary side of the ductus. When this occurs with any of the bioptome held coils, the coil is withdrawn completely out of the ductus and into the delivery sheath. Often with careful and meticulous manipulations, the long delivery sheath containing the bioptome catheter and coil can be re-advanced through the ductus and even into the descending aorta, where the extrusion process is restarted. If the sheath cannot be re-advanced through the ductus, the still grasped coil is withdrawn out of the delivery sheath, out of the body and back into the "loader". The delivery process is restarted beginning with the repositioning of the sheath across the ductus.

When a satisfactory loop of coil has been formed at the pulmonary end of the ductus, the sheath is withdrawn the final few millimeters off the tip of the coil and the bioptome jaws still grasping the coil. At the same time, the bioptome and coil are advanced just enough to relax any tension on the coil. This allows the stiff 0.052″ coil purposefully to angle and shorten as it "coils" and retracts against the pulmonary end of the ductus. While the stiff coil still is attached to the bioptome, it frequently aligns as a circular tube in the PA view and appears as a "donut" in the ampulla with the "hole" aligned with the lumen of the ductus. A repeat descending-aorta aortogram is performed as a final verification of the position and degree of occlusion of the ductus. Prior to the purposeful release, the coil still could be withdrawn within the ductus slightly for "fine" repositioning. With the outer, larger, 6- or 7-French sheath already in place in the pulmonary artery, even the acutely angled coil along with the smaller delivery sheath could be pulled back into the outer sheath. When satisfied with the position of the coil and the degree of occlusion, the bioptome jaws are opened to release the coil. As the tension and control are taken off the coil with the release, the coil often significantly changes its position in the ductus, realigning even 90° in its orientation. Fortunately, this usually represents a better "seating" in the ductus for ductal occlusion.

The bioptome-controlled technique provides as much, or better, control and retrievability of the standard coil as does the manufactured Detachable™ (or Jackson™) coil. The bioptome control technique not only allows, but makes the prograde venous approach preferable. The bioptome control technique is slightly more cumbersome and requires a larger delivery "catheter" than the manufactured detachable coil. Once the coil has been extruded all of the way out of the delivery sheath during delivery, it is difficult to withdraw the coil back into the 4- or 5-French delivery sheath, even though it is still grasped with the bioptome. By the use of the larger 6- or 7-French diameter, long outer sheath to delivery the 4- or 5-French delivery sheath to the pulmonary artery, this problem does not exist and, in turn, makes the procedure very safe. The addition of the long sheath(s) and the bioptome does add some additional expense to the procedure.

0.052 inch Gianturco coils

The larger 0.052″ coils were discussed along with the bioptome control delivery technique, but they deserve some special mention. The 0.052″ coil (Cook Inc., Bloomington, IN) is not only larger in the *coil wire* diameter, but the coils are constructed from a significantly heavier gauge wire and are significantly stiffer than any other Gianturco™ coils. As a consequence, when released, these coils tend to resume their tightly wound shape and form into fairly rigid circular "donuts" or cylinders of coil no matter where they are implanted. Because of their very rigid coiling characteristics, they routinely are delivered using the bioptome control technique as described previously in this chapter. The 0.052″ coils in the US are labeled according to (1) the length of the stretched out wire and (2) the diameter of the formed coil, with no mention of the number of coil loops formed in the labeling. The 0.052″ coils are available in 6, 8, 10 and 12 mm diameter coils with the stretched out length of the coil wires increasing with the coil diameter. The stretched lengths of the coil wires vary between 8 and 15 cm, and provide a varying number of loops of the coil. There are five different 0.052″ coils available (Table 27.1):

Table 27.1 0.052 inch Gianturco coils

Stretched coil length (cm)	Coil diameter (mm)	Number of loops
8	6	4.2
8	8	3.2
10	8	4.0
15	10	4.8
15	12	4.0

The stronger 0.052″ coil is not distorted significantly by external vascular pressure. Once implanted the 0.052″ coils do not change their configuration significantly nor are they pushed through an orifice smaller than their diameter as a consequence of persistent vascular *pressure* against them. The stronger coil provides improved fixation in the patent ductus, making them very useful for the larger PDA. Although these coils tend to resume their cylindrical configuration in the ductus, they also tend to orient obliquely in the ampulla of the ductus and as a consequence have a very high closure rate with only the one coil.

Because of the larger size of the coil wire and the standard use of the bioptome-controlled delivery technique, the 0.052″ coil requires a slightly larger internal diameter delivery system for implant. This is compensated for by the use of a long, thin-walled delivery sheath for the delivery of the 0.052″ coil and allows their use even in small infants. The one major disadvantages of a 0.052″ coil is that if the coil does embolize and/or otherwise have to be retrieved once it is completely out of the delivery sheath, it requires the use of *at least* a 7-French long sheath for retrieval. When an embolized coil is retrieved, it usually is grasped somewhere along the *length* of the coil rather than *exactly* at one end. Grasping the coil along its length requires the coil to be folded on itself, in order to be withdrawn into any sheath. In order to both fold the coil and to withdraw the double strands of the "folded" 0.052″ coil into a sheath/catheter, a significantly larger lumen than the original 4- or 5-French is required. If retrieval is necessary from a pulmonary artery, the larger retrieval sheath *must be* delivered to the pulmonary artery and the coil withdrawn *completely into the sheath* while the coil and tip of the sheath are still in the pulmonary artery and before attempting withdrawal of the coil through the right heart, and especially through the tricuspid valve.

In the event of a residual leak through the 0.052″ coil, additional 0.038″ or 0.035″ coils are delivered through a 4-French retrograde arterial catheter using a "free-release" delivery to finalize the ductus closure. Usually a coil with a diameter that will fit within the loop of the implanted 0.052″ coil is used for the additional implant. The 0.052″ coils are very stable within the ductus, so the ductus can be crossed and additional coils can be added relatively safely after the release of the original 0.052″ coil from the bioptome.

To deliver the additional coil, the retrograde angiographic catheter is replaced with a 4-French snare *catheter* (Microvena™ Corporation, White Bear Lake, MN). A small diameter teflon or hydrophilic Terumo™ Glide wire (Medi-Tech™ BSC, Watertown, MA) is used to manipulate through the 0.052″ coil in the PDA and into the pulmonary artery. The 4-French "snare" catheter or Terumo™ Glide catheter is advanced over the wire, through the 0.052″ coil and into the pulmonary artery. A 0.038″ or 0.035″ "free-release" Gianturco™ coil is delivered through this catheter. One loop of the retrograde delivered coil is formed in the pulmonary artery. As the catheter is withdrawn into the 0.052″ coil/residual leak, the retrograde coil is extruded and is coiled inside and intertwining with the larger diameter 0.052″ coil. With any persistent leak, this process is repeated.

When using the large, stiff 0.052″ coil for PDA occlusion, particularly in very small patients, extra precautions are taken in order to avoid obstruction of adjacent structures. When too much coil is placed on the pulmonary side of the ductus, the pulmonary loops potentially can obstruct the LPA partially. This occurs either by extension of the coil loops into the origin of the LPA and/or from *extrinsic compression* of the origin of the LPA by the mass of stiff coil in the adjacent ductus. In a small infant with a very flat ampulla, the multiple aortic loops can extend into the aortic lumen and potentially cause aortic obstruction.

The rare combination of a patent ductus and an anomalous right subclavian artery (RSCA) potentially creates a unique problem when using the larger 0.052″ coils. As the coil is extruded from the sheath on the aortic side of the ductus, the coil loops can form in the origin of the anomalous RSCA, which is very close to the aortic end of the ductus. The coil may still appear in a reasonable position on fluoroscopy alone. Only careful *angiography* during the delivery confirms the compromising position of the coil.

Simultaneous delivery of double or triple coils

In the absence of one of the newer and more suitable devices for occlusion of the very large PDA, several unique techniques for the delivery of two or even three coils simultaneously through one or multiple delivery systems have been devised. For either technique, the ductus is defined angiographically and measured exactly as with any other coil occlusion procedure.

The delivery through a single delivery system is an extreme modification of the bioptome-controlled delivery technique. The tips of two, or even three, 0.052″ coils are grasped simultaneously in the jaw of a single 7-French bioptome and then delivered simultaneously and side by side through an 8- or 9-French sheath[18]. With a very large ductus (over 6 mm in its narrowest diameter) the ductus is crossed from the pulmonary artery to the descending aorta with an end-hole catheter. A stiff exchange wire is passed through the catheter and the catheter is removed. A long, 8- or 9-French sheath/dilator set with an attached back-bleed valve and side arm flush system is advanced over the wire until the tip of the sheath is well into the descending aorta. An 8-French sheath is used when two coils are to be used and a 9-French sheath when three coils are to be used. The dilator and wire are removed and the sheath cleared of all air and/or clots.

The tips of two or three 0.052″ coils or a combination of 0.052″ and 0.038″ coils all are "prepared for grasping" exactly as prepared when a 3-French bioptome is used. A 7-French bioptome is passed through an 8- or 9-French short sheath, which must be at least as long as the stretched-out and straightened longest coil that is being used. The bioptome is passed from proximal to distal end through the short sheath and the short sheath is withdrawn back on the shaft of the bioptome. The prepared tips of the two (or three) coils can be intertwined together with only one of the tips grasped by the bioptome or, preferably, the prepared tips of the two or three separate coils are held close together and grasped side-by-side in the single large bioptome jaw. The 8- or 9-French short sheath is advanced over the bioptome jaw, which is holding the tips of the coils, which are still extending out of the tip of their original loaders. With the tips held tightly in the jaw, the two or three coils are drawn out of their respective separate loaders and side by side into the 8- or 9-French short sheath, which will act as the loader for the multiple coils side by side. Once the coils are withdrawn completely into the short sheath, the distal end of the short sheath is introduced into the valve of the long sheath and seated in the flange within the valve apparatus at the proximal end of the long sheath. The bioptome is advanced into the short sheath, which pushes the attached coils from the short "loader" sheath into the long sheath. This maneuver advances the coils side by side in the sheath ahead of the bioptome. The thickness of the multiple coils side by side keeps them from folding, kinking or coiling within the large long sheath.

The enclosed coils and bioptome within the sheath are observed closely as the distal ends of the coils approach the distal tip of the sheath. As the bioptome catheter is advanced, the coils are extruded together from the distal end of the long sheath and into the descending aorta. Exactly as with the delivery of a single coil, two, three or more loops of each of the multiple coils are formed in the descending aorta. With this delivery technique, all of the simultaneously delivered coils can be of the same length and diameter or they can be of variable lengths and/or diameters. Different lengths and/or diameters of each coil have the theoretical advantage of forming a more irregular and compressed "knot" of coils rather than possibly forming three parallel rings from three coils of equal length and diameter.

When the desired number of loops of coil have been extruded into the descending aorta, the long sheath and the bioptome catheter along with the coils are withdrawn together until the mass of coil loops "seats" in the aortic ampulla of the ductus. The "mass" of coils in the ductus ampulla offers significant resistance to any further withdrawal of the sheath/bioptome combination. At this point, the tip of the sheath should be just at, or into, the pulmonary end of the ductus.

The position of the coils is confirmed with a descending aorta angiogram injecting immediately adjacent to and just distal to the ductus. If the position of the coils or the degree of occlusion of the ductus does not appear satisfactory, the entire system can be re-advanced or withdrawn slightly to better seat the coils in the ampulla. If the position of the coils is totally unsatisfactory, or if the sheath with the partially extruded coils pulls through the ductus into the pulmonary artery, the coils are withdrawn back into the long delivery sheath. An aortogram is repeated after each repositioning of the sheath and coils. When the coils appear secure and their position is satisfactory in the ductus, the bioptome is advanced further very slightly and the sheath is withdrawn simultaneously, which, in turn, pushes the still straight portion of the coils which *remained in the she*ath out of the delivery sheath and allows approximately 1/2 to 2/3 of a loop of each coil to begin to form at the pulmonary artery end of the ductus. The bioptome is fixed at this position and the sheath is withdrawn off the coils on the pulmonary side of the ductus, but not completely off the jaws of the bioptome. As the sheath is withdrawn, the bioptome is advanced just enough to allow the coils on the pulmonary side of the ductus to curve and begin coiling on the pulmonary side of the ductus. When satisfied with the amount of coil that remains on the pulmonary side of the ductus, the sheath is withdrawn completely off the jaws of the bioptome, as the bioptome catheter is advanced slightly forward. This allows all of the "pulmonary" ends of the coils to loop acutely against the pulmonary artery end of the ductus. The seating and occlusion are confirmed with a repeat aortogram. If not satisfactory or if the mass of coils pulls through a very large ductus, the coils are still held by the bioptome and can be withdrawn back into the 9-F sheath. When the position is satisfactory, the bioptome jaw is opened, releasing the two or three coils.

This simultaneous delivery of several coils through a single sheath obviously requires the use of a significantly larger sheath and represents a fairly complex loading procedure. An alternative technique for delivering more than one coil to the ductus simultaneously is to use several separate, (and smaller!) delivery catheters (sheaths) for each of the separate coils[19]. This requires separate punctures for each delivery system, but allows the delivery of the coils simultaneously from either the retrograde or the venous approach or from both approaches simultaneously. The use of multiple delivery catheters/sheaths permits the simultaneous use of coils of different lengths and/or diameters. Delivery through separate delivery systems provides more control over the coils but, at the same time, requires the coordination of several separate operators for each system. When multiple coils are delivered simultaneously but separately, the delivery technique is the same as for the delivery of individual coils by that particular technique. Bioptome-controlled coil delivery usually is used for multiple, simultaneous coil delivery.

The Amplatzer™ Duct Occluder

The Amplatzer Duct Occluder™ (AGA Medical Corp., Golden Valley, MN) is specifically designed for transcatheter closure of the patent ductus and is very suitable for the larger PDA[20]. In addition to its being designed specifically for occlusion of the ductus and its easy retrievability, the Amplatzer Duct Occluder™ now has the very significant added advantage of being the only device specifically approved for transcatheter PDA occlusion by the US FDA. The Amplatzer Duct Occluder™ is a modification of the Amplatzer™ ASD occluder *concept*. Like the Amplatzer™ ASD device, it is constructed of a weave or mesh of 72 separate, 0.007″ "memory" Nitinol™ wires. The PDA occluder self-expands into a slightly tapered, fat, tubular device, which is designed to fix within, and occlude, the patent ductus by expanding and actually *stretching into* the walls of the lumen of the ductus. For some unexplained reason, the tubular portion of the Amplatzer™ PDA device tapers 2 mm from the largest to the narrowest diameter except in the one smallest sized device (5–4 mm device) which tapers only 1 mm. The distal, or aortic, end of the body of the device has the larger diameter and, in addition, has a thin extra rim or "skirt" which extends 2 mm *circumferentially* around the tubular central body at the aortic end of the device, which, in turn, creates a thin retention disk at the "aortic end" of the device. As a result, the rim or skirt is 4 mm larger in total *diameter* than the largest diameter of the tubular body of the device.

The devices are labeled according to the diameters at each end of the central tubular "hub". with the larger diameter listed first. The body or tubular portion of the device is 5 mm in length for the smallest, 5–4 mm diameter device, 7 mm in length for the 6–4 and 8–6 mm diameter devices, and 8 mm long for the 10–8 through 16–14 mm diameter devices. Each device has polyester disks sewn within (across) the tubular "hub" and within the distal retention disk to promote occlusion and enhance eventual thrombosis in the device. There is a metal micro sleeve "receiver pin" attached to, and recessed into, the center of the narrowest (proximal or pulmonary) end of the tapered tubular body of the device. The micro sleeve has a female thread recessed within it. A microscrew at the end of the delivery cable, which is identical to the attachment for the Amplatzer™ ASD devices, attaches within this micro sleeve on the device.

The 5–4, 6–4 and 8–6 mm devices are delivered through a 5- or 6-French special long sheath, the 10–8 and 12–10 mm devices through a 6- or 7-French sheath, and the 14–12 and 16–14 mm devices through a 7–French sheath.

Delivery technique for the Amplatzer™ Duct Occluder

The ductus is identified and measured *accurately* from an aortogram in the descending aorta exactly as for the other devices. The Amplatzer Duct Occluder™ device is chosen so that the larger diameter of the tubular body of the occluder (the "size" of the device) is 1–2 mm *larger* than the *narrowest* diameter of the ductus. When the ductus is at all reactive and/or "contractile", the *largest* diameter of this narrowest area is used! An end-hole catheter is manipulated from the right heart, into the pulmonary artery, through the ductus and into the descending aorta. The catheter is replaced with a 0.035″ exchange length guide wire. An Amplatzer™ long PDA delivery sheath/dilator that is appropriate for the size of the device being used is passed over the pre-positioned wire into the descending aorta, the dilator and wire are removed slowly, and the sheath is cleared of air and flushed thoroughly.

The appropriate device for the particular ductus is soaked in flush solution. The special delivery cable is passed through the small teflon loader sleeve that comes with each device and the screw tip of the cable is positioned in the small attach/release sleeve within the narrow end of the device. The delivery cable is attached by turning the device in a clockwise direction while the cable is fixed in position. The device should rotate very easily as it is being screwed onto the cable. The device is screwed onto the cable until it stops turning and then is backed off (unscrewed) in a counterclockwise direction for 1/8 turn. While the skirt end of the device is gripped with one hand and pulled away from the attached cable, the device is placed beneath the surface of a flush solution in a bowl on the table. The device is stretched into a long thin strand by the traction in opposite directions and, while continuously flushing the loader, the device is withdrawn into the loader by pulling on the delivery cable while pushing the *loader* toward and over the proximal end of the device.

While continuing the flush on the loader, the loader with the enclosed device is introduced into the proximal end of the pre-positioned sheath. The delivery cable is advanced into and through the loader, being extremely careful not to rotate the delivery cable in either direction during this introduction. Advancing the cable advances the Amplatzer™ Duct Occluder straight into the sheath and eventually to the end of the sheath. Again extra care is taken ***not*** to *rotate* the delivery cable in either direction while the device is being advanced through the sheath. Rotation of the delivery cable counterclockwise could release the device prematurely, and rotation clockwise potentially tightens the device so much that it cannot be "unscrewed" and released when desired.

While observing closely on fluoroscopy, the sheath tip is withdrawn just to the aortic end of the ductus while the delivery cable is advanced just enough to expose the retention disk (skirt) of the Duct Occluder™ in the descending aorta. With the "skirt" and just the *very distal portion* of the hub exposed, the entire system of delivery sheath, delivery cable and attached device carefully and slowly is withdrawn together as a unit until the retention disk is seated in the aortic ampulla of the ductus. This position is determined on the lateral fluoroscopy by comparing with the lateral aortogram of the ductus and by the sensation of resistance to further withdrawal of the device. When there is any question about this position and/or the appropriateness of the size of the device, a repeat aortogram is performed with the injection performed immediately adjacent and just distal to the aortic end of the ductus to verify the exact position. When the position is correct, the delivery cable is fixed in place with slight tension on the cable while the *sheath alone* is withdrawn out of the ductus and off the device. Withdrawal of the sheath extrudes the tapered tubular portion of the Amplatzer™ Ductus Occluder within the narrowest portion of the ductus and allows the device to expand into the walls of the ductus. A repeat descending aortogram adjacent to the device is performed to verify the device position in the ductus and the degree of occlusion. If the device is not in the correct position and/or if there is too much residual leak, the device can be withdrawn easily and safely into the sheath and repositioned or even withdrawn completely out of the body. When the position and degree of occlusion are satisfactory the device is released by unscrewing the cable in a counterclockwise direction using the small pin vise attached to the proximal end of the cable. The device is observed under fluoroscopy during the release to be sure that there is no distortion of the device, the device is not turning with the unscrewing, and it releases easily.

The Amplatzer™ Duct Occluder is a safe and relatively easy device to deliver and has a high rate of immediate ductal occlusion. The advantages of the Amplatzer™ Duct Occluder are its relative simplicity of use, its applicability for the occlusion of large and perhaps the very largest PDA, and its ability to be withdrawn/retrieved any time before its purposeful release. It appears to be the only device to date which is able to occlude a very large, high-flow, high-pressure PDA with a reasonable degree of safety and security. It also utilizes the smallest delivery system for a dedicated and/or true PDA device. The size of the delivery system does increase somewhat proportionately to the size of the PDA device for the larger PDA, however, even the *largest* Amplatzer™ Duct Occluder requires only an 8-French delivery sheath.

The delivery sheaths and delivery cables are not very flexible, making the passage through tight curves difficult, and occasionally resulting in kinking of the sheath when the dilator is removed from the sheath. Because of this, the Amplatzer PDA Occluder™ may not be applicable in the very small infant with a very large PDA with the present sheath. The Amplatzer™ PDA device can be delivered through other, more flexible long sheaths, which overcome the problem of kinking with the AGA sheaths.

There are several potential problems with the Amplatzer™ Duct Occluder. The tubular portion tapers or narrows toward the pulmonary artery end of the device, which encourages the *extrusion* of the device toward the aorta after its release. Since it has no "skirt" or retention ring on the pulmonary end of the device, the combination of the absent retention ring and the slight taper of the device *toward* the pulmonary end of the ductus together make its initial fixation rather precarious. This configuration in conjunction with even a transient, but significant increase in pressure in the pulmonary artery before the device had "grown" securely into the tissues of the wall of the ductus, could allow the device to dislodge and embolize into the aorta. Because of these same features, the Amplatzer™ ductus device is particularly precarious for use in the ductus that is "reactive", where the ductal walls can, and actually do, dilate and contract very significantly. This phenomenon is common in small infants, but does occur even in older patients[21]. Possibly (hopefully) with more experience with the use of the Amplatzer™ Duct Occluder, modifications in the design, including a non-tapered central hub and a retention "skirt" at both ends of the device, will be produced.

The smallest available 5–4 device precludes its use for the very tiny PDA. The 7 mm length and the shape of the Amplatzer™ Duct Occluder make it less satisfactory for the very short, "window" PDA in any size patient and any type of ductus in very small patients because of the resultant protrusion of the hub into the pulmonary artery and/or the retention disk into the lumen of the aorta. The new Eccentric Amplatzer™ PDA Occluder, which is in clinical trials, should circumvent these problems in the future. The Amplatzer™ Duct Occluder is expensive compared to a Gianturco™ coil, even when the costs of any of the adjunct equipment used for the controlled delivery of the Gianturco™ coils are included.

From the very controlled, but limited, experience in the US investigational trial and the vast clinical experience worldwide, the Amplatzer™ PDA device, even with its shortcomings, now appears to be the safest and most suitable device for the large majority of patients with the larger PDA. With FDA approval for PDA occlusion in the United States, the current higher risk and very complex procedures used to circumvent the lack of availability of a truly appropriate device for PDA occlusion are now unnecessary, even in the United States.

Gianturco-Grifka Vascular Occulsion Device (GGVOD)

The Gianturco-Grifka Vascular Occluding Device (GGVOD™) (Cook Inc., Bloomington, IN) was developed initially as a patent ductus occluding device, but eventually was approved by the US FDA for the occlusion of large tubular "vascular structures"[22]. Although it utilizes "spring coil wire" to fill the occlusion bag, the GGVOD™ is not strictly a variation of a "Gianturco™ coil" occluder. The GGVOD™ was developed during the era of the Rashkind™ PDA Occluder when the Rashkind Device™ was in clinical trials and, at the time, was the only device available for transcatheter PDA closure. In concept, the GGVOD™ was considered to be a device that would be usable in every PDA, but, unfortunately, it turned out that it is not suitable for the *majority* of PDAs[23].

With a better knowledge of the marked variation in the sizes and shapes of the PDA and with further work on the GGVOD™, it became apparent that the GGVOD™ is usable only for the occlusion of long tubular or "finger-like" vascular structures including the PDA with that configuration. By coincidence, the one type of PDA which the Rashkind™ PDA device was *not* particularly suitable for, was the long tubular PDA. Because of that, the GGVOD™ was the ideal *complementary* device along with the Rashkind™ device to allow closure of all PDAs. However, by the time the GGVOD™ was approved and became available commercially, the Rashkind™ device had all but disappeared and the Gianturco™ coils were in widespread use for most routine PDA occlusions. These circumstances placed the GGVOD™ in an even smaller but still definite niche for use in the PDA.

The GGVOD™ is a nylon "bag" or "sack" which comes in 3, 5, 7 and 9 mm diameters. The "bags" are oblong and actually somewhat flat rather than circular in their transverse diameter. The size or "diameter" of each occluder is the broadest cross-sectional diameter of the "sack". The sacks themselves are not radio-opaque, however they do have a small radio-opaque marker at the proximal end where the sack attaches to the pusher catheter. To create an occlusive "mass", the sack is packed with a very long length of spring guide, "filler" wire. Each filler wire has a specific length for each different diameter of the sack. Unlike a standard spring guide wire, the spring filler wire does not have a core wire within it. This results in an extremely flexible (or floppy) length of wire, which in turn, conforms to almost any contour within the bag. When tightly filled with the specific length of wire, the sack forms a tense, space occupying mass, which conforms to the contour of the vessel containing the sack. In addition to the specific length of wire, each GGVOD™ comes with a very elaborate and rather complex attach/delivery/release system. The GGVOD™ device and delivery system are delivered to the ductus through a long, 8-French sheath.

The "bag" of the GGVOD™ comes attached to a special delivery catheter. Each filler wire for the specific bag is already positioned within the delivery catheter with the distal end of the filler wire fixed within the bag. The delivery catheter is contained within a tightly fitting outer "release catheter". The bag (sack) and distal end of the delivery catheter/wire are enclosed in a short segment of peal-away sheath. At the proximal end of the catheter, the delivery catheter has a special, multipart handle, the purpose of which is to release the filler wire from an attached pusher wire once the bag is in position and filled.

The ductus is visualized angiographically and accurate measurements of the various diameters *and the total length* of the ductus are determined. The ductus that is suitable for occlusion with the GGVOD™ must be tubular and have approximately parallel walls for the majority of its length. The length of the ductus should be at least one and one-half times its maximum diameter. The size of the GGVOD™ used should be 2 mm larger in diameter than the largest diameter of the tubular area of the ductus in the area where the device is to be implanted.

An end-hole venous catheter is passed prograde from the pulmonary artery, through the ductus, into the descending aorta and positioned well distal to the ductus. This catheter is replaced with a 0.035" exchange length guide wire. An 8-French long sheath/dilator set with an incorporated sheath back-bleed valve and a distal tip marker band on the sheath is passed over the wire, through the ductus and into the descending aorta. The tip of the sheath should extend well into the descending aorta beyond the aortic ampulla of the ductus. The wire and dilator are removed and, after the sheath has been cleared of all air and/or clots, it is placed on a continuous flush.

The peal-away sheath is introduced into the hub of the pre-positioned long sheath. The combined delivery and release catheters are advanced together into the peal-away sheath, which, in turn, advances the sack into the long sheath. The peal-away sheath is removed and the combined delivery and release catheters are advanced in the pre-positioned sheath until the sack of the GGVOD™ has reached the distal end of the long sheath. The long sheath, along with the contained GGVOD™ *system*, is withdrawn until the "bag" (still within the sheath) is still in the aorta, but just *distal* and adjacent to the aortic ampulla of the ductus. The distance between the end of the delivery catheter and the distal radio-opaque marker determines the exact location of the sack in the aorta. While fixing the combined delivery and release catheters in place, the long sheath is withdrawn off of the bag with the bag still positioned in the descending aorta adjacent to the ductus. Two or three loops of the filler wire are advanced into the bag. These initial loops of wire within the bag provide a means of visualizing the "limits" of the bag, demonstrating its eventual diameter and location in the aorta, but at the same time, the wire does not fill the bag completely or tensely. The entire system is withdrawn until the *partially* filled bag is centered in the *tubular portion* of the ductus. A retrograde aortogram is performed adjacent to the ductus to verify the exact position of the bag in the ductus. When the position is satisfactory, the remainder of the filler wire is fed into the bag until the junction/attachment of the filler and pusher wires is past the hub and the filler wire is completely within the bag as visualized on the fluoroscopy. An aortogram is repeated to determine the exact position in, and degree of sealing of, the ductus. At any time up to this point in the procedure, the filler wire can be withdrawn partially or even completely in order to reposition or even remove the bag.

Once satisfied with the position, the degree of occlusion *and* that the filler wire is completely within the bag, the special handle at the proximal end of the pusher wire is activated, which then releases the pusher wire from the filler wire in the bag. Once the pusher wire is released, it is withdrawn into the delivery catheter. The release *catheter* is advanced over the delivery catheter until the tip of the release catheter is flush against the visible marking ring on the neck of the bag. The inner cannula (delivery catheter) is withdrawn forcefully against the release catheter, which pulls the flared tip of the delivery catheter out of the bag, releasing the bag in place. This withdrawal of the inner catheter from the bag may take considerable force and is fairly "violent". Care must be taken ***not*** to advance the outer release catheter at all while withdrawing the inner catheter out of the bag. If the outer release catheter pushes forward, it can easily push the GGVOD™ out of the ductus into the aorta.

There are some advantages of the GGVOD™ for PDA occlusion. The first advantage is that it is available in the United States. Even the largest GGVOD™ is delivered through an 8-French long sheath and can be delivered from either the venous (preferred) or retrograde arterial approach. The GGVOD™ is very useful for the *tubular ductus* and particularly the larger high-flow ductus because of its very tight fit within the lesion. In most cases there is complete occlusion of the ductus by the end of the procedure when using the GGVOD™. During the implant procedure, the filler wire can be withdrawn out of the "sack" and back into the catheter, emptying the sack and allowing repositioning of the sack or, if necessary, complete removal of the sack and system at any time prior to the purposeful release of the wire. With experience, the GGVOD™ can be used in a long, but not *exactly* tubular ductus.

There are several significant disadvantages of the GGVOD™ for PDA occlusion. The most important disadvantage is that it is applicable to only the longer tubular shaped ductus. The GGVOD™ also requires an 8-French delivery sheath even for the smaller devices. This is problematic in the very small infant where tight curves within the heart are encountered, and in any small child when the *arterial* delivery route is necessary. The delivery/release mechanism is very complex and requires meticulous attention to the printed details of the technique in order to prevent errors in the delivery/release. Particular attention must be paid to the sizing of the device for the defect. If the bag is undersized for the ductus, it does not compress against the walls of the ductus and will not hold in place. If the bag is significantly oversized for the ductus, it cannot expand completely, and all of the filler wire, which has a specific length for each bag, does not fit into the bag. If this is not recognized before the release of the wire, it leaves a portion of the filler wire dangling freely in the pulmonary artery or even back into the right ventricle. Finally, once the sack is released, the filled sack is very difficult to retrieve with a catheter. Even if the sack can be grasped with a retrieval device and withdrawn to the vessel entry site, it usually requires at least a cut-down at the local site over the vessel in order to withdraw the sack out of the vessel and the surrounding tissues. Because of the extreme importance of the fine details in order to successfully perform this technique, these details are listed below in a tabular "cook-book" form.

Components of the GGVOD system

- A long, 8-French, valved outer delivery sheath with a distal marker band.
- The nylon "sack" or "bag"—in 3, 5, 7 and 9 mm sizes (diameters).
- An inner, stiff walled, pusher (delivery) catheter to which the bag is attached.
- A long, variable length (according to bag size) detachable, and very flexible, spring filler wire within the pusher catheter.
- A stiffer pusher wire (attached to the proximal end of the filler wire and extending out of the proximal end of the pusher catheter).
- A second, stiff, "bag release" catheter which is pre-positioned *over* the pusher catheter.
- A complex attach/release system, which joins all of these components.
- A short length of 8-French "peal-away" sheath which comes positioned over the distal ends of the two catheters and the attached bag.

Details of the seven major steps for the GGVOD delivery

Step 1: The long delivery sheath is positioned through the ductus into the descending aorta.

- The ductus is crossed from the pulmonary artery to the descending aorta with an end-hole catheter.
- A second catheter from the retrograde arterial approach is placed adjacent to the aortic end of the ductus.
- The end-hole catheter is replaced with a 0.035″ stiff exchange wire.
- The special 8-French, valved long delivery sheath/dilator set with a distal sheath tip marker is passed over the wire until the *sheath tip* is in the descending aorta beyond the ampulla of the ductus.
- The dilator and wire are removed, the system is cleared of air and clot and flushed.

Step 2: The sack and delivery system are introduced into the long sheath.

- All of the components of the GGVOD system are inspected.
- The sack, which is attached to the pusher catheter and the wire/delivery/release system, is introduced into the pre-positioned long sheath as a unit through the short "peal-away" sheath.
- The short "peal-away" sheath is removed ("pealed off the catheter").
- The sack with the attached delivery system is advanced to the tip of the sheath (but still within the tip of the sheath) to a position in the descending aorta just distal to the ductus.

Step 3: The sack is positioned in the aorta and partially filled with filler wire.

- With the pusher catheter held in place, the sheath is withdrawn off the sack (the sack is still distal to the ductus). The sack itself is invisible but the attaching band on the *proximal neck* of the sack is radio-opaque and visible.

• While observing on fluoroscopy, several loops of the "filler" wire are advanced into the sack very loosely by advancing the stiff pusher *wire* 5–10 centimeters. The sack is *not* packed tightly with the filler wire at this point.

Step 4: The partially filled sack is withdrawn to the precise position in the ductus for the implant.

• The entire system, with the partially filled (and now visible) sack is withdrawn as a unit until the sack is within the tubular portion of the ductus.

• The position of the sack is checked with a small aortogram through the second catheter positioned adjacent to the ductus in the descending aorta.

Step 5: The filler wire is pushed into the sack.

• When the sack is in the proper position, the remainder of the filler wire is fed *completely* into the sack. This is checked on fluoroscopy, making sure that the connection point of the filler wire with the pusher wire is completely *within the sack*. The connecting point is identified by a difference in X-ray densities along the wire at the connection point.

• The exact sack position in the ductus and the degree of occlusion are checked by another aortogram.

Step 6: The pusher wire is separated from the filler wire.

• When sure the filler wire is completely within the sack and while observing on fluoroscopy, the *wire* release mechanism is activated by pushing the two side rings on the "handle" forward. This detaches the pusher wire from the filler wire.

• When sure the pusher wire is detached from the filler wire, the *pusher wire* is withdrawn into the pusher catheter —this releases and separates the pusher *wire* from the sack. This withdrawal of the pusher wire is performed very slowly—until absolutely sure that the pusher wire is separated completely from the filler wire.

Step 7: The pusher catheter is separated from the sack.

• The stiffer, middle *release catheter* (which is over the pusher catheter, but within the sheath), is advanced snugly against the neck of the sack.

• With the *release catheter* tip *held securely and exactly in place* against the sack and fixed in position against the tabletop outside of the body, the inner *"pusher" catheter* is withdrawn forcibly from the neck of the sack. (If the *release catheter* moves *at all*, the position of the sack likely will move with it!!)

• The forceful withdrawal of the "pusher catheter" releases the sack entirely from the delivery system and allows the delivery system to be withdrawn from the occluder.

The major disadvantage of the GGVOD™ is the difficulty in retrieving it if it embolizes. The bulk created by intact, filled GGVOD™ devices with all but the smallest sack is too large to withdraw through a percutaneous entrance into a vessel. One alternative is to "open" the sack, withdraw the filler wire completely from the sack and then retrieve the empty sack by itself. The embolized sack, which will be lodged in a vessel, is "opened" by biting or "nibbling" at the surface of the filled sack with a bioptome until a tear is made in the fabric. Once the sack has been "opened" even slightly, usually one or more loops of the filler wire will extrude through the opening. An exposed loop of wire is grasped with a bioptome, a Grabber™ or a Jaws™ catheter and pulled the rest of the way out of the sack and into a retrieval catheter/sheath. The empty sack itself is not visible, however, the metal "attaching ring" at the neck of the sack is visible and provides the general location of the sack. The empty sack is grasped with a Grabber™ or bioptome and withdrawn separately into at least an 8-French sheath. This retrieval process usually is a long and tedious procedure. It always is better to prevent the embolization by abiding by the meticulous attention to the detail of the implant procedure.

PFM "Duct-Occlud™" PDA Occluder

In Europe, there is another coil and delivery system that was designed specifically for PDA closure[24]. The Duct-Occlud™ devices (PFM Medical, Cologne, Germany) are available in several different shapes and multiple sizes along with different thickness and stiffness of the coil material. The standard Duct-Occlud™ device is a spiral coil pre-shaped into a "double cone" or a "double disk" of relatively heavy, stainless steel, coil wire material. The two cones or disks are attached at the center, giving the device a dumbbell or dual wheel shape respectively. The two wider ends of the device are positioned at each end of the ductus while the narrow connection sits in the narrowest portion of the ductus. The Duct-Occlud S™ version is a single cone shape. It is manufactured from larger and stiffer loops of medical grade stainless steel coil wire with the more proximal loops wound back in a reverse direction into and around what would have been the center of the "double cone".

Unlike the Gianturco™ coils, the Duct-Occlud™ device has *no* enmeshed fibers to promote thrombosis, but rather it depends upon the tight windings and rigidity of the coils and the thrombogenicity of the metal of the coils themselves to occlude flow and seal the ductus. The standard versions of the device resulted in a relatively high incidence of residual leak through the center of the device. With the Duct-Occlud S™, the coil windings are tightened and stiffened with reportedly even better closure. The standard Duct-Occlud™ is available in 4–7 mm distal coil diameters while the Duct-Occlud S™ is available in 7, 9 and 11 mm distal coil diameters. Both types have a 3 mm coil diameter at the center segment.

The Duct-Occlud™ device comes with the Occlu-Grip™, which is an elaborate attach/release mechanism providing complete control and retrievability of the device until it is *purposefully* released. The Occlu-Grip™ is a long stainless steel, reusable, control handle, which is available in 24 and 36 cm lengths (depending upon which length Duct-Occlud™ is used). The Occlu-Grip™ contains an attached long Nitinol™ "mandril" wire and the attach/release mechanism for the Duct-Occlud™. The Duct-Occlud™ device comes from the manufacturer with the mandril passing through the Duct-Occlud™ coil to produce a straight configuration of the occluder. The control handle allows both the controlled, purposeful withdrawal of the mandril from within the coil and a precisely controlled advancement of the coil during delivery. The withdrawal of the mandril as the coil is advanced allows the Duct-Occlud™ device to assume its "natural" spiral configuration.

There also are specific delivery and angiographic catheters available with the Duct-Occlud™ delivery systems. The Duct-Occlud™ Occlu-Cath™ delivery catheters are PTFE material and have a gold "marker band" 0.2 mm from the distal tip to enhance X-ray visibility. These special delivery catheters are available in a 4-French size for the Standard Duct-Occlud™ or a 5-French size for the reinforced, Duct-Occlud S™ device. The Occlu-Cath™ for both devices are available in 75 cm and 90 cm lengths. In addition to the special delivery catheters, the Duct-Occlud™ is available with Occlu-Marker™ catheters. These are special pigtail angiographic catheters that contain three narrow radio-opaque bands at the distal end. These bands are exactly 10 and 20 mm apart (measured from top to top or bottom to bottom of the bands) and are used as very accurate calibration marks for the precise measurement of the ductus. The Occlu-Marker™ catheters are available in 50 and 75 cm lengths in 4-French and 90 cm length in a 5-French diameter. Other comparable more "generic", but similar catheters, may be substituted for the Occlu-Cath™ and the Occlu-Marker™ during the delivery of the Duct-Occlud™.

Technique for delivery of the Duct-Occlud device

The exact size and shape of the ductus are determined from an aortogram in the descending aorta adjacent to the ductus. This is performed with the Occlu-Marker™ catheter or with a comparable angiographic catheter and a calibration system. A Duct-Occlud™ device is chosen that is twice the diameter of the narrowest portion of the ductus. The standard Duct-Occlud™ is available in sizes up to 7 mm, and the Duct-Occlud S™ is recommended for the ductus over 2.5 mm in narrowest diameter. The appropriate diameter and length Occlu-Cath™ delivery catheter for the particular coil is passed from the pulmonary artery, through the ductus and into the descending aorta. The straightened Duct-Occlud™ device is introduced into the Occlu-Cath™ and advanced to the distal end of the Occlu-Cath™, which is positioned in the descending aorta. The distal (aortic) loops of the Duct-Occlud™ coil are formed in the aorta by advancing the distal slide mechanism of the Occlu-Grip™ forward to the predetermined position on the rail. The entire system including the delivery catheter, the partially extruded coil and the Occlu-Grip™ device are withdrawn into the ductus until the distal coil loops have pulled snugly into the aortic ampulla of the ductus. The Duct-Occlud™ coil is fixed in place as the catheter and Occlu-Grip™, *together*, are withdrawn until one or two loops of the proximal coil are formed on the pulmonary end of the ductus. A repeat aortogram is performed. At this point in the procedure, if not satisfied with the position and/or degree of occlusion, the Duct-Occlud™ device can be withdrawn partially or completely and either repositioned or removed and a more satisfactory device substituted. When satisfied with the position and the degree of occlusion, the slide mechanism is moved to the final position, deploying the remaining pulmonary and/or central loops of coil. When satisfied with the position the release mechanism is activated. A final aortogram is performed 10–15 minutes after deployment and the catheters are removed.

The Duct-Occlud™ has the advantage of complete retrievability any time during deployment. With the newer Duct-Occlud S™ devices, there is reportedly a high incidence of complete occlusion at the time of implant. The standard Duct-Occlud™ device has the disadvantages of not having a good rate of immediate closure along with no ideal procedure for adding a second Duct-Occlud™ in order to complete the occlusion during the same procedure. The Duct-Occlud™ device along with the Occlu-Grip™ delivery system is much more expensive than the Gianturco™ coil, even including the adjunct delivery techniques for the Gianturco™ coils and even when considering the reusability of the Occlu-Grip™ delivery catheter.

Nit-Occlud™ PDA occlusion system

The Nit-Occlud™ PDA occluder is an extensive modification of the Duct-Occlud™ device and delivery system, which was introduced for PDA occlusion recently (PFM Medical, Cologne, Germany). The Nit-Occlud™ probably will replace, or may have already replaced, the Duct-Occlud™ entirely. The coils of the Nit-Occlud™ are very similar in *design* to the Duct-Occlud S™ devices with a "double opposing cone" shape to fix in the ductus, however the Nit-Occlud™ devices are manufactured of Nitinol™ wire with a graduated stiffness from the aortic disk to the more proximal (pulmonary) disk. The stiffer aortic "disk" provides resistance to the device pulling through the ductus from the aortic end during and after delivery, while the more flexible central and proximal "disk" windings allow the coils of the device to conform to the many shapes of the ductus. The Nit-Occlud™ devices are labeled according to the maximum diameters of the distal and proximal coils ("disks") in that order. Like the Duct-Occlud™ devices, the Nit-Occlud™ devices have no intertwined fabric and depend upon the metal of the devices and the tight windings of the coils to provide the occlusion.

Each device comes pre-attached to a long, flexible, Nitinol™ wire introducer, which, in turn, is mounted on a special delivery handle. Unlike the delivery handle of the previous Duct-Occlud™ device, the Nit-Occlud™ handle is plastic and disposable. Even with the variable flexibility within each device, the Nit-Occlud™ devices are available in four different sizes/configurations in order to conform to the size and shape of almost any ductus.

The Nit-Occlud™ Flex is the smallest of the Nit-Occlud™ devices. The coils of the Nit-Occlud™ Flex are entirely flexible and are available in 4 × 4, 5 × 4 and 6 × 5 mm sizes, with the first number being the size of the aortic or distal "disk". The Nit-Occlud™ Flex devices are delivered through special 4-French implantation sheaths. The Nit-Occlud™ Med are the middle range of the Nit-Occlud™ devices, they have more reinforced aortic coils and are delivered through a 5-French implantation sheath. The Nit-Occlud™ Med devices are available in 7 × 6, 9 × 6 and 11 × 6 mm sizes, with the first number being the diameter of the aortic "disk". Both the Nit-Occlud™ Flex and the Nit-Occlud™ Med are pre-attached to an 85 cm long introducer and are pre-loaded into a short "transporter" sheath. The Nit-Occlud™ Flex comes with a 4-F implantation sheath and the Nit-Occlud™ Med comes with a 5-French long implantation sheath manufactured by PFM™. The sheaths have a shapable distal end and a radio-opaque "marker band" just proximal to the distal tip. Both devices are introduced into the delivery sheath from their transporter sheath similarly to the introduction of a detachable coil into the delivery catheter.

The Nit-Occlud™ Stiff devices are the largest of the standard Nit-Occlud™ devices and have an extra reinforced, aortic disk. The Nit-Occlud™ Stiff devices are available in 10 × 6, 12 × 6 and 14 × 6 mm sizes and come pre-loaded in a 5-French long sheath, which, in turn, is advanced to the ductus through a larger French sized long sheath. The larger long delivery sheath is not part of the Nit-Occlud™ total set and must be obtained separately. The fourth type of Nit-Occlud™ device is the Nit-Occlud™ Double Disk device, which is designed for the short, "window" type ductus. This device has reinforced disks at both ends with both "disks" being flatter and larger in diameter. The more flexible "waist" between the two disks is shorter and narrower in diameter. The diameters of the aortic disks of these devices are similar to those of the aortic disks of the Nit-Occlud™ Stiff devices. The Nit-Occlud™ Double Disks are pre-loaded in a 5-F delivery sheath, which is delivered to the ductus through a larger French sized long sheath.

Delivery of the Nit-Occlud™ devices

The delivery of the Nit-Occlud™ devices is almost identical to the delivery from the venous/pulmonary approach of the Duct-Occlud™ or of a controlled-release delivery of large coils. The ductus is measured accurately using the PFM™ Occlud-Marker™ or another valid calibration system with a descending aorta aortogram with the injection performed just distal to the aortic end of the ductus. When Occlu-Marker™ catheters are used, the "pigtail" angiographic catheter can remain positioned in the descending aorta for the purpose of obtaining repeated, small, selective positioning angiograms throughout the steps of the implant. The device size is chosen so that the distal, aortic coils are at least 2 mm larger in diameter than the *aortic end* of the *ductus*, but still will fit within the ampulla of the ductus and allow the narrowest portion of the device to seat in the pulmonary end of the ductus. The narrowest coils of the device should be at least 3–4 mm *larger* in diameter than the narrowest diameter of the ductus. The type of Nit-Occlud™ device is chosen according to the size and configuration of the ductus.

An end-hole catheter is advanced from the main pulmonary artery, through the ductus and into the descending aorta and is replaced with a long exchange length wire. The long delivery sheath/dilator, which is appropriate in diameter for the device that is being used, is advanced over the wire to the descending aorta and the wire and then the dilator are removed. The sheath is cleared meticulously of all air and/or clots. The appropriate device is introduced into and advanced through the long delivery sheath by advancing the delivery system into the long sheath while visualizing the position of the device on intermittent fluoroscopy until the distal end of the elongated device just reaches the tip of the sheath. Screwing the more distal, "rounder" ball counterclockwise on the shaft of the delivery handle while observing the device on fluoroscopy deploys the aortic "disk" in small very controlled steps. When the aortic coil (disk) is fully deployed, the entire combination of the device, delivery system and long sheath are withdrawn until the aortic disk is seated in the aortic end of the ductus and within the aortic ampulla. A small descending aortogram is performed to confirm the position.

When satisfied with the position of the "aortic disk", the ball slowly is screwed counterclockwise while simultaneously withdrawing the long sheath very slightly. This extrudes the center and proximal portions within and on the pulmonary side of the ductus. A small selective aortogram is repeated to verify the position. When satisfied with the position and the degree of immediate occlusion, the more proximal, flatter "ball" on the handle is screwed counterclockwise to release the device. At any time during the positioning and delivery of the device until this purposeful release, the Nit-Occlud™ device can be withdrawn very safely back into the delivery sheath, repositioned or even totally withdrawn from the body. If the device should embolize once it has been released, it can be recovered from an unwanted position similar to the foreign body recovery of any other large coil.

The Nit-Occlud™ device has had successful clinical use in Europe and has had a very successful FDA, IDE pilot trial in the United States, with 100% occlusion after six months. The Nit-Occlud™ appears to be a nice complement to the already approved Amplatzer™ PDA Occluder. Hopefully the Nit-Occlud™ device can achieve a 510-K, predicate device approval for PDA occlusion in the United States without an unnecessarily prolonged and repeat "investigative device exemption (IDE)" trial.

Angled Amplatzer PDA Occluder™

Recently, AGA™ Medical Corp (Golden Valley, MN) has introduced an "eccentric" or angled version of the Amplatzer™ PDA Occluder[25]. This is a modification of the original Amplatzer™ PDA Occluder to accommodate the PDA particularly in the very small patient, the PDA with little length and/or a PDA with a steep angle off the aorta. The distal "retention disk" of the angled device is eccentric at the wide (aortic) end of the tubular central hub of the device and angled 32° off the long axis of the device. The angled "retention disk" is 4 mm wide at the cephalad area of the disk while the inferior or caudal edge of the retention disk is 9 mm long and extends almost like an "apron" off the caudal edge of the central tubular hub. The aortic retention disk itself is slightly concave in order to conform better to the contour of the lumen of the aorta. This configuration permits the eccentric occluder to fit precisely into an angled, relatively flat, aortic ampulla of a ductus. There is a small platinum marker on the most inferior (caudal) edge of the angled retention disk to help orient the device properly during delivery.

The Amplatzer™ Angled PDA Occluder, like the standard Amplatzer™ PDA Occluder, has a tapered central "hub" and has no retention "skirt" at the pulmonary end. It is anticipated that this will prove to be an even greater problem in the large, relative short ductus and particularly in younger patients where the ductus is likely to be more "reactive".

The Amplatzer™ Angled PDA Occluder, similarly to the standard Amplatzer™ PDA Occluder, is manufactured with a weave of 72 separate 0.007″ Nitinol™ wires and contains polyester patches within the retention disk and the central "hub". The Angled PDA Occluders are labeled identically to the standard Amplatzer™ PDA Occluders with the diameters of the distal end and the proximal end of the *"central tubular"* portion of the devices indicating the size of the device. There presently are four sizes of the Angled PDA devices available to the medical community outside of the United States—a 6/4, an 8/6, a 10/12 and a 12/10 device. These devices are introduced through a 6- or 7-French long delivery sheath.

An even newer version of the Amplatzer™ Angled PDA Occluder has been developed with double the number (144) and finer (0.004″) Nitinol™ wires in the mesh. The newer Angled PDA Occluder™ contains no polyester occlusion disks within the device, relying on the tighter weave and greater number of wires to promote occlusion and thrombosis. The absence of the polyester occlusion disks along with the finer Nitinol™ wires allows the newer Angled PDA Occluder™ to be delivered through a smaller delivery sheath. Both types of Angled PDA Occluders™ have a small, platinum, radio-opaque marker at the "6 o'clock" position on the retention disk to help verify the orientation of the device.

The attach/release/delivery mechanism of the eccentric device is similar to that of the original Amplatzer™ PDA device, however the delivery is significantly different from the original Amplatzer™ PDA device since the angled device must be specifically, and precisely, oriented in relation to the PDA and aorta. Unlike the Amplatzer™ Perimembranous *VSD Occluder*, which has a mechanism in the delivery system for "automatically" orienting the device properly as it is extruded, the angled PDA device has no such mechanism. As a consequence, the entire device is extruded in the *descending aorta* in order to orient the platinum marker on the retention disk to a position that is close to "6 o'clock" as seen on the PA fluoroscopy. The totally extruded device, *along with* the delivery cable and sheath, is rotated clockwise as the combination is moved to and fro slightly. Once the open device has been oriented properly with the "marker" at 6 o'clock, the tubular body of the device is withdrawn back into the delivery sheath leaving only the retention disk exposed in the aorta. While maintaining the retention disk in its proper orientation, the sheath and the exposed disk are withdrawn together until the retention disk seats in the ampulla of the ductus. Thereafter the delivery of the Angled PDA device is identical to the delivery of the standard Amplatzer™ PDA Occluder.

Like the original device, the angled device can be withdrawn and repositioned any time up until the point of purposeful release. In order to achieve the proper orientation of the angled device before release, the withdrawal and repositioning of the angled PDA device is necessary more often than with the standard Amplatzer™ PDA Occluder. Although in trials to date there have been no problems with this device, since the angled occluder is designed to be used in the much shorter PDA and the PDA with "angled" walls, the absence of a pulmonary retention disk potentially is an even greater problem than with the non-angled PDA Occluder™.

The Angled Amplatzer PDA Occluder™ has undergone animal trials in the US and outside of the United States and it has had several very successful clinical trials, and now is in clinical use outside of the US. It, presumably, is to enter a larger, regulated FDA IDE trial in the United States, or hopefully, and more logically, with the approval of the standard Amplatzer™ PDA Occluder, the Angled PDA Occluder will receive an FDA, 510-K approval as a modification of the original Amplatzer™ PDA Occluder.

"Double-umbrella" occlusion of the PDA

The Rashkind PDA Umbrella™ device not only clearly established the feasibility and safety of transcatheter PDA occlusion but also clearly demonstrated the utility of "double-umbrella" devices for PDA occlusion. A "double-umbrella" device, with its very low profile, still probably is the preferable device for the very short "window" type ductus. In addition to the Rashkind™ device, a number of different "umbrella" devices, which were designed more specifically for the occlusion of atrial septal defects, have been used to occlude the patent ductus. The smaller sizes of the earlier Clamshell™ ASD device, its successors the CardioSEAL™, the STARFlex™ devices and even the Amplatzer™ ASD devices have been used in special circumstances and/or under extenuating or high-risk situations for PDA occlusions[26,27]. The Sideris Button™ PDA occlusion device is an umbrella type device. It is a modification of the Sideris Button™ ASD occlusion device and was used for PDA occlusion in one combined US and international trial and used extensively for clinical PDA occlusions outside of the US[28]. The small Amplatzer™ ASD device, the Amplatzer™ Cribriform ASD device and the Amplatzer™ PFO devices could have applicability for a short, shallow ductus similar to the use of the CardioSEAL™ device for those defects while the Amplatzer™ muscular VSD device is applicable for the more tubular PDA[29].

CardioSEAL™/STARFlex™ devices for the PDA

The CardioSEAL™ and STARFlex™ ASD devices (Nitinol Medical Technologies, Boston, MA) presently require the use of a 10-French delivery sheath for delivery of the 17–28 mm devices so are suitable for the occlusion of the PDA only in a larger patient. The preparation and the loading of these devices for their use in a PDA are identical to their preparation and loading for the ASD. The delivery procedure for these ASD devices to the PDA is identical to the delivery of the original 17 mm Rashkind™ device for PDA occlusion. An end-hole catheter is advanced prograde from the venous system through the right heart, pulmonary artery, the PDA and into the descending aorta. The catheter is replaced with a stiff, exchange length, spring guide wire. The 10-French, long dilator/sheath delivery set is delivered into the descending aorta over the pre-positioned wire, the dilator and wire are removed and the sheath is cleared passively of all air and/or clots. A second angiographic catheter is introduced retrograde and positioned in the descending aorta adjacent to the PDA for angiography during the device delivery.

CardioSEAL/STARFlex delivery technique to the PDA

The appropriate sized ASD device is attached to the delivery wire of the delivery catheter and pulled into the "front loader" for the device exactly as for an ASD occlusion. Keeping the long sheath and the loader on a flush, the loader is introduced into the hub of the long sheath and the delivery catheter with the device is advanced in the long sheath. The combination is advanced to approximately the area of the right atrium. From there, the delivery rod is advanced into the hub of the *delivery catheter* while the catheter and sheath are fixed in this position. This advances the delivery wire with the device within the sheath and away from the end of the stiffer delivery catheter, allowing the more flexible delivery wire to advance through the curves of the right ventricle, pulmonary artery, ductus and descending aorta. The delivery wire with the device is advanced slowly until the distal umbrella of the device begins to open in the descending aorta. The sheath/catheter/device, all together are withdrawn slightly—until the tip of the sheath is within one centimeter of the aortic end of the ductus. The delivery wire is advanced further until the distal umbrella has opened completely in the descending aorta. The various positions of the device in relation to the ductus at the various stages of this delivery are checked easily and repeatedly with small angiograms with injections through the second (retrograde) catheter.

Once the distal umbrella is open completely, the entire system—sheath/catheter/device—is withdrawn until the open device begins to "funnel" into the aortic ampulla of the ductus. This is confirmed with a repeat aortogram. With the distal umbrella "seated" in the ampulla, the delivery catheter, delivery wire and the device are fixed in place while the *sheath alone* is withdrawn completely off the proximal umbrella. This allows the proximal umbrella to open on the pulmonary side of the ductus. The sheath is re-advanced over the delivery wire and against the opened "pulmonary" umbrella. This forces the proximal umbrella to open further, pushes it against the pulmonary end of the ductus and prevents dislodgment as the position is being checked. The position of the device in the ductus is confirmed by an additional aortogram injecting immediately adjacent to the distal device on the aortic side of the ductus. When the device is in a satisfactory position, the release mechanism is activated, the delivery wire withdrawn into the sheath and the sheath is withdrawn away from the device.

A final aortogram confirms the position in the ductus and the degree of sealing by the device. A small amount of residual leak, circuitously around and/or between the two umbrellas, is acceptable and usually closes with time. However, a through and through, jet-like, residual leak is not likely to close and has the potential for creating hemolysis. Any such residual leak is closed with another (different?) device while the patient is still in the catheterization laboratory.

Sideris PDA Button Device

The Sideris ASD Button Device™ (Sideris, Athens, Greece) was modified for use in the PDA with the addition of a second, more proximal attaching "knot" on the suture loops of the occluder to allow the counter occluder to "button" a variable distance from the occluding umbrella. The two knots allow some adjustment of the distance between the "occluder umbrella" and the "counter occluder" to accommodate the different lengths of a patent ductus. The "umbrella" material is a 1/16th inch thick sheet of polyurethane foam and the crossed "frame" of the umbrellas is made of teflon-coated stainless steel spring coil wires. The Sideris™ ductus button device is available in sizes from 15 to 40 mm in diameter in 5 mm increments. The devices are delivered through a 7- or 8-French long sheath. A device at least twice the narrowest diameter of the ductus is used for the occlusion.

Delivery of the Sideris PDA Button Device

After sizing the defect angiographically and choosing the size of the device that will be used, the long sheath of the appropriate diameter for the device being used is advanced from the pulmonary artery, through the ductus and into the high descending aorta as described for other devices. The most proximal buttoning loop on the umbrella of the device is attached to a "safety thread", which passes through a hollow delivery wire which, in turn, passes through a 7-French end-hole pusher catheter. The ductus occluder is folded away from the attach/delivery wire and pusher catheter by hand and manually folded/compressed into the proximal end of the sheath. The folded umbrella is pushed through the sheath with a 7-French end-hole catheter until it reaches the aortic end of the sheath. The "attaching" or "safety" thread passes from the center of the device through a hollow "loader wire" or tube, which, in turn, passes through the end-hole catheter. The umbrella is pushed entirely out of the sheath into the descending aorta by advancing the pusher catheter, which, in turn, allows the umbrella to open completely in the descending aorta. The delivery catheter and retaining thread are withdrawn together with the open umbrella until the open umbrella is against the tip of the sheath. With the open umbrella pulled against the end of the delivery sheath, the entire system is withdrawn until the disk (umbrella) of the Button™ occluder is pulled against the aortic ampulla of the ductus. While continuously holding tension on the retaining thread and the hollow loader wire together, the pusher catheter is withdrawn out of the sheath. The counter occluder is mounted over the retaining thread/loader wire and introduced into the sheath. It is pushed through the long sheath over the thread and the loader "wire" with the original end-hole pusher catheter.

Once the counter occluder is at the end of the sheath, tension is maintained on the retaining thread/loader wire while the sheath is withdrawn. This exposes the counter occluder in the pulmonary artery. The counter occluder is pushed forward by the end-hole pusher catheter along (over) the taut retaining thread/loader wire until it "pops" over the second, more proximal, "knot" on the thread loop at the center of the occluder. This maneuver "buttons" the counter occluder to the device. The buttoning process is visualized on fluoroscopy and, in addition, it often is palpable as the counter occluder "buttons" onto the occluder. If the ductus is known to be short and/or the umbrella appears loose, the counter occluder is pushed further over the first, more distal "knot" which is closer to the occluder on the central thread loops. When satisfied with the position of the device and counter occluder, the distal tie on the long retaining thread is cut outside of the body and the hollow loader/guide wire is withdrawn from over the retaining thread. The retraining thread is removed by pulling *one strand* (free end) of the thread through the sheath while allowing the other end to pull into the catheter and then out of the "eye" of the thread loop on the occluder. This releases the device in the ductus.

The Sideris™ device reportedly has the advantage of being usable in the larger and short PDA and yet deliverable through a 7-, or at most, 8-French sheath. It, reportedly, is completely retrievable until the retaining thread is removed during the very last step after completing the implant. The fabric of the Sideris PDA™ occluder is polyurethane which, in the Rashkind PDA™ device, had a history of shrinking markedly, and in the Rashkind ASD™ device of not only shrinking, but also of "recanalizing" in multiple areas. The Sideris PDA™ device has been changed several times, but still, like the CardioSEAL™ and the present STARFlex™ devices, is a square "plug" for a round hole and like the other umbrella devices, is not approved for PDA occlusion in the United States.

"Double-umbrella" PDA occlusion—conclusion

In spite of the large delivery system required, a double umbrella is suited very well for short "window" type ductus of moderate to large sizes. The currently available "double-umbrella" devices are too flimsy to remain in place in a very large, high-flow ductus. There is no question that there is a place for a more robust and round(er) "double umbrella" type occluder similar to the Amplatzer™ Cribriform ASD device for the short, "window" PDA. Hopefully, developments in this area will continue in the future and even eventually be approved specifically for PDA occlusions in the United States.

Sideris Frameless PDA Occluder

Dr Sideris has reported using "frameless" occluding patches in atrial septal defects and in perimembranous ventricular septal defects, and has extended the use of these devices to the PDA. The frameless "patches" are made from a thin sleeve, or covering of a sheet of polyurethane, which is fashioned over an inflated balloon. For use in the PDA, pre-formed clot from the patient's own blood is applied to the balloon surface beneath the patch before implant into the PDA. The deflated balloon with the patch in place over it is delivered from the venous route through a long 9–12-French sheath (depending upon the size of the PDA) to, and through, the ductus. The balloon with the patch is inflated to a size appropriate for the particular ductus and then is withdrawn tightly against and into the aortic end of the ductus. It is unclear whether the "frameless" patch is held in place in the ductus by a second balloon inflated on the pulmonary side of the ductus and/or by tension applied to the balloon/patch from outside of the body by the retaining/retrieval string.

After as little as 23 hours, the balloon within the patch is deflated and withdrawn, leaving the "frameless" patch in place and attached to the aortic side of the ductus. Reportedly, the patch was successful in 9 patients and totally occluded even the very large PDA without any complications of the procedure and/or from the patch. Like the "frameless" ASD and VSD patches, this concept appears very exciting, but requires a well controlled and monitored trial before it can be endorsed to replace the more conventional devices in clinical use.

Complications—transcatheter PDA occlusion

Considering the multiple devices, the rapid introduction of new devices and techniques for transcatheter PDA occlusion and the continued necessity of often having to use a less than ideal device for PDA occlusions, there are remarkably few complications and very few permanent sequelae from the PDA occlusion devices and the implant procedures. There has been one death reported related to an attempted transcatheter PDA occlusion. This death was early in the experience with a new device and was only one death in the tens of thousands of transcatheter PDA occlusion procedures that have been performed with the multiple different and developing devices.

The most common "complication" of the transcatheter techniques is the immediate, incomplete closure of the ductus. With changes in the available devices and persistence on the part of operators, this now rarely occurs. A residual leak following the implant of a single Gianturco™ coil was common. When a residual leak persists 10–15 minutes after the implant of the coil, additional coils now are added during the same catheterization procedure until there is no detectable "jet-like" leak through the coils. The Rashkind™ PDA device had an unacceptable incidence of residual leaks immediately after the initial implant. Many of these leaks closed with time or were closed with an additional device. The Rashkind™ device is no longer in use, but when a patient appears with a residual leak when seen in a late follow-up of the Rashkind™ PDA devices, the patient is encouraged to undergo a completion of the PDA closure with a coil and/or one of the other devices that are now available for PDA occlusion. The complete closure of the ductus is important to prevent the subsequent complications of hemolysis and/or late endocarditis.

Embolization of the Gianturco™ coil was a fairly common event with the "free release" delivery technique and still occurs occasionally, even with the various "control" techniques for delivery of these coils. When a Gianturco™ coil does embolize, it is retrieved as described in Chapter 12. An embolized coil is an embarrassment to the operator, but should cause no permanent sequelae. The highest incidence of embolizations of PDA devices occurred early in the experience with the Rashkind™ PDA device and some of the devices which embolized early in the experience were removed at the time of surgical repair of the ductus. Later in the experience with the Rashkind™ device, most of the embolized PDA devices were removed in the catheterization laboratory and another device implanted in the ductus during the same procedure. There were, however, isolated Rashkind™ PDA devices that embolized to the lungs in several patients and were left in a distal pulmonary artery with no acute or long-term consequences identified.

Embolization also has occurred with the Gianturco-Grifka Bag™ and with the Amplatzer™ PDA device. Even these can be retrieved in the catheterization laboratory. During a retrieval procedure, particularly with the larger devices, extreme care must be taken not to damage other intravascular and/or intracardiac structures during the retrieval. The total number of embolized devices still is small compared to the number of transcatheter PDA occlusion procedures performed, and most embolized devices now are retrieved in the catheterization laboratory.

Vascular complications as a consequence of the delivery of the current devices for PDA occlusion are extremely rare and, for the most part, avoidable. The introduction of the larger delivery systems from the venous approach prevents arterial damage. Meticulous care and handling of the venous introductory sites prevent the majority (all!) of the venous complications. The greatest potential for a vascular complication occurs when an embolized device that cannot be refolded or re-collapsed must be retrieved. This requires the introduction of an even larger sheath and often, in the "turmoil" of a complex recovery procedure, less attention is paid to the introductory site of the large recovery sheath and/or not a large enough sheath is introduced to accommodate the partially folded/collapsed device. In the past, the Porstmann Device™ resulted in frequent arterial complications from the delivery procedure itself since it required an arterial cut-down for the introduction of an extremely large arterial introductory system. This device is no longer in much (or any) use.

The necessity of the patient having to undergo a surgical repair of the PDA because of the "failure" of the transcatheter occlusion attempt represents a more serious complication of a transcatheter device closure of a PDA. Most of the failures in the past, which required subsequent surgery, were a consequence of embolization of the implanted device away from the ductus. The Rashkind™ PDA device had a relatively high incidence of "failures" because the necessarily large, stiff delivery system prevented the delivery of the device to the ductus and/or once delivered, the device would embolize because of the somewhat precarious implant/release procedure. The Rashkind™ PDA device is no longer in use and this complication is far less likely with any of the current devices, particularly when there is a choice of device to suit the size and characteristics of the particular ductus.

There are a number of reports of acute and often severe hemolysis occurring when there is a residual, high-velocity flow through any type of device following PDA occlusion. This was more common with the Rashkind™ devices and still occurs following coil or Amplatzer™ PDA implants in the PDA. The treatment of hemolysis that is due to a high-velocity flow through a device is either to complete the occlusion of the PDA with one or more additional devices or, in the worst case, to remove the device. Rarely the hemolysis subsides with only supportive management, but this cannot be relied upon as a management strategy. These patients require very close observation until the hemolysis subsides completely and/or the cause is corrected.

There also are reports of bacterial endocarditis developing on devices positioned in the ductus, but to date, only on devices with a residual leak. Patients who develop endocarditis on a ductus device require intensive intravenous antibiotic therapy followed by surgical removal of the device.

Encroachment on the proximal left pulmonary artery and/or into the aortic lumen by a Rashkind™ device, by a "wad" of Gianturco™ coils and by an Amplatzer™ PDA device has been demonstrated by echocardiogram. Although very mild gradients have been reported, to date, *significant* encroachment with *hemodynamic* compromise in any area has not been documented. If and when a significant obstruction develops in either a branch pulmonary artery or in the aorta, it can be treated eventually and easily with balloon dilation with or without an intravascular stent implant.

As with all complications, the best treatment is prevention. Most of the complications of transcatheter PDA occlusion are avoidable particularly with the use of the newer devices and techniques. The incidence of complications is minimized (eliminated!) by paying careful attention to the details of each procedure and by utilizing the occasional "extra precautions" during the delivery of a particular device. When a complication of transcatheter PDA occlusion does occur, the consequences of the complication are minimized by early recognition and treatment.

Speculation—conclusion

As of the twenty-first century, the accepted, standard treatment of the patent ductus arteriosus is transcatheter occlusion of the PDA with one of the available occlusion devices. Worldwide, the available devices make essentially every patent ductus in patients after the neonatal period applicable for device closure. In the United States, catheter occlusion of the PDA still is compromised somewhat by the regulatory denial of the existence of some of the catheter procedures and, in turn, the restrictions on the use of some of the additional, now proven more effective and safer devices. Even with these restrictions and the resultant occlusion procedures, which are more complex than necessary, the present catheter occlusion procedures in all patients past small infancy are superior to the trauma and morbidity of surgery for the correction of the persistent patent ductus.

Hopefully, catheterizing physicians everywhere eventually will be able to choose the safest and most appropriate device to suit the particular anatomy, size of the PDA and the particular patient. Just a choice of the occlusion devices already developed and demonstrated to be safe, simplifies the procedures and makes each individual procedure significantly safer. Unquestionably, further miniaturization of the equipment and improvements in both the equipment and techniques will continue in the years to come. Assuming these newer devices achieve timely approval for use, they will make the transcatheter closure of the ductus arteriosus even simpler and safer and relegate surgical closure of the PDA only to historical significance.

References

1. Krichenko A *et al.* Angiographic classification of the isolated, persistently patent ductus arteriosus and implications for percutaneous catheter occlusion. *Am J Cardiol* 1989; **63**(12): 877–880.
2. Porstmann W, Wierny L, and Warnke H. Der Verschluss des D.a.p. ohne Thorakotomie (1 Mitteilung). *Thoraxchirurgie* 1967; **15**: 199.
3. Porstmann W *et al.* Catheter closure of patent ductus arteriosus, 62 cases treated without thoracotomy. *Radiol Clin North Am* 1971; **9**: 203–218.
4. Wang YW. [Percutaneous transfemoral plug closure of patent ductus arteriosus in 100 cases]. *Zhonghua Xin Xue Guan Bing Za Zhi* 1993; **21**(3): 158–160, 187.
5. Rashkind WJ and Cuaso CC. Transcatheter closure of patent ductus arteriosus: successful use in a 3.5 kilogram infant. *Pediatr Cardiol* 1979; **1**: 3–7.
6. King TD and Mills NL. Nonoperative closure of atrial septal defects. *Surgery* 1974; **75**: 383–388.
7. Rashkind WJ. Therapeutic interventional procedures in congenital heart disease. *Radiol Diagn (Berl)* 1987; **28**(4): 449–460.
8. Wallace S *et al.* Therapeutic vascular occlusion utilizing steel coil technique: clinical applications. *Am J Roentgenol* 1976; **127**(3): 381–387.
9. Cambier PA *et al.* Percutaneous closure of the small (less than 2.5 mm) patent ductus arteriosus using coil embolization. *Am J Cardiol* 1992; **69**(8): 815–816.
10. Lloyd TR *et al.* Transcatheter occlusion of patent ductus arteriosus with Gianturco coils. *Circulation* 1993; **88**(4 Pt 1): 1412–1420.
11. Uzun O *et al.* Transcatheter occlusion of the arterial duct with Cook detachable coils: early experience. *Heart* 1996; **76**(3): 269–273.
12. Dalvi B *et al.* New technique using temporary balloon occlusion for transcatheter closure of patent ductus arteriosus with Gianturco coils. *Cathet Cardiovasc Diagn* 1997; **41**(1): 62–70.
13. Sommer RJ *et al.* Use of preformed nitinol snare to improve transcatheter coil delivery in occlusion of patent ductus arteriosus. *Am J Cardiol* 1994; **74**(8): 836–839.
14. Hays MD, Hoyer MH, and Glasow PF. New forceps delivery technique for coil occlusion of patent ductus arteriosus. *Am J Cardiol* 1996; **77**(2): 209–211.
15. Kuhn MA and Latson LA. Transcatheter embolization coil closure of patent ductus arteriosus—modified delivery for enhanced control during coil positioning. *Cathet Cardiovasc Diagn* 1995; **36**(3): 288–290.
16. Hijazi ZM and Geggel RL. Transcatheter closure of large patent ductus arteriosus (> or = 4 mm) with multiple Gianturco coils: immediate and mid-term results. *Heart* 1996; **76**(6): 536–540.
17. Grifka MR and Jones TK. Transcatheter closure of large PDA using 0.052″ Gianturco coils: controlled delivery using a bioptome catheter through a 4 French sheath. *Catheter Cardiovasc Interv* 2000; **49**(3): 301–306.
18. Kumar RK *et al.* Bioptome-assisted simultaneous delivery of multiple coils for occlusion of the large patent ductus arteriosus. *Catheter Cardiovasc Interv* 2001; **54**(1): 95–100.
19. Hijazi ZM and Geggel RL. Results of anterograde transcatheter closure of patent ductus arteriosus using single or multiple Gianturco coils. *Am J Cardiol* 1994; **74**(9): 925–929.
20. Masura J *et al.* Catheter closure of moderate- to large-sized patent ductus arteriosus using the new Amplatzer duct occluder: immediate and short-term results. *J Am Coll Cardiol* 1998; **31**(4): 878–882.
21. Lozier JS and Cowley CG. Reactivity of the ductus arteriosus: Implications for transcatheter therapy. *Catheter Cardiovasc Interv* 2004; **61**(2): 268–270.
22. Grifka RG *et al.* New Gianturco-Grifka vascular occlusion device. Initial studies in a canine model. *Circulation* 1995; **91**(6): 1840–1846.
23. Grifka RG. Transcatheter PDA Closure Using the Gianturco-Grifka Vascular Occlusion Device. *Curr Interv Cardiol Rep* 2001; **3**(2): 174–182.
24. Neuss MB *et al.* Occlusion of the neonatal patent ductus arteriosus with a simple retrievable device: a feasibility study. *Cardiovasc Intervent Radiol* 1996; **19**(3): 170–175.
25. Ewert P *et al.* First closure of a large patent ductus arteriosus in an infant with an angulated nitinol plug. *Catheter Cardiovasc Interv* 2002; **57**(1): 88–91.
26. Bialkowski J *et al.* Percutaneous closure of window-type patent ductus arteriosus: using the CardioSEAL and STARFlex devices. *Tex Heart Inst J* 2003; **30**(3): 236–239.
27. Pedra CA, Sanches SA, and Fontes VF. Percutaneous occlusion of the patent ductus arteriosus with the Amplatzer device for atrial septal defects. *J Invasive Cardiol* 2003; **15**(7): 413–417.
28. Rao P *et al.* Transcatheter occlusion of patent ductus arteriosus with adjustable buttoned device. Initial clinical experience. *Circulation* 1993; **88**(3): 1119–1126.
29. Demkow M *et al.* Transcatheter closure of a 16 mm hypertensive patent ductus arteriosus with the Amplatzer muscular VSD occluder. *Catheter Cardiovasc Interv* 2001; **52**(3): 359–362.

28 Transcatheter atrial septal defect (ASD) occlusion

Introduction

Transcatheter occlusion of an atrial septal defect (ASD) with a double umbrella devices was reported by King and Mills in 1974[1]. The King–Mills™ ASD devices were rigid, quite cumbersome and required a *very* large delivery system. The size of the delivery system required a fairly extensive cut-down on the femoral and/or iliac vein for the introduction of the device. Because of the large size of the delivery system and the extensive cut-down, the King–Mills device was not practical for transcatheter use even in adult patients, much less in children. Although the device worked very well in the first five patients, further use of this device was never pursued. Four of the patients treated with this device are still alive and doing well 31+ years later with no complications definitely related to the devices. One elderly patient died nine years after implant with a non-related illness and causes not related to the device. These patients provide an excellent perspective about the long-term consequences of catheter-delivered devices positioned in the atrial septum[2].

The next major interest in catheter closure of atrial septal defects surfaced independently in 1977 with Rashkind[3]. In addition to a septostomy balloon and a separate PDA occlusion device, Dr Rashkind developed a single disk, Rashkind ASD Occluding Device™. This was a six legged, hexagonal, single umbrella with a disk of thin polyurethane foam, which attached to the atrial septum by tiny "fishhooks" at the tips of three alternate support legs. The delivery system for the Rashkind™ ASD device (USCI Angiographics, Billerica, MA) had an elaborate "centering" mechanism which together with the device, required the use of a 16-French delivery sheath. The Rashkind ASD Device™ began clinical trials in 1981 and a few atrial septal defects were closed in a few very selected patients. In spite of the centering mechanism, the tiny attaching hooks frequently and prematurely hooked to unwanted structures within the left atrium before the septum was engaged and resulted in a significant number of erroneously implanted devices. In addition, the polyurethane material of the umbrella tended to shrink away from the frame resulting in incomplete closures. As a consequence of the size of the delivery system, the hooks and, finally, the development of leaks after implant, the clinical trial using the Rashkind ASD Device™ was abandoned by the investigators almost as soon as it began, and this device never had very extensive use.

The concept of the Rashkind™ double-umbrella *PDA* device and the feasibility of device closure of an ASD demonstrated by both the King–Mills and the original hooked Rashkind *ASD*™ devices stimulated the development of the double-umbrella, Clamshell™ ASD occlusion device by Dr Lock and the engineers at USCI™ (USCI Angiographics, Billerica, MA)[4]. This device began the first extensive, FDA regulated, multicenter clinical IDE trial of an ASD occlusion device, beginning in 1991. In this trial, the Clamshell™ device was used to close the secundum ASD as well as multiple other intracardiac defects, including muscular ventricular septal defects and surgically created fenestrations.

The Clamshell™ ASD Occlusion Device, similar to the Rashkind™ PDA occluder (USCI Angiographics, Billerica, MA), was a "double-umbrella" device with two opposing umbrellas joined at their centers. The fabric of the umbrellas was woven dacron instead of polyurethane, which was used on the Rashkind devices, and there was an additional, single "hinge" or joint at the center of each of the legs of the Clamshell™ device. The extra hinges contributed to greater flexibility of the devices, added the tendency for each opened leg to bend toward the opposite umbrella and, in turn, contributed to a more secure "clamping" against the surface of the atrial septum.

The Clamshell™ umbrella had no centering mechanism so that the implanted device could position itself entirely to one edge of an ASD. As a consequence, the device that was used, had to be at least *twice* as large in diameter as the ASD being closed. The Clamshell™ umbrellas were available in 17, 23, 28, 22 and 40 mm sizes. All sizes of the Clamshell™ devices were delivered through an 11-French delivery sheath. During the time of the clinical trial of the device, the majority of the larger Clamshell devices developed a fracture of at least one leg. Although the fractures did not result in adverse *clinical* events and in spite of a reasonable success at closing atrial septal defects with a good safety record, the Clamshell™ device eventually was abandoned and withdrawn from any use. The fairly large clinical trial of the Clamshell™ ASD device before it was abandoned, demonstrated unequivocally that non-surgical, transcatheter ASD closure was a safe and reasonable alternative to the "time-honored" surgical repair of atrial septal defects[5]. The Clamshell™ device also now has provided over a decade of follow-up of still another catheter-delivered device implanted on the atrial septum and in several other locations within the heart.

The success of the Clamshell™ device in the multiple locations and then its abrupt withdrawal from availability created a compelling incentive and stimulation for the developers of the original Clamshell™ device as well as many other innovators/inventors to develop new and different devices and techniques for the non-surgical closure of atrial septal defects. As a consequence, new and different devices for the correction of atrial septal defects as well as all of the other abnormal communications by non-surgical, transcatheter techniques have blossomed during the past decade.

There now are several successful ASD occlusion devices, including the STARFlex™ (NMT Medical Inc., Boston, MA), the Sideris Button™ (Pediatric Cardiology Custom Medical Devices, Athens, Greece), the Helex™ (W. L. Gore & Associates, Flagstaff, AZ) and the Amplatzer™ ASD occlusion devices (AGA Medical Corp., Golden Valley, MN), which are in clinical use throughout the world outside of the United States. As of this writing, the Helex™ is the only device in a trial in the US for occlusion of atrial defects and the Amplatzer™ ASD Occluder is the only one of the several ASD devices that has FDA approval for the elective closure of ASDs in the United States. At least four other ASD occlusion devices have CE approval for use in Europe.

During this period of time, several other devices were developed for the occlusion of atrial septal defects, they were used in trials in the US and/or used clinically in Europe but, because of unsatisfactory results, already have been *abandoned* for any clinical use. The most notable of these were the Atrial Septal Defect Occluding System™ (ASDOS) (Sulzer Osypka, Rheinfelden, Germany)[6,7] and the Angel Wings™ devices (Microvena Corp., White Bear Lake, MN)[8]. In spite of these less than satisfactory results, even these devices and techniques did continue the interest and lead to the further development of occluder devices.

Technique for transcatheter device occlusion of ASD—general

Now, centrally located secundum atrial septal defects, in children past infancy and in adults of any age, potentially are suitable for transcatheter closure. When a patient is considered a candidate for transcatheter occlusion of any defect in the catheterization laboratory, strict "operating room" sterile precautions are observed from the moment the patient enters the catheterization laboratory and until the catheters are removed. With the ASD, or any catheter-implanted occlusion device, a "foreign body" is being implanted in the patient. The "fresh foreign body" sitting exposed in the circulation definitely increases the chance for endocarditis in the presence of any bacteremia.

General anesthesia is used for many occlusion procedures of the ASD with catheter-delivered devices primarily because the use of transesophageal echocardiographic (TEE) guidance during the implant procedure, and particularly with the relatively long duration of the use of TEE during the procedure. In addition, general anesthesia helps to ensure that the patient does not move at the critical moment during the deployment and implant of any device regardless of the implant guidance. Otherwise there is nothing particularly special about the delivery of an ASD device that requires general anesthesia, and the more routine use of intracardiac echo (ICE) to guide the implant (instead of TEE) may preclude the use of general anesthesia.

Once the access for all catheters is established, patients are given 100 units/kg of intravenous heparin. Their activated clotting time (ACT) is followed periodically throughout the procedure, trying to keep the ACT above 275–300 seconds. At the end of the procedure, the heparin is *not reversed* unless the patient has prolonged, uncontrolled bleeding from the vessel entry sites and/or the ACT still is over 600 seconds, or if the ACT is over 800 seconds, regardless of visible bleeding. When heparin is reversed, it should be reversed "conservatively" in order not to produce a hypercoagulable state. Although the procedures are performed in a "surgery-like" sterile environment, patients who receive the implant of a device are given a therapeutic dose of an intravenous cephalosporin (or equivalent antibiotic) at the time of device implant and three subsequent doses at six hourly intervals for prophylaxis against endocarditis. The patients are discharged on one 81 mg or one 325 mg aspirin per day (depending on body size), which is continued for six months following implant. In the majority of patients, no other anticoagulation therapy is used post-implant. When an occlusion device is used for the occlusion of a patent foramen ovale (PFO), particularly in a significantly older patient, many operators utilize an additional antiplatelet aggregating medication and/or coumadin anticoagulation for 3–6 months following the implant of these devices. PFO occlusion is covered separately in Chapter 29. Bacterial endocarditis prophylaxis is recommended for six months following implant until, presumably, full endothelialization of the device is completed.

Transthoracic echo (TTE) is used to establish the clinical diagnosis of an atrial septal defect as well as to determine the *approximate size of the defect*, the general location in the septum, and the presence of septal rims around the defect in patients with suspected ASDs[9]. In order to be useful for this screening, the TTE must be performed with the *specific intent* of providing this information and these measurements must be performed as precisely as possible. An echo report that states: "*there is an atrial septal defect*" or "*a large atrial defect with a 2.6:1 shunt*" unfortunately represents totally inadequate, semi-useless information! The TTE should be able to identify atrial septal defects that definitely are *unsuitable* for transcatheter closure because of their size and/or location (very large, eccentrically located, sinus venosus and/or primum ASD) as well as to exclude other intracardiac defects, which might represent a contraindication to transcatheter ASD closure. In order to be useful in determining whether a patient should be taken to the catheterization laboratory specifically for closure of the ASD, the echo must identify the size of the defect, the location of the defect and the adequacy of the septal rims around the defect, however, *TTE cannot* determine the *precise size* and the *absolute* suitability of the ASD for transcatheter closure.

A transesophageal echocardiogram (TEE) or intracardiac echocardiogram (ICE) is far more accurate at sizing and localizing the ASD, however, even the TEE or ICE does not correlate accurately enough with the size of the defect determined with a sizing balloon in the defect, which represents the *final* determination of suitability for device closure. This final suitability of the ASD for catheter closure is determined *in the cardiac catheterization laboratory* with very accurate balloon sizing along with TEE or ICE interrogation of the defect. There are several different balloon catheters and techniques used for sizing atrial septal defects. The types of sizing balloons and techniques that are most appropriate for particular defects/devices are discussed as a group and with the particular devices.

The applicability of each atrial septal defect for closure with a catheter-delivered device depends upon its absolute size relative to the overall size of the atrial septum, the location of the defect in the septum, and the type of closure device(s), which is(are) available. In general, transcatheter closure of atrial defects is limited to secundum atrial septal defects, which have some septal rim circumferentially around the defect. Experience has shown that a 10–25° absence of anterior–superior septal rim (subaortic) still is consistent with closure using some of the catheter-delivered devices. The precise size of the defect which can be occluded with a device and exactly how much rim is necessary are determined to a large extent by the type of ASD occlusion device that is available.

The femoral vein/inferior vena cava (IVC) approach is used with all of the devices that are currently available and/or are in trials for transcatheter occlusion of the ASD. The inferior vena cava usually is accessed by introduction of the catheter through a femoral vein, although a transhepatic approach can be used when neither femoral vein is accessible or patent. The angle of the atrial septum is approximately 45° in relation to the long axis of the body/IVC, which is the minimum angle for implanting most of the devices.

Because of the angle that the atrial septum forms between the atria, all catheters, wires and sheaths that are introduced from the neck and superior vena cava (SVC) approach, tend to align *parallel* to the septum as they enter the right atrium and/or cross into the left atrium. Although an atrial septal defect *can be crossed* easily from an internal jugular/superior vena cava approach, the parallel alignment with the septum of the delivery catheters causes the left atrial component of all of the ASD devices currently in use to deploy absolutely perpendicular to the septum. Since none of the "left atrial components" of any of the ASD occlusion devices can be pulled very tightly against the septum in order to align them flush against the septum during their attempted implant from the SVC, the approach from the SVC is not used for the delivery and implant of the currently available ASD occlusion devices.

If there is total ileo-femoral interruption and/or occlusion, the next most satisfactory approach for transcatheter occlusion of an ASD is through a transhepatic approach. The transhepatic approach is described in detail in Chapter 4 ("Catheter Introduction"). The *angle* of approach to the atrial septum from the transhepatic introduction of a catheter actually is better for device implant than the angle from the femoral approach! The transhepatic approach provides a direct, almost perpendicular angle to the plane of the atrial septum and can be used safely for the delivery of even large devices through as large as 12-French sheaths. The transhepatic approach is *not* used commonly for any catheterization procedure and the potential for serious "access" complications may be greater from this approach. As a consequence, the transhepatic approach is not used *routinely* and/or electively in spite of its "better angle" of approach to the septum/atrial septal defect.

Most of the ASD occluding devices are delivered to the atrial septum through a long sheath, which provides a large, somewhat flexible, delivery "tube" or "conduit" with a large lumen but, at the same time, without a concomitant too large an outside diameter. The long sheath delivery technique of intravascular devices initially was developed for transcatheter closure of the Rashkind™ PDA devices in order to deliver the large devices around curves and through the right heart en route to the PDA[10]. The same system was adapted for delivery of the Clamshell™ ASD devices and has been carried over for the delivery of most of the current ASD devices. Several potentially serious complications, which occurred as a consequence of air and/or clot embolizations from the wires, catheters and/or long delivery sheaths in the systemic circulation, were experienced during their very early use, however, now the proper techniques for the prevention of these complications are well established.

Once it is determined from the echocardiogram that an atrial septal defect *appears* suitable for transcatheter ASD occlusion, vascular sheaths are introduced into both femoral veins. Since all of the current sizing balloons require a 9- or 10-French sheath and most of the larger ASD occlusion devices are delivered through 9–12-French long sheaths, a 9–11-French short sheath (depending upon the estimated size of the defect and the type of occluder to be used) is placed in the right femoral vein at the beginning of the case. A 6- or 7-French sheath for an additional angiographic "marker" catheter which remains in the heart during the entire implant procedure is introduced into the left femoral vein. If intracardiac echo (ICE) is to be used to control the delivery of the device, an 11-French sheath is introduced into the left femoral vein instead of and/or in addition to the 6-French venous sheath. When the ICE catheter is introduced from the left femoral vein, it is helpful to have an introductory sheath for the ICE catheter that is at least 30 cm in length in order to guide the stiff and large ICE catheter through and past the more acutely angled left iliofemoral venous system. One femoral artery is cannulated with a small indwelling "Quick Cath" or a 4- or 5-French dilator to establish a line for the continuous monitoring of the arterial pressure.

A detailed right heart catheterization usually is performed to confirm the presence of the ASD, to verify the magnitude of shunting and to exclude associated defects. An angiogram with injection in the pulmonary artery with the angiographic recording continued to visualize the "recirculation" of the contrast through the pulmonary veins and left atrium is very useful to visualize the flow through the ASD and to exclude other unsuspected intracardiac defects, which might interfere with or prohibit the ASD occlusion. Occasionally a 6- or 7-French angiographic "marker" catheter, which is introduced into the *left* femoral vein, is advanced from the right heart through the ASD and into the mouth of the right upper pulmonary vein. One of the X-ray tubes (preferably the lateral) is placed in a "Left anterior oblique (LAO)–cranial" angulation (approximately 60° LAO and 45° cranial) and an angiocardiogram is recorded in this position with the anticipation of producing an "on-edge" view of the atrial septum. This angiogram *roughly* outlines the approximate size of the atrial defect and *roughly* demonstrates the position of the ASD in the septum. The orientation of the heart in the thorax of each patient is different and the location of each ASD on the septum changes the angle that will "cut the defect on edge" exactly. As a consequence, the exact angulation that cuts the atrial septal defect exactly on edge, is significantly different in each patient. If the information appears necessary and when the septum is not aligned on edge optimally by the first angiocardiogram, appropriate changes in the angulation of the X-ray tube(s) are made and the angiocardiograms are repeated. Usually moving the angled tube more toward the straight lateral *away* from the steeper, four-chambered "LAO" view aligns the septum and the septal defect more precisely in the presence of an atrial septal defect. This pulmonary vein/left atrial angiocardiogram also helps to demonstrate or rule out additional and/or remote separate atrial septal defects.

When the pulmonary vein/left atrial angiogram is performed, the particular LAO–cranial angle that cuts the defect "on edge" helps to demonstrate the optimal X-ray angle, which can be used during most of the delivery procedure for the device. A freeze-frame "road map" of a good single frame of the angiocardiogram of the ASD "on edge" is stored for future reference. For the delivery of the device, the same degree of LAO angulation is maintained on the lateral tube. The lateral tube can be rotated from the cranial–LAO to the *caudal*–LAO position. This angle maintains an "edge view" of the septum while at the same time moving the "can" of the image intensifier away from the transesophageal echocardiographer. The other X-ray tube is positioned in the AP or slight RAO position. The second fluoroscopy view provides the side-to-side orientation and position of the device during its delivery. This projection is particularly useful when there is any difficulty in aligning the device on the septum during the delivery of the device. The angiocardiographic catheter is withdrawn out of the pulmonary vein, but can remain positioned in the body of the left atrial cavity just on the left side of the atrial septum. The angiographic catheter can remain in this position throughout most of the delivery of the device unless it must be removed in order to replace it with the ICE catheter through the same sheath.

Before advancing the necessary catheter, wire and/or balloon across the defect and into the left atrium and/or pulmonary veins, the TEE or the ICE probe is introduced into the patient first in order to size the ASD accurately without any distortion from the catheters. For most patients to be able to tolerate the TEE probe for the duration of an ASD occlusion procedure and to remain absolutely still during the critical stages of the procedure, general anesthesia is used for the ASD occlusion procedure. In a rare patient, TEE can be carried out without general anesthesia using heavy supplemental sedation along with topical cocaine or other topical anesthesia sprayed in the oral and posterior pharynx just before introduction of the probe. Unfortunately, the patients who absolutely cannot tolerate the TEE probe are not predictable ahead of time, so when the TEE is used, general anesthesia is the rule. On the other hand, the ASD can be closed with sedation and local anesthesia in most patients when ICE is used to control the implant. For supplemental sedation, liberal doses of intravenous ketamine and/or versed are used in children in addition to the usual demerol–phenergan premedication. In the older teens and adults, intravenous versed is used more often than ketamine for the supplemental sedation because of the reported "nightmares" from ketamine during the recovery from the "deep sedation".

The echocardiographer usually introduces the TEE probe from the patient's left side at the head of the catheterization table. The patient's mouth is propped open with a special mouth splint and the tip of the echo probe is passed gently through the posterior pharynx. Forming a curve transiently on the tip of the TEE probe with the built-in "deflector" helps in passing the probe through the posterior oral pharynx. Once past the posterior oral pharynx, the probe is allowed to straighten and usually is advanced easily from there down the esophagus. Its position is verified from the echo images obtained from the TEE probe itself and by the fluoroscopic image of the large probe within the thorax and behind the heart.

Alternatively to the use of the TEE probe, the physician performing the catheterization introduces the ICE catheter into the sheath in the left femoral vein. By using the slightly longer sheath (30 cm) in the left femoral vein, the sheath extends cephalad to the bifurcation of the inferior vena cava (IVC). This makes the introduction of the large and somewhat stiff ICE catheter around the often acute curves and past the side branches in the pelvis much easier and safer. If the longer sheath is *not* used, a slight deflection is formed on the tip of the ICE catheter as it is introduced into the vein and the tip of the ICE catheter is viewed *continuously* with fluoroscopy as it is maneuvered gently from the femoral vein, through the iliac vein and IVC and into the right atrium.

Once the TEE or ICE probe is in position, the particular echo probe is manipulated to obtain a good image of the entire atrial septum. The atrial septal defect, the rims around the defect and the length of the septum in the longitudinal and anterior–posterior planes all are interrogated and measured accurately with the TEE or ICE before additional catheters and wires are advanced through the defect. The atrial septum and surrounding structures are scrutinized to determine the suitability of the ASD for transcatheter closure, and any other abnormalities are excluded that might contraindicate or interfere with the device closure of the ASD.

One structure that often is not apparent on standard TTE and is looked for specifically with TEE or ICE, is a large and/or long redundant Eustachian valve. A large Eustachian valve does not preclude transcatheter occlusion of the ASD, but certainly can complicate the delivery and/or can compromise the results of the implant because of its proximity to the atrial defect. The Eustachian valve usually is visualized on TEE or ICE as a thin, usually very loose strand of tissue flapping in the low right atrium/inferior vena cava area. Rarely the Eustachian valve is a fairly rigid and dense structure, which appears almost as a separate septum caudally across the right atrium. The tissue of a large and long Eustachian valve can extend up to, and across the orifice of the atrial septal defect. The problems caused by a Eustachian valve that is close to the ASD, and the specific handling of the tissue during device delivery, are discussed separately under the delivery techniques for the CardioSEAL/STARFlex™ (NMT Medical Inc., Boston, MA) and Amplatzer™ ASD devices (AGA Medical Corp., Golden Valley, MN).

Once all of the measurements have been performed and the atrial septum and surrounding tissues have been interrogated with TEE or ICE, balloon sizing of the atrial defect is carried out in order to determine the *exact* dimensions of the defect. Balloon sizing also represents the best method of excluding additional, separate defects in the atrial septum.

Balloon sizing of the atrial septal defect

Before the more extensive manipulation in the left heart for the balloon sizing with any type of sizing balloon and the later introduction of the larger sheaths, and if it was not give previously, the patient is given 100 U/kg of intravenous heparin. If a smaller venous sheath was used in the *right* femoral vein for the diagnostic catheterization, the *right* venous sheath is replaced with a 9–11-French, short sheath with a back-bleed valve and side flush/pressure port. This sheath is cleared of air, attached to a flush system and placed on a slow, continuous flush. A *wire* back-bleed valve with a wire flush port is attached to an end-hole catheter that will accept a 0.035″ guide wire. The catheter is attached to the catheter flush/pressure system through the wire back-bleed valve and flushed thoroughly. This catheter is introduced through the larger right femoral vein sheath and advanced through the right heart, through the ASD and positioned securely in a left upper pulmonary vein. The more cephalad the vein and the straighter the course from the IVC to that vein, the better the support will be for the sizing balloon. An exchange length, Super Stiff™ 0.035″ guide wire (Boston Scientific, Natick, MA) with a short floppy tip is passed through the catheter into a very distal position in the pulmonary vein. The catheter is left in place over the wire and kept on a continuous flush until just before the introduction of the sizing balloon.

The *balloon* and *balloon lumen* of the sizing balloon are flushed thoroughly with a 1:5 dilution of contrast to flush solution and cleared of all air. As slight negative pressure is applied to the balloon lumen, the balloon is rewrapped around the shaft of the catheter while rotating the catheter counterclockwise. While continually flushing around the wire, the original catheter, which is still over the wire, is slowly and carefully withdrawn out of the body, leaving the wire in place in the pulmonary vein. The wire back-bleed/flush valve is placed on the *catheter lumen* of the sizing balloon catheter and maintained on a slow, continuous flush as the sizing balloon catheter is introduced over the wire. The short sheath is maintained on a continuous flush through its side port as the sizing balloon is introduced and as long as the balloon catheter is within the sheath. The sizing balloon is advanced over the pre-positioned wire into the cardiac silhouette. Both the lumen of the *catheter shaft* of the sizing balloon and the short sheath are kept on a slow flush. The previously positioned angiographic catheter can remain in position through the atrial defect and adjacent to the wire, over which the balloon is advanced.

There are three general techniques for "balloon sizing" of an atrial septal defect, two of which measure the "static" diameter of the defect. Both of the "static" techniques use a very large angioplasty-like or "sausage" shaped "static" balloon which is inflated and remains in the defect during the measurement. These "static" balloons are inflated while exactly straddling the defect, and the diameter of the defect is determined by measuring the circumferential indentation or "waist" on the balloon caused by the circumference of the defect (Figure 28.1). The Amplatzer™ "static" sizing technique/balloons (AGA Medical Corp., Golden Valley, MN) usually are used to measure the *stretched* diameter of the defect while the NuMED™ "static" sizing balloons (NuMED Inc., Hopkinton, NY) are used to measure the non-stretched diameter of the defect.

The balloon material of the Amplatzer™ "static" sizing balloons is more elastic, it expands progressively with increasing volume of fluid and pressure in the balloon and is used to purposefully *stretch* the defect and then provides a more ***"stretched"*** static diameter of the defect. The NuMED™ "static" sizing balloon is a very non-compliant balloon, which is available in multiple sizes, is inflated in the defect at a very low pressure (zero pressure!) and, in turn, has a very soft consistency in order to provide a ***"non-stretched"***, static diameter of the defect. Unlike the earlier, but still occasionally used, "pull through"

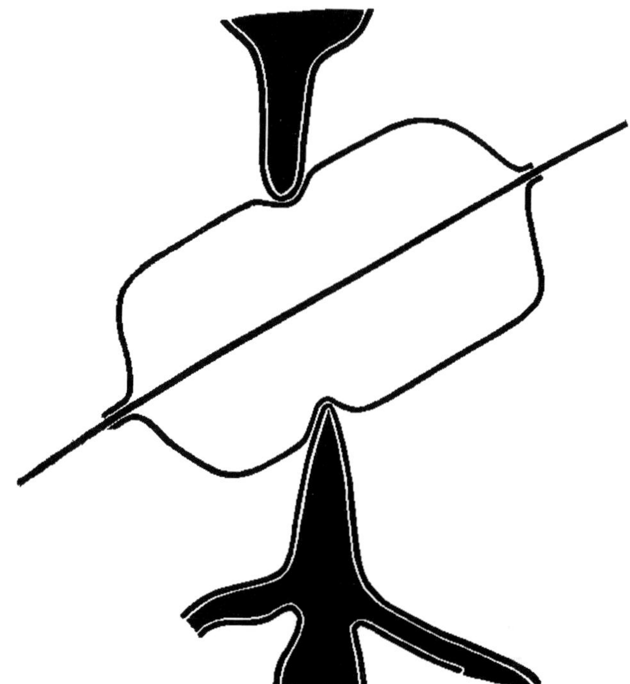

Figure 28.1 "Waist" formed on a static sizing balloon across atrial septal defect (ASD).

"occlusion" balloons used for sizing, neither of the *static* sizing balloons is withdrawn through, or moved purposefully within the defect but rather positioned exactly within, and straddling the atrial septal defect during the sizing. The Amplatzer™ and the NuMED™ sizing balloons are positioned in an identical fashion and the angulation of the X-ray tubes adjusted appropriately and identically for both types of static balloon sizing. Although the two different types of static balloons are positioned across the defect in an identical manner, the techniques for sizing and the measurements obtained are different for the two balloons. Both measurements are accurate but provide different information.

The third balloon sizing technique utilizes the repeated withdrawal of large, soft, spherical, latex, Equalizer™ balloons (Medi-Tech, Boston Scientific, Natick, MA) through the defect. The Equalizer™ balloons are a recent replacement for the earlier and similar "Occlusion" balloons (Medi-Tech, Boston Scientific, Natick, MA), which no longer are available. The spherical "occlusion" type balloon is pulled gently and repeatedly through the defect while repeatedly changing the diameter of the balloon by changing the volume of fluid in the balloon. The diameter of the defect is determined from the measured diameter of the balloon that *just* pulls through the defect or from a circumferential indentation ("waist") created on the balloon as it pulls into and/or through the defect. The exact techniques and equipment for the two "static" and one "pull through" sizing procedures are described in detail in the following sections.

"Static sizing balloon" sizing of the ASD

When sizing the atrial defect with either of the "static" balloon techniques, a short tipped 0.035″ *Super Stiff*™ wire (Medi-Tech, Boston Scientific, Natick, MA) is necessary to support and maintain the sizing balloon in a secure and steady position precisely within the atrial septal defect. A Super Stiff™ exchange wire is positioned across the atrial defect and well into a left upper pulmonary vein. The catheter lumen of the static sizing balloon is maintained on a slow continuous flush through a wire back-bleed/flush port valve, which is attached to the hub of the catheter. The sizing balloon is advanced over the previously positioned wire into the area of the defect as seen on fluoroscopy and TEE or ICE.

While observing on fluoroscopy and TEE or ICE, the balloon is inflated *very gently and slowly* while watching for the circumferential indentation ("waist") on the balloon (*see* Figure 28.1). Because of the mobility and lack of "visibility" of the septum on fluoroscopy, the sizing balloon frequently must be deflated and repositioned slightly either forward or backward in order to position the "waist" as close to the center of the balloon as possible. The balloon is deflated each time before repositioning it within the septal defect. In order to advance the sizing balloon in the defect over the wire, the wire is fixed in place at the vein and the balloon is pushed forward on the wire, but, to withdraw the sizing balloon in the septum, the *wire* is pushed securely into the balloon catheter, while the forward push on the balloon is relaxed. This causes the balloon to "milk" back on the wire similar to "withdrawing" an angioplasty balloon in a vessel, although the balloon may have to be withdrawn over the wire very slightly. The balloon repositioning in the septum is repeated until the septum indents the balloon at the center of the length of the balloon.

The balloon/ASD are visualized on the TEE or ICE and color flow Doppler™ applied to the signal. This echo image provides a measurement of the diameter of the "waist" on the surface of the balloon, which represents the diameter of the defect. The Doppler™ color flow image demonstrates when the balloon is inflated sufficiently to stop all flow through the defect and clearly demonstrates any additional defects in the atrial septum. If there are separate defects, the echo/Doppler™ flow will demonstrate the size of the additional defect and the distance from the defect that is occluded with the balloon.

When inflated sufficiently to create a waist on the balloon, both types of static sizing balloon clearly identify the exact plane of the septum and the location of the defect on the septum as seen on the fluoroscopy, and verify that there are no additional atrial defects. The amount of inflation of the static sizing balloon and the amount of volume/pressure delivered to the balloon depend upon which type of static sizing balloon is being used. Both types of static balloon are discussed in detail subsequently in this chapter.

With the balloon partially inflated, the angulation of the X-ray tubes is changed in order to align the balloon in its longest diameter and to align the "waist" on the balloon exactly on edge so that there is no overlap of the two ends of the balloon over the waist. The change in angulation often is considerable and the changes in the angulation of the X-ray tubes often must be tried several times to achieve the exact, proper perpendicular angulation to the balloon. When aligned correctly, the "waist" on the balloon appears as a thin line, perpendicularly across the long axis of the balloon with no obliquity of the "line" around the balloon and no overlapping shadows of the two inflated ends of the balloon. This angle represents the plane that is exactly perpendicular to the septum at the level of the defect. The extra effort to obtain this exact view is justified in order to obtain the precise measurements of the defect on fluoroscopy and to provide the *exact angle* of the plane of the septum that will be used during the implant of the device.

A left atrial angiogram through the angiographic catheter (which still can be through the defect into the left atrium and adjacent to the balloon) is performed to verify the atrial septal angulation, the defect position and orientation and to look for additional defects. A slow flush around the wire through the *catheter* lumen of the sizing balloon is continued during the entire sizing process.

Amplatzer™ sizing balloon—*stretched* ASD diameter

The Amplatzer™ sizing balloon (AGA Medical Corp., Golden Valley, MN) can be used to provides a static non-stretched and/or a static ***stretched*** diameter of the ASD. The Amplatzer™ sizing balloon has the configuration of a very large angioplasty balloon, but the material of the balloon is a very thin, 0.002″ stretchable, polyurethane membrane, which makes the balloons very elastic and very compliant. The AGA™ sizing balloon is mounted on a 7-French nylon catheter which passes over a 0.035″ wire and through a 9- (10-French easily) French sheath. The Amplatzer™ sizing balloons are 4 cm long and available in only in two sizes—24 and 34 mm diameter. The 24 mm sizing balloon is used for defects up to 16 mm in diameter as measured by TEE or ICE and the 34 mm sizing balloon used for all defects *larger than* 16 mm diameter on the TEE or ICE measurements. The balloon material allows a gradual, progressive increase in the diameter of the balloon (up to 42 mm with the larger balloon!) with a progressively increasing filling volume. In order to reach the maximum diameters of the balloon when using the larger Amplatzer™ sizing balloon, the balloon must be inflated with *90 +cc* of fluid!

In order to obtain the ***stretched*** diameter of the atrial septal defect, the Amplatzer™ sizing balloon is inflated until a *distinct* circumferential indentation or "waist" appears around the balloon and all flow around the balloon is stopped as determined by color flow Doppler™. The Amplatzer™ sizing balloon generates a significant circumferential wall pressure when inflated with the volume at which the waist appears and, in turn, purposefully *stretches* the edges of the atrial defect as the balloon "waist" approximates the diameter of the defect. When the waist is created in this balloon, the atrial defect can be stretched several millimeters. This *stretched* diameter is used to determine the exact size of the Amplatzer™ ASD occlusion device that should be used[11].

The AGA™ sizing balloon has metal, radio-opaque, calibration bands, which are imbedded in the wall of the catheter shaft *just proximal* to the balloon. These marks are spaced at 2, 5 and 10 mm distances from each other when measured from *inside to inside* of two adjacent bands. To use these bands for the calibration, they must be aligned exactly perpendicular to the X-ray beam and, in turn, create *distinct, thin, straight lines* across the catheter shaft. On the small diameter catheter shaft, this often is difficult to determine. When not aligned properly, the bands appear oval or circular, in which case, any measurements of distances between bands will not be accurate for calibration. The X-ray tubes are angled to align both the balloon and the bands perpendicular to the X-ray beam before the measurements are made. As with any other measurements in the catheterization laboratory, the width of the shaft of a catheter is too inaccurate to be of any use as the reference calibration for large diameter defects. As an alternative, a separate catheter with aligned "calibration" marks or an accurate calibration system built into the X-ray system is used as the reference for the measurements of the atrial defect.

In order to "stretch size" the defect accurately for the Amplatzer™ ASD devices with the AGA™ sizing balloons, it is important that in addition to occluding the defect, a distinct waist develops around the balloon and enough of a waist is produced around the balloon to fix the balloon in the defect and occlude any flow adjacent to the balloon. The AGA™ sizing balloon purposefully and often stretches the defect significantly larger than the static non-stretched diameter visualized by TEE or ICE. The AGA™ sizing balloons also tend to make an oval or even an elliptical defect round when a distinct waist is created! Since the fixation of the Amplatzer™ ASD device depends upon the round, "central hub" of the device actually *stretching into* the defect, this measured *"stretched diameter"* is desirable and is the measurement used to choose the size of the appropriate Amplatzer™ ASD occlusion device. The diameter of the waist on the AGA™ sizing balloon as measured on an accurately calibrated biplane angiogram and/or TEE or ICE represents the "stretched diameter" of the defect and also the exact size of the device to be used.

Originally as a double check for the accuracy of the X-ray/echo measuring systems, the exact volume of fluid that was used to fill the AGA™ sizing balloon *at the stretched diameter* of the ASD was recorded. After the measurements within the heart were recorded, the balloon was deflated and withdrawn out of the body over the wire. The measurements from within the heart were confirmed outside of the body by reintroducing the exact same quantity of fluid into the AGA™ balloon that was used during the measurement within the heart, and the inflated diameter with that exact volume checked with a provided AGA™ "sizing plate". The "sizing plate" is a metal or (now) plastic plate with multiple holes in the plate, which are very accurate in size and with the size of the holes increasing in diameter in one mm increments. This technique has the problem of not being able to know which hole in the plate re-creates the exact diameter of the "waist" in the balloon even though the exact volume is known. The sizing plate is seldom used when modern X-ray equipment and TEE or ICE are available.

The size of the Amplatzer™ device that is used is *the same diameter as the waist* on the balloon at its "stretched" diameter as measured on X-ray and/or TEE or ICE. When there is a discrepancy between the X-ray and the echo measurements, both measurements are repeated. With persistent discrepancies, the operator must choose the measurements with which he(she) has the most confidence or err on the side of the larger measurement. With the Amplatzer™ ASD device, when the device obviously is too large or if, at the other extreme, it readily pulls through the defect, the device can be withdrawn and a more appropriate sized device reintroduced, with the only "adverse event" being the cost of the wasted device.

The Amplatzer sizing balloons also can be used to obtain a non-stretched diameter. Using color flow Doppler™ simultaneously with the balloon inflation, the balloon is inflated only until there is no residual flow through the defect and/or around the balloon on color flow Doppler™. This diameter of the balloon is recorded as the defect diameter. Usually no waist is created in the balloon and the diameter will be slightly smaller than when measured during the appearance of the waist. The size of the Amplatzer ASD Occluder™ that is chosen should be the same or the next size larger than the measured balloon when using the non-stretched sizing.

NuMED™ sizing balloon—*non-stretched* ASD diameter

The NuMED™ sizing balloon (NuMED Inc., Hopkinton, NY) usually is used to provide a static, but ***non-stretched*** diameter of the atrial defect. The NuMED™ sizing balloon is a very thin walled, very low-pressure, relatively non-compliant, "angioplasty" balloon which is used for very accurate, *non-stretched*, static measurements of the defects. These sizing balloons inflate at such a low pressure that the "waist" in the balloon can be created *without* distorting or stretching the atrial septum *at all*. The NuMED™ balloons exert such a delicate force that a waist can be created in a partially inflated NuMED™ sizing balloon by a *hole in a single sheet of bond paper* without tearing that hole in the paper! The NuMED™ balloons are available in three and four centimeter lengths and in diameters between 10 and 40 mm (in 5 mm increments). There now are 5 & 6 cm lengths in the 30+ mm diameter balloons. A NuMED™ sizing balloon with a balloon diameter that is approximately *two times* the TEE or ICE diameter of the ASD is used in the measurement of the *non-stretched*, static, ASD diameter. The much larger balloon–to-defect size is used to ensure that the waist is created in the sizing balloon with the balloon only partially inflated and at *essentially "zero" pressure* in the balloon. When the NuMED™ sizing balloons are inflated to their *full* diameters, the wall tension of these balloons increases and they become tense and, when inflated close to their full diameters, these balloons are capable of stretching and *dilation* rather than a precise, non-stretched "sizing"!

The diameter of the "waist" achieved with the NuMED™ balloon inflated at "zero" pressure, when properly aligned and when there is no residual flow, represents the *non-stretched*, static balloon diameter of the atrial defect (*see* Figure 28.1). Once the waist is apparent in the partially inflated balloon, the orientation of the septum is identified by the angle the balloon makes with the septum. If there is residual flow adjacent to the balloon and the flow is not through a completely separate defect, and/or when the separate angiographic catheter still is passing through the defect adjacent to the balloon, the angiographic catheter is withdrawn into the right atrium and/or slightly more fluid is introduced into the balloon until the Doppler™ flow around the balloon stops.

The NuMED™ balloons also have metal calibration bands embedded in the shaft of the catheter, however, the bands are 1.0 and 1.5 cm apart and they are embedded in the shaft of the catheter *within* the area of the balloon. These marks also are accurate for calibration only when they are aligned exactly perpendicular to the X-ray beam and when they appear as distinct, short *straight lines*. These bands are measured from *inside to inside* of the adjacent bands. The bands in the NuMED™ sizing balloons are on a very thin part of the shaft of the catheter, which makes it very difficult to align them precisely on edge. It is more accurate to use the calibration marks of a separate, properly aligned, angiographic "marker" catheter or the calibration dots built into the X-ray system as the calibration for the measurements.

A *non-stretched*, static balloon sizing technique for the atrial septal defect is used primarily with the CardioSEAL™ (NMT Medical Inc., Boston, MA) and the STARFlex™ devices (NMT Medical Inc., Boston, MA), but it can also be used for all of the other ASD occlusion devices. If the NuMED™ balloon is used with the Amplatzer™ ASD device, either a balloon that is close to the diameter of the defect is inflated at a higher pressure or a device is used that is 2–4 mm (1–2 sizes) larger than the non-stretched diameter obtained with the NuMED™ balloon. The softer, NuMED™ static sizing balloons have the advantages of: (1) giving a very accurate and reproducible, *non-stretched* diameter of the defect; (2) conforming to the shape of the defect and, in turn, demonstrating oblong or odd shapes of the ASD; and (3) not stretching the ASD at all during the sizing procedure, possibly allowing for the use of a smaller occluder.

"Occlusion balloon" or "pull through" sizing of the ASD

Until the introduction of the static sizing balloons, the large Medi-tech™ "Occlusion" balloons (Medi-Tech, Boston Scientific, Natick, MA) or the balloon on the large Swan™ floating balloon catheters were used for the sizing of the ASD for the Clamshell™ device, and early in the experience with all of the other ASD occlusion devices. As discussed earlier, the original "Occlusion" balloons (Medi-Tech, Boston Scientific, Natick, MA) are no longer available and have been replaced by the Equalizer™ balloons (Medi-Tech, Boston Scientific, Natick, MA). Similar to the earlier "Occlusion" balloons, the Equalizer™ balloons are available in 20, 27, 33 and 40 mm diameters, however, the Equalizer™ balloons are advertised to be introduced through a minimum of 14 to 16+ French sheaths (as opposed to the 9- or 10-French sheaths for the "Occlusion" balloons)! Fortunately, with some folding of the balloon, balloons up to 33 mm can be introduced and withdrawn through an 11-French sheath.

The "occlusion" balloon, "pull through" sizing technique is still used by some centers for the sizing of the ASD. The Occlusion/Equalizer™ balloons are spherical balloons made of latex, which were designed to be inflated and then withdrawn into "an orifice" to occlude the orifice and/or channel mechanically and totally while measuring the *effects* of the occlusion on the hemodynamics. They were designed to *occlude*, and as a consequence, are not ideal or often even satisfactory for *measuring* the precise dimensions or diameters of defects. Two different techniques are used with these "occlusion" balloons to "measure" the defects.

With one technique, an occlusion balloon that is much larger than the diameter of the defect as it is withdrawn into the defect and a "waist" is produced in the balloon which is measured similar to the static balloon technique. A standard, exchange length, 0.035", spring guide wire, which is a *standard* more flexible guide wire, is positioned in a left upper pulmonary vein using a technique identical to the technique for placing the stiffer wires for the static balloon sizing. A less rigid wire is used purposefully with the "occlusion balloon" techniques in order to allow the "occlusion balloon" to move freely from side-to-side in order for it to "center" in the defect as it is withdrawn into the defect and to avoid fixation against one edge of the defect by the wire, the balloon catheter and/or the "corner" or junction of a balloon where it is attached to the catheter.

A latex Medi-tech™ Occluding balloon (Boston Scientific, Natick, MA), which is *at least twice the diameter* that was measured by TEE or ICE as the diameter of the ASD, is used for the sizing with this technique and this type of balloon. The deflated occlusion balloon is advanced entirely into the left atrium over the *more flexible and non*-stiff wire. The catheter lumen of the balloon catheter is maintained on a slow flush through a wire back-bleed/flush valve exactly as with the static balloons. The occlusion balloon is inflated with 3–5 ml of a solution of very diluted contrast (1:5). This small amount of fluid fills the balloon only partially so that the walls are very soft and compliant. The partially filled occlusion balloon is pulled back slowly to the atrial septum while observing the balloon on fluoroscopy and/or on TEE or ICE for the appearance of a circumferential indentation (waist) on the balloon as it enters the atrial defect. As the balloon is pulled into the defect and "seats" in the defect an *indentation or "waist"* develops on the more proximal surface of the large, soft balloon. These large occlusion balloons assume the tapered shape of a "hot air" balloon with the "waist" created by the edges of the defect appearing along the conical sides of the balloon as the sides of the balloon widen (Figure 28.2). If a waist is not seen and/or the balloon pulls completely through the defect, the balloon is deflated, re-advanced back in the left atrium and filled with slightly more fluid, and the withdrawal into the defect is repeated very gently until a waist forms on the balloon and the balloon is held up in the defect. The diameter of the waist on the balloon is recorded both on TEE or ICE and on a stored image of a biplane fluoroscopy/angiography image. The measurement of this waist represents the *stretched* diameter of the defect, and usually is slightly larger than the measurement obtained with a NuMED™ static sizing balloon technique.

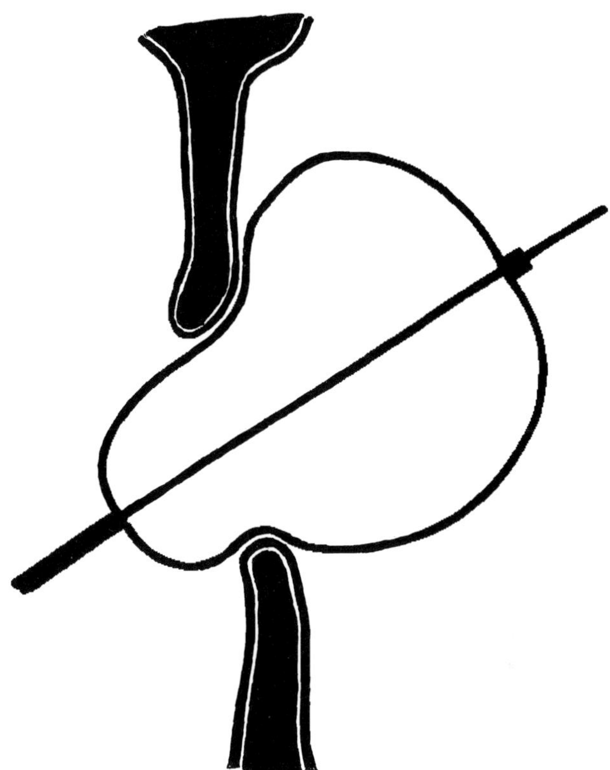

Figure 28.2 "Waist" produced by the rim of the atrial septal defect on a very large *and soft* "occlusion" balloon as it is pulled into the defect.

The second, more standard, method, also using the Medi-tech™ "Occlusion" balloon catheter (Boston Scientific, Natick, MA), is performed using an occlusion balloon that is only *slightly larger* than the ASD diameter that is measured by TEE or ICE echo. The size of the occlusion balloon used for this technique is chosen to *correspond exactly in diameter* to the expected diameter of the defect as measured by the TEE or ICE. The different diameters of the "occlusion" balloon are measured as the balloon is filled with diluted contrast (1:5 dilution) in incremental inflations of 0.2–0.5 ml of fluid added sequentially to the balloon—all *outside of the body* before the balloon is introduced. The exact diameter of the Occlusion/Equalizer™ balloon is measured with each incremental increase in fluid volume up to a 6 ml volume. The balloon of the "occlusion" balloon catheter, which has been "calibrated" in this manner, is deflated and advanced over the previously positioned *soft* exchange wire and into the left atrium. Depending upon the preceding angiocardiographic and TEE or ICE estimates of the ASD size, the balloon is inflated with the amount of dilute contrast that was measured to produce a diameter of the balloon that is exactly equivalent to the size of the ASD. The balloon catheter is withdrawn very gently over the wire toward the right atrium while holding the wire "loosely" so the balloon/wire can move from side to side. During this slow, careful withdrawal, the balloon is observed on the fluoroscopic image for any indication of the balloon catching on and/or being distorted by the edges of the ASD.

If the balloon pulls through the ASD easily with this inflation volume and maneuver, the balloon is deflated and is re-advanced over the wire into the left atrium. An additional 0.5 ml of diluted contrast is added to the balloon and the withdrawal of the balloon into the defect is repeated. The entire procedure is repeated until the sizing balloon *just* begins to catch *within* the defect during the withdrawal and, in the process, occludes the defect as seen by color flow Doppler™ on the TEE or ICE. If the balloon does not catch, even when it is inflated to the maximum pre-measured diameter of the balloon, the original "occlusion" balloon is replaced with a larger sized "occlusion" balloon, the calibration of the balloon and this "sizing" during the gentle withdrawal of the balloon repeated with gradually increasing volumes of instilled fluid in the balloon until the balloon just catches in the septal defect (Figure 28.3). The sequential, increasing diameters with the increasing volumes of fluid in the larger occlusion balloon must be calibrated separately before the ASD measurements by this withdrawal technique.

Although it may be more convenient to leave the angiographic catheter in place through the defect during the sizing with the *occlusion* balloons, it is imperative that *no other catheter remains crossing through the ASD* while the *pull-through sizing* is being performed with an *"occlusion"* balloon. An additional catheter crossing through the atrial septal defect can pass transversely across the ASD and in doing so, create a rigid "band" or "splint" across the lumen, which, in turn, prevents even a much smaller sized balloon from pulling through the defect than the size actually necessary to occlude the defect (Figure 28.4).

In order to obtain additional left atrial angiograms with the "occlusion/sizing" balloon in place, the appropriate sized, inflated occlusion balloon, which is pulled into the defect and "seals" against the edges of the defect, is deflated slightly and advanced a small distance into the left atrium. This "releases" it from the septum. The additional angiographic catheter from the opposite femoral vein is re-advanced through the ASD and back into the left atrium adjacent to the partially moved occlusion/sizing balloon. The occlusion/sizing balloon then is reinflated with its measured "occluding volume", withdrawn back into the ASD and pulled "firmly" against the septum and catheter through the defect. The left atrial/right upper pulmonary vein angiogram is repeated with the occlusion/sizing balloon now occluding the ASD. This demonstrates the adequacy of the sizing and the angle of the septum in relation to the sizing balloon. Of equal importance, the

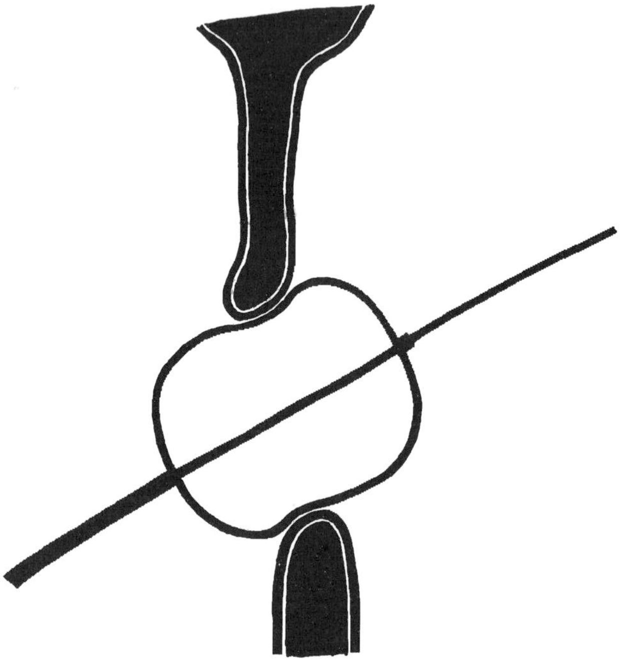

Figure 28.3 Symmetrical and very minimal waist created in an "occlusion" balloon, which is inflated to the exact diameter of the defect, during its withdrawal through the ASD.

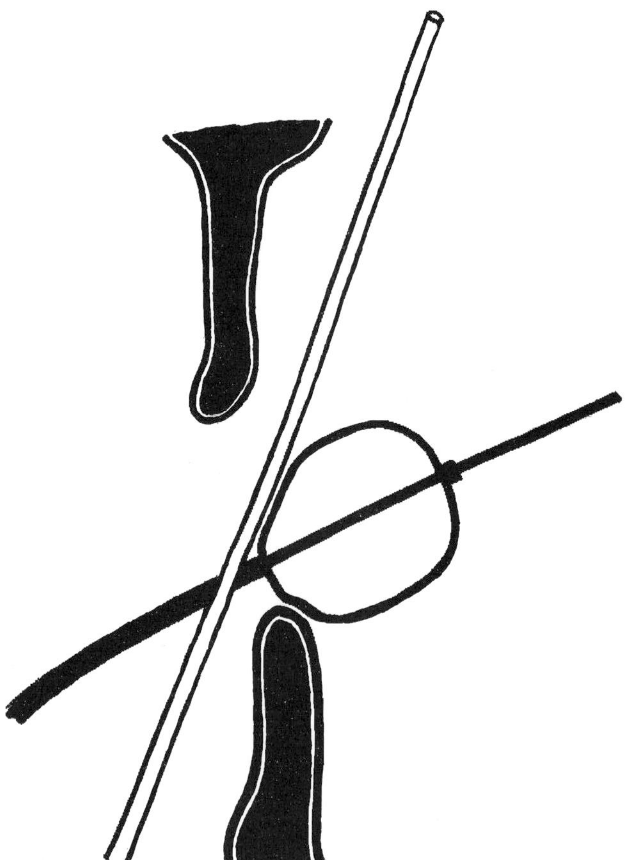

Figure 28.4 An additional catheter crossing an atrial defect during occlusion balloon sizing. The second catheter obstructs the passage of even a small "pull-through" occlusion sizing balloon.

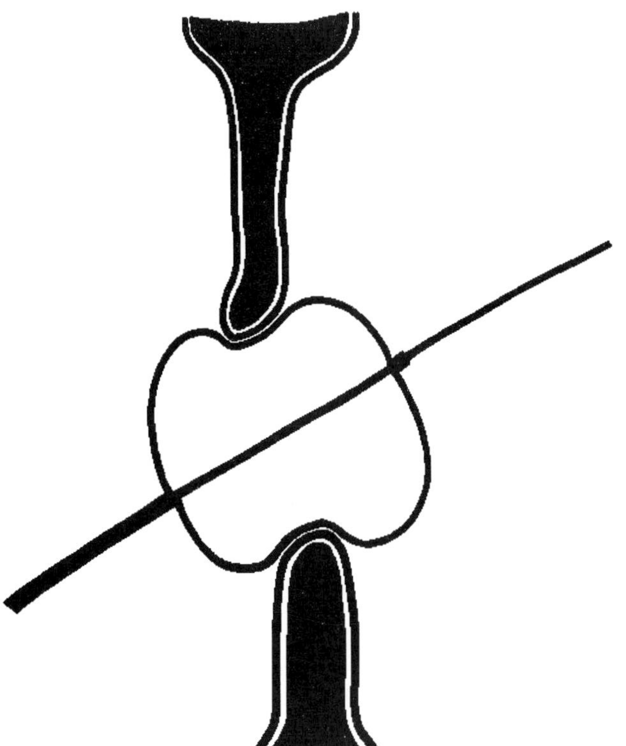

Figure 28.5 Indentation (or transient "waist") in an occlusion balloon during withdrawal through a defect that is smaller than the balloon. Usually a balloon that is too large for the defect but at the same time somewhat soft, "pops" through the defect and the waist can be visualized only very transiently.

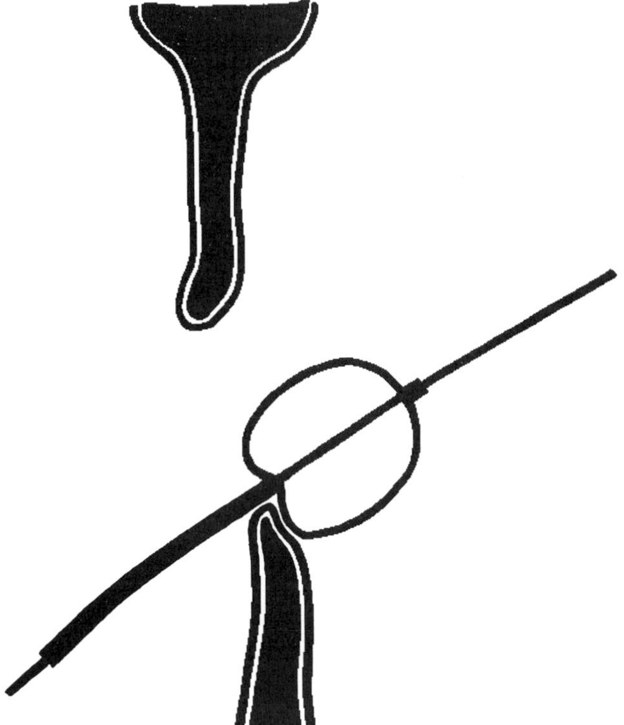

Figure 28.6 The acute angle at the attachment of the surface of the balloon to the shaft of the catheter on the Occlusion/Swan type balloons catching on the edge of the septum and giving the impression of a much smaller defect.

angiogram should demonstrate the presence of any additional even very small ASD and/or if the ASD is very peculiar in shape and possibly cannot be occluded with either a "square" or an absolutely "circular" device.

There are major problems with using the "occlusion sizing" balloons and their "withdrawal" into and through the defect for sizing atrial septal defects. First, an "occlusion" balloon that is significantly larger in diameter than the defect but, at the same time still *soft*, can pull through the defect and in doing so produce a "waist" in the balloon that is very fleeting and can easily be missed, which, in turn, gives the impression of a much larger defect (Figure 28.5). Secondly, the edge of the inflated Occlusion/Equalizer™ sizing balloon where the balloon is attached at the proximal junction of the balloon to the catheter shaft is *perpendicular* to the catheter shaft. This creates a 90° angle off the proximal edge of the attachment of the balloon, where it extends off the shaft of the catheter. This acute angle pulled to one side of the defect by tension on the spring guide wire passing through the defect, catches on the edge of an ASD rather than pulling *into* the ASD and, in turn, gives a false impression that the ASD is much smaller than it actually is (Figure 28.6). This problem is even greater in the presence of a stiff guide wire. The third problem with these latex Occlusion/Equalizer™ balloons when used for the sizing of atrial septal defects is that the balloon walls are fairly tense even when filled with less than their maximum inflation volume. As the balloons pull into, and through the defect repeatedly, the Occlusion/Equalizer™ balloons actually tend to stretch and *enlarge the ASD openings* with each "sizing pull-through".

With all of the sizing balloon techniques and balloons, when the defect forms the waist on the balloon, the septum adjacent to the balloon is carefully inspected by TEE or ICE to verify that there is an adequate rim of septum all around the ASD. Once the defect is sized very accurately and its position and suitability determined, the balloon is deflated and the sizing balloon catheter is withdrawn over the wire. The wire remains in the left upper pulmonary vein for the subsequent delivery of the delivery sheath for the ASD occlusion device.

ASD occlusion devices

Amplatzer™ ASD Device

The success of the Clamshell™ device (United States Catheter, Inc. [USCI] BARD, Glens Falls, NY)[12] and then its subsequent, abrupt withdrawal from availability for clinical use, stimulated the development of several new devices for the occlusion of the ASD. The most successful of these newer ASD occlusion devices is the Amplatzer™ ASD Occlusion device (AGA Medical Corp., Golden Valley, MN)[13]. This device has two retaining disks, which are positioned on the opposite sides of the defect, however, the design and whole concept for occlusion with this device are different from any of the previous ASD occlusion devices[14].

The entire device is a unique and complex "weave" of fine 0.007″ Nitinol™ memory metal wires, which in its "relaxed" state at body temperature, forms two, circular, flat disks joined to each other at the center by a *slightly* smaller diameter, slightly thicker circular hub. The broad central "hub" is part of the contiguous "weave" of the Nitinol™ metal wire. Both of the "disks" and the "hub" have a separate single thin layer disk of thin polyester fabric sewn within the circumference of the hub and each of the two "end" disks. The polyester disks prevent flow through the device, enhance thrombosis within the device and, in turn, promote closure of the defect. The device is available in multiple sizes with the diameter of the central "hub" representing the size of the Amplatzer™ ASD Occlusion device. As the diameter of the device (the hub) increases in diameter, the two "retaining" disks on each side of the hub increase in diameter proportionately with increasing sizes of the device.

The central "hub" is the principal occluding and retaining portion of the Amplatzer™ ASD device. The "hub" is designed to completely fill and actually *stretch* into the edges of the atrial defect. The only purpose of the two end retaining "disks" is to help align and hold the device stable within the atrial defect, particularly during delivery and implant of the device and for a short time after implant. The central hub stretches into the entire circumference of the atrial defect, and, in turn, represents the ultimate "centering mechanism" within an atrial septal defect. The Amplatzer™ devices are available in the United States in sizes from 4 mm to 38 mm, the devices between the 4 and 20 mm increasing in size in one mm increments, while the devices between the 20 and 38 mm are available in 2 mm increments between each size.

The purpose of the disks at each "end" of the Amplatzer™ ASD Occlusion devices are to stabilize the device on the septum within the atrial defect during and immediately after implant. The left atrial "disk" also serves to prevent the device from pulling through the defect as it is being implanted in the septum. The "left" atrial disk is 14 mm larger in *diameter* than the central hub or waist, which provides a 7 mm circumferential rim around the hub on the left side of an ASD. The central hub fixes the device in the septum after implant but also serves to center the device on the septal defect during implant. The right atrial disk of the standard Amplatzer™ ASD Device™ is 12 mm larger in *diameter* than the central "hub", which provides a 6 mm circumferential rim around the hub on the right side of the ASD. For the attachment to the delivery system, there is an attach/release, screw *socket* in a small metal "post" recessed into the center of the right atrial disk. There is a similar, but closed, small metal "post" at the center of the left sided disk where the weave of Nitinol™ wires join together.

The atrial septal defect, the entire atrial septum and, in particular, the rims all around the defect are interrogated by TEE or ICE with, and without, the sizing balloon in the defect; however, the size of the device that is used is chosen to equal the exact ***stretched*** diameter of the atrial defect. If the defect is balloon-sized without stretching, a device that is 1–2 millimeters *larger* than the non-stretched balloon diameter is used. The slightly larger diameter of the device (central hub) compared to the non-stretched diameter, actually holds the device in place once implanted and, at the same time, occludes the defect by stretching tightly against the inner circumference of the edges of even an eccentric and/or mobile atrial defect. With this fixation method, with the large range of sizes and with the larger sizes of devices that are available, considerably larger atrial septal defects can be occluded with the Amplatzer™ atrial septal device than with any of the previous ASD occlusion devices. The maximum diameter of the atrial septal defect and/or the length/width of the atrial septum itself can be the limiting factor for the use of the Amplatzer™ device as long as there is a circumferential rim of atrial septum of at least 6 mm for the smaller devices and 7–8 mm for the very large devices all around the defect. When the defect diameter is measured by TEE or ICE with the balloon inflated in the defect and a sufficient rim still is present around most of the defect, the defect should be applicable for device closure within the range of available device sizes. There *must be* a fairly sturdy rim of at least 7–8 mm *inferiorly* and adjacent to (above) the atrioventricular valves in order that the retaining disks do not encroach on either of the atrioventricular valves and interfere with the valve function. The absence of part of the *anterior (aortic) rim* is of less significance. Unless there is a very extensive (long) absence of the aortic rim, the "hub" of the device as it fills the defect is pushed against the adjacent aorta in the area of the absent rim of the septum, and the edges of the retaining "disks" at each end of the device "wrap around" the aortic wall in that area.

The absence of rim against the *posterior* wall of the atria is a more significant problem area for this device and with all of the other ASD occluders. This also is an area that is particularly difficult to visualize accurately by TEE or angiography, but is seen quite well with ICE. A deficient rim of septal tissue in this posterior area always should be suspected when the defect is located far posterior in the septum. In the posterior septal area, the atrial septum aligns perpendicular to the posterior atrial walls. With the absence of septal rim in that area, the edge of the defect *is* the posterior wall of the two atria where they meet and, in turn, is *flat* and perpendicular to the plane of the septum. In the absence of a posterior rim, the two "disks" of the Amplatzer™ device, even when pushed in that direction by the centering hub, have nothing to "grasp" and/or wrap around. A significant posterior defect without a posterior rim probably is not suitable for transcatheter closure with this, or any other currently available device.

Technique for ASD occlusion with the Amplatzer ASD occluder™

For occlusion with the Amplatzer™ ASD device, the procedure is performed with combined fluoroscopic and TEE or ICE guidance. When TEE is used, the procedure is performed under general anesthesia, while the use of ICE allows the occlusion to be performed with local anesthesia and various degrees of sedation. Once the percutaneous lines have been established, the patient is given heparin intravenously in a dose of 75–100 mg/kg, or a dose calculated according to the measured ACT of the patient. An Amplatzer™ sizing balloon (AGA Medical Corp., Golden Valley, MN), is used to measure the exact "diameter" of the ASD, which will determine which Amplatzer™ device will be used. An end-hole catheter, which accepts at least a 0.035″ wire, is introduced through a 9- or 10-French short sheath previously positioned in the right femoral vein, advanced through the right atrium, through the ASD and into a *left upper* pulmonary vein. With the same meticulous precautions for the prevention of air and/or clots that is used with all maneuvers on the left side of the circulation, a 0.035″ Super Stiff™ exchange guide wire with a short floppy tip (Medi-Tech, Boston Scientific, Natick, MA) is introduced through a wire back-bleed/flush valve on the catheter and advanced through the catheter and well into the pulmonary vein. The catheter remains over the wire and on a continual flush until just before the AGA™ sizing balloon is introduced over this wire for the sizing of the ASD as described above.

When the sizing balloon has been flushed and cleared of all air, the end-hole catheter is removed over the wire, the wire back-bleed valve is placed on the AGA™ sizing balloon, the balloon catheter placed on a flush over the wire and the sizing balloon is advanced to a position where the balloon is straddling the atrial septum. The AGA™ sizing balloon is inflated with a dilution of 1:5–1:8, contrast to flush solution, while observing on fluoroscopy for the formation of a distinct waist on the balloon and/or for the complete cessation of any flow through the septum as observed by Doppler™ on the TEE or ICE. Which "end-point" in the inflation is the operator's choice—each technique was discussed previously. The diameter of the balloon/waist is measured by angiography and TEE or ICE. The cessation of flow on color Doppler™ before the development of a waist on the balloon is the non-stretched diameter, while once a distinct waist is formed on the balloon, the diameter of the waist represents the *stretched* diameter of the ASD. Both of these measurements usually are 25–30% larger than the measurement of the defect by TEE or ICE before the balloon sizing.

By modifying the usual sizing technique that is usually used with the NuMED™ balloon (NuMED Inc., Hopkinton, NY), the NuMED™ sizing balloons *can* be used for sizing the ASD during a closure with an Amplatzer™ device. When the NuMED™ sizing balloon is used to measure the size of an atrial defect for the implant of the Amplatzer™ devices, the sizing balloon should be 10–15 mm *larger* in diameter than the *non-balloon sized diameter* of the ASD as measured by TEE or ICE. The balloon again is centered across the ASD and inflated with dilute contrast until a waist appears on fluoroscopy and until all flow across the ASD is stopped as observed on TEE or ICE. When inflated at "zero" pressure, the NuMED™ sizing balloon does not stretch the defect at all. The device that is used following the "zero-pressure" measurement with the NuMED™ balloon, should be at least 3–4 mm larger than the *non-stretched* diameter of the ASD obtained with the Amplatzer™ or the NuMED™ balloon. On the other hand, when the NuMED™ sizing balloon is inflated to its full diameter and/or with any measurable pressure in the balloon, the non-compliant material of the balloon does generate pressure and will stretch the ASD. When the NuMED™ balloon is inflated purposefully with some pressure, a *stretched* diameter, which is comparable to the Amplatzer™ sizing balloon diameter, is obtained and the device used should be the same size as the measured diameter of the waist on the balloon.

In the presence of very large defects with very thin surrounding rims, there is a growing trend purposefully ***not*** to stretch the defects "at all" during the balloon sizing. Using this technique the balloon is inflated only until the flow across the defect and around the balloon is stopped as demonstrated by color Doppler™ (and *before* a waist is observed). The device is chosen the same size or 1–2 mm larger than the non-stretched diameter of the defect. When this sizing technique is used, the *hub* of the device no longer necessarily creates the very firm fixation of the device in the septum by stretching against the rim of the defect, but rather the fixation of the device also becomes *dependent upon the rims* of the right and left atrial disks clamping the septum between, them very much like fixation with the double-umbrella type of occluders for atrial septal defects. The maximum centering of the device by the "waist" of the hub allows the narrower rims to hold the device very securely *once it is in place*. If this sizing and fixation technique is to become more standard, it would be desirable to have both the right and left disks of the same size and possibly slightly larger in diameter relative to the central waist.

The Occlusion (now Equalizer™) balloons (Medi-Tech, Boston Scientific, Natick, MA) formerly were used for sizing the ASD for closure with the Amplatzer™ device using the techniques described earlier in this chapter. The Medi-tech™ balloons may be slightly more suitable for the Amplatzer™ ASD device than for the CardioSEAL/STARFlex™ devices, since the "sizing" of the atrial defect with the Occlusion/Equalizer™ balloons does tend to *stretch* the defect during the sizing procedure and gives a "stretched" as opposed to a "static" diameter of the defect. Because of the problems with the occlusion balloon "pull-through" sizing technique, which were described earlier in this chapter, and now with the availability of the "static" sizing balloons, occlusion balloons seldom are used anymore for the sizing of an ASD.

In spite of the radically different designs of the devices, the Amplatzer™ device is delivered through a long sheath with a delivery technique that is very similar to the delivery of the initial "umbrella" ASD devices. The delivery sheaths, which are manufactured by AGA™ (AGA Medical Corp., Golden Valley, MN), are available in multiple French sizes according to the increasing size of the device that is being used. The smallest Amplatzer™ ASD devices pass through 6-French sheaths while the very large devices require up to a 12-French sheath. The AGA™ sheaths have a detachable Lure-Lock™ back-bleed valve with a side flush port; however, only the delivery catheters up to 8-French can be introduced *through* the back-bleed valve when it is attached to the delivery *sheath*. When using a delivery catheter larger than 8-French, the back-bleed valve/flush port is attached to the loader with only the delivery cable passing through the valve. The distal portion of the AGA™ sheath has a long, smooth 45° curve, which corresponds roughly to the course from the right atrium to the left atrium.

Many operators now modify the distal tip of the AGA™ ASD delivery sheath in order to improve the apposition of the left atrial "disk" on the septum as the device is extruded from the sheath. This is accomplished by cutting the tip of the sheath at a 35° to 45° angle off the long axis with the angle directed to the left of the distal curve of the sheath as the sheath is pointing away from the operator. With this angle formed at the tip of the sheath, as the left atrial disk is extruded from the sheath, it is deflected roughly at this angle of the tip of the sheath and, in turn, often aligns more parallel to the surface of the atrial septum.

The AGA™ delivery sheaths have several inherent problems. Not being able to have the back-bleed valve on the sheath when the larger devices are being introduced has already been alluded to. The sheaths do not have a distal "marker band" at the tip, which makes the sheaths difficult to see in large patients. These sheaths cannot be "molded" or formed into more desirable or appropriate curves, and they have a tendency to kink when maneuvered at all, and particularly when any torque is applied to them.

An alternative to the use of AGA™ delivery sheaths for the delivery of the Amplatzer™ ASD device is to use a long RB-MTS™ sheath (Cook Inc., Bloomington, IN) with a modified Hausdorf-Lock™ curve (Cook Inc., Bloomington, IN) at the distal end of the sheath. These sheaths have a built-on back-bleed valve/flush port, a radio-opaque marker band at the distal tip, and a special double curve, which bends first toward the *patient's* left (operator's right), and secondarily, cephalad, dorsally and even to the patient's right as the tip of the sheath is facing away from the operator. The pre-formed, Hausdorf™ curve on the sheath tends to align the partially opened device more parallel to the plane of the septum and, in turn, alleviates some of the manipulations of the Amplatzer™ devices within the atrium to achieve this alignment.

The Hausdorf™ modification of the Cook™ long delivery sheaths are only available in 10–12-French sizes, and these pre-formed sheaths have a discrete, fixed length between the proximal and distal curves which is *not* suitable for patients of all sizes nor even all secundum defects in all locations. The distance between the two distinct curves in the Hausdorf™ sheath is almost as critical as the lengths of the various curves on the selective coronary catheters for different sized patients. The "Hausdorf™ curve" must be adjusted for the *size* of each individual patient and/or heart. Heat can be applied to the sheath/dilator to form specific, fairly fixed, "Hausdorf™ type" curves on the standard, smaller diameter, RB-MTS™ sheaths as well as to modify the distance between the "manufactured" Hausdorf™ curves in the larger sheaths in order to have them suit the size of the patient better. In spite of their shortcomings, the Hausdorf™ curves on sheaths still are the most satisfactory for the delivery of all sizes of Amplatzer™ ASD devices. This author uses the modified Hausdorf™ sheaths for the delivery of all ASD occlusion devices.

Regardless of which introductory sheath is being used, before the sheath/dilator is introduced over the wire, the *dilator* is placed on a continuous flush through a wire back-bleed device and the valve on the side port of the sheath (if there is one) is *closed* and *not* maintained on a flush. The long sheath/dilator set is advanced over the wire until the tip of the *dilator* reaches just to the area of the *inferior vena cava–right atrial junction* as seen on fluoroscopy. ***The next few steps potentially are the most dangerous***

in the entire procedure. If the proper precautions are not observed for the removal of all air and clot from the delivery systems, the patient is very likely to experience a systemic embolic event during the subsequent exchanges of catheters and wires and/or the introduction of the device through the long sheath.

The dilator is withdrawn slowly from the sheath over the wire and the sheath is allowed to clear passively of any air and/or clot. This must be performed very *meticulously*. For the smaller AGA™ sheaths, which can have the back-bleed valve attached on the sheath, this is accomplished and, at the same time, is well controlled through the side port of the back-bleed valve on the sheath. For the larger AGA™ sheaths, which have no back-bleed valve attached, this is accomplished by allowing passive back bleeding through the open end of the sheath (around the contained delivery wire) and before the back-bleed valve/flush adaptor can be attached to the long sheath. When the dilator is removed from the larger Amplatzer™ delivery sheaths, on which the Amplatzer™ back-bleed valve cannot be attached, there is *no* real control over the bleeding from the sheath and/or of air being sucked into the sheath until some type of back-bleed/flush adaptor can be introduced over the wire and attached to the sheath. The back-bleed valve must be available immediately, introduced onto, advanced over the wire and attached on the sheath very expediently while the patient's respirations are controlled to prevent any deep inspiratory effort. Once cleared of any air or clot, the sheath is flushed thoroughly through the side port of the back-bleed valve. The RB-MTS™/Hausdorf™ sheaths in all sizes (commercial or home-made) do have a built-on back bleed valve, which obviates the problem of bleeding (and potential air entry) which occurs while changing/attaching the back-bleed valves on the larger AGA™ sheaths.

Once cleared of any possible air and/or clot, the sheath is placed on a continuous flush while the tip of the sheath still is in the right atrium. The delivery *sheath* alone is advanced into the left atrium over the wire, which still is in a left upper pulmonary vein. When the tip of the sheath is well into the left atrium, as seen on fluoroscopy and TEE or ICE, the wire is removed slowly from the sheath. Once the *wire is out of the sheath*, the side port on the hub of the sheath is allowed to bleed back to free it of air and/or clot. When the sheath does *not* bleed back passively, the valve of the back-bleed valve is covered very *tightly* with a gloved finger and *gentle* suction is applied to the side port on the hub of the sheath as the tip of the sheath is moved to and fro and/or rotated slightly within the left atrium. This movement of the sheath should free the tip of the sheath from either a small pulmonary vein or any other obstruction, and allow free bleeding back through the side port. Once the sheath *unequivocally* is cleared of any air and/or clot and only when it is bleeding back freely, is the side port of the sheath begun on a slow flush while the device is prepared for delivery.

The Amplatzer™ devices have a special pusher/delivery cable. The distal end of the cables terminates in a tiny attaching screw, which screws into the hub on the right atrial side of the device. The delivery cables come with a detachable plastic torquing device, which attaches to the proximal end of the cables by a small locking screw. This torque device is used to provide a solid grip on the cables for turning the cables during the release of the Amplatzer™ device. The very *proximal ends* of the *delivery cables* also have a tiny *female screw connector*, which is identical to the connectors present on the "right side" of the devices.

Each AGA™ delivery system comes with a special "loading sheath", which is a short, straight, segment of sheath of the same French size as the long delivery sheath. The loader sheath has a female Lure-lock connector at its proximal end and a male Lure-lock connector fixed on the shaft of the loader approximately 15 mm proximal to the distal tip of the loader. The detachable back-bleed valve/flush port, which comes with the delivery system, is attached to the proximal end (female Lure-lock) of the loader. The pusher/attach/release cable is introduced through the back-bleed valve and advanced through the loader from the proximal to the distal end. The loader is withdrawn back over the cable toward the proximal end of the cable.

The Amplatzer™ ASD device is attached to the delivery/pusher cable by screwing the very fine screw at the distal tip of the delivery cable *clockwise* into the screw socket at the center of the proximal disk of the device. To attach them, the small screw at the tip of the delivery cable is positioned precisely in line with the small hub, advanced gently into the female screw socket on the device, and the device is spun clockwise very *gently* while holding the cable steadily. The device is rotated clockwise continuously and very gently until it stops screwing onto the cable. The device rotates 4–6 times before it is screwed completely onto the cable. The device should screw very easily onto the cable and at no time should *any* force be used while rotating the device or cable. Once the device stops turning on the cable, the device is "unscrewed" with a very slight counterclockwise rotation of approximately one-quarter turn.

The device is soaked in a basin of flush solution and, while keeping the device in the basin under the surface of fluid and while continually flushing the loading sheath through the side port, the delivery cable with the attached device is pulled forcefully into the loader, which, in turn, collapses and draws the device into the loader. It helps to apply counter tension to the left atrial disk of the device by pulling it away from the loader while the delivery cable is pulled in the opposite direction toward the loader. The traction on the device in the opposite directions stretches and elongates the device and allows it to pull into the loader more easily. As tension is applied in the opposite directions to the device, the Amplatzer™ ASD occluder is stretched into a long, relatively thin, almost "braid" of the Nitinol™ wires, which can be withdrawn into the loader in this configuration. The flushing of the side port is continued with the tip of the loader under the surface of the fluid until no more bubbles of air are seen coming from the distal end of the loader.

With the smaller devices, the loader is introduced through an AGA™ back-bleed valve attached to the long sheath. For the larger devices, the AGA™ back-bleed valve must be removed from the long delivery sheath and while continually flushing the loader from a separate back-bleed/flush valve, the tip of the loader is introduced quickly into the open end of the long sheath. When the back-bleed on the AGA™ sheath is removed for the introduction of the larger devices, there can be a significant back-flow of flush/blood from the long sheath and/or air can be sucked *into* the long sheath until the tip of the loader is introduced into the sheath. Any bleeding from the sheath and/or potential for air entry into the sheath is minimized by using a second and separate back-bleed valve/flush system on the long sheath and/or by having the loader ready and immediately adjacent to the sheath before even beginning to remove the back-bleed valve from the long sheath. The male Lure-lock on the loader is attached carefully to the female Lure-lock at the proximal end of the long AGA™ delivery sheath. Currently, the tolerances of the Lure-lock connections on the AGA™ sheaths are somewhat poor, resulting in the connection not tightening securely and often continuing to rotate indefinitely. As the male Lure-lock connection of the loader is screwed onto the female Lure-lock of the long sheath, it is very important that while rotating the loader, the delivery cable extending out of the proximal end of the loader *rotates along with the loader* in a 1:1 relationship. If the cable does not rotate *exactly with the loader* as the loader is screwed onto the sheath, the device within the loader ***is being unscrewed***. Once the loader is attached securely to the proximal end of the long sheath, the delivery cable is advanced into the loader (and sheath), which advances the occluder device from the loader into the sheath. The flush on the side arm of the loader is continued as the device is advanced.

The problems with excessive bleeding and the poor fit of the Lure-lock™ connection on the AGA™ sheath are obviated completely with the use of the RB-MTS™ sheath (Cook Inc., Bloomington, IN). However, when either the RB-MTS or the Hausdorf™ sheath (Cook Inc., Bloomington, IN) is used, the AGA™ loader must be modified before the occluder is withdrawn into the loader. The *male* Lure-lock™ connector at the distal end of the shaft of the AGA™ loader is amputated just proximal to the Lure-lock™ connector before the Amplatzer™ cable is passed through the loader and/or before the device is withdrawn into the loader. Removing the male Lure-lock™ connector is necessary to allow the tip of the loader to be introduced completely through the *chamber* of the built-in back-bleed valve on the sheath and to "seat" all of the way into the proximal end of the sheath within the valve chamber. The modification is necessary because of the "deeper" chamber in the back-bleed valve housing of the RB-MTS™ sheaths. Cutting the distal Lure-lock™ connector from the loader results in a loading sleeve which has only the female Lure-lock™ connector at the proximal end of the loader. Once the device is pulled into the cut-off end of the loader and while the loader is on a *continuous flush*, the cut-off end of the loader is introduced through the valve of the RB-MTS™ or Hausdorf™ sheath, into the valve chamber and seated securely into the proximal end of the sheath. Flush is continued through the side ports of both the loader *and* the long sheath while the loader is introduced into the sheath. The flushing of both the loader and the delivery sheath is continued as the cable along with the device is advanced into the sheath.

Once the device has been advanced 10 cm or more into the sheath with either loader and/or delivery system, the loader is withdrawn and removed from the proximal end of the pusher/delivery cable. The flush is maintained on the long sheath as the pusher/delivery cable along with the device is advanced through the long sheath, which previously was positioned across the atrial septal defect. As the device is advanced through the sheath and during its implant in the atrial defect, it is observed on both fluoroscopy and TEE or ICE. The long sheath is maintained on a slow continuous flush. It is extremely important ***not*** *to rotate, nor torque* the delivery cable in either direction separately from the sheath as the device is being advanced within the sheath and/or during any of the maneuvers of the device and/or sheath required during the device delivery. Any separate counterclockwise rotation of the cable "unscrews" and potentially can release the device prematurely. An occasional, very slight and gentle clockwise torque on the cable ensures that the device is not being unscrewed, but a vigorous clockwise rotation of the cable can tighten the device—possibly so tightly that it forms a peculiar "cobra" configuration when extruded and/or cannot be released after deployment. Rotating the sheath clockwise without a *simultaneous clockwise rotation of the cable, unscrews* the device, while a counterclockwise rotation of the sheath without simultaneous counterclockwise rotation of the cable screws the device on tighter!

As the device reaches the tip of the sheath as visualized on fluoroscopy, the long sheath is withdrawn enough to be sure that the tip of the sheath is free from either a

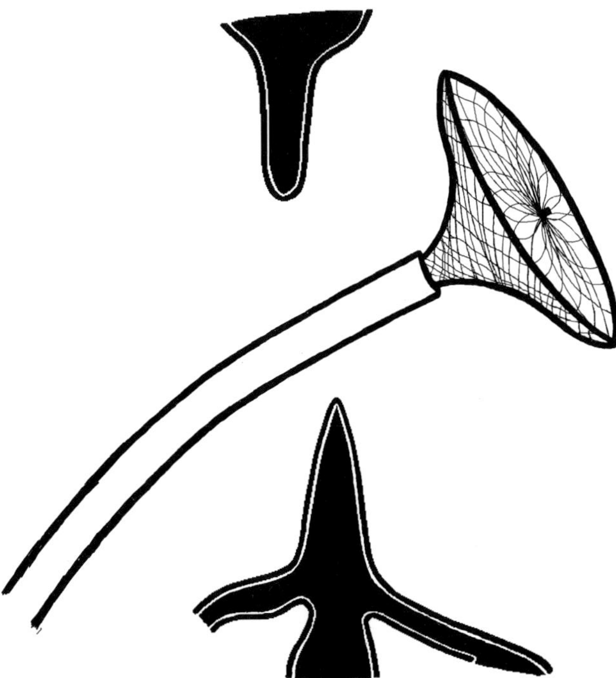

Figure 28.7 Full deployment of the *left atrial disk* of an Amplatzer™ device within the body of the left atrium.

pulmonary vein or the posterior atrial wall. As the delivery cable is advanced further and the sheath is withdrawn slightly, the left atrial disk of the device begins to extrude out of the end of the sheath. The delivery cable at the proximal end of the sheath is held and maintained very firmly in position against the hub of the sheath in order to prevent the *entire* Amplatzer™ occluder from suddenly "squirting" out of the tip of the sheath once it begins to extrude. The subsequent maneuvers with the sheath and device are observed on both fluoroscopy and TEE or ICE.

The sheath is withdrawn off the device and into the body of the left atrium as the left atrial disk is extruded and allowed to open fully with an undistorted configuration (Figure 28.7).

If the left atrial disk does *not* open completely as seen on fluoroscopy but instead, maintains a "mushroom" configuration even as the "waist" of the device begins to extrude out of the sheath, the entire system (sheath, wire and device), as a single unit, is pushed together back into, and against the posterior–lateral wall of the left atrium. This helps to flatten the left atrial disk. If the left atrial disk does not flatten even with this maneuver, it is withdrawn into the sheath, the direction of the sheath and the delivery cable is changed slightly, and the extrusion of the left atrial disk is repeated. If the disk cannot be "flattened" with repeated attempts, the device probably is too large for the particular left atrium and should not be used. When the left atrial disk is extruded fully and expanded into a flat configuration, the central waist begins to open partially as well. This forms a "funnel" configuration of the exposed portion of the central hub of the device with the widest portion adjacent to the left atrial "disk" and the narrower end into the tip of the sheath (and the atrial septal defect). The cable still must be fixed firmly together with, and against the sheath to prevent a spontaneous, rapid, full extrusion of the remainder of the occluder. The opened left atrial disk visualized on fluoroscopy should be on edge in the lateral/left anterior oblique view and en fas in the posterior–anterior/right anterior oblique view.

Because of the orientation of the angle of the delivery sheath to the septum and particularly with the AGA™ sheaths (modified or not), the device often does *not* align very well in relation to the septum as visualized on either fluoroscopy and/or on TEE or ICE and the left atrial disk of the device can appear almost *perpendicular* to the septum in some views. The orientation of the device on the septum often can be improved by slight rotation (usually clockwise) of the sheath (*always together with the device and cable!*) while observing closely on fluoroscopy and TEE or ICE. In order to transmit the rotation of the sheath from outside of the skin to the tip of the sheath, the sheath and cable must be moved forward and backward together very slightly as they are rotated, similar to the rotation of a torque catheter. The rotation usually is clockwise (posteriorly) but occasionally a counterclockwise (anteriorly) rotation is necessary to free the opened left atrial disk and allow it to align properly. Rarely, the abnormal orientation of the device is not corrected by maneuvers of the sheath/cable/device and the AGA™ sheath becomes twisted during the rotation. If the sheath becomes twisted or kinked significantly, the device is withdrawn into the sheath and out of the body and the sheath is replaced.

If the sheath is twisted only slightly, there are several maneuvers that can be attempted in order to correct the abnormal positioning. First, the deployment of the device can be continued with the comforting knowledge that the device can be withdrawn even after it has been deployed completely but erroneously. Alternatively, the device is withdrawn into the sheath completely, the orientation of the sheath is changed and the deployment of the device is restarted from the beginning. The final solution is to withdraw the device into, and completely out of the sheath, replace the delivery sheath over an exchange wire, and begin all over with a new and/or different shaped delivery sheath.

When choosing a new sheath, the use of the RB-MTS™ sheath with the Hausdorf™ type curve at the tip eliminates many of the problems of the device orientating abnormally toward the septum during the device extrusion and withdrawal into the atrial defect with the Amplatzer™ sheath. The proximal curve of the Hausdorf™ sheath directs the distal end of the sheath toward the left atrium while the distal, secondary curve

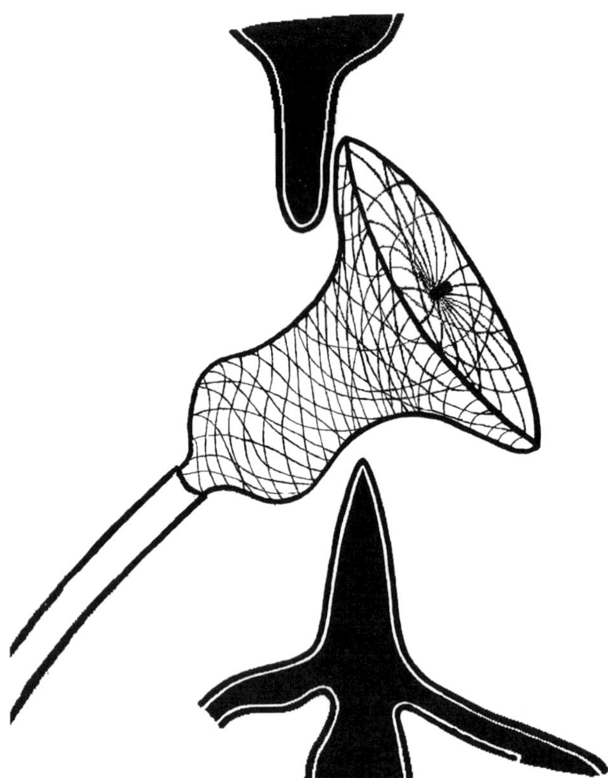

Figure 28.8 Central hub of the Amplatzer™ occluder opening *only partially* within the defect before the right atrial disk begins to open.

directs the tip of the sheath posteriorly, toward the *right-posterior* wall of the left atrium. As the left atrial disk is extruded from the Hausdorf™ sheath, it aligns (almost automatically) en fas in the PA X-ray view and on edge in the LAT–LAO view which, in turn, is parallel to the plane of the septum as seen on both fluoroscopy and TEE or ICE.

Once the device is aligned properly, the sheath, cable and partially extruded device are withdrawn together until *one edge* of the device as seem on TEE or ICE begins to approximate any part of the atrial septum. The delivery cable is advanced slightly while the sheath is withdrawn simultaneously allowing the central hub of the device to extrude partially. The central hub does not open completely until the right-sided disk opens on the right side of the septum but the central hub does elongate through the defect (Figure 28.8).

As a consequence, once the *central hub* ***begins*** *to open*, the sheath and delivery cable, along with the device, are withdrawn toward the septum while the *sheath alone* simultaneously is withdrawn further over the cable and off the device *in one smooth, continuous, fairly rapid motion* without stopping to examine/admire the various intermediate positions in order *to deploy the entire device in the one motion*. The *smooth* deployment of the central hub along with the right atrial disk *all in one motion* usually adjusts the orientation and fixes the Amplatzer™ device securely in the septum. By initially pulling the partially extruded and "funneled" hub into the defect, and at the same time allowing the central hub to open further, the hub centers and secures the device in the defect, while the right atrial disk is opening on the right side of the septum. As this occurs, the left atrial disk becomes centered better on the septum and is pulled against the left atrial side of the septum, which fixes the device securely in the septum. When the device is sized appropriately and is not too large, the device usually clamps securely on both sides of the septum as both sides are extruded.

Once the left sided disk is aligned appropriately and/or even when the alignment of the device to the septum and to the atrial defect appears poor initially during the deployment, if it is decided to persist with the deployment, the absolute and rapid "centering" effect by the fully expanded central hub, combined with the absolutely round shape and the relatively broad rim of the left atrial disk beyond the hub, means that the left atrial disk usually does *not* pull through the atrial defect with this rapid deployment maneuver! One major advantage of the Amplatzer™ ASD Occluder is that any time before its purposeful release from the delivery cable, the device can be withdrawn and repositioned if the operator is not entirely satisfied with the position in the defect.

While the delivery cable is still attached to the device and particularly while the tip of the sheath still is close to the device, the device usually does not appear to align very well immediately after both disks have opened (Figure 28.9). Once the device is deployed in the atrial defect, the withdrawal of the sheath alone is continued until the tip of the sheath reaches the inferior vena cava. The withdrawal of the sheath alone allows the cable more mobility, which, in turn, allows the cable to align more perpendicularly to the device and releases *some* of the angled torsion on the device created by the cable.

Occasionally, a very precise and controlled deployment of the Amplatzer™ device is possible when there are good rims circumferentially around the defect and the left atrial disk does align exactly parallel to the septum as it is extruded from the tip of the delivery sheath, in which case the device/cable/sheath are all withdrawn together until the left atrial disk is touching the septum (Figure 28.10).

When comfortable by both fluoroscopic and TEE or ICE criteria that the distal (left atrial) disk is aligned flat against and parallel to the atrial septum, and when no part of the left atrial disk has prolapsed through the septum, tension on the cable is relaxed very slightly while the sheath is withdrawn off the remainder of the central hub and the beginning of the right atrial disk. The slight relaxation of the tension on the delivery cable allows the remainder of the central hub to expand and "center" within the defect as the initial portion of the right atrial

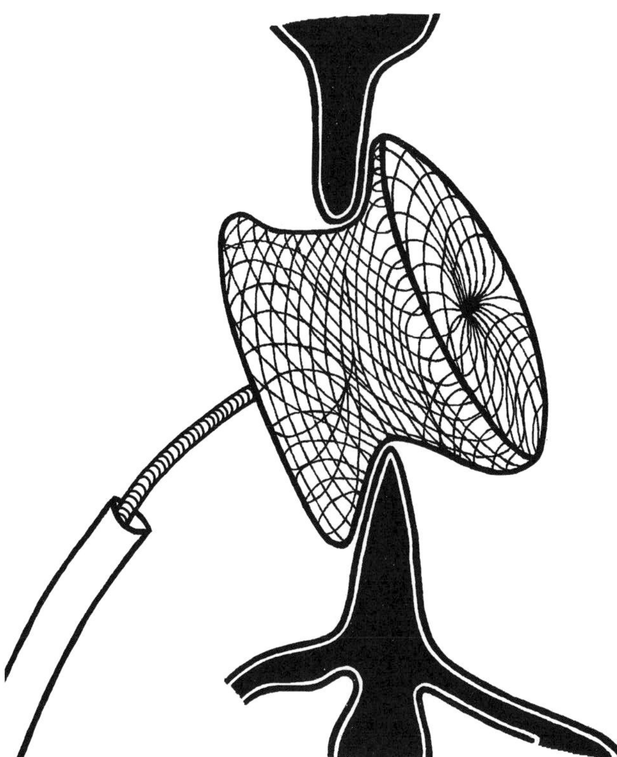

Figure 28.9 Device fully deployed but still attached to cable. Torsion from cable keeps device from aligning exactly, but central hub is opened fully and fixes the device in the septal defect.

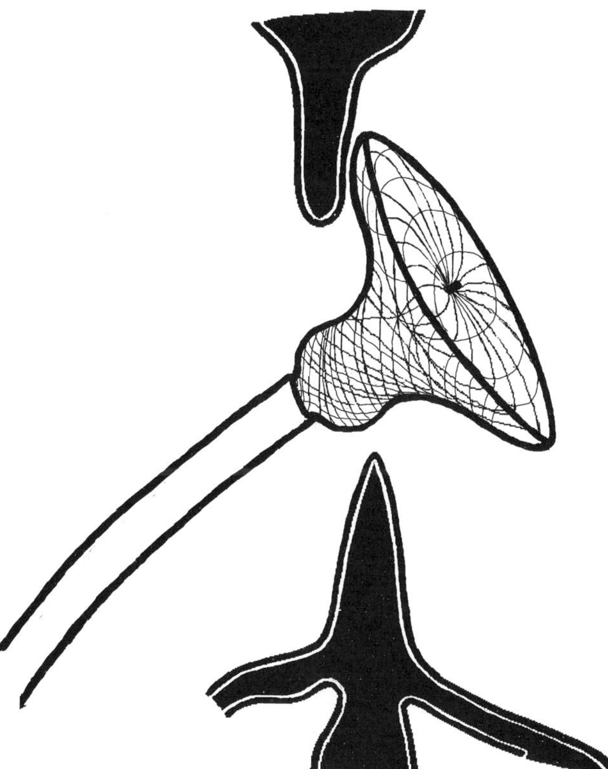

Figure 28.10 Left atrial disk of Amplatzer™ ASD occluder opened fully and pulled back against atrial septum during *stepwise* opening of device.

"disk" begins to extrude. As the sheath is withdrawn further, the cable is advanced in order to deploy the right atrial disk against the right side of the septum while the hub expands completely and fixes the device securely in the septum. Although with such an exact initial alignment of the left atrial disk against the septum, the Amplatzer™ device can be deployed in these more methodical steps, usually, the deployment of the left disk, the central hub, the withdrawal into the defect and the deployment of the right disk, still are performed as one continuous, fairly rapid motion as described earlier with no distinct pauses between the steps.

Occasionally, with an elliptical defect and/or a defect located eccentrically on the septum, the device repeatedly pulls through the septum as long as the central hub is deployed only partially. In that circumstance, the device is withdrawn entirely into the sheath, the sheath is re-advanced into the left atrium, and the deployment is restarted with a different orientation of the sheath/device/left atrial disk. It also occasionally is helpful to deploy more of the central hub/beginning right atrial disk before pulling the entire system into the defect and then to complete the remainder of the deployment of the device rapidly as described above. The properly sized and deployed central hub fills the defect while it centers the device in the defect absolutely and, in turn, prevents *any* edge of the left atrial disk from prolapsing through the defect.

There are some adjunct procedures that are utilized particularly for the deployment of the larger Amplatzer™ ASD occluders in very large atrial septal defects. In order to use the larger devices and these techniques, the total length/diameter of the septum must be large enough to accommodate the total diameter of the retention disks of the device, remembering that the left atrial disk on the 38 and 40 mm devices is 16 mm larger *in diameter* than the hub (stated device size). One technique, which is almost automatic with the use of the Hausdorf™ sheath, is to begin the deployment of the left atrial disk with the tip of the sheath against the right-posterior "roof" of the left atrium near the entrance of the right upper pulmonary veins. As the left disk opens, it aligns en fas as a flat circle in the posterior–anterior X-ray projection and exactly on edge in the lateral or left anterior oblique projection. This orientation usually aligns the device exactly parallel with the atrial septum and the defect, and makes the subsequent deployment straightforward.

A slightly more extreme technique to help align the large devices with the septum is to begin the deployment by opening the left atrial disk *in* the *left* upper pulmonary vein. This technique relies on the fact that the *folded* and elongated very large, Amplatzer™ devices will extend all of the way from the left upper pulmonary veins, across the left atrium and through the atrial defect. The left atrial disk is held in the pulmonary vein with forward pressure on the delivery cable while the sheath is withdrawn to deploy the remainder of the device "across" the left atrium and the defect by the rapid withdrawal of the sheath. The fixation of the left atrial disk in the left upper pulmonary vein also maintains a better *alignment* across the defect from the left posterior atrial wall (pulmonary vein) and relies upon the relatively short depth of the left atrium to allow the right atrial disk to open completely on the right side of the septum while the left atrial disk is in and/or near the left upper pulmonary veins. As soon as the right atrial disk opens, it pulls the left atrial disk out of the vein and allows the left atrial disk to "spring" open and against the left side of the defect while the entire cable/device is relaxed and withdrawn slightly!

When neither of the two previous adjunct techniques is effective at aligning the device better in the defect, a final technique employs the use of a separate stiff venous catheter, dilator or even balloon-sizing catheter to *push* directly against and/or stabilize the anterior "leading" edge of the left atrial disk back into the left atrium while the remainder of the disk is being deployed. This requires the introduction of a separate, large, stiff catheter from an additional venous puncture site. The stiff dilator which comes with the long sheath, and particularly when it is reinforced with the stiff end of a guide and/or deflector wire within it, makes a good "pusher" against the edge of the disk. While the edge of the left atrial disk, which potentially is prolapsing through the defect, is pushed and "held" on the left side of the septum, the remainder of the device is deployed as usual and then the "holding" catheter is withdrawn. Once the device is extruded fully, it is interrogated using TEE or ICE for its proper seating in the defect, before the device is released.

Once both disks have been deployed and the delivery sheath has been withdrawn to the area of the inferior vena cava–right atrial junction to allow the delivery cable maximal flexibility and freedom to bend within the right atrium, the device is tested for its fixation in the septum. Fluoroscopically, the properly positioned right and left atrial disks eventually should align *parallel to the previously visualized plane of the atrial septum.* When the cable still is attached and even with the sheath withdrawn to the inferior vena cava, the two opened disks *usually* do *not* align exactly parallel to the septum and/or even to each other as viewed on fluoroscopy and/or echo (*see* Figure 28.9). The two disks at the more cephalad portion of the septum usually are spread apart by the tension from the still attached cable and the extension of the disks around the aorta in that area. When properly deployed and viewed on the fluoroscopy or the TEE or ICE image, no portion of either disk should appear "folded" or bent toward the center of the device or the opposite disk, no portion of the left sided disk should extend past the edge of septal tissue into the right atrium, all of the right atrial disk should be on the right side of the septum, and *septal tissues should be seen "sandwiched" between the right and left atrial disks* all of the way around the circumference of the device when interrogated with multiple echo views.

Because of its circular configuration and tight fit within the defect, and in spite of the alignment on the septum not appearing ideal, when the Amplatzer™ device is sized correctly, the properly implanted device immediately becomes fixed very securely within the defect. When the device is sized *too large* for the defect, both disks of the device assume a "fatter" appearance immediately after implant and the "hub" of the device initially does not expand to the full potential diameter that it had when the device was open outside of the body. As the device seats in the septum over hours (or days), the hub continues to expand to its nominal diameter and the right and left atrial disks flatten progressively.

At the same time, when an accurately sized device is positioned properly in the septal defect and before release, the completely opened disks of the device should *not* appear *extremely fat* and certainly should not have the configuration of "double opposing mushrooms". This fat, mushroom configuration of the disks indicates that the device is excessively over-sized and probably should be replaced with a smaller device. The Nitinol™ metal of the Amplatzer™ ASD occluders eventually and inevitably will flatten to its initial flat configuration with time, but only as the hub of the device stretches the edges of the atrial defect markedly and/or *necroses* the edges of the septum (or anything else in its path) as the device continues to expand against the edges of the defect and the disks stretch toward their flattened configuration.

At the other extreme, if both disks of the device appear *very flat* on fluoroscopy and/or echo immediately after the device is implanted on the septum and before the release of the device, the device position should be scrutinized *extremely carefully.* Disks which appear very flat *immediately* after both disks are opened indicates either, that the device is undersized significantly for the defect or that both the right and left atrial disks are *on the same side* of the septum in the area where the disks are very flat and close together. When the Amplatzer™ ASD device is in proper position, even a thin rim of atrial septum, which is "sandwiched" between the two disks of the device, will separate the right and left atrial disks slightly from each other. The device is scrutinized on TEE or ICE from all angles and *circumferentially round the entire device* for the appearance of the rim of septal tissue between the disks. Often, at the aortic and cephalic edge of the septum, there is no rim of septal tissue and the aorta itself is "sandwiched" between the disks, which then are splayed apart in that area.

When satisfied with the configuration and the position on the septum by both fluoroscopy and by TEE or ICE, the security of the fixation in the septum is "tested" by means of a moderately vigorous, to and fro, push–pull on the delivery cable/device—the so called "Minnesota wiggle". When both disks are positioned properly on and fixed securely in the septum and as traction is applied to the cable and the device, which is fixed securely in the septum, the right and left atrial disks separate from each other with each *pull*. As the disks are separated, the rim of septal tissue that is between the disks is seen even more clearly on the TEE or ICE. As the cable is *pushed* during the "wiggle", the right and left atrial disks are pushed together, but still should have some distance between the opposing edges of the disks and should not push through and/or away from the septal defect. The entire circumference of the device is scrutinized with the TEE or ICE during the "wiggle" to verify that the septal rim is "sandwiched" between the two disks all of the way round the device. A small hand angiogram, with an injection through the separate catheter positioned close to or against the right sided disk of the device demonstrates the alignment of the device relative to the septum and helps to demonstrate if part of either disk is on the wrong side of the septum.

Rarely, as the left atrial disk and the central hub are extruded from the sheath, the left atrial side does not form a "disk", but rather extrudes in an elongated, spiral or "cobra" configuration. This abnormal configuration usually persists even after the hub and right disk are completely out of the delivery sheath. The exact etiology of this deformation probably is related to how the "wires" of the Nitinol™ weave expand from their elongated configuration relative to each other and/or may be related to excessive torquing of the device and cable while they were still within the sheath. Usually patience is all that is necessary and the device gradually resumes its normal configuration. If the abnormal configuration persists, the device and sheath are moved forward slightly and/or the device is withdrawn into the sheath and the deployment repeated. Rarely, even with repeated withdrawal and redeployment, the deformity persists. In that case the sheath is advanced back into the left atrium over the device and the device is withdrawn out of the body. If the device still has the deformed configuration after it is withdrawn from the sheath, the device is manually elongated by traction on both hubs and then released to allow it to re-form its "resting", flat configuration. In this operator's experience, the device always has resumed its normal configuration with this maneuver outside of the body. Once it returns to its normal shape, the same device can be reloaded and redeployed successfully.

A major advantage of the Amplatzer™ ASD device is that any time before it is released *purposefully*, it very easily can be withdrawn back into the delivery sheath. If the device is not sized accurately, if it is malpositioned in the defect, or if it pulls through the defect *at any stage* of the delivery, the device easily can be withdrawn back into the sheath. The sheath then can be repositioned through the defect where the same device can be reimplanted or the original device is removed completely and a new device delivered through the same sheath. If necessary for any reason, the withdrawal into the sheath and redeployment can be accomplished multiple times. However, the more times a device is pulled into the sheath and redeployed, the more likely the sheath is to be distorted, the delivery cable unwound from the device and/or the device distorted permanently.

Once the device is fixed securely within the septum with a satisfactory position of the device in the septal defect and there is no significant residual leak, the device/cable is prepared for release. The torquing hub is attached firmly to the proximal end of the delivery cable by introducing the end of the delivery cable as far as possible into the open hole in the torquing hub, and then tightening the small set screw that is on the side of the torquing hub onto the cable. The device is uncoupled from the delivery cable by many, rapid, counterclockwise turns of the delivery cable using the torquing device. It usually takes 6 to 7 complete counterclockwise turns of the cable to unscrew the delivery cable from the proximal hub of the device. During all of the time when the device is being unscrewed, the device/cable should be observed on fluoroscopy or, preferably, recorded on biplane stored fluoroscopy to be sure that the device is not bound abnormally to the cable and/or is not being distorted in the septum during the unscrewing process. As the device unscrews completely and becomes free of the cable, it usually moves away from the cable and realigns its position significantly, as it reorients itself more properly into the plane of the septum (Figure 28.11). This movement can be quite extensive and sudden. After the device is released and reoriented on the septum, the position of the device and the presence of any residual leaks are scrutinized by TEE or ICE.

In order to offset the pressure effects of the shunt volume, which has become "trapped" suddenly in the left heart (and left atrium in particular) and until the total circulation has had time to "redistribute this volume", patients with very large defects and/or minimal circumferential rims are given 0.25–0.5 mg/kg of furosemide intravenously immediately prior to the implant of the device. The heparin given during the case is *not* reversed at the end of the case. All patients are given an intravenous dose of a cephalosporin at the time of the implant of the device and two or three more intravenous doses at intervals of 6 or 8 hours before discharge from the

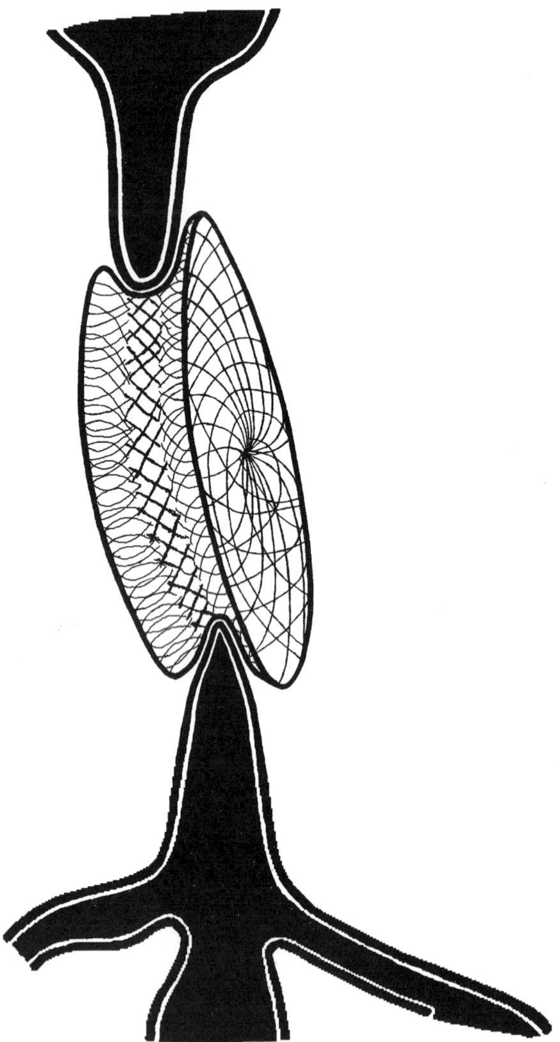

Figure 28.11 Amplatzer™ ASD device fully deployed and released. Torsion from cable is released. Device flattens and aligns exactly on septum with the central hub opened fully and fixing the device in the septal defect.

hospital. The patients are discharged on aspirin, 81 mg/day, which is to be continued for 6 months and with instructions to utilize bacterial endocarditis prophylaxis at times of high risk to bacteremia during that same 6 months.

In the United States, the Amplatzer ASD™ device underwent a regulated FDA, IDE clinical trial and completed a one-year follow-up of the implanted devices in early 2001. The Amplatzer™ ASD occlusion devices received FDA approval for the elective transcatheter occlusion of the secundum ASD in the US in September of 2001, and the final notification of approval was received in December 2001. This is the first implantable intracardiac device ever approved by the FDA for elective clinical use specifically in a congenital heart lesion and in pediatric patients.

Excessive Eustachian valve and the Amplatzer™ device

Although the Amplatzer™ ASD device has no legs that can spring open into the right atrium and that, in turn, could catch on a redundant Eustachian valve, there still are potential problems with the delivery of the Amplatzer™ ASD devices in the presence of excessive Eustachian valve tissue. The redundant Eustachian valve tissue usually is seen as a very flexible structure, which flops in and out of the echo field adjacent to the atrial septum and atrial septal defect. The most common problem with the Amplatzer™ ASD device and the Eustachian tissues occurs as the delivery cable is being unscrewed during the release of the cable from the device. The moderately rough surface of the rotating, exposed cable can tangle with the Eustachian tissue and, when it does, it winds the redundant tissue around the delivery cable. When the cable becomes entangled during the release of the device, the Eustachian tissue sometimes can be untangled by rotating the cable in a *clockwise* direction *after* the release of the device, although this can wind the Eustachian tissue even tighter around the cable and wind it in both directions. When the Eustachian tissue becomes entangled around the cable, the sheath is advanced over the cable and the cable is withdrawn forcefully *into the delivery sheath along with part of the Eustachian valve.*

As with most complications, prevention of the problem is preferable. When the Eustachian tissue is noticed in close proximity to the device and cable and *after* the secure deployment of the device, the long sheath is re-advanced carefully over the cable and back against the surface of the right atrial disk before the cable is unscrewed from the device. The sheath covers the cable, "separates" the rotating cable from the Eustachian valve tissues and prevents cable entrapment.

Very extensive, redundant Eustachian tissue also can become entangled in the mesh of the central hub and/or proximal (right atrial) disk of the device, particularly as the device is rotated and/or as the open mesh of the right atrial disk is extruded. If the Eustachian tissue remains entangled on the device and is unrecognized, it creates a partial "diaphragm" across the entrance of the inferior vena cava. The amount of obstruction from this tissue depends upon the density and extent of the Eustachian tissue.

When the Eustachian tissue remains attached to the *device* after the release of the device, the entangled Eustachian tissue can be separated from the device using a large angioplasty or static sizing balloon. The balloon catheter is maneuvered between the Eustachian tissue and device using TEE or ICE guidance and once positioned between the tissues, the balloon is inflated. This maneuver may have to be repeated several times to free the

Eustachian tissues totally. It always is prudent to avoid the entanglement when Eustachian tissue is present.

In every case of a potential occlusion of an ASD with a catheter-delivered device, the right atrium should be scrutinized thoroughly for long and/or redundant Eustachian valve tissue by TEE or ICE. When encountered, the Eustachian valve tissue can be trapped and "moved away" from the defect with a deflector catheter as described later in this chapter in the discussion of the CardioSEAL™ and STARFlex™ devices, where the Eustachian valve is even more of a problem.

Retrieval of the Amplatzer™ ASD device

One of the major advantages of the Amplatzer ASD Device™ is the ability to be withdrawn back into the delivery sheath, easily, and at any time, before the *purposeful* release of the device from the delivery cable. This withdrawal back into the sheath and redeployment of the device can be repeated many times if necessary. This of course holds true, not only for repositioning the device on the septum, but for removing the device completely if a perfect implant on the septum is not achieved or if the device pulls completely through the septum. The withdrawal is accomplished by placing tension on the delivery cable while the sheath is *advanced* simultaneously over the device and while withdrawing the device. These maneuvers re-elongate the device similar to the procedure for its loading.

Occasionally, the distal end of the delivery sheath becomes distorted (accordioned) with repeated withdrawal and redeployment of the device and eventually even the still attached, but deployed and malpositioned Amplatzer™ device cannot be withdrawn into the original, distorted sheath. The Amplatzer™ system has a unique recovery wire/sheath/dilator exchange system for just such an occurrence. The *proximal* end of every standard Amplatzer™ delivery cable has a small hub with a female screw socket in the hub, which is identical to the socket in the hub on the device. This screw socket allows a second *delivery cable* to be attached to the proximal end of the original cable, which, in turn, produces an "exchange length" delivery cable! The *dilator* of the *recovery* sheath/dilator has an extra large lumen and distal opening, which accommodates the diameter of the delivery *cable*.

The "exchange length" cable allows the original damaged sheath to be withdrawn over the "exchange cable" and completely out of the body while the device still is open *and attached* to the original part of the cable within the heart. Once the damaged sheath is removed, the "recovery" sheath/dilator with the larger lumen of the special dilator is advanced over the "exchange cable" to a position adjacent to the still attached device. The dilator is removed from the new sheath over the cable and the system is cleared meticulously of air and/or clot by allowing free back-flow from the sheath. The back-bleed/flush valve is reintroduced over the "exchange" cable, attached to the new sheath and the system is flushed. With the new sheath in place, the still attached Amplatzer™ occlusion device is readily withdrawn into the new, undamaged sheath.

Once the device has been released from the cable, retrieval of the Amplatzer™ device still is possible, but not as easily, nor as predictably, as before its release[15]. The possibility of a device embolization should always be included in the "pre-catheterization" discussion with the patient/parents. Along with the potential for embolization, the possible need for surgical retrieval should always be presented to the patient/parents.

The key element to retrieval of an embolized Amplatzer™ ASD occluder is to re-catch the device *by the central metal attachment "post"* on the right atrial disk of the device. This is accomplished using a 10 mm Microvena™ snare and snare catheter passed through a very large diameter long sheath. The long sheath that is used for the retrieval of an Amplatzer™ ASD occluder should be ***at least*** two French sizes larger than the original delivery sheath and the retrieval sheath should be as stiff as possible. A long sheath that is even larger than two French sizes larger than the original delivery sheath is even more advantageous. If the fully released device is not still on the septum or, at least, is not in an orientation within the heart and/or great artery with the right atrial "hub" facing the retrieval catheter, the errant device must be reoriented in the vessel or chamber using another catheter and/or wire in order to make the central "post" accessible to the loop of the snare. This reorientation is performed with a separate catheter, often approaching the device from the superior vena cava or even an artery when the device is lodged on the left side of the septum. The orientation of the device can be changed using an active deflector wire and/or a bioptome forceps to grasp an edge of the device in order to turn and/or hold it while the right sided post is grasped by the snare, which has been introduced through the large, long recovery sheath. Once the device has been turned to an appropriate orientation, it is helpful to "impale" the device with a straight, stiff, guide wire passed through and through the mesh of the device in order to fix the device in the particular more favorable location and orientation.

When an Amplatzer™ atrial septal occluder has embolized into, or is lodged in, either ventricle, a very gentle attempt is made to grasp any part of the device with a bioptome in order to withdraw the device out of the ventricle with "teasing" maneuvers. *Absolutely no force* must be used in this attempt. If the device cannot be withdrawn gently through the atrioventricular valve, it may be possible to manipulate it in the ventricle until it moves through, or can be drawn through, the semilunar valve and into the great vessel off the ventricle. In the great artery the device still must be turned/reoriented until the right-sided "post" is accessible to the snare catheter and the long sheath. The ASD occluder always should be withdrawn into the long sheath before attempting to withdraw it through a ventricle.

Once the metal post has been grasped securely with the snare, the device is withdrawn to the tip of the long sheath and withdrawn into the sheath. When the snare loop tightens on the attachment post of the device, the central "post" on the device becomes positioned *next to*, and parallel to the tip of the snare catheter. This creates a distinct "offset" of the small hub (post) on the device next to the tip of the snare catheter. This small offset frequently requires significant extra manipulations of the snare catheter and sheath together in order to maneuver the "shelf" created by the offset of the snare along with the grasped "post" of the device into the sheath. Making a small longitudinal slit in the tip of the long sheath before its introduction into the body has been suggested as beneficial for this maneuver. Occasionally, because of a curve on the sheath and/or the curved course through the body to approach the errant device, the grasped, offset post on the device cannot be centered enough to be withdrawn into the sheath alone even with very extensive manipulations. When this problem is *anticipated*, it is avoided by first introducing the *snare catheter* into and through the ***dilator*** of the new large, long "recovery" sheath *after* first modifying the tip of the dilator. The distal tip of the standard, large French sized, long *dilator*, which comes with the sheath, is excised in small increments until the *lumen* of the excised tip of the dilator at its distal end just will accommodate the snare catheter. The snare catheter is passed through this modified dilator and the combined snare catheter/dilator is introduced into the large, long sheath. An alternative to modifying the tip of the dilator of the recovery sheath is to use the dilator from one of the larger AGA™ "replacement" long sheath/dilator sets, which already have a large central opening.

Passing the snare catheter through the dilator serves two functions. First it "centers" the snare catheter within the lumen of the large sheath and allows the offset of the snared hub of the device to be drawn into the sheath without catching on the edge of the tip of the sheath. The dilator within the sheath also adds significant additional support to the long sheath and prevents or reduces the accordion effect on the shaft of the sheath when strong traction is necessary to withdraw the device into the sheath. Once the "attaching post" on the device is manipulated into the tip of the long sheath, the device can be withdrawn and folded into the larger sheath much like it was when it still was attached to the delivery cable. Once within the sheath, it is withdrawn out of the body.

If the right sided central post of the errant device cannot be grasped, the device is grasped by an edge of one of the disks with a bioptome catheter and re-manipulated/re-orientated until the "post" becomes accessible to the snare. Trying to withdraw the device when it has been grasped anywhere except by the central hub, markedly distorts the device and makes the narrowest profile of the collapsed device significantly larger and unreasonable to be withdrawn into any sheath, even if it is 4 or 5 French sizes larger than the original delivery sheath. This type of retrieval of an Amplatzer™ device probably should not be attempted, in which case surgical retrieval is the most reasonable option.

As with any other device that embolizes to a pulmonary artery, the *retrieval sheath* must be advanced into at least the main pulmonary artery before attempting to capture the device *and* the errant device must be withdrawn completely into the sheath before it is withdrawn out of the pulmonary artery. A partially (or fully!) opened device should not be dragged through the right ventricle (and tricuspid valve). Unless the operators are extremely skilled at foreign body removal and extremely patient, when the device embolizes to the right ventricle, left ventricle or pulmonary artery it is judicious to have the device removed surgically.

There have been several very rare occurrences of premature release of the Amplatzer™ ASD device related to inadvertent unscrewing of the device while manipulating the delivery cable and sheath and/or due to a "defect" in the attaching screw at the end of the delivery cable. The premature release resulted in the embolization of several devices, but no permanent complications. The screw has been changed and this should eliminate this problem when the device is used properly. The delivery cable has been "unwound" during unusually vigorous use, but this does not occur with standard use.

There are several pending modifications of the Amplatzer™ ASD delivery systems which should improve the delivery and make the delivery and implant of the Amplatzer™ ASD device even easier and safer. A new, reinforced sheath has been developed, which can be torqued and advanced without kinking, and presumably will not "accordion" as readily when devices are withdrawn into it. The new sheath is available with an angled distal tip to orient the device and to align it better with the septum as it is extruded from the sheath. The use of the Hausdorf™ modification of the RB-MTS™ sheaths was mentioned earlier under delivery techniques and certainly obviates many of the problems of the current AGA™ sheaths.

CardioSEAL™ and STARFlex™ ASD Occluders

The CardioSEAL™ and STARFlex™ Septal Occluders (NMT Medical Inc., Boston, MA) are second and third generation, respectively, double-umbrella, ASD occluding devices modeled after the original Clamshell™ ASD Device (USCI BARD, Glens Falls, NY). Each umbrella frame still has four legs and the umbrella material of both devices is a smooth, woven dacron fabric. Otherwise, these two devices represent extensive modifications of the original Clamshell™ in both materials and design[16]. The metal frame of both the CardioSEAL™ and STARFlex™ umbrellas is manufactured from a cobalt-based alloy, MP35n, which, compared to stainless steel, is less corrosive, more flexible and is a non-ferrous metal. In order to provide even more flexibility to the legs and, at the same time, greater "compression" against the septum, each leg of both the CardioSEAL™ and the STARFlex™ devices is manufactured of a slightly thinner wire and *each* leg has two hinges, or joints, compared to the single joint on the legs of the Clamshell™ device. The combination of material and/or the leg changes eliminated the *early* leg fractures and markedly reduced the number of leg fractures altogether. Similar to the earlier Clamshell™ device, the two umbrellas of both the CardioSEAL™ and STARFlex™ devices are attached at the center and fold away from each other into a narrow profile for delivery. The only difference between the CardioSEAL™ and the STARFlex™ devices is the addition of four very fine Nitinol™ *spring* "centering" wires on the STARFlex™ devices. Each fine Nitinol™ centering wire extends from the tip of a leg on one umbrella to the tip of the nearest leg on the opposite umbrella.

CardioSEAL™ and STARFlex™ devices are available in 17, 23, 28 and 33 mm sizes. Originally there was a 40 mm device, however, the legs at that length did not have sufficient strength to compress them securely against the septum, and its use has been discontinued. The "size" of the devices represents the maximum diameter, tangentially from the tip of one leg to the tip of the *opposite* leg, measured across the center of the device. The original CardioSEAL™ devices all required an 11-French long sheath for delivery. The newer "front-loading" adaptation of both the CardioSEAL™ and STARFlex™ devices allows a downsizing to a 10-French delivery sheath for the 17–28 mm devices. The larger sized devices *can be introduced* into a 10-French sheath, but the devices are very tight within a 10-French sheath and advancing the devices through a 10-French sheath is very difficult, if not impossible. As a consequence, an 11-French sheath is recommended for the delivery of all of the 28 & 33 mm devices. Like the earlier Clamshell™ device, the CardioSEAL™ device has *no* specific centering mechanism so that a ratio of the device diameter to the defect diameter of 2:1 is recommended for ASD occlusion with the CardioSEAL™ device. The STARFlex™ device has extra Nitinol™ spring centering wires. These centering wires, however, are more useful for centering *after*, as opposed to *during*, implant, and as a consequence, the 2:1 ratio for the device to defect diameter still is recommended for the STARFlex™ device. With their increased flexibility and the extra joints in the legs, which tend to fold the legs even *more toward the septum during the deployment*, the sizing of the ASD for an occlusion with either the CardioSEAL™ or the STARFlex™ device is even more critical.

The CardioSEAL™ and the STARFlex™ devices underwent a regulated, multicenter, FDA clinical IDE trial for ASD closure. The CardioSEAL™ device also underwent a high-risk, protocol trial for closure of other intracardiac defects. The CardioSEAL™ was replaced by the newer designed STARFlex™ modification for ASD occlusions. The CardioSEAL™ device received FDA, Humanitarian Device Exemption (HDE) approval in the United States for the closure of a patent foramen ovale associated with systemic embolic events (and which have failed medical management!), and a standard use approval for the closure of surgical fenestrations which are created purposefully during "Fontan" type intracardiac repairs and for the closure of muscular interventricular septal defects. The use of the CardioSEAL™ device for the closure of the patent foramen ovale requires *notification* of the local Institutional Review Board (IRB). At the same time, the HDE approval is an *approval* for human use and does ***not*** require an IDE *protocol* for these uses. The procedures for each of the "approved uses" of the CardioSEAL™ device are covered in detail in other chapters (29 & 30) under each one of the particular defects, while its use in the secundum ASD is discussed in this chapter in conjunction with the implant techniques for the STARFlex™ device. Currently, the STARFlex™ device is not available in the United States. It was used in one controlled, clinical trial for post-infarct VSD occlusions but apparently this has been abandoned. Both the CardioSEAL™ and the STARFlex™ devices have CE mark approval for occlusion of the ASD as well as other intracardiac defects, and are in clinical use for ASD occlusions throughout much of the world except the United States[17].

Technique for CardioSEAL™ and STARFlex™ ASD implants

Similar to the implant of the Amplatzer™ ASD device and most other atrial septal occlusion devices, the delivery and implant of the device is guided using fluoroscopy with the concomitant use of either transesophageal echo (TEE) or intracardiac echo (ICE). All procedures performed with TEE are performed under general, endotracheal anesthesia while, when ICE is used to guide the implant of the device, some cases can be performed under deep sedation. If the procedure is expected to be at all long and/or complicated, an indwelling Foley™ catheter is placed the patient's urinary bladder at the onset of the procedure. In the patient undergoing an ASD occlusion with a CardioSEAL™ and/or a STARFlex™ device, a 9–11-French short sheath is introduced into the right femoral vein, a 6- or 7-French sheath is introduced into the left femoral vein, and a Quick-Cath™ or a blunt tipped, 5-French dilator introduced into a femoral artery. If ICE is used to control the implant, an 11-French, 30 cm long sheath is introduced (instead of, or in addition to, the 6- or 7-French sheath!) into the left femoral vein.

An end-hole catheter is introduced into the sheath in the right femoral vein and an angiographic "marker" catheter introduced into the sheath in the left femoral vein. The "right heart" pressures and the right heart saturation "sweep" are acquired with either one or a combination of these catheters. The atrial septum and the atrial defect(s) are interrogated with the TEE or ICE, and preliminary echo measurements of the defect and the rims around the defect are recorded before the catheters are advanced through the defect.

When an angiographic "visualization" of the atrial septum is desired, the angiographic catheter then is manipulated through the ASD and into the right upper pulmonary vein. The end-hole catheter is advanced through the ASD and well into a left upper pulmonary vein. One of the X-ray tubes is angled into an approximate 45° LAO–45° Cranial angulation and an angiogram is recorded with injection into the right upper pulmonary vein. The angiogram with this angulation should "cut" the atrial septum on edge on the angiogram and provide an angiographic picture of the size and approximate location of the ASD. Often, this angle of the X-ray tube does not profile the ASD adequately, in which case the X-ray tube angle is changed appropriately and the angiogram repeated.

Once the optimal angiogram has been recorded and the measurements of the atrial defect have been recorded by echo (and angiogram if performed), an exchange length, 0.035″ Super Stiff™ guide wire with a short floppy tip is introduced into the end-hole catheter through a wire back-bleed/flush valve and wedged into a left upper pulmonary vein. The end-hole catheter is maintained over the wire and on a continuous flush until immediately before the sizing balloon is introduced. Once a NuMED™ sizing balloon (NuMED Inc., Hopkinton, NY) with a maximum diameter of approximately twice the measured diameter of the ASD as determined by TEE/ICE and/or angiography, has been prepared, the end-hole catheter is withdrawn off the wire and the sizing balloon is introduced through the short sheath and over the Super Stiff™ wire. The sizing balloon is maintained on a flush over the wire through a wire back-bleed/flush device and advanced until it straddles the ASD. A static, *non-stretched* balloon sizing of the ASD is performed in order to obtain the diameter of the defect for occlusion with either the CardioSEAL™ or the STARFlex™ device. The balloon is inflated partially and at *"zero pressure"* until a malleable, circumferential waist appears around the balloon. If necessary, the angle of the X-ray tube is adjusted to "cut" this waist and the atrial septum more precisely on edge. This waist on the partially inflated balloon is measured angiographically and by TEE or ICE as the non-stretched diameter of the ASD.

When using either the CardioSEAL™ or the STARFlex™ devices, the device chosen for an ASD occlusion should be at least twice the non-stretched, static balloon *sized* diameter of the atrial septal defect. The CardioSEAL™ and STARFlex™ devices both require at least 6–7 mm (measured by TEE or ICE) of atrial septal rim circumferentially around most of the atrial defect, in order to provide the legs some tissue to attach to and to hold the device in place. Inferior–caudally, the rim above both of the atrioventricular valves must be at least the length of the *radius* of the particular device being used in order to accommodate the maximum length of a leg of the device (which corresponds to the radius of the device) without touching either atrioventricular valve. If a CardioSEAL™ or STARFlex™ device is positioned eccentrically, a leg can extend the full length of that leg past the rim or edge of the ASD. When the defect is otherwise fairly central and there is sufficient rim everywhere else, the aortic (anterior–superior) rim can be deficient for 10–15° of the circumference of the rim of the atrial septal defect.

Once the defect is accurately measured and the device is chosen for the particular defect, an appropriate French sized, long sheath is chosen for the delivery of the CardioSEAL™ or STARFlex™ device. A 10-French long sheath is used for the 17 and 23 mm devices while an 11-French long sheath is used for the delivery of the 28 and 33 mm CardioSEAL™ and STARFlex™ devices. A long, large (10–11-French) delivery sheath/dilator set is prepared especially for the delivery of an ASD device. Most of the long sheath/dilator sets that are supplied from the manufacturers either are absolutely straight or have a 180° "transseptal" curve on them. These curves on the sheaths/dilators should be re-formed to more appropriate curves for the delivery of any ASD device. The preferred curve for the delivery of either a CardioSEAL™ or STARFlex™ device to an ASD is a gentle 45° curve just proximal to the distal end of the sheath, with a second "third-dimensional", fairly tight, 45° posterior-superior-leftward curve (as the tip of the sheath faces away from the operator) superimposed distally on the first curve at the very end of the sheath. The more proximal curve directs the sheath from the IVC, leftward, through the ASD and toward the lateral wall of the left atrium, while the distal and posterior curve at the tip of the sheath directs the tip toward the *right* posterior-superior left atrium.

This particular combination of curves now is a vailable commercially preformed as the Hausdorf-Lock™ modification of the RB-MTS™ sheaths (Cook Inc., Bloomington, IN). It is available in 85 cm lengths and in 10–12-French diameters. Unfortunately, the manufactured Hausdorf™ curves all have the same fixed distance between the more proximal and the very distal curves on the end of the sheath. The specificity of this complex curve for a particular ASD depends on the lengths of the curves corresponding to the lengths in the particular heart. As mentioned above, the curves on the sheath/dilator can be formed/changed after heating and with experience and/or trial and error can be formed to fit the specific patient. Delivery sheaths with the "Hausdorf™" curve frequently are used for the delivery of all ASD occlusions devices, but are particularly important for delivery of the CardioSEAL™ and STARFlex™ devices.

Before the long sheath/dilator for the delivery of the device is introduced into the vein, the long delivery sheath/dilator is passed through a short, stiff, *14+-French*, ***"recovery"***, sheath while outside of the patient. A short, thin-walled, 14+-French, metal cannula makes the ideal recovery sheath. The 14+-French, short sheath (or metal cannula) is withdrawn over the long sheath, and positioned back against the hub of the long sheath. The short "recovery" sheath remains there throughout the procedure and is not advanced over the long sheath nor introduced into the skin during a normal ASD device delivery. This larger diameter, short, pre-placed, "recovery" sheath is introduced into the skin and vessel only for the event that it is necessary to remove an incompletely folded CardioSEAL™ or STARFlex™ device from the femoral vein. Otherwise, the larger diameter, short "recovery sheath" remains back at the proximal hub of the long sheath and completely out of the skin/vessel.

After the waist on the static balloon has been measured angiographically and by TEE or ICE, to determine the diameter of the defect, and once the long sheath has been prepared for the device delivery, the sizing balloon is withdrawn carefully from the ASD over the Super Stiff™ wire, which remains positioned in a left upper pulmonary vein. The original short sheath in the right femoral vein is withdrawn over the wire along with the sizing balloon catheter. The long delivery sheath is flushed through the side port of the back-bleed valve and then the stopcock of the side port on the *long sheath* is turned *off*. The *wire* back-bleed/flush valve from the sizing catheter is attached to the *dilator* of the long sheath/dilator set and the side port of the *wire* back-bleed device, which is on the *dilator* is maintained on a continuous flush while the sheath/dilator set is introduced over the wire and advanced into the skin and the vein.

With the *dilator* maintained on continuous flush and the valve of the side port of the sheath *closed* and *not* on a flush, the long sheath/dilator set is advanced over the wire until the tip of the *dilator* is visualized on fluoroscopy just at the area of the *inferior vena cava–right atrial junction*. As mentioned earlier in the discussion of the Amplatzer™ ASD Occluder, ***the next few steps potentially are the most dangerous in the entire procedure***. If the proper steps are not taken for removing all air and/or clot from the delivery system, the patient is very likely to experience a systemic embolic event during the subsequent exchanges of catheters and wires and/or the introduction of the device through the long sheath.

With the tip of the Hausdorf™ *dilator (and sheath)* still in the *right atrium* and the *dilator* still on continuous flush, the dilator is withdrawn *slowly* and carefully until the tip of the dilator is within 10 centimeters of the proximal end (and hub) of the long delivery sheath. The tip of the dilator, still within the sheath, easily is palpated within the sheath as the dilator is being withdrawn out of the subcutaneous tissues and past the surface of the skin. When the tip of the dilator reaches a position outside of the skin but still within the sheath, the flush on the *dilator* is *stopped*. With the flush on each part of the system stopped, the dilator is withdrawn very slowly over the wire out of the last 10 centimeters of the sheath and completely out of the back-bleed valve of the sheath. If there is any, even slight obstruction at the tip of the sheath and/or if the dilator is withdrawn too fast even with the wire passing through a back-bleed/flush valve, air *usually will be* sucked around the tip of the dilator and, in turn, into the lumen of the sheath around the wire as the dilator is withdrawn! When there is no back-bleed valve on the *dilator*, air easily can be sucked into the dilator (and sheath) around the wire during the entire time as the dilator is being withdrawn from the sheath.

Once the dilator is withdrawn completely out of the sheath over the wire, the sheath again, meticulously and *passively*, is cleared of air and/or clot. While watching the fluid column within the tubing on the side port of the long sheath very closely, the stopcock of the side port is opened very carefully and allowed to bleed back *passively* to empty all potential air and/or clots from within the long sheath and the valve chamber of the sheath. Extreme care is taken as the stopcock initially is opened just barely to ensure that fluid and/or air are *flowing* ***out of***, and are ***not*** *being sucked into* the sheath by negative intrathoracic pressure. Realizing that a 10- or 11-French sheath can hold 10–12 ml of air and/or clot, the sheath is allowed to bleed back passively until a column of blood with no air bubbles mixed in it flows freely out of the side port. During the clearing of the sheath, the hub of the sheath is rotated around, elevated (off the table top if possible) and tapped briskly to dislodge air bubbles which *always* will be lodged within the ***chamber of the back-bleed valve*** regardless of how well it was cleared and/or how thoroughly the sheath and dilator were flushed originally before the dilator was introduced into the sheath!

If fluid and/or blood do *not* flow freely out of the side port of the sheath, the stopcock is turned off immediately. Suction ***never*** is applied to the side port *at any time when there is a wire and/or catheter passing through the back-bleed valve* of a sheath. If suction is applied to the side port, a vacuum is created in the sheath and chamber of the back-bleed valve. When there is a wire/catheter passing through the valve, the path of least resistance to the vacuum is *through the back-bleed valve* around the wire and any suction results in more air being sucked into the sheath around the wire! If fluid and/or blood do not flow *passively* out of the side port of the sheath, deep hand pressure is applied over the patient's upper abdomen and/or the anesthesiologist provides positive airway pressure as the closely observed stopcock is carefully reopened. Both maneuvers increase intra-abdominal and intrathoracic pressures and usually result in air, fluid and/or blood flow *out* of the side arm of the sheath.

If there still is no passive back flow from the sheath, possibly because of low venous pressure and/or an obstructed tip of the sheath, first the sheath is withdrawn slightly and the side port is again opened carefully under close observation. If passive back bleed is not obtained with any of these maneuvers, the sheath is *removed* completely out of the body over the wire leaving the wire in place. The removed sheath is inspected outside of the body for kinks and/or clots, flushed thoroughly *outside of the body*, the introduction of the sheath/dilator restarted and the clearing of the sheath repeated until successful.

Once absolutely sure that the sheath *with the tip of the sheath still in the right atrium* has been cleared completely of air and/or clot, the sheath is placed on a continuous flush through the side port of the back-bleed valve. The sheath alone is then advanced carefully over the wire through the atrial defect and deep into the left atrium. Occasionally there is a slight resistance or "catch" as the wide, blunt tip of the sheath catches on the rim of the defect, especially with a small atrial septal defect. In the event of any resistance, the sheath is moved to and fro and rotated very slightly as it is advanced. The sheath never should be pushed forward forcibly. If the sheath cannot be advanced into the left atrium *easily*, the dilator with a back-bleed valve on full flush is reinserted over the wire and into the sheath. The sheath/dilator combination is advanced into the left atrium, the dilator removed and the sheath cleared of air even more meticulously than just described.

When the sheath is well within the left atrium as visualized on fluoroscopy and/or by TEE/ICE, the wire is withdrawn *slowly*. Again, when the wire is completely out of the sheath, the sheath is allowed to bleed back passively as described above and again cleared of any potential air and/or clot. If there is no passive back flow from the side arm of the sheath after the wire is withdrawn completely, the back-bleed *valve* on the hub of the sheath is covered firmly with a gloved finger in order to "seal" the valve very tightly. With the valve sealed tightly with the finger, *gentle* suction is applied to the side port until there is a good, free flow of *only blood* from the side arm. Once the sheath is full of blood, after *suction is stopped* and before flushing, it is a good idea to "vent" the back-bleed valve by introducing the tip of a dilator or the tip of a small forceps into the "leaflets" of the back-bleed valve to partially "open" it while letting it bleed back passively and to continue the venting while beginning the flush into the side port of the sheath. If none of these techniques results in a good flow of fluid/blood from the side port of the sheath, a new wire is introduced and advanced very carefully through the sheath to the level of the inferior vena cava, the wire is fixed in this position, the sheath is removed over the wire and replaced, starting from the very beginning of the procedure. Once cleared in the left atrium, the sheath is flushed thoroughly and maintained on a slow flush, remembering that a long 10- or 11-French sheath has a capacity of 12+ ml of fluid, air and/or clot!

Placing the valve and the side port of the sheath under "water" in a basin of fluid during the entire loading and introduction procedure has been advocated to prevent air from entering the sheath through the valve and around the wire. This does prevent air from being sucked into the valve and sheath from outside, but does not eliminate any air which already—and almost always—is trapped within the valve "chamber" of the sheath after the dilator is removed, it does not eliminate air introduced through the dilator and/or delivery catheter, nor does it prevent any air which already is present in the sheath from being flushed into the left heart! This "under-water" technique only instills a sense of false security.

The location of the tip of the sheath in the left atrium is confirmed on fluoroscopy and by TEE/ICE. If there still is any question about the location of the tip of the sheath and particularly when there is concern that it is trapped in the atrial appendage or in a pulmonary vein, a slow hand injection of 5–10 ml of contrast, followed by 10–15 ml of flush solution is performed through the sheath in order to verify the exact position of the tip of the sheath. After this hand angiogram, the sheath is flushed thoroughly and the side arm of the sheath is maintained on the slow, continuous flush while the device and delivery catheter are prepared.

With the Hausdorf™ curve on the sheath and after the tip is withdrawn out of the appendage or left pulmonary vein, the preformed posterior curve at the tip of the sheath deflects the tip toward the posterior wall of the left atrium and/or even toward the *right*-posterior-superior aspect of the left atrium near the right upper pulmonary veins. The position of the sheath passing through the septum is seen clearly on fluoroscopy and verified with TEE/ICE. The TEE/ICE also shows clearly how the course of the distal sheath in the left atrium tends to run tangentially or even parallel to the plane of the septum. This alignment to the septum becomes very important as the device eventually is withdrawn to, and against, the septum during delivery.

Once the sheath is in position in the left atrium for the device delivery, the appropriate CardioSEAL™ or STARFlex™ device and delivery system are opened, inspected and prepared for the device introduction. The loader, delivery catheters and delivery systems are identical for the CardioSEAL™ and STARFlex™ devices. A delivery rod entering the proximal end of the catheter is at the proximal end of, and controls the to-and-fro movement of the central delivery wire, which extends out of the distal end of the catheter. There is a locking nut proximal to a Tuohy™ side port adaptor on the proximal end of the delivery catheter which, when tightened, prevents the delivery rod (and wire) from moving either in or out of the catheter *at all*. This locking nut is *attached* to the Tuohy™ side port/flush mechanism. The side flushing port at the proximal end of the delivery catheter allows only a very slow flush of the entire length of the delivery catheter around the delivery rod/wire through the side port of the Tuohy™.

For attaching (and releasing) the device to the delivery wire/catheter there is a molded plastic, slide-tumbler with a flat, plastic, plate-like, locking mechanism on the proximal end of the delivery rod. When the tumbler, which is at the proximal end of the delivery rod, slides forward, it pushes a "locking pin" out of a tiny "retaining" sleeve at the distal end of the delivery wire. Withdrawing the tumbler withdraws the pin into the tiny sleeve. The flat, plastic, locking plate, which lies flat on one side of the tumbler, locks the tumbler (and pin) in place by two small protuberances on the tumbler, which fit into two holes on the locking plate. The locking plate is raised slightly off the tumbler to unlock the tumbler and allow the tumbler with the attached control wire to move forward or backward. The plastic locking plate does not deform easily when it is elevated off the tumbler during the attachment or the release of the device, however, it can be distorted and not function subsequently if raised too high and/or forcefully off the surface of the tumbler. The locking plate is elevated just enough to release the tumbler.

The loading of the current CardioSEAL™ and STARFlex™ ASD devices are totally different from the loading technique for the Clamshell™ and the earlier CardioSEAL™ devices. The CardioSEAL™ and STARFlex™ ASD devices both now use the same "front-loading" system and technique. The current delivery catheters no longer have the large metal "delivery pod" at the distal end of the delivery catheter, and the device actually is not loaded into the delivery catheter at all but into a loader and from there directly into the long pre-positioned delivery sheath.

The attach/release mechanism for both the CardioSEAL™ and STARFlex™ ASD devices still is the so-called overlapping "ball-to-ball" (or pin-to-pin) mechanism within a tiny constraining sleeve. It is similar to the Clamshell™ and earlier CardioSEAL™ attach/release mechanisms except that the tiny ball on the attach/release wire now withdraws to *just within* the ***tip*** of the tiny sleeve. On the earlier versions of the pin-to-pin mechanism for the CardioSEAL™ device, when the tumbler was locked, the ball on the delivery wire was pulled deep within the sleeve. The deep recess of the tiny ball into the sleeve did provide a very secure lock on the ball of the device, but at the same time, it did not allow any mobility and/or angulation of the pin on the device (and/or the device) when it was attached to the tip of the delivery catheter. With the current devices, the ball on the attach/release wire is recessed *precisely and just within the tip* of the sleeve when the tumbler is retracted "fully". As a consequence, the pin attached to the device (along with the device) can angle within the sleeve as much as 45° off the long axis of the catheter with the device still attached very securely. If the ball at the tip of the pin on the device does retract deep within the small sleeve when the device is attached, the delivery catheter is defective and should not be used.

The lumen of the delivery catheter is flushed free of air through the side port of the Tuohy™ "Y" adaptor on the delivery rod. After flushing, the locking nut is loosened and the delivery *rod* is advanced into the catheter so that the distal delivery *wire* with the attached distal sleeve extends all the way beyond the end of the catheter. A very gentle, *long* curve is formed on the exposed delivery wire. The curve on the wire is approximately 30° off the long axis and is approximately 20 cms in length. This curve is longer and gentler than the curves formed at the end of the long sheath. This curve is formed on the wire so that the curve on the wire conforms to the gentle curvature of the sheath passing from the right atrium into the left atrium and maintains this same curve after the sheath is withdrawn completely off the device during delivery to the ASD. The catheter is inspected for proper function of the attach/release tumbler in advancing the release pin/ball in and out of the sleeve, for the free movement of the delivery rod through the loosened lock nut, and for the free movement of the rod/wire within the catheter. The small sleeve is carefully inspected to be sure that the sleeve is fixed firmly to the delivery wire and that the ball on the pin in the sleeve is positioned just within the tip of the sleeve when the proximal slide tumbler is withdrawn fully and is in the locked position.

The selected occluder device is opened, inspected and soaked in saline. The device comes attached to a

Quick-loader™. The Quick-loader™ is a thin-walled, semi-clear plastic tube with a *10-French* internal diameter and a small lucent funnel which is fixed on the proximal end of the loading tube. The thin-walled loading tube is contained within a thick transparent Lucite casing. This Lucite casing only serves to reinforce the thinner tubing of the Quick loader™ during the loading. A single, long loading suture passes through the Quick-loader™, out through the proximal (funnel) end of the loader, through all four of the "eyelets" at the tips of the legs of the *distal* umbrella of the device, and back through the proximal end of the loader. The loading suture is tied through a plastic button at the distal end of the loader.

Loading into the Quick-loader™ is accomplished by pulling the attached device into the loader with the attached "loading" suture. The properly operating Quick-loader™ system requires very little traction on the sutures to draw the device into the loader. If excessive tension is applied to the suture as the CardioSEAL™ or STARFlex™ device is pulled into the loader, the excessive traction can over-extend and distort the hinge/spring mechanism of the central hinge of the device, with the disastrous result that the device does not open properly when delivered. This almost always is the case when the larger sized CardioSEAL™ and STARFlex™ devices are used with the Quick-loader™ and, as a consequence, the manufacturer's supplied Quick-loader™ now only is used for the 17–23 mm devices by this operator. A modified loader that is much less traumatic to the devices than the manufacturer's system, is used for the 33 mm and even the 28 mm devices, and is described subsequently.

The tiny attaching "ball" is fixed permanently on the exposed end of the short pin that is *on the central hinge of the proximal* umbrella. To attach the device to the delivery system, the tiny ball on the *delivery/release wire* is extended partially out of the sleeve by advancing the tumbler mechanism at the proximal end of the delivery catheter. The tiny "ball" on the *device* is positioned beside the *wire* to which the ball on the *delivery system* is attached and is introduced into the tiny sleeve. While maintaining the ball on the device within the sleeve, the ball on the delivery/release wire is withdrawn into the sleeve by withdrawing the tumbler at the proximal end of the catheter. The ball on the device will be locked into the tiny sleeve when the protuberance on the tumbler snaps into the small hole on the plastic latch. The attached *wires* of the two tiny balls now overlap each other and pass adjacent to the wire of the opposite ball all within the tiny sleeve. The "compression" by the small inner diameter of the tiny sleeve keeps the ball of the device from sliding out of the sleeve past the ball on the delivery/release wire. The ball on the device is not released until the delivery/release wire (and attached ball on the wire) is advanced purposefully out of the sleeve. At the same time, with the proper positioning of the two tiny balls within the sleeve, the device moves freely, angling from side to side at the end of the delivery wire/sleeve.

When using the manufacturer's Quick-loader,™ the device, which now is attached to the delivery catheter and has the suture passing through the loader, is re-moistened with flush solution. Traction is applied to the button at the ends of the suture which passes through the Quick-loader™ while equal traction is applied *straight* and in the opposite direction to the delivery catheter. Just enough traction is applied to fold the four distal legs of the device, through which the suture passes, symmetrically away from the catheter and toward the funnel of the Quick-loader™. A slow continual flush of saline is injected into the "funnel" while the device is pulled straight into the Quick-loader™ by the suture. The flush "lubricates" the device and helps to prevent air from becoming trapped within the device and loader. As the suture is pulled further, the tips of the legs of the distal umbrella, which are folded toward the funnel, are pulled into the open end of the funnel. With further gentle traction on the button/suture, as the device is pulled into the loader, the distal legs are compressed together very tightly. With further traction on the suture, the folded, distal umbrella is pulled into the tubular portion of the loader while the *proximal*, following, umbrella is pulled into the funnel and the proximal legs are folded in the opposite direction by the funnel (toward the delivery catheter) as the device is pulled further into the funnel.

Continued, straight traction is applied to the "button" (and suture) while the tension is released and a slight push toward the loader is applied to the attached catheter. This completely folds, compresses and pulls/pushes the device entirely into the tubular portion of the loader. Only *mild traction* on the loading suture *ever* should be necessary to fold the umbrellas and draw the device into the loader during the loading into a *properly sized Quick-loader.*™ Whenever *any* resistance is encountered while pulling the device into the loader, the alternative loader should be used. When there is no extra resistance, the folded device is pulled/pushed to the distal tip of the thin sleeve of the Quick-loader™. In the loader the two apposing umbrellas of the device now are folded 180° away from each other for delivery.

It also is *very important* that, during *all* of the steps of the device introduction into the loader, the device is pulled *straight* into the Quick-loader™ with *no twisting or rotating* of the loader, the suture or the device. Any rotation of the device/loader during loading can twist the adjacent legs of the device over each other within the loader. Any twisting of the legs over each other potentially prevents proper opening of the device during delivery.

The 33 mm and the original 40 mm device were always very difficult to pull into the manufacturer's

Quick-loader™, and when these devices are pulled into the Quick-loader,™ the devices frequently become distorted. This is understandable since the Quick-loaders™ for all of the NMT™ devices have a 10-French internal diameter while the larger sized devices repeatedly have been demonstrated to be *extremely tight* when advanced within a 10-French delivery sheath (which actually has a looser internal diameter tolerance than the loader!). No attempt any longer is made at using the Quick-loader™ for the larger sizes of either the CardioSEAL™ or the STARFlex™ devices, and an alternative loading technique to the Quick-loader™ now *always* is used for the 33 mm and even the 28 mm device sizes. With the use of the "alternative" loader, there has been no distortion of any of the devices after delivery!

As an "alternative" front-loader, a short piece of 11-French sheath is substituted for the Quick-loader™. This is a technique devised by the author before the introduction of the Quick-loader™. A segment of 11-French sheath is cut to a length slightly longer than the tubular portion of the Quick-loader™. The proximal, cut-off, end of the short segment of sheath is "flared" by rotating the tip of a large forceps around within the lumen of the "cut-off" end of the segment of sheath. This creates a *slight* "funnel" at one end of the short segment of sheath. The loading suture, which passes from the tips of the legs of the distal umbrella, through the Quick-loader™ and is tied at the "button", is cut as close to the *button* as possible. The two free ends of the suture, which still are attached to the device, are withdrawn completely out of the Quick-loader™. The free ends of the loading suture then are threaded into the flared end of the short segment of sheath, advanced through the segment of sheath, and grasped securely at the distal end of the short sheath with a hemostat.

The device is attached to the catheter exactly as described above. By pulling on the hemostat (similar to the pull on the "button" with the standard loader) while holding the delivery wire attached to the proximal side of the device, the distal legs of the device are folded toward and pulled by the suture into the flared end of the short segment of sheath. With a continual pull on the suture and while manually compressing the fabric on the distal umbrella and then folding the proximal legs away from the sheath with the operator's fingers, both the distal and the proximal legs pull very *easily* into the short segment of sheath. Once the device is within the short segment of sheath, the short segment of sheath performs similar to the Quick-loader™, with the exception that the complex (and unreliable) loader-flush system cannot be attached to the "alternative" (short sheath) loader.

Once the device is completely within the manufacturer's loader, the tip of the delivery catheter is advanced over the rod/delivery wire into the proximal end of the Quick-loader™ until the tip of the delivery catheter is 1–2 mm away from the folded tips of the proximal legs of the contained and folded device within the loader. When the segment of short sheath is substituted for the loader, the tip of the delivery catheter is advanced into the proximal end of the short sheath in exactly the same way. The relationship of the proximal end of the device and the tip of the catheter is visible through the short segment of sheath by holding it up to a light source. Once the tip of the catheter is adjacent to the tips of the proximal legs of the device within either "loader", the locking nut at the proximal end of the delivery catheter is tightened securely onto the delivery rod. This fixes the delivery rod/wire firmly to the delivery catheter and keeps the rod/wire from moving within the catheter.

The two strands of the loading suture still are attached to the distal arms of the device within the loader (or short segment of sheath). One strand of the suture is cut adjacent to the end of the loader, and the suture is withdrawn slowly from the loader/device. The catheter and the loader containing the device are flushed continuously through the delivery catheter and from the *distal* end of the loader/short segment of sheath while tilting and briskly tapping the loader. Once the loader and device are completely free of air, the device is ready for introduction into the sheath.

The delivery *catheter* comes with a separate, large plastic "Tuohy" side-port flushing system, which is positioned loosely over the shaft of the *catheter*. When the standard Quick-loader™ is used, this side port can be advanced over the shaft of the catheter to the end of the delivery catheter and attached to the wide (proximal) end of the "funnel" of the Quick-loader™. The side port of this flush system is attached to a *freely flowing* flush while the Tuohy™ valve is tightened onto the shaft of the catheter. This *theoretically* flushes the device and loader and keeps it free of air while the device is being introduced into the delivery sheath. However, this is *not* necessarily, nor reliably, the case. Often small bubbles remain trapped in the loader in the area of the device in spite of the continuous flush. Since this Tuohy™ flush system adds further complexity to the system and it does not provide a *guarantee* against air bubbles, while at the same time, it does provide a sense of *false security*, some operators have abandoned the use of this added cumbersome and inefficient flush system and remove it completely from the catheter before beginning the loading of the device. It cannot be used and always is removed if the modified (short sheath) loader is used. If the extra flush system is used with the Quick-loader™, flush is continued through the side port while the Tuohy™ valve on the shaft of the catheter is loosened slightly at this time.

The long delivery sheath previously positioned in the left atrium is placed on a vigorous flush. While flushing the *delivery sheath* vigorously and while observing continuously and closely that no air enters the loader, the distal end of the loader sleeve (or short segment of sheath) is introduced *just* into the back-bleed valve at the proximal end of the previously positioned long delivery sheath. As the loader is introduced just into the valve, the vigorous flushing of the long sheath forces fluid (and any trapped air) *back* through, and out of, the loader (or short sheath). This flush is allowed to continue backward, out of the valve of the long sheath for several seconds. Once the loader is cleared and has only flush solution running freely out of its *proximal end*, the *delivery catheter* is placed on a continual flush. The flush through the delivery catheter is very slow through its tight lumen. The tip of the loader or short sheath is advanced further into the valve and through the valve chamber until it stops as it becomes "seated" within the slight flare at the proximal end of the delivery sheath (within the valve chamber). With continual flushing of the sheath and delivery catheter, the delivery catheter is advanced carefully 6–8 cm into the loader (or short segment of sheath). This advances the entire device and the tip of the delivery catheter completely out of the loader and into the long delivery sheath. The loader (or short segment of loading sheath) is withdrawn several millimeters (only!) within the back-bleed valve chamber of the long sheath, but at this point, the loading sheath is ***not*** withdrawn out of the valve. When the extra Tuohy™ side flush port is not used with the manufacturer's loader or the short segment of sheath is used as the loader, flush solution returns vigorously through the loader (or short segment of sheath) as soon as the device is advanced out of the loader into the sheath and the loading sleeve is withdrawn the minimal distance within the valve chamber of the long sheath. This backward flush provides an additional assurance that all air has been forced out of the valve chamber and long sheath. Once the loading sleeve is thoroughly flushed, the delivery catheter is advanced further to be sure that the tip of the delivery catheter is out of the loader and completely into the sheath. The loader (or short segment of sheath) then is withdrawn back onto the proximal end of the delivery catheter.

While still flushing the catheter and while intermittently observing the sheath within the heart on fluoroscopy and TEE/ICE, the *catheter* and the device are advanced together within the sheath only until the device on the fluoroscopic screen is seen within the sheath at approximately *the junction of the inferior vena cava with the right atrium*. The patient empirically is given supplemental sedation and/or anesthesia in an amount sufficient to ensure that he/she does not move for the next five to ten minutes. The primary X-ray tube is positioned into the previously determined angle that cut the septum optimally on edge during the balloon sizing.

Holding the sheath and delivery catheter tightly together, the locking nut that fixes the *delivery rod* to the *delivery catheter* is loosened. Holding the delivery *catheter and sheath together*, the delivery rod/wire with the attached device is advanced very carefully within the sheath until the tips of the distal legs of the attached device reach the end of the sheath. The device/delivery wire and/or catheter moving within the sheath are visible very clearly on the fluoroscopic screen and even quite well on the TEE/ICE image. When the device reaches the tip of the sheath, there usually is 10–15 cm of delivery wire between the end of the delivery catheter and the device. The locking nut is retightened on the delivery rod, refixing the relationship of the rod/wire together with the delivery catheter. The device within the sheath and the atrial septal defect are visualized simultaneously on TEE/ICE.

With the sheath fixed securely in position, the catheter (now fixed in relation to the delivery rod/wire) together with the wire/device is advanced very slowly while observing both by TEE/ICE and on fluoroscopy. The distal legs begin to open as the device is pushed out of the tip of the sheath. As the legs open, the device and its relationship to the intracardiac structures are visible very clearly on the TEE/ICE. If the legs do not open symmetrically and particularly, if they are visualized still to be within a pulmonary vein or the atrial appendage, the sheath along with the catheter and device is withdrawn and/or rotated slightly to allow the legs to open freely within the left atrium. With the legs free in the *posterior* left atrium, the catheter with the delivery rod/wire combination is advanced until the *central hinge* mechanism of the device, which connects the two umbrellas and is very visible on fluoroscopy, becomes aligned with the distal tip of the sheath. This allows the distal legs to open fully.

The distal umbrella should open perpendicularly to the shaft of the catheter/sheath as seen on fluoroscopy and confirmed by the TEE/ICE. These opened legs align at a fairly steep angle to the surface of the atrial septum (and the defect). If not already positioned in that direction, the sheath with the device is rotated posteriorly and toward the *patient's right*. The Hausdorf™ curve on the sheath helps to achieve this position. The tips of the open, distal legs of the device, which are closest to the septum (toward the patient's right) begin to fold or bend partially away from the catheter/sheath as they touch against the posterior/superior septum (Figure 28.12).

The legs of the proximal, right atrial umbrella are visible on fluoroscopy, folded within the sheath and still not pulled back to the right side of the septum. TEE/ICE demonstrates the relationship of the tips of the extended legs to the atrial septum better, as well as showing the distance of these legs and the center of the device to the atrial defect. With the distal legs extended fully, the lock nut on the delivery catheter remains tightened on the delivery rod. While holding the sheath and catheter firmly fixed

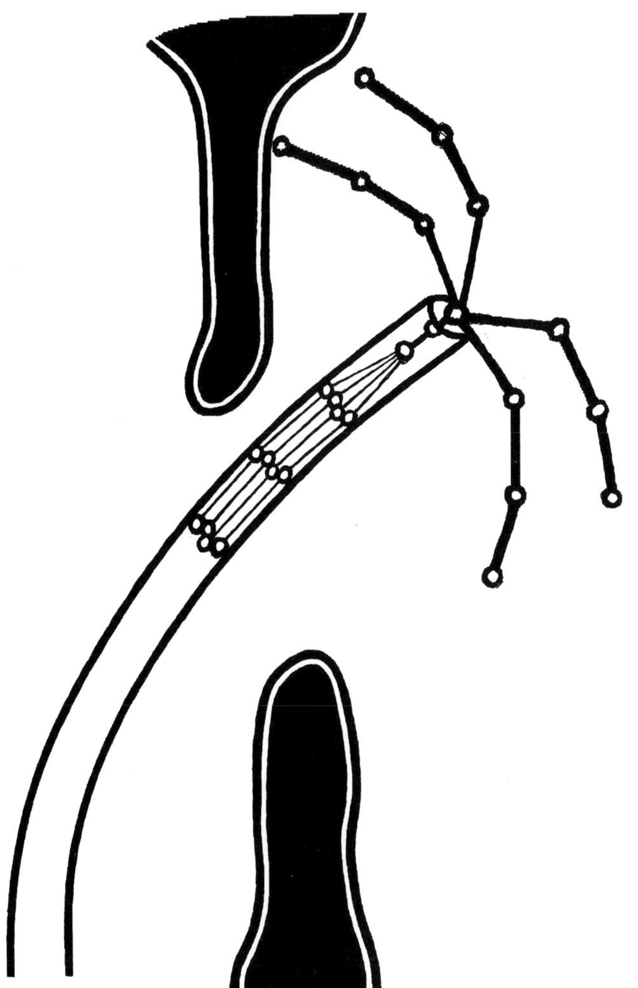

Figure 28.12 Left atrial umbrella of a CardioSEAL™ device opened in the left atrium. Device is very malaligned with the atrial septum. Folded right atrial umbrella still within the sheath does not extend to the right side of the septum.

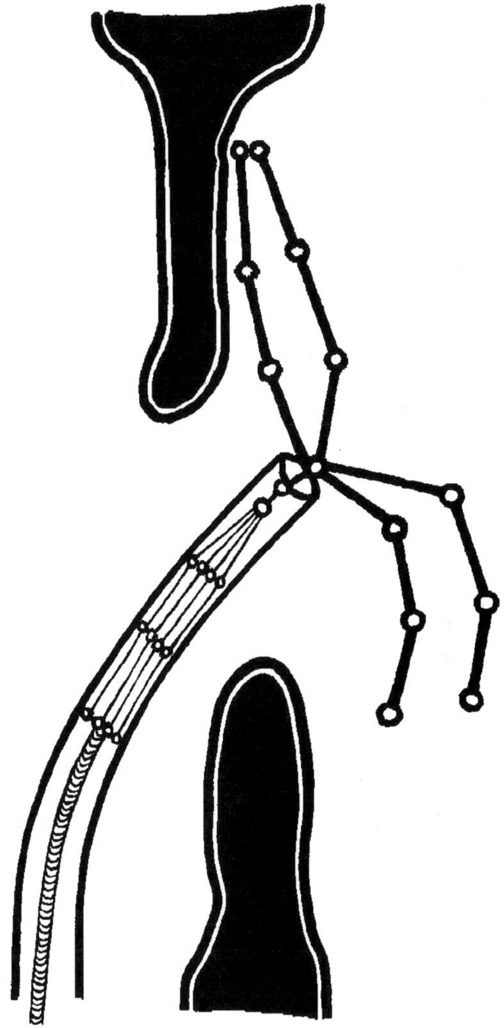

Figure 28.13 More cephalad legs of left atrial umbrella of a CardioSEAL™ device beginning to "bow" as device is withdrawn along septal surface and more into defect. The position of the legs of the right atrial umbrella, which are still folded within the sheath but are extending to the right side of the septum, are visible on fluoroscopy/angiography.

together at the hub of the sheath, the combination sheath, delivery catheter, delivery wire, and attached device, all together are withdrawn slowly along the posterior–superior septum toward the atrial defect. The device and its relationship to the septum are observed very carefully with both fluoroscopy and TEE/ICE. As the device is withdrawn, the distal legs, which are touching the septum, begin to bow and/or bend away from the sheath and often, create a steep angle to the other open legs of the device. The right atrial disk is visible still folded within the sheath, which in turn, demonstrates the relationship of the tips of the legs of the right atrial umbrella to the right side of the defect (Figure 28.13). The simultaneous TEE/ICE image clearly demonstrates the open legs, their proximity to the atrial septum, and their relationship to the atrial septal opening. Often the device still appears almost perpendicular to the surface of the atrial septum.

The entire system is withdrawn slowly until a tip of one leg of the left atrial umbrella, which already is against the septum, approaches within **4–5** mm of the edge of the atrial *defect* as seen on TEE/ICE. The TEE/ICE shows the angle of the device against the septum and how far away the remaining left atrial legs are from the septum. TEE/ICE will show the atrial septal tissues and *may* help to determine whether the tips of the *proximal* device, still folded within the sheath, have reached the *right* side of the septum (*see* Figure 28.13). A small, hand injected, angiocardiogram is performed through the additional angiographic catheter which is positioned through, and just on the left atrial side of, the atrial septal defect. The tip of this additional catheter may be against the proximal surface of the opened distal umbrella of the device. The angiocardiogram confirms whether the tips of the legs of the *proximal* umbrella, which are still folded within the sheath, have reached the *right* side of the plane of the septum and verifies the position of the open distal umbrella against the septum (*see* Firgure 28.13). If the right sided umbrella is not quite far enough to the right of the septum in order to ensure that the right legs will open on the right of the septum, the sheath/catheter/device, with TEE/ICE imaging, are withdrawn carefully together and/or rotated slightly and the angiocardiogram repeated.

Once the tips of the right legs are far enough through the ASD and positioned so they clearly will open on the right side of the septum, the angiographic catheter is withdrawn into the right atrium. The delivery *catheter* (with the delivery rod/wire and device) is fixed in place against the tabletop and/or the patient's leg and the sheath alone is withdrawn *well* off the proximal legs of the device. This allows the proximal (right atrial) legs to spring open. Usually the device reorients slightly and aligns better with the septum when the sheath is well away from the device (Figure 28.14). With the two "umbrellas" open on the opposite sides of the septum, the device is in a relatively secure position before its purposeful release. It is tested with *very* slight, gentle to-and-fro motion on the delivery catheter/wire. The device position is checked by TEE/ICE and a repeat angiocardiogram performed through the additional venous catheter. If there is a gross malposition of the device, at this point with the device still attached, the device still is retrievable, albeit with some difficulty.

A technique used during the earlier trials and which remains as an alternative technique for positioning the CardioSEAL™ or the STARFlex™ device on the septum and over the defect is to begin the positioning and deployment of the device with the sheath in or *near the left upper* pulmonary veins. With this technique, the tip of the sheath is withdrawn out of the pulmonary vein and the distal (left atrial) umbrella is deployed as described above. The entire system is withdrawn from the mid left atrium slowly toward the septum and the atrial defect while observing on TEE/ICE and fluoroscopy. The device is withdrawn until just the *tip* of the *very first* of the open distal legs approaches and barely *touches* the septum as seen on the TEE/ICE. This usually is the most cephalad leg of the device. Usually, but not reliably, this leg bends slightly away from the septum on fluoroscopy as it touches it. At this time, all of the distal (open) legs still should be on the *left* atrial side of the septum while the tips of the proximal legs, which still are folded within the sheath, should be through the defect, and on the *right* side of the atrial septum. The correct position can be verified by performing an angiocardiogram through the additional venous catheter which was previously positioned through the defect on the *left* atrial side of the atrial septum and adjacent to (touching!) the proximal side of the opened distal umbrella. The TEE/ICE confirms that all of the legs of the open left atrial umbrella still are on the left side of the septum. The angiocardiogram demonstrates that the folded legs of the right atrial umbrella are far enough through the defect to open on the right atrial side of the septum. When the correct position of all the legs is confirmed to the satisfaction of the operator, the second venous catheter is withdrawn into the right atrium and the right atrial umbrella of the device deployed by withdrawing the sheath off the right sided legs of the device while fixing the delivery catheter/delivery rod/device in place.

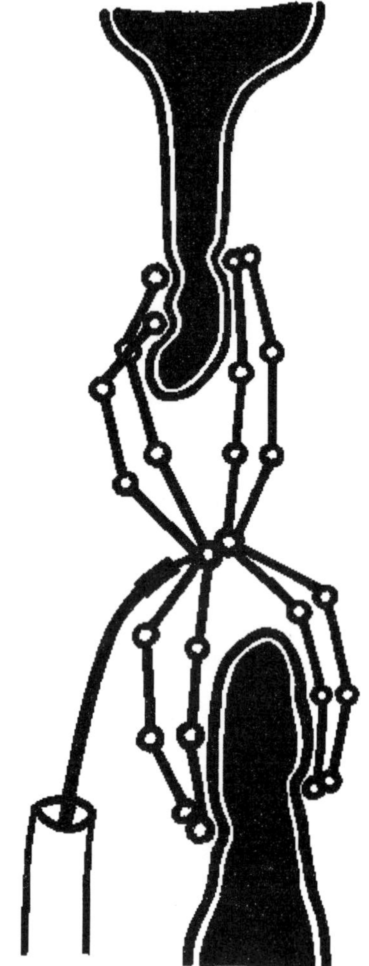

Figure 28.14 Both umbrellas of CardioSEAL™ device opened on septum—device still attached to delivery cable.

Before the right atrial legs are opened and/or when one or more of the left atrial legs pulls through the defect and/or the right atrial legs do not appear to extend far enough through the defect to be able to open on the right atrial side of the septum, the sheath, catheter and device, all together, can be re-advanced back into the left atrium. This can be accomplished *only before the right atrial umbrella is deployed*. When free in the left atrium and as viewed on fluoroscopy and TEE/ICE, the combination of sheath/ catheter/device with only the left atrial disk open is rotated slightly as a "unit" in order to produce a better orientation of the left atrial disk in relation to the septum, and the positioning process repeated. If the device pulls through the defect completely with all of the left legs open but before any of the right atrial legs are opened, an attempt can be made at withdrawing the delivery catheter along with the distal legs of the attached device back into the sheath and then to re-advance the sheath with the totally enclosed device back through the defect into the left atrium. If any one of these steps cannot be performed, the device is withdrawn through the sheath and out of the body.

Exact positioning on the septum is confirmed by TEE/ICE before release of the device. Until this step in the procedure, the device can be withdrawn, at least partially, back into the delivery sheath and is retrievable with only moderate difficulty. However, once the device has been released, the retrieval of a CardioSEAL™ or STARFlex™ device is very difficult. Occasionally, and particularly if the device embolizes through the right ventricle to the pulmonary artery, or, even worse into the left ventricle, catheter retrieval usually is not a reasonable option, even if potentially possible. In that circumstance, the device should be retrieved surgically and the defect closed surgically. Fortunately, even with embolization into a ventricle, the embolized device usually does not compromise hemodynamic stability so that the surgical retrieval does not require an emergent, life-saving procedure.

When the correct position in the defect and on the septum is confirmed with TEE/ICE, the device is ready for release. When satisfied that all of the legs are on the proper sides of the septum, the sheath is fixed in place while *very gentle* traction is applied to the delivery rod/wire. The slide-tumbler, attach/release mechanism at the proximal end of the catheter is activated by raising the lever or "plate" on the tumbler and pushing the tumbler forward. The fixed device often turns and/or springs away from the attaching wire and often "swings" to and fro on the mobile septum. Usually after release, the device aligns better with the atrial septum and often the CardioSEAL™ and usually the STARFlex™ devices "self center" very nicely on the defect. The proper position on the septum is rechecked with TEE/ICE, observing specifically for the relationship of all of the legs of both umbrellas to each other and to their proper side of the septum. TEE/ICE/ Doppler interrogation identifies the integrity of the closure or any persistent leaks.

The X-ray tube that was used to measure the defect with the balloon and/or during the deployment of the device is repositioned to align the device precisely on edge. A selective angiocardiogram is performed with an injection of a large bolus of contrast into the right atrium. This demonstrates the right side of the device on the septum very clearly and, by observing the flow of the contrast through the left heart during recirculation, the left atrial side of the device is visualized fairly well. Re-manipulation of the angio-catheter from the right atrium, to the right ventricle and into the pulmonary artery is potentially dangerous and unnecessary and there is a significant risk of dislodging a freshly implanted device by nudging it with an inadvertent bend and/or twist of the proximal shaft of the catheter. The "recirculation" image after an injection into the pulmonary artery is not significantly better for identifying residual leaks than the recirculation images from a large bolus injection in the right atrium.

In an effort to lessen the pressure effect of the acute "trapping" of the shunt volume load in the left heart following the sudden, successful closure of atrial septal defects, patients are given 0.25–0.5 mg/kg of furosemide intravenously just before or immediately after the device is implanted. This dose is repeated in 6–8 hours in patients with very large defects or "precariously" implanted devices. The catheters are removed and hemostasis achieved by pressure over the puncture sites. Since a "foreign body" has been implanted, these patients are treated with antibiotic prophylaxis primarily against *Staphylococcus aureus* and appropriately for the size of the patient for 24 hours.

Pecularities of the STARFlex™ ASD Occluder

Because of the need for some type of "centering mechanism" on either the Clamshell™ or CardioSEAL™ ASD devices, the manufacturer developed the STARFlex™ ASD device to address this short-coming[16]. The STARFlex™ ASD device actually represents a very minimal modification of the CardioSEAL™ device. Except for the new "centering mechanism", all of the major features of the STARFlex™ device are identical to those of the CardioSEAL™ device. The "centering mechanism" consists of four, very fine, Nitinol™ *micro spring* wires, which extend from the tip of a leg on one umbrella to the tip of the nearest leg on the opposing umbrella. When the device is opened in the atrial septal defect, the tiny spring wires create a "sling" from the tip of a leg on one side of the septum, through the edge of the defect, to the tip of the nearest leg on the other umbrella on the opposite side of the septum. These tiny micro spring wires are stretchable enough to allow the legs to be folded the 180° away from each other for delivery without "over-stretching" the micro spring wires. Yet when both umbrellas of the device are opened in a defect, the four "slings" theoretically are strong enough to push the tips of each of the legs of the umbrella toward the center of the device/defect from all four "quadrants" around the circumference of the ASD and, in doing so, effectively center the device in the ASD.

With several minor exceptions, the loading and delivery of the STARFlex™ devices are identical and were discussed with the previously described technique for the delivery of the CardioSEAL™ and STARFlex™ devices. When the STARFlex™ devices are opened and inspected, the fine Nitinol™ micro spring wires are inspected in particular to be sure that they are not damaged (overstretched and/or "unwound") and that they are not entangled with the legs, hinges, fabric or sutures on the devices. Keeping these tiny wires free and untangled is particularly important during the loading of the STARFlex™ device into the Quick-loader™ or the modified loader. When one of the tiny micro wires becomes tangled, the micro spring wire can be released easily by relaxing any tension on the device and then gently lifting the trapped wire away from its abnormal attachment with the tip of a small forceps.

The second, and only other major difference between the STARFlex™ and the CardioSEAL™ device occurs during the extrusion of the distal legs of the device during the delivery procedure. As the distal legs are opened, the *central hinge* mechanism of the device is *kept* well ***within*** the tip of the sheath so that the most proximal segments of the legs of the device rest against the tip of the sheath, and the fine centering springs wires, which now extend from the tips of the distal legs back to the tip of the sheath, do *not* flex or bend the open legs unduly back toward the sheath (Figure 28.15). If the central hinge mechanism extends beyond the tip of the sheath, tension is placed on the tips of the left atrial legs, which curves the tips of the legs of the open umbrella almost perpendicularly toward the septum and reduces the effective diameter of the device as it is being pulled back toward the septum (Figure 28.16). The extreme of this tension on the legs causes the left atrial umbrella to assume a configuration that resembles more the shape of a parachute or "jellyfish" umbrella (Figure 28.17). This configuration prohibits proper seating over the atrial septal defect. If this configuration occurs, the sheath is advanced very slightly forward over the delivery catheter/wire in order to withdraw the central hinge mechanism of the device back within the tip of the sheath and press the tip of the sheath against the most central segment of the distal legs—hopefully pushing the open legs to a more perpendicular position.

When the left atrial disk is deployed properly, the micro springs extend straight from the tip of the sheath to the straight legs of the left atrial disk. As the entire system is withdrawn, the micro springs are stretched across the edges of four quadrants of the atrial defect and, in the process, tend to center the device on the septum during delivery (Figure 28.18). The micro spring wires are not very sturdy and cannot be relied on to center the device against a strong lateral force of the remainder of the delivery system. Otherwise the withdrawal of the device against the septum and the device deployment are the same as for the CardioSEAL™ device.

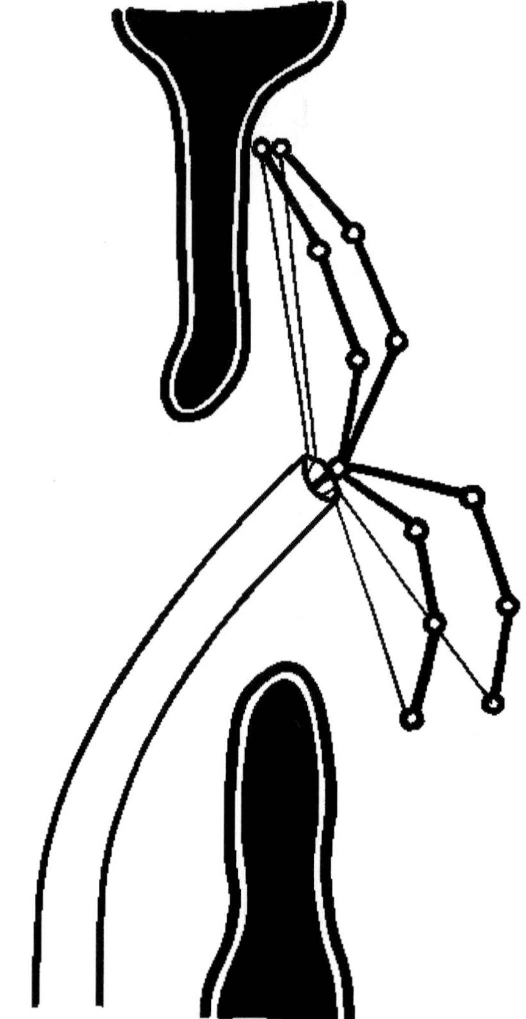

Figure 28.15 Left atrial legs of STARFlex™ device opened properly in left atrium with centering micro springs stretched taut and left atrial legs still extended straight.

Excellent safety and efficacy were demonstrated in clinical trials in Europe and the STARFlex™ achieved CE mark approval. Since then the STARFlex™ device has had successful clinical use in Europe[18]. In the United States, the STARFlex™ was introduced into FDA monitored clinical trials in late 1998. The total number of patients required in order to provide statistical data for the US FDA trial was completed by early 2000. The clinical trial was stopped while the follow-up data were being accumulated and reviewed by the FDA. While the data were in review, a "supplemental use" of the device briefly was available to the original investigators for use to treat

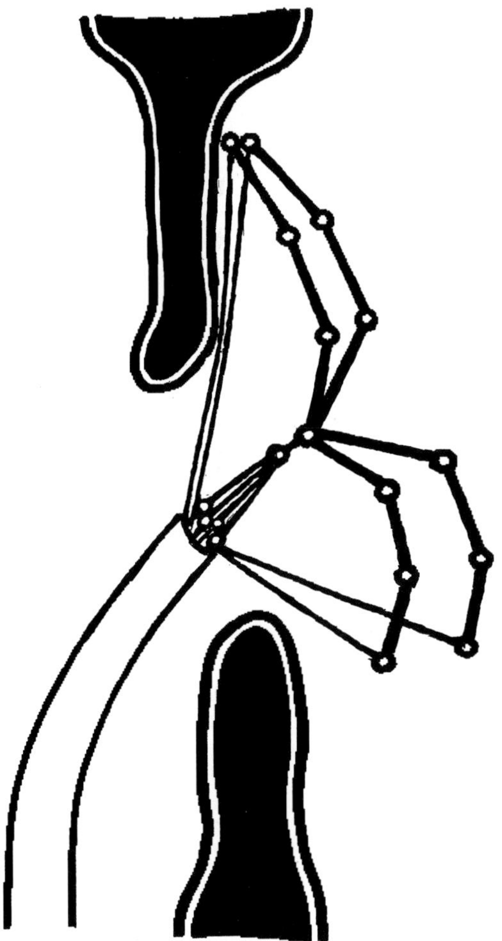

Figure 28.16 Sheath withdrawn too early off right atrial legs and too far within left atrium, causing the micro springs to create central and rightward tension on the tips of the left atrial legs.

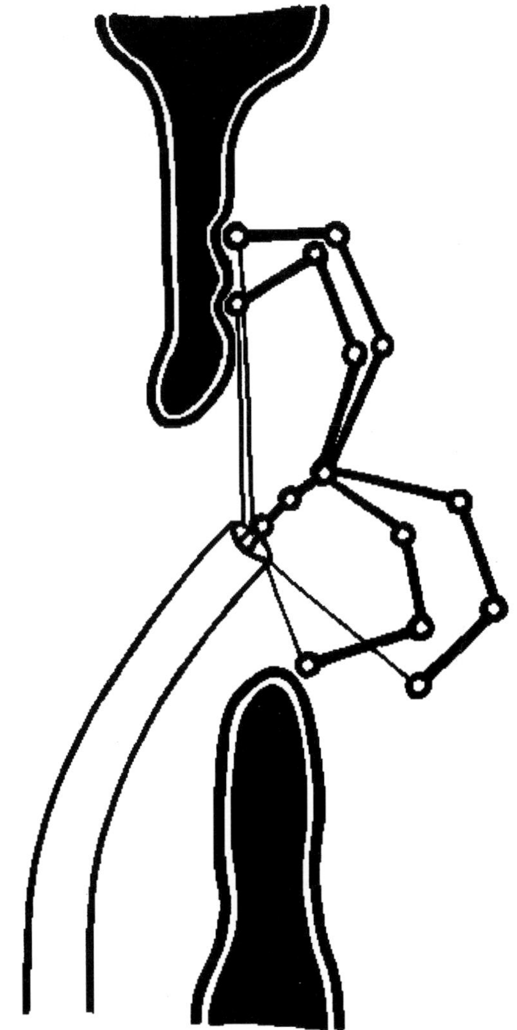

Figure 28.17 Extreme malformation of the left atrial disk of STARFlex™ device when the whole device is extended too far out of sheath. The left atrial legs are folded back even further into a "jellyfish" umbrella configuration.

appropriate patients on a modified protocol, however, this essentially has disappeared in the United States.

The immediate and total occlusion of the ASD is improved with the STARFlex™ device compared to the CardioSEAL™ device, however there still were at least 5–10% with residual leaks after successful implant. In addition, after apparent, totally successful implants and *total occlusions* of the defect with the 40 mm STARFlex™ device, several of these large STARFlex™ devices embolized away from the ASD within several hours after implant. This occurred only with the 40 mm devices. Further investigation indicated that the finer MP-35N metal of the longer legs of the 40 mm devices probably was not strong enough to support the device against the sudden significant pressure difference between the two atria, which occurs when the shunt is stopped suddenly following occlusion of the larger defects. The 40 mm device eventually was abandoned for use for closing the large isolated ASD.

As a consequence of the problem with the 40 mm STARFlex™ device, two new devices of the same materials were developed and tested in animals. These ASD occlusion devices each had *six* arms on each umbrella and the umbrellas were 38 and 43 mm in diameter. The extra arms on each side created a sturdier device and the six arms created a hexagonal configuration, which covered a much larger area for a given device diameter. In spite of the extra, and longer arms and the increased fabric, these new devices still were delivered through 11- and 12-French sheaths. Unfortunately, these larger, six-armed STARFlex™ devices still are not available even in investigative trials for the occlusion of the significantly larger ASD or any other defects in the United States.

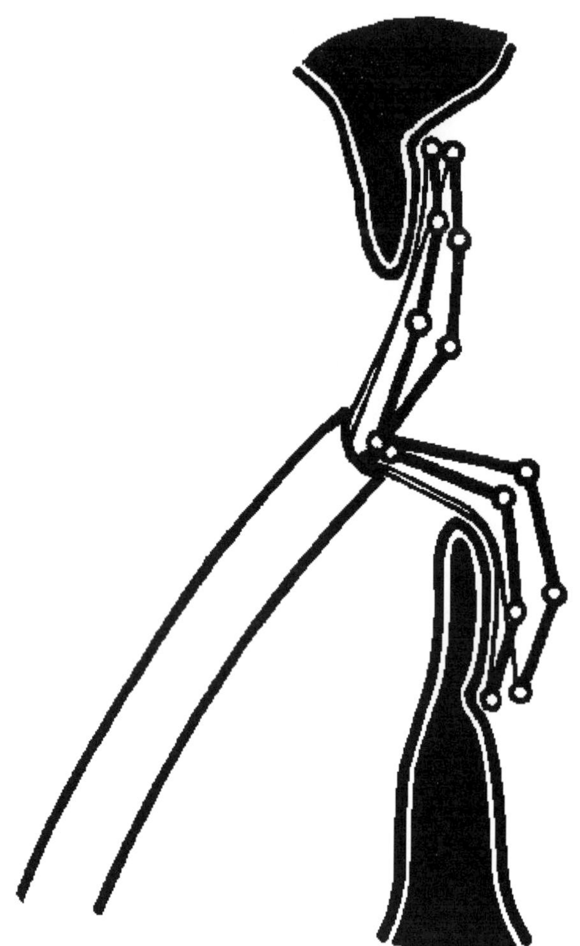

Figure 28.18 Sheath withdrawn properly off STARFlex™ device, allowing the micro springs to *help* "center" the device in the atrial defect and yet not folding the legs too tightly backward on themselves.

Eustachian valve and the delivery of the CardioSEAL™ and STARFlex™ ASD devices

The presence of a large and redundant Eustachian valve creates a significant problem during the delivery of the CardioSEAL™ and STARFlex™ devices. Because of the "pull" toward the inferior vena cava on the delivery catheter and when the delivery sheath is withdrawn off the *right* atrial legs of these "true umbrella" devices during the delivery of the device, the initial opening of the "spring mounted" right atrial legs begins far out into the body of the right atrium and/or actually toward (into!) the inferior vena cava. When there is a large flap of Eustachian valve tissue extending close to the ASD and, as the right-sided legs spring open, the legs very easily and very likely catch on the Eustachian valve tissues. The larger the device (the longer the legs) and/or the larger/longer the Eustachian valve, the greater is the chance of this occurring. The legs catching on the Eustachian valve tissue prevents the right atrial legs from opening completely and results in the trapped legs protruding out into the cavity of the right atrium. The tethered portion of the Eustachian valve along with the attached right atrial umbrella also potentially and selectively "funnels" desaturated inferior vena caval blood selectively under the device toward the left atrium.

This *potential* problem should be recognized easily and is preventable. In every case, the right atrium and the area of the atrial septal defect are scrutinized very carefully by TEE or ICE for the presence of redundant and/or long Eustachian valve tissue. The large Eustachian valve readily is recognized on the TEE/ICE image as a thin structure, which flaps freely and consistently in the right atrium close to, or even in front of, the atrial septal defect. The Eustachian valve can have thicker tissues and/or can have an attachment to the septum giving it the appearance of a "septum" across the right atrium. When excessive Eustachian tissue is recognized, a 6-French, EPT DX, Unidirectional, Steerable, Diagnostic Electrophysiology (EP) "mapping" catheter (Boston Scientific, Natick, MA) with a two-dimensional, controllable, deflecting curve at the tip is introduced through an additional venous sheath. These deflectable EP catheters allow the formation of a 180° curve, or loop, at the tip of the catheter, which once formed, can be locked in position. The straight deflector catheter is advanced from the inferior vena cava into the right atrium and advanced cephalad beyond the free end of the Eustachian valve. While observing on fluoroscopy as well as TEE or ICE, a tight curve is formed on the "deflector catheter" in order to trap the free end of the Eustachian valve. Once the "flapping tissue" of the Eustachian valve is trapped, the "flapping" structures on the echo image disappear and/or are moved by the deflector catheter[19]. The deflected curve on the catheter is locked in position, and the curved catheter with the trapped Eustachian valve is withdrawn toward the inferior vena cava and away from the atrial septal defect. It usually takes only a few attempts to trap the Eustachian tissues with the curved deflector catheter. The Eustachian valve is held in this position away from the septum while the device is delivered to the atrial septal defect. Once the device is in place, the curve on the EP catheter is relaxed which, in turn, releases the Eustachian valve tissue. The released Eustachian valve tissues then may flap against the right side of the device which, however, causes no problems.

When the Eustachian valve is not recognized or cannot be "retracted" satisfactorily with the deflector catheter and does become caught on the device, the Eustachian tissues still can be freed from the device using a sizing balloon and/or a large angioplasty balloon. An end-hole catheter is advanced from the inferior vena cava into the right atrium, manipulated very carefully and very close to the device, then past the device and from there, into the superior vena cava. The spatial relationship of the catheter to the device and the Eustachian tissue is determined with fluoroscopy *and* TEE or ICE. When the catheter has passed between the trapped leg(s) of the device and the Eustachian tissue, the catheter is replaced with an exchange length, spring guide wire. A large diameter sizing or angioplasty balloon is advanced over the wire and maneuvered very gingerly to a position adjacent to the device. A single inflation of the balloon usually is sufficient to separate and release the trapped leg(s) from the tissues. If not, the deflated balloon is moved along the wire and/or the wire is repositioned all together and the inflation repeated. There have been occasions where the legs of the device became trapped on the Eustachian valve but the legs were left trapped with the legs (and presumably, the umbrella) extending out into the body of the right atrium with no reported adverse effects. However, it appears advisable to avoid the entrapment by prevention or to accomplish the separation of the legs from the Eustachian tissue during the same procedure.

Retrieval of the cardioSEAL™ and STARFlex™ devices

With the CardioSEAL™ and the STARFlex™ ASD devices, like all catheter-delivered devices, there are occasional malpositioned devices and even displaced and embolized devices. Contingencies are available for their retrieval. The ease (or difficulty) of retrieval depends a great deal upon at what particular stage of the delivery/implant the device becomes malpositioned. With the CardioSEAL™ and the STARFlex™ devices this is particularly true.

For all of the 28 mm and larger devices and before the long delivery sheath is introduced into the vein for the routine delivery of a CardioSEAL™ or STARFlex™ device, a long sheath/dilator is passed through a short, stiff 14+-French *"rescue"* or *"recovery"* sheath. Either a short, stiff, 14-French sheath or a short, thin-walled, 14-French, metal cannula with a hub makes an ideal "rescue" or "recovery" sheath! The short 14+-French, "rescue" sheath is withdrawn over the sheath, back to the hub of the long sheath and remains there throughout the standard procedure. This short "recovery" sheath serves as a supplemental and external support sheath for the withdrawal out of the vessel and through the skin for a device that has been opened but still is held by the delivery wire and/or grasped by a retrieval catheter. For the standard CardioSEAL™ or STARFlex™ delivery, the long delivery sheath is introduced into the vessel similarly to any other device delivery, but with the short "rescue" sheath, which is positioned over it, remaining back at the hub of the long sheath. The short recovery sheath is not introduced into the skin or the vessel unless a retrieval of an opened device is necessary.

When only the distal legs of the CardioSEAL™ or STARFlex™ devices are deployed and the device still is attached to the delivery catheter/wire, the entire device can be withdrawn most, if not all of, the way back into the delivery sheath by pulling the delivery catheter/wire back while fixing the sheath against the device. The smaller devices usually can be withdrawn completely into the sheath. With the larger devices, the very distal segment of the arms (beyond the last "wrist" joint) often fold out and hang over the outside of the end of the sheath and further attempts at withdrawing the device only buckles and/or accordions the long sheath. In order to remove the partially withdrawn device from the vessel, first the skin and subcutaneous tissues around the long delivery sheath are infiltrated liberally with local anesthesia and the skin incision is extended slightly around the long sheath. The short 14-French "recovery" sheath is introduced into the vein over the 11-French long sheath with a smooth, fast, rotating motion. The long sheath with the legs of the umbrella still hanging out of the distal end of the sheath is withdrawn into the inferior vena cava until the tip of the long sheath approximates the tip of the short "rescue" sheath. The very flexible, exposed parts of the legs hanging out of the tip of the delivery sheath tend to become folded *away from the tip of the sheath* as it is being withdrawn through the more peripheral vein even before they reach the short recovery sheath. When the legs are folded away from the tip of the sheath, the flexible legs do not catch on, or damage venous structures as the long sheath is withdrawn. Pulling the sheath, delivery catheter and attached device against the stiff, short "recovery" sheath, very effectively completes the folding, and allows the still extended legs to be pulled into the short sheath and out of the body.

When both proximal and distal umbrellas have been deployed, but the device still is attached to the delivery wire/catheter, the devices usually still can be withdrawn partially into the tip of the long sheath. This maneuver, of course, everts the proximal umbrella 180° away from its original position/direction in the sheath. As a consequence, it requires considerably more force to withdraw even part of the device into the sheath. The delivery *catheter* is re-advanced over the delivery cable and against the pin connector of the device to add support to the shaft of the long sheath. The combination of catheter, delivery wire and deployed device are withdrawn against and, as much as possible, into the long sheath, which, of course, in doing so, destroys the device. When applying this force, the full length of the long sheath must be observed intermittently for distortion and damage to the long sheath. The force required to pull the device into the long sheath may be greater than the wall strength of the sheath, and result in the long sheath "accordioning" on itself. If the device does not pull into the long sheath, the short 14-French "recovery" sheath is introduced into the vein as described above. The long sheath with the partially collapsed legs extending out of the tip of the sheath is withdrawn carefully down the inferior vena cava and iliac vein to the tip of the short sheath. As the partially exposed legs of the device are withdrawn through the veins, they tend to fold and *taper away* from the tip of the sheath and away from the direction of withdrawal. The exposed, tapering and flexible legs do not create much resistance to the withdrawal and do not traumatize the vessel wall significantly. Once pulled against the short sheath, the entire combination usually folds into and can be pulled completely into the short recovery sheath.

When retrieving a device after both umbrellas have been deployed, all of the device legs may not withdraw completely into a standard "plastic", 14-French recovery sheath and begin to "accordion" the short recovery sheath as well. Usually, even in this circumstance, enough of the device is covered within the short sheath to allow the combination to be withdrawn out of the vessel with minimal extra force and minimal vessel/subcutaneous tissue trauma.

If the device cannot be withdrawn into the larger diameter recovery sheath or out of the skin and/or the device becomes free from the delivery catheter in the iliac area (either released purposefully or if the device breaks loose), the "free" device usually will not "embolize" centrally from a more peripheral vein. The angles created by the exposed legs folding away from the femoral area as the device is withdrawn into the iliac vein also result in the legs flaring out *toward* the central circulation and heart. This angle of the legs fortuitously serves to fix the device very securely in the peripheral venous location and prevents the device from "floating" back to the heart even when released (purposefully or accidentally).

In the event that the device does become free, the delivery catheter is withdrawn through and out of the delivery sheath as well as the larger diameter short "recovery" sheath. A relatively stiff exchange length guide wire is introduced through the delivery sheath and advanced adjacent to and past the errant device. Once this wire is in place, the original delivery and the "recovery" sheaths are withdrawn and replaced with a significantly *larger diameter long* sheath/dilator (14–16-French). After the new large sheath is introduced and its dilator is withdrawn, the *dilator* then is modified specifically to help support the long sheath during the subsequent recovery of the device.

The entire *taper* at the tip of the large dilator, which was part of the large sheath/dilator set, is excised but excised only enough so that it does not become shorter than the long sheath. This produces a *dilator* with a squared off tip and with the much larger lumen of the shaft of the dilator exposed. The "excised" dilator is reintroduced over the wire and back into the large, long sheath. The tip of the modified dilator is advanced to just within the tip of the sheath. Together, the sheath and the enclosed modified dilator create a very thick and strong walled "retrieval sheath". A retrieval device (basket or snare) is introduced through this combination of now "open-ended" dilator and the large sheath. The device is captured with the appropriate retrieval device and withdrawn forcefully into the new much larger and stronger sheath/dilator combination. As the captured device is withdrawn into the sheath, the dilator can be withdrawn into the sheath along with the device.

When a CardioSEAL™ or STARFlex™ occlusion device is displaced and/or embolizes remotely after it is released from the delivery catheter, then the retrieval falls into the category of a very complex "foreign body" recovery. The general principles for the retrieval of free-floating foreign bodies are covered in detail in Chapter 12. How, and ***whether***, the errant device can be retrieved depends upon both the location where the device stops and what retrieval equipment is available. Fortunately, when these devices do embolize, they usually pass completely through the respective atrio-ventricular valves and/or the right or left ventricle and move on through the ventricle to the respective great artery *without* producing any hemodynamic compromise. In these positions the device usually is very stable and represents no immediate danger to the organ(s) adjacent to where it sits and to the patient in general. This allows the organization of a relatively "elective" retrieval!

When a CardioSEAL™ or STARFlex™ device embolizes to the pulmonary artery, the *major* immediate *decision* is whether even to attempt the retrieval in the catheterization laboratory or to send the patient directly for a surgical retrieval and closure of their defect. When either a CardioSEAL™ or a STARFlex™ ASD device is to be retrieved from the pulmonary artery by a transcatheter procedure, it *must be* withdrawn *through the ventricle* through a very large, long retrieval sheath, which must be positioned in the main or even the involved branch pulmonary artery before grasping the errant device. A partially collapsed and exposed CardioSEAL™ or STARFlex™ umbrella ***never*** should be withdrawn into and/or through a ventricle with even a small *part* of the device exposed outside of the sheath! The device absolutely must be withdrawn ***completely*** *into the sheath* before any attempt is made to withdraw it through the right ventricle. When even a part of a single leg of one of these devices extends out of the end of the sheath, it almost guarantees that the device will become tangled in the tricuspid valve apparatus. A device tangled in a ventricle and, at the same time, firmly attached to a retrieval device and partially within a sheath usually cannot be released from the retrieval device nor pulled out of the ventricle without destroying the atrioventricular valve! When a device that is irreversibly attached to a retrieval catheter becomes trapped in an atrioventricular valve, the otherwise elective, controlled thoracotomy retrieval of the errant device suddenly has been converted into an acute, open-heart surgical emergency!

If the decision is made to attempt catheter retrieval, and once a *very* large, long sheath has been positioned in the pulmonary artery, a basket retrieval device probably has the best chance of both grabbing and partially collapsing a large umbrella enough to withdraw it into a very large sheath. Although the device can be captured relatively easily with the basket retrieval device, the downside of this device in this situation is that, once captured, if the basket with the device cannot be drawn completely into the sheath, the device often cannot be released from the basket! This leaves the patient with the umbrella in the pulmonary artery, but now with the umbrella "permanently" attached to the retrieval catheter passing through the entire right heart and extending out of the body—again creating a much more urgent and complex surgical situation.

A retrieval snare represents an alternative retrieval device and technique that may be preferable for the retrieval of an ASD device from the pulmonary artery. This still requires that the device be withdrawn completely into the sheath before it is withdrawn through the pulmonary artery. By grasping a single leg or several adjacent legs of the device, the crumpled umbrella is "elongated" as it is pulled out of the tissues. This elongation of the umbrella may facilitate withdrawing the umbrella into a *very large* diameter, *reinforced*, long sheath. If the device in the pulmonary artery cannot be withdrawn into the sheath completely, it usually can be released from the snare more reliably and, in turn, the *catheter* retrieval abandoned more easily and safely.

In the majority of cases, when a large CardioSEAL™ or STARFlex™ device embolizes into and/or through a ventricle, surgical retrieval is recommended. This makes the positioning and eventual release of these devices for ASD occlusions even more critical.

Helex™ ASD device

A more recent addition in the United States to the armamentarium for the closure of the atrial septal defect is the Helex™ device (W. L. Gore & Associates, Flagstaff, AZ). This is an entirely new concept with new design features to overcome some of the shortcomings of the other devices[20]. The deployed device is basically round. This shape conforms more to the shape of the usual ASD and to the shape of the atrial septum. It has no sharp edges and a very low profile after implant. The Helex™ device is delivered through a 9-French delivery "catheter" *without* the use of an additional long sheath and it is totally retrievable even after full deployment of the device and even after its "release" onto the septum from the "rigid" portion of the delivery catheter.

The Helex™ ASD device is a long strip or "curtain" of expanded polytetrafluoroethylene (ePTFE) fabric (W. L. Gore & Associates, Flagstaff, AZ). The "frame" of the device is a long Nitinol™ memory wire, which passes through a thin tubular fold along one edge of the long ePTFE "curtain". The Nitinol™ wire has an attachment loop and an eyelet at one end, a dense "central eyelet" at its center and a third "eyelet" at the distal end of the long wire. When in its "relaxed state" at body temperature, the Nitinol™ wire forms a very flat spiral or "helix", the outer circumferences of which forms two round circular disks at each end of the "helix". The "circular disks" are positioned on each side of the septum and connected through the atrial defect by the remainder of the spiral of the Nitinol™ wire and covering ePTFE material. The circular curtain of ePTFE fabric attached to this wire frame forms the two "end" disks. The continuous "curtain", when deployed over, and through, an atrial defect, covers the opening of the ASD with a "disk" on each side of the opening while the material of the "curtain" passing through the defect, adds additional occlusive material. The center of the "helix", along with the attached fabric, which runs through the defect between the two outer disks, acts as a partial centering mechanism.

The Helex™ comes in multiple sizes from 15 to 35 mm diameters in 5 mm increments. It is recommended that a ratio of device diameter to defect diameter of 1.7:1, or, preferably, 2:1 be used in choosing the size of the Helex™ device to be used. The Helex™ device comes from the manufacturer in its "relaxed", opened, circular, "helix" configuration and attached to the delivery system. The delivery system includes an outer, 9-French delivery catheter that has a ~90° curve at its distal end. This curve facilitates passage of the catheter from the right to the left atrium and produces a better alignment of the device against the septum during the extrusion of the device. Within the delivery catheter there is an inner control catheter, which, in turn, has a central "mandril", both of which pass completely through the delivery catheter. There also is a nylon retrieval cord which passes from the outside of the proximal end of the control catheter, through the entire length of the control catheter adjacent to the mandrel to the distal end of the control catheter, through the proximal eye on the device and then back to *connect to* the distal end of the shaft of the control catheter.

The diagnostic "catheterization" procedure for the atrial septal defect is the same as for other ASD occlusion devices. General anesthesia is used primarily because of the concomitant use of TEE for the implant. As with the other ASD occlusion devices, intracardiac echo (ICE) during the delivery and implant may obviate the need for TEE and, in turn, general anesthesia. An arterial monitoring line and *two* venous catheters are used. The right heart catheterization is performed to quantitate the ASD and rule out associated defects. An angiographic "marker" catheter is introduced from the left groin and an angiocardiogram is performed with an injection into the right upper pulmonary vein or in a right pulmonary artery, with one X-ray tube positioned in a shallow LAO–Cranial view in an attempt to cut the septum on edge. "Non-stretched" atrial defects are sized with a NuMED™ "static" sizing balloon (NuMED Inc., Hopkinton, NY) introduced through the right groin similarly to the sizing described previously for the CardioSEAL/STARFlex™ devices. The atrial defect size is measured radiographically and by TEE or ICE, while the sizing balloon is inflated in the defect.

The Helex™ device is delivered from the manufacturer attached to the delivery system in the "deployed" state with the circular Helex™ extending just beyond the tip of the delivery catheter. The Helex™ must be loaded into the delivery system before use. The delivery system is flushed through a Tuohy™ valved/side port attached at the proximal end of the delivery catheter and then placed on a continuous flush during the loading of the device. With the device placed in a bowl of flush solution and held completely "under water", the mandrel is advanced out of the delivery catheter in small, 5–7 mm increments. As the mandrel is advanced in this manner the most proximal part of the circular Helex™ straightens away from the tip of the catheter while the fold in the "curtain" covers the mandrel. As each 1–2 cm are straightened, the inner control catheter along with the mandrel and the straightened portion of the device are withdrawn into the delivery catheter until the still curved part of the device again touches the end of the delivery catheter. Each time the device is straightened and withdrawn back into the delivery catheter, entrapped air bubbles are squeezed out of the fabric and flushed out of the system by the continuous flush. Once the bubbles are cleared, the mandrel is advanced again, straightening an additional segment of the device and the straightened segment is withdrawn into the catheter. The procedure is repeated until the entire device is elongated, "straightened" around the mandrel and withdrawn completely into the delivery catheter.

Once completely within the delivery catheter and when the catheter has been flushed thoroughly, the delivery catheter is introduced through a short, 9-French sheath in the right femoral vein and advanced through the right atrium and manipulated into the left atrium. The delivery catheter with the loaded device within it is advanced directly through the defect and into the left atrium without the use of an additional long sheath. By eliminating the need for the long sheath delivery technique *many* of the potential sources of air/clot embolization are reduced. The angiographic catheter from the opposite groin is positioned in the left atrium at this time.

The position of the delivery catheter in the left atrium is confirmed on the TEE or ICE image. The deployment of the Helex™ device begins by advancing both the mandrel *and* the inner control catheter together several centimeters out of the tip of the outer delivery catheter, which is positioned in the left atrium. The mandrel then is withdrawn the same distance, allowing the Nitinol™ frame of the device to bow away from the mandrel and begin to coil. The inner control catheter and mandrel (and device) again are advanced 1–2 cm and the mandril withdrawn the same distance, uncoiling more device. This procedure is repeated until the *centering eye* on the wire of the device (at the center of the Helex™) reaches the tip of the delivery catheter. This "eye" should be clearly visible on fluoroscopy.

At this point, the angiographic catheter is withdrawn until its tip is just within the defect. The delivery catheter with the half opened device, is withdrawn until the now deployed left atrial "disk" touches and is pulled very gently against the septum as seen by fluoroscopy and TEE/ICE. A small, forceful, hand injected angiocardiogram is recorded through the separate angiographic catheter to confirm the position of the left atrial disk on the septum. Similarly to the deployment of the other devices, the left atrial disk usually does *not* lie exactly flat on the septum. The angiographic catheter is withdrawn out of the defect.

At this point, the inner control catheter and mandrel are held in place while, first, the outer *delivery catheter* is withdrawn several *centimeters* into the right atrium. The mandrel, alone, then is withdrawn 1–2 cm, which allows the right atrial "disk" of the device to begin to uncoil away from the mandrel on the right side of the septum. Again, by slowly and meticulously advancing the inner control catheter and mandrel together and then alternately, withdrawing the mandrel the same distance, the entire right atrial "disk" is deployed. The distal end of the inner control catheter is radio-opaque and is seen as it is advanced toward the deployed disk. All of this time the left atrial disk is observed on fluoroscopy and TEE/ICE and maintained firmly against the left side of the septum. The complete deployment of the right atrial "disk" is recognized on fluoroscopy when the opaque tip of the inner *control catheter* reaches the right atrial disk and the complete circles of two wire "disks" approximate each other on the opposite sides of the septum. Simultaneous with this appearance, the *proximal* eyelet of the device becomes positioned at the end of the catheter and closely approximates the other two eyelets. The "locking" wire with the mandrel within the inner delivery catheter still appears straight *within the mandrel* and should be passing through all three eyelets.

The angiographic catheter is maneuvered adjacent to the right atrial disk and a repeat angiocardiogram recorded. If the device does not appear to be in the proper position, or if there is a residual leak, the device is moved and repositioned slightly on the septum by rotating the delivery catheter slightly while it still is attached to the device. If the device is out of position completely with one or the other "disk" prolapsing through the defect, or the device pulls completely through the defect, the device is withdrawn back into the catheter. This is accomplished by repeating the exact procedures used when initially *loading* the device into the delivery catheter (reversing the device extrusion procedure). Once the device is back in the delivery catheter, the delivery catheter is repositioned into the left atrium and the delivery procedure repeated with the same device, or the whole system is withdrawn through the short sheath and the procedure started with a more appropriate device.

Once the device is in the proper position as seen by TEE/ICE and/or angiography, preparations are made to activate the locking mechanism. The outer *delivery* catheter is advanced over the inner control catheter until the tip of the outer catheter is against the center of the right atrial "disk". The red cap that holds the retrieval cord at the proximal end of the control catheter is removed and, while holding the *outer delivery catheter and mandrel in place*, the inner control catheter is withdrawn 1–2 cm and then re-advanced back against the proximal (right atrial) device. This maneuver loosens the retrieval cord and provides a loop of this cord at the distal end of the control catheter. The red cap is reattached to the control catheter to secure the proximal end of the retrieval cord outside of the body.

While recording on biplane angiography and observing the entire device and delivery catheter very closely, the inner control catheter is pushed against the proximal eyelet of the device while the outer delivery catheter (only) is withdrawn 2–3 cm off the inner control catheter, following which the mandrel is withdrawn out of the device. This often takes a moderate amount of pull on the mandrel and requires a simultaneous very firm and precise fixation of both the delivery catheter and the inner control catheter in order to prevent the device from being pushed or pulled through the septum while the mandrel is pulled forcefully during this release. As the mandrel releases, it "pops" free and pulls back into the catheter and several centimeters away from the device. At the same time, the relatively straight inner catheter tends to move forward and, in turn, has the possibility of displacing the entire system/device cephalad slightly. The previously short straight locking wire, which still is within the distal end of the inner control catheter, now assumes a slight "curve". This curve remains on the end of the catheter while the locking wire still is within the control catheter and as long as the catheter still is against the device. When satisfied that the three eyelets still are "in line" and that the now slightly curved locking wire is passing through all three eyelets, the inner control catheter is withdrawn just enough to "uncover" the locking wire. This allows the locking wire to form a tight loop on the proximal side of the device and pulls the three eyelets together while also releasing the device from the delivery system. The device usually repositions abruptly as the locking loop forms. This repositioning usually is into an even more secure position and alignment on the septum. Even after this "release", the device still can be moved on the septum and in turn, repositioned slightly if desired.

The mandrel serves no more function and is removed completely from the system. The device still is "tethered" loosely to the delivery catheter by the safety suture passing through the eyelet at the proximal end of the Nitinol™ "frame" wire of the device. The *outer* delivery catheter carefully is advanced back against the device over this safety suture. Once the catheter is against the device, the device can be moved slightly on the septum by rotating the delivery catheter (which turns the curved tip) a small amount. If the device comes loose from the septum and/or cannot be placed in a satisfactory position over the defect, it still is attached by the safety suture and is completely retrievable as long as the safety suture remains in place through the proximal eyelet.

Once satisfied that the device is in a secure position and is occluding the defect sufficiently, the retrieval cord (safety suture) is removed. If the mandrel was not removed completely before, it is removed before removing the retrieval cord. With the outer delivery catheter loosely against the device, the red locking cap is removed and the inner control catheter is slowly withdrawn. This pulls on the end of the retrieval cord that is attached to the distal end of the catheter and withdraws the other, loose end through the outer catheter, through the eyelet and away from the device.

Retrieval of the Helex™ ASD device

After full deployment and *release* from the delivery catheter, but before the withdrawal of the inner catheter and retrieval cord, the long suture running through the proximal eyelet of the device still attaches the Helex™ device to the inner catheter. If not satisfied with the placement and/or the degree of occlusion by the device and/or if the Helex™ dislodges from the defect while it is being observed/manipulated after release from the delivery catheter, the Helex™ device still can be retrieved using the retaining suture. The device is withdrawn back into the delivery catheter by traction placed together on the suture and the inner control catheter. Traction on the suture and the inner control catheter pulls the most proximal eyelet at the very proximal end of the spiral device back into the delivery catheter, and with some effort the entire device usually can be "uncoiled" and withdrawn into the catheter. As the device is pulled into the delivery catheter it uncoils into its "loaded" straight configuration. As it is uncoiling, the device appears to "snap apart" approximately every centimeter as it uncoils. Even if the device does not withdraw completely into the delivery catheter, it is straightened as it is withdrawn into the femoral vein with the catheter and it can be withdrawn along with, but outside of, the catheter through the short venous introductory sheath.

Even after the retrieval cord is withdrawn, the Helex™ still can be retrieved. The original delivery catheter is replaced with a larger diameter (11-French or larger) long sheath for the retrieval. If the device is still positioned on the septum with the proximal eyelet facing the right atrium, a snare retrieval catheter is used to grasp the device, preferably around the eyelet. If the eyelet is grasped, the device is "uncoiled" exactly as when pulling on the retrieval cord. If an end or eyelet cannot be grasped, the Nitinol™ frame is grasped anywhere along its circumference with a bioptome or grabber retrieval device. When a loose "end" of the device is grasped, the device is withdrawn similarly to using the retrieval cord. When any other area of the Nitinol™ "frame" is grasped and pulled forcefully, the "coiled" configuration of the device begins to unravel and frequently it "unlocks" the device as it straightens. Even when it cannot be uncoiled, the flexible wire frame of the Helex™ can be bent and pulled completely into a very large diameter sheath. With the ability to pull an errant device completely into the retrieval sheath, it is reasonably safe to retrieve a Helex™ device from a pulmonary artery when the large sheath can be positioned through the right ventricle and into the pulmonary artery before the device is grasped.

Sideris ASD Button Occluder

The Sideris ASD "Button" Device™ (Pediatric Cardiology Custom Medical Devices, Athens, Greece) is yet another ASD occlusion device. The Button™ device has been in multiple international trials throughout the world and has had extensive clinical use for over a decade outside of the United States. The Button™ ASD occluder currently has CE approval for clinical use in Europe[21]. The ASD Button Device™ has had at least one US FDA clinical pilot trial but, like most ASD devices at the present time, is available for ASD closure in the US only in investigational trials. This device began as a single square of 1/16″ thick polyurethane foam sewn onto an "X" shaped skeleton or frame of two, equal length, crossed pieces of stiff, 0.018″ teflon-coated, spring guide wire[22]. The length of the wires of the frame determines the size of the device. Each of the wires of the frame has a 2 mm floppy portion at each end. The two wires of the frame are attached at their centers to make the "crossed" frame of the left atrial "occluder disk" or umbrella with the foam disk sewn to the frame. The left atrial disk or "occluder" is held against the septum by a separate "counter occluder" piece. The counter occluder originally was a single bar of relatively stiff spring guide wire but now is a narrow rhomboid of similar wire, which is covered with polyurethane. The counter occluder is held against the occluder umbrella by a unique connecting or "buttoning" mechanism.

With the initial "Button" device, there was a suture knot or "spring button" on one small, 2 mm loop of suture attached to the center of the proximal (right atrial) side of the left atrial "occluder disk". The fourth generation device has two suture knots situated between three small suture loops in line at the center of the proximal side of the occluder. The suture knots form the "buttons" for the attachment of the device. The counter occluder has a small piece of latex, which forms a plug *attached* to the center of the wire bar of the *counter occluder*. The latex plug on the counter occluder has a hole in it, which forms the "button hole" for the "buttons" on the occluder. A "through-and-through" "control suture" passes through the latex plug, through a length of a fine hollow "loading wire", through the most proximal suture loop on the "occluder", and then passes back through the "loading wire" and the latex plug at the proximal end of the hollow "loading" wire. The latex plug on the counter occluder along with the counter occluder is advanced over the control suture and loading wire with an end-hole, "pusher" catheter. When the counter occluder, which is advancing over the loading wire, reaches the defect and the occluding umbrella, the latex plug is pushed forcefully with the pusher catheter and *over* the two knots or "buttons" on the occluder to "button" the counter occluder to the occluder.

The left atrial occluder, the attaching mechanism and the counter occluder all have been modified over the past decade, now through four or five "generations" of the device[23]. The buttons were made radio-opaque on the second-generation device. The attaching mechanism on the occluder now has two radio-opaque knots on triple suture loops. The knots or "buttons" are between each of the small loops and each are 4 mm apart. The counter occluder now is a narrow rhomboid of two strands of the teflon-coated wire and is covered with a rhomboid-shaped piece of polyurethane foam. The counter occluder now is pushed over both "buttons" for a more secure attachment. The first four generations of Button™ ASD devices had no centering mechanism and required a 2:1, device to defect diameter ratio. The fourth generation ASD Button™ device is available in 25–60 mm diameters in five millimeter increments (only up to 55 mm are available in the US). The fourth generation device now also is delivered with an additional, over the wire delivery technique. There are several recent additional modifications of what is still the fourth generation device. The most recent modification has an additional large loop of spring wire attached to the center of the proximal side of the occluder to facilitate centering, and has a round disk of polyurethane on the original "X" frame. This most recent modification is called the "COD™" (Centering On Demand™) Button device.

As with most of the other ASD devices, the Button™ ASD device is delivered to the ASD through a long sheath using fluoroscopic and TEE or ICE guidance. A long sheath with a back-bleed valve/flush port is used and the same precautions for clearing the sheath of air and clots are used as are used with the other devices. The earlier generations of this device were very flexible and compressible. Because of this and the compressibility of the polyurethane foam, they could be folded to a very small diameter and, in turn, delivered through a much smaller sheath than any of the other tested ASD occlusion devices at the time. The newer generation devices still have square umbrellas of polyurethane, but with a larger or thicker counter occluder and with the additional centering wires, they are not as compressible. Depending upon the size of the occluder, an 8–11-French long delivery sheath is now required for their delivery.

The exact size of the ASD now is measured by a static, non-stretched, balloon sizing technique, which is described previously and in detail under the description of the CardioSEAL/STARFlex™ technique. After the defect is sized accurately with the balloon, the sizing balloon is replaced with the long delivery sheath/dilator over the exchange wire, which is positioned in the left upper pulmonary vein. The dilator and then the wire are removed cautiously and separately, observing precautions to prevent the introduction of any air. When "the over the wire" technique is to be used, the floppy tip of an exchange length 0.021" Amplatz™ wire is advanced through the sheath/dilator and positioned into a left upper pulmonary vein before the *dilator* is removed. The wire remains in this position through the sheath during the delivery and implant of the occluder device.

The occluder (left atrial disk) and the counter occluder are delivered separately, however, both components are delivered through the same long sheath. A very long loop of 0.008" nylon "control suture" passes from proximally to distally through a long, metal, hollow "loading wire" which eventually extends through the entire length of the sheath. The control suture then passes through the most proximal, small loop or eye at the end of the "button" sutures (at the center of the right side of the "occluder") and then back through and out of the proximal end of the long, hollow "loading wire". The attaching suture "eye" is proximal on, and in line with, the buttons at the center of the left sided occluder umbrella.

The corners of the occluder are folded manually toward and into the hub of the long sheath or into a short segment of sheath of the same size, which is used as a loader in order to introduce the device through a back-bleed valve. The entire device is introduced into the proximal hub of the long sheath. If the "over the wire" technique is used, the proximal end of the wire, the distal end of which is positioned in the pulmonary vein, is passed through the fabric at the center of the "occluder" before the "occluder" is folded into the loader/delivery sheath. The wire passes through a small hole pierced immediately adjacent to the central, cross pieces of the frame of the occluder. An end-hole "pusher" catheter is advanced over the long, "hollow wire" which contains the control suture attached to the "button loop". The pusher catheter is advanced over the "hollow wire", the long suture and the extra "guide wire" (if used) until the tip of the pusher catheter is up against the center of the folded "occluder". The pusher catheter, which now contains the "hollow wire" with the control suture, is advanced into the delivery sheath behind the folded "occluder". It also is advanced over the long exchange Amplatz™ wire (Cook Inc., Bloomington, IN), if the "over the wire" delivery is used. The folded occluder is pushed through the long sheath with the pusher catheter until the occluder is pushed *completely out of the sheath* and into the left atrium, where it opens and "hangs" loosely. The control suture within the hollow wire is withdrawn firmly against the tip of the delivery sheath, which, in turn, pulls the open left atrial "occluder" against the end of the sheath. The long wire, which is fixed in a left upper pulmonary vein as part of the "over the wire" addition to the delivery system, keeps the occluder more or less in line with the septum and away from the mitral valve after it is pushed out of the long sheath and free into the left atrium and before the occluder is pulled back against the atrial septum.

When pulled back against the tip of the sheath with the control suture, the occluder (left atrial disk) aligns perpendicular to the end of the sheath. The sheath, with the occluder against it, is pulled back against the septum and, in doing so, the device should cover the atrial defect. When satisfied with the position by TEE/ICE and/or an angiocardiogram performed through a separate catheter, the pusher catheter is withdrawn from the long delivery sheath while tension is maintained continually on the control suture (and thus the "occluder") against the septum. Once the pusher catheter has been removed, the central latex *plug* on the *counter occluder* is loaded over the hollow "loading wire" with the contained control suture, but adjacent to the long Amplatz™ guide wire (if the over the wire technique is being used). The counter occluder is angled lengthwise and parallel to the control suture/

loading wire by manual manipulation, introduced into the sheath and then pushed to the end of the sheath with the original pusher catheter. All of the time during the introduction and delivery of the counter occluder, traction must be maintained on the control suture/hollow wire in order to maintain the "occluder" disk against the septum. While the occluder device, pusher catheter, control suture and loading wire are fixed in position the sheath is withdrawn off the counter occluder, which allows the counter occluder to realign perpendicular to the delivery wire. The sheath and the pusher catheter are re-advanced over the still taut, control suture/wire and up against the now perpendicular counter occluder. With a firm push on the sheath and pusher catheter while the control suture is held taut, the latex plug of the counter occluder is pushed over the two suture "buttons", which are on the suture loops that are attached to the proximal side of the "occluder". The counter occluder is advanced over the buttons one at a time until the counter occluder is seen and felt to snap over both "buttons". This locks the counter occluder to the occluder and fixes the occluder on the septum. Since the occluder and counter occluder both are very flexible and still are attached to the control suture, at any time up to this point in the procedure, the whole device can be withdrawn back into the sheath and out of the body by pulling the control suture/wire back into the sheath.

Once satisfied with the position and the stability of the device, the pusher catheter and then the "hollow wire" over the control suture are withdrawn off the control suture. The "over the wire" Amplatz™ wire, which passes through the fabric at the center of the occluder, is withdrawn. *One* of the two ends of the loop of control suture is pulled while the other end is released and fed into the introductory sheath. This pulls the entire length of suture through and out of the eye on the occluder and away from the entire device, releasing the device onto the septum. The device and septum are interrogated by TEE/ICE. When satisfied with the position and the degree of occlusion, the delivery sheath and other catheters are removed. The patient is given four doses of intravenous antibiotics over 24 hours and then discharged on 82 mg of aspirin per day for six months.

The trials of the earlier generations of Button™ devices had a high incidence of residual (or recurrent) leak and of embolization from poor fixation and/or "unbuttoning" of the device. Because of early problems of "unbuttoning" and, in turn, embolization of the device, the Button™ device underwent several significant changes, and now it is in its fifth generation of change since it underwent the initial, authorized, FDA pilot study. The fifth generation "Button™" device has been used in many patients in many centers throughout the rest of the world outside of the United States, and in a few patients in trials in the US. The current generation Button™ device has not undergone an FDA IDE clinical trial with any independent, outside, quality control monitoring.

The Button™ device has several advantages. It reportedly is less expensive than the other devices. Because of the flexibility of the arms of the Button™ devices, the devices are retrievable fairly easily even after distal embolization. The earlier generation devices could be delivered through significantly smaller delivery sheaths. However, even the current "generation" Button™ devices have significant disadvantages. The Button™ devices are not as robust as any of the other devices, they are square devices and coupled with the lack of an effective centering mechanism during delivery on the first four generation devices, they require at least a 2:1 ratio of device diameter to defect diameter for a secure implant. The polyurethane fabric on other types of occlusion devices had a tendency to shrink away from the support arms and leave gaps in the space in the angles between the arms. The earlier generation Button™ devices had a problem with "unbuttoning" and embolizing after implant, however, this reportedly has been corrected.

Retrieval of "Button" devices

One advantage of the design and *materials* of the Button™ devices is their relative ease of retrievability. There is control of the device, even after both the occluder and the counter occluder are deployed and attached to the septum and until the time that the control suture purposefully is withdrawn. The device can be withdrawn off the septum and back into the delivery sheath at any time during delivery and implant before the control suture is withdrawn. Even if the device pulls (or falls) out of the septal defect completely, the control suture maintains control of the device within the right atrium. If the device cannot be withdrawn out through the original delivery sheath, the control suture holds the device in a safe area where it can be grasped with a specific retriever device.

If the Button™ device cannot be withdrawn into the original sheath and/or if it displaces or embolizes after the withdrawal of the control suture, it still is retrievable with a catheter technique. A separate long sheath, which is several sizes *larger* in diameter than the introducer sheath, is introduced and advanced to the area where the loose device has lodged. When the displaced device is in the right atrium and still attached to the control wire, the larger long sheath is positioned adjacent to the still controlled device. A separate retrieval catheter/device is chosen that can grasp the device most effectively and according to the location and orientation of the device. The retrieval catheter is passed through the long, larger sheath, the errant device grasped and withdrawn into the long sheath and out of the body. Because of the more flexible materials of the Button™ devices, they usually can be distorted enough to be withdrawn completely into the larger long sheath regardless of how they are "captured" with the retrieval catheter. If the device has embolized into a pulmonary artery, the sheath must be advanced to the main pulmonary artery and if the device embolized systemically, the long sheath/dilator for retrieval is introduced into a femoral artery.

Guardian Angel™ ASD Occlusion Device

The Guardian Angel™ device (ev3, Plymouth, MN) is a new device developed partially on the concept of the earlier Angel Wings™ device (Microvena Corp., White Bear Lake, MN)[8]. The Guardian Angel™ device is a double-disk device with each of the two disks or umbrellas supported on an *outer*, rigid, Nitinol™ frame. The outer frames of the Guardian Angel™ "umbrellas" have an octagonal shape and no external eyelets at any of the corners of the octagons. This configuration eliminates the previous sharp corners of the Angel Wings™ device and creates disks that are almost "circular" in shape. The octagonal shape of the Guardian Angel™ device conforms to the more "circular" atrial septal defects, which it is designed to close. There are no *radial* support arms, however, the two fabric disks are attached to each other near the center of the device, but now with four sutures on the fabric disks, equally spaced from the centers of the disks. The connecting sutures vary in their distance from the center of the device according to the size of the defect/device and serve as an effective centering mechanism. The separate connecting sutures allow the device to collapse more easily than the circular suture of the original Angel Wings™ device.

The atrial septal defect is identified and sized using identical procedures to those used for the CardioSEAL/STARFlex devices. The Guardian Angel™ ASD occlusion device also is delivered through a large, previously positioned, delivery sheath similar to most of the other ASD occlusion devices. The long sheath is positioned in the left atrium using all of the precautions described previously with the other ASD devices. The Guardian Angel™ device is attached to the delivery catheter by four long sutures, each of which makes a loop through the corner of one quadrant of the proximal "umbrella" of the device. As the sutures are tightened, four alternate "corners" of the proximal "octagon" are drawn together similarly to the way in which the corners of the CardioSEAL™ are pulled together by the loading sutures. With continued traction, the proximal disk is collapsed further and withdrawn into the loader, and then, as further traction is applied to the sutures and the device is pulled further into the loader, the distal disk folds away from the tip of the loader and eventually is pulled into the loader.

Similar to the other devices for occlusion of atrial septal defects, as the device is advanced out of the long pre-positioned delivery sheath, the distal umbrella is extruded into the left atrium first. At the same time, the connected portion of the right atrial disk becomes withdrawn partially out of the tip of the long sheath by the expansion of the left atrial disk. This forms a slight funnel toward the tip of the sheath (and the septum), which serves to center the device in the defect. The long sheath and the device are withdrawn together as the center of the right-sided disk is being exposed. This draws the left atrial disk against the septum while the partially exposed portion of the right atrial disk serves to center the left atrial disk over the defect. The sheath alone then is withdrawn off the remainder of the device, which deploys the right atrial disk on the right side of the septum. The device still is attached to the delivery system by the four sutures and, if the position is not correct or the device pulls through the septum, the device can be withdrawn into the delivery sheath with these sutures.

Aside from this sparse amount of information, there are no published details on the loading, delivery and available sizes of this device. There also is no reported clinical experience with this device, but presumably, the more collapsible frame makes the device more retrievable even after it is released and the "rounder" shape and lack of rigid corners will prevent erosion into tissues, which was a problem with the Angel Wings™ devices. Presumably, the Guardian Angel™ device will enter regulated clinical trials in the not too distant future.

Sideris "frameless" occlusion procedure

Dr Sideris has reported a technique for the patching of both atrial and ventricular septal defects using a transcatheter procedure, but without the necessity of any implantable "frame" for the patch[24]. Reportedly, this technique is applicable to all sizes of atrial septal defects and can be used regardless of the amount of rim surrounding the defect. This procedure is unique and innovative but has not had any monitored and/or controlled use. What is known about the device and technique by this author is discussed in Chapter 32 under new, unique and potential future devices.

Multiple atrial septal defects

The presence of multiple atrial septal defects, particularly if the defects are remote from each other, previously represented absolute exclusion criteria for the use of atrial septal defect occlusion devices *during the protocol IDE* trials in the United States. In countries where the devices are in routine clinical use and, now in the US where several devices are out of "protocol trials", multiple defects have been closed during the same procedure and/or at sequential procedures using a variety of the ASD occlusion devices that are in use.

The exact approach to the closure of multiple defects depends upon several factors. The size of each of the defects and how close they are to each other determines whether both openings can be closed with one larger device overlapping both defects, or whether two (or more) separate devices are necessary. The size of the patient determines whether the particular septum can accommodate one very large device to cover multiple defects. Finally, the types of device that are available and being used in a particular center determine whether one device can be used to overlap two separate defects.

The size, exact location and adjacent structures of the multiple defects are documented with angiography, TEE or ICE in conjunction with the sizing balloons. Often it is helpful (necessary) to place separate static sizing balloons in each separate defect while visualizing and measuring the separate defects on both TEE/ICE and on the X-ray images on the fluoroscopy screen. When using two (or more) sizing balloons and in order to introduce a separate angiographic catheter and/or an ICE catheter, at least one additional venous sheath is introduced in addition to the number of sizing balloons that are in place.

Two separate, precisely sized, smaller devices placed over two separated holes may be preferable to attempting the occlusion with one *very* large (and over-sized) device. There is a greater chance of complete occlusion of several defects that are separated some distance from each other by using separate smaller (correctly sized) devices than with one large device. The one large device may be oversized for the septum, can encroach on adjacent (and vital) structures and still may not overlap both atrial defects *completely*. The ASD occlusion devices with small central hubs are better at overlapping several and/or even multiple *small, adjacent* defects that are within 5–8 mm of the major opening. The ASD occlusion devices with a large diameter central "hub" and/or a broad central connection for self-centering are less likely to overlap defects separated more than 5 mm from each other. When devices with large central hubs are used for multiple defects that are more than 4–5 mm from each other, two separate, smaller devices usually are used. When the separate atrial defects are very close to each other, a single, inflated, sizing balloon may "compress" the adjacent defects together and eliminate shunting, or a sizing balloon that is inflated to stretch-size one defect can disrupt a thin strip of tissue that is separating two adjacent defects and, in turn, coalesce the two defects into one larger opening. In either of those circumstances a single device with a "centering hub" that "stretches" into the major (or communicated) defect is used to occlude both defects. When two atrial defects are separated by a 3–4 mm strip of atrial septal tissue, the two defects can be joined by purposefully incising the strip of tissue with a blade catheter in order to form one larger, more central defect, which can then be occluded with one large device.

When two devices are used, particularly if the defects are fairly close together, the two separate delivery sheaths are placed across the two separate defects at the onset of the occlusion procedure. The delivery of the two sheaths initially prevents dislodgement of a device that was placed earlier while trying to position the second delivery system adjacent to the first device on the septum. The two devices can be *implanted* either in sequence or simultaneously. During "simultaneous" implants, the left atrial "disks" ("umbrellas") of both (or more) devices are opened in the left atrium *one at a time*. The position of the open left atrial disks in the left atrium are adjusted by to-and-fro movement of the delivery systems until the two left atrial umbrellas (disks) are adjacent to, and overlap each other, while still free in the left atrium. The two delivery systems with the attached devices adjacent to each other are withdrawn *together* and when the left atrial umbrella (disk) of *one* of the devices touches the septum, the right atrial umbrella of *that* device is opened. The second device is withdrawn against the first device and the right atrial disk of the second device opened. All of this simultaneous maneuvering of the devices is visualized on biplane fluoroscopy and TEE or ICE. The two devices create a challenging image for the echocardiographer. Usually when there is a significant discrepancy in the size of the defects, the devices purposefully are implanted separately and in succession, with the smaller device implanted first so that the larger device will overlap the smaller device on both sides of the septum rather than "butting" up against the edge of the other device.

Complications of ASD devices/occlusion procedures

Remarkably, significant complications are very infrequent as a result of the use of catheter-delivered ASD occlusion devices. One of the most serious potential hazards, which can result in permanent sequelae, is the embolization of air and/or particulate matter to a vital systemic organ (brain or heart!) during the delivery and implant of the devices. With all of the ASD occlusion devices, there are considerable wire, catheter, device and/or large sheath manipulations in the "systemic side" of the circulation. The patients receive systemic heparin to reduce (*but not eliminate!*) the chance of thrombi forming in catheters and sheaths and on the wires and devices. In addition, all sheaths and catheters are cleared meticulously of air and clot during each exchange of sheath/

dilator, wire, catheter and device and then the sheaths and catheters are maintained on a constant flush to keep them free of clots. Meticulous, extra precautions are taken to prevent the introduction of any air during each separate phase of every implant procedure. Hopefully, all of the various potential sources of air entering into the delivery systems have been experienced previously and now are understood so that adequate precautions can be taken to prevent them. These precautions were discussed in detail in the discussions of the delivery techniques for each of the various devices. These preventive measures and precautions for the exclusion of air *must* remain an essential part of each ASD occlusion procedure, no matter how "routine" these procedures become.

The delivery and implant of all of the catheter-delivered ASD occlusion devices require the introduction of, and at least a moderate amount of intravascular manipulation of, large and/or stiff wires, sheaths/dilators and/or delivery catheters. The large introductory sheaths for the sizing balloons, devices and the ICE catheters create a constant potential for complications at the introductory sites including bleeding, hematomas, localized aneurysms and fistulas. Although these local complications may not be totally preventable, meticulous attention to the details of the introductory technique and to the care of the introductory site when achieving hemostasis can reduce their incidence.

The intravascular maneuvering of large, stiff wires, sheaths and delivery catheters certainly creates the potential for vascular perforation. The larger, stiffer sheaths/dilators should always be advanced over a wire that has been positioned previously through a softer and more maneuverable catheter. ICE and delivery catheters are advanced through sheaths that are introduced over prepositioned catheters and then wires.

The very stiff exchange wires used to support the delivery of the sizing balloons and large sheaths have some potential complications of their own. The short, relatively stiff, "soft" tips of these wires can easily perforate vascular structures if the wires are not controlled very carefully. The very stiff wires, which pass through long and/or fairly acute curves within the vascular system, tend to assume their "straightened" configuration spontaneously on their own and, in doing so, "back out" of their secure distal locations. Once in position, these stiff wires must be held in place manually and purposefully. When a stiff wire does back out of its distal position, the bare wire alone *should not* be pushed back into its more distal location. First, an end-hole catheter is introduced over the wire and *the catheter* is manipulated back into the secure distal location. If a very stiff wire is advanced on its own, it very easily can perforate the wall of a chamber or vessel and potentially cause a pericardial and/or a pleural bleed. If a catheter and/or sheath are advanced over the wire that is in the pericardium, tamponade definitely will follow.

All of the implanted ASD devices expose a finite amount of fabric and/or metal to the circulation and all of the materials impart varying degrees of irregularity to the surfaces of the devices. This results in the potential for thrombus formation on all of these devices. Although there have been sporadic reports of thrombi being seen on both the right and left surfaces of various ASD occluding devices, these fortunately have been extremely rare, and associated with permanent adverse events even more rarely.

When implanting any device, it appears prudent to create the lowest possible profile and the best possible conformity of the device to the surface of the septum immediately after implant by paying attention to how the device sits on the septum, not just whether it stays put or not. All of the patients with catheter-implanted ASD devices are treated with heparin anticoagulation during the implant procedure and at least aspirin "antiplatelet" therapy after discharge. Some centers advocate the use of additional platelet ADP receptor antagonists for an additional three to six months, but no study has demonstrated the efficacy of this. Each device should be scrutinized for masses (thrombi) on the surface as well as for residual leaks at follow-up. Any "mass" on the surface is treated with vigorous systemic anticoagulation until the mass disappears or the mass is determined not to be a thrombus or until the device is removed.

Each of the ASD occluder devices has its own idiosyncrasies in terms of complications. Each of the ASD occlusion devices has the potential for dislodgement and embolization during and after implant. This complication and the potential retrieval of the embolized devices were discussed previously under the sections on each individual device, and are not repeated here. Remarkably, when ASD devices have embolized, none of them have resulted in significant hemodynamic compromise even when a large device passed through or lodged in a ventricle. The major adverse event from an embolized ASD device is that the patient may have to undergo surgical removal of the errant device (and the closure of the ASD). Although no "fun" for the patient, and the purpose of the implant procedure was to avoid surgery, surgery for the closure of an ASD is *not* a catastrophe and still is considered an "accepted alternative therapy" for the closure of an ASD. What would be a relatively uncomplicated surgical retrieval of a device and straightforward closure of an ASD *can be made* significantly more complicated and serious by an ill-advised attempt at retrieval of an embolized device—particularly if the device embolized to the pulmonary artery and/or into either ventricle.

Erosion through adjacent structures has occurred following occlusions with several different ASD occlusion devices. The ASDOS™ and the Angel Wings™ devices, which were the two devices most responsible for this complication, were withdrawn from clinical use and are not discussed in this text. Several cases of pericardial effusion (± tamponade) have occurred with the Amplatzer™ ASD device and the CardioSEAL/STARFlex™ devices. These events are extremely rare and were due to erosion through the wall of the atrium into adjacent areas. More information still is necessary to determine why the very few Amplatzer™ and CardioSEAL/STARFlex™ devices caused the erosion while thousands of other, presumably identical, devices caused no such problems. Until such information is available, each patient should be observed very specifically for any signs of effusion/tamponade following implant of any ASD occlusion device. Most of these erosions occurred within the first 24 hours after implant, but late erosion has been reported as long as 3 years following the implant.

Fractured legs were found fairly frequently during routine follow-up evaluations of the earlier Clamshell™ devices. Although these fractures did not produce any documented, significant adverse events with over 12 years of follow-up, the Clamshell™ devices also were removed from the market. The Clamshell™ device was extensively re-engineered in design and materials into, first the CardioSEAL™, and then the STARFlex™ devices. Even these devices have had fractures of the legs, but with a markedly decreased incidence of fractures and with a much later appearance of the few fractures that did occur. The fractures in the CardioSEAL™ and STARFlex™ devices did not occur until after the devices were fixed securely on the septum, and on close follow-up, these later fractures have had no clinical implications, but should be noted and reported to the manufacturer.

The right atrial legs of the CardioSEAL/STARFlex™ devices can be entrapped by long and/or redundant Eustachian valve tissue during and after implant. This event and its prevention are discussed earlier in the chapter along with the CardioSEAL™ and STARFlex™ delivery techniques. This problem should be avoidable during the delivery of the devices by holding the Eustachian valve away from the septum during implant. If the Eustachian valve does become trapped inadvertently, the device can be "freed" from the entrapping tissue with a separate balloon dilation catheter as described earlier in the discussion of the CardioSEAL/STARFlex™ devices. An alternative to freeing the trapped Eustachian tissue immediately is to do nothing further at the time of implant! If the device legs remain malpositioned over time and particularly if the trapped Eustachian valve is creating any right to left shunt, release of the entrapped Eustachian tissue with a dilation balloon can be performed even after several months, when the device should be seated far more securely in the atrial septum.

Conclusion

The ASD occluding devices discussed in this chapter are those devices that have been developed and/or already are in clinical use. Some ASD occlusion devices, like the King–Mills™ device, the Rashkind™ ASD device, the Clamshell™ ASD device, the ASDOS™ and the Angel Wings™ devices have come and gone and are only of historical interest. Several of the ASD occlusion devices discussed in this chapter not only are available but currently are accepted as the standard of care for the treatment of atrial septal defects in most of the world outside of the United States.

FDA approval of the Amplatzer™ ASD device in the United States in 2001 set an entirely new precedent for the FDA as the first purely elective, implantable device approved, specifically for a congenital heart defect in children. The CardioSEAL™ device received a restricted FDA approval in the United States for closure of the patent foramen ovale, but not specifically for the ASD. Several other ASD occlusion devices are in, and/or have undergone successful clinical FDA, IDE trials in the United States and are awaiting FDA decisions for clinical use. With some understanding of the uniqueness of both the lesion and the pediatric and congenital patients, a reasonable decision from the FDA could result in the availability by the time of this publication of at least one more of these devices being approved for the elective transcatheter device closure of the secundum ASD in the United States.

Similar to the way the King–Mills™ ASD device and the original Rashkind™ hooked ASD device led to the development of the current ASD devices, these current devices undoubtedly will stimulate the future development of more effective and even safer catheter-delivered ASD occluders. Along with that, hopefully a more enlightened and expedient approval process will evolve so that even in the United States pediatric and congenital heart patients can benefit from their availability. As already has occurred with the correction of the PDA, surgical repair of most centrally located ASDs *should be* relegated to the annals of historical medicine at least by the end of this decade.

References

1. King TD and Mills NL. Nonoperative closure of atrial septal defects. *Surgery* 1974; **75**: 383–388.
2. Mills NL and King TD. Late follow-up of nonoperative closure of secundum atrial septal defects using the King–Mills double-umbrella device. *Am J Cardiol* 2003; **92**(3): 353–355.
3. Rashkind WJ and Cuaso CC. Transcatheter closure of atrial septal defects in children. *Proc Assoc Europ Pediatr Cardiol* 1977; **13**: 49.

4. Lock JE *et al*. Transcatheter closure of atrial septal defects. Experimental studies. *Circulation* 1989; **79**(5): 1091–1099.
5. Latson LA *et al*. Transcatheter closure of ASD—early results of multicenter trial of the Bard clamshell septal occluder. *Circulation* (Supp) 1991; **84**(II-544): 2161.
6. Hausdorf G *et al*. Transcatheter closure of secundum atrial septal defects with the atrial septal defect occlusion system (ASDOS): initial experience in children. *Heart* 1996; **75**(1): 83–88.
7. Sievert H *et al*. Transcatheter closure of atrial septal defect and patent foramen ovale with ASDOS device (a multi-institutional European trial). *Am J Cardiol* 1998; **82**(11): 1405–1413.
8. O'Laughlin MP. Microvena atrial septal defect occlusion device—update 2000. *J Interv Cardiol* 2001; **14**(1): 77–80.
9. Hellenbrand WE *et al*. Transesophageal echocardiographic guidance of transcatheter closure of atrial septal defect. *Am J Cardiol* 1990; **66**(2): 207–213.
10. Rashkind WJ *et al*. Nonsurgical closure of patent ductus arteriosus: clinical application of the Rashkind PDA Occluder System. *Circulation* 1987; **75**(3): 583–592.
11. Gu X *et al*. A new technique for sizing of atrial septal defects. *Catheter Cardiovasc Interv* 1999; **46**(1): 51–57.
12. Kreutzer J *et al*. Healing response to the Clamshell device for closure of intracardiac defects in humans. *Catheter Cardiovasc Interv* 2001; **54**(1): 101–111.
13. Sharafuddin M *et al*. Transvenous closure of secundum atrial septal defects: preliminary results with a new self-expanding nitinol prosthesis in a swine model. *Circulation* 1997; **95**: 2162–2168.
14. Bjornstad PG *et al*. Interventional closure of atrial septal defects with the Amplatzer™ device: first clinical experience. *Cardiol Young* 1997; **7**(3): 277–283.
15. Levi DS and Moore JW. Embolization and retrieval of the Amplatzer septal occluder. *Catheter Cardiovasc Interv* 2004; **61**(4): 543–547.
16. Kreutzer J *et al*. Acute animal studies of the STARFlex system: a new self-centering cardioSEAL septal occluder. *Catheter Cardiovasc Interv* 2000; **49**(2): 225–233.
17. Carminati M *et al*. A European multicentric experience using the CardioSeal and Starflex double umbrella devices to close interatrial communication holes within the oval fossa. *Cardiol Young* 2000; **10**(5): 519–526.
18. Hausdorf G *et al*. Transcatheter closure of atrial septal defect with a new flexible, self-centering device (the STARFlex Occluder). *Am J Cardiol* 1999; **84**(9): 1113–1116, A10.
19. McMahon CJ *et al*. Steerable control of the eustachian valve during transcatheter closure of secundum atrial septal defects. *Catheter Cardiovasc Interv* 2000; **51**(4): 455–459.
20. Zahn EM *et al*. Development and testing of the Helex septal occluder, a new expanded polytetrafluoroethylene atrial septal defect occlusion system. *Circulation* 2001; **104**(6): 711–716.
21. Rao PS *et al*. International experience with secundum atrial septal defect occlusion by the buttoned device. *Am Heart J* 1994; **128**(5): 1022–1035.
22. Sideris EB *et al*. Transvenous atrial septal defect occlusion in piglets with a "buttoned" double-disk device. *Circulation* 1990; **81**(1): 312–318.
23. Rao PS *et al*. Results of transvenous occlusion of secundum atrial septal defects with the fourth generation buttoned device: comparison with first, second and third generation devices. International Buttoned Device Trial Group. *J Am Coll Cardiol* 2000; **36**(2): 583–592.
24. Sideris EB *et al*. From disk devices to transcatheter patches: the evolution of wireless heart defect occlusion. *J Interv Cardiol* 2001; **14**(2): 211–214.

29 Occlusion of the patent foramen ovale (PFO), atrial baffle fenestrations and miscellaneous intracavitary communications

Occlusion of the patent foramen ovale

The patent foramen ovale (PFO) usually is a very small *potential* opening in the atrial septum where the septum primum has not completely sealed the embryologic reopening of the ostium secundum in the septum secundum (Figure 29.1). In a PFO, as apposed to an atrial septal defect, the septum primum tissue, which constitutes the "valve of the foramen", is sufficient in size to cover the entire ostium secundum, but at the same time has not *sealed* the opening on the left side of the septum. Under the conditions of normal hemodynamics with higher left atrial than right atrial pressures, the septum primum is forced against the foramen by the higher left atrial pressure and there is no actual *persistent* opening through the foramen. However, with any, even transient increase in *right atrial* pressure, this flap or "valve" can be pushed from right to left, pushed *away* from the septum and forced open. This results in the shunting of blood (and anything else in the right atrium) from the right atrium to the left atrium.

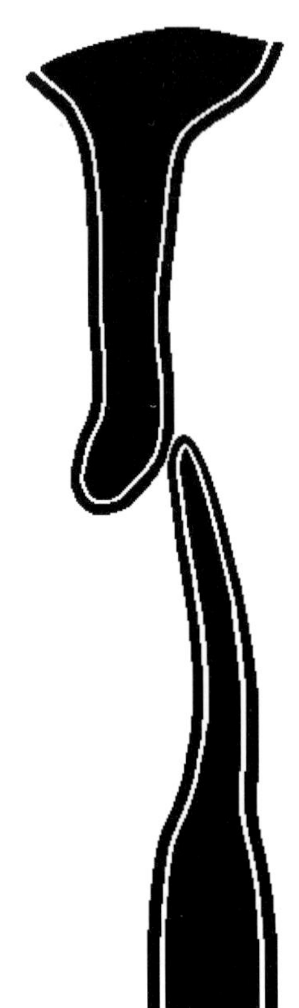

Figure 29.1 "On edge" view—"typical" patent foramen ovale with a short flap of septum primum.

The septum primum tissue of the "valve of the foramen" usually is considered to be very thin, mobile and to cover a small area. This very simplified stereotype of the patent foramen ovale is a very erroneous misconception of what often is a far more complex structure. Often, the tissues of the septum are thickened, tough and non-malleable, particularly in the older patient. The non-sealed septum primum often covers not only the original ostium secundum defect, but extends as a long hammock-like "flap" far cephalad onto the left side of the intact septum secundum and even up onto the wall of the aorta. This flap can create a long "tunnel" from the right atrial to the left atrial side of the septum (within the atrial septum!), which still can have a large potential opening into the left atrium at the top of the flap. When the long septum primum flap is lying against the septum secundum, the opening as visualized is small or even closed and, in turn, the PFO is conceived to be a very "small opening" (Figure 29.2a). The "probe patent" opening in the foramen, which is found in 15–25% of humans at postmortem examinations, indeed often is only 1–2 mm in diameter, however, in patients referred for PFO closure because of "cryptogenic" strokes, the balloon sized (but non-stretched!) potential *opening* is always greater than 5 mm and usually greater than 10 mm in diameter when the "flap" is pushed from right to left whenever the right atrial pressure exceeds the left atrial pressure (Figure 29.2b). Often, the "valve" of the foramen becomes redundant and develops an "aneurysm" of the

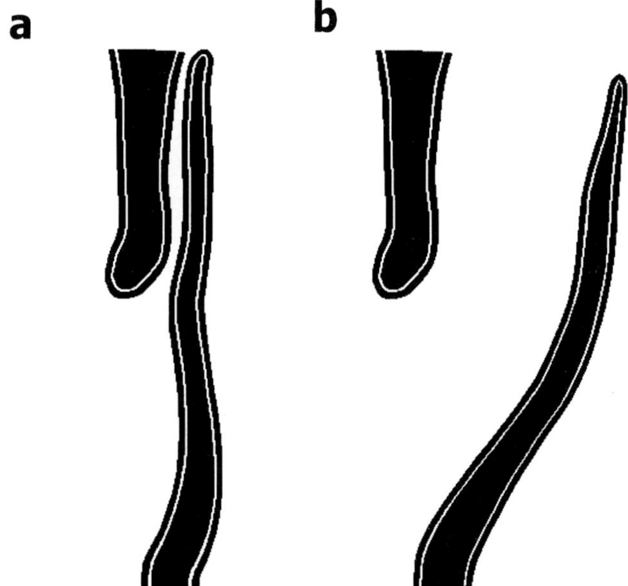

Figure 29.2 "On edge" view of atrial septum. (a) The long flap of a septum primum covering a patent foramen ovale. The flap effectively "seals" the foramen in the conditions of "usual" hemodynamics. (b) The long flap of septum primum pushed away from the foramen in the septum and opening the foramen ovale very widely as a consequence of elevated right atrial pressures.

atrial septum. A large, redundant septum primum can have several additional openings or "fenestrations" in it.

Indications for closure of the patent foramen ovale

Surgical closure of the PFO in patients with a documented PFO and who have suffered a cryptogenic stroke has been a recognized option as an alternative to chronic (lifetime) anticoagulation for many decades. Surgical closure requires an "open-heart" procedure with a thoracotomy, which makes this approach a somewhat extreme option that has risks of its own and, as a consequence, was not utilized too often. Closure of the PFO with a catheter-delivered device was documented to be feasible and safe in the clinical trials of several catheter-delivered ASD devices in the early 90s[1]. The ability to have a PFO closed with a catheterization procedure that was associated with very little risk or discomfort, made the option of PFO closure much more appealing to both the patients and the physicians caring for them.

As a consequence of the very successful PFO closures with several devices in both the clinical ASD trials and the high-risk trials for miscellaneous defects in the US, as well as the extensive use of multiple approved devices for PFO closure in Europe and, finally, with an intense appeal for a "PFO device" in the United States (US), the US FDA approved the CardioSEAL™ device and subsequently the Amplatzer™ PFO device for a humanitarian device exemption (HDE) use for the closure of the PFO in the US in 2000. This HDE approval is restricted to the closure of PFOs in patients who have a cryptogenic stroke and/or other embolic ischemic event with either a subsequent ischemic event and/or "failed medical management". The devices also are approved under the same HDE for closure of "fenestrations" in baffles in patients who have undergone "fenestrated Fontan" operations and for the closure of muscular ventricular septal defects. The HDE usage is not a protocol study, but it is required by the FDA that the local institutional review board (IRB) is "notified" of the intent to use the particular device for the particular group of patients. There is no specific protocol to follow nor specific follow-up of the patients required by the FDA.

The "subsequent ischemic event" and the "failed medical management" are not defined too precisely. Presumably, in a moral society, this does not require a second major stroke and/or loss of some other organ/function before the device "officially" can be used! Similarly, "failed medical management" presumably does not mandate a massive gastrointestinal or intracranial bleed to qualify for use of a device. Failure of medical management is interpreted as an inability to take the required medications and/or an interference with a reasonable life style and/or occupation. Thus "failure" would include the use of chronic warfarin anticoagulation in any active teenager, in any person involved in a very physical, violent or traumatic occupation and/or professional or recreational sport activity and any patients sensitive to the necessary medications.

Once the two devices became available for PFO closure under the HDE use and not in "protocol studies" in the US and, with the relative simplicity and safety of the procedure compared to surgery, interest in the closure of the PFO for cryptogenic stroke skyrocketed with both the physicians *and the affected patients*. The accepted standard therapy for patients with cryptogenic stroke in many centers in the US and around the world now is closure of the PFO with a catheter-delivered device.

In addition to those patients with a PFO and a documented prior embolic phenomenon who "officially" qualify for device closure of the PFO under the HDE criteria, there are many other patients with serious medical problems directly or indirectly related to a patent foramen ovale, who now are referred for occlusion of the PFO and are closed using the device that is approved for closure of muscular ventricular septal defects. Deep sea divers, both recreational and professional, with a PFO develop severe "bends" with particularly severe CNS problems from the systemic nitrogen bubble emboli[2]. Many professional facilities/employers will not license individuals for deep water diving in the presence of a PFO. There are other patients who undergo closure of a PFO because of cyanosis following a pneumonectomy[3], cyanosis secondary to right ventricular malfunction associated with congenital heart defects and/or chronic obstructive pulmonary disease[4], cyanosis with a right to left shunt following a right ventricular myocardial infarct[5], or cyanosis associated with platypnea-orthodeoxia[6]. The cyanosis/hypoxemia in all of these patients can be eliminated by closure of the PFO, and many of these patients are referred for device closure because they also represent a higher risk for surgery. There also is a group of patients with intractable migraine headaches that appear to be related to a PFO. A large number of the patients who are referred for device closure of the PFO and who have had one or more documented embolic events, also have a significant and/or long history of severe, even incapacitating, migraine headaches[7]. Approximately 80% of those patients who had headaches before the closure of their PFO, stop having, or have markedly decreased migraine headaches after the closure of the PFO. A few patients have been treated with a PFO closure with their migraine headaches being their primary indication.

The documentation of a patent foramen ovale is not always straightforward or easy. The thin flap of the septum primum with the appearance of apparent intermittent separation between the septum primum and the septal wall and/or even a "drop-out" in the echo image in the area of the foramen often can be seen on a transthoracic echo (TTE) and/or even a transesophageal echo (TEE). The appearance of the "drop-out" in the septum secundum or in the flap of the septum primum, alone, does not confirm the presence of a *patent* foramen ovale, and under normal circumstances no flow is seen in either direction through the foramen when using Doppler interrogation. The "gold standard" for diagnosis of a PFO is with the use of an injection of "contrast" or "micro bubble" into the right heart, which is performed during a Valsalva maneuver while recording the left heart structures on echo. TEE is considered more sensitive than TTE, however, obtaining a satisfactory Valsalva maneuver during a TEE can be very problematic. During the echo and simultaneously with the injected "contrast" reaching the right atrium, the patient must perform a Valsalva maneuver which is synchronized with the injection, or the patient's breathing must be stopped by an anesthesiologist and/or an additional person must apply deep, sustained, abdominal compression as the "micro bubbles" reach the right atrium[8]. Unfortunately, these "enhancements" for raising intrathoracic pressure at the exact and appropriate time during the "contrast bubble" studies are not "automatic". In fact, when not timed precisely and/or if the exact area that should be imaged becomes displaced out of the visualized field during the maneuver, it can totally mask the presence of a significant right to left shunt. A strong Valsalva maneuver that is performed too early after the peripheral "contrast" injection, can prevent the blood flow (and the contrast material) into the thorax and heart. In addition the sensitivity of the "bubble study" can be compromised by the location of the peripheral venous injection that is used for the "micro bubble" solution. Flow into the right atrium from the superior vena cava (following injections into an arm vein) normally is directed *away* from the opening of a PFO in the atrial septum by the opposing blood flow from the inferior vena cava. As a consequence, all of the blood (and "micro bubbles") from the superior vena cava actually can be diverted away from the septum even with an appropriately timed Valsalva. At the same time, because injections into the lower extremity are very inconvenient, they seldom are used and when used, unless the injection is into a more central portion of the inferior vena cava, the co-ordination of the injections with the "breath holding" is even more difficult.

Because of the inconsistencies of TTE for the detection of right to left shunt through a PFO as well as the inconvenience and the discomfort of TEE itself, several alternative procedures are utilized to detect right to left shunts and/or the actual patency of a PFO. Standard ear oximetry with an optical ear sensor recorded during Valsalva and/or in conjunction with a venous injection of Cardio Green dye and a Valsalva maneuver both have an increased sensitivity over TTE, but are not as selective as TEE at detecting a PFO with shunting[9]. Transthoracic echo using second harmonic imaging to enhance the contrast of the "micro bubbles" following the injection of "contrast" material during a Valsalva maneuver appears markedly improved over standard TTE, and closer in sensitivity to TEE for documenting the presence of right to left shunting at the atrial level[10]. This technique has not gained widespread use for this purpose as yet.

Transcranial Doppler (TCD) has been demonstrated to be as effective as TEE at detecting right to left shunting at the atrial level during a Valsalva maneuver, and now often is used to screen for the presence of a PFO[11]. The TCD signal is measured over the right middle cerebral artery during the injection of a solution of agitated blood/saline into a peripheral vein and along with a Valsalva maneuver. The timing of the Valsalva with the injection is still critical, but the patient requires no sedation and/or anesthesia and does not have the discomfort and respiratory compromise of the TEE probe so that a much better Valsalva maneuver can be achieved. Transcranial Doppler probably will replace TEE in *screening* for the presence of a *right to left shunt* in patients with a cryptogenic stroke, but the documentation of the right to left shunt by the TCD does not *localize* the level of shunting. If the TCD is positive, the patient still will need a TEE with contrast with a good Valsalva to absolutely establish the presence of a PFO before being taken to the catheterization laboratory for definitive therapy.

Device closure of the patent foramen ovale

Each variation in the anatomy of the particular PFO changes the technique for the catheter closure with a device. Virtually all of the devices used for occlusion of atrial septal defects as well as several devices designed either specifically for occlusion of a PFO or for the occlusion of some other defects have been used for occlusion of the patent foramen ovale as well as for closure of the surgical fenestrations in the "Fontan" baffles. Some of these devices required modification to better suit the anatomy of the PFO/fenestrations and/or more effectively to prevent the right to left shunting, which is predominant in these lesions. The delivery technique, implant procedures and, particularly, the precautions for the prevention of air and/or clot embolization are similar, if not more stringent, than the procedures used for ASD occlusion with the same devices.

As with closure of an ASD with a catheter-delivered device, transesophageal echo (TEE) or intracavitary echo (ICE) using an additional intravascular echo catheter usually is used for the positioning and the implant of the device for PFO occlusion. As of this writing, the ICE catheter still requires an 11-French venous sheath *in addition* to the delivery sheath and any other venous catheter! In addition to the guiding of the actual implant of the device, either TEE or ICE is essential for identifying the presence of a large Eustachian valve/Chiari network, which can reach the opening of the foramen and, in turn, complicate the implant of a device in the atrial septum[12]. The Eustachian valve/Chiari networks usually cannot be recognized angiographically and seldom are seen on TTE. The special handling of the Eustachian valve when present was covered in detail in Chapter 28. Static balloon sizing of the defect is extremely beneficial (if not essential!), not only for the sizing of the defect but for determining the "shape" of the PFO and the "malleability" of the septum primum. Angiography through an additional venous catheter is valuable in the sizing/shaping as well as a complement (replacement) to the echo during implant.

The patent foramen ovale has unique characteristics, which are different in *each* individual patient and which dictate which device and technique is used for the particular lesion. The *differences* in the various devices designed specifically for the occlusion of the PFO/fenestrations and the use of devices that were designed more for ASD occlusions for the occlusion of PFO/fenestrations, are discussed in this chapter and compared to their use in the occlusion of ASDs. Each of the specific devices that is available either commercially and/or in an investigational clinical trial is discussed separately.

Many of the patients undergoing PFO closure have been on coumadin anticoagulation because of embolic events prior to referral for the procedure. The coumadin is stopped 2–3 days prior to the catheterization. Patients who are scheduled to undergo a device closure of a patent foramen ovale, a fenestration and/or an atrial septal defect, are started on 82 mg of aspirin one week prior to the procedure if they were not on it previously. In the catheterization laboratory, the patient's activated clotting time (ACT) is measured as soon as the first vascular access (arterial or venous) is secured. Unless the initial ACT is very prolonged, each patient is given 100 mg/kg of heparin once the measured ACT is available. During the catheterization/occlusion procedure the patient's ACT is monitored in order to keep the value above 275–300 seconds. The heparin anticoagulation is not reversed at the end of the procedure. The bleeding at the puncture sites is controlled with manual pressure (often prolonged) over the site. The patient is started on intravenous antibiotics as soon as the device is delivered and two additional doses of the antibiotic are given at eight hourly intervals thereafter. The patients are observed in an intensive care or recovery ward until they are awake following the anesthesia and are observed in the hospital for 12 or more hours. This usually requires overnight observation (as opposed to a discharge at 1:00 or 2:00 am). Patients who undergo device implant are discharged on 82 mg aspirin a day orally and this is continued for six months. Unless they were on other anticoagulants before the procedure and/or at the request of their referring physician, the patients are not started on any other anticoagulants after the device implant.

Unfortunately, the anatomy of the PFO that is associated with cryptogenic strokes, usually does not fit the "typical" description of a PFO, which is stereotyped as a small opening at the edge of a thin "valve" of the septum primum, which covers the foramen ovale (*see* Figure 29.1). Most (all!) of the patients referred for a PFO closure following a systemic embolic event have an opening which *potentially* is quite large[13]. In addition, the actual opening often is covered by a large and thickened flap or "valve" of the septum primum, which in addition creates a long and/or large diameter tunnel (*see* Figure 29.2, a & b). The tissues of the foramen and the septum primum appear to become thicker and more ridged with the increasing age of the patient. The PFO often is associated with an aneurysm of the atrial septum itself. Because of the marked heterogeneity of the PFO, each lesion is studied thoroughly by TEE or ICE, angiography (through a separate catheter) *and* with a static balloon sizing before the occlusion procedure is begun.

The interatrial septum is interrogated with TEE or ICE. The TEE or ICE usually demonstrates the area of the foramen and the characteristics of the "valve" of the foramen including its length, its thickness and its extension onto the left side of the septum and/or onto the wall of the aorta. The echo alone does *not* demonstrate the maximum diameter of the true opening through the defect even during an adequate Valsalva maneuver. The TEE and ICE also are invaluable at identifying long redundant and/or thickened Eustachian valve tissues, which can extend over and/or even attach to the foramen ovale and, as a consequence, can interfere with the delivery of the device.

After the TEE or ICE interrogation, a calibrated angiographic catheter is introduced into a femoral vein through an additional venous sheath. This catheter is manipulated along the right side of the atrial septum and positioned just *within* the foramen. The position is verified with the TEE or ICE. A biplane angiocardiogram is recorded with the X-ray tubes in the straight PA and lateral views and performed using a relatively small injection directly into the foramen. This angiogram usually defines the characteristics of the foramen very well and demonstrates the "tunnel-like" characteristics even better. Occasionally the defect/tunnel can be "cut on edge" better with some angulation of one or both of the X-ray tubes. A mild left anterior oblique (LAO) plus cranial angulation of the lateral X-ray tube often elongates and profiles the "tunnel" better.

Once an angiogram with the optimal tube angulation is obtained, the tip of the angiographic catheter can remain within the foramen. An end-hole catheter with a wire back-bleed valve and flush/pressure side port attached at the proximal end of the catheter is introduced into the right femoral vein through a 9–11-French short sheath. The end-hole catheter is advanced through the foramen, past the angiographic catheter and manipulated deep into a *left upper* pulmonary vein. The end-hole catheter is maintained on a continuous flush through the wire back bleed/flush port and an exchange length, short tipped 0.035″ Super Stiff™ wire (Medi-Tech, Boston Scientific, Natick, MA) is introduced through the wire back-bleed valve, advanced to the tip of the catheter and into the pulmonary vein. A 20 mm diameter NuMED™ sizing balloon (NuMED Inc., Hopkinton, NY) is flushed with a 1:5 dilution of contrast until it is clear of all air. Once the sizing balloon is fully prepared, the end-hole catheter is withdrawn over the wire and the wire back-bleed valve/flush port is attached to the hub of the catheter lumen of the NuMED™ sizing balloon and placed on a continuous flush. The NuMED™ sizing balloon catheter is introduced into the short sheath and advanced over the wire until it is positioned precisely within the foramen ovale. The balloon is inflated very slowly and at "no pressure" while observing the diameter *and the shape* of the balloon. The balloon often must be repositioned forward or backward slightly to position the balloon exactly straddling the length of the defect, and even a 3 cm long balloon occasionally is not long enough to span the entire length of the "tunnel". Even at a "no pressure" inflation the balloon usually expands to a minimum of 10 mm diameter at the narrowest diameter.

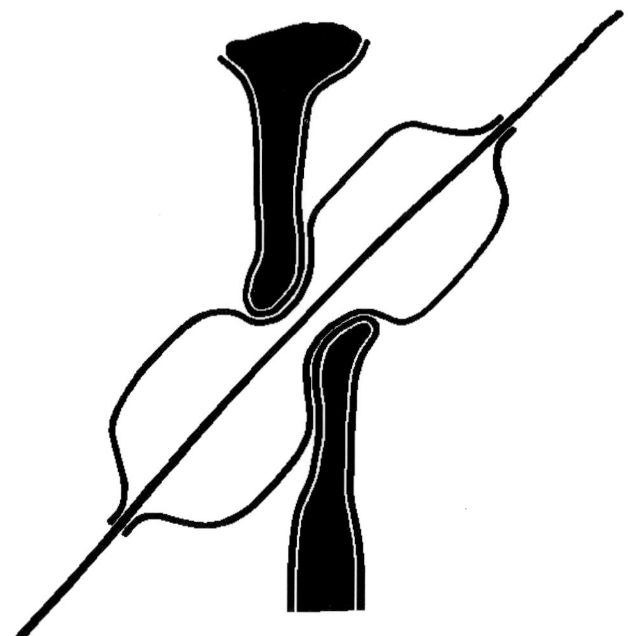

Figure 29.3 "On edge" view—static sizing balloon positioned across a short, discrete PFO.

When there is a relatively discrete opening in the foramen and there is no long flap and/or tunnel, a single, discrete waist develops circumferentially around the balloon at the *single* location corresponding to the discrete opening in the foramen (Figure 29.3). When the flap of the septum primum is long and loose, the zero pressure sizing clearly demonstrates the potentially very large opening (Figure 29.4). Often however, the balloon will have several separate indentations along the opposite sides of the balloon with these indentations at some distance from each other. These separate indentations in the balloon demonstrate the length, the shape and the entrance and exit sites of the "tunnel" of the PFO through the septum (Figure 29.5). An angiogram is repeated by injecting into the "tunnel" or tract of the PFO adjacent to the balloon. This angiogram verifies the length, the diameters and the ends or openings of the "tunnel" very clearly. The length and diameter(s) of the waist(s) are measured accurately from this angiogram. The same measurements of the balloon inflated within the defect are made using TEE or ICE imaging.

When there is a single, discrete waist around the balloon and/or the indentations along the opposite sides of the balloon are separated *less than 5 mm* from each other (*see* Figure 29.3), the PFO occlusion device is delivered

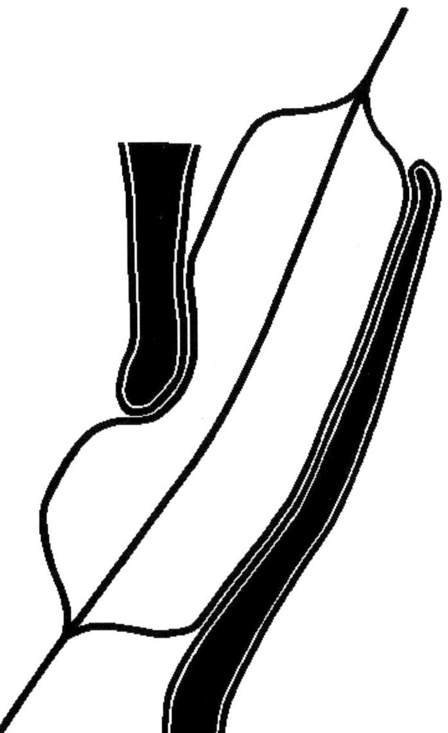

Figure 29.4 "On edge" view—sizing balloon in large diameter PFO; the sizing balloon demonstrating the wide patency of the "tunnel" and the very large *potential* opening of the foramen.

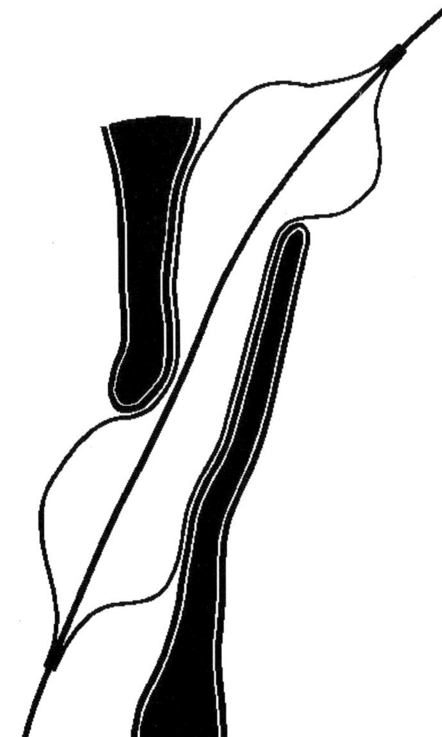

Figure 29.5 "On edge" view—the sizing balloon within a long, irregular and "stiff", tunnel-like PFO demonstrating the length and shape of the tunnel.

through the existing openings of the PFO. The size of the device that is used is determined by both the maximum diameter of the opening during sizing and by the length of the valve (septum primum) of the foramen. The goal is to cover and compress the entire valve of the foramen between the two opposing sides (disks) of the device.

If the indentations on the opposite sides of the balloon are separated by more than 7–10 mm, a transseptal puncture is used to deliver the PFO occlusion device through the valve (septum primum) of the foramen. When there is a long and thick tunnel, the short central attach mechanism connecting the two disks of the CardioSEAL™, the STARFlex™ the CARDIA™ and even the Amplatzer™ PFO devices do not extend completely through the "tunnel" to even reach the right side of the septum while still collapsed within the sheath (Figure 29.6).

If opened in this position, the right sided disk or umbrella cannot deploy and/or open at all on the right side of the septum. If a PFO occlusion device is implanted in this position the right sided legs/umbrella would be within the tunnel and provide no resistance to right to left forces in order to prevent the entire device from dislodging and embolizing to the left atrium. On the other hand, if the device is withdrawn further into a resistant tunnel and deployed *in* and/or *through* the length of a long tunnel, the left atrial legs and/or disks deploy partially (or totally)

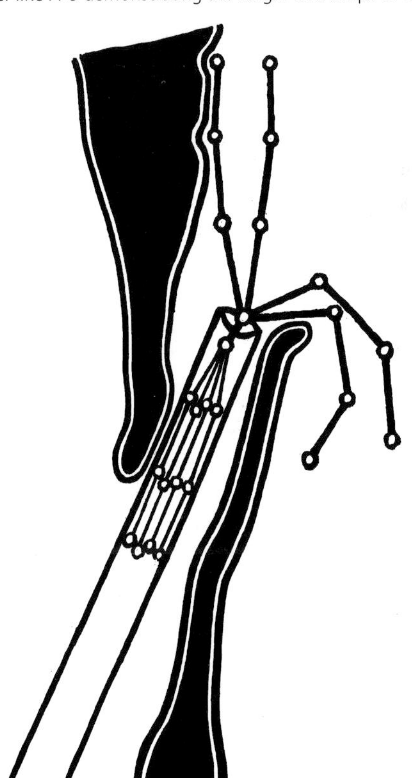

Figure 29.6 "On edge" view—CardioSEAL™ device pulled into long stiff tunnel. The left atrial disk is distorted and hanging out into the left atrium while the right atrial disk, which is still folded in the sheath, still is not on the "right side" of the septum.

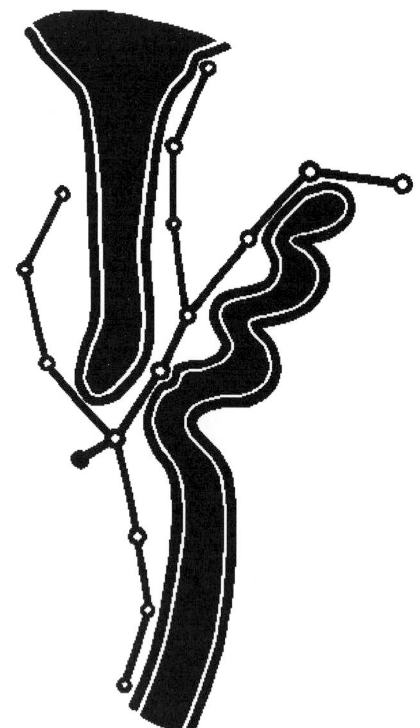

Figure 29.7 "On edge" view—CardioSEAL™ device further into the tunnel but still deployed improperly *within* a tunnel-like patent foramen ovale. The device is expanded incompletely and irregularly as a consequence.

within the tunnel and remain incompletely opened (Figure 29.7). As a consequence, the legs and/or disks, which are trapped within the tunnel, push the septum primum away from the septal surface and neither side of the device can lie flat on the septal surface on one and/or both sides of the septum. A device in this position will occlude the tunnel, but will create a huge mass within the septum.

Devices available for PFO occlusion

Although the CardioSEAL™ device (NMT Technologies, Boston, MA) was originally designed for ASD occlusion, the two double disks attached by a single, narrow, central "post" or hinge and the absence of any "centering mechanism" make it ideal for closure of the PFO (much better than for the closure of ASDs). The CardioSEAL™ device received an FDA, Humanitarian Device Exemption (HDE) approval in the United States for the occlusion of the patent foramen ovale in patients who have had a systemic embolic event and who have "failed medical management". The CardioSEAL™ also is approved for the closure of the purposeful fenestrations in the baffles of patients who have undergone a cavopulmonary and/or "Fontan" type of repair, for inadvertent residual leaks postoperatively, and for the closure of muscular ventricular septal defects.

The Amplatzer™ PFO Occluder (AGA Medical Corp., Golden Valley, MN) is a modification of the Amplatzer™ ASD device specifically for use in closure of the PFO. The broad central, occluding "hub" of the Amplatzer™ ASD device is replaced in the Amplatzer™ PFO device with a very narrow and flexible central connecting waist between two large, flat Nitinol™ outer disks. In addition, the right-sided disk on the Amplatzer™ PFO device is slightly larger than the left sided disk in order to compensate for more dominant right to left "forces" and flow. The specific modification of the Amplatzer™ PFO device gives it the same favorable characteristics for PFO occlusion as the "double-umbrella" CardioSEAL™ Devices with their narrow waists. The Amplatzer™ PFO device also has FDA, HDE approval for PFO occlusions under the same conditions as the CardioSEAL™ device.

In Europe and the rest of the world outside of the United States, there are several other devices available and used for PFO occlusion in addition to the CardioSEAL™ ASD and the Amplatzer™ PFO devices. The STARFlex™ (NMT, Boston, MA) modification of the CardioSEAL™ ASD device probably is used more commonly for PFO occlusions than the CardioSEAL™ device in Europe. The Helex™ ASD device (W. L. Gore & Associates, Flagstaff, AZ) also has been used to occlude the PFO. The Sideris Reverse Button™ (Pediatric Cardiology Custom Medical Devices, Athens, Greece) and the CARDIA™ (Cardia Inc., Burnsville, MN) are two devices that were designed specifically for PFO occlusion and have had extensive use outside of the United States. These other ASD/PFO occlusion devices are not available in the US for occlusion of the PFO, except under investigational protocols and/or for isolated emergency or humanitarian use.

CardioSEAL™ occlusion of the patent foramen ovale

The CardioSEAL™ ASD occlusion device (NMT, Boston, MA) is ideally suited for the occlusion of the *stereotype* PFO and the small fenestrations (whether purposeful or inadvertent) in baffles or patches in postoperative patients. The two, very flat, opposing double, and somewhat "malleable" umbrellas are connected by a very narrow, short, central hinge mechanism. The two umbrellas, once deployed, lie very flat on the opposite surfaces of the atrial septum (particularly with the fenestrations) while the small central spring mechanism fits nicely within the orifice of small defects and pulls the two umbrellas tightly against the two relatively flat opposite surfaces of the septum/baffle. At the same time, the spring mechanism of each arm of the separate umbrellas allows each umbrella to conform to "irregularities" in the less than flat surfaces of the septum. The CardioSEAL™ devices now are front-loaded into the delivery sheath. For occlusion of the PFO and fenestrations, the 17 and 23 mm CardioSEAL™ devices are delivered through a 10-French sheath while the 28 mm and larger devices are delivered through an 11-French sheath.

When the "stereotypic", short, "non-tunnel" PFO is identified anatomically by TEE, angiography, balloon sizing and "shaping", the occlusion is fairly straightforward. A device is used that is *at least twice* the diameter of the maximum diameter of the defect as determined by the static balloon sizing. The 28 mm or the 33 mm CardioSEAL™ devices are used for the *majority* of PFO occlusions. The extra size of the device allows a firm seating on the right as well as the left side of the defect as well as a "covering" of the flap of the foramen even if there is a short "tunnel". After the defect is sized and "shaped", the sizing balloon is withdrawn over the stiff exchange wire, which remains fixed in a left upper pulmonary vein. The short sheath in the right femoral vein is withdrawn over the wire with the balloon catheter.

A wire back-bleed device is placed on the dilator of a 10- or 11-French long sheath/dilator set that is appropriate for the chosen device, and while outside of the body the long sheath/dilator set is passed through a short 14-French sheath, which immediately is withdrawn back to the hub of the long sheath. The short sheath over the delivery sheath serves as an emergency retrieval sheath should a CardioSEAL™ have to be retrieved after it has been deployed on the septum. The dilator is placed on a continuous flush and the long sheath/dilator set is introduced over the previously positioned wire and advanced through the defect until the tip of the sheath is in the *left atrium*. The flush on the dilator is continued and with the tip of the *sheath* maintained in the *left* atrium, the dilator alone is removed slowly over the wire. The flush on the dilator is stopped just as the tip of the dilator (within the sheath) reaches outside of the puncture site at the skin. The dilator is removed very slowly the rest of the way out of the sheath and with the sheath tip still secure in the left atrium, the wire is withdrawn from the sheath. The sheath is allowed to bleed back passively through the side port to clear it of all air and/or clots. This is performed at least as meticulously as during a device occlusion of an ASD since, as opposed to the ASD, the PFO has a greater potential for right to left shunt from the right atrium to the systemic system! Once the sheath unequivocally is free of air and/or clot, the sheath is placed on a continuous flush. The short 14-French sheath is still over the long sheath but remains against the proximal hub of the long sheath and is *not* introduced into the vessel.

The appropriately sized device is loaded and introduced into the long sheath identically to the procedures used for a CardioSEAL™ occlusion of an ASD (described in detail in Chapter 28). There are, however, several significant differences in the delivery, deployment and implant of the CardioSEAL™ device for closure of the stereotypic PFO compared to the CardioSEAL™ occlusion of an ASD. Once any unusual anatomy of the PFO has been ruled out, the typical PFO closure is relatively straightforward and there is a much greater margin of safety for the size of the device used and the delivery procedure itself than with the occlusion of a secundum ASD with the CardioSEAL/STARFlex™ devices. The left atrial umbrella is opened completely and freely in the left atrium and then the entire delivery system with the device is withdrawn *very firmly against* the septum. The device is pulled firmly against the septum until all of the left atrial legs actually oppose the surface of the septum as seen on both fluoroscopy and TEE or ICE (Figure 29.8). The left atrial legs should begin to evert slightly as they pull into the defect before the opening of the right atrial umbrella is started. This is in stark contrast to the delivery of the CardioSEAL™ device for the closure of the usual ASD, where only the tip of one of the left atrial legs is allowed to *touch* the septum, and that with no force at all, before the right atrial legs are opened!

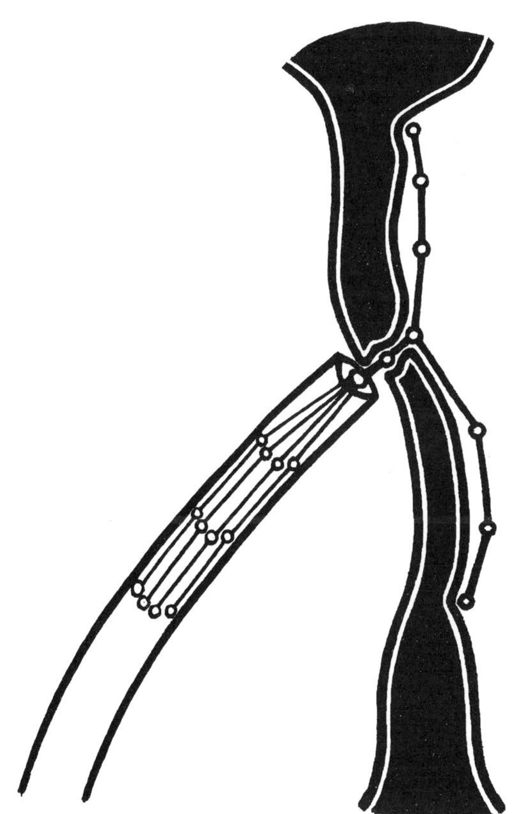

Figure 29.8 "On edge" view—CardioSEAL™ device pulled firmly and properly against left side of a "typical" short PFO.

When the entire left side of the CardioSEAL™ device is pulled tightly against/into the septum during the PFO closure, a biplane angiocardiogram is recorded through the second venous catheter, which now is positioned with the catheter tip *in the defect and under the open left sided umbrella* of the device. This verifies the exact position of the device before opening the right atrial umbrella and, in particular, demonstrates the relation of the tips of the right legs, which are still contained within the sheath, to the plane of the right side of the septum. The stability of the partially opened device against the septum/PFO before release allows more reliance on angiographic guidance for the PFO occlusion. When satisfied by both angiography and/or TEE/ICE that the right legs are well on the right side of the septum the sheath alone is withdrawn to deploy the right legs of the device. Once the right atrial umbrella is open in the typical PFO, the fixation of the device on the septum is tested before device release by fairly vigorous to-and-fro motion on the delivery catheter/wire. When the device is secure in the defect, the release tumbler is advanced, releasing the device. There usually is a significant "reorientation" of the device on the septum with the release. With the usual PFO, the CardioSEAL™ device seats very flat on the septum after release (Figure 29.9).

Although not as necessary for PFO occlusions, the Hausdorf™ modification of the Cook™ MTS™ sheath is equally suitable for the delivery of devices to the PFO as to the ASD. The Hausdorf™ sheath does align the left atrial disk better with the plane of the septum after it has been extruded into the left atrium. Since the left atrial umbrellas can be pulled forcefully into the PFO, this better alignment usually is not necessary.

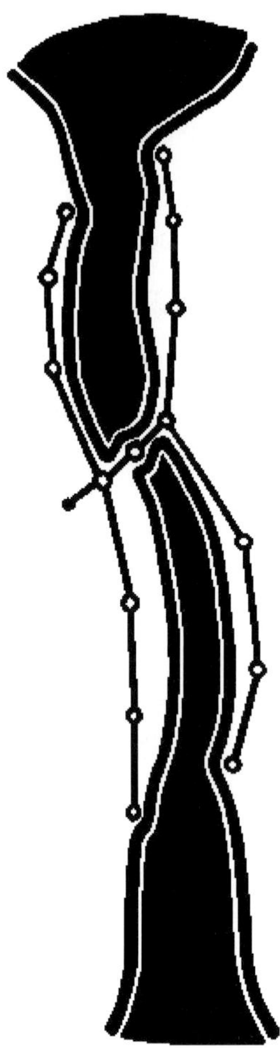

Figure 29.9 "On edge" view—CardioSEAL™ device deployed properly over a short, "typical" PFO and on the septum.

When a long flap of the septum primum (the "valve of the foramen") creates a long tunnel through the atrial septum, this tunnel creates a potential and very significant challenge for a device closure of this type of PFO (*see* Figure 29.2). A torque-controlled venous catheter, which is introduced from the femoral route, ordinarily "falls" across the stereotypic PFO, which has a relatively short flap of septum primum. Often, but not always, some difficulty is encountered in maneuvering from right to left atrium through the "tunnel" PFO defects. Any difficulty in crossing the defect represents a "clue" that there is something unusual about the PFO, and probably that there is some degree of a "tunnel" type of defect. TEE or ICE will demonstrate a slit-like channel between the right atrial and left atrial ends of the defect and demonstrates the *exit* opening(s) of the tunnel into the left atrium. The TEE/ICE provides a "relaxed" measurement of the opening into the left atrium, which may appear very small or even closed with the patient breathing normally. However, when used in conjunction with a Valsalva maneuver, the TEE/ICE documents the presence of the right to left shunt through a small or even apparently closed defect. An angiocardiogram with a small hand injection of contrast through a catheter, with the tip of the catheter positioned just within the right side of the foramen, defines a "tunnel" type of patent foramen ovale very nicely. The angiogram demonstrates the tunnel-like defect and the course through the tunnel to the exit(s) into the left atrium. The tunnel often appears as a large pouch between the two sides of the septum. At the same time, a left atrial and/or pulmonary vein angiogram provide(s) no information about the PFO.

The definitive information about the size, length and configuration of the "tunnel" is obtained with a very low-pressure, static sizing balloon. Pulling a Swan™ floating type balloon (Edwards Lifesciences, Irvine, CA) or an Occlusion™ type of balloon (Boston Scientific, Natick, MA) through the defect also is ***of absolutely no use*** for *sizing* the PFO and, in fact, will provide misleading information. With the balloon deflated, the Swan™ or Occlusion™ type of balloon catheter advances readily through the flap of the PFO and into the left atrium.

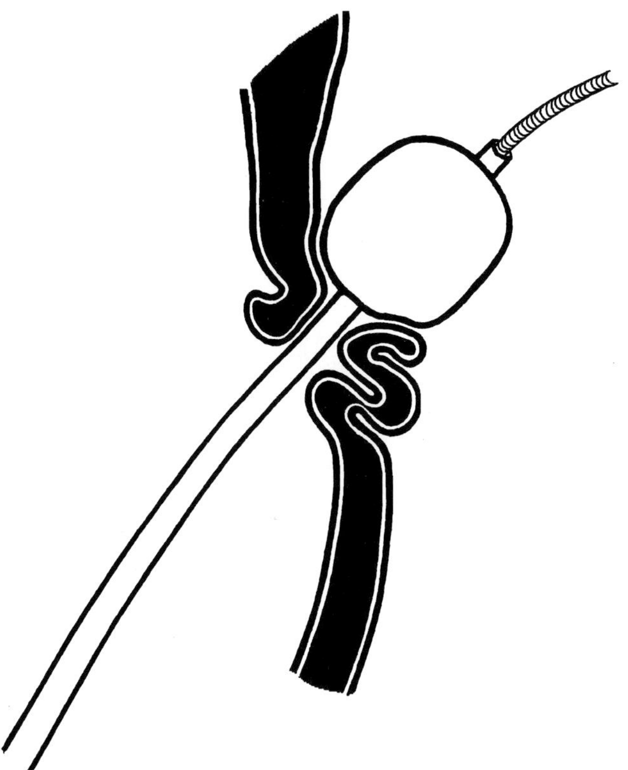

Figure 29.10 "On edge" view—small "Swan™ type" balloon pulling large flap of PFO closed, *suggesting* a very small opening.

However, even with the spherical balloon minimally inflated, when withdrawn back toward the septum, this type of balloon as it is withdrawn, pulls the flap of the septum primum (valve of the foramen) closed against the septum secundum (Figure 29.10). Rather than the balloon pulling into or through the defect and demonstrating its diameter, this type of balloon very effectively closes the opening in the defect, which, in turn, suggests a very small PFO opening even when the opening is very large. This gives totally misleading information about the size and the anatomy of the defect. If a small device is implanted on a long mobile flap of septum primum tissue that is covering a large opening, the right sided disk will have nothing to attach to and in all likelihood will embolize.

This catching of a spherical "Swan™ type" balloon on the septum, in fact, has been utilized to tear the septum *open* purposefully by some catheterizing physicians who are uncomfortable with the transseptal technique[14]. The "Occlusion" or Swan™ balloon, which is caught on the septum primum flap of the septum, is pulled forcefully through the defect in order to purposefully partially avulse the valve of the foramen. This "septostomy" "prepares" the PFO for the delivery of a device directly through the defect without the "necessity" of performing a transseptal puncture. This balloon septostomy-like technique for opening the PFO further is *not* advocated by this author. To perform the "septostomy preparation" of the defect, the deflated Swan™ type balloon catheter is passed over the wire and through the "tunnel" of the PFO. The balloon is inflated in the left atrium and withdrawn forcefully through the septum, performing a mild or "minimal septostomy". The "pull through" presumably straightens and shortens the course of the channel through the septum and opens up the true (or larger) diameter of the defect. This technique should work in the presence of a relatively "soft" septum with a fairly short "tunnel" (where it may not even be necessary), and the septostomy certainly facilitates the use of a larger, more appropriate sized device for the PFO closure. This "pull through" preparation of the foramen is of no benefit in the very thick septum associated with a long "tunnel" in which the devices become very deformed if not delivered through a transseptal puncture.

Any PFO, and particularly when a "tunnel" configuration is suspected, is sized and "shaped" with a NuMED™, static, "no pressure", sizing balloon, which is inflated directly within the "tunnel". The offset *indentations,* which appear on the opposite sides of the soft NuMED™ static balloon when the balloon is inflated within a long defect, provide additional essential information about the length and configuration of the tunnel as well as the accurate measurements of the diameters of various areas at the ends and within the tunnel (*see* Figure 29.5). A selective angiocardiogram through a second venous catheter, which is positioned in the defect adjacent to the static sizing balloon, provides even more detail about the length, diameters and configuration of these defects.

The "tunnel" created between the caudal right sided opening and the more cephalad left sided opening passing from the right to the left atrium within the septum (beneath the valve of the foramen) can be as long as *two to three centimeters*. When sized and "shaped" with the very low pressure *static* balloon inflated within the tunnel, the "very small openings" suggested by the TEE, ICE and/or a "pull through" sizing balloon, frequently are as large as 10–12 mm in diameter at both ends or throughout the length of the tunnel! The angiocardiogram through the catheter in the tunnel clearly demonstrates the anatomy and creates "landmarks" which are used during the deployment of an occlusion device. Small, hand angiocardiograms, injecting through the additional angiographic catheter within the "tunnel" during the deployment of the device, very clearly demonstrate the anatomic relationships for accurate positioning of the occlusion device. The angiographic catheter is withdrawn from the "tunnel" just before the right side of the occlusion device is deployed.

In older adult patients and those patients with arrhythmias and/or chronic cardiac failure, the atrial tissues usually are thicker and stiffer. When closure of the PFO is

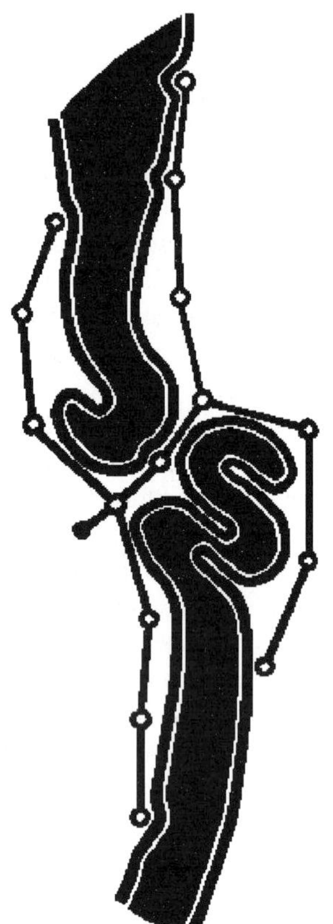

Figure 29.11 "On edge" view—edge of a long septum primum flap "folded" under a CardioSEAL™ device implanted through the compliant "tunnel", still leaving a "mass" under the device.

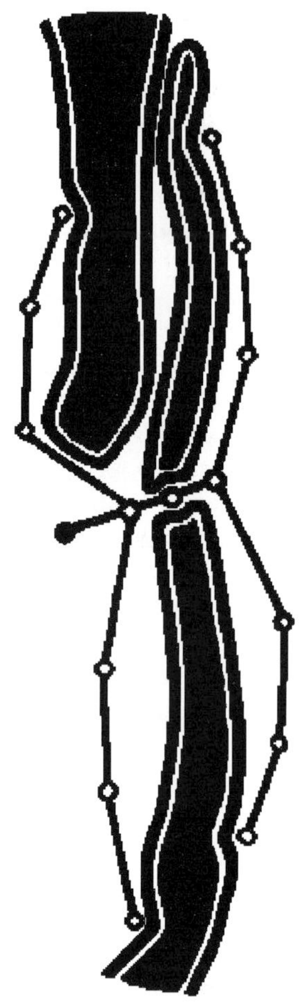

Figure 29.12 "On edge" view—CardioSEAL™ device clamped firmly on septum after *transseptal closure* of long "tunnel" PFO.

attempted through an existing "tunnel", the tissues do not fold and/or "crumple" smoothly between the umbrellas or disks on the two sides of the septum. The very long flaps of the valve and/or these thicker tissues of the tunnel walls cannot be compressed together from the opposite ends by the two disks of any of the available devices. The "umbrella" or "disk" at each end of such a rigid "tunnel" inverts partially into the tunnel. The partial inversion into the tunnel may allow the device to reach completely through the tunnel but, at the same time, does not allow one or both of the "disks" of the device to lie flat on the septum (Figure 29.11). Even though a very large device completely covers the opening on the left side of the septum, the length of the "non-collapsing" tunnel does not allow the central hub to extend completely through the "tunnel" and, in turn, prevents the proximal side of the device from opening *completely* on the right side of the septum. When a device is "stretched" through the length of the tunnel, both ends of the device are everted and extend out of the ends of the tunnel away from the atrial septum. As a consequence, the device cannot open into its normal flat configuration and forms an irregular mass within the "tunnel" (*see* Figure 29.7).

Rather than traversing the length of the tunnel with the delivery sheath, the preferred technique for the closure of a PFO with a "tunnel" that is longer than 5–7 mm or any "tunnel" in an older patient where the tissues are thicker and stiffer, is to cross the septum primum using a transseptal puncture[15]. The transseptal puncture is performed through the septum primum 4–5 mm caudal to the limbus of the foramen. The delivery of the device through the puncture site allows the device to lie flat on both sides of the septum with the legs extending completely over the length of the tunnel as well as over the openings at both ends of the patent foramen (Figure 29.12).

The transseptal puncture through the ostium primum of the PFO is guided by *both* angiography and TEE/ICE. A standard 8- or 9-French, 69 cm long transseptal set is used for the transseptal procedure. The tip of the long transseptal sheath/dilator set is straightened into a gentle 45° curve similar to the curve for delivery of the ASD devices. The 11-French long sheaths for device delivery are available only in 75 or 85 cm lengths and cannot be used for the transseptal *puncture*. When the sheath/dilator set/needle are in position for the puncture, the position of the needle tip on the septum primum and its relationship to the "tunnel" are verified by TEE or ICE, which is being used for the implant procedure. The TEE/ICE image helps to position the puncture site just *below the limbus* of the foramen by demonstrating a "tenting" of the septum primum by the tip of the needle before the puncture and ensures that the needle does not just slide through the existing foramen. The transseptal puncture otherwise is identical to a standard *transseptal procedure*. Once the tip *of the sheath* is well into the left atrium, the needle is withdrawn separately and the dilator very carefully is cleared of air. With a straighter, smooth curve on the sheath/dilator, the combination often points at, and in turn, almost falls into a left upper pulmonary vein with minimal extra manipulation. If the sheath/dilator does not enter the pulmonary vein without any extra effort, the dilator is withdrawn very slowly and the sheath meticulously cleared of any air or clot.

Once the sheath is cleared and flushed, an 8- or 9-French, end-hole catheter is attached to a continuous flush through a wire back-bleed/flush device on its hub, advanced into and through the sheath (which also is kept on a flush) and the catheter is maneuvered deep into a left upper pulmonary vein. A short tipped, exchange length, Super Stiff™ wire (Boston Scientific, Natick, MA) is advanced through the catheter well into the pulmonary vein. The end-hole catheter and the original transseptal sheath are withdrawn over the wire and out of the body. The wire back-bleed device is placed on the *dilator* of the long 11-French sheath/dilator set that is to be used for the delivery of the device and the dilator is placed on a continuous flush. As with the standard delivery, the long 11-French sheath/dilator set outside of the body is introduced into a 14-French short sheath, which is withdrawn back to the hub of the long sheath. The long sheath/dilator set then is introduced over the previously positioned wire and advanced through the septum and into the pulmonary vein, all of the time keeping the dilator on a continuous flush. When passing through the smaller puncture hole from the transseptal, the sheath and dilator are advanced as the one unit, through the puncture hole in the septum primum and into the left atrium. This can take a little extra forward force, and care must be taken that the sheath/dilator set is not advanced too far into the atrial wall or the vein so that it becomes wedged and does not allow a free back flow from the dilator after the wire is removed. The wire is withdrawn slowly from the dilator while continuing the flush through *the dilator* around the wire. Once the wire has been removed completely, the flush is discontinued. The dilator is withdrawn very slowly from the sheath while observing the side port of the wire back-bleed/flush port on the hub of the dilator for bleeding. There ***should be*** a slight, but continuous, drip of fluid and/or blood from the side port of the back-bleed device on the dilator as it is withdrawn from the sheath. This ensures that air is not being sucked into the sheath through the dilator while the dilator is withdrawn. If there is no back flow from the side port on the dilator, the sheath and dilator are withdrawn together very minimally, in order to withdraw them out of a pulmonary vein and allow back flow to occur through the dilator.

An alternative technique to assure that no air or clot remains in the sheath, is to withdraw the dilator from the sheath over the wire while maintaining the dilator on a vigorous flush through the wire back-bleed/flush valve as it is withdrawn until the dilator tip reaches the skin surface. Once the dilator tip reaches the skin, the flush is stopped, the wire back-bleed valve is opened and/or withdrawn off the dilator, and the dilator is allowed to bleed back passively until it is out of the valve of the sheath. Once the dilator is removed, the sheath then is allowed to bleed back *passively* from the side port with the wire still in place. The wire, which extends beyond the end of the sheath, tends to keep the end of the sheath from occluding within the walls of the pulmonary vein or against the wall of the left atrium. When this technique is used, the side port on the sheath is opened very carefully to allow the back bleeding. Fluid and/or blood should drip from the side port of the sheath as the sheath is withdrawn. Suction ***never*** is applied to the side arm of a sheath with a wire passing through the back bleed valve. With *any* resistance to the suction applied to the side arm of the sheath, air always will be sucked through the valve and *into* the sheath around the wire!

Once the large delivery sheath is in place securely in the left atrium and completely clear of air, the loading, delivery and implant of the CardioSEAL™ device is identical to the technique for the more stereotype PFO. The transseptal delivery allows the left atrial umbrella to pull flat against the septum with even greater force before opening the right atrial umbrella. When the right atrial umbrella opens, both sides of the device lie very flat on the septum with no "mass" of septal tissues bunched up under the device (*see* Figure 29.12).

Because of the reported higher incidence of cryptogenic strokes in the presence of both an atrial septal aneurysm and a PFO, many operators now try to "eliminate" the aneurysm along with the PFO closure by including the aneurysm under the umbrellas of the device. The initial identification of atrial septal aneurysms often occurs during the transesophageal echocardiography obtained during the PFO occlusion procedure (Figure 29.13). When the aneurysm is to be treated, the occlusion device should be large enough to cover most of the aneurysm tissue and compress it between the two sides of the device, although some operators feel that even partial inclusion of the aneurysm within the device is sufficient. The goals are to eliminate the mobility of the aneurismal tissue in order to

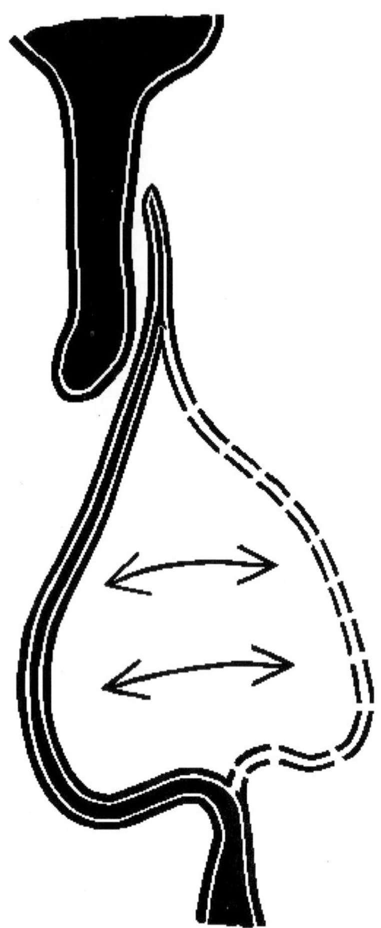

Figure 29.13 "On edge" view—aneurysm of the atrial septum in conjunction with a patent foramen ovale.

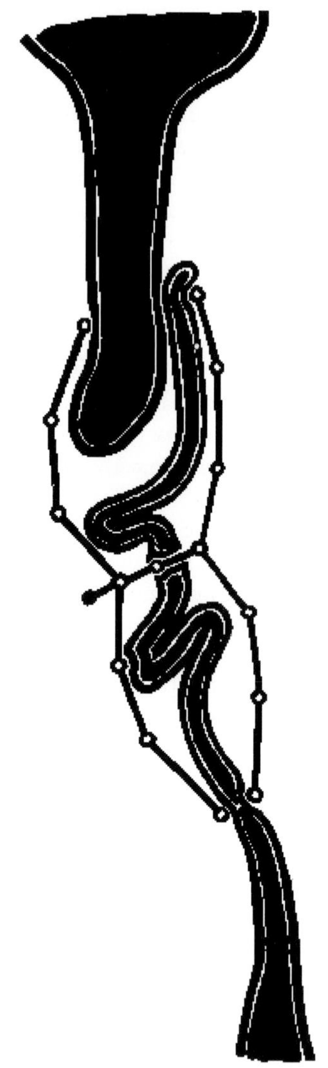

Figure 29.14 "On edge" view—aneurysm of the atrial septum in conjunction with a patent foramen ovale closed with a CardioSEAL™ device using a transseptal technique.

eliminate any potentially thrombogenic residual "pockets" within the "tunnel" of the PFO as well as to close the opening in the PFO.

The transseptal approach also is used for closing the PFO associated with an aneurysm. The puncture site through the septum primum is made nearer to the center of the aneurysm but still close enough to the left atrial opening(s) of the PFO so that the legs of the left atrial umbrella (disk) extend over, and close, the PFO opening(s) as well as cover the aneurysm (Figure 29.14).

Occasionally, and particularly with an aneurysm of the atrial septum in association with the PFO, there are two or more openings in the septum. When there are multiple openings in the septum, it must be determined whether one large single device is sufficient to occlude all of the openings or whether two or more PFO/ASD devices are necessary to cover all defects. The use of a static sizing balloon through the largest (primary) opening of the multiple defects demonstrates the distance from the edge of the balloon to the edge of the aneurysm and the distance between several or multiple orifices as seen on TEE/ICE. The second venous angiographic catheter is passed through the primary or secondary orifice into the left atrium and is used for angiography during the balloon sizing to help make these decisions. With several large openings in the septum, two or more sizing balloons are used simultaneously through the defects to define the exact sizes and relative positions of the defects to each other. Unfortunately, multiple defects frequently are around the periphery of the aneurysm and, as a result, close to edges of the septum and/or valvular structures. When there is no septal rim and/or it appears that impingement on a valve is probable, device closure is not indicated.

When the defects are close together, they usually can be closed with one large device. The single device is placed in the most central of the multiple defects. With widely separated, multiple defects, especially when they are larger defects, then more than one device is necessary to completely close all of them. Occasionally when two defects are close together and separated by only several mm of atrial tissue, the two defects are "coalesced" into one opening with a "stretched" sizing balloon or even using an angioplasty balloon. Then the defect is closed as a larger ASD.

When two or more devices are used, the devices are implanted "simultaneously". The two (or more) delivery sheaths are positioned through the separate openings before introducing either device. This avoids the necessity of having to manipulate a large sheath adjacent to a freshly implanted device. If the devices that are used are of different sizes, the implant of the smaller device is begun first. The left atrial disk of the first (smaller) device is opened in the left atrium and withdrawn against the septum. With the first device held firmly against the septum, the left atrial disk of the second (larger) device is opened and withdrawn against the first disk and left side of the septum. With traction on both delivery systems and devices, the right atrial disk of the first (smaller) device is opened on the right side of the septum, followed immediately by the opening of the right disk of the second device. This effectively compresses the smaller device within the larger device.

An alternative technique for the delivery of two devices simultaneously is to open both sides of the smaller device before beginning to deploy the second (larger) device. This alternative technique requires less simultaneous manipulations of skilled personnel and appears to be equally effective. It is important that the smaller device is implanted first in order that the smaller device is "clamped" within the larger device in order to prevent the smaller device from protruding over an edge of the larger device and, in doing so, creating a steep angle off the septum.

CardioSEAL™ closure of purposeful postoperative surgical fenestrations and/or inadvertent baffle leaks

Purposeful fenestrations frequently are created in the baffles of cavopulmonary repairs for "single ventricles", and leaks left inadvertently often are present at the edges of these same baffles and the baffles of venous switch ("Mustard" and/or "Senning") repairs of transpositions of the great arteries. The locations of the fenestration and/or baffle leaks are identified angiographically and by TEE or ICE. Once the defect is located, the X-ray tubes are positioned to align the defect(s) as precisely on edge as possible. The fenestrations and inadvertent residual leaks in baffles often are a problem for device closure because of their unusual locations on, or at the *edge* of, the baffle/patch, the direction of the necessary access to the particular location, and the location of the defects close to other structures (valves) within the heart. The actual implant of the device usually is fairly straightforward if the associated problems can be overcome. A knowledgeable and cooperative surgeon, who is considering the subsequent catheter closure by the cardiologist, places the purposeful fenestrations thoughtfully and with the subsequent catheter approach as part of the decision where to place the opening. These correctly placed fenestrations should be angled with consideration for the *usual* or *available venous access* with a catheter. The purposeful fenestrations almost always are 3–5 mm in diameter. They are punched or cut out of the baffle material which, by the time of most device closures, has become very stiff and rigid.

The process of permanently occluding these defects begins with a test occlusion of the defect with a balloon catheter to determine the effects on the acute hemodynamics of the patient. With occlusion of the defect, the patient's saturation should increase while the systemic blood pressure and systemic venous pressure should remain nearly the same without significantly dropping or rising, respectively. When a *static* sizing balloon can be used for this test occlusion, information about the size and the "configuration" of the defect is obtained along with the changes in the hemodynamics. An angiocardiogram is performed on the "left" (systemic) as well as the right side of the defect in order to obtain complete information about adjacent critical intracardiac structures (remnants of the original atrial septum, A-V valves, etc.!). Although a TEE/ICE image is not essential for the *actual implant* of the device, the area on both sides of the fenestration should be interrogated by echo for adjacent structures (valves especially), which could be interfered with by the device.

Once the defect is located, tested for the hemodynamic consequences of closure, sized and all adjacent structures identified, an end-hole catheter is manipulated through the defect and into the pulmonary veins and/or as far into the "left atrial" chamber as possible. When the end-hole catheter is positioned in a pulmonary vein, a *short* tipped, exchange length Super Stiff™ wire is passed through the catheter to a position as far distally in the vein as possible. Since many of these defects are directed anteriorly, the catheter often goes preferentially and directly into the ventricle or cephalad and anterior into the area of the original right atrial appendage.

The tip of the catheter, which is passing through the defect, often can be directed "forcefully" away from vital structures by the use of a *transseptal needle* used as a torque device, which remains completely ***within*** a shorter end-hole catheter. The tip of the transseptal needle remains back, *within* the *tip* of the catheter *all of the time* with no desire to "puncture" with the needle during the deflection procedure. The curve at the tip of the needle, the stiffness and the ability to "torque" or redirect the tip of the transseptal needle very precisely and purposefully with a *"one to one"* response are used to redirect or turn the tip of the catheter purposefully by turning the needle once the catheter is through the pre-existing defect. Once the tip of the catheter is pointed in the desired direction by the needle, the catheter is advanced off the needle and the needle withdrawn completely.

When the pulmonary veins cannot be entered and/or are not in a reasonably straight direction from the fenestration/baffle leak, a *long* floppy tipped Super Stiff™ wire (Boston Scientific, Natick, MA) is passed through the catheter and positioned in the "left-sided" atrium across the defect in a location that is away from the A-V valves and is in a minimally arrhythmogenic position. When the wire cannot be positioned in a pulmonary vein, of the two alternate locations, an atrial appendage is preferable to a ventricle for the subsequent sheath delivery. When the wire is in a ventricle, it will be through an atrioventricular valve, which can create a major problem for the positioning of the sheath for the delivery of the device. Because of the small size of the defects, the peculiar angles of these defects and the relative rigidity of the tissues, *both* the sheath and the dilator are advanced over the pre-positioned stiff wire into the left side of the defect. This often takes considerable effort and forceful "drilling" of the sheath over the dilator. Occasionally it is necessary to place an *11-French* long dilator within the long *10-French MTS sheath* (Cook Inc., Bloomington, IN) in order to create a *very tight* fit of the sheath over the dilator. Once the tip of the sheath is positioned in the left sided atrium, the dilator and then the wire are removed cautiously from the sheath and the sheath meticulously is cleared of air and/or clot as described before for PFO closures.

Once these fenestrations or baffle leaks are crossed with the delivery sheath, the occlusion is performed using the most suitable of the *available* PFO devices. Unless the tip of the delivery sheath cannot be kept away from an atrioventricular valve, the delivery of an occlusion device to a fenestration is reasonably "straightforward". Except for the occasional constraints in the area where the left sided umbrella is opened, there are minimal differences in the device delivery, extrusion and implant for the fenestration occlusions compared to the PFO occlusion. Because of the small openings of the fenestrations, the relatively rigid tissue of the baffle and the proximity of adjacent structures, the smallest possible occlusion device is preferred. Because of the unusual angles of the fenestrations and/or the venous approach to the fenestration, the opened left side of the device often approaches the baffle at a very acute angle and must be pulled against the baffle with considerable force, which often is an even more forceful pull on the device against these defects than used in PFO closures. Because of the rigidity of the tissues of the baffles, the small size of the defects and particularly with the CardioSEAL™ device, the device seldom pulls "through" the fenestrations even when using a very significant withdrawal force on the delivery system and/or when there is a marked distortion of the device and baffle.

Because of the force required to pull the device into, and align it with the baffle for the "right side" to open completely on the "right" side of the baffle, the baffle itself often is distorted and pulled away from its original "road mapped" position during the deployment of the device. If this distortion in the position/location of the baffle is not recognized and verified with angiograms through the second catheter or by the TEE or ICE imaging, the device easily can be opened completely on the "left" side of the baffle. A separate catheter for performing angiograms in conjunction with the TEE or ICE imaging is essential in order to delineate the position of the device on the baffle as well as the position of any adjacent critical intracardiac structures *during* the deployment of a device for occlusion of a fenestration.

It is particularly important to identify structures that are very close to the left (systemic) side of the defect and to open the left atrial side of the device away from these structures. A valve that is very close to the fenestration, dictates the type of occluding device that can be used. A device that "extrudes" out of the tip of the delivery sheath like the Amplatzer™ PFO device is more applicable when the left side is adjacent to a valve than a device like the CardioSEAL™ device, where the legs "spring" open some distance away from the tip of the delivery sheath.

During the maneuvers to position the "right side" of the device, small hand angiocardiograms, injecting within the defect and/or immediately adjacent to the right side of the defect, can be performed *through the delivery sheath* when a second catheter is not available in the area. Angiograms performed adjacent to the device and performed through a separate venous angiographic catheter, however, allow positioning of the angiographic catheter immediately adjacent to the defect and a better (larger) bolus of contrast, and, in turn, provide better quality and more information.

One very significant variation in the purposeful "surgical fenestrations" is the communication created between an "external conduit" Fontan and the original right atrium. Instead of a discrete hole through an area of a direct side-to-side anastomosis of the external conduit to the lateral wall of the right atrium, some surgeons interpose a short 3–5 mm diameter segment of tubular shunt material to create the "fenestration". If the small segment of the "tubular shunt" fenestration is short enough, it is handled like a fenestration in an unusually thick walled baffle. However, if the small "tubular" fenestration has significant length to it, a Gianturco-Grifka™ bag, an Amplatzer™ Plug, VSD or PDA device, or a large, controlled-release coil are considered for the occlusion of these lesions.

Inadvertent baffle and/or patch leaks often present an even greater problem for device closure than purposefully created fenestrations. These defects are not created on purpose and, as a consequence, they never are positioned with *any* consideration for a subsequent transcatheter closure. They frequently are along suture lines at the edge of the baffle/patch where it attaches to the atrial wall and/or very anteriorly in the base of the atrial appendage. The location at the edge of the baffle/patch creates an acute angle between the baffle/patch and the adjacent wall. The persistent opening usually is just at this angle, particularly on the "left" side of the baffle/patch. In spite of this, most of these defects form enough of a "flat" surface to allow closure with one of the PFO occlusion devices or their modifications. Some of these residual leaks are in such inaccessible locations that none of the "umbrella" or "double-disk" devices are applicable. Occasionally the defects in those circumstances have been occluded with the large 0.052" Gianturco™ coils *using a controlled release bioptome system*. The filaments of fiber potentially extending as far as 9 mm away from the coil and into the sluggish venous blood flow, always should be a consideration before using a Gianturco™ type coil in this location.

A static sizing balloon is even more useful in these non-purposeful baffle/patch leaks, to determine not only the exact size but also the shape of the defect and any distortion/restriction of the areas on both sides of the defect by the adjacent tissues. As with the purposeful fenestrations, the tissues usually are rigid and some force can be used when "seating" the device in the defect. As long as there is clearance from adjacent vital intracardiac structures, *larger* devices usually are used for inadvertent baffle leaks than for the purposeful, precise diameter, fenestrations. The positioning of the wire, the sheath and the delivery of the device are individualized to correspond to the peculiarities of the residual leak but usually are similar to the closures of purposeful surgical fenestrations.

Internal jugular vein device delivery for PFO, fenestrations or baffle leaks

All of the discussion concerning device closure of the PFO and fenestrations implies that the most desirable and usual approach is from the femoral veins and that there is at least one patent *femoral* vein for access. If both ilio-femoral systems and/or the inferior vena cava are occluded, the PFO, fenestrations and residual patch/baffle leaks can be approached from the internal jugular vein[16]. Because of the angle of approach from the neck, the access across a PFO, fenestration or baffle leak usually is somewhat difficult, although occasionally the peculiar angle and/or location of the fenestrations that were created "randomly" by the surgeons and/or inadvertent leaks make(s) the neck approach *preferable* to the femoral approach even when the femoral veins are patent. With all of these baffle/patch defects, a very significant pull and/or torsion can be placed on the device during implant in comparison to the occlusion of an ASD. The ability to apply extra torsion helps to compensate for a poor angle of approach to these defects when closing them from the neck/internal jugular vein.

In spite of the often bizarre angle of approach to the PFO and/or baffle leak when the catheter is introduced from the neck, the existing defects essentially always can be crossed using a combination of special preshaped and/or "angled" catheters and deflector and/or torque-controlled wires. A catheter that is introduced from the neck usually must be redirected and/or deflected 180° in order to pass under the septum secundum and through a PFO. Once the defect is crossed with a wire and/or an end-hole catheter, the original wire/catheter is replaced with a long floppy tipped, Super Stiff™ wire, which is advanced across the defect into the left atrium and looped around in the atrium until the stiff portion of the wire crosses the defect and is advanced well into the left atrium. The course from the neck to the left atrium is "straightened" by the stiff wire, however, this does create a course of the wire/catheter which aligns almost parallel to the septum and/or baffle and points the wire directly at the A-V valve on the left side of the baffle.

A fairly tight, right angle curve is preformed at the tip of the long delivery sheath/dilator with the hope of aligning the tip of the sheath more perpendicularly to the septum and away from the A-V valve once the wire and dilator are removed and at the time of device delivery. The long delivery sheath/dilator usually follows the wire across the defect into the left atrium and in doing so, the defect is propped open somewhat. Because of the very acute angle against the surface of the baffle and/or of the native septum when coming from the neck, a larger device is used than otherwise would be necessary for the occlusion of a PFO or fenestration of comparable size. This allows more torsion on, and distortion of, the device *and* baffle/septum when pulling the device forcefully into the defect during the implant. The remainder of the delivery and implant for each particular device are the same as from the femoral approach. Since the orientation of the fenestration or baffle/patch leaks in the postoperative patient is infinitely variable, an approach from the neck actually is the preferred access to these lesions when the opening in the baffle/patch is orientated facing cephalad.

Transhepatic access for PFO, fenestrations and baffle leak occlusions

In the presence of occluded femoral access and when unable to cross the defect and/or deliver the device from the superior vena cava approach, the transhepatic approach offers straight access to the atrial septum and/or wall of a baffle. Large devices introduced through as large as 11-French sheaths can, and are, delivered successfully and safely through this route[17]. In the PFO, the tissues of the septum are not as rigid or as resistant to pulling and distortion as they are in postoperative baffles. For this reason, in the absence of the femoral approach, the transhepatic approach is preferable to the internal jugular approach for the transcatheter closure of a PFO using any of the currently available devices. The technique is similar to the transhepatic closure of the ASD, which is described in detail in Chapter 28.

STARFlex™ ASD device closure of PFO, fenestrations and baffle leaks

The STARFlex™ ASD Device (NMT Medical Inc., Boston, MA) has had limited use in these defects in the United States and then, only in one high-risk protocol study. The identification, sizing of the defects and the delivery of the device for use in the PFO and/or fenestrations are identical to those when using the CardioSEAL™ device. The preliminary data from the limited use indicate little difference between the delivery, implant and/or the effectiveness of the STARFlex™ compared to the CardioSEAL™ in closing a PFO or fenestrations/baffle/leaks. The centering wires of the STARFlex™ device theoretically do tend to pull the tips of the legs more firmly against the septum, which could be an advantage for the tight closure of the PFO, particularly on a septum with a very "irregular" surface.

Amplatzer™ PFO occluder closure of PFO, fenestrations and baffle leaks

The Amplatzer™ PFO device is designed specifically for PFO and fenestration closures[18]. The original Amplatzer™ *ASD* occluder, on the other hand, usually is not satisfactory for occlusion of a PFO or fenestrations because of its large diameter central hub or "waist" relative to the smaller "disks" at each end of the hub. The closure of a defect with an Amplatzer™ *ASD* device depends upon the large diameter, central "hub" of the device pushing circumferentially against the edges of the defect to seal the leak. The relatively narrow "rims" of the disks at each end of the hub are not designed as part of the "closure apparatus" and, at the same time, are not broad enough to hold a device within a distensible and/or a long PFO that has very eccentrically located and widely separated openings into each atrium. In addition, with the off-set walls of even a "partial tunnel" PFO, the central hub has nothing to stretch against, with the result that there is very poor or no fixation of the Amplatzer™ ASD device to the "edges" of a PFO.

The Amplatzer™ PFO devices are designed specifically for the anatomy of the PFO. They are made of the same material (a fine Nitinol™ memory wire) and with a similar weave to the Amplatzer™ ASD devices. The central joining "hub" or waist of the Amplatzer™ PFO device, however, is very narrow and *flexible* while the two outer "rims" are much larger and actually create two large diameter, right and left atrial *disks* similar to the other "double-umbrella" devices. On the two larger Amplatzer™ PFO devices, the *right* atrial disk is slightly larger than the left atrial disk to account for the often higher right atrial pressures and the predominantly *right to left* shunting of these defects. Both the right and left atrial disks of the smaller, 18 mm Amplatzer™ PFO device are 18 mm in diameter. The diameter of the *right* atrial disk represents the labeled size of these devices. The Amplatzer™ PFO devices presently are available with a 35, a 25 and an 18 mm right atrial disk. These have corresponding left atrial disks of 25, 18 and 18 mm respectively. The two disks of the PFO devices are connected by a very narrow, fixed diameter, slightly flexible and eccentric central connecting "hub" or waist. The connecting hub is 3 mm long, somewhat stretchable and attached slightly eccentrically to the two disks. The size of the Amplatzer™ PFO device and the technique for delivery that is used for the occlusion of the PFO are determined by the diameter and the anatomy of the defect to be closed.

The closure mechanism of the PFO using the Amplatzer™ PFO devices resembles the closure of defects using the "double-umbrella" devices more closely than the occlusion mechanism of the original Amplatzer™ ASD device. The two, large right and left atrial disks compress the lesion between the two *opposing disks* to accomplish the closure, rather than by the expansion of the central hub into the defect, as is the case in the Amplatzer™ ASD device.

The Amplatzer™ PFO devices are delivered through a 7-, 8- or 9-French, Amplatzer™ long delivery sheath for the 18, 25 and 35 mm devices, respectively. The equivalent sized Hausdorf™ modification of the Cook™ sheaths are equally suitable for the delivery of the Amplatzer™ PFO devices, but for the occlusion of the PFO probably do not contribute much to the procedure. Similar criteria to those which are used for the CardioSEAL™ device, are used to determine whether the Amplatzer™ PFO device is delivered directly through the PFO "channel" or whether the device should be delivered through a transseptal puncture. With the much easier retrievability of the Amplatzer™ PFO device, the delivery through a "questionable tunnel" can be attempted more freely with the Amplatzer PFO device than with the CardioSEAL™ device. The Amplatzer™ PFO device has the great advantage that if it does not implant in an ideal position when an implant in a "tunnel" is attempted, the device *easily* can be withdrawn and reintroduced after performing a transseptal puncture through the septum primum.

Depending upon the anatomy of the PFO, the delivery sheath/dilator is advanced over a wire through the defect and into the left atrium, identically to the technique for the delivery of the sheath when using a CardioSEAL™ device. All of the meticulous precautions concerning the removal of air and clots from the sheath are carried out exactly as with any of the ASD devices. Once the sheath is in position, the Amplatzer™ PFO device is attached to the delivery cable, withdrawn into the short loader sheath, introduced into the delivery sheath and advanced to the end of the long sheath, which is positioned in the left atrium.

The delivery and implant of the Amplatzer™ PFO device is more like the delivery of a CardioSEAL™ device than it is to the delivery of the Amplatzer™ ASD devices. The left atrial disk is extruded completely into the left atrium and the entire delivery system with the opened left atrial disk is withdrawn until the left atrial disk is flat against the PFO and the left side of the septum. The delivery cable is fixed in place, fixing the left disk against the septum while the sheath is withdrawn off the remainder of the device. This extrudes, first, the narrow central connecting waist and then the right-sided disk. The security of the fixation of the device in the septum is verified by gingerly pushing and pulling the cable with the device in a to-and-fro motion, while the device still is attached to the cable. After the proper and secure position has been verified, the device is released by unscrewing the delivery cable in a counterclockwise direction.

Amplatzer™ PFO devices have the same capability as the Amplatzer™ ASD devices of being withdrawn easily back into the delivery sheath *at any time before* the purposeful release of the device from the delivery cable. This allows easy repositioning and/or total withdrawal of the device even after both sides of the device are deployed completely in the PFO and/or on the septum.

The Amplatzer™ PFO device produces occlusion both by covering the orifices of the defect at both ends and by compressing the tissues between the two opposing "disks". The very persistent memory characteristics of the Nitinol™ materials of the Amplatzer™ device makes the Amplatzer™ PFO device less desirable for implant with a "tunnel" PFO unless it is delivered using a transseptal technique. Although the device easily can be deployed in a long tunnel of a PFO, the deployed configuration of the Amplatzer™ PFO device initially will be distorted markedly as it conforms to the shape of the tunnel. The memory of the Nitinol™ metal of the device, however, will continue to exert force against adjacent, distorted tissues until the device resumes its *original* "flat, double disk" "resting" configuration. In reassuming this shape, the device potentially can erode into and/or through any tissues that are in its way until it eventually reaches its "resting", flat opposing disks, configuration. This erosion could be through the aortic or atrial wall as well as only atrial tissues! When delivered transseptally in order to close a "tunnel" PFO, the Amplatzer™ PFO device™ functions similarly to the CardioSEAL™ device in compressing the septum primum against the septum secundum.

The current Amplatzer™ PFO device is not particularly well suited for the closure of baffle fenestrations or baffle leaks. The 18 mm PFO device will close the opening, but even the 18 mm device is unnecessarily large for most fenestrations, particularly for the right-sided disk to fit into, and conform to the usually small, systemic venous channels. The 4 mm Amplatzer™ *ASD* device has been effective in closing fenestrations in baffles[19]. For the closure of many fenestrations, even the 4 mm central hub is oversized for the small opening of the fenestration, and since the rigid rim of the fenestration does not allow the hub to expand, in turn, the end "disks" of the ASD device cannot flatten out as they do within a stretchable septal opening. It probably will be only a matter of a short time before a more appropriate Amplatzer™ device is developed specifically for the size and anatomy of very small fenestrations/baffle leaks!

The CARDIA™ device

The CARDIA™ device (Cardia, Burnsville, MN) is a later generation and significantly different version of the PFO STAR™ device, which was used extensively in Europe for closure of the PFO. The CARDIA™ device currently is in clinical use in Europe and in an investigational trial in the US for PFO closure. CARDIA™ devices are "double umbrellas", similar in *design* to the old Rashkind™ PDA device, however, the CARDIA™ is manufactured from completely different materials and the disk on each side has six evenly spaced legs. Each CARDIA™ device has two opposing hexagonal fabric "umbrellas" mounted on a frame of crossing metal wire arms. The 6 "arms" of the frame, supporting each hexagonal umbrella, actually are three crossing "bows" of flexible, Nitinol™ wires attached to each other at their centers. Each of the wire "bows" actually is a *braid* of multiple strands of extremely fine Nitinol™ wires. The "bows" of each umbrella are curved slightly from the center toward the opposite umbrella so that the two disks compress against each other (and the septum). The free end of each of the stiff Nitinol™ "arms" is "blunted" with a smooth metal tip, hopefully to prevent their digging into tissues. The fabric of the CARDIA™ occluder "umbrellas" is small, thin, hexagonal sheets of Ivalon™. The two opposing umbrellas are attached to each other by short posts at the central, crossing points of the arms. The posts are either 3 or 5 mm in length to accommodate different thicknesses of the septum. At the center on the right atrial side of the right atrial (proximal) disk there is a short pin with a tiny polished ball at the tip of the pin for attachment to the delivery system. The CARDIA™ device is available with both the 3 and the 5 mm central post in 20, 25, 30 and 35 mm sizes. The size represents the maximum diameter of the umbrella when measured from tip to tip of an arm.

The CARDIA™ device comes as a CARDIA™ PFO kit, which includes a special delivery cable/device and a short translucent loader. The delivery cable is a 5-French bioptome that has been modified to hold the device uniquely. Each jaw of the bioptome has a tiny notch on the most distal "lip" of the jaw, which creates a small hole at the tip of the jaws when they are closed. The tiny hole accommodates the diameter of the attachment pin of the device very loosely, but does not allow the tiny "ball" at the tip of the pin to pass through the hole. This hole in the closed jaws allows free rotation of the device, but not much angulation. In addition to the hole in the jaws, there is a very secure locking screw mechanism at the proximal end of the "bioptome" catheter, which is adjacent to the open–close mechanism of the handle. The locking mechanism locks the jaws closed *very securely* over the pin of the device, preventing any inadvertent release of the device. The translucent loader has a slight flair at each end. In addition to the "kit" a separate, short 12-French sheath with a back-bleed valve/flush port is used in the loading of the Cardia™ device into a long delivery sheath.

The delivery cable is passed from proximal to distal first through the short 12-French sheath, through the short translucent loader, and then the device is attached to the delivery cable. The proximal umbrella of the attached device is compressed and folded manually toward the loader with the operator's fingers and withdrawn into the distal end of the translucent loader by withdrawing the delivery cable into and through the loader. As the delivery cable is withdrawn still further into the translucent loader, the arms of the distal umbrella fold away from the loader, and the entire device is pulled into the translucent loader, now with the two umbrellas of the device folded away from *each other*. Once the device is completely within the loader, the short 12-F sheath is pushed tightly into the proximal, also flared end of the loader and the delivery cable along with the attached and folded device are withdrawn out of the loader and into the short 12-F sheath. The translucent loader is discarded. The short 12-F sheath containing the device is flushed thoroughly through the side port of the sheath and is now used to introduce the device into the long delivery sheath.

CARDIA™ devices are delivered through a prepositioned long 11–13-French MTS™ sheath identical to the delivery of a CardioSEAL™ device. All of the precautions necessary to avoid air in the system are applicable to the CARDIA™ device, loading and delivery system. The technique for crossing the PFO in the presence of a "tunnel-type" PFO is probably more critical than for the CardioSEAL™ and the Amplatzer™ devices. The legs of the CARDIA™ devices are flexible from the center, but the individual legs do not bend or flex at any point, which makes them less "moldable" and less conforming to a constraining tunnel than the other two devices. If wedged into a long, potentially large diameter, tunnel the legs of the CARDIA™ device will tend to splint the tunnel open. Once the long sheath is in position either through the PFO and/or transseptally and cleared of all air as described previously under the delivery of a CardioSEAL™ device, the side ports of the long sheath and the short 12-F sheath both are placed on a continuous, vigorous flush while the short sheath is introduced into the valve of the long sheath. With the short sheath seated through the valve and securely against the proximal end of the long sheath, the delivery cable is advanced into the short sheath, which, in turn, advances the CARDIA™ device into the long sheath. The short sheath is withdrawn out of the proximal end of the long sheath and back over the delivery cable. Thereafter the delivery of the CARDIA™ PFO device is identical to the delivery of a CardioSEAL™ device.

The distal (left atrial) legs are deployed completely into the left atrium by a combination of advancing the delivery cable and withdrawing the sheath. The entire system (sheath, cable and partially opened device) is withdrawn back against the septum until the left atrial legs are seen, on both fluoroscopy and TEE/ICE, to "flex" away from the septal surface. With the delivery cable fixed in that position, the sheath alone is withdrawn which, in turn, allows the right-sided legs to open on the right atrial side of the septum. When satisfied with the position and fixation on the septum, the locking mechanism at the proximal end of the delivery cable is unscrewed and the "jaws" are opened, releasing the device.

The arms of the CARDIA™ device are very flexible and allow the easy withdrawal of the device back into the delivery sheath before the device is released, even after *both disks have been deployed* and *without* destroying the device! However, if the CARDIA™ device is withdrawn back into the sheath after deployment of the proximal umbrella, the proximal (right atrial) disk *is everted* within the long sheath. The short introducing sheath is reintroduced into the proximal end of the long sheath and the device is withdrawn from the long sheath and *back into the short sheath* in order to withdraw it through the valve of the long delivery sheath. Once out of the long sheath, the device is delivered from the short sheath and released from the delivery cable. The loading procedure is repeated, starting from the very beginning of the procedure with reattachment.

In spite of the flexibility of the legs of the device, it does clamp securely on the septum, but, at the same time, it is not as "robust" as the CardioSEAL™ or the Amplatzer™ PFO devices. As with the Amplatzer™ PFO device, the Nitinol™ metal will attempt to conform over time to the original "resting" configuration of the device, regardless of what structures may be in the way. The particular advantages and disadvantages of the CARDIA™ PFO devices, compared to the well-tested CardioSEAL™ and Amplatzer™ PFO devices, are yet to be demonstrated.

Sideris Inverted Button™ device for PFO/fenestration closures

The standard Sideris Button™ ASD Occluder (Pediatric Cardiology Custom Medical Devices, Athens, Greece) was designed specifically for left to right shunts and depended somewhat on the higher left atrial pressure to secure the left atrial disk against the left atrial septal surface. With a significant right to left shunt through the atrial septum, the left atrial disk of a *standard* Sideris™ ASD occluder acts more like a sail or "parachute", which can pull the device off the septum in the presence of a right to left shunt. To overcome this problem, the Button™ ASD occluder was redesigned as the Inverted Button™ occluder (Pediatric Cardiology Custom Medical Devices, Athens, Greece) specifically for right to left shunts[20]. The Inverted Button™ occluder differs from the fourth generation Button™ ASD occluder exactly as the name implies by having the small attaching loops and knots placed *on the counter occluder* and the latex attaching plug placed on the "occluder". In addition, the order in which the components of the device are delivered is reversed, with the counter occluder delivered into the left atrium and the "occluder" in the right atrium buttoned against it. As a result, the sides of the septum on which the disk occluder and the counter occluder are placed are reversed compared to the standard Button™ ASD occluders. The Inverted Button Occluder™ is only available with a 25 mm diameter right-sided disk occluder. The Inverted Button Occluder™ is delivered through an 8- or 9-French sheath.

With the Sideris Inverted Button™, the Sideris Standard Button™ and the Sideris Double Disk Button™, the peculiarities of each individual PFO still exist and must be taken into consideration when closing a PFO. None of the Button™ devices are suited any better than the other PFO devices for the long "tunnel" PFO unless they are delivered transseptally. However, since the deployed Buttons™ are not as rigid and are more "compressible" than most of the other devices, they may "wad up" more compactly within a "tunnel" similar to the old Rashkind™ PDA device in a "tubular" PDA. There has been no experience of this reported to date.

The appropriate long delivery sheath for the Inverted Button Device™ is advanced to the left atrium either through the opening in the PFO or transseptally, depending upon the anatomy. For the delivery of the Inverted Button™, the *counter occluder* is attached to the control suture, which is contained within the long hollow wire. The pusher catheter is advanced over the hollow wire containing the control suture and up to the counter occluder while all of these still are outside of the body. The counter occluder with the pusher catheter and control suture/hollow wire are introduced into the pre-positioned delivery sheath and advanced with the pusher catheter to the left side of the PFO through the sheath. The counter occluder is extruded out of the sheath into the left atrium by both pushing the pusher catheter forward while simultaneously withdrawing the delivery sheath back into the right atrium. The control suture in the hollow wire along with the counter occluder is pulled against the left side of the septum by placing traction on the control suture. The control suture is held taut while the pusher catheter is withdrawn out of the sheath over the suture within the hollow wire. The tip of the delivery sheath is maintained in the center of the right atrium.

The latex "button" attached at the center of the disk occluder is introduced over the control suture and hollow wire. By manually compressing the corners of the occluder forward, the occluder is introduced into the delivery sheath following the "button". Using the pusher catheter again, the occluder disk is pushed through the sheath to the right atrium and out of the end of the sheath. The occluder opens towards the septum as it exits the tip of the sheath. Once the occluder is fully open, it is pushed forcefully against the right side of the septum by advancing the pusher catheter and the delivery sheath together, and while applying counter traction on the control suture and the counter occluder.

This "buttons" the occluder to the counter occluder, which is held tightly against the opposite side of the septum by the traction on the control suture. When satisfied with the "buttoning" of the occluder to the counter occluder, the pusher catheter, sheath and long hollow wire are removed. A "right sided" angiogram is performed with an injection through a separate catheter positioned adjacent to the "occluder". When satisfied with the position and degree of occlusion by the device, the control suture is withdrawn by pulling on one end of the suture while advancing the other end of the suture, which pulls it through and out of the attaching eye on the occluder and releases the device on the septum.

In defects with bidirectional shunting, neither the original ASD Button™ occluder nor the Inverted Button™ occluder was satisfactory. The occluding device could blow away from the side that had the occluder as a result of the flow through the defect against the underside of the opened disk pushing it away from the septum. To overcome this, a standard 30 mm diameter Button™ occluder with the attached spring knots is used on the left side of the septum. Instead of the usual counter occluder, however, the right-sided *occluder disk* of the Inverted Button™ occluder is used on the right side of the septum, creating a "double-umbrella" Button™ occluder similar in concept to the CardioSEAL and STARFlex™ devices. The disks on both sides of the septum apparently solve the problem of the devices being blown off the septum and embolizing in the presence of bidirectional shunting. The Inverted Button™ Device has been used for the occlusion of fenestrations. The delivery and implant of the device in these lesions is similar to the delivery for closure of the PFO. The standard 28 mm diameter occluder of the Inverted Button™ device, however, like the larger Amplatzer™ PFO occluder, is large and potentially obstructive for any "right-sided channel" within most of the "lateral tunnels". Smaller Inverted Buttons™ should solve this problem. There is still too little documented experience with the use of this device in fenestrations and inadvertent baffle/ patch leaks.

The Helex™ device for PFO and fenestration occlusions

The Helex™ ASD device (W. L. Gore & Associates, Flagstaff, AZ) recently was introduced into clinical use in Europe with a CE mark for transcatheter closure of the ASD and the PFO; it has undergone a pilot FDA, IDE trial and is just beginning an FDA monitored IDE clinical trial in the United States for the closure of the ASD. The delivery and implant of the Helex™ device for the ASD and PFO are identical and are described in detail in Chapter 28 ("ASD Occlusions"). The preliminary infomation about the Helex™ used for PFO occlusions appears encouraging, although the numbers and duration of implants are far too small and short to come to any conclusions[21].

Conceptually, the Helex™ device is ideally suited for PFO occlusion. The left and right atrial "disks" are large enough to incorporate and compress an atrial septal aneurysm and to cover even multiple openings in an aneurysm/atrial septum. At the same time the central part of the Helex™, which connects the two "disks" and lies within the defect, should fit nicely within the stereotype PFO. The Helex™ itself may not conform to the long, "tunnel-like" configurations within the atrial septum without distorting either the device and/or the "tunnel" significantly. The distance within a long, rigid "tunnel" potentially may either prevent both "end disks" from forming completely or the locking wire from catching all of the eyelets for a firm fixation within the septal tunnel. More experience is necessary before any final conclusions can be drawn about the suitability of this device for *all varieties* of PFO.

There is no mention, to date, of the use of this device for post-surgical fenestrations and/or leaks. The device is available with various sized disks and the connecting component compresses very tightly, so a small Helex™ device should fit easily into small fenestrations without significant distortion and without compromising the channel or adjacent structures on either side of a baffle. If the locking mechanism can attach within the defects with their very small, rigid disks, the 15 mm device should be very suitable for the closure of fenestrations in patients with small systemic venous channels.

Gianturco coils™ for the occlusion of fenestrations

In 1996, during one of the FDA enforced lapses in the availability of the double-umbrella or double-disk devices for transcatheter occlusion of intracardiac defects, there was one report on the use of the standard, non-controlled, Gianturco coil™ for occlusion of the fenestration after "Fontan" surgery[22]. An 8 mm diameter, 10 cm long, 0.038", free-release coil was used in each case. This allowed two full loops of coil on each side of the defect. Although the technique was acutely successful in four patients, there has been no reported medium or long term follow-up, and four patients do not make a series to approve or to condemn a particular technique.

The controllable attach/release systems that now are available for Gianturco™ coils, make the *deployment* of a coil in this circumstance potentially less hazardous. The "double-umbrella devices" fix on the baffle and occlude by the mechanical compressive forces of the opposing umbrellas, thrombosis within (or under) the devices, and by the devices becoming covered with micro thrombi and eventually endothelium. The coils, on the other hand, occlude by the formation of extensive thrombi *on* the metal coils and the fibers that are embedded in the wires of the coil. These fibers *extend and dangle out* into the adjacent blood flow *as much as 9 mm off the surface* the coils. In areas of high-velocity blood flow such as the aorta and even in the pulmonary artery, this potential gross thrombus formation on the surface of the coils has not caused any *recognizable* problem (although any tiny and/or transient embolic materials could travel from the area of the ductus to the lungs or lower half of the body and could go unnoticed). At the same time, there are concerns about an exaggeration of such thrombus formation on both sides of a baffle in the very sluggish venous circulation found in both the systemic and pulmonary venous channels on both sides of the "Fontan" channel. In addition, even after successful deployment, the fixation of a coil on a rigid, partially or totally non-endothelialized surface of a baffle is inherently unstable compared to any of the "umbrella" or double-disk devices that actually clamp onto the surface. The more rigid, 0.052" coils would make this fixation more secure, however, coils currently are not recommended for the occlusion of surgically created "fenestrations" in the venous circulation(s).

A controlled-release coil may be more appropriate for occlusion of the *inadvertent* baffle and/or patch leaks. These inadvertent leaks usually are located at the edge of the baffle or patch and often are deep in a "crevice" out of the main stream of the venous blood flow. The areas where these leaks do occur often make them very difficult (impossible) to occlude with one of the "umbrella" type devices, particularly with the larger and stiffer delivery systems for the "umbrellas". The controlled-release coils are easier to deliver to these locations than the "umbrella devices", and once the defect is occluded, the "thrombi" on the fibers of the coil hopefully are out of the flow of the active circulation. Coil occlusion of this type of lesion probably is reasonably safe when occlusion of the defect is necessary. Now, with the HDE availability of the CardioSEAL™ umbrellas for fenestrations (and hopefully other devices soon to follow), a residual defect in a very difficult location would be the only indication for the closure of a purposeful baffle fenestration with anything except one of the more secure and potentially less thrombogenic devices.

Complications of transcatheter occlusions of the patent foramen ovale, fenestrations and baffle leaks

The complications of the occlusions of the PFO, fenestrations and baffles in the catheterization laboratory are similar to the complications for the occlusions of ASDs, which were covered in detail in Chapter 28. The likelihood of several of the complications occurring, however, is slightly different. The risk of *device embolization* is far *less* during PFO and/or fenestration occlusions (and should be zero), assuming that the proper device is used, correct techniques are utilized, and that all of the equipment functions properly. At the same time, since most of the PFO/fenestration defects are associated with predominantly or potentially *right to left* shunts, the potential for air/clot embolization to the systemic arterial system is even greater than during ASD occlusions. The same precautions for preventing air and/or clot in the sheaths and catheters are utilized, but even more stringently, than for the ASD occlusion procedures. These precautions are equally important during all of the manipulations in the *systemic venous* side of the circulation for the PFO/fenestration occlusion procedures.

Except for this greater risk of air and/or clot embolization to the systemic circulation while manipulating in the systemic venous circulation, the only other complications, which are *unique* to the *procedures* for PFO occlusion compared to the procedures for the closure of ASDs, are the potential complications of a transseptal procedure, which would be performed during the occlusion of a long tunnel PFO. The complications of the transseptal procedure and the prevention of those complications are covered in detail in Chapter 8.

Although not a complication of the *procedure per se*, poor and/or unusual position or "seating" of a device on the septum or baffle and/or in the defect is more common following the occlusions of a PFO or fenestration than following the successful implant of a device in a secundum ASD. When using an Amplatzer™, a CARDIA™ or a Sideris Inverted Button™ device, they all can be withdrawn back into the delivery sheath fairly readily and either withdrawn completely or repositioned and re-implanted when the abnormal position is recognized *before* the occlusion device is *released*. The CardioSEAL™ and STARFlex™ devices, on the other hand, are more difficult to pull out of the septum once both disks are deployed, and when withdrawn into the sheath the devices are destroyed. The CardioSEAL™ and the STARFlex™ devices cannot be withdrawn completely into the delivery sheath and out of the vascular system unless the larger diameter, short "recovery" sheath is pre-positioned over the long delivery sheath at the onset of the procedure, as described earlier in this chapter and in Chapter 28 under ASD occlusion with the STARFlex™ device. The problem of device malposition is minimized (or eliminated) by the use of proper and proven techniques for the implant of the devices. When a device does not lie flat on the septal surface, it may be more prone to residual leak and/or thrombus formation on the surface of the device.

All of the devices used to close both the ASD and the PFO have had a very small incidence of thrombi noted on the devices during early and late follow-up. In addition, all the devices have had rare, but definite, recurrent, central nervous system and/or other embolic events. At the same time, no correlation has been shown between the thrombi on the devices and recurrent central nervous system events[23]. A very few devices have been removed surgically because of the finding of thrombi, but the majority have been treated medically and the thrombi resolved with anticoagulation therapy. Most of the devices also have had a variable incidence of residual leak with some minor correlation between residual leaks and the recurrent central nervous system events. Unfortunately, these adverse events and complications have not had a multifactorial analysis to correlate with the particular device, the technique of implant, the configuration on the septum and/or in the defect, the residual leaks, any pre-existing clotting factors and the type of anticoagulation following implant.

There have been extremely rare, isolated reports of cardiac perforation/erosion by an implanted device[24]. Hopefully this complication can be prevented by the proper choice of device for the particular lesion. Endocarditis has been reported on the devices on two occasions[25,26]. Careful screening of the patients for infection before the implant, the use of strict ("surgical") sterile techniques and antibiotic prophylaxis during the implant procedure, avoiding any elective interventions and/or the religious use of antibiotic prophylaxis during the six months immediately following the implant should be sufficient to avoid this complication.

The future of catheter-delivered devices for the occlusion of PFO/fenestrations

Outside of the United States, multiple catheter-delivered devices have been demonstrated to be effective, and they are in widespread use for the occlusion of a PFO and/or fenestrations in patches/baffles. With the HDE approval by the FDA in the United States of the CardioSEAL™ and the Amplatzer™ PFO devices for the occlusion of the PFO, postoperative fenestrations and patch/baffle leaks, these lesions now are closed routinely in the cardiac catheterization laboratory in cardiovascular centers in the US and the rest of the world. In spite of this acceptance and the widespread use of these devices for occlusion of the PFO, the first randomized trials to try to determine the true efficacy of the closure of the PFO for the prevention of embolic strokes now are ongoing.

As new and improved devices for ASD occlusion are developed, improvements in the devices, the size of the delivery systems, the ease and safety of the delivery and in the immediate occlusion rate for PFO occlusions should occur simultaneously. Presumably, with positive results from the randomized trials, the FDA will bless these improvements with approval for use in the United States and without unique "restrictions" for their use.

References

1. Lock J *et al.* Clamshell umbrella closure of atrial septal defects: initial experience (abstr). *Circulation* 1989; **80**(II): 592.
2. Moon RE, Camporesi EM, and Kisslo JA. Patent foramen ovale and decompression sickness in divers. *Lancet* 1989; **1**(8637): 513–514.
3. Begin R. Platypnea after pneumonectomy. *N Engl J Med* 1975; **293**(7): 342–343.
4. Begin R *et al.* Patent foramen ovale and hypoxemia in chronic obstructive pulmonary disease. *Eur J Respir Dis* 1981; **62**(6): 373–375.
5. Manno BV *et al.* Right ventricular infarction complicated by right to left shunt. *J Am Coll Cardiol* 1983; **1**(2 Pt 1): 554–557.
6. Landzberg MJ *et al.* Orthodeoxia-platypnea due to intracardiac shunting—relief with transcatheter double umbrella closure. *Cathet Cardiovasc Diagn* 1995; **36**(3): 247–250.
7. Wilmshurst P and Nightingale S. Relationship between migraine and cardiac and pulmonary right-to-left shunts. *Clin Sci (Lond)* 2001; **100**(2): 215–220.
8. Belkin RN *et al.* Comparison of transesophageal and transthoracic echocardiography with contrast and color flow Doppler in the detection of patent foramen ovale. *Am Heart J* 1994; **128**(3): 520–525.
9. Karttunen V *et al.* Ear oximetry: a noninvasive method for detection of patent foramen ovale: a study comparing dye dilution method and oximetry with contrast transesophageal echocardiography. *Stroke* 2001; **32**(2): 448–453.
10. Kuhl HP *et al.* Transthoracic echocardiography using second harmonic imaging: diagnostic alternative to transesophageal echocardiography for the detection of atrial right to left shunt in patients with cerebral embolic events. *J Am Coll Cardiol* 1999; **34**(6): 1823–1830.
11. Droste DW *et al.* Right-to-left-shunts detected by transesophageal echocardiography and transcranial Doppler sonography. *Cerebrovasc Dis* 2004; **17**(2–3): 191–196.
12. McMahon CJ *et al.* Steerable control of the eustachian valve during transcatheter closure of secundum atrial septal defects. *Catheter Cardiovasc Interv* 2000; **51**(4): 455–459.
13. Kerut EK *et al.* Patent foramen ovale: a review of associated conditions and the impact of physiological size. *J Am Coll Cardiol* 2001; **38**(3): 613–623.
14. Chintala K *et al.* Use of balloon pull-through technique to assist in CardioSEAL device closure of patent foramen ovale. *Catheter Cardiovasc Interv* 2003; **60**(1): 101–106.
15. Ruiz CE, Alboliras ET, and Pophal SG. The puncture technique: a new method for transcatheter closure of patent foramen ovale. *Catheter Cardiovasc Interv* 2001; **53**(3): 369–372.
16. Sader MA *et al.* Percutaneous transcatheter patent foramen ovale closure using the right internal jugular venous approach. *Catheter Cardiovasc Interv* 2003; **60**(4): 536–539.
17. Shim D, Lloyd TR, and Beekman RH 3rd. Transhepatic therapeutic cardiac catheterization: a new option for the pediatric interventionalist. *Catheter Cardiovasc Interv* 1999; **47**(1): 41–45.
18. Han YM *et al.* New self-expanding patent foramen ovale occlusion device. *Catheter Cardiovasc Interv* 1999; **47**(3): 370–376.
19. Cowley CG *et al.* Transcatheter closure of fontan fenestrations using the Amplatzer septal occluder: initial experience and follow-up. *Catheter Cardiovasc Interv* 2000; **51**(3): 301–304.
20. Rao PS, Chandar JS, and Sideris EB. Role of inverted buttoned device in transcatheter occlusion of atrial septal defects or patent foramen ovale with right-to-left shunting associated with previously operated complex congenital cardiac anomalies. *Am J Cardiol* 1997; **80**(7): 914–921.
21. Sievert H *et al.* Patent foramen ovale closure in patients with transient ischemia attack/stroke. *J Interv Cardiol* 2001; **14**(2): 261–266.
22. Sommer RJ *et al.* Transcatheter coil occlusion of surgical fenestration after Fontan operation. *Circulation* 1996; **94**(3): 249–252.
23. Krumsdorf U *et al.* Incidence and clinical course of thrombus formation on atrial septal defect and patent foramen ovale closure devices in 1,000 consecutive patients. *J Am Coll Cardiol* 2004; **43**(2): 302–309.
24. Trepels T *et al.* Cardiac perforation following transcatheter PFO closure. *Catheter Cardiovasc Interv* 2003; **58**(1): 111–113.
25. Bullock AM, Menahem S, and Wilkinson JL. Infective endocarditis on an occluder closing an atrial septal defect. *Cardiol Young* 1999; **9**(1): 65–67.
26. Goldstein JA *et al.* Infective endocarditis resulting from CardioSEAL closure of a patent foramen ovale. *Catheter Cardiovasc Interv* 2002; **55**(2): 217–220; discussion 221.

30 Transcatheter closure of ventricular septal defects

Introduction

Transcatheter (non-surgical) closure of ventricular septal defects (VSD) has been a goal of pediatric cardiologists for decades. The large majority of congenital ventricular septal defects are outlet, perimembranous septal defects or the inlet defects associated with endocardial cushion defects. The close proximity to the aortic and/or the atrioventricular valve apparatus of these ventricular septal defects has, in general, prevented the use of the available transcatheter occlusion devices for the catheter correction of these particular defects. On the other hand, the more remote location of most of the muscular interventricular septal defects away from vital valve structures makes them ideal lesions for device closure. The difficulty of surgical closure of muscular interventricular septal defects, which results in a higher failure rate, a higher morbidity and even a higher mortality, makes these defects even more inviting to the interventional cardiologist.

Transcatheter closure of muscular ventricular septal defects was accomplished using the Rashkind™ patent ductus arteriosus (PDA) occluding device[1]. This device also was utilized to close post-surgical peri-patch leaks in perimembranous ventricular septal defects and in a few acquired ventricular septal defects, which occurred after acute myocardial infarction. Although, in most cases, the delivery technique and the implant of the device were successful, the PDA devices were too small for most muscular interventricular septal defects, resulting in significant residual leaks and/or actual embolization of the device. A still larger version of the PDA device did overcome some of the deficiencies of the standard PDA device for use in ventricular septal defects. The development and use of the Clamshell™ ASD device with its much larger sizes and the extra hinge mechanism on the arms resulted in more successful transcatheter closure of the muscular VSD, however, it did not solve all of the problems with this procedure[2]. The subsequent development and availability of the CardioSEAL™ ASD device, the STARFlex™ ASD device and finally the Amplatzer™ VSD device have led to even further improvements in the techniques and a significant improvement in the results of catheter device closure of *congenital* muscular VSDs.

There is an almost infinite variety of congenital muscular ventricular septal defects. The muscular defects vary from tiny defects, with no hemodynamic significance, to very large defects, which result in a functional single ventricle. The muscular VSDs occur as single isolated defects, as several separated muscular defects, or even as multiple, so-called "Swiss cheese" defects. The muscular ventricular septal defect(s) may be the only defect(s) or they can be associated with other intracardiac defects, including other both outlet and inlet ventricular septal defects. The muscular defects can occur in any location in the muscular septum.

Almost all of the congenital muscular interventricular septal defects are amenable to closure using a transcatheter device/procedure. The most favorable defects for a transcatheter occlusion technique are located in the apical, mid and anterior muscular septum. The exact technique used for transcatheter muscular defect closure depends upon the location of the defect in the muscular septum, the particular device(s) available at that time and somewhat upon the operator's preference. The decision to close these defects with a catheter technique does not depend upon the presence and location of the defect alone. The net hemodynamic effect *of the muscular VSD* is the primary consideration. When a patient is undergoing surgery for other intracardiac defects, the accessibility to the muscular defects in relation to the other cardiac defects being repaired should be considered. When a hemodynamically significant muscular defect is in a location that would require a ventriculotomy to accomplish a surgical repair, transcatheter VSD closure should be utilized in spite of the planned surgery for any other lesions[2].

The interventricular septal defects that occur following an acute myocardial infarct are muscular defects, however, these defects present some unique problems for catheter closure. Post-myocardial infarct septal defects usually are very significant hemodynamically and they are in an ideal *location* for a transcatheter closure. However, the particular clinical circumstances of these patients represent a major and frustrating challenge for transcatheter therapy. During the first few days/weeks after the infarct, when these patients are the sickest and in the greatest need for having the defect closed, the myocardial tissue damage is still evolving. As a consequence, the ventricular septal defects are still enlarging with continued tissue necrosis at the margins of the infarct (and the ventricular septal defect!). Even after a successful device implant, the necrosis continues with further disintegration of the supporting tissue around the edges of the device. This produces a reopening of the defect and/or, frequently, results in embolization of the devices. When these patients can be stabilized and the closure of these defects can be postponed for three or more weeks, the results are very satisfactory.

Technique for occlusion of a muscular VSD with a CardioSEAL™ ASD device

The CardioSEAL™ ASD device has approval from the US Food and Drug Administration (FDA) for the closure of muscular interventricular septal defects. This approval for use was based on the success and safety of the Clamshell™ and the CardioSEAL™ devices used for this indication in a high-risk trial, in some specific humanitarian use cases, and because of the abysmal results from the attempts at surgical closure of these same defects. The technique described here is for the CardioSEAL™ ASD occlusion device, but the principle can be applied to several other occlusion devices available and/or in trials at this time.

The technique for muscular VSD closure requires the use of a somewhat complex "through-and-through" wire "rail system", which passes through the defect and out of a separate vascular access on the opposite "side" of the defect. The precise technique that is used for muscular VSD closure depends upon the exact location of the defect in the muscular septum, the particular device that is available and somewhat on the operator's preference. The technique described here is applicable primarily to the apical and mid muscular defects. The same delivery technique can be used for a residual, postoperative peri-patch VSD, which is located somewhat caudally on the septum and away from the semilunar and atrioventricular valves. For the delivery of the CardioSEAL™ device to the mid or apical muscular septum, the through-and-through wire passes from the internal jugular vein through the defect and back out of the vascular system through either a systemic vein or a peripheral artery. The jugular vein to femoral vein approach to the mid and/or apical muscular VSD with *delivery of the device* from the jugular vein/right ventricle side of the defect is preferred by most operators and is described first in this section.

The transcatheter closure of a ventricular septal defect requires not only several operators with special skills and training, but also a very sophisticated biplane catheterization laboratory and a large inventory of consumable supplies. In spite of the complexity of the procedure, transcatheter treatment is the preferred therapy for these particular defects. Because of the required remote and separate access sites (e.g. simultaneous femoral and jugular), in order to perform the transcatheter VSD closure, a minimum of two, and preferably three, skilled operators are involved during each procedure. Although it is possible to accomplish the closure of a muscular VSD under only deep sedation, it is preferable to have the patient intubated and under controlled, general anesthesia, since the procedures often are very long and much of the manipulation and precise maneuvering are from the jugular approach. With all of the manipulations that are performed immediately adjacent to the face during the occlusion of a muscular VSD, it is very hard to maintain a sterile field in the neck area and for a long time in a patient who is only sedated.

Unlike the transcatheter ASD closure, the catheter closure of a VSD is not *as* dependent on the use of simultaneous echo during the positioning, release and final implant of the device. Echo, however, is invaluable in determining the relationship of the "disks" and other components of the device to the A-V valves and valve apparatus prior to release of the device. Transesophageal echo (TEE) provides excellent images of these structures. However, when the delivery of the device is from the jugular approach, the "head" end of the table becomes very crowded with the anesthesiologist, the anesthesiologist's equipment, the echocardiographer and the TEE probe all along with one or two cardiologist(s) manipulating catheters from the jugular approach. Transthoracic echocardiographic guidance using an apical image often is preferable to transesophageal echo because of these logistics. The major disadvantage of the use of transthoracic echo for muscular VSD closure is the presence of the transthoracic probe and the *echocardiographer's hands* in the fields of the X-ray beams.

With the apical and mid muscular locations of the defects, the device usually is delivered to the defect from the right internal jugular vein–superior vena cava approach which, however, still requires additional vascular access through one femoral vein and a femoral artery. The diagnostic catheterization is accomplished from a femoral vein. Access to the left ventricle can be with a retrograde catheterization through the aortic valve or, preferably, via the left atrium/mitral valve through an existing interatrial communication or, when there is no pre-existing atrial communication, through a long sheath, transseptal atrial puncture. The venous, transatrial septal approach allows the routine use of larger diagnostic angiographic catheters in the left ventricle, provides the best direction and/or angle for the manipulation of a catheter from the left ventricle through the apical and/or mid muscular VSD, and permits the presence of a separate, retrograde angiographic catheter, which is introduced through a single and smaller arterial puncture, to be positioned in the left ventricle during the entire implant procedure.

Blood for an activated clotting time (ACT) is drawn at the onset of the procedure when the first vascular access is obtained on any patient undergoing closure of a muscular VSD. As soon as the transseptal puncture is completed and/or the left atrium is entered through a pre-existing opening in the septum, the patient is given systemic heparin in a dose of 75–100 mg/kg depending upon the initial ACT. With the extensive manipulations required in the "systemic" circulation, the ACT is monitored periodically throughout the procedure and maintained between 275 and 350 seconds with repeat boluses of heparin throughout the procedure.

When the "left sided" catheter is introduced from the femoral *venous* approach and after crossing the atrial septum and passing through the mitral valve into the left ventricle, the 180° curve, which is pre-formed on the long sheath, forms one long, smooth, concave curve, which directs the tip of the sheath anteriorly and medially toward the ventricular septum. This smooth, entirely concave curve facilitates the subsequent catheter manipulation through the VSD, particularly when using controllable deflector wires, which actively deflect only toward the concavity of the curve. A second left ventricular catheter is introduced through the retrograde arterial approach. The second left ventricular catheter is essential in order to perform "positioning" angiocardiograms when the other left ventricular catheter and/or the device is within the defect.

After the atrial transseptal procedure, the left heart hemodynamics are acquired and angiocardiograms for visualization and accurate measurements of the VSD are performed through a 7- or 8-French angiographic catheter. The standard, rigorous precautions to avoid air and/or clots in the transseptal sheath are utilized with all sheath/dilator/device exchanges during the procedure. The angiographic catheter from the transseptal approach is manipulated to the apex of the left ventricle. Preferably this is a calibrated "marker" catheter, which can be used for the reference measurements as well as the injections. A high-quality left ventricular angiocardiogram is performed in order to visualize and accurately measure the VSD. The exact angulation of the X-ray tubes that will cut the VSD precisely on edge will vary from defect to defect and from patient to patient. One X-ray tube is positioned in approximately a 30° LAO with a 45° cranial angulation for the first angiogram. These angles are the most likely to align the muscular portion of the ventricular septum and the muscular ventricular septal defect(s) on edge. If the septum and defect(s) are not cut precisely on edge with the initial angles of the X-ray tubes, the X-ray tube angulation is adjusted appropriately and the angiocardiogram is repeated to obtain the "ideal cut" of the defect. Once the ventricular defect is aligned precisely on edge, the same X-ray tube angles are used as the working positions of the X-ray tubes during the occlusion procedure. The best angiogram of the defect, along with the specific angles of that view, are saved as the reference view with a frame of this angiogram displayed during subsequent maneuvers as a "road map" during the steps of the VSD closure.

Once the defect(s) is/are clearly visualized and the determination made to proceed with a transcatheter occlusion, the additional access routes are established. The right internal jugular vein is entered percutaneously. A short, 9-French sheath/dilator system with an attached valved back-bleed/flush system is introduced into the jugular vein. The sheath and back-bleed valve/side port are carefully cleared of air and attached to the flush/pressure system. Because of the nature of muscular ventricular septal defects and the usually "hidden" location of the defects within the trabeculae on the right ventricular side of the septum, in most cases the defects are crossed initially with a catheter passing through the defect from the left ventricle to the right ventricle.

When a transseptal puncture is used for the diagnostic catheterization, the long transseptal *sheath* is advanced from the left atrium into the left ventricle over the original angiographic catheter. The angiographic catheter is withdrawn through the transseptal sheath and the sheath again meticulously cleared of air and/or clots by allowing passive back bleeding through the side port of the sheath. Once cleared, the side port of the sheath is attached to the pressure/flush system and placed on a continuous slow flush. If not already present, a separate retrograde angiographic catheter, which will be utilized for the repeat angiocardiograms during the occlusion procedure, is advanced into the left ventricle in addition to the transseptal sheath.

The original angiographic catheter that was in the long transseptal sheath is replaced with a 7-French, Swan-Ganz™ end-hole floating balloon catheter (Arrow International Inc., Reading, PA). Although almost any catheter can be deflected and/or manipulated from the left ventricle through a muscular interventricular defect, an *inflated floating balloon* catheter is preferable for this step in the procedure with the goal that the inflated balloon will pass through the *largest orifice* of the defect. Before introduction into the long sheath, the distal several centimeters of the balloon catheter are heated and/or "pulled" between the thumb and forefinger in order to preform a 180° curve on the distal end of the catheter, which will help direct the balloon tip toward the interventricular septum and the defect once it is "floating" freely beyond the tip of the long sheath. Occasionally the inflated balloon catheter immediately is "sucked" completely through the VSD by the high velocity/volume of the left to right flow of the blood through the defect. More often, even the inflated balloon must be manipulated specifically through the defect with the help of some type of deflector wire. Either an active deflector wire or a pre-formed deflector wire is used to direct the tip of the inflated balloon catheter toward the defect. When a deflection technique is necessary, the transatrial entry into the left ventricle becomes even more advantageous because of the net "concave" course of the catheter toward the interventricular septum when entering the ventricle from the mitral valve.

A standard 0.035" Amplatz™ controllable deflector wire (Cook Inc., Bloomington, IN) with a 5 or 10 mm tip curve (depending upon the size of the patient/ventricle) is advanced to the tip of the balloon catheter within the left ventricle. With the balloon inflated, the curve on the tip of the wire/catheter is formed. By slight rotation of the sheath, catheter and wire and by varying the degree of curve formed on the deflector wire, the balloon is directed anteriorly/posteriorly and/or cephalad/caudal along the septum and precisely toward the VSD. The location of the VSD should be displayed simultaneously on the "roadmap" angiogram in the same views. When directed exactly at the VSD, the balloon catheter is advanced off the deflector wire while maintaining the same curve and the same position/direction on the deflector wire. This maneuver is repeated until the balloon passes into and through the VSD. Occasionally, even when the balloon pops precisely into the ampulla at the left ventricular end of the defect, the balloon will have to be deflated *slightly* to allow it to pass into, and completely through, the defect.

The balloon catheter tip can be directed even more precisely with the stiff end of a teflon-coated, standard spring guide wire that has been pre-curved outside of the body (as described in Chapter 6) into a three-dimensional curve that corresponds to the expected curve of the catheter passing from the left atrium, through the mitral valve, into the left ventricle and against the exact area of the septum of the VSD. The stiff end of the wire allows the formation of a complex "3-dimensional" curve that bends the catheter from right to left as well as with a secondary bend anteriorly or posteriorly. Once the curve is formed in the wire, the wire is introduced and advanced to the end of the balloon catheter. With the proper curve, the balloon catheter will point precisely at the VSD. With the balloon inflated and the wire fixed in position, the balloon is advanced off the wire into the defect. If the curves that were formed on the wire do not direct the balloon catheter precisely toward the defect, the wire is withdrawn from the catheter, re-formed to better fit the particular anatomy and then reintroduced to the tip of the catheter. As with the controllable deflector wire, once seated precisely in the ampulla of the defect, the balloon often must be deflated slightly to allow passage completely through the defect.

Even when the inflated or even partially inflated balloon does pass into and/or *through* the defect, it should pass preferentially into and/or through the largest opening in the defect. This, in turn, helps ensure that the device will be placed in the largest opening of the VSD. Once the balloon has passed into the defect and, preferably, well into the right ventricle, the balloon catheter is maintained in this position while the deflector wire is withdrawn. When the balloon seats in the left ventricular side of the defect but will not pass into, and/or through it into the right ventricle, a very floppy tipped, torque-controlled, guide wire can be advanced through the balloon catheter and into the right ventricle. A repeat or partial further inflation of the balloon, which is "seated" in the defect, helps to maintain the balloon catheter in position in the defect during the exchange and maneuvers with the wires.

With the inflated balloon seated at, or just in, the VSD, the deflector wire is removed carefully and replaced with a very floppy tipped torque-controlled guide wire or a curved tipped Terumo™ Glide wire. The wire is advanced through the balloon catheter and manipulated through the defect and further into the right ventricle. The wire is advanced as far as possible into the right ventricle or right ventricle/pulmonary artery in order to ensure that the *stiff portion* of the wire has passed completely through the defect. The wire must be secure enough to advance the balloon catheter (with or without the balloon inflated) over this wire and completely into the right ventricle.

Occasionally the balloon catheter will not follow the wire into the right ventricle. In that circumstance, the wire alone is manipulated further within the right heart. The wire is advanced, preferably, into the pulmonary artery. When the wire alone crosses the defect and enters the pulmonary artery without the inflated balloon, there is a much greater likelihood that the wire has passed through a minor or secondary VSD opening and not through the major defect and/or through minor trabeculae and/or chordae within the right ventricle.

Occasionally the maneuvering of the catheter from the left ventricle through the VSD can be accomplished only with a *non-balloon* torque-controlled catheter. A specifically pre-curved, standard end-hole catheter is passed through the long sheath and directed into the VSD with the assistance of guide and/or deflector wires. When the balloon is *not* used for this passage, there, again, is a greater likelihood that the catheter will *not* pass through the *largest* opening in the defect. When the inflated balloon catheter is not used to traverse the ventricular defect, angiography along with a sizing balloon and/or echocardiography is used to verify that the center or the largest opening of the defect has been traversed. A soft, static sizing balloon provides the best information about which "orifice" was traversed, the size of the defect and the "configuration" of the entire defect.

The mid and apical muscular interventricular septal defects can be crossed using the retrograde approach to the left ventricle from a femoral artery. This does not provide as satisfactory an angle for the approach to the apical and mid muscular septum as provided by the transatrial approach to the ventricle through the mitral valve. As a consequence, the retrograde arterial approach usually requires the presence of the catheter in the artery for a significant time and/or extensive manipulations with the larger catheter in the artery. When the retrograde approach is used to cross the ventricular septal defect, a second arterial catheter (or a separate catheter introduced transseptally!) will be necessary in order to obtain angiograms *during* the implant procedure. The retrograde approach is the preferred approach to the *anterior, intramural muscular septal defects,* which are discussed later in this chapter.

Once an end-hole catheter has passed through the defect and is secure in the right ventricle, a second operator introduces an end-hole, *floating balloon catheter* through the previously introduced sheath in the jugular vein. The balloon catheter with the balloon inflated is advanced from the right atrium into the right ventricle. The inflated floating balloon catheter passing through the tricuspid valve helps to ensure that the catheter from the jugular vein passes through the *central largest orifice of the tricuspid valve* and not around a chorda of the tricuspid valve and, in turn, ensures that the through-and-through wire and eventual delivery sheath from the jugular vein pass through this central orifice. Once in the right ventricle the balloon catheter that was introduced from the jugular vein is "floated" into the pulmonary artery. Often, a snare (Microvena Corp., White Bear Lake, MN) can be introduced through the end-hole balloon catheter, but if not, the balloon catheter is positioned well into the pulmonary artery and is exchanged over a long guide wire for a true "snare catheter" (Microvena Corp., White Bear Lake, MN).

While one operator manipulates the snare catheter from the jugular vein, a separate operator passes a 0.035", soft tipped, exchange length guide wire through the catheter that is passing through the VSD. The wire and/or catheter is advanced further into the right ventricle and manipulated from the right ventricle into the pulmonary artery. Simultaneously the operator manipulating the catheter from the jugular approach opens the loop of a 20 or 25 mm diameter snare in the pulmonary artery and encircles the free end of the wire that is coming from the left ventricle and through the ventricular septal defect. The wire alone, which is passing through the VSD, is snared in the pulmonary artery with the snare catheter that was introduced from the jugular vein.

Occasionally, the wire that is passing through the VSD, passes preferentially into the right atrium. When the wire passes to the right atrium, it very likely has passed under some chordae of the tricuspid valve, which will *not* allow the subsequent, smooth passage of a sheath from the jugular vein to the VSD. This is particularly true when a Terumo™ Glide™ wire (Terumo Medical Corp., Somerset, NJ) is used to cross the ventricular septal defect. Although the Terumo™ wires usually pass through the septum more readily than other wires, they also are more likely to find their way through very small openings or even *create their own* opening as they are advanced through the ventricular septum. The Terumo™ wire is only used to cross the VSD when previous attempts with a standard soft tipped, torque-controlled, spring guide wire are unsuccessful.

When the wire traversing the VSD passes directly into the *right atrium,* it should be withdrawn back out of the atrium into the ventricle and manipulated from the VSD purposefully toward the right ventricular outflow tract and pulmonary artery. The snare catheter, which was advanced from the jugular vein, already is passing through the tricuspid valve, right ventricle and into the main pulmonary artery. A large snare is opened in the main pulmonary artery. With the two catheter shafts more or less parallel in that area, an open Microvena™ snare (Microvena Corp., White Bear Lake, MN) aligns perpendicular to the long axis of the pulmonary artery with the loop of the snare encircling the entire lumen of the right ventricular outflow tract. The tip of the exchange wire, which is passing through the VSD, is withdrawn slightly into the RV outflow tract, then re-advanced through the open loop of the snare, where it can be grasped readily with the snare. Once the wire is grasped in the pulmonary artery, it is withdrawn very carefully through the tricuspid valve and out through the jugular venous sheath.

Even when a floating balloon catheter was used to cross the tricuspid valve from the jugular venous approach, extra care must be taken in withdrawing the snare/wire combination back through the tricuspid valve to be sure that no chordae of the tricuspid valve have been entrapped. Even when the withdrawal from the ventricle to the atrium meets no resistance, the wire still can course around a chorda of the tricuspid valve. Once the wire coursing through the VSD is withdrawn into the jugular vein, there should be a *straight* course of the wire from the VSD to the jugular vein. A bent and/or circuitous course from the ventricular septal defect to the right atrium/jugular vein indicates that the wire is trapped around and/or through a chorda and, in turn, will not allow a straight, smooth introduction of the delivery sheath. If either of these positions is present, the wire is released from the snare catheter and the snare catheter alone is withdrawn through the tricuspid valve into the right atrium. If the actual *snare catheter* was used from the jugular vein to capture the VSD wire during these maneuvers, it is replaced with the end-hole *floating balloon* catheter and the balloon catheter is floated through the tricuspid valve (hopefully through a different area of the valve) and once again into the pulmonary artery. The snare is introduced through the end-hole balloon catheter and/or the balloon catheter in the pulmonary artery again is exchanged for a snare catheter.

If the standard soft tipped spring guide wire that is passing through the VSD cannot be manipulated into the pulmonary artery, the wire is replaced with a floppy tipped torque-controlled wire and the manipulations repeated. If the wire through the VSD still cannot be manipulated into the pulmonary artery, the end-hole, Swan™ floating balloon catheter from the jugular vein is re-advanced through the tricuspid valve, but instead of manipulating it into the pulmonary artery, the tip of the balloon catheter is advanced into the body/apex of the right ventricle. The snare is introduced into the balloon catheter, which now is positioned in the cavity of the right ventricle, and an attempt is made to snare the wire and/or the balloon catheter in the right ventricle just as it is passing through the VSD into the right ventricle. The relatively straight floating balloon or snare catheter, which is introduced through the tricuspid valve from the jugular vein, usually follows an almost direct course through the tricuspid valve toward the *apex* of the right ventricle and, in turn, aligns the 90° off-set of the opened Microvena™ snare loop almost *en fas to the septum* and the defect. The orientation of the single loop of the Micro-vena™ snare, however, may align parallel to the wire coming through the VSD and, in turn, be counter productive to snaring the wire passing through the VSD. When this occurs, an Ensnare™ (MD TECH, Gainesville, FL) with its three, interlaced "flower leaf" loops is preferable for snaring the tip of the wire in the ventricle.

A final alternative, when the wire cannot be snared in the pulmonary artery or in the right ventricle with the snare introduced through the balloon catheter, is to snare the wire coming through the VSD with a snare introduced directly through the long delivery sheath. A floating balloon catheter is advanced from the jugular vein straight into the apex of the right ventricle. A stiff, exchange length wire with a long floppy tip is pre-curved in order to form a 180° curve at the *transition portion* of the wire and a 360° curve at the soft tip. The 180° curve of the pre-curved exchange wire is positioned in the apex of the ventricle through the end-hole balloon catheter. A long delivery sheath that will accommodate the device that is to be used, is pre-curved outside of the body to correspond to the course from the jugular vein, through the right atrium/tricuspid valve to the location of the VSD within the right ventricle. The short sheath in the jugular vein is replaced over the pre-curved stiff wire with the long delivery sheath/dilator, which is introduced into the jugular vein and advanced over the stiff guide wire into the right ventricle. The *sheath* alone is advanced over the dilator to the apex of the ventricle while the wire and long dilator are removed from the delivery sheath. After the sheath is cleared of any air and/or clot, the snare catheter is advanced through the long sheath directly to the apex of the right ventricle, where the snare cautiously is opened in the right ventricle and manipulated around the wire/catheter passing through the VSD. The wire passing through the VSD is grasped with the snare and the snared wire and/or catheter is drawn into the large, long delivery sheath. This technique prevents the possibility of damage to the tricuspid valve as the snare/wires are being withdrawn through the tricuspid valve. The course of the wire/sheath from the jugular vein to the ventricular defect still should be relatively straight.

By whichever technique the wire through the VSD was grasped and once the wire is snared and is pulled into the right atrium, additional wire is fed from the femoral vein entry site while the snared distal end of the wire *along with the catheter* that has crossed the VSD are withdrawn through the jugular sheath and out of the vascular system at the neck. This creates a through-and-through wire/catheter from the jugular vein, to the right atrium and right ventricle, through the defect to the left ventricle, back to the left atrium, across the atrial septum to the right atrium and out through the femoral vein (Figure 30.1). The catheter that has been advanced through the ventricular septal defect with the wire is maintained over the wire and is allowed to follow the snared wire *into the sheath.* The catheter over the wire prevents laceration of intracardiac structures by the "sawing" effect of the rough surface of the spring guide wire as it is being fed into the femoral sheath and withdrawn through the jugular vein. When the tip of the end-hole *catheter*, which was introduced from a femoral vein, appears outside of the proximal end of the sheath at the jugular puncture site, the original standard exchange guide wire is removed from the now, *through-and-through catheter* and replaced with a 0.035" Super Stiff™ exchange length guide wire (Medi-Tech, Boston Scientific, Natick, MA) with a long floppy tip.

If a second left ventricular catheter has not yet been introduced from a femoral artery, it is introduced at this time. It is advanced retrograde from a femoral artery into the left ventricle. As an alternative, the second catheter in

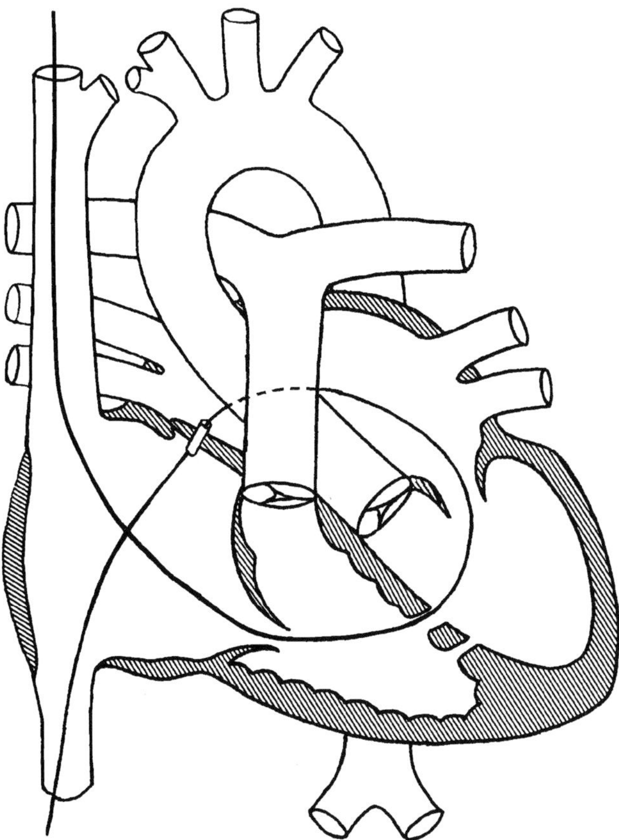

Figure 30.1 Venovenous through-and-through wire for mid and apical muscular ventricular septal defects: from the jugular vein, to the right atrium and right ventricle, through the ventricular septal defect, to the left ventricle, back to the left atrium, across the atrial septum to the right atrium and out through the femoral vein.

the left ventricle could be introduced prograde through a second femoral venous puncture and a second atrial transseptal puncture. The additional left ventricular catheter is necessary for small, but frequent injections of contrast, which are repeated during the device delivery, positioning and implant procedure. The approach with a second transseptal puncture avoids the prolonged time with a catheter in an artery for operators who are very comfortable with the transseptal procedure.

A sizing and test occlusion of the VSD usually is performed using a NuMED,™ low-pressure, sizing balloon (NuMED Inc., Hopkinton, NY). A wire back-bleed/flush valve is attached to the hub of the sizing balloon and placed on a continuous flush. The sizing balloon is introduced over the through-and-through Super Stiff™ wire through the 9- or 10-French sheath in the jugular vein. As the sizing balloon is introduced into the jugular vein, the "through-and-through catheter" which has passed from the femoral vein, transseptally into the left ventricle and through the VSD, is withdrawn simultaneously from the femoral vein introductory site as the tip of the sizing balloon is being introduced over the same wire from the jugular vein. The tips of the sizing balloon from the jugular vein and the catheter from the femoral vein are maintained with the tips "touching" each other as the sizing balloon is introduced. The deflated NuMED™ balloon is advanced over the through-and-through wire, through the right heart and into the ventricular septal defect until the sizing balloon straddles the defect. The shaft of the NuMED™ sizing balloon is maintained on a continual flush all of the time. The catheter over the wire from the femoral venous end of the wire is maintained across the mitral valve and into the left ventricle with its tip still against the tip of the sizing balloon catheter in order to protect the intracardiac tissues from the bare wire.

The NuMED™ sizing balloon is inflated in the center of the defect with a *very low* pressure ("no pressure") inflation. The waist in the balloon clearly demonstrates the size, location and *configuration* of the ventricular septal defect as well as any constrictions within the right ventricle that are created by the catheters/wires passing through chordae abnormally. When the balloon is inflated in the defect, an angiocardiogram is performed through the separate pre-positioned left ventricular angiographic catheter. The angiocardiogram is recorded in the same previously determined optimal angles of the X-ray tubes for visualizing the defect on edge. The angiocardiogram with the balloon inflated demonstrates clearly if there is more than one defect and/or if the catheter/balloon has crossed an accessory opening and is not passing through the major defect. This type of balloon "sizing" provides valuable information about the length of the defect, the course through the right ventricular trabeculae, and the relationship of the defect to the mitral and tricuspid valve apparatuses. If there is an additional defect, its distance from the balloon-occluded defect is determined from the angiocardiogram with the sizing balloon inflated. When there are one or more additional defects, it can be determined from this angiogram whether all of the defects can be "covered" on the left ventricular surface with one device or whether two or more devices will be necessary to occlude all of the defects.

It is helpful while the sizing balloon is inflated in the defect, to obtain an echocardiogram (transthoracic or transesophageal) while the balloon is in the defect. This not only provides a separate measurement of the size of the defect but, of more importance, is more likely to detect additional holes which are *very close* to the central defect and/or to show if the balloon is not through the central and/or largest hole. The echo at this time also helps the echocardiographer to become oriented to the anatomy in the area where the device will be implanted, to rule out other, even small defects and to look for other intracardiac structures (valves!), which might be affected by the device. The echo provides measurements of the distance of additional defects or other, non-radio-opaque intracardiac structures from the balloon-occluded defect.

An earlier, less satisfactory but still occasionally used method of sizing the VSD is to use the original Swan™ floating balloon or a similar but larger "occlusion balloon" from Medi-Tech™ (Medi-Tech, Boston Scientific, Natick, MA). These balloons are passed over the through-and-through wire and are inflated on the left ventricular side of the septum. From there, they are pushed (or pulled depending upon from which direction they were introduced over the wire) into the defect to occlude it. An angiocardiogram is obtained with the inflated balloon against the defect to confirm occlusion and that there is only one defect. The balloon then is deflated in small (0.2 ml) increments until the balloon is pulled over the wire through the defect and into the opposite ventricle. An angiogram is recorded of this "pull through" and this partially deflated size of the Swan™ balloon is measured from the angiogram to provide some additional information about the size and location of the defect. Withdrawing a balloon through the defect from the right ventricle to the left ventricle is very unreliable because the balloon frequently becomes entrapped in the trabeculae of the right ventricle, which, in turn, gives a false impression of both the size and the real location of the defect.

After the sizing with a static balloon and *while* the deflated NuMED™ sizing balloon is being withdrawn from the VSD and right heart, the original catheter passing over the wire from the left ventricle is re-advanced from the opposite end of the through-and-through wire. The tip of the catheter is maintained touching the tip of the NuMED™ sizing balloon as the NuMED™ balloon is withdrawn into the right ventricle, right atrium and out through the jugular vein.

Using the angiographic measurements from balloon sizing, and the measurements from the simultaneous echo, a CardioSEAL™ device (NMT, Boston, MA) is chosen which is at least two to two and a half times the size of the minimum diameter of the lumen of the defect. The device should not be over-sized significantly unless there is an additional adjacent ventricular septal defect that is close enough to the primary defect to be occluded with a single larger device. An over-sized device is more apt to encroach on the atrioventricular valves and/or the valve apparatus within the body of the ventricle. The long arms of an excessively over-sized device could interfere with ventricular function by "splinting" the ventricle open in systole and could contribute to late arm fractures of the devices.

Once the measurements have been obtained and the appropriate device chosen, the device delivery system is prepared. An 11-French long transseptal type sheath with a proximal hemostasis/flush valve and a radio-opaque marker band at the distal end of the sheath is prepared. The distal end of the long 11-French sheath is reshaped from its manufactured 180° curve, "transseptal" configuration into an approximately 30° curve to correspond to the course of the wire from the jugular vein, through the right atrium, tricuspid valve, right ventricle and through the ventricle defect. This is accomplished by "cold pulling" the sheath/dilator between the fingers repeatedly, by soaking the combined sheath/dilator in boiling water or by holding the combination in the jet of a "heat gun" while forming the desired curve. When the curve is formed with either of the heat techniques, the newly formed sheath/dilator immediately is cooled in a flush solution at room temperature to "set" the new curve. Once the new curve is formed and while still outside of the body, the dilator is withdrawn out of the sheath completely in order to verify that the desired curve actually is formed on the *sheath* without the support of the dilator. The appropriate curve usually is approximately 30–60° off the long axis of the sheath. Once it is established that the sheath has the correct curve, the dilator is reinserted into the long sheath.

With the defect delineated and sized, all of the catheters and the through-and-through wire in position, and the long 11-French sheath properly prepared, the short 9-French jugular sheath is removed over the through-and-through wire. The pre-curved 11-French long sheath/dilator set is introduced into the jugular vein over the through-and-through wire. The long *dilator* should have a wire back-bleed valve/flush port attached to the hub of the dilator, and this flush port is kept on a slow, continuous flush. The catheter from the femoral vein end of the wire still is present over the wire with its tip in the superior vena cava or right atrium. The long sheath/dilator set is advanced carefully over the wire into the right atrium until the tip of the long dilator approximates the tip of the catheter coming from the other end of the wire. The sheath/dilator carefully is advanced through the right heart to the VSD while the end-hole diagnostic catheter simultaneously is withdrawn over the wire, just ahead of the dilator tip and into the ventricular septal defect.

The wire is fixed in position and the sheath/dilator is advanced through the defect into the left ventricle while simultaneously withdrawing the opposing catheter until the tip of the *dilator* approaches the left ventricular free wall. Echo guidance is helpful in determining this. The stiff dilator often is directed toward the left ventricular apex and the long sheath/dilator can create an acute kink in even the Super Stiff™ wire unless the wire is observed carefully and manipulated from both ends to direct the tip of the dilator purposefully more cephalad. Once the tip of the *sheath* has passed through the VSD, the dilator and wire are fixed in position, while the *sheath alone* is advanced over the dilator and just to the tip of the dilator. These positions and catheter relationships are confirmed with a repeat left ventricular angiocardiogram and/or by the echocardiogram. When satisfied that the tip of the *sheath* is *well* within the left ventricle, the dilator alone carefully and slowly is withdrawn into the sheath over the wire, all of the time carefully observing on the fluoroscopy the course of the sheath within the right ventricle and VSD. As the dilator is withdrawn into the sheath, the diagnostic end-hole catheter, which was introduced from the opposite end of the wire, again simultaneously is advanced over the wire, into and well within the tip of the long sheath. The tip of the sheath is maintained in the cavity of the left ventricle, being careful not to withdraw or to advance the sheath at all. While observing the sheath on fluoroscopy, the dilator carefully is withdrawn over the wire and completely out of the long sheath. As the dilator is withdrawn within the sheath, the end-hole catheter, which is over the wire and was introduced from the other end of the wire, is advanced further into the sheath keeping the tip of the catheter and the tip of the dilator approximated within the sheath. The catheter within the sheath protects the edge of the tip of the sheath from the wire and, in turn, prevents damage to the sheath as the wire is being withdrawn from the heart. It also serves as a "safety factor" for reinserting the through-and-through wire in the event that the tip of the sheath inadvertently becomes dislodged back into the right ventricle and/or becomes kinked after the stiff wire and dilator are removed. Special care is taken *not* to advance or withdraw the sheath during the process of removing the dilator. Advancing the sheath without the dilator within it is very likely to kink the sheath in the area of its curve in the ventricle. Withdrawing the sheath even slightly, straightens the sheath, which, in turn, can pull the tip of the sheath out of the septal defect and back into the right ventricle. After the dilator is withdrawn, the sheath is allowed to bleed back passively to clear it of any air or clot. Once cleared, the sheath position is verified angiographically with a hand injection of contrast through the sheath itself or through the pre-positioned separate catheter in the left ventricle. The sheath passing through the ventricular septal defect also is visualized by transthoracic or transesophageal echocardiogram at this time.

Once the long dilator is removed, the through-and-through exchange *wire* is withdrawn carefully through the catheter passing from the opposite end of the wire so that the floppy end of the Super Stiff™ wire is withdrawn out of the end-hole catheter in the femoral vein. As the through-and-through, Super Stiff™ wire is being withdrawn from one end, an equal length of the opposite end of the same wire is fed *simultaneously* into the catheter/sheath from the other end. All of the time the sheath is observed carefully on fluoroscopy and readjusted only *minimally* to prevent forward movement and/or unusual tension on the sheath while the stiff wire is being removed. The diagnostic end-hole catheter still should be passing over the wire coming from the left ventricle and should remain well within the distal end of the delivery sheath after the wire has been removed. If the sheath inadvertently is withdrawn into the right ventricle as the dilator and wire are being manipulated, the end-hole catheter, which is well within the distal end of the sheath, allows the reinsertion of the through-and-through wire without all of the complex snaring and other double-wire manipulations. This catheter is left in place within the distal end of the sheath until the device approaches (touches) it during the delivery of the device.

If the delivery sheath tip slips out of the defect at any time during the wire manipulations and/or device delivery, the through-and-through wire is reinserted into the end-hole catheter in the femoral vein and withdrawn out through the proximal, valved, end of the long sheath. The *long dilator* for the sheath is reinserted into the sheath over the wire *before* any attempt is made at repositioning the sheath back through the defect. Attempting to advance the long sheath without the dilator within the sheath almost certainly will kink the sheath at the curvature of the sheath where it passes through the right ventricle/VSD. If the sheath does kink, the sheath is removed over the through-and-through wire and replaced with a new sheath/dilator set. A kink in the sheath prevents the folded CardioSEAL™ device (NMT Medical Inc., Boston, MA) from passing the kink or, if the device does advance past the kink, it can damage the device in the process.

After the dilator and the wire are removed and once the sheath is across the VSD and the sheath tip still is well into the left ventricular cavity without kinks, the CardioSEAL™ device and the delivery catheter are opened and inspected. The delivery rod is advanced all of the way into the proximal end of the delivery catheter. This, in turn, advances the delivery cable out of the end of the delivery catheter. A long smooth, approximately 70°, curve is formed on the entire exposed portion of the delivery cable. This curve corresponds to the angle of approach of the device to the right ventricular septal surface. The appropriate sized CardioSEAL™ device is opened and inspected. The "front loader", which comes attached to the device, is used for *28 mm and smaller* CardioSEAL™ devices. A single suture passes through the distal end of the "front loader" device, out through the funneled proximal end of the loader and, in turn, through the ends of the distal legs of the device. The pin on the proximal side of the device is attached to the attach/release pin/sleeve at the tip of the delivery cable. The device is withdrawn into the "front loader" by tension placed on the suture passing through the loader and the device while counter tension is applied to the end of the delivery cable. The tension on the attached sutures folds the distal umbrella away from the delivery catheter and toward the loader. The folded distal umbrella folds further as it is withdrawn completely into the funnel of the loader. As the proximal umbrella of the device "follows" into and enters the "cone" of the loader, the proximal legs of the device are folded proximally by manual compression. Once the device is within the loader completely, the rigid, thick Plexiglas™ "cover" is withdrawn from the front loader. The delivery catheter is advanced over the delivery cable and into the proximal end of the loader until the tip of the catheter within the loader is 1–2 mm from the tips of the folded proximal legs of the device. The loader with the enclosed device is flushed thoroughly to clear it of all air.

As with all of the other uses of the CardioSEAL™ devices, when a 28 mm or larger device is used, a segment of 11-French sheath is cut off and substituted for the manufacturer's front-loading device (as described in Chapter 28) in order to allow loading without damaging the device by the necessarily excessive tension on the ends of the device when introduced into the standard loader.

The long sheath is fixed securely against the skin at the jugular entry site and placed on a vigorous flush. While observing the sheath continuously on fluoroscopy, particularly in the area where it passes through the curve into and through the right ventricle and VSD, the "front-loader" apparatus (or short segment of 11-French sheath) with the contained folded CardioSEAL™ device is introduced carefully and slowly through the back-bleed valve of the long sheath until it is against the proximal hub of the sheath and until the loader will not advance further. At the same time, the loader should not be *forced* into the shaft of the sheath at the distal end of the loader. With the loader fixed in this position and the sheath still on a flush, the delivery catheter and device are advanced through and out of the loader and into the sheath. The loader is withdrawn 1–2 mm while flush is continued on the side port of the long sheath. This ensures that any air that is trapped in the chamber of the back-bleed valve is flushed back out of the chamber and not into the patient.

While continuing a flush on the side port of the sheath, the device and delivery catheter are advanced through the straight segment of the long sheath (to approximately the area of the mid right atrium). The *delivery catheter and the sheath* are fixed and maintained very carefully as a single unit at this position. While ensuring that the sheath and delivery catheter are not advancing or withdrawing at all, the delivery rod, which controls the delivery cable and the attached device, is advanced into the proximal end of the delivery catheter. This advances the distal end of the delivery cable, with the device attached to it, away from the tip of the catheter and further into the sheath. As the device approaches the area of the right ventricle within the sheath it meets the tip of the end-hole catheter which was introduced from the other end of the wire and which still is within the distal end of the sheath. The end-hole catheter is withdrawn from within the sheath simultaneously as the device is advanced to the end of the sheath, keeping the tip of the catheter just ahead of the distal legs of the device.

As the device is advanced carefully and slowly through the sheath, small adjustments in the position of the sheath usually are necessary. A forward adjustment in the sheath position often is necessary to keep the tip of the sheath well within the left ventricle. The straightening effect of the relatively stiff device/cable advancing within the sheath tends to withdraw the tip of the sheath. On the other hand, as the device/cable are pushed into the sheath, the sheath may be advanced as well, in which case, the sheath may have to be withdrawn slightly to prevent the tip of the sheath from being pushed too far into the left ventricle and, in turn, kinking the more proximal sheath. These maneuvers often need to be repeated alternately as the device is advanced. The other catheter is withdrawn completely out of the tip of the sheath just before the tips of the distal legs of the device reach the tip of the sheath.

After verifying the position by fluoroscopy, angiocardiogram and/or echo, the delivery rod with the attached device is advanced in a very controlled, slight forward motion while *simultaneously* and very minimally, the tip of the sheath is withdrawn away from the free wall of the left ventricle. This deploys the distal legs of the device slowly into the apex of the left ventricular cavity. When the central hinge mechanism of the device reaches the tip of the sheath, the distal legs are out of the sheath completely. Even with the distal arms fully deployed into the left ventricle, they may not open fully as they frequently become trapped against the left ventricular free wall and/or the papillary muscles of the mitral valve. The deployment and further positioning of the device are observed continuously on fluoroscopy and intermittently by echocardiogram. It is important to verify the position of the open legs in the left ventricle and/or any distortion of the device from the delivery system by repeated angiocardiograms through the second catheter in the left ventricle.

Once the central hinge mechanism is just beyond the end of the sheath, the combination of the sheath, catheter and device, as one unit, is withdrawn very slightly until the deployed distal legs open freely (as close as possible to perpendicular to the sheath) in the cavity of the left ventricle. If the device appears to be away from the LV free wall, free from other interventricular structures and still is not open fully and, at the same time, the central hinge of the device still is not in the defect, the delivery rod along with the device is held in place while the sheath alone is re-*advanced* against just the center of the opened distal umbrella. This pushes the sheath slightly over the distal legs, partially collapsing/closing them. The combination sheath/catheter/device with the partially closed legs is withdrawn together very slightly. This slight repositioning usually frees the distal (left) legs of the device. The sheath alone is withdrawn very slightly, allowing the distal legs to open fully again. Once the distal legs are fully and freely deployed, *the entire sheath/catheter/device combination* is withdrawn further into the VSD. As the device pulls into the VSD, the fully deployed distal legs begin to fold away from the tip of the sheath. They bend, first against the septum, and then into the "conical" left ventricular "ampulla" of the VSD. Once the distal legs have formed this configuration, the exact location of the device is verified by an angiocardiogram and/or the echocardiogram. The central hinge of the device, which is still within or just barely out of the sheath, should be positioned in the mid portion or even slightly to the right ventricular side of the ventricular defect.

When the central hinge mechanism of the device is confirmed to be in the narrowest area of the VSD, the delivery catheter, delivery rod, and device are fixed in position while the *sheath alone* is withdrawn. This withdraws the sheath off the proximal (right ventricular) legs and deploys the proximal device in the right ventricle. Since these legs frequently will be entrapped in the coarse muscular trabeculae in the body/apex of the right ventricle, they often do not open fully to the usual 90° off the perpendicular of the long axis of the catheter. Once the correct position of the device is verified by another angiocardiogram with injection in the left ventricle, the release mechanism is activated, leaving the device in the VSD. The degree of closure is verified by a left ventricular angiocardiogram and by interrogation with the echocardiogram/Doppler. The various catheters are *not* removed until the degree of closure is verified and the presence of an additional significant ventricular defect, which might need another device, is excluded.

If there is a *significant* residual leak through the original defect and/or if more than one significant muscular defect exists and was not covered and closed by the single device, it is preferable to cross the additional defect with a floating balloon catheter and to occlude the additional defect(s) during the same catheterization. The optimal working angles of the X-ray tubes for the procedure already are set, all of the catheters are in place and the anatomy is acutely in the mind of the operators. Unlike the freshly placed devices in atrial septal defects, the freshly placed device in the VSD is fixed securely in place and will not be displaced by careful manipulation through and/or around it. During a second (or additional) device implant, the first device also serves as a fixed landmark for positioning of the additional device(s) on the septum.

The most significant manipulation in closing an additional defect is the crossing of the second defect with an end-hole catheter and re-catching the wire on the right side of the septum. The wire passing through the additional ventricular defect occasionally can be snared through the long delivery sheath, which already is in place in the right ventricle. The repeat wire snaring is performed in the pulmonary artery or in the right ventricle similar to the original procedure. When the long sheath/dilator is reintroduced into the right ventricle over a second, reintroduced through-and-through wire, it may follow a new, separate "tract" through different right ventricular trabeculae to the VSD. The additional implant during the same procedure does *not* require a *proportionate* increase in the necessary fluoroscopy time or the volume of contrast that would be necessary during a repeat occlusion performed as a completely separate procedure.

Once the implant of devices is completed, a final large volume angiocardiogram in the left ventricle is performed to verify the occlusion and/or to help quantitate any residual shunt. Once the operator is comfortable that the defect(s) are maximally and adequately occluded, the catheters are removed. The patient is given intravenous antibiotics for 24 hours following the implant and maintained on 82 mg of aspirin per day for six months. The patient is discharged the following day with no particular imposed limitations or restrictions because of the device(s).

When the risks of the surgical repair of the muscular ventricular defects along with the less than satisfactory results are weighed against the risks and difficulties of the catheterization technique, the transcatheter approach is a safer, more successful procedure with far less morbidity than the comparable surgery. In the collaborative study of the Clamshell device, the successful VSD closure with the Clamshell was excellent, with minimal morbidity or mortality in over thirty patients[2]. However, because of the complexity of the procedure and the equipment involved, transcatheter closure of ventricular septal defects is limited to relatively few centers that are very active in therapeutic catheterizations.

Femoral arterial approach for creation of the through-and-through wire

Some operators introduce the "left sided" catheter from a femoral artery to form the through-and-through loop instead of the introduction of both catheters from the venous system. This approach becomes almost *required* if there is congenital or acquired interruption of the inferior vena cava and/or bilateral obliteration of femoral venous access. When entering the left ventricle from the femoral *arterial* approach and after passing around a left aortic arch, the natural curve on the catheter entering the left ventricle is directed posteriorly and laterally, which is exactly away from the septum (and muscular septal defect). Special pre-formed catheters and/or complex double (or triple) wire curves are necessary just to overcome this "anti septal" course before beginning to manipulate the catheter and/or wire across the VSD from the left ventricle. The necessary deflection of the catheter *away* from the natural *concavity* of the curvature of the catheter within the ventricle prohibits the use of the *controllable* deflector wires for this manipulation. The catheter that is used to cross the septum frequently is a right Judkins™ coronary catheter or a catheter with a specially pre-formed "S" curve, either of which, after the catheter has passed around the arch with the tip of the catheter in the ventricle, tends to point the tip anteriorly and medially toward the septum. When these catheters and/or a Swan™ floating balloon catheter are used for the manipulation from the left ventricle into the defect and to the right ventricle, they usually are used in conjunction with specifically curved, rigid deflector wires, which have similar three-dimensional curves formed on them before they are introduced into the catheter. Except in the circumstance of absence of femoral venous access and/or for operators with little experience and/or who are otherwise uncomfortable with the atrial transseptal procedure, there are no advantages to the arterial approach for this part of the procedure, and the arterial approach requires much more procedural time and manipulation with a catheter/sheath in the arterial introductory site.

Once the Swan™ balloon or other end-hole catheter has been manipulated through the ventricular septal defect from the arterial approach, the wire/catheter is snared in the pulmonary artery from the internal jugular vein approach as described earlier, creating a through-and-through wire "rail" from the jugular vein to the right atrium and right ventricle, through the ventricular septal defect to the left ventricle, to the left ventricular outflow tract and the aorta and eventually out through the femoral artery (Figure 30.2). The delivery of the device from the internal jugular vein is the same as when the catheter/wire passing through the defect is introduced from the transseptal/left atrium approach.

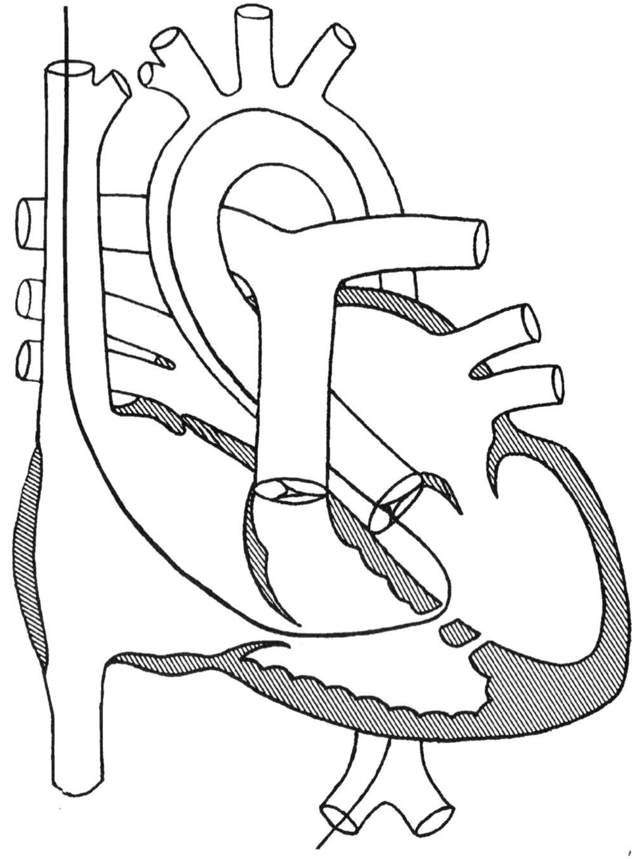

Figure 30.2 Arteriovenous through-and-through wire for mid and apical muscular ventricular septal defects: from the jugular vein to the right atrium and right ventricle, through the ventricular septal defect to the left ventricle, to the left ventricular outflow tract and the aorta and eventually out through the femoral artery.

Delivery of the device to the defect from the left ventricular side of the defect from the femoral vein and transseptal approach

An even more marked variation in the delivery of the CardioSEAL™ device to the muscular ventricular defect is the introduction of the delivery *sheath* and then the delivery of the device *from* the *left* ventricular side of the ventricular defect. With this technique the through-and-through wire is created using the femoral *vein* and the same right internal jugular *vein* approaches for the initial catheter introductions. Once the through-and-through wire is established, the sizing balloon is introduced from the jugular vein and the sizing of the defect performed exactly as with the previous approaches.

However, once the sizing is completed, the sizing balloon is removed from the jugular vein. The Swan™ balloon that was used to cross the septum is withdrawn completely off the wire and out of the venous system from the femoral vein. The Swan™ balloon catheter is reintroduced over the through-and-through wire, but from the right *internal jugular* vein. The Swan™ catheter is advanced over the through-and-through wire from the jugular vein, through the right heart, through the VSD and into the left ventricle. The Swan™ catheter remains with the tip on the left side of the septum to help protect the right-sided cardiac structures from the "sawing" motions of the long wire. Once the through-and-through wire is in place and the catheter is over the wire from the internal jugular vein, an 85 cm (or longer!) long sheath is preformed for the delivery of the device from left ventricular approach. The original "transseptal" curve of an *extra long* 11-French delivery sheath/dilator is formed into a 360° (or even tighter) loop with an additional, separate slight anterior curve on the distal part of the 360° curve. The specially formed and extra-long sheath is introduced into the *femoral* vein over the through-and-through wire and advanced through the inferior vena cava, right atrium, the atrial septum, the mitral valve and into the left ventricle. While simultaneously withdrawing the Swan™ catheter from the opposite (jugular vein) end of the wire, the long sheath/dilator is advanced over the wire from the left ventricle through the VSD until the tip of the *sheath* has passed into the right *atrium* and/or at least *several centimeters* into the *right* ventricle.

Once the *sheath* is in the proper position, the dilator is withdrawn from the sheath very slowly and carefully while simultaneously the Swan™ catheter with the balloon deflated is re-advanced over the wire in order to follow the tip of the dilator *into* the sheath as the dilator is withdrawn. With the now > 360° curve on the sheath, extreme care must be taken not to move the sheath either forward or backward while the dilator is being withdrawn from the sheath. Once the dilator is removed completely and the Swan™ catheter is "retrograde" as far into the distal end of the long sheath (as far back as the left atrium at least) as possible, the long, through-and-through, Super Stiff™ wire is withdrawn completely from the long sheath so that the floppy tip of the Super Stiff™ wire will be withdrawn through the heart. The sheath is allowed to bleed back to clear it completely of air or clot and then placed on a slow continuous flush.

The delivery cable in the CardioSEAL™ delivery catheter is extended as far as possible out of the delivery catheter and a long smooth curve formed on the exposed distal delivery cable to correspond to the 360° curve on the delivery sheath. The appropriate CardioSEAL™ device is attached to the cable, loaded into the "front loader" (or 11-French short sheath) and with the tip of the delivery catheter positioned against the proximal legs of the device in the loader, the tip of the loader is introduced into the hub of the long sheath at the *femoral* vein. The delivery catheter with the device close to the tip of the delivery catheter is advanced within the delivery sheath from the femoral vein until the tip of the distal legs of the device are approximately at the *atrial* septum. From there, the *delivery catheter and the sheath* are fixed in place while the *delivery rod* is advanced into the delivery catheter. This advances the delivery cable and the device within the sheath. The device is advanced slowly and carefully around the entire 360° curve of the sheath while watching and controlling the sheath very closely during all of this maneuvering. The end-hole catheter, which is over the wire and into the sheath from the distal or jugular vein end of the long sheath, is withdrawn simultaneously. With the long curve through the multiple intracardiac structures, there is considerable opportunity for the sheath to push forward and kink and/or to partially straighten out and, in doing so, pull the tip of the sheath back out of the defect and into the left ventricle. Multiple delicate, small to-and-fro adjustments of the sheath often are necessary while the device is being advanced.

The device is advanced all of the way to the tip of the sheath as the catheter from the opposite end of the wire is withdrawn simultaneously. At this point, a left ventricular angiocardiogram is performed to verify that the entire length of the folded distal legs ***including*** *the central hinge point* of the device are completely on the ***right*** ventricular side of the *narrowest area* of the ventricular septal defect. In addition, it is essential to be sure that the *distal* legs of the device, which are still within the sheath, appear well away from the tricuspid valve apparatus. With this confirmed, a slight forward push is applied to the delivery rod/catheter while the sheath only is withdrawn slowly but completely off the distal (*right* ventricular) legs of the device. The legs that are opening in the trabeculae of the right ventricle usually do not open completely on this side of the septum. A repeat left ventricular angiocardiogram is performed to confirm that the opened side of the device still is *completely* on the right ventricular side of the defect and the central hinge is still within, or to the *right of*, the narrow area of the defect. When satisfied with this position, the delivery catheter is pushed forward and the sheath alone is withdrawn off the proximal (left ventricular) legs of the device. Once all four of these legs spring open completely, the sheath is re-advanced firmly against the center of the left ventricular umbrella. This forward force applied to the sheath pushes the device tightly into the defect. A repeat left ventricular angiocardiogram confirms the position and degree of occlusion of the defect. Once satisfied with the position, the release mechanism is activated.

There are several reported advantages to this approach for the delivery of a device for VSD occlusion. When the large delivery sheath is introduced from the femoral vein, a much smaller sheath can be used in the jugular vein. This may be important in small infants, although the jugular vein usually is larger than the femoral vein. The left ventricular approach offers a better angle of approach to the muscular ventricular septal defects when the defect angles cranially in its course from the right ventricle toward the left ventricle. There also is the theoretical possibility of readjusting the "seating" of the device in the defect after both sides of the device are open. The readjustment is performed before the release of the device by pushing the tip of the sheath forcefully against the still attached device after both sides of the device have been opened. During this maneuver, the more proximal curve of the sheath is "buttressed" against the free wall of the left ventricle as the tip of the sheath pushes against the left ventricular side of the device to push it further into the defect. However, it is unlikely that the device can be pushed significantly further into the defect once the right ventricular legs are open and entangled in the right ventricular trabeculae.

There are several significant disadvantages of the delivery approaching from the left ventricular side. These include much less control over the long sheath during the device delivery along with a much greater chance of pulling the tip of the sheath out of the defect during the passage of the device through the sheath to the defect. With the much longer and greater curve in the long delivery sheath, there is a significant chance of kinking the long sheath during the various wire, dilator and device manipulations. Probably the greatest disadvantage of the left ventricular approach/delivery is that, if the device is not far enough into and/or slips back into the left side of the defect as the right (distal) legs are opened, it cannot be re-advanced and/or repositioned back into the defect without withdrawing the device completely into and frequently all of the way out of the sheath and starting the procedure all over.

Device delivery from the arterial and left ventricle approach

The arterial approach described for the creation of the through-and-through wire, also can be used for the delivery of the sheath and then the device from the left ventricular side of the defect and the retrograde *arterial* approach. Since the long sheath must pass from the femoral artery, retrograde around the aortic arch and back into the left ventricle before crossing the defect, for an adult sized patient an even longer delivery sheath than the longest standard (85 cm) long sheaths often must be specially ordered. With the CardioSEAL™ devices larger than 28 mm, this approach requires the introduction of an 11-French sheath and for the smaller CardioSEAL™ devices, a 10-French sheath into the femoral artery. Once within the artery, considerable manipulation with the *sheath* itself is required within the artery. The necessity of the manipulations of this large sheath directly in the artery, particularly in younger and smaller patients, obviates all possible advantages of this approach for delivery of the CardioSEAL/STARFlex™ devices.

For the retrograde delivery technique, the defect is crossed as described previously for positioning the through-and-through wire from the arterial approach. The through-and-through wire is created with the left ventricular end of the wire entering from the femoral artery instead of from the femoral vein, right heart and through the atrial septum. The other end of the wire exits from either the jugular vein or from a femoral vein after being snared in the pulmonary artery as described previously. Once the through-and-through route is established, a Super Stiff™ wire is substituted for the original through-and-through wire as described previously. The jugular venous access is preferable for the stiff through-and-through wire, but the tight, more circuitous curves from the VSD, back through the right heart to the femoral vein are less important when the device is to be delivered from the left ventricular side. After the through-and-through wire is secured in place, the Swan™ balloon or other end–hole catheter used initially to cross the ventricular defect is removed from the arterial (retrograde) end and reintroduced over the opposite (venous) end of the through-and-through wire. The Swan™ balloon or other end-hole catheter is advanced through the ventricular defect and as far along the wire into the left ventricle as possible, and even out into the aorta if possible. This catheter again protects the various intracardiac structures from the "sawing" by the wire during the subsequent, often extensive manipulations to pass the large sheath retrograde to, and through, the defect.

An "S" shaped curve is pre-formed at the distal end of the extra-long sheath. The "distal" portion of the "S" is pre-shaped with as acute and/or as tight a curve as possible formed on this distal portion. This curve is formed to conform to the course of the through-and-through wire as it passes around the arch, into the left ventricle and through the defect. The curve around the arch to the left ventricle is fairly long and smooth while the curve following the course from the long axis of the left ventricle into the ventricular septal defect is approximately 90° and in the opposite direction—i.e. the need for the "S" curve on the delivery sheath. The arterial introductory site and surrounding area are re-infiltrated with an additional *very liberal* amount of local anesthesia. The large, pre-formed sheath/dilator is introduced into the artery over the through-and-through wire and advanced retrograde around the arch, into the left ventricle to, and through, the VSD. As the tip of the dilator approaches the Swan™ or other end-hole catheter, which is over and approaching from the other end of the through-and-through wire, the end-hole catheter is withdrawn proportionately off the wire allowing the tip of the long dilator to remain against the tip of the withdrawing end-hole catheter. The large sheath/dilator must be advanced far enough into the *right* ventricle so that the tip of the *sheath* is at least several *centimeters* beyond the narrowest portion of the VSD into the right ventricle or, preferably, even into the right atrium. The tip of the sheath must be far enough into the right ventricle to accommodate the entire length of the folded distal legs of the device ***and** the central hinge mechanism*, all on the right side of the narrowest portion of the defect.

The manipulations of the large sheath/dilator through the artery, through the very tight curves in the course to the defect, through the defect and, finally, the right ventricular trabeculae are the most difficult and hazardous portions of the procedure from this approach. Once the dilator is advanced as far as possible into the right ventricle, the *sheath* is advanced over the dilator to the tip of the dilator. This position is confirmed with a left ventricular angiocardiogram through a second left ventricular catheter. The second catheter in the left ventricle is introduced from a second arterial puncture and a retrograde approach or from an atrial transseptal approach, but the second catheter in the left ventricle should be in place before beginning manipulations with the large retrograde sheath.

Once the tip of the *sheath* is far enough into the right ventricle, the dilator very carefully and slowly is withdrawn over the wire and out of the sheath while the Swan™ (or other end-hole catheter), which is introduced from the other end of the wire, simultaneously is advanced over the wire, into the distal end of the sheath and as far back into the sheath as possible (around the aortic arch!). Once the sheath is in position with the end-hole catheter from the distal end well within it, the through-and-through wire is withdrawn very carefully completely out of the system so that the floppy end of the Super Stiff™ wire is withdrawn through the heart. Extra care is taken not to move the sheath forward or backward during the dilator and/or wire withdrawal. Even slight movement of the sheath through all of the various tight curves can easily kink the sheath. The end-hole catheter retrograde within the distal end of the sheath serves to protect the end of the sheath from the "cutting" effect of the wire and as a "safety system" for replacing this wire should the sheath slip out of the VSD and/or kink during the various manipulations.

With the sheath in place, the loaded device is introduced into the sheath at the femoral arterial access site. The device is advanced to the defect, delivered and released exactly as with the left ventricular approach to the delivery with the long sheath coming from the transseptal venous route. Because of the tighter and compound bends in the course of the long sheath, the passage of the device around the arch and into the defect is more difficult. Even greater attention must be paid to the sheath and its position to prevent even the slightest withdrawal out of the defect while at the same time avoiding kinking. This approach for the delivery of a VSD device is more applicable to the more anterior muscular defects and those that occur after the surgical repair of an outlet VSD, but even in those defects the hazards and difficulty of the retrograde, left ventricular delivery of the CardioSEAL™ device to a ventricular septal defect outweigh any advantages of this approach. The retrograde left ventricular approach is more reasonable with the Amplatzer™ VSD device, which requires a considerably smaller delivery sheath.

Transcatheter closure of high anteroseptal intramural muscular VSDs

Most of these intramural ventricular septal defects persist and/or redevelop after the closure and/or baffle repair of malalignment ventricular septal defects (e.g. in TOF, Truncus, PA/VSD & TGA/VSD). In order to create a smooth channel and to avoid placing sutures in the aortic valve, the surgeon commonly attaches the cephalad end of the interventricular patch to the spongy, muscular wall of the right ventricle (RV) instead of to the fibrous septum, leaving a small residual opening at the cephalad end of the patch. With healing, retraction of scar tissue and the continued flow through these defects over time, the defects actually continue to open further with "excavation" through the muscular septum. There occasionally are naturally occurring muscular defects in this same area.

Unlike the other muscular interventricular septal defects, the left ventricular opening of these defects usually is high on the left ventricular outlet septum just below the aortic valve, while the outlet on the right ventricular side can exit anywhere along the right ventricular side of the septum, particularly deep within the right ventricle. An initial left ventricular angiocardiogram is performed in the PA and lateral view. It usually is necessary to re-angle the X-ray tubes to position the unusual, long channel of the defect in its longest profile and to show the relationship of the left ventricular end of the defect to the aortic valve. The ideal angle for viewing these anterior and intramural defects "on edge" often is more of a cranial–straight lateral than the cranial–LAO, which is used for the other muscular defects. Occasionally these defects are visualized best with a straight lateral and/or minimal LAO angulation of the lateral X-ray tube. The X-ray tubes often need to be re-angled into a different plane several times in order to demonstrate the particular anatomy of the right ventricular exit site.

As with the closure of other muscular ventricular septal defects, a through-and-through wire is created through the defect. The site for the introduction of the venous catheter is determined from the angiocardiograms. In these higher, more anterior defects, the straighter course for access to the right ventricular side of the septal defect often is from the femoral venous approach rather than from the jugular approach. Because the left ventricular opening of these defects is in the high, left ventricular outflow tract, the entrance angle to enter the left ventricular opening of the defect is far less acute when the defect is approached *through the aortic valve* than when it is approached from the inflow of the left ventricle. As a consequence, the most expedient technique for entering into the anterior intramural defect often is from the retrograde arterial approach.

A long (125 cm) "right coronary" Judkins™ catheter (or other catheter with a long "right coronary curve") is passed retrograde into the left ventricular apex. The tip of the catheter is rotated to the right (medially) and anteriorly as the tip of the catheter is withdrawn along the septum. With this maneuver, the tip of the catheter usually drops into the left ventricular end of the ventricular septal defect and often can be advanced a centimeter or more into the defect. A small hand injection of contrast through the retrograde catheter positioned in the defect defines the anatomy of the defect very well. With the tip of the catheter secured in the defect, an exchange length, very floppy tipped, torque-controlled wire is advanced through the catheter and manipulated into and through the relatively long channel of the ventricular septal defect. It usually is easier to cross the defect with a Glide™ wire, however, the Glide™ wire easily *perforates* thin muscular tissues and passes through other areas of the septum adjacent to the defect, creating a new "channel"! It is preferable to exit the VSD as high (cephalad) on the right ventricular side of the septum as possible when there are multiple right ventricular exits. The higher on the right side of the septum the wire exits, the easier is the subsequent passage of the large, long delivery sheath into the defect on the right side of the septum from the femoral venous approach.

Once the floppy tipped wire has been manipulated through the defect, the wire is advanced to the right ventricular outflow tract and into the pulmonary artery. An end-hole floating balloon (Swan™) catheter is introduced from a femoral vein through a 9-French short sheath and *floated* through the tricuspid valve into the right ventricle and to the pulmonary artery. Similar to the approach across the tricuspid valve for the "snaring" procedures in all of the other VSD closures, the floating balloon catheter is preferred for this passage through the tricuspid valve in order to assure passage through the largest central opening in the valve. A Microvena™ snare (Microvena Corp., White Bear Lake, MN) or Ensnare™ (MDTECH (Medical Device Technologies), Gainesville, FL) is introduced through the end-hole floating balloon catheter or the balloon catheter is replaced over an exchange wire with a true snare catheter in the pulmonary artery and the snare introduced through that catheter. The floppy tip of the exchange wire, which had been manipulated through the VSD, is snared in either the right ventricular outflow tract or the pulmonary artery. Once snared, the wire is withdrawn carefully into the inferior vena cava. If there is any resistance to the withdrawal of the wire through the tricuspid valve and/or the course of the wire from the right ventricle to the inferior vena cava is even slightly circuitous and *not* straight, the intracardiac structures should be visualized with a transthoracic or transesophageal echocardiogram to be sure that vital right ventricular and/or tricuspid valve structures have not been trapped. The wire is withdrawn further only when the wire is free of the tricuspid valve apparatus and not passing through a narrow chordal opening. If there is even the suggestion of entanglement in any of the tricuspid valve structures, the wire is released from the snare. The floppy tipped wire is re-advanced into the pulmonary artery while the snare catheter is withdrawn back out of the femoral vein and an end-hole Swan™ floating balloon catheter is manipulated to the pulmonary artery through a different area of the tricuspid valve. The snare wire can be delivered and manipulated through the Swan™ catheter, although there is less torque control over the Swan™ catheter. Once the wire is snared and easily withdrawn through the tricuspid valve and into the inferior vena cava in a straight course, the distal end of the exchange wire is exteriorized through the femoral vein sheath.

This creates a through-and-through wire from the femoral artery, retrograde through the defect, right ventricle, right atrium and out through the femoral vein (Figure 30.3). Once the through-and-through (rail) wire is established, traction is maintained on both ends of the wire while the retrograde *catheter* is advanced over the wire and maneuvered through the defect and into and through the right heart. The retrograde arterial catheter is advanced over the rail wire until the tip of the *catheter* is exteriorized through the femoral vein sheath. The

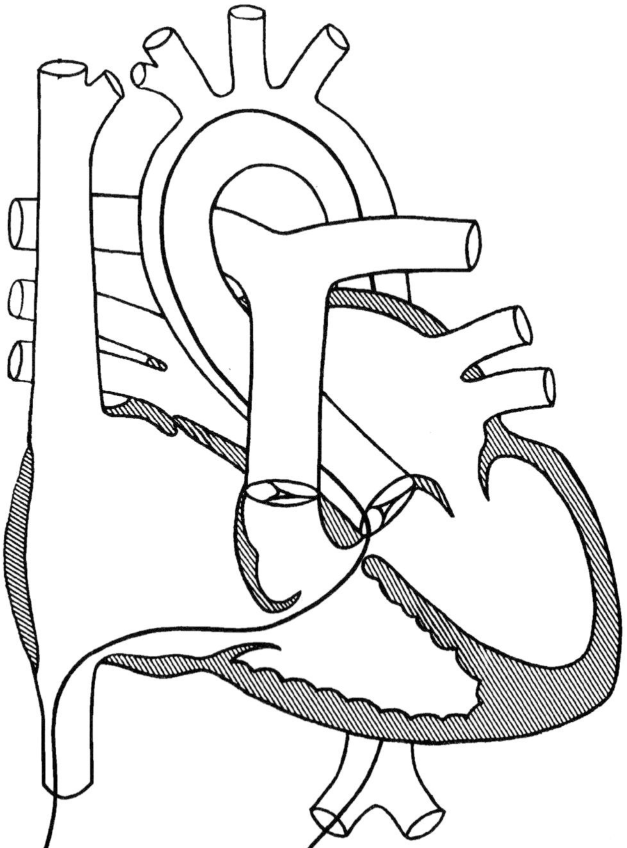

Figure 30.3 Arteriovenous through-and-through wire for high muscular or perimembranous VSD: from the femoral vein, to the right atrium, right ventricle, through the VSD, to the left ventricle (outflow), to the aorta and out through the femoral artery.

original floppy tipped torque wire is replaced through the "through-and-through" catheter with a 0.035″ Super Stiff™ exchange length wire.

If the snared wire could not be withdrawn easily through the tricuspid valve and/or was not straight in its course to the femoral vein after several attempts, the femoral vein approach is abandoned and the floating balloon catheter and then the snare catheter are introduced from the jugular vein. The through-and-through wire is created from the jugular vein through the defect and out through the femoral *artery*. The device delivery from the jugular vein approach to the defect is similar to the technique from the femoral vein for these more anterior defects.

The initial entry into, and passage through the VSD occasionally is accomplished from the femoral *venous* route, obviating the need for any retrograde manipulations to cross the defect. With *congenital* anterior muscular defects, in particular, a long, pre-curved Judkins™ right coronary catheter is manipulated from the right ventricle into the pulmonary artery. While counterclockwise torque is applied to the catheter, it is withdrawn across the pulmonary valve into the right ventricular outflow tract, where the tip of the catheter often falls into the right ventricular end of the anterior muscular VSD. If the tip does not enter the VSD, the maneuver is repeated one or more times, each time changing the torque and, in turn, the angle of the tip of the catheter slightly until it does drop into the right ventricular end of the VSD. Once the tip is "seated" within the VSD, a hand injection angiocardiogram is performed in the defect to confirm the catheter position. A very floppy tipped, torque-controlled wire is advanced into the venous catheter and manipulated through the VSD. Once it passes completely through this anterior VSD, the wire usually continues out into the ascending aorta and from there, the wire can be manipulated into the descending aorta. Once the floppy tipped wire is anywhere in the aorta, it can be snared with a snare catheter introduced from a femoral artery. The wire *and* the tip of the prograde *catheter* are exteriorized through the femoral artery. The floppy tipped wire within the through-and-through *catheter* is replaced with a 0.035″ Super Stiff™ exchange length wire. If the delivery sheath is to be delivered from the venous route, an end-hole catheter is introduced and advanced over the *arterial end* of the through-and-through wire simultaneously as the original "through-and-through" venous catheter is withdrawn from the opposite end of the wire. The retrograde catheter over the wire is advanced through the defect and into at least the right atrium as the original venous catheter is withdrawn completely off the wire and out of the introductory sheath.

At this point in the procedure, an additional left ventricular catheter is introduced. The additional catheter will be used for selective left ventricular angiograms during the sizing of the defect and the very critical positioning during the delivery of the device. The second left ventricular catheter can be introduced either retrograde from an additional arterial puncture or from the venous approach through an atrial transseptal puncture.

Once the through-and-through Super Stiff™ exchange wire is in place, a NuMED™ (NuMED Inc., Hopkinton, NY) sizing balloon is introduced over the *venous* end of the wire. The sizing balloon is advanced over the through-and-through wire while the arterial catheter on the wire from the opposite end simultaneously is withdrawn so that the tips of the two catheters remain approximated during the introduction of the sizing balloon catheter. Both the shafts of the sizing balloon catheter and the retrograde catheter are maintained on a constant flush through wire back-bleed valves, which are attached to the hubs of the catheters. The sizing balloon is advanced across the defect while the original retrograde catheter remains over the arterial end of the wire touching the tip of the sizing balloon catheter. This catheter over the wire now protects the aortic valve and other intravascular structures from the cutting effect of the stiff wire. The sizing balloon is inflated using a *very* low (zero) inflation pressure within the channel of the ventricular defect. If necessary the X-ray tubes are re-angled in order to align the tubes perpendicular to the longest axis of the balloon. The "soft" inflation of the balloon clearly defines the diameters, length and the often irregular course of the intramural defect as well as the very important relationship of the left ventricular end of the defect to the aortic valve.

A left ventricular angiogram is performed while the sizing balloon is inflated in the defect. The various diameters and lengths of the defect are measured on the angiographic screen as well as by echocardiography. The most critical measurements are the diameter of the left ventricular inlet end of the defect and the distance within this end of the defect from the aortic valve to the *narrowest area* of the defect. These measurements determine the maximum length of the arms of the *left side* of the CardioSEAL™ device and/or the bulk of any other device that can be accommodated completely *within* the defect without extending out of the defect into the left ventricular outflow tract and/or compromising the aortic valve.

Once the operator is satisfied that there is sufficient distance from the center of the defect to the aortic valve to allow the "left ventricular" arms or "side" of an appropriate device to open within the defect without encroaching on the aortic valve, the procedure to close the defect is continued. The approach for the delivery of the long sheath for the device delivery depends upon the individual patient's anatomy and which particular device is to be used. Introduction of the long delivery sheath from the *venous* approach usually is possible and preferable.

The delivery sheath required for the size of the particular CardioSEAL™ device being used is chosen and prepared for the introduction of the device. This requires a 10-French long sheath for the 17–28 mm devices and an 11-French sheath for the 33 mm device. As with the introduction of all other CardioSEAL™ devices, a short 14-French "recovery" sheath is placed over the long sheath/dilator while still outside of the body. The introduction of the long sheath from the internal jugular venous or the retrograde arterial approach is identical to the introduction for the closure of any other muscular VSD. The distal end of the long sheath/dilator is *precurved* according to the curves and bends that will be formed along the course from the introductory site to, and through, the defect from whichever introductory site is used.

When the long delivery sheath is to be introduced from the femoral venous approach, the original "transseptal" curve on the long MTS™ sheath is straightened to a slow, smooth, 10–20° curve at the distal end. The dilator is placed on a continuous flush through a wire back-bleed/flush valve. As this delivery sheath/dilator is introduced from the femoral vein, the retrograde catheter that is positioned over the wire is withdrawn simultaneously and synchronously, keeping the tip of the withdrawing catheter and the tip of the advancing dilator together. Once the sheath/dilator has passed from the right ventricle, completely through the VSD and into the left ventricle, the sheath/dilator follows the wire/catheter across the aortic valve and into the ascending aorta. The sheath is advanced over the dilator far enough to position the tip of the *sheath* well above the aortic valve. As long as the large, long sheath positioned across the aortic valve does not create significant aortic regurgitation *and* the patient remains hemodynamically stable, the sheath remains in the aorta during the introduction of the device into, and to the end of, the sheath. As the long dilator is removed from the sheath, the retrograde catheter, which is over the other end of the through-and-through wire, is re-advanced behind the dilator tip and into the distal end of the sheath. As before, this catheter retrograde within the distal end of the sheath helps to keep the wire from cutting into the sheath, keeps the sheath from kinking, and serves as a safety route for the reintroduction of the through-and-through wire if the sheath should pull into or through the defect.

When the tip of the long sheath is positioned in the ascending aorta, the tip of the sheath also is positioned directly under the head vessels! *Extreme* caution must be used to clear the sheath of all air and/or clots as the dilator and wire are removed. As the dilator is withdrawn, the tip of the retrograde catheter is advanced within the sheath as far as the area of the right atrium. As the dilator is withdrawn slowly from the sheath, the aortic pressure is used to bleed and clear the sheath passively through the side port of the sheath. After the sheath is cleared, it is attached to a pressure/flush system and placed on a slow, steady flush. With the sheath on a continuous flush, the through-and-through wire slowly is withdrawn completely out of the body in the direction such that the floppy end of the wire is withdrawn through the heart and vasculature.

While keeping the long sheath on a continuous flush, the CardioSEAL™ occlusion device attached to the delivery cable/catheter is introduced into the long sheath exactly as with the other VSD delivery techniques. The CardioSEAL™ device used should be at least twice the diameter of the narrowest portion of the defect, but more importantly, the legs on the left side of the device *cannot be longer* than the distance from the narrowest portion of the defect to the left ventricular end of the defect and/or the aortic valve. The combination catheter/cable/device is advanced to approximately the area of the tricuspid valve. The tip of the distal legs of the folded CardioSEAL™ device should be touching or almost touching the tip of the retrograde catheter, which still is within the sheath. The sheath and delivery catheter are fixed in position and the delivery rod is advanced into the delivery catheter while the retrograde catheter is withdrawn simultaneously and proportionately. This advances the delivery cable/device away from the distal end of the delivery catheter while the tip of the retrograde catheter positioned within the sheath in the aorta helps to stabilize the long sheath while the device is advanced through the sheath. As the *tips of the left sided legs* of the device reach *just **within** the tip* of the sheath, the tip of the retrograde catheter drops out of the sheath into the aorta.

Once the device reaches the tip of the sheath, the sheath is withdrawn until the tip of the sheath drops back to a position in the left ventricular out-flow tract just below the aortic valve and/or just barely within the left ventricular opening of the VSD. Angiograms are repeated in the aortic root and/or the immediate subaortic area through the second retrograde catheter to demonstrate clearly and precisely the relationship of the aortic valve to the distal tips of the left sided device, which is still folded within the sheath. When absolutely certain that the left sided legs are below and clear of the aortic valve, the delivery catheter and cable are fixed in this position and the sheath is withdrawn off the left ventricular side of the device. With the device partially open, a repeat angiogram in the subaortic area is performed. If the partially open legs remain away from the aortic valve, yet still are completely outside of the left ventricular end of the defect, the entire sheath/delivery catheter/cable/device is withdrawn together until the left ventricular side of the device has been withdrawn into the left ventricular side of the defect and the center hinge of the device is within, or even on the right side of, the narrowest portion of the defect.

The sheath alone is withdrawn further until the tip of the sheath reaches and exposes the central hinge mechanism of the device. Once the central area is in the proper position, further withdrawal of the sheath exposes the entire left sided umbrella and allows it to open freely within the defect. The sheath, delivery catheter, cable and device all are withdrawn *as a unit* until the arms of the left side of the device are *completely within* the defect *and* the central hinge mechanism of the device is in, or slightly on the right ventricular side of, the narrowest area of the VSD. This position and the relationship of the left ventricular arms of the device away from the aortic valve are confirmed with a repeat left ventricular angiocardiogram. Until this stage of the procedure, if the device position is not satisfactory and/or if the device is dangerously close to the aortic valve, the sheath/delivery catheter/ delivery cable/partially open device still can be withdrawn further into the defect. If the position of the device still is totally unsatisfactory, the device can be withdrawn into the sheath and completely out of the patient, although the tips of the distal legs may not withdraw completely into the sheath, and have the possibility of catching on the tricuspid valve as the combination is withdrawn within the ventricle.

When satisfied with the position within the defect and *absolutely certain* that the open, left sided legs are within the defect and away from the aortic valve, the catheter/delivery cable is held in place while the sheath is withdrawn off the proximal (right ventricular) arms of the device. Once both sides of the CardioSEAL™ device have been opened, the device no longer is retrievable from this location by a catheter technique, which reinforces the need for very accurate measurements *before* beginning to deploy the device. The final position and degree of closure of the defect with the device completely open is confirmed with a repeat left ventricular angiocardiogram. The release mechanism of the device is activated.

Left ventricular, retrograde arterial approach for closing intramural antero-septal muscular ventricular septal defects

The arterial approach for placement of the long delivery sheath occasionally is preferable for the anterior muscular and in particular the residual intramural ventricular septal defects following a previous surgical repair. The atrial transseptal approach from the femoral *vein* to the left ventricular side of the defect is *not* suitable for closure of the muscular defects in the *anterior* septum, which precludes this approach to these defects. If the femoral or jugular venous sheath cannot be maintained without it kinking within the anteroseptal ventricular defects and/or the left sided umbrella cannot be opened initially from the venous approach without compromising the aortic valve, these defects are closed using a retrograde approach to the left ventricular end of the defect.

A through-and-through wire from the femoral artery through the defect to the femoral or jugular vein is established as described previously. The distal end of the long delivery sheath is pre-curved to confirm to the concave course from the femoral artery, around the arch and through the aortic valve. The very tip of the sheath/dilator then is curved in the *reverse direction* to form a long "shepherd's crook" curve at the tip in order to enter the VSD. After the introduction of very liberal local anesthesia around the arterial introductory site, the large, long sheath is introduced into the femoral *artery* and advanced retrograde over the through-and-through wire across the aortic valve to the left ventricular end of the defect, as described earlier for the mid muscular VSD closure via the retrograde approach.

When the retrograde approach is used, the large, long delivery sheath enters through the femoral artery with all of the potential arterial complications and the greater problems with control of the long sheath. The retrograde approach can only be used in a relatively long intramural defect in order to ensure that the device opens completely within the defect. When delivered retrograde, the actual final position of the *left ventricular (subaortic!) legs* of the CardioSEAL™ device cannot be determined definitively until the device is opened fully and no longer is retrievable! The operator must be absolutely sure that the proximal (left sided) legs are well away from the aortic valve while the legs are still in their folded configuration within the sheath before the sheath is withdrawn off them.

Amplatzer™ ventricular septal defect occluder for muscular interventricular defects

The Amplatzer™ VSD Occluders (AGA Medical Corp., Golden Valley, MN) are a specific modification of the Amplatzer™ ASD Occluders (AGA Medical Corp., Golden Valley, MN) to make them applicable for the muscular VSD[3,4]. The Amplatzer™ VSD Occluder is designed to conform more to the shape and physiology of the mid and/or apical muscular VSD. The Amplatzer™ VSD Occluders up to 10 mm in diameter are manufactured from 0.004″ Nitinol™ memory metal wire, while the larger diameter devices are manufactured from 0.005″ wire, and they all have a "basket-like" weave of the Nitinol™ memory wires, which is similar to the Amplatzer™ ASD Occluders. The central connecting (occluding) hub of the Amplatzer™ VSD devices measures 7 mm in length for devices up to 14 mm in diameter (size) and 10mm in length for devices between 16 and 24 mm in diameter. All of the muscular VSD occluders have polyester patches sewn into each of the two end disks and across the hub to enhance immediate occlusion.

The diameter of the central hub (or waist) represents the "size" of the device and ranges from 6 to 24 mm in 2 mm increments. The central hub has small rims (or lips) at *each* end, giving the Amplatzer™ muscular VSD device the shape of a "spool" for sewing thread. The rim on the distal, "left ventricular" side of the device extends 4 mm beyond the hub circumferentially around the hub and, in turn, is 8 mm larger in *diameter* than the hub while the rim on the proximal, "right ventricular" side extends 3 mm away from the hub circumferentially around the hub and, in turn, is 6 mm larger in *diameter* than the hub. The Amplatzer™ muscular VSD devices are delivered through 6–10-French long delivery sheaths.

The narrowest diameter of the VSD determines the diameter of the device that is used. The size of the device is chosen several millimeters larger than the narrowest diameter of the defect. Although the Amplatzer™ VSD device is secured in place primarily by the expanded hub stretching against the walls of the defect and not by the rims at each end of the hub, the narrow rims at both ends of the device add to the security of the implant and aid in holding the device in place during the positioning and implant of the device. The same screw-on attach/release mechanism and the same delivery cables and sheaths are used for the Amplatzer™ VSD device as for the Amplatzer™ ASD devices. As is the case with the delivery of the Amplatzer™ ASD devices, RB-MTS™ sheaths (Cook Inc., Bloomington, IN), which can be pre-shaped into special curves, are very useful for the delivery of the Amplatzer™ muscular VSD devices. The RB-MTS™ sheaths can be pre-formed more readily into the desired curves and they do not kink as readily as the Amplatzer™ delivery sheaths.

The muscular ventricular septal defect is visualized angiographically and by echo exactly as for catheter closure using the CardioSEAL™ device as described earlier in this chapter. The angiographic appearance of the defect usually appears significantly larger than the actual sized dimension of the defect. In most cases, the basic technique for the positioning of the long sheaths and the delivery of the Amplatzer™ VSD device is similar to that described previously in this chapter for the CardioSEAL™ device. A catheter is advanced from the femoral vein, across the atrial septum (by transseptal puncture when necessary), to the left atrium, left ventricle, through the VSD to the right ventricle and into the pulmonary artery. Any end-hole torque-controlled catheter and/or torque-controlled wire can be used to enter and cross the VSD, however an end-hole floating balloon catheter (Arrow International Inc., Reading, PA) has a greater chance of passing through the *largest area* of the VSD. Once a catheter has passed through the VSD and into the pulmonary artery, a separate floating balloon catheter is introduced from the jugular vein and "floated" through the tricuspid valve and right ventricle to the pulmonary artery. A snare is introduced through this catheter, or the balloon catheter in the pulmonary artery is replaced over an exchange length wire with a specific snare catheter; snare catheters are more controllable than floating balloon catheters. A floppy tipped wire is passed through the catheter that is crossing the ventricular defect, and is snared in the pulmonary artery with the snare that was introduced from the internal jugular vein. The snared wire is withdrawn through the right ventricle, the right atrium and out through the internal jugular vein, creating a through-and-through wire with all of the precautions described earlier.

An AGA™ (AGA Medical Corp., Golden Valley, MN) or NuMED™ (NuMED Inc., Hopkinton, NY) sizing balloon is introduced over the internal jugular end of the wire and is advanced into the VSD in order to measure the diameter and determine the shape of the VSD. When the NuMED™ balloon is used it is inflated until some resistance to the inflation is encountered in order to "stretch" the defect slightly. Because of the course of the VSD through the septum and, in turn, overlapping structures within the defect, the balloon-sized muscular septal defect, even with the "stretching" of the defect, frequently is significantly smaller than the angiographically measured defect. The AGA™ balloon initially produces a slightly "stretched" diameter of the defect while the NuMED™ balloon gives a more accurate representation of the size and configuration of the defect before pressure is applied to the balloon and it is stretched. An Amplatzer™ muscular VSD occluding device that is 1.5–2 mm larger than the stretched diameter and/or angiographic diameter of the defect as measured in diastole is used for the occlusion.

The sizing balloon is withdrawn and the original short sheath in the internal jugular vein is removed from the jugular vein over the through-and-through wire and replaced with the 6–9-French special Amplatzer™ delivery sheath/dilator (AGA Medical Corp., Golden Valley, MN) or a comparable sized RB-MTS™ sheath (Cook Inc., Bloomington, IN), with the size of the device determining the size of the delivery sheath being used. The devices larger than 12 mm require 7–8-French sheaths, while the devices over 20 mm require an 8–10-French sheath. Using a delivery sheath one French size larger than that "recommended" by the manufacturers facilitates the delivery of the device! As an extra safety precaution, the Swan™ balloon or other end-hole catheter that initially was used to cross the VSD from left to right ventricle and that is still in place over the wire in the left or right ventricle, is advanced to the tip of the AGA™ or RB-MTS™ delivery sheath/dilator as it is introduced into the vein over the wire. The delivery sheath/dilator is advanced into the right ventricle, through the VSD and well into the left ventricle (frequently against the left ventricular free wall) as the catheter over the wire from the left ventricle is withdrawn simultaneously. The sheath is advanced over the dilator to the tip of the dilator and then the dilator is withdrawn out of the sheath over the wire. When the size of the sheath allows it, the retrograde catheter, which is over the wire from the opposite end of the wire, is advanced into the distal end of the long delivery sheath as the dilator is withdrawn and advanced back into the sheath as far as at least the area of the right atrium. After the dilator is withdrawn, the sheath is cleared meticulously of any air and/or possible clots by allowing it to bleed back *passively* from the pressure in the left ventricle. Once the retrograde catheter is secure within the delivery sheath, the through-and-through wire is withdrawn completely out of the system, and again the catheter is allowed to bleed back until it is free of any air or clot before attaching it to a flush system.

With some defects it is desirable to have the sheath tip pointing toward the apex of the left ventricle rather than across the left ventricular cavity. In this circumstance, rather than attempting to advance the retrograde catheter into the delivery sheath, the retrograde catheter is used to push the apical curve of the through-and-through wire into the apex of the ventricle as the wire exits the ventricular septal defect and passes across the left ventricle. This directs the wire that is passing through the defect to the apex of the left ventricle before the delivery sheath and dilator are advanced through the defect. This does not provide protection from the "sawing" of the wire as it is withdrawn, nor the extra safety factor of having the retrograde catheter still within the delivery sheath during the time when the device is being advanced within the sheath.

The Amplatzer™ VSD device is removed from its packaging and soaked in saline. The flush/back-bleed valve is attached to the loader and the delivery cable is passed through the valve and the short loading sleeve. Once the device is thoroughly soaked, the hub of the device is screwed onto the delivery cable with a *clockwise* turning of the device until the device stops turning freely on the screw of the cable. Once it stops, the device is turned *counterclockwise*, but only 1/4 turn. While still "under water" in the flush solution and while flushing through the side port of the valve on the loader, the device is held with one hand while traction is placed on the delivery cable in the opposite direction. Traction at the opposite ends of the device elongates the device into a thin "tube" and allows it to be withdrawn easily into the loading sleeve. Once the device is completely within the loading sleeve, the sleeve is flushed thoroughly with the tip of the sleeve under the surface to the water until no bubbles appear from the tip of the loader. The loading sleeve with the contained device is introduced into the proximal end of the delivery sheath, keeping both the delivery sheath and the loader on a constant flush. The delivery cable is advanced into the loader, which, in turn, advances the compressed and collapsed device into the long sheath. While the device is being advanced into, and through, the sheath, special care is taken *not to twist* or *rotate* the delivery cable in either direction. Counterclockwise turning of the cable unscrews the cable from the device and can cause its premature release within the sheath, while a forceful, continuous clockwise torque on the cable can tighten the cable in the device so excessively that it cannot be unscrewed later when desired. Occasional gentle clockwise torsion is applied to the cable as it is advanced to ensure that the device does not become unscrewed prematurely. As the delivery cable is advanced, the device advances toward the VSD.

When the Swan™ or other end-hole catheter is still within the distal end of the delivery sheath and as the device is advanced within the sheath, the device approaches the tip of the catheter within the sheath while the Swan™ catheter is withdrawn proportionately until the Swan™ is withdrawn completely out of the tip of the sheath. The end-hole catheter retrograde within the sheath provides easy access for replacing the through-and-through wire in the event that the sheath should kink and/or be withdrawn out of the VSD while the device is being advanced.

The tip of the sheath is maintained in the left ventricle, and by advancing the attached delivery cable in very small increments, the device is advanced until just the distal "rim" of the device and the very beginning of the hub are extruded from the distal end of the sheath and the left ventricular rim and the hub begin to open into the cavity of the left ventricle. If there is any distortion and/or failure of expansion of the distal rim or the hub, the sheath with the attached device is repositioned slightly within the left ventricle. This is accomplished by moving the sheath and the delivery cable forward or backward together as a unit and/or by withdrawing the cable/device slightly back into the sheath until the distal components of the device become completely free. Once free, the device/cable is advanced until the distal rim is fully expanded and free in the ventricle and the hub expands further. With the distal rim fully opened and the hub partially opened, the sheath, delivery cable and device are withdrawn as a unit, until the opened distal rim of the device is pulled against and into the left ventricular "ampulla" of the defect. The partially or non-expanded central hub of the device is still within the delivery sheath, and with the left disk in this position the hub should be positioned exactly over the central, narrowest portion of the VSD. The position of the device is confirmed by repeat left ventricular angiograms, injecting through the separate retrograde catheter, and/or by visualizing the device on echo. Once in the optimal position, while fixing the cable (and device) in this position, the sheath alone is withdrawn over the cable and off the device, which allows the entire central hub and then the proximal rim to deploy and fixes the device securely in the VSD.

When the device appears in the proper position, the device, cable, and sheath are moved to-and-fro slightly to ensure a tight fixation of the device within the defect. A repeat left ventricular angiocardiogram is performed to confirm the position and determine the degree of occlusion by the device. With satisfactory positioning and occlusion, the device is released by unscrewing the delivery cable in a counterclockwise direction until the devise pops free from the cable. As occurs with the ASD devices, as the cable is released, the device frequently changes its orientation markedly. A repeat left ventricular angiocardiogram is performed in order to verify the position of the device in the defect and the degree of occlusion, and to be sure that there are no additional muscular defects.

At any time during the positioning in the defect and before its purposeful release, if the Amplatzer™ VSD device does not appear secure and/or actually pulls through the VSD, it can be withdrawn entirely back into the long delivery sheath by holding the sheath in place while pulling on the delivery cable with mild to moderate force. Once back within the sheath, an attempt should be made to advance the sheath with the contained device back through the defect. When the sheath can be repositioned across the defect, the same device can be re-extruded, hopefully in a different and more satisfactory position. If the sheath with the contained device cannot be repositioned across the defect, the device is withdrawn completely out of the delivery sheath and the process for positioning the sheath across the defect is started over, with the passage of the catheter/wire through the defect from the left ventricle.

After the successful implant of the device and when there is a significant residual leak, the location and size of the residual leak will determine the course of action. If the residual leak is immediately adjacent to, or through, the first device, the procedure is concluded. This type of residual leak usually closes within a short time and, in any event, is not optimal for a second Amplatzer™ VSD device. If the residual leak is a result of an additional defect somewhat separate from the first device, as with the use of any other device, an attempt is made at closing this additional defect with an additional device during the same catheterization. The X-ray tubes already are aligned in the proper positions for the location of the defect(s), the exact anatomy has just been determined and is fresh in the operator's mind, and the catheters already are in position within the heart. The first occlusion device also serves as a fixed landmark in the ventricular septum for the implant of additional devices.

Delivery of the Amplatzer VSD occluder™ to mid and apical muscular ventricular septal defects via the retrograde and left ventricle approach

The significantly smaller delivery sheath that is required for the Amplatzer™ VSD device makes the retrograde delivery of the Amplatzer™ VSD device a more viable option than when using the CardioSEAL™ device[5]. The VSD is crossed and a through-and-through wire established from the femoral artery, through the left ventricle, through the defect and to the femoral or jugular vein, exactly as described previously in this chapter for the retrograde delivery of the CardioSEAL™ device. The appropriately sized AGA™ or a comparable sized RB-MTS™ long delivery sheath is introduced into the femoral artery and advanced retrograde to the VSD exactly as the long delivery sheath for the retrograde delivery of the CardioSEAL™ device.

From the retrograde approach into the left ventricle, the through-and-through wire tends to align parallel to the septum and, in turn, perpendicular to the *channel* of the apical and/or muscular VSD. This orientation creates a very acute angle as the wire crosses the muscular septal defect, and, in turn, creates some difficulty during the positioning of the Amplatzer™ delivery sheath through the defect and during the eventual implant of the device. Only after the catheter/wire forms a relatively *smooth curve* from the left ventricle into and through the defect is the catheter removed over the wire and replaced with the AGA™ or RB-MTS™ delivery sheath/dilator. Because of the acute bends and curves that form in the long sheath during the retrograde approach, RB-MTS™ or Flexor™ sheaths (Cook Inc., Bloomington, IN) are preferred to AGA™ VSD delivery sheaths for the retrograde left ventricular approach to the muscular VSD. The RB-MTS™ sheaths are easier to pre-curve into specific curves, and the Flexor™ sheaths have an almost total resistance to kinking.

Whichever long sheath is used, since the acuteness of the angle of approach is very likely to kink the sheath when the wire and dilator are removed, it is even more desirable to maintain an end-hole catheter prograde over the wire from the venous end of the wire. As the dilator is withdrawn from the sheath, the prograde catheter is advanced simultaneously and proportionately into the distal end of the sheath, keeping the tip of the dilator and the tip of the catheter together as the dilator is withdrawn. This protects the tissues and tip of the sheath from the "sawing" of the wire, helps to keep the long delivery sheath from kinking and provides access for the replacement of the through-and-through wire if the sheath should kink and/or becomes displaced. Once the dilator is withdrawn, the venous catheter is positioned within the sheath (entering from the tip of the sheath), and verifying that the sheath is not kinked, the through-and-through wire is withdrawn from the sheath.

In order to prevent the AGA™ delivery sheath from kinking during the actual device delivery, a separate 0.018″ stiff wire or a Terumo™ wire (Terumo Medical Corp., Somerset, NJ) is passed into the AGA™ sheath and advanced to the tip of the sheath. This wire remains within the sheath, *adjacent to the Amplatzer™ device* and delivery cable, in order to provide extra support for the sheath as the device is being delivered and until the device reaches the distal end of the delivery sheath. The extra wire is removed just before the *extrusion* of the device from the sheath.

The long delivery sheath, which is introduced retrograde from the left ventricle, must remain far enough into the right ventricle to allow the distal flange of the Amplatzer™ VSD device to open entirely in the right ventricle and the central hub to open within the defect without the device being pulled back through the defect by the acute angulations. Once both sides of the device are deployed and before the device is released, a left ventricular angiogram is performed to verify the position of the device in the defect and the degree of occlusion of the defect. This is performed, preferably, through a separate catheter in the left ventricle, but occasionally can be accomplished through the side port on the delivery sheath.

The Amplatzer™ VSD device, like the other Amplatzer™ devices, has the advantage of being able to be withdrawn at *any time* before its purposeful release. When the device that is delivered retrograde is extruded completely out of the sheath, but while it still is attached to the cable, the device creates an acute angle with the delivery cable, and special care must be taken not to dislodge the device while "unscrewing" it. Once released, the position and degree of occlusion are verified by a repeat left ventricular angiogram and by echocardiogram. Residual leaks or additional defects are handled exactly as with the other approaches to catheter closing of the muscular VSD.

Retrograde only delivery of the Amplatzer VSD device to mid and apical muscular ventricular septal defects

The Amplatzer™ VSD device can be delivered retrograde to the mid muscular VSD *without* the use of a through-and-through wire and/or the associated venous access. When this is accomplished expediently, this technique *can* shorten the duration of the VSD occlusion procedure significantly[5]. On the other hand, if the sheath cannot be advanced through the defect satisfactorily and/or the device cannot be seated securely in the defect, the delivery procedure must be started all over using the through-and-through wire technique. The retrievability of the Amplatzer™ device up until the moment of release provides a safety factor and allows the retrograde only approach to be attempted.

For the retrograde only delivery, a Swan™ balloon catheter (Arrow International Inc., Reading, PA), a preformed right Judkins™ or a "Cobra" catheter is passed retrograde across the aortic valve into the left ventricular apex. An "S" curve is formed on the tip of the Swan™ catheter before it is introduced into the artery. Using the Swan™ catheter, the balloon is inflated and with moderate manipulations usually the balloon at least will "seat" in the left ventricular "ampulla" of the VSD, even if it does not pass through it into the trabeculae of the right ventricle. It may be necessary to assist this maneuver with a preformed "S" shaped rigid deflector wire. With the right Judkins™ or "Cobra" catheter, the muscular VSD is entered from the left ventricle by rotating the tip of the catheter medially and anteriorly onto the septum as the tip of the catheter is withdrawn from the apex toward the outflow tract within the left ventricle. As it is withdrawn, the catheter tip usually will slip into the ampulla of the VSD. The catheter is advanced as far as possible into the VSD and, if possible, through the VSD and into the right ventricle.

A torque-controlled, exchange length wire with a long and very floppy tip is passed through this catheter and maneuvered further through the VSD. This wire is advanced far enough into the right ventricle to secure the *stiff portion* of the wire well across the VSD and into the right ventricle. The floppy portion of the wire will not support the passage of any type of delivery sheath/dilator into and through the defect. Only the stiff portion of the wire has the capability of supporting the advancing of a stiff delivery sheath/dilator through the defect. This often requires the formation of a large loop of the floppy tip and distal portion of the wire within the right ventricle and/or even back into the right atrium. There usually is some problem and considerable manipulation required to secure the *stiff portion* of the wire far enough into the right ventricle to support the advancing of a long, relatively stiff, delivery sheath/dilator through the acute angle from the left ventricle into the VSD and from there into the right ventricle. With all retrograde approaches to the VSD, the wire tends to align parallel to the septum and, in turn, absolutely perpendicular to the VSD channel. This very acute angle as the wire crosses the septal defect makes it very difficult to advance the stiff portion of the wire and/or the sheath/dilator far enough into the right ventricular side of the defect without some "fixation" of the wire from the right ventricular side. Only after the *stiff portion* of the wire is secured completely across the defect is the catheter removed over the wire and replaced with the long delivery sheath/dilator. Even when the wire is far enough into the ventricle, often it will not support the passage of the stiff, relatively straight AGA™ delivery sheath/dilator around the acute angle, through the defect and far enough into the right ventricle for the delivery and implant of the device.

Once the sheath/dilator has passed into and through the ventricular defect, the acute angle of approach at the junction of the left ventricular wall to the VSD has an even higher likelihood of kinking the sheath when the dilator is removed. In order to prevent the sheath from kinking during device delivery, a separate 0.018″ stiff wire is introduced into the AGA™ sheath adjacent to the device and delivery cable similar to the technique during retrograde delivery when a through-and-through wire was used. Without the support of either the smooth curves of a through-and-through wire and/or a venous catheter advanced retrograde within the distal end of the sheath as the wire is removed, the AGA™ sheath, in particular, becomes very vulnerable to kinking.

In addition to not kinking, the sheath must remain far enough into the *right* ventricle to allow the distal flange of the Amplatzer™ VSD device to open entirely in the right ventricle and the central hub of the device to open within the defect without the acute angulations pulling the device back through the defect. Once completely delivered, the device, before release, still creates an acute angle to the delivery catheter and is on significant tension. In addition to the technical problems of delivery, the retrograde approach always has the potential problems of arterial damage from the extensive, repeated manipulations of the relatively large, stiff delivery sheath directly in the artery. In spite of the problems, the retrograde approach with the Amplatzer VSD occluder™ has been successful and should be considered, particularly if there is a problem with the usual venous access sites.

Catheter closure of anterior–muscular intramural ventricular septal defects using the Amplatzer ventricular septal occluder™

The technique for the delivery of the Amplatzer™ VSD device to the anterior–muscular intermural muscular septal defects is similar to the delivery of the CardioSEAL™ device to these defects, but the procedure is considerably easier and safer with the Amplatzer™ VSD device. If for no other reason, the Amplatzer™ VSD device is safer because of the much smaller delivery sheath required when using the arterial approach for the delivery of the device. The defect is identified, crossed retrograde with a catheter from the femoral artery, and a through-and-through wire to a systemic vein is established using the previously described techniques. The device used is determined from the size of the defect. The device should be 2–3 mm larger than the *narrowest measured diameter* of the defect. The AGA™ delivery sheath or a specially formed, RB-MTS™ sheath is positioned across the defect from either the femoral venous or femoral arterial approach, as described earlier in this chapter for the CardioSEAL™ device. The course of the wire/sheath to these anterior muscular defects usually is much straighter and results in less kinking of the sheath from either access compared to the course to the mid muscular defects.

The long femoral *venous* sheath/dilator is advanced over the through-and-through wire, through the ventricular defect and into the ascending aorta. The dilator and wire are withdrawn very slowly and the sheath cleared meticulously of all air and/or clots. The device is advanced to a position just within the tip of the sheath. The sheath is withdrawn into the left ventricular outflow tract just proximal to the aortic valve in a similar fashion to the delivery of the CardioSEAL™ device. With the Amplatzer™ VSD device, only the left ventricular flange or rim of the device is opened in the left ventricular out-flow tract. The still mostly folded device within the sheath is withdrawn until the distal (left) ventricular flange of the device is *within the left ventricular end* of the defect and the hub of the device, which still is within the sheath, is in the area of the narrowest portion of the VSD. The position of the device is confirmed with a left ventricular angiogram. The delivery cable is fixed in position while the long sheath is withdrawn, allowing the central hub to expand within the center of the defect. When the position is satisfactory, while holding the delivery cable in the exact position, the sheath is withdrawn completely off the device, opening the entire device within the defect. With the Amplatzer™ VSD device, if the position is not satisfactory even after the entire device is open, the device still can be withdrawn into the delivery sheath for repositioning and/or completely removed from the long sheath. This capability adds a significant safety factor to the catheter occlusion of these defects with Amplatzer™ VSD devices. When in the proper position, the device is released by a counterclockwise rotation of the delivery cable.

The angle of entry into the left ventricular end of the anterior intramural muscular defect from the retrograde approach is much more favorable than the angle to enter the mid or apical muscular defects. A catheter and/or wire passing retrograde from the aorta into these defects passes through the defect in almost a straight line from the aorta. If the retrograde arterial approach is used for the delivery of the Amplatzer™ devices to the left ventricle end of these anterior or intramural defects, it still is preferable to use a through-and-through wire and to deliver the device through a preformed, long, RB-MTS™ sheath, which is pre-shaped similarly to the sheath for the delivery of the CardioSEAL™ device. The venous end of the wire is introduced from either the femoral or the internal jugular vein, depending upon the "straightest" course to the right ventricular side of the defect. The retrograde delivery sheath is advanced through the defect and positioned well into the right ventricular cavity.

As the distal (right ventricular) side of the Amplatzer ™ device is being positioned and opened, the device is positioned as far as possible toward the *right* ventricular end of the narrowest area of the tunnel-like defect, but still far enough toward the *left* ventricular end of the device to secure the device once released. The position is confirmed with a left ventricular angiocardiogram. The still folded proximal (left ventricular) end of the device, which is still within the sheath, must be well away from the aortic valve even in its elongated, folded position. If this distance away from the aortic valve is not possible, the device should not be delivered. If necessary, the device is withdrawn completely, the sheath repositioned and/or a different size device and/or approach utilized. The Amplatzer™ VSD occluder can be repositioned even after it has been entirely opened by withdrawing the device completely back into the sheath. If the sheath can be re-advanced further into the defect, the same device can be redeployed in the more favorable position. If the sheath, with the contained device, cannot be re-advanced on its own, the device is withdrawn out of the sheath and the sheath repositioned, beginning from the start of the procedure.

Coil closure of muscular interventricular septal defects

Before the availability of either the CardioSEAL™ or the Amplatzer™ VSD devices, some smaller muscular ventricular septal defects were occluded with Gianturco™ coils (Cook Inc., Bloomington, IN) using one of the controlled-release mechanisms[6]. Coil occlusion of a muscular VSD still has the one advantage of requiring a much smaller delivery system than is possible with any of the other devices. Also, for the delivery of a coil to a muscular ventricular defect, a through-and-through wire is not absolutely necessary, although a through-and-through wire may be necessary to initially cross the defect and/or to position the delivery catheter/sheath across the defect *from the right to the left ventricle* for a venous delivery of a sizing balloon and/or the coil. The venous approach is necessary in the smaller patient when sizing of the defect with a balloon is required, since the smallest sizing balloons require an 8-French sheath. A *separate* retrograde catheter, in addition to the delivery catheter, is essential in order to be able to perform left ventricular angiography for the very critical positioning of the coil during implant, regardless of which approach is used to deliver the coil.

For the retrograde delivery of a coil to the muscular VSD, once the defect has been identified angiographically, it is entered from the left ventricle with an end-hole Swan™ balloon catheter delivered retrograde from the femoral artery. The Swan™ balloon catheter is manipulated as far into and/or through the defect as possible. With the Swan™ balloon catheter fixed in or through the defect, a floppy tipped wire is passed through the balloon catheter. The wire is manipulated far enough through the defect and right ventricle and into the right atrium or pulmonary artery to have several centimeters of the *stiff portion* of the wire beyond the defect in the right ventricle. Often, an accurate diameter of the very small defect can be determined from the angiocardiogram and/or an echocardiogram, and further sizing of the defect with a balloon is unnecessary. In that situation, the retrograde closure can proceed after the wire is placed in a very secure position across the defect. When the defect appears large and/or cannot be accurately sized from the angiocardiogram, sizing is carried out with a small NuMED™ sizing balloon.

In much larger patients and with the wire in a secure position across the defect, the small NuMED™ sizing balloon is introduced into the femoral artery through an 8-French sheath and advanced retrograde through the left ventricle and into the ventricular septal defect. The balloon is inflated in the defect and the narrowest portion measured radiographically. The angles of the X-ray tubes are adjusted to elongate the balloon and the VSD in their longest axes. A repeat left ventricular angiocardiogram is performed through a separate left ventricular catheter. This documents the closure of the defect with the sizing balloon and rules out additional defects. The sizing balloon is withdrawn over the wire, paying particular attention to keeping the wire in its secure position well through the defect.

In smaller patients who cannot tolerate the larger sheath and considerable manipulation in the artery, and where sizing still is considered necessary, sizing with a balloon is performed from the venous approach after forming a through-and-through wire "rail" as described earlier in this chapter for VSD sizing with other devices.

The 0.052″ Gianturco™ coil (Cook Inc., Bloomington, IN) with a bioptome controlled attach–release is preferred for VSD closure. The Jackson™ controlled-release coil (Cook Inc., Europe) has been used but even the largest Jackson™ coil is significantly less "robust" than the 0.052″ coils. A 4-French delivery *catheter* through a 4-French sheath can be used for the Jackson™ controlled-release coils. Although a 4-French long *sheath can* be used with the bioptome-controlled delivery of a 0.052″ coil, a 5-French sheath provides a smoother delivery and allows easier withdrawal of a totally extruded coil back into the sheath. The long delivery sheath for the retrograde delivery of the 0.052″ coils is introduced into the femoral artery through short sheaths one to two French sizes larger than the long delivery sheath.

The long sheaths and/or the delivery catheters for the *retrograde delivery* of the coils are "pre-curved" into a "shepherd's crook" curve to conform to the course around the arch, into the left ventricle and then into the defect. Preforming the delivery sheath helps to maintain the sheath/coil in the defect during the coil delivery. The distal end of the long sheath/dilator and/or the catheter is heated in boiling sterile water or in the hot "jet" of a heat gun. A long 180° curve is formed in the distal part of the sheath/dilator or catheter to correspond to the course from the descending aorta around the arch and into the apex of the left ventricle. Once this first curve is formed, a secondary curve, which faces 90° away from the concavity of the original curve, is formed at the very tip of the sheath or catheter so that the final configuration resembles a "shepherd's crook". The lengths of the various curves depend upon the size of the patient and the distance from the aortic arch/aortic valve to the left ventricular entrance of the muscular VSD.

When the defect has been sized accurately, the delivery catheter or sheath/dilator for the coil is introduced over the retrograde wire and advanced completely through the defect. It is advisable to have the tip of the delivery catheter or sheath at least 1.5–2 cm *into the right ventricle*. The longer the coil being used, the further the delivery sheath/catheter must be into the right ventricle. With the delivery sheath/dilator securely in place, first the dilator, then the wire are withdrawn slowly while observing the course and position of the sheath on fluoroscopy. *Very slight* forward or backward adjustments of the sheath may be necessary to compensate for the removal of the straightening effect of the dilator and/or straight portion of the stiff wire in the sheath as the dilator and the wire are removed. As and after the dilator is removed, the sheath is allowed to bleed back passively from the pressure within the right ventricle. When completely clear of air and/or clot, the long sheath is attached to a continuous slow flush. Once the long delivery sheath/catheter is in place, a left ventricular angiogram is repeated, since the tension on the relatively stiff sheath often can distort the original anatomy.

The coil is attached to the 3-French bioptome and withdrawn into the special loader as described previously in Chapter 27 for the controlled delivery of a coil for the occlusion of a PDA. The coil attached to the bioptome is introduced into the pre-positioned long sheath and advanced to the VSD, while again observing the course and the tip of the sheath very closely and continuously on fluoroscopy. As the relatively stiff coil–bioptome is advanced around the aortic arch and passes through the curves from the left ventricle to the VSD, the delivery sheath tends to straighten and/or be pushed forward. The long sheath is adjusted repeatedly with *very slight* forward or backward movements to keep the sheath tip well within the defect while at the same time not kinking the sheath in one of the curves by advancing it against resistance at the tip. The coil is advanced to the tip of the delivery sheath. The majority of the coil, which still is within the sheath, should be *beyond* the narrowest portion and on the right ventricular side of the defect.

The coil is advanced out of the delivery sheath by very slowly advancing the bioptome catheter while simultaneously withdrawing the long sheath very slightly. The coil begins to coil in the trabeculae of the right ventricle. If the first loop of the coil appears too far into the ventricle, the bioptome catheter and coil are withdrawn into the sheath, the sheath withdrawn slightly and the process restarted. Ideally the first full loop of the coil will form just on the right ventricular side of the narrowest portion of the defect. Because of the complex trabeculations in the right ventricle, this first loop may be elongated or stretched out around a trabecula, but the more proximal portion of the exposed loop should be adjacent to the narrow portion of the defect. The position of the coil within the right ventricle and the defect is verified with a left ventricular angiogram while injecting as close as possible to the VSD. With the bioptome-controlled and/or the Jackson™ coils, the coil can be withdrawn and this right ventricular loop of the coil adjusted many times until the operator is satisfied with the security of the loop on the right side of the defect. Once a right ventricular loop is secured adjacent to the defect, the delivery sheath is withdrawn slowly as the bioptome catheter is advanced. This extrudes the remainder of the coil into the left ventricular "ampulla" of the VSD. At any time until just before the coil is extruded completely out of the sheath and/or if the operator is not satisfied with the position or "looping" of the coil, the sheath can be re-advanced over the coil in order to withdraw the coil back into the sheath and re-advance the sheath back into the defect. With the bioptome-controlled system, once the very proximal end of the coil which is grasped in the bioptome jaws is extruded *completely out of the sheath*, the coil usually forms an acute angle off the long axis of the bioptome, which makes it difficult, if not impossible, to withdraw the coil back into the sheath after that stage of the extrusion. All adjustments of the coil should be made before this final millimeter of extrusion. Once the 0.052″ coil is completely extruded, it re-forms its original tight coil configuration and usually seats very tightly into the ampulla of the muscular VSD. The proper position of the coil in the defect and the degree of occlusion are verified with another left ventricular angiogram with the injection in the vicinity of the VSD. Once satisfied with the fixation and degree of occlusion, the device is released.

Ten minutes after the coil implant, a large-volume left ventricular angiocardiogram is performed to verify the exact position of the coil and the degree of closure of the defect. Often there will be a "smoke-like" leak through the fibers of the coil at this stage. This type of residual leak closes over a short time. If, on the other hand, there is a relatively large and/or a jet-like leak, the residual leak needs addressing with an additional occlusion device to secure complete closure *during the same catheterization procedure*. As with closure of the muscular VSD with the other devices, the location and orientation of the defect have been clearly defined and the arterial and venous lines already are in place for an additional coil during the same catheterization. Of more importance, a residual, high-pressure, *jet-like* leak through a coil is likely to persist and result in hemolysis, which, in turn, very likely will necessitate immediate re-intervention.

The approach to the residual leak is the same as for the original defect. The defect is recrossed, usually with a preformed catheter and a Terumo Glide™ wire followed by an end-hole catheter and/or sheath from the left ventricular to the right ventricular side. There is *almost no* chance of dislodging the original 0.052″ coil with further manipulation through and/or around it. The original coil is entangled in the right ventricular trabeculae and very rapidly becomes fixed very firmly in the defect. The second (or more) coil(s) is(are) implanted with a similar technique to the first coil with a controlled-release system, although a 0.038″ coil may be adequate for a small residual leak and actually "nest" better within the larger original 0.052″ coil. The loop of coil on the right side of the defect intertwines in the original coil and creates a firm fixation during the deployment of the rest of the coil. Once the additional coil has been implanted, the same process of reassessment is carried out as after the first coil.

Coils to close muscular ventricular septal defects can be delivered from the venous/right ventricular approach. This is a safer delivery approach, however, this approach usually requires the extra effort of crossing the defect initially from the left ventricle, and the creation of a through-and-through wire in order to position the delivery sheath/catheter coming from the right ventricle. When the coil is delivered from the right side, most of the coil is delivered onto the left side of the defect, leaving only one to one and a half loops on the right ventricular side.

Catheter occlusion of post-acute myocardial infarction ventricular septal defects

Anterior and inferior myocardial infarcts occasionally result in the development of a large muscular interventricular septal defect as a consequence of a "blow out" of the necrotic septum. These defects usually are very large with a resultant very large left to right shunt and uncontrolled heart failure. The appearance of a new, large VSD in an otherwise very ill, but previously stable patient often results in an acute cardiovascular collapse and requires some immediate intervention performed as a life-saving procedure. Until the development of the large, catheter-delivered "umbrella" devices, surgical intervention was the only alternative available and still may be preferable early after the infarction. Surgery on these patients, however, is associated with a very high mortality, high morbidity and a high incidence of recurrence of the VSD. Because of these factors the concept of a catheter-delivered closure device initially was very appealing and now is being attempted in multiple institutions and with multiple devices.

Unfortunately, acute myocardial infarct patients are extremely ill, requiring ventilation, massive cardiac drug therapy and often even support with balloon-pump and/or other left ventricular assist devices. This alone makes them extremely poor candidates and very difficult patients for either catheter or surgical intervention. The patients often require emergency, life-saving intervention within hours, or at most days, of the acute myocardial infarct. The timing of the intervention and the nature of the VSD at this stage of the infarct compound the problems of any type of closure of the defects. The acute infarct is an *evolving process* with necrotic and/or necrosing tissues, particularly around the rim or margins of the newly developed ventricular defect. Some of these defects are very large, precluding the use of even the largest available catheter-delivered devices. Within the first three weeks of the acute infarct, the tissues are very friable and do not hold sutures and/or catheter-delivered occlusion devices very well. Finally, the acute myocardial infarct patient is admitted to a coronary care unit in an adult hospital, which often has only single-plane catheterization laboratory facilities, and although expert in the care of the acute myocardial infarct, have no experience with and/or none of the equipment for the implant of transcatheter occlusion devices. The optimal biplane catheterization laboratory facilities with the necessary "expendable" equipment and the majority of the experience with transcatheter VSD closures are in the pediatric catheterization laboratories, which may be in a separate hospital. This adds additional logistical problems to the catheter treatment of these very ill patients.

Initially, the "large", 17 mm, Rashkind™ PDA device (USCI BARD, Glens Falls, NY) was used in a high-risk study to attempt closing the acute post myocardial infarct VSD[1]. The success of these procedures was very marginal. The patients were stabilized enough to be taken to the catheterization laboratory and the devices could be delivered, however, many of the implanted devices dislodged within minutes to hours after implant. It also became apparent that device implants within two, or even three weeks of the acute infarct were destined to fail, primarily owing to the on-going tissue necrosis from the underlying infarction process and the fact that the Rashkind™ PDA device was not large enough for most of these defects. At the same time, there were successful implants in patients who had been stabilized for three to four weeks after their infarct and/or who had had an emergency surgical repair, but who had a recurrence of their VSD leading to the transcatheter closure. By "natural selection", these were smaller defects, which were of less hemodynamic significance by the time of the catheter procedure. Although acute, early and absolute emergency attempts at closing these defects still are necessary and desirable, because of the earlier bad experiences with the Rashkind™ devices, considerable effort is still made to stabilize these patients medically, even utilizing left ventricular assist device support until at least three weeks following their infarct before attempting a transcatheter closure. There is a trend for treating the patient who is unstable with a new ventricular septal defect associated with an acute myocardial infarct with an early surgical repair, and then if there is persistence or a recurrence of the defect, closing that defect with a catheter-delivered device[7].

As the timing of when to close these defects was being determined through experience, the larger double-umbrella, Clamshell™ ASD devices (USCI BARD, Glens Falls, NY) became available. These replaced the Rashkind™ devices in the high-risk protocols for use in the post-myocardial infarct VSD[8], however, after only a few attempts at closing acute ventricular septal defects with the Clamshell™ device, the Clamshell™ device was withdrawn from clinical use because of leg fractures in the devices used in ASDs. The Clamshell™ device eventually was replaced with the CardioSEAL™ device (NMT Medical Inc., Boston, MA) and then the STARFlex™ device (NMT Medical Inc., Boston, MA), which still has some use for post-myocardial infarct VSD closure[9].

The CardioSEAL™ and STARFlex™ devices are usually delivered from the jugular venous approach over a through-and-through venous to venous or venous to arterial "rail" wire. Because of the complexity of the combined intracardiac manipulations and the need for precise *depth perception* during the procedure, along with the very precarious status of these patients, a biplane fluoroscopy/X-ray system is essential in order to expedite the procedure.

The acute ventricular septal defect in the post-infarct patient usually is very large when visualized by echocardiogram and/or angiographically. The goal in closing these acute infarct defects is to include not only the defect under the "patch", but also to include as much of the surrounding necrotic tissue as possible. When using either the CardioSEAL™ or STARFlex™ devices, little or no time is spent in balloon sizing the larger defects in unstable patients. Rather, in the majority of cases the 40 mm device was used for the implant in an attempt to extend the legs well beyond the margins of the defect. If the defect itself is greater than 15–18 mm in diameter by echo and/or angiographically, there is little chance that the standard CardioSEAL™ or STARFlex™ devices will remain in place, and the use of these devices probably should not be tried in defects of that size or larger.

When the defect is satisfactory in size, a through-and-through wire is established from the jugular vein to either a femoral vein or a femoral artery, as described earlier in this chapter. The long introductory sheath/dilator is introduced over a through-and-through wire from the jugular vein, advanced from the right atrium, to the right ventricle, to the VSD and positioned across the defect in the left ventricle. The dilator is removed, the sheath cleared meticulously and the CardioSEAL/STARFlex™ device delivered as previously described. The left sided legs are opened in the left ventricle and withdrawn into the defect similarly to the technique for congenital apical muscular defect closures. The device, the defect, and particularly the margins of the defect are scrutinized critically by echo and angiographically when the left sided legs are opened and in position against the defect and before the right-sided legs are opened. The right legs are opened *only* after the device appears secure in the defect while minor traction is being applied to the still attached device. In contrast to the congenital muscular VSD, once the device is delivered and stays in place, little further attention is paid to its exact position and/or any residual leak during this initial catheterization. Post-myocardial infarct defects usually are so large that a successful and stable implant, even with only a partial occlusion, usually provides significant improvement in the patient's hemodynamic status, while further manipulation around these freshly implanted devices can easily dislodge them. If a CardioSEAL™ or STARFlex™ device embolizes in these very ill patients, surgical intervention usually is necessary to retrieve it. With the availability of the Amplatzer™ muscular VSD occluders, a new investigational six-legged and larger STARFlex™ device, and finally the new Amplatzer™ Post Myocardial Infarct Muscular VSD (PIMVSD) Occluders, new attempts to close the larger and more acute defects are ongoing.

For a time, there were new *6-legged*, STARFlex™ devices (NMT, Boston, MA), which were used in a limited high-risk clinical trial for post-myocardial ventricular septal defects. Except for the two additional legs, these devices were identical to the earlier STARFlex™ devices. They were available in 38 and 43 mm diameters and were delivered through only a 12-French long sheath. The six legs on each umbrella provided a "rounder" configuration to each umbrella, which, in turn, allowed a greater coverage area over an essentially "round" defect, and the six legs provided a sturdier fixation against the septum than an equivalent sized four leg "square" device. The loading, delivery and implant of the 6-legged device is identical to the delivery of the previous CardioSEAL™ and STARFlex™ devices. The double opposing true *umbrella* devices have the theoretical advantage for the closure of post-myocardial infarct ventricular septal defects of clamping onto the surface of the healthier tissues surrounding and slightly away from the defect, as opposed to pushing into the soft, necrotic tissues for their fixation. The fine Nitinol™ centering spring wires on the STARFlex™ devices do "self center" the device over the defect once it is implanted and, at the same time, without putting further pressure on the necrotic tissues. Theoretically this self-centering mechanism continues to center the device even when the defect enlarges and/or changes shape. The 6-legged STARFlex™ devices appeared to be the most appropriate devices for use in the very large post-myocardial infarct VSD, however, because of the bureaucracy involved and the requirements of the US FDA for a new trial for even these minor changes in the devices, these devices probably never will be available for clinical use.

There now is a *special*, larger Amplatzer™ post-myocardial infarct muscular VSD™ (PIMVSD™) occluder (AGA Medical Corp., Golden Valley, MN), which is a variation of the standard Amplatzer™ muscular VSD device[10]. It is similar in design to the standard Amplatzer™ muscular VSD device, with a central hub and small rims or flanges at each end of the hub. In these special PIMVSD™ occluders, the hub is 10 mm in length and both the right and left ventricular rims extend 5 mm circumferentially around the hub, making both end disks 10 mm larger in diameter than the central hub. The PIMVSD™ devices are available in device sizes of 16 through 24 mm in 2 mm increments. The size of the PIMVSD™ device represents the diameter of the central hub. As with all of the Amplatzer™ devices, the seating of the device in the defect and the closure of the defect depend upon the central "hub" portion of the defect actually filling and exerting some pressure around the inner circumference of the defect rather than by the rims or "flanges" at each end either sealing the defect and/or holding the device in place. The Amplatzer™ PIMVSD™ device that is used for these defects is 2–3 mm larger than the stretched diameter of the defect, which limits the use of this device to defects 22 mm or smaller in diameter if the device is to be "over-sized" for the defect by even 2 mm. The over-sizing of the device for the size of the defect may cause excessive pressure on the already friable, necrotic rim of the defect and aggravate the continuing necrosis and enlargement of the defect. Because of these two factors, the accurate sizing of the defect becomes more critical. As a consequence, sizing by echocardiogram, angiography and/or the AGA™ sizing balloon is recommended for the use of the special PIMVSD™ device in these defects.

Once the defect has been sized accurately by echo, angiocardiogram and preferably with a sizing balloon, an Amplatzer™ PIMVSD™ occluder that is 3–4 mm larger than the diameter of the defect is used to close the defect. For the post-myocardial VSD, the large Amplatzer™ PIMVSD™ device can be delivered from either the jugular or femoral venous approach, although the angle to, and the angle of the device against the septum as it is being deployed in the more common apical defects usually are better from the jugular venous approach. The angle to the higher, more mid and/or anterior muscular defects, on the other hand, often is more favorable when approaching from the femoral vein. Although the course through the right ventricle is more circuitous coming from the femoral vein, the tip of the sheath aligns more perpendicularly to the septum after it has passed through the more anterior defect.

A 12-French AGA™ or equivalent long delivery sheath/dilator is advanced through the right ventricle, through the VSD and into the left ventricle over a previously positioned, jugular or femoral vein to femoral artery or femoral vein, through-and-through "rail" wire. The AGA™ delivery sheath is relatively stiff, straight and cannot be "preformed", so the tip often does not align even close to perpendicular to the septum from either access route. As with the delivery of other Amplatzer™ devices, an RB-MTS™ with a preformed curve to suit the defect can be used to deliver the Amplatzer™ PIMVSD™ occluder.

The delivery of the device through a long delivery sheath is similar to the closure of other muscular defects, except that with the more friable tissues, great care must be taken not to pull the device through the defect and/or enlarge the defect as the hub and right sided flange are being deployed. Once deployed, the position in the defect is scrutinized by echo and a left ventricular angiocardiogram. When satisfied with the device's position and its stability, a counterclockwise unscrewing of the cable releases the delivery cable from the device. The Amplatzer™ PIMVSD™ device, like the other Amplatzer™ occluders, has the advantage of being fully retrievable at any time up until its purposeful release. On the other hand, the continued pressure that the Amplatzer™ PIMVSD™ device exerts around the rim of the already weakened tissues may actually enlarge the defect within a short time and make this device less satisfactory for the acute post-myocardial infarct VSD over the long run.

The current maximum size of the PIMVSD™ occluder is 24 mm in diameter. Some of the immediate post-infarct VSDs, which need immediate attention, are larger than can be occluded with a 24 mm device, and closure of these larger defects has been accomplished with a larger Amplatzer™ Atrial Septal Occluder[11]. Although occasionally effective, these devices with their very short waist (or hub) are not ideally suited for the thick muscular septum, and should only be considered for this use in an extreme emergency.

Transcatheter closure of these post-myocardial infarction ventricular septal defects remains a continuing challenge, but does appear to have a better outcome than the surgical alternative. Transcatheter closure appears particularly useful in the post-infarct ventricular septal defect that has undergone surgical repair, but that has a significant residual and/or recurrent ventricular defect, and in those patients who can be stabilized for three to four weeks following the initial event.

Transcatheter closure of post-traumatic ventricular septal defects

Severe blunt trauma to the chest, in addition to multiple other injuries, can result in rupture of the interventricular septum. The VSD may appear as the only lesion or as part of multiple cardiac injuries[12]. The rupture usually is in the apical muscular septum, which often requires a ventriculotomy for surgical repair. In addition, these patients can be very unstable hemodynamically and usually are not good candidates for an open-heart surgical repair on cardiopulmonary bypass because of their multiple additional injuries. As a consequence, these patients are ideal candidates for transcatheter closure of their ventricular septal defect[13,14].

Because of the co-existing injuries and instability of these patients, the patient with a post-traumatic interventricular septal defect is handled similarly to the patient with a post-infarction muscular septal defect. The defect is defined angiographically and by TEE. Once identified, it is preferable to cross these defects from the left ventricle to the right ventricle using a floating balloon catheter, as described earlier in this chapter. These defects frequently have multiple outlets through the trabeculae on the right ventricular side of the septum. The inflated, floating balloon catheter has the best chance of passing through the largest and most important of these defects. If the wire/catheter passing through the defect does *not* pass through the major and largest orifice on the right side, sizing can result in an undersized device, and if the occlusion device is implanted in the smaller orifice there is less chance of occluding the defect successfully.

Once the defect is crossed, a through-and-through wire "rail" with the right-sided wire exiting from the internal jugular vein is created, as described earlier in this chapter for the closure of the standard muscular VSD. It is particularly important to size (and shape!) these defects with a sizing balloon and to perform a left ventricular angiogram through a separate left ventricular catheter with the sizing balloon *inflated* in order to verify the degree of occlusion and identify separate and/or more important defects. Because of their extreme compliance and ability to conform to any unusual shape at almost zero pressure, NuMED™ sizing balloons are preferred for the sizing and shaping of these particular muscular septal defects. A sizing balloon is used that is approximately twice the size of the defect as estimated by angio and/or TEE in order to allow the balloon to conform loosely to the defect and at the same time fill the defect without enlarging it. The walls or rim of the post-traumatic VSD are more likely to be very irregular, but at the same time, unlike the post-infarct VSD, are composed of fairly rigid tissues, which should support any type of device. The anatomy of the defect will determine the preferential device for the occlusion. The Amplatzer™ Muscular VSD Occluder is preferred when the configuration of the circumference of the defect is more or less round and when there is only one major opening on the right ventricular side of the defect. If, on the other hand, the defect is very irregular or elongated and/or has two or more large openings on the right side of the septum, the STARFlex™ occluder is preferable. The "double umbrella" with the narrow waist has a better chance of overlapping the entire defect and occluding it with one device.

The long sheath/dilator for the delivery of either type of occlusion device to the traumatic VSD is introduced from the internal jugular vein over the through-and-through wire as described earlier. After advancing the particular device through the sheath and opening the left ventricular (distal) disk (umbrella) in the left ventricle, the entire system is withdrawn into the defect and the remainder of the device deployed with angiographic and TEE control to determine the positioning and degree of occlusion during and after the deployment of the occluder, exactly as with other muscular ventricular septal defects.

Although post-traumatic ventricular septal defects are rare, when they do occur they should be considered for transcatheter closure, which can be accomplished safely and early in the course of the lesion.

Transcatheter closure of perimembranous ventricular septal defects

Perimembranous interventricular septal defects are one of the most common defects of all congenital heart diseases. Isolated perimembranous ventricular septal defects are far more common than all of the various muscular interventricular septal defects added together. Perimembranous and/or outlet ventricular septal defects also occur very commonly as part of many complex congenital heart lesions. As a consequence, there always has been a keen interest in a catheter approach to the closure of these defects. While both the CardioSEAL™ device and the Amplatzer™ VSD device are very effective and safe for closing almost all congenital *muscular ventricular septal defects*, neither is satisfactory or safe for occlusion of most perimembranous defects.

Although the anatomy of isolated perimembranous ventricular septal defects appears relatively "simple" or straightforward compared to most of the other congenital heart defects, their location in the immediate subaortic area of the left ventricular outflow tract with little, or no, tissue between the cephalad edge of the defect and the aortic valve and with the atrioventricular conduction system running on the left ventricular surface of the defect, creates unique problems for any occlusions using a catheter-delivered device. Until recently, all of the extensively tested septal closure devices required some amount of firm, circumferential rim surrounding the defect for the legs or "flanges" of the devices to extend onto and/or push against in order to create the fixation and/or attachment of the devices.

Often, the perimembranous ventricular septal defect develops a membranous aneurysm on the right side of the defect, resulting in partial closure of the defect. The aneurysms have one or even many secondary orifices that are located some distance away from the left ventricular ampulla of the defect and, in turn, away from the aortic annulus/leaflets. The Rashkind™ PDA[15,16], the Clamshell™ ASD, the CardioSEAL™ ASD, the Sideris™ Button[17], the Gianturco™ Coil[18], the Gianturco-Grifka™ Bag and the Amplatzer™ VSD devices have all been used for closure of the perimembranous VSD, particularly with an associated aneurysm of the VSD—and all with some, but not consistent, success. All of these attempts at closure with the various earlier devices still represent a very small and inconsistent percentage of the total number of perimembranous ventricular septal defects.

The attempts and partial successes with the various available devices along with a general continued interest in transcatheter closure of the perimembranous ventricular septal defect resulted in the development of the Amplatzer™ perimembranous VSD occlusion devices specifically for the perimembranous ventricular septal defect. This device is beginning phase II clinical trials in the US and has completed trials, has CE approval and has been in extensive use in Europe and much of the rest of the world.

The eccentric Amplatzer™ membranous ventricular septal defect occluder and delivery system

Dr Kurt Amplatz and the AGA™ Corporation (Golden Valley, MN) modified the basic shape of their previous occlusion devices quite extensively to develop an eccentric Amplatzer™ Membranous VSD occluder[19]. In its clinical use so far, the device appears relatively safe and does *not* appear to interfere with the aortic valve function for most perimembranous ventricular septal defects[20], and even some residual subaortic ventricular septal defects following a prior surgical repair. The eccentric device is suitable for perimembranous ventricular septal defects that have at least 1 mm of subaortic rim between the cephalad rim of the defect and the aortic annulus, and perimembranous defects with large septal aneurysms. The narrower the cephalad, subaortic rim of the defect, the more precarious is the *implant* of the device, although usually the properly orientated and sized Amplatzer™ Membranous VSD device sits within the left ventricular opening (ampulla) of the defect and away from the aortic valve even when virtually no subaortic rim exists.

Before being considered for transcatheter closure, the ventricular septal defect is examined angiographically and by transesophageal echocardiography. The diameter of the left ventricular opening or "ampulla", the diameter of the narrowest diameter of the defect, the presence and configuration of any associated "septal aneurysm", and the *size*, number and location of openings in the aneurysm are defined. The exact location of the defect in relation to the aortic valve on the left side and the tricuspid valve/aneurysmal tissue on the right side are identified.

The Amplatzer™ Membranous VSD device currently is manufactured from the same, fine 0.004″ super elastic Nitinol™ wire, which is formed into a mesh or weave, but with a completely different design of the "hub" and "disks". The Amplatzer™ Membranous VSD occluder comes with a special new braided delivery sheath (AGA Medical Corp., Golden Valley, MN) and a special delivery/pusher *catheter* (AGA Medical Corp., Golden Valley, MN), which permits precise directional postioning of the device. The central "hub" of the device is only 1.5 mm long and is available in diameters ranging between 4 and 18 mm in 2 mm increments. The "left ventricular" or "distal" retention disk is very eccentric, with only a 0.5 mm rim along the cephalad edge of the device. This almost absent rim on the cephalad edge of the left side of the device extends into a 5 mm rim around the sides and caudally, giving the left sided rim of the Amplatzer™ Membranous VSD device the appearance of a "bib" hanging from the hub of the device. The most caudal area of the "left" disk (6 o'clock position) contains a small platinum marker to indicate the orientation of the device during implant. The right-sided disk is symmetrical, with a 2 mm rim circumferentially around the central hub and with a recessed attach–release micro screw, which is similar to the micro screw at the center of the other Amplatzer™ occluders, except that one part of the outer circumference of the micro screw housing is *flattened*. The left sided disk has a "central" hub without a micro screw.

The Amplatzer™ TorqVue™ Delivery system (AGA Medical Corp., Golden Valley, MN), which comes with the Amplatzer™ Membranous VSD occluder, consists of the original delivery/attach/release cable, a special delivery/pusher catheter and a new delivery sheath reinforced with wire braid. The delivery/pusher catheter and the delivery sheath both have a fixed, gentle 180° curve preformed into their distal ends. The tip of the delivery/pusher catheter has a circular metal "ring" fixed at its tip, into which the attach–release micro screw housing inserts. The ring at the tip of the pusher catheter has a flattened segment within its inner circumference. The flattened segment is situated on the convex (outer) side of the built-in curve of the delivery/pusher catheter. The fixed, preformed, curves of the delivery/pusher catheter and delivery sheath together maintain this flattened surface within the distal ring at the tip of the pusher catheter orientated on the outer, or convex, curve of the catheter during delivery.

The *housing* of the attach–release micro screw, which is attached to the "right ventricular" disk (side) of the device, has a flattened area on the cephalad, outer surface of the housing, which matches exactly with the flattened area within the tip of the delivery/pusher catheter. When the Amplatzer™ Membranous VSD device is orientated with the long portion of the left sided retention disk pointing *caudally*, the flattened surface on the micro screw housing is on its *cephalad* surface and "points" in the opposite direction from the platinum marker located on the caudal, long edge of the left ventricular disk of the device. When the housing of the micro screw inserts into the ring at the tip of the delivery/pusher catheter, the corresponding flattened areas within the ring and on the outside of the housing of the micro screw ensure that the device orients into its proper orientation in the VSD when delivered *properly and carefully*.

Specifics for the delivery of the Amplatzer™ Membranous VSD device

Delivery of the Amplatzer™ Membranous VSD device is controlled with transesophageal echo visualization *and* repeated left ventricular angiocardiograms. Left ventricular angiograms are recorded in the PA and lateral views and with additional LAO–cranial and RAO–caudal angulation views in order to determine the best angulation to cut the *left ventricular orifice* of the ventricular septal defect precisely on edge. The X-ray tubes are positioned with the angulations that best visualize the defect on edge. If not already in place, the transesophageal echo probe is introduced and the anatomy verified by echo.

The Amplatzer™ Membranous VSD device is delivered prograde from a right ventricular approach through a catheter introduced from a femoral vein. However, the defect initially is crossed with a *retrograde* catheter—usually with a Judkins™ or Amplatz™ right coronary catheter. The preformed right coronary catheter is advanced retrograde from the aorta into the cavity or apex of the left ventricle. As the catheter is withdrawn along the ventricular septum from the cavity of the left ventricle into the outflow tract, the tip is rotated medially and posteriorly. As the tip of the catheter approaches just below the aortic valve, this usually directs the tip of the preformed "right coronary" catheter *into* the left ventricular orifice of the perimembranous VSD. As the tip of the catheter enters the VSD, the tip moves significantly toward the patient's right. It may take several attempts at withdrawing the tip along the septum for it to "drop" into the VSD. The location of the tip of the catheter is verified with a small injection of contrast through the catheter.

Once the catheter tip is well into the VSD, a very floppy tipped, torque-controlled wire or a floppy Amplatzer™ "noodle" wire (AGA Medical Corp., Golden Valley, MN) with at least a 90° curve preformed at the tip is advanced through the retrograde catheter, into, then through the VSD and into the right ventricular outflow tract (RVOT). From the RVOT, the wire is manipulated directly toward the pulmonary artery. The wire may tend to *loop* into the *body or apex* of the right ventricle before it passes to the pulmonary artery. If the wire does loop into and through the body of the right ventricle, the wire usually also is passing around chordae/trabeculae in the ventricle, which, in turn, will prevent the creation of a straight course of the wire and eventually the delivery catheter from the VSD to the inferior vena cava. When the wire, which is passing through the VSD, repeatedly passes into the body of the ventricle, the original retrograde catheter or an end-hole floating balloon catheter is advanced over the wire and through the VSD. With the tip of the catheter in the right ventricle, this usually helps to direct the *curved* wire toward the pulmonary artery. If not, an active deflector wire is used to deflect the tip of the *catheter*, which has passed through the VSD into the RVOT, toward the pulmonary artery. Once the tip of the catheter is deflected, the catheter is advanced off the deflector wire and into the pulmonary artery and/or the deflector wire is replaced in the now turned catheter with the floppy tipped wire and the floppy wire is advanced into the pulmonary artery.

Although a Terumo™ Glide™ wire (Terumo Medical Corp., Somerset, NJ) passes through the ventricular defect and into the pulmonary artery more readily, the Glide™ wire is *not* recommended for this procedure. Glide™ wires easily *perforate through* tissues when advanced out of the tip of a catheter, particularly when the tip of the catheter is up against the tissues, and in doing so, the Glide™ wires create their own tract rather than passing through the true natural openings. When that happens, the catheter and/or the delivery sheath/dilator cannot be advanced through the tiny "created" opening.

When the tip of the wire that is passing through the VSD is free in the pulmonary artery, a floating balloon (Swan™) catheter is introduced from a *femoral vein* and advanced from the right atrium, through the tricuspid valve and right ventricle and into the pulmonary artery. The floating balloon catheter helps to ensure that the catheter passes through the *largest central opening* of the tricuspid valve and ***not*** through and/or around chordal attachments. A 20 mm Microvena™ Gooseneck™ snare (Microvena, Corp., White Bear Lake, MN) is introduced into the end-hole floating balloon catheter or the balloon catheter is replaced over an exchange wire with a specific snare catheter and the snare is introduced through the specific snare catheter. The wire that is passing through the VSD and into the pulmonary artery is snared in the pulmonary artery. The snared wire is withdrawn carefully from the pulmonary artery, carefully through the tricuspid valve and out through the femoral vein, creating a through-and-through wire "rail" through the VSD. The course of this wire passing from the VSD through the right ventricle to the inferior vena cava should be relatively *straight*. If the wire has a circuitous or "S" shaped course, it indicates that the wire is passing under a chorda in the right ventricle, in which case it will not allow the long delivery sheath for the Amplatzer™ Membranous VSD device to orient properly when passed through that course. If the through-and-through wire does not have a straight course from the VSD to the inferior vena cava, the wire is released from the snare, withdrawn into the right ventricle and repositioned in the pulmonary artery. The end-hole floating balloon catheter is reintroduced from the femoral vein, re-floated through the tricuspid valve and the snaring and creation of the through-and-through wire "loop" is repeated until the wire has a straight course.

Once the course of the wire through the VSD and tricuspid valve is correct, the retrograde catheter is advanced over the through-and-through wire, through the VSD and right heart and out through the femoral vein, creating a "through-and-through catheter". The initial floppy tipped torque wire is replaced through the through-and-through catheter with an exchange length Amplatzer™ fixed core soft tipped "noodle" wire (AGA Medical Corp., Golden Valley, MN) or a *standard*, exchange length, 0.035" teflon-coated wire.

The initial short femoral venous sheath is removed over the through-and-through wire. As the retrograde catheter is withdrawn back into the vein, the 7-, 8- or 9-French (depending on the device size being used) long, special Amplatzer™ TorqVue™ delivery sheath/dilator with a 180° tip curve (AGA Medical Corp., Golden Valley, MN) is introduced into the femoral vein over the through-and-through wire and advanced over the wire while simultaneously withdrawing the retrograde catheter. The through-and-through wire is kept fairly taught and the tip of the retrograde catheter and the tip of the delivery sheath/dilator are kept "kissing" during this entire introduction of the sheath/dilator. As the retrograde catheter is withdrawn, the delivery sheath/dilator is advanced through the right ventricle, through the defect, to the left side of the VSD and into the aorta until the tip of the *sheath* is in the ascending aorta.

The dilator is withdrawn back into the TorqVue™ sheath to a position well within the right ventricle or even the right atrium. With the tip of the sheath fixed in this position in the aorta, a degree of slack is created in the through-and-through wire by pushing only the wire forward from the femoral artery. This creates a 3–4 mm gap of loose wire between the tip of the retrograde catheter and the tip of the sheath. The delivery sheath is withdrawn until the tip of the sheath drops just below the aortic valve in the left ventricular outflow tract (but *not* into the VSD). The retrograde catheter is advanced with the loose segment of wire to follow the tip of the sheath into the left ventricular outflow tract. While maintaining considerable slack on the wire, the retrograde catheter is pushed forward to advance the tip toward the body of the left ventricular cavity. The catheter with the loop of wire following the tip of the catheter is pushed forward toward and into the *apex* of the left ventricle while simultaneously the tip of the sheath is torqued counterclockwise and advanced with the tip of the retrograde catheter. As the catheter and wire advance toward the apex, the 180° curve of the TorqVue™ delivery sheath, which is being advanced simultaneously, should turn and advance toward the apex along with the tip of the catheter.

Alternatively, once the tip of the TorqVue™ sheath has been withdrawn into the left ventricular outflow tract, the retrograde catheter, alone, is advanced to the apex of the left ventricle over a long, loose loop of the through-and-through wire, which is being advanced simultaneously out of the tip of the sheath. Once the tip of the retrograde catheter is fixed securely within the left ventricular apex along with the free length of the through-and-through wire extending from the tip of the sheath at the VSD to the tip of the retrograde catheter at the apex, the long delivery sheath is advanced carefully while torquing it slightly counterclockwise over the free segment of the wire and into the left ventricular apex. Because of the relative stiffness of the TorqVue™ sheath and particularly in smaller patients, this maneuver may take several attempts and possibly the exchange of the original retrograde catheter for a stiffer catheter in order to fix the loop of wire in the apex as the sheath is advanced over the wire. It is not infrequent for the patient to develop left bundle branch block, second and/or even complete heart block during these maneuvers! In the event of any of these arrhythmias, all catheter/wire/sheath maneuvers are stopped until the original normal rhythm returns. When a conduction disturbance is created and when catheter/wire/sheath manipulations are resumed, a different maneuver/technique is used.

The position of the TorqVue™ sheath in the left ventricular apex is critical for the success of the procedure and *must be* achieved before an attempt is made to deliver the Amplatzer™ Membranous VSD device. When the TorqVue™ sheath is positioned in the apex of the left ventricle, a smooth 180° curve is formed from the right ventricle, through the VSD to the apex of the left ventricle. The convex surface of the curve in the sheath faces cephalad and, in turn, the convex surface of the delivery/pusher catheter with the flat segment of the ring within its distal tip also will be facing cephalad when it is advanced within the curve of the TorqVue™ sheath. This orientation forces the Amplatzer™ Membranous VSD device to be properly oriented with the long "lip" of the left ventricular disk with its marker pointing caudally when properly attached to the delivery/pusher catheter. If the TorqVue sheath remains in the aorta and does not pass into the apex of the ventricle, the con*cavity* of the curve of the sheath will be facing cephalad. As a consequence, the marker and the longer area of the left ventricular disk on the Amplatzer™ Membranous VSD device will point *cephalad* if it is delivered through the sheath, while the sheath is directed into the aorta. The proper positioning of the tip of the TorqVue™ sheath into the apex of the left ventricle often is the most difficult part of the delivery and implant of the Amplatzer™ membranous VSD occluder.

Once the tip of the sheath is positioned in the apex and with the tip of the retrograde catheter positioned adjacent to the tip of the sheath, the through-and-through wire is withdrawn carefully through the retrograde catheter and the dilator is withdrawn from the TorqVue™ delivery sheath. The delivery sheath and the retrograde catheter are cleared of air/clot passively by allowing them to bleed back from the left ventricular pressure and then placed on a continuous flush. The retrograde catheter is withdrawn to the high left ventricular outflow tract and an angiocardiogram obtained through this catheter. This angiogram demonstrates the relationships of the long sheath, the VSD and the aortic valve to each other. The X-ray tubes are repositioned as necessary to place the left ventricular end of the VSD as much on edge as possible.

The size of the Amplatzer™ Membranous VSD device usually is chosen with the intent of implanting the hub of the device *in the actual defect* with the "lip" or rim extending onto the left ventricular side of the ventricular defect. In order to fix a device in that location, the central hub should be 1–2 mm larger in diameter than the largest measurement of the left ventricular orifice of the defect as determined by either echo or angiographic measurement of the left ventricular side (opening) of the ventricular defect. Measurement of the openings in the right-sided aneurysmal tissue is *not* the measurement taken for the narrowest defect diameter when the device is to be implanted in the actual ventricular defect.

When there is a significant aneurysm of the ventricular septal defect and with one or more smaller openings in the aneurysm, the device can be implanted totally *within the aneurysm*. The technique for implant into the aneurysm is discussed subsequently in this section.

To load the Amplatzer™ Membranous VSD device, the delivery *cable* is passed through the delivery/pusher *catheter* and both the cable and the delivery/pusher catheter are passed through the loader. The device is screwed onto the delivery cable similarly to the other Amplatzer™ occlusion devices. Once attached to the cable, the cable/device is withdrawn to the tip of the delivery/pusher catheter. The flat area within the ring at the tip of the delivery/pusher catheter is aligned with the flat area on the surface of the attach–release screw housing on the device, and this screw housing (hub on the device) is withdrawn into the tip of the delivery/pusher catheter. Often a slight "snap" or "give" is felt as the two fix together properly. With the screw housing on the device pulled tightly into the tip of the delivery catheter by pulling the cable forcefully into the delivery/pusher catheter, the proximal end of the delivery cable is clamped firmly against the proximal hub of the delivery/pusher catheter to hold the cable and catheter in a secure fixed relationship. A hemostat can be clamped on the cable against the hub of the catheter or the torquer "unscrew–release" device can be advanced over the cable and tightened on the cable against the proximal hub of the delivery/pusher catheter. In either case, the cable must be clamped very tightly against the hub while the device is pulled tightly into the tip of the delivery/pusher catheter. This will hold the device and the delivery/pusher catheter tightly together and fixes the orientation of the device to the delivery/pusher catheter.

The device, which is attached to the cable, and the delivery/pusher catheter are withdrawn together into the loader, and the loader is flushed and introduced into the previously positioned long delivery sheath. The device on the delivery cable/delivery/pusher catheter is advanced to the tip of the sheath, which is positioned in the left ventricular apex. The 180° curve of the delivery/pusher catheter follows the similar 180° curve of the TorqVue™ sheath and, in turn, orients the pusher catheter and the device properly. The entire system—device/cable/pusher catheter/sheath—is withdrawn very carefully into the left ventricular outflow tract just caudal to the VSD. The left ventricular "disk" is extruded by partially advancing the delivery cable/pusher catheter *together* and by simultaneously withdrawing the sheath several millimeters further. The proximal ends of the delivery/pusher catheter and the sheath must be held very firmly together as, once the extrusion begins, the device forcefully tends to "pop" all of the way out of the sheath. When the initial position of the delivery sheath begins in the apex of the left ventricle and the device and the pusher catheter are maintained together, the "caudal marker" on the left sided disk should be oriented correctly and caudally.

If the "caudal marker" on the left disk of the Amplatzer™ Membranous VSD device is not oriented *caudally* in the outflow tract, the sheath is re-advanced over the left disk of the device and the combination re-advanced to the apex of the left ventricle. The combination is withdrawn to the left ventricular outflow tract and the left disk then is re-extruded in the left ventricular outflow tract and its orientation rechecked. If it is still not oriented properly, the sheath is re-advanced over the device again and the process repeated until the device does orient properly.

The position of the left sided disk and its relationship to the aortic valve and the VSD are verified by trans-esophageal echo and by an angiogram through the retrograde catheter, which now should be positioned high in the left ventricular outflow tract. When the left ventricular disk is deployed properly, the "waist" should be *minimally* deployed. The entire system is withdrawn together until the left ventricular disk enters the left ventricular side of the VSD. The delivery/pusher catheter and the delivery sheath still must be held together very firmly otherwise, as the device begins to deploy further, the entire hub and right side of the device also tend to "pop out" of the delivery sheath completely. This withdrawal of the delivery sheath and partially exposed device must be very gentle and careful since the left sided disk does not offer much resistance to being pulled completely through the defect. As soon as the properly orientated, left sided disk enters the VSD and it is away from the aortic valve as seen on the echo, the delivery cable and delivery/pusher catheter are fixed in position while the delivery sheath alone is withdrawn off the "hub", off the right sided disk of the device and back into the right ventricle. This deploys the device properly in the VSD. The position in the VSD, away from the aortic valve and the absence of any new aortic regurgitation are verified by echo. A repeat left ventricular outflow tract angiogram is performed and the retrograde catheter is withdrawn into the aortic root, where an additional aortogram is recorded to rule out distortion of the aortic valve and/or any aortic regurgitation.

When the Amplatzer™ Membranous VSD device is in the proper position and not interfering with the aortic valve, the clamp on the proximal end of the delivery cable is released and slight traction is placed on the delivery/pusher catheter while fixing the delivery cable in place. Hopefully this will allow the delivery/pusher catheter to pull proximally off the proximal hub/screw attachment of the device and allow the device, now only attached to the cable, to reorient slightly. When the device remains in the proper position, the delivery cable is unscrewed counterclockwise to release the device. Occasionally the delivery/pusher catheter does not "pop" free easily from the hub of the device either before or after the device is unscrewed. When that occurs, the delivery/pusher catheter is wiggled and pulled back slightly while pushing the delivery cable forward very slightly in order to push the attach–release sleeve on the device out of the "ring" on the pusher catheter.

If the tip of the delivery sheath pulls back into the VSD before the left sided disk begins to open and/or if the sheath position does not begin in a proper direction toward the left ventricular apex, the sheath and contained pusher catheter can twist and change the orientation of the convex curve of the sheath/catheter combination. This in turn changes the orientation of the left sided device so that the platinum marker will not be directed caudally (between 5 & 7 o'clock) when the left sided disk is extruded.

When the exposed left sided disk along with the sheath/delivery/pusher catheter cannot easily be rotated together, the remainder of the entire device is extruded into the outflow tract, the combined delivery sheath/pusher catheter rotated together to reorient the left sided disk, and then the right sided disk and part of the "hub" are withdrawn back into sheath. When the left disk *does* reorient successfully by this maneuver, the sheath, delivery/pusher catheter and device are withdrawn into the defect, the position of the left disk verified angiographically and by TEE and the right disk reopened on the right side of the defect by withdrawing the sheath alone. If the device cannot be orientated with the marker on the left disk positioned between 5 and 7 o'clock, the device is withdrawn completely and the procedure restarted from the beginning. Similarly, if there is any interference with the aortic valve apparatus, unusual extension of the device into either the left or right ventricular outflow tract, interference with the tricuspid valve or any degree of conduction block, the device is withdrawn into the sheath and the procedure either restarted or abandoned.

In the presence of a large aneurysm associated with a "perimembranous" ventricular septal defect, there is an alternative occlusion technique for the implant of the Amplatzer™ Membranous VSD occluder. The VSD occluder can be implanted completely within the aneurysm with the "waist" of the device positioned across the "exit" opening in the aneurysm. The ventricular septal defect is crossed and a through-and-through wire is created exactly as described previously. Once the delivery sheath has passed through the aneurysm, the VSD and into the aorta, a repeat angiogram is performed in the left ventricular outflow tract adjacent to, or, *preferably in*, the ventricular septal defect. With the opening(s) in the aneurysm partially occluded by the sheath passing through it or one of them, this angiogram should fill the aneurysm with contrast and demonstrate more precisely all of the opening(s) from the aneurysm into the right ventricle. The opening in the aneurysm around the sheath is measured and the size and location of other openings defined from the angiogram and by TEE. Unless there is a separate "exit opening" in the aneurysm that is much larger and *not* the one the sheath is passing through, a device is chosen that is 3–4 mm larger than the "exit opening" in the aneurysm that the sheath *is* passing through. When there are multiple openings in the aneurysm that are close to each other, a single Amplatzer™ Membranous VSD device within the aneurysm should cover all of the openings.

The manipulation of the sheath from the aorta to the apex of the left ventricle and the initial extrusion of the device in the left ventricular outflow tract are identical to the procedure for delivery into the left ventricular orifice of the ventricular defect. When the extruded left sided disk is oriented properly, the delivery sheath, the pusher/delivery catheter and the device are withdrawn together. Since the device and particularly the left sided disk that will be implanted *into* the aneurysm, usually is smaller than the device for implant into the true defect, the opened left disk usually pulls through the left ventricular opening of the defect and into the aneurysm. When properly sized, the left sided disk fixes within the aneurysm against the "exit opening". The position and degree of occlusion are checked with a repeat angiogram through the retrograde catheter (into the aneurysm, or at least, into the mouth of the aneurysm) and by TEE. When satisfied with the position within the aneurysm and with the degree of occlusion, the sheath is withdrawn off the device, opening the waist into the "exit opening" in the aneurysm, and the right sided disk on the right ventricular side of the opening. Often the right sided disk initially remains somewhat compressed and distorted. The degree of occlusion is visualized by a repeat angiogram and by TEE interrogation. When satisfied with the occlusion and position of the device, the clamp on the proximal cable is released, the pusher catheter withdrawn and the cable unscrewed by rotating it counterclockwise until the device releases.

The Amplatzer™ Membranous VSD occluder has had a fairly extensive clinical usage outside of the United States in patients with significant shunts and/or symptoms. The device appears very versatile and relatively safe for the large majority of perimembranous ventricular septal defects in patients past infancy. There have been several reports of malposition of the device and a greater than one percent incidence of permanent, complete heart block in the early experience. A much larger and well-controlled experience with the device and a significantly longer follow-up are necessary to determine the precise limitations and safety of this device for the routine closure of the perimembranous VSD. Certainly even a 1% incidence of complete heart block is unacceptable.

Experimental Sideris™ "frameless" catheter-delivered device closure of perimembranous interventricular septal defects

Dr Sideris has reported the use of "frameless" occluders (Pediatric Cardiology Custom Medical Devices, Athens, Greece) for the successful occlusion of the ASD, the PDA and the VSD. The "frameless" device uses an inflated latex balloon covered with a thin sheet, or layer, of polyurethane foam to fix the "frameless" patch in place within the defects. The balloon fills the defect temporarily, but functions only as a "frame" to hold the polyurethane patch in place until it has adhered securely to the rim of the defect by tissue ingrowth into the patch. The sheet of polyurethane foam, all by itself, becomes the "patch" after the balloon is deflated. Most of the experiences reported with the Sideris "frameless" devices have been with the ASD devices but it has had successful use in the perimembranous and malalignment VSD.

With the framless ASD device, the implanting balloon, when inflated, has a diameter slightly larger than the diameter of the defect. The balloon is covered with the polyurethane foam "cup" over the entire balloon with the shaft of the balloon catheter passing into the opening in the "cup". The balloon with the covering patch is pulled into, and seated in, the defect with the patch circumferentially pulled against the rim of the defect by the large balloon. The balloon with the ASD "patch" is held securely in this position in the defect by traction applied to the proximal shaft of the balloon catheter, which is fixed outside of the body at the femoral venous puncture site. There is a second balloon, which is proximal to the distal balloon on the catheter shaft. The second balloon inflates on the right side of the septum but apparently does not contribute significantly to maintaining the "patch" in place. There is a "safety thread" passing from outside of the body, through a corner of the patch and back outside of the body. Traction is maintained on the balloon (from outside of the body against the patient's leg) for up to 48 hours! After 48 hours, the two balloons are deflated and withdrawn, leaving the polyurethane "patch" in place on the septal defect. When satisfied with the position of the patch and the fixation of the patch in the defect, the safety thread is withdrawn from the patch.

For closure of a perimembranous VSD with the "frameless" device, the VSD is crossed and a through-and-through wire created, similarly to the technique for the

Amplatzer™ Membranous VSD occluder. The precise details of the loading and delivery of the frameless device to the defect and how the exact size is chosen are not available.

The "frameless" VSD occluder uses the same concept as the frameless ASD occluder, with the polyurethane foam adhering to, and occluding the defect within 24–48 hours. On the frameless VSD occluder, instead of the catheter-applied traction to the outside of the body, there is a counter occluder attached to the balloon. The balloon with the polyurethane covering is inflated with a diluted contrast solution. The inflated balloon is seated on the left side of the membranous ventricular septal defect, occluding the defect, while the counter occluder holds the balloon/patch in place from the opposite side of the defect. The counter occluder positioned on the right side of the defect holds the balloon in place long enough and securely enough for the polyurethane to adhere to the rim of the defect by fibroblast ingrowth into the fabric. The balloon spontaneously deflates over a period of days as the diluted contrast elutes out of the latex balloon. By the time the balloon deflates, the polyurethane foam is adherent to the rim of the VSD and creates a patch, reportedly sealing the defect. The deflated balloon remains attached, but flattened under the "patch".

These experimental "frameless" devices may prove clinically *practical* over time for safe, perimembranous VSD closure, and certainly they represent the ingenuity and imagination that will eventually lead to the catheter closure of all perimembranous ventricular septal defects. This type of patch would seem ideal for implant *within* a large aneurysm of the ventricular septal defect and should avoid all of the problems of atrioventricular block of any degree.

Complications of transcatheter closure of ventricular septal defects

Because the procedures are so complex, transcatheter closure of ventricular septal defects (VSD) has an even greater potential for the complications that are common to all extensive intracardiac manipulations. There are more *left heart manipulations* and a higher complexity of these manipulations with the multiple exchanges of wires, sheaths, catheters and devices than with any other intracardiac procedure. As a consequence, the risks of introducing systemic air and/or clot at some point during the procedure are much greater. The treatment of these embolic complications is prevention, which, in turn, requires constant vigilance and attention to each small detail of each procedure for clearing the sheaths, catheters and delivery systems of all air and/or clots.

There also are complications unique to transcatheter VSD occlusion related to the delivery systems, the delivery techniques and the devices themselves. The VSD occlusion procedures require the establishment of a "through-and-through" wire. Establishing the "wire rail", in itself, requires extensive intracardiac manipulation with wires, catheters and snares. The actual snaring and withdrawing of the wires through the heart has the potential for snagging and damage to cardiac valves. This damage is prevented by the use of very gentle manipulations whenever manipulating the snared wires. Even the rubbing and/or the tension of the through-and-through wire against tissues creates a "sawing effect" and can damage the cardiac valves and/or intracardiac conduction system. The conduction damage can cause bundle branch or even complete heart block. These problems are minimized (prevented!) by maintaining a catheter over the wire at all times and by avoiding any tightening of the "loops" in the wire as it passes through the heart.

The VSD devices require the introduction and manipulation of stiff and often large sheaths. The size of the delivery sheaths alone, if not handled very "gently", can compromise the access vessels, particularly when access is from an arterial approach. The stiff sheaths have the potential of tearing any cardiac valve as they are advanced through the valves. If resistance is encountered during the introduction of the sheath/dilator, the combination probably is not passing through the true orifice of the valve and is caught on a narrow angle and/or chorda of the valve or even can be perforating the valve leaflet. This damage is prevented by utilizing very soft tipped wires and/or floating balloon catheters to cross the defects and/or valves and by *never forcing* a stiff sheath/dilator through valves and/or valve structures. In the worst case scenario where the resistance to the sheath/dilator introduction is not solved by changing the tension and, in turn, direction of the through-and-through wire through the valve, the wire is removed and repositioned through the valve before the delivery dilator/sheath is introduced!

The stiff sheaths also create hemodynamic instability without actually damaging the valves by holding the cardiac valves open when a sheath is positioned across the valve. When recognized and not allowed to persist, the hemodynamic compromise usually produces no permanent sequelae. The hemodynamic compromise, however, can complicate the procedure and the potential is there for permanent damage if the compromise is not recognized by constant intra-arterial monitoring and then rectified.

The occlusion devices themselves have potential problems unique to the individual devices. Catheter-implanted devices always have the potential for embolization. This potential is prevented, or at least minimized, by careful attention to the details of the procedure, including precise sizing and localization of the defects before choosing and delivering an occlusion device. This often entails balloon sizing, the use of an additional catheter for angiography during the implant and both echo and angiographic imaging. Once deployed completely, and even before their release, the double-umbrella devices cannot be retrieved safely through a catheter. A particularly precarious position for the device probably is an indication for the use of a different type of device.

VSD devices all have the potential of interfering with adjacent valves. The muscular VSD devices have the potential for opening in the chordae of either the tricuspid or the mitral valve. Because of the way the legs open perpendicularly and away from the septum, the CardioSEAL™ and STARFlex™ devices have the greatest potential for catching atrioventricular valvular structures while they are being implanted, but this can occur with any device. The use of a different type of occlusion device and/or a change in the positioning of the device as verified by angiography and/or echo during implant should prevent any significant interference with the atrioventricular valve apparatus.

Essentially all occluding devices in any type of ventricular septal defect are between a high and a low-pressure system, which creates the potential for hemolysis. Hemolysis occurs following device implant when there is a high-pressure jet of blood passing through and/or immediately adjacent to the freshly implanted device. The more secure the "seating" of the occluding device, the less the chance of a residual "jet-like" lesion being present. Once a ventricular septal occluder is implanted and hemolysis does occur, the patient is observed and treated medically with supportive therapy whenever possible. With persistence and/or certainly progression of the hemolysis, the persistent lesion must be eliminated either with the implant of an additional device or with the surgical removal of the occluder device and closure of the defect completely.

Closure of a perimembranous ventricular septal defect entails the implant of a device immediately adjacent to the aortic valve with the very real potential for interfering with the function of the aortic valve and/or permanently damaging the aortic valve. This potential has been reduced significantly, but not entirely eliminated by the design and implant technique of the Amplatzer™ Membranous VSD device. During the implant of a perimembranous VSD occluder, the integrity of the aortic valve function is visualized by echo and tested by aortic root and left ventricular angiography before the release of the occlusion device. If there is even a suggestion of encroachment on the aortic valve, the device is removed and the procedure is abandoned and/or reattempted with a different device. Whenever possible, the implant of the device *within the aneurysm* of the ventricular septal defect should prevent this complication.

The perimembranous ventricular septal defect occluder, which is implanted in the orifice of the defect, also is positioned very close to (against) the atrioventricular conduction tissues. Left bundle branch block and/or complete heart block have been encountered during and after these implants. If an "electrical" block occurs during implant, the device, at the very least, is removed and/or repositioned until the block resolves. A prolonged degree of, or certainly permanent complete heart block at any time during the procedure is an indication to abandon the particular device or the procedure altogether. The long-term effects on the atrioventricular conduction system of a device in the perimembranous septal area are still unknown. The early experience suggests that a finite percentage of complete heart block is created, which may not be possible to avoid entirely! This, of course, could be a major problem with this particular device.

Although attempted for over one and a half decades, the use of catheter-delivered devices for closure of the post-myocardial infarct VSD is still in its "infancy" and evolving. The severity of the illness of the patients and evolving nature of the defects have made the procedure very complex and the risks of the procedure inherently very high. The improvements in the devices that are available, the greater familiarity with the techniques for closure of muscular ventricular septal defects, and the better support for the patients all have decreased but not eliminated the inherent risks of the procedure because of the precarious status of the patients.

Unquestionably, with the continued improvement in the current devices and techniques, the development of new devices for the occlusion of ventricular septal defects and with the increasing experience in the use of these devices, complications related to the devices and the procedures in all categories of patient should become less frequent. In spite of device improvements, continual vigilance and precise attention to the details of the procedure always will be necessary to reduce complications to a minimum, or hopefully even to eliminate them.

References

1. Lock JE *et al.* Transcatheter closure of ventricular septal defects. *Circulation* 1988; **78**(2): 361–368.
2. Bridges ND *et al.* Preoperative transcatheter closure of congenital muscular ventricular septal defects. *N Engl J Med* 1991; **324**(19): 1312–1317.
3. Amin Z *et al.* New device for closure of muscular ventricular septal defects in a canine model. *Circulation* 1999; **100**(3): 320–328.
4. Thanopoulos BD *et al.* Transcatheter closure of muscular ventricular septal defects with the amplatzer ventricular septal defect occluder: initial clinical applications in children. *J Am Coll Cardiol* 1999; **33**(5): 1395–1399.

5. Hijazi ZM. Device closure of ventricular septal defects. *Catheter Cardiovasc Interv* 2003; **60**(1): 107–114.
6. Chaudhari M *et al*. Transcatheter coil closure of muscular ventricular septal defects with Gianturco coils. *J Interv Cardiol* 2001; **14**(2): 165–168.
7. Schiele TM *et al*. Transcatheter closure of a ruptured ventricular septum following inferior myocardial infarction and cardiogenic shock. *Catheter Cardiovasc Interv* 2003; **60**(2): 224–228.
8. Landzberg M and Lock JE. Transcatheter management of ventricular septal rupture after myocardial infarction. *Semin Thorac Cardiovasc Surg* 1998; **10**(2): 128–132.
9. Pienvichit P and Piemonte TC. Percutaneous closure of postmyocardial infarction ventricular septal defect with the CardioSEAL septal occluder implant. *Catheter Cardiovasc Interv* 2001; **54**(4): 490–494.
10. Holzer R *et al*. Transcatheter closure of postinfarction ventricular septal defects using the new Amplatzer muscular VSD occluder: Results of a U.S. Registry. *Catheter Cardiovasc Interv* 2004; **61**(2): 196–201.
11. Chessa M *et al*. Transcatheter closure of congenital and acquired muscular ventricular septal defects using the Amplatzer device. *J Invasive Cardiol* 2002; **14**(6): 322–327.
12. Tiao GM *et al*. Cardiac and great vessel injuries in children after blunt trauma: an institutional review. *J Pediatr Surg* 2000; **35**(11): 1656–1660.
13. Bauriedel G *et al*. Transcatheter closure of a posttraumatic ventricular septal defect with an Amplatzer occluder device. *Catheter Cardiovasc Interv* 2001; **53**(4): 508–512.
14. Cowley CG and Shaddy RE. Transcatheter treatment of a large traumatic ventricular septal defect. *Catheter Cardiovasc Interv* 2004; **61**(1): 144–146.
15. Rigby ML and Redington AN. Primary transcatheter umbrella closure of perimembranous ventricular septal defect. *Br Heart J* 1994; **72**(4): 368–371.
16. Vogel M, Rigby ML, and Shore D. Perforation of the right aortic valve cusp: complication of ventricular septal defect closure with a modified Rashkind umbrella. *Pediatr Cardiol* 1996; **17**(6): 416–418.
17. Sideris EB, Haddad J, and Rao PS. The role of the "Sideris" devices in the occlusion of ventricular septal defects. *Curr Interv Cardiol Rep* 2001; **3**(4): 349–353.
18. Kalra GS *et al*. Transcatheter closure of ventricular septal defect using detachable steel coil. *Heart* 1999; **82**(3): 395–396.
19. Gu X *et al*. Transcatheter closure of membranous ventricular septal defects with a new nitinol prosthesis in a natural swine model. *Catheter Cardiovasc Interv* 2000; **50**(4): 502–509.
20. Hijazi ZM *et al*. Catheter closure of perimembranous ventricular septal defects using the new Amplatzer membranous VSD occluder: initial clinical experience. *Catheter Cardiovasc Interv* 2002; **56**(4): 508–515.

31 Purposeful perforation of atretic valves, other intravascular structures and recanalization of totally obstructed vessels

Introduction

The opening of atretic valves or other imperforate vascular structures has always been necessary in the therapy of congenital heart disease. Until the era of aggressive pediatric cardiac catheterization laboratory interventions, all perforations and/or openings of valvular or total vascular occlusions were accomplished exclusively by surgery. The atrial transseptal procedure was the first examples of a purposeful perforation of a cardiac or vascular structure by a catheterization procedure[1]. The early transseptal perforations were for diagnostic purposes only, with no therapeutic intent and with the specific intent of *not* leaving a permanent opening. The atrial transseptal procedure now is a standard, accepted procedure and is described in detail in Chapter 8 ("Transseptal Technique").

The transition from a perforation that was intended *not* to remain open to a perforation that is performed specifically for a therapeutic purpose and is performed with the intention that the perforation remains open, occurred with the blade/balloon septostomy procedures. The intact atrial septum was perforated with a transseptal needle and some type of dilator, catheter and/or sheath. The small atrial septal opening that was created by the perforation was enlarged by a blade septostomy procedure to create a permanent opening[2]. The blade septostomy procedure following a transseptal puncture still is an established, standard approach for the creation of an interatrial communication in a previously intact septum. The blade atrial septostomy is a separate, established procedure and is described in detail in Chapter 14 ("Blade and Balloon Atrial Septostomy"). The blade septostomy procedure established that a permanent opening could be created in a previously totally intact vascular structure in the catheterization laboratory.

Following the blade septostomy, the next major development in the therapeutic procedures that was accepted in the pediatric/congenital environment was balloon dilation of stenotic valves and other vascular structures[3]. It did not take much imagination to envision the extension of the dilation of the stenotic pulmonary valve to the perforation, and then the dilation, of the atretic pulmonary valve. Beginning more than a decade ago, crude and relatively dangerous perforations of atretic pulmonary valves were accomplished with variable and unpredicatable results using various forms of stiff needles and/or wires along with, essentially, "brute force"[4]. It took several more years after the first publications about these crude perforation techniques and considerable innovation before laser and later, radio-frequency (RF) energy was introduced to perform the initial perforation[5–8].

Perforation of the atrial septum with radio-frequency energy

The ability of radio-frequency energy to drill into, and actually perforate, tissues became apparent somewhat inadvertently during electrophysiologic ablation procedures in the cardiac catheterization laboratory. Specific catheters and a modified RF generator then were developed in order to *purposefully perforate* tissues. Since there was no "predicate procedure" for the perforation of valvular tissue in the United States, the RF perforation system was developed as an alternative to a transseptal needle puncture of the atrial septum, with the RF perforation providing the advantage of requiring less force and, in turn, providing more control over the puncture. The RF perforation of the atrial septum also had the advantage of being able to approach and puncture the septum from a greater variety of, and much steeper, angles than could be accomplished with a needle puncture. After several years, much persistence and dedicated effort, radio-frequency perforation of the atrial septum was established and approved by the FDA in the United States in 2001. This procedure is described in detail in Chapter 8.

During the same period of time, perforation of the atretic pulmonary valve in the catheterization laboratory had been documented as an effective and safe procedure, and became the standard of care throughout the world *except* in the United States. With the availability of RF generators for septal puncture in the United States, the capability of performing RF perforation of the atretic pulmonary valve both "legally" and more safely became possible in the United States. The RF procedure for perforation of an atretic pulmonary valve now represents the standard of care for the perforation, even in the United States.

Perforation of pulmonary valve atresia from the right ventricle

Pulmonary valve atresia with intact ventricular septum is associated with various degrees of underdevelopment/ hypoplasia of the right ventricle. These infants usually have a patent ductus as their sole source of pulmonary blood supply and a patent foramen ovale or small atrial septal defect as the sole access for the systemic venous blood back into the systemic circulation. In the current era, the ductus patency is maintained initially with an infusion of prostaglandin. However, in order to survive any length of time, these infants require the minimum of a more dependable pulmonary blood supply and, often, an open atrial communication to allow the systemic venous blood returning to the right atrium to rejoin the systemic circulation. Ideally and in the presence of a moderate sized right ventricle and tricuspid valve, opening the pulmonary valve will allow prograde pulmonary blood flow from the right ventricle, the systemic venous blood is returned to the "functioning" circulation and, at the same time, the very high pressure in the right ventricle is decompressed. In reality, because of the usual small size of the right ventricle (and tricuspid valve) and the very low compliance of the right ventricle, the opening of the pulmonary valve alone often is not satisfactory as the total palliation in these patients.

Opening the pulmonary valve does "vent" the right ventricle, which decreases the right ventricular pressure and does allow some prograde flow into the pulmonary bed, however, most infants with this lesion also require an additional systemic to pulmonary shunt to provide adequate pulmonary flow. In the presence of a very small right ventricle, these patients also require the creation of a larger and more permanent atrial septal opening to "vent" the systemic venous blood into the effective systemic cardiac output. In the past, these interventions were accomplished by the combination of a balloon atrial septostomy performed in the catheterization laboratory, a surgical systemic to pulmonary artery shunt and a surgical valvotomy (or valvectomy) plus or minus a right ventricular outflow tract (RVOT) overhaul to allow prograde flow from the right ventricle to the pulmonary artery and, at the same time, accomplish the "venting" of the very high right ventricular pressure. When prograde flow to the pulmonary artery that is sufficient to maintain systemic cardiac output can be established by opening the pulmonary valve, then closure of the atrial communication rather than opening it must be considered! This is discussed subsequently.

In addition to the immediate palliation for these patients, this combination of the valvotomy and/or RVOT overhaul and the systemic to pulmonary artery shunt results in significant growth of the hypoplastic right ventricle in many of the patients. The right ventricular growth converts these patients from future "single-ventricle repairs" into potential candidates for an eventual two, or at least, one and one half ventricle repair. Several recent developments in the cardiac catheterization laboratory make it possible to accomplish the opening of the pulmonary valve, the establishment of a more permanent systemic to pulmonary connection and, if necessary, the atrial septostomy all in the catheterization laboratory without subjecting the patient to any surgical intervention. The combination of procedures, accomplished by one method or another, now is the recommended approach for virtually all infants with pulmonary atresia and intact ventricular septum who do *not* have extensive fistulous communications between the right ventricle, coronary arteries and aorta, and almost regardless of the size of the right ventricle at the time of presentation.

Perforation and dilation of the atretic pulmonary valve in the catheterization laboratory eliminates the most dangerous part of the *surgical* palliation of pulmonary atresia with intact ventricular septum. A puncture of the atrial septum with a long transseptal needle is an established procedure for crossing an intact atrial septum. The structure of the pulmonary valve in pulmonary valve atresia is a "plate-like" fusion of the leaflets, which is not dissimilar to a "septum". It has been demonstrated repeatedly in the past, that if a sharp "instrument" can be directed *precisely* at this "plate" and pushed with *enough force*, the plate can be perforated like a septum. Once perforated, the plate-like valve can be dilated.

Perforation of the atretic pulmonary valve has been attempted using specially curved transseptal needles, using the stiff ends of spring guide wires or the end of a Mullins™ deflector wire (Argon Medical Inc., Athens, TX) with, or without, the small "protective ball" amputated from the tip of the wire. The valve was approached for these "brute force" perforations from the right ventricle when using the transseptal needle. When using a stiff wire for the perforations, the atretic pulmonary valve was approached either through the right ventricle or retrograde through the patent ductus to the pulmonary artery and to the valve. Valve perforations with each of these "instruments", and from both approaches, *occasionally* were successful. Unfortunately, the force and "push" that were necessary to penetrate the valve, often pushed the supporting catheter, which contained the stiff needle and/or the retrograde wire, backwards and away from the plate-like valve rather than causing the perforating instrument to puncture the valve. When the guide or support catheter was pushed away, it prevented the perforation, or even worse, displaced the sharp instrument away from the center of the "plate-like" valve and into the perivalvular area. A puncture into the adjacent areas resulted in perforation into the pericardium and/or an adjacent chamber/vessel, often with catastrophic results.

Experimental, and recently, clinical experience demonstrated the feasibility of "drilling" through tissue, and more specifically pulmonary valve tissue, with laser or radio-frequency (RF) energy. Both energy sources have demonstrated considerable success in penetrating the valve. When this is followed by a balloon dilation of the valve, very adequate pulmonary valve openings are achieved allowing unobstructed prograde blood flow into the pulmonary artery. The amount of this prograde flow then is dependent on the size of the tricuspid valve, the potential volume and the compliance of the right ventricle.

Laser energy was the first energy source to be used in clinical trials in Europe[5–7]. The laser energy is delivered through a fine fiberoptic strand or "wire" to a very specific area, and proved very successful at perforating the atretic pulmonary valve in patients with pulmonary valve atresia by essentially vaporizing the tissue in front of the beam. The laser beam, unfortunately, also *easily* continues to perforate any tissues in its path beyond and/or adjacent to the valve. The laser energy was successful at perforating an opening in the atretic pulmonary valve in approximately 80% of the small number of patients in whom it was tried initially. The opening allowed the passage of a guide wire through the valve and subsequent dilation of the valve.

Although successful in perforating the valve, the laser system has several disadvantages in addition to the poor controllability of the depth of penetration. The Excimer Laser™ generator is large and very expensive. Unless the particular pediatric cardiac catheterization laboratory works in conjunction with an adult catheterization laboratory and/or performs many laser-assisted pacemaker lead extractions, the capital expense of the laser generator "just" for the very few pulmonary atresia patients who present to even large pediatric cardiac centers, cannot be justified easily. In addition to the ease of perforating *unwanted* structures within the heart with the laser, the intense laser energy also carries a risk of "stray" laser beams in the area of the patient, which can create retinal damage to the operators and other employees in the catheterization laboratory. As a consequence, all personnel in the laboratory are required to wear special, somewhat cumbersome, protective eye wear. The fiberoptic laser "wires" are expensive and finally, and absolutely the greatest deterrent to operators in the US until very recently: there was no laser "*wire*" that was approved for use outside of specific protocols in the United States.

As an excellent alternative to laser energy, radio-frequency energy delivered through a very fine insulated wire can also be used to perforate atretic tissues, and the atretic pulmonary valve in particular. The RF energy is less powerful for perforating structures, but it is considerably more controllable than the laser energy. A radio-frequency generator for perforation is considerably less expensive and less complex than any laser generator. In addition, radio-frequency generators are commonly available in pediatric and congenital catheterization laboratories, where they are used for the ablation of abnormal intracardiac "electrical" conduction tracts. However, the current, and now standard RF "ablation" generator, which is low impedance and uses low-voltage (30–50 volts), high-power (30–50 watts) sustained (60–90 second) energy for the "ablation" of tissues *without perforation*, requires significant electrical modifications to convert the generator into a high-impedance, high-voltage (150–180 volts), low-power (3–5 watts) and short-duration (1–2 second) energy generator, which is necessary for "perforation".

The special BMC Radio Frequency Perforation System™ (Baylis Medical Co. Inc., Montreal, Canada) is a generator that is designed and dedicated specially for "perforation". The generator now is available commercially (even in the US) and is reasonably priced. This generator has built into it the necessary high-voltage, low-power and short-duration pulses of energy that are necessary to generate the high impedance necessary for perforation. A single use RF perforating "catheter" matched to the RF generator along with an "injection" coaxial catheter and a connecting cable are available as "perforating kits" to be used with the specific RF generator. The total RF generator and the "catheter kit" are approved for "intravascular perforation", even in the United States.

The disposable "kit" consists of the Nykanen Radio Frequency Perforation Catheter™ and a special Coaxial Injectable Catheter™ (Baylis Medical Co. Inc., Montreal, Canada). The "perforation catheter" is a 0.024", 265 cm long, teflon "catheter" tightly bound over a 0.016" conductance *wire*. Only the distal 1.5 mm and several mm of the proximal bare wire are exposed. The teflon over the wire provides an insulated coating to the wire and produces a relatively stiff, "pushable" shaft for the combination. The distal region of the "catheter" is flexible and can be bent or pre-formed into a specific curve for easier maneuverability. This allows the perforating "catheter" to be maneuvered similarly to a fine torque-controlled guide wire. The proximal end of the teflon "catheter" has no "hub" but attaches to a removable connecting cable, which, in turn connects it to the generator. The "coaxial injectable catheters" are thin walled 0.035" or 0.038" diameter, 145 cm long catheters with a distal radio-opaque marker and a floppy, distal 10 cm tip. The inner diameters of the two catheters are 0.024" and 0.027", respectively. These catheters also have removable hubs so that the coaxial catheter and the contained perforation catheter together can act as a "thick guide wire" *over which* other catheters (balloon catheters) can be introduced.

Technique for perforation of the pulmonary valve in patients with pulmonary atresia and intact ventricular septum

The diagnosis of pulmonary atresia with or without a ventricular septal defect usually is made clinically in the newborn period with confirmation by echocardiographic evaluation. By the time these infants are seen by a cardiologist, they usually already are receiving prostaglandin to keep the ductus arteriosus open, and this provide the infants with some pulmonary flow. Rarely infants with pulmonary atresia and intact ventricular septum arrive in the catheterization laboratory at several months of age, having had a naturally persistent ductus arteriosus and/or a previously created systemic to pulmonary artery surgical shunt as palliation. As opposed to patients with pulmonary atresia and an intact ventricular septum, patients with pulmonary valve atresia *and a ventricular septal defect* often have extensive systemic to pulmonary collateral flow to the lungs and/or, occasionally, a large persistent patent ductus arteriosus and, as a consequence, these patients can survive to an older age with no prior intervention.

A cardiac catheterization laboratory that has very high-quality, ***biplane*** X-ray imaging and angulation capabilities for the X-ray tubes, is necessary for these perforation procedures. Because of the precarious nature of these infants, the extensive catheter manipulation required and the potential for inadvertent occlusion of the ductus arteriosus during the procedure, these infants are intubated and ventilated before starting the catheterization. Any patient in whom a purposeful perforation is considered, is type and cross-matched for one or two units of fresh whole blood. If the replacement of blood becomes necessary, the clotting factors as well as the oxygen carrying capacity of *whole blood* are desirable. When an RF perforation is anticipated, a large "grounding plate" is placed under the back of the patient at the very beginning of the procedure. The grounding plate is attached to the RF generator via the conductive cable as the patient is being positioned on the catheterization table. Percutaneous access to at least one femoral vein and a femoral artery is established.

In the catheterization laboratory, the diagnosis is confirmed and the details of the right ventricular and pulmonary artery anatomy are defined with selective biplane right ventricular (outflow tract!) and aortic angiography. The angiograms not only define the anatomy of the valve, but demonstrate any right ventricular to coronary artery fistulae in patients with pulmonary atresia with an intact ventricular septum. In these patients, who usually do have a good pulmonary artery in the presence of coronary artery to RV fistulae, a right ventricular (RV) dependent coronary circulation *must be excluded* before valve perforation is considered. The laser or RF techniques for valve perforation also are used in patients with pulmonary atresia and a ventricular septal defect, but only when there is a well-developed main pulmonary artery and the RF catheter/wire or laser wire, which is advanced from the ventricle, can be advanced *into* the right ventricular infundibulum and supported exactly at and against the "valve" area. Whether using laser (which has only recently become available in the US) or RF energy, the techniques for pulmonary valve perforation are similar.

Radio-frequency perforation of the pulmonary valve from the right ventricular approach in patients with pulmonary atresia and intact ventricular septum

The technique for pulmonary valve perforation using the radio-frequency perforating system, which is designed specifically for RF tissue perforation and is available around the world (even in the United States), is described in detail in this chapter. In addition to quality, biplane angiograms in the right ventricular outflow tract, a biplane angiogram of the main pulmonary artery is necessary to visualize the valve annulus from the pulmonary side. It is desirable to position a catheter in the main pulmonary artery against the pulmonary side of the atretic pulmonary valve. The catheter in the pulmonary artery is introduced retrograde and passed into the pulmonary artery through either the patent ductus arteriosus or a previously placed shunt. The ductus in the newborn, and particularly when the infant is on prostaglandins, is very "mushy", friable and often tortuous. Force never should be used in crossing the ductus. If the ductus cannot be crossed readily and almost inadvertently, a biplane aortogram is performed in the descending aorta with the injection of contrast immediately adjacent and/or slightly distal to the aortic end of the ductus. This aortogram will determine the exact course of the ductus and will define the pulmonary artery/pulmonary valve more precisely. Occasionally, even with the course of the ductus clearly defined, it is necessary first to cross the ductus with a small, soft tipped, torque-controlled wire and then to advance a multipurpose angiographic catheter over this wire into the pulmonary artery. The catheter itself in the pulmonary artery serves as a constant "target" during the perforation from the right ventricle, and is used for repeated angiography in the pulmonary artery during the perforation.

If a catheter cannot be placed in the pulmonary artery, at the very least there must be some capability of obtaining *repeated*, good quality, *biplane* angiographic imaging of the main pulmonary artery/pulmonary valve. When the pulmonary artery cannot be entered reasonably, the pulmonary artery imaging is obtained from the contrast injected in the aorta and the flow through the ductus, through a previous shunt or through collaterals. The tip of the angiographic catheter for these injections in the aorta is maintained immediately adjacent to or actually in the origin of the vessel(s) providing the pulmonary flow in order that the maximum contrast reaches the pulmonary artery with each injection.

In the very rare instance where there is no demonstrable systemic to pulmonary artery flow, the biplane imaging of the pulmonary artery is obtained from a biplane pulmonary *vein* wedge angiocardiogram. This technique is satisfactory only if the main pulmonary artery can be visualized adequately and repeatedly by this technique. The use of repeated pulmonary vein wedge angiograms to visualize the pulmonary arteries requires the presence of an additional venous catheter situated in the vein wedge position throughout the entire perforation procedure.

Biplane "freeze frame" images from the right ventricular angiogram, which demonstrate the right ventricular outflow and the atretic pulmonary valve areas most satisfactorily, are displayed as "road maps" for the subsequent catheter positioning. After the pulmonary artery is visualized angiographically and/or the retrograde catheter is placed in the pulmonary artery adjacent to the pulmonary valve, a 4- or 5-French, pre-shaped "right coronary" or "cobra" guiding catheter is advanced into the right ventricle and manipulated very carefully and precisely into the right ventricular outflow tract (RVOT). This "guiding" catheter is maneuvered until it is against the center of the atretic valve in the right ventricular outflow tract. The specific guiding catheter that is used depends upon the size and, particularly, the right ventricular anatomy of each individual patient. The angle at the tip of the particular guiding catheter, which is positioned in the RVOT, should point the tip of the catheter directly at the other catheter in the pulmonary artery and/or at the center of the atretic valve *in both the PA and lateral views* as seen on previous angiograms. Several different shaped guiding catheters often must be tried in order to position the tip of the guiding catheter pointing precisely in the *exact* direction in *both X-ray planes*. As much time and effort is taken as is necessary to achieve this precise positioning before proceeding with the perforation. Any misalignment in either plane very likely will result in perforation out of the vascular channels and into the pericardium. When the right ventricular catheter tip appears to be in the ideal, proper position, a repeat, small, not too forceful, hand injected, biplane angiocardiogram is performed through this catheter. This angiogram demonstrates the outflow tract and valve even better and illustrates clearly any distortion to the area created by the catheter itself. When the tip of the catheter is aligned precisely, these images are displayed as the new "road map".

If none of the available pre-shaped guiding catheters can be positioned precisely in a direct line to, and against, the valve, the guiding catheter is withdrawn. The tip of the catheter is softened by immersing it in sterile, boiling water. Once softened, a different, more appropriate curve is formed at the tip. After reshaping the guiding catheter, it is reintroduced and positioned properly against the valve.

Alternatively or in addition, a Mullins™ deflector wire outside of the body is pre-shaped with very *smooth* curves to correspond to the desired course from the right atrium, to the right ventricle, to the right ventricular infundibulum and finally against the atretic valve. All of the bends on the wire are formed "tighter" than the existing curves through the right heart to allow for some straightening of the wire as it passes within the guiding catheter. When a Mullins™ wire is used to hold the guiding catheter tip in place, the guiding catheter must be at least one French size larger in order to accommodate both the Mullins™ wire and the perforating catheter side by side within the lumen of the guiding catheter.

The Mullins™ wire is introduced into the pre-shaped and previously positioned catheter through a Tuohy™/ side port back-bleed valve. The wire is advanced within the catheter to a position just *within* the distal tip of the catheter. The purpose of the Mullins™ wire is to redirect and maintain the guiding catheter in its position against, and pointing directly at, the *center* of the atretic valve while the perforating wire/catheter is introduced. Again, it is even more important that once this considerably stiffer combination is positioned against the valve a repeat small biplane angiogram is performed through the guiding catheter to demonstrate any further distortion of the area.

Once the catheters are in place, preferably on both sides of the valve, the RF perforation catheter, which has been advanced through the BMC coaxial catheter while they still are outside of the body, is introduced into the guiding catheter that is pre-positioned in the right ventricular outflow tract against the atretic valve. The perforating/ coaxial catheter is introduced through a wire back-bleed flush valve or a Tuohy™ side port adaptor attached to the hub of the guiding catheter. Otherwise, with the significantly larger lumen of the guiding catheter than the diameter of the perforating/coaxial catheter and with the high pressure in the right ventricle, there will be significant bleeding into and externally out of the catheter around the perforating catheter through the hub of the guiding catheter. The guiding catheter is cleared of blood by allowing it to bleed back passively through the Tuohy™ valve and then placed on a continuous flush. Any blood that remains in the catheter can clot, and potentially represents an embolus. The Tuohy™ type side port adaptor also allows contrast injections through the side port into the guiding catheter and around the perforating/coaxial catheters. If a Mullins™ wire is used to support the guiding catheter, a second Tuohy™ side port valve is "piggy-backed" onto the angled side port of the first Tuohy™. The R-F wire is passed through the first Tuohy™ adaptor, which is attached directly to the guide catheter. The Mullins™ wire is introduced through the second Tuohy™ valve, which is attached to the angled port of the first Tuohy™.

The perforating catheter, which is within the coaxial catheter, is advanced to the tip of the guiding catheter. An alternative technique in a small, very tight RVOT is to introduce only the "perforation catheter" into the guiding catheter without the covering coaxial catheter. The "perforating catheter" alone is more flexible and causes less displacement of the precisely positioned guiding catheter. In this circumstance, the coaxial catheter can be introduced and advanced over the perforating catheter *after* the valve has been perforated. Once the perforation catheter is in the RVOT at the tip of the pre-positioned guiding catheter, a repeat biplane angiogram of the RVOT/pulmonary valve is performed to verify that the catheter in the RVOT is still pointing exactly at the center of the pulmonary valve. If the tip of the guiding catheter is displaced at all away from the *center* of the atretic valve, the guiding catheter with the contained perforating catheter is readjusted by very slight torque and/or to-and-fro motion. The biplane angiogram is repeated to verify the exact relationships after any readjustment.

When the tip of the guiding catheter is in position and pointing in the precise direction, the proximal end of the wire of the perforation catheter is attached to the generator with the BMC™ connecting cable. The tip of the RF perforation catheter is advanced just barely out of the tip of the guiding catheter and *into the tissue* of the atretic valve. The flush on the side port of the catheter is stopped. The generator is set for a one second duration and 5 watts power. While continuously observing the tip of the perforating catheter on *biplane* stored fluoroscopy or slow frame rate *biplane* cine angiography, a single burst of RF energy is delivered while simultaneously holding, but not advancing, the tip of the perforating catheter against the valve. Usually this is sufficient for the perforating catheter to pass through the valve into the pulmonary artery. If not, the positioning of the guide and perforating catheter tips is rechecked on biplane fluoroscopy. If the positions are still not ideal, the perforating catheter is withdrawn within the tip of the guiding catheter while the guiding catheter repositioned. When the guiding catheter is in the exact position, the perforating catheter tip is re-advanced into the valve tissues. When both catheters are in the precise position, the RF energy is reapplied to the perforating catheter while again holding the tip of the perforating catheter *against* the valve without pushing forcefully. This process is repeated until the perforating catheter advances through the valve "plate" and into a "free" position within the pulmonary artery just beyond the valve while no energy is being applied. Any advancing of the tip of the perforating catheter within the pulmonary artery must be with no energy applied, as any RF energy applied to the tip will allow the tip to perforate any structure (wall!) in its vicinity! The exact position of the tip of the perforating catheter in the pulmonary artery is verified with a biplane pulmonary artery angiogram before proceeding further.

Once the tip of the perforating catheter has entered the pulmonary artery freely, the perforating catheter is advanced *with no energy applied* as far as possible distally into the branch pulmonary artery or through the patent ductus into the descending aorta. When the perforating catheter is *well into* the pulmonary artery or the descending aorta, the coaxial catheter is advanced over the perforating catheter to the tip of the perforating catheter. The subsequent maneuvers depend upon the associated anatomy and the position of the perforating/coaxial catheters after they are advanced following the perforation.

If the perforating/coaxial catheters pass into the descending aorta, together they are snared there with a snare catheter, which is introduced retrograde from the femoral artery. With traction held on the perforating/coaxial catheter with the snare catheter, the guide catheter is removed from the femoral vein over the combined perforating/coaxial catheter and replaced with a 2–4 mm diameter low-profile dilation balloon. When passed over the combined perforating/coaxial catheter, this requires a balloon catheter with a catheter lumen that will accommodate a 0.035″ guide wire. An alternative technique, when the perforating/coaxial catheters pass into the descending aorta, is to withdraw the perforating catheter from the coaxial catheter and exchange it for a stiff 0.014″ or 0.016″ exchange length "coronary" guide wire. This exchange of the perforating catheter for wire is performed while the guiding catheter still is in position in the RVOT and the snare is around and gripping the *coaxial catheter* loosely. If the coaxial catheter begins to withdraw or buckle while the new, stiffer wire is introduced into it, the distal end of the coaxial catheter is grasped firmly with the snare in the descending aorta. This supports the passage of the stiffer exchange guide wire through the relatively flimsy coaxial catheter as it passes through the tortuous course from the inferior vena cava through the right heart, pulmonary artery and ductus to the descending aorta.

Once the stiffer, smaller exchange wire emerges from the tip of the coaxial catheter in the descending aorta, this *wire* alone is grasped securely with the retrograde snare. The snared distal end is withdrawn into the femoral area or even out through the femoral artery sheath. Either way, a very secure "through-and-through" or "rail" wire system is created. The coaxial and the guiding catheters are removed over the fixed wire. The through-and-through wire allows simultaneous strong traction from the two ends of the wire which, in turn, allows a very forceful forward push on the balloon dilation catheter without the catheter and/or the wire buckling in the right ventricle as the balloon passes through the tight valve. With the traction applied at both ends of the exchange wire, the very low profile 2–4 mm diameter coronary balloon is passed over the wire and advanced through the "plate" of the pulmonary valve to initiate a sequential dilation of the valve.

After the dilation with the initial, small coronary balloon, the balloon is exchanged over the same "rail" wire for a larger dilating balloon. Dilation balloons of progressively increasing size are used until a balloon that is appropriate in diameter for a single balloon pulmonary valve dilation of the particular valve annulus can be introduced.

An alternative technique, which can be used when there is a patent ductus that can be traversed easily, is to position a retrograde snare catheter instead of an angiographic catheter in the pulmonary artery before and during the actual perforation of the valve. Instead of maneuvering the original retrograde angiographic catheter into the pulmonary artery, a 4-French Microvena™ snare catheter is passed retrograde through the patent ductus into the pulmonary artery. The standard snare catheter often is easier and safer to position in the pulmonary artery than an angiographic catheter. A floppy, soft tipped, torque-controlled wire is advanced totally atraumatically from the aorta through the ductus and against the atretic pulmonary valve. The end-hole snare catheter then advances easily over this previously positioned wire. A small 5 or 10 mm diameter snare (depending upon the diameter of the pulmonary annulus) is opened in the annulus of the pulmonary valve on the main pulmonary artery side of the valve. The properly sized snare aligns perpendicular to the long axis of the pulmonary artery, around and outlining the *circumference* of the valve annulus. The "circle" of the snare serves as a very clear "target" for the perforation with the RF catheter. As soon as the RF catheter with the coaxial catheter has advanced through the valve tissue, the perforating catheter also will be through the loop of the snare in the pulmonary artery! If there is any difficulty passing the coaxial catheter along with the RF perforating catheter through the new "puncture", the RF perforating catheter alone can be advanced through the valve and grasped with the snare. Once the RF catheter is snared securely, traction is placed on the RF catheter and the coaxial catheter is drawn into the descending aorta with the snare. Either the coaxial catheter or a balloon dilation catheter is advanced over this fixed RF catheter and through the valve as described previously.

If a retrograde angiographic catheter is positioned from the aorta, through the ductus and into the pulmonary artery, and the perforating catheter is *not* manipulated on its own from the pulmonary artery through the ductus into the descending aorta after the perforation of the valve, the retrograde angiographic catheter in the pulmonary artery is replaced with a snare catheter. Again, because of the frequent tortuosity and "mushy" nature of the ductus in these patients, the ductus is crossed with a very soft tipped torque wire and the snare catheter is advanced through the ductus over this wire. Once the snare is open in the main pulmonary artery, the perforating wire/catheter almost automatically will be *through* the loop of the snare! The perforating catheter is grasped with the snare in the pulmonary artery and withdrawn into the descending aorta through the ductus, as described above.

The worst-case scenario is when there is no patent ductus, or when present, the ductus cannot be crossed from either direction. In that case, the perforating catheter, immediately after perforating the valve, is manipulated as far as possible into a *distal* right or left branch pulmonary artery. With the guiding catheter still positioned in the RVOT and forced against the pulmonary valve over the perforating catheter, the coaxial catheter is advanced over the perforating catheter, through the valve and to the tip of the perforating catheter/wire. With the guiding and coaxial catheters *both* fixed in these positions, the perforating catheter/wire is withdrawn carefully and replaced with a 0.014–0.018" (depending upon which coronary dilation balloons are available) stiff, exchange length, "coronary" guide wire. The guide wire is advanced out of the tip of the coaxial catheter until the long floppy tip of the guide wire is "balled up" *completely* in a distal pulmonary artery branch. This "wadding up" of the floppy tip is essential in order to ensure that the *stiff portion* of the guide wire will be across the valve and well out *into* the *branch* pulmonary artery.

Once the stiffer exchange guide wire is in this secure position in the distal pulmonary artery, the guide catheter and then the coaxial catheter are removed over the guide wire and replaced with a *very low-profile*, 2–3 mm diameter, "coronary" dilation balloon. Occasionally, even the very low-profile balloon will not follow over the wire through the thick valve tissue. In that circumstance, the balloon is withdrawn over the wire and replaced with a larger guiding catheter that can accommodate the low-profile balloon. The guiding catheter is manipulated very gingerly over the wire through the right ventricle and up against the pulmonary valve. With the guiding catheter as an additional support, the low-profile balloon is passed over the wire, through the guiding catheter and through the valve.

The sequential dilation of the valve is started over this wire. Once the "waist" in the initial balloon has been eliminated, the balloon is removed over the wire and replaced with a slightly larger, 3–5 mm balloon. The balloons are replaced sequentially until a balloon is introduced that is appropriate in size for a single-balloon valve dilation, according to the annulus diameter of the pulmonary valve. Occasionally, the initial smaller wire must be exchanged for a larger and stiffer wire to support the larger balloons, which will not pass through the *guiding catheter*.

Laser technique for perforation of the pulmonary valve in pulmonary atresia with intact ventricular septum—from the right ventricular approach

Excimer Laser™ energy has been used for the perforation of the atretic pulmonary valve outside of the United States for over a decade, but the lack of a small laser catheter approved by the US FDA precluded its use in the US until recently[6,7]. The Excimer Laser uses ultraviolet light with a wavelength of 308 nm to ablate tissues in the path of the laser light. The laser energy is generated with a VCX-300 Excimer Laser System (Spectranetics, Colorado Springs, CO), which often is available in an interventional catheterization laboratory for laser lead extractions. The recent approval by the US FDA of the Point 9™ Extreme Excimer Laser catheter (Spectranetics, Colorado Springs, CO) for the treatment of total occlusions of peripheral and coronary arteries in humans has made this very small laser catheter available for use for selected congenital lesions in the US. The Point 9™ Laser catheter is a 0.9 mm diameter, fairly flexible catheter, consisting of multiple layers of optical fiber strands, which run the length of the catheter and through which the laser energy is delivered. The bundled fibers surround an open lumen, which accepts a 0.014″ wire.

The Point 9™ Laser catheter is advanced to the atretic pulmonary valve through a pre-positioned guiding catheter that has a *lumen* of at least 1 mm (3-French) diameter. The specific guide catheter that is optimal for the particular patient varies with the size and anatomy of each individual patient. The guide catheter should have preformed curves at the distal end that correspond to the course from the inflow to the outflow of the particular right ventricle. The guide catheter is maneuvered into the narrow outflow tract of the right ventricle to a position as close to the center of the "plate" of the atretic valve as possible. The Point 9™ Laser catheter is delivered over a stiff 0.014″ guide wire with a fine floppy tip as well as through the guiding catheter. The floppy tip of the guide wire extends beyond the tip of the laser catheter and often loops back on itself in the right ventricular outflow tract as the Point 9™ catheter is maneuvered to the atretic valve. As the tip of the Point 9™ catheter approaches the valve, the wire is withdrawn into the laser catheter.

Once positioned against the "plate" of the valve, 45 microJoules, at 15 kV and 25 Hz, of laser energy are delivered through the catheter in one second bursts. The tip of the catheter usually passes through the atretic tissue with 1 or 2 bursts of energy with each burst penetrating approximately 100 microns. If there is *any* forward push applied to the catheter during the delivery of the energy, the laser catheter will continue through any tissue in front of it including out of the vascular space! Once the tip of the laser catheter has advanced through the atretic tissue into the main pulmonary artery, the guide wire is advanced out of the catheter and preferably into the descending aorta through the ductus. Once the wire is successfully through the "valve" the remainder of the procedure is identical to the procedure using RF energy.

Laser energy has the disadvantages of requiring a large and expensive generator, which may not be available in all congenital heart catheterization laboratories, and the potential of retinal injury to surrounding personnel from the "scatter" of the high-intensity ultraviolet light. Until more experience shows a distinct advantage of laser over RF energy, the RF systems now appear preferable for pulmonary valve perforation in congenital heart lesions.

Technique for perforation of the pulmonary valve in pulmonary atresia with intact ventricular septum retrograde through the patent ductus from the pulmonary arterial approach

When there is significant difficulty or even the absolute impossibility of positioning the guiding catheter properly in the right ventricular outflow tract (RVOT) and/or there also is an easily crossed patent ductus, the perforation of the pulmonary valve in patients with pulmonary atresia with intact ventricular septum can be performed from the pulmonary artery side of the valve using a retrograde approach through the ductus[9]. Before the availability of the current and safer "burning" techniques to perform the perforation, stiff wires in association with the use of "brute force" had been used to push through the atretic pulmonary valves into the right ventricular outflow tract from the pulmonary artery approach. Because the "target" area of the right ventricular outflow tract is small and very narrow, the strong force (push), which necessarily had to be applied to the retrograde catheter, could easily displace the direction of the catheter tip with the result that this technique had a very high likelihood of perforation into the pericardium instead of into the right ventricle. The retrograde perforation of the pulmonary valve is far more reasonable with the availability of RF wires and RF energy for the perforation.

When the guiding catheter cannot be positioned in the RVOT with the tip of the catheter directed *precisely* at the valve in *both* X-ray planes, the retrograde approach for perforating the valve should be considered. The retrograde perforation still requires that a catheter is positioned in the RVOT for the purpose of performing selective biplane angiography even if the catheter cannot be directed precisely at the valve. The RVOT must be visualized very clearly, precisely and repeatedly with biplane imaging during a retrograde perforation. The right ventricular outflow tract usually tapers to a very fine tip or point just below the atretic valve. As a consequence, the RVOT presents a much smaller "target" when perforating from the pulmonary artery toward the RVOT.

With a prograde venous catheter positioned in the RVOT, a Swan™ floating balloon catheter (Arrow International Inc., Reading, PA) is introduced retrograde into the femoral artery and advanced retrograde through the patent ductus and into the pulmonary artery with or without a pre-positioned floppy tipped wire through the ductus. With some retrograde "push" applied to the Swan™ catheter, the balloon is inflated in the main pulmonary artery directly in the pulmonary valve annulus and against the atretic valve. The inflated balloon in conjunction with the usual course through the ductus usually orients the lumen of the Swan™ catheter parallel to the long axis of the pulmonary artery and also often points the end hole of the Swan™ catheter directly toward the blind RVOT. The precise direction of the tip of the catheter that is seated in the atretic pulmonary valve is changed in order to point the lumen exactly toward the RVOT by varying the amount of "push" and/or torque on the Swan™ catheter. When the tip of the Swan™ catheter is pointing in the exact direction, the RF perforating wire/catheter is advanced through the Swan™ catheter to its tip, until the RF perforating wire is positioned against the atretic pulmonary valve. The relative relationships of the tip of the Swan™ and the RF catheter to the RVOT are verified with a small selective biplane angiocardiogram in the RVOT. The angle of the Swan™ catheter/perforating catheter together also can be adjusted slightly by minimal to-and-fro motion on the shaft of the Swan™ catheter while the perforating catheter is passing through it. When the tip of the Swan™ catheter/perforating wire/catheter is "aimed" *exactly* at the small, blind RVOT, the RF perforating wire/catheter is advanced until the tip of the wire is embedded in the "valve" tissue. The position is rechecked with a repeat small selective biplane angiocardiogram in the RVOT, and adjustments to align the Swan™ catheter again are made as necessary. Since the RVOT "target" is so small, perforation from the retrograde approach is not attempted unless the perforating wire/catheter tip and the narrow RVOT are aligned ***exactly***. When the RF perforating wire/catheter is pointing *precisely* at the RVOT, and only then, is the RF energy applied while the perforating wire/catheter is held in the valve adjacent to the small RVOT.

Instead of the retrograde Swan™ catheter, a preformed, end-hole only catheter can be used for the retrograde perforation. The tip of a non-Swan™ type catheter is harder to keep exactly aligned in the *center* of the pulmonary valve on the pulmonary side of the atretic valve. This can be accomplished eventually with patience and often multiple exchanges of catheters with different curves at the tip.

Once the perforation wire/catheter is through the atretic pulmonary valve and free in the RVOT, a 5 or 10 mm Microvena™ snare wire is introduced through the catheter in the RVOT and the tip of the perforating wire/catheter snared in that location. Occasionally, in very small infants, only the perforating wire without the covering "coaxial catheter" can be passed through the lumen of a small Swan™ catheter. In that circumstance the RF perforating wire alone is advanced through the valve after the perforation and grasped with the snare in the RVOT. If possible, the snared wire and/or catheter is withdrawn through the ventricle and tricuspid valve and exteriorized through the femoral vein but, once the perforating wire/catheter is held securely, the Swan™ balloon catheter is withdrawn from the femoral artery over the proximal end of the perforating wire/catheter and is replaced over the perforating wire/catheter with either the coaxial catheter or a 4-French, multipurpose, end-hole catheter with a tapered tip. This step is unnecessary if the original retrograde catheter for the perforation was a non-Swan™ end-hole catheter. With traction held on the tip of the perforating wire/catheter in the right ventricle with the snare catheter, the coaxial or tapered end-hole catheter is advanced over the perforating wire/catheter, retrograde through the ductus and then push–pulled across the pulmonary valve using traction at both ends of the perforating wire/catheter. Once the end-hole, retrograde catheter is in the RV, the snare around the wire is loosened enough to allow the *catheter* to pass over the perforating wire/catheter and through the snare. The perforating wire/catheter is withdrawn out of the femoral artery catheter and replaced with a floppy tipped, exchange length wire. If necessary during this exchange, the snare is tightened over the end-hole catheter that is passing through the pulmonary valve to hold the catheter in place.

Snaring the distal end of the catheter in the RVOT supports the retrograde passage of the stiffer exchange wire through the ductus, the pulmonary artery, the perforated pulmonary valve and into the right ventricle.

Once the tip of the exchange wire is through the valve and in the right ventricle, the floppy tip of the *wire* is grasped in the right ventricle with the snare and the combination wire and catheter is pulled back, and very carefully through the tricuspid valve. Extra care is taken not to catch on the tricuspid valve structures and/or to pull too vigorously through the tricuspid valve. If the combination cannot be pulled *easily* through the valve, the snare is opened, releasing the grip on the wire. The retrograde *catheter* is withdrawn partially off the tip of the wire and back toward the pulmonary valve. The floppy tip of the wire alone is re-grasped with the snare, which is still within the right ventricle, and a repeat attempt is made to withdraw the snare catheter with the grasped retrograde wire back through the tricuspid valve and into the right atrium.

If the snare/wire still catches on the tricuspid valve, the wire is released from the snare and the snare loop withdrawn completely into the snare catheter. The snare catheter is withdrawn into the right atrium. A very careful attempt then is made at manipulating the retrograde catheter/wire, which is passing through the pulmonary valve, through the tricuspid valve and back into the right atrium. The catheter may "bind" in the thick, tight pulmonary valve structure and care must be taken to prevent it from buckling and pulling out of the recently perforated valve! If the wire is maneuvered to the right atrium, the tip of the wire is re-snared in the right atrium.

If the wire/catheter cannot be maneuvered back to the right atrium, the snare catheter is manipulated through a different area of the tricuspid valve and back into the right ventricle, and/or an end-hole Swan™ balloon catheter is introduced from the femoral vein and used to cross the tricuspid valve into the right ventricle from the right atrium and then the Swan™ catheter is used as the snare delivery catheter. When an inflated Swan™ balloon advances across the small tricuspid valve, there is a better chance that the balloon will pass through the largest orifice of the tricuspid valve, and the snare wire can be used through the Swan™ catheter. The small size of the hypoplastic tricuspid valve and/or the tricuspid valve regurgitation, however, may prevent a Swan™ balloon catheter from "floating" into the right ventricle.

Once the floppy tip of the wire is grasped with the snare in the right ventricle with either catheter that has passed through a different area of the tricuspid valve, the retrograde exchange wire is pulled carefully into the right atrium. From the right atrium, the exchange wire is exteriorized through the femoral vein sheath, creating a through-and-through femoral vein to femoral artery wire.

The remainder of the procedure is the same as when the perforation of the atretic pulmonary valve was from the prograde approach. Sequential dilations of the pulmonary valve are accomplished introducing the dilation balloons from the *femoral vein* over the through-and-through wire, as described previously.

Once the pulmonary valve is open and there is prograde access to the pulmonary artery, the necessity for further palliation of the patient in the catheterization laboratory during the same procedure is determined in the laboratory at that time. Following a perforation and dilation of the pulmonary valve in patients with pulmonary atresia and intact ventricular septum, there almost always is a question about the adequacy of the right ventricular volume and the need for a systemic to pulmonary shunt and/or an atrial septostomy. These patients usually were dependent upon the patent ductus for most of the pulmonary flow and all have an existing patent foramen ovale/atrial septal defect; however, usually one or both of these sources of blood flow is/are inadequate.

Once the infant stabilizes after the valve perforation/dilation and there *is* adequate pulmonary flow, then further clinical assessment determines the need for an atrial septostomy. In the presence of a very small right ventricular cavity and/or persistent very high right ventricular end diastolic and/or systolic pressures, the right ventricle often is not capable of accommodating an adequate diastolic volume from the systemic venous blood return. The resultant small right ventricular systolic volume then will be inadequate to provide enough forward blood flow through the lungs to the left heart to sustain an adequate systemic output. In the absence of an adequate opening or "vent" at the atrial level, the systemic venous blood pools in the systemic venous vascular bed and right atrium, the right atrium becomes massively dilated with the systemic venous return, and the cardiac output remains low. When this occurs acutely in the catheterization laboratory, a balloon or blade and balloon atrial septostomy is performed during the same catheterization.

At the same time, when the patient does have even a marginal systemic cardiac output without significant right atrial/hepatic congestion after the pulmonary valve perforation, atrial septostomy is not performed during the initial catheterization. Some elevation of the right atrial pressure may augment the right ventricular filling of these small ventricles. When an atrial septostomy is performed, it lowers the right atrial pressure, and in turn, may compromise right ventricular filling! By eliminating this extra filling pressure and volume, the potential growth of the right ventricle also may be compromised. The balloon or a blade/balloon atrial septostomy always can be performed hours, days or weeks later if the systemic output decreases and/or the right atrium and liver become distended.

In addition to the question of adequate return of the systemic venous blood to the systemic output, the adequacy of the net pulmonary flow is assessed before the infant leaves the catheterization laboratory. After the valve has been opened successfully, the adequacy of the forward flow through the opened valve, the effect of the pulmonary regurgitation on the net forward flow and how much of the pulmonary flow still is from the ductus are determined from the angiograms. If a catheter intervention to increase the pulmonary flow is even considered, a catheter is advanced either prograde or retrograde across the ductus, prostaglandin is stopped and the infant observed in the laboratory for 30 minutes or longer. When the ductus remains patent after the prostaglandin has been stopped, no further intervention is considered at that time. When the ductus patency and flow are prostaglandin dependent, the 30 minutes usually are sufficient time for the prostaglandin effect to wear off and for the ductus to close functionally. When the net prograde pulmonary flow is insufficient after the ductus closes, the infant will become significantly desaturated and/or hypoxic. The choices at that time are to restart prostaglandin and terminate the case with plans for a subsequent surgical shunt or to consider the implant of a stent in the patent ductus arteriosus as a means of establishing a more permanent systemic to pulmonary artery "shunt". With the newer, pre-mounted, flexible, small stents this is a much more viable option.

The technical details of the atrial septostomy procedures are discussed in Chapters 13 and 14 and the technique for stenting the patent ductus are discussed in Chapter 25. Until far more definitive data are available about which ventricles grow after the pulmonary valve is open and which patients have adequate pulmonary flow with the ductus closed, the decisions for further catheter intervention are "on-the-spot", somewhat arbitrary judgment decisions in the catheterization laboratory during each individual case, but usually some type of an augmented systemic to pulmonary shunt, if not an atrial septostomy, is required.

Perforation of the pulmonary valve in patients with pulmonary atresia and an associated ventricular septal defect

Hausdorf and associates extended the use of radiofrequency perforation of the plate-like pulmonary valve to perforation of the "muscular tract" between the right ventricular outflow tract (RVOT) and the main pulmonary artery for the attempted palliation of ten patients with pulmonary atresia and a ventricular septal defect[10]. The distance between the RVOT and the main pulmonary artery varied between 1.2 and 12 mm. Except for two newborns, their ten patients were much larger and older patients, some even years past the newborn period. All of the patients except the two newborns had either significant systemic to pulmonary collaterals or a surgically placed systemic to pulmonary artery shunt as their source of pulmonary artery blood flow.

Because patients with pulmonary atresia and a ventricular septal defect have either a very tortuous patent ductus arteriosus and/or present at a later age with no ductus arteriosus, perforation of the atretic pulmonary valve without the use of a through-and-through wire usually is necessary in these patients. Before being considered for valve perforation, patients with pulmonary atresia and a ventricular septal defect should have an adequate diameter, main pulmonary artery documented angiographically. This angiographic anatomy is obtained from biplane angiograms in the aorta adjacent to the "source" vessels for the pulmonary flow, from selective biplane injections into aortopulmonary collaterals, or even from biplane pulmonary vein wedge angiograms. The "indirect" angiographic pictures of the main pulmonary artery are stored as "road maps".

After the anatomy of the main pulmonary artery and its precise location are identified, an end-hole "guiding" catheter is pre-shaped to conform to the course from the right atrium to the right ventricular outflow tract (RVOT). This guiding catheter must be manipulated into the right ventricular infundibulum with the tip directed exactly in the direction of the pulmonary artery as visualized on the biplane "road maps". It may be possible to advance the tip of the guiding catheter only to the proximal, or inflow end, of the infundibulum. The RF perforating catheter is advanced through and out of the tip of the guiding catheter. With occasional good fortune or even luck, the very thin perforating catheter passes through the infundibulum until it is close to, or against, the area of a tiny atretic valve structure. When this occurs, the course through the traversed infundibulum tends to align the tip of the perforating catheter more directly at the center of the stump of the atretic main pulmonary artery segment. The position is verified with biplane angiography, injecting through the guiding or a separate venous catheter.

With the tip of the RF wire pushed against the atretic tissues and in the precise direction of the pulmonary artery as visualized in both PA and LAT X-ray planes, RF energy is applied for several seconds. The perforating wire is advanced in short steps toward the pulmonary artery *between* bursts of RF energy, and the RF energy re-applied. Very rarely, the RF perforating catheter is advanced in very short distances *during* the application of the energy while observing the course through the tissue *very carefully*. Once through the atretic tissues and into the pulmonary artery, the perforating catheter is advanced without energy applied to it into a distal pulmonary artery branch and distally as far as is possible. The tract of the RF wire from the RVOT to the pulmonary artery is examined carefully to verify that the wire is in the *center* of the muscular tract in both planes. The procedure then is similar to a pulmonary atresia with intact ventricular septum where the ductus arteriosus was not traversed, although maneuvering through the tract of RVOT tissue usually is even more difficult.

More often, in patients with pulmonary atresia and a ventricular septal defect, the perforating catheter/wire cannot be advanced beyond the tip of the guiding catheter positioned at the *proximal end* of the infundibulum. If, on *biplane* imaging, the guiding catheter is pointing directly toward, although still some distance away from, a pulmonary artery of an adequate diameter, the RF energy is utilized to perforate through the infundibulum, to the area of the "valve", and then through the remaining tissues into the pulmonary artery. This is performed with very short bursts of RF energy and small advances of the perforating catheter/wire between the applications of energy. Between each advance, the position of the perforating catheter/wire and its orientation toward the valve is rechecked with small, selective, hand injected, biplane angiograms in both planes of imaging and injecting through the guiding catheter or an adjacent venous catheter in the outflow tract. The attempted perforation is continued only as long as the perforating catheter/wire stays on a direct course to the valve and the patient exhibits no hemodynamic deterioration during the procedure. Once the valve is crossed, the wire positioning and dilation procedure are the same as previously described for pulmonary atresia with intact ventricular septum *without* a patent ductus. After the communication has been established and the tract partially dilated, usually the tract is maintained open with an intravascular stent.

Purposeful perforation of other vascular structures or total vessel obstructions

Pediatric and congenital catheterization laboratory interventionalists who are very comfortable with transseptal atrial puncture have extended the needle puncture technique of the transseptal procedure to the perforation of multiple other structures, some for diagnostic purposes and others in order to create permanent openings.

Puncture of surgically created interatrial baffles and/or patches were the logical extension of the standard atrial transseptal procedure. The venous approach usually is used, however, for baffles and some patches, the needle tip is positioned and directed very differently according to the orientation of the patch or baffle[11]. Usually, more force must be applied to the needle/transseptal set to penetrate the thicker structures of a baffle/patch. The extra force required increases the risk of the perforating needle continuing forward beyond or on the "other side" of the desired perforation into unwanted structures. The use of an RF perforating catheter through a special transseptal sheath/dilator set (Baylis Medical Co. Inc., Montreal, Canada) eliminates the extra force (and in turn, extra risk) necessary for these "transseptal" perforations. Unfortunately, RF perforation is not applicable through patches and/or baffles that are made of synthetic (non-tissue) materials.

In addition to the native atrial septum, patches in the interatrial septum and baffles within the atria, the transseptal needle and set are used to perforate and, in turn, re-cannulate totally occluded vascular channels. The transseptal needle requires a relatively straight line of access or "straight shot" from the site of catheter introduction to the site being "re-cannulated" in order to transmit the forward force from outside of the body, along the needle and to the needle tip at the puncture site. When forward force is applied within any significant, "non-contained" curve in the course of the needle, the force applied to the proximal needle causes the needle to "bow" proximally and, in turn, the forward force is dissipated into the curve rather than being delivered to the tip, and the direction of the tip is changed significantly.

Even with this limitation, the transseptal needle has been used successfully to puncture and rebuild long (5–6 cm!) total obstructions in multiple different vascular channels (*see* Chapter 24, "Venous Stents"). These include total obstructions in the native superior vena cava, the superior limbs of intracardiac venous baffles, totally disconnected right pulmonary arteries in postoperative "hemi-Fontan" patients[12], aortic coarctations with a discrete membranous interruption, and all varieties of ilio-femoral/IVC total venous obstruction[13]. The access for these punctures is from the femoral, jugular or hepatic vein approach depending upon the vessel, the location and orientation of the obstruction and which approach provides the *straightest* route to *and through* the obstruction.

The availability of the radio-frequency perforating systems has extended the possible sites of vascular obstruction that might be perforated and reconstituted. With the flexibility of the RF perforating catheter (wire), and since little or no forward "force" is required for the perforation, RF perforating catheters can traverse a very tortuous route to the site to be perforated. Perforating RF catheters (wires) readily pass around relatively acute curves and, in turn, can approach the area to be punctured from sharp or acute angles. The use of the RF wire allows the perforation of the atrial septum[14], atrial baffles and other vascular structures from a variety of venous access sites. As long as contact is *maintained* against the surface to be punctured by the RF perforating catheter, the RF energy will penetrate native tissues.

The usual interatrial septum is aligned parallel to, and even away from, a catheter that is introduced from the superior vena cava (SVC). The curved tip of a transseptal needle, even with an added curve formed on the shaft of the needle, often cannot engage the interatrial septum from a superior vena cava approach. Even when a very curved needle does "catch" on the septum from the SVC approach, the straight direction necessary to apply forward force to the tip of the needle for perforation is not possible. Using the RF perforation system, a pre-formed guiding catheter or special RF transseptal set with nearly a right angle curve at the tip can be introduced from the jugular vein/superior vena cava approach and then the catheter/set is rotated until the pre-formed curve at the tip of the catheter positions the tip against, and nearly perpendicular to, the interatrial septum. The RF perforation wire and coaxial catheter are advanced through the guiding catheter and just against the septum. The RF energy is applied as the RF perforation wire and coaxial catheter are advanced through the septum with virtually no force. Once the RF perforation wire and catheter are in the left atrium, they are exchanged through the coaxial catheter for a stiffer exchange length wire, and then whatever sheath/catheter system is desired.

Excimer Laser™ energy also has been used to perforate other totally occluded structures in addition to atretic pulmonary valves. In our institution, a very scarred-in distance of 5–6 mm between the side of the main/right pulmonary artery and the totally disconnected stump of the proximal left pulmonary artery was perforated successfully with a laser catheter on a compassionate use basis. The left pulmonary artery had been totally disconnected as a consequence of multiple prior surgeries. Both of the vessels were encased in dense scar tissue. The convex, cephalad and left side of the main/right pulmonary artery just at the origin of the right pulmonary artery was *parallel* to the side of the disconnected proximal LPA. The perforation was performed through the convex, left side of the main/right pulmonary artery, through scar tissue surrounding the walls of the two adjacent vessels and through the side and into the discontinuous LPA. After perforation, the tract between the two vessels could be dilated and an intravascular stent implanted in the channel to maintain the patency.

Laser energy has the advantage of greater perforating capability. The RF energy for perforation is more controllable and is readily available in more catheterization laboratories. The RF techniques now are used for almost all of the applications for which laser perforations previously were utilized in previous studies even outside of the United States.

The dedicated RF perforating system with the RF perforating catheter has extended the type and number of obstructed structures that can be opened or recommunicated in the catheterization laboratory. RF perforation already has been used to reconnect a chronic total left pulmonary artery obstruction[15]. In that patient, the distal left pulmonary artery became totally isolated four years earlier following an even earlier surgical patch repair of the artery. The intravascular course to the obstruction was the usual intracardiac tortuous course to a left pulmonary artery. The distal pulmonary artery beyond the obstruction was identified by pulmonary vein wedge angiography. The obstruction could not be crossed with any type of mechanical wire probing but was crossed with a 2-French RF catheter using 11 watts of power delivered for 11 seconds.

When a totally obstructed vascular structure is encountered, maximum information should be obtained about the length and course of the obstruction as well as the status and size of the chamber or vessel lumen that is open at both ends or on both sides of the obstruction. This information is acquired from magnetic resonance imaging *and* with biplane angiography before a perforation through the obstruction is considered. In branch pulmonary artery occlusions, information about the distal vessel is obtained angiographically from the flow into the obstructed vessel through shunts, systemic to pulmonary collaterals and/or from pulmonary vein wedge angiograms. The length and the course of the obstruction are "road mapped" and placed in the longest axis of the biplane review screens.

A guiding catheter is chosen which, when placed in the proximal end of the obstruction, aligns the tip of the catheter parallel to the long axis of the two discontinuous segments of the obstructed vessel. Changing the guiding catheter, changing the curve of the guiding catheter and/or the use of a Mullins™ wire within the guiding catheter adjacent to the RF perforating catheter are used to accomplish the *precise direction* of the guiding catheter. The RF perforating catheter is passed through the tip of the pre-positioned guiding catheter and engaged in the proximal end of the obstruction. The guiding catheter, the tip of the RF perforating catheter and the entire length of the obstruction are visualized in both X-ray planes with biplane fluoroscopy or biplane cine imaging while the RF energy is delivered to the RF catheter. The tip of the RF perforating catheter is advanced only between the applications of RF energy, and must follow a precise "road mapped" course through the obstructed area and toward the area of the previously visualized "lumen" at the other end of the obstruction.

If the RF perforating catheter begins to detour away from this precise course at all, the RF energy is not applied and the RF catheter is withdrawn. The "tract" created is visualized with a biplane angiogram performed with a *very small contrast injection* through the guiding catheter. This angiogram demonstrates any new and/or erroneous "tract" that has been created with the RF catheter. If the tract is precisely in line between the two portions of the vessel, the RF catheter is advanced back into the tract and the energy delivery repeated. If the newly created tract is angling away from the distal vessel but is not outside of the vessel, the guiding catheter is repositioned into the proper direction and the process restarted. If the new tract extended out of the vessel, extravasation of contrast will be seen. With a small amount of contained extravasation, the patient remains stable, particularly the post-operative patient, who usually will have extensive scarring around the vessel. In the presence of significant extravasation, the perforation attempt is abandoned at least temporarily. The area is observed intermittently on fluoroscopy for at least 30 minutes as long as the patient remains stable.

If the extravasation continues to increase, occlusion of the newly created tract with a micro coil is carried out. The fine delivery catheter for the micro coil is delivered directly into the tract through the already positioned guiding catheter. A small, "straight" micro occluding coil is used for the occlusion, as described in Chapter 26.

If there is no extension of the extravasation and/or once the extravasation is stable, the guiding catheter is repositioned to redirect the RF catheter in the more appropriate direction and the RF perforation restarted. As long as the patient remains clinically stable and there still is a desire to open the obstruction, the process is continued until the distal segment of the vessel is entered. Once the distal vessel is entered, the coaxial catheter is advanced over the RF perforating catheter and the RF perforating catheter is withdrawn. The position in the distal vessel is confirmed angiographically through the coaxial catheter. Once the position in the distal segment is verified, a stiff exchange guide wire is advanced through the coaxial catheter and positioned as far distally in the vessel as possible. The exchange guide wire must be *small* enough in diameter to accommodate a small "coronary" balloon dilation catheter. The newly created communicating tract is dilated sequentially as described previously. Once the perforated tract is enlarged to the diameter of the adjacent vessel, intravascular stents are implanted to maintain the new communication.

Recannulation of total venous occlusions

Acute total venous occlusion usually is a result of an acute thrombus formation in a vein that has sluggish flow and/or has been damaged by surgical or catheter intervention, including chronic indwelling intravenous catheters and infusions. Occlusions of small veins usually go unrecognized until access to the specific vein is desired at a later time. Acute occlusions of large, central veins present with the acute onset of venous congestion "upstream" from the obstruction. The most notable examples are the appearance of the "superior vena cava syndrome" with distention of the head, neck and arm veins and swelling of the head and face when the superior vena cava becomes obstructed, or lower extremity venous congestion and edema when the iliofemoral and/or inferior vena cava become(s) obstructed.

Venous occlusions usually involve very large thrombi and should be addressed when they occur (or are recognized) and very aggressively. The goal is to remove the thrombus along with the cause of thrombus if possible. The fresh venous thrombus is crossed with a standard guide and/or Terumo™ wire. If an indwelling venous line is in place, the line is removed. Once the thrombus is crossed, it is macerated and the debris from the maceration withdrawn with a mechanical thrombectomy device/catheter, as described in Chapter 12. Once the debris has been removed, any remaining clot is compressed against the vessel wall with an angioplasty balloon and/or intravascular stent. The balloon used should be the size of the unobstructed vein or the diameter of adjacent non-involved veins. If there is a discrete narrowing and/or narrowing of a surgical anastomosis in the vein as the source of the thrombus, the stenotic lesion is treated with dilation and the implant of an intravascular stent.

When not recognized and/or not treated acutely, venous thrombi result in permanent chronic venous occlusions. Even long, chronic, total occlusions of peripheral as well as central veins frequently can be traversed and recanalized using long needles and/or stiff wires in conjunction with finely tapered dilators, as described in Chapter 21. This is accomplished relatively blindly using "brute force" to penetrate through the obstructions. The perforation of the obstruction usually is directed by aiming for a catheter or wire that is positioned in the vessel at the opposite end of the obstruction.

It appears that the directional control of the Safe Steer Wire™ (Intraluminal Therapeutics Inc., Carlsbad, CA) combined with a radio frequency source of energy in the Safe Cross System™ (Intraluminal Therapeutics Inc., Carlsbad, CA) adds purposeful directional control to recannulations, while the RF energy produces a more controlled perforation and, as a unit, it reduces the "force" necessary to recanalize totally occluded vascular tracts[16]. The Safe Steer Wire™ uses optical coherence reflectometry to distinguish between thrombus and the viable tissues of the vascular wall in order to navigate the wire only within the limits of the vascular walls. The addition of radio-frequency energy delivered through the same "wire" provides the penetrating ability of the Safe Cross System™. The Safe Cross System™ has been used successfully for recanalization of totally occluded coronary arteries, totally occluded intravascular stents and totally occluded peripheral vessels[17].

Recently intravascular ultra sound (IVUS) has been added to the armamentarium to help identify the true lumen during the recanalization of totally occluded coronary arteries[18]. Both the Safe Cross System™ and the use of IVUS potentially could be used in the treatment of the vascular obstructions (both arterial and venous) that are encountered in pediatric and congenital heart patients and present exciting challenges for new developments in the pediatric/congenital cardiac catheterization laboratory.

Recannulation of total acute arterial occlusions

Acute occlusion of a femoral artery during, and/or immediately following, a retrograde arterial catheterization is not an uncommon complication of cardiac catheterization in pediatric and congenital heart patients. Arterial occlusions, like most other complications, are best treated by prevention. The meticulous handling of the arterial access sites to prevent complications is discussed in Chapter 4. However, particularly during interventional procedures that require the introduction of large sheaths and/or catheters into sometimes relatively small arteries, compromise of the artery may be inevitable. Occlusion of an artery may be manifest with any of a very wide spectrum of signs and symptoms. A totally obstructed artery can manifest as only a decreased pulse in the involved extremity, as decreased (or absent) capillary perfusion in the extremity, as an absent pulse with a cool and pale extremity or, in the worst case, as a cold, very pale and painful extremity. The latter, more extreme signs of obstruction obviously need immediate attention, while various degrees of urgency are applied to the treatment of the "lesser" signs of obstruction. When any degree of arterial compromise is recognized, it should be treated *at that time*. Usually, even decreased peripheral pulses in the involved extremity indicate an artery that is totally occluded by thrombus although, because of collateral flow around the obstruction, the totally occluded artery may not cause acute *symptoms*. Any arterial occlusion eventually may result in claudication, growth retardation of the extremity and/or loss of a potential access site for a future and essential intervention.

The initial management of an acute arterial occlusion is to continue or initiate treatment with intravenous heparin in therapeutic doses for one to two hours while observing the extremity closely. With return of the pulse/perfusion, the heparin is discontinued. If the pulse/perfusion does not return to normal and/or if there is *any* deterioration in the pulse/perfusion of the extremity, further more vigorous intervention is recommended. One alternative, more aggressive courses of management is to begin intravenous thrombolytic therapy with streptokinase, urokinase or rtPA, which is covered in Chapters 2 and 4. When the pulse and perfusion return with thrombolytic therapy, the thrombolytic infusion is stopped while continuing intravenous heparin for at least another 24 hours. The situation becomes more complicated when thrombolytic therapy is initiated but is not effective and/or there is progression of the signs of obstruction in spite of the thrombolytic. In that situation, surgical or catheter intervention is required. However, following the use of a thrombolytic, mechanical intervention can be very hazardous. This has led some centers to proceed with catheter recannulation of the artery immediately when the initial heparin therapy was not effective.

When mechanical intervention in the catheterization laboratory is instituted, heparin therapy is continued. In the infant and small child, the involved femoral artery can be approached with a catheter/wire introduced from the *venous* system, advanced prograde through the left heart, into the aorta, manipulated to the descending aorta and eventually, the involved artery. The entry into the left heart is through a pre-existing PFO/ASD or through a transseptal atrial puncture. The prograde approach allows the introduction of multiple and larger catheters and their use for longer periods of time without compromise of an additional artery. The prograde approach does hinder the precise control over the tip of the catheter/wire somewhat and requires the availability of very long exchange wires, and long diagnostic and balloon dilation catheters.

In larger adolescent and adult patients, the approach to the involved femoral artery is usually from the contralateral femoral artery or even from a brachial artery. The catheters and/or balloon dilation catheters used are much smaller relative to the vessel in the larger patient, and the turn into the contralateral femoral artery is less acute, making the manipulations from another introductory *artery* less traumatic in the larger patient. Also the available catheters and/or balloon dilation catheters often are not long enough to allow a prograde approach in the larger patient, where the catheter would have to extend from a femoral vein to the heart, loop through the left heart and then back to a femoral artery.

Whichever route is used, first an angiogram is obtained with an injection in the descending aorta proximal to the obstruction in order to identify the area of obstruction and to provide a "mirror image" view of the uninvolved, opposite iliofemoral arterial system as a representation of the normal vessel anatomy. With the lesion localized, an end-hole catheter is manipulated selectively into the involved vessel and a floppy tipped guide wire and/or a straight Terumo™ wire is used to probe through the fresh obstruction (clot ± spasm) as the catheter is advanced along with the wire. Once successfully probed, the catheter is replaced over the wire with an appropriately sized, low-profile, balloon angioplasty catheter. In the infant and small child coronary artery balloons are ideal in size and have very long catheter shafts. In smaller patients the initial catheter is replaced over the wire with the appropriate coronary balloon and/or the wire and catheter are replaced with a fixed wire, coronary angioplasty balloon catheter. The obstructed area is dilated to a diameter equal to the normal, comparative, ipsilateral vessel. A repeat small angiogram is performed to visualize the degree of opening and whether further repeat dilations are necessary. Once the lumen is open and flow established, the balloon and wires are removed. The patients are maintained on intravenous heparin for at least an additional 24 hours.

Complications of "purposeful perforations"

The purposeful perforation techniques are designed to do just that—perforate! The only, very slight, differences between the desired, purposeful perforation and an inadvertent, catastrophic, erroneous perforation are the meticulous attention to the details of the planned perforation, total awareness of the anatomy adjacent to the structure being perforated and the *very early* recognition of the *beginning* of an abnormal course of the perforating device. A purposeful perforation that goes astray completely usually results in a perforation of the external wall of a vascular structure into the pericardium, pleura and/or peritoneum and, as a consequence, results in a major adverse event.

Awareness, and, in turn, prevention are the best treatments of inadvertent perforations. Repeated *biplane* angiographic visualization of the anatomy, before and during the purposeful perforation, continually verifies the direction and location of the perforating device. Any deviation in the desired direction of the perforating device necessitates a redirection of the device or termination of the procedure.

When either the fine tip of a transseptal needle or the tip of a 2-French RF wire ***alone*** perforates through the wall of a vascular structure, an extremely small opening is created. These small perforations, if recognized and if nothing larger is pushed through the opening, often seal on their own. When an erroneous perforation occurs in a patient who has had previous surgery, the area almost always is encased in dense scar with no "space" for "extravasation" and, in turn, is "self sealing". In "native" (not previously operated) areas and/or when the pressure in the vascular structure that is perforated is very high (e.g. the right ventricle in pulmonary atresia with intact ventricular septum or the left atrium with severe mitral stenosis), sealing of the perforation usually does not occur, and certainly the perforation cannot be relied upon to seal on its own. The abnormal perforations also cannot seal if the abnormal course is not recognized and a larger catheter/dilator is advanced through the initial tiny erroneous opening.

When an abnormal perforation occurs, the surgical and anesthesia services are notified immediately of a pending emergency case. When extravasation continues through an erroneous perforation, the opening occasionally can be "tamponaded" by the inflation of a Swan™ or angioplasty type balloon within the vessel or chamber adjacent and/or proximal to the site of perforation. This can be accomplished only in vascular channels that are not the sole vascular supply to a vital structure. If available, a "covered stent" can be used to "cover the area" in the wall of a perforated vessel. When a small perforation is recognized while the perforating wire/needle is still in the opening, occasionally a micro coil can be used through a coaxial catheter over the wire/needle to occlude the perforation. Rarely one of the vascular occlusion devices (a coil, umbrella or an Amplatzer™ device) can be placed in the abnormal opening to seal a larger opening. Each unexpected perforation creates its own separate circumstances and should be anticipated before attempting a desired perforation.

Even as attempts are made to "tamponade" or occlude the leaking perforation, a blood infusion with the previously "typed and crossed" whole blood is started. The area into which the blood is draining (pericardium, pleura) is tapped and an adequate sized drain secured in the space. When significant blood loss continues, the withdrawn blood is returned to the patient by autotransfusion through a filtered blood administration set. The patient is prepared for surgical intervention as expediently as possible.

Another, somewhat rare complication during pulmonary valve perforations in newborn patients is the premature and unexpected closure of the ductus arteriosus due to the manipulations through the ductus during the procedure. When the ductus is the sole source of pulmonary blood flow, the closure of the ductus results in progressive hypoxemia and acidosis and can lead to death. The likelihood of spontaneous occlusion of the ductus occurring is reduced by minimizing the manipulations through the ductus, accurately maintaining and/or increasing the prostaglandin infusion to the patient, and maintaining the infant's fluid volume. In the event of a spontaneous closure of the ductus, the rate of the prostaglandin infusion is increased and an attempt is made to cross the ductus gently with a fine, floppy tipped guide wire. If the ductus can be crossed expediently with the wire, the implant of a stent in the ductus to maintain its patency should be considered. The definitive treatment once intractable ductus occlusion occurs, however, usually is an emergency surgical shunt.

Conclusion

As with all interventional therapeutic catheter procedures, the definite risks of each procedure must be weighed against the potential benefits of the procedure. Consideration of the alternative procedure should include the risks of the alternative procedure. Cardiac lesions undergoing purposeful catheter perforations are all very complex, and the alternative surgical procedures for these lesions all carry significant risks. The purposeful transcatheter perforation of most lesions in an experienced catheterization laboratory are more than justified and are considered as the first-line of therapy.

References

1. Ross J Jr, Braunwald E, and Morrow AG. Transseptal left atrial puncture; new technique for the measurement of left atrial pressure in man. *Am J Cardiol* 1959; **3**(5): 653–655.
2. Park SC *et al.* A new atrial septostomy technique. *Cathet Cardiovasc Diagn* 1975; **1**(2): 195–201.
3. Kan JS *et al.* Percutaneous transluminal balloon valvuloplasty for pulmonary valve stenosis. *Circulation* 1984; **69**: 554.
4. Latson LA. Nonsurgical treatment of a neonate with pulmonary atresia and intact ventricular septum by transcatheter puncture and balloon dilation of the atretic valve membrane. *Am J Cardiol* 1991; **68**(2): 277–279.
5. Parsons JM, Rees MR, and Gibbs JL. Percutaneous laser valvotomy with balloon dilatation of the pulmonary valve as primary treatment for pulmonary atresia. *Br Heart J* 1991; **66**(1): 36–38.
6. Qureshi SA *et al.* Transcatheter laser-assisted balloon pulmonary valve dilation in pulmonic valve atresia. *Am J Cardiol* 1991; **67**(5): 428–431.
7. Redington AN, Cullen S, and Rigby ML. Laser or radiofrequency pulmonary valvotomy in neonates with pulmonary atresia and intact ventricular septum—description of a new method avoiding arterial catheterization. *Cardiol Young* 1992; **2**: 387–390.
8. Rosenthal E *et al.* Radiofrequency-assisted balloon dilatation in patients with pulmonary valve atresia and an intact ventricular septum. *Br Heart J* 1993; **69**(4): 347–351.
9. Coe JY *et al.* Transaortic balloon valvoplasty of the pulmonary valve. *Am J Cardiol* 1996; **78**(1): 124–126.
10. Hausdorf G, Schneider M, and Lange P. Catheter creation of an open outflow tract in previously atretic right ventricular outflow tract associated with ventricular septal defect. *Am J Cardiol* 1993; **72**(3): 354–356.
11. El-Said HG *et al.* 18-year experience with transseptal procedures through baffles, conduits, and other intra-atrial patches. *Catheter Cardiovasc Interv* 2000; **50**(4): 434–439; discussion 440.
12. McMahon CJ, El-Said HG, and Mullins CE. Transcatheter creation of an atriopulmonary communication in the Hemi-Fontan or Glenn circulation. *Cardiol Young* 2002; **12**(2): 196–199.
13. Ing FF *et al.* Reconstruction of stenotic or occluded iliofemoral veins and inferior vena cava using intravascular stents: re-establishing access for future cardiac catheterization and cardiac surgery. *J Am Coll Cardiol* 2001; **37**(1): 251–257.
14. Justino H, Benson LN, and Nykanen DG. Transcatheter creation of an atrial septal defect using radiofrequency perforation. *Catheter Cardiovasc Interv* 2001; **54**(1): 83–87.
15. Fink C *et al.* Transcatheter recanalization of the left main pulmonary artery after four years of complete occlusion. *Catheter Cardiovasc Interv* 2001; **53**(1): 81–84.
16. Cordero H *et al.* Initial experience and safety in the treatment of chronic total occlusions with fiberoptic guidance technology: optical coherent reflectometry. *Catheter Cardiovasc Interv* 2001; **54**(2): 180–187.
17. Lee PY *et al.* Percutaneous recanalization of chronic subclavian artery occlusion using optical coherence reflectometry-guided radiofrequency ablation guidewire. *Catheter Cardiovasc Interv* 2003; **60**(4): 558–561.
18. Matsubara T *et al.* IVUS-guided wiring technique: promising approach for the chronic total occlusion. *Catheter Cardiovasc Interv* 2004; **61**(3): 381–386.

32 Special innovative or new, therapeutic catheterization procedures and devices

Percutaneous pulmonary valve implant

A transcatheter-delivered valve mounted within a stent and a technique for its delivery were devised and developed by Dr Philip Bonhoeffer in conjunction with Alan Tower of the NuMED™ Corporation[1]. The Bonhoeffer™ valve and technique introduce an exciting new era to the catheter treatment of congenital heart patients. Although not yet a "routine" procedure, this unique device and technique for the implant of a prosthetic valve into the right ventricular outflow tract/pulmonary artery have been demonstrated to be, not only doable, but an effective and safe procedure[2]. This technique should become an integral part of the armamentarium of the interventional cardiologist for use in congenital heart lesions.

There are a large number of patients with congenital heart disease who have very significant pulmonary valve regurgitation as a result of prior surgical and/or interventional procedures on the pulmonary valve and/or right ventricular outflow tract (RVOT). These prior procedures include all surgical patches/reconstructions of the RVOT, surgical ventricular to pulmonary artery conduits (including the RVOT in the Ross™ procedure), most, if not all, surgical pulmonary valvotomies and possibly even balloon dilation of the pulmonary valve—all regardless of the original underlying lesion. There is an increasing number of these patients who, over time, have developed severe right ventricular dilation and significant right ventricular failure as a consequence of the pulmonary valve regurgitation (with or without residual stenosis). The current standard therapy for these patients who have pulmonary valve regurgitation and significant right ventricular failure is the *surgical* implant and/or replacement of a *valved* conduit. Most of these patients already have had at least several prior major surgical procedures, and all of the valved conduits that are implanted have their own relatively short (relative to the life span of the patient) duration of functional competence. These factors make the prospect of repeat surgery even less palatable and the idea of replacing the valve at least once percutaneously during a cardiac catheterization, a very desirable alternative.

The Bonhoeffer™ valve is a glutaraldehyde-preserved valve, which is harvested from a bovine jugular vein and mounted within a Cheatham-Platinum™ (C-P™) stent (NuMED Inc., Hopkinton, NY). The stent/valve is mounted on a specially designed balloon dilation/delivery catheter (NuMED Inc., Hopkinton, NY) and is delivered percutaneously from a femoral vein puncture. The balloon delivery catheter is specially manufactured with a 16-French shaft and a 20 mm (or desired diameter less than 20 mm) BIB™ delivery balloon (NuMED Inc., Hopkinton, NY), a transparent, thin-walled, plastic "covering" sheath which extends from the shaft of the catheter over the entire catheter/balloon/stent/valve, and a special 18-French "carrot" dilator tip which is incorporated onto the tip of the delivery catheter just distal to the balloon.

The candidates for percutaneous valve replacement are large adolescent and adult patients with predominantly pulmonary valve regurgitation and a fixed diameter pulmonary valve annulus and/or RVOT. At the present time these valves are suitable only when the valve annulus/RVOT is *no larger* than 22 mm in diameter. The stent/valves are best suited for implant in previous RVOT *conduits*, which provide some length as well as the fixed diameter of the outflow tract. The valves can be implanted in smaller outflow tracts, however an attempt is made to dilate the stent/valve up to 18–20 mm in diameter in order to create the *optimal diameter* for the *function* of the valve within the stent and to accommodate the total cardiac output of most full grown adult patients. The presence of associated stenosis and/or calcification in the original valve/valve annulus do/does not, necessarily, represent a contraindication to the implant of a percutaneous pulmonary valve implant; however, any stenotic area where the valve is to be implanted always should be pre-dilated to within 2 mm of the proposed implant diameter of the valve in order to ensure that the percutaneous stent/valve can be expanded to its functional diameter.

Before the patient is even considered for a stent/valve implant, the area of the pulmonary annulus and the RVOT where the valve is to be implanted are imaged and measured *very accurately* using biplane angiography. The measurements for the seating of the stent/valve are very critical and are made using a very accurate and reliable calibration system for the measurements, as described in Chapter 11. Often, the angles of one or both of the X-ray tubes must be changed in order to orient the area of implant precisely on edge and to obtain the most accurate measurements of this area. At the same time, it usually is more "comfortable" and convenient to perform the valve implant in the straight PA and lateral views. If necessary, "road map" images are obtained in these views to be used for the implant in addition to the views used for the measurements.

Once the angiograms have been obtained, the measurements are verified and even before the stent/valve is opened from its sterile packaging, a 0.035" Super Stiff™ delivery wire with a short floppy tip (Medi-Tech, Boston Scientific, Natick, MA) is positioned as far distally as possible into a branch pulmonary artery. The wire must be positioned so that only the stiff portion of the wire remains positioned across the RVOT and that the wire is in a very secure and stable position. This Super Stiff™ wire must be able to support the passage of the large, stiff, delivery balloon/catheter on which the stent/valve is mounted through the often curved and/or circuitous course to the RVOT. Since these patients almost always have very large dilated right ventricles, marked pulmonary valve regurgitation and often tricuspid valve regurgitation, the manipulation of any catheter into a satisfactory distal pulmonary artery location for this positioning of the wire represents a significant challenge in each of these procedures. Any extra time spent in achieving a *very secure* position of the wire in a very distal branch pulmonary artery, is time well spent during the catheterization procedure. Once the wire is in place the catheter that was used for the delivery of the wire is left in place over the wire and kept on a slow continuous flush through a wire back-bleed valve to protect the ventricle and valve structures from the rough surface of the wire, to keep clots from forming on the wire, and to allow repositioning of the wire should it work its way backward while the stent/valve is being prepared. Although not essential, it simplifies the procedure to introduce a separate angiographic catheter from a separate vein and position it in the area of the proposed stent/valve implant. Although angiograms can be performed with injection through the protective sheath over the balloon/stent once it has been withdrawn off the balloon/stent/valve, these angiograms cannot be performed before the sheath is withdrawn, and the limited angiograms through the sheath and around the catheter never are as satisfactory as an angiogram obtained with a power injection through a separate catheter in the area.

Once the wire is in place, the packaged valve is opened, inspected and the valve is checked for its competency. The tissue valve comes mounted within a 40 mm long C-P™ stent. The stent/valve is packaged in the *dilated* configuration with the stent/valve opened to a 20 mm diameter. Before the stent/valve is used, it is washed sequentially four, or more, times, each time in a separate, fresh solution of normal saline or Ringer's lactate. During the wash, the valve function is tested. The stent is pulled longitudinally through the flush solution so that the solution enters one of the open ends of the stent. When the fluid enters from the distal (pulmonary artery) end of the stent, the flow of the fluid entering the stent closes the valve and should not allow the fluid to pass through it. When the stent/valve is filled with fluid and is held upright (vertically) with the *distal* end up, the fluid within the stent/valve is held within the stent/valve like a cup. When the stent is pulled through the fluid in the opposite direction (from proximal to distal), the fluid passing into the stent opens the valve completely and allows the fluid to flow freely through it.

Once the Super Stiff™ delivery wire is in place and the valve has been tested, the valve/stent is mounted on the delivery balloon/catheter. First, a separate, deflated, 8 or 10 mm diameter, 4 cm long, but very smooth, standard angioplasty balloon is passed gently through the fully expanded valve/stent from the proximal to the distal end and the balloon is inflated carefully, but to its designated diameter and pressure. The stent/valve then is compressed (crimped) circumferentially over the inflated balloon very carefully, in slow, sequential steps moving circumferentially around the stent until the stent with the contained valve is compressed fairly tightly over the 8 or 10 mm balloon. This balloon is deflated and *very carefully* withdrawn from the valve/stent. The withdrawal must be very meticulous in order not to catch the valve nor put any tension on the valve leaflets within the stent since the surface of the deflated balloon, which was previously inflated, will be rough and the balloon is being withdrawn *against* the opening direction of the valve mechanism. The large special balloon delivery catheter for the stent/valve then is introduced into the partially compressed stent/valve, paying very careful attention to inserting the tip of the balloon delivery catheter into the *proximal* (right ventricular) end of the stent/valve. As a "reminder", the stent valve has *blue* sutures around its *distal* (pulmonary artery) end to correspond to the "blue carrot" dilator tip of the introducer balloon/catheter.

The stent/valve is centered exactly over the BIB™ delivery balloon and again circumferentially and firmly but carefully, slowly and sequentially compressed and crimped over the deflated balloon. Once the stent/valve is compressed tightly on the balloon, the clear protective sheath is advanced off the more proximal shaft of the delivery catheter to cover the balloon/stent/valve. The initial introduction of the protective sheath over the proximal end of the stent is performed very meticulously with manual compression of the tip of each of the struts of the stent in order to be sure that each separate tip passes inside of the protective sheath as it is advanced onto the stent. The protective sheath is advanced until it abuts the *proximal* end of the "carrot" dilator tip. The valve/stent then is ready for introduction and delivery. There are two separate marks on the shaft of the catheter, which correspond to the two separate positions of the proximal end of the protective sheath when the tip of the sheath is entirely over, or withdrawn completely off the stent/valve. These marks are embedded in the walls at the proximal end of the shaft of the delivery catheter. The protective sheath is not radio-opaque, so these marks represent the only way of verifying the position of the protective sheath in relation to the stent/valve.

The catheter that was utilized for positioning the wire and the short introductory sheath are removed over the wire, being very careful to maintain the wire in its secure distal position in the pulmonary artery. Once the short sheath and catheter are removed, the skin incision and subcutaneous tissues over the wire are enlarged enough to accommodate the circumference of a *22-French system* over the wire. The skin/subcutaneous tract/vein are predilated with a separate 22-French short dilator. A dilator that is larger than the delivery catheter is used to ensure the easy passage of the mounted stent/valve/balloon through the skin/subcutaneous tissues and the wall of the vein at the introductory site. The dilator is removed over the wire and the stent/valve on the special balloon delivery catheter is introduced over the wire and through the dilated tract. With careful observation of the tip and the course of the wire on fluoroscopy, the mounted stent/valve is advanced over the wire to the area of implant. This part of the procedure can be very difficult, as even the 0.035" Super Stiff™ wire may not support the stent/valve/balloon delivery catheter adequately. Advancing the catheter/stent/valve usually pushes the combination to the "outer circumference" of the curved path to the position in the outflow tract. Pushing the catheter/stent/valve a short distance over the wire and then alternately withdrawing the shaft of the wire an equally short distance (*without* allowing the tip of the wire to withdraw!) usually allows the catheter/stent/valve to be "inched" forward over the wire and into position.

Once the balloon/valve/stent has reached the area of implant, a biplane angiogram is performed and compared with the baseline, "road map" angiogram in the same views. Often the large and stiff catheter/stent/valve over the wire will change the relative position of structures in the area. Any necessary adjustments of the balloon/valve/stent position compared to the exact location for implant are made and then the protective sheath is withdrawn off the valve. The protective sheath is not visible on fluoroscopy, however its position is checked by the calibrated marks at the proximal end of the delivery catheter. After the protective sheath is withdrawn, a repeat angiogram is performed to ensure that the withdrawal of the sheath did not change the relative position of the balloon and stent in relation to the desired position for implant. When the stent appears to be in the precise, desired position and the measurements appear satisfactory, the inner balloon of the BIB™ dilation balloon is inflated. Once the inner balloon is inflated completely, the position in the annulus area is rechecked with a repeat angiogram, the position of the stent/valve adjusted, and the outer balloon inflated to fix the stent/valve in position. The BIB™ balloon is inflated at least one more time to ensure full dilation and fixation of the stent in the annulus.

Subsequent maneuvers depend upon the degree of "fixation" of the stent/valve in the annulus. A repeat angiogram is performed through the second catheter (or the protective sheath) to verify the location and fixation of the stent/valve. When the stent is fixed in a satisfactory position, the balloon/delivery catheter is withdrawn very carefully over the wire and out of the stent/valve. This is a very critical part of the procedure as the deflated BIB™ delivery balloon has a *very* rough and irregular surface and easily catches on the valve and/or the supporting stent. It frequently must be "teased" out of the stent/valve. It may be possible to re-advance the protective sheath at least partially over the balloon as the balloon is deflating within the stent/valve. Once over the balloon, the smooth surface of the sheath provides a separation between the rough balloon and the valve. When the original pulmonary/RVOT annulus was only a few mm smaller than the expanded diameter of the stent/valve, the withdrawal is even more precarious and must be performed very cautiously.

Once the delivery balloon/catheter has been withdrawn from the stent, the second angiographic catheter is manipulated gently through the stent/valve and a repeat pulmonary artery angiogram is recorded. If a second catheter is not utilized, the balloon/delivery catheter is withdrawn over the wire and replaced with an end-hole, multipurpose catheter or a Multi-track™ catheter (B. Braun Medical Inc., Bethlehem, PA), which then is re-advanced carefully through the valve to the pulmonary artery distal to the valve. Repeat hemodynamics are measured and a repeat pulmonary artery angiogram recorded with the injection of the contrast performed distal to the valve. If the stent/valve appears at all precarious in its freshly implanted position, the hemodynamic/anatomic assessment of the valve postimplant is performed by echo/Doppler interrogation only, without any attempt to cross the freshly implanted stent/valve with a catheter.

Annulus/outflow tract "reduction" with a "banded" self-expanding covered stent

In its present configuration, the Bonhoeffer™ stent/valve is suitable only for patients with a rigid, fixed diameter, outflow tract of 20 mm or less. To overcome this problem, a unique catheter-delivered self-expanding covered stent/internal band has been developed and tested in animals to percutaneously reduce the diameter of the widely dilated pulmonary artery/RVOT[3,4]. It has been tested with a self-contained bovine jugular vein valve and as an internal stent/band only device. The basis of this device is a self-expanding, covered, Nitinol™ stent, which has a central, open tubular portion of a fixed diameter and with both ends of the tubular device widely flared (AMF, Groupe Lepine, Lyon, France). The entire stent is covered with a 0.3 mm polytetrafluoroethylene (PTFE) membrane (Zeus Inc., Orangeburg, SC) to make the walls impervious. The central tubular portion creates a lumen with a fixed diameter of 18 mm while both of the distal ends "flare" away from the central portion and are capable of expanding up to 30 mm in diameter. The very wide diameter of the ends allows fixation of the stent/band into much larger diameter areas in an aneurysmal vessel/outflow tract. The expanded device has the appearance of a large "dumbbell" with a large lumen extending from end to end through its center. This configuration allows the creation of a circumferential band with a fixed lumen, which is the diameter of the central portion, while the expanded ends fix the stent/band into very large, aneurysmally dilated right ventricular outflow tracts/pulmonary arteries (RVOT/PA) and occlude flow from around the central lumen by the PTFE covering. This covered stent/band can be implanted either as only the tubular covered stent/band or can have a bovine jugular vein valve incorporated into the tubular portion of the central lumen for a "one-stage" outflow tract reduction–valve implant procedure.

Most patients with significant pulmonary regurgitation do have some remnant of the original and/or a tissue pulmonary valve, which may or may not be stenotic. Even in a markedly aneurysmal pulmonary artery/right ventricular outflow tract, when there is any residual stenosis of the outflow tract, the stenosis is pre-dilated before the implant of the stent/band with or without the incorporated bovine valve. The minimal diameter of the outflow tract must allow the full expansion of the valve segment of the stent/band device and the eventual valve.

When the stent/band is implanted with no incorporated valve, it creates a fixed, rigid diameter of the RVOT with a maximum diameter of 18 mm. This tubular "band" is ideal for the subsequent percutaneous implant of a Bonhoeffer™ stent/valve in its present configuration. The compressed stent/band is delivered percutaneously from the femoral vein, over a pre-positioned Super Stiff™ wire. The band portion of the self-expanding stent is centered in the area where the valve is to be implanted and the entire stent/band is extruded from the delivery sheath. As the stent/band is extruded, the ends flare to their predetermined wide diameters with the central area fixed at the diameter of the band. The wide diameters of the ends of the self-expanding stent fix the stent/band in place, while the central tubular area serves as an eventual site to fix a stent/valve. The covering of the flared ends of the stent funnel the entire flow through the lumen of the central, "banded" area. When the valve is implanted separately, the valved stent is delivered with the enclosed bovine valve and is implanted in this tubular portion of the stent/band approximately two months after the "stent/band" was placed.

Percutaneous valve implant in the aortic position

The bovine jugular vein valve mounted within a stent also provides the possibility for a "percutaneous" aortic valve replacement. This concept has been tried in animals and performed at least once in a human[5–7]. The percutaneous aortic valves are mounted in much shorter and stronger stents. There still are problems in placing such a stent/valve in the aortic position, which are significantly greater than in the pulmonary position. The stent/valve implanted in the aortic root must not occlude the orifices of the coronary arteries. In most cases, particularly in the older adult patient, dilation of the aortic sinuses displaces the orifices of the coronary arteries far laterally and away from a stent placed in the aortic annulus. In addition to the problem of the coronary ostia, the very large stent/valve delivery system is introduced into an artery, which at the present size and configuration of the stent/valve requires a surgical cut-down on the femoral or even iliac artery. An alternative is the delivery of the stent-mounted valve prograde through a transseptal puncture, the mitral valve and the left ventricle. Although the larger delivery system can be introduced percutaneously into a vein, it then requires the extensive manipulation of the large and stiff delivery system/stent/valve through a circuitous course through the left heart. The aortic roots of patients with aortic regurgitation usually are markedly dilated and far larger in diameter than the currently available bovine or other tissue valves. At the same time the percutaneous aortic valve is placed within the thickened (calcified) original valve, which reduces the diameter significantly and allows a very secure implant.

In spite of the present obstacles, this concept for a transcatheter replacement of the aortic valve appears very promising for future developments.

Prospective catheterization laboratory completion of lateral tunnel/Fontan circuits

In spite of the lack of prospective and/or planned commercial development in this area, the most innovative uses of covered stents in humans to date have been in pediatric/congenital heart lesions. Covered stents were used to "rebuild" disrupted intra-atrial, venous channels/baffles in several complex patients with single ventricles who had undergone "Fontan" cavopulmonary type single ventricle repairs, and where the baffles and/or venous channels were disrupted and leaking significantly. Two very different types of covered stent were used initially for this purpose in two similar, very sick patients, and both under very extenuating circumstances. The covered stents were placed in disrupted lateral tunnel channels to percutaneously repair the "tunnels". The covered stents extended from the inferior vena cava, at the caudal end of the right atrium, through the area of the "true" right atrium and superiorly into the base of the caval–pulmonary anastomosis with the right pulmonary artery. In doing so the channels that were created with the covered stents directed all of the systemic venous flow from the inferior cava to the pulmonary arteries and eliminated all of the intra-atrial leaking[8].

With some collaborative cardiology–surgery "pre-planning" in prospective studies and with very little change in either the surgical or the catheterization procedure, the use of covered stents in "Fontan" patients is being extended to provide an elective final phase of the "Fontan completion" in the catheterization laboratory[9,10]. The "catheter completion" still requires further improvements in the design of the covered stents and a specifically "pre-planned" second stage, "bi-directional Glenn", using one of two different proposed methods.

When performing the bi-directional Glenn, the surgeon creates a contiguous "floor" or, at the most, a very small restrictive opening, between the caudal surface of the right pulmonary artery and the most cephalic "roof" of the right atrium. Ideally, the circumference of this "roof" and the orifice of the inferior vena cava into the right atrium both are outlined with opaque sutures to assist the later catheter steps in the procedure. A wide open interatrial communication (common atrium!) also must be ensured at the time of the bi-directional Glenn anastomosis. For the "completion" of the Fontan in the catheterization laboratory, the "roof/floor" of the right atrium/right pulmonary artery is punctured with a "transseptal" type puncture from either the right atrium into the pulmonary artery or from the superior vena cava/pulmonary artery into the right atrium, and the opening is dilated to a diameter 2–3 mm smaller than the diameter of the stent/graft which will be implanted. A channel is created from the inferior vena cava to the opening in the right pulmonary artery with a large, long, specifically manufactured, covered stent, which is implanted extending from the cephalic, newly created opening in the floor of the right pulmonary artery, through the cavity of the right atrium and caudally, well into the inferior vena cava. This creates a separate, confined inferior caval to pulmonary artery channel. This technique requires relatively little change in the "second-stage" surgical procedure, but is very challenging for the interventionist in the catheterization laboratory. The interposed covered stent must create a channel large enough in diameter to carry two thirds of the systemic venous blood flow and, after the "stent" shrinks in length during the implant, still be long enough to extend *exactly* from the IVC through the right atrium and into the pulmonary artery. An even greater challenge for this procedure is generated by the subsequent eventual *growth of the patients*. The new "tube graft" must be large enough in diameter to accommodate the increasing volume in blood flow and the growth of the patient and the patient's heart, in particular the *length* of the right atrium! The diameter of some stent grafts *may* be adjustable with subsequent balloon dilation, but the implant length is fixed—or possibly it could shrink—with further dilation of the stent that creates the channel!

An alternative technique requires an open-heart, surgical procedure on bypass by the surgeon with opening of the right atrium at the earlier "Glenn" stage, but currently makes the procedure more suitable for patients of all sizes and makes the final stage, which is performed in the catheterization laboratory by the interventionist, much more straightforward. During the surgical "bidirectional Glenn" stage of the procedure, the surgeon ensures that there is an adequate intra-atrial communication and then establishes the *complete* lateral tunnel, caval–pulmonary baffle within the right atrium, however, with *two very significant variations* from the standard lateral tunnel. First, a large (15–20 mm) window or "fenestration". Which communicates with the right atrium, is created in the medial wall of the baffle of the lateral tunnel. Secondly, the cephalad end of the newly created lateral tunnel is *attached* to the caudal surface of the *intact* right pulmonary artery, but *no opening or communication is made* between the right atrium/lateral tunnel and the pulmonary artery at the time of the bidirectional "Glenn" surgical procedure—i.e. the inferior vena cava/right atrial blood flow is *not* opened into the pulmonary artery and, as a consequence, the patients function as though they only have had the bidirectional Glenn anastomosis!

For the "completion" of the "Fontan" the interventional cardiologist in the catheterization laboratory punctures through the intact roof/floor between the right atrium and the right pulmonary artery, into the right pulmonary artery at the cephalad end of the lateral tunnel, dilates the tunnel to right pulmonary artery communication and implants a large diameter, but short stent (covered?) to widen the opening and to keep this newly created channel open. This stage of the procedure is performed from a percutaneous femoral venous approach. The large "fenestration" that the surgeon has created in the medial wall of the lateral tunnel is closed with a percutaneous atrial septal occlusion device! The advantage of this version of the "Fontan completion" would be that the native tissue of the "lateral tunnel" will grow in "diameter" to accommodate the patient's growth and increased blood flow with the growth. The partial native tissue lateral tunnel also has a better chance of accommodating the growth of the patient in "length" as occurs with the current lateral tunnel, cavopulmonary anastomoses.

The capability of having custom-designed, large, covered stents, which are made to fit specific lesions/patients, would make it conceivable to perform a conversion of a failed, classic, right atrial to pulmonary artery "Fontan" to a lateral tunnel cavopulmonary "Fontan" in the catheterization laboratory. These special covered stents could be modifications of the aortic "stent grafts", which already are used for the catheter treatment of aortic aneurysms[11]. The stent graft would have to be built to the specific dimensions of each individual patient (e.g. length of RA, diameter of IVC–RA junction and proposed SVC–PA diameters).

In the catheterization laboratory, first the original atrial septum/septal patch would require reopening widely in order to allow the coronary sinus blood to return back into the circulation once the "lateral tunnel" is completed. The cephalic end of the catheter-implanted, stent graft "lateral tunnel" could be implanted in the original direct right atrial to pulmonary artery connection or a puncture could be performed from the most cephalic portion of the stump of the right atrium through the bottom (caudal surface) of the *adjacent* right pulmonary artery and then the cephalic end of the custom "lateral tunnel" stent graft implanted directly into the pulmonary artery. The stent graft would form a tunnel through the right atrium between the inferior vena cava and the right pulmonary artery similar to the catheterization "completion" of the "Fontan" described above. If the cephalad end of the catheter-implanted "lateral tunnel" was *not* implanted through the original connection between the right atrium and pulmonary artery connection, then this original right atrial to pulmonary artery connection would be occluded separately with a catheter-delivered device. The superior vena cava still would need connecting to the pulmonary artery.

Once the cephalic end of the stent graft, which passes through the right atrium to the right pulmonary artery, was anchored into the right pulmonary artery, the superior vena cava still would have its native connection to the right atrium and be draining past the pulmonary artery, around and outside of the stent graft, with the result that the superior vena cava blood still would pass through the atrial septal defect into the systemic output. An additional puncture would be necessary from the superior vena cava into the top (cephalad surface) of the right pulmonary artery. A second, short, 18–20 mm diameter *covered* stent would be implanted in this communication, which would divert all of the superior vena caval blood into the pulmonary artery. Since the surrounding area would be so densely scarred from two previous cardiac surgeries (at least one systemic to pulmonary shunt and/or a "Glenn" plus the original "Fontan"), this extra vascular vessel-to-vessel puncture would not result in a significant extravasation of blood into the surrounding thorax. Although "catheterization revision" would represent a very extensive procedure in the catheterization laboratory, with the proper equipment, it should be very doable and still would be less of a procedure than the current surgical revision of a classic "Fontan".

Perforation of vessel walls with creation of a vessel-to-vessel communication and/or shunt

Dr Kurt Amplatz reported the possibility of percutaneously creating communications between native, vascular structures using a modification of the Nitinol™ mesh, Amplatzer™ occluders from a preliminary study in animals. Dr Chigogidze from the Bakuolev Scientific Center of Cardio-Vascular Surgery in Russia also has performed some animal work on the successful percutaneous creation in the cardiac catheterization laboratory of vascular shunts between adjacent major vascular structures. Communications were created between adjacent venous structures, the aorta and vena cava, the pulmonary artery and the superior vena cava and even between the aorta and a pulmonary artery. The minute details of the procedure are not available to this author, however, the general concept was presented and represents a very exciting development in the area of transcatheter therapy[12].

Tiny intravascular magneto-mechanical devices are placed in the adjacent vessels ostensibly to pull the vessels together and to direct a flexible "kinetic" needle as it punctures from one vessel to the other. Once the magnets are in place in the adjacent vessels, a puncture from one vessel into the adjacent vessel is performed with the special "kinetic" needle attached to a flexible wire. The exact mechanism of the needle puncture is unclear. Once the needle has entered the adjacent vessel, it is captured with a snare catheter and the needle with the attached wire is withdrawn through the peripheral entry site of this vessel. The exteriorization of this wire creates a through-and-through "rail" wire. A large sheath/dilator set is advanced over the wire and pulled through the new communication between the vessels. Presumably, the presence of the large sheath/dilator within the newly created openings in the walls of both of the vessels prevents exsanguination from the now large puncture sites in the walls of these vessels.

Once the sheath has passed through the puncture site into the adjacent vessel, the dilator is removed over the wire. A specially prepared, Nitinol™ *self-expanding*, covered, stent graft, which is flared widely at both ends, is implanted in the area between the two vessels by withdrawing the sheath off the stent graft. The Nitinol™ stent graft is covered with polyurethane and has a central diameter of the desired opening between the two vessels. Once implanted, the covered stent creates a channel between the two vessels while at the same time sealing the openings in the walls of the vessel.

Reportedly, vena cava to portal vein, superior vena cava to pulmonary artery and aorta to pulmonary artery communications all have been created successfully in animals! In addition, with an extension of this technique, a normal heart in an animal was converted to a completed "Fontan" circuit by the creation of: (1) a superior vena cava to right pulmonary artery communication with one stent graft (i.e. a "Glenn" shunt); (2) exclusion of the main pulmonary artery trunk and the pulmonary valve from the circulation by a covered stent which bridged across the main pulmonary artery from the right to the left pulmonary artery; and (3) the completion of the "Fontan atrial lateral tunnel" with a covered stent, which extended from the inferior vena cava and through the right atrium, connecting into the right pulmonary artery/superior vena caval channel. To date, these procedures have been performed only in animals, but the concept certainly is an exciting evolution into the immediate future of interventional cardiology.

Completion of the first stage "Norwood" procedure for hypoplastic left heart syndome in the catheterization laboratory

By the combination of implanting a stent in the ductus arteriosus to maintain its patency and the implant of "flow restrictors" in the proximal branch pulmonary arteries to reduce pulmonary artery flow and pressure, Drs Boucek and Chan in conjunction with AGA Medical Corporation (AGA Medical Corp., Golden Valley, MN) have developed a procedure for the initial palliation of patients with hypoplastic left heart syndrome entirely in the cardiac catheterization laboratory[13].

The special flow restricting devices (AGA Medical Corp., Golden Valley, MN) are very similar to the Amplatzer™ Intravascular Plugs (AGA Medical Corp., Golden Valley, MN), however the flow restrictors have holes of a specific diameter passing through the devices. After very accurate sizing of both the proximal right and left pulmonary arteries, flow restrictors that are several millimeters larger in diameter than each pulmonary artery are placed precisely in each proximal branch pulmonary artery. If the flow restrictor devices are undersized, they can migrate distally and/or change their orientation in the vessel and totally obstruct flow to the entire lung and/or a major branch. If the flow restrictor is too large for the particular vessel, the openings in the central portion of the device may not open entirely or sufficiently to allow any flow through the device.

Once the flow restrictors are placed in the separate right and left pulmonary arteries, the ductus arteriosus is stented with a self-expanding stent, which again, is several millimeters larger in diameter than the existing ductus. The stent also must be long enough to cover all of the ductal tissue, but at the same time not so long as to interfere with the pulmonary valve and/or compromise the entrance of the transverse aortic arch into the descending aorta at the area of the ductus. Presently, the Precise™ or Smart™ stents (Cordis Corp., Miami Lakes, FL) or the Protégé™ stents (ev3, Plymouth, MN) appear to be the most suitable for this use. The Protégé™ stents have the advantage of having a separate attach–release mechanism, which allows withdrawal or repositioning of the stent up until the moment of final deployment. Because of the limited lengths of these stents that are available, occasionally several stents must be overlapped in the ductus to cover all of the ductal tissue adequately.

At present, the flow restrictor devices are custom manufactured for the specific investigational study and are not available commercially. The procedure is technically very challenging in small sick hypoplastic left heart syndrome patients, however, certainly it is less traumatic than the comparable "standard" surgical "first stage Norwood" procedure. As the equipment is developed and improves, this innovative approach should replace the initial surgery for many (most) of these patients.

Radio-frequency tissue desiccation

Sigwart introduced the concept of "ablation" of an abnormal portion of the ventricular septum for the treatment of obstructive hypertrophic cardiomyopathy by the subselective infusion of alcohol into a septal perforating coronary artery[14]. The relief of the obstruction is accomplished by the purposeful creation of a *localized* myocardial infarction in the abnormal septal tissues. The procedure is very effective for the relief of left ventricular outflow tract obstruction, however the procedure seldom is used in pediatric patients and, as a consequence, is technically very challenging for the majority of physicians who perform therapeutic interventions primarily on *pediatric and/or congenital* heart patients. The alcohol septal ablation procedure definitely is not without some significant complications.

More recently the ablation of left ventricular septal tissue has been performed using radio-frequency (RF) energy. "Excavation" of the left ventricular outflow tract with reduction of the gradient across the outflow tract has been accomplished using an RF catheter with an 8 or 10 mm electrode tip, a high output 100-w RF generator (Boston Scientific, Natick, MA), which is set at 60 watts for 1 minute with the tip cooled with a continuous saline flush of 300 to 600 ml/hour while the RF is active. The catheter tip, which is deflected against the tissue while the energy is applied, is drawn along the area of abnormal muscle in the outflow tract in order to create a channel or groove in the tissues. The RF energy apparently "excavates" the area of the septum by desiccation of the tissues without any resultant adverse effects from the disseminated (embolized) materials (gases?). This particular use of radio-frequency energy is very new and the long-term effects/consequences certainly are not known.

Hypertrophic cardiomyopathy with left ventricular obstruction is a relatively rare lesion in the pediatric population, however, if RF energy is effective in relieving and sustaining the relief of the left sided muscular obstruction, then this procedure should have extensive application for the innumerable congenital heart patients who have *muscular right ventricular outflow tract obstruction* with or without other lesions.

Sideris "frameless" transcatheter patch occlusion devices

The latest, and completely different entry into the procedures and devices for the occlusion of intracardiac defects are the Sideris™ "frameless" Transcatheter Patches (Pediatric Cardiology Custom Medical Devices, Athens, Greece), which were developed to eliminate the perceived problems of the metal frames that are present in all of the current intracardiac occlusion devices[15]. The Sideris "Patches" and techniques are based on experimental information that the porous material of polyurethane foam, when firmly fixed in place against a surface within the circulation for the *relatively* short time of 23–48 hours, stimulates *adhesions*, which adhere to tissues securely enough to hold the patch in place permanently in that length of time. The fixation is secure enough to withstand displacement from the pressures/flow within or through an intracardiac defect[16,17]. This has been demonstrated in animal models and is reported to be successful in atrial septal defects, ventricular septal defects and very large patent ductus in humans.

ASD frameless patch device

The occlusion of atrial septal defects with a "frameless" patch was performed in animals and, on a compassionate use basis, in humans outside of the United States[18]. The delivery system consists of two relatively large, inflatable spherical latex balloons attached in series, immediately adjacent to each other, at the distal end of a triple lumen, end-hole catheter (Pediatric Cardiology Custom Medical Devices, Athens, Greece). The most distal balloon, which communicates with one lumen of the catheter, is covered *completely* with a "sleeve patch" or "sack", which is composed of a thin layer of polyurethane foam. The sheet of foam is wrapped over the distal balloon so that the "open end" of the folded patch extends proximally against the second, more proximal balloon. The second balloon is mounted on the triple lumen catheter immediately proximal to the first balloon and communicates with the second lumen. The central (third) lumen of the catheter extends through the distal end of the catheter and, in turn, through the center of the patch and allows the balloons/patch to be delivered over a wire.

The polyurethane patch has a radio-opaque suture running through the proximal margins of the patch for radiographic visualization of the general area of the patch. During implant and while the patch is "fixing" on the septum, there also is a very long loop of "retrieval" nylon suture passing through an edge of the "patch" material. Both ends of this suture extend from the patch, which is positioned in the atrial septum, and exit out of the body in the inguinal area adjacent to the catheter. This suture serves as a retrieval mechanism should the patch not adhere to the particular area after the balloon is deflated.

The atrial defect is measured very accurately with a static sizing balloon. A short tipped, stiff exchange length guide wire is positioned across the defect and into a left upper pulmonary vein similarly to the delivery of other ASD occlusion devices. A large, long sheath/dilator that will accommodate the delivery balloon with the covering patch is advanced over a wire to the area of the right atrium, the dilator alone is removed and the sheath is cleared passively of air/clot and placed on a continuous flush. The special balloon catheter carrying the collapsed polyurethane "patch" on the deflated latex balloon is introduced over the wire, into the large, long sheath, advanced out of the sheath and into the *left atrium* over the wire. The two ends of the long suture, which is attached to the "patch" material, extend back through the long sheath, along the side of the shaft of the balloon catheter and out of the proximal end of the long sheath. The distal balloon with the "patch" covering it is inflated to a diameter "several" millimeters larger than the measured diameter of the defect. The inflated distal balloon, which is covered with the "patch", is pulled back against and into the defect by withdrawing the balloon catheter while observing the balloon and septum on TEE or ICE. If the balloon/patch pulls through the defect, the balloon is deflated, re-advanced into the left atrium, refilled with slightly more fluid and repositioned back against/into the septal defect. The position and degree of occlusion are confirmed with TEE/ICE. If there still is leakage around the balloon, the balloon is inflated even further. Once the distal balloon is against the septum and completely occluding the defect, the second, more proximal balloon is inflated. This balloon inflates in the right atrium and helps to "stabilize" the distal, left atrial balloon with the "patch" against the rim of the defect. The "patch" material, which is covering the distal balloon, now should be in firm contact with the entire rim of the atrial septal defect. The polyurethane sheet of material is wrapped around the balloon and the catheter, but not fastened to the shaft of the catheter. Because of the extensive stretchability of the polyurethane foam and of the latex balloons, only three sizes of balloon/patch combinations reportedly are suitable for all defects.

The constant pressure of the polyurethane against the septum, which is necessary for the fixation of the polyurethane "patch", is accomplished by continual tension against the distal balloon, which is maintained on the shaft of the balloon *catheter* by fastening the proximal shaft of the catheter against the skin "outside" of the vasculature system for 48 hours! The second large latex balloon, which is inflated on the right side of the septum, helps to stabilize the "patch" in position against the rim of the atrial septal defect for the 48 hours, but does not hold the distal balloon against the septum.

Enough traction is applied to the balloon/delivery catheter at the skin surface to maintain the distal (left atrial) balloon against, and partially into, the atrial defect without pulling the balloon through the defect. The balloon catheter is fixed securely against the patient's leg at the puncture site with several sutures in order to maintain the "traction" on the catheter/balloon against the atrial septum. The patient is returned to the hospital ward but is kept at *strict bed rest* with their leg extended straight for 48 hours. All of this time the two balloons are inflated within the heart and the proximal end of the balloon catheter extends out of the femoral puncture site under some tension! The patient is returned to the catheterization laboratory in 24 hours to check the balloons' position and stability. When the distal balloon remains in its proper position, it moves only in synchrony with the atrial septal motion and should not be "bobbling" in the left atrium.

After 48 hours the patient is returned to the catheterization laboratory. The tension is released from the catheter at the skin puncture site and the left atrial balloon, which is covered with the "patch", is deflated. This allows the originally spherical patch material to collapse and shrink into a flat, but crumpled "patch" across the atrial defect while the deflated and collapsed balloon now is positioned on the *right* atrial side of the patch. The area is interrogated by TEE for any residual leak or displacement of the patch. When comfortable with the position and fixation of the patch, the more proximal balloon is deflated and the balloon catheter with the two deflated balloons is withdrawn very gently away from the septum. The septum and the now free "patch" again are interrogated with the TEE/ICE for security on the septum, position and any leak. When satisfied with the implant, the long "retaining" suture is withdrawn slowly and carefully from the "patch" material by pulling one end while releasing the opposite end of the suture.

Because the "patch" material is pushed against the inner edge of the atrial defect and adheres to the septum by that contact, theoretically, atrial defects that have no rim and which are very large, can be occluded with this device. Further multicenter, monitored trials of this device with controlled rigid follow-up are necessary to establish the utility of this very innovative but radical approach to ASD closure.

Frameless VSD patch

The same "frameless" patch concept has been reported for the closure of perimembranous ventricular septal defects (VSD). The patch is similar (identical?) to the frameless patches for atrial septal defects (Pediatric Cardiology Custom Medical Devices, Athens, Greece). The ventricular septal defect is crossed from the left ventricle into the right ventricle and a through-and-through wire "rail" created exactly as described for other techniques for perimembranous ventricular defect closures (Chapter 30). Once the "rail" is created, the frameless VSD device, which is mounted on the latex balloon, is delivered through a long sheath introduced from the femoral vein and pre-positioned across the VSD. In the report on the VSD patches, the patches are pre-soaked in the patient's blood, which accelerates the development of adhesions, and the duration of the traction against the patch necessary to fix the patch in place is only 23 hours. The frameless patch has been used with reported success in a number of patients outside of the United States[19]. This is another innovative concept with some very favorable points, but like the frameless ASD patch, the VSD patch also requires a well controlled trial before it becomes an accepted procedure.

Frameless PDA patch

The same concept used for the frameless ASD and VSD patches has been applied successfully to occlude the large patent ductus arteriosus (PDA)[20]. Like the VSD patch, the PDA patch is pre-clotted and only requires 23–24 hours of balloon fixation before the implanting/fixation balloons can be removed. Also, like the other devices, the PDA frameless patch has not been used in the United States or in any regulated and/or controlled clinical trials.

Dr Sideris has been experimenting with several "surgical glues" in addition to the pre-clotting to enhance and accelerate fixation of the patches to the tissues, which in turn would eliminate the undesirable relatively long period of fixation and immobilization of the patients. The frameless patches certainly are imaginative and possibly indicative of the potential for transcatheter occlusion therapy in the future.

The future of interventional/therapeutic catheterizations

The various procedures and devices described in this chapter provide a glimpse into the future of transcatheter therapeutic procedures for pediatric and congenital heart patients. Although all of these ideas may not evolve into clinically useful procedures, they do illustrate the continued imagination and innovation of the current pediatric/congenital interventionists and provide a challenge for the future. Patient care certainly will continue to be improved, not only by procedures performed by catheterization rather than surgery, but also by collaborative and/or "hybrid" surgical/catheterization procedures[21].

References

1. Bonhoeffer P *et al.* Percutaneous replacement of pulmonary valve in a right-ventricle to pulmonary-artery prosthetic conduit with valve dysfunction. *Lancet* 2000; **356**(9239): 1403–1405.
2. Khambadkone S *et al.* Percutaneous pulmonary valve implantation for right ventricular outflow tract lesions after congenital heart surgery. *Cardiol Young* 2003; **13**(Suppl 1 (Abstracts '03 AEPC)): 32 (Abstract #92).
3. Boudjemline Y *et al.* Percutaneous pulmonary valve replacement in large right ventricular outflow tract: an experimental study. *Cardiol Young* 2003; **13**(Suppl 1 (abstracts of '03 AEPC meeting)): 30 (Abstract #84).
4. Boudjemline Y *et al.* Percutaneous pulmonary valve replacement in a large right ventricular outflow tract: an experimental study. *J Am Coll Cardiol* 2004; **43**(6): 1082–1087.
5. Boudjemline Y and Bonhoeffer P. Percutaneous implantation of a valve in the descending aorta in lambs. *Eur Heart J* 2002; **23**(13): 1045–1049.
6. Boudjemline Y *et al.* Percutaneous implantation of a biological valve in the aorta to treat aortic valve insufficiency—a sheep study. *Med Sci Monit* 2002; **8**(4): BR 113–116.
7. Cribier A *et al.* Percutaneous transcatheter implantation of an aortic valve prosthesis for calcific aortic stenosis: first human case description. *Circulation* 2002; **106**(24): 3006–3008.
8. Richens T *et al.* Interventional treatment of lateral tunnel dehiscence in a total cavopulmonary connection using a balloon expandable covered stent. *Catheter Cardiovasc Interv* 2000; **50**(4): 449–451.
9. Konertz W *et al.* Modified hemi-Fontan operation and subsequent nonsurgical Fontan completion. *J Thorac Cardiovasc Surg* 1995; **110**(3): 865–867.
10. Hausdorf G, Schneider M, and Konertz W. Surgical preconditioning and completion of total cavopulmonary connection by interventional cardiac catheterization: a new concept. *Heart* 1996; **75**(4): 403–409.
11. Diethrich EB. AAA stent grafts: current developments. *J Invasive Cardiol* 2001; **13**(5): 383–390.
12. Chigogidze NA, Avaliani MV, and Cherkasov VA. New percutaneous technology of vascular shunting. *Cardiol Young* 2003. **13**(Suppl 1 (abstracts of '03 AEPC meeting)): 30 (abstract #86).
13. Mitchell MB *et al.* Mechanical limitation of pulmonary blood flow facilitates heart transplantation in older infants with hypoplastic left heart syndrome. *Eur J Cardiothorac Surg* 2003; **23**(5): 735–742.
14. Sigwart U. Non-surgical myocardial reduction for hypertrophic obstructive cardiomyopathy. *Lancet* 1995; **346**(8969): 211–214.
15. Sideris EB *et al.* From disk devices to transcatheter patches: the evolution of wireless heart defect occlusion. *J Interv Cardiol* 2001; **14**(2): 211–214.
16. Sideris EB *et al.* Transcatheter patch occlusion of experimental atrial septal defects. *Catheter Cardiovasc Interv* 2002; **57**(3): 404–407.
17. Sideris EB *et al.* Transcatheter atrial septal defect occlusion in piglets by balloon detachable devices. *Catheter Cardiovasc Interv* 2000; **51**(4): 529–534.
18. Sideris A *et al.* Transcatheter patch correction of atrial septal defects: experimental validation and early clinical experience. *Cardiol Young* 2000; **10**: 13.
19. Sideris EB *et al.* Transcatheter patch occlusion of perimembranous ventricular septal defects. *J Am Coll Cardiol* 2003; **41**(6 Suppl B): 473.
20. Sideris A *et al.* Accelerated transcatheter patch occlusion of large patent ductus arteriosus. *Cardiol Young* 2003; **13**(Suppl 1 (Abstracts of '03 AEPC)): 35 (abstract #99).
21. Bacha EA *et al.* New Therapeutic Avenues with Hybrid Pediatric Cardiac Surgery. *Heart Surg Forum* 2004; **7**(1): 33–40.

33 Endomyocardial biopsy

Introduction

Transcatheter endomyocardial biopsies are utilized to obtain specimens of myocardium from hearts that are suspected of being diseased and/or damaged. Transcatheter biopsies have replaced open and direct transthoracic puncture of the myocardium. Biopsies using catheter techniques were introduced over four decades ago, and although the equipment has been refined, the procedure is little changed[1]. Biopsies are performed to establish the diagnosis of myocarditis[2,3], to monitor the course of treatment of myocarditis[4], to differentiate different types of cardiomyopathies[5,6], to confirm cardio-toxicity of drugs[7], to follow the course of therapy and/or to detect rejection in cardiac transplant patients[8] and even to obtain specimens of very specific, localized tissues[9]. With the frequency of pediatric transplants, endomyocardial biopsy has become one of the more frequent procedures performed in major pediatric/congenital catheterization laboratories.

Because endomyocardial biopsies are performed so frequently, they often are considered "routine" or "minor" procedures and often are taken "lightly" by the operators and catheterization laboratory staff. In reality, endomyocardial biopsy potentially is one of the more dangerous procedures performed in the cardiac catheterization laboratory. With each biopsy sample, the forceful mechanical jaws of the bioptome catheter purposefully "bite" into the myocardium, each time with the potential of "biting" all of the way through the muscle, through the wall of the heart or through a chorda of the tricuspid valve! In addition, the patients who are undergoing biopsy frequently are the sickest of the patients brought to the catheterization laboratory. The patients undergoing biopsy often have obstructed systemic venous routes to the heart as a result of numerous previous indwelling lines and/or previous catheterizations/biopsies. As a consequence, the venous access for the biopsy can be complicated or often totally obstructed so that, because of the vascular access, the endomyocardial biopsy becomes one of the more challenging and time-consuming procedures in the cardiac catheterization laboratory.

A myocardial biopsy usually is accomplished in the cardiac catheterization laboratory and accompanied by at least a minimal hemodynamic evaluation, which includes estimates of cardiac output by Fick and/or thermodilution determinations. The hemodynamic data are usually obtained before the tissue biopsies are performed. Transplant patients also undergo a complete angiographic study of their coronary arteries at least on an annual basis. The coronary arteriography usually is performed after the tissue samples are obtained.

Some institutions perform the biopsies using only echocardiographic guidance[10], in which case the biopsies can be performed in a specific procedure room that does not contain X-ray equipment, in the intensive care unit and/or even in the patient's hospital room[11]. When the biopsy is performed in other than the catheterization laboratory and echo only guidance is used, the jugular approach using special sheaths, which are long enough to reach the ventricle but not as long as the standard long transseptal sheaths, becomes the preferred approach[12].

Like the performance of a balloon atrial septostomy using echo guidance only, the manipulation of the bioptome into the ventricle is more difficult, but once the bioptome is in the desired chamber, the localization of the jaws of the forceps on a specific area of the myocardial surface and the visualization of the tissues that are immediately adjacent to the forceps are more precise. When not performed in the catheterization laboratory, the accurate hemodynamic assessment and/or the coronary angiography cannot be obtained during the same procedure. In addition, in the rare event of a cardiac perforation during the biopsy, the facilities for complex resuscitations including a pericardiocentesis and/or the rapid placement of a pericardial drain usually are not as available. The performance of a biopsy in the catheterization laboratory does not preclude the use of the echo simultaneously!

Equipment for endomyocardial biopsy

A biplane X-ray system is recommended, if not essential, for fluoroscopic-guided endomyocardial biopsies. In order to localize the tip of the bioptome catheter spatially within the heart in "three dimensions" the two planes of fluoroscopy are necessary. A single-plane only, X-ray system can be used for myocardial biopsies, but only with the capability of rapidly rotating the X-ray tube at least 90° around the thorax in order to obtain the perpendicular plane for the precise positioning of the bioptome jaws. Even with the rotation capability, a single-plane system is far less than satisfactory. If, in the rotated (angled) position of the X-ray tube, the bioptome is not in a satisfactory position and it is repositioned while the X-ray tube is in the rotated position, then the position of the tip of the bioptome has changed relative to the original position of the X-ray tube. The positioning of the bioptome must be started all over! Without actually viewing the bioptome in two views, the precise location of the bioptome jaws in the plane perpendicular to the one visualized is only a guess.

Although there is some directional control over a curved bioptome catheter and/or long sheath, the resistance to torque within the vascular system prevents a true one-to-one relationship between the degree of rotation of the shaft of the sheath/bioptome to the degree of rotation of the distal tip of the bioptome. The final, three-dimensional spatial position of the tip of a curved sheath and/or bioptome catheter is determined by visualizing the catheter tip in two, roughly perpendicular, X-ray planes and extrapolating the "three-dimensional" position within the cardiac chamber from the two planes.

For added safety, and particularly in very high-risk cases, either transthoracic echo (TTE) or transesophageal echo (TEE) can be used in conjunction with the fluoroscopy to guide the forceps of the bioptome within the specific cardiac chamber while the samples are being obtained. As mentioned previously, some centers even perform the biopsies at the patient's bedside using only TTE to guide the bioptome to the site of biopsy[13,14]. These biopsies have been carried out without complications with the echocardiogram providing a clear image of the endocardial surface and of all immediately adjacent structures *once the bioptome* catheter is positioned in the ventricle.

All bioptome catheters that are used currently are single use, disposable catheters. Many companies, including Argon Medical Inc., Athens, TX, Cook Inc., Bloomington, IN, CERES Medical Systems, L.L.C., Stafford, TX and Cordis Corp., Miami Lakes, FL manufacture disposable bioptome (biopsy forceps) catheters, and several sizes of bioptome are available from most of the manufacturers. Each bioptome "catheter" consists of a small, articulated pair of jaws at the distal end of the bioptome with a flexible "cable catheter" connecting the jaws to an "activating handle" at the proximal end. The jaws on the bioptome open to approximately 180° by moving the two sliding, side rings on the handle forward and away from the central fixed ring on the central shaft of the handle. Standard bioptome catheters are available in 5- through 7-French sizes and most are at least 100 cm long.

There is a very tiny, 3-French bioptome with a totally different "activating handle" available from Cook Inc., Bloomington, IN. The smaller the French size of the bioptome catheter, the smaller are the "jaws" of the bioptome and, in turn, the smaller the possible "bite" and/or the specimen, which is acquired. Because of this, the 3-French sized bioptome is used for myocardial biopsies almost exclusively in very small infants.

Although initially almost all biopsies were performed from the jugular approach, most pediatric and congenital cardiac catheterization laboratories are arranged physically for optimal access to the patient's vascular system from the *inguinal* area. As a consequence, for a myocardial biopsy performed in the pediatric/congenital cardiac catheterization laboratory, the usual and preferred approach is from a femoral vein. The femoral approach not only is more convenient for the operators, but certainly is more comfortable and less frightening for the sedated patient than a jugular venous approach. Although the desirable approach and majority of biopsies are performed from the femoral vein, a catheterization laboratory that performs myocardial biopsies must be prepared to utilize a jugular vein, a brachial vein, a systemic artery or even a transthoracoabdominal puncture into the hepatic veins when both the iliofemoral and the cephalad venous systems are occluded.

The bioptome forceps is delivered to the ventricular site for the biopsy through a special, long, pre-curved, transseptal type sheath, which has a back-bleed valve with a flush side port. Delivering the bioptome through a long sheath, which is positioned initially in the ventricle, eliminates the cumbersome, repeated and often unsuccessful maneuvering of the bioptome catheter alone, reduces the chance of perforation with the stiff bioptome catheter, and lessens the chance of the bioptome forceps catching on vital intraventricular structures when the "jaws" are opened freely in the ventricle.

The use of the long sheath/dilator for the delivery of the bioptome is similar to the guiding catheter system originally developed by Lurie for delivering the bioptome directly to the ventricular cavity[15]. The sheath for a biopsy must be long enough to reach the site of the biopsy (ventricle) but usually does not have to be as long as a standard transseptal sheath, and definitely must be shorter than the bioptome catheter being used. A radio-opaque marker band at the distal tip of the sheath is useful, if not essential. The radio-opaque band helps to visualize the exact position of the *tip of the sheath* especially when the bioptome catheter is positioned within the sheath. The improved visibility of the tip of the sheath provided by the radio-opaque band reduces the fluoroscopy time. The long sheath used to deliver the biopsy catheter must be fairly "kink resistant", since some manipulations of the sheath itself are required within the ventricle. Several manufacturers now provide sheaths of special lengths, in a variety of diameters specifically for biopsies from the usual femoral vein approach. These include Cook Inc., Bloomington, IN, Cordis Corp., Miami Lakes, FL and Daig Corp., Minnetonka, MN.

All except the most stoical patients require some sedation in order to undergo a myocardial biopsy procedure. The standard premedication/sedation/anesthesia that is used in the particular catheterization laboratory along with the liberal use of local anesthesia at the introductory site for the catheter usually is sufficient for a myocardial biopsy performed from the femoral approach. Since most of these procedures require only a relatively short time in the vessels and with the greater than usual chance of causing a cardiac perforation, extra, systemic heparin usually is not utilized. In patients who are undergoing evaluation of the coronary arteries along with the biopsy, the biopsy is performed first and then systemic heparin is added after the biopsy samples are obtained, but before the extensive systemic arterial catheter manipulation.

Although the biopsy procedures usually are relatively short, a small indwelling arterial line often is introduced for more precise monitoring of the patient during these procedures, particularly when access for the biopsy is a problem and/or the patient's clinical status is precarious. In most catheterization laboratories, when meticulous technique and a 21- or 20-gauge teflon cannula is used for the indwelling arterial line, the introduction of a small femoral arterial cannula is a straightforward and very benign procedure without complications. At the same time, since the potential for cardiac perforation is greater with myocardial biopsy than any other procedure in the catheterization laboratory, the continually *monitored and visualized* curve of the arterial pressure from the indwelling arterial line provides a very early *predictor* of impending trouble compared to an intermittently sampled blood pressure obtained with an extremity cuff, which will provide only a *late indicator* of serious trouble that had begun significantly earlier. When a perforation does occur, the arterial line becomes essential for monitoring the patient during the resuscitation. It also is far better to have the arterial line in place before the event occurs and/or while preventing further hemodynamic deterioration than attempting to obtain arterial access with the patient in shock! When an arterial line is *not* used, the cuff blood pressure should be monitored *more frequently* and much more attention must be paid to each of the readings from the cuff blood pressure, to the monitored heart rate, and to the displayed electrocardiogram for any even subtle changes that might indicate a perforation and/or the accumulation of a pericardial effusion.

Transthoracic echo (TTE) guidance is used by some centers either alone or in conjunction with fluoroscopy for the positioning of the bioptome jaws within the ventricle for each "bite". Even bedside biopsies from the jugular approach using TTE guidance alone have been advocated. The echo theoretically demonstrates more clearly if the jaws are against a thin or otherwise "wrong" area of myocardium and/or entangled on interventricular structures such as the tricuspid valve apparatus and chordae. The performance of the biopsy at the bedside from the jugular approach and using "echo only" almost prohibits the concomitant use of a long pre-curved sheath pre-positioned in the ventricle for the introduction of the bioptome catheter. In a "bedside environment", it is very difficult to maintain the sterility of the longer sheath extending from the neck and to manage the clearing and adequate flushing of the sheath. When the jugular route is used, the bioptome frequently is delivered directly into the ventricle from a short sheath fixed in the jugular introductory site, which eliminates the direct course to the ventricle and the protection of the ventricular structures provided by the long sheath. Bedside biopsies also preclude the sophisticated monitoring that is available routinely in the catheterization laboratory.

Even if the echo machine is not used during the actual tissue sampling, an echo machine always should be available in the catheterization laboratory. In the event of any instability in the patient's condition, a pericardial effusion can be ruled out or documented definitively and immediately and, in turn, treated rapidly, depending on the echo findings.

Preparing the sheath and bioptome catheter for the biopsy

The distal end of the long sheath is pre-curved outside of the body and before the sheath is introduced into the patient into a *three-dimensional curve* which conforms to the proposed course of the sheath from the *particular vascular access site* (in a vein or peripheral artery), into the desired ventricle and to the thickest area of the myocardium within the accessed ventricle. These "three-dimensional" curves that are formed are similar to those described by Lurie for his special bioptome and delivery catheters (Cordis Corp., Miami Lakes, FL)[16]. The curves that are formed on the sheath vary for each patient according to the size of the patient, the size and "location" of the heart, the introductory (vascular access) site for the sheath and the desired area of the myocardium that is to be biopsied. As a consequence, the specific curves that are necessary for each patient/procedure are not commercially available and must be formed individually for each biopsy procedure. A curve that is "tighter" than actually desired to direct the bioptome to the site for biopsy, is formed on the sheath/dilator in order to allow for some straightening of the sheath when it is in the warm circulation and when the shaft of the bioptome catheter is introduced into the sheath.

When forming the curves on the sheath/dilator outside of the body and when manipulating the sheath within the vascular system, extra precautions must be taken not to *kink* the sheath. The curves on the sheath are formed and/or changed *only* with the long dilator still positioned completely within the sheath. To form the curves, the sheath/dilator combination is "softened" either by heating the sheath/dilator combination in sterile boiling water or in a jet of hot air from a "heat gun". Once the sheath/dilator is "softened" in the heat, the sheath/dilator manually is shaped into the desired curves and then immersed in cold flush solution to "fix" the curves on the sheath/dilator combination. Minor curves can be formed on the sheath/dilator by repeatedly "cold pulling" the tip of the sheath/dilator combination between the thumb and forefinger while simultaneously forming the desired curve. The "cold-pulled" curves usually cannot be formed as tight as the curves formed after heating the sheath/dilator. Once the curves on the combined sheath/dilator are formed, the dilator temporarily is withdrawn from the sheath outside of the body in order to verify that the exact desired curves have been formed specifically on the *sheath* and not just on the dilator.

Curves that correspond to the "three-dimensional" curves on the sheath are also formed on the distal end of the shaft (or "cable") of the bioptome catheter. The curves on the distal shaft of the bioptome catheter (cable) are formed by manual, gradual and *smooth bending* (but *not* pulling!) of the shaft of the cable of the bioptome "catheter" in the areas where the curves are desired. Like the curves on the sheath, in order to compensate for some straightening within the body, the curves on the cable are formed slightly tighter than the expected curved course through the intravascular route to the site for the biopsy. At the same time, care must be taken not to create *any* sharp "angles" in the woven, wire shaft of the bioptome cable and not to "over-curve" the "cable" of the bioptome to the point that the jaw mechanism of the bioptome no longer will function. Continued, adequate function of the jaws only is assured by testing the jaw mechanism after only partially forming an initial very slight bend of the ultimately desired curve and then retesting the jaws each time before tightening the curve any further. This sequence is repeated until either the desired curves are formed or until there is even the slightest resistance to the smooth function of the jaws. Once the cable of the shaft of the bioptome catheter is pre-curved, the operation of the jaws is retested several times while manually forming different temporary bends on the more proximal catheter. A slight "over-curving" or kinking in the shaft of the bioptome catheter shaft can prohibit the opening and/or closing of the jaws.

Technique of myocardial biopsy from the femoral vein approach

For a right ventricular biopsy from the femoral vein approach, the curves on both the sheath and the bioptome are formed as visualized in the posterior–anterior projection first to correspond to the smooth curve of approximately 90° from the inferior vena cava, through the tricuspid valve and into the right ventricle. In the body, this curve passes from the *patient's* right toward the *patient's* left side. The second (three-dimensional) curve is formed at the very distal end of the first curve on both the sheath/dilator and on the distal shaft of the biopsy catheter. This secondary curve is formed to direct the tip posteriorly and toward the interventricular septum in the right ventricle, which with the curved sheath or catheter tip facing *away from the operator* will be a relatively sharp curvature to the *left* of the tip of the sheath (and the operator).

Once the desired hemodynamics are obtained, an end-hole catheter is positioned in the pulmonary artery, an exchange length guide wire is introduced through the end-hole diagnostic catheter, and the catheter is withdrawn over the wire. If a closed-ended angiographic catheter was used for the diagnostic catheterization, the catheter is withdrawn, the original catheter is replaced with an end-hole catheter and the end-hole catheter and then the wire are advanced through the right ventricle and into the pulmonary artery. Once the wire is in place, the end-hole catheter and the short sheath are removed. The long sheath/dilator that has been pre-curved for the biopsy is introduced over the wire. With the wire positioned in the pulmonary artery, the sheath/dilator is advanced over the wire until the tip of the dilator is well into the right ventricle or even into the pulmonary artery. The *sheath* is advanced over the dilator until the tip of the sheath and the tip of the dilator are together. While keeping the tip of the sheath securely in the right ventricle, the dilator and then the wire are withdrawn out of the sheath. Once the wire and the dilator have been removed, the sheath is allowed to bleed back passively through the side port, paying particular attention that all entrapped air and/or clot is removed from the back-bleed valve apparatus itself. Usually blood is "pumped" vigorously from the right ventricle, which both verifies the location of the tip of the sheath and thoroughly clears the long sheath. Once cleared of all air (and clots!) the side port of the sheath is attached to a flush/pressure system, the sheath is flushed thoroughly and then placed on a slow continuous flush. Except for intermittent, short checks of the pressure through the sheath, the sheath is maintained on a steady slow flush.

A less desirable and slightly more precarious way of introducing the sheath into the right ventricle is to advance the exchange wire into the superior vena cava instead of the pulmonary artery and then initially to advance the *pre-curved* biopsy sheath/dilator into the *high* right atrium. The wire is removed and the *dilator* is cleared of air and clot. In the right atrium, passive bleeding back through the dilator is not as brisk as from the right ventricle, and gentle suction on the hub of the dilator may be necessary to obtain blood return through the dilator. Once cleared of air and/or clot, the dilator is attached to the flush/pressure system and the combination sheath/dilator withdrawn from the SVC through the right atrium while gently rotating the tip anteriorly and to the patient's left. When adequate curves have been formed at the distal end of the sheath/dilator, the combination "falls" almost automatically from the right atrium into the right ventricle as the tip of the sheath/dilator is withdrawn through the right atrium. When the tip of the dilator drops into the right ventricle as confirmed by the appearance of a right ventricular pressure through the dilator, the dilator is fixed in position while the sheath is advanced over the dilator to the tip of the dilator. The dilator is withdrawn slowly from the sheath and the sheath is cleared passively of air and clot as described above.

If the sheath/dilator combination does not "fall" into the ventricle as the combination is withdrawn from the high to the low right atrium, no further attempt is made to maneuver the combination of sheath/dilator into the ventricle. The sheath/dilator combination is stiff and the dilator has a sharp distal tip, which easily can perforate myocardium if *pushed* excessively. When the tip of the dilator does not "fall" into the ventricle during withdrawal from the superior vena cava, the dilator is withdrawn slowly from the sheath and the sheath meticulously cleared of air and/or clot. If the venous pressure is low and/or particularly if there is any airway obstruction, there is significant danger of the patient sucking air into the sheath rather than blood flowing freely from the sheath when the tip of the sheath is in the right atrium. The stopcock on the side port of the sheath is opened very cautiously with the anticipation of having to close it instantaneously if there is negative pressure and any suggestion of fluid/air being drawn *into* the side arm/flush port of the sheath. When there is any negative pressure from within the vascular space and there is any tendency for air to be sucked into the side arm/sheath, the side port is kept closed and capped with a syringe. The end (valve) of the sheath is covered very tightly with a gloved fingertip, the side port stopcock is opened to the syringe and *very gentle* suction is applied intermittently to the side port with the syringe. When a vacuum is created and no blood is aspirated, the suction on the syringe is released slowly. The sheath is rotated and/or withdrawn slightly and while still covering the back-bleed valve tightly, gentle suction again is applied to the syringe on the side port until blood flow through the side port is obtained easily —*all of the time* keeping the valve at the end of the sheath covered tightly with the finger. Once the sheath is cleared completely of air/clots, it is attached to the pressure flush system and placed on a continuous flush.

From the right atrium, a very brief attempt is made at torquing and advancing the cleared sheath alone, very slightly and *very gingerly* into the right ventricle. The sheath, alone, very easily can be kinked, particularly when the tip of the sheath impinges against any structure within the heart, and/or any forward pressure is applied concomitantly to the sheath against even minimal resistance. Again, *unless* the sheath *"falls"* easily into the ventricle, it generally is more judicious to introduce an end-hole catheter that is the same French size as the sheath and to maneuver the *sheath/catheter* combination into the ventricle than it is to attempt any *significant* maneuvers into the ventricle with the sheath alone.

The catheter is maintained on a continuous slow flush as it is introduced into the sheath and until it advances well *beyond* the tip of the sheath. An active tip deflector wire (Cook Inc., Bloomington, IN) or a static Mullins™ deflector wire (Argon Medical Inc., Athens, TX) can be used within the catheter to deflect the tip of the catheter, which is beyond the tip of the sheath, toward the right ventricle. The deflector is bent approximately 90° and the catheter is rotated to point anteriorly and to the patient's left (toward the tricuspid valve). Occasionally the sheath must be rotated simultaneously with the catheter in order to "aim" the tip of the catheter at the tricuspid valve. Once the tip of the catheter is aimed toward the tricuspid valve, the deflector wire is held in place, the catheter is advanced further out of the sheath, off the still deflected wire and into the right ventricle. Once the catheter is secured within the ventricle, the sheath is advanced over the catheter to the desired position in the ventricle. Occasionally, both the sheath and catheter advance together over the wire and into the right ventricle. Once the tip of the *sheath* is in the ventricle, the preformed curve on the sheath will help to maintain the tip of the sheath in the correct position in the ventricle for the biopsy. The deflector wire and then the catheter are withdrawn from the sheath and the sheath again carefully cleared passively of air/clots.

Once within the ventricle, the *pre-curved* sheath is maneuvered with fluoroscopic and/or echo visualization very *cautiously* into the desired position against the presumed thicker areas of the ventricular myocardium. The precise thickness of the area of the myocardium can be visualized with echo. When the "squared-off" single opening of the tip of the sheath is positioned against the ventricular myocardium, it may not be possible to withdraw blood, fluid or any entrapped air from the sheath, and as a consequence it is important that the sheath is cleared passively and completely before being maneuvered *against* the myocardium of the ventricle for the introduction of the bioptome. A large, long sheath can hold as much as 8–10 ml of air! The introduction of a significant amount of air during a myocardial biopsy is an additional risk to the procedure, which is second only to the risk of perforation. Once cleared of air, the sheath is kept on a slow flush during all of the subsequent positioning within the ventricle.

The pre-curved bioptome with the jaws of the bioptome closed is introduced into the pre-positioned and pre-curved sheath and advanced under continual fluoroscopic observation to just within the tip of the sheath. The sheath is kept on a slow but continuous flush through the side port as the bioptome is introduced into and advanced within the sheath. As the stiffer (often straighter!) bioptome catheter is advanced within the sheath, the tip of the sheath often is seen on fluoroscopy to move away from the original position on the myocardial surface. As this occurs, the sheath is allowed to retract away from the myocardium by relaxing the forward push on the sheath, and once the bioptome reaches the tip of the sheath, the combination of the sheath and bioptome is re-advanced against the myocardial surface. Again the position against the endocardium and the thickness of the myocardium in front of the bioptome can be verified with echo. This is particularly important in patients who have any malpositioning of the cardiac silhouette and/or those who have had multiple prior biopsies. The handle mechanism of the bioptome is activated to the "open" position with the "jaws" at the very tip, but still *within* the tip of the sheath. This activation of the jaws of the bioptome also tends to withdraw the tip of the sheath slightly. The jaws of the bioptome themselves, while still *within the tip of the sheath* do not open, but, as the bioptome jaws are advanced out of the tip of the sheath, the "pre-activation" of the handle results in the jaws opening fully while the jaws are immediately adjacent to the tip of the sheath and just as the jaws exit the tip of the sheath. With the tip of the sheath pre-positioned adjacent to the myocardium, the open jaws immediately dig into the endocardium, which is adjacent to the tip of the sheath, without passing through any of the cavity of the ventricle. This technique allows the jaws to be directed to very precise sites on the myocardium, and since the *open jaws* are not advanced any distance through the cavity of the ventricle, the possibility of "biting" unwanted (and possibly vital) structures such as the chordae of the tricuspid valve is reduced by this technique of pre-positioning the sheath. Adjacent and/or trapped structures can usually be visualized on echo.

The bioptome with the jaws wide open together with the sheath is pushed forward against the endocardium within the ventricle and the jaws of the bioptome are closed tightly on the tissue. When the jaws are in adequate approximation to the tissues, some resistance is felt to the closure of the jaws. The bioptome catheter is withdrawn as the sheath simultaneously is maintained or advanced slightly against the myocardium by a slight forward push on the sheath. There usually also is some resistance felt and then a sudden jerk backwards of the shaft of the bioptome catheter as the closed bioptome jaws are withdrawn away with the grasped endomyocardial tissue. With the sheath still on a slow flush and the jaws of the bioptome maintained tightly closed, the bioptome is withdrawn slowly and completely out of the sheath. The sheath is maintained on a flush while keeping it in the same position in the ventricle.

Once out of the sheath, the closed jaws of the bioptome are positioned over a sterile Petri dish and the jaws are opened. The sample of tissue from the "bite" is removed from the bioptome jaws and flushed onto the sterile Petri dish using a "jet" of flush solution squirted through a needle attached to a syringe full of flush solution. Depending upon the particular laboratory and the studies desired, five to seven *good* tissue samples are required for each biopsy study[17]. Once the bioptome is removed after each "bite", the sheath is repositioned slightly to a different site on the myocardium by careful, gentle torque and minimal, to-and-fro motion of the sheath alone within the ventricle while, at the same time, being very careful not to push the sheath forward too forcefully. Once the sheath is in a new and satisfactory position as visualized on fluoroscopy and/or echo, the bioptome is reintroduced and the tissue sampling repeated in a similar fashion.

If the sheath alone cannot be repositioned adequately within the ventricle there are several helpful procedures to achieve a new, different position. Once the bioptome catheter is reintroduced into the sheath, the sheath and the bioptome catheter together can be maneuvered more liberally within the ventricle. The extra support provided by the bioptome within the sheath allows more control over the movement, and the bioptome cable provides some resistance to the kinking of the sheath.

When the sheath/bioptome catheter together cannot be maintained in an adequate position, a fine, preformed, 0.017″ Mullins static, deflector wire (Argon Medical Inc., Athens, TX) can be used to help reposition the sheath more selectively. The lumen of the pre-curved bioptome sheath, which already is in the ventricle, must be sufficiently larger than the shaft of the bioptome catheter in order to allow the wire and the shaft of the bioptome to have room side by side within the long sheath. The 0.017″ Mullins™ deflector wire is pre-curved outside of the body similar to the curving of the bioptome cable to conform to the desired "three-dimensional" course from the venous entry site to the *new site* that is desired for the biopsy. The distal "RA to RV" and "posterior" curves are formed on the wire significantly "tighter" than the actually desired curves to allow for straightening of the wire by the sheath/bioptome. The wire is introduced adjacent to the bioptome catheter through the back-bleed valve of the sheath. The wire can be introduced into the sheath after a bioptome catheter already is in place within the sheath or the bioptome can be introduced after the wire is in place and has "repositioned" the sheath. An "active deflector wire" (Cook Inc., Bloomington, IN) can also be used to deflect the sheath; however, an even larger sheath is necessary to accommodate the larger "gauge" of the active deflector wire. In addition, with an active deflector wire, the deflection only can be created in a single dimension and only in the direction of the concavity of the curve from the right atrium to the right ventricle. A final method of repositioning the sheath is to replace the bioptome in the sheath with a standard catheter that is the same size as the sheath and then to use one of the deflector wires within the catheter to reposition the tip of the sheath. Once the sheath is repositioned, the catheter is removed and the bioptome is reintroduced, both very carefully. Unless the curves on the bioptome are re-formed, the bioptome easily can displace the sheath once again as the stiffer bioptome is reintroduced.

Right ventricular biopsy from the jugular approach

Biopsies from the neck were routine during the early development of biopsy techniques. The jugular approach is preferable when the biopsy is performed at the patient's bedside using echo guidance only. The jugular approach is still used electively in the catheterization laboratory in many centers and the jugular approach becomes absolutely necessary when the femoral venous access is occluded and/or when a particular site is desired in the ventricle for the biopsy. The approach from the neck is less convenient for the catheterizing physicians in most catheterization laboratories because of the physical arrangement of the X-ray equipment, and the neck approach is more uncomfortable for the patient during and after the procedure. At the same time, some physicians in the catheterization laboratory prefer the jugular venous approach for routine biopsies in spite of these disadvantages.

Unless the patient is very *stoical and extremely cooperative*, general anesthesia and/or very heavy "conscious sedation" is used when biopsies are performed from the neck in pediatric and congenital patients. When the neck approach is used, the patient's head must be maintained turned away (restrained) from the venous entrance site, much of the "activity" of the biopsy catheter manipulation is performed immediately adjacent to the patient's face and the face and head must be kept covered during the whole procedure.

Once the jugular vein is entered, the approach to the tricuspid valve and the *ventricle* itself is "straighter", more direct and more "controllable" than the approach from the groin. The major differences are the distance from the skin to the right ventricle, the greater danger of air aspiration through the sheath because of this shorter distance and the different "pre-curves" that are formed at the distal ends of the biopsy sheath and biopsy catheter. The curves on the sheath and/or bioptome catheter are somewhat of a "mirror image" to the curves when coming from the groin, but in order to approach the *septal wall* of the right ventricle from the superior vena cava, the angle *within* the ventricle is more acute. The initial curves formed on the sheath and bioptome catheter, in turn, are more acute. To correspond to the course from the neck/right atrium into the mid right ventricle, a 150–180° curve is formed initially at the distal end of the sheath/dilator. This curve is similar in shape to the standard "transseptal" curves provided by the manufacturers on the long MTS™ sheaths (United States Catheter, Inc. [USCI] Angiographics, Billerica, MA; Cook Inc., Bloomington, IN), but always must be "tightened" to a more acute curve compared to the manufacturer's curves. The secondary or "third-dimensional curve", which is formed at the end of the initial curve in order to direct the tip posteriorly in the ventricle, is formed in the opposite direction of the curve formed on the sheath when the bioptome is introduced from the inferior vena cava. When the distal end and tip of the initial curve of the sheath/dilator and/or bioptome are pointing away from the operator, the secondary curve should direct the tip of the sheath posteriorly toward the septal surface of the right ventricular cavity i.e., when the tip of the long sheath is facing away from the operator and toward the *operator's* left, the secondary curve is formed directed posteriorly or dorsally in the chest.

In spite of entering the right atrium from the opposite direction, the sheath that is introduced from the superior vena cava is introduced or maneuvered into the right ventricle over a pre-positioned wire similarly to when the sheath is introduced from the femoral vein/inferior vena cava. The wire is pre-positioned in the pulmonary artery through a separate end-hole catheter introduced from the jugular vein and advanced into the pulmonary artery. The long sheath/dilator combination or the sheath introduced over an end-hole catheter of the same French size is advanced over the wire until the tip of the dilator or catheter is well within the right ventricle or into the pulmonary artery. The tip of the sheath is advanced to the tip of the dilator or catheter. The sheath is fixed in position and the dilator or catheter is withdrawn from the sheath followed by the wire. The sheath is cleared passively of all air and/or clot similarly to the introduction from the femoral approach.

Rarely, the end-hole catheter and then the wire from the jugular vein are advanced through the atrium and into the inferior vena cava. The pre-curved sheath/dilator or sheath/catheter is advanced over the wire into the inferior vena cava and the pre-curved sheath "withdrawn" into the right ventricle from there. The dilator or catheter and wire are withdrawn from the sheath. The sheath is cleared of air and/or clot while in the inferior vena cava. This may require gentle suction on the side port of the sheath while sealing the valve of the sheath with a gloved finger. Once cleared and on a continuous flush, the pre-curved sheath alone is withdrawn from the inferior vena cava until the tip of the curved sheath "flips" into the right ventricle. With any or all of these maneuvers performed from the jugular vein, extreme care is necessary to prevent air entry into the delivery system because of the shorter distance and more direct transmission of negative pressures from the heart to the venous entrance site.

Even the standard, special biopsy sheaths are unnecessarily long for the approach from the jugular vein. As a consequence, manipulation of the sheath and bioptome catheter by the catheterizing physician is necessarily from a very awkward position. The proximal end of the long sheath will be significantly cephalad to the patient's head, well beyond the cephalad (head) end of the catheterization table, frequently immediately adjacent to the (unsterile) suspension arms of the X-ray system and with no place to "rest" or even temporarily to release the proximal end of the sheath from the operator's grip. Without specially manufactured shorter sheaths, this requires at least two very well coordinated catheterizing physicians working together in this area to prevent contamination of the catheters, sheaths and site as well as to prevent the introduction of air into the system.

Left ventricular biopsy

Usually, the right heart biopsies are sufficient for tissue diagnosis[17]. Occasionally, because of unique myocardial problems, a left heart biopsy is desired. This is accomplished preferably by a prograde approach through an atrial transseptal puncture or alternatively and rarely, when there is no reasonable access to the venous system, from the retrograde arterial approach.

For the prograde, atrial transseptal approach, a standard Mullins Transseptal Set™ is used. The transseptal sheath should have an internal diameter large enough to accommodate the bioptome catheter *plus* some type of deflector wire(s) adjacent to the bioptome. The sheath, bioptome and any deflector wires are pre-curved with a tighter than normal, 270°, "transseptal curve" *plus* a short, relatively sharp anterior curve at their tips. The curves on all of the items are formed in proportion to the patient's size, the cardiac size and the cardiac position within the thorax. The anterior curve is formed on the distal end of the exaggerated "transseptal" curve of the sheath by bending (forming) the distal tip anterior when the tip of the sheath is facing away from the operator and curving to the operator's right (anteriorly when the proximal "transseptal" curve is facing the patient's left when approached from the femoral area). The exaggerated manufactured "transseptal curve" directs the sheath/bioptome into the left ventricle and medially while the anterior curve deflects the sheath/bioptome toward the septal wall of the left ventricular cavity.

For operators who are comfortable with the atrial transseptal procedure, the prograde transseptal approach to the left ventricle for a myocardial biopsy is no more difficult or significantly more hazardous than the standard right ventricular biopsy from a venous approach. There are, in fact, several advantages of a left ventricular biopsy from the atrial transseptal approach to the left ventricle compared to the "routine" right ventricular biopsy. Generally, the myocardium of the left ventricle is thicker and it is easier to position the bioptome against an area of the myocardium that is away from vital intraventricular structures in the left ventricle than it is in the right ventricle. From the venous and atrial transseptal approach, large bioptome catheters can be used in conjunction with a deflector wire without compromise of an artery by the large sheath. All of the necessary curves to the biopsy site from the femoral venous approach essentially are *concave curves*. This allows the use of *active* deflector wires within the sheath adjacent to the bioptome to help position the bioptome more precisely. The curved bioptome catheters are easier to control with all concave curves and with the static deflector wires than when there is an associated complex curve in the "reverse" direction.

The technique for acquiring the samples during left ventricular biopsies is similar to the right ventricular biopsy. Because of the longer sheaths, the transseptal procedure itself and the more precise preformed curves necessary to create a firm apposition against the left ventricle walls, transseptal left ventricular biopsies often are considered more difficult. Left ventricular biopsies do require more stringent precautions for clearing the sheaths and catheters of even infinitesimal amounts of air and/or clot since all of the maneuvering of the catheters, sheaths and/or bioptomes will be within the systemic circulation. Particular attention must be paid to prevent the introduction of air into the sheath each time a sample is withdrawn through, and out of, the back-bleed valve of the long sheath. Fortunately, *as long as the tip of the sheath bounces freely and away from the endocardium even intermittently*, the high pressure in the left ventricle usually *pumps* the sheath free of air and/or clot.

Once the sheath/dilator has entered the left atrium through the transseptal puncture, the special preformed curve almost automatically directs the set into the left ventricle and toward the septal wall of the left ventricle. If the sheath/dilator set does not advance easily into the left ventricle, the dilator is withdrawn, the sheath, which is in the left atrium, is cleared of air and/or clots and placed on a continuous flush. An end-hole catheter that is the same French size as the sheath/dilator is placed on a continuous flush through a wire back-bleed device, advanced through the sheath and, with the catheter extending beyond the tip of the sheath, the catheter is maneuvered into the left ventricle using either a torque-controlled guide wire or with the use of deflector wires, as described in Chapter 8. Once the catheter is in the left ventricle, the tip of the catheter, still on a flush, is deflected against the ventricular wall to a position where the biopsy can be obtained. This is accomplished with an active or a static deflector wire. Once the catheter is in position, the catheter is maintained on a vigorous flush and the sheath, also still on a flush, is advanced over the catheter to the end of the catheter and against the endocardial surface. With the catheter and sheath still on a vigorous flush, first the catheter and then the deflector wire are withdrawn from the sheath.

When the tip of the sheath is pressed tightly against the endocardium there can be no passive bleeding back from the sheath and nothing can be withdrawn through the sheath to "clear" it, however, when the catheter and sheath were being maintained on a vigorous flush during the previous maneuvers, the sheath would be full of flush and contain no air or clots. The side arm of the sheath is maintained on a flush while an appropriately pre-curved bioptome catheter is introduced into the sheath and advanced to the endocardial surface of the left ventricle. The biopsy is carried out identically to the right ventricular biopsies but the sheath is kept on a continuous flush during both the introduction and withdrawal of the bioptome catheter between samples.

When the sheath needs to be redirected slightly to a different location on the endocardial surface, this is accomplished using a deflector wire introduced into the sheath adjacent to the bioptome catheter. If a more significant readjustment of the position is necessary, the sheath is withdrawn back into the ventricular cavity, the end-hole catheter is reintroduced and the catheter is maneuvered to the new location using some combination of deflector wires. Once the desired position is achieved with the tip of the catheter, the long sheath is re-advanced over the catheter exactly as with the initial positioning. All of the time when there is no passive back bleeding, the sheath and/or catheter must be maintained on a vigorous flush.

Retrograde arterial approach for myocardial biopsy

The retrograde approach for a myocardial biopsy is utilized only when there is no venous access at all or, possibly, when a left ventricular biopsy is desired and there is no *femoral* venous access. Whenever venous access is available to the right ventricle and/or to an atrial transseptal puncture, the venous route is employed for myocardial biopsies.

For the retrograde approach, a significantly longer sheath is necessary to delivery the bioptome catheter from the femoral artery, around the aortic arch, across the aortic valve and into a very secure position against the septal wall within the left ventricle. In order not to compromise the artery any more than necessary, usually a smaller bioptome is used for biopsies performed through the retrograde arterial approach. At the same time, when using the retrograde approach, the use of a rigid (static) deflector wire will usually be necessary and, as a consequence, the sheath must be one or two French sizes larger than the bioptome that is to be used, in order to accommodate a deflector wire *adjacent to the bioptome* catheter within the sheath.

The sheath/dilator, static deflector wires and distal end of the bioptome catheter, all are pre-curved before introduction into the artery to correspond to the course around the arch, into the left ventricle and with a separate very distal curve in order to approximate the appropriate wall of the left ventricle of each individual patient. These curves are formed outside of the body and again, are preformed "tighter" than the visualized curves within the body. The distal end of an extra long (75 or 85 cm) MTS™ sheath/dilator set first is straightened. A fairly tight, 180° curve is formed on the sheath/dilator 4–10 cm proximal to the tip of the *sheath* (depending on the height of the patient and the length of the patient's ascending aorta), which leaves the distal 4–8 cm of the sheath straight. This allows the 180° curve to be positioned at the top of the aortic arch while the more distal, straightened end of the sheath extends through the ascending aorta to a position well into the cavity of the left ventricle. The tightness of this 180° curve and the length of the straightened segment are determined according to the size of the patient and the length of the ascending aorta in each individual patient.

In order to obtain samples from the medial or septal surface of the left ventricle, a second, relatively acute "outward" curve (on the outer or *convex* side of the more proximal curve) is formed at the tip of the straight portion at the distal end of the sheath. The second curve then will be directed away from the primary 180° concave curve on the sheath. This distal curve gives the sheath/dilator a "shepherd's crook" configuration and functions to deflect the tip of the sheath away from the cavity and toward the *septal wall* of the ventricle once the dilator is removed.

A similar but slightly "tighter" combination of the same curves with the same compound "shepherd's crook" type of distal configuration is formed on the distal end of the bioptome catheter. The opening and closing of the bioptome jaws must be tested several times as the compound curves are formed on the bioptome catheter. Any static deflector wire that is to be used during the retrograde biopsy also has similar, but slightly tighter curves formed on it. The more precise the curves that are preformed on the sheath, bioptome catheter and static deflector wires, the more readily and precisely the sheath with the bioptome will "engage" on the desired area of the left ventricular myocardium. "Active" deflector wires are not suitable to assist in the positioning of the sheath during the retrograde approach unless the biopsy is to be obtained from the posterolateral wall of the ventricle.

To perform a retrograde left ventricular biopsy, first an end-hole catheter is advanced retrograde from a femoral artery entry site, around the aortic arch and into the left ventricle. A stiff, exchange length spring guide wire with a *long* floppy tip (Medi-Tech, Boston Scientific, Natick, MA) is passed through the catheter and positioned securely in the left ventricular cavity with the floppy tip looped back on itself toward or into the left ventricular outflow tract. The end-hole catheter and the short introductory sheath are removed over the wire and the preformed long sheath/dilator combination for the biopsy is advanced over the exchange wire as far as possible into the ventricle. The *sheath* is advanced to the tip of the dilator. The wire is withdrawn slowly from the dilator. The dilator is allowed to bleed back passively to clear it of any air and/or clot and then the dilator is withdrawn slowly out of the sheath. The sheath is allowed to bleed back *passively* through the side port of the back-bleed valve. Usually, because of the left ventricular pressure, this "back bleeding" is very brisk. Occasionally, when the tip of the pre-curved, end-hole only sheath is positioned tightly against the wall of the ventricle, it will be occluded against the wall and there is no passive back bleeding. When the tip of the sheath is occluded and not recognized, a "vacuum" is created in the sheath and dilator as the dilator is withdrawn. When the dilator does not bleed back during the withdrawal, it allows a large column of air to be sucked through the dilator into the sheath as the dilator is withdrawn. Under *this* circumstance the sheath never should be flushed and/or should anything be introduced into the sheath until there is free back bleeding of blood only from the side arm of the sheath! If there is no passive back bleeding from the sheath, the sheath must be withdrawn and/or rotated very slightly *until* vigorous back bleeding occurs. Only when there is a free flow of blood from the proximal end of the sheath is the sheath attached to the flush/pressure system and placed on a slow flush.

To avoid this problem with air in the sheath, both the sheath and dilator are placed on a vigorous flush before being introduced into the artery over the wire. The flush is continued on both the sheath and the dilator but continued very vigorously on the dilator as the wire and then the dilator are withdrawn very slowly. This technique should keep the sheath full of fluid and prevent the vacuum as the dilator is withdrawn.

The preformed bioptome catheter is advanced through the long sheath into the left ventricle with the sheath maintained on a continuous flush. Just as the jaws of the bioptome approach the tip of the sheath, the opening mechanism is activated so that just as the jaws are advanced beyond the tip of the sheath, they open immediately adjacent to the tip of the sheath. The jaws are pushed into the endocardium by continuing to advance the precurved sheath/bioptome catheter forward together. Once the open jaws are forced against the tissues, the jaws are closed, withdrawn slowly back into the tip of the sheath and then completely out of the sheath to remove the sample. The sheath is maintained on a continuous flush during the entire acquisition of the tissue samples as well as during the introduction and withdrawal of the bioptome catheter. In addition, the sheath is allowed to bleed back around the bioptome each time the catheter is withdrawn and then the flush is continued as the bioptome is introduced into the sheath.

Post-biopsy care

Once the necessary hemodynamic/anatomic information and the biopsy specimens have been obtained, the catheters are removed and hemostasis achieved by selective pressure over the catheter introductory site(s). The patient is observed in the catheterization laboratory for at least 15 minutes, which usually corresponds to the time necessary to obtain hemostasis. Even when the patient remains absolutely stable hemodynamically during this time, it is desirable to perform a quick, screening, transthoracic echo of the pericardial space before the patient leaves the catheterization laboratory. It always is more expedient to treat a perforation/pericardial effusion early and in the catheterization laboratory than later after the patient has left the laboratory. Except when either a retrograde left heart biopsy was performed, or very large sheaths were used in the veins, or when there is an extensive left heart coronary study, or, of course, unless there is a known complication, the biopsy patient usually can be discharged after 6–8 hours of in-hospital observation. This usually corresponds to the time when the biopsy reports are available and the patient's medications are adjusted accordingly.

Complications of myocardial biopsy

Although complications rarely occur during myocardial biopsies, any complication of cardiac catheterization can occur with a myocardial biopsy procedure. Because of the repeated withdrawal and reintroduction of the bioptome catheter into the long biopsy sheaths, the introduction of air and/or clot through the sheath is very easy and, as described, extreme attention must be paid to prevent this problem, particularly during left heart biopsies.

The most obvious, very serious complication of a myocardial biopsy is perforation of the myocardium along with cardiac tamponade and all of the other possible consequences of cardiac perforation, including shock, central nervous system damage and even death. As with all complications, *prevention* is the best treatment and with biopsies, prevention is accomplished best by strict attention to the meticulous details of the technique. Unfortunately, when "purposefully and repeatedly chewing" into the myocardium and when repeated enough times in any one patient or by any one operator, a perforation eventually is almost inevitable, regardless of the care and precision of the technique. The next best treatment to prevention is the continual expectation and anticipation of a perforation with rapid recognition and immediate therapy of the perforation when it does occur, preferably before the long sheath for the biopsy has been removed. An indwelling arterial pressure line during the procedure provides the very earliest indication of a perforation and cardiac tamponade. A perforation should be considered whenever there is any deterioration in the patient's hemodynamic status during or immediately after the procedure, and can be diagnosed rapidly with a transthoracic echocardiogram in the catheterization laboratory.

Treatment is to secure (or re-establish if the biopsy line was removed!) a large venous access line while the pericardium is being tapped and drained with the insertion of a large size pericardial drain. Circulating volume replacement is initiated with normal saline or lactate (not the flush solution containing heparin!) and plasma expanders until whole blood is available. When the hemopericardium is large and/or continues to accumulate, the blood from the pericardial drainage is filtered and autotransfused to the patient while fresh whole blood is obtained and the patient is prepared for surgery. If recognized immediately and treatment is begun early, usually the patient's vital signs can be maintained until the perforation can be closed definitively.

Damage to the tricuspid valve apparatus with the creation of a flail tricuspid valve leaflet has been reported in patients undergoing transcatheter myocardial biopsies in as many as 6–10% of procedures, although actual damage to the valve structures during a procedure are reported very rarely[18,19]. There appears to be a decrease in the incidence of tricuspid valve damage when the bioptome is delivered to the right ventricle through a pre-curved long sheath that is pre-positioned in the ventricle and when using echocardiography to guide the bioptome[10,20]. Certainly, prevention of tricuspid valve/valve apparatus damage is the only effective treatment. Prevention is accomplished most effectively by the very precise positioning of the bioptome forceps, being sure that the forceps are against the myocardium during *each and every* "bite". The combination of both biplane fluoroscopy and echocardiography provides the most accurate positioning, but does add to the expense and complexity of the procedure.

References

1. Sakakibara S and Konno S. Endomyocardial biopsy. *Jpn Heart J* 1962; **3**: 537–543.
2. Fenoglio JJ Jr *et al*. Diagnosis and classification of myocarditis by endomyocardial biopsy. *N Engl J Med* 1983; **308**(1): 12–18.
3. Schmaltz AA and Kandolf R. Myocarditis in childhood: results of a decade's research—biopsy studied. *Klin Padiatr* 2001; **213**(1): 1–7.
4. Mason JW, Billingham ME, and Ricci DR. Treatment of acute inflammatory myocarditis assisted by endomyocardial biopsy. *Am J Cardiol* 1980; **45**(5): 1037–1044.
5. Ferrans VJ *et al*. Ultrastructural studies of myocardial biopsies in 45 patients with obstructive or congestive cardiomyopathy. *Recent Adv Stud Cardiac Struct Metab* 1973; **2**: 231–272.
6. Lorell B, Alderman EL, and Mason JW. Cardiac sarcoidosis. Diagnosis with endomyocardial biopsy and treatment with corticosteroids. *Am J Cardiol* 1978; **42**(1): 143–146.
7. Billingham ME *et al*. Adriamycin cardiotoxicity: endomyocardial biopsy evidence of enhancement by irradiation. *Am J Surg Pathol* 1977; **1**(1): 17–23.
8. Caves PK *et al*. Percutaneous transvenous endomyocardial biopsy in human heart recipients. Experience with a new technique. *Ann Thorac Surg* 1973; **16**(4): 325–336.
9. Colvin EV, Lau YR, and Samdarshi TE. Vegetation biopsy using transesophageal echocardiography guidance: a technique to aid in diagnosis of culture-negative endocarditis. *Cathet Cardiovasc Diagn* 1996; **37**(2): 215–217.
10. Miller LW *et al*. Echocardiography-guided endomyocardial biopsy. A 5-year experience. *Circulation* 1988; **78**(5 Pt 2): III99–102.
11. Appleton RS *et al*. Endomyocardial biopsies in pediatric patients with no irradiation. Use of internal jugular venous approach and echocardiographic guidance. *Transplantation* 1991; **51**(2): 309–311.
12. Goldstein JA. Novel long-neck sheath for endomyocardial biopsy. *Cathet Cardiovasc Diagn* 1998; **43**(3): 352–356.

13. French JW, Popp RL, and Pitlick PT. Cardiac localization of transvascular bioptome using 2-dimensional echocardiography. *Am J Cardiol* 1983; **51**(1): 219–223.
14. Weston MW. Comparison of costs and charges for fluoroscopic- and echocardiographic-guided endomyocardial biopsy. *Am J Cardiol* 1994; **74**(8): 839–840.
15. Lurie PR, Fujita M, and Neustein HB. Transvascular endomyocardial biopsy in infants and small children: description of a new technique. *Am J Cardiol* 1978; **42**: 453–457.
16. Lurie PR. Revision of pediatric endomyocardial biopsy technique. *Am J Cardiol* 1987; **60**(4): 368–370.
17. Baandrup U, Florio RA, and Olsen EG. Do endomyocardial biopsies represent the morphology of the rest of the myocardium? A quantitative light microscopic study of single v. multiple biopsies with the King's bioptome. *Eur Heart J* 1982; **3**(2): 171–178.
18. Braverman AC *et al.* Ruptured chordae tendineae of the tricuspid valve as a complication of endomyocardial biopsy in heart transplant patients. *Am J Cardiol* 1990; **66**(1): 111–113.
19. Huddleston CB *et al.* Biopsy-induced tricuspid regurgitation after cardiac transplantation. *Ann Thorac Surg* 1994; **57**(4): 832–836; discussion 836–837.
20. Williams MJ *et al.* Tricuspid regurgitation and right heart dimensions at early and late follow-up after orthotopic cardiac transplantation. *Echocardiography* 1997; **14**(2): 111–118.

34 Phlebotomy, pericardial and pleural drainage

Phlebotomy ("exchange phlebotomy", erythrophoresis)

Cyanotic congenital heart patients with polycythemia often require a phlebotomy during and/or separate from a cardiac catheterization. The large majority of patients with polycythemia have complex cardiac defects and/or an Eisenmenger's complex with significant right to left shunting and with moderate to marked desaturation. The human body's physiologic response to systemic desaturation is to increase the oxygen carrying capacity of the blood. This it does by producing more red blood cells. An increased number of red cells does deliver more oxygen to the tissues, but at the same time increases the viscosity of the blood which, then, slows the velocity of blood flow. When the hematocrit increases to more than 65%, the viscosity of the blood begins to increase exponentially with the blood flow through the vessels and to the tissues slowing proportionately to the increase in hematocrit. The slowing in the blood flow is far out of proportion to any gain in oxygen carrying capacity by the increased red cell mass so that the net oxygen delivery to the tissues is reduced.

When patients become significantly polycythemic, they develop increased cyanosis, increasing fatigue, dyspnea, listlessness and headaches. The level of the hematocrit at which these signs and symptoms develop varies from patient to patient, but in any one patient, it often is a very reproducible level. Older patients often can determine when their hematocrit has increased to the level that they need therapy even before the hematocrit is measured.

At a hematocrit over 70%, the blood flow becomes very sluggish and prone to thrombosis. In the presence of this lowered threshold for intravascular thrombosis from the polycythemia, even a slight degree of dehydration further aggravates the viscosity and can precipitate major intravascular thrombotic events. In addition to the changes in blood flow, many clotting factors in the blood become deranged because of the proportionate decrease in plasma volume. As a treatment for the multiple adverse effects of significant polycythemia, polycythemic patients are treated by a phlebotomy with a volume replacement with an equal volume of iso-osmotic *colloidal* solution. The colloid replacement usually is either a 5% solution of pooled human albumin in normal saline, a 5% solution of pooled human plasma proteins, or Hetastarch. The albumin is available as Buminate 5% solution, Plasbumin-5 or Albuminar-5. The pooled plasma proteins are available as Plasmanate™. The albumin solutions and the plasma protein solutions both are iso-osmotic with human plasma. This treatment is offered when the patient's spun venous hematocrit approaches 65–70% and/or when the patients exhibit signs or symptoms from their polycythemia.

The amount of whole blood to be withdrawn during a phlebotomy is determined by the formula:

$$\text{Vol} = \{(\text{Hct}_1 - \text{Hct}_2)/\text{Hct}_1\} \times \text{TBV}$$

where Vol = the volume of blood to be removed, Hct_1 = the initial hematocrit, Hct_2 = the desired hematocrit and TBV = estimated blood volume of the patient (90–100 ml/kg of body weight). The exact volume of blood withdrawn from the patient is replaced, ml for ml with a *colloidal* volume replacement fluid, using either plasma, albumin, Plasmanate or Hetastarch. Hetastarch is the only non-blood product colloidal replacement fluid.

Normal saline and/or Ringer's lactate has been used to replace the removed blood volume during a phlebotomy, but these isotonic fluids are diuresed so rapidly that the circulating *volume* cannot be maintained adequately, nor is the circulating volume sustained for any period of time. Many patients who had the blood replaced with only normal saline or Ringer's lactate, developed acute systemic hypotension with an aggravation of their right to left shunting, further desaturation, the development of acidosis, shock, cardiovascular collapse and even death. This sequence of events gave the "phlebotomy" procedure itself a very bad reputation with many "authorities" actually declaring the procedure too dangerous and contraindicated.

A phlebotomy does not have to be performed in a cardiac catheterization laboratory, although if the laboratory is available and/or the patient is undergoing a catheterization anyway, it is the ideal and most convenient location to perform the procedure. If not performed in a cardiac catheterization laboratory, the phlebotomy must be performed in a "special procedure" area where full monitoring and *full resuscitation* equipment are available. The patient undergoing a phlebotomy requires monitoring with an electrocardiogram, saturation monitoring with a pulse oximetry and frequent blood pressures with at least a frequently cycled, cuff blood pressure apparatus or in more precarious cases, an indwelling arterial line.

The "phlebotomy" with colloid replacement represents an "exchange transfusion" involving the withdrawal of thickened whole blood and replacing the blood that is removed, with an equal volume of the colloidal fluid. A large bore intravenous cannula/catheter is introduced into at least one large vein. Since all of these patients have significant right to left shunting, very meticulous precautions are necessary to prevent the introduction of even minute amounts of air and/or the development of clots during the entire phlebotomy procedure. Unfortunately, the volume and rate of blood/fluid exchanged is too great to allow the use of air filters in the intravenous lines. The blood withdrawal and the colloidal fluid replacement can be performed through a single intravenous line, and, in fact, there are special phlebotomy/exchange "sets" now commercially available. These sets have a series of either two or three, three-way stopcocks attached to the "withdrawal" syringe. This creates a closed system with a port into a sealed container for the "discard" blood, a port for the inflow of the plasma/colloid from a sealed and "de-aired" reservoir, and an optional third port from a sealed reservoir to introduce flush solution. The flush solution is isotonic saline or Ringer's lactate, *without* dextrose and with 3 units of heparin/ml added to the flush solution. Once the "set" or a self-fabricated, similar system is set up and thoroughly cleared of air, the most distal stopcock is attached to a common line going from the stopcocks to the patient.

The larger the vein and the larger the intravenous cannula, the more effective is the blood withdrawal/replacement. The procedure becomes even more efficient when two separate, large, vascular lines can be accessed. With the use of two separate lines, the colloid fluid is introduced through one line while the blood is withdrawn simultaneously through the other line. With two separate lines, there is no "mixing" and/or diluting of the discard (withdrawn) blood and the introduced (colloid) fluid in the "common line" during each exchange of an increment of blood out and fluid in. Theoretically, there is more uniform mixing within the patient's circulation of the fluid introduced through two separate lines, with less chance of the just introduced colloid fluid being withdrawn undiluted from the single vessel. In patients who undergo a phlebotomy during and/or in conjunction with a heart catheterization, optimal efficiency is achieved by withdrawing the blood from the indwelling arterial line while introducing the colloidal replacement fluid through a large venous catheter.

The amount of blood withdrawn/replaced with *each syringe* withdrawal/fluid infusion varies with the size of the patient and the status of the patient. The blood is exchange in 5–10 ml increments in very small patients and/or patients who are in "heart failure", while it can be exchanged in as much as 50 ml increments in adult sized patients who are very stable. In patients where the polycythemia is secondary to obstruction to pulmonary flow ("tetralogy" type physiology or pulmonary vascular disease), the exchange of blood also is performed at a slower rate. In those patients, as the thicker blood is diluted, the systemic resistance drops faster than the comparable increase in the pulmonary blood flow.

As the blood is withdrawn and the fluid is replaced, a separate nurse or technician maintains an accurate tabulation of the number of syringes of blood withdrawn and the number of syringes of fluid reintroduced. This is critically important, particularly when two separate lines are being used and there is a greater chance of the withdrawal getting ahead of the re-infusion or vice versa.

Once the phlebotomy/exchange is completed, the patient is observed with heart rate, ECG, blood pressure and pulse oximetry monitoring for at least four hours before being discharged. During this time the patient is ambulated purposefully several times while under close observation to be sure there is no aggravation of postural hypotension by the dilution of the blood volume. It often takes hours for the circulating hemoglobin/hematocrit to equilibrate following a phlebotomy with colloid exchange so that a repeat hematocrit *immediately* after the procedure is of little use. Some older, cyanotic patients require a phlebotomy as often as every three months although many go 6–12 months between phlebotomies.

Pericardial drainage

A pericardiocentesis often is not considered a catheterization laboratory procedure. Pericardial drainage can be a purely elective procedure, or, at the opposite extreme, a very acute emergency procedure. The urgency of the pericardiocentesis depends upon the etiology of the effusion and the presentation of the patient. Patients with pericardial effusions can present with the effusion as an "incidental" finding with a large heart on chest X-ray or non specific S-T changes on an echocardiogram, with or without vague symptoms related to low cardiac output and/or chest discomfort. At the opposite extreme, pericardial effusions present with signs and symptoms of acute cardiovascular collapse due to cardiac tamponade. In any situation, a pericardial tap and drainage is a *serious procedure* with definite inherent risks. In all circumstance, it involves inserting a needle, relatively blindly, through the chest wall into the often relatively narrow and/or isolated pericardial space surrounding the heart. When the puncture is over the area of the right atrium, the heart wall is very thin below the site of the needle puncture. In addition to the underlying thin wall of the right atrium, the puncture can be over (and potentially into) the right or left ventricle, and/or the coronary arteries can lie on the epicardial surface of the heart just beneath the visceral pericardium.

When the heart is in a normal position, has a normal orientation and is in a patient of "normal" size and "habitus", the site for the usual pericardiocentesis is at the left chondroxiphoid junction. The goal is to enter the anterior–inferior pericardium over the area of the right ventricle. Occasionally pericardial punctures for loculated inferior and/or posterior effusions are made over the apical area of the cardiac silhouette or, in extreme cases, from posterior. Malpositions of cardiac chambers due to individual chamber enlargement, mesocardia and dextrocardia, of course, require a different approach to suit the anatomy and the location of the effusion.

Although not *absolutely* necessary in all situations, a pericardiocentesis is performed most safely and most expeditiously *in the cardiac catheterization laboratory*. The environment of the cardiac catheterization laboratory intrinsically is sterile. In addition, acute pericardial effusions, with or without tamponade, unfortunately do occur as a complication of a cardiac catheterization secondary to cardiac perforation. As a consequence, the catheterization laboratory "automatically" is totally prepared for a pericardiocentesis both in equipment and "experience" and under all circumstances.

Of equal importance, biplane fluoroscopic equipment is available in the catheterization laboratory to provide actual visualization of the cardiac silhouette and the course of needles, wires and catheters toward and within the cardiac silhouette. The necessary disposable equipment for a pericardiocentesis is available readily and immediately in the catheterization laboratory. Monitoring and emergency equipment for any type of cardiovascular emergency including even opening the chest, along with personnel experienced with the use of this equipment are also available immediately in the catheterization laboratory. Most catheterization laboratories have echocardiographic equipment present *in the laboratory* and with most pediatric cardiologists, this results in echocardiographic support being available automatically and immediately.

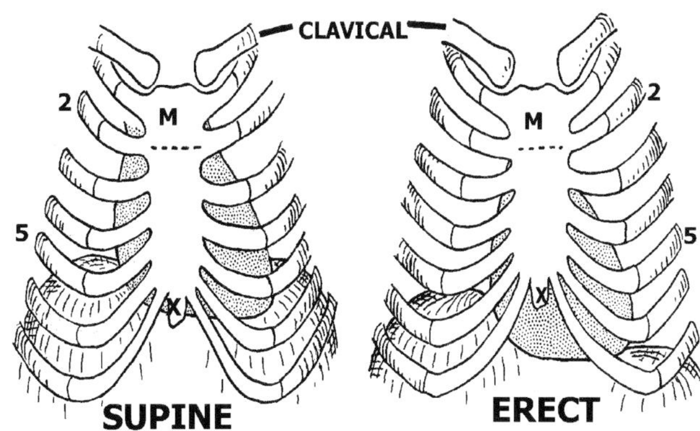

Figure 34.1 The position of the cardiac silhouette in the thorax comparing the supine to the erect position of the patient. M, the manubrium; X, the xyphoid; the numbers 2 & 5 indicate the respective ribs.

Another factor favoring the catheterization laboratory for pericardiocentesis in that the catheterization laboratory personnel are accustomed to moving expeditiously when it is required in an emergency procedure. It usually is more expedient to move a sick patient with an effusion to the catheterization laboratory to perform the procedure than it is to arrange for all of the support and equipment necessary for the procedure to be moved to the area where the patient happens to be "residing".

Although most modern catheterization tables do not have the capability of tilting of the catheterization table itself cranially or caudally, usually various "wedge" cushions, which are used otherwise to create unusual patient positions on the table, are available in the catheterization laboratory. A tall "pillow" or wedge is placed under the head, neck and thorax of the patient to position the patient into a steep, "semi-sitting" position. This position helps to both "lower" the cardiac mass caudally in the thorax and to "float" the heart more cephalad in the pericardial fluid and away from the area of puncture (Figure 34.1). Once the patient is secured in the "sitting" position, the posterior–anterior (PA) X-ray tube is angled caudally to an angle perpendicular to the anterior chest wall. The X-ray image then will correspond to the straight PA view even thought the patient is in the "sitting" position. This, in turn, provides an accurate equivalent of a straight PA X-ray view of the thorax and cardiac silhouette. At the same time, the lateral X-ray tube can be raised to provide a simultaneous lateral view of the chest and cardiac silhouette.

Expendable equipment

There must be the capability of creating a large and secure sterile field around the proposed area of puncture. Disposable, single-hole, paper drapes with the adhesive around the opening of the drape are the most satisfactory for the immediate area around the puncture site. A transparent "Steri-drape" or an "eye-hole" drape serves this function for the small local area around the puncture site. It is important to have a drape with an opening that has self-adherent adhesive about it. With the patient propped up at an angle, without an adhesive or self-adherent opening, the drape will slide on the patient's chest and contaminate the sterile field.

In addition to the local sterile area, the overall sterile field should be large enough to allow the manipulation of long wires without the danger of a wire which has passed into the pericardium becoming contaminated by the other end of the wire flopping off the sterile field. Large operating room or catheterization laboratory "lap" drapes are useful to create a large enough sterile field.

Short bevel, thin-walled needles, which are identical to the needles for percutaneous vessel entry, are ideal for pericardiocentesis in small and average sized patients. The 21-gauge needle is used for the infant, small and/or very thin child while the 19-gauge needle is sufficient for all, except *extremely* large or obese patients. Similarly, the wires used for percutaneous vascular access are ideal for the pericardiocentesis. Because of the "perpendicular" angle in the approach to the pericardial space compared to the "parallel" angle to a small peripheral vessel for vascular introductions, "J" wires are more suited for pericardiocentesis than straight wires. A very floppy tipped 0.018″ or a 0.021″, 5 mm diameter "J" tipped wire is used through the 21-gauge needle and a very floppy tipped 0.021″ or a 0.025″ 1 cm "J" tipped wire is used through the 19-gauge needle. Occasionally a floppy tipped, torque-controlled wire of the same diameters is useful for selective manipulation within the pericardial space.

For an acute, new effusion, almost any catheter that has multiple side holes will serve to drain the pericardium. A standard multipurpose, an angiographic or a pig-tail catheter can be used. There are special pediatric pericardiocentesis sets (Cook Inc., Bloomington, IN) and special, short, pig-tail, Lock™ catheters (Cook Inc., Bloomington, IN), which are designed specifically for pericardial drainage[1,2]. In addition to being very short, these special drainage catheters have the side holes arranged only on the convex and concave surfaces of the distal catheter shaft. In this way, the holes are not occluded by the opposing pericardial surfaces when the pericardial surfaces collapse toward each other as the fluid in the space decreases. These special pericardial catheters are the most satisfactory for any chronic drainage.

There also are special pericardial drainage sets, which contain the necessary syringes, specimen tubes and a closed system of tubing, stopcocks and a collection bag for the fluid. These sets make collection of the fluid much more efficient and are particularly useful for the prevention of contamination of personnel and/or the environment of the room during the collection of the fluids. The sets are justified in any institution performing more than an extremely rare pericardial or pleural drainage. For chronic drainage, the pericardial drain is attached to a Pleura-Evac Suction™ system.

Technique of pericardiocentesis and/or drainage

The patient undergoing either an elective or an emergency pericardiocentesis is type and cross-matched for fresh whole blood. Ideally, the patient is positioned on the catheterization table with a 45° "wedge" cushion and/or pillows under his head, shoulders and thorax so that the patient is in a "semi-sitting" position. Monitoring of at least two leads of an ECG, the pulse oximetry, and an automatically cycled, cuff blood pressure is established.

The chest, from the *suprasternal notch* in the neck, down to the *umbilicus* on the abdomen and from one *anterior axillary line* to the other is scrubbed and painted with Betadine. The apex of the angle at the left costal–xiphoid angle is draped with a "Steri-drape™" or a precut "brachial" drape with the angle of the left costal–xiphoid junction positioned in the center of the opening. The remaining area over the patient caudal to the xiphoid area is draped with a "lap" drape or a combination of separate towels and drapes. Two percent xylocaine is injected with a 25-gauge needle very superficially, *subcuticularly* into the skin in the angle between the xiphoid and the left inferior costal margin. In order to facilitate the removal and exchange of the needles from the syringe, syringes with a *"slip lock" tip connection* are used on all of the syringes used during this procedure.

A small, superficial "skin wheal" is formed with the infiltration of xylocaine. Once the subcuticular infiltration is completed, the needle is withdrawn and the 25-gauge needle on the syringe containing the xylocaine is replaced with a standard 21- or 19-gauge "percutaneous" needle of the size appropriate for the patient. A 21-gauge needle is used for infants and small children and a 19-gauge needle for the larger patient. Occasionally an 18-gauge, 10 cm long, or even a Chiba™ needle will be necessary to penetrate to the pericardium in very large patients or patients with a very thick chest wall. The need for a longer needle can be determined by a quick examination of the thorax in the posterior–anterior (PA) and lateral (LAT) views on fluoroscopy. A metal instrument tip is placed on the anterior chest wall at the proposed puncture site and the thorax is viewed in the PA and LAT plane fluoroscopy. The distance from the tip of the instrument to the cardiac silhouette determines the necessary length of the needle.

The 21-, 19- or 18-gauge "percutaneous" needle, which is attached to the syringe containing the local anesthesia, is introduced into the skin in the previously superficially anesthetized area in the angle between the xiphoid and the left costal margin. Once the tip of the needle is completely beneath the skin, the plunger of the syringe is withdrawn slightly to apply continual negative pressure (suction) to the syringe/needle. The needle is advanced into the subcutaneous tissues in the costoxiphoid angle at the left sternal rib junction. The needle is advanced one or two millimeters at a time with continued negative pressure on the syringe and aiming the needle toward the patient's left axilla. Each time the needle is advanced one or two millimeters and assuming there is no fluid or blood return into the needle/syringe, the vacuum on the syringe is released and 0.1 to 0.2 ml of the local anesthesia is injected into the tissues. Suction is reapplied to the syringe and the needle is advanced further into the tissues. With each advance of the needle and assuming no fluid or blood returns into the needle/syringe while the vacuum is applied to the needle, a small additional amount of local anesthesia is injected through the needle.

The needle attached to the syringe is introduced slowly, step-wise and vertically (perpendicularly to the skin) in the space just below the inferior margin of the adjacent rib while, all of the time, attempting to gently angle the *proximal end of the syringe* caudally and slightly to the *patient's right*. This angulation, in turn, will direct of tip of the needle in a more cephalad direction toward the left shoulder. The needle/syringe will remain more or less perpendicular to the skin surface until the tip of the needle passes just below the lower (caudal) edge of the rib. As the needle tip passes under the *dorsal* margin of the rib, the tip of the needle is redirected more cephalad and laterally toward the left shoulder. With the alternating negative pressure and infiltration of local anesthesia, the needle, slowly and meticulously is introduced into the anterior chest cavity beneath the ribs, directing it posteriorly and toward the left shoulder/axilla (which also should be in the direction of the cardiac silhouette). The direction of the needle is guided by visualizing both the needle and the heart on fluoroscopy and with transthoracic echocardiography.

The *overall shadow* of the heart and pericardium as well as the needle are visualized on biplane fluoroscopy as the needle is advanced into the tissues. However, the fluoroscopy does not distinguish the fluid in the pericardial space from the wall of a cardiac chamber within the overall cardiac silhouette. The fluoroscopy is the most effective in directing the needle toward the gross outline of the cardiac silhouette and away from the pleural space. This visualization is particularly important in very large patients or in patients with a very thick chest wall.

The introduction of the needle *into the pericardial space* is guided by transthoracic echocardiography in conjunction with the fluoroscopy. The transthoracic echocardiographic transducer is placed on the chest wall over the apex of the heart (under the drapes but out of the sterile field) as soon as the needle is introduced below the skin. The walls of the cardiac chambers, the pericardium and the fluid in the pericardial space are visualized clearly on the echo. The tip of the needle usually is not visualized well as it enters the skin or continuously as it passes through the subcutaneous tissues but, once the tip of the needle approaches the pericardium, it is visualized clearly and will demonstrate the entrance of the needle into the fluid in the pericardial space. The angle of the transthoracic echo transducer is adjusted in order to visualize the pericardial space and the tip of the needle continuously as the needle approaches and enters the effusion. Control of the puncture with echo-imaging is particularly important in cases where the "target" effusion is small with a small and/or thin anterior effusion in the area where the needle is being directed.

The echo clearly demonstrates when the needle "indents" the parietal pericardium before entering the fluid in the pericardial space. When the needle "indents" the parietal pericardium inward and pushes the *intact* parietal pericardium into and through the pericardial fluid and *against the visceral pericardium on the heart surface,* this is seen clearly on the echo before the needle punctures the parietal pericardium. This simultaneous visualization will help to prevent puncturing directly from the parietal pericardium, through the visceral pericardium and into the surface of the heart and/or a cardiac chamber. The echo clearly demonstrates when the needle enters the pericardial space.

As the needle is advanced through the parietal pericardium into the pericardial space, usually there is a sensation of a slight "give" as the needle enters the pericardial space and fluid begins to return into the syringe, which is maintained on negative pressure during the introduction of the needle. The syringe containing the xylocaine is removed immediately from the needle and replaced with an empty syringe. If the needle passes through the pericardial space and touches the surface of the myocardium, there usually is a sensation of movement or "scratching" felt (or even seen) on the needle and/or of the loosely held syringe. Simultaneous with this sensation, there may be extra and/or irregular cardiac beats and/or S-T changes noted on the monitored ECG. With any of these indicators of myocardial contact, the needle/syringe is withdrawn slightly and after reassessing the anatomy by fluoroscopy and echo, the needle is redirected into the pericardial space.

Before the availability of echo-imaging and, still, in an emergency in the absence of an echo-machine, a precordial electrocardiographic (ECG) lead is attached to a *metal hub* of the pericardiocentesis needle during the needle puncture into the pericardium. While the tip of the needle is in the skin and subcutaneous tissues, a standard chest lead electrocardiogram will be recorded. However, when the needle tip passes through the pericardial space and contacts the myocardium, the ECG lead displays ST-T wave changes and/or ectopic beats as the indicator that the needle is through the pericardial space and touching the myocardium.

As the needle enters the pericardium with continual negative pressure applied to the syringe, pericardial fluid enters the syringe. The characteristics of this fluid depend upon the etiology of the effusion and can confirm the proper location of the puncture. When the fluid is either clear or "milky", it is obvious that the "pericardial" puncture is into the correct location. On the other hand, if the fluid that is withdrawn is hemorrhagic, the fluid itself does not distinguish between hemorrhagic pericardial fluid, blood from within the heart, blood from a laceration on the surface of the heart or blood from the laceration of a coronary artery by the pericardiocentesis needle! When a bloody effusion is withdrawn and the tip of the needle appears to be in the pericardial space on the echo-image, the location of the tip of the needle is verified by a slow injection of several tenths of a ml of agitated fluid through the needle while observing the area of the tip of the needle on the echocardiogram. When the needle is properly in the pericardial fluid, the echo-image shows a swirl of "bubbles" within the fluid in the pericardial space during the injection. If the needle is not in the pericardial space, the tiny fluid injection may not help to distinguish the exact location of the needle tip.

When the pericardial tap is performed in the catheterization laboratory using fluoroscopic guidance, several tenths of a ml of contrast can be injected *gently and slowly* through the needle while observing the area of the needle tip on *fluoroscopy*. When the needle is correctly in the pericardium, the contrast diffuses laterally into the pericardial space as it is diluted with the pericardial fluid. If the tip of the needle is in a cardiac chamber, the contrast rapidly flows away from the area along with the flow of the blood. If the tip of the needle is embedded in the myocardial tissues or in other tissues, a small stain of contrast is created in the tissues in the area—generally with no adverse effect on the patient.

If the needle tip does penetrate a heart chamber, it is placed on slight negative pressure and withdrawn slowly out of the cardiac chamber and into the pericardial space while observing the needle tip on echo and/or fluoroscopy. The puncture into a cardiac chamber with a *small* needle *usually* does not create a problem. Puncture through the atrial wall, however, *can* lacerate the wall and initiate a rapid accumulation of blood into the pericardial space, actually increasing the cardiac tamponade. If the needle is not withdrawn into the pericardial space on the way out of the chamber and comes back into the subcutaneous tissues and/or out of the skin, the pericardial space is observed by echo for five minutes or more before restarting the procedure. The pericardial puncture is restarted using a different angle and/or in a different location after the period of observation and after reassessing the anatomy and direction of puncture. However, if the pericardial fluid is increasing rapidly after the initial puncture, the repeat pericardial tap is started immediately.

When it is confirmed that the needle is properly within the pericardial space and the fluid is withdrawn easily while the syringe containing the local anesthesia is still attached, the needle is held steadily and the syringe with the xylocaine is replaced with a clean syringe. Enough fluid is withdrawn into the clean syringe for the desired laboratory analysis. After the samples are obtained or, if there is no free flow of fluid, the needle is held firmly in position, the syringe carefully is removed from the needle hub and a very floppy tipped, straight, or a "J" tipped, spring guide wire is introduced through the needle into the pericardial space.

The wire is advanced as far as possible into the pericardium while observing its course on the posterior–anterior and lateral *fluoroscopy* as well as on echo. The echo usually only shows fleeting glimpses of the wire coursing into the pericardial space parallel to, and outside of the myocardium and often cannot follow the course of the wire within the pericardium/cardiac chambers. When the course of the wire on fluoroscopy is very wide, lateral and very inferior and/or posterior, it helps to confirm that the wire is in the pericardial space. However, even such apparently obvious biplane *fluoroscopic* images can be misleading. In the presence of a very large and/or displaced heart, the wire can make a wide and/or posterior loop all *within* the cardiac chambers, giving the impression of passing within the pericardial space. Usually, when a wire is introduced directly into a *cardiac chamber* from a sub-xiphoid "pericardial" puncture, it follows a course more anteriorly into the right atrium and/or the pulmonary artery.

If the wire in the pericardium does not pass readily into the posterior–inferior pericardial space, an attempt is made to manipulate the wire further under fluoroscopic visualization by looping the wire in the pericardial space until the *loop* of the wire passes into the posterior/inferior space. A "J" tipped spring guide wire should be used for any extensive manipulations within the pericardium. All manipulations of the wire are with continuous fluoroscopic and echocardiographic guidance.

Once the operator is sure that the wire is well into the pericardial space, the needle is removed and the "tract" through the subcutaneous tissues and down to the pericardial surface is dilated enough to accommodate the drainage catheter and/or sheath which is to be placed into the pericardial space. The tissues in this area are relatively thick, they are adjacent to costochondral ligaments and/or cartilage and, as a consequence, it is fairly difficult to penetrate them with a drainage catheter and/or sheath/dilator without some pre-dilation. The dilation can be performed by using either a small "mosquito" forceps, a Medi-cut™ plastic cannula, a dilator with a finely tapered, "feathered" tip and/or a combination of several of these. When the wider diameter, proximal portion of the hub of the tapered plastic cannula of a 20- or 18-gauge Medi-Cut™ needle is introduced deep into the tissues, it makes an excellent dilator. A standard but very finely tapered or "feather tipped" dilator or sheath/dilator combination also is very effective as a subcutaneous dilator to form a tract into the pericardium.

When resistance is met during this dilation, the course of the wire through the skin and subcutaneous tissues is visualized on fluoroscopy to be sure the wire in the "tract" has not kinked. If kinked, the wire is withdrawn *very slightly*, if necessary to "exteriorize" the kink. Occasionally the tissues are so tough that none of the plastic materials will function as a dilator. In that situation, the "tract" around the wire is opened superficially with a number 11 scalpel blade and then blunt dissected with a sharp "mosquito" forceps, dissecting along the course of the wire. Once the "tract" is opened slightly with the forceps, the plastic Medi-Cut™ dilator or fine tipped dilator is advanced through the tract over the wire. Once the tract is dilated, usually a short sheath/dilator is introduced into the pericardial space and the sheath is left in place to facilitate the introduction and exchange of various drainage catheters. When a standard catheter introducer sheath is used, these all come with the appropriate dilator and a back-bleed valve.

From the combination of the clinical history and the nature of the fluid obtained through the needle, a decision is made whether the pericardial tap will be a "one-time" acute tap or whether an indwelling drain is to be left in place in the pericardial space. When a drain is to be left in place and when the sheath/dilator combination is used to dilate the tract, the sheath is advanced over the dilator, the dilator removed and either the drainage catheter is introduced directly through the sheath or the sheath itself is used to drain the pericardium. If no drain is to be left in place, a short *sheath*/dilator set with a hemostasis valve initially is introduced over the wire into the pericardial space. The dilator is withdrawn from the sheath over the wire. A multipurpose or pig-tail, end and side hole catheter is passed over the wire through the sheath, into the pericardial space and, with the help of the wire and under fluoroscopic and echocardiographic visualization, the catheter is manipulated as far as possible into the posterior/inferior area of the space. The wire is removed and the fluid aspiration is begun. If samples for the laboratory were not obtained through the needle, the first fluid samples withdrawn are sent for bacteriologic, virologic and histologic examination.

In general, the pericardial aspiration is continued until no more fluid can be withdrawn and/or the pericardial space is empty as visualized by the echocardiogram. In the case of a massive, chronic effusion with a volume or a liter or more, no more than two thirds of the fluid is removed until the equivalent volume of fluid is administered intravenously into the vascular system and the patient is given time to allow the fluid shifts to equilibrate. A massive pericardial effusion with signs of tamponade results in constriction and "third spacing" of the circulating volume. As a consequence, the rapid removal of a very large amount of chronic pericardial fluid can result in cardiovascular collapse if the circulating volume is not replaced and/or allowed to redistribute.

Once the pericardial space is emptied and if no drain is to be left in place, the soft tipped wire is reintroduced through the catheter, the draining catheter is withdrawn over the wire, and the wire and then the sheath are withdrawn from the pericardium. A sterile dressing is applied loosely over the site to soak up any persistent drainage through the tract. Pressure over the area is not necessary and, in fact, has no effect on continued drainage from the pericardium.

Alternative access site to the pericardium

Occasionally, and particularly in the patient who has had previous cardiac surgery, the pericardial effusion will be loculated and/or well away from the anterior, subxiphoid area. In these circumstances a different approach for the pericardial tap is necessary and usually an approach from over the apex of the heart is utilized. In these same patients, both the pleura and pericardium usually have significant adhesions, which, in turn, reduce the possibility of pneumothorax and/or lung puncture from an apical pericardial puncture. It is even more imperative that these procedures are performed in the catheterization laboratory where biplane fluoroscopy is available in addition to the echocardiographic guidance.

The patient is positioned, monitored and prepped and draped in a similar fashion to the sub-xiphoid approach with the exception that an area in the anterior axillary line in the 5th or 6th left intercostal space is the central area of the skin preparation. The exact area for puncture is determined from the fluoroscopic image of the heart and the location of the effusion on the echocardiogram. The administration of local anesthesia, the puncture through the chest wall into the pericardium and the insertion of wires and drains into the apical area of the pericardium are similar to the sub-xiphoid approach.

Chronic pericardial drainage

When the effusion is recurrent and/or anticipated to be recurrent, a drain is left in place following the acute pericardial tap. There now are commercially available special, short, Lock™ "pig-tail" drain catheters for this purpose[2]. These special drains, in addition to having a very short shaft, have all of the holes in the catheter only along the convex or concave surface of the "pig-tail" curve. With this arrangement of the holes, even as the pericardial fluid decreases, the holes within the pericardial space remain perpendicular to the surfaces of the pericardium and are not occluded by the pericardial surfaces.

Once the majority of the fluid has been drained acutely, in order to introduce the chronic drain, a "J" tipped or very floppy tipped torque-controlled spring guide wire is introduced through the sheath and/or acute drainage catheter and advanced deep into the pericardial space. It is preferable that the wire is positioned posterior–inferiorly for optimal pericardial drainage. The acute drainage catheter and sheath are withdrawn over the wire and replaced directly over the wire with a 7- or 8-French special short, chronic pericardial drainage catheter. The special drainage catheter is attached to a "water seal" drain. The skin puncture site and the drainage catheter are coated in Betadine paste, the drain secured with tape and an Oxicel dressing applied over the area. The pericardial drain can be left in place for one, two, or more days; however, the drainage catheter through the skin does create a tract for the introduction of bacteria directly into the pericardium.

Percutaneous pericardial drainage into the pleura

A unique percutaneous solution has evolved for establishing drainage of fluid from the pericardium into the pleura in patients with chronic and/or recurring pericardial effusions[3]. By draining the pericardial fluid directly into the pleural space, an "internal" drain of the pericardial fluid is created without the necessity of pericardial tubes passing externally. This "internal drainage" concept eliminates the chronic direct access to the pericardium from the skin and utilizes the fact that the pleural space is able to reabsorb fluid far more rapidly than the pericardial space.

A needle and then a spring guide wire are introduced into the fluid in the pericardial space from the sub-xiphoid approach as described above. The spring guide wire and then a 6- or 7-French dilator is directed posterior–laterally into the caudal (inferior) pericardial space. This directs the tip of the dilator roughly toward the left pleural space. Several ml of contrast are injected into the pericardial space in order to outline the parietal pericardium. The initial spring guide wire is replaced with a 0.035″ Super Stiff™ guide wire with a long floppy tip (Boston Scientific, Natick, MA). This stiff guide wire is advanced as far as possible into the pericardial space and the dilator is removed over the wire.

A 20 mm diameter angioplasty balloon with very short shoulders is introduced into the pericardiocentesis opening and advanced into the pericardial space directly over the wire. While maintaining the wire well into the pericardial space, the balloon is withdrawn until it is straddling the parietal pericardium, but not far enough back to be into the subcutaneous tissues and/or between the rib in front of the pericardium. The position of the balloon is verified on echo as well as with the fluoroscopy. With the balloon withdrawn firmly in this position, the balloon is inflated. A discrete "waist" appears in the balloon at the level of the parietal pericardium and should disappear with further inflation of the balloon as the "window" is created in the pericardium. The extra stiff wire helps to control the balloon so that it does not pull back into the subcutaneous tissues or squirt further into the pericardial space during the inflation, and the inflation often must be stopped to reposition the balloon precisely across the plane of the parietal pericardium. Once in the precise location the inflation/deflation is repeated 2 to 4 times before removing the balloon over the wire. After the balloon is withdrawn, it is replaced over the wire with a sheath/dilator or a pericardial drainage catheter and an angiogram with an injection of a small amount of contrast into the pericardium is performed. This angiogram usually demonstrates some "spilling" of the contrast into the pleural space.

The percutaneous balloon pericardiotomy procedure has been modified using an Inoue™ balloon[4]. The Inoue™ balloon provides a large diameter balloon with "short shoulders", however, the deflated balloon itself requires a 14-French introductory tract and the central "waist", which is built into the balloon, obligatorily is very close to the "shoulders", making it difficult to keep the proximal end of the balloon out of the subcutaneous tract and the chest wall when the balloon is inflated in the parietal pericardium. In spite of these potential problems the results have been as satisfactory as when a single standard angioplasty balloon is used.

A double-balloon technique[5] of percutaneous balloon pericardiotomy has been used to facilitate better positioning of the dilation balloons exactly in the parietal pericardium. The pericardium is entered using the previously described needle puncture technique. Once a spring guide wire has been introduced into the pericardial space through the needle, the needle is replaced with a 6-French sheath dilator set. The dilator and the original single wire are removed and replaced with two 0.035″ Super Stiff™ wires with long floppy tips, which are advanced separately deep into the pericardial space through the sheath. The sheath is removed over the two wires. Once the sheath has been removed, the two wires usually take widely divergent courses in the pericardial space, separating from each other at the parietal pericardium. A tract through the intercostal space is enlarged either with a large dilator or with a 4 or 5 mm diameter, high-pressure, angioplasty balloon passed over one of the wires. Once the "tract" is dilated, two separate 10 or 12 mm angioplasty balloons are introduced over the separate wires and advanced to a position where they straddle the parietal pericardium, which can be determined by the position where the balloons separate from each other and as seen on echo. The positions of the balloons are verified by inflating the balloons at very low pressures while examining the balloons for the location of the "waists" that are created on the balloons. When the balloons are centered across the parietal pericardium, the balloons are inflated to their full pressure and/or until the "waists" in the balloons disappear.

The evaluation and follow-up management following the Inoue™ or the double-balloon pericardiocentesis is the same as for the single-balloon technique. Unfortunately most of the chronic effusions are a consequence of lethal underlying diseases and there is no long-term follow-up for this procedure. The risks, morbidity and complications are minimal and certainly are less than for the creation of a comparable surgical pericardial window.

Acute pericardial tamponade as a consequence of a cardiac catheterization

When a cardiac or intrapericardial vascular perforation/tear occurs in the cardiac catheterization laboratory, it results in an acute hemorrhagic pericardial effusion. The effusion accumulates very rapidly and acutely compromises the patient's hemodynamic status. Any time a patient has a sudden clinical and/or hemodynamic deterioration during a diagnostic or a therapeutic procedure in the catheterization laboratory, a pericardial effusion with acute pericardial tamponade *always* must be considered and immediately must be confirmed or ruled out. The patient's blood pressure drops (often precipitously), the pulse pressure decreases and the pressure curve often demonstrates a paradoxical arterial pulse with an exaggeration of the normal drop in arterial blood pressure with inspiration. Usually an inspiratory decline in systolic pressure, which is greater than 10 mmHg, indicates cardiac tamponade. An overall decrease in blood volume can diminish this effect on the systemic blood pressure.

On fluoroscopy the cardiac silhouette may increase visibly in size and/or the movements of the edges of the cardiac silhouette decrease, however, there may be no visible change in heart size and/or motion. The venous pressure and end-diastolic pressure increase but in a patient who already may have been in some cardiac failure, these changes initially can be very subtle. Even without any of these "confirmatory" signs, any patient who deteriorates suddenly in the catheterization laboratory is investigated immediately with echocardiographic interrogation of the pericardial space and of the chamber contractility for the possibility of an acute pericardial tamponade. The possibility of an acute bleed into the pericardium with resultant acute cardiac tamponade is the primary reason for having an echocardiographic machine present in the cardiac catheterization laboratory at all times. A delay of even a few minutes that would be necessary to locate and retrieve an echo machine that was located outside of the catheterization laboratory, could easily mean the difference between a successful resuscitation and a catastrophic event resulting in permanent sequelae.

In the presence of a new pericardial effusion demonstrated on the echocardiogram an emergent pericardiocentesis is performed. During the seconds to few minutes before the pericardiocentesis, the patient is given a rapid infusion of intravenous fluids. Although the infusion probably will increase systemic venous pressure further, the extra fluids will augment the systemic cardiac output. In the remote event that an echo-machine is not available *immediately*, the emergent pericardiocentesis is performed on the basis of the clinical signs of tamponade. The same general procedure as for the elective pericardial tap is utilized, however, in the emergent situation, the tap is performed far more expediently than a "scheduled" pericardiocentesis. The patient's position on the catheterization table is *not* changed. The xiphoid area of the patient's chest is prepped and draped very rapidly, and the pericardiocentesis is carried out immediately with the help of fluoroscopy and/or echo when available for directing the needle toward the pericardium. There is less opportunity for "double checking" needle and wire positions during an emergency pericardiocentesis.

In the presence of tamponade due to a cardiac perforation, there will be *blood* under pressure in the pericardial space and blood will be forced back into the aspirating syringe and/or squirt out of an open needle as the needle punctures into the pericardial space. In this circumstance, the location of the tip of the needle in the pericardial space cannot be confirmed by the nature of the "fluid" or by the pressure of the fluid in the pericardium. The position of the tip of the needle is confirmed rapidly by echo visualization of the needle tip, by a small biplane angiogram with injection through the pericardiocentesis needle and/or by significant clinical/hemodynamic improvement in the patient's status as the blood is withdrawn from the space. Once sure that the needle tip is in the pericardium, the blood from the pericardium is aspirated as rapidly as possible through the needle, but at the same time, collected carefully in large sterile syringes. When the effusion accumulates faster than it can be aspirated with the needle and the needle *unequivocally is in the pericardial space* (by echo and/or angio), the needle is replaced with a larger, more permanent pericardial drain. A wire is passed quickly through the needle. A quick visualization by fluoroscopy will demonstrate the course of the wire and help to confirm that the wire is in the pericardial space and demonstrate the location of the wire in the pericardium. Once the location of the wire in the pericardium is confirmed, the needle is withdrawn over the wire and replaced with a tapered, large end and side hole catheter. The aspiration of blood is continued until either the patient stabilizes and the blood stops accumulating, or the patient has the pericardium opened surgically.

In the event of an acute tamponade in the catheterization laboratory, the congenital heart surgeon is notified as soon as the problem is recognized. Immediate preparation is made for fluid, and preferably, whole blood replacement. Intravenous normal saline, Ringer's lactate and/or a collodial volume expander is administered through the venous catheter and/or additional venous lines while awaiting whole blood. An infusion of isoproterenol increases ventricular contractility, drops systemic vascular resistance and, in turn, will increase systemic output transiently in the face of tamponade as long as the overall vascular volume is maintained and/or increased. If whole blood or packed cells were prepared in advance of the catheterization procedure specifically for the patient, the blood is acquired from the blood bank and administered as rapidly as possible. If blood and/or blood products specifically for the patient are not available, a sample of the patient's blood is sent for emergent type and crossmatching. In the presence of continued massive blood loss and in the absence of immediately available, stored blood for replacement, the blood from the pericardium is autotransfused back to the patient's vascular system through the venous line and a blood filter. This is the reason for initially collecting all blood drained from the pericardium in large sterile syringes. During any such resuscitation, regardless of how efficiently the resuscitation is performed, the patient will become acidotic. The blood gases are checked at least every 5 to 10 minutes and bicarbonate is administered accordingly.

Any re-accumulation of the pericardial blood is monitored by echocardiogram. If the accumulation does not stop, is not decreasing significantly with the aspiration and/or if there is difficulty in decompressing the pericardium because of the rate of bleeding into the pericardium, the patient should undergo an emergent open thoracotomy by the surgeons. The surgeon performs this thoracotomy in order to not only drain the pericardium, but to identify and repair the perforation. The thoracotomy can be performed in the catheterization laboratory, but if the patient can be stabilized in the catheterization laboratory and transferred expediently, the thoracotomy is performed more expeditiously in the operating room, where all of the equipment and experienced help for a thoracotomy are available to the surgeons. The insertion of a larger tube to expedite the aspiration prior to the thoracotomy is indicated only if there is an unavoidable delay in proceeding with the thoracotomy.

Pleural drainage

The needle drainage of fluid from the pleural space usually is not quite as serious and/or as complicated as drainage of the pericardium. Pleural fluid usually accumulates more slowly and should be suspected from the increasing respiratory effort of the patient along with subtle changes in their heart rate and blood pressure. Pleural fluid is identified clinically by decreased breath sounds and dullness to percussion over the area of the fluid on physical exam. These signs and symptoms usually occur significantly before there is any symptomatic compromise of the patient. The exceptions to this are in the surgical recovery room with immediate or recently postoperative patients or, in the cardiac catheterization laboratory, following a major intrathoracic, vascular perforation or laceration. In postoperative patients when existing chest drainage tubes become clotted, blood accumulation in the pleura can be very rapid and requires urgent attention. The fluid and its exact location are confirmed by standard and/or decubitus chest X-ray views. In the recovery room, acute pleural fluid accumulation is anticipated in all postoperative patients and handled expeditiously there. With significant fluid in the pleural space, the volume of fluid creates a large distance from any intrathoracic or sub-diaphragmatic intra-abdominal organs that might be in the area and, in turn, makes an X-ray/fluoroscopic guided needle puncture into the area of the pleural fluid fairly safe. As a consequence thoracocentesis for pleural effusions usually is performed at the bedside.

Unfortunately, acute and sometimes massive bloody pleural effusions occasionally are *generated* in the catheterization laboratory when a pulmonary artery or other intrathoracic vascular structure tears. In the event of an acute pleural bleed, the catheterization laboratory must be capable of not only performing a thoracocentesis, but a thoracocentesis under very acute, emergent and unanticipated circumstances. Because of this, the catheterization laboratory must be prepared for, and proficient in, performing thoracocentesis at any time.

This complication is suspected whenever a patient undergoing major, intrathoracic manipulations and/or therapeutic procedures during a catheterization develops hemodynamic instability associated with respiratory distress. A "haziness" or even a total opacity in the lung field of the involved chest rapidly becomes apparent on the posterior–anterior fluoroscopy. The lateral fluoroscopy demonstrates a fluid level with the density of the fluid in the posterior aspect of the involved chest cavity.

Usually the operator has some indication about the event that precipitated the bleeding into the pleura and, in turn, some ideas of the site/source of bleeding. Simultaneous with the preparations to evacuate the effusion, an aggressive attempt at identifying the exact site of bleeding should be made. If the pleural effusion occurs in a temporal relationship to the purposeful puncturing of a structure, the dilation of a particular vessel or even the probing of a particular area, that particular area is the most suspect and is investigated angiographically. If it is not in place already, an angiographic catheter is manipulated back into the suspected area and a small selective angiogram is performed. The problem area is identified by the extravasation of contrast from the involved vessel/area into the surrounding lung parenchyma and/or the adjacent pleura. When the culprit area is in a *branch vessel*, a balloon angioplasty or a "static sizing" balloon is maneuvered into this vessel and inflated at a low pressure in an attempt to occlude flow to the area, isolate the area of the laceration/perforation from the circulation, and/or "tamponade" the bleeding vessel. Obviously, this temporary occlusion is not possible in a main pulmonary artery and/or in a cardiac chamber.

As soon as bleeding into the pleural space is identified, preparations immediately are made to obtain replacement blood for the patient. Acute pleural bleeding can be massive. If stand-by, "pre-cross matched" blood is not available, a sample of the patient's blood is sent for emergent type and cross-matching. A patient who develops a hemothorax in the catheterization laboratory, fortunately, already has at least one venous access line. Intravenous normal saline, Ringer's lactate and/or a colloidal volume expander are started until blood is available. As with an acute pericardial bleed, the cardiovascular surgeon is notified at the onset of the problem.

The radiographically dense area on the chest fluoroscopy localizes the area of the collection of blood and provides a visual "target" for a thoracocentesis. Usually, when bleeding into the pleura occurs in the catheterization laboratory, the patient is supine, on his back, sedated and/or anesthetized, and has one or more catheters entering his body from the femoral and/or the jugular areas. These factors make it unreasonable to elevate the patient into a "sitting position" for an ideal thoracocentesis positioning. As a consequence, in the catheterization laboratory, the pleural puncture is performed with the patient supine. The area of the fluid collection in the involved chest is localized by direct visualization on the biplane fluoroscopy. With the patient supine, a "fluid level" of the pleural fluid "layers out" posteriorly in the involved chest and identifies the area on the rib cage for the thoracocentesis. Percussion of the area helps to confirm the "fluid level" on the involved side.

Usually the patient with an acute pleural effusion in the catheterization laboratory is sedated and/or anesthetized and, since the thoracocentesis is very emergent, local anesthesia usually is not administered. When the procedure is more "elective" and/or the patient is sedated only lightly, then local anesthesia is administered. For the local anesthesia, the *skin* and *superficial subcutaneous* tissues in the interspace between two ribs that are in the middle of the fluid area (posteriorly in the chest) as visualized on the lateral fluoroscopy are infiltrated with 2% xylocaine anesthesia using a small 25-gauge needle. The entire chest around the anesthestized area is scrubbed and draped. A large gauge (18- or 16-gauge), short beveled needle is placed on a syringe containing the local anesthesia. The needle is inserted into the anesthestized skin starting at the *cephalad* edge of the rib which is immediately caudal to the infiltrated *interspace*. With alternating small injections of local anesthesia and then negative pressure applied to the syringe, the needle is "marched" up and over the top of the rib and into the adjacent interspace. By staying close to the top (cephalad) edge of the rib, the intercostal artery, which runs under the caudal edge of the rib, is avoided during the puncture. With the needle close to the cephalad surface of the rib and while continuing the negative pressure on the syringe, the needle is advanced into the interspace. Every few millimeters, as the needle is advanced into the interspace without fluid (blood) return, the negative pressure on the syringe is alternated with small injections of local anesthesia until the needle enters the pleural space.

As the needle "pops" into the fluid in the pleural space, blood from the effusion is withdrawn into the syringe. When blood is withdrawn, the syringe containing the local anesthesia is replaced with a sterile, large syringe and the blood is withdrawn through the needle and collected thereafter in multiple large, sterile syringes. If there is a very large accumulation of blood to start with and/or if the blood is continuing to accumulate, a large 0.038″ long floppy tipped Super Stiff™ guide wire is passed through the needle. The needle is replaced over the wire with a very large sheath–dilator set. The dilator and wire are removed and either the sheath itself or a very large diameter catheter with multiple side holes is passed through the sheath and used to withdraw the blood.

If the hemothorax initially accumulated very rapidly and/or is massive in volume with an associated acute hemodynamic collapse of the patient, then a large "chest tube" with a trocar may be used initially for the thoracocentesis rather than a needle. The involved area is identified on fluoroscopy. The skin and subcutaneous tissue in an interspace between two ribs in the center of the involved area (as identified on fluoroscopy) are infiltrated extensively with local anesthesia and then scrubbed and draped. An incision approximately 1 cm long is made in the skin and subcutaneous tissues which were anesthestized. Blunt dissection with a forceps is carried out into the subcutaneous tissues between the ribs. A 22–28-French chest tube with its contained sharp obturator then is forced through the incision and pushed into the pleural cavity. Once the chest tube/obturator is well into the pleural cavity, the obturator is withdrawn several centimeters into the chest tube until the tip of the obturator is withdrawn well within the tip of the softer chest tube. The chest tube, with the obturator withdrawn away from the tip of the tube, is directed posteriorly and pushed into the pleural cavity as far as possible. When the chest tube is well within the pleural cavity, the combination chest tube/obturator is directed cephalad or caudal and posteriorly toward the area of the largest collection of blood and the obturator is removed completely. The chest tube is secured in the skin and subcutaneous tissues around the tube with a large "purse string" suture around the tube. The "purse string" tightened in the skin around the tube is necessary not only to help keep the tube in place but to prevent air from being sucked into the thorax around the tube.

The thoracocentesis itself relieves the intrathoracic pressure and the respiratory effort should improve immediately. When no "cross-matched" blood is available for immediate replacement and in the face of continued, massive blood loss, the blood is withdrawn from the pleura into syringes and is auto-transfused back into the patient, preferably through a blood filter.

If the source of the blood loss had not been located and stopped earlier and/or if the bleeding persists *after the patient is stabilized* with the chest tube and replacement fluid/blood, a renewed effort is made to find the true or major source of the persistent bleeding. The very best way to stabilize the patient is to stop the bleeding at the site of injury to the vessel/chamber. When the vessel with the bleeding site is a branch vessel, an end-hole catheter is positioned proximally in the vessel and a hand injection angiogram is performed to identify the precise area of tear/rupture. Once identified, a floppy tipped guide wire is advanced very gently and carefully well *past* the area of tear or rupture. An angioplasty balloon or a "static sizing" balloon is advanced over the guide wire and is inflated at a very low pressure at the exact site of rupture/tear in the vessel. The inflated balloon will stop the bleeding from that vessel. Even if the bleeding stops with this maneuver, all of the preparations for blood replacement and surgical intervention should continue. The chest tube is attached to active suction and/or to a water seal suction system. The chest cavity is drained of all pleural blood and maintained on the water seal drain to prevent a pneumothorax.

If the patient was heparinized, the heparin is reversed with protamine until the ACT drops to < 125 seconds. Once the patient has remained stable with no further bleeding into and/or from the pleura for at least thirty minutes, the previously inflated and "tamponading" balloon is deflated very slowly and only partially. The chest drain is checked for any re-accumulation of blood. If there is *no* new drainage and the pleural space remains dry after thirty minutes, the balloon is deflated completely and withdrawn over the wire to a site that is just proximal to the site of bleeding, but not out of the vascular system and with the wire remaining in place beyond the lesion. The patient is observed for at least an additional sixty minutes. When there still is no further bleeding into the chest, the balloon and then the wire are removed very gingerly from the offending vessel. The chest tube is left in place and the patient observed very closely in an intensive care unit for at least 24 hours before the chest tube is removed.

With any re-accumulation of blood in the pleura at any stage during and/or after the deflation of the "tamponading" balloon, the balloon is reinflated and the patient is taken to the *operating room* for a thoracotomy for the surgical control of the tear/perforation. Control of bleeding from tears in previously operated patients often requires a lobectomy or even a pneumonectomy, so maximum attempts are made to control the bleeding in the catheterization laboratory, including the total occlusion of significant vessels when necessary. This is discussed in some detail in Chapters 17 and 23.

Thoracocentesis for pneumothorax

The treatment of a pneumothorax also usually is not considered a cardiac catheterization laboratory procedure, however a pneumothorax may be *created* in the catheterization laboratory and then it will require emergency therapy there. The possibility of creating a pneumothorax is always present during internal jugular and subclavian approaches for the introduction of lines and/or catheters and/or during any pericardiocentesis or thoracocentesis. Often the amount of air that is introduced is very small and inconsequential, causing no symptoms and only being discovered incidentally as a lucent area in the thorax, noted on fluoroscopy when the particular line or catheter is being introduced. A more significant pneumothorax must be suspected whenever a patient undergoing any of these particular procedures develops acute and/or sudden respiratory distress. In the catheterization laboratory, the diagnosis is confirmed readily on fluoroscopy by the appearance of a new, large, lucent area within one side of the chest cavity. If the patient continues to suck air into the chest cavity from the puncture, the other, more opaque structures within the thorax, including the entire mediastinum, will shift away from the area of lucency as a tension pneumothorax develops.

If the needle that initiated the pneumothorax is still in place in the thorax, suction is applied to the needle with a large syringe or the "wall suction" apparatus in the catheterization laboratory until the respiratory distress and the area of lucency within the chest disappear. If the needle had been removed before the pneumothorax was discovered, a new needle is introduced directly into the area of lucency and the air evacuated. The needle introduction for this procedure is identical to the needle introduction for a thoracocentesis, but directed over the highest (usually anterior) part of the area of the lucency. When an acute pneumothorax occurs during a "puncture" in the catheterization laboratory, it only requires the acute evacuation of the air and usually does not need a chronic drain.

Complications of phlebotomy with colloidal volume exchange, pericardiocentesis and thoracocentesis

Although a phlebotomy often is considered a minor procedure, it does carry very significant risks, not the least of which is the death of the patient! When the procedure is performed properly, this is an extremely unlikely event. It certainly occurred more commonly when the thickened blood was withdrawn rapidly and was replaced only with saline, Ringer's and/or nothing! Death from a phlebotomy should be preventable with colloid volume replacement, by performing the procedure relatively slowly and with careful monitoring of the patient during and after the procedure.

Whenever an intravenous line is present in a cyanotic patient, the possibility of air and/or thrombus entering the systemic circulation along with all of the potential resultant catastrophic events is always present. Every possible precaution is taken at clearing the entire system of air at the onset, maintaining the system "sealed" and, when not actually removing blood or infusing colloid fluid, keeping the system on a constant flush of isotonic, heparinized fluid. There is essentially no danger of "over-flushing" these patients or danger of putting them into any type of "pulmonary edema", so extra flush is utilized liberally.

There definitely is a shift of blood and fluids between the patient's intravascular and extravascular spaces during and following a phlebotomy/fluid exchange. This shift hopefully is accommodated for by the colloid fluid replacement. The period of monitored observation following the phlebotomy/fluid exchange allows for the patients to re-equilibrate his/her circulating volume and/or be treated for orthostatic hypotension and any other problems from this.

All of the volume expanders used to replace the blood in the phlebotomy/exchanges except the Hetastarch are human blood products, and as such carry the risk of blood born infections, especially hepatitis C. In their preparation, the sources of the blood are screened, the individual samples are tested for known infective agents, and all of the pooled blood products are heated at 60° for a period of time to attempt to eradicate any infective agents; however, none of the colloidal blood expanders are *completely* safe from this standpoint. Although this risk is extremely small, it is a risk that must be explained to each patient.

Pericardiocentesis and thoracocentesis usually are the treatment of a complication, but complications also can occur as a consequence of these procedures. As with all other procedures, prevention by the precise attention to the details of the technique is the best treatment. In the case of the pericardiocentesis, even this occasionally is not sufficient to prevent inadvertent puncture into the cardiac chambers or into a coronary artery on the surface of the heart. Certainly, performing the pericardial tap in the cardiac catheterization laboratory under fluoroscopic guidance along with echocardiography adds to the safety of the procedure.

Complications of pericardiocentesis are more frequent and usually more serious than complications of thoracocentesis. Complications of pericardiocentesis usually result in bleeding into the pericardium and as a consequence, even patients undergoing elective pericardiocentesis are cross-matched for replacement whole blood before the procedure. Puncture through the pericardial space and into cardiac chambers was mentioned during the description of the procedure. Punctures of the right ventricle (with the needle only) usually seal spontaneously. An attempt is made to direct all pericardial taps toward the free wall of the ventricle rather than the wall of the right atrium. If a ventricular puncture does not seal spontaneously and/or if a large dilator or catheter inadvertently is advanced through the puncture site into the ventricle, then a large, rapidly accumulating, pericardial bleed occurs which, in turn, requires an even more urgent (and correct) pericardiocentesis. The location of the wire that is introduced through the needle must be verified with absolute certainty by fluoroscopy and echocardiography before larger dilators, sheaths and/or drainage catheters are introduced into the pericardium (or, when not verified correctly, into a cardiac chamber!).

A puncture of the wall of the right atrium, even with only the needle, has a greater chance of *lacerating* an opening in the wall of the atrium and creating a massive bleed into the pericardium. When this occurs, the treatment is a repeat pericardiocentesis, but into the correct location and being absolutely sure that wires introduced through the pericardiocentesis needle are in the pericardium and not in the right atrium before larger dilators or catheters are passed over them.

Laceration of a surface coronary artery is unlikely but also, probably totally fortuitous and unavoidable. This complication is more likely when the heart is malpositioned and/or the approach for the pericardial puncture is from the apex. It also is more likely to occur when there is a small amount of effusion, a narrow pericardial space and/or the surface of the heart is close to the site of puncture.

Pneumothorax is the most likely complication of a thoracocentesis. Pneumothorax should be avoidable by careful attention to the location of the thoracocentesis in relation to the pleural fluid. A pneumothorax that occurs during a thoracocentesis is treated by attaching the thoracocentesis tube to a water seal drain and/or by performing a repeat thoracocentesis and attaching the new tube to a water seal drain. Pneumothorax also can occur during a pericardiocentesis, particularly when the pericardiocentesis is from the apical approach and/or when an unusual angulation of the needle is required to reach a loculated effusion. If a pneumothorax occurs during a pericardiocentesis, it is treated with a thoracocentesis and a water seal drain.

References

1. Park SC *et al.* Experience with a newly developed pericardiocentesis set. *Am J Cardiol* 1990; **66**(20): 1529–1531.
2. Lock JE *et al.* Chronic percutaneous pericardial drainage with modified pigtail catheters in children. *Am J Cardiol* 1984; **53**(8): 1179–1182.
3. Palacios IF *et al.* Percutaneous balloon pericardial window for patients with malignant pericardial effusion and tamponade. *Cathet Cardiovasc Diagn* 1991; **22**(4): 244–249.
4. Chow WH *et al.* Inoue balloon pericardiotomy for patients with recurrent pericardial effusion. *Angiology* 1996; **47**(1): 57–60.
5. Hsu KL *et al.* Percutaneous balloon pericardiotomy for patients with recurrent pericardial effusion: using a novel double-balloon technique with one long and one short balloon. *Am J Cardiol* 1997; **80**(12): 1635–1637.

35 Complications of diagnostic and therapeutic cardiac catheterizations

Introduction

Cardiac catheterizations generally are considered safe procedures, but no matter how "simple" and/or "straightforward" an individual catheterization procedure appears, *all* catheterization procedures involve definite risks with potentially severe consequences. The complications of cardiac catheterizations occur during all steps of the catheterization procedure and involve all structures of the circulation. In general, but not necessarily, the risks of complications occurring in pediatric and congenital patients with heart disease increase with the severity of the illness of the patient, increase with the increasing complexity of the procedure performed and increase in an inverse proportion to the size of the patient. In spite of significant improvements in equipment, techniques and the skills of the physicians who are performing cardiac catheterizations, the percentage of complications is as frequent in the present era as a decade ago. When the "simpler" diagnostic cardiac catheterizations now are performed, they are performed on more complicated and/or sicker patients. In addition, the majority of cardiac catheterizations that are now performed are for the purpose of therapeutic procedures, all of which have inherently higher risks for complications.

The complications of all catheterization procedures, both diagnostic and therapeutic, are more common during the "learning phases" of the procedures. The "learning phases" apply both to the early experience of individual catheterizing physicians while they learn a new procedure and/or to catheterization laboratories where the procedures and techniques are being introduced initially. The "learning curve" also applies to the development and use of *new products and procedures* by otherwise experienced catheterizing physicians and/or in laboratories. The more skilled, experienced and meticulous the catheterizing physicians who perform the catheterizations are, the less likely is a complication to occur. These factors are even more apparent in the therapeutic catheterization procedures where the procedures often are more complicated, they involve large and complex intravascular equipment, and they require the smooth synchronization of many knowledgeable people in the catheterization laboratory.

In spite of maximum skill, optimum technique and all possible precautions, complications still do occur during and/or from diagnostic as well as from therapeutic cardiac catheterizations. The complications that occur during therapeutic catheterizations tend to occur with a greater frequency and often with worse consequences compared to the complications from diagnostic cardiac catheterizations. All of the "routine" manipulations of catheters, which are utilized to position catheters during a diagnostic procedure, are also required and usually are even more involved and difficult during therapeutic catheterizations. Significantly larger and stiffer catheters and wires are used for the introduction and delivery of the therapeutic devices. The maneuvering of the larger, more complex intravascular equipment requires more vigorous and potentially more traumatic manipulations. The therapeutic procedures frequently involve the *purposeful* overstretching, perforating, cutting and/or tearing structures and/or the deposit of foreign bodies within the heart, all of which can cause major complications. The complications unique to a particular therapeutic device and/or procedure are covered in detail in the preceding separate chapters on each device and/or procedure.

Most of the reports on the complications of cardiac catheterization in pediatric and congenital patients are in reports from one or more decades ago[1,2]. The best statistical data about the incidence of complications from therapeutic catheterizations in congenital heart patients is from the VACA data and from the several smaller collaborative studies on new devices[3]. The VACA data now are more than ten years old and are "ancient history" because of the improved equipment, newer procedures and newer and improved devices that have appeared since those data were collected. The more recent information about complications has been accumulated from the data in several collaborative investigational studies of new devices, from isolated reports, from "I blew it" sessions at interventional meetings, from anecdotal comments and/or from personal communications and/or experiences. There are numerous more recent reports of complications and their management in the adult "coronary" and "peripheral" literature and some of these complications are applicable to pediatric and congenital patients.

In all catheterization procedures, the ideal treatment of a complication is the *prevention* of the complication before it occurs. The more information that is available about a specific patient and the patient's cardiac defects prior to a cardiac catheterization, the better the chance of preventing and/or successfully treating a complication. Prevention is accomplished by individually using very careful and meticulous techniques as well as by utilizing established, safe procedures whenever possible. Continued awareness of the possibility of a complication during any procedure along with the early recognition of the complication when it does occur are critical in order that therapy begins before the problem becomes irreversible. Once a complication occurs, the preparation of an experienced catheterization laboratory staff for the optimal management of the complication and the *immediate availability* of surgical and anesthesia support are essential in order to ensure a successful outcome for the patient.

The complications discussed in this chapter are the more "general or non-specific" complications that occur during both diagnostic and therapeutic cardiac catheterizations. These complications are organized starting with the more "peripheral" vascular complications and working toward the more central circulation, which includes the major, general and/or systemic complications. This order of presentation does not necessarily correlate with the frequency or the severity of the complications. Many (most) of the complications that are related to a *specific procedure and/or device* are discussed in detail in the chapters dealing with those specific techniques, procedures and/or devices.

Peripheral vascular (femoral, brachial, axillary) injury

The most common adverse events and complications occurring from cardiac catheterization procedures in pediatric and congenital patients are related to the vascular access sites. Problems with the vascular access sites occur with both the arteries and the veins. Although these complications can be very serious, many "adverse events" of the vascular access sites are self-limited and/or create no permanent sequelae. The complications from arterial access sites usually are more serious and are more likely to lead to recognizable, permanent sequelae. Most of the complications that are related to either the arterial and venous access sites are covered in detail in Chapters 4 and 9 and are not repeated in this chapter.

Local bleeding at the introductory site post-catheterization is relatively common, and although alarming usually only represents a minor adverse event from a cardiac catheterization. Bleeding from the arterial or venous puncture can cause an ecchymosis and/or local pain upon motion and/or palpation of the area. Arterial bleeding results in acute swelling and/or obvious external blood loss which comes to the catheterizing physician's attention and will be treated expeditiously. Venous bleeding, on the other hand, can go undetected, becoming extensive and even extending into the retroperitoneal, perineal and/or the intramuscular spaces in the thigh. This more extensive bleeding can be very painful and cause extensive discoloration, but even then *usually* causes no permanent sequelae.

The exception is when there is extensive bleeding into the perivascular ("third") spaces in the lower extremity, particularly in infants. Blood accumulating in the perivascular spaces causes compression of the adjacent veins to the extent that venous flow is obstructed with a resultant further increase in the pressure in the tissues. This "third spacing" of the blood causes a vicious cycle of increased pressure–more venous obstruction–more pressure with eventual tissue ischemia and necrosis. The skin of the extremity initially becomes very blue to even purple and the whole extremity is swollen. The skin of the swollen extremity usually still has some capillary refill after the skin color is blanched with a finger compression. If not treated immediately, the blueness of the skin darkens and appears almost black and the capillary refill is lost.

Prevention of third-space accumulation of blood is essential. With any signs of lower extremity swelling and/or discoloration, all potential sources of blood extravasation into the extremity are investigated and eliminated. Any potentially constricting dressings that are more central to the swelling are removed. The extremity is elevated well above the level of the trunk while, at the same time, not flexing the inguinal area at all. Pressure applied in the inguinal area to maintain hemostasis is "titrated" with just enough pressure to prevent bleeding, but not enough to obstruct venous flow in the involved vein. Extreme cases of "third spacing" have required fasciotomies to relieve the pressure and/or have had leeches applied to the surface of the extremity. The leeches actually extract blood from the tissues and simultaneously inject hirudin locally. Again, close observation of the puncture sites, careful techniques for applying pressure to provide hemostasis, and patience usually prevent this complication.

Complications of catheters and catheter manipulations

When not handled and/or manipulated properly, the various catheters, indwelling lines, wires and devices all can result in complications. These complications are primarily the result of kinking, knotting, actually breaking and/or dislodgement of one of the intravascular tools. There are rare instances of manufacturing flaws; however, most of the complications of catheter manipulations are iatrogenic and are preventable by the use of proper, meticulous techniques. The potential problems with catheter and wire manipulations are discussed in Chapters 5 and 6, while the complications related to the specific devices are discussed in detail in the specific chapters dealing with those devices.

Peripheral nerve injury

Brachial plexus injuries occur more frequently during therapeutic catheterization procedures. These injuries are a consequence of the long duration of the more complex diagnostic and/or of the therapeutic procedures and the unusual and stretched positions in which the arms are placed, in order to visualize specific areas of the heart/ great vessels. In order to visualize the specific areas being treated adequately, very unusual and extreme angles of the X-ray tubes often are necessary during the catheterization of complex lesions and/or during the procedures and, as a consequence, extreme extension and/or abduction of the arms is/are necessary in order to move the arm and/or shoulder out of the field of view. Extreme extension of the arms stretches the brachial plexus over the head of the humerus and when this hyperextension is extreme and/or the extension of the extremity lasts for any duration, the brachial plexus becomes over-stretched and can be injured quite easily. Although this particular injury to the nerve *usually* is transient with resultant pain and weakness of the extremity, it can result in permanent paresis or even paralysis of the arm.

A similar injury to the brachial plexus occurs from a sudden and/or violent, extreme abduction–extension of the shoulder as occurs if an arm of a heavily sedated/ anesthetized patient suddenly and violently falls off the side of the catheterization table—e.g. if the restraint on the patient's arm is released at the end of a catheterization procedure before the patient is awake enough to control his (her) extremities before the patient is transferred off the narrow catheterization table!

Although most of the brachial plexus injuries are transient, the temporary disability from them can last for several months and can be debilitating. Once there is a stretch injury, the only treatment is time and passive rehabilitation. Stretch injuries of the brachial plexus can be avoided, or certainly minimized, by careful positioning and supporting of the arms in a non-stretched position. When the patient's arms must be extended and/or stretched out of a particular X-ray field of view, this should be for as short a period of time as possible. When the unusual angulation of the X-ray tubes and an extended arm position are necessary over any prolonged time, the arms are relaxed from the extended position and exercised passively *at least every hour*. Once the catheterization is completed, loose restraints also must be maintained on the patient's arms as long as the patient is on the catheterization table and/or until the patient is fully awake and in full control of his senses and motor function.

Brachial plexus, inguinal and/or brachial nerve injury also can occur from direct punctures of the nerve with, or without, the infiltration of local anesthesia, during attempted percutaneous access into the adjacent vessels. The nerve injuries as a consequence of isolated punctures during percutaneous catheter introductions have been transient with no permanent sequelae. Localized nerve injuries were more severe in the past when cut-downs were performed in those same areas. The cut-downs involved considerable stretching, displacing and even cutting of the nerves during the mechanical dissection. Hopefully, trauma from local dissection during a cut-down is an event of the past. In the event that a cut-down should be necessary, awareness of the proximity of the nerve plexus and avoiding the area should prevent these injuries.

Central vascular injury

In addition to the trauma at the introductory site, perforation of the more central vessels occurs during wire and/or catheter manipulations. This problem is more common in the venous system than in the central arteries. The veins have thinner walls with multiple small branching vessels, which are entered inadvertently, frequently and very easily. The combination of lack of awareness of the exact location of the tip of the catheter combined with a relatively small extra forward force on the catheter or wire, results in a perforation and/or disruption of the more central veins. This is particularly true in the pelvic and abdominal vessels and when the venous catheter is introduced from the left inguinal area. Most (all!) venous injuries are preventable.

When it is recognized that the catheter has extended out of the vein and further extensive catheter manipulation is *not continued* in the area, a perforation of the wall of a vein usually causes minimal extravasation of blood and few or no symptoms. Uncontrolled continued probing or pushing of the catheter when it is outside of the vein will exacerbate the extravasation of blood. Even an extensive extravasation can go unnoticed or, at the other extreme, the patient may have significant pain corresponding to the area of the extravasation either during the procedure and/or upon awakening from the catheterization. Even with a larger extravasation of blood from a large vein in the pelvic/abdominal region, there rarely is any compromise of the circulating blood volume or the cardiac output, nor is special intervention for the extravasation required. A large venous tear, even without hemodynamic compromise, usually results in the eventual loss of that venous channel.

Perforations and/or tears of the venous system occur more often during therapeutic catheter procedures. The wires, sheaths and delivery catheters are larger and stiffer, far more extensive manipulations with wires and catheters are required than during a diagnostic catheterization, and often several sheaths/catheters must be introduced into a single vein. The therapeutic procedures have the additional problem of large, rough and/or sharp devices occasionally being free or exposed in the venous system. These can result in vein perforations and tears, particularly when the device must be moved or removed.

Central systemic arterial injury

Although injuries to the central arteries in congenital heart patients are very rare during diagnostic catheterizations, perforation and tearing of the central arteries are more frequent during therapeutic catheterization procedures. The majority of congenital heart patients who undergo cardiac catheterizations are relatively young and have "healthy" vascular *tissues*. As a consequence, the problems with ruptured intravascular plaques and dissection of the walls of atherosclerotic vessels are not present in these patients (yet!). However, puncture and/or tear of the wall of the aorta with a wire and/or a stiff catheter still can occur during extensive intravascular manipulations, particularly with the use of active deflector wires and/or in small infants. Usually the rigid tip of a wire and/or a catheter pushes away from, or slides off the wall of an artery rather than penetrating it. However, when the tip of the catheter is forced against the wall of the vessel and, at the same time, the shaft of the catheter is *constrained* and/or in a particularly tight area of the vessel while forward force is applied to the catheter, this leaves no room for the catheter tip or the catheter shaft to move or buckle away from the wall. The continued forward force on the catheter/wire, in turn, results in the tip penetrating the area. This was discussed in detail and illustrated in Chapter 6, Figure 6.1 (a) and (b). The larger, much stiffer wires used during therapeutic procedures increase the chance of such perforations. This problem is avoided by close observation of the wire/catheter relationship, by avoiding restricted or constrained areas during such manipulations, and by never pushing a wire forcefully out of the tip of a catheter into the central circulation. The perforation of an artery with wires and/or catheters is uncommon during cardiac catheterizations in congenital heart patients and should be avoidable with the use of meticulous and careful techniques.

The one procedure that does have a greater potential for central arterial injury is during the selective catheterization of the *coronary arteries* even in younger congenital patients. Selective coronary catheterizations are performed with commercially available, preformed "selective coronary" artery catheters. These catheters have specially formed tips, which are designed specifically for the selective cannulation of the coronary vessels, but at the same time, have fairly *rigid* curves with relatively hard tips on the catheters. The majority of even very experienced pediatric interventionalists usually are less familiar with the idiosyncrasies of the coronary arteries and the use of the special coronary artery catheters than their adult contemporaries. If not manipulated very gently and skillfully, these preformed "coronary" catheters often penetrate deeply into, and/or extend far past the orifice of, the coronary artery. This can totally occlude the coronary artery in a small patient. The rigidity of these curves at the tip of the catheter also can cause the tip of the catheter to excavate the endothelium and, in turn, obstruct the very small coronary artery. In addition to the occlusion and/or injury of the coronary arteries by the catheters themselves during the catheterizations, the coronaries easily are obstructed by "debris" of any sort coming from or off the catheter (air or clot) or even by the spasm of the vessel wall due to irritation/disruption by the tip of a catheter or wire. Occlusion of a coronary artery results in ischemia and/or infarction of the myocardium distal to the obstruction.

With *any evidence* of ischemia on the monitored electrocardiogram during catheter manipulation in or about the coronary arteries, the catheter is withdrawn immediately out of the coronary. If the ischemia does not resolve immediately, a small angiocardiogram is recorded with the contrast injection performed *adjacent* to the orifice of the vessel with the suspected damage. If injury to the wall of the coronary artery is noted, the cardiovascular surgeon and, if readily available, an experienced adult cardiac interventionist is notified immediately. When spasm of the vessel is suspected, with or without injury, intra-arterial nitroglycerine is administered adjacent to the orifice of the involved coronary artery through the catheter. Avoiding selective manipulations in the coronary arteries unless there is a specific need to perform a therapeutic procedure in the coronary artery is the best treatment.

The presence of a "hooded coronary" orifice should be suspected, and whenever possible excluded, in any patient who is undergoing a dilation of the aortic valve before the dilation is performed. When the coronary artery arises deep in the sinus of the valve, a *fully opened* and redundant leaflet of the valve has the potential of folding into the sinus and covering the coronary orifice completely during diastole. The "tethering" of the leaflet by the valvular aortic stenosis holds the redundant leaflet away from the coronary orifice. Once the valve is dilated successfully, the tethering is "released" and the redundant leaflet flops over, covering the orifice of the coronary artery during diastole, which, in turn, results in marked myocardial ischemia. The only management is recognition, prevention and/or immediate surgical intervention to "re-tether" the leaflet away from the orifice of the coronary artery.

Arterial spasm at the introductory site into an artery was discussed in Chapters 4 and 9 under peripheral artery injuries. Spasm around a catheter also can occur in small central arteries when a catheter inadvertently is wedged into a small artery. When a catheter does become gripped by spasm of an artery, the manipulation of the catheter is stopped immediately and the patient is given further sedation, fluids and vasodilators until the vessel relaxes and before attempting to withdraw the catheter. If a catheter is moved forcefully when an artery is in spasm over the catheter, the artery can be disrupted.

The greatest danger and highest incidence of injury to the central systemic arteries now are a consequence of the purposeful dilation of the aorta, with or without the concomitant implant of an intravascular stent. The normal wall of a high-pressure, systemic artery has some elasticity and with this, the capacity to stretch or dilate slightly to absorb the systolic pulse wave. When an artery is dilated very significantly beyond its nominal, largest diameter, and thus its ability to stretch, the maximum diameter of the intima and media of the normal arterial wall is exceeded, which, in turn, causes these layers of the vessel wall to tear. Successful balloon dilation of congenital and acquired *stenotic lesions* of the aorta and central arteries requires significant over-dilation, over-stretching and/or tearing *of the abnormal, narrowed tissue* in the area of the stenosis of the vessel, while hopefully at the same time not over-dilating and/or tearing the normal tissues of the artery that are adjacent to the stenosis. When the stenosis is due to an abnormal membrane across the artery, as found in a classic coarctation of the aorta or due to a build-up of thickened abnormal tissues as in Takayasu's aortitis, significant over-dilation of *only the abnormal tissues* with probable local "tearing" of these tissues is expected to be effective at relieving the stenosis. If, on the other hand, the narrowed area is a diffuse hypoplasia of the *vessel itself* with no discrete abnormal tissues, and/or if the diameter of the dilation balloon significantly exceeds the diameter of the adjacent normal vessel, then the normal wall of the vessel tears, resulting in, at the very least, a thinning of the normal arterial wall. The thinned arterial wall can develop an aneurysm and/or can rupture through the area of weakness.

The best treatment of arterial tears and/or aneurysms is their prevention. The major technique of prevention is avoiding over-dilation to any more than 10–15% of the diameter of the *smallest adjacent normal* vessel. The stenosis in the relatively large diameter vessels and the adjacent vessels must be measured *extremely accurately* using true calibration grids and/or calibrated marks on catheters as accurate reference sources, and not using the diameter of a relatively small catheter for any large vessel measurement.

The balloon dilation of many systemic arterial lesions now involves the associated implant of an intravascular stent. The balloon expandable stent has the advantage of being able to dilate the stenosis to the *exact diameter of the adjacent normal vessel* while, at the same time, the stent prevents *any* rebound or recoil stenosis of the dilated lesion. The artery is dilated to *exactly* the desired diameter of the vessel without the need for any "over-dilation" to compensate for recoil. This avoids *any* significant over-dilation of the adjacent *normal* vessel, which must be used to achieve a result when dilation alone is used.

When a tear of a systemic artery does occur, it requires urgent management. When recognized during or shortly after the dilation procedure and while the balloon is still in place or, at least, still in the vascular system near the area of the tear, the balloon is positioned across the area of the tear and reinflated at a very low pressure, but to the full diameter of the balloon within the lesion. This inflation is performed in order to occlude the leak in the wall of the artery, while at the same time, ***not*** dilating the vessel any further. If the balloon had been removed before the tear was recognized, the wire at least still should be in place past the lesion. In that circumstance, a new and slightly larger diameter dilation balloon is introduced into the artery, positioned across the tear and inflated at low pressure in the area of the tear. The inflated balloon also occludes all of the flow through the particular vessel, which can limit the possible duration of such a balloon inflation/tamponade. While positioning and inflating the balloon, blood and/or fluid transfusion is started while more blood is acquired, the patient is prepared for a thoracocentesis and for immediate transfer to the operating room to repair the tear or rupture. An acute rupture of the aorta carries up to a 60% mortality.

A "covered stent" that could cover the area of the tear within the aorta is an appealing concept for the definitive treatment of an acute rupture of the aorta in the catheterization laboratory. However, this requires *immediate* access to a wide variety and multiple sizes of "covered" stents. No large diameter covered stent is commercially available as yet in the United States for pediatric/congenital heart patients, much less widely stocked in pediatric or congenital catheterization laboratories. The acuteness of the vessel tear does not allow the time necessary to individually "hand make" a covered stent for the specific lesion unless the operator is very experienced and accomplished at this procedure from other uses of covered stents.

Aneurysms that are discovered at the site of a prior arterial dilation, but which are not discovered until later during follow-up, represent a perplexing and still unsolved problem. This is true particularly for the aneurysm following dilation of coarctation of the aorta. Some of these aneurysms are very small and discrete and have not progressed over at least a decade of observation. These probably can be observed yearly or every two years with repeat MRI or CT studies as long as they remain unchanged. However, any aneurysm that is large and/or is growing, is referred for surgical repair/resection.

Although intravascular stents prevent some problems by eliminating the need for over-dilation of the artery, some of the current stents used in the arteries actually create complications that are inherent in the design of the stents themselves. These complications are discussed in more detail in Chapter 25, involving the use of stents in coarctation of the aorta. Movement or displacement of a stent during deployment in an artery or the aorta usually is more of a nuisance than a complication. The displaced stent is repositioned and fixed back in the lesion or, when it cannot be moved back into the lesion, it is implanted in an adjacent normal vessel where it will do no harm.

A potentially more dangerous problem occurs with the J & J™ P _ _ 8 and P _ _ 10 series stents when they are expanded on a large balloon to the larger diameters with a single inflation of the *large diameter* balloon. The balloon first assumes a "dumbbell" shape as only the two ends of the balloon/stent initially expand. This causes the sharp tips at the ends of the stents to protrude radially, almost perpendicularly, off the balloon with the initial expansion and, in turn, to puncture radially into the wall of the vessel with the further expansion of the balloon. This can result in small, radial rows of tiny punctures into or through the arterial wall at each end of the stent and/or the formation of an aneurysm. This problem probably can be prevented by a step-wise dilation of the stent and by expanding the stent on a balloon that has an effective dilating length that is *shorter* than the stent. The initial inflation during a step-wise dilation inflates the stent *initially* to a smaller and, in turn, more uniform diameter, which prevents the ends from flaring. The sequential dilation in a large diameter lesion can only be accomplished by the use of the BIB™ (balloon in balloon) delivery balloon, which expands the stent (including the middle of the stent) to half of the ultimate diameter at the first stage and then, still on the same balloon, expands the stent to its full diameter. The sequential expansion with the BIB™ balloon also avoids the creation of the radial sharp tips from the severe "dumbbelling" of the balloon. The problem of the ring of sharp tips can also now be avoided by the use of newer stents of different designs, which do not have sharp distal tips. All of the problems of arterial injury due to the expansion of stents are discussed and illustrated in Chapter 22.

Pulmonary artery injury

Damage to the pulmonary arteries in congenital heart patients during cardiac catheterizations is more common than damage to the systemic arteries. The native pulmonary arteries have much thinner walls and can be torn and/or perforated more readily than the thicker walled systemic arteries. There are far more lesions that require therapeutic intervention in the pulmonary arteries than in the systemic vessels. The complicated anatomy of the pulmonary arteries in congenital heart patients along with acute angles and turns into and within the branch pulmonary arteries, require far more extensive manipulations than are necessary in the systemic arteries. Finally, for balloon dilations and the implant of stents, often very large, stiff wires and large diameter sheaths must be manipulated and positioned in these very acutely angled, fragile pulmonary arteries. The complications related specifically to dilation and/or stent implants in the pulmonary arteries are covered in more detail in Chapters 17 and 23, respectively.

Because of the complex anatomy of the pulmonary arteries, extensive and complex manipulations with guide and deflector wires are necessary to enter specific areas. A wire tip exiting the tip of a catheter, which is forced and constrained against the wall of the vessel or wedged in a blind corner in a vessel, very easily can be pushed *through* the pulmonary vessel wall. This problem was discussed earlier in this chapter and illustrated in Chapter 6. The active deflection of the tip of a catheter in the confined space of a pulmonary artery can force the tip of the catheter through the thin wall of the pulmonary artery even more easily than in the systemic arteries. Problems of perforating pulmonary arteries with wires and/or deflectors are avoided by having a thorough knowledge of the anatomy in the particular vessels prior to any extensive catheter/wire/sheath manipulations. The anatomy is delineated most specifically by selective biplane angiography. Once the anatomy has been defined very clearly, then, wires and catheters can be manipulated more purposefully, skillfully and safely to the known selected site.

Even after the wires, catheters and/or sheaths are positioned successfully in the distal pulmonary arteries, there still are significant continued risks for damage to the pulmonary arteries. The mere presence of a relatively large sheath, catheter and/or balloon positioned for any length of time in a relatively small branch pulmonary artery can result in enough occlusion of flow to cause stasis and, in turn, *thrombosis* in the vessel distal to the catheter/long sheath. Thrombosis is more likely if the vessel is totally occluded by the catheter/sheath, when the sheath/catheter is not on a *continuous flush* and/or when the patient has not received systemic heparin. Recognition of this potential problem and avoiding the combination of circumstances is the best treatment. If a thrombus is noted on angiograms, the area is treated with a selective, localized infusion of heparin or a thrombolytic.

Stiff wires, which are positioned far distally in the pulmonary artery branches/capillaries in order to support the delivery of sheaths/balloons/stents, easily and frequently do perforate the distal capillary bed in the distal pulmonary arteries. When a perforation of a distal pulmonary artery and/or rupture of a capillary bed occurs, the immediate management depends upon the underlying pathology, the speed in recognizing the perforation, the size of the involved vessel, the size of the perforation and the pulmonary artery pressure in that vessel immediately proximal to the puncture/perforation. A distal puncture with a small wire in a pulmonary artery with a normal proximal pulmonary artery pressure often goes unnoticed and only appears as a slight extravasation of contrast into the pulmonary parenchyma during a subsequent angiocardiogram. These small perforations usually are self-limited. A larger perforation, a tear and/or a perforation/tear in a vessel with a high pressure results in an acute bleed into the lung parenchyma and from there into the pleura of the involved lung. Usually the patient coughs and has some respiratory compromise as an early sign of extravasation of a significant amount of blood into the lung parenchyma. A radio-opaque density appearing in the lung parenchyma in the area of perforation and/or an accumulation of fluid in the pleura on fluoroscopy is diagnostic of a perforation.

If the tear/perforation is in a pulmonary artery that is exposed to high pressure and/or the blood in the pleura is accumulating rapidly following a perforation, aggressive treatment is begun immediately in the catheterization laboratory. Perforations usually are secondary to a wire puncture and occur far distally in the pulmonary vessel/lung parenchyma. In spite of the wire being "suspect" as the cause of the perforation, the wire is ***kept in place*** in the peripheral location and ***not withdrawn***. If a perforation of this sort continues to bleed, an end-hole only catheter is advanced over the wire, wedged into the site of the perforation, and *then* the wire is withdrawn. The size/degree of the perforation/leak is visualized with a small, low-pressure, hand injection of contrast through this catheter. For a small "end vessel" perforation, a small Gianturco™ coil is advanced through the catheter and wedged into the vessel, usually with immediate and total cessation of the bleeding. An actual tear of a larger and/or more proximal vessel usually requires more extensive management.

The balloon dilation of pulmonary arteries with, or without, intravascular stent implants carries significant additional risks. These risks vary according to the etiology of the stenosis, the location of the stenosis and how high the pulmonary artery pressure is in the location of the tear. The patients with the lowest risks are the patients with pulmonary artery stenosis who have had prior surgery on, or in the area of, the involved pulmonary artery at least a year earlier, and those with only slightly elevated pulmonary artery pressures in the area.

When a major pulmonary artery tear occurs, it usually occurs with a balloon dilation of the vessel and it often is more central in the larger vessels and, in turn, creates a more acute problem. If recognized early enough, the exchange guide wire still should be in place distal to the lesion in the particular involved branch pulmonary artery and/or the balloon still is in place over the wire at the area of the tear, or at least, in the proximity of the tear. The balloon is positioned adjacent to and/or slightly proximal to the area of the tear and inflated to full diameter but at a *low pressure*. The goal is to occlude the involved vessel and/or to cover and seal the tear. If the wire and/or the balloon is/are not still in place, an exchange length guide wire and then a dilation or a sizing balloon that is slightly larger in diameter than the torn vessel are advanced as rapidly as possible into the involved pulmonary artery and the balloon is inflated at just enough pressure to occlude the involved pulmonary artery and/or seal the site of bleeding.

While the balloon is being positioned, or at least as soon as the balloon is in place in the pulmonary artery, the pleural space is tapped to drain the accumulated blood. A drain is left in place in the pleura in order to be able to determine the rate of any continued accumulation of blood. The patient is stabilized with the replacement of blood as necessary and is observed for at least 30 minutes with the vessel occluded. If the bleeding into the pleura does not stop with the balloon inflated in the involved major vessel, the patient is taken to the operating room with the balloon still in place.

When the bleeding does stop with the balloon occlusion of the vessel and the patient remains stable, the balloon is slowly deflated, but is kept in the pulmonary artery for 30 to 60 minutes while watching the vital signs for any deterioration and observing the drain in the pleura for any signs of recurrent bleeding. If there is no re-accumulation of blood in the lung parenchyma, pleura or from the drain, the balloon is withdrawn carefully back into the more proximal pulmonary artery. Once the balloon is withdrawn, a *small*, low-pressure, but selective, angiogram is performed in the pulmonary artery proximal to the site of the tear. This angiogram establishes, or rules out, further bleeding from that site at that time. No further manipulation will be performed in the involved pulmonary artery during this same catheterization procedure when the bleeding has stopped. When the bleeding has stopped for at least 30 minutes of further observation, the balloon is withdrawn over the wire, replaced with a smooth, small end-hole catheter and the wire removed gingerly. If, on the other hand, the patient resumes bleeding from the perforation/tear as the balloon is deflated, the balloon is reinflated, and a second longer attempt is made at "tamponading" the area. When the bleeding cannot be stopped with the tamponading balloon and/or once the tamponading balloon is deflated, the patient is taken to the operating room for surgical repair of the tear (or a partial pneumonectomy!).

The highest risk patients for pulmonary disruption are those with *congenital* branch pulmonary artery stenosis, particularly those with multiple, generalized, obliterative pulmonary arterial lesions with systemic or suprasystemic central pulmonary artery pressures. These lesions are very tight, they are in small, friable, branch pulmonary vessels and they are not surrounded by any "protective" postsurgical scar tissue. With this combination of circumstances, these patients represent almost a "no-win" situation for intervention. A very conservative dilation alone produces no change in the stenosis. Over-dilation of the lesion and especially the adjacent vessel is very likely to result in rupture of the vessel.

Intravascular stents implanted *very conservatively* in these multiple branch pulmonary artery stenoses provide the best opportunity for opening these lesions, but still can have all of the problems of dilation alone. When the pulmonary artery pressures are extremely high and the vessel does open successfully *without* rupturing from either the dilation or the stent, then the isolated segment of lung, which previously was hypoperfused beyond the lesion, becomes markedly hyperperfused after a successful dilation, which results in localized pulmonary edema of that segment of lung. This usually can be managed medically as discussed in Chapters 17 & 23.

In the event of the rupture of a small and/or distal pulmonary artery, the angioplasty balloon is reinflated in the vessel to a full diameter, but at a low pressure that is just enough to occlude flow through the vessel. When the bleeding can be stopped, the inflation of the balloon is maintained for 30–60 minutes, after which the balloon is deflated slowly. If the bleeding does not subside and/or recurs when the balloon is deflated, either a covered stent is placed within the torn area of the vessel or the more central vessel just proximal to the tear is occluded with a catheter-delivered occlusion device. The use of a covered stent over the area depends upon the immediate availability of a covered stent of the appropriate size or the "hand manufacturing" of a suitable covered stent. Commercial covered stents in sizes appropriate for central pulmonary arteries are restricted from availability in the US by the FDA and the "hand manufacture" of an appropriate covered stent takes time and experience. Occlusion of the vessel just proximal to the tear may involve a significantly large branch pulmonary artery and large segment of lung, but in the absence of an appropriate covered stent, the alternative is the surgical removal of at least the involved *lobe* of the lung, if not the entire lung.

Similarly, when pulmonary edema occurs in a small segment of lung and the edema cannot be controlled with diuretics, positive pressure ventilation and/or the opening of additional segments of the lung with dilation and/or stents, the vessel supplying the involved segment of lung is occluded with a catheter-delivered device as distally as possible in the particular vessel. In either of these circumstances, that segment of functional lung is lost. The alternative is a surgical attempt at repair of the culprit vessel, which, unfortunately, usually involves a lobectomy, which includes the involved segment.

Another group of patients who are at very high risk for pulmonary artery rupture are patients who have had very *recent* surgery on the pulmonary artery in the area to be dilated. "Healing" occurs in 6–8 weeks, but significant "protective" scarring does not occur for 6 or probably 12 months. Proline™ sutures do not resorb immediately and the suture lines can be stretched immediately after a surgical patch and/or anastomosis. As a consequence the newly sutured areas can be dilated to the nominal diameter of the artery *reasonably* safely within a few days of the surgery. From two weeks to three months postoperatively, the healing of the tissues at the suture lines is at its weakest and, during that time, will not withstand any over-dilation beyond the nominal diameter of the vessel. Whenever possible, dilation of any vessels with or without the implant of stents is avoided during this postoperative healing period.

Pulmonary edema can develop in whole lobes of a lung or even in an entire lung following a successful dilation of a very tight stenosis of one branch pulmonary artery in a patient with a marked elevation of the pressures in the non-stenotic pulmonary arteries. The "unprepared" vascular bed in the segment beyond the previous obstruction suddenly receives a very high-pressure and markedly increased flow. This occurs with a successful dilation with, or without, the implant of a stent. In the large vessels involving major segments of lung, the localized pulmonary edema usually can be controlled medically, but occasionally even requires positive pressure ventilation. In the circumstance when a large isolated segment and/or even a whole lung is in pulmonary edema, it is helpful if any adjacent segments of the lung, which have branch stenoses, and/or an entire contralateral lung, which is involved with the stenoses, can be dilated with stent implants during the same procedure. Opening stenotic areas in vessels that supply additional segments of the lung, redistributes the flow and lowers the central pulmonary artery pressure, which, in turn, decreases the pressure, flow and the pulmonary edema in the initially involved segment(s).

Initially, the only stents available for use in the *central* pulmonary arteries were the rigid, J & J™ Palmaz™ P _ _ 8 series of stents. These larger intravascular stents generated some complications unique to the stents themselves and to the necessary delivery techniques to the pulmonary arteries. There still are no dilation balloons that are *ideal* for the delivery of these large diameter stents to the central pulmonary arteries. The straight, rigid stents frequently had to be implanted in a curved vessel or, if not the vessel itself, delivered around a curved course in the approach to the implant site. Most of the larger balloons were longer than the stents and/or had long "shoulders" which extended beyond the ends of the stents. The balloon/stent discrepancies caused displacement of the stents on the balloons and displacement away from the very precise, critical implant locations during inflation in these curved locations as well as frequent rupture of the balloons within the stents during implant. These complications are discussed in detail in Chapter 23.

The rigidity of the stents and the very sharp ends of these stent struts were the major culprits for all of these problems. When the stents were inflated to the larger diameters with the initial balloon inflation on a large balloon, the sharp tips of the stents flared out radially. These radially flared tips punctured the inflating balloon itself, particularly when implanted on a curve. In addition, the sharp tips punctured any adjacent balloon and/or even the vessel wall. Puncture of the inflating balloon caused entrapment of the balloon within the stent and, at the very least, displacement of the stent.

To decrease the problems with the P _ _ 8 stents, they were expanded on balloons slightly *shorter* than the stent, the stents were expanded sequentially using either BIB™ balloons in larger patients or, whenever possible in smaller patients, the stents were expanded sequentially using two separate balloons of sequentially increasing diameters. Most problems from punctures of balloons now can be avoided by the use of newer, more flexible stents with smoother (non-puncturing) ends and the implant of larger stents with BIB™ balloons.

When a balloon is punctured and becomes entrapped in a stent, the most critical factor for recovery is to maintain a good wire position through and peripheral to the stent. After a small puncture is detected, the balloon is attached to the pressure injector and an attempt is made to purposefully over-inflate the balloon at a very high rate and pressure. When the puncture is very tiny, the rapid pressure inflation allows some further expansion of the balloon/stent in spite of the puncture. Whenever possible, the large delivery sheath is advanced over the wire/balloon and into the stent after any expansion of the stent. If the stent is not expanded enough to allow the sheath to be advanced into it, the sheath is pushed against the most proximal end of the stent and used as a "buttress" against the stent while withdrawing the ruptured balloon from within the stent. Once the original balloon is removed, it is replaced with a different and shorter balloon and the implant completed.

The "closed-cell" design of the J & J P _ _ 8 stents (Johnson & Johnson, Warren, NJ) blocks access to ("jails") any side branches of the pulmonary artery (or other vessel) that arise off the vessel in the area where the stent is implanted. This usually does not interfere with flow, but does prevent future catheter access into those branch vessels. The "open-cell" design of the Intra Therapeutics™ stents (ev3, Plymouth, MN) allows access through the side of the stent and should be considered when placing stents in vessels where further access to the side vessel is considered essential. Each side "cell" of these particular stents allows dilation up to a diameter as large as 12 mm through the side cell.

The BIB™ balloons (NuMED Inc., Hopkinton, NY) helped to prevent stent displacement and puncture of stents. Unfortunately, their favorable qualities are somewhat overshadowed by their very large, deflated profiles, which require very large delivery sheaths, and when deflated their large profile becomes very irregular and rough, making them difficult to remove from the stent. This can cause stent displacement even after an ideal implant. The best treatment of this complication is prevention by the use of an even larger, long delivery sheath that can be advanced into the freshly implanted stent over the balloon as it is *deflating*, as described in Chapters 22–25. Of even greater immediate significance, the BIB balloons are being withheld from shipment to the United States while the FDA "investigates" their use in conjunction with the C-P™ stents (NuMED Inc., Hopkinton, NY).

Vena caval injury

The venae cavae, like the pulmonary arteries, are thin walled and are vulnerable to perforation. Fortunately, the cavae are large vessels and are relatively immune to direct injury during cardiac catheterizations in the congenital heart patient. Perforation and/or tear of the cavae are more likely to occur when there is an unrecognized anomalous vein, and catheter maneuvers are attempted forcefully and blindly before the exact anatomy is determined. The use of the *active deflections* of catheters to overcome the anomalous course of the veins before the exact anatomy of the vein is visualized also leads to venous damage.

Central venous perforations usually go unrecognized unless the catheter and/or wire is advanced *far* out of the vein into a very unusual location. Perforation with a wire of either of the venae cavae results in an extravasation of blood, but this usually goes unnoticed unless an angiocardiogram is recorded in the area of perforation. Even this may go unnoticed until the angiograms are reviewed *in detail* after the catheterization. With an extensive extravasation from a cava puncture/tear, the patient may develop pain in the area during and/or after the procedure. The treatment is observation and support for any discomfort and/or replacement of any depleted circulating volume.

Total disruption of the inferior vena cava can, and has, occurred in small infants during balloon septostomies, during the forceful removal of a balloon angioplasty catheter trapped by spasm of the vena cava and/or during the forceful attempted extraction of an embolized device trapped in the cava. In spite of total disruption of the cava, the patient frequently remains hemodynamically stable and often asymptomatic! The major sequela is that the inferior vena cava will be occluded totally at subsequent attempts at catheterization.

Total occlusions of the inferior or superior vena cava can occur without prior disruption of the vessel. The central vein occlusions occur predominantly from the propagation of thrombi from a more peripheral vein and, particularly, in the setting of a previous indwelling venous line left in place following catheterizations and/or surgical procedures. When a total occlusion of the inferior cava occurs, it usually causes no signs or symptoms as long as the renal veins are spared. Superior vena cava obstruction, on the other hand, often exhibits marked signs of obstructed venous drainage from the head and upper body with swelling of the upper trunk and head and, in severe cases, hydrocephalus.

When caval obstruction is encountered, an attempt is made to re-cannulate the obstruction, dilate the tract through the obstruction and rebuild the vessel with intravascular stents, as described in Chapter 31. The sooner treatment is instituted after the obstruction occurs, the greater the likelihood of a successful reconstruction of the large veins.

Injury to cardiac chambers

Injury to an atrial chamber

Catheter and/or wire manipulation in the atrium frequently results in atrial ectopic beats and/or occasionally, sustained atrial arrhythmias, presumably from the direct trauma to the atrial wall and/or conduction tissues within the atrial wall/septae. The arrhythmias are discussed as a separate section later in this chapter.

Perforation of the wall of the atrium during wire or specific catheter manipulations is uncommon in spite of large loops of a catheter and/or wire, which frequently and purposefully are formed in the atria during manipulations to maneuver catheters, sheaths and/or devices into the ventricles. During the formation of these loops, the tip of the catheter/wire is pushed into the wall of the atrium while a loop is being formed on the back of the catheter/wire. If the shaft of the catheter/wire just proximal to the tip is trapped and/or constrained in a fixed position as the catheter/wire is pushed, the shaft of the catheter cannot move away (back) and, as a consequence, the tip can move only forward *through the wall*, as described previously with vessel perforations!

In addition to the catheter/wire manipulations, wires are used as deflectors within catheters within the atrium and/or are extruded out of catheters in the atrium in order to enter specific locations. All of the dangers and complications that occur in other vascular areas from the use of active deflector wires and/or from the use of free wires beyond the tips of catheters are identical for these similar uses of wires in the atrium. Deflector wires very commonly are used to maneuver from the atrium to the ventricle. The tip of a catheter that is looped in the atrium can easily become trapped in the atrial appendage. When a catheter tip is trapped in the appendage *and* this position is not recognized *and* then the catheter is deflected with an active deflector wire, the catheter tip catches on, and digs into, the appendage and can tear the tissues. This is avoided by awareness of the potential problem, close fluoroscopic observation during any deflection and by the use of passive, or preformed deflector wires within atrial chambers. The preformed, curved deflector wire causes the tip of the catheter to "back away" from a wall and/or a confined area within the atrium as the curved tip of the wire approaches and deflects the tip of the catheter.

Wires extruded out of the tip of the catheter can easily be forced through the atrial wall when the tip of the catheter is embedded in the wall and when the tip of the catheter is not able to move away from the wall freely. Again this is prevented by awareness of the potential problem and by close fluoroscopic observation whenever a wire is being advanced out of a catheter.

Perforations of the wall of the heart occurring during a purposeful needle or radio-frequency transseptal puncture represent a unique cause of perforation of the atrium. Although undesired perforation of the aorta or the atrial wall is the most feared complication of the transseptal procedures, this particular atrial perforation is preventable by using established techniques and biplane fluoroscopy and paying attention to the details of the procedure. The details of the transseptal procedure along with the potential complications and the management of those complications are discussed in detail in Chapter 8 and are not repeated here.

The Rashkind™ balloon atrial septostomy (BAS) is the oldest of the intracardiac interventional procedures, yet it still is one of the crudest and most dangerous to perform. The septostomy procedure itself and the equipment for the septostomy have changed very little in the four decades of use since the introduction of the procedure[4]. The Rashkind™ procedure and the details of the complications resulting from the Rashkind™ "pull through" are discussed in Chapter 13. During the Rashkind™ septostomy, the inflated balloon is yanked purposefully, very forcefully and rapidly from the left atrium, through the atrial septum into the right atrium, *purposefully tearing* the interatrial septum (only!) to make a larger opening. There is *no measurable* control on the amount of force used to pull the balloon, or the speed with which the balloon is pulled and/or the distance which it is pulled, all of which leaves many opportunities for serious errors.

If the balloon is not inflated with a large enough volume and/or the balloon is not pulled forcefully enough through the septum, the procedure does not provide a permanent atrial communication. If the balloon is inflated to a diameter that is too large for the patient/left atrium, the left atrium can rupture. If the balloon is not positioned correctly to begin the pull, the left atrial appendage, the right atrial appendage, the mitral valve or the tricuspid valve can be avulsed! If the balloon is pulled too far, the IVC can be pulled off the right atrium. As a "bonus complication", the balloon can rupture, resulting in the embolization of a non-opaque piece of latex to *anywhere* in the body!

The most important safety factors for this procedure are the meticulous attention to the details of the technique, the use of biplane fluoroscopy and the experience of the operator—which only can be learned through experience on patients! The alternative technique of using a *dilation* balloon to open the atrial septum avoids many of the hazards of the Rashkind BAS, but does not appear to be as effective as a standard "Rashkind" septostomy, particularly in the small infant.

The Park™ blade atrial septostomy (BBAS), although appearing more formidable to the inexperienced operator, actually adds safety to the atrial septostomy procedure, particularly in the presence of a thicker, tougher atrial septum[5]. The open blade is still pulled forcefully from the left atrium through the septum to the right atrium, but this "pull-through" is very slow and is *controlled very precisely*. The blade pull-through can be started with the blade partially open and then repeated with a successively more extended opening of the blade. Once the septum is incised, then when the subsequent BAS is performed, less force is required on the "uncontrolled" balloon pull through. The greatest hazard to the blade septostomy procedure is the introduction of air and/or clot through the blade catheter itself and/or the long sheath through which the blade catheter is introduced. This is preventable by meticulous and proper techniques, which are described in Chapter 14.

The transcatheter occlusion of atrial septal defects (ASD) with devices (Chapters 28 and 29) has generated some new and unique complications of cardiac catheterization. Malposition of the ASD occlusion device on the septum can cause the device to interfere with the function of one or both of the atrio-ventricular valves, or can cause occlusion of a pulmonary vein, the coronary sinus and/or even the superior vena cava. These are potentially very serious complications of the ASD occlusion devices, but fortunately, are very rare. The treatment of these complications is avoiding them to begin with. The positioning of the device during deployment is guided by meticulous, transesophageal or intracardiac echo performed by experienced operators. If the device cannot be positioned on the septum and away from all of these structures with the initial deployment, the device is withdrawn into the delivery catheter and repositioned on the septum. If the original device cannot be positioned properly, either a different ASD device is attempted for the occlusion or the catheter occlusion procedure is abandoned. When a device is delivered and then found to interfere with either of the A-V valves, the device must be removed either in the catheterization laboratory or surgically.

Actual embolization of the occlusion device away from the septum after the device has been released from the delivery catheter can occur and has occurred. Embolization of the ASD device results from the presence of inadequate atrial rims around the defect, poor sizing of the device, poor positioning of the device during deployment or a combination of these causes. This occurs most frequently when attempting to close defects that are unsuitable for device closure with the particular device. If the embolized device is still within the right or left atrium, it occasionally can be retrieved with a catheter retrieval device, however, if the device has passed into the right or left ventricle, or through the right ventricle, then surgical removal is recommended. These complications and their management are discussed in detail in Chapters 28 and 29.

Ventricular chamber injury

There is almost infinite potential for "injury" to the ventricles. Catheters routinely are introduced into the ventricles for pressure measurements and angiocardiograms and are advanced through the ventricles in order to reach the great arteries. The ventricles are inconsistent in size and shape and their inner surfaces are "spongy" and irregular, with multiple recesses within their walls (trabeculae, papillary muscles, chordae) in which catheters, wires and/or devices can become trapped.

When there is any question about the exact anatomy within a ventricular cavity, the location of the catheter in the ventricle and/or when a catheter does not advance as expected through the ventricle, a *biplane* angiocardiogram is *recorded* to define the anatomy precisely before proceeding with any further manipulation. This can be a full volume ventricular angiocardiogram, however, when there is a question about the location of the catheter, the injection preferably should be a *small volume*, forceful *hand injection* through the catheter with the tip of the catheter positioned in the questionable location and with biplane *recording* of the injection.

The most common "ventricular perforation" during diagnostic cardiac catheterizations in congenital heart patients is "myocardial staining", which occurs during selective high-pressure injections of contrast into the ventricles. When the tip of the catheter is wedged into the myocardium and/or is driven into the myocardium with the high-pressure injection, contrast extravasates into the tissues during the pressure injection[6]. If the catheter is wedged deeply enough into the myocardium, the extravasation can extend completely through the myocardium and into the pericardium. The blood in the pericardium is visible on fluoroscopy because the contrast from the extravasated injection will be mixed with the extravasated blood.

An intramyocardial injection produces a "stain" in the muscle tissue, which usually is only an "embarrassment" to the catheterizing physician and causes the patient no known permanent sequelae. This benign consequence from an intramyocardial injection is not guaranteed! The intramyocardial injection, in addition to a pericardial effusion, may produce arrhythmias and/or cause a depression of myocardial function[6]. Permanent small scars and even "aneurysms" in the myocardium can develop by liquefaction of the hematoma in the myocardium[7]. When a large extravasation extends into the pericardium, the effusion can create pericardial tamponade.

The best treatment of the intramyocardial injection, as for all complications, is prevention of the event. Careful positioning of a catheter for the ventricular injections and small, hand, but at the same time *forceful*, test injections through the catheter after it is positioned and just prior to attaching the catheter to the pressure injector are the most important means of preventing intramyocardial injections.

The ventricular myocardium is very sensitive to mechanical stimulation and prone to serious arrhythmias. Bundle branch block and even complete heart block are common, although fortunately, *usually* transient "arrhythmias" occurring as a consequence of ventricular wall "injury" during catheter manipulations. These "electrical" blocks can occur during very common, standard and well controlled catheter manipulations within either ventricle. The conduction bundles in the ventricles course superficially along the septal wall of the ventricles. The "trauma" from what appeared to be a relatively minor bump or bounce of a catheter against the conduction system can result in a bundle branch block or even complete heart block.

When a second- or third-degree conduction block is created, catheter manipulations are stopped at least temporarily and the patient's rhythm is allowed to recover. When complete heart block is created, the patient's heart rate, blood pressure and oxygenation all must be monitored very closely. The bundle branch blocks usually are transient and resolve spontaneously within several minutes. Once the rhythm returns to normal the catheterization procedure is resumed, but usually with a different catheter and/or approach to the ventricular manipulation. Often a floating balloon catheter is substituted for a torque-controlled catheter for the subsequent catheter manipulations in the ventricle.

When complete heart block persists for more than several minutes and/or with any deterioration in the patient's hemodynamics, a bolus of isuprel is administered intravenously to stimulate the ventricular rate. Decadron usually is administered intravenously as a "tissue anti-inflammatory" agent. A transvenous, pacing catheter is introduced into the ventricle if normal conduction does not return with the above medications and/or there is any deterioration in the patient's hemodynamic status. The other arrhythmias are discussed later in this chapter in a separate section.

Wires frequently are used in the ventricle to manipulate catheters into specific locations in the ventricle, to manipulate from the ventricle to a great artery and/or to support catheters/devices within the ventricle. When a guide wire is advanced out of the tip of a catheter that is pressed against the wall of the ventricle, even the "soft" tip of a wire can easily penetrate the myocardium *unless* the tip of the *catheter* is able to move *easily away* from the wall of the ventricle. Guide wires with stiffer tips and Terumo Glide™ wires are even more prone to penetrate the myocardium. Whenever a wire is advanced out of the tip of a catheter that is positioned in a ventricle, the wire and the catheter are observed very carefully to ensure that the tip of the catheter does "back away" from the wall of the ventricle as the tip of the wire is advanced out of the tip of the catheter, and that the floppy tip of the wire follows a "floppy" and freely moving course through the *cavity* of the ventricle. If the wire meets resistance as it is advanced and/or when the tip of the wire moves in synchrony with the ventricular motion and in a very fixed or confined course, the wire is in the myocardial tissues and not free within the cavity!

Similarly, when a *catheter* in a ventricle is deflected with an active deflector wire, the strong deflection force delivered to the tip of the catheter can easily dig into and/or "excavate" through myocardial tissues. Because the active deflector wire requires a very strong force applied at the control handle of the deflector system in order to deflect the tip of the catheter, there is no way to determine from the "feel" of this force whether the force applied to the handle is meeting the resistance of just the stiffness of the catheter or the resistance of the catheter digging into the myocardium! The catheter tip is observed very closely to ensure that the tip is moving freely within the cavity during any active deflection.

All ventricular punctures and/or perforations during catheter manipulations are even more common in infants where the cardiac structures are much smaller (particularly compared to the image on the fluoroscopy screen!), the anatomy often is bizarre and ill defined, and where the tissues are much less compacted and, in turn, much less resistant to perforation. This combination of factors contributes to catheters and/or wires being pushed or "deflected" directly through blind corners or recesses in the ventricles. This type of perforation is avoided by a thorough knowledge of the anatomy determined from a preceding biplane angiogram, combined with very knowledgeable, precise and skillful manipulations of the catheters. For added safety, smaller and more malleable catheters should be used in infants. Floating balloon diagnostic catheters are less controllable but may be slightly safer in small infants and are preferable for less experienced operators in infants and small children.

Endomyocardial biopsy is a very common procedure in most cardiac catheterization laboratories. In spite of this, an endomyocardial biopsy potentially is one of the most hazardous procedures performed in the cardiac catheterization laboratory. There is a significant chance of cardiac perforation, damage to the atrioventricular valve apparatus and/or air or clot embolization with each "bite" during the procedure. Frequently, six or more "bites" are obtained during any one procedure, incurring the same risks each time. In spite of these risks, but because the biopsies are performed so often and repeatedly in the same patients, the biopsy procedures often are taken less seriously by the operators and catheterization laboratory staff.

With each sample ("bite") during a biopsy procedure, first a stiff and relatively large sheath is maneuvered into the ventricular chamber using a guide wire and/or deflector system. The sheath purposefully is pushed firmly against (into!) the ventricular wall. The relatively stiff bioptome is advanced through the sheath and the bioptome and sheath are pushed against the myocardium. While the sheath and bioptome are pushed firmly into the myocardial wall, the jaws of the bioptome are opened as it is pushed beyond the end of the sheath into the myocardium. The forward push is maintained as the jaws of the forceps are closed. This purposefully digs a piece of myocardium out of the heart wall! This procedure is repeated six or more times—hopefully changing the position of the sheath/bioptome slightly with each subsequent sample. The wall thickness in the area and/or any chordae that might happen to be in the area, actually cannot be seen on fluoroscopy at any time during this sampling! The "safety" in the procedure depends upon directing the sheath and bioptome to an area of the wall that is *expected* to be thicker and assuming that by opening the bioptome against the wall it will open adjacent to and/or behind any chordae. These structures occasionally can be seen with a transthoracic echo, but this imaging modality usually is not used for a "routine biopsy".

As with the therapeutic catheterization procedures in all other vascular areas, the therapeutic procedures in the ventricles and/or on the valves of the ventricles necessitate far more extensive manipulations in the ventricles than do diagnostic catheterizations. These more extensive manipulations also are with larger and stiffer wires, catheters and sheaths and, in turn, are even more likely to result in complications than are similar manipulations during diagnostic catheterizations.

A ventricular perforation during a therapeutic procedure is more likely to occur in the left ventricle than in the right ventricle. Perforation of the right ventricular wall occurs more often during catheter/wire manipulations as the catheters and wires are being advanced through the ventricle in order to perform procedures in the pulmonary arteries as opposed to actual procedures in the right ventricle. Left ventricular perforations can occur as catheters/wires are being manipulated in and/or through the left ventricle, particularly during active deflection of catheters, however, more frequently, serious perforations of the left ventricle occur during therapeutic procedures on either the mitral or the aortic valve.

During balloon valvuloplasties of both the aortic and mitral valves, the distal ends of stiff guide wires, or an acutely curved stiff portion of the stiff guide wires, which support the balloons, are positioned in the left ventricular cavity. A perforation of the ventricular wall can occur during the positioning of these wires, but is more likely to occur during the inflation of the valvuloplasty balloon in the valve. As the balloons are inflated in the valve, they become very rigid. As they inflate this very rigid structure can be squeezed forcefully and rapidly *out of* the valve and into the ventricular cavity. This potentially forces the wire and/or tip of the balloon through the apex of the ventricle.

The best treatment, as usual, is prevention by the very careful, meticulous preparation and positioning of the proper wire(s) for the dilation. Super Stiff™ wires with a long floppy tip (Medi-Tech, Boston Scientific, Natick, MA) are used for both the aortic and the mitral valves. The Super Stiff™ wire provides better overall control of to-and-fro motion of the balloon in the valve during its inflation while the smooth curve in the apex prevents the balloon tip on the wire from perforating the myocardium if the balloon does "squirt" into the ventricle. The long floppy tip curled in the ventricular cavity is less traumatic to the intracavitary structures. A tight "pig-tail" is formed at the very floppy tip of the wire and a smooth 180° curve is formed just at the transition area between the stiff and floppy portions of the wire. The "pig-tail" at the distal end of the wire prevents the tip of the wire from digging into the ventricular wall. The smooth curve in the transition zone of the wire is positioned deep in the ventricle close to the apex during the valve dilation to keep the balloon/wire from perforating the apex.

When a perforation of the ventricle does occur, this is one of the most serious acute complications in the catheterization laboratory. It requires the efficient mobilization of all resources of the catheterization laboratory and the cardiovascular operating room for the successful management of this complication. Blood loss from the ventricle into the pericardium usually is rapid and massive and results in rapid tamponade and cardiovascular collapse. The operating room is notified of the perforation immediately. Blood and/or fluid replacement is initiated immediately while an emergency pericardiocentesis is carried out with fluoroscopic and echocardiographic guidance. A large diameter drainage catheter is placed in the pericardium through the pericardiocentesis site and preparations are made for auto-transfusion of the blood withdrawn from the pericardial space. In rare instances, a very small ventricular perforation from a puncture by a wire only will seal on its own, especially in the right ventricle. However, unless the perforation unequivocally is known and/or determined to be a small puncture from a wire only and particularly in the left ventricle, the patient is referred to the operating room for surgical repair of the opening as soon as they are stabilized. Occasionally the patient must be moved rapidly while they are being stabilized/resuscitated.

Large, broad and tense loops of stiff wires in the ventricles by themselves and/or even within catheters during therapeutic procedures, can cause stretching of the wall of the ventricular chamber and/or hold the atrio-ventricular valves open. These loops usually do not result in permanent injury to the ventricle but can compromise the patient's hemodynamics significantly. The stretching of the wall by a stiff loop of wire/catheter restricts the ventricular contractility directly while the propped open A-V valve creates free regurgitation. The combined effects decrease cardiac output acutely and/or cause a significant vagal response with bradycardia and hypotension. The problem is corrected acutely by relieving the tension on the wire and/or removing the wire completely. Occasionally, however, it is more expedient to consider completing the manipulation/procedure very rapidly while "tolerating" the temporarily decreased function rather than "automatically" withdrawing the wire. If the procedure can be completed without progressive deterioration in the patient, continuing the maneuver avoids the necessity of totally repositioning the wire, catheter and/or device and starting all over from the beginning of the procedure.

The use of catheter-delivered occlusion devices has generated some new problems and complications in the ventricles. The most serious of these problems in the ventricles is for an errant device to become entangled in the ventricular cavity—particularly in the atrio-ventricular valve apparatus. This occurs, not only with occlusion devices used in ventricular septal defects (VSD), but with atrial septal defect/patent foramen ovale (ASD/PFO) occlusion devices or even patent ductus arteriosus (PDA) occlusion devices. The entrapment of a VSD device in a ventricle usually is the consequence of the device becoming dislodged and/or malpositioned during its implant in the muscular ventricular septum. The double-umbrella devices (CardioSEAL and STARFlex) are *less* likely to be dislodged from a muscular ventricular defect once implanted. However, as these devices are opened in the ventricle and/or if they do dislodge, they are the most likely to be entangled in the valvular apparatus within the ventricle because of their multiple protruding arms. The Amplatzer VSD device has no "protruding" ends or arms and if it dislodges, it is more likely to tumble freely in the ventricle and to embolize to the great artery arising from the ventricle.

The ASD devices can become lodged in the ventricle as a result of embolization from the atrium. Embolization of the ASD device can occur during the device deployment or hours later, after an apparently successful implant. Remarkably, when such an embolization occurs, even the larger devices with multiple extended arms tend to tumble completely through the ventricle and into the great artery off the ventricle! The embolized device then lodges in a great artery as the vessel narrows more peripherally. When an ASD device does lodge in the ventricle, an attempt is made to grasp it with a bioptome forceps or snare catheter and to "tease" it *very gently* out of the ventricle. When *any* resistance is encountered during a very gentle attempt to withdraw the errant device from the ventricle, the device is released from the retrieval device and referred for removal surgically under direct visualization.

The usual way that any of the devices become *lodged* in the ventricle is iatrogenic, when an attempt is made to pull an open, or partially open, device through the ventricle from the pulmonary artery. With the VSD and ASD devices, this only occurs when one of these devices has embolized through the ventricle into the pulmonary artery. When an embolized device is grasped in the pulmonary artery with a foreign body retrieval catheter, it is erroneous and dangerous to attempt withdrawing the grasped device out of the pulmonary artery without first collapsing it completely into a long sheath. If any device is to be retrieved from the pulmonary artery, it first *must be* withdrawn *completely* into a large, long sheath while still in the pulmonary artery. No exposed part of a device extending out of a sheath should be withdrawn through the ventricle.

When an umbrella or coil that was used in an attempt to occlude the PDA becomes entrapped in the ventricle, the complication also is iatrogenic. With the PDA devices, the deployed, *open* devices have been pulled through the PDA and into the pulmonary artery (PA) and/or have embolized from the PDA to the PA after a successful implant. The device either is still held by the delivery catheter or is grasped with a retrieval forceps in the PA. As with ASD devices that embolize to the pulmonary artery, when a misguided attempt is made to withdraw the still open PDA device back through the ventricle, the device commonly becomes entangled in the tricuspid valve apparatus during the withdrawal. This is equally true for the coil occlusion devices as for the other PDA devices. Any embolized device that is positioned in the pulmonary artery must be withdrawn *completely* into a long sheath before being withdrawn through the ventricle. An occlusion device that is entangled firmly in a ventricle should be removed surgically to prevent permanent damage to the valve.

Valvular damage

The most common "injury" to a valve during cardiac catheterization is the creation of valvular incompetence as a consequence of a purposeful dilation of a stenotic valve. Some degree of valve insufficiency is expected and is produced by the majority of balloon dilations of valves. Careful attention to the appropriate balloon diameter(s) to annulus diameter ratio for the particular valve being dilated minimizes the creation of excessive regurgitation. However, when a thickened stenotic valve is torn open by a dilation balloon, there is no absolute control over where the valve splits and very little control on how far it splits. The use of a smaller balloon relative to the annulus diameter *may* be less likely to create as much valvular regurgitation, but, at the same time, is less likely to open the stenotic valve sufficiently. The creation of significant, unwanted valve regurgitation is a known, but accepted small risk of balloon dilation of all valves.

The significance of valvular regurgitation as a result of balloon dilation of a particular valve depends upon which valve is involved and, obviously, on how much valve regurgitation is produced. Pulmonary valve regurgitation appears to be well tolerated, even to the point that wide open pulmonary valve regurgitation is considered part of the results of a successful pulmonary valve dilation. The significance of tricuspid regurgitation depends not only upon the amount of regurgitation, but also upon the underlying condition and the level of the right ventricular pressure. Mild or moderate tricuspid regurgitation in the presence of a normal right ventricular pressure appears to be tolerated well for many years, if not indefinitely. Severe tricuspid regurgitation and/or tricuspid regurgitation in the presence of high right ventricular pressures usually require surgical intervention for repair or valve replacement.

Significant aortic and/or mitral valve regurgitation is not well tolerated and eventually requires surgical intervention, usually with valve replacement. In order to avoid any regurgitation of the aortic or mitral valves, far more conservative balloon dilations of these valves are performed. As a consequence, a mild or even a moderate residual obstructive gradient along with no, or minimal, valve regurgitation is accepted as a "good result" when dilating the aortic and/or mitral valves.

Puncture of valve leaflets can occur while crossing a semilunar valve during a retrograde arterial catheterization. Although valve perforation can occur while crossing a normal semilunar valve in a large patient, valve perforation is more common in very small patients and/or in the presence of aortic valve stenosis. Rather than any particular skill, the passage of a catheter and/or a wire retrograde across a semilunar valve depends more upon the "chance" passage of that wire and/or catheter through the center of the valve while the valve transiently is in the open position. The smaller the valve orifice, the more difficult it is to cross. Crossing the aortic valve usually requires multiple "probes" with the wire and/or catheter in the direction of the valve, hoping that the wire and/or catheter will pop through the center of the orifice when the valve is in the open position. These probes with the catheter and/or wire are "blind probes". The exact valve cannot be *visualized* on fluoroscopy and the forward probing with the catheter and/or wire cannot be timed to coincide with the microsecond when the valve is open. Even a "freeze frame" image of the central opening in one fluoroscopy plane, often has no correlation to the location of the opening in the corresponding view in the perpendicular plane. As a consequence, the majority of the forward probes with wires and/or catheters bounce into the sinuses of the valve and/or against the closed valve leaflets. With vigorous (or impatient!) probing with a wire or catheter that is at all stiff, or even with a very soft tipped wire as it exits the tip of a catheter when the tip of the catheter is very close to the closed valve, the wire or catheter can easily perforate the delicate valve leaflet. Perforation of a leaflet with just a wire results in a tiny leakage of the valve, and can go unnoticed unless a balloon or larger catheter is passed through the same tract. If a balloon dilation is performed with the balloon in the tract *through the tissue* of the *leaflet*, massive valve regurgitation is created.

The treatment, again, is prevention. Extra *soft, floppy* tipped wires and rapid, but very gentle, "probing" with the catheter and/or wire are used to cross the semilunar valve. *Rapid, multiple,* short and *very gentle* retrograde probes with a very *soft tipped* wire or a soft catheter have a much greater chance of crossing through the valve orifice than any chance with slow meticulous "aiming" and pushing forcefully at the valve. The "soft tip" of a standard guide wire, in actuality, is quite stiff, particularly as the tip of the wire is being advanced just out of the tip of a catheter. Similarly, the soft end of the Glide™ wires are stiff and even more capable of perforation through valve tissues when pushed forcefully against the valve.

In order to "visualize" the exact course through the aortic valve orifice, it is very helpful to advance a catheter and/or guide wire *prograde* through the aortic valve *before* attempting the retrograde crossing. The prograde catheter/wire is introduced through a pre-existing atrial septal defect or through an atrial transseptal puncture and advanced through the aortic valve with a floating balloon catheter and/or deflector wires. The prograde catheter/wire will pass through the orifice of the aortic valve and provide a visible demonstration of the exact course of the tract through the *orifice* of the valve in both the AP and lateral planes of the fluoroscopy. The tip of the retrograde catheter/wire then can be "tracked" meticulously and gently following along the exact course of the prograde catheter, through the precise orifice and into the ventricle. This is particularly useful when there is a tight stenosis and very small orifice of the aortic valve.

Atrioventricular (A-V) valve tears and/or avulsion are primarily a consequence of interventional procedures. Tears can occur in either A-V valve and occur as a result of a catheter/guide wire and, subsequently, a dilation balloon passing erroneously through chordae, clefts or unrecognized perforations in the valve leaflets. When a balloon is inflated in the abnormal position, the valve structure is torn as a direct consequence of the dilation in the constrained abnormal location. Tears in both A-V valves and/or valve structures also occur after a successful and uneventful dilation of *a more distal structure* is completed and as a balloon is withdrawn through the more proximal valve apparatus. A new, deflated, angioplasty balloon, which is folded or wrapped manually or commercially outside of the body, has a very smooth profile which can easily pass through an *abnormal* and tight location in an atrioventricular valve (for example, between tricuspid valve chordae). When the same balloon is inflated in the more distal structure (e.g. in the pulmonary valve, pulmonary artery or even the aortic valve), the balloon is well away from the atrioventricular valve and the inflation itself does not tear and/or otherwise harm the valve. However, after the dilation in the more distal location, the deflated balloon now has a much larger, irregular and rougher deflated profile. When the rough profile of the deflated balloon is withdrawn through the tight, abnormal location in the atrioventricular valve, it easily catches on, and tears, the A-V valve tissues. Again, prevention is the only real treatment of this problem. The use of a floating balloon catheter to cross the A-V valve prograde initially is the most absolute way of crossing through the central and/or larger orifice of the A-V valve and avoiding the small clefts and/or chordal spaces.

The straightening of long loops of the wire/balloon catheter during the inflation of the balloon also can tear the valve apparatus. The most common example of this is the tearing of the mitral valve during a prograde dilation of the aortic valve. The course of the wire from the systemic venous system, across the atrial septum, through the mitral valve, left ventricle and finally across the aortic valve, forms a fairly tight 360° loop. Unless the balloon in the aortic valve is well out of the ventricle, the part of the loop traversing the ventricle and mitral valve is straightened along with the balloon. Anything in the path of this straightening, particularly in the confined area through the mitral apparatus, is likely to tear. Careful passage of the original catheter through the central orifice of the mitral valve from the left atrium into the left ventricle using a floating balloon catheter, maintaining a long sheath all of the way to the apex of the left ventricle, and the more distal positioning of the balloon on the wire across the aortic valve will minimize the risk of a mitral valve tear.

Tears in atrioventricular valves and/or valve apparatuses can go unnoticed during the procedure and only become apparent on assessment of overall cardiac function during subsequent angiocardiograms and/or echocardiograms. The treatment of valve tears, again, is prevention. Very careful attention must be paid to the "route" of the catheter/wire being advanced through or across valves. If there is any resistance to the passage through the valve with the catheter/wire and/or with the subsequent dilation balloon, the relationship of the wire/catheter/balloon to the valve and the valve apparatus is examined carefully by echo and/or angiocardiogram. If the valve apparatus cannot be visualized clearly and/or there is any question of passage through an abnormal location in a valve, the wire is removed and repositioned across the valve. When a valve is torn significantly, surgical repair is the only "correction".

Rupture of a valve annulus occurs very rarely from the balloons during balloon dilation of valves. When an annulus rupture does occur, it usually is a result of using a balloon, or balloons, for the valve dilation, which is/are significantly larger than the *stretchable* annulus diameter of the valve. This is particularly true when the valve dilation is performed using high-pressure balloons. There are established, general criteria for balloon to annulus ratios for the dilation of pulmonary, aortic and mitral valves, whether using single or multiple balloons. The specific criteria for each valve are discussed in detail in the earlier chapters dealing with the specific valve dilations. The criteria for balloon size in relation to annulus diameter are based on a wide general past experience for both safe and effective dilations, but not on any absolute scientific "tests" of balloon sizes for valve dilations. The balloon to annulus ratio *is* dependent upon very accurate measurements of the valve annulus diameter. The criteria that are available, however, are different for each patient according to different valvular anatomy, associated vessel abnormalities, and the characteristics of the vascular supporting tissues of the individual patients. The final result of a balloon dilation of a valve often is a compromise between a satisfactory relief of the gradient versus "pushing the limit" of maximum safe balloon size for the particular annulus.

Myocardial damage

Specific or discrete damage to the myocardium has been mentioned previously under injuries to chambers and/or valves. In addition to the visible sequelae of these injuries, an elevation in the cardiac enzyme troponin I also provides an indicator of more generalized myocardial injury. However, elevations of serum troponin I to greater than 0.4 nanograms per liter occur from many diagnostic catheterizations and very frequently follow interventional procedures in pediatric and congenital heart patients even without any particular "adverse event" occurring during the procedure[8,9]. The procedures with electrocardiographic indication of myocardial injury during the procedure and the more extensive interventional procedures have higher elevations of troponin I. With the exception of the patient with other obvious "myocardial injury", elevated troponin I does not appear to correlate to the procedure or to be associated with any long-term sequelae.

Pericardial effusion

Pericardial effusions and/or eventual tamponade are a potential consequence of any central chamber and/or central vascular puncture or tear that occurs within the pericardial cavity. The occurrence of a pericardial effusion is always considered in the event of any deterioration in a patient's condition during manipulations with catheters, wires, sheaths and/or devices within the heart or great vessels. Chapter 33 is devoted to the diagnosis and management of pericardial effusions and the subject is not repeated here.

Cardiac arrhythmias

Transient/"benign" arrhythmias

Many cardiac "arrhythmias" are encountered during the manipulations of cardiac catheters in the heart. Congenital heart patients undergoing diagnostic cardiac catheterizations usually are "young" and although they have markedly deformed hearts, for the most part, they have relatively healthy myocardium. As a consequence, most of the arrhythmias generated by the manipulations of catheters in congenital heart patients are transient, self-limited and require no active treatment to revert back to the original rhythm. There are a few arrhythmias that do require some active treatment, but then, readily convert back to, and remain in, the original rhythm. These arrhythmias generally do not recur after the catheterization and, presumably, those that revert on their own and even those that convert with treatment in the catheterization laboratory, result in no permanent sequelae.

Sinus bradycardia secondary to excessive vagal stimulation probably is the most common "arrhythmia" seen during the cardiac catheterization of congenital heart patients. This is manifest by a significant slowing of the heart rate, plus or minus some drop in blood pressure, but with the patient still in a sinus mechanism with normal atrioventricular (A-V) electrical conduction on the monitored ECG. This common sinus bradycardia must be distinguished from bradycardia due to higher degrees of A-V block including complete atrioventricular block, which may be permanent and certainly is more serious. Respiratory depression from the sedatives and analgesics used to medicate the patients commonly causes vagal stimulation, which then results in sinus bradycardia. This is very common, particularly in infants. This sinus bradycardia responds to tactile stimulation of the patient and/or a few breaths given to the patient with an Ambu™ bag. If there is no response to the stimuli and respiratory support, the patient is given atropine intravenously and observed until the return of a normal heart rate or while investigating other causes of the bradycardia.

Another common cause of bradycardia results from "stretching" of intracardiac tissues by a loop or even just a broad curve of a catheter and/or wire within a cardiac chamber. This is particularly common when extra stiff wires/catheters are "looped" 180–360° in the atrium and/or when very large loops or "bows" are formed in the stiff wires and/or catheters in their course through the ventricles. This bradycardia resolves with the relief of the stress or tension on the catheter/wire or by the removal of the loops or bows in the catheter/wire. Occasionally, this bradycardia is "accepted" or "tolerated" temporarily by the catheterizing physician for several seconds, or even minutes, when the particular loop in the wire is critical for the delivery of a particular catheter or device to a more distal and difficult area. During this time, the patient's blood pressure and oxygenation must be monitored very critically, and with any continued deterioration of these parameters, the catheter loops are withdrawn. This sinus bradycardia resolves once the underlying mechanical cause of the bradycardia is eliminated and also responds to the administration of atropine.

Sinus bradycardia and even various degrees of A-V block occur, and are expected, during balloon dilation of the cardiac valves. This *bradycardia* presumably is a consequence of the stretch on the tissues along with the total obstruction of the cardiac output during the balloon inflation. This sinus bradycardia is minimized by very rapid inflation/deflation of the balloons during valve dilations. The use of double, or even triple, balloons for valve dilations also minimizes the bradycardia/hypotension by creating gaps or spaces between the inflated balloons, which allows some forward flow even during full inflation of the balloons and, in turn, decreasing the obstruction of flow through the orifice while the balloons are inflated. The two (or three) balloons also allow a more rapid inflation/deflation of each separate, smaller balloon, which obstructs flow for less time. Usually, unless there has been absolutely no relief of the obstruction, even severe degrees of bradycardia and associated hypotension recover spontaneously once the balloon is deflated. However, an appropriate dose of atropine should be drawn up into a syringe and ready to administer rapidly before any balloon dilation of a valve is performed. Occasionally, following a balloon dilation of a valve, in addition to the atropine, several chest compressions of the heart are necessary while the heart rate and blood pressure are recovering.

Bundle branch block, high degrees of atrioventricular block or even complete atrioventricular block can occur concurrently with the hypotension/bradycardia during the actual inflation of the balloon in any of the valves. These conduction blocks presumably are due to the pressure from the inflated balloon(s) against the atrioventricular conduction bundles and, in turn, direct trauma to the conduction tissues. The true atrioventricular blocks are always more serious and are not necessarily self-limited. In the event of a complete block, the catheter manipulations are stopped, the catheter(s) is/are removed from the area and the patient is allowed to recover from the conduction block before resuming the procedure. Atropine frequently is given in an attempt to speed up the *sinus mechanism* and hopefully the overall heart rate, however, this does not treat the cause of the atrioventricular block directly. The cause of the A-V block needs to be determined so that if, and when, the block resolves and the procedure is resumed, that particular maneuver can be avoided. More prolonged and specific resuscitative efforts may be necessary when complete A-V block occurs. With persistence of a high degree of A-V block, a temporary pacemaker is introduced through the venous access and the patient paced electronically until an adequate spontaneous heart rate resumes.

Right or left bundle branch block occurs as a consequence of either direct trauma from a catheter "bumping" against the conduction bundle and/or from loops of catheters and/or wires pressing against the conduction bundle. Bundle branch block is a common "transient arrhythmia" seen during catheter manipulations within the heart, it causes no change in the measurable hemodynamics, and no attempt is made to treat the block. The occurrence of bundle branch block is minimized by gentle, directed manipulation of catheters through the ventricular chambers and, whenever possible, the avoidance of tense loops of wires within the cardiac chambers. The use of floating balloon catheters for manipulation through the ventricular chamber presumably reduces the direct trauma to the ventricular wall and, in turn, the development of bundle branch block. When an isolated bundle branch block occurs, usually there is no immediate hemodynamic consequence, however, the catheter manipulations are stopped *temporarily* to allow the conduction system to recover.

Tachyarrhythmias which are precipitated in the catheterization laboratory usually are acute in onset and do result in some hemodynamic compromise. Supraventricular tachycardia secondary to catheter manipulation within an atrium is quite common. The heart rate becomes extremely fast and there is a sudden drop in systemic blood pressure as a result of the tachycardia. These tachycardias often stop on their own or they are stopped by further manipulation of the catheter against the wall of the atrium or by the formation of a large loop with the catheter within the atrium. The large loops presumably stretch the atrium, producing a vagal reaction. This usually stops the supraventricular tachycardias. When the additional catheter manipulations are not successful in stopping the tachycardia, particularly when the tachycardia produces a significant drop in the systemic blood pressure, the patient is given a very rapid bolus of 0.2 mg/kg (up to 12 mg total) of adenosine through the catheter. Catheter-induced supraventricular tachycardias usually and readily are converted by the additional catheter manipulations and/or the adenosine. If the patient does not convert readily, the tachycardia may, in actuality, be atrial flutter or even fibrillation. When catheter induced, even these arrhythmias usually can be converted electrically with a DC shock of 0.5 watts/kg of body weight applied across the thorax crossing the area of the heart. Electrical cardioversion also occasionally is necessary for any of the supraventricular tachycardias.

Ventricular extrasystoles, often even occurring in short runs of multiple ventricular extra beats, are very common during catheter and/or wire manipulations within a ventricle and frequently are "taken for granted" in the usual, *younger* congenital heart patients. The progression of these ventricular extra beats into a sustained ventricular tachycardia and/or ventricular fibrillation is extremely rare in this group of patients, probably because the usual congenital patient is younger and has a basically "healthy myocardium". However, this "protection" from sustained tachycardia should not be assumed in any patient. There is no "protection" present in patients who have failing hearts, in cardiomyopathy at any age, and in older patients with congenital heart disease. These patients readily can convert into sustained ventricular tachycardia and/or fibrillation, which are discussed subsequently in this chapter.

Major, life-threatening arrhythmias

Although any arrhythmia occurring in the catheterization laboratory is potentially serious, as discussed previously, most are transient and require no treatment. At the same time, all of the previously mentioned "simple" arrhythmias do become very serious and even life-threatening when they become sustained and/or do not respond to "simple" therapy.

Sinus bradycardia usually is self-limited and/or responds to minimal therapy, however, sinus bradycardia may be secondary to serious hemodynamic and/or metabolic problems. Untreated, severe sinus bradycardia can progress into a subsequent cardiac arrest, particularly in critically ill patients where a marked, sudden reduction in cardiac output occurs when crossing stenotic areas and/or valves. Acute cardiac tamponade often presents with bradycardia. This always must be considered with the appearance of bradycardia, particularly when the sinus bradycardia does not respond completely and quickly to catheter stimulus and/or atropine. In addition to respiratory depression precipitated by medications, hypothermia and/or acidosis also cause sinus bradycardia, which can progress to eventual cardiac arrest. In these circumstances, the underlying cause must be corrected before the bradycardia will respond to therapy. Very rarely, a temporary pacemaker is required for persistent bradycardia, even when it is *not* due to complete heart block. Unfortunately, when not due to block, pacing alone often is not beneficial.

Complete heart block can, and occasionally does, develop during any maneuvers with cardiac catheters within the cardiac chambers. Complete heart block in the catheterization laboratory usually is due to a catheter, wire or an implanted device bumping or pressing against the atrioventricular conduction bundle. As is the case in the prevention of bundle branch block, floating balloon catheters probably are less likely to traumatize the tissues and produce complete heart block when passing through a ventricle. In all patients with *ventricular inversion*, the atrioventricular conduction bundles lie very superficially in the tissues, are very susceptible to even minor trauma and, as a consequence, have an increased susceptibility for developing complete atrioventricular block. As a consequence, the use of a floating balloon catheter is recommended *whenever* manipulating a catheter through either ventricle in patients with ventricular inversion. When complete heart block occurs in any patient regardless of what maneuver is being performed, the maneuver is stopped and the catheter withdrawn from the area. The patient is given intravenous isoproterenol to accelerate the ventricular rate. An intravenous bolus of Decadron™ is administered empirically with the goal of reducing local inflammation/edema in the tissues in the area of the bundle. With persistence of the block and significant bradycardia, a transvenous pacemaker lead is introduced and positioned in the ventricle.

Although premature ventricular contractions and even short runs of ventricular tachycardia are very common and usually are self-limited during cardiac catheterizations in younger congenital heart patients, sustained ventricular tachycardia/fibrillation can occur with any manipulation within a ventricle in any patient. Progression into sustained ventricular arrhythmias is anticipated in patients with "sick" and/or "older" myocardium and/or during very extensive catheter and/or wire manipulations within a ventricle. Extra attention is paid to them, and to stopping or preventing these premature ectopic beats in older or other vulnerable patients. A sustained ventricular arrhythmia usually results in some, if not significant, compromise of the patient's hemodynamics.

When multiple premature ventricular contractions are encountered in a particularly vulnerable patient, the patient is given a bolus of one mg/kg of intravenous xylocaine just prior to extensive manipulations, and particularly before therapeutic procedures involving the ventricle.

Once a sustained ventricular arrhythmia occurs, the most effective treatment is immediate electrical cardioversion beginning with 0.5 watts/kg shock applied across the heart over the patient's thorax. The patient simultaneously is given a bolus of one mg/kg of intravenous xylocaine and any underlying metabolic abnormalities are corrected. If the tachycardia/fibrillation continues, the electrical cardioversion is repeated with a 0.5 watts/kg incremental increase in the current with each repeated shock up to 2 watts/kg. The bolus of xylocaine can be repeated in 5–10 minutes. The DC defibrillator must be available for immediate use during every catheterization with it turned on and the voltage set according to the patient's weight at the onset of each catheterization. In particularly high-risk patients, the paddles are prepared with conducting paste prior to beginning the ventricular manipulations or radio-lucent electrical defibrillator leads are placed on the patient and attached to the defibrillator at the onset of the catheterization procedure.

In a cardiac catheterization laboratory equipped to perform electrophysiologic catheter studies, a pacing catheter can be introduced and used to "over-drive pace" the patient out of either an atrial or a ventricular tachyarrhythmia.

Respiratory complications

The patient's airway is a constant potential for complications. A major additional advantage of the use of general anesthesia for cardiac catheterizations is the presence of the anesthesiologist helping with, and/or actually responsible for, the patient's respiratory status. Patients with any inherent upper airway obstruction tend to obstruct their airway totally when given deep sedation. In very ill patients, hypoxia from the respiratory obstruction can lead to rapid hemodynamic deterioration and even cardiac arrest if not managed expeditiously. Even when airway obstruction does not cause hypoxia, it results in marked negative swings in intrathoracic pressures, which distort *all* pressure measurements and recordings and significantly increase the risk of air being sucked into the circulation through sheaths and/or catheters. Extending the patient's oral pharynx, introducing an oral pharyngeal tube into the airway and/or even intubating the patient are the usual treatments, in that sequence, for upper airway obstruction depending upon the severity of the obstruction.

Even the endotracheal intubation can be a "double-edged sword" in the management of airway obstruction. The endotracheal tube immediately gives the operator a sense of security about the airway but, by itself, the endotracheal tube is not a "cure" for all airway problems. The tube itself can *cause* airway obstruction with resultant hypoxia and hypercarbia. The endotracheal tube, which is managed by the catheterizing physician, can become detached from the respirator tubing, it can become kinked and/or compressed, or the tip of an endotracheal tube can rest on the carina or down in one bronchus. These are physical problems with the endotracheal tube, which should be obvious by proper care and close inspection of the respirator tubing and the endotracheal tube, from changes in the respirator/anesthesia machine pressures and/or from the location of the tube visualized on the fluoroscopic image of the thorax.

Generalized bronchospasm is another major souse of respiratory distress. It usually, but not always, is in a patient with underlying bronchospastic disease, the consequence of an acute allergic reaction and/or of a concomitant lower respiratory infection. In children with congenital heart disease, bronchospasm usually is *not* a consequence of "heart failure". Regardless of etiology, the initial treatment of significant bronchospasm is with an inhaled beta agonist such as albuterol. The albuterol is administered directly into the airway utilizing an ultrasonic nebulizer. While the initial treatment is carried out, the underlying cause of the bronchospasm is investigated and treated more specifically in addition to the nebulization therapy.

Generalized pulmonary edema and/or acute unilateral or localized pulmonary edema certainly can occur in the catheterization laboratory. Bilateral, diffuse pulmonary artery edema is usually a consequence of underlying cardiac disease with either severe left heart inflow obstruction (obstructed pulmonary veins, cor triatriatum, mitral stenosis) or severe functional failure of the systemic ventricle. Generalized pulmonary edema is anticipated and treated with diuretics, positive pressure ventilation, other medical treatment of cardiac failure and/or an interventional procedure aimed directly at the cause of the pulmonary edema.

Unilateral and/or localized pulmonary edema frequently follows the sudden relief of a discrete area of severe obstruction more proximally in the involved pulmonary artery. The more severe the obstruction, the higher the central pulmonary artery pressure proximal to the obstruction and/or the more successful is the relief of the isolated area of obstruction, the more likely it is that the patient will develop a unilateral and/or localized pulmonary edema. Very severe localized pulmonary edema can progress into hemorrhagic pulmonary edema and/or the accumulation of a pleural effusion. Treatment includes anticipation of the problem. An attempt is made to distribute the flow/pressure as widely as possible throughout the lungs by initially performing only a partial dilation of the obstruction of a single area and completing the dilation of as many additional areas of obstruction as possible during the same catheterization. Partial dilation of each area allows less flow to the areas and dilating additional areas allows more flow to multiple areas, in turn, lowering the more central pulmonary artery pressure. Localized/unilateral pulmonary edema also is treated with diuretics and positive pressure ventilation.

Pneumothorax

Pneumothorax occurs during internal jugular and/or subclavian vein punctures for catheter introduction or during pericardiocenteses. The pleural space is just caudal to the puncture site for the internal jugular vein and just posterior to the subclavian vein. Even in experienced hands, the needle tip easily can stray into the lung parenchyma and result in a pneumothorax. Awareness of these very close relationships and taking specific efforts to avoid the pleura are the best treatment. The diagnosis is suspected when air is heard sucking into the open puncture needle, air returns into an aspirating syringe attached to the puncture needle and/or the patient begins having respiratory distress during one of these punctures. When suspected and looked for specifically, the pneumothorax is confirmed by fluoroscopy of the chest. Pneumothorax is confirmed by a lucent area in the thorax with a shift of the visible "tissue" structures away from the area of lucency on fluoroscopy or an X-ray. The pneumothorax may be small and self-limited, causing no symptoms and requiring no treatment, to the other extreme of a large pneumothorax that causes severe respiratory distress and must be treated immediately. Treatment with a thoracocentesis and usually a water seal drain in the pleural space is required when there is a significant accumulation of pleural air associated with symptoms of respiratory distress. The treatment is described in detail in Chapter 34.

Pleural fluid

Pleural fluid secondary to the underlying cardiac and/or a pulmonary problem can be present before the cardiac catheterization begins. When there is a significant amount of pleural fluid present at the onset of a cardiac catheterization, the pleural fluid is drained *prior to proceeding* with the catheterization procedure in order to make the patient's respirations more comfortable and in order to obtain more valid hemodynamics during the catheterization. The drainage of pleural fluid requires a thoracocentesis and/or an indwelling chest tube for continued drainage.

New pleural fluid appearing during a catheterization almost always is blood and is the result of a puncture and/or tear of a vessel or a cardiac chamber outside of the confines of the pericardium—usually a pulmonary artery or vein. This is an extremely rare complication of a *diagnostic* catheterization, but if unsuspected and/or unrecognized can be lethal. The consequence of the pleural fluid depends on the amount and the rate of accumulation of the pleural fluid, which, in turn, depends upon the site and size of the tear. The accumulation of a large amount of fluid (blood) in the pleural space interferes with respirations, but the loss of circulating blood volume usually is the most immediate and obvious problem.

The treatment of a new accumulation of pleural fluid is a combination of identifying the site of the blood loss into the pleura, stopping this blood loss and the acute replacement of the drained fluid (including autotransfusion of the drained blood when necessary). An emergency thoracocentesis with the insertion of a chest tube is performed in the catheterization laboratory, and the surgeons and the operating room are notified of the potential need of their services.

The catheterizing physician should have some suspicion from the preceding events in the catheterization laboratory as to the location of a tear or puncture. The exact location and size are confirmed with a selective angiogram into the suspected vessel. Once identified, the feeding pulmonary artery is temporarily occluded with a balloon catheter. When a localized vessel can be occluded successfully without simultaneously destroying a large segment of functioning lung, it is occluded permanently either with coils or with a more specific occlusion device. Preferably, when there is a large area of lung involved distal to the tear and when an appropriate sized covered stent is available, a covered stent is placed over the torn area within the vessel. All of the time the blood drained form the pleura is replaced with bank blood and/or by auto-transfusion to maintain the patient's hemodynamic stability. The diagnosis and management of hemothorax is covered in detail in Chapter 34.

Gastric over distention

Although technically not a respiratory complication, a massive amount of air in the patient's stomach can cause respiratory distress, particularly in small infants. A crying and/or gasping infant or child swallows large amounts of air. Even larger amounts of air are introduced into the stomach when a patient receives multiple positive breaths of air during ventilation with a face mask. Large volumes of air in the stomach push the diaphragm cephalad, compressing the lungs and, in turn compromise normal inspirations. This "minor problem" should be considered in an infant who is uncomfortable with associated respiratory distress and with a stomach full of air visualized on fluoroscopy. This "complication" is remedied easily when it is treated by emptying the stomach with a nasogastric tube.

Air embolization

Air entering the circulation is a constant potential problem with many potential sites and sources for the air to enter. The consequence of air in the circulation depends upon the amount of air introduced and the *destination* of the air in the circulation. The consequence of air can be as "minor" as an "embarrassing bubble" bouncing around in a "right sided" cardiac chamber, to the other extremes of a massive stroke, cardiac arrest and/or death when the air reaches the systemic circulation. The only definitive and reliable treatment of air in the circulation is prevention. Prevention is possible by the knowledge of how and where air can enter the circulation and the meticulous, detailed, attention to eliminating all of these potential routes of entry. In congenital heart patients, because of the numerous intracardiac and intravascular communications with the resultant constant, or potential, "right to left" shunting, *any "lumen" introduced into any location* in the circulation is a potential source of a catastrophic systemic embolization.

In spite of the overwhelming advantages of indwelling sheaths in vessels during catheterizations, an indwelling sheath also represents the most likely site for the introduction of free air into the circulation. This is equally true of sheaths ***with*** a back-bleed valve/flush port on them as it is for the "open" sheaths. No matter how well the sheath and dilator of a sheath/dilator set are flushed outside of the body, there *always* will be more air trapped in the *valve chamber* of the sheath after the dilator is either introduced into or withdrawn from the sheath. As the tip of the dilator is introduced into a valve on a sheath, a very slight gap is created in the "valve leaflets" adjacent to the dilator. This tiny opening is enough to allow air to enter the "chamber" instantaneously between the valve and the shaft of the dilator. Unless the hub of the dilator also is sealed, fluid flows out of either or both ends of the dilator, allowing more air to pass adjacent to the back-bleed valve and into the valve chamber. The larger the diameter of the sheath/dilator set, the greater is the volume of air trapped in the chamber.

Once the sheath/dilator is introduced into a vessel and after the dilator is removed, unless the sheath *and the chamber of the back-bleed valve* are emptied very specifically and purposefully of all air *after the dilator is removed*, air *will* remain in the valve "chamber" of the sheath. With the first "flush" of the sheath and/or the passage of a catheter through the sheath, this air is flushed directly into the circulation! Once a dilator or catheter is removed, the valve chamber is always emptied *passively* unless the valve itself can be sealed very tightly with a gloved finger placed *tightly over* the *entire flat* surface of the valve. In the presence of any resistance to flow into the tip of the sheath and/or when there is a wire or a catheter passing through the valve, any suction on the side port of a back-bleed valve on the sheath preferentially will suck air through the valve and *into* the sheath! In a low-pressure venous system, the valve port of the sheath must be drained passively and even more thoroughly. When the valve chamber is being emptied, the *side port* is positioned facing up and the valve chamber is tapped gently to loosen any bubbles adhering to the inside of the valve chamber as the sheath is drained.

If *any suction* is applied to the side port when there is a wire or catheter passing through the back-bleed valve, *air will be* ***sucked into*** the sheath through the valve. If this is a long and/or large diameter sheath with only a wire through the sheath/valve, as much as 12 ml of air can be sucked into the sheath! When either a dilator or a catheter is withdrawn out of a sheath through the back-bleed valve, a potential *vacuum* is created in the sheath. When a catheter or dilator is withdrawn over a wire and with the proximal end of the catheter or a dilator *open to air*, air will be sucked in through the catheter or dilator lumen and can *fill* the sheath! Even when the proximal end of the catheter or dilator is closed, air can still be sucked into the sheath through the valve *around* the dilator or catheter by the vacuum created in the sheath. The catheter and/or dilator are withdrawn *very slowly* in order to allow blood to follow the tip of the catheter/dilator back into the tip of the sheath, still with the proximal end of either the sheath or the dilator sealed tightly. When there is sufficient intravascular pressure *and* the tip of the sheath is *free*, a catheter or dilator with the proximal end open can be withdrawn slowly enough to allow blood to drip out of the proximal end of the catheter or dilator (and around a wire, if present) as the catheter or dilator is withdrawn from the sheath. Again, a long, large diameter sheath can fill with as much as 12 ml of air, which if not cleared, will be flushed into the circulation!

More obvious sources of air getting into the circulation are through the proximal end of a sheath which is open and the open proximal end of a catheter, when the distal tip of the sheath or catheter is positioned in a low- or *negative-pressure vascular bed*, for example in the systemic veins and/or right atrium in the presence of significant respiratory obstruction. With severe *inspiratory* obstruction, as much as *minus 50 mmHg* of negative intravascular pressure can be generated in the systemic venous system. In that circumstance and in the presence of even a small direct communication with atmospheric pressure in the room, massive amounts of air can be sucked into the circulation. The shorter the length and/or the larger the diameter of the sheath/catheter that is providing communication with the air, the greater is the risk of air entry from this source. When a sheath is inadvertently opened in the presence of marked intrathoracic *negative pressure*, enough air can be sucked into the venous circulation to create a large enough "air lock" to occlude all forward blood flow through the right heart. This type of air entry was a much more frequent problem when the short introductory sheaths routinely did *not* have attached, or even attachable, back-bleed valves. This massive amount of air entry still remains possible when a detachable back-bleed valve is removed temporarily from the indwelling sheath or when the side port of the back-bleed valve is opened.

Air, of course, also can be *injected* directly along with medications, flush solutions and/or contrast media when there is a major breakdown in technique and/or equipment. The individuals who inject anything through the flush system and/or directly into the catheter/sheath are responsible for clearing air from syringes, connectors and tubing, but the physician performing the catheterization ultimately is responsible for preventing air from entering a catheter and/or an indwelling line going into the patient. Fluid and/or blood always must be bled back or withdrawn from any catheter and/or tubing before it is attached to a flush line or an injector. Pressurized containers for injection (flush bags, injector syringes) are checked routinely and repeatedly for the presence of any air *and always* are positioned vertically with the exit port of the container always facing downward when attached to the tubing and/or catheter for infusion/injection.

It is possible for small amounts of air to enter the circulation from ruptured balloons on either angioplasty and/or floating balloon catheters. It often is difficult (impossible!) to remove *all* of the air during even the most meticulous preparation of an angioplasty balloon. Occasionally the balloons of floating balloon catheters are filled with room air rather than carbon dioxide (CO_2) and/or the CO_2, unknowingly, diffuses from the balloon and/or the "reservoir" system for the CO_2, which, in turn, replaces the CO_2 with room air in the balloon. Although the amount of air from either of these sources usually is small, when balloons rupture, they often are in very critical locations, just proximal to vital organs—particularly, anywhere in the systemic circulation proximal to the coronary arteries and/or the carotid arteries, where even a small amount of air potentially is catastrophic. Even a small "bubble" of air can create an "air lock" and prevent any blood flow in a small vessel.

Prevention of air entering the circulation is the best (only!) treatment. CO_2 is used to fill all "gas-filled" balloons, regardless of which "side" of the circulation the balloon is to be used in. By meticulous attention to proper procedures and techniques, it is possible to prevent air from entering the circulation in all other circumstances. Once the air has entered the circulation, it occasionally is "treatable", but only if the air is visible and "trapped" in a chamber or vessel and not occluding that vessel. When a significant amount of air enters the circulation and becomes trapped, the bolus of air is visible very clearly as a radio-lucent area bouncing around in the highest area of the circulation (e.g. the right atrial appendage, right ventricular outflow tract). In this event, the patient's thorax is positioned to orient the area with the trapped "bubble" as high (up) as possible while directing a catheter specifically into the radio-lucent area. An attempt is made to position the tip of the catheter precisely in the "bubble" and then to withdraw as much of the air as possible before the air can disseminate throughout the circulation.

Once free air has entered the circulation, disseminated and reached vital organs there is very little definitive therapy available. Often, with the patient sedated or anesthetized and unless the amount of air is massive, an air embolus to a vital organ may not cause any adverse signs *during the catheterization* and only becomes apparent when the patient awakens (or doesn't awaken!). The exception is free air in the coronary arteries. A small "bubble" of air lodged in a coronary artery obstructs the flow acutely and results in acute ischemia with ST-T wave changes, bradycardia, depressed cardiac function and even cardiac arrest. Although the "bubble(s)" in the coronary often are not visible, the sequence of known manipulations of catheters and/or sheaths immediately preceding the cardiac event along with the sequence of cardiac events should be sufficient to diagnose air in the coronary as the most probable cause of the deterioration. Treatment consists of prolonged and vigorous, external cardiac message along with the maintenance of an adequate circulating volume, adequate ventilation and maintenance of the acid–base balance. It can take as long as 30–45 minutes of sustained mechanical cardiopulmonary resuscitation to resuscitate a patient after air has entered the coronary arteries.

The brain is probably the most catastrophic destination for free air that has entered the circulation. *Very tiny* amounts of air *possibly* cause no permanent sequelae, but may be the cause of headaches, somnolence and/or transient changes in mentation following a cardiac catheterization. Larger air emboli are assumed to be the culprit when a patient awakens from a cardiac catheterization with a significant central nervous deficit but subsequently the patient does recover significantly over several days *and/or* when free air had been seen to enter the systemic circulation sometime during the catheterization. When prevention of CNS air is not successful, the treatment is usually limited to supportive therapy and "tincture of time"!

Thrombi/emboli

Thrombi and particulate matter, like air, represent a constant potential for embolization to the vital organs in the systemic circulation during *all* cardiac catheterization procedures in patients with congenital heart disease. Thrombi can pre-exist within vessels or cardiac chambers of any patient and can develop spontaneously anyplace and anytime around wires and/or in catheters and sheaths within the circulation. Any thrombus represents a potential embolus to a vital organ! Thrombi form at the site of vascular injury (introductory sites into vessels, "abrasions" or "bumps" by wires and catheters, and injected irritants), in any areas of stasis in the blood flow and on the surface of any "foreign material" within the circulation.

Some "injury" to the intima of the vasculature probably occurs with all movements of catheters, wires or sheaths within the vasculature. Significant stasis of blood flow occurs more frequently in areas where the blood flow already was sluggish (e.g. systemic venous circulation in a P/O "Fontan" circulation), when blood flow is obstructed in small diameter vessels/areas by catheters, sheaths and/or devices, and within the lumens of catheters and sheaths. There always is a "dead space" around wires within catheters and around all catheters and wires within sheaths. If the catheter/sheaths are not flushed adequately (continuously!) blood accumulating in these dead spaces is very prone to thrombus formation. The surfaces of all catheters, wires and sheaths, themselves, represent "foreign" materials, which potentially are thrombogenic when positioned in the circulation, regardless of "coatings". Finally, the formation of thrombi in all of these circumstances or on any materials is enhanced when the patient is polycythemic and/or dehydrated.

As is the case with air emboli, prevention of thrombi formation and, in turn, prevention of the embolization of particulate matter is the most effective, and the only totally satisfactory, treatment of particulate embolic complications. Adequate hydration to reduce stasis in the flow of blood in patients undergoing cardiac catheterization is accomplished with supplemental intravenous fluids administered before and during the procedure. Significant polycythemia is treated with a phlebotomy performed at the onset of the procedure *before* catheters are introduced and manipulations are begun. The phlebotomy should always include a fluid replacement with a volume of *colloidal* fluid equivalent to the blood volume withdrawn. Trauma to the intima of the vessels/chambers is minimized by proper equipment and techniques for catheter introductions and manipulations. In order to avoid unnecessary and/or prolonged obstruction of blood flow, catheters and/or sheaths are positioned in narrowed or constricted locations for the minimal time possible. Except when pressures actually are being recorded and/or blood samples are being withdrawn, the lumens of catheters and sheaths are maintained on a constant flush through side port/back-bleed valves. It is particularly important to maintain the constant flush *around wires* that remain passing through catheters and/or sheaths.

Systemic heparinization is recommended for most, if not all, patients undergoing cardiac catheterizations. Patients are given 75–100 mg/kg of intravenous heparin once the sheath/catheters have been introduced into the patient. The heparin helps to prevent thrombi from forming in and/or on catheters, wires and sheaths and may help to prevent thrombi at the traumatized introductory sites for the sheaths/catheters. When heparin is used, a blood activated clotting time (ACT) is measured periodically and heparin administered periodically to keep the ACT above 275–300 seconds.

When a fresh thrombus is detected in a vessel (e.g. a pulmonary artery, a peripheral vein or a systemic artery), whenever possible, intravenous heparin is administered directly into the involved vessel and the ACT is maintained above 300 seconds. If the thrombus persists and/or progresses and particularly with signs of compromise of tissues, a mechanical thrombectomy is performed or thrombolytic therapy is administered either locally into the involved vessel and/or systemically. There are very favorable results from the use of both modalities in congenital heart patients. These are discussed in Chapters 2, 4, and 9.

Renal injury

There are numerous reports of renal injury due to contrast medium given during adult cardiac catheterizations, and contrast-related nephropathy is reportedly the third leading cause of renal failure in adults[10]. Although these renal problems can occur in pediatric/congenital patients undergoing cardiac catheterization, fortunately, they are extremely rare in this population of patients. When renal damage does occur during a cardiac catheterization, it usually is a consequence of the combination of some underlying renal disease in the particular patient *and* the use of an excessive amount of contrast medium during the catheterization. Occasionally an idiosyncrasy to the contrast agent will cause renal damage. Although large volumes of contrast per body weight frequently are used during cardiac catheterizations in very complex congenital heart patients, these procedures usually also are very long in duration and the patients receive extra amounts of infused "flush" solution very liberally during the long procedure. The newer non-ionic and iso-osmolar contrast agents also ***probably*** have decreased the incidence of recognizable renal damage, although this has not been documented in any controlled study. Renal damage during a catheterization is manifest by hematuria, a decrease in the urine output along with a concomitant increase in the creatinine and blood urea nitrogen.

As with other complications, prevention is the best treatment for renal damage. The catheterizing physician must be aware of any underlying renal problems, which are more common in patients with congenital heart disease. Contrast medium should be used judiciously and the 4 ml/kg "rule of thumb" for the maximum amount of contrast used during a catheterization should be observed during any single procedure whenever possible. This "rule" was generated from a vast experience with the clinical use of contrast agents, but it was not based on any actual controlled trials, and it originated several decades ago, when the ionic, hyper-osmolar contrast agents were the only ones available. There still are *no controlled experimental studies* to document that the old 4 ml/kg "rule of thumb" *still is not true* in spite of the facts that the current contrast agents are "non-ionic" and "iso-osmolar", and there are many anecdotal reports of the use of more than 4 ml/kg during any one procedure. The volume of contrast used during any procedure should be monitored closely, and when more than 4 ml/kg are used there must be a valid reason, not just sloppy technique. When a volume of contrast medium greater than 4 ml/kg is used, the additional contrast should be used only during extra-long procedures where the contrast has sufficient time to be cleared by the kidneys. When large volumes of contrast are used during a catheterization procedure, the patients are given extra saline and/or lactate flush solution during the procedure. In addition, an intravenous dose of 0.5 mg/kg of furosemide is given arbitrarily during and/or immediately after the procedure. In adult patients with severely compromised renal function, fenoldopam, a selective dopamine 1 receptor agonist, seems to have a beneficial effect at preventing radiocontrast induced nephropathy when administered at 0.03–0.1 microgram/kg/min before and during the catheterization[11].

When hematuria and/or an increase in blood urea nitrogen/creatinine occurs during and/or after a cardiac catheterization, the patient initially is maintained on the supplemental intravenous fluids until these laboratory values return to normal or, at the other extreme, when signs of actual renal shut down occur. Renal shutdown very rarely occurs secondary to excessive volumes of a contrast agent, but if renal shutdown should occur, it is treated like any other renal shutdown with fluid restriction and, when necessary, even dialysis.

Central nervous system injury

A significant central nervous system (CNS) injury is probably the most dreaded complication of a cardiac catheterization. Central nervous system injuries can be localized or generalized. CNS injuries can be manifest from the one extreme with a minimal consequence such as transient somnolence to the other extreme of seizures, paralyses, coma and even death. Generalized central nervous system injury occurs as a consequence of extreme hypoxia, hypotension, reactions to contrast agents, reaction to anesthetics and/or other medications or a combination of any of the above. Rarely some of these causes of central nervous system injury are not anticipated and, even when anticipated, cannot be prevented.

Cerebrovascular injury as a consequence of air and/or particulate embolization from material from within sheaths or catheters, off wires as a consequence of extensive catheter/wire manipulation in the systemic circulation and/or in the presence of right to left shunting was discussed previously under air and thrombotic complications. Doppler studies have shown an almost continual microembolization to the brain during all catheter/wire manipulations and the flushing of catheters within the systemic (or potentially systemic) circulation[12]. The consequences of any emboli to the brain include all neurologic phenomena including headache, somnolence, seizures, all degrees of paresis, paralysis, expressive aphasia, visual loss and even coma and death.

Prevention of all types of central nervous system injury is the *only effective* therapy. All potential sources of central nervous system injury that are known or suspected are avoided or corrected *before* the event occurs. There are encouraging results from the use of acute thrombolytic therapy *immediately* after a documented *thrombotic* stroke. This therapy depends upon the rapid confirmation of the diagnosis and the equally rapid initiation of therapy by a qualified neurologist and/or neurovascular radiologist working in close coordination with the congenital cardiac catheterization facility. The pediatric interventionist alone should not attempt this type of therapy.

Generalized systemic reactions/complications

In addition to the numerous complications involving the more specific organs and systems of the body, there are generalized reactions that occur and can threaten the patient's life.

Blood loss–hypotension–shock

Significant, gradual blood loss from the usual catheter introductory sites is a preventable complication and should not occur in the twenty-first century during a *diagnostic* cardiac catheterization. Vascular cut-downs with their often obligatory loss of blood are no longer used for many cardiac catheterizations in congenital heart patients. Hemostasis valves with flush ports are available for all sheaths used for cardiac catheterization, so even during multiple catheter exchanges there should be a minimal blood loss.

The most frequent current cause of blood loss at the catheter introductory site occurs as a result of the inadvertent disconnection of the hub of the catheter and/or indwelling arterial pressure line from the connecting tubing of the pressure and flush systems. A disconnected catheter and/or indwelling line can result in a rapid loss of blood from within the vascular system, particularly from within a high-pressure chamber or vessel. Lure™ lock connectors are used where lines do not have to be repeatedly disconnected and reconnected. Otherwise, tightly fitting, slip lock connectors are used, however, only with continual, close observation of the area of the connectors. ***All*** of the personnel in the laboratory must be aware of the potential problem of these connections coming loose. Catheterizing physicians must assure the tightness of the connections when they detach and reattach lines and/or catheters for samples and/or injections. The scrub and circulating nurses in the room constantly must be aware of loose connections of the lines and/or the appearance of an accumulation of blood on the "field". The recording technician/nurse in the "control room" as well as the nurses/technicians within the catheterization laboratory immediately must recognize the disappearance of any monitored pressure(s) during the case and notify the catheterizing physician immediately.

Bleeding into the subcutaneous tissues adjacent to the introductory sites of the catheters can also occur very easily during the procedure. The bleeding comes from any earlier puncture attempts that were unsuccessful or from puncture sites into vessels that are dilated to a larger diameter opening than the diameter of the sheath that is introduced into the opening in the vessel. Since the skin areas and subcutaneous tissues adjacent to the introductory sites are covered with opaque sterile drapes, a significant amount of subcutaneous bleeding can easily go unnoticed under the drapes and can continue for a long period of time.

Another cause of localized tissue bleeding occurs when, after a successful puncture of a vessel with a needle with continued good blood return into the needle, the wire cannot be introduced into the vessel. The blood continues to return into the needle during multiple repeated attempts at introducing the wire. When the operator finally abandons that particular *puncture*, but does *not hold pressure* for an adequate period of time, the bleeding *at the surface of the skin* stops, but the bleeding from the vessel continues deep into the subcutaneous tissue, in spite of no visible "surface" bleeding. This source of local bleeding is prevented by patience by the operator in applying pressure to achieve hemostasis for several minutes after *each* successful puncture, but failed cannulation, of a vessel.

Local bleeding into the tissues also occurs following a *through-and-through puncture* of the anterior and posterior walls of the vessel. The cannulation of the vessel with the wire is accomplished as the tip of the needle is *withdrawn* through the *back* wall of the vessel and enters the lumen successfully during the withdrawal of the needle from "behind" the vessel. The lumen of the vessel then is cannulated with the sheath/dilator passing over the wire through only the puncture site in the *anterior wall* of the vessel. The sheath then seals the "anterior" opening in the vessel, but leaves the posterior puncture site open and bleeding. In order to prevent this type of bleed during the procedure, local pressure is applied for an extra period of time over the entire introductory site when a through-and-through needle puncture is recognized.

Local subcutaneous bleeding is more common in patients who are overweight with abundant, loose, soft tissues around the vessel puncture sites and in patients who have been on chronic anticoagulation. Although bleeding into the surrounding tissue is more common in these patients, it can occur in *any* patient. Local, continued bleeding into the perivascular tissues is more common following arterial punctures, but can occur following venous punctures. Even when this "internal" bleeding into the local subcutaneous tissues is extensive, it *usually* is not life-threatening, but does result in a significant accumulation of blood in the soft tissues of the extremity and adjacent trunk and does result in ugly and uncomfortable hematomas and/or ecchymoses. Heat applied locally and analgesics for the pain are the only "therapy" required for this type of local bleeding.

Subcutaneous bleeding can continue after the catheterization procedure is completed and the patient has left the catheterization laboratory. The superficial "skin" bleeding is stopped quickly with pressure over the site, but if pressure is not continued diligently for an extended period of time, particularly in the "higher-risk" patients mentioned above, the subcutaneous bleeding may continue until the developing hematoma tamponades itself with a very large accumulation of blood and a massive, ugly ecchymosis.

Acute internal blood loss into any body cavity can occur from the puncture and/or tear of any vessel or chamber during the manipulations of both diagnostic and therapeutic catheters. The site, severity and the management of the bleeding, depend upon the location and size of the tear/perforation. Treatment of the resultant circulatory collapse from the blood loss out of the vascular space must occur concurrently with the investigation and treatment of the local bleeding site. The recognition and management of massive blood loss during such perforations is covered earlier in this chapter under vessel and chamber perforations.

Late bleeding occurs from single or multiple, purposeful or inadvertent, puncture sites and/or from previously unrecognized disruption of a peripheral or more central vessel. Again, this is particularly likely when the patient is anticoagulated acutely during the procedure, in chronically anticoagulated patients and/or in association with thrombolytic therapy for a known vessel occlusion. The late bleeding can be internal and/or superficial and cannot be predicted unless the previous puncture/disruption of the vessel was recognized during the procedure and the complication anticipated. A significant late bleed into virtually any body *cavity or space*, usually results in pain and/or discomfort for the patient and particularly pain in the area where the blood is collecting. Any complaint of pain in a post-catheterization patient should be investigated thoroughly with this complication in mind. These investigations may include needle taps into a cavity where the pain is localized. Management usually is observation and blood replacement as necessary. A persistent bleed from a high-pressure vessel or chamber requires urgent angiographic documentation of the site of the bleeding and subsequent definitive intervention by a catheter and/or surgery.

Hematologic complications

Severe symptoms can result from significant anemia, which occurs as a result of an insidious blood loss during a cardiac catheterization, particularly in small infants. This usually occurs in infants who have a low hemoglobin/hematocrit at the start of the catheterization *and* in those who otherwise have a precarious circulation. Although the blood loss may not be rapid enough and/or a large enough acute volume loss to compromise the hemodynamics of the patient suddenly and obviously, a drop in the hemoglobin/hematocrit from a marginally low to a very low starting value is sufficient to aggravate cardiac failure and/or hypoxemic spells in a previously compensated patient. Small amounts of, but persistent, blood loss and the multiple blood samples obtained during a catheterization procedure can drop the circulating hemoglobin significantly in infants and small children. The catheterizing physician must be aware of the occasional necessity of blood replacement for other than hypovolemic shock.

Hemolysis with a significant drop in circulating hemoglobin can and does occur following the implant of some intracardiac devices. Significant hemolysis has been reported predominantly following the implant of occlusion devices placed in a patent ductus arteriosus when there is an incomplete closure of the ductus. Hemolysis develops when there is a residual very high-velocity flow through and/or adjacent to any rigid foreign intravascular structure. The hemolysis results in anemia, hemoglobinemia and hematuria, and can be significant enough to cause transient renal shut down, require urgent transfusions and/or urgent re-intervention for the incompletely closed ductus. There should be a high index of suspicion for hemolysis whenever a "jet" of flow remains adjacent to/through an implanted device, and the appearance of hematuria following a catheterization. The presence of hemoglobinuria plus free hemoglobin and an increase in the reticulocyte count in the blood confirm the diagnosis and provide an indication of the severity of the hemolysis.

The best treatment is prevention by closing the ductus completely during the initial occlusion procedure. When there is a residual leak with a persistent "jet" of blood/contrast through and/or adjacent to the original occlusion device, an additional device should be added at that time. If hemolysis does occur, the patient is supported with blood replacement and intravenous infusion of a supplemental maintenance volume of fluid to ensure a high renal blood flow. If the hematuria does not subside quickly, the patient is taken back to the catheterization laboratory to complete the occlusion of the ductus or is taken to the operating room for removal of the device and closure of the ductus.

Hypothermia

All patients undergoing cardiac catheterization are susceptible to systemic hypothermia. Systemic hypothermia can result in acidosis, which further complicates hypoxia and/or low cardiac output, and if not treated can precipitate a cardiovascular collapse. The smaller and/or the more debilitated the patient is, the greater the likelihood of developing serious hypothermia. Patients undergoing cardiac catheterization are naked, they are in a very cool environment unless specific measures are taken to warm the catheterization room, and they are surrounded by wet coverings. The procedure rooms of most cardiac catheterization laboratories are kept very cool in order to keep the electronic equipment (and the operators) cool during the procedure. The undressed patient is covered with a "drape" of a single, thin layer, often of paper. Large areas of the drape become wet and the moisture or actual fluid frequently penetrates through the drape to the patient's skin, where it enhances evaporation and cooling of the patient. Repeated and/or continuous "flushes" of room temperature (cold) flush solution are infused into the patient throughout the procedure. As a consequence of these combined factors, the core temperature of the sedated/anesthetized patient is lowered very rapidly. Small infants and/or debilitated patients, in particular, but even many larger patients, cannot maintain their body temperature under these circumstances without extra specific support of their body temperature.

The *core temperature* of all patients undergoing cardiac catheterization should be monitored. This is absolutely essential in small and/or debilitated patients and during long procedures. Specific warm-air circulators under the drapes, warming pads or, as a last resort, external heat lamps, are used to warm the patient externally in the catheterization laboratory. In addition, for the small infant and the debilitated patient, the room temperature of the catheterization laboratory is raised (often to an uncomfortable temperature for the operators) in order to maintain the patient's core temperature. When possible, intravenous fluids are passed through a warmer before the fluid is infused into the patient.

Hypoxia, acidosis

Hypoxia of any degree represents decreased oxygenation of the tissues and eventually leads to acidosis with decreased function of all tissues. In cyanotic patients, some hypoxia is present before the catheterization procedure even begins, but usually is compensated for very well. Although compensated for and tolerated, any pre-existing hypoxia does decrease the threshold of the patient for further hypoxia and for the development of acidosis. Severely cyanotic and/or otherwise precarious patients often receive supplemental oxygen throughout the catheterization in an attempt to avert further hypoxia. A further drop in systemic saturation can be caused by any compromise of the patient's airway/ventilation, a decrease in the systemic resistance, or, in the presence of an intracardiac/great artery communication, an increase in the pulmonary resistance.

Pulse oximetry is monitored continuously on all patients undergoing cardiac catheterization, and an indwelling arterial line is maintained in most patients for drawing saturations and blood gases. Any decrease in the patient's saturation requires immediate investigation and correction of the cause *before* the hypoxia progresses. While the cause of the increasing hypoxia is being investigated, supplemental oxygen is administered and/or increased by nasal cannulae, a facemask or an endotracheal airway. An arterial blood gas is obtained and should help to distinguish between respiratory and metabolic causes of the hypoxia to direct to appropriate therapy.

Allergic reactions

The potential for a systemic allergic reaction is always present during a cardiac catheterization. Allergic reactions in the catheterization laboratory most frequently are due to contrast agents, but can be caused by any medication including local anesthetics, sedatives, general anesthetics, antiarrhythmic medications and antibiotics. Fortunately, allergic reactions are rare in pediatric/congenital heart patients, but with the increasing age and multiple repeated catheterizations in this population, allergic reactions probably will be an increasing problem. The allergic reactions may be as simple as a mild skin rash and/or a few cutaneous hives or as serious as an anaphylactic reaction with severe bronchospasm and/or shock.

Prevention of allergic reactions again is the best treatment. The catheterizing physician should be familiar with the patient's past history of "allergy". Agents and medications to which a patient has a history of an "allergic reaction" are avoided whenever possible, no matter how mild and unlikely the reaction seemed from the history. When a patient has a history of an allergic reaction to iodine-containing foods and/or more specifically to a contrast agent, but at the same time, specific angiographic anatomic information is critical for the management of the patient, the patient is pre-treated to prevent a recurrent reaction. The patient is premedicated with an intravenous antihistamine (benadryl 1–1.5 mg/kg) and given an intravenous dose of a rapid-acting steroid (dexamethasone 0.5 mg/kg) at the onset of the catheterization. Thirty minutes after the administration of the antihistamine and steroid, the patient is given a test injection (0.25–0.5 ml) of the contrast agent. Assuming there is no reaction from the test injection, the contrast agent is used to obtain the essential anatomic information, but should be used sparingly. The patient is given a repeat dose of both the antihistamine and the steroid at the end of the catheterization procedure and observed in the hospital for 12–24 hours after the procedure.

In the event of an unanticipated, acute allergic reaction occurring during the catheterization procedure, the same antihistamine and steroid are given intravenously and immediately at the onset of the reaction. In the event of an anaphylactic type reaction, *additional* general resuscitative measures are begun immediately. These measures include a colloid volume infusion, intravenous norepinephrine in a dose of 0.1 microgram/kg, and appropriate therapy for any associated bronchospastic reaction as described previously in this chapter.

Infections

Both local and/or systemic infections can result from a cardiac catheterization. These infections do not appear until days, or even weeks, after the procedure has been completed. Local infections at the site of the catheter introduction were far more common when a "cut-down" approach was the standard technique for introducing catheters[13]. The cut-downs resulted in moderately large and deep incisions through which considerable manipulation was performed. The incisions in the inguinal area were in a particularly precarious location for contamination during and after the catheterization, especially in infants still wearing diapers. Local infections manifest first with redness, then swelling and eventually the development of a purulent exudate and dehiscence of the incision. The use of rigid sterile precautions along with percutaneous techniques for the introduction of catheters essentially has eliminated local infections at the catheter introductory site.

Systemic infections with bacteremia and/or endocarditis still do occur, but fortunately, very rarely. Many of the current diagnostic and therapeutic procedures are very long procedures and they involve the repeated handling, introduction and exchange of multiple catheters, wires and devices into the circulation. The therapeutic procedures often include the permanent implant of a device that represents a "foreign body" as a nidus for infection in the circulation. All of these factors contribute to the potential for the introduction of and "seating" of bacteria in the body.

Some patients coming to the catheterization laboratory have been in the hospital in the intensive/recovery room and/or in the operating room prior to coming to the catheterization laboratory and arrive with indwelling lines that have been in place for days or weeks and likely are colonized with "hospital" strains of bacteria. These patients represent an even greater risk of developing serious systemic infections and are treated vigorously with antibiotics during and following the catheterization. The specific antibiotic is determined from the patient's previous antibiotic regimens and/or from specific cultures.

Prevention of infections is accomplished by the use of rigid, "operating room" sterile techniques during all catheterization procedures and the administration of prophylactic intravenous antibiotics for 24 hours following the implant of any device or following any extremely long and/or complicated catheterization[14]. When an antibiotic is used prophylactically, it should protect against skin organisms. Any patient who develops a fever more than 12 hours after a catheterization procedure is suspected of having an infection related to the catheterization procedure until proven otherwise. These patients require continued in-hospital observation and investigation with repeated white blood counts and repeated blood cultures to establish or rule out bacteremia. With signs of progressive sepsis, intravenous antibiotics are begun either after 3–6 cultures are drawn or after any positive blood culture is obtained. The surgical explant of an implanted device must be considered in order to treat a documented post-catheterization systemic infection successfully.

Elevation in a patient's body temperature occurring within several hours after a cardiac catheterization *usually* is a result of either a pyrogenic contaminant, relative dehydration of the patient and/or atelectasis. These elevations in the patient's temperature usually resolve with time, anti-pyretics, further awakening of the patient and rehydration of the patient. Unless the elevated temperature persists or recurs, the patient does not require immediate investigation for infection; however, if these elevations in temperature persist or become more severe, they must be investigated thoroughly and treated appropriately.

Malignant hyperthermia

Malignant hyperthermia can occur in the catheterization laboratory, particularly when halothane and/or succinylcholine are used in patients receiving general anesthesia. This is an autosomal dominant condition, which results in a rapid and marked rise in body temperature, tachycardia, tachypnea, respiratory and metabolic acidosis, cyanosis and eventually generalized muscle rigidity and myoglobinuria. It occurs in association with several forms of myopathy but also as an isolated condition. The best treatment is prevention by obtaining a careful patient and family history for any unexplained fevers, muscle cramps, previous reactions to anesthesia and/or increased serum CK values. With any history even suggestive of a hyperthermic reaction, halothane and succinylcholine unequivocally are avoided.

In any patient and at the very first signs and/or symptoms of rapidly increasing body temperature associated with the signs and symptoms mentioned above, dantrium (dantrolene sodium) is administered rapidly intravenously, starting with 1 mg/kg, increasing to 10 mg/kg and continuing until symptoms subside. Supportive therapy including stopping any anesthetic agent, ventilation with 100% oxygen, correcting acidosis, extra intravenous fluid and external cooling are administered simultaneously. With a documented past history of a malignant hyperthermic reaction, the patient is treated with prophylactic 1 mg/kg of intravenous dantrium prior to the catheterization, regardless of what anesthetic is to be used during the catheterization.

Dantrium for infusion is supplied in vials of a sterile lyophilized mixture of 20 mg dantrium, 3000 mg mannitol and enough sodium hydroxide to produce a solution with a pH of 9.5 when mixed with 60 ml of sterile *water for injection*. Precipitation of the solution will result if mixed with dextrose and/or sodium chloride solution. Because of the highly alkaline pH, dantrium must be administered through a very secure and freely flowing intravenous line.

Death

The death of a patient is the complication most feared by the patient and/or parent, but fortunately, very rarely occurs as a result of a catheterization procedure *per se*. The severity of the patient's underlying illness and/or the increasing complexity of the catheterization procedure that is performed, do increase the risk of a patient dying as a result of the catheterization. Death results from the progression of any one or several of the complications that have been mentioned previously in this chapter. Fortunately, in spite of the *potential* for death occurring during *any* cardiac catheterization, continued attention to proper techniques and the prevention of known causes of complications, reduce the likelihood of a patient dying to a very low percentage.

Conclusion

An extensive listing and detailed descriptions of the innumerable "general" complications that can occur during any cardiac catheterization are presented in this chapter. There are many other complications related to very specific procedures and devices, which are discussed in the separate chapters dealing with those particular procedures and devices. Although the complications can occur during and/or as a consequence of any cardiac catheterization regardless of how "simple" or complicated the catheterization procedure is, the occurrence of complications actually is small and most of the complications can be prevented.

Complications are prevented primarily by a thorough knowledge of the innumerable causes of complications, and then by the utilization of meticulous attention to the details of performing established techniques and procedures. When prevention is not totally successful, there are management strategies discussed in detail in this chapter for the complications that do occur. These management techniques can nullify and/or minimize the permanent sequelae of the complications. The number and seriousness of the potential complications may seem overwhelming; however, the likelihood of complications in a cardiac catheterization that is performed safely and properly are very small. The potential for a complication occurring during a cardiac catheterization should not dissuade a qualified operator from carefully performing any *indicated* diagnostic and/or therapeutic procedure.

References

1. Stanger P *et al.* Complications of cardiac catheterization of neonates, infants, and children. A three-year study. *Circulation* 1974; **50**(3): 595–608.
2. Fellows KE *et al.* Acute complications of catheter therapy for congenital heart disease. *Am J Cardiol* 1987; **60**(8): 679–683.
3. Allen HD and Mullins CE. Results of the Valvuloplasty and Angioplasty of Congenital Anomalies Registry. *Am J Cardiol* 1990; **65**: 772–774.
4. Rashkind WJ. Atrial septostomy in congenital heart disease. *Adv Pediatr* 1969; **16**: 211–232.
5. Park SC *et al.* A new atrial septostomy technique. *Cathet Cardiovasc Diagn* 1975; **1**(2): 195–201.
6. Kawai C and Abelmann WH. Transient myocardial damage secondary to extravasation of contrast material during left ventricular angiocardiography. *Circulation* 1964; **30**: 897–901.
7. Vandenberg R. *et al.* Aneurysm of the right ventricle caused by selective angiocardiography. *Circulation* 1964; **30**: 902–906.
8. Kannankeril PJ, Wax DF, and Pahl E. Elevations of troponin I after interventional cardiac catheterization. *Cardiol Young* 2001; **11**(4): 375–378.
9. Kannankeril PJ, Pahl E, and Wax DF. Usefulness of troponin I as a marker of myocardial injury after pediatric cardiac catheterization. *Am J Cardiol* 2002; **90**(10): 1128–1132.
10. D'Elia JA *et al.* Nephrotoxicity from angiographic contrast material. A prospective study. *Am J Med* 1982; **72**(5): 719–725.
11. Kini AS *et al.* A protocol for prevention of radiographic contrast nephropathy during percutaneous coronary intervention: effect of selective dopamine receptor agonist fenoldopam. *Catheter Cardiovasc Interv* 2002; **55**(2): 169–173.
12. Yang Y *et al.* Characterization of ultrasound-detected cerebral microemboli in patients undergoing cardiac catheterization using an *in vitro* middle cerebral artery model. *Catheter Cardiovasc Interv* 2001; **53**(3): 323–330.
13. Leaman DM and Zelis RF. What is the appropriate "dress code" for the cardiac catheterization laboratory? *Cathet Cardiovasc Diagn* 1983; **9**(1): 33–38.
14. Heupler FA Jr *et al.* Infection prevention guidelines for cardiac catheterization laboratories. Society for Cardiac Angiography and Interventions Laboratory Performance Standards Committee. *Cathet Cardiovasc Diagn* 1992; **25**(3): 260–263.

Index

Note: page numbers in *italic* type refer to figures; those in **bold** type refer to tables.

D